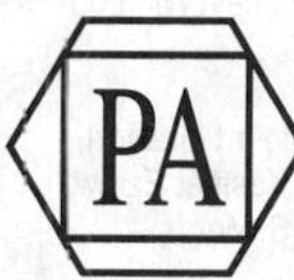

Physician Assistant's Drug Handbook

Foreword by

J. Dennis Blessing, PhD, PA-C
The University of Texas Medical Branch

Springhouse Corporation
Springhouse, Pennsylvania

Staff

Senior Vice President, Editorial
Patricia Dwyer Schull, RN, MSN

Publisher
Donna O. Carpenter, ELS

Clinical Director
Ann M. Barrow, RN, MSN, CCRN

Art Director
John Hubbard

Managing Editor
Andrew T. McPhee, RN, BSN

Drug Information Editor
Lisa Truong, RPh, PharmD

Senior Editor
Naina Chohan

Editors
Laini Berlin, Suzanne L. McHugh

Clinical Editors
Theresa P. Fulginiti, RN, BSN, CEN; Eileen Gallen, RN, BSN; Jane Bliss-Holtz, DNSc, RN,C; Pamela S. Messer, RN, MSN; Suzanne E. Omrod, RN, MSN; Kimberly A. Zalewski, RN, MSN, CEN

Associate Acquisitions Editor
Louise E. Quinn

Copy Editors
Brenna H. Mayer (manager), Karen C. Comerford, Beth Pitcher, Pamela Wingrod

Designers
Arlene Putterman (associate art director), Joseph John Clark, Elaine Kasmer Ezrow, Donald G. Knauss, Donna S. Morris

Typographers
Diane Paluba (manager), Joyce Rossi Biletz

Manufacturing
Deborah Meiris (director), Patricia K. Dorshaw (manager), Otto Mezei (book production manager)

Editorial Assistants
Carrie R. Cameron, Carol A. Caputo

Indexer
Deborah K. Tourtlotte

The clinical procedures described and recommended in this publication are based on research and consultation with medical, pharmaceutical, and legal authorities. To the best of our knowledge, these procedures reflect currently accepted practice; nevertheless, they can't be considered absolute and universal recommendations. For individual application, all recommendations must be considered in light of the patient's clinical condition and, before the administration of new or infrequently used drugs, in light of the latest package-insert information. The authors and publisher disclaim responsibility for adverse effects resulting directly or indirectly from the suggested procedures, from undetected errors, or from the reader's misunderstanding of the text.

A member of the Reed Elsevier plc group

Visit our Web site at www.springnet.com

PADH-010399
ISSN: 1522-4848
ISBN: 0-87434-975-3

Contents

Clinical reviewers and consultants

Steven R. Abel, RPh, PharmD, FASHP
Head, Department of Pharmacy Practice
Purdue University
Indianapolis

Ann Curran Brown, PA-C
Certified Physician Assistant
Media, PA

Michael F. Bullano, PharmD
Pharmacoeconomics and Health Outcomes Research Fellow
University of Pennsylvania Medical Center
Philadelphia

Lawrence Carey, RPh, PharmD
Clinical Pharmacist Coordinator
Jefferson Home Infusion Service
Philadelphia

David M. DiPersio, PharmD, BCPS
Clinical Pharmacist, Critical Care
Vanderbilt University Medical Center
Assistant Clinical Professor
University of Tennessee
Nashville

Teresa S. Dunsworth, PharmD, BCPS
Clinical Associate Professor of Clinical Pharmacy
West Virginia University School of Pharmacy
Morgantown

Susan Epp, PA-C, NCCPA, MPAS
Physician Assistant
Broadlawns Medical Center
Des Moines, IA

Cynthia A. Gobin, PharmD
Clinical Assistant Professor
Temple University School of Pharmacy
Philadelphia

Mildred D. Gottwald, PharmD
Assistant Clinical Professor
University of California
Department of Clinical Pharmacy
San Francisco

Kenneth R. Harbert, PhD, CHES, PA-C
Chairman, Department of Physician Assistant Studies
PCOM
Philadelphia

Bridget A. Haupt, PharmD
Director of Pharmacy Services
Children's Seashore House
Philadelphia

Barbara Kannewurf, RPh, PharmD
Clinical Pharmacist
Professional Consultants Limited
Stafford, VA

James A. Koestner, PharmD
Clinical Pharmacist, Surgical Intensive Care Unit
Vanderbilt University Medical Center
Nashville, TN

Henry R. Lemke, MMS, PA-C
Program Director, PA Studies
UNT Health Science Center
Fort Worth, TX

Randall A. Lynch, RPh, PharmD
Assistant Director, Pharmacy Services
Presbyterian Medical Center
Philadelphia

Mary Y. Ma, BA, PharmD, FASHP
Antimicrobial Clinical Specialist
Veterans Affairs Medical Center
Los Angeles

Carrie A. McCoy, RN, MSN, CEN
Associate Professor of Nursing
Northern Kentucky University
Department of Nursing
Highland Heights

Steven Meisel, PharmD
Assistant Director of Pharmacy
Fairview Southdale Hospital
Edina, MN

George Melko, PharmD
Clinical Pharmacist
Jefferson Home Infusion Service
Philadelphia

Keith M. Olsen, PharmD, FCCP
Associate Professor of Pharmacy
University of Nebraska Medical Center
Omaha

Christy Owens, PharmD
Clinical Services Coordinator
York Prescription Benefits – Yale New Haven (CT) Health

Robert Owens, PharmD
Clinical Pharmacy Specialist
Medical Center of Delaware
Newark

Larry A. Pfeifer, RPh, MS
Chief Pharmacist
Gillis W. Long Hansen's Disease Center
Carville, LA

Cathy Pollard-Colombo, PA-C, CIC
TB Coordinator; Infection Control Practitioner
Bronx-Lebanon Hospital
Bronx, NY

Jack Runyan, PhD, PA-C
Director, Physician Assistant Studies
University of Texas–Pan American
Edinburg

Brenda K. Shelton, RN, MS, CCRN, AOCN
Critical Care Clinical Nurse Specialist
The Johns Hopkins Oncology Center
Baltimore

Joel Shuster, PharmD
Clinical Associate Professor
Temple University School of Pharmacy
Clinical Pharmacist
Medical College of Pennsylvania
Philadelphia

Gary Smith, RPh, PharmD
Clinical Manager, Asthma Disease Management
Express Scripts/Value Rx
Plymouth, MN

Dawn M. Specht, RN, MSN, CEN, CCRN, PHRN
Clinical Nurse Specialist; Critical Care/Neuroscience
The Cooper Health System: Cooper Hospital
Camden, NJ

Lori H. Syed, PharmD
Pharmacy Administration Specialty Resident
University of California, San Francisco

Rein Tideiksaar, PhD, PA-C
Director
Sierra Health Services, Inc.
Las Vegas

Janice Tramel, NP/PA-C
Associate Director
University of Southern California (Los Angeles) School of Medicine–PA Program

Kenneth K. Wieland, PharmD
Clinical Coordinator Pharmacy Department
Chestnut Hill Hospital
Philadelphia

Foreword

When I became an educator, I took 2 years away from clinical practice to work on a Master's degree. When I returned, I was shocked at how much my knowledge of drugs had slipped. Although I had previously prescribed drugs confidently, I was amazed at my weakened recall of familiar drugs. I was also surprised at the number of new drugs that had become available of which I had limited or no knowledge and no practical experience. I joked with colleagues about needing to leave an examination room to look up basic drug information.

Like many of my colleagues, I found it frustrating to continually refer to large, seemingly "comprehensive" references available for drug information. Researching them for specific drugs inevitably proves time consuming and burdensome. I remember wishing for a text that would allow me to quickly review and update critical drug information. What I needed was a resource that was informative, user-friendly, easy to read, succinct, and clinically applicable.

I believe the *Physician Assistant's Drug Handbook* is that resource. It's designed specifically for physician assistants and includes all the prescribing information you'll need in an easy-to-read style, together with additional information not included in other drug handbooks.

The design of the book facilitates its use in a busy, clinical setting. Almost every drug can be easily found through the alphabetical listing by generic name or through the index, which also lists trade names and drug indications. Each entry presents complete and up-to-date information in a consistent format. *Italics* and icons draw attention to dosage adjustments and drug interactions. Up-front chapters review pharmacology, drug administration considerations in pediatric and geriatric populations, and effective prescribing practices. An extensive section on major pharmacologic classes is an invaluable aid when comparing drugs within a class.

The appendices add much to this book's usefulness, each of which offers important information that's hard to find elsewhere. The handbook also contains a color photoguide to more than 300 commonly used pills, which can help you identify medications brought in by a patient.

Take a few minutes to review this book for yourself. I think you'll agree that it's an excellent resource. Students will also find it to be an excellent supplement for their studies and clinical rotations.

Ultimately, I know you'll find the *Physician Assistant's Drug Handbook* to be a key resource in your quest for providing quality care. Part of that quality lies in our knowledge of the drugs we prescribe and prescription writing that's appropriate and 100% accurate. This book can play an integral role in that ongoing effort.

J. Dennis Blessing, PhD, PA-C
Associate Professor
The University of Texas Medical Branch
Galveston, Texas
Editor-in-Chief
Physician Assistant

Common abbreviations

Abbreviation	Meaning
AIDS	acquired immunodeficiency syndrome
ALT	alanine aminotransferase
AST	aspartate aminotransferase
ATP	adenosine triphosphate
AV	atrioventricular
b.i.d.	twice a day
BUN	blood urea nitrogen
cAMP	cyclic 3′, 5′ adenosine monophosphate
CBC	complete blood count
CK	creatine kinase
CNS	central nervous system
COPD	chronic obstructive pulmonary disease
CPR	cardiopulmonary resuscitation
CSF	cerebrospinal fluid
CV	cardiovascular
CVA	cerebrovascular accident
CVP	central venous pressure
DIC	disseminated intravascular coagulation
DNA	deoxyribonucleic acid
ECG	electrocardiogram
EEG	electroencephalogram
FDA	Food and Drug Administration
g	gram
G	gauge
G6PD	glucose-6-phosphate dehydrogenase
GI	gastrointestinal
GU	genitourinary
HIV	human immunodeficiency virus
h.s.	at bedtime
I.M.	intramuscular
INR	International Normalized Ratio

Abbreviation	Meaning
IU	International Unit
I.V.	intravenous
kg	kilogram
L	liter
LD	lactate dehydrogenase
m^2	square meter
mm^3	cubic millimeter
MAO	monoamine oxidase
mcg	microgram
mEq	milliequivalent
mg	milligram
MI	myocardial infarction
ml	milliliter
ng	nanogram (millimicrogram)
NSAID	nonsteroidal anti-inflammatory drug
OTC	over-the-counter
P.O.	by mouth
P.R.	per rectum
p.r.n.	as needed
PT	prothrombin time
PVC	premature ventricular contraction
q	every
q.i.d.	four times a day
RBC	red blood cell
RDA	recommended daily allowance
RNA	ribonucleic acid
SA	sinoatrial
S.C.	subcutaneous
SIADH	syndrome of inappropriate antidiuretic hormone
S.L.	sublingually
T_3	triiodothyronine
T_4	thyroxine
t.i.d.	three times a day
WBC	white blood cell

1 How to use the *Physician Assistant's Drug Handbook*

The *Physician Assistant's Drug Handbook* provides exhaustively reviewed, completely updated drug information on virtually every drug in current clinical use. It covers all aspects of drug information from fundamental pharmacology to specific management of toxicity and overdose. It also includes several unique features—individual entries that describe major pharmacologic classes, a comprehensive listing of indications that includes clinically approved but unlabeled uses, and specific recommendations for use in renal failure.

Introductory chapters

Chapter 2 explains, in a general way, how drugs work. It also discusses adverse reactions and gives general guidelines about drug use in pregnancy and the presence of drugs in breast milk. Chapter 3 discusses the unique issues related to administering drugs to pediatric and geriatric patients. Chaper 4 discusses how to take an effective medication history and write a proper prescription.

Generic drug entries

The individual drug entries provide detailed information on virtually all drugs in current clinical use, all arranged alphabetically by generic name for easy access. This edition includes entries for drugs recently approved. A guide word at the top of each page identifies the generic drug presented on that page. Each generic entry is complete where it falls alphabetically and does not require cross-referencing to other sections of the book.

In each drug entry, the generic name (with alternate generic names following in parentheses) precedes an alphabetically arranged list of current trade names. (An asterisk signals products available only in Canada.) Several drugs available solely as combinations (such as acetaminophen and oxycodone hydrochloride [Percocet]) are listed in an appendix.

Next, the pharmacologic and therapeutic classifications identify the drug's pharmacologic or chemical category and its major clinical uses. Listing both classifications helps the reader grasp the multiple, varying, and sometimes overlapping uses of drugs within a single pharmacologic class and among different classes. If appropriate, the next line identifies drugs regulated under the jurisdiction of the Controlled Substances Act of 1970. These drugs are divided into the following groups, or schedules:

- Schedule I (C-I): High abuse potential and no accepted medical use—for example, heroin marijuana, and LSD.
- Schedule II (C-II): High abuse potential with severe dependence liability—for example, narcotics, amphetamines, dronabinol, and some barbiturates. Emergency telephone orders for limited quantities of these drugs are authorized but the prescriber must provide a written signed prescription order to the pharmacy within 72 hours.
- Schedule III (C-III): Less abuse potential than schedule II drugs and moderate dependence liability—for example, nonbarbiturate sedatives, nonamphetamine stimulants, anabolic steroids, and limited amounts of certain narcotics. Telephone orders are permitted for these drugs.
- Schedule IV (C-IV): Less abuse potential than schedule III drugs and limited dependence liability—for example, some sedatives, antianxiety agents, and nonnarcotic analgesics. Telephone orders are permitted for these drugs.
- Schedule V (C-V): Limited abuse potential. Primarily small amounts of narcotics, such as codeine, used as antitussives or antidiarrheals. Under federal law, limited quantities of certain C-V drugs may be purchased without a prescription directly from a pharmacist if allowed under specific state statutes. The purchaser must be at least age 18 and must furnish suitable identification. All such transactions must be recorded by the dispensing pharmacist.

The pregnancy risk category identifies the potential risk to the fetus. Categories listed were determined by application of the Food and Drug Administration (FDA) definitions to available clinical data in order to define a drug's potential to cause birth defects or fetal death. These categories, labeled A, B, C, D, and X, are listed below with an explanation of each. Drugs in category A usually are considered safe to use in pregnancy; drugs in category X usually are contraindicated.

- A: Adequate studies in pregnant women have failed to show a risk to the fetus in the first trimester of pregnancy—and there is no evidence of risk in later trimesters.
- B: Animal studies have not shown an adverse effect on the fetus, but there are no adequate clinical studies in pregnant women.
- C: Animal studies have shown an adverse effect on the fetus, but there are no adequate studies in humans. The drug may be useful in pregnant women despite its potential risks.
- D: There is evidence of risk to the human fetus, but the potential benefits of use in pregnant women may be acceptable despite the risks, such as when the drug is needed in a life-threatening situation or for a serious disease for which safer drugs cannot be used or are ineffective.
- X: Studies in animals or humans show fetal abnormalities, or adverse reaction reports indicate evidence of fetal risk. The risks involved clearly outweigh potential benefits.
- NR: Not rated.

Pregnancy risk classifications were assigned for all appropriate generic drugs according to the above criteria.

How supplied lists the preparations available for each drug (for example, tablets, capsules, solution, or injection), specifying available dosage forms and strengths.

Indications, route, and dosage presents all clinically accepted indications for use with general dosage recommendations for adults and children; dosage adjustments for specific patient groups, such as the elderly or patients with renal or hepatic impairment, are included when appropriate. (Note that additional information may be found in the *Special considerations* section.) A preceding open diamond signals a clinically accepted but unlabeled use. Dosage instructions reflect current clinical trends in therapeutics and should not be considered as absolute and universal recommendations. For individual application, dosage must be considered according to the patient's condition.

Pharmacodynamics explains the mechanism and effects of the drug's physiologic action.

Pharmacokinetics describes absorption, distribution, metabolism, and excretion of the drug; it specifies onset and duration of action, peak levels, and half-life as appropriate.

Contraindications and precautions lists conditions that are associated with special risks in patients who receive the drug.

Interactions specifies the clinically significant additive, synergistic, or antagonistic effects that result from combined use of the drug with other drugs. The interacting agent is italicized.

Effects on diagnostic tests lists significant interference with a diagnostic test or its result by direct effects on the test itself or by systemic drug effects that lead to misleading test results.

Adverse reactions lists the undesirable effects that may follow use of the drug; these effects are arranged by body systems (CNS, CV, EENT, GI, GU, Hematologic, Hepatic, Metabolic, Musculoskeletal, Respiratory, Skin, and Other). Local effects occur at the site of drug administration (by application, infusion, or injection); adverse reactions not specific to a single body system (for example, the effects of hypersensitivity) are listed under Other. Throughout, the most common adverse reactions (those experienced by at least 10% of people taking the drug in clinical trials) are in *italic* type; less common reactions are in roman type; life-threatening reactions are in ***bold italic*** type; and reactions that are both common and life-threatening are in **BOLD CAPITAL** letters. At the end of this section, Note signals a list of severe and hazardous reactions that mandate discontinuation of the drug.

Overdose and treatment summarizes the clinical manifestations of drug overdose and recommends specific treatment as appropriate. Usually, this segment recommends emesis or gastric lavage, followed by activated charcoal to reduce the amount of drug absorbed and possibly a cathartic to eliminate the toxin. This section specifies antidotes, drug therapy, and other special care, if known. It also specifies the effects of hemodialysis or peritoneal dialysis for dialyzable drugs.

Special considerations offers detailed recommendations specific to the drug for preparation and administration; for patient education during therapy; and for use in geriatric, pediatric, and breast-feeding patients. Also included are recommendations for monitoring the effects of drug therapy, for preventing and treating adverse reactions, for promoting patient comfort, and for storing the drug. Considerations that are common to all members of the drug's pharmacologic class are listed only in the relevant *pharmacologic class* entry. If specific considerations are unknown for geriatric, pediatric, or breast-feeding use of the drug, or if known information appears in the pharmacologic class entry or in the generic entry, these headings are omitted. For example, if the *Indications, route, and dosage* section lists detailed instructions for use in children and no additional considerations apply, the generic entry omits the heading *Pediatric use*. However, relevant information that applies to all drugs in the drug's pharmacologic class may exist in the pharmacologic class entry. Cross-references to pharmacologic class entries are denoted in italics.

Pharmacologic class entries

Listed alphabetically as a separate section, 39 entries describe the pharmacology, clinical indications and actions, adverse effects, and special implications of drugs that belong to a major pharmacologic group. The reader can compare the effects and uses of drugs within each class. Pharmacologic class entries list special considerations common to all generic members and include geriatric, pediatric, and breast-feeding use. If specific considerations are unknown, these headings are omitted.

Representative combinations at the end of each class entry lists major combinations of generic drugs in the class with other generics of the same or of another class, followed by trade names of products that contain each combination of generics.

Photoguide

This extensive section provides full-color photographs of more than 300 of the most commonly prescribed tablets and capsules in the United States. Shown in actual size, the tablets and capsules are organized alphabetically for quick reference.

Graphic enhancement

Selected charts and tables compare uses, effects, or dosages of drugs within a class.

Appendices

The appendices provide a charted summary of physician assistants' prescribing authority by state, a summary of combination analgesic drugs, a chart about topical drugs, an immunization schedule, formulas for calculating creatinine clearance, therapeutic drug monitoring guidelines, therapeutic management guidelines, and key pharmaceutical companies' contact numbers and Web site addresses.

Index

The index lists both the generic and trade names, diseases, and pharmacologic classes.

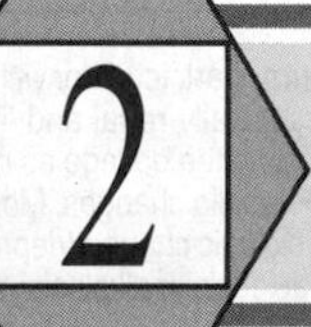

Overview of pharmacology

Administration of a drug provokes a series of physicochemical events within the body. The first event, when a drug combines with cellular drug receptors, is known as the drug *action.* The result of this action is known as the drug *effect.*

Depending on the number of cellular drug receptors affected by a given drug, a drug effect can be local, systemic, or both. A local effect follows application to the skin; however, transdermal absorption can produce systemic effects. Moreover, local effects can follow systemic absorption. The antipeptic ulcer drug cimetidine acts solely by blocking histamine receptor cells in the parietal cells of the stomach. This is known as a local drug effect because the drug action is limited to one area and does not spread to other parts of the body. However, diphenhydramine produces a systemic effect in that it blocks histamine receptors in widespread areas of the body. Thus, local drug effects are specific to a limited number of organ systems, whereas systemic drug effects are generalized and affect different and diverse organ systems.

Drug properties

Drug absorption, distribution, metabolism, and excretion make up a drug's pharmacokinetic profile. This branch of pharmacology also describes a drug's onset of action, peak concentration level, duration of action, and bioavailablity.

Absorption

Before a drug can act within the body, it must be absorbed into the blood—usually after oral administration, the most commonly used route. For a drug that is contained in a tablet or capsule to be absorbed, the dosage form must disintegrate and dissolve in gastric juices. Absorption can only occur after a drug is dissolved. Most absorption of orally administered drugs occurs in the small intestine, where the mucosal villi provide extensive surface area. Once absorbed and circulated in the blood, the drug is bioavailable, or ready to produce an effect. Complete or partial absorption depends on the drug's physicochemical effects, its dosage form, route of administration, interactions with other substances in the GI tract, and various patient characteristics. These factors also determine the speed of absorption. Thus, oral solutions and elixirs, which bypass the need for disintegration and dissolution, are usually absorbed more rapidly. Some tablets have enteric coatings that prevent disintegration in the acidic environment of the stomach; others may have coatings of varying thickness that delay it.

Drugs administered I.M. must first be absorbed through the muscle into the blood. Rectal suppositories must dissolve to be absorbed through the rectal mucosa. I.V. drugs, which are injected directly into the blood, are completely and immediately bioavailable.

Distribution

After absorption, a drug moves from the bloodstream into various fluids and tissues within the body. Patient variations can greatly alter the amount of drug that is distributed throughout the body. For example, a given dose must be distributed to a larger volume in an edematous than a nonedematous patient; the amount of drug may sometimes need to be increased. The dose should be decreased when the edema is corrected. Conversely, in an extremely dehydrated patient, the drug is distributed to a much smaller volume, so the dose must then be decreased. The total area to which a drug is distributed is known as volume of distribution.

Patients who are particularly obese may present another problem when considering drug distribution. Drugs such as digoxin, gentamicin, and tobramycin are not well distributed to fatty tissue. Therefore, dosage based on actual body weight may lead to overdose and serious toxicity. Sometimes, dosage is based on lean body weight, which may be estimated from actuarial tables that give average weight range for height.

Metabolism

Most drugs are metabolized in the liver. Hepatic disease may affect one or more of the liver's metabolic functions. Therefore, the metabolism of a drug may be increased, decreased, or unchanged in patients with hepatic disease. These patients should be monitored closely for drug effect and toxicity.

The rate of drug metabolism varies with the individual. In some patients, drugs are metabolized so rapidly that their blood and tissue levels prove therapeutically inadequate, whereas the rate of metabolism is so slow in others that normal doses produce toxic results.

Excretion

The body eliminates drugs by metabolism (usually hepatic) and excretion (usually renal). Drug excretion refers to the movement of a drug or its metabolites from the tissues back into circulation and from the circulation into the organs of excretion. Although most drugs are excreted by the kidneys, some can be removed via the lungs, exocrine glands (sweat, salivary, or mammary), liver, skin, and intestinal tract. Drugs may also be removed artificially by direct interventions such as hemodialysis.

Other modifying factors

An important factor that influences a drug's action and effect is its *binding to plasma proteins,* especially albumin, and other tissue components. Because only a free, unbound drug can act in the body, binding influences effectiveness and duration of effect. Protein binding can be affected by malnutrition, renal failure, and other protein-bound drugs. When protein binding occurs, drug dosage may need to be modified.

The *patient's age* also affects drug action and effect. Elderly patients often have decreased hepatic function, less muscle mass, and diminished renal function. They need lower doses and sometimes longer dosage intervals to avoid toxicity. With similar consequences, neonates have underdeveloped metabolic enzyme systems and inadequate renal function. These patients require highly individualized dosages and careful monitoring.

Another factor influencing drug action is *underlying disease.* For example, acidosis may cause insulin resistance. Genetic diseases, such as G6PD deficiency and hepatic porphyria, may turn drugs into toxins with serious consequences. Patients with G6PD deficiency may develop hemolytic anemia when given sulfonamides or other drugs. If given a barbiturate, a genetically susceptible patient can develop an acute porphyria attack. Also, patients who have highly active hepatic enzyme systems (for example, rapid acetylators), when treated with isoniazid, can develop hepatitis from the rapid intrahepatic buildup of a toxic metabolite.

Drug administration issues

Factors related to the administration of a drug can also influence a drug's action within the body. The dosage form of the drug is important. Some tablets and capsules are too large to be swallowed by ill patients. Although an oral solution may be substituted, it produces higher drug blood levels than a tablet because the liquid is more easily and completely absorbed. When a potentially toxic drug (such as digoxin) is given, the increased amount absorbed could cause toxicity. Sometimes a change in dosage form requires a change in dosage itself.

Routes of drug administration are not therapeutically interchangeable. For example, diazepam is readily absorbed orally but is slowly and erratically absorbed I.M. However, gentamicin must be given parenterally because oral administration yields blood levels inadequate to treat systemic infections.

Improper storage can alter a drug's potency. Most drugs should be stored in tight containers and protected from direct sunlight and extremes in temperature and humidity to avoid deterioration. Some may require special storage conditions such as refrigeration.

The timing of drug administration is important. The administration of an oral drug during or shortly after meals may decrease the amount absorbed. This is not clinically significant with most drugs and may sometimes be desirable with drugs such as aspirin. However, penicillins and tetracyclines should not be given with meals because certain foods can inactivate their action. If the effect of food on a drug is uncertain, consult with the pharmacist.

Consider the patient's age, height, and weight. This information may be required when calculating the dosage for many drugs, and should be available in the patient's chart, together with current laboratory data (especially renal and liver function studies) for adjusting the dosage as needed.

Watch for metabolic changes. Monitor the patient for any physiologic change (depressed respiratory function, acidosis or alkalosis) that might alter drug effect.

Know the patient's history. Obtain a comprehensive family history, when possible. Ask about past reactions to drugs, possible genetic traits that might alter drug response, and the current use of other medications. Multiple drug therapy can cause drug interactions that can dramatically change the effects of many drugs.

Drug interactions

When one drug administered in combination with or shortly after another drug alters the effect of either or both drugs, this is known as a *drug interaction.* Usually, the effect of one drug is increased or decreased. For instance, a drug may inhibit or stimulate the metabolism or excretion of the other, or it may release another from plasma protein-binding sites, freeing it for further action.

Combination therapy is based on drug interaction. A drug, for example, may be given to potentiate another's action. Probenecid, which blocks the excretion of penicillin, may be given with penicillin to maintain adequate blood levels of penicillin for a longer period. In most cases, two drugs with similar actions are given together precisely because of the additive effect that results. For instance, aspirin and codeine, both analgesics, are commonly given in combination because together they provide greater pain relief than either alone.

Drug interactions are sometimes used to prevent or antagonize specific adverse reactions. Hydrochlorothiazide and spironolactone, both diuretics, are commonly administered in combination because the former is potassium depleting, whereas the latter is potassium sparing.

However, not all drug interactions are beneficial. Multiple drugs can interact to produce effects that are undesirable and sometimes hazardous. Harmful drug interactions decrease efficacy or increase toxicity. For example, in a patient taking both diuretics and lithium, the diuretics may cause an increase in serum levels of lithium, resulting in lithium toxicity. Such a drug effect is known as antagonism. Drug combinations that produce these effects should be avoided. Another inhibiting effect occurs when a tetracycline is administered with calcium- or magnesium-containing drugs or foods (such as antacids or milk). These combine with tetracycline in the GI tract and cause inadequate absorption of tetracycline.

Adverse reactions

Any drug effect other than what is therapeutically intended is called an adverse reaction. It may be expected and benign or unexpected and potentially harmful. Mild, but *predictable,* adverse reactions are sometimes called adverse effects; one such example is drowsiness caused by antihistamines. During hay fever season, a patient may have to contend with this drowsiness to obtain relief from symptoms of hay fever. In this case, the dosage may be adjusted up or down to balance therapeutic effects with adverse effects.

An adverse reaction may be tolerated for a necessary therapeutic effect, or it may be hazardous and unacceptable and require discontinuation of the drug. Some adverse reactions subside with continued use. For example, the drowsiness associated with paroxetine and the orthostatic hypotension associated with prazosin usually subside after several days, as the patient develops a tolerance to these effects. However, many adverse reactions are dose-related and lessen or disappear only if the dosage is reduced. Although most adverse reactions are not therapeutically desirable, an occasional one can be put to clinical use. An example is the drowsiness associated with diphenhydramine, which makes it useful as a mild hypnotic.

Hypersensitivity, also known as drug allergy, is the result of an antigen-antibody immune reaction that occurs when a drug is given to a susceptible patient. The most dangerous hypersensitivity is penicillin allergy, which can be fatal.

Idiosyncratic reactions occur rarely. These are highly unpredictable, individual, and unusual reactions. The best known idiosyncratic drug reaction is aplastic anemia caused by chloramphenicol. This reaction only occurs in 1 out of 40,000 patients, but can be fatal. A common idiosyncratic reaction is extreme sensitivity to very low doses of a drug, or insensitivity to higher-than-normal doses.

To resolve adverse reactions, monitor minor changes in the patient's clinical status because these may be an early indication of pending toxicity. Listen to the patient's complaints about his reactions to a drug, and consider each complaint objectively. Adverse reactions may be reduced in many ways. Dosage reduction or a rescheduling of the same dose may be helpful. For example, pseudoephedrine may produce stimulation that will not be problematic if the drug is given early in the day; similarly, the drowsiness associated with antihistamines or tranquilizers can be harmless if the dose is taken at bedtime. It is important that the patient be informed of the expected adverse reactions so that he won't become worried or stop taking the drug. The patient should always report any unusual or unexpected adverse reactions promptly.

Recognizing drug allergies or serious idiosyncratic reactions can be lifesaving. Ask the patient about other drugs he has taken or is taking and if unusual reactions have occurred. If a patient claims to be allergic to a drug, ask him to relate exactly what happens after taking the drug. He may be referring to a harmless adverse effect such as upset stomach as an allergic reaction, or he may have a true tendency toward anaphylaxis. Record and report clinical changes during the patient's hospital stay. If a severe adverse reaction is suspected, withhold the drug and check with the pharmacist.

Toxic reactions

Chronic drug toxicities are usually caused by the cumulative effect and resulting accumulation of the drug in the body. These effects may be extensions of the desired therapeutic effect; for example, glyburide normalizes blood glucose when given in usual doses but in larger doses can produce undesired hypoglycemia.

Drug toxicities typically occur when drug blood levels rise because of impaired metabolism or excretion. For example, blood levels of theophylline rise when hepatic dysfunction impairs metabolism of the drug. Similarly, digoxin toxicity can follow impaired renal function because digoxin is eliminated from the body almost exclusively by the kidneys. Toxic blood levels also occur after excessive dosage. Tinnitus is usually a sign that the safe dose of aspirin has been exceeded.

Most drug toxicities are predictable and dose-related; fortunately, most are also readily reversible once the dosage is adjusted. Monitor patients carefully for physiologic changes that might alter drug effect. Watch especially for impaired hepatic and renal function. Warn the patient about signs of pending toxicity, and tell him what to do if a toxic reaction occurs. Also, be sure to emphasize the importance of taking a drug exactly as prescribed. Warn the patient about serious problems that could arise if he changes the dose or dosage schedule.

Drugs and pregnancy

Since the thalidomide tragedy of the late 1950s—when thousands of malformed infants were born after their mothers used the mild sedative-hypnotic during pregnancy—use of drugs during pregnancy has been a source of serious medical concern and controversy. To identify drugs that may cause such teratogenic effects, preclinical drug studies always include tests on pregnant laboratory animals. These tests point out gross teratogenicity but do not clearly establish safety. Because different species react to drugs differently, animal studies do not eliminate possible teratogenic effects in humans. For example, the preliminary studies on thalidomide gave no warning of teratogenic effects, and it was subsequently released for general use in Europe.

Although the placental barrier was believed to protect the fetus from drug effects, it really isn't much of a barrier. Except for drugs with exceptionally large molecular structures, such as heparin, virtually every drug administered to a pregnant woman crosses the placenta and enters the fetal circulation. Theoretically, heparin could be used in a pregnant woman without harming the fetus—but even heparin carries a warning for cautious use during pregnancy. Conversely, because a drug crosses the placenta doesn't necessarily mean it's harmful to the fetus.

Only one factor—the stage of fetal development—seems to be clearly related to exaggerated risk during pregnancy. During two stages of pregnancy—the first and third trimesters—the fetus is especially vulnerable to damage from maternal use of drugs. During these times, *all* drugs should be given with extreme caution.

The most sensitive period for drug-induced fetal malformation is the first trimester, when fetal organs are undergoing organogenesis. All drugs, except those labeled as category A or B, should be withheld during this time unless the mother's health is in jeopardy. Theoretically, even aspirin may be harmful to the fetus. Stress that all self-prescribed drugs during early pregnancy should be avoided.

The last trimester is also a sensitive period with regard to the fetus. After birth, the neonate must rely on his own metabolism to eliminate any remaining drug. Because his detoxifying systems are not fully developed, residual drug may take a long time to be metabolized—and thus may induce prolonged toxic reactions. Consequently, drugs should be used only when absolutely necessary during the last 3 months of pregnancy.

However, in some conditions pregnant women must continue to take certain medications. A woman with a seizure disorder that is well controlled with an anticonvulsant should continue taking the drug even during pregnancy. The potential risk to the fetus is outweighed by the mother's need. The relative risk to the fetus is expressed by the drug's pregnancy risk category.

Follow these guidelines to avoid indiscriminate and potentially harmful use of drugs during pregnancy:

- Before a drug is prescribed for a woman of childbearing age, ask for the date of her last menstrual period and if she may be pregnant. If a drug is a known teratogen, some manufacturers may recommend special precautions to ensure that the drug not be given until pregnancy is ruled out.
- Especially during the first and third trimesters, tell pregnant patients to avoid all drugs except those essential to maintain the pregnancy or maternal health.
- Topical drugs are not exempt from the warning against indiscriminate use during pregnancy. Many topically applied drugs can be absorbed in large enough amounts to be harmful to the fetus.
- When a pregnant patient needs a drug, prescribe the safest possible drug in the lowest possible dose to minimize potential effects to the fetus.
- Tell pregnant patients to seek medical approval before taking any drug or herbal or "natural" agents.

Drugs and lactation

Most drugs taken by a breast-feeding woman appear in breast milk. Levels of drug in breast milk tend to be high when drug blood levels are high, usually after each dose has been taken. Therefore, advise the patient to breast-feed before taking her medication and not afterward.

Sometimes breast-feeding may continue with medical approval. However, it should be temporarily replaced with bottle-feeding when tetracyclines, chloramphenicol, sulfonamides (during first 2 weeks postpartum), oral anticoagulants, iodine-containing drugs, or antineoplastics are being used.

To protect the infant, a breast-feeding woman should avoid taking drugs indiscriminately. She should first check with her health care provider or pharmacist to be sure of taking the safest drug at the lowest dose.

Patient education

Use the following guidelines to educate the patient so that he or she obtains maximal therapeutic benefits and avoids adverse reactions, accidental overdose, or potentially harmful changes in drug effectiveness during therapy:

- Tell the patient to store the drug in its original container, at room temperature (unless directed otherwise), in a place that is not accessible to children or exposed to sunlight. Avoid storage in the bathroom medicine cabinet, in the kitchen in close proximity to heat, or in the glove compartment or trunk of a car, where extremes of temperature and humidity will cause the drug to deteriorate.
- Instruct the patient to learn the trade and generic names of all drugs he is taking and to inform his regular health care professional about their use. Before taking a drug, tell him also to report unusual reactions experienced in the past, any allergies to foods and other agents, special medical problems, and medications taken over the past few weeks, including OTC or herbal medicines. (This might be the appropriate time to tell the patient that herbal agents may cause toxic reactions; although some may have therapeutic use, these agents have not been fully evaluated and are not strictly regulated.)
- Inform the patient to always read the label before taking a drug, to take it exactly as prescribed, and never to share prescription drugs.
- Instruct the patient to check the expiration date before taking the drug.
- Warn the patient not to change brands of a drug without medical approval to avoid potentially harmful changes in effectiveness. Certain generic preparations are not equivalent in effect to brand-name preparations of the same drug.
- Caution the patient never to mix different drugs in a single container, remove a drug from its original container, or remove the label. Relying on memory to identify a drug and specific directions for its use is hazardous.
- Instruct the patient to safely discard drugs that are outdated or no longer needed and to keep them out of reach of children and pets.
- Advise the patient to inform the health care professional about use of drugs before undergoing any surgery (including dental surgery).
- Stress the importance of informing the physician assistant, nurse, or pharmacist about any adverse reactions experienced during drug therapy.
- Instruct the patient to call the health care professional, poison control center, or pharmacist immediately if he or someone else has taken an overdose. Keep their phone numbers handy together with other emergency numbers. Also, have syrup of ipecac available at home to induce vomiting, but only if advised to do so by these professionals.
- Tell the patient to have all prescriptions filled at the same pharmacy. The pharmacist can warn against possible harmful drug interactions.
- Tell the patient to have a sufficient supply of drugs when traveling. He should carry them with him and not stow them in his luggage.
- Advise the patient to teach his children about safety and medicines. Tell him to show the children what a medicine container looks like and to never refer to medicine as candy. Instruct him to treat vitamins, especially those containing iron, as medicines.

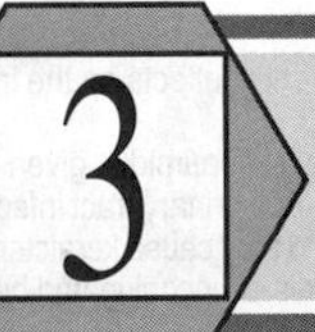

Pediatric and geriatric drug therapy

Drug action and its adverse effects may vary substantially among pediatric and geriatric patients, as opposed to those in the general adult population. Developmental differences or immature or declining body systems can exaggerate these variations and make a drug's effects less predictable and sometimes even risky. These variations must be kept in mind when administering a drug to a patient with particular developmental considerations.

This chapter outlines special considerations for drug therapy for pediatric and geriatric patients.

Pediatric drug therapy

Providing drug therapy to children and adolescents is challenging. Physiologic differences, including those in vital organ maturity and body composition, between children and adults can significantly influence a drug's effectiveness.

Physiologic changes affecting drug action

A child's absorption, distribution, metabolism, and excretion processes undergo profound changes that affect drug dosage.

Absorption

Drug absorption in children depends on the form of the drug, its physical properties, other drugs or substances (such as food) taken simultaneously, physiologic changes, and the presence of disease.

The pH of neonatal gastric fluid affects drug absorption because it is neutral or slightly acidic and becomes more acidic as the infant matures. For example, nafcillin and penicillin G are better absorbed in an infant than an adult because of low gastric acidity.

Several infant formulas or milk products may increase gastric pH and impede absorption of acidic drugs. If possible, oral medications should be given on an empty stomach.

Gastric emptying time and transit time through the small intestine—which is longer in children than in adults—can affect absorption. Also, intestinal hypermotility (as in diarrhea) can diminish absorption.

A child's comparatively thin epidermis allows increased absorption of topical drugs.

Distribution

As with absorption, changes in body weight and physiology during childhood can significantly influence a drug's distribution and effects. In a premature infant, body fluid makes up about 85% of total body weight; in a full-term infant, 55% to 70%; and in an adult, 50% to 55%. Extracellular fluid (mostly blood) constitutes 40% of a neonate's body weight, compared with 20% in an adult. Intracellular fluid remains fairly constant throughout life and has little effect on drug dosage.

Extracellular fluid volume influences a water-soluble drug's concentration and effect because most drugs travel through extracellular fluid to reach their receptors. Children have a larger proportion of fluid to solid body weight, so their distribution area is proportionately greater.

Because the proportion of fat to lean body mass increases with age, the distribution of fat-soluble drugs is more limited in children than in adults. Consequently, a drug's lipid or water solubility affects the dosage for a child.

Binding to plasma proteins. Because of a decrease in albumin concentration or intermolecular attraction between drug and plasma protein, many drugs are less bound to plasma proteins in infants than in adults.

Moreover, preparations that bind plasma proteins may displace endogenous compounds, such as bilirubin or free fatty acids. Conversely, an endogenous compound may displace a weakly bound drug. For example, displacement of bound bilirubin can cause a rise in unbound bilirubin, which can lead to increased risk of kernicterus at normal bilirubin levels.

Because only an unbound, or free, drug has a pharmacologic effect, alteration of the protein-bound to unbound active drug ratio can significantly influence its effect

Several diseases and disorders, such as nephrotic syndrome and malnutrition, can also decrease plasma protein and increase the concentration of an unbound drug, thus intensifying the drug's effect or producing a toxic effect.

Metabolism

A neonate's ability to metabolize a drug depends on the integrity of the hepatic enzyme system, the intrauterine exposure to the drug, and the nature of the drug itself.

Certain metabolic mechanisms are underdeveloped in neonates. Glucuronidation is a metabolic process that renders most drugs more water soluble, thereby facilitating renal excretion. This process is insufficiently developed to permit full pediatric doses until the infant is age 1 month. Thus, chloramphenicol may cause gray syndrome in a neonate, illustrating the infant's inability to metabolize the drug. Use of chloramphenicol in neonates, therefore, requires decreased dosage and monitoring of blood levels.

Conversely, intrauterine exposure to drugs may induce precocious development of hepatic enzyme mechanisms, increasing the infant's capacity to metabolize potentially harmful substances.

Older children can metabolize drugs such as theophylline more rapidly than adults because of their increased hepatic metabolic activity. Larger doses than those recommended for adults may be required.

Also, preparations given concurrently to a child may alter hepatic metabolism and induce production of hepatic enzymes. Phenobarbital can induce hepatic enzyme production and accelerate metabolism of drugs given concurrently.

Excretion
Renal excretion of a drug is the net effect of glomerular filtration, active tubular secretion, and passive tubular reabsorption. Because so many drugs are excreted in the urine, the degree of renal development or presence of renal disease can profoundly affect a child's dosage requirements.

If a child is unable to excrete a drug renally, drug accumulation and possible toxicity may result unless the dosage is reduced.

Physiologically, an infant's kidneys differ from an adult's in that they have a high resistance to blood flow and receive a smaller proportion of cardiac output; exhibit incomplete glomerular and tubular development and short, incomplete loops of Henle (glomerular filtration reaches adult values between 2½ and 5 months; tubular secretion may reach adult values between 7 and 12 months); have low glomerular filtration rate (penicillins are eliminated by this route); demonstrate decreased ability to concentrate urine or reabsorb various filtered compounds; and have a reduced ability of the proximal tubules to secrete organic acids.

Special administration considerations
Biochemically, a drug displays the same mechanisms of action in all individuals. However, the response of a drug can be affected by a child's age and size as well as the maturity of the target organ. To ensure optimal drug effect and minimal toxicity, consider the following factors when prescribing drugs for pediatric patients.

Adjusting pediatric dosages
When calculating pediatric dosages, avoid using formulas that modify adult dosages: A child is not a scaled-down version of an adult. Pediatric dosages should be calculated on the basis of either body weight (mg/kg) or body surface area (mg/m^2).

Reevaluate dosages regularly to ensure necessary adjustments as the child develops. Although body surface area provides a useful standard for adults and older children, it should not be used in premature or full-term infants. Use the body weight method instead. Don't exceed the maximum adult dosage when calculating amounts per kilogram of body weight (except with certain drugs such as theophylline).

Obtain an accurate maternal drug history—prescription and OTC drugs, vitamins, and herbal agents or other health foods taken during pregnancy. Drugs passed through breast milk can also have adverse effects on the breast-feeding infant. Before a drug is prescribed for a breast-feeding woman, the potential effects on the infant should be studied.

For example, sulfonamides given to a breast-feeding mother for a urinary tract infection appear in breast milk and may cause kernicterus at lower-than-normal levels of unconjugated bilirubin.

Administering oral medications
Consider the following when prescribing oral medications for a pediatric patient.

If the patient is an infant, administer an oral medication in the liquid form if possible. For accuracy, the preparation should be measured and given by syringe; never in a vial or cup. The patient's head should be lifted to prevent aspiration of the medication, and his chin pressed down to prevent choking. The drug may also be placed in a nipple to allow the infant to suck the contents.

If the patient is a toddler, explain how he is to take the medication. If possible, have the parents enlist the child's cooperation. Medication should not be mixed with food or called "candy," even if it has a pleasant taste. The child should drink liquid medication from a calibrated medication cup rather than from a spoon: It's easier and more accurate. If the preparation is available only in tablet form, it should be crushed and mixed with a compatible syrup. (Check with the pharmacist or a reference source to verify that the tablet can be crushed without compromising its effectiveness.)

If the patient is an older child who can swallow a tablet or capsule by himself, have him place the medication on the back of his tongue and swallow it with water or fruit juice. Remember, milk or milk products may interfere with drug absorption.

Administering I.V. infusions
In infants, use a peripheral vein or a scalp vein in the temporal region for I.V. infusions. The scalp vein is safest in that the needle is not likely to be dislodged; however, the head must be shaved around the site. Temporary disfigurement may also result from the needle and infiltrated fluids. For these reasons, the scalp veins are not used as commonly today as in the past.

The extremities are the most accessible insertion sites; however, because patients tend to move about, keep the following precautions in mind:

- Protect the insertion sites to prevent catheter or needle dislodgment.
- Place clamps out of the child's reach and secure any connections.
- Provide a simple explanation to the child who is restrained while asleep to allay anxiety and maintain trust.

During an I.V. infusion, check the child's condition. Flow rate may vary if a pump isn't used. Flow should be adequate because some drugs (calcium, for example) can be irritating at low flow rates. Infants, small children, and children with compromised cardiopulmonary status are particularly vulnerable to fluid overload with I.V. medication administration. Ensure that a limited amount of fluid is infused in a controlled manner, use a volume-control set and an infusion pump or syringe.

Administering I.M. injections
I.M. injections are the preferred route of administration when a drug cannot be given by other parenteral routes and rapid absorption is necessary.

The vastus lateralis muscle is the preferred injection site in children under age 2; in older children, either the ventrogluteal area or the gluteus medius muscle can be used. To select the correct needle size, consider the patient's age, muscle mass, and nutritional status and the drug's viscosity; record and rotate injection sites. Explain to the patient that the injection will hurt or pinch, but that the medication will help him. Restrain him during the injection, if needed, and comfort him afterward.

Administering topical medications and inhalants
Consider the following when administering topical medications or inhalants.

Use eardrops warmed to room temperature; cold drops can cause considerable pain and possibly vertigo. To administer drops, turn the child on his side, with the affected ear up. If the child is under age 3, pull the pinna down and back; if he is age 3 or over, pull the pinna up and back.

Avoid using inhalants in young children: Obtaining their cooperation is difficult. Before attempting to administer medication through a metered-dose nebulizer to an older child, explain the inhaler to him.

Then have him hold the nebulizer upside down and close his lips around the mouthpiece. Have him exhale, pinch his nostrils shut and, when he starts to inhale, release one dose of medication into his mouth. Tell the patient to continue inhaling until his lungs feel full. Most inhaled agents are not useful if taken orally; if you doubt the patient's ability to use the inhalant correctly, don't use it.

Use topical corticosteroids cautiously because delayed growth in children has been associated with chronic steroid use. When topical corticosteroids are used on the diaper area of infants, avoid covering this area with plastic or rubber pants, which will act as an occlusive dressing and enhance systemic absorption.

Administering parenteral nutrition
Administer I.V. nutrition to patients who are unable to take adequate food orally and those with hypermetabolic conditions who need supplementation, including premature infants and children who have burns or other major trauma, intractable diarrhea, malabsorption syndromes, and emotional disorders (such as anorexia nervosa).

Before fat emulsions are given to infants and children, however, the potential benefits must be weighed against possible risks. Their use is limited by the child's ability to metabolize them; for example, a child with a diseased liver cannot efficiently metabolize fats.

Some fats, however, must be supplied both to prevent essential fatty acid deficiency and to permit normal growth and development. A minimum of calories (2% to 4%) must be supplied as linoleic acid—an essential fatty acid found in lipids. In infants, fats are essential for normal neurologic development.

Fat solutions may decrease oxygen perfusion and may adversely affect children with pulmonary disease. Minimize this risk by providing only the minimum fat needed for essential fatty acid requirements and not the usual intake of 40% to 50% of the child's total calories.

Fatty acids can also displace bilirubin bound to serum albumin, causing an increase in free, unconjugated bilirubin and an increased risk of kernicterus. However, fat solutions may interfere with some bilirubin assays and cause falsely elevated levels. To prevent this, obtain a blood sample 4 hours after lipid infusion; or if the emulsion is introduced over 24 hours, centrifuge the blood sample before the assay is performed.

Geriatric drug therapy
When prescribing drug therapy for elderly patients, consider the physiologic and pharmacokinetic changes that may alter appropriate drug dosage or cause common adverse reactions or compliance problems.

Physiologic changes affecting drug action
As a person ages, gradual physiologic changes occur. Some of these age-related changes may alter the therapeutic or toxic effects of medications.

Body composition
Proportions of fat, lean tissue, and water in the body change with age. Total body mass and lean body mass tend to decrease; the proportion of body fat tends to increase.

Depending on the individual, these changes in body composition affect the relationship between a drug's concentration and distribution in the body.

For example, a water-soluble drug such as gentamicin is not distributed to fat. Because there's relatively less lean tissue in an elderly person, more drug remains in the blood.

GI function
In elderly patients, decreases in gastric acid secretion and GI motility slow the emptying of stomach contents and the movement of intestinal contents through the entire tract. Furthermore, research suggests that elderly patients may have more difficulty absorbing medications. This is an especially significant problem with drugs having a narrow therapeutic range, such as digoxin, in which any change in absorption can be crucial.

Hepatic function
The liver's ability to metabolize certain drugs decreases with age. This is caused by diminished blood flow to the liver, which results from the age-related decrease in cardiac output and from the diminished activity of certain liver enzymes. When an elderly patient takes certain sleep medications such as flurazepam, the liver's reduced ability to metabolize the drug may produce a hangover effect the next morning.

Decreased hepatic function may cause more intense drug effects due to higher blood levels, longer-lasting drug effects due to prolonged blood levels, and greater incidence of drug toxicity.

Renal function

Although an elderly person's renal function is usually sufficient to eliminate excess body fluid and waste, the ability to eliminate some medications may be reduced by 50% or more.

Many medications commonly used by elderly patients, such as digoxin, are excreted primarily through the kidneys. If the kidneys' ability to excrete the drug is decreased, high drug blood levels may result. Digoxin toxicity, therefore, is relatively common in elderly patients who are not receiving a reduced digoxin dosage that accommodates decreased renal function.

Drug dosages can be modified to compensate for age-related decreases in renal function. The drug dosage may be adjusted with the help of laboratory tests, such as BUN and serum creatinine, so that the patient receives the expected therapeutic benefits without the risk of toxicity. Observe the patient for signs or symptoms of toxicity.

Special administration considerations

Aging is usually accompanied by a decline in organ function that can profoundly affect drug distribution and clearance. This physiologic decline is likely to be exacerbated by a disease or chronic disorder. Together, these factors can significantly increase the risk of adverse reactions, drug toxicity, and noncompliance. Be aware of these changes when prescribing a drug to a geriatric patient.

Adverse reactions

Compared with younger people, elderly patients experience twice as many adverse drug reactions as a result of greater drug consumption, poor compliance with drug regimens, and numerous physiologic changes.

Signs and symptoms of adverse drug reactions—confusion, weakness, and lethargy—are often mistakenly attributed to senility or disease. If the adverse reaction isn't identified, the patient may continue to receive the drug. Furthermore, he may receive unnecessary additional medication to treat complications caused by the original drug. This can sometimes result in a pattern of inappropriate and excessive drug use.

Although any drug can cause adverse reactions, most of the serious reactions in the elderly are caused by relatively few agents. Be particularly alert for toxicities resulting from diuretics, antihypertensives, digoxin, corticosteroids, anticoagulants, sleeping aids, and OTC drugs.

Diuretic toxicity

Because total body water content decreases with age, normal dosages of potassium-wasting diuretics, such as hydrochlorothiazide and furosemide, may result in fluid loss and even dehydration in an elderly patient.

These diuretics may deplete serum potassium, causing weakness in the patient, and they may raise blood uric acid and glucose levels, complicating preexisting gout and diabetes mellitus.

Antihypertensive toxicity

Many elderly people experience light-headedness or fainting when using antihypertensive medications, partly in response to atherosclerosis and decreased elasticity of the blood vessels. Antihypertensive drugs lower blood pressure too rapidly, resulting in insufficient blood flow to the brain. This may cause dizziness, fainting, or even stroke.

Consequently, dosages of antihypertensive drugs must be carefully individualized. In elderly patients, too aggressive treatment of high blood pressure may do more harm, so treatment goals should be reasonable. Although bringing blood pressure down to 120/85 mm Hg may be appropriate in a young hypertensive patient, a more reasonable goal for an elderly hypertensive patient might be 150/95 mm Hg.

Digoxin toxicity

As the body's renal function and rate of excretion decline, digoxin levels in the blood may build to toxic levels, causing nausea, vomiting, diarrhea, and—most serious—arrhythmias. Try to prevent severe toxicity by monitoring serum levels and by observing the patient for early signs or symptoms, such as appetite loss, confusion, or depression.

Corticosteroid toxicity

Elderly patients on corticosteroids may experience short-term effects, including fluid retention and psychological manifestations ranging from mild euphoria to acute psychotic reactions. Long-term toxic effects such as osteoporosis can be especially severe in elderly patients who have been taking prednisone or related steroidal compounds for months or even years. To prevent serious toxicity, carefully monitor patients on long-term regimens. Observe them for subtle changes in appearance, mood, and mobility; signs of impaired healing; and fluid and electrolyte disturbances.

Anticoagulant effects

Elderly patients taking anticoagulants are at an increased risk for bleeding, especially when they also take NSAIDs. Observe INRs carefully, and monitor these patients for bruising and other signs of bleeding.

Sleeping aid toxicity

Sedatives or sleeping aids may cause excessive sedation or residual drowsiness. Keep in mind that ingestion of alcohol may exaggerate such depressant effects, even if the sleeping aid was taken the previous evening.

OTC drug toxicity

When aspirin, aspirin-containing analgesics, and other OTC NSAIDs are used in moderation, toxicity is minimal, but prolonged ingestion may cause GI irritation—even ulcers—and gradual blood loss resulting in severe anemia. Prescription NSAIDs may cause similar problems, especially in the elderly. Although anemia from chronic aspirin consumption can affect all age groups, elderly patients may be less able to compensate because of their already reduced iron stores. Acetaminophen, long marketed for its safety, may cause toxicity when taken with alcohol.

Laxatives may cause diarrhea in elderly patients who are extremely sensitive to such drugs as bisacodyl. Chronic oral use of mineral oil as a lubricating laxative may result in lipid pneumonia from aspiration of small residual oil droplets in the patient's mouth.

Noncompliance

Poor compliance can be a problem with patients of any age. A significant number of hospitalizations result from noncompliance to medical regimen. However, in elderly patients, specific factors linked to aging—such as diminished visual acuity, hearing loss, forgetfulness, the common need for multiple drug therapy, and socioeconomic factors—can combine to make compliance a special problem. Approximately one-third of elderly patients fail to comply with their prescribed drug therapy. They may fail to take prescribed doses or to follow the correct schedule or they may take medications prescribed for previous disorders, discontinue medications prematurely, or use medications that are to be given on an as needed basis indiscriminately. Elderly patients may also have multiple prescriptions for the same medication and, therefore, inadvertently take an overdose.

Review the patient's medication regimen with him. Make sure he understands the medication amount and the time and frequency of doses. Also, explain how he should take each medication—that is, with food or water or by itself.

Provide the patient whatever help is needed to avoid drug therapy problems. Suggest that he use drug calendars, pill sorters, or other aids to help him comply with his prescribed drug regimen, and refer him to the pharmacist if he needs further information.

4 Effective prescribing practices

Two components of drug therapy are essential for prescribers: taking a detailed medication history and writing prescriptions appropriately and accurately. A careful medication history can help identify the use, dosage, effectiveness, potential interactions, and adverse reactions for each drug used.

Proper prescription writing practices are essential in providing comprehensive patient care and ensuring patient safety. They also reduce the legal liability of the prescriber, making errors and misunderstandings less likely.

Taking a medication history

Before prescribing a drug for a patient, conduct a complete assessment of the patient's condition and medication history. Assess the patient's knowledge about drug therapy and its effectiveness. A beneficial outcome to current or past drug use improves the patient's health status and overall quality of life. Interview the patient during the hospital admission or in an outpatient setting. Include specific questions about the patient's background that can significantly influence drug therapy, including questions about allergies, medical history, habits, socioeconomic status, lifestyle and beliefs, sensory deficits, and specific prescription and OTC drugs being taken, including herbal agents.

Allergies

The patient may have allergic reactions to drugs or foods. Obtain specific information about the drug name; a description of the reaction; its situation, time, and setting; and contributing factors, such as concurrent use of stimulants, tobacco, alcohol, or illegal drugs or a significant change in nutritional patterns. Tell the patient to describe the allergic reaction to help determine whether the reaction is an adverse effect or a dislike of taking the drug.

Allergies to foods can also affect drug therapy. Shellfish allergies, for instance, can contraindicate use of drugs that contain iodine or are byproducts of shellfish. Patients with allergies to eggs can't receive vaccines that are derived from chick embryos.

Medical history

When gathering the medical history, note the presence of chronic disorders and record the date of diagnosis, initial and current treatment, and the primary health care provider's name.

Careful attention to the patient's medical history can reveal important problems associated with drug therapy, such as conflicting and incompatible drug regimens. A patient who doesn't have a family physician to oversee and coordinate all care may seek the care of several specialists who may prescribe drug therapy without knowledge of other drugs being taken by the patient. You may find it helpful to contact the patient's pharmacist for a detailed list of medications the patient is taking.

Habits

Consider the patient's dietary habits and nontherapeutic use of drugs. Certain foods can directly influence the effectiveness of a drug. A patient receiving the anticoagulant warfarin, for instance, should not increase his intake of green leafy vegetables because they contain vitamin K, which can antagonize warfarin's anticoagulant effect.

Nontherapeutic uses of drugs can also affect a patient's health and impair the effectiveness of drug therapy. Consider the use of alcohol, tobacco, caffeine, and illegal drugs, such as marijuana, cocaine, or heroin. If the patient uses alcohol, note the frequency of use and the amount and type of alcohol consumed. Carefully document the intake of stimulants such as caffeine because these agents can adversely affect a patient's CV and CNS status. Record the type of stimulant used, frequency of intake, and amount consumed.

For the patient who uses tobacco, document the number of years the patient has smoked or chewed, type of tobacco used, and the quantity, frequency, and brand of tobacco product used each day.

Defining a patient's use of illicit drugs may be difficult. However, if such use is suspected, encourage the patient to discuss his use openly and honestly, emphasizing that these drugs have profound effects that may cause serious drug interactions. If the patient admits using illicit drugs, document the type of drug used, amount and frequency of use, and preferred route of administration.

Socioeconomic status

The patient's age, educational level, occupation, and insurance coverage may be important for compliance. The patient's age determines the individuals (parents or family members) to be included in the plan of care and the level of information appropriate for patient teaching.

Knowing the patient's educational background and occupation is helpful when selecting appropriate interventions, planning a drug regimen that fits the patient's daily routine, and encouraging compliance. Knowledge of the patient's insurance status may help you anticipate the need for financial assistance and counseling. Remember that noncompliance commonly results from an inability to afford the medications the patient has been prescribed.

Lifestyle and beliefs

Support systems, marital status, childbearing status, attitudes toward health and health care, whether the health care system is used, and daily activity

COMPONENTS OF A PROPERLY WRITTEN PRESCRIPTION

Prescriptions contain certain basic information and should be filled out properly to avoid misunderstandings. Here's an example of a correctly written prescription.

Lakeview Hospital
2000 N. Main Street
Lewistown, N.J. 00265

PATIENT'S NAME Kelly R. Weaver

ADDRESS 1000 Limerick Lane
Dresher, N.J. 00265

DATE 2/15/99

ADDRESSOPLATE OR COMPLETE ABOVE

This Rx NOT VALID For Schedule Drugs

Synthroid 0.2mg tab

Disp: #30

Sig: i tab P.O. daily

Refill 3 William Jackson PA-C

IN ORDER FOR A BRAND NAME PRODUCT TO BE DISPENSED, THE PRESCRIBER MUST HANDWRITE, "BRAND NECESSARY" OR "BRAND MEDICALLY NECESSARY" IN THE SPACE ABOVE.

Pharmacy will dispense a generic equivalent (under the formulary system) unless the particular drug is encircled.

PRESCRIBER'S PRINTED NAME William Jackson, PA-C

patterns may affect the plan of care for a patient and the likelihood of compliance. For example, an 18-year-old single parent who has dropped out of high school, is on medical assistance, and has no family support will probably require more teaching and assistance to gain compliance than a 40-year-old affluent professional with a great deal of family support, who understands the reasons for using the drug, and can afford the cost of therapy.

Sensory deficits

Any sensory deficit can significantly shape an appropriate plan of care. Impaired vision, paralysis of one or more extremities, loss of a limb, or loss of sensation in an extremity can impair the patient's ability to administer a subcutaneous injection, break a scored tablet, or open a medication container. Color blindness may cause difficulty in distinguishing between two medications. Hearing impairment can complicate effective patient instruction.

Always evaluate sensory deficits fully before planning drug therapy.

Special monitoring

Some drugs require special monitoring, such as monitoring the blood glucose or checking the radial pulse. Make sure the patient knows how to accurately perform special monitoring procedures. Discuss the effects of drug therapy with the patient and determine if new symptoms or unforeseen adverse reactions have developed. Noting the patient's pattern of administration may provide insight into why a particular drug regimen succeeds or fails.

OTC drugs

A comprehensive drug history should also include determining OTC drug use. OTC drugs include a wide range of products, from nutritional supplements to herbal or natural products to homeopathic remedies. Many OTC drugs can inhibit or potentiate the effects of a prescribed drug. For example, aspirin potentiates the anticoagulant effects of warfarin. Include dosage and frequency information as well as the type of product used.

Cognitive status

A patient's intact cognitive abilities ensure that he can understand and implement the actions necessary for compliance. During the interview, note whether the patient is alert and oriented, able to interact appropriately with people, and exhibits appropriate conversation. Consider whether the patient can think clearly and express his thoughts coherently. Finally, check short- and long-term memory because the patient will need both to follow the prescribed drug regimen.

If such an evaluation identifies cognitive deficits, determine the probable cause, which can range from a transient drug-related effect to permanent neurologic impairments. Then determine whether the patient can comply with the prescribed drug regimen. If compliance isn't possible, find another way to ensure that the patient receives the prescribed therapy.

Effective prescription writing

The physician assistant can write prescriptions in accordance with state laws governing such practice. It is important that the prescription be correctly and safely written. (See *Components of a properly written prescription.*)

Prescription components

Write a prescription legibly, and include the following components: patient's full name and address, date of the prescription, prescribed drug name, dosage form (if more than one formulation exists), total amount of the drug to be dispensed, amount of each dose, administration route, administration schedule or time, number of times the prescription can be refilled, and your signature and credentials.

Prescription writing practices

Some examples of effective prescription writing practices to ensure the accurate interpretation of your written prescriptions include these:

- Never abbreviate the names of drugs; abbreviations can be misinterpreted and the wrong drug given by mistake.
- Don't abbreviate the word "unit"; a sloppy, handwritten "U" or "u" could look like a zero and cause a tenfold drug overdose error.
- Don't use ambiguous abbreviations that could be misinterpreted, such as O.D., which could represent "once daily" or "right eye." When the accurate interpretation of an abbreviation is in question, write out the abbreviation completely.
- Avoid the unnecessary use of a decimal point and zero after a whole number. For instance, write "4 mg," not "4.0 mg." If the decimal point isn't seen, a tenfold drug overdose error could occur.
- Always place a zero before the decimal point when the quantity is less than 1. For instance, write "0.2 ml," not ".2 ml."
- Write instructions (including the reason the drug is being prescribed) on the prescription to prevent misinterpretation of the order and reduce the risk of error.

Keep in mind that medication errors often stem from poorly written prescriptions. To prevent such errors from occurring, write clearly and precisely, and review all parts of the form before signing the prescription. Besides enhancing patient safety and ensuring a beneficial outcome to treatment, a properly written prescription may also serve as an important legal protection.

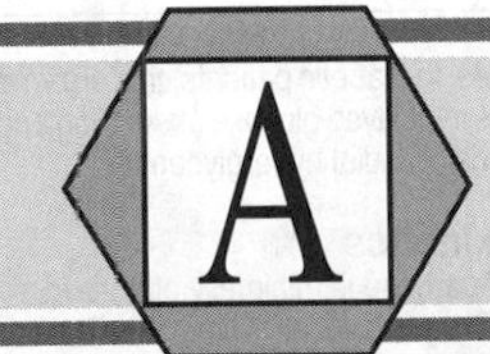

abciximab
ReoPro

Pharmacologic classification: antiplatelet aggregator
Therapeutic classification: platelet aggregation inhibitor
Pregnancy risk category C

How supplied
Available by prescription only
Injection: 2 mg/ml

Indications, route, and dosage
Adjunct to percutaneous transluminal coronary angioplasty or atherectomy (PTCA) for the prevention of acute cardiac ischemic complications in patients at high risk for abrupt closure of the treated coronary vessel
Adults: 0.25 mg/kg as an I.V. bolus administered 10 to 60 minutes before start of PTCA, followed by a continuous I.V. infusion of 10 mcg/minute for 12 hours.

Pharmacodynamics
Platelet aggregation inhibiting action: As the Fab fragment of the chimeric human-murine monoclonal immunoglobulin antibody 7E3, abciximab binds selectively to platelet glycoprotein (GP IIb/IIIa) receptors and inhibits platelet aggregation.

Pharmacokinetics
- *Absorption:* Abciximab is only given I.V.
- *Distribution:* Unknown.
- *Metabolism:* Unknown.
- *Excretion:* Unknown.

Contraindications and precautions
Contraindicated in patients with hypersensitivity to any component of drug or to murine proteins and in those with active internal bleeding, recent (within 6 weeks) clinically significant GI or GU bleeding, history of CVA within 2 years or CVA with significant residual neurologic deficit, bleeding diathesis, thrombocytopenia (less than 100,000/mm^3), recent (within 6 weeks) major surgery or trauma, intracranial neoplasm, intracranial arteriovenous malformation, intracranial aneurysm, severe uncontrolled hypertension, or history of vasculitis. Also contraindicated when oral anticoagulants have been administered within past 7 days, unless PT is 1.2 times control or less, or when I.V. dextran is being used before PTCA or is intended to be used during PTCA.

Use cautiously in patients who are at increased risk for bleeding, including those who weigh less than 165 lb (75 kg), are over age 65, have history of GI disease, or are receiving thrombolytics. Conditions that also increase the risk of bleeding include PTCA within 12 hours of onset of symptoms for acute MI, prolonged PTCA (lasting over 70 minutes), or failed PTCA. Heparin anticoagulation used in conjunction with abciximab may also contribute to the risk of bleeding.

Interactions
Antiplatelet agents, heparin, NSAIDs, other anticoagulants, and *thrombolytics* increase the risk of bleeding. Monitor patient closely.

Effects on diagnostic tests
None reported.

Adverse reactions
CNS: confusion, hypesthesia.
CV: bradycardia, *hypotension,* peripheral edema.
EENT: abnormal vision.
GI: *nausea, vomiting.*
Hematologic: anemia, *bleeding,* leukocytosis, ***thrombocytopenia.***
Respiratory: pleural effusion, pleurisy, pneumonia.
Other: pain.

Overdose and treatment
There has been no report of overdosage in humans. Discontinue infusion after 12 hours to avoid effects of prolonged platelet receptor blockade.

☑ Special considerations
- Patients at risk for abrupt closure, and thus candidates for drug therapy, include those undergoing PTCA with at least one of the following conditions: unstable angina or a non-Q-wave MI, an acute Q-wave MI within 12 hours of symptom onset or the presence of two type B lesions in the artery to be dilated, one type B lesion in the artery to be dilated in women age 65 or older or diabetic patients, one type C lesion in the artery to be dilated, or angioplasty of an infarct-related lesion within 7 days of MI.
- Drug should be used with aspirin and heparin.
- Keep epinephrine, dopamine, theophylline, antihistamines, and corticosteroids readily available if anaphylaxis occurs.
- Inspect solution for particulate matter before administration. If opaque Hparticles are visible, discard solution and obtain new vial. Withdraw necessary amount of drug for bolus injection through a sterile, nonpyrogenic, low-protein-binding 0.2- or 0.22-millipore filter into a syringe. Administer bolus 10 to 60 minutes before procedure.
- Withdraw 4.5 ml of drug for continuous infusion through a sterile, nonpyrogenic, low-protein-bind-

ing 0.2- or 0.22-micron filter into a syringe. Inject into 250 ml of sterile 0.9% NaCl or 5% dextrose and infuse at 17 ml/hour for 12 hours through a continuous infusion pump equipped with an in-line filter. Discard unused portion at the end of the 12-hour infusion.

- Administer drug in a separate I.V. line; do not add other medications to the infusion solution.
- Monitor closely for bleeding. Bleeding associated with abciximab therapy falls into two broad categories: bleeding observed at the arterial access site for cardiac catheterization and internal bleeding involving the GI tract, GU tract, or retroperitoneal sites.
- Institute bleeding precautions. Maintain patient on bed rest for 6 to 8 hours following sheath removal or drug discontinuation, whichever is later. Minimize or avoid, if possible, arterial punctures, venous punctures, and I.M. injections, and avoid use of urinary catheters, nasotracheal intubation, nasogastric tubes, and automatic blood pressure cuffs.

Patient education

- Instruct patient to report bleeding promptly.

Pediatric use

- Safety and effectiveness in pediatric patients have not been established.

Breast-feeding

- It is unknown if drug occurs in breast milk or is absorbed systemically after ingestion. Use cautiously.

acarbose

Precose

Pharmacologic classification: alpha-glucosidase inhibitor
Therapeutic classification: antidiabetic
Pregnancy risk category B

How supplied

Available by prescription only
Tablets: 50 mg, 100 mg

Indications, route, and dosage

Adjunct to diet to lower blood glucose in patients with non-insulin-dependent diabetes mellitus whose hyperglycemia cannot be managed by diet alone or by diet and a sulfonylurea

Adults: Initially, 25 mg P.O. t.i.d. with the first bite of each main meal. Subsequent dosage adjustment made at 4- to 8-week intervals based on 1-hour postprandial glucose levels and tolerance. Maintenance dosage is 50 to 100 mg P.O. t.i.d. depending on patient's weight. Maximum dosage for patients weighing 132 lb (60 kg) or less is 50 mg P.O. t.i.d.; for patients weighing over 132 lb, maximum dosage is 100 mg P.O. t.i.d.

Pharmacodynamics

Antidiabetic action: The ability of acarbose to lower blood glucose results from a competitive, reversible inhibition of pancreatic alpha-amylase and membrane-bound intestinal alpha-glucoside hydrolase enzymes. In diabetic patients, this enzyme inhibition results in delayed glucose absorption and a lowering of postprandial hyperglycemia.

Pharmacokinetics

- *Absorption:* Acarbose is minimally absorbed.
- *Distribution:* Drug acts locally within the GI tract.
- *Metabolism:* Metabolized exclusively within the GI tract, principally by intestinal bacteria with some metabolized action caused by digestive enzymes.
- *Excretion:* Within 96 hours, 51% of dose is excreted in feces as unabsorbed drug. The fraction of drug that is absorbed is almost completely excreted by the kidneys. Plasma elimination half-life of acarbose is about 2 hours. Drug accumulation does not occur with t.i.d. oral dosing.

Contraindications and precautions

Contraindicated in patients with hypersensitivity to drug, diabetic ketoacidosis, cirrhosis, inflammatory bowel disease, colonic ulceration, or partial intestinal obstruction and in those predisposed to intestinal obstruction. Also contraindicated in patients with chronic intestinal diseases associated with marked disorders of digestion or absorption and in those with conditions that may deteriorate because of increased gas formation in the intestine. Avoid drug in patients with serum creatinine levels exceeding 2 mg/dl and in breast-feeding or pregnant women.

Use cautiously in patients with mild to moderate renal impairment.

Interactions

Concomitant therapy with *calcium channel blocking agents, corticosteroids, estrogens, isoniazid, nicotinic acid, oral contraceptives, phenothiazines, phenytoin, sympathomimetics, thiazides, other diuretics,* and *thyroid products* may cause hyperglycemia or hypoglycemia when withdrawn. Monitor patient's blood glucose levels. *Intestinal adsorbents* (*activated charcoal*) and *digestive enzyme preparations containing carbohydrate-splitting enzymes* (*amylase, pancreatin*) may reduce the effect of acarbose. Do not administer concomitantly. When acarbose is used with a *sulfonylurea* or *insulin*, it may increase the hypoglycemic potential of these agents. Monitor patient's blood glucose level closely.

Effects on diagnostic tests

Acarbose therapy, particularly in doses over 50 mg t.i.d., may cause elevations of serum transaminases and, in rare cases, bilirubin.

Adverse reactions

GI: *abdominal pain, diarrhea, flatulence.*
Other: elevated serum transaminase levels.

Overdose and treatment

Unlike sulfonylureas or insulin, acarbose overdosage does not result in hypoglycemia. An overdose may result in transient increases in flatulence, diarrhea, and abdominal discomfort, which quickly subside.

☑ **Special considerations**

- Drug alone does not cause hypoglycemia. However, when given in combination with a sulfonylurea or insulin, it may increase the hypoglycemic potential of the sulfonylurea. Monitor patient receiving both drugs closely. If hypoglycemia occurs, treat with oral glucose (dextrose), whose absorption is not inhibited by acarbose, rather than sucrose (cane sugar). Severe hypoglycemia may require I.V. glucose infusion or glucagon administration. Dosage adjustment in acarbose and sulfonylurea may be required to prevent further episodes of hypoglycemia.
- During periods of increased stress, such as infection, fever, surgery, or trauma, patient may require insulin therapy. Monitor patient closely for hyperglycemia in these situations.
- Monitor patient's 1-hour postprandial plasma glucose levels to determine therapeutic effectiveness of acarbose and to identify appropriate dose. Thereafter, glycosylated hemoglobin should be measured every 3 months. Treatment goals include decreasing both postprandial plasma glucose and glycosylated hemoglobin levels to normal or near normal by using the lowest effective dose of acarbose either as monotherapy or in combination with sulfonylureas.
- Monitor serum transaminase levels every 3 months during first year of therapy and then periodically thereafter in patients receiving doses exceeding 50 mg t.i.d. Abnormalities may require dosage adjustment or withdrawal of drug.

Patient education

- Tell patient to take drug with the first bite of each of three main meals daily.
- Make sure patient understands that therapy relieves symptoms but does not cure disease.
- Stress importance of adhering to specific diet, reducing weight, exercising, and following personal hygiene programs. Explain how and when to perform self-monitoring of blood glucose level, and teach recognition of and intervention for hyperglycemia.
- If a sulfonylurea agent is also taken, teach patient recognition of and intervention for hypoglycemia. Tell patient to treat symptoms of low blood glucose with a form of dextrose rather than with products containing table sugar.
- Advise patient to carry medical identification regarding diabetic status.

Pediatric use

- Safety and effectiveness in pediatric patients have not been established.

Breast-feeding

- It is not known whether drug is excreted in breast milk. Acarbose should not be given to breast-feeding women.

acebutolol

Sectral

Pharmacologic classification: beta-adrenergic blocker
Therapeutic classification: antihypertensive, antiarrhythmic
Pregnancy risk category B

How supplied

Available by prescription only
Capsules: 200 mg, 400 mg

Indications, route, and dosage

Hypertension
Adults: 400 mg P.O. either as a single daily dose or divided b.i.d. Patients may receive as much as 1,200 mg divided b.i.d.

Ventricular arrhythmias
Adults: 400 mg P.O. daily divided b.i.d. Increase dosage to provide an adequate clinical response. Usual daily dosage is 600 to 1,200 mg.

◊ ***Angina***
Adults: Initially, 200 mg b.i.d. Increase up to 800 mg daily until angina is controlled. Patients with severe angina may require higher doses.

✦ ***Dosage adjustment.*** Reduce dosage in the elderly and patients with impaired renal function. Avoid doses over 800 mg/day in the elderly.

Pharmacodynamics

Antihypertensive action: Exact mechanism of the antihypertensive effect is unknown. Drug has cardioselective beta-adrenergic blocking properties and mild intrinsic sympathomimetic activity.

Antiarrhythmic action: Drug decreases heart rate and prevents exercise-induced increases in heart rate; it also decreases myocardial contractility, cardiac output, and SA and AV nodal conduction velocity.

Pharmacokinetics

- *Absorption:* Acebutolol is well absorbed after oral administration. Peak plasma levels occur at about 2½ hours.
- *Distribution:* Drug is about 26% protein-bound; minimal quantities are detected in CSF.
- *Metabolism:* Acebutolol undergoes extensive first-pass metabolism in the liver; peak levels of its major active metabolite, diacetolol, occur at about 3½ hours.
- *Excretion:* From 30% to 40% of a given dose of acebutolol is excreted in urine; rest occurs in feces and bile. Half-life of acebutolol is 3 to 4 hours; half-life of diacetolol is 8 to 13 hours.

Contraindications and precautions

Contraindicated in patients with persistent severe bradycardia, second- and third-degree heart block, overt cardiac failure, and cardiogenic shock. Use cautiously in patients at risk for heart failure and in patients with bronchospastic disease, diabetes, hyperthyroidism, and peripheral vascular disease.

Interactions
Acebutolol may potentiate hypotensive effects of *other antihypertensive agents*; it also may alter *insulin* or *oral antidiabetic* dosage requirements in stable diabetic patients. Hypotensive effects of acebutolol may be antagonized by *indomethacin, NSAIDs,* and *alpha-adrenergic stimulants* such as those contained in *OTC cold remedies.*

Effects on diagnostic tests
Drug may cause positive antinuclear antibody titers.

Adverse reactions
CNS: depression, dizziness, fatigue, headache, hyperesthesia, hypoesthesia, impotence, insomnia.
CV: bradycardia, chest pain, edema, ***heart failure,*** hypotension.
GI: abdominal pain, constipation, diarrhea, dyspepsia, flatulence, nausea, vomiting.
Respiratory: ***bronchospasm,*** cough, dyspnea.
Skin: rash.
Other: arthralgia, myalgia.

Overdose and treatment
Clinical signs of overdose include severe hypotension, bradycardia, heart failure, and bronchospasm.

After acute ingestion, empty stomach by emesis or gastric lavage; follow with activated charcoal to reduce absorption. Then provide symptomatic and supportive treatment.

☑ Special considerations
Besides those relevant to all *beta-adrenergic blockers,* consider the following recommendation.
- Do not discontinue drug abruptly.

Patient education
- Advise patient to report wheezing promptly.

Pediatric use
- Safety and efficacy in pediatric patients have not been established.

Breast-feeding
- Both acebutolol and its metabolite, diacetolol, occur in breast milk; breast-feeding is not recommended for women receiving drug.

acetaminophen
Acephen, Anacin-3, Bromo-Seltzer, Tempra, Tylenol, Valorin

Pharmacologic classification: para-aminophenol derivative
Therapeutic classification: nonnarcotic analgesic, antipyretic
Pregnancy risk category B

How supplied
Available without a prescription
Tablets: 120 mg, 160 mg, 325 mg, 500 mg, 650 mg
Tablets (chewable): 80 mg, 120 mg, 160 mg
Capsules: 325 mg, 500 mg
Suppositories: 80 mg, 120 mg, 125 mg, 300 mg, 325 mg, 650 mg
Solution: 48 mg/ml, 80 mg/ml*, 100 mg/ml, 80 mg/5 ml, 120 mg/5 ml, 130 mg/5 ml, 160 mg/5 ml, 167 mg/5 ml, 500 mg/15 ml
Suspension: 48 mg/ml, 80 mg/ml*, 80 mg/5 ml*, 100 mg/ml, 160 mg/5 ml
Granules: 80 mg/packet
Oral powders: 80 mg, 160 mg

Indications, route, and dosage
Mild pain; fever
Adults and children over age 12: 325 to 650 mg P.O. or P.R. q 4 to 6 hours p.r.n. Maximum dose should not exceed 4 g daily. Maximum dosage for long-term therapy is 2.6 g daily.
Children age 11 to 12: 480 mg/dose q 4 to 6 hours.
Children age 9 to 10: 400 mg/dose q 4 to 6 hours.
Children age 6 to 8: 320 mg/dose q 4 to 6 hours.
Children age 4 to 5: 240 mg/dose q 4 to 6 hours.
Children age 2 to 3: 160 mg/dose q 4 to 6 hours.
Children age 12 to 23 months: 120 mg/dose q 4 to 6 hours.
Children age 4 to 11 months: 80 mg/dose q 4 to 6 hours.
Children age 3 months or less: 40 mg/dose q 4 to 6 hours.

Pharmacodynamics
Mechanism and site of action is unclear and may be related to inhibition of prostaglandin synthesis in the CNS.

Analgesic action: Analgesic effect may be related to an elevation of the pain threshold.

Antipyretic action: Drug is believed to exert its antipyretic effect by direct action on the hypothalamic heat-regulating center to block the effects of endogenous pyrogen. This results in increased heat dissipation through sweating and vasodilation.

Pharmacokinetics
- *Absorption:* Drug is absorbed rapidly and completely via the GI tract. Peak plasma concentrations occur in ½ to 2 hours, slightly faster for liquid preparations.
- *Distribution:* Drug is 25% protein-bound. Plasma concentrations do not correlate well with analgesic effect, but do correlate with toxicity.
- *Metabolism:* Approximately 90% to 95% is metabolized in the liver.
- *Excretion:* Acetaminophen is excreted in urine. Average elimination half-life ranges from 1 to 4 hours. In acute overdose, prolongation of elimination half-life is correlated with toxic effects. Half-life over 4 hours is associated with hepatic necrosis; over 12 hours is associated with coma.

Contraindications and precautions
No known contraindications. Use cautiously in patients with history of chronic alcohol abuse because hepatotoxicity has occurred after therapeutic doses. Also use cautiously in patients with hepatic or CV disease, renal function impairment, or viral infection.

Interactions
Concomitant use of acetaminophen may potentiate the effects of *anticoagulants* and *thrombolytic*

drugs, but this effect appears to be clinically insignificant. *Antacids* and *food* delay and decrease the absorption of acetaminophen. Combined *caffeine* and acetaminophen may enhance the therapeutic effect of acetaminophen. Concomitant use of *phenothiazines* and acetaminophen in large doses may result in hypothermia. *Anticonvulsants* and concomitant use of *isoniazid* with acetaminophen may result in an increased risk of hepatotoxicity.

Effects on diagnostic tests
Acetaminophen may cause a false-positive test result for urinary 5-hydroxyindoleacetic acid.

Adverse reactions
Hematologic: hemolytic anemia, neutropenia, leukopenia, ***pancytopenia, thrombocytopenia*** (rare).
Hepatic: jaundice, ***severe liver damage*** (with toxic doses).
Skin: rash, urticaria.
Other: hypoglycemia.

Overdose and treatment
In acute overdose, plasma levels of 300 mcg/ml 4 hours postinjection or 50 mcg/ml 12 hours postinjection are associated with hepatotoxicity. Clinical manifestations of overdose include cyanosis, anemia, jaundice, skin eruptions, fever, emesis, CNS stimulation, delirium, methemoglobinemia progressing to depression, coma, vascular collapse, seizures, and death. Acetaminophen poisoning develops in stages:

Stage 1 (12 to 24 hours after ingestion): nausea, vomiting, diaphoresis, anorexia.

Stage 2 (24 to 48 hours after ingestion): clinically improved but elevated liver function tests.

Stage 3 (72 to 96 hours after ingestion): peak hepatotoxicity.

Stage 4 (7 to 8 days after ingestion): recovery.

To treat toxic overdose of acetaminophen, empty stomach immediately by inducing emesis with ipecac syrup if patient is conscious or by gastric lavage. Administer activated charcoal via nasogastric tube. Oral acetylcysteine (Mucomyst) is a specific antidote for acetaminophen poisoning and is most effective if started within 10 to 12 hours after ingestion, but it can help if started within 24 hours after ingestion. Administer a Mucomyst loading dose of 140 mg/kg P.O., followed by maintenance doses of 70 mg/kg P.O. every 4 hours for an additional 17 doses. Doses vomited within 1 hour of administration must be repeated. Remove charcoal before giving acetylcysteine because it may interfere with absorption of this antidote.

Acetylcysteine minimizes hepatic injury by supplying sulphydryl groups that bind with acetaminophen metabolites. Hemodialysis may be helpful to remove acetaminophen from the body. Monitor laboratory parameters and vital signs closely. Provide symptomatic and supportive measures (respiratory support, correction of fluid and electrolyte imbalances). Determine plasma acetaminophen levels at least 4 hours after overdose. If plasma acetaminophen levels indicate hepatotoxicity, perform liver function tests every 24 hours for at least 96 hours.

☑ Special considerations
- Acetaminophen has no significant anti-inflammatory effect. Even so, studies have shown substantial benefit in patients with osteoarthritis of the knee. Therapeutic benefits may stem from the analgesic effects of drug.
- Many OTC products contain acetaminophen. Be aware of this when calculating total daily dose.
- Patients unable to tolerate aspirin may be able to tolerate acetaminophen.
- Monitor vital signs, especially temperature, to evaluate drug's effectiveness.
- Assess patient's level of pain and response before and after drug administration.
- Store rectal acetaminophen suppositories in refrigerator.

Patient education
- Instruct patient in proper administration of prescribed form of drug.
- Advise patient on chronic high-dose drug therapy to arrange for monitoring of laboratory parameters, especially BUN, serum creatinine, liver function tests, and CBC.
- Warn patient with current or past rectal bleeding to avoid using rectal acetaminophen suppositories. If they are used, they must be retained in the rectum for at least 1 hour.
- Warn patient that high doses or unsupervised chronic use of acetaminophen can cause liver damage. Use of alcoholic beverages increases the risk of liver toxicity.
- Tell patient to avoid use for self-medication of a fever above 103° F (39° C), a fever persisting longer than 3 days, or a recurrent fever.
- When prescribing buffered acetaminophen effervescent granules, consider sodium content for sodium-restricted patients.
- Tell patient not to take NSAIDs together with acetaminophen on a regular basis.
- Warn patient to avoid taking tetracycline antibiotics within 1 hour after taking buffered acetaminophen effervescent granules.
- Tell patient not to use drug for arthritic or rheumatic conditions without medical approval. Drug may relieve pain but not other symptoms.
- Tell adult patient not to take drug for over 10 days without medical approval.
- Tell patient on high-dose or long-term therapy that regular follow-up visits are essential.

Geriatric use
- Elderly patients are more sensitive to drug. Use with caution.

Pediatric use
- Children should not take more than five doses per day or take drug for over 5 days unless prescribed.

Breast-feeding
- Drug is excreted into breast milk in low concentrations. No adverse effects have been reported.

acetazolamide

acetazolamide sodium

Ak-Zol, Diamox, Diamox Sequels

Pharmacologic classification: carbonic anhydrase inhibitor
Therapeutic classification: antiglaucoma agent, anticonvulsant, diuretic, altitude sickness agent (prevention and treatment)
Pregnancy risk category C

How supplied

Available by prescription only
Tablets: 125 mg, 250 mg
Capsules (extended-release): 500 mg
Injection: 500 mg

Indications, route, and dosage

Preoperative management of acute angle-closure glaucoma
Adults: 250 mg P.O. q 4 hours; 250 mg b.i.d. P.O.; or for short-term rapid-relief therapy, I.V. administration of 500 mg, which may be repeated in 2 to 4 hours, if necessary, followed by 125 to 250 mg P.O. q 4 hours.
Edema in heart failure
Adults: 250 to 375 mg P.O. daily in morning.
Children: 5 mg/kg P.O. or I.V. daily in morning.
Drug-induced edema
Adults: 250 to 375 mg P.O. as single daily dose for 1 to 2 days alternating with 1 drug-free day.
Open-angle glaucoma, secondary glaucoma
Adults: 250 mg to 1 g P.O. or I.V. daily, divided q.i.d.
Prevention or amelioration of acute mountain sickness
Adults: 500 to 1,000 mg P.O. in divided doses taken preferably 48 hours before ascent and continued for at least 48 hours after arrival at the high altitude.
Myoclonic seizures, refractory generalized tonic-clonic (grand mal) or absence (petit mal) seizures, mixed seizures
Adults: 375 mg P.O. or I.V. daily up to 250 mg q.i.d. Initial dosage when used with other anticonvulsants usually is 250 mg daily.
Children: 8 to 30 mg/kg P.O. or I.V. daily, divided t.i.d. or q.i.d.
◊ ***Diuresis and alkalization of urine in the treatment of toxicity associated with weakly acidic drugs***
Adults: 5 mg/kg I.V. p.r.n.
Children: 5 mg/kg I.V. or 150 mg/m^2 I.V. once daily (in morning) for 1 to 2 days alternated with 1 drug-free day.
◊ ***Prevention of cystine or uric acid nephrolithiasis***
Adults: 250 mg P.O. h.s.
◊ ***Periodic paralysis***
Adults: 250 mg P.O. b.i.d. or t.i.d. Maximum dose, 1.5 g daily.

Pharmacodynamics

Antiglaucoma action: In open-angle glaucoma and perioperatively for acute angle-closure glaucoma, acetazolamide and acetazolamide sodium decrease the formation of aqueous humor, lowering intraocular pressure.

Anticonvulsant action: Inhibition of carbonic anhydrase in the CNS appears to slow down abnormal paroxysmal discharge from the neurons.

Diuretic action: Acetazolamide and acetazolamide sodium act by noncompetitive reversible inhibition of the enzyme carbonic anhydrase, which is responsible for formation of hydrogen and bicarbonate ions from carbon dioxide and water. This inhibition results in decreased hydrogen concentration in the renal tubules, promoting excretion of bicarbonate, sodium, potassium, and water; because carbon dioxide is not eliminated as rapidly, systemic acidosis may occur.

Altitude sickness agent: Acetazolamide shortens the period of high-altitude acclimatization; by inhibiting conversion of carbon dioxide to bicarbonate, it may increase carbon dioxide tension in tissues and decrease it in the lungs. The resultant metabolic acidosis may also increase oxygenation during hypoxia.

Pharmacokinetics

- *Absorption:* Acetazolamide is well absorbed from the GI tract after oral administration.
- *Distribution:* Drug is distributed throughout body tissues.
- *Metabolism:* None.
- *Excretion:* Excreted primarily in urine via tubular secretion and passive reabsorption.

Contraindications and precautions

Contraindicated in patients with hypersensitivity to drug; in long-term therapy for chronic noncongestive angle-closure glaucoma; and in those with hyponatremia or hypokalemia, renal or hepatic disease or dysfunction, adrenal gland failure, and hyperchloremic acidosis. Use cautiously in patients with respiratory acidosis, emphysema, diabetes, or COPD and in those receiving other diuretics.

Interactions

Acetazolamide alkalinizes urine and thus may decrease excretion of *amphetamines, flecainide, procainamide,* and *quinidine.* Acetazolamide may increase excretion of *salicylates, phenobarbital,* and *lithium,* lowering plasma levels of these drugs and possibly necessitating dosage adjustments.

Effects on diagnostic tests

Because it alkalinizes urine, acetazolamide may cause false-positive proteinuria in Albustix or Albutest. Drug may also decrease thyroid iodine uptake.

Adverse reactions

CNS: confusion, drowsiness, paresthesia.
EENT: hearing dysfunction, transient myopia, tinnitus.
GI: anorexia, altered taste, diarrhea, nausea, vomiting.

GU: hematuria, polyuria.
Hematologic: ***aplastic anemia,*** hemolytic anemia, leukopenia.
Skin: rash.
Other: asymptomatic hyperuricemia, hyperchloremic acidosis, hypokalemia.

Overdose and treatment

Specific recommendations are unavailable. Treatment is supportive and symptomatic. Acetazolamide increases bicarbonate excretion and may cause hypokalemia and hyperchloremic acidosis. Induce emesis or perform gastric lavage. Do not induce catharsis because this may exacerbate electrolyte disturbances. Monitor fluid and electrolyte levels.

☑ Special considerations

- Suspensions containing 250 mg/5 ml of syrup are the most palatable and can be made by a pharmacist. These remain stable for about 1 week. Tablets will not dissolve in fruit juice.
- Reconstitute powder by adding at least 5 ml sterile water for injection.
- Direct I.V. administration is preferred if drug must be given parenterally.

Patient education

- Warn patient to use caution while driving or performing tasks that require alertness, coordination, or physical dexterity because drug may cause drowsiness.

Geriatric use

- Observe elderly and debilitated patients closely because they are more susceptible to drug-induced diuresis. Excessive diuresis promotes rapid dehydration, leading to hypovolemia, hypokalemia, and hyponatremia and may cause circulatory collapse. Reduced dosages may be indicated in these patients.

Breast-feeding

- Safety of drug in breast-feeding women has not been established.

acetylcholine chloride

Miochol

Pharmacologic classification: cholinergic agonist
Therapeutic classification: miotic
Pregnancy risk category NR

How supplied

Available by prescription only
Ophthalmic solution: 1%

Indications, route, and dosage

To produce miosis during surgery
Adults and children: 0.5 to 2 ml of 1% solution instilled gently in anterior chamber of eye. Drug is used during ophthalmic surgery to cause rapid, complete miosis.

Pharmacodynamics

Miotic action: The cholinergic activity of acetylcholine causes contraction of the sphincter muscles of the iris, resulting in miosis and contraction of the ciliary muscle, leading to accommodation. It also acts to deepen the anterior chamber and vasodilates conjunctival vessels of the outflow tract.

Pharmacokinetics

- *Absorption:* Action begins within seconds.
- *Distribution:* Unknown.
- *Metabolism:* Probably local, by cholinesterases.
- *Excretion:* Duration of activity is 10 to 20 minutes.

Contraindications and precautions

Contraindicated in patients with hypersensitivity to drug or its components.

Interactions

None reported.

Effects on diagnostic tests

None reported.

Adverse reactions

CV: bradycardia, hypotension.
EENT: corneal edema, clouding, decompensation.
Respiratory: breathing difficulties.
Other: diaphoresis, flushing.

Overdose and treatment

Overdose is extremely rare after ophthalmic use but may cause miosis, flushing, vomiting, bradycardia, bronchospasm, increased bronchial secretion, sweating, tearing, involuntary urination, hypotension, and seizures. Flush eyes with 0.9% NaCl solution or sterile water. If drug was accidentally swallowed, vomiting is usually spontaneous; if not, induce emesis with activated charcoal or a cathartic. Treat accidental dermal exposure by washing the area twice with water. Epinephrine may be used to treat adverse CV reactions.

☑ Special considerations

- Solutions of acetylcholine chloride are unstable; prepare solution immediately before use. Discard unused solution and one that is not clear and colorless.
- If the center rubber plug seal does not go down or is already down when reconstituting, do not use the vial.
- Do not gas-sterilize vial. Ethylene oxide may produce formic acid.

acetylcysteine

Mucomyst, Mucosil, Parvolex*

Pharmacologic classification: amino acid (L-cysteine) derivative
Therapeutic classification: mucolytic, antidote for acetaminophen overdose
Pregnancy risk category B

How supplied

Available by prescription only

Solution: 10%, 20%
Injection:* 200 mg/ml

Indications, route, and dosage

Acute and chronic bronchopulmonary disease, tracheostomy care, pulmonary complications of surgery, diagnostic bronchial studies
Administer by nebulization, direct application, or intratracheal instillation.
Adults and children: 1 to 2 ml of 10% or 20% solution by direct instillation into trachea as often as hourly; or 3 to 5 ml of 20% solution or 6 to 10 ml of 10% solution administered by nebulizer q 2 to 3 hours. For instillation via percutaneous intratracheal catheter, administer 1 to 2 ml of 20% solution or 2 to 4 ml of 10% solution; via tracheal catheter to treat a specific bronchopulmonary tree segment, administer 2 to 5 ml of 20% solution. For diagnostic bronchial studies (administered before procedure), administer 1 to 2 ml of 20% solution or 2 to 4 ml of 10% solution for two or three doses.

Acetaminophen toxicity
Adults and children: Initially, 140 mg/kg P.O., followed by 70 mg/kg q 4 hours for 17 doses (a total of 1,330 mg/kg) or until acetaminophen assay reveals nontoxic level.

Alternatively, may be administered I.V.: Loading dose 150 mg/kg I.V. in 200 ml D_5W over 15 minutes, followed by 50 mg/kg I.V. in 500 ml D_5W over 4 hours, followed by 100 mg/kg I.V. in 1,000 ml D_5W over 16 hours.

Pharmacodynamics

Mucolytic action: Drug produces its mucolytic effect by splitting the disulfide bonds of mucoprotein, the substance responsible for increased viscosity of mucus secretions in the lungs; thus, pulmonary secretions become less viscous and more liquid.

Acetaminophen antidote: Mechanism by which acetylcysteine reduces acetaminophen toxicity is not fully understood; it is thought that acetylcysteine restores hepatic stores of glutathione or inactivates the toxic metabolite of acetaminophen via a chemical interaction, thereby preventing hepatic damage.

Pharmacokinetics

- *Absorption:* Most inhaled acetylcysteine acts directly on the mucus in the lungs; the remainder is absorbed by pulmonary epithelium. Action begins within 1 minute after inhalation and immediately upon direct intratracheal instillation; peak effect occurs in 5 to 10 minutes. After oral administration, drug is absorbed from the GI tract.
- *Distribution:* Unknown.
- *Metabolism:* Drug is metabolized in the liver.
- *Excretion:* Unknown.

Contraindications and precautions

Contraindicated in patients hypersensitive to drug. Use cautiously in elderly or debilitated patients with severe respiratory insufficiency.

Interactions

Activated charcoal adsorbs orally administered acetylcysteine, preventing its absorption.

Acetylcysteine is incompatible with *oxytetracycline, tetracycline, chlortetracycline, erythromycin lactobionate, amphotericin B, ampicillin, iodized oil, chymotrypsin, trypsin,* and *hydrogen peroxide*; drug should be administered separately.

Effects on diagnostic tests

None reported.

Adverse reactions

CV: hypotension, hypertension, tachycardia.
EENT: *rhinorrhea.*
GI: *nausea, stomatitis, vomiting.*
Respiratory: ***bronchospasm*** (especially in asthmatic patients).
Other: clamminess, chest tightness, fever.

Overdose and treatment

No information available.

☑ Special considerations

- Acetylcysteine solutions release hydrogen sulfide and discolor on contact with rubber and some metals (especially iron, nickel, and copper); drug tarnishes silver (this does not affect drug potency).
- Solution may turn light purple; this does not affect safety or efficacy of the drug. Use plastic, stainless steel, or other inert metal when administering drug by nebulization. Do not use hand-held bulb nebulizers; output is too small and particle size too large.
- After opening, store in refrigerator or use within 96 hours.
- Monitor cough type and frequency; for maximum effect, instruct patient to clear airway by coughing before aerosol administration. Many clinicians pretreat with bronchodilators before administration of acetylcysteine. Keep suction equipment available; if patient has insufficient cough to clear increased secretions, suction will be needed to maintain open airway.
- When used orally for acetaminophen overdose, dilute with cola, fruit juice, or water to a 5% concentration and administer within 1 hour.
- Do not place directly in the chamber of a heated (hot pot) nebulizer.

Patient education

- Warn patient of unpleasant odor (rotten egg odor of hydrogen sulfide), and explain that increased amounts of liquefied bronchial secretion plus unpleasant odor may cause nausea and vomiting; have patient rinse mouth with water after nebulizer treatment.

Geriatric use

- Elderly patients may have inadequate cough and be unable to clear airway completely of mucus. Keep suction equipment available and monitor patient closely.

Pediatric use

- Drug may be given by tent or croupette. A sufficient volume (up to 300 ml) of a 10% or 20% solution should be used to maintain a heavy mist in the tent for the time prescribed. Administration may be continuous or intermittent.

Breast-feeding
- It is unknown if drug is excreted in breast milk.

activated charcoal
Actidose-Aqua, Charcoaid, Charcocaps, Insta-Char

Pharmacologic classification: adsorbent
Therapeutic classification: antidote, antidiarrheal, antiflatulent
Pregnancy risk category NR

How supplied
Available without a prescription
Tablets: 325 mg, 650 mg
Tablets with 40 mg simethicone: 200 mg
Tablets (delayed-release) with 80 mg simethicone: 250 mg
Capsules: 260 mg
Powder: 30 g, 50 g
Suspension: 0.625 g/5 ml, 0.7 g/5 ml (50 g), 1 g/5 ml, 1.25 g/5 ml

Indications, route, and dosage
Flatulence or dyspepsia
Adults: 600 mg to 5 g P.O. as a single dose, or 975 mg to 3.9 g t.i.d. after meals.
Poisoning
Adults and children: Five to ten times the estimated weight of drug or chemical ingested. Dose is 30 to 100 g in 250 ml water to make a slurry.

Give orally, preferably within 30 minutes of ingestion. Larger doses are necessary if food is in the stomach. Drug is used adjunctively in treating poisoning or overdose with acetaminophen, amphetamines, antimony, aspirin, atropine, arsenic, barbiturates, camphor, cocaine, cardiac glycosides, glutethimide, ipecac, malathion, morphine, opium, oxalic acid, parathion, phenol, phenothiazines, phenytoin, poisonous mushrooms, potassium permanganate, propoxyphene, quinine, strychnine, sulfonamides, or tricyclic antidepressants.

Activated charcoal may be given 20 to 60 g q 4 to 12 hours (gastric dialysis) to enhance removal of some drugs from the bloodstream. Monitor serum drug level.

◇ To relieve GI disturbances (halitosis, anorexia, nausea, vomiting) in uremic patients
Adults: 20 to 50 g daily.

Pharmacodynamics
Antidote action: Drug adsorbs ingested toxins, thereby inhibiting GI absorption.

Antidiarrheal action: Activated charcoal adsorbs toxic and nontoxic irritants that cause diarrhea or GI discomfort.

Antiflatulent action: Activated charcoal adsorbs intestinal gas to relieve discomfort.

Pharmacokinetics
- *Absorption:* Drug is not absorbed from the GI tract.
- *Distribution:* None.
- *Metabolism:* None.
- *Excretion:* Excreted in feces.

Contraindications and precautions
No known contraindications.

Interactions
Milk products decrease the effectiveness of activated charcoal. Actvated charcoal inactivates *syrup of ipecac* and also adsorbs and inactivates many oral medications when used concomitantly, including orally administered *acetylcysteine*; charcoal should be removed by gastric lavage before *acetylcysteine* is administered.

Effects on diagnostic tests
None reported.

Adverse reactions
GI: black stools, constipation, nausea.

Overdose and treatment
No information available.

☑ Special considerations
- Do not give activated charcoal by mouth to a semiconscious or unconscious patient; instead, administer the drug through a nasogastric tube.
- Because activated charcoal adsorbs and inactivates syrup of ipecac, give only after emesis is complete.
- Activated charcoal is most effective when used within 30 minutes of toxin ingestion; a cathartic is commonly administered with or after activated charcoal to speed removal of the toxin/charcoal complex.
- Do not give in ice cream, milk, or sherbet; dairy products reduce the adsorptive capacity of drug.
- Powder form is most effective. Mix with tap water to form consistency of thick syrup. A small amount of fruit juice or flavoring may be added to make mixture more palatable.
- Dose may need to be repeated if patient vomits shortly after administration.
- Prolonged use (over 72 hours) may impair patient's nutritional status.
- If administering drug for indications other than poisoning, be sure to give other medications 1 hour before or 2 hours after activated charcoal.
- Activated charcoal may be used orally to decrease colostomy odor.

Patient education
- Tell patient to call poison information center or hospital emergency department before taking activated charcoal as an antidote.
- If patient is using activated charcoal as an antidiarrheal or antiflatulent, instruct patient to take medications 1 hour before or 2 hours after activated charcoal. For antidiarrheal use, advise patient to report diarrhea that persists after 2 days of therapy, fever, or flatulence that persists after 7 days.
- Warn patient that activated charcoal turns stools black.
- Advise patient not to mix drug with milk products, which may lessen its effectiveness.

acyclovir (acycloguanosine)

acyclovir sodium

Zovirax

Pharmacologic classification: synthetic purine nucleoside
Therapeutic classification: antiviral
Pregnancy risk category C

How supplied

Available by prescription only
Tablets: 400 mg, 800 mg
Capsules: 200 mg
Oral suspension: 200 mg/5 ml
Injection: 500 mg/vial, 1 g/vial
Ointment: 5%

Indications, route, and dosage

Initial and recurrent mucocutaneous herpes simplex virus (HSV type 1 and HSV type 2) or severe initial genital herpes or herpes simplex in immunocompromised patient

Adults and children over age 12: 5 mg/kg, given at a constant rate over 1 hour by I.V. infusion q 8 hours for 7 days (5 days for genital herpes).

Children under age 12: 250 mg/m² given at a constant rate over 1 hour by I.V. infusion q 8 hours for 7 days (5 days for genital herpes).

◊ ***Treatment of disseminated herpes zoster***

Adults: 5 to 10 mg/kg I.V. q 8 hours for 7 to 10 days. Infuse over at least 1 hour.

Treatment of initial genital herpes

Adults: 200 mg P.O. q 4 hours while awake (total 5 capsules daily). Continue treatment for 10 days.

Treatment of acute herpes zoster infections

Adults: 800 mg P.O. five times daily for 7 to 10 days. Initiate therapy within 48 hours of rash onset.

Intermittent therapy for recurrent genital herpes

Adults: 200 mg P.O. q 4 hours while awake (a total of five capsules daily). Treatment should continue for 5 days. Initiate therapy at first sign of recurrence.

Chronic suppressive therapy for recurrent genital herpes

Adults: 400 mg P.O. b.i.d. for up to 1 year.

Genital herpes; non-life-threatening herpes simplex infection in immunocompromised patients

Adults and children: Apply sufficient quantity of ointment to adequately cover all lesions q 3 hours, six times daily for 7 days.

Treatment of acute varicella (chickenpox) infections

Adults and children age 2 and older weighing over 88 lb (40 kg): 800 mg P.O. q.i.d. for 5 days.

Children age 2 or older weighing below 88 lb: 20 mg/kg P.O. q.i.d. for 5 days.

Immunocompromised patient

Adults and children over age 12: 10 mg/kg I.V. over 1 hour q 8 hours for 7 days.

Children under age 12: 500 mg/m² I.V. over 1 hour q 8 hours for 7 days.

Herpes simplex encephalitis

Adults and children over age 6 months: 10 mg/kg I.V. q 8 hours for 10 days; usual daily dose is 30 mg/kg.

✦ ***Dosage adjustment.*** In patients with renal failure, adjust normal oral dosage (200 to 400 mg) to 200 mg q 12 hours if creatinine clearance drops below 10 ml/minute/1.73 m². For normal dosages exceeding 400 mg, refer to package insert.

In patients with renal failure, give 100% of the I.V. dose q 8 hours if creatinine clearance exceeds 50 ml/minute/1.73 m²; 100% of the dose q 12 hours if it ranges between 25 and 50 ml/minute/1.73 m²; 100% of the dose q 24 hours if it ranges between 10 and 25 ml/minute/1.73 m²; and 50% of the dose q 24 hours if it falls below 10 ml/minute/1.73 m².

Pharmacodynamics

Antiviral action: Acyclovir is converted by the viral cell into its active form (triphosphate) and inhibits viral DNA polymerase.

In vitro, acyclovir is active against herpes simplex virus type 1, herpes simplex virus type 2, varicella-zoster virus, Epstein-Barr virus, and cytomegalovirus. In vivo, acyclovir may reduce the duration of acute infection and speed lesion healing in initial genital herpes episodes. Patients with frequent herpes recurrences (more than six episodes a year) may receive oral acyclovir prophylactically to prevent recurrences or reduce their frequency.

Pharmacokinetics

- *Absorption:* With oral administration, acyclovir is absorbed slowly and incompletely (15% to 30%). Peak concentrations occur in 1½ to 2 hours. Absorption is not affected by food. With topical administration, absorption is minimal.
- *Distribution:* Distributed widely to organ tissues and body fluids. CSF concentrations equal approximately 50% of serum concentrations. About 9% to 33% of a dose binds to plasma proteins.
- *Metabolism:* Drug is metabolized inside the viral cell to its active form. About 10% of dose is metabolized extracellularly.
- *Excretion:* Up to 92% of systemically absorbed acyclovir is excreted as unchanged drug by the kidneys by glomerular filtration and tubular secretion. In patients with normal renal function, half-life is 2 to 3½ hours. Renal failure may extend half-life to 19 hours.

Contraindications and precautions

Contraindicated in patients with hypersensitivity to drug. Use cautiously in patients with underlying neurologic problems, renal disease, or dehydration and in those receiving nephrotoxic drugs.

Interactions

Concomitant use with *probenecid* may result in reduced renal tubular secretion of acyclovir, leading to increased drug half-life, reduced elimination rate, and decreased urine excretion. This reduced clearance causes more sustained serum drug levels. Concomitant use with *zidovudine* may result in increased levels of acyclovir, causing toxicity.

Effects on diagnostic tests
Serum creatinine and BUN levels may increase.

Adverse reactions
CNS: *encephalopathic changes (lethargy, obtundation, tremor, confusion, hallucinations, agitation,* ***seizures, coma***), headache, malaise.
GI: diarrhea, *nausea, vomiting.*
GU: hematuria, *transient elevations of serum creatinine levels.*
Hematologic: bone marrow hypoplasia, leukopenia, megaloblastic hematopoiesis, thrombocytosis, ***thrombocytopenia.***
Skin: itching, rash, transient burning and stinging, pruritus, urticaria, vulvitis.
Other: *inflammation, phlebitis* (at injection site).

Overdose and treatment
Overdose has followed I.V. bolus administration in patients with unmonitored fluid status or in patients receiving inappropriately high parenteral dosages. Acute toxicity has not been reported after high oral dosage. Hemodialysis results in 60% decrease in plasma concentration of the drug.

Clinical effects of overdose include signs of nephrotoxicity, including elevated serum creatinine and BUN levels, progressing to renal failure.

☑ Special considerations
- Drug should not be administered S.C., I.M., by I.V. bolus, or ophthalmically.
- I.V. dose should be infused over at least 1 hour to prevent renal tubular damage.
- Solubility of acyclovir in urine is low. Ensure that the patient taking the systemic form of drug is well hydrated to prevent nephrotoxicity.
- Monitor serum creatinine level. If level does not return to normal within a few days after therapy begins, may increase hydration, adjust dose, or discontinue drug.
- Encephalopathic signs are more likely in patients who have experienced neurologic reactions to cytotoxic drugs.

Patient education
- Warn patient that although drug helps manage the disease, it does not cure it or prevent it from spreading to others.
- For best results, tell patient to begin taking drug when early infection symptoms (such as tingling, itching, or pain) occur.
- Instruct patient who is taking ointment to use a finger cot or rubber glove and to apply about a ½" ribbon of ointment for every 4 square inches of area to be covered. Ointment should thoroughly cover each lesion. Warn patient to avoid getting ointment in the eye.
- Instruct patient to avoid sexual intercourse during active genital infection.

Geriatric use
- Administer drug cautiously to elderly patients because they may suffer from renal dysfunction or dehydration.

Pediatric use
- Safety and effectiveness of oral and topical acyclovir in children have not been established. I.V. acyclovir has been used with only a few children. To reconstitute acyclovir for children, do not use bacteriostatic water for injection containing benzyl alcohol.

adenosine
Adenocard

Pharmacologic classification: nucleoside
Therapeutic classification: antiarrhythmic
Pregnancy risk category C

How supplied
Available by prescription only
Injection: 3 mg/ml in 2-ml and 5-ml vials

Indications, route, and dosage
Conversion of paroxysmal supraventricular tachycardia (PSVT) to sinus rhythm
Adults: 6 mg I.V. by rapid bolus injection (over 1 to 2 seconds). If PSVT is not eliminated in 1 to 2 minutes, give 12 mg by rapid I.V. push. Repeat 12-mg dose if necessary. Single doses over 12 mg are not recommended.

Pharmacodynamics
Antiarrhythmic action: Adenosine is a naturally occurring nucleoside. In the heart, it acts on the AV node to slow conduction and inhibit reentry pathways. Adenosine is also useful for the treatment of PSVT associated with accessory bypass tracts (Wolff-Parkinson-White syndrome).

Pharmacokinetics
- *Absorption:* Drug is administered by rapid I.V. injection.
- *Distribution:* Adenosine is rapidly taken up by erythrocytes and vascular endothelial cells.
- *Metabolism:* Metabolized within tissues to inosine and adenosine monophosphate.
- *Excretion:* Unknown; circulating plasma half-life is less than 10 seconds.

Contraindications and precautions
Contraindicated in patients with hypersensitivity to drug and in those with second- or third-degree heart block or sick sinus syndrome, unless an artificial pacemaker is present, because adenosine decreases conduction through the AV node and may produce first-, second-, or third-degree heart block. These effects are usually transient; however, patients in whom significant heart block develops after a dose of adenosine should not receive additional doses.

Use cautiously in patients with asthma because bronchoconstriction may occur.

Interactions
Higher degrees of heart block occur in patients receiving concomitant *carbamazepine. Dipyridamole* may potentiate the effects of the drug, and smaller doses may be necessary.

Methylxanthines antagonize effects of adenosine. Therefore, patients receiving *theophylline* or *caffeine* may require higher doses or may not respond to adenosine therapy.

Effects on diagnostic tests
None reported.

Adverse reactions
CNS: apprehension, back pain, blurred vision, burning sensation, dizziness, heaviness in arms, lightheadedness, neck pain, numbness, tingling in arms.
CV: chest pain, *facial flushing,* headache, hypotension, palpitations, diaphoresis.
GI: metallic taste, nausea.
Respiratory: *chest pressure, dyspnea, shortness of breath,* hyperventilation.
Other: *throat tightness, groin pressure.*

Overdose and treatment
Because the half-life of adenosine is less than 10 seconds, the adverse effects of overdosage usually dissipate rapidly and are self-limiting. Treat lingering adverse effects symptomatically.

☑ Special considerations
- Rapid I.V. injection is necessary for drug action. Administer directly into a vein if possible; if an I.V. line is used, use the most proximal port and follow with a rapid sodium chloride flush to ensure that drug reaches the systemic circulation rapidly.
- Check solution for crystals, which may occur if solution is cold. If crystals are visible, gently warm solution to room temperature. Do not use solutions that are not clear.
- Discard unused drug because it contains no preservatives.

Patient education
- Warn patient that adverse reactions may occur.

albumin, human (normal serum albumin, human)
Albuminar-5, Albuminar-25, Albutein 5%, Albutein 25%, Buminate 5%, Buminate 25%, Plasbumin-5, Plasbumin-25

Pharmacologic classification: blood derivative
Therapeutic classification: plasma protein
Pregnancy risk category C

How supplied
Injection: 5% (50 mg/ml) in 50-ml, 250-ml, 500-ml, 1,000-ml vials; 25% (250 mg/ml) in 20-ml, 50-ml, 100-ml vials

Indications, route, and dosage
Shock
Adults: Initially, 500 ml (5% solution) by I.V. infusion, may repeat after 30 minutes. Dose varies with patient's condition and response. Do not exceed 250 g/48 hours.
Children: 10 to 20 ml/kg (5% solution) by I.V. infusion, at a rate up to 5 to 10 ml/minute.
Hypoproteinemia
Adults: 1,000 to 1,500 ml 5% solution by I.V. infusion daily, maximum rate 5 to 10 ml/minute; or 200 to 300 ml of 25% solution by I.V. infusion daily, maximum rate 3 ml/minute. Dose varies with patient's condition and response.
Burns
Adults and children: Dosage varies based on extent of burn and patient's condition. Usually maintain plasma albumin level at 2 to 3 g/dl.
Hyperbilirubinemia
Infants: 1 g/kg albumin (4 ml/kg of 25% solution) 1 to 2 hours before transfusion.
◊ *High-risk neonates with low serum protein concentration:* 1.4 to 1.8 ml/kg of 25% solution.

Pharmacodynamics
Plasma volume-expanding action: Albumin 5% supplies colloid to the blood and expands plasma volume. Albumin 25% provides intravascular oncotic pressure at 5:1, causing fluid to shift from interstitial space to the circulation and slightly increasing plasma protein concentration.

Pharmacokinetics
- *Absorption:* Albumin is not adequately absorbed from the GI tract.
- *Distribution:* Albumin accounts for approximately 50% of plasma proteins; it is distributed into the intravascular space and extravascular sites, including skin, muscle, and lungs. In patients with reduced circulating blood volume, hemodilution secondary to albumin administration persists for many hours; in patients with normal blood volume, excess fluid and protein are lost.
- *Metabolism:* Although albumin is synthesized in the liver, liver is not involved in clearance of albumin from plasma in healthy individuals.
- *Excretion:* Little is known about excretion in healthy individuals. Administration of albumin decreases hepatic albumin synthesis and increases albumin clearance if plasma oncotic pressure is high. In certain pathologic states, the liver, kidneys, or intestines may provide elimination mechanisms for albumin.

Contraindications and precautions
Contraindicated in patients with hypersensitivity to drug. Use with extreme caution in patients with hypertension, cardiac disease, severe pulmonary infection, severe chronic anemia, or hypoalbuminemia with peripheral edema.

Interactions
None significant.

Effects on diagnostic tests
Preparations of albumin derived from placental tissue may increase serum alkaline phosphatase level; all products may slightly increase plasma albumin level.

Adverse reactions

CNS: headache.
CV: hypotension, tachycardia, ***vascular overload after rapid infusion.***
GI: increased salivation, nausea, vomiting.
Respiratory: altered respiration, dyspnea, pulmonary edema.
Skin: urticaria, rash.
Other: chills, fever, back pain.

Overdose and treatment

Clinical manifestations of overdose include signs of circulatory overload, such as increased venous pressure and distended neck veins, or pulmonary edema; slow flow to a keep-vein-open rate and reevaluate therapy.

☑ Special considerations

- Solution should be a clear amber color; do not use if cloudy or contains sediment. Store at room temperature; freezing may break bottle.
- Use opened solution promptly, discarding unused portion after 4 hours; solution contains no preservatives and becomes unstable.
- One volume of 25% albumin produces the same hemodilution and relative anemia as five volumes of 5% albumin; reference to "1 unit" albumin usually indicates 50 ml of the 25% concentration, containing 12.5 g of albumin.
- Dilute if necessary with 0.9% NaCl solution or 5% dextrose injection. Use 5-micron or larger filter; do not give through 0.22-micron I.V. filter.
- Be certain patient is properly hydrated before starting infusion; product may be administered without regard to blood typing and crossmatching.
- Avoid rapid I.V. infusion; rate is individualized based on patient's age, condition, and diagnosis. In patients with hypovolemic shock, infuse 5% solution at a rate not exceeding 2 to 4 ml/minute, and 25% solution (diluted or undiluted) at a rate not exceeding 1 ml/minute; in patients with normal blood volume, infuse 5% solution at a rate not exceeding 5 to 10 ml/minute, and 25% solution (diluted or undiluted), at a rate not exceeding 2 to 3 ml/minute. Do not give more than 250 g in 48 hours.
- Monitor vital signs carefully; observe patient for adverse reactions.
- Monitor intake and output, hematocrit, serum protein, hemoglobin, and electrolyte levels to help determine continuing dosage.
- Each liter contains 130 to 160 mEq of sodium before dilution with any additional I.V. fluids; a 50-ml bottle of solution contains 7 to 8 mEq sodium. This preparation was once known as "salt-poor albumin."

Pediatric use

- Premature infants with low serum protein concentrations may receive 1.4 to 1.8 ml/kg of a 25% albumin solution/kg (350 to 450 mg albumin).

albuterol sulfate

Proventil, Proventil HFA, Proventil Repetabs, Proventil Syrup, Ventolin, Ventolin Syrup, Volmax

Pharmacologic classification: adrenergic
Therapeutic classification: bronchodilator
Pregnancy risk category C

How supplied

Available by prescription only
Tablets: 2 mg, 4 mg
Tablets (sustained-release): 4 mg, 8 mg
Syrup: 2 mg/5 ml
Aerosol inhaler: 90 mcg/metered spray
Solution for nebulization: 0.083%, 0.5%
Capsules for inhalation: 200 mcg microfine

Indications, route, and dosage

To prevent and treat bronchospasm in patients with reversible obstructive airway disease
Adults and children age 12 and older: Tablets: give 2 to 4 mg (immediate-release) P.O. t.i.d. or q.i.d.; maximum dosage, 8 mg q.i.d. Alternatively, use sustained-release tablets. Usual starting dosage is 4 mg q 12 hours. Increase to 8 mg q 12 hours if patient fails to respond. Cautiously increase stepwise as needed and tolerated to 16 mg q 12 hours.

Aerosol inhalation: One to two inhalations q 4 to 6 hours. More frequent administration or a greater number of inhalations is not usually recommended. However, because deposition of inhaled medications is variable, higher doses are occasionally used, especially in patients with acute bronchospasm.

Solution for inhalation: 2.5 mg t.i.d. or q.i.d. by nebulizer.

Capsules for inhalation: 200 mcg inhaled q 4 to 6 hours using a Rotohaler inhalation device.
Children age 6 to 11: Administer 2 mg P.O. t.i.d. or q.i.d.
Children age 2 to 5: Administer 0.1 mg/kg P.O. t.i.d., not to exceed 2 mg t.i.d.
✦ ***Dosage adjustment.*** In adults over age 65, give 2 mg P.O. t.i.d. or q.i.d.
To prevent exercise-induced bronchospasm
Adults and children age 12 and older: Two inhalations 15 minutes before exercise.

Pharmacodynamics

Bronchodilator action: Albuterol selectively stimulates beta-adrenergic receptors of the lungs, uterus, and vascular smooth muscle. Bronchodilation results from relaxation of bronchial smooth muscles, which relieves bronchospasm and reduces airway resistance.

Pharmacokinetics

- *Absorption:* After oral inhalation, albuterol appears to be absorbed gradually (over several hours) from the respiratory tract; however, dose is mostly swallowed and absorbed through the GI tract. Onset of action occurs within 5 to 15 minutes, peaks in ½ to 2 hours, and lasts 3 to 6 hours. After oral administration, albuterol is well-absorbed through

the GI tract. Onset of action occurs within 30 minutes and peaks in 2 to 3 hours. Drug effect lasts 4 to 6 hours with immediate-release tablets and 12 hours with extended-release tablets.
- *Distribution:* Albuterol does not cross the blood-brain barrier.
- *Metabolism:* Drug is extensively metabolized in the liver to inactive compounds.
- *Excretion:* Albuterol is rapidly excreted in urine and feces. After oral inhalation, 70% of a dose is excreted in urine unchanged and as metabolites within 24 hours; 10% in feces. Elimination half-life is about 4 hours. After oral administration, 75% of a dose is excreted in urine within 72 hours as metabolites; 4% in feces.

Contraindications and precautions
Contraindicated in patients with hypersensitivity to drug or any component of its formulation. Use cautiously in patients with CV disorders, including coronary insufficiency and hypertension; in patients with hyperthyroidism or diabetes mellitus; and in those who are unusually responsive to adrenergics.

Interactions
Concomitant use of orally inhaled albuterol with *epinephrine* and other orally inhaled *sympathomimetic amines* may increase sympathomimetic effects and risk of toxicity. Serious CV effects may follow concomitant use with *MAO inhibitors* and *tricyclic antidepressants.*

Propranolol and *other beta-adrenergic blockers* may antagonize the effects of albuterol.

Effects on diagnostic tests
Albuterol may decrease the sensitivity of spirometry used for the diagnosis of asthma.

Adverse reactions
CNS: *tremor, nervousness,* dizziness, insomnia, *headache, hyperactivity,* weakness, CNS stimulation, malaise.
CV: *tachycardia, palpitations,* hypertension.
EENT: dry and irritated nose and throat (with inhaled form), nasal congestion, epistaxis, hoarseness, taste perversion.
GI: heartburn, *nausea, vomiting,* anorexia.
Respiratory: **BRONCHOSPASM,** cough, wheezing, dyspnea, bronchitis, increased sputum.
Other: muscle cramps, hypokalemia (with high doses), increased appetite, hypersensitivity reactions.

Overdose and treatment
Clinical manifestations of overdose include exaggeration of common adverse reactions, particularly angina, hypertension, hypokalemia, and seizures.

To treat, use selective beta-adrenergic blockers (such as metoprolol) with extreme caution; these may induce asthmatic attack. *Dialysis is not appropriate.* Monitor vital signs and electrolyte levels closely.

☑ Special considerations
Besides those relevant to all *adrenergics,* consider the following recommendations.
- Small, transient increases in blood glucose levels may occur after oral inhalation.
- Serum potassium levels may decrease after I.V. and inhalation therapy administration, but potassium supplementation is usually unnecessary.
- Effectiveness of treatment is measured by periodic monitoring of patient's pulmonary function.

Patient education
- Instruct patient in proper use of inhaler. Tell him to read directions before use, that dryness of mouth and throat may occur, and that rinsing with water after each dose may help.

— *Administration by metered-dose nebulizers:* Shake canister thoroughly to activate; place mouthpiece well into mouth, aimed at back of throat. Close lips and teeth around mouthpiece. Exhale through nose as completely as possible; then inhale through mouth slowly and deeply while actuating the nebulizer to release dose. Hold breath 10 seconds (count "1-100, 2-100, 3-100," until "10-100" is reached); remove mouthpiece, and then exhale slowly.

— *Administration by metered powder inhaler:* Caution patient not to take forced deep breath, but to breathe with normal force and depth. Observe patient closely for exaggerated systemic drug action.

— *Administration by oxygen aerosolization:* Administer over 15- to 20-minute period, with oxygen flow rate adjusted to 4 L/minute. Turn on oxygen supply before patient places nebulizer in mouth. Lips need not be closed tightly around nebulizer opening. Placement of Y tube in rubber tubing permits patient to control administration. Advise patient to rinse mouth immediately after inhalation therapy to help prevent dryness and throat irritation. Rinse mouthpiece thoroughly with warm running water at least once daily to prevent clogging. (It is not dishwasher-safe.) After cleaning, wait until mouthpiece is completely dry before storing. Do not place near artificial heat (dishwasher or oven). Replace reservoir bag every 2 to 3 weeks or as needed; replace mouthpiece every 6 to 9 months or as needed.

Note: Replacement of bags or mouthpieces may require a prescription.
- Tell patient that repeated use may result in paradoxical bronchospasm. He should discontinue drug and call immediately.
- Tell patient to call if troubled breathing persists 1 hour after using medication, if symptoms return within 4 hours, if condition worsens, or if new (refill) canister is needed within 2 weeks.
- Tell patient to wait 15 minutes after using inhaled albuterol before using adrenocorticoids (beclomethasone, dexamethasone, flunisolide, or triamcinolone).
- Warn patient to use only as directed, and not to use more than prescribed amount or more often than prescribed.

Geriatric use
- Lower dose may be required because elderly patients are more sensitive to sympathomimetic amines.

Pediatric use

• Safety and efficacy of extended-release tablets in children under age 12 or immediate-release tablets in children under age 6 have not been established.

Breast-feeding

• Because it is unknown if albuterol is excreted in breast milk, alternative feeding methods are recommended.

alclometasone dipropionate

Aclovate

Pharmacologic classification: topical adrenocorticoid
Therapeutic classification: anti-inflammatory
Pregnancy risk category C

How supplied

Available by prescription only
Cream, ointment: 0.05%

Indications, route, and dosage

Inflammation of corticosteroid-responsive dermatoses

Adults: Apply a thin film to affected areas b.i.d. or t.i.d. Gently massage until the medication disappears, or apply a thick layer and cover with an occlusive dressing and tape and leave in place for 1 to 4 days. Repeat p.r.n.

Pharmacodynamics

Anti-inflammatory action: Drug stimulates the synthesis of enzymes needed to decrease the inflammatory response. Alclometasone is a group VI nonfluorinated topical glucocorticoid with less anti-inflammatory activity than hydrocortisone 0.2% or greater. It is similar in potency to desonide 0.05% and fluocinolone acetonide, 0.01%. Applied topically, alclometasone may be used for refractory lesions of psoriasis and other deep-seated dermatoses such as localized neurodermatitis.

Pharmacokinetics

• *Absorption:* Amount absorbed depends on amount of drug applied and on nature of the skin at the application site. It ranges from about 1% in areas with thick stratum corneum (such as the palms, soles, elbows, and knees) to as high as 36% in areas of the thinnest stratum corneum (face, eyelids, and genitals). Absorption increases in areas of skin damage, inflammation, or occlusion. Some systemic absorption of topical steroids may occur, especially through the oral mucosa.

• *Distribution:* After topical application, drug is distributed throughout the local skin. If drug is absorbed into the circulation, it is rapidly removed from the blood and distributed into muscle, liver, skin, intestines, and kidneys.

• *Metabolism:* After topical administration, drug is metabolized primarily in the skin. The small amount that is absorbed into systemic circulation is metabolized primarily in the liver to inactive compounds.

• *Excretion:* Inactive metabolites are excreted by the kidneys, primarily as glucuronides and sulfates, but also as unconjugated products. Small amounts of the metabolites are also excreted in feces.

Contraindications and precautions

Contraindicated in patients hypersensitive to corticosteroids.

Interactions

None reported

Effects on diagnostic tests

None reported.

Adverse reactions

EENT: cataracts, glaucoma (if used around eyes for a prolonged period).
Skin: burning, pruritus, irritation, dryness, erythema, folliculitis, acneiform eruptions, perioral dermatitis, hypopigmentation, hypertrichosis, allergic contact dermatitis; *secondary infection,* maceration, atrophy, striae, miliaria (with occlusive dressings).
Other: ***hypothalamic-pituitary-adrenal axis suppression,*** Cushing's syndrome, hyperglycemia, glycosuria.

Overdose and treatment

No information available.

☑ Special considerations

Recommendations for use of alclometasone, care and teaching of patient during therapy, and use in elderly patients and children, and during breast-feeding are the same as those for all *topical adrenocorticoids.*

aldesleukin (interleukin-2, IL-2)

Proleukin

Pharmacologic classification: lymphokine
Therapeutic classification: immunoregulatory
Pregnancy risk category C

How supplied

Available by prescription only
Injection: 22 million IU/vial

Indications, route, and dosage

Metastatic renal cell carcinoma; ◇ metastatic melanoma

Adults: 600 000 IU/kg (0.037 mg/kg) I.V. q 8 hours for 5 days (a total of 14 doses). After a 9-day rest, repeat the sequence for another 14 doses. Repeat courses may be administered after a rest period of at least 7 weeks from hospital discharge.
◇ *Adults:* Continuous I.V. infusion of 18 million IU/m^2 for two 5-day cycles with a 5- to 8-day rest between cycles.
◇ *Adults:* 18 million IU S.C. daily for 5 days.

* Canada only ◇ Unlabeled clinical use

Pharmacodynamics
Immunoregulatory action: Aldesleukin is a lymphokine, a highly purified immunoregulatory protein synthesized using genetically engineered *Escherichia coli.* The drug produced is similar to human IL-2: it enhances lymphocyte mitogenesis, stimulates long-term growth of IL-2-dependent cell lines, enhances lymphocyte cytotoxicity, induces both lymphokine-activated and natural killer cell activity, and induces the production of interferon gamma.

Pharmacokinetics
• *Absorption:* Onset is rapid after I.V. administration.
• *Distribution:* Peak serum levels are proportional to dose. About 30% of drug rapidly distributes to plasma; the balance is rapidly distributed to the liver, kidneys, and lungs. Initial studies indicate that the distribution half-life is 13 minutes after a 5-minute I.V. infusion.
• *Metabolism:* Drug is metabolized by the kidneys to amino acids within the cells lining the proximal convoluted tubules.
• *Excretion:* Drug is excreted through the kidneys by peritubular extraction and glomerular filtration. Peritubular extraction ensures drug clearance as renal function diminishes and serum creatinine increases. Elimination half-life is 85 minutes.

Contraindications and precautions
Contraindicated in patients hypersensitive to drug or any component of the formulation and in those with abnormal cardiac (thallium) stress test or pulmonary function tests or organ allografts. Retreatment is contraindicated in patients who experience the following adverse effects: pericardial tamponade; disturbances in cardiac rhythm that were uncontrolled or unresponsive to intervention; sustained ventricular tachycardia (five beats or more); chest pain accompanied by ECG changes, indicating MI or angina pectoris; renal dysfunction requiring dialysis for 72 hours or more; coma or toxic psychosis lasting 48 hours or more; seizures that were repetitive or difficult to control; ischemia or perforation of the bowel; GI bleeding requiring surgery.

Use with extreme caution in patients with cardiac or pulmonary disease or seizure disorders.

Interactions
Patients receiving *antihypertensives* may be at increased risk for hypotension. Concomitant use with *corticosteroids* may decrease antitumor effectiveness of aldesleukin. Aldesleukin may enhance the toxicity of *hepatotoxic, nephrotoxic, cardiotoxic,* or *myelotoxic drugs.* Because aldesleukin can alter CNS function, use cautiously with *psychotropic agents.*

Effects on diagnostic tests
No direct laboratory test interference has been reported. Toxic effects of drug may be seen in decreasing hepatic, renal, and thyroid function tests; abnormal serum electrolytes; or abnormal cardiac or pulmonary function tests.

Adverse reactions
CNS: *headache, mental status changes, dizziness, sensory dysfunction, special senses disorders, syncope, motor dysfunction,* ***coma,*** fatigue.
CV: *hypotension, sinus tachycardia, arrhythmias, bradycardia,* ***PVCs,*** *premature atrial contractions,* ***MI, heart failure, cardiac arrest,*** myocarditis, endocarditis, ***CVA,*** pericardial effusion, thrombosis, ***capillary leak syndrome (CLS).***
EENT: conjunctivitis.
GI: *nausea, vomiting, diarrhea, stomatitis, anorexia, bleeding, dyspepsia, constipation.*
GU: *oliguria, anuria, proteinuria, hematuria, dysuria,* urine retention, urinary frequency.
Hematologic: *anemia,* **THROMBOCYTOPENIA, LEUKOPENIA,** *coagulation disorders,* leukocytosis, eosinophilia.
Hepatic: *jaundice,* ascites, hepatomegaly, *elevated bilirubin, serum transaminase, and alkaline phosphatase levels.*
Respiratory: *pulmonary congestion, dyspnea, pulmonary edema,* ***respiratory failure, pleural effusion, apnea, pneumothorax,*** tachypnea.
Skin: *pruritus, erythema, rash, dryness, exfoliative dermatitis,* purpura, alopecia, petechiae.
Other: *elevated BUN and serum creatinine levels; hypomagnesemia; acidosis; hypocalcemia; hypophosphatemia; hypokalemia; hyperuricemia; hypoalbuminemia;* hypoproteinemia; hyponatremia; hyperkalemia; arthralgia; myalgia; *fever; chills; weakness; malaise;* edema; *infections of catheter tip, urinary tract, or injection site; phlebitis;* **SEPSIS;** *weight gain* or loss; *abdominal, chest, or back pain.*

Overdose and treatment
Administration of high doses will produce rapid onset of expected adverse reactions, including cardiac, renal, and hepatic toxicity.

Drug toxicity is dose-related. Treatment is supportive. Because of short serum half-life of drug, discontinuation may ameliorate many of the adverse effects. Dexamethasone may decrease the toxicity of drug but may also impair effectiveness.

☑ Special considerations
• Perform standard hematologic tests, including CBC, differential, and platelet counts; serum electrolytes; and renal and hepatic function tests before therapy. Also obtain chest X-ray. Repeat daily during drug administration.
• Discontinue drug if moderate to severe lethargy or somnolence develops because continued administration can result in coma.
• Patients should be neurologically stable with a negative computed tomography scan for CNS metastases. Drug may exacerbate symptoms in patients with unrecognized or undiagnosed CNS metastases.
• Renal and hepatic impairment occur during treatment. Avoid administering other hepatotoxic or nephrotoxic drugs because toxicity may be additive. Also be prepared to adjust dosage of other drugs to compensate for this impairment. Dosage modification because of toxicity is usually accomplished by holding a dose or interrupting therapy

rather than by reducing the dose to be administered.

• Severe anemia or thrombocytopenia may occur. Packed RBCs or platelets may be necessary.

• Treat CLS with careful monitoring of fluid status, pulse, mental status, urine output, and organ perfusion. Central venous pressure monitoring is necessary.

• Because fluid management or administration of pressor agents may be essential to treat CLS, use cautiously in patients who require large volumes of fluid (such as patients with hypercalcemia).

• To avoid altering the pharmacologic properties of drug, reconstitute and dilute carefully, and follow manufacturer's recommendations. Do not mix with other drugs or albumin.

• Reconstitute vial containing 22 million IU (1.3 mg) with 1.2 ml sterile water for injection. Do not use bacteriostatic water or 0.9% NaCl injection because these diluents cause increased aggregation of drug. Direct the stream at the sides of the vial and gently swirl to reconstitute. Do not shake.

• Reconstituted solution will have a concentration of 18 million IU (1.1 mg)/ml. Reconstituted drug should be particle-free and colorless to slightly yellow.

• Add the correct dose of reconstituted drug to 50 ml D_5W and infuse over 15 minutes. Do not use an in-line filter. Plastic infusion bags are preferred because they provided consistent drug delivery in early clinical trials.

• Vials are for single-use only and contain no preservatives. Discard unused drug.

• Powder for injection or reconstituted solutions must be stored in the refrigerator. After reconstitution and dilution, drug must be administered within 48 hours. Be sure that solutions are returned to room temperature before administering drug to patient.

• Preliminary studies indicate that a high percentage of patients (over 75%) develop nonneutralizing antibodies to aldesleukin when treated with the every-8-hour dosing regimen. A small number (less than 1%) develop neutralizing antibodies. The clinical significance of this finding is not yet known.

• Aldesleukin has been investigated for various cancers, including Kaposi's sarcoma, metastatic melanoma, colorectal cancer, and malignant lymphoma.

Patient education

• Make sure patient understands the serious toxicity that is associated with drug. Adverse effects are expected with normal doses, and serious toxicity may occur despite close clinical monitoring.

Pediatric use

• Safety and effectiveness have not been established in children under age 18.

Breast-feeding

• It is unknown if drug is excreted in breast milk. Consider risk and benefit and decide whether to discontinue drug or breast-feeding because of risk of serious adverse effects to the infant.

alendronate sodium

Fosamax

Pharmacologic classification: osteoclast-mediated bone resorption inhibitor
Therapeutic classification: antiosteoporotic
Pregnancy risk category C

How supplied

Available by prescription only
Tablets: 10 mg, 40 mg

Indications, route, and dosage

Osteoporosis in postmenopausal women

Adults: 10 mg P.O. daily taken with water at least 30 minutes before first food, beverage, or medication of the day.

Prevention of osteoporosis in postmenopausal women

Adults: 5 mg P.O. daily taken with water at least 30 minutes before first food, beverage, or medication of the day.

Paget's disease of bone

Adults: 40 mg P.O. daily for 6 months taken with water at least 30 minutes before first food, beverage, or medication of the day.

Pharmacodynamics

Antiosteoporotic action: At the cellular level, alendronate suppresses osteoclast activity on newly formed resorption surfaces, which reduces bone turnover. Bone formation exceeds bone resorption at bone remodeling sites and thus leads to progressive gains in bone mass.

Pharmacokinetics

• *Absorption:* Alendronate is absorbed from the GI tract. Food or beverages can decrease bioavailability significantly.

• *Distribution:* Distributed to soft tissues but is then rapidly redistributed to bone or excreted in urine. Protein binding is about 78%.

• *Metabolism:* Drug does not appear to be metabolized.

• *Excretion:* Excreted in the urine.

Contraindications and precautions

Contraindicated in patients with hypersensitivity to any component of drug, hypocalcemia, or severe renal insufficiency (creatinine clearance below 35 ml/minute).

Use cautiously in patients with active upper GI problems, such as dysphagia, symptomatic esophageal diseases, gastritis, duodenitis, or ulcers, and in patients with mild to moderate renal insufficiency (creatinine clearance between 35 and 60 ml/minute).

Interactions

Antacids and *calcium supplements* interfere with absorption of alendronate. Instruct patient to wait at least 30 minutes after taking alendronate before consuming other drugs. *Aspirin* and *NSAIDs* increase risk of upper GI adverse reactions with alendronate doses above 10 mg daily. Monitor patient closely. *Hormone replacement therapy* is not recommended when used in treatment of osteoporosis concomitantly with alendronate because of lack of clinical evidence regarding effectiveness.

Effects on diagnostic tests
None reported.

Adverse reactions
CNS: headache.
GI: abdominal pain, nausea, dyspepsia, constipation, diarrhea, flatulence, acid regurgitation, esophageal ulcer, vomiting, dysphagia, abdominal distention, gastritis.
Other: musculoskeletal pain, taste perversion.

Overdose and treatment
Hypocalcemia, hypophosphatemia, and upper GI adverse events, such as upset stomach, heartburn, esophagitis, gastritis, or ulcer, may result from oral overdosage. Although specific information is lacking regarding the treatment of overdosage with alendronate, administration of milk or antacids (to bind alendronate) should be considered. Dialysis is not beneficial.

☑ Special considerations
- Hypocalcemia must be corrected before drug therapy begins. Other disturbances of mineral metabolism (such as vitamin D deficiency) should also be corrected before initiating therapy.
- When drug is used to treat osteoporosis in postmenopausal women, disease is confirmed by low bone mass findings on diagnostic studies or history of an osteoporotic fracture.
- Drug is indicated for patients with Paget's disease who have alkaline phosphatase levels at least twice the upper limit for normal, in those who are symptomatic, or in those at risk for future complications from the disease.
- Monitor patient's serum calcium and phosphate levels throughout therapy.

Patient education
- Stress importance of taking each tablet with glass of water first thing in the morning at least 30 minutes before ingesting food, beverages, or other medications. Tell patient that waiting for longer than 30 minutes improves absorption of drug.
- Warn patient not to lie down for at least 30 minutes after taking drug to facilitate delivery to stomach and to reduce the potential for esophageal irritation.
- Tell patient to take supplemental calcium and vitamin D if daily dietary intake is inadequate.
- Inform patient about the benefit of weight-bearing exercises in increasing bone mass and the importance of modifying excessive cigarette smoking and alcohol consumption, if these factors are part of patient's lifestyle.

Geriatric use
- Although no overall differences in efficacy or safety were observed in clinical trials between elderly and younger patients, greater sensitivity of some older individuals cannot be ruled out. Use cautiously in this age group.

Pediatric use
- Safety and effectiveness in children have not been established.

Breast-feeding
- Because drug may be excreted in breast milk, do not give to breast-feeding women.

alfentanil hydrochloride
Alfenta

Pharmacologic classification: opioid
Therapeutic classification: analgesic, adjunct to anesthesia, anesthetic
Controlled substance schedule II
Pregnancy risk category C

How supplied
Available by prescription only
Injection: 500 mcg/ml in 2-, 5-, 10-, and 20-ml ampules

Indications, route, and dosage
Analgesic adjunct in the maintenance of general anesthesia with barbiturate, nitrous oxide, and oxygen
Adults: Initially, 8 to 20 mcg/kg I.V., then increments of 3 to 5 mcg/kg I.V. Alternatively, may administer as a continuous infusion of 0.5 to 1 mcg/kg/minute.
Primary anesthetic for induction of anesthesia when endotracheal intubation and mechanical ventilation are required
Adults: Initially, 130 to 245 mcg/kg I.V.; then 0.5 to 1.5 mcg/kg/minute I.V.
Monitored anesthesia care
Adults: Initially, 3 to 8 mcg/kg I.V.; maintenance dose is 0.25 to 1 mcg/kg/minute. Total dose, 3 to 40 mcg/kg I.V.

Pharmacodynamics
Analgesic/anesthetic action: Alfentanil is a potent opiate receptor agonist with a quick onset and short duration of action.

Pharmacokinetics
- *Absorption:* Administered I.V., alfentanil has an immediate onset of action.
- *Distribution:* Redistributed quickly after absorption, drug is highly (over 90%) protein-bound.
- *Metabolism:* Alfentanil is metabolized in the liver. It has a short half-life (about 1.5 hours).
- *Excretion:* Drug is excreted in urine.

Contraindications and precautions
Contraindicated in patients with hypersensitivity to drug. Use cautiously in patients with head injury, pulmonary disease, decreased respiratory reserve, or hepatic or renal impairment.

Interactions
Concomitant use with other *CNS depressants* (*narcotic analgesics, general anesthetics, antihista-*

mines, phenothiazines, barbiturates, benzodiazepines, sedative-hypnotics, tricyclic antidepressants, alcohol,* and *muscle relaxants*) potentiates the respiratory and CNS depression, sedation, and hypotensive effects of alfentanil. Concomitant use with *cimetidine* may also increase respiratory and CNS depression, causing confusion, disorientation, apnea, or seizures.

Drug accumulation and enhanced effects may result if drug is given concomitantly with other drugs that are extensively metabolized in the liver (*rifampin, phenytoin, digitoxin, erythromycin*); combined use with *anticholinergics* may cause paralytic ileus.

Patients who become physically dependent on the drug may experience acute withdrawal syndrome if given high doses of a *narcotic agonist-antagonist* or a single dose of a *narcotic antagonist.*

Severe CV depression may result from concomitant use with *general anesthetics. Diazepam* may produce CV depression when given concomitantly with high doses of alfentanil—administration before or after high doses of alfentanil decreases blood pressure secondary to vasodilation; therefore, recovery may be prolonged.

Alfentanil may produce muscle rigidity involving all the skeletal muscles (incidence and severity are dose-related).

Effects on diagnostic tests
Drug may increase biliary tract pressure with resultant increases in amylase and lipase plasma levels.

Adverse reactions
CNS: anxiety, headache, confusion, sleepiness, sedation.
CV: *hypotension, hypertension, bradycardia, tachycardia,* ***arrhythmias, asystole.***
EENT: blurred vision.
GI: *nausea, vomiting.*
Respiratory: *chest wall rigidity,* ***bronchospasm, respiratory depression,*** hypercapnia, ***respiratory arrest, laryngospasm.***
Skin: pruritus, urticaria.

Overdose and treatment
The most common signs and symptoms of alfentanil overdose are CNS depression, respiratory depression, and miosis (pinpoint pupils). Other acute toxic effects include hypotension, bradycardia, hypothermia, shock, apnea, cardiopulmonary arrest, circulatory collapse, pulmonary edema, and seizures.

To treat acute overdose, first establish adequate respiratory exchange through a patent airway and ventilation as needed; administer a narcotic antagonist (naloxone) to reverse respiratory depression. (Because the duration of action of alfentanil may be longer than that of naloxone, repeated naloxone dosing may be necessary.) Do not give unless patient has clinically significant respiratory or CV depression. Monitor vital signs closely.

Provide symptomatic and supportive treatment (continued respiratory support, correction of fluid or electrolyte imbalance). Closely monitor laboratory parameters, vital signs, and neurologic status.

☑ Special considerations
Besides those relevant to all *opioids,* consider the following recommendations.
- Assisted or controlled ventilation is required.
- Use a tuberculin syringe (or equivalent) to administer small volume of alfentanil accurately; alternatively, use infusion pump for controlled delivery.

Geriatric use
- Lower doses are usually indicated for elderly patients because they may be more sensitive to drug's therapeutic and adverse effects (especially apnea).

Pediatric use
- Safe use in children under age 12 has not been established.

Breast-feeding
- Drug is excreted in breast milk. Administer cautiously to breast-feeding women.

alglucerase (glucocerebrosidase, glucocerebrosidase-beta-glucosidase, glucosylceramidase)
Ceredase

Pharmacologic classification: glycosidase
Therapeutic classification: replacement enzyme
Pregnancy risk category C

How supplied
Available by prescription only
Injection: 80 U/ml, 10 U/ml

Indications, route, and dosage
Long-term endogenous enzyme (glucosylceramidase) replacement therapy in confirmed type I Gaucher's disease
Adults: Dosage should be individualized; initial dose of up to 60 U/kg/infusion may be used. Frequency of infusion may be adjusted based on severity of disease or patient convenience; initial frequency is once q 2 weeks. After response is established, reduce dosage downward for maintenance at intervals of 3 to 6 months.

Pharmacodynamics
Enzymatic action: Drug appears to reduce glycolipid accumulation by acting as a catalyst for the hydrolysis of glucocerebroside to glucose and ceramide—part of the normal degradation pathway for lipids.

Pharmacokinetics
- *Absorption:* After I.V. administration, steady-state enzymatic activity is achieved within 60 minutes.
- *Distribution:* Gaucher's cells in liver, spleen, bone marrow, lung, kidney, and intestine.
- *Metabolism:* Unknown.

• *Excretion:* Unknown.

Contraindications and precautions
No known contraindications. Use cautiously in patients who exhibit hypersensitivity to drug. Pretreatment with antihistamines has allowed continued use in some patients.

Interactions
None reported.

Effects on diagnostic tests
None reported.

Adverse reactions
GI: abdominal discomfort, nausea, vomiting.
Other: chills, slight fever, discomfort, burning, swelling at injection site.

Overdose and treatment
No toxicity detected.

☑ Special considerations
• Infusion should run over 1 to 2 hours and be given once every 2 weeks.
• Monitor response parameters to utilize lowest effective dose.
• There is no age restriction for receiving alglucerase.
• Hemoglobin levels may normalize after 6 months of therapy.
• Improved mineralization of bone may also follow prolonged treatment.
• *Do not shake bottle.* Shaking may denature the glycoprotein and render it biologically inactive.
• Store drug at 39.2° F (4° C). Do not use if the solution is discolored or contains particles.
• Alglucerase is preservative-free. Do not store for subsequent use after opening.
• Prepare fresh solution by diluting the appropriate amount of alglucerase with 0.9% NaCl to a final volume not to exceed 100 ml. Use an in-line particulate filter during administration.

Pediatric use
• There are no age restrictions for the use of alglucerase.

Breast-feeding
• Excretion in breast milk is unknown. Use with caution in breast-feeding women.

allopurinol
Lopurin, Zyloprim

Pharmacologic classification: xanthine oxidase inhibitor
Therapeutic classification: antigout
Pregnancy risk category C

How supplied
Available by prescription only
Tablets (scored): 100 mg, 300 mg

Indications, route, and dosage
Gout, primary or secondary hyperuricemia
Gout may be secondary to diseases such as acute or chronic leukemia, polycythemia vera, multiple myeloma, or psoriasis or after administration of chemotherapeutic agents. Dosage varies with severity of disease; can be given as single dose or divided, but doses larger than 300 mg should be divided.
Adults: Mild gout, 200 to 300 mg P.O. daily; severe gout with large tophi, 400 to 600 mg P.O. daily. Same dose for maintenance in secondary hyperuricemia.
Hyperuricemia secondary to malignancies
Children age 6 to 10: 300 mg P.O. daily (100 mg t.i.d.).
Children under age 6: 150 mg P.O. daily (50 mg t.i.d.).
To prevent acute gouty attacks
Adults: 100 mg P.O. daily; increase at weekly intervals by 100 mg without exceeding maximum dose (800 mg), until serum uric acid level falls to 6 mg/100 ml or less.
To prevent uric acid nephropathy during cancer chemotherapy
Adults: 600 to 800 mg P.O. daily for 2 to 3 days, with high fluid intake.
◇ *Adults:* 350 to 700 mg/m² (allopurinol sodium) I.V. over 24 hours or divided into 4- to 6-hour doses.
Recurrent calcium oxalate calculi
Adults: 200 to 300 mg P.O. daily in single dose or divided doses.
✦ ***Dosage adjustment.*** In adults with creatinine clearance up to 9 ml/minute, give 100 mg q 3 days; 10 to 19 ml/minute, give 100 mg q 2 days; 20 to 39 ml/minute, 100 mg daily; 40 to 59 ml/minute, 150 mg daily; 60 to 79 ml/minute, 200 mg daily; and if it is 80 ml/minute, give 250 mg daily.
◇ ***Stomatitis from fluorouracil***
Adults: Allopurinol mouthwash, 600 mg/day.

Pharmacodynamics
Antigout action: Allopurinol inhibits xanthine oxidase, the enzyme catalyzing the conversion of hypoxanthine to xanthine, and the conversion of xanthine to uric acid. By blocking this enzyme, allopurinol and its metabolite, oxypurinol, prevent the conversion of oxypurines (xanthine and hypoxanthine) to uric acid, thus decreasing serum and urine concentrations of uric acid. Drug has no analgesic, anti-inflammatory, or uricosuric action.

Pharmacokinetics
• *Absorption:* After oral administration, approximately 80% to 90% of a dose is absorbed. Peak concentrations of allopurinol are achieved 2 to 6 hours after a usual dose.
• *Distribution:* Distributed widely throughout the body except in the brain, where drug concentrations are 50% of those found in the rest of the body. Allopurinol and oxypurinol are not bound to plasma proteins.
• *Metabolism:* Drug is metabolized to oxypurinol by xanthine oxidase. Half-life of allopurinol is 1 to 2 hours; of oxypurinol, about 15 hours.
• *Excretion:* 5% to 7% of an allopurinol dose is excreted in urine unchanged within 6 hours of in-

gestion. After this, it is excreted by the kidneys as oxypurinol, allopurinol, and oxypurinol ribonucleosides. About 70% of the administered daily dose is excreted in urine as oxypurinol and an additional 2% appears in feces as unchanged drug within 48 to 72 hours.

Contraindications and precautions
Contraindicated in patients with hypersensitivity to drug and in those with idiopathic hemochromatosis.

Interactions
In patients with decreased renal function, the concomitant use of allopurinol and a *thiazide diuretic* may increase the risk of allopurinol-induced hypersensitivity reactions.

Concomitant use with *azathioprine* and *mercaptopurine* may increase the toxic effects of these drugs, particularly bone marrow depression. Combined use of these drugs requires reduction of initial doses of *azathioprine* or *mercaptopurine* to 25% to 33% of the usual dose, with subsequent doses adjusted according to patient response and toxic effects.

Concomitant use of allopurinol with *cyclophosphamide* may increase the incidence of bone marrow depression through an unknown mechanism. Allopurinol inhibits hepatic microsomal metabolism of *dicumarol*, thus increasing the half-life of dicumarol; patients receiving the two drugs concomitantly should be observed for increased anticoagulant effects.

Concomitant use of allopurinol with *ampicillin* or *amoxicillin* may increase the incidence of rash.

Because allopurinol or its metabolites may compete with *chlorpropamide* for renal tubular secretion, patients who receive these drugs concomitantly should be observed for signs of excessive hypoglycemia.

Concomitant use of *co-trimoxazole* with allopurinol has been associated with thrombocytopenia.

Theophylline clearance can decrease with large doses (600 mg/day), leading to increased plasma theophylline levels.

Effects of diagnostic tests
Increased alkaline phosphatase, AST, and ALT levels have been reported in patients on allopurinol therapy.

Adverse reactions
CNS: drowsiness, headache, paresthesia, peripheral neuropathy, neuritis.
CV: hypersensitivity vasculitis, necrotizing angiitis.
EENT: epistaxis.
GI: nausea, vomiting, diarrhea, abdominal pain, gastritis, dyspepsia.
GU: *renal failure,* uremia.
Hematologic: ***agranulocytosis,*** anemia, ***aplastic anemia, thrombocytopenia,*** leukopenia, leukocytosis, eosinophilia.
Hepatic: altered liver function studies, ***hepatitis, hepatic necrosis,*** hepatomegaly, cholestatic jaundice.
Skin: alopecia, ecchymoses, ***rash*** (usually maculopapular); ***exfoliative, urticarial, and purpuric lesions; Stevens-Johnson syndrome (erythema multiforme);*** severe furunculosis of nose; ichthyosis, ***toxic epidermal necrolysis.***
Other: arthralgia, fever, myopathy, taste loss or perversion, chills.

Overdose and treatment
No information available.

☑ Special considerations
- Rash occurs mostly in patients taking diuretics and in those with renal disorders.
- Monitor patient's intake and output. Daily urine output of at least 2 L and maintenance of neutral or slightly alkaline urine is desirable.
- If renal insufficiency occurs during treatment, reduce allopurinol dose.
- Monitor CBC, serum uric acid levels, and hepatic and renal function at start of therapy and periodically thereafter.
- Acute gout attacks may occur in first 6 weeks of therapy; concurrent use of colchicine or another anti-inflammatory agent may be prescribed prophylactically.
- Minimize GI adverse reactions by administering drug with meals or immediately after. Tablets may be crushed and administered with fluid or food.
- Allopurinol may predispose patient to ampicillin-induced rash.
- Allopurinol-induced rash may occur weeks after discontinuation of drug.

Patient education
- Encourage patient to drink plenty of fluids (10 to 12 8-oz [240 ml] glasses daily) while taking drug unless otherwise contraindicated.
- When using to treat recurrent calcium oxalate stones, advise patient to reduce dietary intake of animal protein, sodium, refined sugars, vitamin C, oxalate-rich foods, and calcium.
- Advise patient to avoid hazardous activities requiring alertness until CNS response to drug is known, because drowsiness may occur.
- Advise patient to avoid alcohol because it decreases effectiveness of allopurinol.
- Tell patient to report all adverse reactions immediately.
- Advise patient to take a missed dose when remembered unless it is time for next scheduled dose and not to double the doses.
- Inform patient to discontinue drug and call immediately at first sign of rash or other signs that may indicate an allergic reaction.

Geriatric use
- Follow dosage recommendations for adults. Watch for renal disorders or impaired renal function and treat according to dosage recommendations for patients with impaired renal function.

Pediatric use
- Do not use drug in children except to treat hyperuricemia secondary to malignancies.

Breast-feeding
• Because oxypurinol and allopurinol are distributed into breast milk, allopurinol should be used with extreme caution in breast-feeding women.

alpha$_1$-proteinase inhibitor (human) (alpha$_1$-PI)
Prolastin

Pharmacologic classification: enzyme inhibitor
Therapeutic classification: replacement protein
Pregnancy risk category C

How supplied
Available by prescription only
Injection: 500-mg and 1,000-mg activity per vial

Indications, route, and dosage
For chronic replacement of alpha$_1$-antitrypsin in patients with clinically demonstrable panacinar emphysema and PiZZ, PiZ (null), or Pi (null) (null) phenotype
Adults: 60 mg/kg I.V. over 30 minutes once weekly to increase and maintain functional alpha$_1$-PI level in the epithelial lining of the lower respiratory tract providing adequate antielastase activity in the lungs of patients with alpha$_1$-antitrypsin deficiency.

Pharmacodynamics
Enzyme inhibiting action: Alpha$_1$-PI inhibits the elastase released by inflammatory cells in the lung parenchyma. Persons with congenital alpha$_1$-antitrypsin deficiency develop emphysema in the third or fourth decade of life as a result of chronic degradation of elastin tissues.

Pharmacokinetics
• *Absorption:* Alpha$_1$-PI must be administered I.V.
• *Distribution:* I.V. alpha$_1$-PI appears to distribute to lung tissues; however, distribution is not well documented.
• *Metabolism:* Half-life is about 4½ days.
• *Excretion:* Unknown.

Contraindications and precautions
Contraindicated in patients with selective immunoglobulin A (IgA) deficiency who have known antibodies against IgA. Use cautiously in patients at risk for circulatory overload.

Interactions
None reported.

Effects on diagnostic tests
None reported.

Adverse reactions
CNS: dizziness, light-headedness.
Hematologic: possible viral transmission, transient leukocytosis.
Other: delayed fever (transient).

Overdose and treatment
No information available.

☑ Special considerations
• Only patients with early evidence of clinically demonstrable panacinar emphysema should be considered for chronic replacement therapy with alpha$_1$-PI. Subjects with the PiMZ or PiMS phenotypes of alpha$_1$-antitrypsin deficiency appear to be at small risk for panacinar emphysema and should not receive treatment with alpha$_1$-PI.
• Alpha$_1$-PI is not indicated for use in patients other than those with PiZZ, PiZ (null) or Pi (null) (null) phenotypes.
• Drug should only be used I.V. May be given at a rate of 0.08 ml/kg/minute or greater.
• Refrigerate at 35° to 46° F (2° to 8° C). Avoid freezing.
• Factors that could diminish alpha$_1$-PI effectiveness or cause adverse effects include improper storage and handling or method of administration, incorrect diagnosis, and individual biological differences.
• Follow manufacturers' directions for use carefully.
• Consider risk of transmitting viruses before prescribing drug. Prophylaxis against hepatitis B is recommended.
• Commercial assays of antigenic activity may be used to monitor alpha$_1$-PI serum levels in patients receiving this agent; however, results of such tests do not reflect the functional activity (potency; the capacity to neutralize pancreatic elastase) of alpha$_1$-PI and cannot be used to determine therapeutic dosage.

Pediatric use
• Alpha$_1$-PI has been used only in adults.

alprazolam
Alprazolam Intensol, Apo-Alpraz*, Novo-Alprazol*, Xanax

Pharmacologic classification: benzodiazepine
Therapeutic classification: antianxiety
Controlled substance schedule IV
Pregnancy risk category D

How supplied
Available by prescription only
Tablets: 0.25 mg, 0.5 mg, 1 mg, 2 mg
Oral solution: 0.1 mg/1 ml, 1 mg/1 ml

Indications, route, and dosage
Anxiety
Adults: Usual starting dose is 0.25 to 0.5 mg P.O. t.i.d. Increase dose p.r.n. q 3 to 4 days. Maximum total daily dosage, 4 mg in divided doses.
✦ ***Dosage adjustment.*** In elderly or debilitated patients or those with hepatic impairment, initial dose is 0.25 mg P.O. b.i.d. or t.i.d.
Panic disorder
Adults: Initially, 0.5 mg P.O. t.i.d. Increase as needed and tolerated at intervals of 3 to 4 days in in-

crements of 1 mg daily. Most patients require more than 4 mg daily; however, dosages from 1 to 10 mg daily have been reported.

◇ ***Agoraphobia***
Adults: 2 to 8 mg/day P.O.

◇ ***Depression, premenstrual syndrome***
Adults: 0.25 mg P.O. t.i.d.

Pharmacodynamics

Anxiolytic action: Alprazolam depresses the CNS at the limbic and subcortical levels of the brain. It produces an antianxiety effect by enhancing the effect of the neurotransmitter gamma-aminobutyric acid on its receptor in the ascending reticular activating system, which increases inhibition and blocks both cortical and limbic arousal.

Pharmacokinetics

- *Absorption:* When administered orally, alprazolam is well absorbed. Onset of action occurs within 15 to 30 minutes, with peak action in 1 to 2 hours.
- *Distribution:* Drug is distributed widely throughout the body. About 80% to 90% of an administered dose is bound to plasma protein.
- *Metabolism:* Alprazolam is metabolized in the liver equally to alpha-hydroxyalprazolam and inactive metabolites.
- *Excretion:* Alpha-hydroxyalprazolam and other metabolites are excreted in urine. Alprazolam's half-life is 12 to 15 hours.

Contraindications and precautions

Contraindicated in patients with hypersensitivity to drug or other benzodiazepines or acute angle-closure glaucoma. Use cautiously in patients with hepatic, renal, or pulmonary disease.

Interactions

Alprazolam potentiates the CNS depressant effects of *phenothiazines, narcotics, barbiturates, alcohol, general anesthetics, antihistamines, MAO inhibitors,* and *antidepressants.*

Concomitant use with *cimetidine* and possibly *disulfiram* diminishes hepatic metabolism of alprazolam, increasing its plasma concentration.

Heavy smoking accelerates alprazolam metabolism, thus lowering clinical effectiveness.

Benzodiazepines may decrease serum levels of *haloperidol.*

Plasma levels of *digoxin* may increase. The effects of alprazolam may decrease with use of *rifampin. Theophylline* may increase the sedative effects of alprazolam.

Effects on diagnostic tests

Alprazolam therapy may elevate liver function test results. Minor changes in EEG patterns, usually low-voltage, fast activity, may occur during and after alprazolam therapy.

Adverse reactions

CNS: *drowsiness, light-headedness,* headache, confusion, tremor, dizziness, syncope, *depression,* insomnia, nervousness.
CV: hypotension, tachycardia.
EENT: blurred vision, nasal congestion.
GI: *dry mouth,* nausea, vomiting, *diarrhea, constipation.*
Skin: dermatitis.
Other: muscle rigidity, weight gain or loss.

Overdose and treatment

Clinical manifestations of overdose include somnolence, confusion, coma, hypoactive reflexes, dyspnea, labored breathing, hypotension, bradycardia, slurred speech, unsteady gait, and impaired coordination.

Support blood pressure and respiration until drug effects subside; monitor vital signs. Flumazenil, a specific benzodiazepine antagonist, may be useful. Mechanical ventilatory assistance via endotracheal tube may be required to maintain a patent airway and support adequate oxygenation. As needed, use I.V. fluids and vasopressors, such as dopamine and phenylephrine, to treat hypotension. If the patient is conscious, induce emesis. Use gastric lavage if ingestion was recent, but only if an endotracheal tube is in place to prevent aspiration. After emesis or lavage, administer activated charcoal with a cathartic as a single dose. Dialysis is of limited value. Do not use barbiturates if excitation occurs because of possible exacerbation of excitation or CNS depression.

☑ Special considerations

Besides those relevant to all *benzodiazepines,* consider the following recommendations.

- Patients receiving prolonged therapy with high doses should be weaned from the drug gradually to prevent withdrawal symptoms. A 2- to 3-month withdrawal may be necessary.
- Lower doses are effective in elderly patients and patients with renal or hepatic dysfunction.
- Anxiety associated with depression is also responsive to alprazolam but may require more frequent dosing.
- Store drug in a cool, dry place away from direct light.

Patient education

- Be sure patient understands potential for physical and psychological dependence with chronic use of alprazolam.
- Instruct patient not to alter drug regimen.
- Warn patient that sudden changes in position can cause dizziness. Advise him to dangle legs for a few minutes before getting out of bed to prevent falls and injury.

Geriatric use

- Lower doses are usually effective in elderly patients because of decreased elimination.
- During initiation of therapy or after an increase in dose, elderly patients who receive drug require supervision with ambulation and activities of daily living.

Pediatric use

- Closely observe neonate for withdrawal symptoms if mother took alprazolam during pregnancy. Use of alprazolam during labor may cause neonatal flaccidity.

• Safety has not been established in children under age 18.

Breast-feeding
• The breast-fed infant of a woman taking alprazolam may become sedated, have feeding difficulties, or lose weight. Avoid use in breast-feeding women.

alprostadil
Prostin VR Pediatric

Pharmacologic classification: prostaglandin
Therapeutic classification: prostaglandin derivative
Pregnancy risk category NR

How supplied
Available by prescription only
Injection: 500 mcg/ml

Indications, route, and dosage
Temporary maintenance of patency of ductus arteriosus until surgery can be performed
Infants: Initial I.V. infusion of 0.05 to 0.1 mcg/kg/minute via infusion pump. After satisfactory response is achieved, reduce infusion rate to the lowest dosage that will maintain response. Maintenance doses vary. Infusion rate should be the lowest possible dose and is usually achieved by progressively halving the initial dose. Rates as low as 0.002 to 0.005 mcg/kg/minute have been effective.

Pharmacodynamics
Ductus arteriosus patency adjunct action: Alprostadil, also known as prostaglandin E_1 or PGE_1, is a prostaglandin that relaxes or dilates the rings of smooth muscle of the ductus arteriosus and maintains patency in neonates when infused before natural closure.

Pharmacokinetics
• *Absorption:* Alprostadil is administered I.V.
• *Distribution:* Distributed rapidly throughout the body.
• *Metabolism:* 68% of dose is metabolized in one pass through the lung, primarily by oxidation; 100% is metabolized within 24 hours.
• *Excretion:* All metabolites are excreted in urine within 24 hours.

Contraindications and precautions
Contraindicated in neonates with respiratory distress syndrome. Use cautiously in neonates with bleeding disorders.

Interactions
None reported.

Effects on diagnostic tests
None reported.

Adverse reactions
CNS: *seizures.*
CV: bradycardia, hypotension, tachycardia, ***cardiac arrest,*** edema.
GI: diarrhea.
Hematologic: *DIC.*
Respiratory: **APNEA.**
Other: *flushing, fever, sepsis, hypokalemia.*

Overdose and treatment
Clinical manifestations are similar to the adverse reactions and include apnea, bradycardia, pyrexia, hypotension, and flushing. Apnea most commonly occurs in neonates weighing below 4.4 lb (2 kg) at birth and usually develops during the first hour of drug therapy.

Treatment of apnea or bradycardia requires discontinuance of the infusion and appropriate supportive therapy, including mechanical ventilation as needed. Pyrexia or hypotension may be treated by reducing the infusion rate. Flushing may be corrected by repositioning the intra-arterial catheter.

☑ Special considerations
• Adding a 500-mcg solution to 50 ml of D_5W or 0.9% NaCl solution provides a concentration of 10 mcg/ml. At this concentration, a 0.01 ml/kg/minute infusion rate will deliver 0.1 mcg alprostadil/kg/minute.
• Drug must be diluted before administration. Discard prepared solution after 24 hours.
• Assess all vital functions closely and frequently to prevent adverse effects.
• Monitor arterial pressure by umbilical artery catheter, auscultation, or Doppler transducer. Slow rate of infusion if arterial pressure decreases significantly.
• In infants with restricted pulmonary blood flow, measure effectiveness of drug by monitoring blood oxygenation. In infants with restricted systemic blood flow, measure effectiveness of drug by monitoring systemic blood pressure and blood pH.
• Apnea and bradycardia may reflect drug overdose. Stop the infusion immediately if they occur.
• Monitor respiratory status during treatment; have ventilatory assistance immediately available.
• Peripheral arterial vasodilation (flushing) may respond to repositioning of the catheter.
• Drug should be administered only by personnel trained in pediatric intensive care.
• Store ampules in refrigerator.

alprostadil
Caverject, Muse

Pharmacologic classification: prostaglandin
Therapeutic classification: corrective agent for impotence
Pregnancy risk category NR

How supplied
Available by prescription only
Sterile powder for injection: 6.15-mcg, 11.9-mcg, 23.2-mcg vials
Urethral suppository pellet: 125 mcg, 250 mcg, 500 mcg, 1,000 mcg

Indications, route, and dosage

Erectile dysfunction due to vasculogenic, psychogenic, or mixed etiology

Adults: Dosages are highly individualized. For injection: initial dose is 2.5 mcg intracavernously. If partial response occurs, increase second dose by 2.5 to 5 mcg, and then increase dosage further in increments of 5 to 10 mcg until patient achieves an erection (suitable for intercourse but not lasting over 1 hour). If initial dose is not effective, increase second dose to 7.5 mcg within 1 hour; then increase dosage further in 5- to 10-mcg increments until patient achieves an erection. Patient must remain in primary health care provider office until complete detumescence occurs. If patient responds, do not repeat procedure for 24 hours. For pellet: start initially with lower doses (125 or 250 mcg). Increases or decreases should be made on separate occasions in a stepwise manner until patient achieves an erection that is sufficient for sexual intercourse.

Erectile dysfunction of pure neurologic etiology (spinal cord injury)

Adults: Dosages are highly individualized. Initial dose is 1.25 mcg intracavernously. If partial response occurs, give second dose of 1.25 mcg and then a third dose of 2.5 mcg; increase dosage further in 5-mcg increments until patient achieves an erection (suitable for intercourse but not lasting over 1 hour). If initial dose is not effective, increase second dose to 2.5 mcg within 1 hour; then increase further in 5-mcg increments until patient achieves an erection. Patient must remain in primary health care provider's office until complete detumescence occurs. If patient responds, do not repeat procedure for 24 hours.

Pharmacodynamics

Corrective action of impotence: A prostaglandin derivative that induces erection by relaxation of trabecular smooth muscle and by dilation of cavernosal arteries. This leads to expansion of lacunar spaces and entrapment of blood by compressing the venules against the tunica albuginea, a process referred to as the corporal veno-occlusive mechanism.

Pharmacokinetics

- *Absorption:* Alprostadil's absolute bioavailability has not been determined.
- *Distribution:* Drug is bound in plasma protein primarily to albumin (81%).
- *Metabolism:* Drug is rapidly converted to compounds that are further metabolized before excretion.
- *Excretion:* Metabolites are excreted primarily in urine; rest are excreted in the feces.

Contraindications and precautions

Contraindicated in patients with hypersensitivity to drug, conditions associated with disposition to priapism (sickle cell anemia or trait, multiple myeloma, or leukemia), or penile deformation (angulation, cavernosal fibrosis, or Peyronie's disease). Do not give to men with penile implants or when sexual activity is contraindicated. Also avoid use in women, children, and newborns. Muse should not be used for sexual intercourse with a pregnant woman unless the couple uses a condom barrier.

Interactions

Anticoagulants increase risk of bleeding from intracavernosal injection site. Monitor patient closely. Safety and efficacy of concomitant use with *vasoactive agents* have not been studied and, therefore, is not recommended. Alprostadil may decrease *cyclosporine's* serum concentration.

Effects on diagnostic tests

None reported.

Adverse reactions

CNS: headache, dizziness, fainting.
CV: hypertension, hypotension, swelling of leg veins.
GU: *penile pain*, prolonged erection, penile fibrosis, penis disorder, penile rash, penile edema, prostatic disorder, testicular and perineal aching, burning of urethra, minor urethral burning.
Respiratory: upper respiratory infection, flu syndrome, sinusitis, nasal congestion, cough.
Other: injection site hematoma, injection site ecchymosis, back pain, localized trauma, localized pain.

Overdose and treatment

Overdosage was not observed in clinical trials with alprostadil. If intracavernous overdose of drug occurs, patient should be under medical supervision until systemic effects have resolved or penile detumescence has occurred. Symptomatic treatment of systemic symptoms is appropriate.

☑ Special considerations

- Patient must have underlying treatable medical causes of erectile dysfunction diagnosed and treated before initiation of therapy.
- Regular follow-up of patients with careful examination of the penis is strongly recommended to detect signs of penile fibrosis. Discontinue drug in patients in whom penile angulation, cavernosal fibrosis, or Peyronie's disease develops.
- Monitor users of Muse for hypotension; titrate drug to the lowest effective dose.
- Female partners of users of Muse may experience vaginal itching and burning.

Patient education

- To ensure safe and effective use, thoroughly instruct patient how to prepare and administer alprostadil before beginning intracavernosal treatment at home. Stress importance for following instructions carefully.
- Tell patient to discard vials with precipitates or discoloration. Reconstituted vial is designed for one use only and should be discarded after withdrawal of proper volume of the solution.
- Instruct patient not to shake the contents of reconstituted vial.
- Stress importance of not reusing or sharing needles or syringes as well as not sharing medication.
- Ensure that patient has the manufacturer's instructions for administration that are included in each package of alprostadil to refer to at home.

• Tell patient that desirable dose will be established in the primary health care provider's office. Patient should not change the dose without medical approval.
• Inform patient that he can expect an erection to occur within 5 to 20 minutes after drug administration and that standard treatment goal is to produce an erection not lasting over 1 hour.
• Inform patient that an erection lasting over 6 hours has been known to occur after alprostadil injection. If this occurs, instruct patient to seek medical attention immediately.
• Tell patient that drug should not be used more than three times weekly, with at least 24 hours between each use. The maximum frequency use of Muse is two administrations per 24-hour period.
• Review possible adverse reactions with patient. Besides priapism, instruct patient to immediately report penile pain that was not present before or that has increased in intensity as well as the occurrence of nodules or hard tissue in the penis.
• Instruct patient to inspect penis daily for signs or symptoms of redness, swelling, tenderness, or curvature of the erect penis, which might suggest an infection. Tell him to call if infection is suspected.
• Remind patient that regular follow-up visits are necessary to evaluate effectiveness and safety of therapy.
• Inform patient that drug does not offer protection from transmission of sexually transmitted diseases and that protective measures continue to be necessary.
• Warn patient that a small amount of bleeding can occur at the injection site. This can increase the risk of transmitting blood-borne diseases, if present, to his sexual partner.
• Inform patient that drug does not offer protection from transmission of sexually transmitted diseases and that protective measures continue to be necessary.
• Caution patient using Muse to use condom when having sexual intercourse with a pregnant partner, and to prevent potential vaginal burning and itching in female partner.

Pediatric use
• Drug is not indicated for use with newborns or children.

Breast-feeding
• Drug is not indicated for use in women.

alteplase (recombinant alteplase, tissue plasminogen activator)
Activase

Pharmacologic classification: enzyme
Therapeutic classification: thrombolytic enzyme
Pregnancy risk category C

How supplied
Available by prescription only
Injection: 20-mg (11.6 million IU), 50-mg (29 million IU), 100-mg (58 million IU) vials

Indications, route, and dosage
Lysis of thrombi obstructing coronary arteries in management of acute MI
Three-hour infusion:
Adults weighing over 143 lb (65 kg): 60 mg in first hour, with 6 to 10 mg I.V. bolus over first 1 to 2 minutes; then 20 mg/hour for an additional 2 hours. Total dose, 100 mg.
Adults weighing 143 lb or less: 1.25 mg/kg given over 3 hours as described above.
Accelerated infusion:
Adults weighing over 148 lb (67 kg): 15 mg I.V. push, 50 mg over 30 minutes, then 35 mg over 60 minutes.
Adults weighing 148 lb or less: 15 mg I.V. push, 0.75 mg/kg over 30 minutes (not to exceed 50 mg), then 0.50 mg/kg over 60 minutes (not to exceed 35 mg).
Pulmonary embolism
Adults: 100 mg by I.V. infusion over 2 hours. Heparin therapy should be initiated at the end of the infusion.
Acute ischemic stroke
Adults: 0.9 mg/kg (maximum dose, 90 mg). Administer 10% of dose as an I.V. bolus over 1 minute; remaining 90% over 1 hour.

Pharmacodynamics
Thrombolytic action: Alteplase is an enzyme that catalyzes the conversion of tissue plasminogen to plasmin in the presence of fibrin. This fibrin specificity produces local fibrinolysis in the area of recent clot formation, with limited systemic proteolysis. In patients with acute MI, this allows for reperfusion of ischemic cardiac muscle and improved left ventricular function with a decreased incidence of heart failure after an MI.

Pharmacokinetics
• *Absorption:* Alteplase must be given I.V.
• *Distribution:* Drug is rapidly cleared from the plasma by the liver; 80% of a dose is cleared within 10 minutes after infusion is discontinued.
• *Metabolism:* Primarily hepatic.
• *Excretion:* Over 85% of drug is excreted in the urine, 5% in feces. Plasma half-life is under 10 minutes.

Contraindications and precautions
Contraindicated in patients with history or evidence of intracranial hemorrhage, suspected subarachnoid hemorrhage, seizure at the onset of stroke, active internal bleeding, intracranial neoplasm, arteriovenous malformation, aneurysm, and severe uncontrolled hypertension (more than 185 mm Hg systolic or 110 mm Hg diastolic). Also contraindicated in patients with a history of CVA, recent (within 2 months) intraspinal or intracranial trauma or surgery, or known bleeding diathesis (see package insert).

Use cautiously in patients with recent (within 10 days) major surgery; in pregnancy and first 10 days postpartum; organ biopsy; trauma (including cardiopulmonary resuscitation); GI or GU bleeding; cerebrovascular disease; hypertension; likelihood of left-sided heart thrombus; hemostatic defects, including those secondary to severe hepatic or renal disease; hepatic dysfunction; occluded AV cannula; severe neurologic deficit (NIH Stroke Scale over 22); signs of major early infarct on a computed tomographic (CT) scan; mitral stenosis; atrial fibrillation; acute pericarditis or subacute bacterial endocarditis; septic thrombophlebitis; diabetic hemorrhagic retinopathy or other hemorrhagic ophthalmic conditions; in those receiving anticoagulants; and in patients age 75 and older.

Interactions

Concomitant use of alteplase with drugs that antagonize platelet function (*aspirin, dipyridamole, abciximab*) is associated with an increased risk of bleeding if administered prior to, during, or after alteplase therapy.

Effects on diagnostic tests

Altered results may be expected in coagulation and fibrinolytic tests. The use of aprotinin (150 to 200 U/ml) in the blood sample may attenuate this interference.

Adverse reactions

CNS: ***cerebral hemorrhage,*** fever.
CV: hypotension, ***arrhythmias,*** edema.
GI: nausea, vomiting.
Hematologic: ***severe, spontaneous bleeding (cerebral, retroperitoneal, GU, GI).***
Other: bleeding at puncture sites, hypersensitivity reactions ***(anaphylaxis).***

Overdose and treatment

No information is available regarding accidental ingestion.

Excessive I.V. dosage can lead to bleeding problems. Doses of 150 mg have been associated with an increased incidence of intracranial bleeding. Discontinue infusion immediately if signs or symptoms of bleeding are observed.

☑ Special considerations

- Expect to begin alteplase infusions as soon as possible after onset of MI symptoms (angina pain or equivalent, greater than 30 minutes duration; angina that is unresponsive to nitroglycerin; or ECG evidence of MI).
- Administer drug within 3 hours after onset of stroke symptoms after exclusion of intracranial hemorrhage by CT scan or other diagnostic imaging methods able to detect the presence of hemorrhage. Treatment should only be performed in facilities that can provide appropriate evaluation and management of intracranial hemorrhage.
- Heparin is usually administered during or after alteplase as part of the treatment regimen for acute MI or pulmonary embolism. The use of anticoagulant or antiplatelet therapy for 24 hours is contraindicated when alteplase is used for acute ischemic stroke.
- Drug therapy for acute ischemic stroke should be discontinued in patients who have not recently used oral anticoagulants or heparin if pretreatment PT exceeds 15 seconds or if an elevated activated partial prothrombin time is identified.
- Monitor ECG for transient arrhythmias (sinus bradycardia, ventricular tachycardia, accelerated idioventricular rhythm, ventricular premature depolarizations) associated with reperfusion after coronary thrombolysis. Have antiarrhythmic agents available.
- Avoid I.M. injections, venipuncture, and arterial puncture during therapy. Use pressure dressings or ice packs on recent puncture sites to prevent bleeding. If arterial puncture is necessary, select a site on the arm and apply pressure for 30 minutes afterward.
- Prepare solution using supplied sterile water for injection. Do not use bacteriostatic water for injection.
- Do not mix other drugs with alteplase. Use 18G needle for preparing solution—aim water stream at lyphilized cake. Expect a slight foaming to occur. Do not use if vacuum is not present.
- Drug may be further diluted with 0.9% NaCl solution injection or D_5W to yield a concentration of 0.5 mg/ml. Reconstituted or diluted solutions are stable for up to 8 hours at room temperature.

Patient education

- Teach patient signs and symptoms of internal bleeding and tell him to report these immediately.
- Advise patient about proper dental care to avoid excessive gum trauma.

aluminum carbonate

Basaljel

Pharmacologic classification: inorganic aluminum salt
Therapeutic classification: antacid, hypophosphatemic agent
Pregnancy risk category NR

How supplied

Available without a prescription
Tablets or capsules: aluminum hydroxide equivalent 500 mg
Suspension: aluminum hydroxide equivalent 400 mg/5 ml

Indications, route, and dosage

Antacid
Adults: 10 ml suspension P.O. q 2 hours p.r.n. or 1 to 2 tablets or capsules q 2 hours p.r.n.
Treatment of hyperphosphatemia and prevention of urinary phosphate stones formation (with low-phosphate diet)
Adults: 1 g P.O. t.i.d. or q.i.d.; adjust to lowest possible dose after therapy is initiated, monitoring diet and serum levels.

Pharmacodynamics

Antacid action: Exerts its antacid effect by neutralizing gastric acid; this increases pH, thereby decreasing pepsin activity.

Hypophosphatemic action: Aluminum carbonate reduces serum phosphate levels by complexing with phosphate in the gut. This results in formation of insoluble, nonabsorbable aluminum phosphate, which is then excreted in feces. Calcium absorption increases secondary to reduced phosphate absorption.

Pharmacokinetics
- *Absorption:* Aluminum carbonate is largely unabsorbed; small amounts may be absorbed systemically.
- *Distribution:* None.
- *Metabolism:* None.
- *Excretion:* Excreted in feces; some may be excreted in breast milk.

Contraindications and precautions
No known contraindications. Use cautiously in patients with chronic renal disease.

Interactions
Aluminum carbonate may decrease absorption of many drugs, including *tetracycline, quinolones, coumarin anticoagulants, phenothiazines* (especially *chlorpromazine*), *chenodiol, antimuscarinics, diazepam, chlordiazepoxide, indomethacin, isoniazid, vitamin A, digoxin, iron salts,* and *sodium or potassium phosphate,* thereby lessening their effectiveness. Separate administration by at least 2 hours. Use with *enterically coated drugs* causes premature drug release.

Effects on diagnostic tests
Aluminum carbonate may interfere with imaging techniques using sodium pertechnetate Tc 99m and thus impair evaluation of Meckel's diverticulum. It may also interfere with reticuloendothelial imaging of liver, spleen, or bone marrow using technetium Tc 99m sulfur colloid. It may antagonize the effect of pentagastrin during gastric acid secretion tests.

Aluminum carbonate may increase serum gastrin levels and decrease serum phosphate levels.

Adverse reactions
CNS: encephalopathy.
GI: *constipation,* intestinal obstruction.
Other: hypophosphatemia, osteomalacia.

Overdose and treatment
No information available. Patients with impaired renal function are at a higher risk of aluminum toxicity to brain, bone, and parathyroid glands.

☑ Special considerations
- When administering suspension, shake well and give with small amounts of water or fruit juice.
- After administration through a nasogastric tube, tube should be flushed with water to prevent obstruction.
- When administering drug as an antiurolithic, encourage increased fluid intake to enhance drug effectiveness.
- Constipation may be managed with stool softeners or bulk laxatives, or administer alternately with magnesium-containing antacids (unless patient has renal disease).
- Monitor serum calcium and phosphate levels periodically; reduced serum phosphate levels may lead to increased serum calcium levels.
- Long-term aluminum carbonate use can lead to calcium resorption and subsequent bone demineralization.

Patient education
- Advise patient to take drug only as directed and not to take more than 24 capsules or tablets or 120 ml (24 tsp) of regular suspension in a 24-hour period. Instruct patient to shake suspension well.
- As needed, advise patient to restrict sodium intake, to drink plenty of fluids, and to follow a low-phosphate diet.
- Advise patient not to switch antacids without medical approval.

Geriatric use
- Because elderly patients commonly have decreased GI motility, they may become constipated from this drug.

Pediatric use
- Use cautiously in children under age 6.

aluminum hydroxide
AlternaGEL, Alu-Cap, Aluminett, Alu-Tab, Amphojel, Dialume, Nephrox

Pharmacologic classification: aluminum salt
Therapeutic classification: antacid, hypophosphatemic agent
Pregnancy risk category C

How supplied
Available without a prescription
Tablets: 300 mg, 500 mg, 600 mg
Capsules: 475 mg, 500 mg
Suspension: 320 mg/5 ml, 450 mg/5 ml, 600 mg/5 ml, 675 mg/5 ml

Indications, route, and dosage
Antacid; hyperphosphatemia
Adults: 500 to 1,500 mg P.O. (tablet or capsule) 1 hour after meals and h.s.; or 5 to 30 ml of suspension p.r.n. 1 hour after meals and h.s.

Pharmacodynamics
Antacid action: Aluminum hydroxide neutralizes gastric acid, reducing the direct acid irritant effect. This increases pH, thereby decreasing pepsin activity.

Hypophosphatemic action: Aluminum hydroxide reduces serum phosphate levels by complexing with phosphate in the gut, resulting in insoluble, nonabsorbable aluminum phosphate, which is then excreted in feces. Calcium absorption increases secondary to decreased phosphate absorption.

Pharmacokinetics
• *Absorption:* Absorbed minimally; small amounts may be absorbed systemically.
• *Distribution:* None.
• *Metabolism:* None.
• *Excretion:* Excreted in feces; some may be excreted in breast milk.

Contraindications and precautions
No known contraindications. Use cautiously in patients with renal disease.

Interactions
Aluminum hydroxide may decrease absorption of many drugs, including *quinolones, tetracycline, phenothiazines* (especially *chlorpromazine*), *coumarin anticoagulants, chenodiol, antimuscarinics, diazepam, chlordiazepoxide, isoniazid, vitamin A, digoxin, iron salts,* and *sodium or potassium phosphate,* thereby decreasing their effectiveness; separate drugs by at least 2 hours. Drug causes premature release of *enterically coated drugs;* separate doses by 1 hour.

Effects on diagnostic tests
Drug therapy may interfere with imaging techniques using sodium pertechnetate Tc 99m and thus impair evaluation of Meckel's diverticulum. It may also interfere with reticuloendothelial imaging of liver, spleen, and bone marrow using technetium Tc 99m sulfur colloid. It may antagonize pentagastrin's effect during gastric acid secretion tests. Drug may also elevate serum gastrin levels and reduce serum phosphate levels.

Adverse reactions
CNS: encephalopathy.
GI: *constipation,* intestinal obstruction.
Other: hypophosphatemia, osteomalacia.

Overdose and treatment
No information available. Patients with impaired renal function are at a higher risk of aluminum toxicity to brain, bone, and parathyroid glands.

☑ Special considerations
• Shake suspension well (especially extra-strength suspension) and give with small amounts of water or fruit juice.
• After administration through nasogastric tube, tube should be flushed with water to prevent obstruction.
• When administering drug as an antiurolithic, encourage increased fluid intake to enhance drug effectiveness.
• Constipation may be managed with stool softeners or bulk laxatives. Also, alternate aluminum hydroxide with magnesium-containing antacids (unless patient has renal disease).
• Periodically monitor serum calcium and phosphate levels; decreased serum phosphate levels may lead to increased serum calcium levels. Observe patient for hypophosphatemia signs and symptoms (anorexia, muscle weakness, and malaise).

Patient education
• Caution patient to take drug only as directed; to shake suspension well or chew tablets thoroughly; and to follow with sips of water or juice.
• As indicated, instruct patient to restrict sodium intake, drink plenty of fluids, or follow a low-phosphate diet.
• Advise patient not to switch to another antacid without medical approval.

Geriatric use
• Because elderly patients commonly have decreased GI motility, they may become constipated from this drug.

Pediatric use
• Use with caution in children under age 6.

Breast-feeding
• Although drug may be excreted in breast milk, no problems have been associated with its use in breast-feeding women.

amantadine hydrochloride
Symmetrel

Pharmacologic classification: synthetic cyclic primary amine
Therapeutic classification: antiviral, antiparkinsonian
Pregnancy risk category C

How supplied
Available by prescription only
Capsules: 100 mg
Syrup: 50 mg/5 ml

Indications, route, and dosage
Prophylaxis or symptomatic treatment of influenza type A virus, respiratory tract illnesses in elderly or debilitated patients
Adults up to age 64 and children age 10 and older: 200 mg P.O. daily in a single dose or divided b.i.d.
Children age 1 to 9: 4.4 to 8.8 mg/kg P.O. daily, divided b.i.d. or t.i.d. Do not exceed 150 mg/day.
Adults over age 64: 100 mg P.O. once daily.

Treatment should continue for 24 to 48 hours after symptoms disappear. Prophylaxis should start as soon as possible after initial exposure and continue for at least 10 days after exposure. Prophylactic treatment may be continued up to 90 days for repeated or suspected exposures if influenza virus vaccine is unavailable. If used with influenza virus vaccine, continue dose for 2 to 4 weeks until protection from vaccine develops.
Treatment of drug-induced extrapyramidal reactions
Adults: 100 to 300 mg/day P.O. in divided doses.
Treatment of idiopathic parkinsonism, parkinsonian syndrome
Adults: 100 mg P.O. b.i.d.; in patients who are seriously ill or receiving other antiparkinsonian drugs, 100 mg/day for at least 1 week, then 100 mg b.i.d., p.r.n. Patient may benefit from as much as

400 mg/day, but doses over 200 mg must be closely supervised.
✦ ***Dosage adjustment.*** In patients with renal dysfunction, base maintenance dosage on creatinine clearance value, as follows:

For syrup, give 200 mg on the first day; for capsules, give 100 mg the first day, and then 100 mg daily if creatinine clearance is between 30 and 50 ml/minute/1.73 m^2; 200 mg on the first day and 100 mg q alternating day if it ranges between 15 and 29 ml/minute/1.73 m^2; and 200 mg q 7 days if it falls below 15 ml/minute/1.73 m^2.

Note: Patients on chronic hemodialysis should receive 200 mg q 7 days.

Pharmacodynamics

Antiviral action: Amantadine interferes with viral uncoating of the RNA in lysosomes. In vitro, amantadine is active only against influenza type A virus. (However, spontaneous resistance commonly occurs.) In vivo, amantadine may protect against influenza type A virus in 70% to 90% of patients; when administered within 24 to 48 hours of onset of illness, it reduces duration of fever and other systemic symptoms.

Antiparkinsonian action: Amantadine is thought to cause the release of dopamine in the substantia nigra.

Pharmacokinetics

- *Absorption:* With oral administration, drug is well absorbed from the GI tract. Peak serum levels occur in 1 to 8 hours; usual serum level is 0.2 to 0.9 mcg/ml. (Neurotoxicity may occur at levels exceeding 1.5 mcg/ml.)
- *Distribution:* Distributed widely throughout body and crosses the blood-brain barrier.
- *Metabolism:* About 10% of dose is metabolized.
- *Excretion:* About 90% of dose is excreted unchanged in urine, primarily by tubular secretion. Portion of drug may be excreted in breast milk. Excretion rate depends on urine pH (acidic pH enhances excretion). Elimination half-life in patients with normal renal function is approximately 24 hours; in those with renal dysfunction, it may be prolonged to 10 days.

Contraindications and precautions

Contraindicated in patients with hypersensitivity to drug. Use cautiously in patients with seizure disorders, heart failure, peripheral edema, hepatic disease, mental illness, eczematoid rash, renal impairment, orthostatic hypotension, and CV disease and in the elderly.

Interactions

When used concomitantly, amantadine may potentiate anticholinergic adverse effects of *trihexyphenidyl* and *benztropine* (when these drugs are given in high doses), possibly causing confusion and hallucinations. Concomitant use with a combination of *hydrochlorothiazide* and *triamterene* may decrease urinary amantadine excretion, resulting in increased serum amantadine levels and possible toxicity.

Concomitant use with *CNS stimulants* may cause additive stimulation. Concomitant use with *alcohol* may result in light-headedness, confusion, fainting, and hypotension.

Effects on diagnostic tests

None reported.

Adverse reactions

CNS: depression, fatigue, confusion, *dizziness*, hallucinations, anxiety, *irritability*, ataxia, *insomnia*, headache, *light-headedness*.
CV: peripheral edema, orthostatic hypotension, ***heart failure.***
GI: anorexia, *nausea*, constipation, vomiting, dry mouth.
Skin: *livedo reticularis* (with prolonged use).

Overdose and treatment

Clinical effects of overdose include nausea, vomiting, anorexia, hyperexcitability, tremors, slurred speech, blurred vision, lethargy, anticholinergic symptoms, seizures, and possible ventricular arrhythmias, including torsades de pointes and ventricular fibrillation. CNS effects result from increased levels of dopamine in the brain.

Treatment includes immediate gastric lavage or emesis induction along with supportive measures, forced fluids and, if necessary, I.V. administration of fluids. Urine acidification may be used to increase drug excretion. Physostigmine may be given (1 to 2 mg by slow I.V. infusion at 1- to 2-hour intervals) to counteract CNS toxicity. Seizures or arrhythmias may be treated with conventional therapy. Patient should be monitored closely.

☑ Special considerations

- To prevent orthostatic hypotension, instruct patient to move slowly when changing position (especially when rising to standing position).
- If patient experiences insomnia, administer dose several hours before bedtime.
- Prophylactic drug use is recommended for selected high-risk patients who cannot receive influenza virus vaccine. Manufacturer recommends prophylactic therapy lasting up to 90 days with possible repeated or unknown exposure.

Patient education

- Warn patient that drug may impair mental alertness.
- Advise patient to take drug after meals to ensure best absorption.
- Caution patient to avoid abrupt position changes because these may cause light-headedness or dizziness.
- If drug is being taken to treat parkinsonism, warn patient not to discontinue it abruptly because that might precipitate a parkinsonian crisis.
- Warn patient to avoid alcohol while taking drug.
- Instruct patient to report adverse effects promptly, especially dizziness, depression, anxiety, nausea, and urine retention.

Geriatric use
• Elderly patients are more susceptible to adverse neurologic effects; dividing daily dosage into two doses may reduce risk.

Pediatric use
• Safety and effectiveness of drug in children under age 1 have not been established.

Breast-feeding
• Drug is excreted in breast milk. Breast-feeding should be avoided during therapy with amantadine.

amcinonide
Cyclocort

Pharmacologic classification: topical adrenocorticoid
Therapeutic classification: anti-inflammatory
Pregnancy risk category C

How supplied
Available by prescription only
Cream, ointment: 0.1%
Lotion: 0.1%

Indications, route, and dosage
Inflammation of corticosteroid-responsive dermatoses
Adults and children: Apply a light film to affected areas b.i.d. or t.i.d. Rub cream in gently and thoroughly until it disappears.

Pharmacodynamics
Anti-inflammatory action: Amcinonide stimulates the synthesis of enzymes needed to decrease the inflammatory response. Amcinonide is a group II fluorinated corticosteroid with much greater anti-inflammatory activity than hydrocortisone 0.25% to 2.5%. The anti-inflammatory actions equal those of betamethasone valerate cream 0.1% and triamcinolone acetonide cream 0.1%.

Pharmacokinetics
• *Absorption:* Amount of drug absorbed depends on the amount applied and on the nature of the skin at the application site. It ranges from about 1% in areas with a thick stratum corneum (such as the palms, soles, elbows, and knees) to as high as 36% in areas of the thinnest stratum corneum (face, eyelids, and genitals). Absorption increases in areas of skin damage, inflammation, or occlusion. Some systemic absorption of topical steroids may occur, especially through the oral mucosa.
• *Distribution:* After topical application, amcinonide is distributed throughout the local skin. Any drug that is absorbed into circulation is removed rapidly from the blood and distributed into muscle, liver, skin, intestines, and kidneys.
• *Metabolism:* After topical administration, drug is metabolized primarily in the skin. The small amount that is absorbed into systemic circulation is metabolized primarily in the liver to inactive compounds.
• *Excretion:* Inactive metabolites are excreted by the kidneys, primarily as glucuronides and sulfates, but also as unconjugated products. Small amounts of the metabolites are also excreted in feces.

Contraindications and precautions
Contraindicated in patients hypersensitive to drug.

Interactions
None significant.

Effects on diagnostic tests
None reported.

Adverse reactions
Skin: burning, pruritus, irritation, dryness, erythema, folliculitis, acneiform eruptions, perioral dermatitis, hypopigmentation, hypertrichosis, allergic contact dermatitis, *secondary infection, maceration, atrophy, striae, miliaria* (with occlusive dressings).
Other: ***hypothalamic-pituitary-adrenal axis suppression,*** Cushing's syndrome, hyperglycemia, glycosuria.

Overdose and treatment
No information available.

☑ Special considerations
Recommendations for use of amcinonide, for care and teaching of patients during therapy, and for use in elderly patients, in children, and during breast-feeding are the same as those for all *topical adrenocorticoids.*

Patient education
• Instruct patient to avoid prolonged use around eyes, genitalia, rectal area, face, axillae, and skinfolds.
• If a dose is forgotten, apply a dose as soon as possible. Do not double doses.

amifostine
Ethyol

Pharmacologic classification: organic thiophosphate
Therapeutic classification: cytoprotective
Pregnancy risk category C

How supplied
Available by prescription only
Injection: 500 mg anhydrous basis and 500 mg mannitol/10 ml vial

Indications, route, and dosage
Reduction of the cumulative renal toxicity associated with repeated administration of cisplatin in patients with advanced ovarian cancer
Adults: 910 mg/m² daily as a 15-minute I.V. infusion, starting within 30 minutes before chemotherapy. If hypotension occurs and blood pressure does not return to normal within 5 minutes of treatment, subsequent cycles should use 740 mg/m².

Pharmacodynamics

Cytoprotective action: Amifostine is dephosphorylated by alkaline phosphatase in tissues to a pharmacologically active free thiol metabolite. The higher concentration of free thiol in normal tissues is available to bind to, and thereby detoxify, reactive metabolites of cisplatin, which can reduce the toxic effects of cisplatin on renal tissue. Free thiol can also act as a scavenger of free radicals that may be generated in tissues exposed to cisplatin.

Pharmacokinetics

- *Absorption:* Not applicable because drug is administered I.V.
- *Distribution:* Amifostine is rapidly cleared from the plasma with a distribution half-life of less than 1 minute. It has been found in bone marrow cells 5 to 8 minutes following administration.
- *Metabolism:* Amifostine is rapidly metabolized to an active free thiol metabolite. A disulfide metabolite is produced subsequently and is less active than the free thiol.
- *Excretion:* Amifostine and the two metabolites have been found to be minimally excreted in the urine.

Contraindications and precautions

Contraindicated in patients hypersensitive to aminothiol compounds or mannitol. Amifostine should not be used in patients receiving chemotherapy for malignancies that are potentially curable (certain malignancies of germ cell origin), except in clinical studies. Also contraindicated in hypotensive or dehydrated patients and in those receiving antihypertensive drugs that cannot be stopped for 24 hours preceding amifostine administration.

Use cautiously in the elderly and in patients with ischemic heart disease, arrhythmias, heart failure, or history of stroke or transient ischemic attacks. Also use cautiously in patients in whom the common adverse effects of nausea, vomiting, and hypotension are likely to have serious consequences.

Interactions

None known although special consideration should be given to the administration of amifostine in patients receiving *antihypertensive medications* or other *drugs that could potentiate hypotension.*

Effects on diagnostic tests

None reported.

Adverse reactions

CNS: loss of consciousness, dizziness, somnolence.
CV: *hypotension.*
GI: *nausea, vomiting.*
Other: flushing or feeling of warmth, chills or feeling of coldness, hiccups, sneezing, hypocalcemia, allergic reactions ranging from rash to rigors.

Overdose and treatment

Although overdosage has not occurred in clinical trials, the most likely symptom is hypotension, which should be managed by infusion of 0.9% NaCl solution and other supportive measures, as clinically indicated.

☑ Special considerations

- Reconstitute each single-dose vial with 9.5 ml of sterile NaCl injection, 0.9% NaCl. The use of other solutions to reconstitute the drug is not recommended. Reconstituted solution (500 mg amifostine/10 ml) is chemically stable for up to 5 hours at room temperature (about 77° F [25° C]) or up to 24 hours under refrigeration (35° to 46° F [2° to 8° C]).
- Drug can be prepared in polyvinyl chloride bags at concentrations of 5 to 40 mg/ml and has the same stability as when it is reconstituted in the single-use vial.
- Inspect vial for particulate matter and discoloration before administration whenever solution and container permit. Do not use if cloudiness or precipitate is observed.
- If possible, stop antihypertensive therapy 24 hours preceding amifostine administration. If antihypertensive therapy cannot be stopped, do not use drug because of risk of severe hypotension.
- Patients receiving amifostine should be adequately hydrated before administration of drug and be kept in a supine position during the infusion.
- Monitor blood pressure every 5 minutes during infusion. If hypotension occurs, requiring interruption of therapy, place patient in Trendelenburg's position and give an infusion of 0.9% NaCl solution using a separate I.V. line. If blood pressure returns to normal within 5 minutes and patient is asymptomatic, infusion may be restarted so that the full dose of drug can be given. If full dose of amifostine cannot be administered, dose of drug for subsequent cycles should be 740 mg/m^2.
- Do not infuse for more than 15 minutes because a longer infusion time has been associated with a higher incidence of adverse reactions.
- Administer antiemetic medication, including dexamethasone 20 mg I.V. and a serotonin 5HT receptor antagonist, before and in conjunction with amifostine. Additional antiemetics may be required based on the chemotherapy drugs administered.
- When amifostine is used with highly emetogenic chemotherapy, monitor fluid balance of patient.
- Monitor serum calcium level in patients at risk for hypocalcemia, such as those with nephrotic syndrome. If necessary, calcium supplements can be administered.

Patient education

- Instruct patient to remain in a supine position during infusion.

Geriatric use

- Drug should be used with caution in elderly patients because safety of administration has not been established in this age-group.

Pediatric use

- Safety and effectiveness in children have not been established.

Breast-feeding

• Breast-feeding should be discontinued if patient is treated with amifostine because it is not known if drug or its metabolites are excreted in breast milk.

amikacin sulfate

Amikin

Pharmacologic classification: aminoglycoside
Therapeutic classification: antibiotic
Pregnancy risk category D

How supplied

Available by prescription only
Injection: 50 mg/ml, 250 mg/ml

Indications, route, and dosage

Serious infections caused by susceptible organisms

Adults and children with normal renal function: 15 mg/kg/day divided q 8 to 12 hours I.M. or I.V. (in 100 to 200 ml D_5W administered over 30 to 60 minutes). Do not exceed 1.5 g/day.

◇ *Adults:* 4 to 20 mg given intrathecally or intraventricularly as a single dose in conjunction with I.M. or I.V. administration.

Neonates with normal renal function: Initially, 10 mg/kg I.M. or I.V. (in D_5W administered over 1 to 2 hours), then 7.5 mg/kg q 12 hours.

Uncomplicated urinary tract infections

Adults: 250 mg I.M. or I.V. b.i.d.

✦ ***Dosage adjustment.*** In renal failure, initially, 7.5 mg/kg. Subsequent doses and frequency determined by blood amikacin concentrations and renal function studies. One method is to administer additional 7.5 mg/kg doses and alter dosing interval based on steady state serum creatinine:

creatinine (mg/dl) × 9 = dosing interval (hours)

Keep peak serum concentrations between 15 and 30 mcg/ml, and trough serum concentrations should not exceed 5 to 10 mcg/ml.

Pharmacodynamics

Antibiotic action: Amikacin is bactericidal; it binds directly to the 30S ribosomal subunit, thus inhibiting bacterial protein synthesis. Its spectrum of activity includes many aerobic gram-negative organisms (including most strains of *Pseudomonas aeruginosa*) and some aerobic gram-positive organisms. Amikacin may act against some organisms resistant to other aminoglycosides, such as *Proteus, Pseudomonas,* and *Serratia;* some strains of these may be resistant to amikacin. It is ineffective against anaerobes.

Pharmacokinetics

• *Absorption:* Poorly absorbed after oral administration and is given parenterally; after I.M. administration, peak serum concentrations occur in 45 minutes to 2 hours.

• *Distribution:* Amikacin is distributed widely after parenteral administration; intraocular penetration is poor. Factors that increase volume of distribution (burns, peritonitis) may increase dosage requirements. CSF penetration is low, even in patients with inflamed meninges. Intraventricular administration produces high concentrations throughout the CNS. Protein binding is minimal. Amikacin crosses the placenta.

• *Metabolism:* Not metabolized.

• *Excretion:* Excreted primarily in urine by glomerular filtration; small amounts may be excreted in bile and breast milk. Elimination half-life in adults is 2 to 3 hours. In patients with severe renal damage, half-life may extend to 30 to 86 hours. Over time, amikacin accumulates in inner ear and kidneys; urine concentrations approach 800 mcg/ml 6 hours after a 500-mg I.M. dose.

Contraindications and precautions

Contraindicated in patients with hypersensitivity to drug or other aminoglycosides. Use cautiously in patients with impaired renal function or neuromuscular disorders, in neonates and infants, and in the elderly.

Interactions

Concomitant use with the following drugs may increase the hazard of nephrotoxicity, ototoxicity, and neurotoxicity: *amphotericin B, loop diuretics, methoxyflurane, polymyxin B, capreomycin, cisplatin, cephalosporins, vancomycin,* and other *aminoglycosides;* hazard of ototoxicity is also increased during use with *ethacrynic acid, furosemide, bumetanide, urea,* or *mannitol. Dimenhydrinate* and other *antiemetics* and *antivertigo drugs* may mask amikacin-induced ototoxicity.

Amikacin may potentiate neuromuscular blockade from *general anesthetics* or *neuromuscular blocking agents* such as *succinylcholine* and *tubocurarine.*

Concomitant use with *penicillins* results in a synergistic bactericidal effect against *Pseudomonas aeruginosa, Escherichia coli, Klebsiella, Citrobacter, Enterobacter, Serratia,* and *Proteus mirabilis.* However, the drugs are physically and chemically incompatible and are inactivated when mixed or given together. In vivo inactivation has also been reported when aminoglycosides and *penicillins* are used concomitantly.

Effects on diagnostic tests

Drug-induced nephrotoxicity may elevate BUN, nonprotein nitrogen, or serum creatinine levels, and increase urinary excretion of casts.

Adverse reactions

CNS: ***neuromuscular blockade.***
EENT: *ototoxicity.*
GU: *nephrotoxicity, azotemia.*
Other: arthralgia, acute muscular paralysis.

Overdose and treatment

Clinical signs of overdose include ototoxicity, nephrotoxicity, and neuromuscular toxicity. Drug can be removed by hemodialysis or peritoneal dialysis. Treatment with calcium salts or anticholinesterases reverses neuromuscular blockade.

* Canada only ◇ Unlabeled clinical use

☑ Special considerations

Besides those relevant to all *aminoglycosides*, consider the following recommendations.

- Because drug is dialyzable, patients undergoing hemodialysis need dosage adjustments.
- Recommendations for care and teaching of patients during therapy and use in elderly patients and breast-feeding women are the same as for all *aminoglycosides*.

Pediatric use

- Because potential for ototoxicity is unknown, amikacin should only be used in infants when other drugs are ineffective or contraindicated. Patient should be closely monitored during therapy.

amiloride hydrochloride

Midamor

Pharmacologic classification: potassium-sparing diuretic
Therapeutic classification: diuretic, antihypertensive
Pregnancy risk category B

How supplied

Available by prescription only
Tablets: 5 mg

Indications, route, and dosage

Hypertension; edema associated with heart failure, usually in patients who are also taking thiazide or other potassium-wasting diuretics
Adults: Usually 5 mg P.O. daily. Dosage may be increased to 10 mg daily, if necessary. Do not exceed 20 mg daily.
◊ ***Lithium-induced polyuria***
Adults: 5 to 10 mg b.i.d.
◊ ***Cystic fibrosis***
Adults: Aerosolized amiloride dissolved in 0.3% NaCl solution.

Pharmacodynamics

Diuretic action: Amiloride acts directly on the distal renal tubule to inhibit sodium reabsorption and potassium excretion, thereby reducing potassium loss.

Antihypertensive action: Amiloride is commonly used in combination with more effective diuretics to manage edema associated with heart failure, hepatic cirrhosis, and hyperaldosteronism. Mechanism of amiloride's hypotensive effect is unknown.

Pharmacokinetics

- *Absorption:* About 50% of an amiloride dose is absorbed from the GI tract. Food decreases absorption to 30%. Diuresis usually begins in 2 hours and peaks in 6 to 10 hours.
- *Distribution:* Amiloride has wide extravascular distribution.
- *Metabolism:* Insignificant.
- *Excretion:* Most of the amiloride dose is excreted in urine; half-life is 6 to 9 hours in patients with normal renal function.

Contraindications and precautions

Contraindicated in patients with elevated serum potassium level (over 5.5 mEq/L). Do not administer to patients receiving other potassium-sparing diuretics, such as spironolactone and triamterene. Also contraindicated in patients with anuria, acute or chronic renal insufficiency, diabetic nephropathy, and hypersensitivity to drug.

Use with extreme caution in patients with diabetes mellitus.

Interactions

Amiloride may potentiate hypotensive effects of other *antihypertensive agents*; this may be used to therapeutic advantage.

Amiloride increases the risk of hyperkalemia when administered with other *potassium-sparing diuretics, angiotensin-converting enzyme inhibitors, potassium supplements, potassium-containing medications* (*parenteral penicillin G*), or *salt substitutes.* Amiloride may reduce renal clearance of *lithium* and increase lithium blood levels.

NSAIDs, such as *indomethacin* or *ibuprofen,* may alter renal function and thus affect potassium excretion.

The renal clearance of *digoxin* may be decreased, along with the inotropic effect.

Effects on diagnostic tests

Transient abnormal renal and hepatic function tests have been noted. Amiloride therapy causes severe hyperkalemia in diabetic patients following I.V. glucose tolerance testing; discontinue amiloride at least 3 days before testing.

Adverse reactions

CNS: *headache,* weakness, dizziness, encephalopathy.
CV: orthostatic hypotension.
GI: *nausea, anorexia, diarrhea, vomiting,* abdominal pain, constipation, appetite changes.
GU: impotence.
Hematologic: ***aplastic anemia,*** neutropenia.
Respiratory: dyspnea.
Other: hyperkalemia, fatigue, muscle cramps.

Overdose and treatment

Clinical manifestations of overdose are consistent with dehydration and electrolyte disturbance.

Treatment is supportive and symptomatic. In acute ingestion, empty stomach by emesis or lavage. In severe hyperkalemia (6.5 mEq/L or more), reduce serum potassium levels with I.V. sodium bicarbonate or glucose with insulin. A cation exchange resin, sodium polystyrene sulfonate (Kayexalate), given orally or as a retention enema, may also reduce serum potassium levels.

☑ Special considerations

Recommendations for use of amiloride and for care and teaching of the patient during therapy are the same as those for all *potassium-sparing diuretics.*

Patient education

- Tell patient to take drug with food because it may cause stomach upset.

• Advise patient to avoid consumption of large quantities of foods that are high in potassium.

Geriatric use
• Elderly and debilitated patients require close observation because they are more susceptible to drug-induced diuresis and hyperkalemia. Reduced dosages may be indicated.

Pediatric use
• Safety and efficacy in children have not been established.

Breast-feeding
• Amiloride is excreted in breast milk in animals; human data are unavailable.

amino acid infusions
Aminosyn, Aminosyn with dextrose, Aminosyn with electrolytes, Aminosyn-PF, Aminosyn (pH6), Aminosyn II, Aminosyn II in dextrose, Aminosyn II with electrolytes, Aminosyn II with electrolytes in dextrose, FreAmine III, FreAmine III with electrolytes, Novamine, Novamine without electrolytes, ProcalAmine, Travasol with electrolytes, Travasol without electrolytes, TrophAmine

amino acid infusions for renal failure
Aminess, Aminosyn-RF, NephrAmine, RenAmin

amino acid infusions for high metabolic stress
Aminosyn-HBC, BranchAmin, FreAmine HBC

amino acid infusions for hepatic failure or hepatic encephalopathy
HepatAmine

Pharmacologic classification: protein substrates
Therapeutic classification: parenteral nutritional therapy and caloric agent
Pregnancy risk category C

How supplied
Available by prescription only
Injection: without electrolytes—1,000 ml (3.5%, 5%, 8.5%, 10%; 10% with 60 mg potassium metabisulfite, 11.4%); 500 ml (5%, 5.5% with sodium bisulfite, 7%, 8.5%, 8.5% with sodium bisulfite, 10%, 10% with sodium bisulfite, 11.4%); 250 ml (5%, 10% with sodium bisulfite, 11.4%)
Injection: with electrolytes—1,000 ml (3% with 50 mg potassium metabisulfite and 3 mEq calcium/L, 3% with potassium metabisulfite, 3.5%, 3.5% with 60 mg sodium hydrosulfite), 500 ml (3.5%, 5.5%, with 3 mEq sodium bisulfite/L, 7% with potassium bisulfite, 8% in 1,000-ml container with potassium metabisulfite, 8.5% with potassium metabisulfite, 8.5% with 3 mEq sodium bisulfite/L)

Indications, route, and dosage
Hepatic encephalopathy in patients with cirrhosis or hepatitis; nutritional support
Adults: 80 to 120 g of amino acids (12 to 18 g of nitrogen)/day. Use formulation specifically for hepatic failure or encephalopathy (HepatAmine). Typically, 500 ml amino acid injection is mixed with 500 ml dextrose 50% in water and administered over 8 to 12 hours. Add electrolytes, vitamins, and trace elements.
Total supportive, or supplemental and protein-sparing parenteral nutrition to maintain normal nutrition and metabolism (amino acid infusions)
Adults: 1 to 1.5 g/kg I.V. daily.
Children: 2 to 3 g/kg I.V. daily.

Note: Individualize dosage to metabolic and clinical response as determined by nitrogen balance and body weight corrected for fluid balance. Add electrolytes, vitamins, trace elements, and nonprotein caloric agents p.r.n.

Pharmacodynamics
Nutritional action: Amino acid infusions provide a substrate for protein synthesis in the protein-depleted patient or enhance conservation of body protein.

Pharmacokinetics
• *Absorption:* Administered directly into vascular system.
• *Distribution:* No information available.
• *Metabolism.* No information available.
• *Excretion:* No information available.

Contraindications and precautions
Contraindicated in patients with anuria and in those with inborn errors of amino acid metabolism, such as maple syrup urine disease and isovaleric acidemia. Also contraindicated in patients with severe uncorrected electrolyte or acid-base imbalances, hyperammonemia, and decreased circulating blood volume.

Use cautiously in neonates (especially with low birth weight), in pediatric patients, and in patients with impaired renal, hepatic, or cardiac function.

Interactions
Concurrent *tetracycline* administration may reduce the protein-sparing effects of infused amino acids.

Because of the potential for incompatibility, other drugs should not be mixed with amino acid solutions. Mixture with *folic acid* precipitates *calcium salts* as *calcium folate.* Mixture with *sodium bicarbonate* may precipitate *calcium* and *magnesium* and decreases the activity of *insulin* and *vitamin B complex* with *vitamin C. Acidic I.V. solutions* for total parenteral nutrition (TPN) may release bicarbonate as gas. When *vitamin K* is indicated, administer it separately. *Supplementary vitamins, electrolytes, trace minerals, heparin,* or *insulin* may be added cautiously when necessary; other medications should not be administered via the central venous catheter. Simultaneous administration with *blood* may cause pseudoagglutination.

Effects on diagnostic tests
None reported.

Adverse reactions
CV: thrombophlebitis, edema, thrombosis.
GI: nausea.
GU: glycosuria, osmotic diuresis.
Hepatic: elevated liver enzyme levels.
Skin: flushing.
Other: hypersensitivity reactions, tissue sloughing at infusion site caused by extravasation, *catheter sepsis, rebound hypoglycemia* (when long-term infusions are abruptly stopped), hyperglycemia, osteoporosis, metabolic acidosis, alkalosis, hypophosphatemia, ***hyperosmolar hyperglycemic nonketotic syndrome,*** hyperammonemia, ***electrolyte imbalances,*** fever, weight gain.

Overdose and treatment
No information available.

☑ Special considerations
- Consult pharmacist about compatibility before combining amino acid infusions with other substances.
- Begin I.V. infusion slowly and increase over 1 to 2 days as tolerated to prevent hyperglycemia. Taper off over 1 to 2 days to prevent rebound hypoglycemia.
- Replace all I.V. equipment (I.V. lines, filter, and bottle) every 24 hours.
- Observe infusion site for signs of infection, drainage, edema, and extravasation. Check for fever or other possible signs of infection or hypersensitivity.
- TPN line should be used solely for providing nutrition, not for collecting blood samples, transfusing blood, or administering drugs.
- Check vital signs at least every 4 hours.
- Monitor intake, output, and pattern as well as caloric intake for significant changes.
- Patient should be weighed daily at the same time (preferably in the morning after urinating), in the same clothing, and on the same scale. After weight is stabilized, weighing patient two or three times weekly is sufficient.
- Patient's fingerstick blood glucose should be tested every 6 hours until infusion rate is stabilized, then twice daily.
- High blood glucose levels may require supplementary insulin to prevent dehydration and coma.
- Essential fatty acid deficiency may result from long-term fat-free I.V. feedings. Providing 500 ml of fat emulsion weekly may be necessary.
- If TPN must be interrupted, administer D_5W or $D_{10}W$ by peripheral vein to prevent rebound hypoglycemia.
- Watch for signs of circulatory overload.
- Regularly monitor the following laboratory values throughout TPN therapy: CBC with differential and platelet count, serum electrolytes, blood glucose, urine glucose and ketones, PT, renal and hepatic function tests, trace elements, and plasma lipids.
- In patients receiving protein-sparing therapy, check BUN determinations daily. If BUN levels increase 10 to 15 mg/dl for more than 3 days, therapy adjustment is usually required.
- Carefully monitor BUN and creatinine ratios. A BUN-to-creatinine ratio exceeding 10:1 may indicate that patient is receiving too much protein per unit of glucose. Reportedly, 100 to 150 g carbohydrate calories per gram of nitrogen are required to use amino acids effectively.
- Frequent, meticulous mouth care is important to prevent parotitis.
- Administer 10 mg of phytonadione weekly to prevent vitamin K deficiency.

Patient education
- Tell patient receiving TPN that he may imagine taste or smell of food. Explain that these sensations are common, and suggest some distracting activity during mealtimes.
- Encourage patient to take special care with oral hygiene. Recommend that a soft toothbrush and a fluoride toothpaste be used and that teeth be flossed daily.
- Inform patient that fewer bowel movements occur while receiving TPN.

Pediatric use
- The effect of amino acid infusions without dextrose on the carbohydrate metabolism of children is unknown.
- Take special precautions in children with acute renal failure and especially in low-birth-weight infants. In these patients, laboratory and clinical monitoring must be extensive and frequent.
- Monitor serum calcium levels frequently to check for signs of bone demineralization.

aminocaproic acid
Amicar

Pharmacologic classification: carboxylic acid derivative
Therapeutic classification: fibrinolysis inhibitor
Pregnancy risk category C

How supplied
Available by prescription only
Tablets: 500 mg
Syrup: 250 mg/ml
Injection: 5 g/20 ml for dilution; 24 g/96 ml for infusion

Indications, route, and dosage
Excessive acute bleeding from hyperfibrinolysis; ◇ amegakaryocytic thrombocytopenia; ◇ missed abortion; ◇ allergic reaction; ◇ dermatides; ◇ prophylaxis for blood transfusion reaction; ◇ connective tissue disease; ◇ rheumatoid arthritis; ◇ idiopathic thrombocytopenia; ◇ agranulocytosis
Adults: 4 to 5 g I.V. or P.O. over first hour, followed with constant infusion of 1 g/hour for about 8 hours

or until bleeding is controlled. Maximum dosage, 30 g/24 hours.

Excessive acute bleeding from hyperfibrinolysis

Children: 100 mg/kg I.V., or 3 g/m² I.V. first hour, followed by constant infusion of 33.3 mg/kg/hour or 1 g/m²/hour. Maximum dosage, 18 g/m² for 24 hours.

Chronic bleeding tendency

Adults: 5 to 30 g/day P.O. in divided doses at 3- to 6-hour intervals.

◊ ***Antidote for excessive thrombolysis due to administration of streptokinase or urokinase***

Adults: 4 to 5 g I.V. in first hour, followed by continuous infusion of 1 g/hour. Continue treatment for 8 hours or until hemorrhage is controlled.

◊ ***Secondary ocular hemorrhage in nonperforating traumatic hyphema***

Adults: 100 mg/kg P.O. q 4 hours for 5 days; maximum, 5 g/dose and 30 g/day.

◊ ***Hereditary hemorrhagic telangiectasia***

Adults: 1 to 1.5 g P.O. b.i.d. for 1 to 2 months followed by 1 to 2 g daily.

Pharmacodynamics

Hemostatic action: Aminocaproic acid inhibits plasminogen activators; to a lesser degree, it blocks antiplasmin activity by inhibiting fibrinolysis.

Pharmacokinetics

- *Absorption:* Aminocaproic acid is rapidly and completely absorbed from the GI tract. Peak plasma level occurs in 2 hours; sustained plasma levels are achieved by repeated oral doses or continuous I.V. infusion.
- *Distribution:* Drug readily permeates human blood cells and other body cells. It is not protein-bound.
- *Metabolism:* Insignificant.
- *Excretion:* Duration of action of a single parenteral dose is less than 3 hours; 40% to 60% of a single oral dose is excreted unchanged in urine in 12 hours.

Contraindications and precautions

Contraindicated in patients with active intravascular clotting or presence of DIC unless heparin is used concomitantly. Injectable form is contraindicated in newborns. Use cautiously in patients with cardiac, renal, or hepatic disease.

Interactions

Concomitant use with *estrogens* and *oral contraceptives containing estrogen* increases risk of hypercoagulability; use with caution.

Effects on diagnostic tests

Drug may elevate serum potassium level in some patients with decreased renal function; it may increase CK, AST, and ALT levels.

Adverse reactions

CNS: dizziness, malaise, headache, delirium, ***seizures,*** hallucinations, weakness.
CV: hypotension, bradycardia, ***arrhythmias*** (with rapid I.V. infusion), generalized thrombosis.
EENT: tinnitus, nasal congestion, conjunctival suffusion.
GI: nausea, cramps, diarrhea.
GU: ***acute renal failure.***
Skin: rash.
Other: malaise, myopathy.

Overdose and treatment

Clinical manifestations of overdose may include nausea, diarrhea, delirium, thrombotic episodes, and cardiac and hepatic necrosis. Discontinue drug immediately. Animal studies have demonstrated subendocardial hemorrhagic lesions after long-term high-dose administration.

☑ Special considerations

- To prepare an I.V. infusion, use 0.9% NaCl injection, D_5W injection, or lactated Ringer's injection for dilution. Dilute doses up to 5 g with 250 ml of solution, doses of 5 g or greater with at least 500 ml.
- Avoid rapid I.V. infusion to minimize risk of CV adverse reactions; use infusion pump to ensure constancy of infusion.
- Monitor coagulation studies, heart rhythm, and blood pressure. Chronic use of drug requires routine CK determinations. Be alert for signs of phlebitis.

Patient education

- Tell patient to change positions slowly to minimize dizziness.
- With long-term use, tell patient that routine CK determinations will be necessary.
- Teach patient signs and symptoms of thrombophlebitis, and advise him to report them promptly.

aminoglutethimide

Cytadren

Pharmacologic classification: antiadrenal hormone
Therapeutic classification: antineoplastic
Pregnancy risk category D

How supplied

Available by prescription only
Tablets: 250 mg

Indications, route, and dosage

Dosage and indications may vary. Check current literature for recommended protocol.

Adrenal hyperplasia from ectopic corticotropin-producing tumors; ◊ ***medical adrenalectomy in postmenopausal metastatic breast cancer;*** ◊ ***prostate cancer; suppression of adrenal function in Cushing's syndrome***

Adults: 250 mg P.O. q.i.d. at 6-hour intervals. Dosage may be increased in increments of 250 mg daily q 1 to 2 weeks to a maximum total daily dose of 2 g.

Pharmacodynamics

Antineoplastic action: Aminoglutethimide interferes with the enzymatic conversion of cholesterol to delta-5-pregnenolone, effectively inhibiting the synthesis of corticosteroids, androgens, and estrogens. Therefore, by suppressing the adrenals, aminoglutethimide inhibits the growth of tumors that need estrogen to thrive.

Pharmacokinetics

• *Absorption:* Aminoglutethimide is well absorbed across the GI tract after oral administration.
• *Distribution:* Drug is distributed widely into body tissues.
• *Metabolism:* Drug is metabolized extensively in the liver.
• *Excretion:* Drug and its metabolites are primarily eliminated through the kidneys, mostly as unchanged drug.

Contraindications and precautions

Contraindicated in patients hypersensitive to drug or glutethimide.

Interactions

Concomitant use of aminoglutethimide with *dexamethasone* decreases the half-life and therapeutic effect of dexamethasone by increasing the metabolism of dexamethasone.

By a similar mechanism, aminoglutethimide may diminish the effects of *warfarin.*

Effects on diagnostic tests

Aminoglutethimide therapy may decrease plasma cortisol, serum thyroxine, and urinary aldosterone levels and may increase serum alkaline phosphatase, AST, and thyroid-stimulating hormone concentrations.

Adverse reactions

CNS: *drowsiness,* headache, dizziness.
CV: hypotension, tachycardia.
GI: *nausea, anorexia,* vomiting.
Hematologic: transient leukopenia, ***agranulocytosis, thrombocytopenia.***
Skin: *morbilliform rash,* pruritus, urticaria.
Other: fever, myalgia, adrenal insufficiency, masculinization, hirsutism, hypothyroidism.

Overdose and treatment

Clinical manifestations of overdose include exaggerated rash, hypotension, nausea, and vomiting.

Treatment usually is supportive and includes induction of emesis, gastric lavage, antiemetics, and symptomatic treatment of abnormal vital signs. Drug is removable by dialysis.

☑ Special considerations

• Drug should be given in divided doses, two or three times daily, to reduce incidence of nausea and vomiting.
• Most adverse effects decrease in incidence and severity after the first 2 to 6 weeks of therapy because of accelerated metabolism of drug with continued use.
• Some recommend routine hydrocortisone supplementation as glucocorticoid replacement (in patients with metastatic breast cancer).
• Adrenal hypofunction may develop under stressful conditions, such as surgery, trauma, or acute illness. Additional steroids may be required to ensure a normal response to stress.
• Aminoglutethimide therapy does not require gradually tapered withdrawal because the adrenal cortex rapidly returns to normal responsiveness following cessation of therapy.
• Up to 50% of patients require mineralocorticoid replacement with fludrocortisone at a dosage of 0.1 mg daily or three times weekly.
• Monitor blood pressure frequently.
• Perform baseline hematologic studies and monitor CBC periodically. Also monitor thyroid function studies because drug may decrease thyroid hormone production.

Patient education

• Emphasize importance of continuing medication despite nausea and vomiting, which usually subside as therapy continues.
• Warn patient that drowsiness may occur. Patient should avoid hazardous activities that require alertness until sedative effect subsides. Tolerance usually develops within 1 month.
• If rash persists for 5 to 8 days when starting therapy, tell patient to call. Therapy may be discontinued temporarily until rash clears.
• Advise patient to stand up slowly to avoid dizziness.

Geriatric use

• Elderly patients are more sensitive to CNS adverse effects and are more likely to be lethargic. Safety precautions are recommended.

Pediatric use

• Drug may induce precocious sexual development in males and masculinization in females.

Breast-feeding

• It is not known whether drug distributes into breast milk. However, because of potential for serious adverse reactions in the infant, breast-feeding during therapy is not recommended.

aminophylline

Phyllocontin, Truphylline

Pharmacologic classification: xanthine derivative
Therapeutic classification: bronchodilator
Pregnancy risk category C

How supplied

Available by prescription only
Tablets: 100 mg, 200 mg
Tablets (controlled-release): 225 mg
Liquid: 105 mg/5 ml
Injection: 250-mg, 500-mg vials and ampules
Rectal suppositories: 250 mg, 500 mg
Rectal solution: 300 mg/5 ml

Indications, route and dosage

Symptomatic relief of acute bronchospasm
Patients not currently receiving theophylline who require rapid relief of symptoms: Loading dose is

6 mg/kg (equivalent to 4.7 mg/kg anhydrous theophylline) I.V. slowly (25 mg/minute or less), then maintenance infusion.
Adults (nonsmokers): 0.7 mg/kg/hour I.V. for 12 hours, then 0.5 mg/kg/hour I.V.; or 3 mg/kg P.O. q 6 hours for two doses, then 3 mg/kg q 8 hours.
Otherwise healthy adult smokers: 1 mg/kg/hour I.V. for 12 hours, then 0.8 mg/kg/hour I.V.; or 3 mg/kg P.O. q 4 hours for three doses, then 3 mg/kg q 6 hours.
Older patients; adults with cor pulmonale: 0.6 mg/kg/hour I.V. for 12 hours, then 0.3 mg/kg/hour I.V; or 2 mg/kg P.O. q 6 hours for two doses, then 2 mg/kg q 8 hours.
Adults with heart failure or liver disease: 0.5 mg/kg/hour I.V. for 12 hours, then 0.1 to 0.2 mg/kg/hour I.V.; or 2 mg/kg P.O. q 8 hours for two doses, then 1 to 2 mg/kg q 12 hours.
Children age 9 to 16: 1 mg/kg/hour I.V. for 12 hours, then 0.8 mg/kg/hour I.V.; or 3 mg/kg P.O. q 4 hours for three doses, then 3 mg/kg q 6 hours.
Children age 6 months to 9 years: 1.2 mg/kg/hour I.V. for 12 hours, then 1 mg/kg/hour I.V.; or 4 mg/kg P.O. q 4 hours for three doses, then 4 mg/kg q 6 hours.
Patients currently receiving theophylline: Aminophylline loading infusions of 0.63 mg/kg (0.5 mg/kg anhydrous theophylline) will increase plasma levels of theophylline by 1 mcg/ml, after serum levels have been evaluated. Some clinicians recommend a loading dose of 3.1 mg/kg (2.5 mg/kg anhydrous theophylline) if no obvious signs of theophylline toxicity are present, then maintenance infusion.

Chronic bronchial asthma
Adults: 400 mg P.O. daily divided t.i.d. or q.i.d.
Children: 16 mg/kg P.O. daily divided t.i.d. or q.i.d.

Monitor serum levels to ensure that theophylline concentrations range from 10 to 20 mcg/ml.

◊ ***Periodic apnea associated with Cheyne-Stokes respirations; left-sided heart failure***
Adults: 200 to 400 mg I.V. bolus.

◊ ***Reduction of severe bronchospasm in infants with cystic fibrosis***
Infants: 10 to 12 mg/kg I.V.

Pharmacodynamics
Bronchodilating action: Aminophylline acts at the cellular level after it is converted to theophylline. (Aminophylline [theophylline ethylenediamine] is 79% theophylline). Theophylline acts by either inhibiting phosphodiesterase or blocking adenosine receptors in the bronchi, resulting in relaxation of the smooth muscle. Drug also stimulates the respiratory center in the medulla and prevents diaphragmatic fatigue.

Pharmacokinetics
• *Absorption:* Most dosage forms are absorbed well; absorption of the suppository, however, is unreliable and slow. Rate and onset of action also depend on the dosage form selected. Food may alter the rate, but not the extent of absorption, of oral doses.
• *Distribution:* Distributed in all tissues and extracellular fluids except fatty tissue.
• *Metabolism:* Drug is converted to theophylline, then metabolized to inactive compounds.
• *Excretion:* Excreted in urine as theophylline (10%).

Contraindications and precautions
Contraindicated in patients with hypersensitivity to xanthine compounds (caffeine, theobromine) and ethylenediamine and in patients with active peptic ulcer disease and seizure disorders (unless adequate anticonvulsant therapy is given). Rectal suppositories are also contraindicated in patients who have an irritation or infection of the rectum or lower colon.

Use cautiously in neonates and infants under age 1, young children, and the elderly and in patients with heart failure, CV disorders, COPD, cor pulmonale, renal or hepatic disease, hyperthyroidism, diabetes mellitus, peptic ulcer, severe hypoxemia, or hypertension.

Interactions
Aminophylline increases the excretion of *lithium.* Concomitant *cimetidine, allopurinol* (high dose), *propranolol, erythromycin, quinolones,* or *troleandomycin* may increase serum concentration of aminophylline by decreasing hepatic clearance. *Phenobarbital, rifampin, phenytoin, carbamazepine, tobacco, marijuana,* and *aminoglutethimide* decrease effects of aminophylline. *Alkali-sensitive drugs* reduce activity of aminophylline. Do not add these drugs to I.V. fluids containing aminophylline.

Effects on diagnostic tests
Aminophylline may alter the assay for uric acid, depending on method used, and increases plasma-free fatty acids and urinary catecholamines. Theophylline levels are falsely elevated in the presence of furosemide, phenylbutazone, probenecid, theobromine, caffeine, tea, chocolate, cola beverages, and acetaminophen, depending on type of assay used.

Adverse reactions
CNS: *nervousness, restlessness,* headache, *insomnia,* ***seizures,*** muscle twitching, irritability.
CV: *palpitations, sinus tachycardia,* extrasystoles, flushing, marked hypotension, ***arrhythmias.***
GI: *nausea, vomiting,* diarrhea, epigastric pain, hematemesis.
Respiratory: tachypnea, ***respiratory arrest.***
Skin: urticaria.
Other: irritation (with rectal suppositories), hyperglycemia, fever.

Overdose and treatment
Clinical manifestations of overdose include nausea, vomiting, insomnia, irritability, tachycardia, extrasystoles, tachypnea, and tonic/clonic seizures. Onset of toxicity may be sudden and severe; arrhythmias and seizures are the first signs. Induce emesis, except in patients with seizures, then use activated charcoal and cathartics. Charcoal hemoperfusion may be beneficial. Treat arrhythmias with lidocaine and seizures with I.V. benzodiazepine; support respiratory and CV systems.

☑ Special considerations

• Before giving loading dose, check that patient has not had recent theophylline therapy.
• Do not combine in fluids for I.V. infusion with the following: ascorbic acid, chlorpromazine, codeine phosphate, dimenhydrinate, dobutamine, epinephrine, erythromycin gluceptate, hydralazine, insulin, levorphanol tartrate, meperidine, methadone, methicillin, morphine sulfate, norepinephrine bitartrate, oxytetracycline, penicillin g potassium, phenobarbital, phenytoin, prochlorperazine, promazine, promethazine, tetracycline, vancomycin, vitamin B complex with C.
• Do not crush controlled-release tablets.
• I.V. drug administration includes I.V. push at a very slow rate or an infusion with 100 to 200 ml of 5% dextrose or 0.9% NaCl.
• GI symptoms may be relieved by taking oral drug with full glass of water at meals, although food in stomach delays absorption. Enteric-coated tablets may also delay absorption. There is no evidence that antacids reduce GI adverse reactions.
• Suppositories are slowly and erratically absorbed; retention enemas may be absorbed more rapidly. Rectally administered preparations can be given when patient cannot take drug orally. Schedule after evacuation, if possible; may be retained better if given before meal. Advise patient to remain recumbent 15 to 20 minutes after insertion.
• Individuals metabolize xanthines at different rates. Adjust dose by monitoring response, tolerance, pulmonary function, and theophylline blood levels. Therapeutic level is 10 to 20 mcg/ml, but some patients may respond at lower levels; toxicity occurs at levels over 20 mcg/ml.
• Plasma clearance may be decreased in patients with heart failure, hepatic dysfunction, or pulmonary edema. Smokers show accelerated clearance. Dose adjustments necessary.

Patient education

• Teach patient rationale for therapy and importance of compliance with prescribed regimen; if a dose is missed, patient should take it as soon as possible, but not double up on doses. Advise patient to avoid taking extra "breathing pills."
• Advise patient of adverse effects and possible signs of toxicity.
• Tell patient not to eat or drink large quantities of xanthine-containing foods and beverages.
• Warn patient that OTC remedies may contain ephedrine in combination with theophylline salts; excessive CNS stimulation may result. Tell patient to seek medical approval before taking *any* other medications.

Geriatric use

• Use reduced doses and monitor the patient closely. Warn elderly patients of dizziness, a common adverse reaction at start of therapy.

Pediatric use

• Drug is not recommended for use in infants under age 6 months.

Breast-feeding

• Drug is excreted in breast milk and may cause irritability, insomnia, or fretfulness in the breast-fed infant.

aminosalicylate sodium (para-aminosalicylate sodium, PAS)

Nemasol Sodium, Sodium P.A.S

Pharmacologic classification: structural analogue of aminobenzoic acid
Therapeutic classification: antitubercular
Pregnancy risk category NR

How supplied

Available by prescription only
Tablets: 500 mg (equivalent to 365 mg of aminosalicylic acid)

Indications, route, and dosage

Adjunctive treatment for tuberculosis
Adults: 3.3 to 4 g (aminosalicylic acid) P.O. q 8 hours or 5 to 6 g q 12 hours. Maximum daily dose is 12 g (aminosalicylic acid). Must be taken with other antitubercular agents.
Children: 75 mg/kg (aminosalicylic acid) P.O. b.i.d. Maximum daily dose, 12 g (aminosalicylic acid). Must be taken with other antitubercular agents.

Pharmacodynamics

Antitubercular action: Drug is thought to suppress growth and reproduction of *Mycobacterium tuberculosis* by competitively inhibiting folic acid formation. Considered adjunctive therapy in tuberculosis, drug inhibits onset of bacterial resistance to the antitubercular drugs streptomycin and isoniazid.

Pharmacokinetics

• *Absorption:* Drug is absorbed rapidly from the GI tract; peak serum levels occur within ½ to 1 hour after ingestion.
• *Distribution:* Widely distributed in various body fluids, especially in pleural and caseous tissue, but achieves low CSF concentration. It is only about 15% bound to protein.
• *Metabolism:* Metabolized in the liver.
• *Excretion:* Over 80% of drug is excreted through the kidneys as metabolites and free acid. Its half-life is about 1 hour; half-life is greatly prolonged (up to 23 hours) in decreased renal function. It is not known if drug is removed by hemodialysis or peritoneal dialysis.

Contraindications and precautions

Contraindicated in patients with hypersensitivity to drug, other salicylates, or sulfonamides.

Use cautiously in patients with peptic ulcer or other GI diseases, severely impaired renal or hepatic function, or G6PD deficiency and in patients with heart failure. Also use cautiously in patients who may become pregnant because drug may be teratogenic.

Interactions
Concurrent use with *coumarin* or *indandione-derivative anticoagulants* may increase the anticoagulant effects of these agents because of decreased hepatic synthesis of procoagulant factors. Dosage adjustments may be necessary during and after aminosalicylate sodium therapy.

Probenecid or *sulfinpyrazone* may decrease renal tubular secretion of aminosalicylate sodium when used concurrently, resulting in increased and prolonged serum concentrations or toxicity. Aminosalicylate sodium dosage adjustments may be necessary during and after concurrent therapy, and patients should be monitored.

Aminosalicylate sodium may impair absorption of *rifampin*. Patients should be advised to take aminosalicylate sodium and rifampin at least 6 hours apart.

Aminosalicylate sodium may impair absorption of *vitamin B_{12}* from the GI tract; requirements for *vitamin B_{12}* may be increased in patients receiving aminosalicylate sodium.

Aminosalicylate sodium may reduce oral absorption of *digoxin*, possibly necessitating increased digoxin doses.

Effects on diagnostic tests
Drug may produce a false-positive test result with copper sulfate tests used for urine glucose determinations; may increase serum values of ALT and AST; may produce an orange turbidity or yellow color with Ehrlich's reagent used for urine urobilinogen determinations; and may cause Schilling test results to be misinterpreted because of impaired absorption of vitamin B_{12}.

Adverse reactions
GI: abdominal pain, nausea, vomiting, diarrhea, anorexia.
Hematologic: hemolytic anemia, leukopenia, ***agranulocytosis, thrombocytopenia.***
Hepatic: ***hepatitis,*** jaundice.
Skin: eruptions of various types.
Other: ***hypersensitivity reactions (fever),*** mononucleosis-like syndrome, goiter or myxedema (with long-term therapy), encephalopathy.

Overdose and treatment
No information available.

☑ Special considerations
- Drug may be taken with or after meals or with an antacid if gastric irritation occurs. If irritation persists, a temporary dose reduction or brief rest period of up to 2 weeks may be helpful. Aminosalicylate sodium may then be restarted in small daily doses and gradually increased to full therapeutic doses. If tolerated, total daily dose may be given as a single dose.
- If crystalluria occurs, the urine should be maintained at neutral or alkaline pH.
- Therapy may have to be continued for 1 to 2 years (and sometimes indefinitely), although shorter treatment regimens have been effective in some patients.
- Patient compliance may be poor because of gastric irritation or hypersensitivity reactions. Children may tolerate aminosalicylate sodium better than adults.
- Urine glucose enzymatic tests (Chemstrip uG, Diastix, or glucose enzymatic test strip) are not affected by aminosalicylate sodium (false-positive results may occur with copper sulfate tests, such as Benedict's solution or Clinitest).
- Drug should be administered with other antitubercular agents.

Patient education
- Instruct patient to take drug with or after meals or with an antacid to minimize possible gastric irritation.
- Stress importance of compliance with the full course of therapy, which may take months or years.
- Emphasize importance of not missing doses and taking them at evenly spaced times. Tell patient that if a dose is missed, it should be taken as soon as possible. However, if it is almost time for the next dose, the missed dose should be skipped to prevent doubling the dose at any one time.
- Advise patient to call if symptoms do not improve within 3 weeks.
- Instruct patient taking rifampin to separate doses of the two drugs by 6 hours.
- Tell diabetic patients that false-positive reactions with copper sulfate urine glucose tests may occur.
- Inform patient about potential adverse reactions, especially hypersensitivity reactions, crystalluria, goiter, myxedema, hemolytic anemia, hepatitis, and infectious mononucleosis-like syndrome.
- Advise patient to keep drug out of direct sunlight or heat and not to use drug if it becomes wet or turns brown or purple.

Breast-feeding
- Drug is excreted in breast milk. However, problems in humans have not been documented.

amiodarone hydrochloride
Cordarone

Pharmacologic classification: benzofuran derivative
Therapeutic classification: ventricular and supraventricular antiarrhythmic
Pregnancy risk category D

How supplied
Available by prescription only
Tablets: 100 mg*, 200 mg
Injection: 50 mg/ml

Indications, route, and dosage
Recurrent ventricular fibrillation and unstable ventricular tachycardia; ◊ supraventricular arrhythmias; ◊ atrial fibrillation; ◊ angina; ◊ hypertrophic cardiomyopathy
Adults: Loading dose of 800 to 1,600 mg P.O. daily for 1 to 3 weeks until initial therapeutic response occurs. Maintenance dosage, 200 to 600 mg P.O. daily. Alternatively, for first 24 hours 150 mg I.V. over

10 minutes (mixed in 100 ml D_5W); then 360 mg I.V. over 6 hours (mix 900 mg in 500 ml D_5W); then maintenance of 540 mg I.V. over 18 hours at a rate of 0.5 mg/minute. After first 24 hours, continue a maintenance infusion of 0.5 mg/minute in a 1 to 6 mg/ml concentration. For infusions greater than 1 hour, concentrations should not exceed 2 mg/ml unless a central venous catheter is used. Do not use for more than 3 weeks.

◊ *Children:* 10 to 15 mg/kg P.O. daily or 600 to 800 mg/1.73 m^2 P.O. daily for 4 to 14 days or until response is seen. Then 5 mg/kg or 400 mg/1.73 m^2; usual maintenance dose is 2.5 mg/kg or 200 mg/1.73 m^2/day.

Conversion from I.V. to P.O.

Adults: Daily dose of 720 mg (rate 0.5 mg/minute): for 1 week, 800 to 1,600 mg daily; 1 to 3 weeks, 600 to 800 mg daily; more than 3 weeks, 400 mg daily.

Pharmacodynamics

Ventricular antiarrhythmic action: Although it has mixed class Ic and III antiarrhythmic effects, amiodarone generally is considered a class III agent. It widens the action potential duration (repolarization inhibition). With prolonged therapy, the effective refractory period increases in the atria, ventricles, AV node, His-Purkinje system, and bypass tracts, and conduction slows in the atria, AV node, His-Purkinje system, and ventricles; sinus node automaticity decreases. Amiodarone also noncompetitively blocks beta-adrenergic receptors. Clinically, it has little, if any, negative inotropic effect. Coronary and peripheral vasodilator effects may occur with long-term therapy. Amiodarone is among the most effective antiarrhythmic agents, but its therapeutic applications are somewhat limited by its severe adverse reactions.

Pharmacokinetics

- *Absorption:* Drug has slow, variable absorption. Bioavailability is about 22% to 86%. Peak plasma levels occur 3 to 7 hours after oral administration; however, onset of action may be delayed from 2 to 3 days to 2 to 3 months—even with loading doses.
- *Distribution:* Distributed widely because it accumulates in adipose tissue and in organs with marked perfusion, such as the lungs, liver, and spleen. It is also highly protein-bound (96%). The therapeutic serum level is not well-defined but may range from 1 to 2.5 mcg/ml.
- *Metabolism:* Metabolized extensively in the liver to a pharmacologically active metabolite, desethyl amiodarone.
- *Excretion:* Main excretory route is hepatic, through the biliary tree (with enterohepatic recirculation). Because no renal excretion occurs, patients with impaired renal function do not require dosage reduction. Terminal elimination half-life—25 to 110 days—is the longest of any antiarrhythmic; in most patients, half-life ranges from 40 to 50 days.

Contraindications and precautions

Contraindicated in patients with hypersensitivity to drug and in those with severe SA node disease resulting in preexisting bradycardia. Unless an artificial pacemaker is present, drug is also contraindicated in patients with second- or third-degree AV block and in those in whom bradycardia has caused syncope. Use with caution in patients already receiving antiarrhythmics, beta-adrenergic blockers, and calcium channel blockers.

Interactions

Concomitant use of amiodarone with *quinidine, disopyramide, tricyclic antidepressants,* or *phenothiazines* may cause additive effects that lead to a prolonged QT interval, possibly resulting in torsades de pointes ventricular tachycardia.

Concomitant use with *warfarin* may cause prolonged PT, as a result of enhanced drug displacement from protein-binding sites. Concomitant use with *digoxin, flecainide, theophylline, cyclosporine, lidocaine, quinidine, phenytoin,* or *procainamide* may lead to increased serum levels of these drugs, resulting in enhanced effects.

Cholestyramine increases elimination of amiodarone. *Cimetidine* increases amiodarone levels. *Phenytoin* decreases amiodarone levels. Concomitant use with *beta-adrenergic* and *calcium channel blocking agents* may cause sinus bradycardia, sinus arrest, and AV block.

Effects on diagnostic tests

Amiodarone alters thyroid function test results, causing increased serum T_4 and decreased T_3 levels. (However, most patients maintain normal thyroid function during therapy.)

Adverse reactions

CNS: peripheral neuropathy, ataxia, paresthesia, tremor, insomnia, sleep disturbances, headache, *malaise, fatigue.*

CV: bradycardia, hypotension, ***arrhythmias, heart failure, heart block, sinus arrest.***

EENT: *corneal microdeposits,* visual disturbances.

GI: *nausea, vomiting,* constipation, abdominal pain.

Hepatic: *altered liver enzymes,* hepatic dysfunction, ***hepatic failure.***

Respiratory: SEVERE PULMONARY TOXICITY (PNEUMONITIS, ALVEOLITIS).

Skin: *photosensitivity,* blue-gray skin pigmentation, solar dermatitis.

Other: hypothyroidism, hyperthyroidism, edema, coagulation abnormalities.

Overdose and treatment

Clinical effects of overdose include bradyarrhythmias. Treatment may involve beta-adrenergic agonists (such as isoproterenol) or artificial pacing to help restore an acceptable heart rate. To treat hypotension, positive inotropic agents (such as dopamine or dobutamine) or vasopressors (such as epinephrine or norepinephrine) may be administered. General supportive measures should be used, as necessary. Drug cannot be removed by dialysis.

☑ Special considerations

- Drug is effective in treating arrhythmias resistant to other drug therapy. However, its high incidence of adverse effects limits its use.

• Divide loading dose into three equal doses, and give with meals to minimize GI intolerance. Maintenance dose may be given once daily but may be divided into two doses taken with meals if GI intolerance occurs.
• Monitor blood pressure and heart rate and rhythm frequently for significant change.
• Periodically monitor hepatic and thyroid function tests. Perform periodic ophthalmologic evaluations to assess corneal microdeposits.
• Monitor for signs and symptoms of pneumonitis, such as exertional dyspnea, nonproductive cough, and pleuritic chest pain. Also check pulmonary function tests and chest X-ray. (Pulmonary toxicity is more common with daily doses exceeding 600 mg.) Pulmonary complications require discontinuation of amiodarone and possibly treatment with corticosteroids.
• Digoxin, quinidine, phenytoin, and procainamide doses should be decreased during amiodarone therapy to avoid toxicity.
• Adverse effects are more prevalent with high doses but usually resolve within about 4 months after drug therapy stops.
• Amiodarone I.V. infusions exceeding 2 hours must be administered in glass or polyolefin bottles containing D_5W.

Patient education
• Advise patient to use sunscreen to prevent photosensitivity, which may result in sunburn and blistering.
• Although corneal microdeposits typically appear 1 to 4 months after therapy begins, only 2% to 3% of patients have actual visual disturbances. To minimize this complication, recommend frequent instillation of methylcellulose ophthalmic solution.

Geriatric use
• Use cautiously in elderly patients because ataxia may occur.

Pediatric use
• Children receiving amiodarone concomitantly with digoxin may experience more acute effects of interaction. Children may experience faster onset of action and shorter duration of effect than adults.

Breast-feeding
• Drug is excreted in breast milk and should not be used in breast-feeding women.

amitriptyline hydrochloride
Amitriptyline, Elavil, Endep, Levate*, Novotriptyn*

Pharmacologic classification: tricyclic antidepressant
Therapeutic classification: antidepressant
Pregnancy risk category D

How supplied
Available by prescription only
Tablets: 10 mg, 25 mg, 50 mg, 75 mg, 100 mg, 150 mg
Injection: 10 mg/ml

Indications, route, and dosage
Depression; ◊ anorexia or bulimia associated with depression; ◊ adjunctive treatment of neurogenic pain
Adults: Initial outpatient, 75 to 150 mg/day P.O. in divided doses or 50 to 150 mg h.s.; inpatient, 100 to 300 mg/day. I.M. dose is 20 to 30 mg q.i.d., which should be changed to oral route as soon as possible. Maintenance dose is 50 to 100 mg/day.
✦ ***Dosage adjustment.*** In elderly or adolescent patients, 10 mg P.O. t.i.d. and 20 mg h.s.

Pharmacodynamics
Antidepressant action: Amitriptyline is thought to exert its antidepressant effects by inhibiting reuptake of norepinephrine and serotonin in CNS nerve terminals (presynaptic neurons), resulting in increased concentrations and enhanced activity of these neurotransmitters in the synaptic cleft. Amitriptyline more actively inhibits reuptake of serotonin than norephinephrine; it carries a high incidence of undesirable sedation, but tolerance to this effect usually develops within a few weeks.

Pharmacokinetics
• *Absorption:* Amitriptyline is absorbed rapidly from the GI tract after oral administration and from muscle tissue after I.M. administration.
• *Distribution:* Distributed widely into the body, including the CNS and breast milk; 96% protein-bound. Peak effect occurs 2 to 12 hours after a given dose, and steady state is achieved within 4 to 10 days; full therapeutic effect usually occurs in 2 to 4 weeks.
• *Metabolism:* Drug is metabolized by the liver to the active metabolite nortriptyline; a significant first-pass effect may account for variability of serum concentrations in different patients taking the same dosage.
• *Excretion:* Mostly in urine.

Contraindications and precautions
Contraindicated during acute recovery phase of MI, in patients with hypersensitivity, and in patients who have received an MAO inhibitor within the past 14 days.

Use cautiously in patients with recent history of MI and in those with unstable heart disease or renal or hepatic impairment.

Interactions
Concomitant use of amitriptyline with *sympathomimetics*, including *epinephrine, phenylephrine, phenylpropanolamine*, and *ephedrine* (commonly found in *nasal sprays*) may increase blood pressure; use with *warfarin* may increase PT and cause bleeding.

Concomitant use with *thyroid hormones, pimozide* or *antiarrhythmic agents* (*quinidine, disopyramide, procainamide*) may increase incidence of arrhythmias and conduction defects.

Amitriptyline may decrease hypotensive effects of *centrally acting antihypertensive drugs*, such as *guanethidine, guanabenz, guanadrel, clonidine, methyldopa*, and *reserpine*. Concomitant use with *disulfiram* or *ethchlorvynol* may cause delirium and tachycardia.

Additive effects are likely after concomitant use of amitriptyline with *CNS depressants*, including *alcohol, analgesics, barbiturates, narcotics, tranquilizers*, and *anesthetics* (oversedation); *atropine* or other *anticholinergic drugs*, including *phenothiazines, antihistamines, meperidine*, and *antiparkinsonian agents* (oversedation, paralytic ileus, visual changes, and severe constipation); or *metrizamide* (increased risk of seizures).

Barbiturates and *heavy smoking* induce amitriptyline metabolism and decrease therapeutic efficacy; *phenothiazines* and *haloperidol* decrease its metabolism, decreasing therapeutic efficacy; *methylphenidate, cimetidine, oral contraceptives, propoxyphene, selective serotonin reuptake inhibitors* (for example, *Prozac*), and *beta blockers* may inhibit amitriptyline metabolism, increasing plasma levels and toxicity.

Effects on diagnostic tests

Amitriptyline may prolong conduction time (elongation of QT and PR intervals, flattened T waves on ECG); it also may elevate liver function test results, decrease WBC counts, and decrease or increase serum glucose levels.

Adverse reactions

CNS: ***coma, seizures,*** hallucinations, delusions, disorientation, ataxia, tremor, peripheral neuropathy, anxiety, insomnia, restlessness, drowsiness, dizziness, weakness, fatigue, headache, extrapyramidal reactions.
CV: ***MI, stroke, arrhythmias,*** heart block, *orthostatic hypotension, tachycardia, ECG changes,* hypertension.
EENT: *blurred vision,* tinnitus, mydriasis, increased intraocular pressure.
GI: *dry mouth,* nausea, vomiting, anorexia, epigastric distress, diarrhea, constipation, paralytic ileus.
GU: urine retention.
Hematologic: ***agranulocytosis, thrombocytopenia,*** leukopenia, eosinophilia.
Skin: rash, urticaria, photosensitivity.
Other: *diaphoresis,* hypersensitivity reaction, edema.

After abrupt withdrawal of long-term therapy: nausea, headache, malaise (does not indicate addiction).

Overdose and treatment

The first 12 hours after acute ingestion are a stimulatory phase characterized by excessive anticholinergic activity (agitation, irritation, confusion, hallucinations, hyperthermia, parkinsonian symptoms, seizure, urine retention, dry mucous membranes, pupillary dilation, constipation, and ileus). This is followed by CNS depressant effects, including hypothermia, decreased or absent reflexes, sedation, hypotension, cyanosis, and cardiac irregularities, including tachycardia, conduction disturbances, and quinidine-like effects on the ECG.

Severity of overdose is best indicated by widening of the QRS complex and usually represents a serum level in excess of 1,000 mg/ml; metabolic acidosis may follow hypotension, hypoventilation, and seizures. Delayed cardiac anomalies and death may occur.

Treatment is symptomatic and supportive, including maintaining airway, stable body temperature, and fluid and electrolyte balance. Induce emesis with ipecac if gag reflex is intact; follow with gastric lavage and activated charcoal to prevent further absorption. Dialysis is of little use. Physostigmine may be cautiously used to reverse the symptoms of tricyclic antidepressant poisoning in life-threatening situations. Treatment of seizures may include parenteral diazepam or phenytoin; treatment of arrhythmias, parenteral phenytoin or lidocaine; and treatment of acidosis, sodium bicarbonate. *Do not give barbiturates;* these may enhance CNS and respiratory depressant effects.

☑ Special considerations

Besides those relevant to all *tricyclic antidepressants,* consider the following recommendations.

- Drug also may be used to prevent migraine and cluster headaches, intractable hiccups and postherapeutic neuralgia.
- Amitriptyline causes a high incidence of sedative effects. Tolerance to sedative effects usually develops over several weeks but may never occur.
- The full dose may be given at bedtime to help offset daytime sedation.
- Oral administration route should be substituted for parenteral route as soon as possible.
- I.M. administration may result in a more rapid onset of action than oral administration.
- Do not withdraw drug abruptly.
- Discontinue drug at least 48 hours before surgical procedures.
- Sugarless chewing gum or hard candy or ice may alleviate dry mouth. Stress the importance of regular dental hygiene because dry mouth can increase the incidence of dental caries.
- Depressed patients, particularly those with known manic depressive illness, may experience a shift to mania or hypomania.

Patient education

- Tell patient to take drug exactly as prescribed and not to double dose for missed ones.
- Advise patient that full dose may be taken at bedtime to alleviate daytime sedation. Alternatively, it may be taken in the early evening to avoid morning "hangover."
- Explain that full effects of drug may not become apparent for up to 4 weeks after initiation of therapy.
- Warn patient that drug may cause drowsiness or dizziness. Tell him to avoid hazardous activities that require alertness until full effects of drug are known.
- Warn patient not to drink alcoholic beverages while taking drug.

• Suggest taking drug with food or milk if it causes stomach upset and using sugarless gum or candy to relieve dry mouth.
• After initial doses, advise patient to lie down for about 30 minutes and raise to upright position slowly to prevent dizziness or fainting.
• Warn patient not to stop taking drug suddenly.
• Encourage patient to report troublesome or unusual effects, especially confusion, movement disorders, rapid heartbeat, dizziness, fainting, or difficulty urinating.
• Tell patient to store drug safely away from children.

Geriatric use
• Elderly patients may be at greater risk for adverse cardiac effects.

Pediatric use
• Drug is not recommended for children under age 12.

Breast-feeding
• Drug is excreted in breast milk in concentrations equal to or greater than those in maternal serum. Approximately 1% of the ingested dose appears in the breast-fed infant's serum. The potential benefit to the mother should outweigh the possible adverse reactions in the infant.

amlodipine besylate
Norvasc

Pharmacologic classification: dihydropyridine calcium channel blocker
Therapeutic classification: antianginal, antihypertensive
Pregnancy risk category C

How supplied
Available by prescription only
Tablets: 2.5 mg, 5 mg, 10 mg

Indications, route, and dosage
Chronic stable angina, vasospastic angina (Prinzmetal's or variant angina)
Adults: Initially, 5 to 10 mg P.O. daily.
Hypertension
Adults: Initially, 5 mg P.O. daily. Adjust dosage based on patient response and tolerance. Maximum daily dose, 10 mg.
✦ ***Dosage adjustment.*** In small, frail, or elderly patients, those receiving other antihypertensives, or those with hepatic insufficiency, give 2.5 mg daily.

Pharmacodynamics
Antianginal/antihypertensive action: Contractility of cardiac muscle and vascular smooth muscle depends on movement of extracellular calcium ions into cardiac and smooth-muscle cells through specific ion channels. Amlodipine inhibits the transmembrane influx of calcium ions into vascular smooth muscle and cardiac muscle, thus decreasing myocardial contractility and oxygen demand. As a peripheral arterial vasodilator, the drug acts directly on vascular smooth muscle to reduce peripheral vascular resistance and blood pressure. It also dilates coronary arteries and arterioles.

Pharmacokinetics
• *Absorption:* After oral administration of therapeutic doses of amlodipine, absorption produces peak plasma concentrations between 6 and 12 hours. Absolute bioavailability has been estimated to be between 64% and 90%.
• *Distribution:* Approximately 93% of the circulating drug is bound to plasma proteins in hypertensive patients.
• *Metabolism:* Drug is extensively metabolized in the liver, with about 90% converted to inactive metabolites.
• *Excretion:* Excreted primarily in urine.

Contraindications and precautions
Contraindicated in patients with hypersensitivity to drug. Use cautiously in patients receiving other peripheral dilators and in those with aortic stenosis, heart failure, or severe hepatic disease.

Interactions
None reported.

Effects on diagnostic tests
None reported.

Adverse reactions
CNS: *headache,* somnolence, fatigue, dizziness, light-headedness, paresthesia.
CV: *edema,* flushing, palpitations.
GI: nausea, abdominal pain.
Other: dyspnea, muscle pain, rash, pruritus.

Overdose and treatment
Symptoms of overdose include nausea, weakness, dizziness, drowsiness, confusion, and slurred speech. Overdose also can cause excessive peripheral vasodilation with marked hypotension and bradycardia, both of which may reduce cardiac output. Junctional rhythms and second- or third-degree AV block also can occur. Massive overdose warrants active cardiac and respiratory monitoring and frequent blood pressure measurements. Treatment of hypotension consists of CV support, including elevation of the extremities and judicious administration of fluids. If hypotension remains unresponsive to these conservative measures, administration of vasopressors (such as phenylephrine) should be considered, with attention to circulating volume and urine output. I.V. calcium gluconate may help reverse the effects of calcium entry blockade. Because amlodipine is highly protein-bound, hemodialysis is not likely to benefit the patient.

☑ Special considerations
• Some patients, especially those with severe obstructive coronary artery disease, have developed increased frequency, duration, or severity of angina or even acute MI after initiation of calcium channel blocker therapy or at time of dosage increase. Monitor patient carefully.

• Because the vasodilation induced by amlodipine is gradual in onset, acute hypotension has rarely been reported after oral administration of amlodipine. However, caution should be exercised when administering drug, particularly in patients with severe aortic stenosis.

Patient education
• Tell patient to take nitroglycerin S.L. as needed for acute anginal symptoms. If patient continues nitrate therapy during titration of amlodipine dosage, urge continued compliance.
• Caution patient to continue taking amlodipine even when feeling better.
• Tell patient to notify primary health care provider about signs of heart failure, such as swelling of hands and feet or shortness of breath.

Geriatric use
• Elderly patients may require a smaller dosage of amlodipine.

Pediatric use
• Safety and effectiveness in children have not been established.

Breast-feeding
• Because it is not known whether amlodipine is excreted in human milk, breast-feeding is not recommended during amlodipine therapy.

amobarbital

amobarbital sodium
Amytal

Pharmacologic classification: barbiturate
Therapeutic classification: sedative-hypnotic, anticonvulsant
Controlled substance schedule II
Pregnancy risk category D

How supplied
Available by prescription only
Tablets: 30 mg, 50 mg, 100 mg
Capsules: 65 mg, 200 mg
Powder for injection: 250-mg, 500-mg vials
Powder (bulk): 15 g, 30 g

Indications, route, and dosage
Sedation
Adults: Usually 30 to 50 mg P.O. b.i.d. or t.i.d. but may range from 15 to 120 mg b.i.d. to q.i.d.
Children: 2 mg/kg P.O. daily divided into four equal doses.
Insomnia
Adults: 65 to 200 mg P.O. or deep I.M. h.s.; I.M. injection not to exceed 5 ml in any one site. Maximum dosage, 500 mg.
Children over age 6: 2 to 3 mg/kg deep I.M. h.s.
Preanesthetic sedation
Adults: 200 mg P.O. 1 to 2 hours before surgery.
Labor
Adults: 200 to 400 mg P.O.; may repeat at 1- to 3-hour intervals. Maximum dose, 1 g.
Anticonvulsant
Adults: 65 to 500 mg by slow I.V. injection (rate not exceeding 100 mg/minute). Maximum dose, 1 g.

Pharmacodynamics
Anticonvulsant action: The exact cellular site and mechanism(s) of action are unknown. Parenteral amobarbital suppresses the spread of seizure activity produced by epileptogenic foci in the cortex, thalamus, and limbic systems by enhancing the effect of gamma-aminobutyric acid (GABA). Both presynaptic and postsynaptic excitability are decreased.

Sedative-hypnotic action: Drug acts throughout the CNS as a nonselective depressant with an intermediate onset and duration of action. Particularly sensitive to this drug is the mesencephalic reticular activating system, which controls CNS arousal. Amobarbital decreases both presynaptic and postsynaptic membrane excitability by facilitating the action of GABA.

Pharmacokinetics
• *Absorption:* Amobarbital is absorbed well after oral administration. Absorption after I.M. administration is 100%. Onset of action is 45 to 60 minutes.
• *Distribution:* Drug is distributed well throughout body tissues and fluids.
• *Metabolism:* Amobarbital is metabolized in the liver by oxidation to a tertiary alcohol.
• *Excretion:* Less than 1% of a dose is excreted unchanged in the urine; rest is excreted as metabolites. The half-life is biphasic, with a first phase half-life of about 40 minutes and a second phase of about 20 hours. Duration of action is 6 to 8 hours.

Contraindications and precautions
Contraindicated in patients with bronchopneumonia or other severe pulmonary insufficiency or hypersensitivity to barbiturates, or porphyria.

Use cautiously in patients with suicidal tendencies, acute or chronic pain, history of drug abuse, hepatic or renal impairment, or pulmonary or CV disease.

Interactions
Amobarbital may add to or potentiate CNS and respiratory depressant effects of other *sedative-hypnotics, antihistamines, narcotics, antidepressants, MAO inhibitors, tranquilizers*, and *alcohol.*

Amobarbital enhances the enzymatic degradation of *warfarin* and other *oral anticoagulants*; patients may require increased doses of the *anticoagulants.* Amobarbital also enhances hepatic metabolism of *digitoxin* (not *digoxin*), *corticosteroids, theophylline* and other *xanthines, oral contraceptives* and other *estrogens*, and *doxycycline.*

Amobarbital impairs the effectiveness of *griseofulvin* by decreasing absorption from the GI tract. Amobarbital may cause unpredictable fluctuations in serum *phenytoin* levels.

Valproic acid, MAO inhibitors, and *disulfiram* decrease the metabolism of amobarbital and can increase its toxicity.

Rifampin may decrease amobarbital levels by increasing metabolism.

Effects on diagnostic tests

Amobarbital may cause a false-positive phentolamine test. The physiologic effects of amobarbital may impair absorption of cyanocobalamin ^{57}Co; it may decrease serum bilirubin concentrations in neonates, epileptic patients, and patients with congenital nonhemolytic unconjugated hyperbilirubinemia. EEG patterns are altered, with a change in low-voltage, fast-activity; changes persist for a time after discontinuation of therapy.

Adverse reactions

CNS: *drowsiness, lethargy, hangover,* paradoxical excitement, somnolence.
CV: bradycardia, hypotension, syncope.
GI: nausea, vomiting.
Hematologic: exacerbation of porphyria.
Respiratory: ***respiratory depression, apnea.***
Skin: rash; urticaria; ***Stevens-Johnson syndrome;*** pain, irritation, sterile abscess at injection site.
Other: ***angioedema,*** physical and psychological dependence.

Overdose and treatment

Clinical manifestations of overdose include unsteady gait, slurred speech, sustained nystagmus, somnolence, confusion, respiratory depression, pulmonary edema, areflexia, and coma. Oliguria, jaundice, hypothermia, fever, and shock with tachycardia and hypotension may occur.

Maintain and support ventilation as necessary; support circulation with vasopressors and I.V. fluids as needed.

Treatment is aimed to maintain and support ventilation and pulmonary function as necessary; support cardiac function and circulation with vasopressors and I.V. fluids as needed. If patient is conscious with a functioning gag reflex and ingestion has been recent, then induce emesis by administering ipecac syrup. Gastric lavage may be performed if a cuffed endotracheal tube is in place to prevent aspiration when emesis is inappropriate. Follow with administration of activated charcoal or sodium chloride cathartic. Measure fluid intake and output, vital signs, and laboratory parameters. Maintain body temperature.

Alkalinization of urine may be helpful in removing amobarbital from the body; hemodialysis may be useful in severe overdose.

☑ Special considerations

Besides those relevant to all *barbiturates,* consider the following recommendations.

- Not commonly used as a sedative or aid to sleeping; barbiturates have been replaced by safer benzodiapines for such use.
- Administer drug orally before meals or on an empty stomach to enhance rate of absorption.
- Reconstitute powder for injection with sterile water for injection. Roll vial in hands; do not shake. Use 2.5 or 5 ml (for 250 or 500 mg of amobarbital) to make 10% solution. For I.M. use, prepare 20% solution by using 1.25 or 2.5 ml of sterile water for injection.
- Administer reconstituted parenteral solution within 30 minutes after opening the vial.
- Do not administer amobarbital solution that is cloudy or forms a precipitate after 5 minutes of reconstitution.
- Administer I.V. dose at a rate no greater than 100 mg/minute in adults or 60 mg/m^2/minute in children to prevent possible hypotension and respiratory depression. Have emergency resuscitative equipment available.
- Administer I.M. dose deep into large muscle mass, giving no more than 5 ml in any one injection site. Sterile abscess or tissue damage may result from inadvertent superficial I.M. or S.C. injection.
- Administering full loading doses over short periods of time to treat status epilepticus may require ventilatory support in adults.
- Assess cardiopulmonary status frequently for possible alterations. Monitor blood counts for potential adverse reactions.
- Assess renal and hepatic laboratory studies to ensure adequate drug removal.
- Monitor PT carefully when patient on amobarbital starts or ends anticoagulant therapy. Anticoagulant dosage may need to be adjusted.

Patient education

- Warn patient of possible physical or psychological dependence with prolonged use.
- Tell patient to avoid alcohol while taking drug.

Geriatric use

- Elderly patients usually require lower doses. Confusion, disorientation, and excitability may occur in elderly patients. Use with caution.

Pediatric use

- Safe use in children under age 6 has not been established. Use of amobarbital may cause paradoxical excitement in some children.

Breast-feeding

- Amobarbital passes into breast milk and may cause drowsiness in the infant. If so, dosage adjustment or discontinuation of drug or of breast-feeding may be necessary. Use with caution.

amoxapine

Asendin

Pharmacologic classification: dibenzoxazepine, tricyclic antidepressant
Therapeutic classification: antidepressant
Pregnancy risk category C

How supplied

Available by prescription only
Tablets: 25 mg, 50 mg, 100 mg, 150 mg

Indications, route, and dosage

Depression
Adults: Initial dosage is 50 mg P.O. b.i.d. or t.i.d; may increase to 100 mg b.i.d. or t.i.d. by end of first week. Increases above 300 mg daily should be made only if this dosage has been ineffective during a trial period of at least 2 weeks. When effec-

tive dosage is established, entire dosage (not exceeding 300 mg) may be given h.s. Maximum dosage in hospitalized patients, 600 mg.

Note: Do not give more than 300 mg in a single dose.

✦ ***Dosage adjustment.*** In elderly patients, recommended starting dose is 25 mg t.i.d.

Pharmacodynamics

Antidepressant action: Drug is thought to exert its antidepressant effects by inhibiting reuptake of norepinephrine and serotonin in CNS nerve terminals (presynaptic neurons), which results in increased concentrations and enhanced activity of these neurotransmitters in the synaptic cleft. Amoxapine has a greater inhibitory effect on norepinephrine reuptake than on serotonin. Drug also blocks CNS dopamine receptors, which may account for the higher incidence of movement disorders during therapy.

Pharmacokinetics

- *Absorption:* Amoxapine is absorbed rapidly and completely from the GI tract after oral administration.
- *Distribution:* Amoxapine is distributed widely into the body, including the CNS and breast milk. Drug is 92% protein-bound. Peak effect occurs in 8 to 10 hours; steady state, within 2 to 7 days. Proposed therapeutic plasma levels (parent drug and metabolite) range from 200 to 500 ng/ml.
- *Metabolism:* Drug is metabolized by the liver to the active metabolite 8-hydroxyamoxapine; a significant first-pass effect may explain variability of serum concentrations in different patients taking the same dosage.
- *Excretion:* Amoxapine is excreted in urine and feces (7% to 18%); about 60% of a given dose is excreted as the conjugated form within 6 days.

Contraindications and precautions

Contraindicated in patients with hypersensitivity, during acute recovery phase of MI, and in those who have received a MAO inhibitor within the past 14 days.

Use cautiously in patients with history of urine retention, CV disease, angle-closure glaucoma, or increased intraocular pressure. Also, use with extreme caution in patients with a history of seizures.

Interactions

Concomitant use of amoxapine with *sympathomimetics*, including *epinephrine, phenylephrine, phenylpropanolamine*, and *ephedrine* (commonly found in *nasal sprays*) may increase blood pressure; use with *warfarin* may increase PT and cause bleeding.

Concomitant use with *thyroid medication, pimozide*, and *antiarrhythmic agents* (*quinidine, disopyramide, procainamide*) may increase the incidence of arrhythmias and conduction defects.

Amoxapine may decrease hypotensive effects of *centrally acting antihypertensive drugs* such as *guanethidine, guanabenz, guanadrel, clonidine, methyldopa*, and *reserpine*.

Concomitant use with *disulfiram* or *ethchlorvynol* may cause delirium and tachycardia.

Additive effects are likely after concomitant use of amoxapine with *CNS depressants*, including *alcohol, analgesics, barbiturates, narcotics, tranquilizers*, and *anesthetics* (oversedation); *atropine* or other *anticholinergic drugs*, including *phenothiazines, antihistamines, meperidine*, and *antiparkinsonian agents* (oversedation, paralytic ileus, visual changes, and severe constipation); or *metrizamide* (increased risk of seizures).

Barbiturates and *heavy smoking* induce amoxapine metabolism and decrease therapeutic efficacy; *phenothiazines* and *haloperidol* decrease its metabolism, decreasing therapeutic efficacy. *Methylphenidate, cimetidine, oral contraceptives, propoxyphene,* and *beta blockers* may inhibit amoxapine metabolism, increasing plasma levels and toxicity.

Effects on diagnostic tests

Amoxapine may prolong conduction time (elongation of QT and PR intervals, flattened T waves on ECG); it also may elevate liver function test results, decrease WBC counts, and decrease or increase serum glucose levels.

Adverse reactions

CNS: *drowsiness, dizziness,* excitation, tremor, weakness, confusion, anxiety, insomnia, restlessness, nightmares, ataxia, fatigue, headache, nervousness, *tardive dyskinesia, EEG changes,* ***seizures,*** extrapyramidal reactions (rare), ***neuroleptic malignant syndrome*** (high fever, tachycardia, tachypnea, profuse diaphoresis).
CV: *orthostatic hypotension, tachycardia,* hypertension, palpitations.
EENT: *blurred vision.*
GI: *dry mouth, constipation,* nausea, excessive appetite.
GU: *urine retention, acute renal failure* (with overdose).
Skin: rash, edema.
Other: *diaphoresis.*

After abrupt withdrawal of long-term therapy: nausea, headache, malaise (does not indicate addiction).

Overdose and treatment

The first 12 hours after acute ingestion are a stimulatory phase characterized by excessive anticholinergic activity (agitation, irritation, confusion, hallucinations, hyperthermia, parkinsonian symptoms, seizures, urine retention, dry mucous membranes, pupillary dilation, constipation, and ileus). This is followed by CNS depressant effects, including hypothermia, decreased or absent reflexes, sedation, hypotension, cyanosis, and cardiac irregularities, including tachycardia, conduction disturbances, and quinidine-like effects on the ECG.

Overdose with amoxapine produces a much higher incidence of CNS toxicity than do other antidepressants. Acute deterioration of renal function (evidenced by myoglobin in urine) occurs in 5% of overdosed patients; this is most likely to occur in patients with repeated seizures after the overdose.

Seizures may progress to status epilepticus within 12 hours.

Severity of overdose is best indicated by widening of the QRS complex, which generally represents a serum level in excess of 1,000 ng/ml; serum concentrations are not usually helpful. Metabolic acidosis may follow hypotension, hypoventilation, and seizures.

Treatment is symptomatic and supportive, including maintaining airway, stable body temperature, and fluid and electrolyte balance; monitor renal status because of the risk of renal failure. Induce emesis with ipecac if patient is conscious; follow with gastric lavage and activated charcoal to prevent further absorption. Dialysis is of little use. Treat seizures with parenteral diazepam or phenytoin (the value of physostigmine is less certain); arrhythmias, with parenteral phenytoin or lidocaine; and acidosis, with sodium bicarbonate. *Do not give barbiturates;* these may enhance CNS and respiratory depressant effects.

☑ Special considerations

Besides those relevant to all *tricyclic antidepressants,* consider the following recommendations.

- Amoxapine is associated with a high incidence of seizures.
- Antidepressants can cause manic episodes during the depressed phase in patients with bipolar disorder.
- The full dose may be given at bedtime to help reduce daytime sedation.
- The full dose should not be withdrawn abruptly.
- Tolerance to sedative effects usually develops over the first few weeks of therapy.
- Drug should be discontinued at least 48 hours before surgical procedures.
- Sugarless chewing gum or hard candy or ice may alleviate dry mouth.
- Tardive dyskinesia and other extrapyramidal effects may occur because of the dopamine-blocking activity of amoxapine. Elderly patients appear to be more susceptible to these effects.
- Watch for gynecomastia in males and females because amoxapine may increase cellular division in breast tissue.

Patient education

- Explain that full effects of drug may not become apparent for at least 2 weeks or more after therapy begins, perhaps not for 4 to 6 weeks.
- Tell patient to take drug exactly as prescribed; however, full dose may be taken at bedtime to alleviate daytime sedation. Patient should not double dose for missed ones.
- Warn patient that because drug may cause drowsiness or dizziness, hazardous activities that require alertness should be avoided until drug's full effects are known.
- Tell patient not to drink alcoholic beverages while taking drug.
- Suggest that patient takes drug with food or milk if it causes stomach upset; dry mouth can be relieved with sugarless gum or hard candy.
- After initial doses, tell patient to lie down for about 30 minutes and rise slowly to prevent dizziness.
- Warn patient not to discontinue drug suddenly.
- Encourage patient to report unusual or troublesome reactions immediately, especially confusion, movement disorders, rapid heartbeat, dizziness, fainting, or difficulty urinating.
- Warn patient of risks of tardive dyskinesia and explain its symptoms.
- Inform patient that exposure to sunlight, sunlamps, or tanning beds may cause burning of the skin or abnormal pigmentary changes.
- Tell patient to store drug safely away from children.

Geriatric use

- Lower doses are indicated because older patients are more sensitive to the therapeutic and adverse effects of drug.
- Elderly patients are much more susceptible to tardive dyskinesia and extrapyramidal symptoms.

Pediatric use

- Drug is not recommended for patients under age 16.

Breast-feeding

- Amoxapine is excreted in breast milk in concentrations of 20% of maternal serum as parent drug and 30% as metabolites. The potential benefits to the mother should outweigh the possible adverse reactions in the infant.

---

amoxicillin/clavulanate potassium

Augmentin, Clavulin*

Pharmacologic classification: aminopenicillin and beta-lactamase inhibitor
Therapeutic classification: antibiotic
Pregnancy risk category B

How supplied

Available by prescription only
Tablets (chewable): 125 mg amoxicillin trihydrate, 31.25 mg clavulanic acid; 200 mg amoxicillin trihydrate, 31.25 mg clavulanic acid; 250 mg amoxicillin trihydrate, 62.5 mg clavulanic acid; 400 mg amoxicillin trihydrate, 62.5 mg clavulanic acid
Tablets (film-coated): 250 mg amoxicillin trihydrate, 125 mg clavulanic acid; 500 mg amoxicillin trihydrate, 125 mg clavulanic acid; 875 mg amoxicillin trihydrate, 125 mg clavulanic acid
Oral suspension: 125 mg amoxicillin trihydrate and 31.25 mg clavulanic acid/5 ml (after reconstitution)
Suspension: 200 mg amoxicillin trihydrate and 28.5 mg clavulanic acid/5 ml (after reconstitution); 250 mg amoxicillin trihydrate and 62.5 mg clavulanic acid/5 ml (after reconstitution); 400 mg amoxicillin trihydrate and 57 mg clavulanic acid/5 ml (after reconstitution)

Indications, route, and dosage

Lower respiratory infections, otitis media, sinusitis, skin and skin structure infections, and

urinary tract infections caused by susceptible organisms
Adults and children weighing over 88 lb (40 kg): 250 mg (based on amoxicillin component) P.O. q 8 hours or one 500-mg tablet q 12 hours. For more severe infections, 500 mg q 8 hours or 875 mg q 12 hours.
Children weighing under 88 lb: 20 to 40 mg/kg/day P.O. (based on amoxicillin component) given in divided doses q 8 hours.

Pharmacodynamics
Antibiotic action: Amoxicillin is bactericidal; it adheres to bacterial penicillin-binding proteins, thus inhibiting bacterial cell wall synthesis.

Clavulanate has only weak antibacterial activity and does not affect mechanism of action of amoxicillin. However, clavulanic acid has a beta-lactam ring and is structurally similar to penicillin and cephalosporins; it binds irreversibly with certain beta-lactamases and prevents them from inactivating amoxicillin, enhancing its bactericidal activity.

This combination acts against penicillinase- and non-penicillinase-producing gram-positive bacteria, *Neisseria gonorrhoeae, N. meningitidis, Haemophilus influenzae, Escherichia coli, Proteus mirabilis, Citrobacter diversus, Klebsiella pneumoniae, P. vulgaris, Salmonella,* and *Shigella.*

Pharmacokinetics
- *Absorption:* Amoxicillin and clavulanate potassium are well absorbed after oral administration; peak serum levels occur at 1 to 2½ hours.
- *Distribution:* Both amoxicillin and clavulanate potassium distribute into pleural fluid, lungs, and peritoneal fluid; high urine concentrations are attained. Amoxicillin also distributes into synovial fluid, liver, prostate, muscle, and gallbladder; and penetrates into middle ear effusions, maxillary sinus secretions, tonsils, sputum, and bronchial secretions. Amoxicillin and clavulanate cross the placenta and low concentrations occur in breast milk. Amoxicillin and clavulanate potassium have minimal protein-binding of 17% to 20% and 22% to 30%, respectively.
- *Metabolism:* Amoxicillin is metabolized only partially. The metabolic fate of clavulanate potassium is not completely identified, but it appears to undergo extensive metabolism.
- *Excretion:* Amoxicillin is excreted principally in urine by renal tubular secretion and glomerular filtration; drug is also excreted in breast milk.

Clavulanate potassium is excreted by glomerular filtration. Elimination half-life of amoxicillin in adults is 1 to 1½ hours; it is prolonged to 7½ hours in patients with severe renal impairment. Half-life of clavulanate in adults is about 1 to 1½ hours, prolonged to 4½ hours in patients with severe renal impairment.

Both drugs are removed readily by hemodialysis and minimally removed by peritoneal dialysis.

Contraindications and precautions
Contraindicated in patients with hypersensitivity to drug or other penicillins and in those with a previous history of amoxicillin-associated cholestatic jaundice or hepatic dysfunction. An oral penicillin should not be used in patients with severe pneumonia, empyema, bacteremia, pericarditis, meningitis, and purulent or septic arthritis. Use with caution in patients with mononucleosis.

Interactions
Concomitant use with *allopurinol* appears to increase incidence of rash from both drugs.

Probenecid blocks tubular secretion of amoxicillin, raising its serum concentrations; it has no effect on clavulanate.

Large doses of penicillins may interfere with renal tubular secretion of *methotrexate,* thus delaying elimination and prolonging elevated serum concentrations of methotrexate.

The effectiveness of *oral contraceptives* may be reduced.

Effects on diagnostic tests
Amoxicillin/potassium clavulanate alters results of urine glucose tests that use cupric sulfate (Benedict's reagent or Clinitest). Make urine glucose determinations with glucose oxidase methods (Chemstrip uG or Diastix or glucose enzymatic test strip). Positive Coombs' tests have been reported with other clavulanate combinations. Amoxicillin/potassium clavulanate may produce a positive direct antiglobulin test (DAT).

Adverse reactions
CNS: agitation, anxiety, insomnia, confusion, behavioral changes, dizziness.
GI: *nausea,* vomiting, *diarrhea,* indigestion, gastritis, stomatitis, glossitis, black "hairy" tongue, enterocolitis, pseudomembranous colitis.
Hematologic: anemia, ***thrombocytopenia,*** thrombocytopenic purpura, eosinophilia, leukopenia, ***agranulocytosis.***
Other: hypersensitivity reactions (erythematous maculopapular rash, urticaria, ***anaphylaxis***), overgrowth of nonsusceptible organisms, vaginitis.

Overdose and treatment
Clinical signs of overdose include neuromuscular sensitivity or seizures. After recent ingestion (4 hours or less), empty the stomach by induced emesis or gastric lavage; follow with activated charcoal to reduce absorption. Amoxicillin/clavulanate potassium can be removed by hemodialysis.

☑ Special considerations
Besides those relevant to all *penicillins,* consider the following recommendations.
- Oral dosage is maximally absorbed from an empty stomach, but food does not cause significant impairment of absorption.
- Suspension is stable for 7 days at room temperature and 14 days in refrigerator after reconstitution.
- When using film-coated tablets, be aware that both dosages contain different amounts of amoxicillin, but the *same amount* of clavulanate; therefore two "250-mg" tablets are not the equivalent of one "500-mg" tablet.

• Because ampicillin/clavulanate potassium is dialyzable, patients undergoing hemodialysis may need dosage adjustments.

Patient education
• Tell patient to chew chewable tablets thoroughly or crush before swallowing and wash down with liquid to ensure adequate absorption of drug; capsule may be emptied and contents swallowed with water.
• Instruct patient to report diarrhea promptly.
• Inform patient to complete full course of medication.

Geriatric use
• In elderly patients, diminished renal tubular secretion may prolong half-life of amoxicillin.

Breast-feeding
• Both amoxicillin and potassium clavulanate are excreted in breast milk; drug should be used with caution in breast-feeding women.

amoxicillin trihydrate
Amoxil, Polymox, Trimox, Wymox

Pharmacologic classification: aminopenicillin
Therapeutic classification: antibiotic
Pregnancy risk category NR

How supplied
Available by prescription only
Tablets (chewable): 125 mg, 250 mg
Capsules: 250 mg, 500 mg
Suspension: 125 mg/5 ml, 250 mg/5 ml, 50 mg/ml (after reconstitution, pediatric drops)

Indications, route, and dosage
Systemic infections, acute and chronic urinary or respiratory tract infections caused by susceptible organisms, uncomplicated urinary tract infections caused by susceptible organisms
Adults: 250 mg P.O. q 8 hours. In adults and children weighing over 44 lb (20 kg) who have severe infections or those caused by susceptible organisms, 500 mg q 8 hours may be needed.
Children: 20 to 40 mg/kg P.O. daily, divided into doses given q 8 hours.

Pediatric drops: children under 13 lb (6 kg), 0.75 ml q 8 hours; 13 to 15 lb (6 to 7 kg), 1 ml q 8 hours; 16 to18 lb (7 to 8 kg), 1.25 ml q 8 hours.

Pediatric drops: children with lower respiratory tract infection only weighing under 13 lb, 1.25 ml q 8 hours; 13 to 15 lb, 1.75 ml q 8 hours; 16 to18 lb, 2.25 ml q 8 hours.

Uncomplicated gonorrhea
Adults: 3 g P.O. as a single dose.
Children over age 2: 50 mg/kg given with 25 mg/kg probenecid as a single dose.

✦ **Dosage adjustment.** In renal failure, patients who require repeated doses may need adjustment of dosing interval. If creatinine clearance is 10 to 50 ml/minute, increase interval to q 6 to 12 hours; if creatinine clearance is less than 10 ml/minute, administer q 12 to 16 hours. Supplemental doses may be necessary after hemodialysis.

Oral prophylaxis of bacterial endocarditis
Consult current American Heart Association recommendations before administering drug.
Adults: 3 g 1 hour before procedure and 1.5 g 6 hours later.
Children: 50 mg/kg 1 hour before procedure and 25 mg/kg 6 hours later. Do not exceed adult dosage.

Pharmacodynamics
Antibacterial action: Amoxicillin is bactericidal; it adheres to bacterial penicillin-binding proteins, thus inhibiting bacterial cell wall synthesis.

Spectrum of action of amoxicillin includes non-penicillinase–producing gram-positive bacteria, *Streptococcus* group B, *Neisseria gonorrheae, Proteus mirabilis, Salmonella,* and *Haemophilus influenzae.* It is also effective against non-penicillinase-producing *Staphylococcus aureus, S. pyogenes, Streptococcus bovis, S. pneumoniae, S. viridans, N. meningitidis, Escherichia coli, Salmonella typhi, Bordetella pertussis, Peptococcus,* and *Peptostreptococcus.*

Pharmacokinetics
• *Absorption:* Amoxicillin is approximately 80% absorbed after oral administration; peak serum concentrations occur at 1 to 2½ hours after an oral dose.
• *Distribution:* Drug distributes into pleural peritoneal and synovial fluids and into the lungs, prostate, muscle, liver, and gallbladder; it also penetrates middle ear, maxillary sinus and bronchial secretions, tonsils, and sputum. Amoxicillin readily crosses the placenta; about 17% to 20% is protein-bound.
• *Metabolism:* Amoxicillin is metabolized only partially.
• *Excretion:* Excreted principally in urine by renal tubular secretion and glomerular filtration; also excreted in breast milk. Elimination half-life in adults is 1 to 1½ hours; severe renal impairment increases half-life to 7½ hours.

Contraindications and precautions
Contraindicated in patients with hypersensitivity to drug or other penicillins. Use with caution in patients with mononucleosis.

Interactions
Concomitant use with *allopurinol* appears to increase the incidence of rash from both drugs.

Concomitant use with *clavulanate potassium* enhances effect of amoxicillin against certain beta-lactamase-producing bacteria.

Probenecid blocks renal tubular secretion of amoxicillin, raising its serum concentrations.

Large doses of penicillins may interfere with renal tubular secretion of *methotrexate,* thus delaying elimination and prolonging elevated serum concentrations of methotrexate.

The effectiveness of *oral contraceptives* may be decreased.

Effects on diagnostic tests
Amoxicillin may alter results of urine glucose tests that use cupric sulfate (Benedict's reagent or Clinitest). Make urine glucose determinations with glucose oxidase methods (Chemstrip uG, Diastix, or glucose enzymatic test strip).

Amoxicillin may falsely decrease serum aminoglycoside concentrations.

Adverse reactions
CNS: lethargy, hallucinations, ***seizures,*** anxiety, confusion, agitation, depression, dizziness, fatigue.
GI: *nausea,* vomiting, *diarrhea,* glossitis, stomatitis, gastritis, abdominal pain, enterocolitis, pseudomembranous colitis, black "hairy" tongue.
GU: interstitial nephritis, nephropathy.
Hematologic: anemia, *thrombocytopenia,* thrombocytopenic purpura, eosinophilia, leukopenia, hemolytic anemia, ***agranulocytosis.***
Other: hypersensitivity reactions (erythematous maculopapular rash, urticaria, ***anaphylaxis***), overgrowth of nonsusceptible organisms, vaginitis.

Overdose and treatment
Clinical signs of overdose include neuromuscular sensitivity or seizures. After recent ingestion (4 hours or less), empty the stomach by induced emesis or gastric lavage; follow with activated charcoal to reduce absorption. Drug can be removed by hemodialysis.

☑ Special considerations
Besides those relevant to all *penicillins,* consider the following recommendations.
- Oral dosage is maximally absorbed from an empty stomach, but food does not cause significant loss of potency.
- Pediatric drops may be placed on child's tongue or added to formula, milk, fruit juice, or soft drink. Be sure child ingests all of prepared dose.
- Suspension and drops are stable for 7 days at room temperature and 14 days in refrigerator after reconstitution.
- Amoxicillin may cause less diarrhea than ampicillin.

Patient education
- Tell patient to chew tablets thoroughly or crush before swallowing and wash down with liquid to ensure adequate absorption of drug; capsule may be emptied and contents swallowed with water.
- Tell patient to report diarrhea promptly.
- Instruct patient to complete full course of medication.

Geriatric use
- Because of diminished renal tubular secretion, half-life may be prolonged in elderly patients.

Breast-feeding
- Drug is distributed readily into breast milk; safe use in breast-feeding women has not been established. Alternative feeding method is recommended during therapy.

amphetamine sulfate

Pharmacologic classification: amphetamine
Therapeutic classification: CNS stimulant, short-term adjunctive anorexigenic agent, sympathomimetic amine
Controlled substance schedule II
Pregnancy risk category C

How supplied
Available by prescription only
Tablets: 5 mg, 10 mg
Capsules: 6.25 mg, 10 mg

Indications, route, and dosage
Attention deficit disorder with hyperactivity
Children age 6 and older: 5 mg P.O. daily. Increase at 5-mg increments weekly until desired response. Dosage rarely exceeds 40 mg/day. Give first dose upon awakening, and additional doses at 4- to 6-hour intervals.
Children age 3 to 5: 2.5 mg P.O. daily, increase at 2.5-mg increments weekly until desired response is achieved.
Narcolepsy
Adults: 5 to 60 mg P.O. daily in divided doses or a single dose.
Children over age 12: 10 mg P.O. daily, with 10-mg increments weekly, p.r.n.
Children age 6 to 12: 5 mg P.O. daily, with 5-mg increments weekly, p.r.n.
Short-term adjunct in exogenous obesity
Adults: 5 to 30 mg daily in divided doses of 5 to 10 mg.

Pharmacodynamics
CNS stimulant action: Amphetamines are sympathomimetic amines with CNS stimulant activity; in hyperactive children, they have a paradoxical calming effect.

Amphetamines are used to treat narcolepsy and as adjuncts to psychosocial measures in attention deficit disorder in children. The cerebral cortex and reticular activating system appear to be their primary sites of activity; amphetamines release nerve terminal stores of norepinephrine, promoting nerve impulse transmission. At high dosages, effects are mediated by dopamine.

Anorexigenic action: Anorexigenic effects are thought to occur in the hypothalamus, where decreased smell and taste acuity decreases the appetite. They may be tried for short-term control of refractory obesity, with caloric restriction and behavior modification.

Pharmacokinetics
- *Absorption:* Drug is absorbed completely within 3 hours after oral administration; therapeutic effects persist for 4 to 24 hours.
- *Distribution:* Distributed widely throughout body, with high concentrations in the brain. Therapeutic plasma levels are 5 to 10 mcg/dl.
- *Metabolism:* Metabolized by hydroxylation and deamination in the liver.

• *Excretion:* Drug is excreted in urine.

Contraindications and precautions

Contraindicated in patients with hypersensitivity or idiosyncrasy to the sympathomimetic amines, symptomatic CV disease, hyperthyroidism, moderate to severe hypertension, glaucoma, advanced arteriosclerosis, or history of drug abuse; within 14 days of MAO inhibitor therapy; and in agitated patients.

Use cautiously in elderly, debilitated, or hyperexcitable patients or in those with suicidal or homicidal tendencies.

Interactions

Concomitant use with *MAO inhibitors* (or *drugs with MAO-inhibiting effects* such as *furazolidone*) or within 14 days of such therapy may cause hypertensive crisis; concomitant use with *antihypertensives* may antagonize their hypertensive effects.

Concomitant use with *antacids, sodium bicarbonate,* or *acetazolamide* may enhance reabsorption of amphetamine and prolong its duration of action, whereas concomitant use with *ammonium chloride* or *ascorbic acid* enhances amphetamine excretion or shortens duration of action.

Use with *phenothiazines* or *haloperidol* decreases amphetamine effects; *barbiturates* counteract amphetamine by CNS depression, whereas *caffeine* or other CNS stimulants produce additive effects.

Amphetamines may alter *insulin* requirements, and may decrease the effectiveness of *guanethidine.*

Effects on diagnostic tests

Amphetamines may elevate plasma corticosteroid levels and also may interfere with urinary steroid determinations.

Adverse reactions

CNS: *restlessness,* tremor, *hyperactivity, talkativeness, insomnia,* irritability, dizziness, headache, chills, dysphoria, euphoria.
CV: *tachycardia, palpitations,* hypertension, ***arrhythmias.***
GI: dry mouth, metallic taste, diarrhea, constipation, anorexia, weight loss.
GU: impotence.
Skin: urticaria.
Other: altered libido.

Overdose and treatment

Symptoms of acute overdose include increasing restlessness, irritability, insomnia, tremor, hyperreflexia, diaphoresis, mydriasis, flushing, confusion, hypertension, tachypnea, fever, delirium, self-injury, arrhythmias, seizures, coma, circulatory collapse, and death.

Treat overdose symptomatically and supportively: If ingestion is recent (within 4 hours) use gastric lavage or emesis; activated charcoal, sodium chloride catharsis, and urinary acidification may enhance excretion. Forced fluid diuresis may help.

In massive ingestion, hemodialysis or peritoneal dialysis may be necessary. Keep patient in a cool room, monitor patient's temperature, and minimize external stimulation. Haloperidol may be used for psychotic symptoms; diazepam, for hyperactivity.

☑ Special considerations

• Avoid administration late in the day (after 4 p.m.) to prevent insomnia.
• Amphetamine capsules should not be used for initial or subsequent titration of dosage; however, once dosage has been established, capsules can be substituted if once-daily dosing is required.

Patient education

• Instruct patient about the potential for drowsiness and to avoid activities such as driving that require alertness.

Pediatric use

• Amphetamines are not recommended for weight reduction in children under age 12; use of amphetamines for hyperactivity is contraindicated in children under age 3. A pediatric elixir is available; temporary suppression of normal growth has followed its long-term use; such use must be monitored carefully.

---

amphotericin B

Abelcet (liposomal amphotericin B), AmBisome, Amphotec, Fungizone

Pharmacologic classification: polyene macrolide
Therapeutic classification: antifungal
Pregnancy risk category B

How supplied

Available by prescription only
Injection: 50-mg lyophilized cake
Oral suspension: 100 mg/ml
Suspension for injection: 5 mg/ml
Cream: 3%
Lotion: 3%
Ointment: 3%

Indications, route, and dosage

Systemic (potentially fatal) fungal infections, caused by susceptible organisms; ◊ fungal endocarditis; fungal septicemia

Adults and children: Some clinicians recommend an initial dose of 1 mg I.V. in 20 ml D_5W infused over 20 minutes. If test dose is tolerated, then give daily doses of 0.25 to 0.30 mg/kg, gradually increasing by 5 to 10 mg/day until daily dose is 1 mg/kg/day or 1.5 mg/kg q alternate day. Duration of therapy is dependent upon the severity and nature of infection.

Liposomal amphotericin B: 5 mg/kg given as a single infusion, administered at a rate of 2.5 mg/kg/hour. If infusion lasts longer than 2 hours, mix bag q 2 hours.

Sporotrichosis: 0.4 to 0.5 mg/kg amphotericin B daily I.V. for up to 9 months. Total I.V. dosage of 2.5 g over 9 months.
Aspergillosis: Total I.V. dosage of 3.6 g over 11 months.
◊ ***Fungal meningitis***
Adults: Intrathecal injection of 25 mcg/0.1 ml diluted with 10 to 20 ml of CSF and administered by barbotage two or three times weekly. Initial dose should not exceed 50 mcg.
◊ ***Coccidioidal arthritis***
Adults: 5 to 15 mg into joint spaces.
◊ ***Candidal cystitis***
Adults: Bladder irrigations in concentrations of 5 to 50 mcg/ml instilled periodically or continuously for 5 to 7 days.
Oropharyngeal candidiasis
Adults and children: 100 mg/ml oral suspension q.i.d. swish and swallow.
Topical fungal infections (3% cream, lotion, ointment)
Adults and children: Apply liberally and rub well into affected area b.i.d. to q.i.d.
Cutaneous or mucocutaneous candidal infections
Adults and children: Apply topical product b.i.d., t.i.d., or q.i.d. for 1 to 3 weeks; apply up to several months for interdigital or paronychial lesions.
◊ ***Sinus irrigation***
Adults: 1 mg/ml
◊ ***Histoplasmal pulmonary and intrapleural effusion***
Adults: 15 to 20 mg with 25 mg hydrocortisone sodium succinate.
◊ ***Pulmonary coccidioidomycosis***
Adults: Via intermittent positive pressure breathing device, 5 to 10 mg q.i.d.
◊ ***Ophthalmic candidal infection***
Adults: 0.1 to 1 mg/ml drop suspension q 30 minutes.

Note: Intrathecal and intra-articular uses are unapproved.

Pharmacodynamics

Antifungal action: Amphotericin B is *fungistatic* or *fungicidal,* depending on the concentrations available in body fluids and on the susceptibility of the fungus. It binds to sterols in the fungal cell membrane, increasing membrane permeability of fungal cells, causing subsequent leakage of intracellular components; it also may interfere with some human cell membranes that contain sterols.

Spectrum of activity includes *Histoplasma capsulatum, Coccidioides immitis, Blastomyces dermatitidis, Cryptococcus neoformans, Candida* species, *Aspergillus fumigatus, Mucor* species, *Rhizopus* species, *Absidia* species, *Entomophthora* species, *Basidiobolus* species, *Paracoccidioides brasiliensis, Sporothrix schenckii,* and *Rhodotorula* species.

Pharmacokinetics

- *Absorption:* Drug is absorbed poorly from the GI tract.
- *Distribution:* Distributes well into inflamed pleural cavities and joints; in low concentrations into aqueous humor, bronchial secretions, pancreas, bone, muscle, and parotids. CSF concentrations reach about 3% of serum concentrations. Drug is 90% to 95% bound to plasma proteins; it reportedly crosses the placenta.
- *Metabolism:* Not well defined.
- *Excretion:* Elimination of amphotericin B is biphasic: initial serum half-life of 24 hours, followed by a second phase half-life of about 15 days. About 2% to 5% of drug is excreted unchanged in urine. Amphotericin B is not readily removed by hemodialysis.

Contraindications and precautions

Contraindicated in patients with hypersensitivity to drug. Use cautiously in patients with renal impairment.

Interactions

Concomitant use with *aminoglycosides, cisplatin,* and *other nephrotoxic drugs* should be avoided, when possible, because of added nephrotoxic effects.

Because amphotericin B induces hypokalemia and hypomagnesia, concomitant use with *digoxin* increases the risk of digitalis toxicity. Because of added potassium depletion, concomitant use with *corticosteroids* requires careful monitoring of serum electrolyte levels and cardiac function.

Amphotericin B-induced hypokalemia may enhance effects of *skeletal muscle relaxants.* It potentiates the effects of *flucytosine* and *other antibiotics,* presumably by increasing cell membrane permeability.

Effects on diagnostic tests

Amphotericin B therapy may increase BUN, serum creatinine, alkaline phosphatase, and bilirubin levels.

Amphotericin B may cause hypokalemia and hypomagnesemia and may decrease WBC, RBC, and platelet counts.

Adverse reactions

CNS: *headache,* peripheral neuropathy, ***seizures*** (with systemic form).
CV: hypotension, ***arrhythmias, asystole,*** hypertension (with systemic form).
EENT: hearing loss, tinnitus, transient vertigo, blurred vision, diplopia (with systemic form).
GI: *anorexia, weight loss, nausea, vomiting, dyspepsia, diarrhea, epigastric pain, cramping,* melena, ***hemorrhagic gastroenteritis*** (with systemic form).
GU: *abnormal renal function with hypokalemia, azotemia, hyposthenuria, renal tubular acidosis, nephrocalcinosis;* with large doses, ***permanent renal impairment,*** anuria, oliguria (with systemic form).
Hematologic: *normochromic, normocytic anemia,* ***thrombocytopenia,*** leukopenia, ***agranulocytosis,*** eosinophilia, leukocytosis (with systemic form).
Hepatic: hepatitis, jaundice, ***acute liver failure*** (with systemic form).
Respiratory: dyspnea, tachypnea, ***bronchospasm,*** wheezing (with systemic form).

Skin: maculopapular rash, pruritus without rash (with systemic form); possible dryness, contact sensitivity, erythema, burning, pruritus (with topical administration).
Other: arthralgia, tissue damage with extravasation, *phlebitis, thrombophlebitis, pain at injection site,* myalgia, *fever, chills, malaise, generalized pain,* flushing, ***anaphylactoid reactions*** (with topical administration).

Overdose and treatment
Overdose may affect CV and respiratory function. Treatment is largely supportive.

☑ Special considerations
- Cultures and histologic and sensitivity testing must be completed and diagnosis confirmed before starting therapy in nonimmunocompromised patient.
- Prepare infusion as manufacturer directs, with strict aseptic technique, using *only* 10 ml of sterile water to reconstitute. To avoid precipitation, do not mix with solutions containing sodium chloride, other electrolytes, or bacteriostatic agents such as benzyl alcohol.
- Lyophilized cake contains no preservatives. Do not use if solution contains a precipitate or other foreign particles. Store cake at 35.6° to 46.4° F (2° to 8° C). Protect drug from light, and check expiration date.
- Liposomal amphotericin B when mixed with D_5W may be stored in refrigerator for 15 hours and at room temperature for 6 hours.
- Liposomal amphotericin B should not be mixed with other I.V. solutions.
- For I.V. infusion, use an in-line membrane with a mean pore diameter larger than 1 micron.
- Infuse slowly; rapid infusion may cause CV collapse.
- Do not mix or piggyback antibiotics with amphotericin B infusion; the I.V. solution appears compatible with small amounts of heparin sodium, hydrocortisone sodium succinate, and methylprednisolone sodium succinate.
- Give in distal veins, and monitor site for discomfort or thrombosis; if thrombosis occurs, alternate-day therapy may be considered.
- Vital signs should be checked every 30 minutes for at least 4 hours after start of I.V. infusion; fever may appear in 1 to 2 hours but should subside within 4 hours of discontinuing drug.
- Monitor intake and output and check for changes in urine appearance or volume; renal damage may be reversible if drug is stopped at earliest sign of dysfunction.
- Monitor potassium and magnesium levels closely; monitor calcium and magnesium levels twice weekly; perform liver and renal function studies and CBCs weekly.
- Severity of some adverse reactions can be reduced by premedication with aspirin or acetaminophen, antihistamines, antiemetics, meperidine, or small doses of corticosteroids; by addition of phosphate buffer to the solution; and by alternate-day dosing. If reactions are severe, drug may have to be discontinued for varying periods.
- Use topical products for folds of groin, neck, or armpit; avoid occlusive dressing with ointment, and discontinue if signs of hypersensitivity develop.
- Topical products may stain skin or clothes.
- Store at room temperature. Solution is stable at room temperature and in indoor light for 24 hours or in the refrigerator for 1 week.

Patient education
- Teach patient signs and symptoms of hypersensitivity and other adverse reactions, especially those associated with I.V. therapy. Warn that fever and chills are likely to occur and can be quite severe when therapy is initiated. These symptoms usually subside with repeated doses. Encourage patient feedback during infusion.
- Warn patient that therapy may take several months; teach personal hygiene and other measures to prevent spread and recurrence of lesions.
- Urge patient to adhere to regimen and to return, as instructed, for follow-up.
- Tell patient that topical products may stain skin and clothing; cream or lotion may be removed from clothing with soap and water.

Breast-feeding
- Safety has not been established in breast-feeding patients.

amphotericin B cholesteryl sulfate complex
Amphotec

Pharmacologic classification: polyene macrolide
Therapeutic classification: antifungal
Pregnancy risk category B

How supplied
Available by prescription only
Injection: 50 mg/20 ml, 100 mg/50 ml

Indications, route, and dosage
Invasive aspergillosis in patients in whom renal impairment or unacceptable toxicity precludes use of amphotericin B deoxycholate in effective doses and in those with invasive aspergillosis in whom prior amphotericin B deoxycholate therapy has failed
Adults and children: 3 to 4 mg/kg/day I.V.; may increase to 6 mg/kg/day if no improvement occurs or if fungal infection has progressed. Administer by continuous infusion at 1 mg/kg/hour.

Pharmacodynamics
Fungistatic/fungicidal action: Depends on concentration of drug and susceptibility of fungal organism. Drug binds to sterols in cell membranes of sensitive fungi, resulting in leakage of intracellular contents and causing cell death due to changes in membrane permeability. Also binds to sterols in mammalian cell membranes, which is believed to account for human toxicity.

Spectrum of activity includes *Aspergillus fumigatus, Candida albicans, Coccidioides immitis,* and *Cryptococcus neoformans.*

Pharmacokinetics

• *Absorption:* For an infusion rate of 1 mg/kg/hour and dosage ranges from 3 to 6 mg/kg/day, maximum plasma concentration at end of an infusion ranges from 2.6 to 3.4 mcg/ml.
• *Distribution:* Multicompartmental; steady-state volume increases with higher doses, possibly from uptake by tissues.
• *Metabolism:* Unknown.
• *Excretion:* Unclear; elimination half-life, 27 to 29 hours; increasing doses increase the elimination half-life. Drug may not be removed by dialysis.

Contraindications and precautions

Contraindicated in patients with hypersensitivity to any component of drug unless the benefits outweigh the risk of hypersensitivity.

Interactions

No formal drug interaction studies have been done. However, the following drugs are known to interact with amphotericin B.

Antineoplastic agents enhance renal toxicity, bronchospasm, hypotension. *Corticosteroids* enhance potassium depletion; could predispose the patient to cardiac dysfunction. *Cyclosporine* and *tacrolimus* may possibly increase serum creatinine levels. *Cardiac glycosides* enhance potassium excretion; increases risk of digitalis toxicity. *Flucytosine* may cause synergistic effect and also cause increased toxicity of flucytosine.

Imidazoles (ketoconazole, miconazole, fluconazole, clotrimazole) may cause antagonistic effects, although their significance is not determined.

Nephrotoxic drugs (such as *aminoglycosides, pentamidine)* may enhance renal toxicity. Monitor renal function closely. Amphotericin B–induced hypokalemia may enhance curariform effects of *skeletal muscle relaxants* (such as *tubocurarine*) due to hypokalemia.

Effects on diagnostic tests

None reported.

Adverse reactions

CNS: abnormal thoughts, anxiety, agitation, confusion, depression, dizziness, hallucinations, headache, hypertonia, neuropathy, paresthesia, ***seizures,*** somnolence, stupor.
CV: ***arrhythmias,*** *atrial fibrillation, bradycardia,* ***cardiac arrest, heart failure, hemorrhage,*** hypertension, *hypotension,* phlebitis, syncope, orthostatic hypotension, ***shock, supraventricular tachycardia,*** *tachycardia,* ***ventricular extrasystoles.***
EENT: eye hemorrhage, tinnitus.
GI: anorexia, GI disorder, GI hemorrhage, hematemesis, melena, *nausea,* stomatitis, *vomiting.*
GU: abnormal renal function, hematuria, ***renal failure.***
Hematologic: anemia, agranulocytosis, coagulation disorders, hypochromic anemia, increased PT, leukocytosis, ***leukopenia, thrombocytopenia.***
Hepatic: jaundice, abnormal liver function test results, ***hepatic failure.***
Metabolic: *hypokalemia,* hypocalcemia, hyperglycemia, hypervolemia, hypophosphatemia, hyponatremia, hyperkalemia, *increased creatinine, bilirubinemia,* hypomagnesemia, alkaline phosphatase, BUN, AST, ALT, LD levels.
Musculoskeletal: arthralgia, myalgia.
Respiratory: ***apnea,*** asthma, dyspnea, epistaxis, hemoptysis, hyperventilation, hypoxia, increased cough, lung or respiratory disorders, ***pulmonary edema.***
Skin: pruritus, rash, sweating, skin disorder.
Other: ***allergic reaction; anaphylaxis;*** asthenia; *chills;* edema; *fever;* abdominal, chest, or back pain; peripheral or facial edema; infection, mucous membrane disorder; pain or reaction at injection site; sepsis.

Overdose and treatment

Amphotec is not dialyzable. Amphotericin B deoxycholate overdose has been reported to result in cardiorespiratory arrest. If overdose is suspected, discontinue therapy, monitor clinical status, and administer supportive therapy.

☑ Special considerations

• Pretreatment with antihistamines and corticosteroids or reducing the rate of infusion (or both) may reduce the acute infusion-related reactions.
• Dilute in D_5W and administer by continuous infusion at 1 mg/kg/hour. Perform a test dose before commencing new courses of treatment; infuse a small amount of drug (10 ml of final preparation containing 1.6 to 8.3 mg of amphotericin B) over 15 to 30 minutes and monitor for next 30 minutes. Can shorten infusion time to 2 hours or lengthen infusion time based on patient tolerance.
• Drug is incompatible with NaCl, electrolyte solutions, and bacteriostatic agents.
• Infuse drug over at least 2 hours.
• Don't mix with other drugs. If administered through an existing I.V. line, flush line with D_5W before infusion or use a separate line.
• Store vials at room temperature. Reconstitute 50-mg vial with rapid addition of 10 ml of sterile water for injection, and 100-mg vial with rapid addition of 20 ml sterile water with a sterile syringe and 20G needle. Shake vial gently. Do not use diluent other than sterile water for injection.
• Reconstituted drug is clear or opalescent liquid and is stable for 24 hours refrigerated. Discard partially used vials.
• Don't administer undiluted drug.
• Don't filter or use an in-line filter and don't freeze.
• Monitor vital signs every 30 minutes during initial therapy. Acute infusion-related reactions (fever, chills, hypotension, nausea, tachycardia) usually occur 1 to 3 hours after starting I.V. infusion. These reactions are usually more severe after initial doses and usually diminish with subsequent doses. If severe respiratory distress occurs, stop infusion immediately and don't treat further with drug.

• Monitor intake and output; report changes in urine appearance or volume.
• Monitor renal and hepatic function tests, serum electrolytes (especially potassium, magnesium, and calcium), CBCs, and PT.

Patient education
• Instruct patient to report symptoms of hypersensitivity immediately.
• Warn patient of possible discomfort at I.V. site.
• Advise patient of potential adverse effects, such as fever, chills, nausea, and vomiting. Tell him that these can be severe with initial treatment but usually subside with repeated doses.

Geriatric use
• No unexpected adverse events have been reported.

Pediatric use
• No unexpected adverse events have been reported.

Breast-feeding
• It is unknown if drug is excreted in breast milk. Because of the potential for serious adverse reactions in breast-fed infants, a decision should be made to discontinue breast-feeding or to stop treatment, taking into account the importance of drug to the mother.

ampicillin
Apo-Ampi*, Novo-Ampicillin*, Omnipen, Penbritin*, Polycillin, Principen

ampicillin sodium
Ampicin*, Omnipen-N, Penbritin*, Polycillin-N, Totacillin-N

ampicillin trihydrate
D-Amp, Polycillin, Principen, Totacillin

Pharmacologic classification: aminopenicillin
Therapeutic classification: antibiotic
Pregnancy risk category B

How supplied
Available by prescription only
Capsules: 250 mg, 500 mg
Suspension: 100 mg/ml (pediatric drops), 125 mg/5 ml, 250 mg/5 ml, 500 mg/5 ml (after reconstitution)
Parenteral: 125 mg, 250 mg, 500 mg, 1 g, 2 g
Pharmacy bulk package: 10-g vial
Infusion: 500 mg, 1 g, 2 g

Indications, route, and dosage
Systemic infections, acute and chronic urinary tract infections caused by susceptible organisms
Adults: 250 to 500 mg P.O. q 6 hours.
Children: 50 to 100 mg/kg P.O. daily, divided into doses given q 6 hours; or 100 to 200 mg/kg I.M. or I.V. daily, divided into doses given q 6 to 8 hours.
Meningitis
Adults: 8 to 14 g I.V. divided q 3 to 4 hours for 3 days; then may give I.M. if desired.
Children age 2 months to 12 years: Up to 400 mg/kg I.V. daily for 3 days; then up to 300 mg/kg I.M. divided q 4 hours. May be given concurrently with chloramphenicol, pending culture results.
Uncomplicated gonorrhea
Adults: 3.5 g P.O. with 1 g probenecid given as a single dose.
✦ ***Dosage adjustment.*** Dosing interval should be increased to q 12 hours in patients with severe renal impairment (creatinine clearance 10 ml/minute or less).
Prophylaxis for salmonella in patients infected with human immunodeficiency virus (HIV)
Adults: 50 to 100 mg P.O. q.i.d. for several months.
Prophylaxis for bacterial endocarditis before dental or minor respiratory procedures
Adults: 2 g (I.V. or I.M.) 30 minutes before procedure; then 1 g P.O. of amoxicillin or 1 g I.V. or I.M. 6 hours postprocedure.
Children: 50 mg/kg I.V. or I.M. 30 minutes before procedure; then 25 mg/kg I.V. or I.M. or 25 mg/kg of oral amoxicillin 6 hours postprocedure.

Pharmacodynamics
Antibiotic action: Ampicillin is bactericidal; it adheres to bacterial penicillin-binding proteins, thus inhibiting bacterial cell wall synthesis.

Spectrum of action includes non-penicillinase-producing gram-positive bacteria. It is also effective against many gram-negative organisms, including *Neisseria gonorrhoeae, N. meningitidis, Haemophilus influenzae, Escherichia coli, Proteus mirabilis, Salmonella,* and *Shigella.* Ampicillin should be used in gram-negative systemic infections only when organism sensitivity is known.

Pharmacokinetics
• *Absorption:* Approximately 42% of ampicillin is absorbed after an oral dose; peak serum concentrations occur at 1 to 2 hours. After I.M. administration, peak serum concentrations occur at 1 hour.
• *Distribution:* Ampicillin distributes into pleural, peritoneal and synovial fluids, lungs, prostate, liver, and gallbladder; it also penetrates middle ear effusions, maxillary sinus and bronchial secretions, tonsils, and sputum. Drug readily crosses the placenta; minimally protein-bound (15% to 25%).
• *Metabolism:* Drug is only partially metabolized.
• *Excretion:* Ampicillin is excreted in urine by renal tubular secretion and glomerular filtration. It is also excreted in breast milk. Elimination half-life is about 1 to 1½ hours; in patients with extensive renal impairment, half-life is extended to 10 to 24 hours.

Contraindications and precautions
Contraindicated in patients with hypersensitivity to drug or other penicillins. Use with caution in patients with mononucleosis.

Interactions
Concomitant use with an *aminoglycoside antibiotic* causes a synergistic bactericidal effect against some strains of enterococci and group B strepto-

cocci. However, the drugs are physically and chemically incompatible and are inactivated if mixed or given together.

Concomitant use with *allopurinol* appears to increase incidence of rash from both drugs.

Concomitant use with *clavulanate* results in increased bactericidal effects because clavulanic acid is a beta-lactamase inhibitor.

Probenecid inhibits renal tubular secretion of ampicillin, raising its serum concentrations.

Large doses of penicillins may interfere with renal tubular secretion of *methotrexate*, thus delaying elimination and elevating serum concentrations of *methotrexate*.

The effects of *oral contraceptives* may be decreased.

Effects on diagnostic tests
Ampicillin alters results of urine glucose tests that use cupric sulfate (Benedict's reagent or Clinitest). Make urine glucose determinations with glucose oxidase methods (Chemstrip uG, Diastix, or glucose enzymatic test strip).

Ampicillin may falsely decrease serum aminoglycoside concentrations.

Adverse reactions
CNS: lethargy, hallucinations, ***seizures,*** anxiety, confusion, agitation, depression, dizziness, fatigue.
GI: *nausea,* vomiting, *diarrhea,* glossitis, stomatitis, gastritis, abdominal pain, enterocolitis, pseudomembranous colitis, black "hairy" tongue.
GU: interstitial nephritis, nephropathy.
Hematologic: anemia, ***thrombocytopenia,*** thrombocytopenic purpura, eosinophilia, leukopenia, hemolytic anemia, ***agranulocytosis.***
Other: hypersensitivity reactions (erythematous maculopapular rash, urticaria, ***anaphylaxis***, overgrowth of nonsusceptible organisms, pain at injection site, vein irritation, thrombophlebitis, vaginitis.

Overdose and treatment
Clinical signs of overdose include neuromuscular sensitivity or seizures. After recent ingestion (within 4 hours), empty the stomach by induced emesis or gastric lavage; follow with activated charcoal to reduce absorption. Drug can be removed by hemodialysis.

☑ Special considerations
Besides those relevant to all *penicillins,* consider the following recommendation.
- Administer I.M. or I.V. only when patient is too ill to take oral drug.

Patient education
- Encourage patient to report diarrhea promptly.
- Instruct patient to complete all of the prescribed drug.

Geriatric use
- Because of diminished renal tubular secretion in elderly patients, half-life of drug may be prolonged.

Breast-feeding
- Use cautiously. Ampicillin is distributed readily into breast milk; safety in breast-feeding women has not been established.

ampicillin sodium/sulbactam sodium
Unasyn

Pharmacologic classification: aminopenicillin/beta-lactamase inhibitor combination
Therapeutic classification: antibiotic
Pregnancy risk category B

How supplied
Available by prescription only
Injection: Vials and piggyback vials containing 1.5 g (1 g ampicillin sodium with 500 mg sulbactam sodium) and 3 g (2 g ampicillin sodium with 1 g sulbactam sodium)

Indications, route, and dosage
***Skin and skin-structure infections, intra-abdominal and gynecologic infections caused by susceptible beta-lactamase—producing strains of* Staphylococcus aureus, Escherichia coli, Klebsiella *(including* K. pneumoniae), Proteus mirabilis, Bacteroides *(including* B. fragilis), Enterobacter, *and* Acinetobacter calcoaceticus**
Adults: 1.5 to 3 g I.M. or I.V. q 6 hours. Do not exceed 4 g/day sulbactam sodium.
✦ ***Dosage adjustment.***

DOSAGE IN RENAL FAILURE

Creatinine clearance (ml/min/ 1.73 m²)	Half-life (hr)	Recommended dosage
≥ 30	1	1.5 to 3 g q 6 to 8 hr
15 to 29	5	1.5 to 3 g q 12 hr
5 to 14	9	1.5 to 3 g q 24 hr

Pharmacodynamics
Antibiotic action: Ampicillin is bactericidal; it adheres to bacterial penicillin-binding proteins, thus inhibiting bacterial cell wall synthesis. Sulbactam inhibits beta-lactamase, an enzyme produced by ampicillin-resistant bacteria that degrades ampicillin.

Pharmacokinetics
- *Absorption:* Peak plasma levels occur immediately after I.V. infusion and within 1 hour after I.M. injection.
- *Distribution:* Both drugs distribute into pleural, peritoneal and synovial fluids, lungs, prostate, liver, and gallbladder; they also penetrate middle ear

effusions, maxillary sinus and bronchial secretions, tonsils, and sputum. Ampicillin readily crosses the placenta; it is minimally protein-bound at 15% to 25%; sulbactam is about 38% bound.

• *Metabolism:* Both drugs are metabolized only partially; only 15% to 25% of both drugs are metabolized.

• *Excretion:* Both ampicillin and sulbactam are excreted in the urine by renal tubular secretion and glomerular filtration. It is also excreted in breast milk. Elimination half-life is 1 to 1½ hours; in patients with extensive renal impairment, half-life can be as long as 10 to 24 hours.

Contraindications and precautions

Contraindicated in patients with hypersensitivity to drug or other penicillins. Use cautiously in patients with maculopapular rash.

Interactions

Concomitant use with *probenecid* decreases excretion of both ampicillin and sulbactam; use with *allopurinol* may lead to an increased incidence of rash. The ampicillin component may cause in vitro inactivation of *aminoglycosides* if these antibiotics are mixed in the same infusion container.

Large doses of I.V. penicillins can increase bleeding risks of *anticoagulants* because of a prolongation of bleeding times.

Effects on diagnostic tests

Ampicillin alters results of urine glucose tests that use cupric sulfate (Benedict's reagent or Clinitest). Make urine glucose determinations with glucose oxidase methods (Chemstrip uG, Diastix, or glucose enzymatic test strip).

In pregnant women, transient decreases in serum estradiol, conjugated estrone, conjugated estriol, and estriol glucuronide may occur.

Adverse reactions

GI: *nausea,* vomiting, *diarrhea,* glossitis, stomatitis, gastritis, black "hairy" tongue, enterocolitis, pseudomembranous colitis.

Hematologic: anemia, ***thrombocytopenia,*** thrombocytopenic purpura, eosinophilia, leukopenia, ***agranulocytosis.***

Other: hypersensitivity reactions (erythematous maculopapular rash, urticaria, ***anaphylaxis***), ***overgrowth of nonsusceptible organisms,*** pain at injection site, vein irritation, thrombophlebitis.

Overdose and treatment

Neurologic adverse reactions, including seizures, are likely. Treatment is supportive. Although confirming data are lacking, ampicillin and sulbactam are likely to be removed by hemodialysis.

☑ Special considerations

• I.V. administration should be given by slow injection over at least 10 to 15 minutes or infused in greater dilutions with 50 to 100 ml of a compatible diluent over 15 to 30 minutes.

• For I.V. use, reconstitute powder in piggyback units to desired concentrations with sterile water for injection, 0.9% NaCl injection, 5% dextrose injection, lactated Ringer's injection, 1/6 M sodium lactate injection, 5% dextrose in 0.45% NaCl, or 10% invert sugar.

• If piggyback bottles are unavailable, reconstitute standard vials of sterile powder with sterile water for injection to yield solutions of 375 mg/ml (250 mg ampicillin/125 mg sulbactam). Then immediately dilute an appropriate volume with a suitable diluent to yield solutions of 3 to 45 mg/ml (2 to 30 mg ampicillin/1 to 15 mg sulbactam per ml).

• For I.M. injection, reconstitute with sterile water for injection, or 0.5% or 2% lidocaine hydrochloride injection. To obtain 375 mg/ml solutions (250 mg ampicillin/125 mg sulbactam/ml), add contents of the 1.5-g vial to 3.2 ml of diluent to produce 4 ml withdrawal volume; add 3-g vial to 6.4 ml of diluent to produce 8 ml withdrawal volume.

• Reconstituted solutions are stable for varying periods (from 2 hours to 72 hours) depending on diluent used. Check with pharmacist. For patients on sodium restriction, note that a 1.5-g dose of ampicillin sodium/sulbactam sodium yields 5 mEq of sodium.

Geriatric use

• Because of diminished renal tubular secretion in elderly patients, half-life of drug may be prolonged.

Pediatric use

• Safe use in children under age 12 is not established.

Breast-feeding

• Ampicillin is distributed readily into breast milk; safety in breast-feeding women has not been established. Alternative feeding method is recommended during therapy.

amrinone lactate

Inocor

Pharmacologic classification: bipyridine derivative
Therapeutic classification: inotropic, vasodilator
Pregnancy risk category C

How supplied

Available by prescription only
Injection: 5 mg/ml

Indications, route, and dosage

Short-term management of heart failure

Adults: Initially, 0.75 mg/kg I.V. bolus over 2 to 3 minutes; then, begin maintenance infusion of 5 to 10 mcg/kg/minute. Additional bolus of 0.75 mg/kg may be given 30 minutes after therapy starts. Maximum daily dose is 10 mg/kg.

Pharmacodynamics

Vasodilating action: The primary vasodilating effect of amrinone seems to stem from a direct effect on peripheral vessels.

Inotropic action: The mechanism of action responsible for the apparent inotropic effect is not fully understood; however, it may be associated with inhibition of phosphodiesterase activity, resulting in increased cellular levels of adenosine 3′,5′-cyclic phosphate; this, in turn, may alter intracellular and extracellular calcium levels. The role of calcium homeostasis has not been determined. Clinical effects include increased cardiac output mediated by reduced afterload and, possibly, inotropism.

Pharmacokinetics

- *Absorption:* With I.V. administration, onset of action occurs in 2 to 5 minutes, with peak effects in about 10 minutes. CV effects may persist for 1 to 2 hours.
- *Distribution:* Distribution volume is 1.2 L/kg. Distribution sites are unknown. Protein binding ranges from 10% to 49%. Therapeutic steady-state serum levels range from 0.5 to 7 mcg/ml (ideal concentration: 3 mcg/ml).
- *Metabolism:* Amrinone is metabolized in the liver to several metabolites of unknown activity.
- *Excretion:* In normal patients, amrinone is excreted in the urine, with a terminal elimination half-life of about 4 hours. Half-life may be prolonged slightly in patients with heart failure.

Contraindications and precautions

Contraindicated in patients with hypersensitivity to amrinone or bisulfites. It should not be used in patients with severe aortic or pulmonic valvular disease in place of surgical intervention or during an acute phase of MI.

Interactions

Concomitant use with *disopyramide* may cause severe hypotension.

Effects on diagnostic tests

The physiologic effects of amrinone may decrease serum potassium or increase serum hepatic enzymes.

Adverse reactions

CV: *arrhythmias,* hypotension.
GI: nausea, vomiting, anorexia, abdominal pain.
Hematologic: ***thrombocytopenia*** (based on dose and duration of therapy).
Hepatic: elevated enzymes, hepatotoxicity (rare).
Other: burning at injection site, ***hypersensitivity reactions*** (pericarditis, ascites, myositis vasculitis, pleuritis), fever, chest pain.

Overdose and treatment

Clinical effects of overdose include severe hypotension. Treatment may include administration of a potent vasopressor, such as norepinephrine, as well as other general supportive measures, including cautious fluid volume replacement.

☑ Special considerations

- Administer drug as supplied or dilute in normal or half-0.9% NaCl solution to concentration of 1 to 3 mg/ml. Do not dilute drug with solutions containing dextrose because slow chemical reaction occurs over 24 hours. However, amrinone can be injected into running dextrose infusions through Y-connector or directly into tubing. Use diluted solution within 24 hours.
- Do not administer furosemide in I.V. lines containing amrinone because a chemical reaction occurs immediately.
- Monitor blood pressure and heart rate throughout infusion. Infusion should be slowed or stopped if patient's blood pressure decreases or if arrhythmias (ventricular or supraventricular) occur. Dosage may need to be reduced.
- Monitor platelet counts. A count below 150,000/mm^3 usually necessitates dosage reduction. Thrombocytopenia usually occurs after prolonged treatment.
- Monitor electrolyte levels (especially potassium) because drug increases cardiac output, which may cause diuresis.
- Hemodynamic monitoring may be useful in guiding therapy.
- Monitor liver function tests to detect hepatic damage (rare).
- Observe for adverse GI effects (such as nausea, vomiting, and diarrhea); reduce dosage or discontinue drug.
- Amrinone is prescribed primarily for patients who have not responded to therapy with cardiac glycosides, diuretics, and vasodilators.

Pediatric use

- Safety and effectiveness in children under age 18 have not been established.

Breast-feeding

- Drug may be excreted in breast milk. Safety in breast-feeding women has not been established.

amyl nitrite

Pharmacologic classification: nitrate
Therapeutic classification: vasodilator, cyanide poisoning adjunct
Pregnancy risk category C

How supplied

Available by prescription only
Nasal inhalant: 0.18 ml, 0.3 ml

Indications, route, and dosage

Angina pectoris
Adults: 0.18 to 0.3 ml by inhalation (one glass ampule inhaler), p.r.n.
Adjunct treatment of cyanide poisoning
Adults and children: 0.3 ml by inhalation for 15 to 30 seconds; repeat q 60 seconds until I.V. sodium nitrite infusion and I.V. sodium thiosulfate infusion are available.

Pharmacodynamics

Vasodilating action: Drug reduces myocardial oxygen demand by decreasing left ventricular end-diastolic pressure (preload) and systemic vascular resistance and arterial pressure (afterload). It also increases collateral coronary blood flow. By relaxing vascular smooth muscle, it produces generalized vasodilation. Amyl nitrite also relaxes all other smooth muscle, including bronchial and biliary smooth muscle. In cyanide poisoning, it converts hemoglobin to methemoglobin, which reacts with cyanide to form cyanmethemoglobin.

Pharmacokinetics

- *Absorption:* Inhaled drug is absorbed readily through the respiratory tract; action begins in 30 seconds and lasts 3 to 5 minutes.
- *Distribution:* Not available.
- *Metabolism:* Amyl nitrite, an organic nitrite, is metabolized by the liver to form inorganic nitrites, which are much less potent vasodilators than the parent drug.
- *Excretion:* One-third of the inhaled dose is excreted in urine.

Contraindications and precautions

Contraindicated in patients with hypersensitivity to nitrites, severe anemia, angle-closure glaucoma, orthostatic hypotension, increased intracranial pressure, and in pregnant patients.

Use cautiously in patients with glaucoma, volume depletion, and hypotension.

Interactions

Concomitant use of *alcohol, phenothiazines, beta blockers*, or *antihypertensives* may cause excessive hypotension.

Effects on diagnostic tests

Amyl nitrite therapy alters the Zlatkis-Zak color reaction, causing a false decrease in serum cholesterol levels.

Adverse reactions

CNS: *headache, sometimes with throbbing;* dizziness; weakness.
CV: *orthostatic hypotension, tachycardia,* flushing, palpitations, fainting.
GI: nausea, vomiting.
Hematologic: methemoglobinemia.
Skin: cutaneous vasodilation, rash.
Other: hypersensitivity reactions.

Overdose and treatment

Clinical signs of overdose include methemoglobinemia, characterized by blue skin and mucous membranes, hypotension, tachycardia, palpitations, skin changes, diaphoresis, dizziness, syncope, vertigo, headache, nausea, vomiting, anorexia, increased intracranial pressure, confusion, moderate fever, and paralysis. Hypoxia may lead to metabolic acidosis, cyanosis, seizures, coma, and cardiac collapse. Treat with high flow oxygen and methylene blue. Usual dose of methylene blue for adults and children is 1 to 2 mg/kg I.V. given slowly over several minutes. In severe cases, this dose may be repeated only once; doses exceeding 4 mg/kg may produce methemoglobinemia.

☑ Special considerations

- Drug is rarely used as an antianginal.
- Keep patient sitting or lying down during and immediately after inhalation. Crush ampule (has a woven gauze covering) between fingers and hold to nose for inhalation.
- Monitor for orthostatic hypotension; do not allow patient to make rapid postural changes while inhaling drug.
- Drug is highly flammable; keep away from open flame and extinguish all cigarettes before use.
- Drug is used illegally to enhance sexual pleasure, chiefly by homosexuals. Street names include "Amy" and "poppers."

Patient education

- Explain that ampule must be crushed to release drug.
- Warn patient to use drug only when seated or lying down.

Geriatric use

- Orthostatic hypotensive effects may be more likely to occur in elderly patients.

Pediatric use

- Safety and efficacy have not been established.

Breast-feeding

- It is unknown whether amyl nitrite is excreted in breast milk; risk and benefit must be considered.

anagrelide hydrochloride

Agrylin

Pharmacologic classification: platelet-reducing agent
Therapeutic classification: platelet-reducing agent
Pregnancy risk category C

How supplied:

Available by prescription only
Capsules: 0.5 mg, 1 mg

Indications, route, and dosage

Essential thrombocythemia to reduce the elevated platelet count, risk of thrombosis and to ameliorate associated symptoms

Adults: 0.5 mg P.O. q.i.d. or 1 mg b.i.d. for at least 1 week; then adjust dosage to lowest effective dose required to maintain platelet count below 600,000/mm^3, and ideally to the normal range. Do not increase dosage to more than 0.5 mg/day in any 1 week; do not exceed 10 mg/day or 2.5 mg in a single dose.

Pharmacodynamics

Platelet-reducing action: Mechanism of action still under investigation; reduction in platelet production is thought to result from a decrease in megakaryocyte hypermaturation. Drug inhibits cAMP phosphodiesterase, as well as adenosine diphosphate- and collagen-induced platelet aggregation.

Pharmacokinetics

- *Absorption.* Following oral administration of 1 mg in healthy individuals, peak plasma levels occur in approximately 1 hour. Plasma levels decline to less than 10% of peak levels in 24 hours.

- *Distribution:* Plasma half-life at fasting and at 0.5 mg doses is 1.3 hours. Drug does not accumulate in plasma after repeated administration and bioavailability is modestly reduced by food.
- *Metabolism:* Drug is extensively metabolized before elimination in urine.
- *Excretion:* Eliminated in urine; less than 1% is recovered unchanged in urine.

Contraindications and precautions
Use with caution in patients with CV disease because drug may cause vasodilation, tachycardia, palpitations, and heart failure. Use cautiously in patients with creatinine clearance over 2 mg/dl and in those with liver function tests exceeding 1.5 times the upper normal limits. Interruption of drug use will cause platelet counts to rise within 4 days of discontinuation.

Interactions
Sucralfate may interfere with anagrelide absorption; no other drug interaction studies have been performed.

Effects on diagnostic tests
None reported.

Adverse reactions
CNS: amnesia, *asthenia*, confusion, ***CVA,*** depression, *dizziness, headache,* insomnia, migraine, nervousness, pain, paresthesia, somnolence.
CV: ***arrhythmias, angina pectoris, chest pain,*** CV disease, ***heart failure, hemorrhage,*** hypertension, *palpitations,* orthostatic hypotension, vasodilatation, syncope, ***tachycardia.***
EENT: abnormal vision, amblyopia, diplopia, tinnitus, visual field abnormality.
GI: *abdominal pain,* aphthous stomatitis, constipation, *diarrhea*, dyspepsia, eructation, *flatulence,* GI distress, GI hemorrhage, gastritis, melena, *nausea,* vomiting.
GU: dysuria, hematuria.
Hematologic: anemia, ecchymosis, lymphadenoma, ***thrombocytopenia.***
Metabolic: dehydration.
Respiratory: *dyspnea*, rhinitis, epistaxis, respiratory disease, sinusitis, pneumonia, bronchitis, asthma.
Skin: alopecia, pruritus, rash, skin disorder, urticaria.
Other: anorexia, arthralgia, back pain, chills, *edema,* fever, flulike symptoms, leg cramps, malaise, myalgia, neck pain, photosensitivity.

Overdose and treatment
Monitor patient closely; monitor platelet counts.

☑ Special considerations
- Food has no clinically significant effect on anagrelide.
- During the first 2 weeks of treatment, monitor blood counts, liver and renal function tests.

Patient education
- Tell patient to use drug only as prescribed.
- Inform patient that drug can be taken without regard to meals.
- Instruct patient to report increased bleeding, bruising, or cardiac symptoms.

Geriatric use
- Evaluate use of drug carefully in patients with renal, liver, or CV disease.

Pediatric use
- Safety and efficacy of drug has not been established in patients under age 16.

Breast-feeding
- It is not known if drug is excreted in breast milk. Use with caution.

anastrozole
Arimidex

Pharmacologic classification: nonsteroidal aromatase inhibitor
Therapeutic classification: antineoplastic
Pregnancy risk category D

How supplied
Available by prescription only
Tablets: 1 mg

Indications, route, and dosage
Treatment of advanced breast cancer in postmenopausal women with disease progression following tamoxifen therapy
Adults: 1 mg P.O. daily.

Pharmacodynamics
Antineoplastic action: A potent and selective nonsteroidal aromatase inhibitor, anastrozole significantly lowers serum estradiol concentrations. Estradiol is the principal estrogen circulating in postmenopausal women that has the ability to stimulate breast cancer cell growth.

Pharmacokinetics
- *Absorption:* Anastrozole is absorbed from the GI tract; food affects the extent of absorption.
- *Distribution:* Anastrozole is 40% bound to plasma proteins in the therapeutic range.
- *Metabolism:* Anastrozole is metabolized in the liver.
- *Excretion:* About 11% of anastrozole is excreted in urine as parent drug and about 60% is excreted in urine as metabolites. Half-life is about 50 hours.

Contraindications and precautions
Contraindicated in pregnant women.

Interactions
None reported.

Effects on diagnostic tests
None reported.

Adverse reactions

CNS: *headache,* dizziness, depression, paresthesia.
CV: chest pain, edema.
GI: *nausea,* vomiting, diarrhea, constipation, abdominal pain, anorexia.
Respiratory: dyspnea, increased cough, pharyngitis.
Skin: *hot flashes,* rash, sweating.
Other: *asthenia, pain, back pain,* bone pain, dry mouth, peripheral edema, pelvic pain, vaginal hemorrhage, weight gain, increased appetite, thromboembolic disease, vaginal dryness.

Overdose and treatment

A single dose of anastrozole that results in life-threatening symptoms has not been established. Animal studies with single oral doses that exceeded 100 mg/kg were associated with severe irritation of the stomach (necrosis, gastritis, ulceration, and hemorrhage). There is no specific antidote to overdosage and treatment must be symptomatic. Vomiting may be induced if the patient is alert. Dialysis may be helpful. General supportive care, including frequent monitoring of vital signs and close observation of the patient, is indicated.

☑ Special considerations

- Pregnancy must be excluded before treatment is started with anastrozole.
- Drug should be administered under supervision of qualified staff experienced in the use of anticancer agents.

Patient education

- Instruct patient to report adverse reactions.
- Stress importance of follow-up care.

Pediatric use

- Safety and effectiveness in pediatric patients have not been established.

Breast-feeding

- It is not known whether anastrozole is excreted in breast milk. Drug should not be administered to breast-feeding women.

anistreplase (anisoylated plasminogen-streptokinase activator complex, APSAC)

Eminase

Pharmacologic classification: thrombolytic enzyme
Therapeutic classification: thrombolytic enzyme
Pregnancy risk category C

How supplied

Available by prescription only
Injection: 30 U/single-dose vial

Indications, route, and dosage

Treatment of acute coronary arterial thrombosis

Adults: 30 U by direct I.V. injection over 2 to 5 minutes.

Pharmacodynamics

Enzymatic action: Anistreplase is derived from Lys-plasminogen and streptokinase. It activates the endogenous fibrinolytic system to produce plasmin, which degrades fibrin clots, fibrinogen, and other plasma proteins, including procoagulant factors V and VIII.

Pharmacokinetics

- *Absorption:* Drug is administered I.V.
- *Distribution:* Information not available.
- *Metabolism:* Immediately after injection, anistreplase is deacylated by a nonenzymatic process to form the active streptokinase-plasminogen complex. The half-life of acylated and deacylated anistreplase is 88 to 112 minutes.
- *Excretion:* Unknown. Duration of fibrinolytic activity is 4 to 6 hours and is limited by the deacylation of the anistreplase.

Contraindications and precautions

Contraindicated in patients with history of severe allergic reaction to anistreplase or streptokinase; active internal bleeding, CVA, recent (within the past 2 months) intraspinal or intracranial surgery or trauma, aneurysm, arteriovenous malformation, intracranial neoplasm, uncontrolled hypertension, or known bleeding diathesis.

Use cautiously in patients with recent (within 10 days) major surgery, trauma (including cardiopulmonary resuscitation), GI or GU bleeding, cerebrovascular disease, hypertension, mitral stenosis, atrial fibrillation, acute pericarditis, subacute bacterial endocarditis, septic thrombophlebitis, and diabetic hemorrhagic retinopathy; in pregnancy and first 10 days postpartum; in patients receiving anticoagulants; and in those older than age 75.

Interactions

Concurrent use with *heparin, oral anticoagulants,* and *drugs that alter platelet function* (including *aspirin* and *dipyridamole*) may increase risk of bleeding. Use with *adrenocorticoids, glucocorticoids,* or *chronic therapeutic corticotropin* or *ethacrynic acid* may increase risk of severe hemorrhage.

Antihypertensive agents may increase risk of severe hypotension. *Cefamandole, cefoperazone, cefotetan, plicamycin,* and *valproic acid* may increase risk of severe hemorrhage because of their ability to cause hypoprothrombinemia, inhibit platelet aggregation, or cause irreversible platelet damage. *NSAIDs* or *sulfinpyrazone* may increase the risk of bleeding.

Effects on diagnostic tests

Anistreplase prolongs activated partial thromboplastin time (APTT), PT, and thrombin time; drug remains active in vitro and can cause degradation of fibrinogen in blood samples drawn for analysis. Decreases in the activities of alpha$_2$-antiplasmin, factor V, factor VIII, fibrinogen, and plasminogen have been reported as well as moderate reductions in hematocrit and hemoglobin. Concentrations of fibrinogen- and fibrin-degradation products are increased.

Adverse reactions

CNS: ***intracranial hemorrhage.***
CV: ARRHYTHMIAS, *conduction disorders, hypotension.*
EENT: hemoptysis, gum or mouth hemorrhage.
GI: hemorrhage.
GU: hematuria.
Hematologic: ***bleeding tendency,*** eosinophilia.
Skin: hematoma, urticaria, pruritus, flushing, delayed purpuric rash (2 weeks after therapy).
Other: bleeding at puncture sites, ***anaphylaxis or anaphylactoid reactions*** (rare), arthralgia.

☑ Special considerations

- The following tests may be needed before and after drug administration: APTT, PT, thrombin time, hemoglobin, hematocrit, fibrinogen determination, platelet count, and fibrin-fibrinogen degradation products.
- Coronary angiography may be useful to monitor effectiveness.
- ECG monitoring is recommended to detect arrhythmias associated with acute MI or reperfusion and may help determine effectiveness of treatment.
- Initiate therapy as soon as possible after onset of clinical symptoms of acute MI.
- Monitor vital signs, mental status, and neurologic status.
- Anistreplase is derived from human plasma. No cases of hepatitis or human immunodeficiency virus infection have been reported to date.
- Reconstitute by slowly adding 5 ml sterile water for injection. Direct the stream against the side of the vial, not at the drug itself. Gently roll the vial to mix the dry powder and water. To avoid excessive foaming, *do not shake vial.* Solution should be colorless to pale yellow.
- Do not mix with other medications or further dilute after reconstitution.
- Discard drug that is not administered within 30 minutes of reconstituting.
- To decrease risk of rethrombosis, heparin therapy may be initiated after administration.
- Addition of fibrinolysis inhibitor (for example, aprotinin) or aminocaproic acid to blood samples drawn to obtain specific measurement of fibrinogen will attenuate the degradation of fibrinogen associated with thrombolytic-treated patients.
- Keep patient on strict bed rest and apply pressure dressings to recently invaded sites. To minimize risk of bleeding, avoid nonessential handling or moving of patient, invasive procedures such as biopsies, and I.M. injections.

Patient education

- Instruct patient and caregiver to recognize and report signs and symptoms of internal bleeding.
- Instruct patient about importance of strict bed rest.

Geriatric use

- No age-specific problems have been reported to date. Risk-benefit must be assessed in patients age 75 and over because preexisting conditions increase the risk of hemorrhagic complications.

Pediatric use

- Safety and efficacy have not been established.

Breast-feeding

- It is unknown if drug is excreted in breast milk. Use with caution in breast-feeding women.

anthralin

Anthra-Derm, Drithocreme, Drithocreme HP 1%, Dritho-Scalp, Lasan

Pharmacologic classification: germicide
Therapeutic classification: topical antipsoriatic
Pregnancy risk category C

How supplied

Available by prescription only
Ointment: 0.1%, 0.25%, 0.4%, 0.5%, 1%
Cream: 0.1%, 0.2%, 0.25%, 0.4%, 0.5%, 1%

Indications, route, and dosage

Quiescent or chronic psoriasis
Adults and adolescents: Apply thinly daily or as directed. Start with lowest concentration and increase, p.r.n.

Pharmacodynamics

Antipsoriatic action: Although the mechanism of action is not fully known, it is thought that anthralin decreases the mitotic rate and reduces the proliferation of epidermal cells in psoriasis by inhibiting the synthesis of nucleic protein in psoriatic cell tissue.

Pharmacokinetics

- *Absorption:* Limited absorption with topical use.
- *Distribution:* None.
- *Metabolism:* None.
- *Excretion:* None.

Contraindications and precautions

Contraindicated in patients with hypersensitivity to drug. Do not use on acute or inflammatory eruptions or apply to the face or genitalia. Avoid contact with the eyes or mucous membranes. Use cautiously in patients with renal disease because renal abnormalities may occur.

Interactions

None reported.

Effects on diagnostic tests

None reported.

Adverse reactions

Skin: contact dermatitis, irritation, erythema, discoloration of hair or finger nails.
Other: excessive soreness, spread of psoriasis.
Note: Discontinue drug if sensitization develops.

Overdose and treatment
If accidental oral ingestion occurs, force fluids and contact local or regional poison information center.

☑ Special considerations
- Avoid use of drug on eyes and mucous membranes.
- Drug may stain skin, hair, and fabrics.
- Gloves may be worn when applying drug because drug may stain skin.
- Patients with renal disease and those having extensive or prolonged applications should have periodic urine tests for albuminuria.

Patient education
- Advise patient how to apply drug. At the end of the treatment period, patient should bathe or shower to remove excess cream.
- Tell patient that drug may stain skin, clothing, or bed linens a red-brown to purple-brown color. To prevent staining of clothing and linen, advise him to use protective dressings.
- Advise patient to avoid applying cream to uninvolved scalp areas when shampooing with anthralin.
- Tell patient to always wash hands thoroughly after use.
- Advise patient to avoid applying to normal skin by coating area surrounding lesion with petroleum jelly.
- Advise patient to decrease the frequency of application if redness develops on adjacent normal skin.

Pediatric use
- Safety and efficacy have not been established.

Breast-feeding
- Because drug may be excreted in breast milk, a decision should be made to discontinue breast-feeding or to discontinue the drug, depending on the importance of the drug to the mother.

antihemophilic factor (AHF)
Alphanate, Bioclate, Helixate, Hemofil M, Humate-P, Hyate C, Koate-HP, Kogenate, Monoclate-P, Profilate-HP, Recombinate

Pharmacologic classification: blood derivative
Therapeutic classification: antihemophilic
Pregnancy risk category C

How supplied
Available by prescription only
Injection: Vials, with diluent. Number of units on label. A porcine product is available for patients with congenital hemophilia A who have antibodies to human factor VIII:C.

Indications, route, and dosage
Hemophilia A (factor VIII deficiency)
Adults and children: Dosage is highly individualized and depends on patient weight, severity of deficiency, severity of hemorrhage, presence of inhibitors, and level of factor VIII desired.

One AHF unit equals the activity present in 1 ml normal pooled human plasma less than 1 hour old.

Do not confuse commercial product with blood bank-produced cryoprecipitated factor VIII from individual human donors.

AHF is designed for I.V. use only; use plastic syringe because solution adheres to glass surfaces.

Pharmacodynamics
Antihemophilic action: AHF replaces deficient clotting factor that converts prothrombin to thrombin.

Pharmacokinetics
- *Absorption:* AHF must be given parenterally for systemic effect.
- *Distribution:* AHF equilibrates intravascular and extravascular compartments; it does not readily cross placenta.
- *Metabolism:* AHF is cleared rapidly from plasma.
- *Excretion:* AHF is consumed during blood clotting. Half-life ranges from 4 to 24 hours (average 12 hours).

Contraindications and precautions
Contraindicated in patients with hypersensitivity to murine (mouse) protein or drug. Use cautiously in neonates, infants, and patients with hepatic disease.

Interactions
None significant.

Effects on diagnostic tests
None reported.

Adverse reactions
CV: tightness in chest.
GI: nausea.
Respiratory: wheezing.
Skin: *urticaria.*
Other: *chills, fever,* hypersensitivity reactions, (stinging at injection site, fever, ***anaphylaxis***), risk of hepatitis B and human immunodeficiency virus.

Overdose and treatment
Large or frequently repeated doses of AHF in patients with blood group A, B, or AB may cause intravascular hemolysis; monitor CBC and direct Coombs' test, and if intravascular hemolysis occurs, give serologically compatible type O RBCs.

☑ Special considerations
- Refrigerate concentrate until needed; before reconstituting, warm concentrate and diluent bottles to room temperature. To mix, gently roll vial between hands; do not shake or mix with other I.V. solutions. Keep product away from heat (but do not refrigerate because that may cause precipitation of active ingredient), and use within 3 hours.
- Take baseline pulse rate before I.V. administration. If pulse rate increases significantly during administration, flow rate should be reduced or drug discontinued. Adverse reactions are usually related to too-rapid infusion.

• Monitor coagulation studies before and during therapy; monitor vital signs regularly, and be alert for allergic reactions.
• Prophylactic oral diphenhydramine may be prescribed if patient has history of transient allergic reactions to AHF.
• All products are heat-treated by special method similar to pasteurization to decrease risk of transmitting hepatitis. Patient should be immunized with hepatitis B vaccine to decrease the risk of transmission of hepatitis.

Patient education
• Teach patient how to use, inject, and store prescribed product.
• Advise patient not to take salicylates or other drugs that inhibit platelet formation.

Pediatric use
• Administer cautiously to neonates and older infants because of susceptibility to hepatitis.

anti-inhibitor coagulant complex
Autoplex T, Feiba VH Immuno

Pharmacologic classification: activated prothrombin complex
Therapeutic classification: hemostatic
Pregnancy risk category C

How supplied
Available by prescription only
Injection: Number of units of factor VIII correctional activity indicated on label of vial

Indications, route, and dosage
Prevention and control of hemorrhagic episodes in some patients with hemophilia A in whom inhibitor antibodies to antihemophilic factor have developed; management of bleeding in patients with acquired hemophilia who have spontaneously acquired inhibitors to factor VIII
Adults and children: Dosage is highly individualized and varies among manufacturers. For Autoplex T, give 25 to 100 unit/kg I.V. depending on the severity of hemorrhage. If no hemostatic improvement occurs within 6 hours after initial administration, repeat dosage. For Feiba VH Immuno, give 50 to 100 unit/kg I.V. q 6 or 12 hours until patient shows signs of improvement. Maximum daily dosage of Feiba VH Immuno is 200 unit/kg.

Pharmacodynamics
Hemostatic action: Unknown. It has been suggested that efficacy of anti-inhibitor coagulant complex may be related in part to the presence of the activated factors, which leads to more complete factor X activation in conjunction with tissue factor, phospholipid, and ionic calcium and allows the coagulation process to proceed beyond those stages where factor VIII is needed.

Pharmacokinetics
• *Absorption:* Administered only I.V.
• *Distribution:* Unknown.
• *Metabolism:* Unknown.
• *Excretion:* Unknown.

Contraindications and precautions
Contraindicated in patients with signs of fibrinolysis or DIC and in those with normal coagulation mechanism. Use cautiously in patients with liver disease.

Interactions
Antifibrinolytic agents may alter the effects of anti-inhibitor coagulant complex. Do not use concomitantly.

Effects on diagnostic tests
None reported.

Adverse reactions
CNS: headache.
CV: changes in blood pressure, ***acute MI, thromboembolic events.***
GI: nausea, vomiting.
Hematologic: ***DIC.***
Skin: flushing, rash, urticaria.
Other: fever, chills, hypersensitivity reactions, risk of infection, including viral hepatitis B and HIV.

Overdose and treatment
None reported although high doses may predispose the patient to thromboembolic events. Monitor patient closely and treat symptomatically.

☑ Special considerations
• Administer hepatitis B vaccine before administering drug.
• Keep epinephrine readily available to treat anaphylaxis.
• I.V. use: Warm the drug and diluent to room temperature before reconstitution. Reconstitute according to manufacturer's directions. Use the filter needle provided by the manufacturer to withdraw the reconstituted anti-inhibitor coagulant complex solution from the vial into the syringe; the filter needle should then be replaced with a sterile injection needle for administration. Administer drug as soon as possible. Autoplex T infusions should be completed within 1 hour following reconstitution, Feiba VH Immuno infusions within 3 hours.
• The rate of administration should be individualized according to patient's response. Autoplex T infusions may begin at rate of 1 ml/minute; if well tolerated, may increase infusion rate gradually to 10 ml/minute. Feiba VH Immuno infusion rate should not exceed 2 U/kg.
• If flushing, lethargy, headache, transient chest discomfort, or changes in blood pressure or pulse rate develop because of rapid rate of infusion, stop drug. These symptoms usually disappear with cessation of infusion. Infusion may be resumed at a slower rate.
• Assess patient closely for hypersensitivity reactions.
• Monitor vital signs regularly.

Patient education
- Reassure patient that because of the manufacturing process, risk of transmission of HIV is extremely low.

Pediatric use
- Use with caution in neonates because of risk of thrombosis or hepatitis associated with use of drug.

antithrombin III (heparin cofactor I)
ATnativ, Thrombate III

Pharmacologic classification: glycoprotein
Therapeutic classification: anticoagulant, antithrombotic
Pregnancy risk category B

How supplied
Available by prescription only
Injection: 500 IU, 1,000 IU

Indications, route, and dosage
Prophylaxis and adjunct treatment of thromboembolism associated with hereditary antithrombin III deficiency
Adults, adolescents, and children: Initial dose is individualized to quantity required to increase antithrombin III activity to 120% of normal activity as determined 30 minutes after administration. Usual rate of infusion is 50 to 100 IU/minute I.V., not to exceed 100 IU/minute. Dose is calculated based on anticipated 1% increase in plasma antithrombin III activity produced by 1 IU/kg of body weight using the formula:

$$\text{Dose} = \frac{\left[\begin{matrix}\text{desired}\\ \text{level}\end{matrix} - \begin{matrix}\text{baseline}\\ \text{level}\end{matrix}\right] \times \begin{matrix}\text{body}\\ \text{weight}\\ \text{(kg)}\end{matrix}}{1.4\ \text{kg}}$$

Maintenance: Dose is individualized to quantity required to increase antithrombin III activity to 80% of normal activity and is administered at 24-hour intervals. Dose is calculated as follows:

$$\text{Dose} = \frac{\left[\begin{matrix}\text{desired}\\ \text{level}\end{matrix} - \begin{matrix}\text{baseline}\\ \text{level}\end{matrix}\right] \times \begin{matrix}\text{body}\\ \text{weight}\\ \text{(kg)}\end{matrix}}{\text{actual increase}}$$

produced by 1 IU/kg as determined 30 minutes after administration of initial dose.

Treatment is usually continued for 2 to 8 days except in pregnancy or when used with surgery or prolonged immobilization, when more prolonged administration may be needed.

Pharmacodynamics
Antithrombotic action: Administration of exogenous antithrombin III corrects hereditary antithrombin III deficiency, normalizing coagulation-inhibiting capability and inhibiting formation of thromboemboli. It also inactivates plasmin, but to a lesser extent than the clotting factor.

Pharmacokinetics
- *Absorption:* Drug is administered I.V.
- *Distribution:* Binding to epithelium and redistribution into the extravascular compartment removes antithrombin III from the blood. Special receptors on hepatocytes bind antithrombin III clotting factor complexes, rapidly removing them from circulation.
- *Metabolism:* Unknown.
- *Excretion:* Unknown.

Contraindications and precautions
No known contraindications. Use with extreme caution in children and neonates because safety has not been established.

Interactions
Concurrent administration with *heparin* increases the anticoagulant effect of both; heparin dosage reduction may be necessary.

Effects on diagnostic tests
Plasma levels of antithrombin III may be measured with clotting assays or amidolytic assays using synthetic chromogenic substrates. Immunoassays may not detect all congenital antithrombin III deficiencies.

Adverse reactions
CV: vasodilation, lowered blood pressure.
GU: diuresis.

Overdose and treatment
No information available. Patients with antithrombin III levels of 50% to 210% remained asymptomatic.

☑ Special considerations
- Transmission of viral disease by drug has not been reported to date.
- Determinations of antithrombin III activity should be performed twice daily until the dosage requirement has stabilized, then performed daily, immediately before dose. Functional assays are preferable because quantitative immunologic test results may be normal despite decreased drug activity.
- 1 IU is equivalent to the quantity of endogenous antithrombin III present in 1 ml of normal human plasma.
- Dyspnea and increased blood pressure may result from too-rapid administration (1,500 IU in 5 minutes).
- Heparin binds to antithrombin III lysine-binding sites in a 1:1 molar ratio, which results in increased efficacy of heparin.
- Drug is not recommended for long-term prophylaxis of thrombotic episodes.
- Store drug at 36° to 46° F (2° to 8° C).
- Reconstitute using 10 ml sterile water (provided), 0.9% NaCl, or 5% dextrose. *Do not shake vial.* Further dilution in same diluent solution is acceptable.
- Solutions should be at room temperature for administration and should be used within 3 hours of reconstitution.

Geriatric use
- No specific problems have been reported to date.

Pediatric use
- No specific problems have been reported to date.

Breast-feeding
- Distribution into breast milk is unlikely because of drug's large molecular size. No problems in breast-fed infants have been reported.

apraclonidine hydrochloride
Iopidine

Pharmacologic classification: alpha-adrenergic agonist
Therapeutic classification: ocular hypotensive
Pregnancy risk category C

How supplied
Available by prescription only
Ophthalmic solution: 0.5%, 1%

Indications, route, and dosage
Prevention or control of intraocular pressure elevations after argon laser trabeculoplasty or iridotomy
Adults: Instill 1 drop (1% solution) in the eye 1 hour before initiation of laser surgery on the anterior segment, then 1 drop immediately after surgery.
Short-term adjunctive therapy in patients on maximally tolerated medical therapy who require additional intraocular pressure reduction
Adults: Instill 1 to 2 drops (0.5% solution) in the eye t.i.d.
◊ ***Open-angle glaucoma***
Adults: Instill 1 drop (0.5% solution) in the eye b.i.d. or t.i.d.

Pharmacodynamics
Ocular hypotensive action: Apraclonidine is an alpha-adrenergic agonist that reduces intraocular pressure, possibly by decreasing aqueous humor production.

Pharmacokinetics
- *Absorption:* Onset of action is within 1 hour after instillation, and maximum effect on intraocular pressure reduction occurs in 3 to 5 hours.
- *Distribution:* No information available.
- *Metabolism:* No information available.
- *Excretion:* No information available.

Contraindications and precautions
Contraindicated in patients hypersensitive to apraclonidine or clonidine and in those on concurrent MAO inhibitor therapy. Use cautiously in patients with severe cardiac disease, including hypertension and vasovagal attacks.

Interactions
Topical *beta-adrenergic blocking agents* or *pilocarpine* may produce additive lowering of intraocular pressure.

Effects on diagnostic tests
None reported.

Adverse reactions
CNS: insomnia, irritability, dream disturbances, headache, irritability, paresthesia.
CV: bradycardia, vasovagal attack, palpitations, hypotension, orthostatic hypotension.
EENT: upper eyelid elevation, conjunctival blanching and microhemorrhage, mydriasis, eye burning or discomfort, foreign body sensation in eye, eye dryness and *itching, hyperemia,* conjunctivitis, blurred vision, nasal burning or dryness or increased pharyngeal secretions.
GI: abdominal pain, discomfort, diarrhea, vomiting, taste disturbances, dry mouth.
Skin: pruritus not associated with rash, sweaty palms.
Other: body heat sensation, decreased libido, extremity pain or numbness, allergic response.

Overdose and treatment
No information available.

☑ Special considerations
- Protect stored drug from light and freezing.

Patient education
- Warn patient about the potential for dizziness and drowsiness.

Pediatric use
- Safety and efficacy have not been established.

Breast-feeding
- There is no information regarding the excretion of apraclonidine in breast milk. Consider discontinuing breast-feeding on the day of surgery.

aprotinin
Trasylol

Pharmacologic classification: naturally occurring protease inhibitor
Therapeutic classification: systemic hemostatic
Pregnancy risk category B

How supplied
Available by prescription only
Injection: 10,000 kallikrein inactivator U (KIU)/ml (1.4 mg/ml)

Indications, route, and dosage
Prophylactic reduction of perioperative blood loss and the need for blood transfusion in patients undergoing cardiopulmonary bypass during repeat coronary artery bypass graft surgery or in selected patients undergoing initial coronary artery bypass graft surgery in whom the risk of bleeding is high because of impaired hemostasis or in whom transfusion is unavailable or unacceptable;* ◊ *surgery on aortic arch
Adults: Usual test dose is 10,000 KIU (1.4 mg) I.V.; if no adverse reactions occur within 10 minutes, give loading dose of 2 million KIU (280 mg) I.V. over 20 to 30 minutes while the patient is supine, after induction of anesthesia but before sternotomy; fol-

low loading dose with continuous I.V. infusion of 500,000 KIU/hour (70 mg/hour). Before cardiopulmonary bypass is initiated, 2 million KIU (280 mg) of aprotinin should be added to the priming fluid of the cardiopulmonary bypass circuit by replacement of an aliquot of the priming fluid.

Note: If an allergic reaction occurs during injection or infusion of aprotinin, drug administration should be discontinued immediately. Severe acute hypersensitivity reactions should be treated immediately with appropriate therapy (for example, epinephrine, corticosteroids, maintenance of adequate airway, oxygen, I.V. fluids, antihistamines, maintenance of blood pressure), as indicated.

Pharmacodynamics

Systemic hemostatic action: The precise mechanism by which aprotinin minimizes perioperative bleeding associated with coronary artery bypass graft surgery is unclear but appears to involve effects on platelet function as well as on coagulation and fibrinolysis. Aprotinin may improve hemostasis during and after cardiopulmonary bypass by preserving platelet membrane glycoproteins that maintain the adhesive and aggregative capacity of platelets. In addition, aprotinin inhibits fibrinolysis through inhibition of plasmin and plasma and tissue kallikreins. Because of its effects on kallikrein, aprotinin also inhibits activation of the intrinsic clotting system, a process that initiates coagulation and promotes fibrinolysis.

Pharmacokinetics

- *Absorption:* Not reported.
- *Distribution:* After I.V. injection, aprotinin is rapidly distributed into the total extracellular space, leading to a rapid initial decrease in plasma concentrations. After this phase, a plasma half-life of about 150 minutes is observed, followed by a terminal elimination phase with a half-life of about 10 hours.
- *Metabolism:* No information available.
- *Excretion:* After a single I.V. dose, from 25% to 40% is excreted in urine over 48 hours.

Contraindications and precautions

Contraindicated in patients hypersensitive to beef because drug is prepared from bovine lung.

Interactions

Concomitant use of aprotinin and *heparin* may result in greater prolongation of the whole blood-activated clotting time than heparin alone. However, aprotinin should not be used as a heparin-sparing agent. Aprotinin may inhibit the effects of *fibrinolytic agents.*

Effects on diagnostic tests

Because aprotinin inhibits contact activation of the intrinsic clotting system, therapy with the drug prolongs the results of coagulation assays that depend on contact activation, including the partial thromboplastin time and celite-activated clotting time (ACT) assays.

Aprotinin has resulted in elevated serum creatine levels postoperatively. In most cases, renal dysfunction was not severe and was reversible.

Drug may alter liver function studies and may block the acute hypotensive effect of captopril.

Adverse reactions

CNS: ***cerebral embolism, CVA.***
CV: ***cardiac arrest, heart failure, ventricular tachycardia, MI,*** heart block, *atrial fibrillation,* atrial flutter, hypotension, supraventricular tachycardia.
GU: nephrotoxicity, ***renal failure.***
Respiratory: pneumonia, respiratory disorder, apnea, asthma, dyspnea, ***pulmonary edema.***
Other: hypersensitivity reactions, ***anaphylaxis,*** fever, ***shock,*** sepsis, phlebitis, hemolysis.

Overdose and treatment

Maximum amount of drug that can be safely administered in single or multiple doses has not been determined. Doses up to 17.5 million KIU have been administered within 24 hours without apparent toxicity.

☑ Special considerations

- Aprotinin is recommended only for selected patients undergoing initial coronary artery bypass graft surgery because of the risks of anaphylaxis (should a second procedure be needed) and renal dysfunction associated with aprotinin therapy.
- Although a causal relationship has not been established, use of aprotinin therapy in patients undergoing deep hypothermic circulatory arrest during surgery of the aortic arch may be associated with an increased risk of adverse renal effects or death compared with age-matched historical controls.
- Aprotinin is administered by I.V. injection and I.V. infusion through a central venous line; drug also is added to the priming fluid of the cardiopulmonary bypass circuit. No other drug should be administered concomitantly with aprotinin in the same I.V. line. Rapid I.V. administration of large (loading) doses of aprotinin should be avoided because of the potential for hypotension or anaphylactoid reactions.
- Dosage and potency of aprotinin usually are expressed in KIU, but mg also has been used; 1 mg of drug has a potency of approximately 7,143 KIU.
- Use with caution when administering aprotinin (even in test doses) to patients with prior exposure to drug because of risk of anaphylaxis. In such patients, I.V. administration of an antihistamine shortly before administration of the loading dose of aprotinin is recommended. Patients who experience an allergic reaction to the test dose should not receive additional doses.
- Even after uneventful administration of the test dose or in patients without previous exposure to aprotinin, the full therapeutic dose of aprotinin may cause anaphylaxis.
- A dosage reduction may be necessary in patients with renal failure. Liver damage occurs as often as renal damage.

Pediatric use

- Safety and efficacy in children under age 18 have not been established.

arbutamine hydrochloride
GenESA

Pharmacologic classification: adrenergic agonist
Therapeutic classification: sympathomimetic diagnostic aid
Pregnancy risk category B

How supplied
Available by prescription only
Injection: 20-ml prefilled syringe containing a total of 1 mg (0.05 mg/ml)

Indications, route, and dosage
Single-dose diagnostic aid in patients with suspected coronary artery disease (CAD) who cannot exercise adequately (stress induction with arbutamine is indicated as an aid in diagnosing the presence or absence of CAD)
Adults: Dose is calculated and delivered via the GenESA Device, a closed-loop, computer-controlled, I.V. infusion device. This device initially delivers 0.1 mcg/kg/minute for 1 minute and adjusts dose until maximal heart rate limit (target heart rate set by user) is achieved or to maximum infusion rate of 0.8 mcg/kg/minute (maximum total dose 10 mcg/kg).

Pharmacodynamics
Sympathomimetic diagnostic aid action: By increasing cardiac work through positive chronotropic and inotropic actions, arbutamine acts as a cardiac stress agent to mimic exercise and provoke myocardial ischemia in patients with compromised coronary arteries. Beta-agonist activity provides cardiac stress by increasing heart rate, contractility and systolic blood pressure; alpha-receptor activity decreases the potential for hypotension.

Pharmacokinetics
- *Absorption:* Onset of effect on heart rate is approximately 1 minute after initiation of infusion. Drug is not orally bioavailable.
- *Distribution:* Due to sensitivity limitations of drug assay, pharmacokinetics have been characterized for first 20 to 30 minutes after stopping infusion. Apparent volume of distribution is 0.74 L/kg and plasma half-life is approximately 8 minutes. Drug is 58% bound to plasma proteins.
- *Metabolism:* Metabolized hepatically to methoxyarbutamine.
- *Excretion:* Drug is 75% eliminated by metabolism to methoxyarbutamine, which is then excreted in either a free or conjugated form in the urine. After I.V. infusion, 84% of total dose is excreted in the urine and 9% in the feces within 48 hours.

Contraindications and precautions
Contraindicated in patients with idiopathic hypertrophic subaortic stenosis, history of recurrent sustained ventricular tachycardia, heart failure (New York Heart Association class III or IV), or known hypersensitivity to drug.

Also contraindicated in patients with an implanted cardiac pacemaker or automated cardioverter or defibrillator. Drug contains sodium metabisulfite, a sulfite that may produce an allergic response in susceptible patients.

Avoid use of drug in patients with unstable angina, mechanical left ventricular outflow obstruction (such as severe valvular aortic stenosis), uncontrolled systemic hypertension, cardiac transplant, history of cerebrovascular disease, angle-closure glaucoma, or uncontrolled hyperthyroidism or in those receiving class I agents such as quinidine, lidocaine, or flecaninide.

Interactions
Beta-blocking agents may attenuate arbutamine's effects and should be discontinued at least 48 hours before administration of arbutamine. *Digoxin, atropine, other cholinergic drugs,* and *tricyclic antidepressents* should not be given with arbutamine.

Effect on diagnostic tests
None reported.

Adverse reactions
CNS: anxiety, dizziness, fatigue, headache, hypoesthesia, pain, paresthesia, *tremor.*
CV: *angina pectoris,* **ARRHYTHMIAS,** chest pain, flushing, hypotension, hot flashes, palpitation, vasodilatation.
GI: nausea.
EENT: dry mouth, taste perversion.
Respiratory: dyspnea.
Skin: increased sweating.

Overdose and treatment
Risk of drug overdose is low, given the rapid onset and short half-life of drug and controlled administration. Symptoms of overdose are those of catecholamine excess, such as tremor, headache, flushing, hypotension, dizziness, paresthesia, nausea, hot flashes, angina, increased sweating and anxiety, tachyarrhythmias, hypertension, MI, and ventricular fibrillation.

Management of overdose should include cessation of infusion, establishment of an airway, and adequate oxygenation. Severe signs and symptoms may be treated with I.V. beta blocker such as metoprolol (7.5 to 50 mg), esmolol (10 to 80 mg), or propranolol (0.5 to 2 mg). Sublingual nitrates should be considered if clinically appropriate.

Special considerations
- Monitor blood pressure, heart rate and a diagnostic quality ECG continuously throughout drug infusion with cardiac emergency supplies available.
- Do not dilute drug and administer only via the prefilled syringe using the GenESA Device.
- Before using the GenESA Device, it is essential to read and understand the manufacturer's directions for use.
- Transient prolongation of corrected QT interval, as measured from surface ECG, occurs with administration. However, this does not appear to be associated with an increased incidence of arrhythmias.

• Transient reductions in serum potassium concentrations can occur but rarely to hypokalemic levels.
• Do not administer atropine to enhance drug-induced chronotropic response; coadministration may lead to tachyarrhythmias.
• Safety and efficacy of drug in patients with recent history (within 30 days) of an MI have not been evaluated; do not use drug in these patients.

Patient education
• Tell patient to discontinue use of beta-blocking agents at least 48 hours before test.

Breast-feeding
• It is unknown if drug occurs in breast milk; avoid use in breast-feeding patients.

ardeparin sodium
Normiflo

Pharmacologic classification: low-molecular-weight heparin
Therapeutic classification: anticoagulant
Pregnancy risk category C

How supplied
Available by prescription only
Injection: 5,000 anti-factor Xa U/0.5 ml, 10,000 anti-factor Xa U/0.5 ml

Indications, route, and dosage
Prevention of deep venous thrombosis which may lead to pulmonary embolism following knee replacement surgery
Adults: 50 anti-factor Xa U/kg S.C. q 12 hours for 14 days or until patient is ambulatory, whichever is shorter. Give initial dose the evening of day of surgery or the following morning.

Pharmacodynamics
Anticoagulant activity: Ardeparin is a low-molecular-weight heparin that binds to and accelerates the activity of antithrombin III. This results in an inactivation of factor Xa and thrombin, which prevents the formation of clots. Ardeparin also inhibits thrombin by binding to heparin cofactor II.

Pharmacokinetics
• *Absorption:* Mean peak plasma anti-factor Xa and anti-factor IIa activity is obtained in approximately 3 hours after S.C. injection. Mean absolute bioavailability based on anti-factor Xa activity is 92%.
• *Distribution:* Steady state volume of distribution based on anti-factor Xa activity is approximately 99 ml/kg.
• *Metabolism:* Information not available.
• *Excretion:* Elimination half-life based on anti-factor Xa activity is approximately 3 hours

Contraindications and precautions
Contraindicated in patients with known hypersensitivity to drug, active bleeding, or thrombocytopenia associated with antiplatelet antibodies in the presence of drug. Do not use in patients with known hypersensitivity to pork products.

Use with extreme caution in patients with history of heparin-induced thrombocytopenia and in those with a known hypersensitivity to methylparaben, propylparaben, and sulfites. Use cautiously in patients at increased risk for hemorrhage (bacterial endocarditis) and in those with congenital or acquired bleeding disorders; active ulcerative disease; angiodysplastic GI disease; hemorrhagic stroke; recent eye, spinal, or brain surgery or procedures; severe uncontrolled hypertension; or in patients treated concomitantly with platelet inhibitors. When epidural or spinal anesthesia or spinal puncture is used, patients who are anticoagulated or scheduled to be anticoagulated with low-molecular-weight heparins are at risk of developing epidural or spinal hematomas, which can result in long-term paralysis.

Interactions
Concomitant use of ardeparin with *anticoagulants* and *antiplatelet agents* (including *aspirin, NSAIDs*) increases risk of bleeding.

Effects on diagnostic tests
Ardeparin may decrease platelet count and increase transaminase and serum triglyceride levels.

Adverse reactions
CNS: dizziness, headache, ***CVA,*** insomnia.
CV: chest pain, peripheral edema.
GI: nausea, vomiting.
Hematologic: anemia, ecchymosis, ***hemorrhage, thrombocytopenia,*** hematoma (at injection site)
Skin: pruritus, rash, local reaction.
Other: arthralgia, fever, pain.

Overdose and treatment
Bleeding is the principal sign of ardeparin overdose. Most bleeding can be stopped by discontinuing the drug and applying pressure to the site and replacing hemostatic blood elements if necessary. Protamine sulfate can also be administered. Dose of protamine should be equal to the dose of ardeparin administered (1 mg of protamine neutralizes 100 anti-factor Xa U of ardeparin). If bleeding persists after 2 hours, blood should be drawn and residual anti-factor Xa levels determined. Additional protamine can be administered if clinically important bleeding persists or anti-factor Xa levels remain high. Drug does not appear to be dialyzable.

☑ Special considerations
• Base dosing on actual body weight.
• Ardeparin cannot be used interchangeably (unit for unit) with heparin sodium or other low-molecular-weight heparins.
• Routinely monitor CBC, platelet counts, urinalysis and occult blood in stools throughout therapy. Routine monitoring of coagulation parameters is not required.
• Do not mix with other injections or infusions.
• With patient sitting or lying down, administer drug with deep S.C. injection in the abdomen, avoiding the navel, outer aspect of upper arm, or anterior

thigh. Extrude air and excess medication before administration. The full length of the needle should be introduced into the skin fold held between the thumb and forefinger. Hold skin fold throughout the injection. Rotate injection site.
• Do not give drug I.M to avoid possible occurrence of hematoma at the injection site.

Patient education
• Instruct patient to report abnormal bruising, bleeding, or dark stools.
• Instruct patient to observe for hematoma at injection site.
• Tell patient to avoid use of OTC medications such as aspirin or NSAIDs.

Geriatric use
• No significant difference was seen in patients over age 65 compared with those under age 65.

Pediatric use
• Safety and effectiveness in children have not been established.

Breast-feeding
• It is not known if drug is excreted in breast milk. Use cautiously when administering to breast-feeding patients.

ascorbic acid (vitamin C)
Ascorbicap, Cebid Timecelles, Cecon, Cemill, Cetane, Cevalin, Cevi-Bid, Ce-Vi-Sol, C-Span, Dull-C, Flavorcee

Pharmacologic classification: water-soluble vitamin
Therapeutic classification: vitamin
Pregnancy risk category A (C if exceeds RDA)

How supplied
Available by prescription only
Injection: 100 mg/ml in 2-ml and 10-ml ampules; 250 mg/ml in 10-ml ampules and 10-ml, 30-ml, and 50-ml vials; 500 mg/ml in 2-ml and 5-ml ampules and 50-ml vials; 500 mg/ml (with monothioglycerol) in 1-ml ampules

Available without a prescription
Tablets: 25 mg, 50 mg, 100 mg, 250 mg, 500 mg, 1,000 mg, 1,500 mg
Tablets (effervescent, sugar-free): 1,000 mg
Tablets (chewable): 100 mg, 250 mg, 500 mg
Tablets (timed-release): 500 mg, 750 mg, 1,000 mg, 1,500 mg
Capsules (timed-release): 500 mg
Crystals: 100 g (4 g/tsp), 1,000 g (4 g/tsp, sugar-free)
Powder: 100 g (4 g/tsp), 500 g (4 g/tsp), 1,000 g (4 g/tsp, sugar-free)
Liquid: 50 ml (35 mg/0.6 ml)
Solution: 50 ml (100 mg/ml)
Syrup: 20 mg/ml in 120 ml and 480 ml; 500 mg/5 ml in 5 ml, 10 ml, 120 ml, and 473 ml

Indications, route, and dosage
Frank and subclinical scurvy
Adults: 100 to 250 mg, depending on severity, P.O., S.C., I.M., or I.V. daily or b.i.d., then at least 50 mg/day for maintenance.
Children: 100 to 300 mg, depending on severity, P.O., S.C., I.M., or I.V. daily, then at least 35 mg/day for maintenance.
Infants: 50 to 100 mg P.O., I.M., I.V., or S.C. daily.
Prevention of ascorbic acid deficiency in those with poor nutritional habits or increased requirements
Adults: 45 to 60 mg P.O., S.C., I.M., or I.V. daily.
Pregnant or breast-feeding women: At least 60 to 80 mg P.O., S.C., I.M., or I.V. daily.
Children and infants over age 2 weeks: At least 20 to 50 mg P.O., S.C., I.M., or I.V. daily.
◊ ***Potentiation of methenamine in urine acidification***
Adults: 4 to 12 g daily in divided doses.
◊ ***Adjunctive therapy in the treatment of idiopathic methemoglobinemia***
Adults: 300 to 600 mg P.O. daily in divided doses.

Pharmacodynamics
Nutritional action: Ascorbic acid, an essential vitamin, is involved with the biologic oxidations and reductions used in cellular respiration. It is essential for the formation and maintenance of intracellular ground substance and collagen. In the body, ascorbic acid is reversibly oxidized to dehydroascorbic acid and influences tyrosine metabolism, conversion of folic acid to folinic acid, carbohydrate metabolism, resistance to infections, and cellular respiration. Ascorbic acid deficiency causes scurvy, a condition marked by degenerative changes in the capillaries, bone, and connective tissues. Restoring adequate ascorbic acid intake completely reverses symptoms of ascorbic acid deficiency. Data regarding use of ascorbic acid as a urinary acidifier are conflicting.

Pharmacokinetics
• *Absorption:* After oral administration, ascorbic acid is absorbed readily. After very large doses, absorption may be limited because absorption is an active process. Absorption also may be reduced in patients with diarrhea or GI diseases. Normal plasma concentrations of ascorbic acid are about 10 to 20 mcg/ml. Plasma concentrations below 1.5 mcg/ml are associated with scurvy. However, leukocyte concentrations (although not usually measured) may better reflect ascorbic acid tissue saturation. Approximately 1.5 g of ascorbic acid is stored in the body. Within 3 to 5 months of ascorbic acid deficiency, clinical signs of scurvy become evident.
• *Distribution:* Distributed widely in the body, with large concentrations found in the liver, leukocytes, platelets, glandular tissues, and lens of the eye. Ascorbic acid crosses the placenta; cord blood concentrations are usually two to four times the maternal blood concentrations. Ascorbic acid is distributed into breast milk.
• *Metabolism:* Metabolized in the liver.
• *Excretion:* Ascorbic acid is reversibly oxidized to dehydroascorbic acid. Some is metabolized to in-

active compounds that are excreted in urine. The renal threshold is approximately 14 mcg/ml. When the body is saturated and blood concentrations exceed the threshold, unchanged ascorbic acid is excreted in urine. Renal excretion is directly proportional to blood concentrations. Ascorbic acid is also removed by hemodialysis.

Contraindications and precautions
No known contraindications. Use cautiously in patients with renal insufficiency.

Interactions
Concomitant use of ascorbic acid with *acidic drugs* in large doses (more than 2 g/day) may lower urine pH, causing renal tubular reabsorption of acidic drugs. Conversely, concomitant use with *basic drugs* (for example, *amphetamines* or *tricyclic antidepressants*) may cause decreased reabsorption and therapeutic effect.

Concurrent use of ascorbic acid with *sulfonamides* may cause crystallization. Concomitant use with *iron* maintains it in the ferrous state and increases *iron* absorption in the GI tract, but this increase may not be significant. A combination of 30 mg of *iron* with 200 mg of ascorbic acid is sometimes recommended.

Concomitant use of ascorbic acid with *dicumarol* influences the intensity and duration of the anticoagulant effect; use with *warfarin* may inhibit the anticoagulant effect; use with *ethinyl estradiol* may increase plasma levels of *ethinyl estradiol.*

Smoking may decrease serum ascorbic acid levels, thus increasing dosage requirements of this vitamin.

Salicylates inhibit ascorbic acid uptake by leukocytes and platelets. Although no evidence exists that *salicylates* precipitate ascorbic acid deficiency, patients receiving high doses of *salicylates* with ascorbic acid supplements must be observed for symptoms of ascorbic acid deficiency.

Effects on diagnostic tests
Ascorbic acid is a strong reducing agent; it alters results of tests that are based on oxidation-reduction reactions. Large doses of ascorbic acid (over 500 mg) may cause false-negative glucose determinations using the glucose oxidase method, or false-positive results using the copper reduction method or Benedict's reagent.

Ascorbic acid should not be used for 48 to 72 hours before an amine-dependent test for occult blood in the stool is conducted. A false-negative result may occur.

Depending on the reagents used, ascorbic acid may also cause interactions with other diagnostic tests.

Adverse reactions
CNS: faintness, dizziness (with too-rapid I.V. administration).
GI: diarrhea.
GU: acid urine, oxaluria, renal calculi.
Other: discomfort at injection site.

Overdose and treatment
Excessively high doses of parenteral ascorbic acid are excreted renally after tissue saturation and rarely accumulate. Serious adverse effects or toxicity are uncommon. Severe effects require discontinuation of therapy.

☑ Special considerations
- Administer large doses of ascorbic acid (1,000 mg/day) in divided amounts because the body uses only a limited amount and excretes the rest in urine. Large doses may increase small-intestine pH and impair vitamin B_{12} absorption. The recommended RDA of ascorbic acid is as follows:

Adults: 60 mg/day
Smokers: 100 mg/day
Infants and children: 30 mg/day
Patients on chronic hemodialysis: 100 to 200 mg/day

- Administer oral solutions of ascorbic acid directly into the mouth or mix with food. Effervescent tablets should be dissolved in a glass of water immediately before ingestion.
- Administer I.V. solution slowly.
- Conditions that elevate the metabolic rate (hyperthyroidism, fever, infection, burns and other severe trauma, postoperative states, neoplastic disease, and chronic alcoholism) significantly increase ascorbic acid requirements.
- Reportedly, patients taking oral contraceptives require ascorbic acid supplements.
- Smokers appear to have increased requirements for ascorbic acid because the vitamin is oxidized and excreted more rapidly than in nonsmokers.
- Use ascorbic acid cautiously in patients with renal insufficiency because the vitamin is normally excreted in urine.
- Persons whose diets are chemically deficient in fruits and vegetables can develop subclinical ascorbic acid deficiency. Observe for such deficiency in elderly and indigent patients, patients on restricted diets, those receiving long-term treatment with I.V. fluids or hemodialysis, and drug addicts or alcoholics.
- Overt symptoms of ascorbic acid deficiency include irritability; emotional disturbances; general debility; pallor; anorexia; sensitivity to touch; limb and joint pain; follicular hyperkeratosis (particularly on thighs and buttocks); easy bruising; petechiae; bloody diarrhea; delayed healing; loosening of teeth; sensitive, swollen, and bleeding gums; and anemia.
- Protect ascorbic acid solutions from light.

Patient education
- Teach patient about good dietary sources of ascorbic acid, such as citrus fruits, leafy vegetables, tomatoes, green peppers, and potatoes.
- Inform patient to cover foods and fruit juices tightly and to use them promptly.
- Advise patients with ascorbic acid deficiency to decrease or stop smoking. Replacement ascorbic acid dosages are greater for the smoker.
- Tell patients who are prone to renal calculi, who have diabetes, who are undergoing tests for occult blood in stools, or who are on sodium-restricted di-

ets or anticoagulant therapy to avoid high doses of ascorbic acid.

Pediatric use

- Infants fed on cow's milk alone require supplemental ascorbic acid.

Breast-feeding

- Administer with caution to breast-feeding women because ascorbic acid is distributed into breast milk.

asparaginase

Elspar

Pharmacologic classification: enzyme (L-asparagine amidohydrolase) (cell cycle-phase specific, G1 phase)
Therapeutic classification: antineoplastic
Pregnancy risk category C

How supplied

Available by prescription only
Injection: 10,000-IU vials

Indications, route, and dosage

Dosage and indications may vary. Check current literature for recommended protocol.

Acute lymphocytic leukemia

Adults and children: When used alone, 200 IU/kg daily I.V. for 28 days. When used in combination with other chemotherapeutic agents, dosage is highly individualized.

Pharmacodynamics

Antineoplastic action: Asparaginase exerts its cytotoxic activity by inactivating the amino acid asparagine, which is required by tumor cells to synthesize proteins. Because the tumor cells cannot synthesize their own asparagine, protein synthesis and eventually synthesis of DNA and RNA are inhibited.

Pharmacokinetics

- *Absorption:* Drug is not absorbed across the GI tract after oral administration; therefore, it must be given I.V. or I.M.
- *Distribution:* Drug distributes primarily within the intravascular space, with detectable concentrations in the thoracic and cervical lymph. Drug crosses the blood-brain barrier to a minimal extent.
- *Metabolism:* Metabolic fate of asparaginase is unclear; hepatic sequestration by the reticuloendothelial system may occur.
- *Excretion:* Plasma elimination half-life, which is not related to dose, sex, age, or hepatic or renal function, ranges from 8 to 30 hours.

Contraindications and precautions

Contraindicated in patients with pancreatitis or history of pancreatitis and previous hypersensitivity unless desensitized. Use cautiously in patients with hepatic dysfunction.

Interactions

Concomitant use of asparaginase with *methotrexate* decreases the effectiveness of *methotrexate* because asparaginase destroys the actively replicating cells that *methotrexate* requires for its cytotoxic action. Concomitant use of asparaginase and *vincristine* can cause additive neuropathy and disturbances of erythropoiesis. When asparaginase is used with *prednisone*, hyperglycemia may result from an additive effect on the pancreas.

Effects on diagnostic tests

Asparaginase therapy alters the results of thyroid function tests by decreasing concentrations of serum thyroxine-binding globulin.

Adverse reactions

CNS: confusion, drowsiness, depression, hallucinations, ***intracranial hemorrhage,*** fatigue, ***coma,*** agitation, headache, lethargy, somnolence.
GI: *vomiting, anorexia, nausea,* cramps, weight loss.
GU: *azotemia,* ***renal failure,*** glycosuria, polyuria.
Hematologic: ***anemia, hypofibrinogenemia,*** depression of other clotting factors, ***leukopenia.***
Hepatic: elevated AST and ALT levels, ***hepatotoxicity.***
Skin: *rash, urticaria,* hypersensitivity reactions.
Other: **HEMORRHAGIC PANCREATITIS, ANAPHYLAXIS,** chills, ***death, fatal hyperthermia,*** fever, *hyperglycemia.*

Overdose and treatment

Clinical manifestations of overdose include nausea and diarrhea. Treatment is generally supportive and includes antiemetics and antidiarrheals.

☑ Special considerations

- Reconstitute drug for I.M. administration with 2 ml unpreserved 0.9% NaCl or sterile water for injection. Do not use if precipate forms.
- I.M. injections should not contain more than 2 ml per injection. Multiple injections may be used for each dose.
- For I.V. administration: Reconstitute with 5 ml of sterile water for injection or NaCl injection. Solution will be clear or slightly cloudy. May further dilute with NaCl injection or D_5W and administer I.V. over 30 minutes. Filtration through a 5-micron inline filter during administration removes particulate matter that may develop on standing; filtration through a 0.22-micron filter results in a loss of potency. Do not use if precipitate forms.
- Shake vial gently when reconstituting. Vigorous shaking results in a decrease of potency.
- Refrigerate unopened dry powder. Reconstituted solution should be used within 8 hours.
- Do not use as sole agent to induce remission unless combination therapy is inappropriate. Not recommended for maintenance therapy.
- Drug should be administered in hospital settings with close supervision.
- I.V. administration of asparaginase with or immediately before vincristine or prednisone may increase toxicity reactions.

• Conduct skin test before initial dose. Observe site for 1 hour. Erythema and wheal formation indicate a positive reaction.
• Risk of hypersensitivity increases with repeated doses. Patient may be desensitized, but this does not rule out risk of allergic reactions. Routine administration of 2-unit intradermal test dose may identify high-risk patients.
• Because of vomiting, patient may need parenteral fluids for 24 hours or until oral fluids are tolerated.
• Monitor CBC and bone marrow function. Bone marrow regeneration may take 5 to 6 weeks.
• Obtain frequent serum amylase determinations to check pancreatic status. If elevated, asparaginase should be discontinued.
• Tumor lysis can result in uric acid nephropathy. Prevent occurrence by increasing fluid intake. Allopurinol should be started before therapy begins.
• Watch for signs of bleeding.
• Monitor blood glucose and test urine before and during therapy. Watch for signs of hyperglycemia, such as glycosuria and polyuria.
• Keep epinephrine, diphenhydramine, and I.V. corticosteroids available for treatment of anaphylaxis.

Patient education
• Encourage patient to maintain adequate intake of fluids to increase urine output and facilitate excretion of uric acid.
• Tell patient that because drowsiness may occur during therapy or for several weeks after treatment has ended, he should avoid hazardous activities requiring mental alertness.

Pediatric use
• Drug toxicity appears to be less severe in children than adults.

Breast-feeding
• It is not known if drug occurs into breast milk. However, because of the potential for serious adverse reactions and carcinogenicity in the infant, breast-feeding is not recommended.

aspirin
A.S.A., Ascriptin, Aspergum, Bufferin, Buffinol, Ecotrin, Empirin, Entrophen, Halfprin, Novasen*, ZORprin

Pharmacologic classification: salicylate
Therapeutic classification: nonnarcotic analgesic, antipyretic, anti-inflammatory, antiplatelet
Pregnancy risk category D

How supplied
Available by prescription only
Tablets (enteric-coated): 975 mg
Tablets (extended-release): 800 mg
Tablets (effervescent): 325 mg, 500 mg

Available without a prescription
Tablets: 65 mg, 81 mg, 325 mg (5 grains), 500 mg, 600 mg, 650 mg
Tablets (enteric-coated): 165 mg, 325 mg, 500 mg, 650 mg
Tablets (extended-release): 650 mg
Capsules: 325 mg, 500 mg
Chewing gum: 227.5 mg
Suppositories: 60 mg, 65 mg, 125 mg, 130 mg, 195 mg, 200 mg, 300 mg, 325 mg, 600 mg, 650 mg, 1.2 g

Indications, route, and dosage
Arthritis
Adults: 3.6 to 5.4 g P.O. daily in divided doses.
Children: 80 to 130 mg/kg P.O. daily in divided doses.
Mild pain or fever
Adults: 325 to 650 mg P.O. or P.R. q 4 hours, p.r.n.
Mild pain
Children: 65 mg/kg P.O. or P.R. daily divided q 4 to 6 hours, p.r.n.
Transient ischemic attacks and thromboembolic disorders
Adults: 650 mg P.O. b.i.d. or 325 mg q.i.d.
Reduction of the risk of heart attack in patients with previous MI or unstable angina
Adults: 160 to 325 mg P.O once daily.
Treatment of Kawasaki (mucocutaneous lymph node) syndrome
Adults: 80 to 100 mg/kg P.O. daily in four divided doses. Some patients may require up to 120 mg/kg daily to maintain acceptable serum salicylate concentrations of over 200 mcg/ml during the febrile phase. After the fever subsides, reduce dosage to 3 to 8 mg/kg once daily. Therapy is usually continued for 6 to 10 weeks.
Rheumatic fever
Adults: 4.9 to 7.8 g P.O. daily divided q 4 to 6 hours for 1 to 2 weeks; then decrease to 60 to 70 mg/kg daily for 1 to 6 weeks; then gradually withdraw over 1 to 2 weeks.
Children: 90 to 130 mg/kg P.O. daily divided q 4 to 6 hours.

Pharmacodynamics
Analgesic action: Aspirin produces analgesia by an ill-defined effect on the hypothalamus (central action) and by blocking generation of pain impulses (peripheral action). The peripheral action may involve blocking of prostaglandin synthesis via inhibition of cyclo-oxygenase enzyme.

Anti-inflammatory effects: Although the exact mechanism is unknown, aspirin is believed to inhibit prostaglandin synthesis; it may also inhibit the synthesis or action of other mediators of inflammation.

Antipyretic effect: Aspirin relieves fever by acting on the hypothalamic heat-regulating center to produce peripheral vasodilation. This increases peripheral blood supply and promotes sweating, which leads to loss of heat and to cooling by evaporation.

Anticoagulant effects: At low doses, aspirin appears to impede clotting by blocking prostaglandin synthetase action, which prevents formation of the platelet-aggregating substance thromboxane A_2. This interference with platelet activity is irreversible and can prolong bleeding time. However, at high doses, aspirin interferes with prostacyclin production, a potent vasoconstrictor and inhibitor of platelet aggregation, possibly negating its anticlotting properties.

Pharmacokinetics

- *Absorption:* Aspirin is absorbed rapidly and completely from the GI tract. Therapeutic blood salicylate concentrations for analgesia and anti-inflammatory effect are 150 to 300 mcg/ml; responses vary with the patient.
- *Distribution:* Aspirin is distributed widely into most body tissues and fluids. Protein-binding to albumin is concentration dependent, ranges from 75% to 90%, and decreases as serum concentration increases. Severe toxic effects may occur at serum concentrations greater than 400 mcg/ml.
- *Metabolism:* Aspirin is hydrolyzed partially in the GI tract to salicylic acid with almost complete metabolism in the liver.
- *Excretion:* Excreted in urine as salicylate and its metabolites. Elimination half-life ranges from 15 to 20 minutes.

Contraindications and precautions

Contraindicated in patients with hypersensitivity to drug, G6PD deficiency, bleeding disorders such as hemophilia, von Willebrand's disease, or telangiectasia. Also contraindicated in patients with NSAID-induced sensitivity reactions or in children with chickenpox or flulike symptoms.

Use cautiously in patients with GI lesions, impaired renal function, hypoprothrombinemia, vitamin K deficiency, thrombotic thrombocytopenic purpura, or hepatic impairment.

Interactions

When used concomitantly, *anticoagulants* and *thrombolytic drugs* may to some degree potentiate the platelet-inhibiting effects of aspirin. Concomitant use of aspirin with drugs that are highly protein-bound (*phenytoin, sulfonylureas, warfarin*) may cause displacement of either drug and adverse effects. Monitor therapy closely for both drugs. Concomitant use with other GI-irritant drugs such as *alcohol, steroids, antibiotics,* and other *NSAIDs* may potentiate the adverse GI effects of the aspirin. Use together with caution. Concomitant use with other ototoxic drugs, such as *aminoglycosides, bumetanide, capreomycin, ethacrynic acid, furosemide, cisplatin, vancomycin,* or *erythromycin,* may potentiate ototoxic effects. Aspirin decreases renal clearance of *lithium carbonate,* thus increasing serum lithium levels and the risk of adverse effects. Aspirin is antagonistic to the uricosuric effect of *phenylbutazone, probenecid,* and *sulfinpyrazone.*

Ammonium chloride and other *urine acidifiers* increase aspirin blood levels; monitor for aspirin toxicity. *Antacids* in high doses, and other *urine alkalizers,* decrease aspirin blood levels; monitor for decreased salicylate effect. *Corticosteroids* enhance aspirin elimination. *Food* and *antacids* delay and decrease absorption of aspirin.

Effects on diagnostic tests

Aspirin will cause an increased bleeding time. Aspirin interferes with urinary glucose analysis performed with Diastix, Chemstrip uG, glucose enzymatic test strip, Clinitest, and Benedict's solution, and with urinary 5-hydroxyindoleacetic acid and vanillylmandelic acid tests. Serum uric acid levels may be falsely increased. Aspirin may interfere with the Gerhardt test for urine acetoacetic acid.

Adverse reactions

EENT: *tinnitus, hearing loss.*
GI: *nausea, GI distress, occult bleeding, dyspepsia,* ***GI bleeding.***
Hematologic: leukopenia, ***thrombocytopenia,*** *prolonged bleeding time.*
Hepatic: abnormal liver function studies, hepatitis.
Skin: *rash,* bruising, urticaria, angioedema.
Other: hypersensitivity reactions (***anaphylaxis,*** asthma), ***Reye's syndrome.***

Overdose and treatment

Clinical manifestations of overdose include GI discomfort, oliguria, acute renal failure, hyperthermia, EEG abnormalities, and restlessness as well as metabolic acidosis with respiratory alkalosis, hyperpnea, and tachypnea because of increased CO_2 production and direct stimulation of the respiratory center.

To treat aspirin overdose, empty the patient's stomach immediately by inducing emesis with ipecac syrup if patient is conscious, or by gastric lavage. Administer activated charcoal via nasogastric tube. Provide symptomatic and supportive measures (respiratory support and correction of fluid and electrolyte imbalances). Closely monitor laboratory parameters and vital signs. Enhance renal excretion by administering sodium bicarbonate to alkalinize urine. Use cooling blanket or sponging if patient's rectal temperature is more than 104° F (40° C). Hemodialysis is effective in removing aspirin, but is only used in severely poisoned individuals or those at risk for pulmonary edema.

☑ Special considerations

Besides those relevant to all *salicylates,* consider the following recommendations.

- Enteric-coated products are absorbed slowly and are not suitable for acute therapy. They are ideal for long-term therapy such as for arthritis.
- There is no evidence that aspirin reduces the incidence of transient ischemic attacks in women.
- Avoid giving effervescent aspirin preparations to sodium-restricted patients.
- Stop aspirin therapy 1 week before elective surgery, if possible.
- Moisture may cause aspirin to lose potency. Store in a cool, dry place, and avoid using if tablets smell like vinegar.

Patient education

- Tell parents to keep aspirin out of children's reach; encourage use of child-resistant closures because aspirin is a leading cause of poisoning.
- Advise patients receiving high-dose, long-term aspirin therapy to watch for petechiae, bleeding gums, and signs of GI bleeding.
- Instruct patient to avoid use of aspirin if allergic to tartrazine dye.

• Tell patient to take drug with food or after meals to avoid GI upset.

Geriatric use

• Patients older than age 60 may be more susceptible to the toxic effects of aspirin. Use with caution.
• Effects of aspirin on renal prostaglandins may cause fluid retention and edema, a significant drawback for elderly patients and those with heart failure.

Pediatric use

• Because of epidemiologic association with Reye's syndrome, the Centers for Disease Control and Prevention recommend that children with chickenpox or flulike symptoms not be given aspirin or other salicylates.
• Do not use long-term salicylate therapy in children under age 14; safety has not been established.

Breast-feeding

• Salcylates are distributed into breast milk; avoid use of aspirin during breast-feeding.

astemizole

Hismanal

Pharmacologic classification: H_1-receptor antagonist
Therapeutic classification: antiallergy
Pregnancy risk category C

How supplied

Available by prescription only in the U.S.
Tablets: 10 mg

Available without a prescription in Canada
Tablets: 10 mg

Indications, route, and dosage

Relief of symptoms associated with chronic idiopathic urticaria and seasonal allergic rhinitis

Adults and children age 12 and older: 10 mg P.O. daily.

Pharmacodynamics

Antihistamine action: Astemizole blocks the effects of histamine at H_1 receptors. Astemizole is a nonsedating antihistamine because its chemical structure prevents entry into the CNS.

Pharmacokinetics

• *Absorption:* Drug is rapidly absorbed from the GI tract. Peak plasma levels occur within 1 hour.
• *Distribution:* About 96% of drug is bound to plasma proteins.
• *Metabolism:* Hepatic.
• *Excretion:* Primarily in the feces. Elimination half-life is 1 to 2½ days.

Contraindications and precautions

Contraindicated in patients with known hypersensitivity to astemizole and in those with severe hepatic impairment or who are receiving drugs known to impair the metabolism of astemizole (such as systemic itraconazole, ketoconazole, clarithromycin, erythromycin, troleandomycin, or quinine) because this may result in elevated levels of astemizole leading to QT interval prolongation and serious cardiac events.

Use cautiously in patients with hepatic, renal, cardiac, or lower respiratory tract diseases, especially asthma. Avoid coadministration of astemizole with other antifungals, serotonin reuptake inhibitors, HIV protease inhibitors, grapefruit juice, and other 3A4 inhibitors.

Interactions

Concomitant use with *itraconazole, ketoconazole, clarithromycin, erythromycin, troleandomycin,* and *quinine* produces elevated levels of astemizole which is associated with prolongation of the QT interval and can lead to serious arrhythmias.

Concurrent use with *fluconazole, metronidazole, miconazole I.V., fluoxetine, fluvoxamine, nefazodone, paroxetine, sertraline, ritonavir, indinavir, saquinavir, nelfinavir, zileuton, grapefruit juice,* and *other 3A4 inhibitors* may influence the metabolism of astemizole and is therefore not recommended.

Effects on diagnostic tests

None reported.

Adverse reactions

CNS: headache, nervousness, dizziness, drowsiness.
CV: ***arrhythmias*** (with high plasma levels).
EENT: dry mouth, pharyngitis, conjunctivitis.
GI: abdominal pain, increased appetite, nausea, diarrhea.
Other: arthralgia, weight gain, cholestatic jaundice.

Overdose and treatment

Cases of serious ventricular arrhythmias have been reported with overdoses of 200 mg or more. Careful observation and constant ECG monitoring is recommended. Treatment is supportive. Some patients may require an antiarrhythmic agent.

☑ Special considerations

Besides those relevant to all *antihistamines,* consider the following recommendations.
• Because of its potential for anticholinergic effects, use drug cautiously in patients with lower airway diseases (including asthma) because drying effects can increase the risk of bronchial mucus plug formation.
• Use with caution in patients with hepatic or renal disease. Drug is not believed to be dialyzable.
• Because of potential interactions, obtain a full drug profile, including nonprescription products.
• Astemizole should not be used on an as needed basis for immediate relief of symptoms.

Patient education

• Instruct patient to take drug on an empty stomach at least 2 hours after a meal and to avoid eating for at least 1 hour after each dose.

• Advise patient not to exceed the recommended dose of 10 mg daily or to increase the dose in an attempt to accelerate the onset of effects.

Breast-feeding

• Animal studies indicate that drug may be excreted in breast milk.

atenolol

Tenormin

Pharmacologic classification: beta-adrenergic blocker
Therapeutic classification: antihypertensive, antianginal
Pregnancy risk category D

How supplied

Available by prescription only
Tablets: 25 mg, 50 mg, 100 mg
Injection: 5 mg/10 ml

Indications, route, and dosage

Hypertension

Adults: Initially, 50 mg P.O. as a single daily dose. May increase dosage to 100 mg/day after 7 to 14 days. Higher dosages are unlikely to produce further benefit.

Chronic stable angina pectoris

Adults: 50 mg P.O. once daily; may be increased to 100 mg/day after 7 days for optimal effect. Maximum daily dosage is 200 mg/day.

To reduce risk of CV mortality in patients with acute MI

Adults: 5 mg I.V. over 5 minutes, followed by another 5 mg I.V. 10 minutes later. Initiate oral therapy 10 minutes after the final dose in patients who tolerate the full I.V. dose.

✦ ***Dosage adjustment.*** In patients with renal failure, adjust dosage if creatinine clearance is below 35 ml/minute. In patients with creatinine clearance of 15 to 35 ml/minute/1.73 m^2, give 50 mg/day; in patients with creatinine clearance below 15 ml/minute/1.73 m^2, give 25 mg/day; in patients undergoing hemodialysis, dosage is 25 to 50 mg after each treatment under close supervision.

Pharmacodynamics

Antihypertensive action: Atenolol may reduce blood pressure by adrenergic receptor blockade, thus decreasing cardiac output by decreasing sympathetic outflow from the CNS and by suppressing renin release. At low doses, atenolol, like metoprolol, selectively inhibits cardiac $beta_1$-receptors; it has little effect on $beta_2$-receptors in bronchial and vascular smooth muscle.

Antianginal action: Atenolol aids in treating chronic stable angina by decreasing myocardial contractility and heart rate (negative inotropic and chronotropic effect), thus reducing myocardial oxygen consumption.

Cardioprotective action: The mechanism whereby atenolol improves survival in patients with MI is unknown. However, it reduces the frequency of PVCs, chest pain, and enzyme elevation.

Pharmacokinetics

• *Absorption:* About 50% to 60% of an atenolol dose is absorbed. An effect on heart rate usually occurs within 60 minutes, with peak effect at 2 to 4 hours. Antihypertensive effect persists for about 24 hours.
• *Distribution:* Drug distributes into most tissues and fluids except the brain and CSF; approximately 5% to 15% is protein-bound.
• *Metabolism:* Minimal.
• *Excretion:* Approximately 40% to 50% of a given dose is excreted unchanged in urine; remainder is excreted as unchanged drug and metabolites in feces. In patients with normal renal function, plasma half-life is 6 to 7 hours; half-life increases as renal function decreases.

Contraindications and precautions

Contraindicated in patients with sinus bradycardia, greater than first-degree heart block, overt cardiac failure, or cardiogenic shock. Use cautiously in patients at risk for heart failure and in those with bronchospastic disease, diabetes, and hyperthyroidism.

Interactions

Atenolol may potentiate the antihypertensive effects of other *antihypertensive agents*; it also may alter *insulin* or *oral hypoglycemic* dosage requirements in stable diabetic patients.

Antihypertensive effects of atenolol may be antagonized by *indomethacin, NSAIDs*, and *alpha-adrenergic agents* such as those found in *OTC cold remedies.*

Effects on diagnostic tests

Atenolol may increase or decrease serum glucose levels in diabetic patients; it does not potentiate insulin-induced hypoglycemia or delay recovery of serum glucose to normal levels.

Atenolol also may cause changes in exercise tolerance and ECG; it has reportedly elevated platelet count as well as serum levels of potassium, uric acid, transaminase, alkaline phosphatase, LD, creatinine, and BUN.

Adverse reactions

CNS: *fatigue,* lethargy, vertigo, drowsiness, *dizziness.*
CV: *bradycardia, hypotension,* ***heart failure,*** intermittent claudication.
GI: nausea, diarrhea.
Respiratory: dyspnea, ***bronchospasm.***
Skin: rash.
Other: fever, leg pain.

Overdose and treatment

Clinical signs of overdose include severe hypotension, bradycardia, heart failure, and bronchospasm.

After acute ingestion, empty stomach by emesis or gastric lavage; follow with activated charcoal to reduce absorption. Thereafter, treat symptomatically and supportively.

☑ Special considerations

Besides those relevant to all *beta-adrenergic blockers,* consider the following recommendations.

- Give oral single daily dose at same time each day.
- Drug may be taken without food.
- Dosage may need to be reduced in patients with renal insufficiency.
- I.V. atenolol affords a rapid onset of the protective effects of beta-adrenergic blockade against reinfarction.
- Patients who cannot tolerate I.V. atenolol after an MI may be candidates for oral atenolol therapy. Some evidence suggests that gastric absorption of atenolol may be delayed in the early phase of MI. This may result from the physiologic changes that accompany MI or from the effects of morphine, which is commonly administered to treat chest pain. However, oral therapy alone may still provide benefits. Clinical trials suggest giving 100 mg of atenolol daily P.O. (either as 50 mg b.i.d. or 100 mg once daily) for at least 7 days. In the absence of contraindications, some may continue therapy for 1 to 3 years.
- Although such use is controversial, atenolol has been used as an adjunct treatment for alcohol withdrawal.

Patient education

- Stress importance of not missing doses, but tell patient not to double the dose if one is missed, especially if taking drug once daily.
- Advise patient to seek medical approval before taking OTC cold preparations.

Geriatric use

- Elderly patients may require lower maintenance dosages of atenolol because of increased bioavailability or delayed metabolism; they also may experience enhanced adverse effects.

Pediatric use

- Safety and efficacy in children have not been established; use only if potential benefit outweighs risk.

Breast-feeding

- Safety has not been established. An alternative feeding method is recommended during therapy.

atorvastatin calcium

Lipitor

Pharmacologic classification: 3-hydroxy-3-methylglutaryl-coenzyme A (HMG-CoA) reductase inhibitor
Therapeutic classification: antilipemic
Pregnancy risk category X

How supplied

Available by prescription only
Tablets: 10 mg, 20 mg, 40 mg

Indications, route, and dosage

Adjunct to diet to reduce elevated low-density lipoprotein (LDL), total cholesterol, apo B, and triglyceride levels in patients with primary hypercholesterolemia and mixed dyslipidemia

Adults: Initially 10 mg P.O. once daily. Increase dosage p.r.n. to maximum of 80 mg daily as single dose. Dosage based on blood lipid levels drawn within 2 to 4 weeks after starting therapy.

Alone or as an adjunct to lipid-lowering treatments such as LDL apheresis in patients with homozygous familial hypercholesterolemia

Adults: 10 to 80 mg P.O. once daily.

Pharmacodynamics

Antilipemic action: Inhibits HMG-CoA reductase, an early (and rate-limiting) step in cholesterol biosynthesis.

Pharmacokinetics

- *Absorption.* Rapidly absorbed. Plasma levels peak within 1 to 2 hours. Therapeutic response can be seen within 2 weeks; maximum response within 4 weeks and maintained during chronic therapy.
- *Distribution:* Mean volume of distribution is approximately 565 L. Drug is 98% or more bound to plasma proteins with poor drug penetration into RBCs. Drug is likely to be secreted in breast milk.
- *Metabolism:* Extensively metabolized to orthohydroxylated and parahydroxylated derivatives and various beta-oxidation products. In vitro inhibition of HMG-CoA reductase by orthohydroxylated and parahydroxylated metabolites is equivalent to that of atorvastatin. About 70% of circulating inhibitory activity for HMG-CoA reductase is attributed to active metabolites. In vitro studies suggest the importance of atorvastatin metabolism by cytochrome P450 3A4.
- *Excretion:* Drug and its metabolites are eliminated primarily in bile following hepatic or extrahepatic metabolism; however, drug does not appear to undergo enterohepatic recirculation. Mean plasma elimination half-life of atorvastatin is approximately 14 hours, but the half-life of inhibitory activity for HMG-CoA reductase is 20 to 30 hours because of the contribution of active metabolites. Less than 2% of a dose of atorvastatin is recovered in urine following oral administration.

Contraindications and precautions

Contraindicated in patients hypersensitive to drug or with active hepatic disease or conditions associated with unexplained persistent elevations of serum transaminase levels, in pregnant or breast-feeding women, and in women of childbearing age (except in women not at risk for becoming pregnant).

Use cautiously in patients with history of hepatic disease or heavy alcohol use.

Interactions

Azole antifungals, cyclosporine, erythromycin, fibric acid derivatives, and *niacin* may possibly increase risk of rhabdomyolysis. Avoid concomitant use. Use with *antacids* may cause decreased concentrations of atorvastatin. LDL-cholesterol reduction not affected. *Digoxin* may increase plasma digoxin levels; monitor serum digoxin levels. *Erythromycin* increases plasma concentration of drug. *Oral contraceptives* may increase levels of hormones.

Effects on diagnostic tests
Drug may increase liver function test results.

Adverse reactions
CNS: asthenia, *headache.*
GI: abdominal pain, constipation, diarrhea, dyspepsia, flatulence.
Musculoskeletal: arthralgia, back pain, myalgia.
Respiratory: pharyngitis, sinusitis.
Skin: rash.
Other: accidental injury, allergic reaction, flulike syndrome, *infection.*

Overdose and treatment
There is no specific treatment for atorvastatin overdosage. If overdosage occurs, treat patient symptomatically, and provide supportive measures as required. Because of extensive drug binding to plasma proteins, hemodialysis is not expected to significantly enhance drug clearance.

☑ Special considerations
- Know that drug should be withheld or discontinued in patients with serious, acute conditions that suggest myopathy or those at risk for renal failure secondary to rhabdomyolysis as a result of trauma; major surgery; severe metabolic, endocrine, and electrolyte disorders; severe acute infection; hypotension; or uncontrolled seizures.
- Use drug only after diet and other nonpharmacologic treatments prove ineffective. Patient should follow a standard low-cholesterol diet before and during therapy.
- Before initiating treatment, exclude secondary causes for hypercholesterolemia and perform a baseline lipid profile. Periodic liver function tests and lipid levels should be done before starting treatment, at 6 and 12 weeks after initiation, or after an increase in dosage and periodically thereafter.
- Know that drug may be given as a single dose at any time of day without regard for food.
- Watch for signs of myositis.

Patient education
- Teach patient proper dietary management, weight control, and exercise. Explain their importance in controlling elevated serum lipid levels.
- Warn patient to avoid alcohol.
- Tell patient to report adverse reactions, such as muscle pain, malaise, and fever.
- Warn female patient that drug is contraindicated during pregnancy due to potential danger to the fetus. Advise her to call immediately if pregnancy occurs.

Geriatric use
- Safety and efficacy in patients age 70 and above with drug doses up to 80 mg daily were similar to those of patients below age 70.

Pediatric use
- Experience in children is limited to drug doses up to 80 mg daily for 1 year in eight patients with homozygous familial hypercholesterermia. No clinical or biochemical abnormalities were reported in these patients. None of these patients was below age 9.

Breast-feeding
- Because of the potential for adverse reactions in breast-fed infants, women taking atorvastatin should not breast-feed.

atovaquone
Mepron

Pharmacologic classification: ubiquinone analogue
Therapeutic classification: antiprotozoal
Pregnancy risk category C

How supplied
Available by prescription only
Suspension: 750 mg/5 ml

Indications, route, and dosage
Mild to moderate* Pneumocystis carinii *pneumonia (PCP) in patients who cannot tolerate trimethoprim-sulfamethoxazole
Adults: 750 mg P.O. b.i.d. for 21 days given with food.

Pharmacodynamics
Antiprotozoal action: The mechanism of action of atovaquone against *P. carinii* has not been fully elucidated. In *Plasmodium* species, the site of action appears to be the cytochrome bc_1 complex (Complex III). Several metabolic enzymes are linked to the mitochondrial electron transport chain via ubiquinone. Inhibition of electron transport by atovaquone results in indirect inhibition of these enzymes. The ultimate metabolic effects of such a blockade may include inhibition of nucleic acid and ATP synthesis.

Pharmacokinetics
- *Absorption:* Absorption of atovaquone is limited. However, bioavailability of drug is increased approximately threefold when administered with meals. In particular, fat has been shown to enhance absorption significantly.
- *Distribution:* Drug is extensively bound (99.9%) to plasma proteins.
- *Metabolism:* Atovaquone is not metabolized.
- *Excretion:* Drug undergoes enterohepatic cycling and is primarily excreted in feces. Less than 0.6% is excreted in urine.

Contraindications and precautions
Contraindicated in patients with hypersensitivity to drug. Use cautiously in breast-feeding patients.

Interactions
Use caution when administering concurrently with other highly *plasma-protein-bound drugs* with narrow therapeutic indices because competition for binding sites may occur. *Phenytoin,* however, is not affected. Use with *rifampin* results in a significant decrease in plasma concentrations. Levels of *zi-*

dovudine may be increased, although this may not be clinically significant.

Effects on diagnostic tests
None reported.

Adverse reactions
CNS: *headache, insomnia,* asthenia, anxiety, dizziness.
EENT: *cough,* sinusitis, rhinitis, taste perversion.
GI: *nausea, diarrhea, vomiting,* constipation, *abdominal pain,* anorexia, dyspepsia.
Skin: *rash,* pruritus, *diaphoresis.*
Other: *fever, oral candidiasis, pain,* hypoglycemia, hypotension.

Overdose and treatment
There have been no reports of overdosage from oral administration of atovaquone.

☑ Special considerations
- Drug has not been systematically studied for use in the treatment of more severe episodes of PCP, nor has it been evaluated as an agent for PCP prophylaxis. In addition, the efficacy of atovaquone in patients who are failing therapy with trimethoprim-sulfamethoxazole has not been systematically studied.
- GI disorders may limit absorption of oral form; patients with these disorders may not achieve plasma drug concentrations associated with response to therapy.
- Drug is ineffective for concurrent pulmonary conditions, such as bacterial, viral, or fungal pneumonia or mycobacterial disease.
- Patients with acute PCP should be carefully evaluated for other possible causes of pulmonary disease and treated with additional agents as appropriate.

Patient education
- Instruct patient to take drug with meals because food enhances absorption significantly.

Geriatric use
- Use cautiously in elderly patients because they have a greater frequency of decreased hepatic, renal, and cardiac function.

Pediatric use
- Efficacy of drug has not been studied in children. No children under 4 months participated in phase I safety trials.

Breast-feeding
- It is not known if drug is excreted in breast milk. Therefore, use caution when administering drug to breast-feeding patient.

atracurium besylate
Tracrium

Pharmacologic classification: nondepolarizing neuromuscular blocker
Therapeutic classification: skeletal muscle relaxant
Pregnancy risk category C

How supplied
Available by prescription only
Injection: 10 mg/ml

Indications, route, and dosage
Adjunct to general anesthesia, to facilitate endotracheal intubation, and to provide skeletal muscle relaxation during surgery or mechanical ventilation
Dose depends on anesthetic used, individual needs, and response. Doses are representative and must be adjusted.
Adults and children over age 2: Initially, 0.4 to 0.5 mg/kg by I.V. bolus. Maintenance dose of 0.08 to 0.10 mg/kg within 20 to 45 minutes of initial dose should be administered during prolonged surgical procedures. Maintenance doses may be administered q 15 to 25 minutes in patients receiving balanced anesthesia. Maintenance infusion rate for intensive care unit (ICU) patients who require mechanical ventilation is 11 to 13 mcg/kg/minute.
Children age 1 month to 2 years: Initially, 0.3 to 0.4 mg/kg by I.V. bolus when under halothane anesthesia. Frequent maintenance doses may be needed.

Pharmacodynamics
Skeletal muscle relaxant action: Atracurium produces skeletal muscle paralysis by causing a decreased response to acetylcholine (ACh) at the neuromuscular junction. Because of its high affinity to ACh receptor sites, atracurium competitively blocks access of ACh to the motor end-plate, thus blocking depolarization. At usual doses (0.45 mg/kg), atracurium produces minimal CV effects and does not affect intraocular pressure, lower esophageal sphincter pressure, barrier pressure, heart rate or rhythm, mean arterial pressure, systemic vascular resistance, cardiac output, or central venous pressure. CV effects such as decreased peripheral vascular resistance, usually seen at doses greater than 0.5 mg/kg, are caused by histamine release.

Pharmacokinetics
- *Absorption:* Onset of action is within 2 minutes, with maximum neuromuscular blockade within 3 to 5 minutes. Maximum neuromuscular blockade increases with increasing dose. Repeated administration does not appear to be cumulative, nor is recovery time prolonged. Recovery from neuromuscular blockade under balanced anesthesia usually begins 20 to 35 minutes after dose is injected.
- *Distribution:* Distributed into the extracellular space after I.V. administration. Drug is approximately 82% protein-bound.

• *Metabolism:* In plasma, atracurium is rapidly metabolized by Hofmann elimination and by nonspecific enzymatic ester hydrolysis. The liver does not appear to play a major role.
• *Excretion:* Drug and its metabolites are excreted in urine and feces by biliary elimination.

Contraindications and precautions
Contraindicated in patients with hypersensitivity to drug. Use cautiously in patients with CV disease; severe electrolyte disorder; bronchogenic carcinoma; hepatic, renal, or pulmonary impairment; neuromuscular disease; or myasthenia gravis and in elderly or debilitated patients.

Interactions
The neuromuscular blockade associated with atracurium may be enhanced by concomitant use with many *general anesthetics*, particularly *enflurane* and *isoflurane*, or with *aminoglycoside antibiotics, clindamycin, lincomycin, polymyxin antibiotics, furosemide, lithium, beta-adrenergic blockers, depolarizing neuromuscular blocking agents,* other *nondepolarizing neuromuscular blocking agents, parenteral magnesium salts, quinidine, quinine, procainamide, thiazide diuretics*, and *potassium-depleting drugs.*

Concomitant use of *opioid analgesics* may cause additive respiratory depression and should be used with extreme caution during surgery and immediately postoperatively.

Effects on diagnostic tests
None reported.

Adverse reactions
CV: bradycardia, hypotension, tachycardia.
Respiratory: ***prolonged dose-related apnea,*** wheezing, increased bronchial secretions, dyspnea, ***bronchospasm, laryngospasm.***
Skin: *flushing,* erythema, pruritus, urticaria, rash.
Other: ***anaphylaxis.***

Overdose and treatment
Clinical manifestations of overdose include prolonged respiratory depression or apnea and CV collapse. A sudden release of histamine may also occur.

A peripheral nerve stimulator is recommended to monitor response and to determine the nature and degree of neuromuscular block. Maintain an adequate airway and manual or mechanical ventilation until patient can maintain respiration unassisted.

For treatment of overdose, administer cholinesterase inhibitors, such as edrophonium, neostigmine, or pyridostigmine, to reverse neuromuscular blockade; and atropine or glycopyrrolate to counteract muscarinic adverse effects of cholinesterase inhibitors. Monitor vital signs at least every 15 minutes until patient is stable, then every 30 minutes for next 2 hours. Observe airway until patient has fully recovered from drug effects. Note rate, depth, and pattern of respirations.

☑ Special considerations
• Administer drug by I.V. injection because I.M. injection causes tissue irritation.
• Reduce dose and administration rate in patients in whom histamine release may be hazardous.
• Prior administration of succinylcholine does not prolong duration of action of atracurium, but it quickens onset and may deepen neuromuscular blockade.
• Atracurium has a longer duration of action than succinylcholine and a shorter duration than tubocurarine or pancuronium.
• Drug has little or no effect on heart rate and does not counteract or reverse the bradycardia caused by anesthetics or vagal stimulation. Thus, bradycardia is seen more frequently with atracurium than with other neuromuscular blocking agents. Pretreatment with anticholinergics (atropine or glycopyrrolate) is advised.
• If bradycardia occurs during drug administration, treat with I.V. atropine.
• Alkaline solutions such as barbiturates should not be admixed in the same syringe or given through the same needle with atracurium.
• Peripheral nerve stimulator should be used to monitor responses during ICU administration and may be used to detect residual paralysis during recovery and to avoid atracurium overdose.
• Use drug only if endotracheal intubation, administration of oxygen under positive pressure, artificial respiration, and assisted or controlled ventilation are immediately available.
• To evaluate patient for recovery from neuromuscular blocking effect, observe for ability to breathe, to cough, to protrude tongue, to keep eyes open, to lift head keeping mouth closed, and to show adequate strength of hand-grip. Assess for adequate negative inspiratory force (–25 cm H_2O).
• Until head and neck muscles recover from blockade effects, patient may find speech difficult.
• If indicated, assess for need for pain medication or sedation. Drug does not affect consciousness or relieve pain.

Geriatric use
• Elderly patients may be more sensitive to drug's effects.

Pediatric use
• Safety and efficacy have not been established for children under age 1 month.

Breast-feeding
• It is unknown if drug is excreted in breast milk; therefore, use cautiously in breast-feeding women.

atropine sulfate

Pharmacologic classification: anticholinergic, belladonna alkaloid
Therapeutic classification: antiarrhythmic, vagolytic
Pregnancy risk category C

How supplied

Available by prescription only
Tablets: 0.4 mg, 0.6 mg
Injection: 0.05 mg/ml, 0.1 mg/ml, 0.3 mg/ml, 0.4 mg/ml, 0.5 mg/ml, 0.6 mg/ml, 0.8 mg/ml, 1 mg/ml, and 1.2 mg/ml
Ophthalmic ointment: 0.5%, 1%
Ophthalmic solution: 0.5%, 1%, 2%, 3%

Indications, route, and dosage

Symptomatic bradycardia, bradyarrhythmia (junctional or escape rhythm)
Adults: Usually 0.5 to 1 mg by I.V. push; repeat q 3 to 5 minutes, to maximum of 2 mg. Lower doses (less than 0.5 mg) may cause bradycardia.
Children: 0.02 mg/kg I.V. up to maximum 1 mg; or 0.3 mg/m^2; may repeat q 5 minutes.
Preoperatively for diminishing secretions and blocking cardiac vagal reflexes
Adults and children weighing over 44 lb (20 kg): 0.4 mg I.M. or S.C. 30 to 60 minutes before anesthesia.
Children weighing less than 44 lb: 0.1 mg I.M. for 6.6 lb (3 kg), 0.2 mg I.M. for 8.8 to 20 lb (4 to 9 kg), 0.3 mg I.M. for 22 to 44 lb (10 to 20 kg) 30 to 60 minutes before anesthesia.
Antidote for anticholinesterase insecticide poisoning
Adults and children: 1 to 2 mg I.M. or I.V. repeated q 20 to 30 minutes until muscarinic symptoms disappear.
Hypotonic radiograph of the GI tract
Adults: 1 mg I.M.
Acute iritis, uveitis
Adults: 1 to 2 drops (0.5% or 1% solution) into the eye q.i.d. (in children use 0.5% solution) or a small amount of ointment in the conjunctiva sac t.i.d.
Cycloplegic refraction
Adults: 1 to 2 drops (1% solution) 1 hour before refraction.
Children: 1 to 2 drops (0.5% solution) into each eye b.i.d. for 1 to 3 days before eye examination and 1 hour before examination.

Pharmacodynamics

Antiarrhythmic action: An anticholinergic (parasympatholytic) agent with many uses, atropine remains the mainstay of pharmacologic treatment for bradyarrhythmias. It blocks the effects of acetylcholine on the SA and AV nodes, thereby increasing SA and AV node conduction velocity. It also increases sinus node discharge rate and decreases the effective refractory period of the AV node. These changes result in an increased heart rate (both atrial and ventricular).

Atropine has variable—and clinically negligible—effects on the His-Purkinje system. Small doses (below 0.5 mg) and occasionally larger doses may lead to a paradoxical slowing of the heart rate, which may be followed by a more rapid rate.

As a cholinergic blocking agent, atropine decreases the action of the parasympathetic nervous system on certain glands (bronchial, salivary, and sweat), resulting in decreased secretions. It also decreases cholinergic effects on the iris, ciliary body, and intestinal and bronchial smooth muscle.

As an antidote for cholinesterase poisoning, atropine blocks the cholinomimetic effects of these pesticides.

Pharmacokinetics

• *Absorption:* I.V. administration is the most common route for bradyarrhythmia treatment. With endotracheal administration, atropine is well absorbed from the bronchial tree (drug has been used in 1-mg doses in acute bradyarrhythmia when an I.V. line has not been established). Effects on heart rate peak within 2 to 4 minutes after I.V. administration. Drug is well absorbed after oral and I.M. administration, and peak inhibitory effects on salivation occur in 30 minutes to 1 hour after either route.
• *Distribution:* Drug is well distributed throughout the body, including the CNS. Only 18% of drug binds with plasma protein (clinically insignificant).
• *Metabolism:* Atropine is metabolized in the liver to several metabolites. About 30% to 50% of a dose is excreted by the kidneys as unchanged drug.
• *Excretion:* Drug is excreted primarily through the kidneys; however, small amounts may be excreted in the feces and expired air. Elimination half-life is biphasic, with an initial 2-hour phase followed by a terminal half-life of about 12½ hours.

Contraindications and precautions

Contraindicated in patients with hypersensitivity to drug or sodium metabisulfite, acute angle-closure glaucoma, obstructive uropathy, obstructive disease of GI tract, paralytic ileus, toxic megacolon, intestinal atony, unstable CV status in acute hemorrhage, asthma, and myasthenia gravis.

Ophthalmic form is contraindicated in patients with glaucoma or hypersensitivity to drug or belladonna alkaloids and in those who have adhesions between the iris and lens. Atropine should not be used during the first 3 months of life because of the possible association between cycloplegia produced and development of amblyopia.

Use cautiously in patients with Down syndrome. Ophthalmic form should be used with caution in patients with increased intraocular pressure and the elderly.

Interactions

Concomitant use of atropine and other *anticholinergics* or *drugs with anticholinergic effects* produce additive effects. Coadministration with *amantadine* may result in an increase in anticholinergic adverse effects.

Effects on diagnostic tests

None reported.

Adverse reactions

CNS: *headache, restlessness,* ataxia, disorientation, hallucinations, delirium, *insomnia, dizziness,* excitement, agitation, confusion, especially in elderly patients (with systemic or oral form); confusion, somnolence, headache (with ophthalmic form).
CV: palpitations and bradycardia following low-dose atropine, tachycardia after higher doses (with systemic or oral form); tachycardia (with ophthalmic form).

EENT: photophobia, increased intraocular pressure, *blurred vision, mydriasis,* cycloplegia (with systemic or oral form), ocular congestion with long-term use, conjunctivitis, contact dermatitis of eye, ocular edema, eye dryness, transient stinging and burning, eye irritation, hyperemia (with ophthalmic form).
GI: *dry mouth,* thirst, *constipation,* nausea, vomiting (with systemic or oral form); dry mouth, abdominal distention in infants (with ophthalmic form).
GU: urine retention, impotence (with systemic or oral form).
Hematologic: leukocytosis (with systemic or oral form).
Skin: dryness (with ophthalmic form).
Other: severe allergic reactions, including ***anaphylaxis*** and urticaria (with systemic or oral form).

Overdose and treatment
Clinical signs of overdose reflect excessive anticholinergic activity, especially CV and CNS stimulation.

Treatment includes physostigmine administration, to reverse excessive anticholinergic activity, and general supportive measures, as necessary.

☑ Special considerations
- Observe for tachycardia if patient has cardiac disorder.
- With I.V. administration, drug may cause paradoxical initial bradycardia, which usually disappears within 2 minutes.
- Monitor patient's fluid intake and output; drug causes urine retention and hesitancy. If possible, patient should void before taking drug.
- High doses may cause hyperpyrexia, urinary retention, and CNS effects, including hallucinations and confusion (anticholinergic delirium). Other anticholinergic drugs may increase vagal blockage.
- Adverse reactions vary considerably with dose.

Geriatric use
- Monitor closely for urine retention in elderly males with benign prostatic hyperplasia.

attapulgite
Children's Kaopectate, Diar-Aid, Diarrest, Diasorb, Diatrol, Donnagel, Fowler's*, Kaopectate, Kaopectate Advanced Formula, Kaopectate Maximum Strength, Kaopek, K-Pek, Parepectolin, Rheaban, Rheaban Maximum Strength

Pharmacologic classification: hydrated magnesium aluminum silicate
Therapeutic classification: antidiarrheal
Pregnancy risk category NR

How supplied
Available without a prescription
Tablets: 300 mg, 600 mg*, 630 mg*, 750 mg
Tablets (chewable): 300 mg, 600 mg
Oral suspension: 600 mg/15 ml, 750 mg/5 ml, 750 mg/15 ml*, 900 mg/15 ml*

Indications, route, and dosage
Acute, nonspecific diarrhea
Adults and adolescents: 1.2 to 1.5 g (unless using Diasorb, in which case dosage can be as high as 3 g) P.O. after each loose bowel movement; do not exceed 9 g within 24 hours.
Children age 6 to 12: 600 mg (suspension) or 750 mg (tablet) P.O. after each loose bowel movement; do not exceed 4.2 g (suspension and chewable tablets) or 4.5 g (tablet) within 24 hours.
Children age 3 to 6: 300 mg P.O. after each loose bowel movement; do not exceed 2.1 g within 24 hours.

Pharmacodynamics
Antidiarrheal action: Although its exact action is unknown, it is believed that attapulgite absorbs large numbers of bacteria and toxins and reduces water loss in the GI tract.

Pharmacokinetics
- *Absorption:* Attapulgite is not absorbed.
- *Distribution:* Not applicable.
- *Metabolism:* Not applicable.
- *Excretion:* Drug is excreted unchanged in feces.

Contraindications and precautions
Contraindicated in patients with dysentery or suspected bowel obstruction. Use cautiously in dehydrated patients.

Interactions
Absorption of *oral medications* may be impaired when administered concurrently with attapulgite. Administer attapulgite not less than 2 hours before or 3 to 4 hours after these medications, and monitor for decreased effectiveness.

Effects on diagnostic tests
None reported.

Adverse reactions
GI: constipation.

Overdose and treatment
Because attapulgite is not absorbed, an overdose is unlikely to pose a significant health problem.

☑ Special considerations
- Ensure that patient achieves adequate fluid intake to compensate for fluid loss from diarrhea.
- Drug should not be used if diarrhea is accompanied by fever or blood or mucus in the stool. Discontinue drug if any of these signs occurs during treatment.

Patient education
- Tell patient to take drug after each loose bowel movement until diarrhea is controlled.
- Instruct patient to call if diarrhea is not controlled within 48 hours or if fever develops.

Geriatric use
- Use cautiously and only under medical supervision.

Pediatric use
• Use only under medical supervision in children under age 3.

auranofin
Ridaura

Pharmacologic classification: gold salt
Therapeutic classification: antiarthritic
Pregnancy risk category C

How supplied
Available by prescription only
Capsules: 3 mg

Indications, route, and dosage
Rheumatoid arthritis, ◊ psoriatic arthritis, ◊ active systemic lupus erythematosus, ◊ Felty's syndrome
Adults: 6 mg P.O. daily, administered either as 3 mg b.i.d. or 6 mg once daily. After 4 to 6 months, may be increased to 9 mg daily. If response remains inadequate after 3 months at 9 mg daily, discontinue drug.

Pharmacodynamics
Antiarthritic action: Auranofin suppresses or prevents, but does not cure, adult or juvenile arthritis and synovitis. It is anti-inflammatory in active arthritis. This drug is thought to reduce inflammation by altering the immune system. Auranofin has been shown to decrease high serum concentrations of immunoglobulins and rheumatoid factors in patients with arthritis. However, the exact mechanism of action remains unknown.

Pharmacokinetics
• *Absorption:* When administered P.O., 25% of the gold on auranofin is absorbed through the GI tract. Time to peak plasma concentration is 1 to 2 hours.
• *Distribution:* Drug is 60% protein-bound and is distributed widely in body tissues. Oral gold from auranofin is bound to a higher degree than gold from the injectable form. Synovial fluid levels are approximately 50% of blood concentrations. No correlation between blood-gold concentrations and safety or efficacy has been determined.
• *Metabolism:* The metabolic fate of auranofin is not known, but it is believed that drug is not broken down into elemental gold.
• *Excretion:* 60% of absorbed auranofin (15% of the administered dose) is excreted in the urine and the remainder in the feces. Average plasma half-life is 26 days, compared with about 6 days for gold sodium thiomalate.

Contraindications and precautions
Contraindicated in patients with history of severe gold toxicity, necrotizing enterocolitis, pulmonary fibrosis, exfoliative dermatitis, bone marrow aplasia, severe hematologic disorders or history of severe toxicity caused by previous exposure to other heavy metals.

Use cautiously with other drugs that cause blood dyscrasias or in patients with renal, hepatic, or inflammatory bowel disease; rash; or bone marrow depression. Use of drug in pregnant women is not recommended.

Interactions
Concomitant use of auranofin with *other drugs that may cause blood dyscrasias* can produce additive hematologic toxicity.

Effects on diagnostic tests
Serum protein-bound iodine test, especially when done by the chloric acid digestion method, gives false readings during and for several weeks after gold therapy.

Adverse reactions
CNS: confusion, hallucinations, ***seizures.***
EENT: conjunctivitis.
GI: *diarrhea, abdominal pain, nausea, stomatitis,* glossitis, anorexia, metallic taste, dyspepsia, flatulence, constipation, dysgeusia, ***ulcerative colitis.***
GU: proteinuria, hematuria, ***nephrotic syndrome,*** glomerulonephritis, ***acute renal failure.***
Hematologic: ***thrombocytopenia*** (with or without purpura), ***aplastic anemia, agranulocytosis,*** leukopenia, eosinophilia, anemia.
Hepatic: jaundice, elevated liver enzymes.
Respiratory: interstitial pneumonitis.
Skin: *rash, pruritus, dermatitis,* exfoliative dermatitis, urticaria, erythema, alopecia.

Overdose and treatment
In acute overdose, empty gastric contents by induced emesis or gastric lavage. When severe reactions to gold occur, corticosteroids, dimercaprol (a chelating agent), or penicillamine may be given to aid recovery. Prednisone 40 to 100 mg daily in divided doses is recommended to manage severe renal, hematologic, pulmonary, or enterocolitic reactions to gold. Dimercaprol may be used concurrently with steroids to facilitate the removal of the gold when steroid treatment alone is ineffective. Use of chelating agents is controversial, and caution is recommended. Appropriate supportive therapy is indicated as necessary.

☑ Special considerations
• Discontinue drug if platelet count decreases to below 100,000/mm³.
• When switching from injectable gold, start auranofin at 6 mg P.O. daily.

Patient education
• Emphasize importance of monthly follow-up to monitor patient's platelet count.
• Reassure patient that beneficial drug effect may be delayed for 3 months. However, if response is inadequate after 6 to 9 months, auranofin will probably be discontinued.
• Encourage patient to take drug as prescribed and not to alter the dosage schedule.
• Diarrhea is the most common adverse reaction. Tell patient to continue taking drug if patient experiences mild diarrhea; however, tell him to call immediately if blood occurs in stool.

- Tell patient to continue taking concomitant drug therapy, such as NSAIDs, if prescribed.
- Dermatitis is a common adverse reaction. Advise patient to report rash or other skin problems immediately.
- Stomatitis is another common adverse reaction. Tell patient that stomatitis is often preceded by a metallic taste and advise him to call immediately.

Geriatric use
- Administer usual adult dose. Use cautiously in patients with decreased renal function.

Pediatric use
- Safe dosage has not been established; use in children under age 6 is not recommended.

Breast-feeding
- Drug is not recommended for use during breast-feeding.

azathioprine
Imuran

azathioprine sodium
Imuran

Pharmacologic classification: purine antagonist
Therapeutic classification: immunosuppressive
Pregnancy risk category D

How supplied
Available by prescription only
Tablets: 50 mg
Injection: 100 mg per vial

Indications, route, and dosage
Prevention of the rejection of kidney transplants
Adults and children: Initially, 3 to 5 mg/kg P.O. daily beginning on day of (or 1 to 3 days before) transplantation. After transplantation, dosage may be administered I.V., until patient is able to tolerate oral dosage. Usual maintenance dosage is 1 to 3 mg/kg daily. Dosage varies with patient response.
Severe, refractory rheumatoid arthritis
Adults: Initially, 1 mg/kg (about 50 to 100 mg) P.O. taken as a single dose or in divided doses. If patient response is unsatisfactory after 6 to 8 weeks, dosage may be increased by 0.5 mg/kg daily (up to a maximum of 2.5 mg/kg daily) at 4-week intervals.

Pharmacodynamics
Immunosuppressant action: The mechanism of immunosuppressive activity is unknown; however, drug may inhibit RNA and DNA synthesis, mitosis, or (in patients undergoing renal transplantation) coenzyme formation and functioning. Azathioprine suppresses cell-mediated hypersensitivity and alters antibody production.

Pharmacokinetics
- *Absorption:* Azathioprine is well absorbed orally.
- *Distribution:* Drug and its major metabolite, mercaptopurine, are distributed throughout the body; both are 30% protein-bound. Azathioprine and its metabolites cross the placenta.
- *Metabolism:* Azathioprine is metabolized primarily to mercaptopurine.
- *Excretion:* Small amounts of azathioprine and mercaptopurine are excreted in urine intact; most of a given dose is excreted in urine as secondary metabolites.

Contraindications and precautions
Contraindicated in patients hypersensitive to drug and during pregnancy. Use cautiously in patients with impaired renal or hepatic function.

Interactions
The major metabolic pathway of azathioprine is inhibited by *allopurinol*, which competes for the oxidative enzyme xanthine oxidase; concomitant use with *allopurinol* is potentially hazardous and should be avoided. If concomitant use is unavoidable, dose should be reduced by one-third to one-fourth the usual dose.

Drug may reverse neuromuscular blockade resulting from use of the nondepolarizing muscle relaxants *tubocurarine* and *pancuronium*.

Methotrexate may increase plasma levels of the metabolite 6-MP. Plasma levels of *cyclosporine* may be decreased.

Anemia and severe leukopenia have been reported with concomitant use with *ACE inhibitors*.

Effects on diagnostic tests
Azathioprine alters CBC and differential blood counts, decreases serum uric acid levels, and elevates liver enzyme test results.

Adverse reactions
GI: *nausea, vomiting,* ***pancreatitis,*** steatorrhea, diarrhea, abdominal pain.
Hematologic: **LEUKOPENIA,** ***bone marrow suppression,*** anemia, ***pancytopenia, thrombocytopenia, immunosuppression*** (possibly profound).
Hepatic: ***hepatotoxicity,*** jaundice.
Skin: rash.
Other: arthralgia, alopecia, ***infections,*** fever, myalgia, ***increased risk of neoplasia.***

Overdose and treatment
Clinical signs of overdose include nausea, vomiting, diarrhea, and extension of hematologic effects. Supportive treatment may include treatment with blood products if necessary.

☑ Special considerations
- Monitor patient for signs of hepatic damage: clay-colored stools, dark urine, jaundice, pruritus, and elevated liver enzyme levels.
- If infection occurs, reduce drug dosage and treat infection.
- If nausea and vomiting occur, divide dose or give with or after meals.
- Monitor for unusual bleeding or bruising, fever, or sore throat.

• If used to treat rheumatoid arthritis, NSAIDs should be continued when azathioprine therapy is initiated.
• Hematologic status should be monitored while patient is receiving azathioprine. CBCs, including platelet counts, should be taken at least weekly during the first month, twice monthly for the second and third months, then monthly.
• Chronic immunosuppression with azathioprine is associated with an increased risk of neoplasia.

Patient education
• Teach patient about disease and rationale for therapy; explain possible adverse effects and importance of reporting them, especially unusual bleeding or bruising, fever, sore throat, mouth sores, abdominal pain, pale stools, or dark urine.
• Encourage compliance with therapy and follow-up visits.
• Advise patient to avoid pregnancy during therapy and for 4 months after stopping therapy.
• Tell patients with rheumatoid arthritis that clinical response may not be apparent for up to 12 weeks.
• Suggest taking drug with or after meals or in divided doses to prevent nausea.

azelaic acid cream
Azelex

Pharmacologic classification: naturally occurring saturated dicarboxylic acid
Therapeutic classification: antiacne
Pregnancy risk category B

How supplied
Available by prescription only
Cream: 20%

Indications, route, and dosage
Mild to moderate inflammatory acne vulgaris
Adults: Apply a thin film and gently but thoroughly massage into affected areas b.i.d. (morning and evening).

Pharmacodynamics
Antiacne action: Unknown. Antimicrobial action may be attributed to inhibition of microbial cellular protein synthesis.

Pharmacokinetics
• *Absorption:* Azelaic acid cream minimally penetrates the stratum corneum and other viable skin layers. About 4% of the topically applied drug is systemically absorbed.
• *Distribution:* Minimal.
• *Metabolism:* Azelaic acid cream has negligible cutaneous metabolism.
• *Excretion:* Mainly excreted unchanged in the urine. Half-life after topical dosing is 12 hours.

Contraindications and precautions
Contraindicated in patients with known hypersensitivity to any of its components. Use cautiously in pregnant or breast-feeding women.

Interactions
None reported.

Effects on diagnostic tests
None reported

Adverse reactions
Skin: pruritus, burning, stinging, tingling.

Overdose and treatment
Discontinue therapy.

☑ Special considerations
• Apply drug after thoroughly washing and patting dry affected areas. Wash hands well after drug application.
• Monitor patient with dark complexion for early signs of hypopigmentation after use.
• Discontinue drug if sensitivity or severe irritation develops with drug use, and institute appropriate treatment.

Patient education
• Tell patient to use drug for full prescribed treatment period.
• Instruct patient how to apply drug. Advise against applying occlusive dressings or wrappings to affected areas.
• Tell patient to keep drug away from mouth, eyes, and other mucous membranes. If drug accidently comes into contact with the eyes, instruct patient to wash eyes with abundant water and call if eye irritation persists.
• Advise patient with dark complexions to report abnormal changes in skin color.
• Warn patient that temporary skin irritation may occur when drug is applied to broken or inflamed skin, usually at the start of therapy. However, tell patient to call if it persists.

Pediatric use
• Safety and effectiveness in patients under age 12 have not been established.

Breast-feeding
• Azelaic acid may enter breast milk. Use with caution in breast-feeding women.

azelastine hydrochloride
Astelin

Pharmacologic classification: phthalazinone derivative
Therapeutic classification: antihistamine
Pregnancy risk category C

How supplied
Available by prescription only
Nasal spray: 137 mcg/metered spray

Indications, route, and dosage
Seasonal allergic rhinitis
Adults and children age 12 and older: 2 sprays per nostril b.i.d.

Pharmacodynamics
Antihistaminic action: Exhibits H_1-receptor antagonist activity. In a placebo-controlled study, there was no evidence of an effect of azelastine on cardiac repolarization as represented by QT_c interval.

Pharmacokinetics
• *Absorption:* After intranasal administration, the systemic bioavailability is approximately 40%. Plasma levels peak within 2 to 3 hours.
• *Distribution:* Steady-state volume of distribution is 14.5 L/kg. Plasma protein binding of azelastine and desmethylazelastine are approximately 88% and 97%, respectively.
• *Metabolism:* Drug is oxidatively metabolized to the principal active metabolite, desmethylazelastine, by the cytochrome P450 enzyme system. After intranasal dosing to steady-state, plasma concentrations of desmethylazelastine range from 20% to 50% of azelastine concentrations.
• *Excretion:* Elimination half-life and plasma clearance are 22 hours, and 0.5 L/hour/kg, respectively. Approximately 75% of azelastine is excreted in the feces with less than 10% as unchanged drug. Desmethylazelastine has an elimination half-life of 54 hours.

Contraindications and precautions
Contraindicated in patients with known hypersensitivity to drug or its components.

Interactions
Cimetidine may increase plasma levels of azelastine; avoid concomitant use. Concurrent use of *CNS depressants* and *ethanol* may increase sedation.

Effects on diagnostic tests
None reported.

Adverse reactions
CNS: dizziness, *headache, somnolence.*
EENT: *bitter taste,* dry mouth, epistaxis, nasal burning.
GI: nausea.
Respiratory: pharyngitis, paroxysmal sneezing, rhinitis.
Other: fatigue, weight increase.

Overdose and treatment
No overdosage has been reported with the nasal spray. Acute overdosage with this dosage form is unlikely to result in clinically significant adverse events, other than increased somnolence. Provide general supportive measures if overdosage occurs.

☑ Special considerations
• Know that drug should be used in pregnancy only if the benefit justifies the potential risk to the fetus.
• The imprinted expiration date applies to the product in the bottles with child-resistant screw caps. After the spray pump is inserted into the first bottle of the dispensing package, both bottles of product should be discarded after 3 months.

Patient education
• Warn patient not to drive or perform hazardous activities if somnolence occurs.
• Advise patient not to use alcohol, CNS depressants, or other antihistamines while taking drug.
• Teach patient proper use of nasal spray.
• Instruct patient to replace the child-resistant screw top on the bottle with the pump unit. Prime the delivery system with 4 sprays or until a fine mist appears. Reprime the system with 2 sprays or until a fine mist appears if 3 or more days have elapsed since the last use. The bottle should be stored upright at room temperature with the pump closed tightly. Keep unit away from children.
• Tell patient to avoid getting the spray in the eyes.

Geriatric use
• In clinical trials, adverse events in this patient group were similar to those under age 60.

Pediatric use
• Safety and effectiveness in patients under age 12 have not been established.

Breast-feeding
• It is not known if drug is excreted in breast milk. Use caution when administering to breast-feeding patients.

azithromycin
Zithromax

Pharmacologic classification: azalide macrolide
Therapeutic classification: antibiotic
Pregnancy risk category B

How supplied
Available by prescription only
Capsules: 250 mg
Tablets: 250 mg
Powder for oral suspension: 100 mg/5 ml, 200 mg/5 ml; 300 mg*, 600 mg*, 900 mg*, 1,000 mg
Injection: 500 mg

Indications, route, and dosage
***Acute bacterial exacerbations of chronic obstructive pulmonary disease caused by* Haemophilus influenzae, Moraxella (Branhamella) catarrhalis, *or* Streptococcus pneumoniae; *uncomplicated skin and skin structure infections caused by* Staphylococcus aureus, Streptococcus pyogenes, *or* S. agalactiae; *and second-line therapy of pharyngitis or tonsillitis caused by* S. pyogenes**
Adults and adolescents age 16 and older: Initially, 500 mg P.O. as a single dose on day 1, followed by 250 mg daily on days 2 through 5. Total cumulative dose is 1.5 g.
***Community-acquired pneumonia caused by* Chlamydia pneumoniae, H. influenzae, Mycoplasma pneumoniae, S. pneumoniae; *I.V. form can be used for above infections and those caused by* Legionella pneumophila, M. catarrhalis, *and* S. aureus**

Adults and adolescents age 16 and over: 500 mg P.O. as a single dose on day 1, followed by 250 mg P.O. daily on days 2 to 5. Total dose is 1.5 g. For those who require initial I.V. therapy, 500 mg I.V. as a single daily dose for 2 days, followed by 500 mg P.O. as a single daily dose to complete a 7- to 10-day course of therapy. The timing of the change from I.V. to P.O. therapy should be directed by the health care provider based on patient's clinical response.
***Nongonococcal urethritis or cervicitis caused by* Chlamydia trachomatis**
Adults and adolescents age 16 and older: 1 g P.O. as a single dose.
Pelvic inflammatory disease caused by* Chlamydia trachomatis, Neisseria gonorrhoeae, *or* Mycoplasma hominis *in patients requiring initial I.V. therapy
Adults: 500 mg I.V. as a single daily dose for 1 to 2 days, followed by 250 mg P.O. daily to complete a 7-day course of therapy. The timing of the change from I.V. to P.O. therapy should be directed by the health care provider based on patient's clinical response.
Otitis media
Children over age 6 months: 10 mg/kg P.O. on day 1; then 5 mg/kg on days 2 to 5.
Tonsillitis
Children over age 2: 12 mg/kg P.O. daily for 5 days.
Chancroid
Adults: 1 g P.O. as a single dose.
Disseminated* Mycobacterium avium *complex (MAC) in patients with advanced infection with HIV
Adults: 1.2 g P.O. once weekly alone or in combination with rifabutin.

Pharmacodynamics
Antibiotic action: Azithromycin, a derivative of erythromycin, binds to the 50S subunit of bacterial ribosomes, blocking protein synthesis. It is bacteriostatic or bactericidal, depending on concentration.

Pharmacokinetics
- *Absorption:* Azithromycin is rapidly absorbed from the GI tract; food decreases both maximum plasma concentrations and amount of drug absorbed.
- *Distribution:* Drug is rapidly distributed throughout the body and readily penetrates cells; it does not readily enter the CNS. It concentrates in fibroblasts and phagocytes. Significantly higher levels of drug are reached in the tissues as compared with the plasma. Uptake and release of drug from tissues contributes to the long half-life. With a loading dose, peak and trough blood levels are stable within 48 hours. Without a loading dose, 5 to 7 days are required before steady state is reached.
- *Metabolism:* Drug is not metabolized.
- *Excretion:* Excreted mostly in the feces after excretion into the bile. Less than 10% is excreted in the urine. Terminal elimination half-life is 68 hours.

Contraindications and precautions
Contraindicated in patients with hypersensitivity to erythromycin or other macrolides. Use cautiously in patients with impaired hepatic function.

Interactions
Concomitant administration with *aluminum-* and *magnesium-containing antacids* may result in lower peak plasma levels of azithromycin. Separate administration times by at least 2 hours.

Other macrolides interact with several drugs. Until the effect of azithromycin is known, use cautiously. Macrolides may increase plasma *theophylline* levels by decreasing *theophylline* clearance. Concomitant administration with drugs metabolized by the hepatic cytochrome P450 system (such as *phenytoin, barbiturates, carbamazepine,* and *cyclosporine*) may result in impaired metabolism of these agents and increased risk of toxicity. Clearance of *triazolam* may be decreased, increasing the risk of *triazolam* toxicity. Acute ergot toxicity has been reported when macrolides have been administered with *ergotamine* or *dihydroergotamine.*

Also use cautiously with *warfarin* because other macrolides may increase PT; effect of azithromycin is unknown. Monitor PT carefully.

The possibility that azithromycin, as a macrolide agent, may interact with *astemizole* to cause potentially serious adverse CV effects, should be considered. Thus, concomitant use is to be avoided.

Effects on diagnostic tests
None reported.

Adverse reactions
CNS: dizziness, vertigo, headache, fatigue, somnolence.
CV: palpitations, chest pain.
GI: *nausea, vomiting, diarrhea, abdominal pain,* dyspepsia, flatulence, melena, cholestatic jaundice, pseudomembranous colitis.
GU: candidiasis, vaginitis, nephritis.
Skin: rash, photosensitivity.
Other: angioedema.

Overdose and treatment
No information available. Treat symptomatically.

☑ Special considerations
- Obtain culture and sensitivity tests before giving first dose. Therapy can begin before results are obtained.
- Drug may cause overgrowth of nonsusceptible bacteria or fungi. Watch for signs and symptoms of superinfection.
- Serologic tests for syphilis and cultures for gonorrhea should be taken from patients diagnosed with sexually transmitted urethritis or cervicitis. Drug should not be used to treat gonorrhea or syphilis.
- Reconstitute 500-mg vial with 4.8 ml of sterile water for injection. Shake well until drug is dissolved (yields a concentration of 100 mg/ml). Dilute solution further in at least 250 ml of 0.9% NaCl, 0.45% NaCl, D_5W, or lactated Ringer's solution to yield a concentration range of 1 to 2 mg/ml.

• Infuse 500-mg dose of azithromycin I.V. over 1 or more hours. Do *not* give as a bolus or I.M. injection.

Patient education

• Tell patient to take all of drug prescribed, even if he is feeling better.
• Remind patient that drug should always be taken on an empty stomach because food or antacids decrease absorption. Patient should take drug 1 hour before or 2 hours after a meal and should not take antacids.
• Instruct patient to promptly report adverse reactions.

Geriatric use

• In clinical trials of patients with normal hepatic and renal function, in using the 5-day dosage regimen, no significant pharmacokinetic differences were seen in those between age 65 and 85.

Pediatric use

• Safety and efficacy in children age 16 and younger have not been established.

Breast-feeding

• It is unknown if drug is excreted in breast milk. Use cautiously in breast-feeding women.

aztreonam

Azactam

Pharmacologic classification: monobactam
Therapeutic classification: antibiotic
Pregnancy risk category B

How supplied

Available by prescription only
Injection: 500-mg, 1-g, 2-g vials

Indications, route, and dosage

Urinary tract, respiratory tract, intra-abdominal, gynecologic, or skin infections; septicemia caused by gram-negative bacteria; ◊ adjunct therapy in pelvic inflammatory disease; ◊ gonorrhea

Adults: 500 mg to 2 g I.V. or I.M. q 8 to 12 hours. For severe systemic or life-threatening infections, 2 g q 6 to 8 hours may be given. Maximum dose is 8 g daily. For gonorrhea, give 1 g I.M. single dose.

✦ ***Dosage adjustment.*** In patients with a creatinine clearance of 10 to 30 ml/minute/1.73 m^2, reduce dose by ½ after an initial dose of 1 to 2 g. In patients with a creatinine clearance below 10 ml/minute/1.73 m^2, an initial dose of 500 mg to 2 g should be followed by ¼ of the usual dose at the usual intervals; give ⅛ the initial dose after each session of hemodialysis.

Pharmacodynamics

Antibacterial action: Aztreonam is a monobactam that inhibits mucopeptide synthesis of the bacterial cell wall. It preferentially binds to penicillin-binding protein 3 (PBP3) of susceptible organisms and often causes cell lysis and cell death.

Aztreonam has a narrow spectrum of activity and is usually bactericidal in action. Aztreonam is effective against *Escherichia coli, Enterobacter, Klebsiella pneumoniae, Proteus mirabilis,* and *Pseudomonas aeruginosa.* It has limited activity against *Citrobacter, Haemophilus influenzae, K. oxytoca, Hafnia, Serratia marcescens, E. aerogenes, Morganella morganii, Providencia, Branhamella catarrhalis, Proteus vulgaris,* and *Neisseria gonorrhoeae.*

Pharmacokinetics

• *Absorption:* Absorbed poorly from GI tract after oral administration but is absorbed rapidly and completely after I.M. or I.V. administration; peak concentrations occur in 60 minutes.
• *Distribution:* Drug is distributed rapidly and widely to all body fluids and tissues, including bile, breast milk, and CSF. It crosses the placental barrier and is found in fetal circulation.
• *Metabolism:* From 6% to 16% is metabolized to inactive metabolites by nonspecific hydrolysis of the beta-lactam ring; 56% to 60% is protein-bound, less if renal impairment is present.
• *Excretion:* Aztreonam is excreted principally in urine as unchanged drug by glomerular filtration and tubular secretion; 1.5% to 3.5% is excreted in feces as unchanged drug. Half-life averages 1.7 hours. Drug is excreted in breast milk; it may be removed by hemodialysis and peritoneal dialysis.

Contraindications and precautions

Contraindicated in patients with hypersensitivity to drug. Use cautiously in patients with impaired renal function and in the elderly.

Interactions

When used concomitantly, *probenecid* may prolong the rate of tubular secretion of aztreonam. Synergistic or additive effects occur when the drug is used concomitantly with *aminoglycosides*, or other *beta-lactam antibiotics*, including *piperacillin, cefoperazone, cefotaxime, clindamycin*, or *metronidazole*. Potent inducers of beta-lactamase production (*cefoxitin, imipenem*) may inactivate aztreonam. *Chloramphenicol* is antagonistic; give the two preparations several hours apart.

Use with *clavulanic acid* may be synergistic or antagonistic, depending on organism involved. *Furosemide* increases serum aztreonam levels, but this is clinically unimportant.

Effects on diagnostic tests

Aztreonam therapy alters urinary glucose determinations using cupric sulfate (Clinitest or Benedict's solution).

Coombs' test may become positive during therapy. Drug may prolong PT and partial thromboplastin time and may transiently increase ALT, AST, LD, and serum creatinine levels.

Adverse reactions

CNS: ***seizures,*** headache, insomnia, confusion.
CV: hypotension.

GI: diarrhea, nausea, vomiting.
Hematologic: neutropenia, anemia, pancytopenia, ***thrombocytopenia,*** leukocytosis, thrombocytosis.
Other: hypersensitivity reactions (rash, ***anaphylaxis***), transient elevation of ALT and AST; thrombophlebitis (at I.V. site); discomfort, swelling (at I.M. injection site).

Overdose and treatment

No information is available on the symptoms of overdose. Hemodialysis or peritoneal dialysis increases elimination of aztreonam.

☑ Special considerations

- Drug has also been used to treat bone and joint infection caused by susceptible aerobic, gram-negative bacteria.
- To reconstitute for I.M. use, dilute with at least 3 ml of sterile water for injection, bacteriostatic water for injection, 0.9% NaCl solution, or bacteriostatic 0.9% NaCl solution for each gram of aztreonam (15-ml vial).
- To reconstitute for I.V. use, add 6 to 10 ml of sterile water for injection to each 15-ml vial; for I.V. infusion, prepare as for I.M. solution. May be further diluted by adding to 0.9% NaCl, Ringer's solution, lactated Ringer's solution, 5% or 10% dextrose, or other electrolyte-containing solutions. For I.V. piggyback (100-ml bottles), add at least 50 ml of diluent for each gram of aztreonam. Final concentration should not exceed 20 mg/ml.
- I.V. route is preferred for doses larger than 1 g or in patients with bacterial septicemia, localized parenchymal abscesses, peritonitis, or other life-threatening infections; administer by direct I.V. push over 3 to 5 minutes or by intermittent infusion over 20 to 60 minutes.
- After addition of diluent, shake vigorously and immediately; not intended for multiple-dose use.
- Solutions may be colorless or light straw yellow. On standing, they may develop a slight pink tint; potency is not affected.
- Admixtures of aztreonam and nafcillin, cephradine, or metronidazole are incompatible; in general, do not mix aztreonam with other medications. Check with pharmacy for compatibility.
- Reduced dose may be required in patients with impaired renal function, cirrhosis, or other hepatic impairment.
- Drug may be stored at room temperature for 48 hours or in refrigerator for 7 days.

Patient education

- Tell patient to call immediately if rash, redness, or itching develops.

Geriatric use

- Studies in elderly males (age 65 to 75) have shown that the half-life of aztreonam may be prolonged in elderly patients because of their diminished renal function.

Breast-feeding

- Although drug is excreted in breast milk, it is not absorbed from infant's GI tract and is unlikely to cause any serious problems.

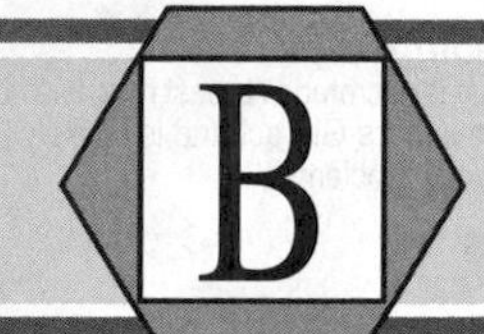

bacillus Calmette-Guérin (BCG), live intravesical

TheraCys, TICE BCG

Pharmacologic classification: bacterial
Therapeutic classification: antineoplastic
Pregnancy risk category C

How supplied

Available by prescription only
TheraCys
Suspension (powder form) for bladder instillation: 81 mg/vial
TICE BCG
Suspension (powder form) for bladder instillation: approximately 50 mg/ampule

Indications, route, and dosage

Treatment of in situ carcinoma of the urinary bladder (primary and relapsed)
Adults: Consult published protocols, specialized references, and manufacturer's recommendations.

Pharmacodynamics

Antitumor action: Exact mechanism unknown. Instillation of the live bacterial suspension causes a local inflammatory response. Local infiltration of histiocytes and leukocytes is followed by a decrease in the superficial tumors within the bladder.

Pharmacokinetics

- *Absorption:* No information available.
- *Distribution:* No information available.
- *Metabolism:* No information available.
- *Excretion:* No information available.

Contraindications and precautions

Contraindicated in immunocompromised patients, in those receiving immunosuppressive therapy, and in those with urinary tract infection or fever of unknown origin. If fever is caused by infection, withhold drug until patient recovers.

Interactions

Concomitant *antimicrobial therapy* for other infections may attenuate the response to BCG live.

Drugs that depress the bone marrow, radiation therapy, and *immunosuppressants* may impair the response to BCG intravesical because these treatments can decrease the patient's immune response. These treatments may also increase the risk of osteomyelitis or disseminated BCG infection.

Effects on diagnostic tests

Tuberculin sensitivity may be rendered positive by BCG intravesical treatment. Determine patient's reactivity to tuberculin before initiating therapy.

Adverse reactions

GI: *nausea, vomiting, anorexia,* diarrhea.
GU: *dysuria, urinary frequency, hematuria, cystitis, urinary urgency,* nocturia, urinary incontinence, *urinary tract infection,* cramps, pain, decreased bladder capacity, renal toxicity, genital pain.
Hematologic: *anemia,* leukopenia.
Hepatic: elevated liver enzyme levels.
Other: hypersensitivity reaction, *malaise, fever, chills,* myalgia, arthralgia, ***disseminated mycobacterial infection.***

Overdose and treatment

Closely monitor the patient for signs of systemic BCG infection and treat with antituberculosis medication.

☑ Special considerations

- Reconstitute drug just before use, only with diluent provided. All persons handling drug should wear masks and gloves.
- Handle drug and all material used for instillation of the drug as infectious material because it contains live attenuated mycobacteria. Dispose of all associated materials (syringes, catheters, and containers) as biohazardous waste.
- The vial of TheraCys should be reconstituted with 3 ml of the supplied diluent. Do not remove the rubber stopper to prepare the solution. Further dilute in 50 ml of sterile, preservative-free NaCl (final volume, 53 ml). A urethral catheter is instilled into the bladder under aseptic conditions, the bladder is drained, and then 53 ml of the prepared solution is added by gravity feed. The catheter is then removed.
- Use strict aseptic technique to administer drug, thus minimizing the trauma to the GU tract and preventing introduction of other contaminants to the area.
- If there is evidence of traumatic catheterization, do not administer drug and delay treatment for at least 1 week. Subsequent treatment may resume as if no interruption of the schedule has occurred.
- Bladder irritation can be treated symptomatically with phenazopyridine, acetaminophen, and propantheline bromide. Systemic adverse reactions that are caused by hypersensitivity can be treated with diphenhydramine hydrochloride.

Patient education

- After instillation, patient should retain the fluid in bladder for 2 hours (if possible). For the first hour, tell patient to lie 15 minutes prone, 15 minutes supine, and 15 minutes on each side. Patient may be up for the second hour.

- For safety, patient should be seated when voiding. Instruct patient to disinfect urine for 6 hours after instillation of drug. Tell patient to add undiluted household bleach (5% sodium hypochlorite solution) in equal volume to voided urine to the toilet; allow to stand for 15 minutes before flushing.
- Tell patient to call if symptoms worsen or if the following occur: blood in the urine, fever and chills, frequent urge to urinate or painful urination, nausea, vomiting, joint pain, rash, or cough.

Pediatric use

- Safe use in children has not been established.

Breast-feeding

- It is not known if drug is excreted in breast milk. Use with caution in breast-feeding women.

bacillus Calmette-Guérin (BCG) vaccine

TICE BCG

Pharmacologic classification: vaccine
Therapeutic classification: bacterial vaccine
Pregnancy risk category C

How supplied

Available by prescription only
Powder for injection: 1 to 8 x 10^8 colony-forming units (CFU) per ml of Tice-University of Illinois strain BCG per ml, equivalent to approximately 50 mg

Indications, route, and dosage

Tuberculosis (TB) exposure
Adults and children over age 1 month: Apply 0.2 to 0.3 ml of prepared vaccine on the cleaned surface of the skin; apply multiple-puncture disk through vaccine. The vaccine should flow into the wound and dry. Keep site dry for 24 hours.

Repeat dosage in all patients who have a negative tuberculin test reaction to 5 tuberculin units (TU) at 2- to 3-month follow-up. Advisory Committee on Immunization Practices (ACIP) and Advisory Committee for the Elimination of Tuberculosis (ACET) suggest revaccination with a full dose at age 1 if skin test reaction is negative to 5 TU.
Neonates under age 1 month: Reduce dosage to one-half by using 2 ml of sterile water when reconstituting.

Pharmacodynamics

Immunostimulant action: BCG vaccine promotes active immunity to tuberculosis. Immunity is not permanent or entirely predictable.

Pharmacokinetics

- *Absorption:* No information available.
- *Distribution:* No information available.
- *Metabolism:* No information available.
- *Excretion:* No information available.

Contraindications and precautions

Contraindicated in patients with hypogammaglobulinemia, in the presence of a positive tuberculin reaction (when meant for use as immunoprophylactic after exposure to TB) in immunosuppressed patients, in those with fresh smallpox vaccinations, in those who have suffered burns, and in patients receiving corticosteroid therapy. Avoid use during pregnancy.

Interactions

Concomitant use of BCG vaccine with *antitubercular drugs* (*isoniazid, rifampin, streptomycin*) inhibits the multiplication of BCG and impairs the efficacy of the vaccine. Concomitant use with *corticosteroids* or *immunosuppressants* may alter the immune response to BCG vaccine and avoid use.

Effects on diagnostic tests

BCG vaccination may affect the interpretation of subsequent tuberculin skin test reactions.

Adverse reactions

Other: osteomyelitis, lymphadenopathy, allergic reaction.

Overdose and treatment

Treatment is with antituberculosis drugs.

☑ Special considerations

- Obtain thorough history of allergies and reactions to immunizations.
- Epinephrine solution 1:1,000 should be available to treat allergic reactions.
- Severe or prolonged reactions may be treated with antitubercular drugs.
- To prepare percutaneous injection, add 1 ml sterile water (without preservatives) to each vial of vaccine. Draw mixture into syringe and expel into ampule three times to ensure adequate mixing.
- If alcohol is used to swab the skin, allow it to evaporate before vaccination. Otherwise, it could inactivate the virus.
- Vaccinate patients with chronic skin diseases in area of healthy skin.
- BCG vaccine is of no value as an immunoprophylactic in patients with a positive PPD test reaction.
- Articles contaminated with this live vaccine must be autoclaved or treated with formaldehyde before disposal.
- Store vaccine at 36° to 46° F (2° to 8° C). Avoid exposure to light.
- BCG vaccine has shown some value in treating various cancers, including malignant melanoma, multiple myeloma, leukemia, bladder cancer, some lung cancers, and some breast tumors. Consult other references and published protocols for appropriate dosage regimens.

Patient education

- Tell patient to expect swollen lymph nodes or a body rash after vaccination. A lesion at the injection site develops within 7 to 10 days of vaccination and may persist for up to 6 months.

• Tell patient to report distressing adverse reactions.
• Tell patient that a tuberculin skin test will be performed 2 to 3 months after vaccination to confirm development of delayed hypersensitivity.

bacitracin

AK-Tracin, Altracin, Baciguent, Baci-IM

Pharmacologic classification: polypeptide antibiotic
Therapeutic classification: antibiotic
Pregnancy risk category C

How supplied

Available without a prescription
Topical: ointment form (500 units/g) and in combination products containing neomycin, polymyxin B, and bacitracin

Available by prescription only
Injection: 50,000-unit vials
Ophthalmic ointment: 500 units/g

Indications, route, and dosage

Topical infections, impetigo, abrasions, cuts, and minor wounds
Adults and children: Apply thin film to cleansed area once daily to t.i.d. for no more than 7 days.
Pneumonia and empyema caused by a staphylococcal infection
Children weighing under 5.5 lb (2.5 kg): 900 units/kg I.M. daily in two or three divided doses.
Children weighing over 5.5 lb: Give 1,000 units/kg I.M. daily in two or three divided doses.
◊ ***Treatment of antibiotic-associated pseudomembranous colitis caused by* Clostridium difficile**
Adults: 20,000 to 25,000 units P.O. q 6 hours for 7 to 10 days.

Pharmacodynamics

Antibacterial action: Bacitracin impairs bacterial cell wall synthesis, damaging the bacterial plasma membrane and making the cell more vulnerable to osmotic pressure. Drug is effective against many gram-positive organisms, including *C. difficile.* Drug is only minimally active against gram-negative organisms.

Pharmacokinetics

• *Absorption:* With I.M. administration, bacitracin is absorbed rapidly and completely; serum concentrations range from 0.2 to 2 mcg/ml. Drug is not absorbed from the GI tract and not significantly absorbed from intact or denuded skin wounds or mucous membranes.
• *Distribution:* Drug is distributed widely throughout all body organs and fluids except CSF (unless meninges are inflamed). Binding to plasma protein is minimal.
• *Metabolism:* Not significantly metabolized.
• *Excretion:* When administered I.M., the kidneys excrete 10% to 40% of dose.

Contraindications and precautions

Contraindicated in patients hypersensitive to drug and in atopic patients. Use cautiously in patients with myasthenia gravis and neuromuscular disease.

Interactions

Systemically administered bacitracin may induce additive damage when given concomitantly with other *nephrotoxic drugs.* It also may prolong or increase neuromuscular blockade induced by *anesthetics* or *neuromuscular blocking agents.*

Effects on diagnostic tests

Urinary sediment tests may show increased protein and cast excretion. Serum creatinine and BUN levels may increase during bacitracin therapy.

Adverse reactions

EENT: slowed corneal wound healing, temporary visual haze (with ophthalmic form), ototoxicity (when topical form is used over large areas for prolonged periods or with systemic use).
Skin: stinging, rash, other allergic reactions; pruritus, burning, swelling of lips or face (with topical form).
GU: ***nephrotoxicity, renal failure.***
Other: *hypersensitivity reactions;* tightness in chest, hypotension; overgrowth of nonsusceptible organisms (with ophthalmic form).

Overdose and treatment

With parenteral administration over several days, bacitracin may cause nephrotoxicity. Acute oral overdose may cause nausea, vomiting, and minor GI upset. Treatment is supportive.

☑ Special considerations

• Culture and sensitivity tests should be done before treatment starts.
• Obtain baseline renal function studies before starting therapy, and monitor results daily for signs of deterioration.
• Patients allergic to neomycin may also be allergic to bacitracin.
• Injectable forms of drug may be used for I.M. administration only. I.V. administration may cause severe thrombophlebitis. Dilute injectable drug in solution containing sodium chloride and 2% procaine hydrochloride (if hospital policy permits). After reconstitution, bacitracin concentration should range from 5,000 to 10,000 units/ml. Inject deeply into upper outer quadrant of buttocks (may be painful). Do not give if patient is sensitive to procaine or para-aminobenzoic acid derivatives.
• Ensure adequate fluid intake and monitor output closely.
• Monitor patient's urine pH. It should be kept above 6 with good hydration, and alkalinizing agents (such as sodium bicarbonate) should be given, if necessary, to limit nephrotoxicity.
• Drug may be used orally with neomycin as bowel preparation or in solution as wound irrigating agent.

Patient education

• Advise patient to discontinue topical use of drug and to call promptly if condition worsens or does not respond to treatment.
• Warn patient with a skin infection to avoid sharing washcloths and towels with family members.
• Instruct patient to wash hands before and after applying ointment.
• Advise patient using ophthalmic ointment to clean eye area of excess exudate before applying ointment. Warn him not to touch tip of tube to any part of eye or surrounding tissue.
• Warn patient that ophthalmic ointment may cause blurred vision. Tell him to stop drug immediately and report symptoms of sensitivity, such as itchy eyelids or constant burning.
• Instruct patient to store ophthalmic ointment in tightly closed, light-resistant container.
• Caution patient not to share eye medications with other persons.

baclofen

Lioresal

Pharmacologic classification: chlorophenyl derivative
Therapeutic classification: skeletal muscle relaxant
Pregnancy risk category C

How supplied

Available by prescription only
Tablets: 10 mg, 20 mg
Intrathecal kit: 500 mcg/ml, 2,000 mcg/ml

Indications, route, and dosage

Spasticity in multiple sclerosis and other spinal cord lesions

Adults: Initially, 5 mg P.O. t.i.d. for 3 days. Dosage may be increased (based on response) at 3-day intervals by 15 mg (5 mg/dose) daily up to maximum of 80 mg daily.

Intrathecal administration

Must be diluted with sterile preservative-free 0.9% NaCl injection.

Adults: Screening phase: Initial intrathecal bolus of 50 mcg in 1 ml over not less than 1 minute. Observe patient for response. A positive response consists of a significant decrease in muscle tone or frequency or severity of spasm. If initial response is inadequate, repeat dose with 75 mcg in 1.5 ml 24 hours after last injection. Repeat observation of patient. If there is still an inadequate response, repeat dosing at 100 mcg in 2 ml 24 hours later. If still no response, patient should not be considered for an implantable pump for chronic baclofen administration. Ranges for chronic doses are 12 to 2,003 mcg/day.

Postimplant dose titration:

If the screening dose produced the desired effect for over 8 hours, the initial intrathecal dose is the same as the test dose; this dose is infused intrathecally for 24 hours. If the screening dose produced the desired effect for less than 8 hours, the initial intrathecal dose is twice the test dose, followed slowly by 10% to 30% increments at 24-hour intervals.

Pharmacodynamics

Skeletal muscle relaxant action: Precise mechanism of action is unknown, but drug appears to act at the spinal cord level to inhibit transmission of monosynaptic and polysynaptic reflexes, possibly through hyperpolarization of afferent fiber terminals. It may also act at supraspinal sites because baclofen at high doses produces generalized CNS depression. Baclofen decreases the number and severity of spasms and relieves associated pain, clonus, and muscle rigidity and therefore improves mobility.

Pharmacokinetics

• *Absorption:* Drug is rapidly and extensively absorbed from the GI tract, but is subject to individual variation. Peak plasma levels occur at 2 to 3 hours. Also, as dose increases, rate and extent of absorption decreases. Onset of therapeutic effect may not be immediately evident; varies from hours to weeks. Peak effect is seen at 2 to 3 hours.
• *Distribution:* Studies indicate that baclofen is widely distributed throughout body, with small amounts crossing the blood-brain barrier. About 30% is plasma protein-bound.
• *Metabolism:* About 15% is metabolized in the liver via deamination.
• *Excretion:* 70% to 80% is excreted in urine unchanged or as its metabolites; remainder, in feces.

Contraindications and precautions

Contraindicated in patients with hypersensitivity to drug. Use cautiously in patients with renal impairment or seizure disorders or when spasticity is used to maintain motor function.

Interactions

Concomitant use with *CNS depressant drugs*, including *alcohol, narcotics, antipsychotics, anxiolytics*, and *general anesthetics*, may add to the CNS effects of drug. Use with *tricyclic antidepressants* or *MAO inhibitors* may cause CNS depression, respiratory depression, and hypotension. Baclofen may increase blood glucose levels and require dosage adjustments of *antidiabetic drug* or *insulin*.

Effects on diagnostic tests

Baclofen therapy increases blood glucose, AST, and alkaline phosphatase levels.

Adverse reactions

CNS: ***CNS depression*** (potentially life-threatening with intrathecal administration), *drowsiness, dizziness,* headache, *weakness, fatigue, hypotonia, confusion,* insomnia, dysarthria, **SEIZURES**.
CV: ***CV collapse*** (secondary to CNS depression), hypotension, hypertension.
EENT: blurred vision, nasal congestion, slurred speech.
GI: *nausea,* constipation, *vomiting.*
GU: urinary frequency.
Hepatic: increased AST and alkaline phosphatase levels.

Respiratory: ***respiratory failure*** (secondary to CNS depression).
Skin: rash, pruritus.
Other: excessive perspiration, hyperglycemia, weight gain, dyspnea.

Overdose and treatment

Clinical manifestations of overdose include absence of reflexes, vomiting, muscular hypotonia, marked salivation, drowsiness, visual disorders, seizures, respiratory depression, and coma.

Treatment requires supportive measures, including endotracheal intubation and positive-pressure ventilation. If patient is conscious, remove drug by inducing emesis followed by gastric lavage.

If patient is comatose, *do not induce emesis.* Gastric lavage may be performed after endotracheal tube is in place with cuff inflated. Do not use respiratory stimulants. Monitor vital signs closely.

☑ Special considerations

- Intrathecal administration should be performed only by qualified individuals familiar with administration techniques and patient management problems.
- Incidence of adverse reactions may be reduced by slowly decreasing the dosage. Abrupt withdrawal can result in hallucinations or seizures and acute exacerbation of spasticity.
- Watch for increased incidence of seizures in patients with epilepsy.
- Watch for increased blood glucose levels in diabetic patients.
- Baclofen is used investigationally to reduce choreiform movements in Huntington's chorea; to reduce rigidity in Parkinson's disease; to reduce spasticity in CVA, cerebral lesions, cerebral palsy, and rheumatic disorders; for analgesia in trigeminal neuralgia; and for treatment of unstable bladder.
- In some patients, smoother response may be obtained by giving daily dose in four divided doses.
- Patient may need supervision during walking. The initial loss of spasticity induced by baclofen may affect patient's ability to stand or walk. (In some patients, spasticity helps patient to maintain upright posture and balance.)
- Observe patient's response to drug. Signs of effective therapy may appear in a few hours to 1 week and may include diminished frequency of spasms and severity of foot and ankle clonus, increased ease and range of joint motion, and enhanced performance of daily activities.
- Discontinue drug if signs of improvement do not occur within 1 to 2 months.
- Closely monitor patients with epilepsy by EEG, clinical observation, and interview for possible loss of seizure control.
- Implantable pump or catheter failure can result in sudden loss of effectiveness of intrathecal baclofen.
- During prolonged intrathecal baclofen therapy for spasticity, approximately 10% of patients become refractory to baclofen therapy requiring a "drug holiday" to regain sensitivity to its effects.

Patient education

- Advise patient to report adverse reactions promptly. Most can be reduced by decreasing dosage. Reportedly, drowsiness, dizziness, and ataxia are more common in patients over age 40.
- Warn patient of additive effects with use of other CNS depressants, including alcohol.
- Caution patient to avoid hazardous activities that require mental alertness.
- Tell diabetic patient that baclofen may elevate blood glucose levels and may require adjustment of insulin dosage during treatment with baclofen. Urge patient to promptly report changes in urine or blood glucose tests.
- Caution patient against taking OTC drugs without medical approval. Explain that hazardous drug interactions are possible.
- Inform patient that drug should be withdrawn gradually over 1 to 2 weeks. Abrupt withdrawal after prolonged use of drug may cause anxiety, agitated behavior, auditory and visual hallucinations, severe tachycardia, and acute spasticity.

Geriatric use

- Elderly patients are especially sensitive to drug. Observe carefully for adverse reactions, such as mental confusion, depression, and hallucinations. Lower doses are usually indicated.

Pediatric use

- Use of oral form is not recommended for children under age 12.
- Safety of intrathecal administration in children under age 4 has not been established.

becaplermin

Regranex Gel

Pharmacologic classification: recombinant human platelet-derived growth factor (rhPDGF-BB)
Therapeutic classification: wound repair agent
Pregnancy risk category C

How supplied

Available by prescription only
Gel: 100 mcg/g in tubes of 2 g, 7.5 g, 15 g

Indications, route and dosage

Treatment of lower extremity diabetic neuropathic ulcers that extend into the subcutaneous tissue and beyond and have an adequate blood supply

Adults: Apply daily in 1/16" even thickness to entire surface of wound. Cover site with a saline-moistened dressing. Remove after 12 hours. Rinse gel from wound with saline or water and cover wound with moist dressing. Continue treatment until complete healing occurs.

When squeezing gel from tubes, length of gel to be applied varies with tube size:

Tube size (g)	Inches	Centimeters
2	ulcer length × ulcer width × 1.3	(ulcer length × ulcer width) ÷ 2
7.5, 15	ulcer length × ulcer width × 0.6	(ulcer length × ulcer width) ÷ 4

Pharmacodynamics

Wound repair action: Recombinant of human platelet-derived growth factor that promotes the chemotactic recruitment and proliferation of cells involved in wound repair and enhances the formation of new granulation tissue.

Pharmacokinetics

- *Absorption:* Minimal systemic absorption, less than 3% in rats.
- *Distribution:* Unknown.
- *Metabolism:* Unknown.
- *Excretion:* Unknown.

Contraindications and precautions

Contraindicated in patients with known hypersensitivity to any component of product or in those with known neoplasms at site of application. Gel is for external use only. If an application site reaction occurs, possibility of sensitization or irritation caused by parabens or m-cresol should be considered.

Interactions

None reported.

Effects on diagnostic tests

None reported.

Adverse reactions

Skin: erythematous rash.

Overdose and treatment

No information available.

☑ Special considerations

- When used as an adjunct to, and not a substitute for, good ulcer care practices including initial sharp débridement, pressure relief, and infection control, gel increases incidence of complete healing of diabetic ulcers. Its efficacy in treating diabetic neuropathic ulcers that do not extend through the dermis into subcutaneous tissue or ischemic diabetic ulcers has not been evaluated.
- Do not use gel in wounds that close by primary intention.
- To apply gel, squeeze the calculated length of gel onto a clean measuring surface, such as wax paper. Then transfer the measured gel from the measuring surface using an application aid.
- Recalculate amount of gel to be applied weekly. If ulcer does not decrease in size by about one-third after 10 weeks or complete healing has not occurred by 20 weeks, reassess continued treatment.
- Use gel in addition to good ulcer care program, including a strict nonweight-bearing program.

Patient education

- Instruct patient to wash hands thoroughly before applying gel.
- Advise patient not to touch tip of tube against ulcer or other surfaces.
- Inform patient to use a cotton swab, tongue blade, or other application aid to apply gel evenly over the surface of the ulcer, producing a thin (1/16″) continuous layer.
- Tell patient to apply drug once daily in a carefully measured quantity. Quantity will change on a weekly basis.
- Tell patient to store gel in the refrigerator, and never to freeze it.
- Inform patient not to use gel after expiration date on the bottom, crimped end of the tube.

Pediatric use

- Safety and effectiveness in patients under age 16 have not been established.

Breast-feeding

- It is not known if drug occurs in breast milk. Use drug with caution when administering to breast-feeding patients.

beclomethasone dipropionate

beclomethasone dipropionate monohydrate

Nasal inhalants
Beconase, Vancenase

Nasal sprays
Beconase AQ, Vancenase AQ

Oral inhalants
Beclovent, Becloforte*, Vanceril

Pharmacologic classification: glucocorticoid
Therapeutic classification: anti-inflammatory, antiasthmatic
Pregnancy risk category C

How supplied

Available by prescription only
Nasal aerosol: 42 mcg/metered spray
Nasal spray: 42 mcg/metered spray
Oral inhalation aerosol: 42 mcg/metered spray

Indications, route, and dosage

Steroid-dependent asthma
Oral inhalation
Adults and children over age 12: Two inhalations t.i.d. or q.i.d. or four inhalations b.i.d. Maximum of 20 inhalations daily.
Children age 6 to 12: One to two inhalations t.i.d. or q.i.d. Maximum of 10 inhalations daily.
Perennial or seasonal rhinitis; prevention of recurrence of nasal polyps after surgical removal
Nasal inhalation
Adults and children over age 12: One spray (42 mcg) in each nostril b.i.d. to q.i.d. Usual total dosage is 168 to 336 mcg daily.

Children age 6 to 12: One spray in each nostril t.i.d. (252 mcg daily).
Nasal spray
Adults and children over age 12: One or two sprays (42 to 84 mcg) in each nostril b.i.d. Usual total dosage is 168 to 336 mcg daily.
Children age 6 to 12: Start with one spray in each nostril b.i.d. (168 mcg daily). If response is inadequate or symptoms more severe, dose can be increased to two sprays per nostril b.i.d. (336 mcg daily).
Nonallergic (vasomotor) rhinitis
Nasal spray
Adults and children over age 12: One or two sprays (42 to 84 mcg) in each nostril b.i.d. Usual total dosage is 168 to 336 mcg daily.
Children age 6 to 12: Start with one spray in each nostril b.i.d. (168 mcg daily). If response is inadequate or symptoms more severe, the dose can be increased to two sprays per nostril b.i.d. (336 mcg daily).

Pharmacodynamics

Anti-inflammatory action: Beclomethasone stimulates the synthesis of enzymes needed to decrease the inflammatory response. The anti-inflammatory and vasoconstrictor potency of topically applied beclomethasone is, on a weight basis, about 5,000 times greater than that of hydrocortisone, 500 times greater than that of betamethasone or dexamethasone, and about 5 times greater than fluocinolone or triamcinolone.

Antiasthmatic action: Beclomethasone is used as a nasal inhalant to treat symptoms of seasonal or perennial rhinitis and to prevent the recurrence of nasal polyps after surgical removal, and as an oral inhalant to treat bronchial asthma in patients who require chronic administration of corticosteroids to control symptoms.

Pharmacokinetics

- *Absorption:* After nasal inhalation, drug is absorbed primarily through the nasal mucosa, with minimal systemic absorption. After oral inhalation, drug is absorbed rapidly from the lungs and GI tract. Greater systemic absorption is associated with oral inhalation, but systemic effects do not occur at usual doses because of rapid metabolism in the liver and local metabolism of drug that reaches the lungs. Onset of action usually occurs in a few days but may take as long as 3 weeks in some patients.
- *Distribution:* Distribution after intranasal administration has not been described. There is no evidence of tissue storage of drug or its metabolites. About 10% to 25% of a nasal spray or orally inhaled dose is deposited in the respiratory tract. The remainder, deposited in the mouth and oropharynx, is swallowed. When absorbed, it is 87% bound to plasma proteins.
- *Metabolism:* Swallowed drug undergoes rapid metabolism in the liver or GI tract to several metabolites, some of which have minor glucocorticoid activity. The portion that is inhaled into the respiratory tract is partially metabolized before absorption into systemic circulation. Drug is mostly metabolized in the liver.
- *Excretion:* Excretion of inhaled drug has not been described; however, when drug is administered systemically, its metabolites are excreted mainly in feces via biliary elimination and to a lesser extent in urine. Biological half-life of drug averages 15 hours.

Contraindications and precautions

Contraindicated in patients hypersensitive to drug and in those experiencing status asthmaticus or other acute episodes of asthma. Use cautiously in patients with tuberculosis, fungal or bacterial infection, herpes, or systemic viral infection.

Interactions

None reported.

Effects on diagnostic tests

None reported.

Adverse reactions

CNS: headache.
EENT: *mild transient nasal burning and stinging,* nasal congestion, sneezing, burning, stinging, dryness, epistaxis, nasopharyngeal fungal infections, hoarseness, fungal infection of throat, throat irritation.
GI: dry mouth, fungal infection of mouth.
Skin: hypersensitivity reactions (urticaria, rash).
Other: ***angioedema, bronchospasm,*** suppression of hypothalamic-pituitary-adrenal function, ***adrenal insufficiency,*** facial edema, wheezing.

Overdose and treatment

No information available.

☑ Special considerations

Recommendations for use of beclomethasone and for care and teaching of patients during therapy are the same as those for all *inhalant adrenocorticoids.*

Pediatric use

- Drug is not recommended for children under age 6.

benazepril hydrochloride

Lotensin

Pharmacologic classification: ACE inhibitor
Therapeutic classification: antihypertensive
Pregnancy risk category C (D in second and third trimesters)

How supplied

Available by prescription only
Tablets: 5 mg, 10 mg, 20 mg, 40 mg

Indications, route, and dosage

Hypertension
Adults: Initially, 10 mg P.O. daily. Titrate dosage as needed and tolerated; maintenance dosage range is 20 to 40 mg daily in one or two equally divided doses.

✦ ***Dosage adjustment.*** In patients with renal failure with creatinine clearance below 30 ml/minute/1.73 m², initial dose is 5 mg P.O. daily. Do not exceed 40 mg daily.

Note: Although rare, angioedema has been reported in patients receiving ACE inhibitors. Angioedema associated with laryngeal edema or shock may be fatal. If angioedema of the face, extremities, lips, tongue, glottis, or larynx occurs, treatment with benazepril should be discontinued and appropriate therapy instituted immediately.

Pharmacodynamics

Antihypertensive action: Benazepril and its active metabolite, benazeprilat, inhibit ACE, preventing conversion of angiotensin I to angiotensin II, a potent vasoconstrictor. Reduced formation of angiotensin II decreases peripheral arterial resistance and aldosterone secretion, which reduces sodium and water retention and lowers blood pressure.

Although the primary mechanism through which benazepril lowers blood pressure is believed to be suppression of the renin-angiotensin-aldosterone system, benazepril has an antihypertensive effect even in patients with low renin levels.

Pharmacokinetics

- *Absorption:* At least 37% of drug is absorbed. After oral administration, peak plasma concentrations are reached within 0.5 to 1 hour.
- *Distribution:* Serum protein binding of drug is about 96.7%; that of benazeprilat, 95.3%.
- *Metabolism:* Benazepril is almost completely metabolized in the liver to benazeprilat, which has much greater ACE inhibitory activity than benazepril, and to the glucuronide conjugates of benazepril and benazeprilat.
- *Excretion:* Drug is excreted primarily in the urine.

Contraindications and precautions

Contraindicated in patients with hypersensitivity to ACE inhibitors. Use cautiously in patients with renal or hepatic impairment.

Interactions

Diuretics and other *antihypertensive agents* increase risk of excessive hypotension. The diuretic may need to be discontinued or benazepril dose lowered. Concomitant use with *lithium* increases serum lithium levels and lithium toxicity. Avoid concomitant use.

Concomitant use of *potassium-sparing diuretics, potassium supplements,* and *sodium substitutes* containing potassium should also be avoided because of risk of hyperkalemia. Concomitant use with *digoxin* may increase plasma digoxin levels. Concomitant use with *allopurinol* may increase risk of hypersensitivity reaction.

Effects on diagnostic tests

ACE inhibitors may cause agranulocytosis and bone marrow depression; however, available data on benazepril are insufficient to show that benazepril does not affect the CBC in the same way. Drug may increase serum creatinine and BUN levels. Elevations of liver enzymes, serum bilirubin, uric acid, and blood glucose have been reported, along with scattered incidents of hyponatremia, electrocardiographic changes, leukopenia, eosinophilia, and proteinuria.

Adverse reactions

CNS: headache, dizziness, anxiety, fatigue, insomnia, nervousness, paresthesia.
CV: symptomatic hypotension, palpitations.
EENT: dysphagia, increased salivation.
GI: nausea, vomiting, abdominal pain, constipation.
Respiratory: dry, persistent, tickling, nonproductive cough; dyspnea.
Skin: hypersensitivity reactions (rash, pruritus), increased diaphoresis.
Other: ***angioedema,*** arthralgia, arthritis, impotence, myalgia, hyperkalemia.

Overdose and treatment

Hypotension is the most common symptom of overdose. No data suggest physiologic maneuvers that might accelerate elimination of benazepril and its metabolite if an overdose occurs. Drug is only slightly dialyzable, but dialysis might be considered in overdosed patients with severely impaired renal function. Angiotensin II could presumably serve as a specific antagonist-antidote, but angiotensin II is essentially unavailable outside of scattered research facilities. Because drug's hypotensive effect is achieved through vasodilation and effective hypovolemia, treatment of benazepril overdose by I.V. infusion of 0.9% NaCl solution is reasonable.

☑ Special considerations

- Blood pressure should be measured when drug levels are at peak (2 to 6 hours after a dose) and at trough (just before a dose) to verify adequate blood pressure control.
- Excessive hypotension can occur when drug is given with diuretics. If possible, diuretic therapy should be discontinued 2 to 3 days before starting benazepril to decrease the potential for excessive hypotensive response. If benazepril does not adequately control blood pressure, diuretic therapy may be reinstituted with care. If the diuretic cannot be discontinued, initiate benazepril therapy at 5 mg P.O. daily.
- Assess renal and hepatic function before and periodically throughout therapy. Monitor serum potassium levels.
- Other ACE inhibitors have been associated with agranulocytosis and neutropenia. Monitor CBC with differential counts before therapy, every 2 weeks for first 3 months of therapy and periodically thereafter.

Patient education

- Advise patient to report signs or symptoms of infection (such as fever and sore throat); easy bruising or bleeding; swelling of tongue, lips, face, eyes, mucous membranes, or extremities; difficulty swallowing or breathing; and hoarseness.
- Because light-headedness can occur, especially during the first few days of therapy, tell patient to rise slowly to minimize this effect and to report symptoms. Tell patient who experiences syncope to stop taking drug and call immediately.

• Inadequate fluid intake, vomiting, diarrhea, and excessive perspiration can lead to light-headedness and syncope. Tell patient to use caution in hot weather and during exercise.
• Tell patient to avoid sodium substitutes; these products may contain potassium, which can cause hyperkalemia in patients on drug therapy.
• Tell female patient of childbearing age about consequences of second- and third-trimester exposure to ACE inhibitors. Explain that these do not appear to result from exposure during the first trimester. Advise her to report suspected pregnancy as soon as possible.
• A persistent dry cough may occur and usually does not subside unless drug is stopped. Advise patient to call if this effect becomes bothersome.

Pediatric use
• Safety and effectiveness in children have not been established.

Breast-feeding
• Minimal amounts of unchanged benazepril and benazeprilat are excreted in breast milk. Exercise caution when administering to breast-feeding women.

bentiromide
Chymex

Pharmacologic classification: para-aminobenzoic acid (PABA) derivative
Therapeutic classification: pancreatic function test
Pregnancy risk category B

How supplied
Available by prescription only
Solution: 500 mg/7.5 ml (170 mg PABA)

Indications, route, and dosage
Screening test for pancreatic exocrine insufficiency; monitoring of adequacy of supplemental pancreatic therapy
Adults and children over age 12: Following overnight fast and morning void, administer a single 500-mg dose P.O., and follow with an 8-oz (240 ml) glass of water.
Children age 6 to 12: Dose is 14 mg/kg followed with an 8-oz (240 ml) glass of water.

Give patient another glass of water 2 hours after dose. An additional two glasses of water are recommended during 2 to 6 hours postdosing.

Pharmacodynamics
Pancreatic function testing action: Following oral administration, bentiromide is cleaved by the pancreatic enzyme chymotrypsin, causing the release of PABA. This test is not conclusive, because a negative result does not rule out pancreatic disease and an abnormal result is only a strong indicator of a problem. Confirmatory tests are required.

Pharmacokinetics
• *Absorption:* Depends on presence of chymotrypsin in the small intestine. PABA is absorbed after hydrolysis of bentiromide by chymotrypsin; the extent of absorption may be altered by other conditions, including gastric stasis, maldigestion, and malabsorption. Mean peak plasma level in healthy adults is about 6 mcg/ml and occurs in 2 to 3 hours. In patients with chronic pancreatitis, mean peak plasma levels are reduced to 3 mcg/ml and occur in 2 to 6 hours.
• *Distribution:* Distribution into body tissues and fluids iss unknown for bentiromide or PABA.
• *Metabolism:* Drug is hydrolyzed in the small intestine and the metabolites are further broken down in the liver.
• *Excretion:* PABA and its metabolites are excreted in urine.

Contraindications and precautions
Contraindicated in patients with hypersensitivity to drug or PABA; such patients may have an anaphylactic reaction. Drug should be used cautiously in pregnant and breast-feeding patients because safety has not been established.

Interactions
When used concomitantly, bentiromide may displace *methotrexate* from PABA binding sites. *Pancreatic enzyme preparations* may yield a false-negative result; they should be discontinued 5 days before testing with bentiromide. PABA interferes with the antibacterial action of sulfa drugs. Therapeutic and toxic effects of salicylates may be increased with concomitant use of PABA.

Effects on diagnostic tests
Drug therapy alters no other tests, but several factors may invalidate bentiromide test results. Drugs such as acetaminophen, benzocaine, chloramphenicol, thiazides, lidocaine, PABA preparations, procainamide, procaine, and sulfonamides are metabolized into arylamines, which increase the PABA content in urine. Foods such as apples, plums, prunes, and cranberries act similarly. All these drugs and foods should be discontinued at least 3 days before testing with bentiromide. If retesting using bentiromide is needed, separate subsequent administration by at least 7 days to avoid interference of test results by prior bentiromide dosings.

Adverse reactions
CNS: headache.
GI: diarrhea, flatulence, nausea, vomiting.
Respiratory: shortness of breath (rare).
Other: weakness.

Overdose and treatment
No information available.

☑ Special considerations
• A pretest urine sample may help determine dietary PABA levels.
• Hydrate patient after administration of bentiromide by giving 250 ml of water immediately and 250 to 750 ml during the next 6 hours.

• Collect patient's urine for exactly 6 hours after administration for analysis.
• Monitor blood glucose for possible adjsutment in diabetic patient during fast.

Patient education

• Tell patient to avoid the medications and foods listed in "Interactions" and "Effects on diagnostic tests" sections for the specified times.
• Tell patient to fast after midnight the night before test.
• Instruct patient to void just before testing to ensure accurate results.

Pediatric use

• Dose for children age 6 to 12 is 14 mg/kg, to a maximum dose of 500 mg.

benzocaine

Americaine, Hurricaine, Lanacane, Maximum Strength Anbesol, Mouth Aid, Orabase Gel, Orajel, Solarcaine

Pharmacologic classification: local anesthetic (ester)
Therapeutic classification: anesthetic
Pregnancy risk category C

How supplied

Available without a prescription
Gel: 20%
Ointment, cream, and dental paste: 1% to 20%
Topical solution: 20%
Topical spray: 20%
Lotion: 0.5% to 8%

Indications, route, and dosage

Local anesthetic for dental pain or dental procedures
Adults and children: Apply topical gel (20%) or dental paste to area p.r.n.
Local anesthetic for pruritic dermatoses, pruritus, or other irritations
Adults: Apply topical preparation (1% to 20%) to affected area p.r.n.
Relief of pain and pruritus in acute congestive and serous otitis media, acute swimmer's ear, and other forms of otitis externa
Adults: 4 to 5 drops (otic) in external auditory canal; insert cotton into meatus; repeat q 1 to 2 hours.

Pharmacodynamics

Analgesic action: Acts at sensory neurons to produce a local anesthetic effect.

Pharmacokinetics

• *Absorption:* No information available.
• *Distribution:* No information available.
• *Metabolism:* No information available.
• *Excretion:* No information available.

Contraindications and precautions

Contraindicated in patients with hypersensitivity to any component of the preparation or related substances and in those with secondary infection in the area or serious burns. Do not use in eyes or in ears with a perforated tympanic membrane or discharge. Use cautiously in patients with severely traumatized mucosa or local sepsis.

Interactions

None significant.

Effects on diagnostic tests

None reported.

Adverse reactions

Skin: urticaria, burning, stinging, tenderness, irritation, itching, erythema, rash.
Other: edema.

Note: Discontinue drug if symptoms of hypersensitivity occur.

Overdose and treatment

Maximum recommended dose is 5 g/day. Overdose is unlikely; however, methemoglobinemia has been reported after topical application for teething pain. Treat symptomatically; if necessary, administer methylene blue 1% 0.1 ml/kg I.V. over at least 10 minutes.

☑ Special considerations

• Use with antibiotic to treat underlying cause of pain because using alone may mask more serious condition.
• Keep container tightly closed and away from moisture.

Patient education

• Tell patient to call if pain lasts longer than 48 hours, if burning or itching occurs, or if the condition persists.
• Instruct patient to keep container tightly closed and away from moisture.
• Advise patient not to eat or chew gum until effect of local anesthetic has worn off to avoid the risk of bite trauma.

Pediatric use

• Excessive use may cause methemoglobinemia in infants. Do not use in children under age 1.

benzonatate

Tessalon Perles

Pharmacologic classification: local anesthetic (ester)
Therapeutic classification: nonnarcotic antitussive
Pregnancy risk category C

How supplied

Available by prescription only
Capsules: 100 mg

Indications, route, and dosage

Cough suppression
Adults and children over age 10: 100 mg P.O. t.i.d.; up to 600 mg daily.

Children under age 10: 8 mg/kg daily P.O. in three to six divided doses.

Pharmacodynamics

Antitussive action: Drug suppresses the cough reflex at its source by anesthetizing peripheral stretch receptors located in the respiratory passages, lungs, and pleura.

Pharmacokinetics

- *Absorption:* Action begins within 15 to 20 minutes and lasts for 3 to 8 hours.
- *Distribution:* Not established.
- *Metabolism:* Not established.
- *Excretion:* Not established.

Contraindications and precautions

Contraindicated in patients hypersensitive to drug or para-aminobenzoic acid anesthetics (procaine, tetracaine).

Interactions

None significant.

Effects on diagnostic tests

None reported.

Adverse reactions

CNS: dizziness, headache, sedation.
EENT: nasal congestion, burning sensation in eyes.
GI: nausea, constipation, GI upset.
Skin: hypersensitivity reactions (rash).
Other: chills.

Overdose and treatment

CNS stimulation from overdose of drug may cause restlessness and tremors, which may lead to chronic seizures followed by profound CNS depression.

Empty stomach by gastric lavage and follow with activated charcoal. Treat seizures with a short-acting barbiturate given I.V; do not use CNS stimulants. Mechanical respiratory support may be necessary in severe cases.

☑ Special considerations

- Monitor cough type and frequency and volume and quality of sputum. Encourage fluid intake to help liquefy sputum.

Patient education

- Instruct patient not to chew or dissolve capsules in the mouth because local anesthesia will result.
- Teach patient comfort measures for a nonproductive cough: limit talking and smoking; use a cold mist or steam vaporizer; use sugarless hard candy to increase saliva flow.

Breast-feeding

- Safe use during breast-feeding has not been established.

benzquinamide hydrochloride

Emete-Con

Pharmacologic classification: benzoquinolizine derivative
Therapeutic classification: antiemetic
Pregnancy risk category NR

How supplied

Available by prescription only
Injection: 50 mg/vial

Indications, route, and dosage

Nausea and vomiting associated with anesthesia and surgery
Adults: 50 mg I.M. (0.5 to 1 mg/kg); may repeat in 1 hour and thereafter q 3 to 4 hours, p.r.n. Or 25 mg (0.2 to 0.4 mg/kg) I.V. as single dose, administered slowly.

Pharmacodynamics

Antiemetic action: Drug probably acts directly at the chemoreceptor trigger zone (vomiting center). Exact mechanism is unknown, but drug has anticholinergic, antihistamine, and antiseritonergic activity.

Pharmacokinetics

- *Absorption:* Unknown. Onset of action occurs in about 15 minutes and duration of action is 3 to 4 hours.
- *Distribution:* Distributed rapidly in body tissues, with highest concentration in the liver and kidneys. About 58% of drug is plasma protein-bound.
- *Metabolism:* Mostly (90% to 95%) metabolized in the liver.
- *Excretion:* About 5% to 10% of drug is excreted unchanged in urine. Metabolites are excreted in urine, bile, and feces.

Contraindications and precautions

Contraindicated in patients with hypersensitivity to drug as well as for I.V. use in patients with CV disease and within 15 minutes of administering preanesthetic or CV drugs.

Interactions

When used concomitantly, benzquinamide may enhance response to *drugs that increase blood pressure* such as *epinephrine.*

Effects on diagnostic tests

Benzquinamide increases free fatty acid serum levels.

Adverse reactions

CNS: *drowsiness,* fatigue, insomnia, nervousness, restlessness, headache, excitation, tremor, twitching, dizziness.
CV: sudden elevation in blood pressure, transient arrhythmias (premature atrial contractions, PVCs, atrial fibrillation) (after I.V. administration); hypertension; hypotension.
EENT: salivation, blurred vision.

GI: anorexia, nausea, dry mouth.
Skin: urticaria, rash, diaphoresis, allergic reactions, flushing.
Other: muscle weakness, hiccups, chills, fever.

Overdose and treatment

Overdosage may manifest itself as a combination of CNS stimulant and depressant effects. Treatment includes providing supportive measures. Use of atropine may be helpful.

☑ Special considerations

- I.M administration is the preferred route. CV adverse reactions are more likely to occur with I.V. administration.
- Reconstitute with 2.2 ml sterile water for injection or bacteriostatic water for injection. Solution remains stable for 14 days at room temperature. Protect stored drug from light.
- Give I.M. injection into large muscle mass; use deltoid muscle only if well developed. Be especially careful to avoid inadvertent I.V. injection.
- Monitor patient's blood pressure. (Patient who is receiving drugs that increase blood pressure may require a lower dose.)

Patient education

- Warn patient that drug may cause dry mouth.

Geriatric use

- Because elderly patients commonly have CV problems, including hypertension, they may require a decreased dose.

Pediatric use

- Drug is not approved for use in children.

benztropine mesylate

Cogentin

Pharmacologic classification: anticholinergic
Therapeutic classification: antiparkinsonian agent
Pregnancy risk category C

How supplied

Available by prescription only
Tablets: 0.5 mg, 1 mg, 2 mg
Injection: 1 mg/ml in 2-ml ampule

Indications, route, and dosage

Acute dystonic reaction
Adults: 1 to 2 mg I.M. or I.V. followed by 1 to 2 mg P.O. b.i.d. to prevent recurrence.
Parkinsonism
Adults: 0.5 to 6 mg P.O. daily. Initially, 0.5 to 1 mg, increased 0.5 mg q 5 to 6 days. Adjust dosage to meet individual requirements. Maximum dosage, 6 mg/day.
Drug-induced extrapyramidal reactions
Adults: 1 to 4 mg P.O. or I.V. daily or b.i.d. Adjust dosage to meet individual requirements. Maximum dosage, 6 mg/day.

Pharmacodynamics

Antiparkinsonian action: Benztropine blocks central cholinergic receptors, helping to balance cholinergic activity in the basal ganglia. It may also prolong effects of dopamine by blocking dopamine reuptake and storage at central receptor sites.

Pharmacokinetics

- *Absorption:* Drug is absorbed from the GI tract.
- *Distribution:* Largely unknown; however, drug crosses the blood-brain barrier and may cross the placenta.
- *Metabolism:* Unknown.
- *Excretion:* Like other muscarinics, benztropine is excreted in the urine as unchanged drug and metabolites. After oral therapy, small amounts are probably excreted in feces as unabsorbed drug.

Contraindications and precautions

Contraindicated in patients with hypersensitivity to drug or its components or acute angle-closure glaucoma and in children under age 3. Use cautiously in hot weather, in patients with mental disorders, and in children over age 3.

Interactions

Concomitant use with *amantadine* may amplify such adverse anticholinergic effects as confusion and hallucinations. Benztropine dosage should be decreased before giving *amantadine.* Concomitant use with *haloperidol* and *phenothiazines* may decrease their effect, possibly reflecting direct CNS antagonism. Concomitant use with *phenothiazines* increases the risk of adverse anticholinergic effects.

Alcohol and other *CNS depressants* increase the sedative effects of benztropine. *Antacids* and *antidiarrheals* may decrease benztropine absorption. Administer benztropine at least 1 hour before administering these agents.

Effects on diagnostic tests

None reported.

Adverse reactions

CNS: disorientation, hallucinations, depression, toxic psychosis, confusion, memory impairment, nervousness.
CV: tachycardia.
EENT: dilated pupils, blurred vision.
GI: dry mouth, *constipation,* nausea, vomiting, paralytic ileus.
GU: urine retention, dysuria.

Some adverse reactions may result from atropine-like toxicity and are dose related.

Overdose and treatment

Clinical manifestations of overdose include central stimulation followed by depression and psychotic symptoms such as disorientation, confusion, hallucinations, delusions, anxiety, agitation, and restlessness. Peripheral effects may include dilated, nonreactive pupils; blurred vision; hot, flushed, dry skin; dryness of mucous membranes; dysphagia; decreased or absent bowel sounds; urine retention; hyperthermia; tachycardia; hypertension; and increased respiration.

Treatment is primarily symptomatic and supportive, as necessary. Maintain a patent airway. If patient is alert, induce emesis (or use gastric lavage) and follow with a sodium chloride cathartic and activated charcoal to prevent further absorption. In severe cases, physostigmine may be administered to block the antimuscarinic effects of benztropine. Give fluids as needed to treat shock, diazepam to control psychotic symptoms, and pilocarpine (instilled into the eyes) to relieve mydriasis. If urine retention occurs, catheterization may be necessary.

☑ Special considerations

Besides those relevant to all *anticholinergics*, consider the following recommendations.

- To help prevent gastric irritation, administer drug after meals.
- Never discontinue drug abruptly.
- Monitor patient for intermittent constipation and abdominal distention and pain, which may indicate paralytic ileus.

Patient education

- Explain that drug's full effect may not occur for 2 to 3 days after therapy begins.
- Caution patient not to discontinue drug suddenly; dosage should be reduced gradually.
- Tell patient that drug may increase sensitivity of eyes to light.

Pediatric use

- Drug is not recommended for use in children under age 3.

Breast-feeding

- Drug may be excreted in breast milk, possibly causing infant toxicity. Avoid use of drug in breast-feeding women. Benztropine may decrease milk production.

bepridil hydrochloride

Vascor

Pharmacologic classification: calcium channel blocker
Therapeutic classification: antianginal
Pregnancy risk category C

How supplied

Available by prescription only
Tablets: 200 mg, 300 mg, 400 mg

Indications, route, and dosage

Treatment of chronic stable angina (classic effort-associated angina) in patients who are unresponsive or inadequately responsive to other antianginals

Adults: Initially, 200 mg P.O. daily; after 10 days, adjust dosage based on patient tolerance and response. Most common maintenance dose is 300 mg daily. Maximum daily dose, 400 mg.

Pharmacodynamics

Antianginal action: Precise mechanism of action is unknown. It inhibits calcium ion influx into cardiac and vascular smooth muscle and also inhibits the sodium inward influx, resulting in reductions in the maximal upstroke velocity and amplitude of the action potential. It is believed to reduce heart rate and arterial pressure by dilating peripheral arterioles and reducing total peripheral resistance (afterload). The effects are dose-dependent. Bepridil has dose-related class I antiarrhythmic properties affecting electrophysiologic changes, such as prolongation of QT and QTc intervals.

Pharmacokinetics

- *Absorption:* Drug is rapidly and completely absorbed after oral administration; peak concentrations occur in 2 to 3 hours.
- *Distribution:* Over 99% of drug is plasma protein-bound.
- *Metabolism:* Metabolized in the liver.
- *Excretion:* Elimination is biphasic. Bepridil has a distribution half-life of 2 hours. Over 10 days, 70% is excreted in urine, 22% in feces as metabolites. Terminal half-life after multiple dosing averaged 42 hours (range, 26 to 64 hours).

Contraindications and precautions

Contraindicated in patients with hypersensitivity to drug; uncompensated cardiac insufficiency, sick sinus syndrome or second- or third-degree AV block unless pacemaker is present; hypotension (below 90 mm Hg systolic); congenital QT interval prolongation; or history of serious ventricular arrhythmias. Also contraindicated in those receiving other drugs that prolong QT interval.

Use cautiously in patients with left bundle-branch block, sinus bradycardia, impaired renal or hepatic function, or heart failure. Drug is not recommended for use in patients within 3 months of an MI.

Interactions

Concurrent administration with *quinidine, procainamide,* or *tricyclic antidepressants* is contraindicated because of additive prolongation of QT interval. Also avoid *potassium-wasting diuretics* because of their potential for causing hypokalemia, which increases risk of serious ventricular arrhythmias. Modest increases in steady-state serum *digoxin* concentrations have also been observed with concurrent use of bepridil, although data are insufficient to determine clinical significance in patients with cardiac conduction abnormalities.

Effects on diagnostic tests

Increased ALT levels and abnormal liver function test results have been observed.

Adverse reactions

CNS: *dizziness,* drowsiness, *nervousness, headache,* insomnia, paresthesia, *asthenia,* tremor.
CV: edema, flushing, palpitations, tachycardia, ***ventricular arrhythmias, including torsades de pointes, ventricular tachycardia, ventricular fibrillation.***
EENT: tinnitus.
GI: *nausea, diarrhea,* constipation, abdominal discomfort, dry mouth, anorexia.
Hematologic: ***agranulocytosis.***

Respiratory: dyspnea, shortness of breath.
Skin: rash.
Other: flu syndrome.

Overdose and treatment

Exaggerated adverse reactions, especially clinically significant hypotension, high-degree AV block, and ventricular tachycardia, have been observed. Treat with appropriate supportive measures, including gastric lavage, beta-adrenergic stimulation, parenteral calcium solutions, vasopressor agents, and cardioversion, as necessary. Close observation in a cardiac care facility for a minimum of 48 hours is recommended.

☑ Special considerations

- Careful patient selection and monitoring are essential. Use the following selection criteria: Diagnosis of chronic stable angina with failure to respond or inadequate response to other therapies, QTc interval less than 0.44 seconds, absence of hypokalemia, hypotension, severe left ventricular dysfunction, serious ventricular arrhythmias, unpacked sick sinus syndrome, second- or third-degree AV block, and no concomitant use of other drugs that prolong the QT interval.
- Monitor serum potassium levels and correct hypokalemia before initiating therapy. Use potassium-sparing diuretics for patients who require diuretic therapy.
- Monitor QTc interval before and during therapy. Reduced dosage is required if QTc prolongation is greater than 0.52 seconds or increases more than 25%. If prolongation of QTc interval persists, discontinue bepridil.
- Beta blockers, nitrates, digoxin, insulin, and oral antidiabetic agents may be used with bepridil.
- Food does not interfere with absorption of bepridil.
- Elderly patients may require more frequent monitoring.
- Use cautiously in patients with renal or hepatic disorders. No clinical data are available.
- If infection is suspected, obtain WBC count.

Patient education

- Instruct patient to recognize signs and symptoms of hypokalemia and the importance of compliance with prescribed potassium supplements.
- Tell patient to report signs or symptoms of infection, such as sore throat and fever.
- Instruct patient to take drug with food or at bedtime if nausea occurs.

Geriatric use

- Recommended starting dose is same as in adult patients; however, more frequent monitoring may be required.

Pediatric use

- Safety and efficacy have not been established.

Breast-feeding

- Drug is excreted in breast milk; risk-benefit must be assessed.

beractant (natural lung surfactant)

Survanta

Pharmacologic classification: bovine lung extract
Therapeutic classification: lung surfactant
Pregnancy risk category NR

How supplied

Available by prescription only
Suspension: 25 mg of phospholipids/ml suspended in 0.9% NaCl in 8-ml single-dose vials

Indications, route, and dosage

Prevention and treatment (rescue) of respiratory distress syndrome (RDS; hyaline membrane disease) in premature infants
Infants: 100 mg of phospholipids/kg of birth weight (4 ml/kg) administered by intratracheal instillation through a 5 French end-hole catheter inserted into the infant's endotracheal tube with the tip of the catheter protruding just beyond the end of the tube above the carina. Shorten the length of the catheter before inserting it through the tube. Beractant should not be instilled into a mainstem bronchus. Use the accompanying dosing chart as a guide.

BERACTANT DOSING CHART

Weight (g)	Total dose (ml)
600 to 650	2.6
651 to 700	2.8
701 to 750	3
751 to 800	3.2
801 to 850	3.4
851 to 900	3.6
901 to 950	3.8
951 to 1000	4
1001 to 1050	4.2
1051 to 1100	4.4
1101 to 1150	4.6
1151 to 1200	4.8
1201 to 1250	5
1251 to 1300	5.2
1301 to 1350	5.4
1351 to 1400	5.6
1401 to 1450	5.8
1451 to 1500	6
1501 to 1550	6.2
1551 to 1600	6.4
1601 to 1650	6.6
1651 to 1700	6.8
1701 to 1750	7
1751 to 1800	7.2

(continued)

BERACTANT DOSING CHART *(continued)*

Weight (g)	Total dose (ml)
1801 to 1850	7.4
1851 to 1900	7.6
1901 to 1950	7.8
1951 to 2000	8

Pharmacodynamics

Surfactant action: Beractant is a natural bovine lung extract containing phospholipids, neutral lipids, fatty acids, and surfactant-associated proteins to which dipalmitoylphosphatidylcholine, palmitic acid, and tripalmitin are added to standardize and to mimic surface tension-lowering properties of natural lung surfactant. Endogenous lung surfactant lowers surface tension on alveolar surfaces during respiration and stabilizes the alveoli against collapse at resting transpulmonary pressures. Drug lowers minimum surface tension, restores pulmonary surfactant, and restores surface activity to the lungs of premature infants with RDS.

Pharmacokinetics

- *Absorption:* Most of the administered dose becomes lung-associated within hours.
- *Distribution:* Across the alveolar surface.
- *Metabolism:* Lipids enter endogenous surfactant pathway of recycling and reutilization.
- *Excretion:* Alveolar clearance of lipid components is rapid.

Contraindications and precautions

No known contraindications.

Interactions

None significant.

Effects on diagnostic tests

None reported.

Adverse reactions

CV: *transient bradycardia,* vasoconstriction, hypotension.
Hematologic: decreased oxygen saturation, hypocapnia, hypercapnia.
Other: endotracheal tube reflux or blockage, pallor, ***apnea.***

Overdose and treatment

Overdose may result in acute airway obstruction. Treatment should be supportive and symptomatic.

☑ Special considerations

- Crackles and moist breath sounds can occur transiently after beractant administration. Endotracheal suctioning or other remedial action is not required unless clear-cut signs of airway obstruction are present.
- There is an increased probability of post-treatment nosocomial sepsis.
- Frequently monitor infant. Transient bradycardia and decreased oxygen saturation have occurred during dosing. Initiate appropriate corrective measures.
- Marked improvements in oxygenation may occur within minutes of administration and significant improvements may be sustained for 48 to 72 hours.
- Ensure proper placement and patency of endotracheal tube before administration. Suction endotracheal tube if needed and allow infant to stabilize before administration of beractant.
- Determine total dose and slowly withdraw entire contents of vial into syringe through at least a 20G needle. Attach premeasured French catheter to syringe and fill with beractant. Discard excess through the catheter so that syringe contains only the total dose to be given.
- To ensure homogeneous distribution of beractant, each dose is divided into quarter doses and administered with the infant in a different position: head and body inclined slightly down, head turned to the right; head and body inclined slightly down, head turned to the left; head and body inclined slightly up, head turned to the right; head and body inclined slightly up, head turned to the left. Four doses may be administered within the first 48 hours of life at intervals not exceeding every 6 hours.
- Refrigerate stored beractant; warm to room temperature before administration (standing, at least 20 minutes; in hand, at least 8 minutes). Do not use artificial warming methods.
- Begin preparation before infant's birth if preventive dose is to be given.

Prevention strategy: Weigh, intubate, and stabilize infant. Dose should be administered as soon as possible after birth, within 15 minutes. Position infant and gently instill first quarter dose through catheter over 2 to 3 seconds; remove catheter and manually ventilate with sufficient oxygen to prevent cyanosis, at a rate of 60 breaths/minute and with sufficient positive pressure to provide adequate air exchange and chest wall excursion.

Rescue strategy: First dose should be given as soon as possible after the infant is placed on a ventilator for management of RDS, preferably by 8 hours of age. Position infant and gently instill first quarter dose through catheter over 2 to 3 seconds; remove catheter and return infant to mechanical ventilator.

Both strategies: Ventilate infant for at least 30 seconds or until stable. Reposition infant and instill next quarter dose. Remaining doses should be instilled using same procedure. After final quarter dose is administered, remove catheter without flushing. Do not suction for 1 hour unless signs of significant airway obstruction occur. Resume usual ventilator management and clinical care once dosing procedure is completed.

Repeat doses: Need for repeat doses is determined by evidence of continuing respiratory distress. Dosage is 100 mg phospholipids/kg based on infant's birth-weight. Infant should not be reweighed.

betamethasone (systemic)
Betnelan*, Celestone

betamethasone sodium phosphate
Betnesol*, Celestone Phosphate, Selestoject

betamethasone sodium phosphate and betamethasone acetate
Celestone Soluspan

Pharmacologic classification: glucocorticoid
Therapeutic classification: anti-inflammatory
Pregnancy risk category NR

How supplied
Available by prescription only
betamethasone
Tablets: 0.6 mg
Syrup: 0.6 mg/5 ml
betamethasone sodium phosphate
Tablets (effervescent): 500 mcg*
Injection: 4 mg (3 mg base)/ml in 5-ml vials
*Enema**: 5 mg (base)
betamethasone sodium phosphate and betamethasone acetate suspension
Injection: betamethasone acetate 3 mg and betamethasone sodium phosphate (equivalent to 3 mg base) per ml (not for I.V. use)

Indications, route, and dosage
(Note: betamethasone acetate suspension should not be given I.V.)
Severe inflammation or immunosuppression
Adults: 0.6 to 7.2 mg P.O. daily.
betamethasone sodium phosphate
Adults: 0.5 to 9 mg I.M., I.V., or into joint or soft tissue daily.
betamethasone sodium phosphate and betamethasone acetate suspension
Adults: 0.5 to 2 ml into joint or soft tissue q 1 to 2 weeks p.r.n.
Adrenocortical insufficiency
Adults: 0.6 to 7.2 mg P.O. daily, or up to 9 mg I.M. or I.V. daily.
Children: 17.5 mcg/kg P.O. daily or 500 mcg/m² P.O. daily in three or four divided doses; or 17.5 mcg/kg/day or 500 mcg/m²/day I.M. in three divided doses q 3 days.
◇ ***Hyaline membrane disease***
Adults: Give 2 ml I.M. daily to expectant mothers for 2 to 3 days before delivery.

Pharmacodynamics
Anti-inflammatory action: Drug stimulates the synthesis of enzymes needed to decrease the inflammatory response. It is a long-acting steroid with an anti-inflammatory potency 25 times that of an equal weight of hydrocortisone. It has essentially no mineralocorticoid activity. Betamethasone tablets and syrup are used as oral anti-inflammatory agents.

Betamethasone sodium phosphate is highly soluble, has a prompt onset of action, and may be given I.V. Betamethasone sodium phosphate and betamethasone acetate (Celestone Soluspan) combine the rapid-acting phosphate salt and the slightly soluble, slowly released acetate salt to provide rapid anti-inflammatory effects with a sustained duration of action. It is a suspension and should not be given I.V. It is particularly useful as an anti-inflammatory agent in intra-articular, intradermal, and intralesional injections.

Pharmacokinetics
• *Absorption:* Drug is absorbed readily after oral administration. After oral and I.V. administration, peak effects occur in 1 to 2 hours. Onset and duration of action of the suspensions for injection vary, depending on their injection site (an intra-articular space or a muscle) and on the local blood supply. Systemic absorption occurs slowly following intra-articular injections.
• *Distribution:* Drug is removed rapidly from the blood and distributed to muscle, liver, skin, intestines, and kidneys. Betamethasone is bound weakly to plasma proteins (transcortin and albumin). Only the unbound portion is active. Adrenocorticoids are distributed into breast milk and through the placenta.
• *Metabolism:* Metabolized in the liver to inactive glucuronide and sulfate metabolites.
• *Excretion:* Inactive metabolites and small amounts of unmetabolized drug are excreted by the kidneys. Insignificant quantities of drug are also excreted in feces. Biological half-life of drug is 36 to 54 hours.

Contraindications and precautions
Contraindicated in patients hypersensitive to drug and in those with viral or bacterial infections (except in life-threatening situations) or systemic fungal infections.

Use with caution in patients with renal disease, hypertension, osteoporosis, diabetes mellitus, hypothyroidism, cirrhosis, diverticulitis, nonspecific ulcerative colitis, recent intestinal anastomoses, thromboembolic disorders, seizures, myasthenia gravis, heart failure, tuberculosis, ocular herpes simplex, emotional instability, and psychotic tendencies.

Interactions
When used concomitantly, betamethasone may decrease the effects of *oral anticoagulants* (rarely); increase the metabolism of *isoniazid* and *salicylates*; and cause hyperglycemia, requiring dosage adjustment of *insulin* or *oral antidiabetic agents* in diabetic patients. Use with *barbiturates, phenytoin,* and *rifampin* may cause decreased corticosteroid effects because of increased hepatic metabolism. Use with *cholestyramine, colestipol,* and *antacids* decreases the effect of betamethasone by adsorbing the corticosteroid, decreasing the amount absorbed.

Betamethasone may enhance hypokalemia associated with *diuretic* or *amphotericin B* therapy. The hypokalemia may increase the risk of toxicity in patients concurrently receiving *cardiac glycosides.*

* Canada only ◇ Unlabeled clinical use

Concomitant use with *estrogens* may reduce the metabolism of corticosteroids by increasing the concentrations of transcortin. The half-life of the corticosteroid is then prolonged because of increased protein binding. Concomitant administration of *ulcerogenic drugs* such as *NSAIDs* may increase the risk of GI ulceration.

Effects on diagnostic tests

Adrenocorticoid therapy suppresses reactions to skin tests; causes false-negative results in the nitroblue tetrazolium tests for systemic bacterial infections; and decreases ^{131}I uptake and protein-bound iodine levels in thyroid function tests.

It may increase glucose and cholesterol levels; decrease serum potassium, calcium, thyroxine, and triiodothyronine levels; and increase urine glucose and calcium levels.

Adverse reactions

Most adverse reactions to corticosteroids are dose- or duration-dependent.
CNS: *euphoria, insomnia,* psychotic behavior, pseudotumor cerebri, vertigo, headache, paresthesia, ***seizures.***
CV: ***heart failure,*** hypertension, edema, ***arrhythmias,*** thrombophlebitis, ***thromboembolism.***
EENT: cataracts, glaucoma.
Endocrine: menstrual irregularities, cushingoid state (moonface, buffalo hump, central obesity).
GI: *peptic ulceration,* GI irritation, increased appetite, pancreatitis, nausea, vomiting.
Skin: delayed wound healing, acne, various skin eruptions.
Other: muscle weakness, osteoporosis, hirsutism, susceptibility to infections; hypokalemia, hyperglycemia, and carbohydrate intolerance; growth suppression in children; ***acute adrenal insufficiency may follow increased stress (infection, surgery, or trauma) or abrupt withdrawal after long-term therapy.***

Note: After abrupt withdrawal: rebound inflammation, fatigue, weakness, arthralgia, fever, dizziness, lethargy, depression, fainting, orthostatic hypotension, dyspnea, anorexia, hypoglycemia. ***After prolonged use, sudden withdrawal may be fatal.***

Overdose and treatment

Acute ingestion, even in massive doses, rarely occurs. Toxic signs and symptoms rarely occur if drug is used for less than 3 weeks, even at large doses. However, chronic use causes adverse physiologic effects, including suppression of the hypothalamic-pituitary-adrenal axis, cushingoid appearance, muscle weakness, and osteoporosis.

☑ Special considerations

Recommendations for use of betamethasone and for care and teaching of patients during therapy are the same as those for all *systemic adrenocorticoids.*
- Investigational use includes prevention of respiratory distress syndrome in premature infants (hyaline membrane disease). Give 6 mg (2 ml) of Celestone Soluspan I.M. once daily 24 to 36 hours before induced delivery.

Pediatric use

- Chronic use of betamethasone in children and adolescents may delay growth and maturation.

Breast-feeding

- Information is incomplete. Risk versus benefits must be determined and reviewed with patient.

betamethasone dipropionate, augmented

Diprolene, Diprolene AF

betamethasone dipropionate

Alphatrex, Diprosone, Maxivate

betamethasone valerate

Betacort* Betaderm*, Betatrex, Beta-Val, Betnovate*, Celestoderm-V*, Ectosone*, Metaderm*, Novobetamet*, Valisone

Pharmacologic classification: topical glucocorticoid
Therapeutic classification: anti-inflammatory
Pregnancy risk category C

How supplied

Available by prescription only
betamethasone dipropionate, augmented
Cream, gel, lotion, ointment: 0.05%
betamethasone dipropionate
Lotion, ointment, cream: 0.05%
Aerosol: 0.1%
betamethasone valerate
Lotion, ointment: 0.1%
Cream: 0.01%, 0.1%

Indications, route, and dosage

Inflammation of corticosteroid-responsive dermatoses
betamethasone dipropionate
Adults and children over age 12: Apply cream, lotion, or ointment sparingly daily or b.i.d. Dosage of Diprolene ointment 0.05% should not exceed 45 g per week. To apply aerosol, direct spray onto affected area from a distance of 6″ (15 cm) for only 3 seconds t.i.d. or q.i.d.
betamethasone valerate
Adults and children: Apply cream, lotion, ointment, or gel in a thin layer once daily to q.i.d.

Pharmacodynamics

Anti-inflammatory action: Drug stimulates the synthesis of enzymes needed to decrease the inflammatory response. Betamethasone, a fluorinated derivative, has the advantage of availability in various bases to vary the potency for individual conditions.

Pharmacokinetics

- *Absorption:* Amount absorbed depends on the potency of the preparation, amount applied, and nature of the skin at the application site. It ranges from about 1% in areas with a thick stratum corneum to as high as 36% in areas with a thin stratum corneum. Absorption increases in areas of skin damage, inflammation, or occlusion. Some systemic absorption of topical steroids occur.

• *Distribution:* After topical application, drug is distributed throughout the local skin. Drug absorbed into circulation is removed rapidly from the blood and distributed into muscle, liver, skin, intestines, and kidneys.

• *Metabolism:* After topical administration, drug is metabolized primarily in the skin. The small amount that is absorbed into systemic circulation is metabolized primarily in the liver to inactive compounds.

• *Excretion:* Inactive metabolites are excreted by the kidneys, primarily as glucuronides and sulfates, but also as unconjugated products. Small amounts of the metabolites are also excreted in feces.

Contraindications and precautions
Contraindicated in patients hypersensitive to corticosteroids.

Interactions
None significant.

Effects on diagnostic tests
None reported.

Adverse reactions
Skin: burning, pruritus, irritation, dryness, erythema folliculitis, acneiform eruptions, perioral dermatitis, hypopigmentation, hypertrichosis, allergic contact dermatitis; *secondary infection, maceration, atrophy, striae, miliaria* (with occlusive dressings).
Other: ***hypothalamic-pituitary-adrenal axis suppression,*** Cushing's syndrome, hyperglycemia, glycosuria (with betamethasone dipropionate).

Overdose and treatment
No information available.

☑ Special considerations
Besides those relevant to all *topical adrenocorticoids,* consider the following recommendation.

• Diprolene ointment may suppress the hypothalamic-pituitary-adrenal axis at doses as low as 7 g daily. Patient should not use more than 45 g weekly and should not use occlusive dressings.

Pediatric use
• Treatment with Diprolene ointment is not recommended in children under age 12.

betaxolol hydrochloride
Betoptic, Betoptic S, Kerlone

Pharmacologic classification: beta-adrenergic blocker
Therapeutic classification: antiglaucoma, antihypertensive
Pregnancy risk category C

How supplied
Available by prescription only
Tablets: 10 mg, 20 mg
Ophthalmic solution: 5 mg/ml (0.5%) in 2.5-ml, 5-ml, 10-ml, 15-m dropper bottles
Ophthalmic suspension: 2.5 mg/ml (0.25%) in 2.5-ml, 5-ml, 10-ml, 15-ml dropper bottles

Indications, route, and dosage
Chronic open-angle glaucoma and ocular hypertension
Adults: Instill 1 to 2 drops in eyes b.i.d.
Management of hypertension (used alone or with other antihypertensives)
Adults: Initially, 10 mg P.O. once daily. After 7 to 14 days, full antihypertensive effect should be seen. If necessary, double dosage to 20 mg P.O. once daily. (Doses up to 40 mg daily have been used.)
✦ ***Dosage adjustment.*** In patients with renal impairment, initial dose is 5 mg P.O. daily. Increase by 5-mg/day increments q 2 weeks to maximum of 20 mg/day.

Pharmacodynamics
Antihypertensive action: Cardioselective adrenergic blocking effects of betaxolol slow heart rate and decrease cardiac output.

Ocular hypotensive action: Betaxolol hydrochloride is a cardioselective $beta_1$ blocker that reduces intraocular pressure (IOP), possibly by reducing production of aqueous humor when administered as an ophthalmic solution.

Pharmacokinetics
• *Absorption:* Essentially complete after oral administration; minimal after ophthalmic use. A small first-pass effect reduces bioavailability by about 10%. Absorption is not affected by food or alcohol.

• *Distribution:* Peak concentrations in plasma occur about 3 hours (range, 1.5 to 6) after a single oral dose. Drug is about 50% bound to plasma proteins.

• *Metabolism:* Hepatic; about 85% of drug is recovered in the urine as metabolites. Elimination half-life is prolonged in patients with hepatic disease, but clearance is not affected, so dosage adjustment in unnecessary.

• *Excretion:* Primarily renal (about 80%). Plasma half-life is 14 to 22 hours.

Contraindications and precautions
Contraindicated in patients with hypersensitivity to drug, severe bradycardia, greater than first-degree heart block, cardiogenic shock, or uncontrolled heart failure.

Interactions
When used concomitantly, ophthalmic betaxolol may increase the systemic effect of *oral beta blockers,* enhance the hypotensive and bradycardiac effect of *reserpine* and *catecholamine-depleting agents,* and enhance the lowering of IOP with *pilocarpine, epinephrine,* and *carbonic anhydrase inhibitors.*

Concomitant use of oral betaxolol with *reserpine* and *catecholamine-depleting drugs* may have an additive effect when administered with a *beta blocker.* Use with *general anesthetics* may cause increased hypotensive effects. Observe carefully for excessive hypotension, bradycardia, or orthostatic hypotension. Use with *calcium channel blocking agents* increases risk of hypotension, left-sided heart failure, and AV conduction disturbances. *I.V. calcium antagonists* should be used with caution. Concomitant use with *beta blockers* may increase the effects of *lidocaine*.

Effects on diagnostic tests
Although oral beta blockers have been reported to decrease serum glucose levels from blockage of normal glycogen release after hypoglycemia, no such effect has been reported with the use of ophthalmic beta blockers.

Oral beta blockers may alter the results of glucose tolerance tests.

Adverse reactions
Ophthalmic form

CNS: insomnia, depressive neurosis.

EENT: *eye stinging on instillation causing brief discomfort,* photophobia, erythema, itching, keratitis, occasional tearing.

Systemic form

CNS: dizziness, fatigue, headache, insomnia, lethargy, anxiety.

CV: bradycardia, chest pain, ***heart failure,*** edema.

GI: nausea, diarrhea, dyspepsia.

Respiratory: dyspnea, pharyngitis, ***bronchospasm.***

Skin: rash.

Other: impotence, arthralgia.

Overdose and treatment
Clinical manifestations of overdose, which are extremely rare with ophthalmic use, may include diplopia, bradycardia, heart block, hypotension, shock, increased airway resistance, cyanosis, fatigue, sleepiness, headache, sedation, coma, respiratory depression, seizures, nausea, vomiting, diarrhea, hypoglycemia, hallucinations, and nightmares. Discontinue drug and flush eye with 0.9% NaCl solution or water. For treatment of accidental substantial ingestion, emesis is most effective if initiated within 30 minutes, providing the patient is not obtunded, comatose, or having seizures. Activated charcoal may be used. Treat bradycardia, conduction defects, and hypotension with I.V. fluids, glucagon, atropine, or isoproterenol; refractory bradycardia may require a transvenous pacemaker. Treat bronchoconstriction with I.V. aminophylline; seizures, with I.V. diazepam.

☑ Special considerations
Ophthalmic use

• Betaxolol is a cardioselective beta-adrenergic blocker. Its pulmonary and systemic effects are considerably milder than those of timolol or levobunolol.

• Ophthalmic betaxolol is intended for twice-daily dosage. Encourage patient to comply with this regimen.

• In some patients, a few weeks' treatment may be required to stabilize pressure-lowering response. Determine IOP during the first 4 weeks of drug therapy.

Systemic use

• Withdrawal of beta blocker therapy before surgery is controversial. Some clinicians advocate withdrawal to prevent any impairment of cardiac responsiveness to reflex stimuli and to prevent any decreased responsiveness to exogenous catecholamines.

• To withdraw drug, dosage should be gradually reduced over at least 2 weeks.

Patient education
Ophthalmic use

• Instruct patient to tilt head back and, while looking up, drop the drug into the lower lid.

• Warn patient not to touch dropper to eye or surrounding tissue.

• Instruct patient not to close eyes tightly or blink more than usual after instillation.

• Remind patient to wait at least 5 minutes before using other eyedrops.

• Advise patient to wear sunglasses or avoid exposure to bright lights.

• Tell patient to shake suspension well before use.

Systemic use

• Advise patient to take drug exactly as prescribed and warn against discontinuing it suddenly.

• Advise patient to report shortness of breath or difficulty breathing, unusually fast heartbeat, cough, or fatigue with exertion.

Geriatric use
• Use with caution in elderly patients with cardiac or pulmonary disease.

Breast-feeding
• Use with caution. After oral administration, betaxolol is excreted in breast milk in sufficient amounts to exert an effect on the breast-feeding infant.

bethanechol chloride
Duvoid, Myotonachol, Urecholine

Pharmacologic classification: cholinergic agonist

Therapeutic classification: urinary tract and GI tract stimulant

Pregnancy risk category C

How supplied
Available by prescription only

Tablets: 5 mg, 10 mg, 25 mg, 50 mg

Injection: 5 mg/ml

Indications, route, and dosage
Acute postoperative and postpartum nonobstructive (functional) urine retention, neurogenic atony of urinary bladder with retention

Adults: 10 to 50 mg P.O. t.i.d., or q.i.d. Or 2.5 to 5 mg S.C. (Use 10 mg S.C. with extreme caution.) *Never give I.M. or I.V.* When used for urine retention, some patients may require 50 to 100 mg P.O. per dose. Use such doses with extreme caution. Test dose: 2.5 mg S.C. repeated at 15- to 30-minute intervals to total of four doses to determine the minimal effective dose; then use minimal effective dose q 6 to 8 hours. Adjust dosage to meet individual requirements.

◊ ***Bladder dysfunction caused by phenothiazines***

Adults: 50 to 100 mg P.O. q.i.d.

◊ ***To lessen the adverse effects of tricyclic antidepressants***

Adults: 25 mg P.O. t.i.d.

◊ ***Chronic gastric reflux***

Adults: 25 mg P.O. q.i.d.

◊ ***Familial dysautonomia***

Children: 0.2 to 0.4 mg/kg S.C. q.i.d. 30 minutes before meals with an oral antacid; then after 2 weeks, give 1 to 2 mg P.O. q.i.d.

◊ ***To diagnose flaccid or atonic neurogenic bladder***

Adults: 2.5 mg S.C.

◊ ***To diagnose cystic fibrosis***

Children over age 1: 1 mg intradermally.

Children age 2 months to 1 year: 0.5 mg intradermally.

Infants from birth to age 2 months: 0.25 mg intradermally.

Pharmacodynamics

Urinary tract stimulant action: Bethanechol directly binds to and stimulates muscarinic receptors of the parasympathetic nervous system. That increases tone of the bladder detrusor muscle, usually resulting in contraction, decreased bladder capacity, and subsequent urination.

GI tract stimulant action: Bethanechol directly stimulates cholinergic receptors, leading to increased gastric tone and motility and peristalsis. Drug improves lower esophageal sphincter tone by directly stimulating cholinergic receptors, thereby alleviating gastric reflux.

Pharmacokinetics

- *Absorption:* Poorly absorbed from the GI tract (absorption varies considerably among patients). After oral administration, action usually begins in 30 to 90 minutes; after S.C. administration, in 5 to 15 minutes.
- *Distribution:* Largely unknown; however, therapeutic doses do not penetrate the blood-brain barrier.
- *Metabolism:* Unknown. Usual duration of effect after oral administration is 1 hour; after S.C. administration, up to 2 hours.
- *Excretion:* Unknown.

Contraindications and precautions

Contraindicated for I.M. or I.V. use and in patients with hypersensitivity to drug or its components; uncertain strength or integrity of bladder wall; mechanical obstructions of GI or urinary tract; hyperthyroidism, peptic ulceration, latent or active bronchial asthma, pronounced bradycardia or hypotension, vasomotor instability, cardiac or coronary artery disease, seizure disorder, Parkinson's disease, spastic GI disturbances, acute inflammatory lesions of the GI tract, peritonitis, or marked vagotonia; or when increased muscular activity of GI or urinary tract is harmful. Use cautiously in pregnant women.

Interactions

Concomitant use with *procainamide* and *quinidine* may reverse the cholinergic effect of bethanechol on muscle. Concomitant use with *ganglionic blockers* such as *mecamylamine* may cause a critical blood pressure decrease; this effect is usually preceded by abdominal symptoms. Additive effects may occur with *cholinergic drugs*, especially *cholinesterase inhibitors.*

Effects on diagnostic tests

Bethanechol increases serum levels of amylase, lipase, bilirubin, and AST and increases sulfobromophthalein retention time.

Adverse reactions

CNS: headache, malaise.
CV: hypotension, reflex tachycardia.
EENT: lacrimation, miosis.
GI: *abdominal cramps, diarrhea,* excessive salivation, nausea, belching, borborygmus.
GU: urinary urgency.
Respiratory: ***bronchoconstriction,*** increased bronchial secretions.
Skin: flushing, diaphoresis.

Overdose and treatment

Clinical signs and symptoms of overdose include nausea, vomiting, abdominal cramps, diarrhea, involuntary defecation, urinary urgency, excessive salivation, miosis, excessive tearing, bronchospasm, increased bronchial secretions, hypotension, excessive sweating, bradycardia or reflex tachycardia, and substernal pain.

Treatment requires discontinuation of drug and administration of atropine by S.C., I.M., or I.V. route. (Atropine must be administered cautiously; an overdose could cause bronchial plug formation.) Contact local or regional poison control center for more information.

☑ Special considerations

- Atropine sulfate should be readily available to counteract toxic reactions that may occur during treatment with bethanechol.
- Never give bethanechol I.M. or I.V. because that could cause circulatory collapse, hypotension, severe abdominal cramps, bloody diarrhea, shock, or cardiac arrest. Give only by S.C. route when giving parenterally.
- For administration to treat urine retention, bedpan should be readily available.
- Give drug on an empty stomach; eating soon after drug administration may cause nausea and vomiting.
- Patients with hypertension receiving bethanechol may experience a precipitous decrease in blood pressure.

bicalutamide
Casodex

Pharmacologic classification: nonsteroidal antiandrogen
Therapeutic classification: antineoplastic
Pregnancy risk category X

How supplied
Available by prescription only
Tablets: 50 mg

Indications, route, and dosage
Adjunct therapy for treatment of advanced prostate cancer
Adults: 50 mg P.O. once daily in morning or evening.

Pharmacodynamics
Antineoplastic action: Drug competitively inhibits the action of androgens by binding to cytosol androgen receptors in the target tissue. Prostatic carcinoma, known to be sensitive to androgens, responds to treatment that either counteracts the effect of androgen or removes its source.

Pharmacokinetics
- *Absorption:* Well absorbed from GI tract.
- *Distribution:* 96% is protein-bound.
- *Metabolism:* Drug undergoes stereospecific metabolism. The S (inactive) isomer is metabolized primarily by glucuronidation. The R (active) isomer also undergoes glucuronidation but is predominantly oxidized to an inactive metabolite followed by glucuronidation.
- *Excretion:* Excreted in urine and feces.

Contraindications and precautions
Contraindicated in patients with hypersensitivity to drug or to any component in the tablet and during pregnancy. Use cautiously in patients with moderate to severe hepatic impairment (drug is extensively metabolized by the liver).

Interactions
Bicalutamide displaces *coumarin anticoagulants* from their protein-binding sites. Monitor PT closely. The anticoagulant dose may need adjustment.

Effects on diagnostic tests
Drug may elevate patient's AST, ALT, bilirubin, BUN, and creatinine levels and decrease patient's hemoglobin and WBC counts.

Adverse reactions
CNS: headache, dizziness, paresthesia, insomnia.
CV: *hot flashes,* hypertension, chest pain, peripheral edema.
GI: *constipation, nausea, diarrhea,* abdominal pain, flatulence, increased liver enzymes, vomiting, weight loss.
GU: nocturia, hematuria, urinary tract infection, impotence, gynecomastia, urinary incontinence.
Hematologic: hypochromic anemia, iron-deficiency anemia.
Respiratory: dyspnea.
Skin: rash, sweating.
Other: *general pain, back or pelvic pain, asthenia, infection,* flu syndrome, hyperglycemia, bone pain.

Overdose and treatment
A single dose of bicalutamide that results in symptoms of an overdose considered to be life-threatening has not been established. There is no specific antidote: Treatment of an overdose should be symptomatic. Vomiting may be induced if patient is alert. Dialysis is not likely to be helpful because bicalutamide is highly protein-bound and is extensively metabolized.

☑ Special considerations
- Bicalutamide is used in combination therapy with a luteinizing hormone–releasing hormone (LHRH) analogue for the treatment of advanced prostate cancer. Treatment should begin at the same time as that with the prescribed LHRH analogue.
- Administer bicalutamide at the same time each day.
- Monitor serum prostate specific antigen (PSA) levels regularly. PSA levels help in assessing patient's response to therapy. Elevated levels require a reevaluation of patient to determine disease progression.
- Monitor liver function studies. When a patient develops jaundice or exhibits laboratory evidence of liver injury in the absence of liver metastases, drug should be discontinued. Abnormalities are usually reversible on drug discontinuation.
- Drug is not indicated for use in women.

Patient education
- Inform patient that drug may be taken without regard to meals.
- Advise patient to take drug at the same time each day.
- Tell patient that bicalutamide is used with other drug therapy. Stress importance of not interrupting or stopping any of these drugs without medical consultation.

Pediatric use
- Safety and effectiveness in children have not been established.

Breast-feeding
- Drug is not indicated for use in women.

biperiden hydrochloride

biperiden lactate
Akineton

Pharmacologic classification: anticholinergic
Therapeutic classification: antiparkinsonian
Pregnancy risk category C

How supplied
Available by prescription only
Tablets: 2 mg

Injection: 5 mg/ml in 1-ml ampule

Indications, route, and dosage

Extrapyramidal disorders

Adults: 2 mg P.O. daily, b.i.d., or t.i.d., depending on severity. Usual dose is 2 mg daily. For treatment of extrapyramidal symptoms induced by drugs, give 2 mg I.M. or slow I.V. q 30 minutes, not to exceed 8 mg in a 24-hour period.

Parkinsonism

Adults: 2 mg P.O. t.i.d. or q.i.d. For prolonged therapy, titrate dose to maximum of 16 mg daily.

Pharmacodynamics

Antiparkinsonian action: Drug blocks central cholinergic receptors, helping to balance cholinergic activity in the basal ganglia. It may also prolong the effects of dopamine by blocking dopamine reuptake and storage at central receptor sites.

Pharmacokinetics

- *Absorption:* Drug is well absorbed from the GI tract.
- *Distribution:* Drug is minimally absorbed; it is metabolized in the liver.
- *Metabolism:* Exact metabolic fate is unknown.
- *Excretion:* Excreted in the urine as unchanged drug and metabolites. After oral therapy, small amounts are probably excreted as unabsorbed drug.

Contraindications and precautions

Contraindicated in patients with hypersensitivity to drug, angle-closure glaucoma, bowel obstruction, or megacolon. Use cautiously in patients with prostatic hyperplasia, arrhythmias, or seizure disorders.

Interactions

Amantadine may amplify the anticholinergic adverse effects of biperiden, such as confusion and hallucinations. Decrease biperiden dosage before *amantadine* administration.

Concomitant use with *haloperidol* or *phenothiazines* may decrease the antipsychotic effectiveness of these drugs, possibly by direct CNS antagonism. Concomitant use with *phenothiazines* increases risk of anticholinergic adverse effects.

Alcohol and other *CNS depressants* increase the sedative effects of biperiden. *Antacids* and *antidiarrheals* may decrease biperiden absorption. Administer biperiden at least 1 hour before these drugs are administered. Plasma levels of *digoxin* may be elevated.

Effects on diagnostic tests

None reported.

Adverse reactions

CNS: disorientation, euphoria, drowsiness, agitation.
CV: transient postural hypotension (with parenteral use).
EENT: blurred vision.
GI: dry mouth, *constipation.*
GU: urine retention.

Note: Adverse reactions are dose-related and may resemble atropine toxicity.

Overdose and treatment

Clinical effects of overdose include central stimulation followed by depression and psychotic symptoms, such as disorientation, confusion, hallucinations, delusions, anxiety, agitation, and restlessness. Peripheral effects may include dilated, nonreactive pupils; blurred vision; hot, dry, flushed skin; dry mucous membranes; dysphagia; decreased or absent bowel sounds; urine retention; hyperthermia; headache; tachycardia; hypertension; and increased respiration.

Treatment is primarily symptomatic and supportive, as necessary. Maintain patent airway. If the patient is alert, induce emesis (or use gastric lavage) and follow with a sodium chloride cathartic and activated charcoal to prevent further absorption of orally administered drug. In severe cases, physostigmine may be administered to block antimuscarinic effects of biperiden. Give fluids, as needed, to treat shock; diazepam to control psychotic symptoms; and pilocarpine (instilled into the eyes) to relieve mydriasis. If urine retention occurs, catheterization may be necessary.

☑ Special considerations

Besides those relevant to all *anticholinergics,* consider the following recommendations.

- When giving drug parenterally, keep patient supine; parenteral administration may cause transient postural hypotension and disturbed coordination.
- When giving biperiden I.V., inject drug slowly.
- Because biperiden may cause dizziness, patient may need assistance when walking.
- In patients with severe parkinsonism, tremors may increase when drug is administered to relieve spasticity.

Patient education

- Tell patient that tolerance to therapeutic and adverse effects can occur with chronic drug use.
- Tell patient that drug may increase sensitivity of the eyes to light.
- Instruct patient to take drug with food to avoid GI upset.

Geriatric use

- Use cautiously in elderly patients. Lower doses are indicated.

Pediatric use

- Drug is not recommended for children.

Breast-feeding

- Drug may be excreted in breast milk, possibly resulting in infant toxicity. It may also decrease milk production. Avoid use of drug in breast-feeding women.

bisacodyl

Biscolax, Dulcagen, Dulcolax, Fleet Laxative

Pharmacologic classification: diphenylmethane derivative
Therapeutic classification: stimulant laxative
Pregnancy risk category B

How supplied
Available without a prescription
Tablets: 5 mg
Suppositories: 10 mg

Indications, route, and dosage
Constipation; preparation for delivery, surgery, or rectal or bowel examination
Adults: 10 to 15 mg P.O. daily. Up to 30 mg may be used for thorough evacuation needed for examinations or surgery. Alternatively, give one suppository (10 mg) P.R. daily.
Children age 6 to 12: 5 mg P.O. daily. Alternatively, give one-half of suppository (5 mg) P.R. daily.

Pharmacodynamics
Laxative action: Bisacodyl has a direct stimulant effect on the colon, increasing peristalsis and enhancing bowel evacuation.

Pharmacokinetics
• *Absorption:* Absorption is minimal; action begins 6 to 8 hours after oral administration and 15 to 60 minutes after P.R. administration.
• *Distribution:* Bisacodyl is distributed locally.
• *Metabolism:* Minimal absorption; bisacodyl is metabolized in the liver.
• *Excretion:* Drug is excreted primarily in feces; some in urine.

Contraindications and precautions
Contraindicated in patients with hypersensitivity, abdominal pain, nausea, vomiting, or other symptoms of appendicitis or acute surgical abdomen and in those with rectal bleeding, gastroenteritis, or intestinal obstruction.

Interactions
Antacids, milk, and *drugs that increase gastric pH levels* may cause premature dissolution of the enteric coating, resulting in intestinal or gastric irritation or cramping.

Effects on diagnostic tests
None reported.

Adverse reactions
CNS: muscle weakness with excessive use, dizziness, faintness.
GI: *nausea, vomiting, abdominal cramps,* diarrhea (with high doses), *burning sensation in rectum* (with suppositories), laxative dependence with long-term or excessive use.
Other: alkalosis, hypokalemia, tetany, protein-losing enteropathy in excessive use, fluid and electrolyte imbalance.

Overdose and treatment
No cases of overdose have been reported.

☑ Special considerations
• Patient should swallow tablets whole rather than crushing or chewing them, to avoid GI irritation. Administer with 8 oz (240 ml) of fluid.

Patient education
• Instruct patient not to take drug within 1 hour of milk or antacid consumption.
• Tell patient to take only as directed to avoid laxative dependence.

Breast-feeding
• Bisacodyl may be used by breast-feeding women.

bismuth subsalicylate

Pepto-Bismol

Pharmacologic classification: adsorbent
Therapeutic classification: antidiarrheal
Pregnancy risk category C (D in third trimester)

How supplied
Available without a prescription
Tablets (chewable): 262 mg
Suspension: 262 mg/15 ml, 524 mg/15 ml

Indications, route, and dosage
Mild, nonspecific diarrhea
Adults: 30 ml or 2 tablets q ½ to 1 hour up to a maximum of eight doses and for no more than 2 days.
Children age 9 to 12: 15 ml or 1 tablet.
Children age 6 to 9: 10 ml or ⅔ tablet.
Children age 3 to 6: 5 ml or ⅓ tablet.
Children's dosage given q ½ to 1 hour up to a maximum of eight doses in 24 hours and for no more than 2 days.

Pharmacodynamics
Antidiarrheal action: Bismuth adsorbs extra water in the bowel during diarrhea. It also adsorbs toxins and forms a protective coating for the intestinal mucosa.

Pharmacokinetics
• *Absorption:* Bismuth is absorbed poorly; significant salicylate absorption may occur after using bismuth subsalicylate.
• *Distribution:* Distributed locally in the gut.
• *Metabolism:* Metabolized minimally.
• *Excretion:* Excreted in urine.

Contraindications and precautions
Contraindicated in patients hypersensitive to salicylates. Use cautiously in patients already taking aspirin or aspirin-containing medications.

Interactions
Bismuth subsalicylate may impair *tetracycline* absorption. Bismuth subsalicylate may impair the uricosuric effect of *sulfinpyrazone* and may increase the risk of *aspirin* toxicity.

Drug may have an additive effect if the patient is also taking *aspirin*.

Effects on diagnostic tests
Because bismuth is radiopaque, it may interfere with radiologic examination of the GI tract.

Adverse reactions
GI: temporary darkening of tongue and stools.
Other: salicylism (with high doses).

Overdose and treatment
Overdose has not been reported. However, overdose is more likely with bismuth subsalicylate; probable clinical effects include CNS effects, such as tinnitus, and fever.

☑ Special considerations
- Monitor hydration status and serum electrolyte levels; record number and consistency of stools.
- If administered by tube, tube should be flushed via nasogastric tube, to clear it and ensure passage of drug to stomach.
- If patient is also receiving tetracycline, administer bismuth at least 1 hour apart; to avoid decreased drug absorption, dosages or schedules of other medications may require adjustment.
- Bismuth subsalicylate has been used investigationally to treat peptic ulcer. Doses of 600 mg t.i.d. may be as effective as cimetidine 800 mg once daily.
- Drug is useful for indigestion without causing constipation; nausea; and relief of flatulence and abdominal cramps.

Patient education
- Advise patient taking anticoagulants or medication for diabetes or gout to seek medical approval before taking drug.
- Instruct patient to chew tablets well or to shake suspension well before using.
- Tell patient to report persistent diarrhea.
- Warn patient that bismuth may temporarily darken stools and tongue.

Breast-feeding
- Small amounts of drug are excreted in breast milk. Patient should seek medical approval before use.

bisoprolol fumarate
Zebeta

Pharmacologic classification: beta-adrenergic blocker
Therapeutic classification: antihypertensive
Pregnancy risk category C

How supplied
Available by prescription only
Tablets: 5 mg, 10 mg

Indications, route, and dosage
Hypertension (used alone or in combination with other antihypertensives)
Adults: Initially, 5 mg P.O. once daily. If response is inadequate, increase to 10 mg once daily. Maximum recommended dosage, 20 mg daily.
✦ ***Dosage adjustment.*** In adults with renal or hepatic dysfunction, start at 2.5 mg P.O.; then increase with caution.

Pharmacodynamics
Antihypertensive action: Mechanism of action has not been completely established. Possible antihypertensive factors include decreased cardiac output, inhibition of renin release by the kidneys, and diminution of tonic sympathetic outflow from the vasomotor centers in the brain.

Pharmacokinetics
- *Absorption:* Bioavailability after a 10-mg oral dose of bisoprolol is about 80%. Absorption is not affected by the presence of food.
- *Distribution:* About 30% of bisoprolol binds to serum proteins.
- *Metabolism:* The first-pass metabolism of bisoprolol is about 20%.
- *Excretion:* Bisoprolol is eliminated equally by renal and nonrenal pathways, with about 50% of dose appearing unchanged in the urine and the remainder appearing as inactive metabolites. Less than 2% of dose is excreted in the feces. The plasma elimination half-life of drug is 9 to 12 hours (slightly longer in elderly patients, in part because of decreased renal function in that population).

Contraindications and precautions
Contraindicated in patients with hypersensitivity to drug and in those with cardiogenic shock, overt cardiac failure, marked sinus bradycardia, or second- or third-degree AV block. Use cautiously in patients with bronchospastic disease.

Interactions
Bisoprolol should not be combined with other *beta-blocking agents*. Patients receiving *catecholamine-depleting drugs*, such as *reserpine* or *guanethidine*, should be closely monitored because the added beta-adrenergic blocking action of bisoprolol may excessively reduce sympathetic activity. In patients receiving concurrent therapy with *clonidine*, bisoprolol should be discontinued for several days before *clonidine* withdrawal.

Effects on diagnostic tests
Drug may produce hypoglycemia and interfere with glucose or insulin tolerance tests.

Adverse reactions
CNS: asthenia, fatigue, dizziness, *headache,* hypoesthesia, vivid dreams, depression, insomnia.
CV: bradycardia, peripheral edema, chest pain.
EENT: pharyngitis, rhinitis, sinusitis.

GI: nausea, vomiting, diarrhea, dry mouth.
Respiratory: cough, dyspnea.
Other: arthralgia.

Overdose and treatment

The most common signs of overdose from a beta-adrenergic blocker such as bisoprolol are bradycardia, hypotension, heart failure, bronchospasm, and hypoglycemia. If overdosage occurs, drug therapy should be discontinued and supportive and symptomatic treatment should be provided.

☑ Special considerations

- Patients with renal or hepatic dysfunction or bronchospastic disease unresponsive to or intolerant of other antihypertensive therapies should start therapy at 2.5 mg daily. A $beta_2$-adrenergic agonist (bronchodilator) should be made available to patients with bronchospastic disease.
- Exacerbation of angina pectoris, MI, and ventricular arrhythmia has been observed in patients with coronary artery disease after abrupt cessation of therapy with beta blockers. It is advisable, even in patients without overt coronary artery disease, to taper therapy with bisoprolol over 1 week, with patient under careful observation. If withdrawal symptoms occur, bisoprolol therapy should be reinstituted, at least temporarily.

Patient education

- Inform diabetic patients subject to spontaneous hypoglycemia or those requiring insulin or oral hypoglycemic agents that bisoprolol may mask some manifestations of hypoglycemia, particularly tachycardia.
- Warn patient not to drive, operate machinery, or perform any other task requiring alertness until reaction to bisoprolol has been established.
- Stress importance of taking drug as prescribed, even when feeling well. Advise patient not to discontinue drug abruptly because serious consequences can occur.
- Instruct patient to call if adverse reactions occur.
- Tell patient to seek medical approval before taking OTC medications.

Pediatric use

- Safety and effectiveness in children have not been established.

Breast-feeding

- It is not known if drug is excreted in breast milk. Use with caution when administering to breast-feeding women.

bitolterol mesylate

Tornalate

Pharmacologic classification: adrenergic, $beta_2$ agonist
Therapeutic classification: bronchodilator
Pregnancy risk category C

How supplied

Available by prescription only
Aerosol inhaler: 370 mcg/metered spray

Indications, route, and dosage

To prevent and treat bronchial asthma and bronchospasm

Adults and children over age 12: For symptomatic relief of bronchospasm, 2 inhalations at an interval of at least 1 to 3 minutes followed by a third inhalation, if needed; to prevent bronchospasm, 2 inhalations q 8 hours. Usually, dose should not exceed 3 inhalations q 6 hours or 2 inhalations q 4 hours. However, because deposition of inhaled medications is variable, higher doses are occasionally used, especially in patients with acute bronchospasm.

Pharmacodynamics

Bronchodilator action: Bitolterol selectively stimulates $beta_2$-adrenergic receptors of the lungs. Bronchodilation results from relaxation of bronchial smooth muscles, which relieves bronchospasm and reduces airway resistance. Some CV stimulation may occur as a result of $beta_1$-adrenergic stimulation, including mild tachycardia, palpitations, and changes in blood pressure or heart rate.

Pharmacokinetics

- *Absorption:* After oral inhalation, bronchodilation results from local action on the bronchial tree, with most of the inhaled dose being swallowed. Onset of action occurs within 3 to 5 minutes, peaks in ½ to 2 hours and lasts 4 to 8 hours.
- *Distribution:* Bitolterol is widely distributed throughout body.
- *Metabolism:* Drug is hydrolyzed by esterases to active metabolites.
- *Excretion:* After oral administration, bitolterol and its metabolites are excreted primarily in urine.

Contraindications and precautions

Contraindicated in patients with hypersensitivity to drug. Use cautiously in patients with ischemic heart disease, hypertension, hyperthyroidism, diabetes mellitus, arrhythmias, seizure disorders, or history of unusual responsiveness to beta-adrenergic agonists.

Interactions

Concomitant use with other *orally inhaled beta-adrenergic agonists* may produce additive sympathomimetic effects. Evidence suggests that cardiotoxic effects may be increased when bitolterol is used with a *theophylline salt* such as *aminophylline.*

Propranolol and *other beta blockers* may antagonize the effects of bitolterol.

Effects on diagnostic tests

Bitolterol therapy may increase AST levels and decrease platelet or leukocyte count. Proteinuria may also occur. Drug may also render spirometry insensitive for the diagnosis of asthma.

Adverse reactions

CNS: *tremor,* nervousness, headache, dizziness, light-headedness.
CV: palpitations, chest discomfort, tachycardia.
EENT: throat irritation, cough.
GI: nausea, vomiting.
Other: dyspnea, hypersensitivity reactions.

Overdose and treatment

Clinical manifestations of overdose include exaggeration of common adverse reactions, especially arrhythmias, extreme tremor, nausea, and vomiting.

Treatment requires supportive measures. To reverse effects, use selective $beta_1$-adrenergic blockers (acebutolol, atenolol, metoprolol) with extreme caution (may induce asthmatic attack). Monitor vital signs and ECG closely.

☑ Special considerations

Besides those relevant to all *adrenergics,* consider the following recommendation.

- Repeated use may result in paradoxical bronchospasm. Discontinue immediately if this occurs.

Patient education

- Tell patient to use drug only as directed and not to exceed the prescribed amount or shorten intervals between doses.
- Teach patient to use drug correctly. Tell patient to ensure proper delivery of dose by cleaning plastic mouthpiece with warm tap water and drying thoroughly at least once daily. Tell him that dryness of mouth and throat may occur, but that rinsing with water after each dose may help.
- Tell patient to call promptly if troubled breathing persists 1 hour after using drug, if symptoms return within 4 hours, if condition worsens, or if new (refill) canister is needed within 2 weeks.
- Tell patient to wait 15 minutes after use of bitolterol before using adrenocorticoid inhaler.
- Give patient instructions on proper use of inhaler:

Administration by metered-dose nebulizers: Shake canister to activate; place mouthpiece well into mouth, aimed at back of throat. Close lips and teeth around mouthpiece. Exhale through nose, then inhale through mouth slowly and deeply, while actuating the nebulizer, to release dose. Hold breath 10 seconds (count "1 to 100, 2 to 100, 3 to 100" to "10 to 100"), remove mouthpiece, then exhale slowly.

Administration by metered powder inhaler: Caution patient not to take forced deep breaths, but to breathe normally. Observe patient closely for exaggerated systemic drug action. Patients requiring more than three aerosol treatments within 24 hours should be under close medical supervision.

Administration by oxygen aerosolization: Administer over 15 to 20 minutes, with oxygen flow rate adjusted to 4 L/minute. Turn on oxygen supply before patient places nebulizer in mouth. (Patient need not close lips tightly around nebulizer opening.) Placement of Y tube in rubber tubing permits patient to control administration. Advise patient to rinse mouth immediately after inhalation therapy to help prevent dryness and throat irritation. Rinse mouthpiece with warm running water at least once daily to prevent clogging. (It is not dishwasher-safe.) Wait until mouthpiece is dry before storing. Do not place near artificial heat (dishwasher or oven). Replace reservoir bag every 2 to 3 weeks or as needed; replace mouthpiece every 6 to 9 months or as needed. Replacement of bags or mouthpieces may require a prescription.

Geriatric use

- Lower doses are indicated in elderly patients, who may be more sensitive to drug's effects.

Pediatric use

- Drug is not recommended for use in children under age 12.

Breast-feeding

- Administer cautiously to breast-feeding women. It is unknown whether drug is distributed into breast milk.

black widow spider (*Latrodectus mactans*) antivenin

Pharmacologic classification: antivenin
Therapeutic classification: black widow spider antivenin
Pregnancy risk category C

How supplied

Available by prescription only
Injection: combination package—1 vial of antivenin (6,000 antivenin units/vial), one 2.5-ml vial of diluent (sterile water for injection), and one 1-ml vial of normal equine (horse) serum (1:10 dilution) for sensitivity testing

Indications, route, and dosage

Black widow spider bite

Adults and children: 2.5 ml (1 vial) I.M. in anterolateral thigh. If symptoms do not subside in 1 to 3 hours, an equal dose may be repeated. Antivenin also may be given I.V. in 10 to 50 ml of 0.9% NaCl solution over 15 minutes (preferred route for severe cases, such as patients in shock or those under age 12).

Pharmacodynamics

Antivenin action: Black widow spider antivenin provides immune globulins that specifically bind black widow spider venom.

Pharmacokinetics

- *Absorption:* I.V. effect is rapid. Concentration peaks 2 to 3 days after an I.M. injection; mean half-life is less than 15 days.
- *Distribution:* Unknown.
- *Metabolism:* Unknown.
- *Excretion:* Unknown.

Contraindications and precautions

Contraindicated in patients hypersensitive to drug when desensitization is not feasible.

Interactions
None significant.

Effects on diagnostic tests
None reported.

Adverse reactions
Other: hypersensitivity reactions, ***anaphylaxis, neurotoxicity.***

Overdose and treatment
No information available.

☑ Special considerations
- Immobilize patient immediately. Splint the bitten limb to prevent spread of venom.
- If possible, hospitalize patient.
- Obtain a thorough patient history of allergies, especially to horses and horse immune serum, and previous reactions to immunizations.
- Test patient for sensitivity (against a control of 0.9% NaCl solution in opposing extremity) before giving antivenin. Give 0.02 ml of the 1:10 dilution of horse serum intradermally. Read results after 10 minutes.

  Positive reaction: Wheal with or without pseudopodia and surrounding erythema. If skin sensitivity test is positive, consider a conjunctival test and desensitization schedule.
- Early use of antivenin is recommended for best results.
- Apply tourniquet above site of I.M. injection if systemic reaction to antivenin occurs.
- Epinephrine solution 1:1,000 should be available to treat allergic reactions.
- Black widow spider venom is neurotoxic and may cause ascending motor convulsions. Watch patient carefully for 2 to 3 days for signs of neurotoxicity.
- A black widow spider bite induces painful muscle spasms. Patient may need analgesia and prolonged warm baths.
- Administer a 10-ml injection of 10% calcium gluconate I.V. to control muscle pain as needed.
- Vital signs should be checked every 30 minutes for 1 to 3 hours.
- Establish when patient received last tetanus immunization; a booster may be recommended at this time.

Patient education
- Inform patient that allergic reactions to the antivenin may cause rash, joint swelling or pain, fever, or difficulty breathing.
- Encourage patient to report unusual effects experienced while hospitalized.
- Explain that residual effects of the spider bite (general weakness, tingling of the extremities, nervousness, and muscle spasm) may persist for weeks or months after recovery from the acute phase.

Breast-feeding
- Advise patient to discontinue breast-feeding temporarily until effects of the venom subside or if symptoms of serum sickness develop.

bleomycin sulfate
Blenoxane

Pharmacologic classification: antibiotic, antineoplastic (cell cycle–phase specific, G_2 and M phase)
Therapeutic classification: antineoplastic
Pregnancy risk category D

How supplied
Available by prescription only
Injection: 15-unit, 30-unit vials

Indications, route, and dosage
Dosage and indications may vary. Check literature for current protocol.

Hodgkin's disease, squamous cell carcinoma, malignant lymphoma, or testicular carcinoma
Adults: 10 to 20 units/m² (0.25 to 0.5 units/kg) I.V., I.M., or S.C., one or two times weekly. After 50% response, maintenance dose of 1 unit daily or 5 units weekly.

Malignant pleural effusion; prevention of recurrent pleural effusions
Adults: 60 units in 50 to 100 ml of 0.9% NaCl solution by intracavitary administration.

◇ ***Tumors of the head and neck***
Adults: 10 to 20 units/m² daily by regional arterial administration for 5 to 14 days.

Pharmacodynamics
Antineoplastic action: The exact mechanism of cytotoxicity of bleomycin is unknown. Its action may be through scission of single- and double-stranded DNA and inhibition of DNA, RNA, and protein synthesis. Bleomycin also appears to inhibit cell progression out of the G_2 phase.

Pharmacokinetics
- *Absorption:* Bleomycin is poorly absorbed across the GI tract following oral administration. I.M. administration results in lower serum levels than those occurring after equivalent I.V. doses.
- *Distribution:* Drug distributes widely into total body water, mainly in the skin, lungs, kidneys, peritoneum, and lymphatic tissue.
- *Metabolism:* Metabolic fate of drug is undetermined; however, extensive tissue inactivation occurs in the liver and kidney and much less in the skin and lungs.
- *Excretion:* Bleomycin and its metabolites are excreted primarily in urine. The terminal plasma elimination phase half-life is reported at 2 hours.

Contraindications and precautions
Contraindicated in patients hypersensitive to drug. Use cautiously in patients with renal or pulmonary impairment.

Interactions
Concomitant use may decrease serum levels of *phenytoin* and *digoxin.*

Effects on diagnostic tests

Bleomycin therapy may increase blood and urine concentrations of uric acid.

Adverse reactions

GI: stomatitis, anorexia, nausea, vomiting, diarrhea.
Respiratory: ***pulmonary fibrosis,*** pulmonary toxicity such as **PNEUMONITIS.**
Skin: *erythema, hyperpigmentation, acne, rash, reversible alopecia, striae, skin tenderness, pruritus.*
Other: *chills,* fever, weight loss, severe idiosyncratic reaction consisting of hypotension, mental confusion, fever, chills and wheezing has occurred in approximately 1% of lymphoma patients.

Overdose and treatment

Clinical manifestations of overdose include pulmonary fibrosis, fever, chills, vesiculation, and hyperpigmentation. Treatment is usually supportive and includes antipyretics for fever.

☑ Special considerations

- To prepare solution for I.M. administration, reconstitute drug with 1 to 5 ml of 0.9% NaCl solution, sterile water for injection, or D_5W.
- For I.V. administration, dilute with a minimum of 5 ml of diluent and administer over 10 minutes as I.V. push injection.
- Prepare infusions of bleomycin in glass bottles because absorption of drug to plastic occurs with time. Plastic syringes do not interfere with bleomycin activity.
- Use precautions in preparing and handling drug; wear gloves and wash hands after preparing and administering.
- Drug can be administered by intracavitary (see manufacturer's recommendation), intra-arterial, or intratumoral injection. It can also be instilled into bladder for bladder tumors.
- Cumulative lifetime dosage should not exceed 400 units.
- Response to therapy may take 2 to 3 weeks.
- Administer a 1- to 2-unit test dose to lymphoma patients before the first two doses to assess hypersensitivity to bleomycin. If no reaction occurs, then follow the dosing schedule. The test dose can be incorporated as part of the total dose for the regimen.
- Have epinephrine, diphenhydramine, I.V. corticosteroids, and oxygen available in case of anaphylactic reaction.
- Premedication with aspirin, steroids, and diphenhydramine may reduce drug fever and risk of anaphylaxis.
- Dosage should be reduced in patients with renal or pulmonary impairment.
- Drug concentrates in keratin of squamous epithelium. To prevent linear streaking, do not use adhesive dressings on skin.
- Allergic reactions may be delayed especially in patients with lymphoma.
- Pulmonary function tests may be useful in predicting fibrosis; they should be performed to establish a baseline and then monitored periodically.
- Monitor chest X-rays and auscultate the lungs.
- Bleomycin is stable for 24 hours at room temperature and 48 hours under refrigeration. Refrigerate unopened vials containing dry powder.

Patient education

- Explain that hair should grow back after treatment is discontinued.

Geriatric use

- Use with caution in patients over age 70 because they are at increased risk for pulmonary toxicity.

Breast-feeding

- It is not known if drug occurs in breast milk. However, because of risk of serious adverse reactions, mutagenicity, and carcinogenicity in infants, breast-feeding is not recommended.

botulinum toxin type A

Botox

Pharmacologic classification: neurotoxin
Therapeutic classification: muscle relaxant
Pregnancy risk category C

How supplied

Available by prescription only
Powder for injection: 100 units/vial

Indications, route, and dosage

Treatment of strabismus

Adults and children age 12 and older: Injections into extraocular muscles should be made only by staff familiar with the technique, which involves surgical exposure of the region as well as electromyographic guidance of the injection needle.

Dosage varies with the degree of deviation (lower doses are used for small deviations). For vertical muscles and for horizontal strabismus of less than 20 prism diopters, the usual dose is 1.25 to 2.5 units in any one muscle. For horizontal strabismus of 20 to 50 prism diopters, dosage is 2.5 to 5 units injected into any one muscle. For persistent VI nerve palsy greater than 1 month's duration, dosage is 1.25 to 2.5 units injected into the medial rectus muscle.

Subsequent doses for recurrent or residual strabismus should not be administered unless 7 to 14 days have elapsed after the initial dose and substantial function has returned to the injected and adjacent muscles. Dosage may be increased to twice the initial dose for patients experiencing incomplete paralysis; patients with adequate response should receive a similar dose. The maximum single dose for any one muscle is 25 units.

Treatment of blepharospasm

Adults: Initially, 1.25 to 2.5 units injected into the medial and lateral pretarsal orbicularis oculi of the upper and lower lids. Effects should be apparent within 3 days and peak in 1 to 2 weeks after treatment. At subsequent treatments, dosage may be doubled if inadequate paralysis is achieved, but exceeding 5 units per site produces no benefit. The effect of each treatment lasts about 3 months. Treatment can be repeated indefinitely.

The monthly cumulative dosage of botulinum toxin type A should not exceed 200 units.

Pharmacodynamics

Neuromuscular blocking action: Drug produces a neuromuscular paralysis by binding to acetylcholine receptors on the motor end plate. It may also inhibit the release of acetylcholine from the presynaptic nerve ending.

Pharmacokinetics

- *Absorption:* Unknown.
- *Distribution:* Unknown.
- *Metabolism:* Unknown.
- *Excretion:* Unknown. However, patients treated for blepharospasm did not require retreatment for an average of 12.5 weeks after injection. Over 50% of patients treated for strabismus maintained improvements over 6 months.

Contraindications and precautions

Contraindicated in patients hypersensitive to drug or its components.

Interactions

Muscle paralysis may be potentiated by concomitant use of *aminoglycoside antibiotics.*

Effects on diagnostic tests

None reported.

Adverse reactions

EENT: *ptosis, vertical deviation* (after treatment of strabismus), *eye irritation, photophobia* (after treatment of blepharospasm), *swelling of eyelid.*
Skin: diffuse rash, ecchymoses.

Overdose and treatment

Information may be obtained from the manufacturer, Allergan Pharmaceuticals, at 1-800-347-5063 (8 a.m. to 4 p.m. Pacific time), or at other times at (714) 724-5954 for a recorded message.

☑ Special considerations

- Store drug in the freezer at or below 23° F (–5° C).
- Reconstitute drug with 0.9% NaCl solution without a preservative. The vacuum in the vial should be noticeable when reconstituting. Inject the diluent into the vial gently because severe agitation can denature the protein.
- Reconstituting with 1 ml produces a concentration of 10 units/0.1 ml; adding 2 ml yields 5 units/0.1 ml. Adding more diluent (such as 4 ml to produce 2.5 units/0.1 ml or 8 ml to yield 1.25 units/0.1 ml) or using different injection volumes are methods commonly used to adjust dosage.
- Reconstituted drug should be clear, colorless, and free from particles. Administer within 4 hours of removal from the freezer; refrigerate until used. Be sure to record the date and time of reconstitution.
- When treating strabismus, injection volume should be 0.05 to 0.15 ml per muscle. When treating blepharospasm, injection volumes are maintained at 0.05 to 0.1 ml per site. Dosage adjustments are made by altering the volume of diluent used to reconstitute the drug.
- When treating strabismus, several drops of an ocular decongestant and a topical anesthetic should be applied before the procedure.
- Prepare injection by drawing slightly more volume than needed into a sterile 1-ml syringe. Expel air bubbles in the barrel of the syringe, and attach an electromyographic injection needle (if treating strabismus), such as a 1½", 27G needle. Expel unnecessary drug (into an appropriate waste container) while checking for leakage around the needle. Be sure to use a new needle and syringe for each injection.

Patient education

- Because many patients with blepharospasm may have been sedentary for extended periods of time, recommend caution as they resume normal activity.
- Explain that muscle paralysis becomes evident 1 to 2 days after injection and increases in intensity over first week. Paralysis lasts for 2 to 6 weeks and eventually resolves.

Pediatric use

- Safety and efficacy in children under age 12 have not been established.

Breast-feeding

- It is not known if drug is excreted in breast milk. Use with caution in breast-feeding women.

bretylium tosylate

Bretylate*, Bretylol

Pharmacologic classification: adrenergic blocker
Therapeutic classification: ventricular antiarrhythmic
Pregnancy risk category C

How supplied

Available by prescription only
Injection: 50 mg/ml

Indications, route, and dosage

Ventricular fibrillation and hemodynamically unstable ventricular tachycardia

Adults: 5 mg/kg undiluted by rapid I.V. injection. If ventricular fibrillation persists, increase dosage to 10 mg/kg and repeat p.r.n. For continuous suppression, administer diluted solution by continuous I.V. infusion at 1 to 2 mg/minute, or infuse diluted solution at 5 to 10 mg/kg over more than 8 minutes q 6 hours.

Other ventricular arrhythmias

Adults: Initially, 5 to 10 mg/kg I.M., undiluted, or I.V. diluted. Repeat in 1 to 2 hours if necessary. Maintenance dose is 5 to 10 mg/kg q 6 hours I.M. or I.V. or 1 to 2 mg/minute I.V. infusion.

◊ *Children:* For acute ventricular fibrillation, initially 5 mg/kg I.V., followed by 10 mg/kg q 15 to 30 minutes, with a maximum total dose of 30 mg/kg; maintenance dose, 5 to 10 mg/kg q 6 hours. For other ventricular arrhythmias, 5 to 10 mg/kg q 6 hours.

Pharmacodynamics

Ventricular antiarrhythmic action: Bretylium is a class III antiarrhythmic used to treat ventricular fibrillation and tachycardia. Like other class III antiarrhythmics, it widens the action potential duration (repolarization inhibition) and increases the effective refractory period (ERP); it does not affect conduction velocity. These actions follow a transient increase in conduction velocity and shortening of the action potential duration and ERP.

Initial effects stem from norepinephrine release from sympathetic ganglia and postganglionic adrenergic neurons immediately after drug administration. Norepinephrine release also accounts for an increased threshold for successful defibrillation, increased blood pressure, and increased heart rate. This initial phase of drug's action is brief (up to 1 hour).

Bretylium also alters the disparity in action potential duration between ischemic and nonischemic myocardial tissue; its antiarrhythmic action may result from this activity.

Hemodynamic drug effects include increased blood pressure, heart rate, and possible cardiac irritability (all resulting from initial norepinephrine release). Drug-induced adrenergic blockade ultimately predominates, leading to vasodilation and a subsequent blood pressure drop (primarily orthostatic). This effect has been referred to as chemical sympathectomy.

Pharmacokinetics

- *Absorption:* Drug is incompletely and erratically absorbed from the GI tract; it is well absorbed after I.M. administration. With I.M. administration, the antiarrhythmic (ventricular tachycardia and ectopy) action of the drug begins within about 20 to 60 minutes but may not reach maximal level for 6 to 9 hours when given by this route (for this reason I.M. administration is not recommended for treating life-threatening ventricular fibrillation).

With I.V. administration, antifibrillatory action begins within a few minutes. However, suppression of ventricular tachycardia and other ventricular arrhythmias occurs more slowly—usually within 20 minutes to 2 hours; peak antiarrhythmic effects may not occur for 6 to 9 hours.

- *Distribution:* Drug is distributed widely throughout the body. It does not cross the blood-brain barrier. Only about 1% to 10% is plasma protein-bound.
- *Metabolism:* No metabolites have been identified.
- *Excretion:* Excreted in the urine mostly as unchanged drug; half-life ranges from 5 to 10 hours (longer in patients with renal impairment). Duration of effect ranges from 6 to 24 hours and may increase with continued dosage increases. (Patients with ventricular fibrillation may require continuous infusion to maintain desired effect.)

Contraindications and precautions

Contraindicated in digitalized patients unless the arrhythmia is life-threatening, not caused by a cardiac glycoside and unresponsive to other antiarrhythmics. Use with caution in patients with aortic stenosis and pulmonary hypertension.

Interactions

Concomitant use of bretylium with other *antiarrhythmic agents* may cause additive toxic effects and additive or antagonistic cardiac effects. Concomitant use with *cardiac glycosides* may exacerbate ventricular tachycardia associated with *digitalis* toxicity. When used concomitantly with *pressor amines* (*sympathomimetics*), bretylium may potentiate the action of these drugs.

Effects on diagnostic tests

None reported.

Adverse reactions

CNS: *vertigo, dizziness, light-headedness, syncope* (usually secondary to hypotension).
CV: SEVERE HYPOTENSION (especially orthostatic), bradycardia, anginal pain, transient arrhythmias, transient hypertension, increased PVCs.
GI: severe nausea, vomiting (with rapid infusion).

Overdose and treatment

Clinical effects of overdose primarily involve severe hypotension.

Treatment includes administration of vasopressors (such as dopamine or norepinephrine), to support blood pressure, and general supportive measures, as necessary. Volume expanders and positional changes also may be effective.

☑ Special considerations

- Administer I.V. infusion at appropriate rate to avoid or minimize adverse reactions.
- For I.M. injection, do not exceed 5-ml volume in any one site and rotate sites.
- Patient should remain supine and avoid sudden postural changes until tolerance to hypotension develops.
- Simultaneous initiation of therapy with a cardiac glycoside and bretylium should be avoided.
- Monitor ECG and blood pressure throughout therapy for any significant change. If supine systolic pressure decreases to less than 75 mm Hg, norepinephrine, dopamine, or volume expanders may be prescribed to elevate blood pressure.
- Monitor patient closely if patient is receiving pressor amines (sympathomimetics) to correct hypotension; bretylium potentiates the effects of these drugs.
- Observe for increased anginal pain in susceptible patients.
- Because bretylium is excreted exclusively by the kidneys, patients with renal impairment require dosage modification. Dosage interval should be increased because the elimination half-life increases threefold to sixfold.
- Subtherapeutic doses (less than 5 mg/kg) may cause hypotension.

• Drug is not a first-line agent, according to American Heart Association advanced cardiac life-support guidelines. With ventricular fibrillation, drug should follow lidocaine; with ventricular tachycardia, drug should follow lidocaine and procainamide.
• Ventricular tachycardia and other ventricular arrhythmias respond to drug less rapidly than ventricular fibrillation.
• Drug is ineffective against atrial arrhythmias.

Breast-feeding
• Safety has not been established.

brimonidine tartrate
Alphagan

Pharmacologic classification: selective alpha$_2$-adrenergic agonist
Therapeutic classification: ophthalmic agent for glaucoma or ocular hypertension
Pregnancy risk category B

How supplied
Available by prescription only
Ophthalmic solution: 0.2%; 5 ml, 10 ml

Indications, route, and dosage
Lowering of intraocular pressure in patients with open-angle glaucoma or ocular hypertension
Adults: 1 drop in affected eye(s) t.i.d., approximately 8 hours apart.

Pharmacodynamics
Ocular antihypertensive action: Brimonidine is an alpha$_2$-adrenergic receptor agonist that reduces aqueous humor production and increases uveoscleral outflow.

Pharmacokinetics
• *Absorption:* After ocular administration, peak plasma concentrations within 1 to 4 hours and declined with a systemic half-life of approximately 3 hours.
• *Distribution:* Not reported.
• *Metabolism:* Systemically, is metabolized primarily by the liver.
• *Excretion:* Systemically, urinary excretion is major route of elimination.

Contraindications and precautions
Contraindicated in patients with hypersensitivity to brimonidine tartrate or benzalkonium chloride and in those receiving MAO inhibitor therapy. Use cautiously in patients with cerebral or coronary insufficiency, CV disease, hepatic or renal impairment, depression, Raynaud's phenomenon, orthostatic hypotension, or thromboangiitis obliterans.

Interactions
Concomitant use with *CNS depressants* may be additive or potentiate their effects. Concomitant use with *beta blockers, antihypertensives,* or *cardiac glycosides* may further decrease blood pressure. Use cautiously with *tricyclic antidepressants* because it may interfere with brimonidine's intraocular pressure-lowering effects.

Effects on diagnostic tests
None reported

Adverse reactions
CNS: anxiety, asthenia, depression, dizziness, *drowsiness, fatigue, headache,* insomnia, muscular pain.
CV: hypertension, palpitations, syncope.
EENT: abnormal vision or taste; blepharitis; *blurring, burning, or stinging;* conjunctival blanching, edema, hemorrhage, discharge, or *follicles;* corneal staining or erosion; eyelid erythema or eyelid edema; *foreign body sensation;* lid crusting; nasal dryness; *ocular hyperemia, allergic reactions, pruritus,* ache or pain, dryness, tearing, or irritation; *oral dryness,* photophobia.
GI: nausea, vomiting, diarrhea.
Respiratory: cough and cold symptoms.

Overdose and treatment
Supportive and symptomatic treatment. Maintain a patent airway.

☑ Special considerations
• Monitor intraocular pressure because loss of effects after first month of therapy may occur.

Patient education
• Tell patient to wait at least 15 minutes after instilling drug to insert soft contact lenses.
• Caution patient of potential for decreased mental alertness; drug may cause fatigue or drowsiness.

Pediatric use
• Safety and effectiveness in children have not been established.

Breast-feeding
• It is unknown if drug is excreted in breast milk. Use with caution.

bromocriptine mesylate
Parlodel

Pharmacologic classification: dopamine receptor agonist
Therapeutic classification: semisynthetic ergot alkaloid, dopaminergic agonist, antiparkinsonism agent, inhibitor of prolactin release, inhibitor of growth hormone release
Pregnancy risk category B

How supplied
Available by prescription only
Tablets: 2.5 mg
Capsules: 5 mg

Indications, route, and dosage
Amenorrhea and galactorrhea associated with hyperprolactinemia; female infertility

Adults: 0.5 to 2.5 mg daily, increased by 2.5 mg daily at 3- to 7-day intervals as tolerated until optimal therapeutic effects are achieved. Maintenance dose is usually 5 to 7.5 mg daily (range, 2.5 to 15 mg daily).

Acromegaly

Adults: Initially, 1.25 to 2.5 mg P.O. daily h.s. for 3 days. An additional 1.25 to 2.5 mg may be added q 3 to 7 days until patient receives therapeutic benefit. Therapeutic dose range varies from 20 to 30 mg daily in most patients. Maximum dosage should not exceed 100 mg daily. Dosages of 20 to 60 mg daily have been administered as divided doses.

Parkinson's disease

Adults: Initially, 1.25 to 2.5 mg P.O. b.i.d. with meals. Dosage may be increased by 2.5 mg daily q 14 to 28 days, up to 100 mg daily or until a maximal therapeutic response is achieved. Safety in dosages over 100 mg daily has not been established.

◊ ***Premenstrual syndrome***

Adults: 2.5 to 7.5 mg P.O. b.i.d. from day 10 of menstrual cycle until onset of menstruation.

◊ ***Cushing's syndrome***

Adults: 1.25 to 2.5 mg P.O. b.i.d. to q.i.d.

◊ ***Hepatic encephalopathy***

Adults: 1.25 mg P.O. daily, increased by 1.25 mg q 3 days until 15 mg is reached.

Pharmacodynamics

Prolactin-inhibiting action: Drug reduces prolactin concentrations by inhibiting release of prolactin from the anterior pituitary gland, a direct action on the pituitary. It may also stimulate postsynaptic dopamine receptors in the hypothalamus to release prolactin-inhibitory factor via a complicated catecholamine pathway. Drug reduces high serum prolactin concentrations and restores ovulation and ovarian function in amenorrheic women and suppresses puerperal or nonpuerperal lactation in women with adequate gonadotropin concentrations and ovarian function. The average time for reversing amenorrhea is 6 to 8 weeks, but it may take up to 24 weeks.

Antiparkinsonism action: Drug activates dopaminergic receptors in the neostriatum of the CNS, which may produce its antiparkinsonism activity. Dysregulation of brain serotonin activity also may occur. The precise role of bromocriptine in treating parkinsonism syndrome requires further study of its safety and efficacy in long-term therapy.

Pharmacokinetics

- *Absorption:* Drug is 28% absorbed when given orally and reaches peak levels in about 1 to 3 hours. Plasma concentrations for therapeutic effects are unknown. After an oral dose, serum prolactin decreases within 2 hours, is decreased maximally at 8 hours, and remains decreased at 24 hours.
- *Distribution:* About 90% to 96% is bound to serum albumin.
- *Metabolism:* First-pass metabolism occurs with over 90% of the absorbed dose. Drug is metabolized completely in the liver, principally by hydrolysis, before excretion. The metabolites are not active or toxic.
- *Excretion:* Primarily through bile. Only 2.5% to 5.5% of dose is excreted in urine. Almost all (85%) of dose is excreted in feces within 5 days.

Contraindications and precautions

Contraindicated in patients with hypersensitivity to ergot derivatives, uncontrolled hypertension, or toxemia of pregnancy. Use cautiously in patients with renal or hepatic impairment and history of MI with residual arrhythmias.

Interactions

Concomitant use of bromocriptine with *drugs that increase prolactin concentrations* (*amitriptyline, butyrophenones, imipramine, methyldopa, phenothiazines,* and *reserpine*) may require increased dosage of bromocriptine.

Bromocriptine may potentiate *antihypertensive agents*, requiring a reduction of their dosage to prevent hypotension.

Alcohol intolerance may result when high doses of bromocriptine are administered; therefore, concomitant ingestion of *alcohol* should be limited.

Effects on diagnostic tests

Transient elevation of BUN, ALT, AST, CK, alkaline phosphatase, and uric acid levels may occur.

Adverse reactions

CNS: *dizziness, headache,* fatigue, mania, lightheadedness, drowsiness, delusions, nervousness, insomnia, depression, ***seizures.***
CV: *hypotension,* ***stroke, acute MI.***
EENT: nasal congestion, blurred vision.
GI: *nausea,* vomiting, *abdominal cramps, constipation,* diarrhea, anorexia.
GU: urine retention, urinary frequency.
Skin: coolness and pallor of fingers and toes.

Overdose and treatment

Overdosage of bromocriptine may cause nausea, vomiting, and severe hypotension. Treatment includes emptying the stomach by aspiration and lavage, and administering I.V. fluids to treat hypotension.

☑ Special considerations

- Examine patient carefully for pituitary tumor (Forbes-Albright syndrome). Use of bromocriptine does not affect tumor size, although it may alleviate amenorrhea or galactorrhea.
- First-dose phenomenon occurs in 1% of patients. Sensitive patients may experience syncope for 15 to 60 minutes but can usually tolerate subsequent treatment without ill effects. Patient should begin therapy with lowest dosage, taken at bedtime.
- Administer drug with meals, milk, or snacks to diminish GI distress.
- Alcohol intolerance may occur, especially when high doses of bromocriptine are administered; therefore, alcohol intake should be limited.
- As an antiparkinsonism agent, drug is usually given with either levodopa alone or levodopa-carbidopa combination.
- Adverse reactions are more common when drug is given in high doses, as in treating parkinsonism.

Patient education

- Advise patient that it may take 6 to 8 weeks or longer for menses to be reinstated and for galactorrhea to be suppressed.
- Tell patient to take first dose where and when she can lie down because drowsiness commonly occurs after initiation of therapy.
- Instruct patient to report visual problems, severe nausea and vomiting, or acute headaches.
- Tell patient to take drug with meals to avoid GI upset.
- Warn patient that the CNS effects of drug may impair ability to perform tasks that require alertness and coordination.
- Advise patient to use a nonhormonal contraceptive during treatment because of potential amenorrheic adverse effects.
- Advise patient to limit use of alcohol during treatment.

Geriatric use

- Use with caution, particularly in patients receiving long-term, high-dose therapy. Regular physical assessment is recommended, with particular attention toward changes in pulmonary function.
- Safety is not established for long-term use at the doses required to treat Parkinson's disease.

Pediatric use

- Drug is not recommended for children under age 15.

Breast-feeding

- Because drug inhibits lactation, it should not be used in women who intend to breast-feed.

brompheniramine maleate

Dimetapp Allergy

Pharmacologic classification: alkylamine antihistamine
Therapeutic classification: antihistamine (H_1-receptor antagonist)
Pregnancy risk category C

How supplied

Available with or without a prescription
Tablets: 4 mg
Elixir: 2 mg/5 ml
Injection: 10 mg/ml

Indications, route, and dosage

Rhinitis, allergies

Adults and children age 12 and older: 4 mg P.O. q 4 to 6 hours. Do not exceed 24 mg in 24 hours.
Children age 7 to 11: 2 mg P.O. q 4 to 6 hours. Do not exceed 12 mg in 24 hours.
Children age 2 to 6: 1 mg P.O. q 4 to 6 hours. Do not exceed 6 mg in 24 hours.

Hypersensitivity

Adults and children age 12 and older: 5 to 20 mg S.C., I.M. or I.V. b.i.d. Do not exceed 40 mg in 24 hours.
Children below age 12: 0.5 mg/kg/day or 15 mg/m²/day S.C., I.M. or I.V. in three to four divided doses.

Pharmacodynamics

Antihistamine action: Antihistamines compete with histamine for histamine$_1$ receptor sites on the smooth muscle of the bronchi, GI tract, uterus, and large blood vessels; by binding to cellular receptors, they prevent access of histamine and suppress histamine-induced allergic symptoms, even though they do not prevent its release.

Pharmacokinetics

- *Absorption:* Absorbed readily from the GI tract; action begins within 15 to 30 minutes and peaks in 2 to 5 hours. A second lower peak effect apparently exists, possibly from drug reabsorption in the distal small intestine.
- *Distribution:* Drug is distributed widely into the body.
- *Metabolism:* Approximately 90% to 95% of drug is metabolized by the liver.
- *Excretion:* Half-life of drug ranges from about 12 to 34½ hours. Brompheniramine and its metabolites are excreted primarily in urine; a small amount is excreted in feces. About 5% to 10% of an oral dose is excreted unchanged in urine.

Contraindications and precautions

Contraindicated in patients with hypersensitivity to drug's ingredients; in those with acute asthma, severe hypertension or coronary artery disease, angle-closure glaucoma, urine retention, and peptic ulcer; and within 14 days of MAO-inhibitor therapy. Use cautiously in patients with increased intraocular pressure, diabetes mellitus, ischemic heart disease, hyperthyroidism, hypertension, bronchial asthma, or prostatic hyperplasia and in the elderly.

Interactions

MAO inhibitors interfere with the metabolism of brompheniramine and thus prolong and intensify their central depressant and anticholinergic effects; additive CNS depression may occur when brompheniramine is given concomitantly with other *CNS depressants,* such as *alcohol, antianxiety agents, barbiturates, sleeping aids,* and *tranquilizers.*

Drug may diminish the effects of *sulfonylureas* and partially may counteract the anticoagulant effects of *heparin.*

Effects on diagnostic tests

Discontinue drug 4 days before performing diagnostic skin tests; it can prevent, reduce, or mask positive skin test response.

Adverse reactions

CNS: dizziness, tremors, irritability, insomnia, *drowsiness, stimulation.*
CV: hypotension, palpitations.
GI: anorexia, nausea, vomiting, *dry mouth and throat.*
GU: urine retention.
Hematologic: ***thrombocytopenia, agranulocytosis.***

Skin: urticaria, rash.
Other: (after parenteral administration) local stinging, diaphoresis, syncope.

Overdose and treatment
Clinical manifestations of overdose may include either those of CNS depression (sedation, reduced mental alertness, apnea, and CV collapse) or of CNS stimulation (insomnia, hallucinations, tremors, or seizures). Anticholinergic symptoms, such as dry mouth, flushed skin, fixed and dilated pupils, and GI symptoms, are common, especially in children.

Treat overdose by inducing emesis with ipecac syrup (in conscious patients), followed by activated charcoal to reduce further drug absorption. Use gastric lavage if patient is unconscious or ipecac fails. Treat hypotension with vasopressors, and control seizures with diazepam or phenytoin I.V. *Do not give stimulants.*

☑ Special considerations
Besides those relevant to all *antihistamines,* consider the following recommendations.
- Drug causes less drowsiness than some antihistamines.
- Store parenteral solutions and elixirs away from light and freezing temperatures; solution may crystallize if stored below 32° F (0° C). Crystals dissolve when warmed to 86° F (30° C).

Patient education
- Instruct patients who self-medicate not to exceed 24 mg/day (for adults and children age 12 and older) or 12 mg/day (for children age 6 to 11).

Geriatric use
- Elderly patients are usually more sensitive to adverse effects of antihistamines and are especially likely to experience a greater degree of dizziness, sedation, hyperexcitability, dry mouth, and urine retention than younger patients. Symptoms usually respond to a decrease in medication dosage.

Pediatric use
- Drug is not indicated for use in newborns; children, especially those under age 6, may experience paradoxical hyperexcitability.

Breast-feeding
- Antihistamines such as brompheniramine should not be used during breast-feeding. Many of these drugs are secreted in breast milk, exposing the infant to risks of unusual excitability, especially premature infants and other neonates, who may experience seizures.

budesonide
Pulmicort Turbuhaler, Rhinocort

Pharmacologic classification: glucocorticosteroid
Therapeutic classification: anti-inflammatory
Pregnancy risk category C

How supplied
Available by prescription only
Nasal inhaler: 32 mcg/metered dose (200 doses per container)
Oral inhalation powder: 200 mcg/dose (200 doses per container)

Indications, route, and dosage
Management of symptoms of seasonal or perennial allergic rhinitis or nonallergic perennial rhinitis
Adults and children over age 6: 2 sprays in each nostril in the morning and evening or 4 sprays in each nostril in the morning. Maintenance dosage should be the fewest number of sprays needed to control symptoms. Doses exceeding 256 mcg/day (4 sprays/nostril) are not recommended.

Note: If improvement does not occur within 3 weeks, discontinue treatment.

Chronic asthma
Adults: 200 to 400 mcg oral inhalation b.i.d. when previously used bronchodilators alone or inhaled corticosteroids; 400 to 800 mcg oral inhalation b.i.d. when previously used oral corticosteroids.
Children age 6 or older: Initially 200 mcg oral inhalation b.i.d. Maximum dose is 400 mg b.i.d.

Pharmacodynamics
Anti-inflammatory action: Precise mechanism of action of glucocorticosteroids like budesonide on allergic and nonallergic rhinitis is not known. Glucocorticosteroids show a wide range of inhibitory activities against multiple cell types (such as mast cells, eosinophils, neutrophils, macrophages, and lymphocytes) and mediators (such as histamine, eicosanoids, leukotrienes, and cytokines) involved in allergic and nonallergic, irritant-mediated inflammation.

Pharmacokinetics
- *Absorption:* The amount of an intranasal dose that reaches systemic circulation is generally low (about 20%). Oral inhalation has a rapid onset of action.
- *Distribution:* Drug is 88% protein-bound in the plasma; volume of distribution is 200 L.
- *Metabolism:* Drug is rapidly and extensively metabolized in the liver.
- *Excretion:* Eliminated in urine (about 67%) and feces (about 33%).

Contraindications and precautions
Contraindicated in patients hypersensitive to drug or its components and in those who have had recent septal ulcers, nasal surgery, or nasal trauma until total healing has occurred.

Use cautiously in patients with tuberculosis infections; untreated fungal, bacterial, or systemic viral infections; or ocular herpes simplex.

Interactions
Concomitant use of budesonide with other *inhaled glucocorticosteroids* or alternate-day *prednisone* therapy may increase the risk of hypothalamic-pituitary-adrenal suppression.

Ketoconazole may increase plasma levels of budesonide.

Effects on diagnostic tests
None reported.

Adverse reactions
CNS: *headache,* nervousness.
EENT: *nasal irritation, epistaxis, pharyngitis, sinusitis,* reduced sense of smell, nasal pain, hoarseness.
GI: taste perversion, dry mouth, dyspepsia, nausea, vomiting.
Respiratory: *cough,* candidiasis, wheezing, dyspnea.
Skin: facial edema, rash, pruritus, contact dermatitis.
Other: myalgia, hypersensitivity reactions, weight gain.

Overdose and treatment
Acute overdosage is unlikely due to the limited amount of product in each container. Chronic overdosage may produce signs and symptoms of hyperadrenocorticism.

☑ Special considerations
- Replacing a systemic glucocorticosteroid with a topical glucocorticosteroid can result in signs of adrenal insufficiency; in addition, some patients may experience symptoms of withdrawal, such as joint or muscular pain, lassitude, and depression.
- Patients previously treated for prolonged periods with systemic glucocorticosteroids who are subsequently given topical glucocorticosteroids should be carefully monitored for acute adrenal insufficiency in response to stress.
- In patients with asthma or other clinical conditions requiring long-term systemic treatment, a too-rapid decrease in systemic glucocorticosteroids may severely exacerbate symptoms.
- Excessive doses of budesonide or concomitant use with other inhaled glucocorticosteroids may lead to signs or symptoms of hyperadrenocorticism.
- Because glucocorticosteroids can affect growth, monitor children closely, weighing benefits of therapy against the possibility of growth suppression.
- Patients using budesonide for several months or longer should be examined periodically for evidence of *Candida* infection or other signs of adverse effects on the nasal mucosa.

Patient education
- Warn patient not to exceed prescribed dosage or to use for long periods because of risk of hypothalamic-pituitary-adrenal axis suppression.
- Have patient follow these instructions for the nasal inhaler: After opening aluminum pouch, use within 6 minutes. Shake canister well before using. Blow nose to clear nasal passages. Tilt head slightly forward; insert nozzle into nostril, pointing away from septum; hold other nostril closed; inspire gently; and spray. Shake canister again and repeat in other nostril. Store with valve downward. Do not store in area of high humidity. Do not break, incinerate, or store canister in extreme heat; contents under pressure.
- Instruct patient to hold the inhaler upright when loading Pulmicort Turbuhaler, not to blow or exhale into the inhaler nor shake it while loaded, and to hold inhaler upright while orally inhaling the dose. Place the mouthpiece between the lips and inhale forcefully and deeply.
- Assure patient that drug rarely causes nasal irritation or burning; advise patient to call if such symptoms recur.
- Warn patient to avoid exposure to chickenpox or measles, if at risk for contacting these diseases, and to consult primary health care provider immediately if exposed.
- Teach patient good nasal and oral hygiene.
- Tell patient to call if condition worsens or if symptoms do not improve within 3 weeks.
- Inform patient that effects are not immediate; response requires regular use.
- Inform patient that with use of oral inhaler improvement in asthma control can occur within 24 hours, with maximum benefit anticipated between 1 to 2 weeks and possibly taking longer.
- Advise patient that Pulmicort Turbohaler is *not* indicated for relief of acute bronchospasm.

Pediatric use
- Safety and effectiveness of drug for treating seasonal or perennial allergic rhinitis in children under age 6 have not been established. Drug is not recommended for treatment of nonallergic rhinitis in children because adequate numbers of such children have not been studied.

Breast-feeding
- Use cautiously when administering drug to breast-feeding women.

bumetanide
Bumex

Pharmacologic classification: loop diuretic
Therapeutic classification: diuretic
Pregnancy risk category C

How supplied
Available by prescription only
Tablets: 0.5 mg, 1 mg, 2 mg
Injection: 0.25 mg/ml

Indications, route, and dosage
Edema (heart failure, hepatic and renal disease); ◇ postoperative edema; ◇ premenstrual syndrome; ◇ disseminated cancer
Adults: 0.5 to 2 mg P.O. once daily. If diuretic response is not adequate, give a second or third dose at 4- to 5-hour intervals. Maximum dosage is 10 mg/day. Give parenterally when oral route is not feasible. Usual initial dose is 0.5 to 1 mg I.V. over 1 to 2 minutes or I.M. If response is not adequate, give a second or third dose at 2- to 3-hour intervals. Maximum dosage is 10 mg/day.
◇ Pediatric heart failure
Children: 0.015 mg/kg every other day to 0.1 mg/kg daily. Use with extreme caution in neonates.

Pharmacodynamics

Diuretic action: Loop diuretics inhibit sodium and chloride reabsorption in the proximal part of the ascending loop of Henle, promoting the excretion of sodium, water, chloride, and potassium; bumetanide produces renal and peripheral vasodilation and may temporarily increase glomerular filtration rate and decrease peripheral vascular resistance.

Pharmacokinetics

- *Absorption:* After oral administration, 85% to 95% of dose is absorbed; food delays oral absorption. I.M. bumetanide is completely absorbed. Diuresis usually begins 30 to 60 minutes after oral and 40 minutes after I.M. administration; peak diuresis occurs 1 to 2 hours after either. Diuresis begins a few minutes after I.V. administration and peaks in 15 to 30 minutes.
- *Distribution:* Drug is about 92% to 96% protein-bound; it is unknown whether bumetanide enters CSF or breast milk or crosses the placenta.
- *Metabolism:* Drug is metabolized by the liver to at least five metabolites.
- *Excretion:* Excreted in urine (80%) and feces (10% to 20%). Half-life ranges from 1 to 1½ hours; duration of effect is about 2 to 4 hours.

Contraindications and precautions

Contraindicated in patients with hypersensitivity to drug or sulfonamides (possible cross-sensitivity), in those with anuria or hepatic coma, and in patients in states of severe electrolyte depletion.

Use cautiously in patients with hepatic cirrhosis and ascites and in those with depressed renal function.

Interactions

Bumetanide potentiates the hypotensive effect of most other *antihypertensive agents* and of other *diuretics*; both actions are used to therapeutic advantage.

Concomitant use of bumetanide with *potassium-sparing diuretics* (*spironolactone, triamterene, amiloride*) may decrease bumetanide-induced potassium loss; use with other *potassium-depleting drugs* such as *steroids* and *amphotericin B* may cause severe potassium loss.

Bumetanide may reduce renal clearance of *lithium* and increase lithium levels; lithium dosage may require adjustment.

Indomethacin and *probenecid* may reduce the diuretic effect of bumetanide, and their combined use is not recommended; however, if there is no therapeutic alternative, an increased dose of bumetanide may be required.

Concomitant administration of bumetanide with *ototoxic* or *nephrotoxic* drugs may result in enhanced toxicity.

Effects on diagnostic tests

Drug therapy alters electrolyte balance and liver and renal function tests.

Adverse reactions

CNS: dizziness, headache, vertigo.
CV: volume depletion and dehydration, orthostatic hypotension, ECG changes, chest pain.
EENT: transient deafness, tinnitus.
GI: nausea, vomiting, upset stomach, dry mouth, diarrhea, pain.
GU: ***renal failure,*** premature ejaculation, difficulty maintaining erection, oliguria.
Hematologic: azotemia, ***thrombocytopenia.***
Skin: rash, pruritus, diaphoresis.
Other: hypokalemia; hypochloremic alkalosis; asymptomatic hyperuricemia; weakness; arthritic pain; fluid and electrolyte imbalances, including dilutional hyponatremia, hypocalcemia, hyperglycemia, and glucose intolerance impairment; muscle pain and tenderness.

Overdose and treatment

Clinical manifestations of overdose include profound electrolyte and volume depletion, which may cause circulatory collapse.

Treatment of drug overdose is primarily supportive; replace fluid and electrolytes as needed.

☑ Special considerations

Besides those relevant to all *loop diuretics,* consider the following recommendation.

- Give I.V. bumetanide slowly, over 1 to 2 minutes, for I.V. infusion; dilute bumetanide in D_5W, 0.9% NaCl solution, or lactated Ringer's solution; use within 24 hours.

Geriatric use

- Elderly and debilitated patients require close observation because they are more susceptible to drug-induced diuresis. Excessive diuresis promotes rapid dehydration, hypovolemia, hypokalemia, and hyponatremia in these patients, and may cause circulatory collapse. Reduced dosages may be indicated.

Pediatric use

- Safety and efficacy in children under age 18 have not been established.

Breast-feeding

- Drug should not be used by breast-feeding women.

buprenorphine hydrochloride

Buprenex

Pharmacologic classification: narcotic agonist-antagonist, opioid partial agonist
Therapeutic classification: analgesic
Controlled substance schedule V
Pregnancy risk category C

How supplied

Available by prescription only
Injection: 0.3 mg/ml in 1-ml ampules

Indications, route, and dosage

Moderate to severe pain

Adults and children over age 13: 0.3 mg I.M. or slow

I.V. q 6 hours p.r.n. May repeat 0.3 mg or increase to 0.6 mg per dose if necessary. S.C. administration is not recommended.

◊ *Adults:* 25 to 250 mcg/hour via I.V. infusion (over 48 hours for postoperative pain)

◊ *Adults:* 60 to 180 mcg via epidural injection.

◊ ***Reverse fentanyl-induced anesthesia***
Adults: 0.3 to 0.8 mg, I.V. or I.M., 1 to 4 hours after the induction of anesthesia and about 30 minutes before the end of surgery.

◊ ***Circumcision***
Children age 9 months to 9 years: 3 mcg/kg I.M. along with surgical anesthesia.

Pharmacodynamics

Analgesic action: Exact mechanisms of action of buprenorphine are unknown. It is believed to be a competitive antagonist at some and an agonist at other opiate receptors, thus relieving moderate to severe pain.

Pharmacokinetics

- *Absorption:* Absorbed rapidly after I.M. administration. Onset of action occurs in 15 minutes, with peak effect 1 hour after dosing.
- *Distribution:* About 96% of drug is protein-bound.
- *Metabolism:* Drug is metabolized in the liver.
- *Excretion:* Duration of action is 6 hours. Drug is excreted primarily in the feces as unchanged drug with approximately 30% excreted in urine.

Contraindications and precautions

Contraindicated in patients with hypersensitivity to drug. Use cautiously in elderly or debilitated patients and in patients with head injuries, increased intracranial pressure, and intracranial lesions; respiratory, kidney, or hepatic impairment; CNS depression or coma; thyroid irregularities; adrenal insufficiency; prostatic hyperplasia; urethral stricture; acute alcoholism; delirium tremens; or kyphoscoliosis.

Interactions

If administered within a few hours of *barbiturate anesthetic* such as *thiopental*, buprenorphine may produce additive CNS and respiratory depressant effects and, possibly, apnea.

Reduced doses of buprenorphine are usually necessary when drug is used concomitantly with other *CNS depressants* (*narcotic analgesics, antihistamines; phenothiazines, barbiturates, benzodiazepines, sedative-hypnotics; alcohol*), *tricyclic antidepressants*, and *muscle relaxants*, which may potentiate the respiratory and CNS depression, sedation, and hypotensive effects of the drug; use with *general anesthetics* may also cause severe CV depression.

Patients who become physically dependent on this drug may experience acute withdrawal syndrome if given an *antagonist*. Use with caution and monitor closely.

Use with caution if a patient is also to receive *MAO inhibitors*.

There is one report of respiratory and CV collapse in a patient who received *diazepam* and buprenorphine in usual doses, given concomitantly.

Effects on diagnostic tests

None reported.

Adverse reactions

CNS: *dizziness, sedation, headache,* confusion, nervousness, euphoria, *vertigo,* ***increased intracranial pressure.***
CV: *hypotension,* bradycardia, tachycardia, hypertension.
EENT: *miosis,* blurred vision.
GI: *nausea,* vomiting, constipation, dry mouth.
GU: urine retention.
Respiratory: ***respiratory depression,*** hypoventilation, dyspnea.
Skin: pruritus, *diaphoresis.*

Overdose and treatment

To date there has been limited experience with overdosage. Safety of buprenorphine in acute overdosage is expected to be better than that of other opioid analgesics because of its antagonist properties at high doses. Overdose may cause CNS depression, respiratory depression, and miosis (pinpoint pupils). Other acute toxic effects might include hypotension, bradycardia, hypothermia, shock, apnea, cardiopulmonary arrest, circulatory collapse, pulmonary edema, and seizures.

To treat acute overdose, first establish adequate respiratory exchange via a patent airway and ventilation as needed; administer a narcotic antagonist (naloxone) to reverse respiratory depression. Because the duration of buprenorphine is longer than that of naloxone, repeated naloxone dosing is necessary. Naloxone should not be given unless the patient has clinically significant respiratory or CV depression. Monitor vital signs closely.

Naloxone does not completely reverse buprenorphine-induced respiratory depression; mechanical ventilation and higher than usual doses of naloxone and doxaprane may be indicated.

Provide symptomatic and supportive treatment (continued respiratory support, correction of fluid or electrolyte imbalance). Closely monitor laboratory parameters, vital signs, and neurologic status.

☑ Special considerations

Besides those relevant to all *opioid (narcotic) agonist-antagonists,* consider the following recommendations.

- Adverse effects of drug may not be as readily reversed by naloxone as are those of pure agonists.
- Buprenorphine 0.3 mg is equal to 10 mg morphine or 75 to 100 mg meperidine in analgesic potency; duration of analgesia is longer than either.

Patient education

- Teach patient to avoid activities that require full alertness.
- Instruct patient to avoid alcohol and other CNS depressants.

Geriatric use

• Administer with caution; lower doses are usually indicated for elderly patients, who may be more sensitive to the therapeutic and adverse effects of these drugs.

Breast-feeding

• It is unknown if drug is excreted in breast milk; use with caution.

bupropion hydrochloride

Wellbutrin, Wellbutrin SR

Pharmacologic classification: aminoketone
Therapeutic classification: antidepressant
Pregnancy risk category B

How supplied

Available by prescription only
Tablets: 75 mg, 100 mg
Tablets (sustained-release): 100 mg, 150 mg

Indications, route, and dosage

Depression

Adults: Initially, 100 mg P.O. b.i.d. If necessary, increase after 3 days to usual dosage of 100 mg P.O. t.i.d. If no response occurs after several weeks of therapy, consider increasing dosage to 150 mg t.i.d. For sustained-release tablets, start with 150 mg P.O. q morning; increase to target dose of 150 mg P.O. b.i.d. as tolerated as early as day 4 of dosing. Maximum dose is 400 mg/day.

Pharmacodynamics

Antidepressant action: Mechanism of action is unknown. Bupropion does not inhibit MAO; it is a weak inhibitor of norepinephrine, dopamine, and serotonin reuptake.

Pharmacokinetics

• *Absorption:* Animal studies indicate that only 5% to 20% of the drug is bioavailable. Peak plasma levels are achieved within 2 to 3 hours.
• *Distribution:* At plasma concentrations up to 200 mcg/ml, drug appears to be about 80% bound to plasma proteins.
• *Metabolism:* Probably hepatic; several active metabolites have been identified. With prolonged use, the active metabolites are expected to accumulate in the plasma and their concentration may exceed that of the parent compound. Bupropion appears to induce its own metabolism.
• *Excretion:* Primarily renal; elimination half-life of parent compound in single-dose studies ranged from 8 to 24 hours.

Contraindications and precautions

Contraindicated in patients with hypersensitivity to drug or seizure disorders and who have taken MAO inhibitors within previous 14 days. Also contraindicated in patients taking Zyban, or those with history of bulimia or anorexia nervosa because of a higher incidence of seizures. Use cautiously in patients with recent MI, unstable heart disease, and renal or hepatic impairment.

Interactions

Concomitant administration with *levodopa, phenothiazines, MAO inhibitors,* or *tricyclic antidepressants* or recent and rapid withdrawal of *benzodiazepines* may increase the risk of adverse effects, including seizures.

Animal studies suggest that bupropion may induce drug-metabolizing enzymes.

Effects on diagnostic tests

None reported.

Adverse reactions

CNS: *headache,* ***seizures,*** anxiety, *confusion,* delusions, euphoria, hostility, impaired sleep quality, *insomnia, sedation, tremor,* akinesia, akathisia, *agitation, dizziness,* fatigue.
CV: ***arrhythmias,*** hypertension, hypotension, palpitations, syncope, *tachycardia.*
EENT: *auditory disturbances,* blurred vision.
GI: *dry mouth,* taste disturbance, increased appetite, *constipation,* dyspepsia, *nausea, vomiting, weight loss, anorexia, weight gain,* diarrhea.
GU: impotence, menstrual complaints, urinary frequency, decreased libido, urine retention.
Skin: pruritus, rash, cutaneous temperature disturbance, *excessive diaphoresis.*
Other: arthritis, fever, chills.

Overdose and treatment

Signs of overdose include labored breathing, salivation, arched back, ptosis, ataxia, and seizures.

If the ingestion was recent, empty the stomach using gastric lavage or induce emesis with ipecac, as appropriate; follow with activated charcoal. Treatment should be supportive. Control seizures with I.V. benzodiazepines; stuporous, comatose, or convulsing patients may need intubation. There are no data to evaluate the benefits of dialysis, hemoperfusion, or diuresis.

☑ Special considerations

• Consider the inherent risk of suicide until significant improvement of depressive state occurs. High-risk patients should have close supervision during initial drug therapy. To reduce risk of suicidal overdose, prescribe the smallest quantity of tablets consistent with good management.
• Many patients experience a period of increased restlessness, especially at initiation of therapy. This may include agitation, insomnia, and anxiety. In clinical studies, these symptoms required sedative-hypnotic agents in some patients; about 2% had to discontinue drug.
• Antidepressants can cause manic episodes during the depressed phase in patients with bipolar disorder.
• Clinical trials revealed that 28% of patients experienced a weight loss of 5 lb (2.3 kg) or more. This effect should be considered if weight loss is a major factor in patient's depressive illness.

Patient education

- Advise patient to take drug regularly as scheduled, and to take each day's dosage in three divided doses to minimize risk of seizures.
- Warn patient to avoid the use of alcohol, which may contribute to the development of seizures.
- Advise patient to avoid activities that require alertness and coordination until CNS effects of drug are known.
- Tell patient not to chew, divide, or crush sustained-release tablets.
- Instruct patient not to take Zyban in combination with Wellbutin, nor should he take other medications, including OTC medications, without medical approval.

Pediatric use

- Safety in children under age 18 has not been established.

Breast-feeding

- Because of the potential for serious adverse reactions in the infant, breast-feeding during therapy is not recommended.

bupropion hydrochloride

Zyban

Pharmacologic classification: aminoketone
Therapeutic classification: nonnicotine aid to smoking cessation
Pregnancy risk category B

How supplied

Available by prescription only
Tablets (sustained-release): 150 mg

Indications, route, and dosage

Aid to smoking cessation treatment

Adults: 150 mg daily P.O. for 3 days; increased to maximum of 300 mg daily P.O. given as two doses of 150 mg taken at least 8 hours apart.

Note: Therapy is started while patient is still smoking; approximately 1 week is needed to achieve steady-state blood levels of drug. Patient should set target cessation date during second week of treatment.

Pharmacodynamics

Smoking cessation action: Bupropion is a relatively weak inhibitor of the neuronal uptake of norepinephrine, serotonin, and dopamine, and does not inhibit MAO. The mechanism by which drug enhances the ability to abstain from smoking is unknown.

Pharmacokinetics

- *Absorption:* Following oral administration, peak plasma concentrations are achieved within 3 hours.
- *Distribution:* Volume of distribution from a single 150-mg dose is estimated to be 1,950 L. Bupropion is 84% bound to plasma proteins at concentrations up to 200 mcg/ml.
- *Metabolism:* Drug is extensively metabolized in the liver mainly by the P-450 2B6 isoenzyme system to three active metabolites.
- *Excretion:* Mean elimination half-life of drug is thought to be about 21 hours. Following oral administration, 87% of a dose is recovered in the urine and 10% in the feces. The fraction of a dose excreted unchanged is 0.5%.

Contraindications and precautions

Contraindicated in patients with seizure disorders or with a current or prior diagnosis of bulimia or anorexia nervosa because of potential for seizures. Concurrent administration of MAO inhibitors is contraindicated; at least 14 days must elapse between discontinuation of an MAO inhibitor and starting bupropion therapy. Concurrent administration of Wellbutrin, Wellbutrin SR, or others medications containing bupropion is contraindicated because of potential for seizures. Also contraindicated in patients known to be allergic to drug or to its formulation.

Interactions

Bupropion is metabolized to hydroxybupropion by the CYP2B6 isoenzyme. Therefore, *drugs that affect enzyme metabolism,* such as *orphenadrine* and *cyclophosphamide,* may cause an interaction.

Because bupropion is extensively metabolized, coadministration of other drugs may effect its activity. Certain drugs may induce the metabolism of bupropion such as *carbamazepine, phenobarbital,* and *phenytoin,* whereas others such as *cimetidine* inhibit the metabolism of bupropion.

Studies have indicated that acute toxicity of bupropion is enhanced by the *MAO inhibitor, phenelzine.*

Some clinical data suggest a higher incidence of adverse reactions in patients receiving concurrent administration with *levodopa.* If concurrent use is necessary, give small initial doses of buproprion and gradually increase dose.

Concurrent administration of bupropion and agents such as *antipsychotics, antidepressants, theophylline,* and *systemic steroids,* or treatment regimens *(abrupt withdrawal of benzodiazepines)* that lower seizure threshold should be undertaken with extreme caution.

Effect on diagnostic tests

None reported.

Adverse reactions

CNS: agitation, dizziness, hot flashes, *insomnia,* somnolence, tremor.
CV: ***complete AV block***, hypertension, hypotension, tachycardia.
EENT: *dry mouth,* taste perversion.
GI: anorexia, dyspepsia, increased appetite.
GU: impotence, polyuria, urinary frequency and urgency.
Metabolic: edema, weight gain.
Musculoskeletal: arthralgia, leg cramps and twitching, myalgia.
Respiratory: bronchitis, ***bronchospasm.***
Skin: dry skin, pruritus, rash, urticaria.
Other: allergic reactions, neck pain.

Overdose and treatment

Hospitalization is recommended for overdoses. If patient is conscious, induce vomiting with syrup of ipecac. Activated charcoal may also be administered every 6 hours for first 12 hours. Perform ECG and EEG monitoring for first 48 hours. Provide adequate fluid intake and obtain baseline tests.

If patient is stuporous, comatose, or experiencing seizures, airway intubation is recommended before undertaking gastric lavage. Gastric lavage may be beneficial within first 12 hours after ingestion because drug absorption may not be complete. Although diuresis, dialysis, or hemoperfusion is sometimes used to treat drug overdose, there is no experience with their use in managing bupropion overdose. Based on animal studies, seizures can be treated with an I.V. benzodiazepine and other supportive measures.

Special considerations

- Because drug use is associated with a dose-dependent risk of seizures, do not exceed 300 mg daily for smoking cessation.
- If patient has not made progress towards abstinence by week 7 of therapy, stop therapy because it is unlikely that he will quit smoking.
- Dose need not be tapered when stopping treatment.

Patient education

- Stress importance of combining behavioral interventions, counseling, and support services with drug therapy.
- Inform patient that risk of seizures is increased if he has a seizure or eating disorder (bulimia or anorexia nervosa), exceeds the recommended dose, or takes other medications containing bupropion.
- Instruct patient to take doses at least 8 hours apart.
- Inform patient that drug is usually taken for 7 to 12 weeks.
- Advise patient that, although he may continue to smoke during drug therapy, it reduces his chance of breaking the smoking habit.
- Tell patient that drug and nicotine patch should only be used together under medical supervision because his blood pressure may increase.

Geriatric use

- Experience in patients age 60 and older was similar to that in younger patients.

Pediatric use

- Safety and efficacy have not been established.

Breast-feeding

- Drug and its metabolites are secreted in breast milk. Because of the potential for serious adverse reactions in the infant, a choice must be made between breast-feeding and drug therapy.

buspirone hydrochloride

BuSpar

Pharmacologic classification: azaspirodecanedione derivative
Therapeutic classification: antianxiety
Pregnancy risk category B

How supplied

Available by prescription only
Tablets: 5 mg, 10 mg

Indications, route, and dosage

Management of anxiety disorders

Adults: Initially, 5 mg P.O. t.i.d. Dosage may be increased at 3-day intervals. Usual maintenance dosage is 20 to 30 mg daily in divided doses. Do not exceed 60 mg/day.

Pharmacodynamics

Anxiolytic action: Buspirone is an azaspirodecanedione derivative with anxiolytic activity. It suppresses conflict and aggressive behavior and inhibits conditioned avoidance responses. Its precise mechanism of action has not been determined, but it appears to depend on simultaneous effects on several neurotransmitters and receptor sites: decreasing serotonin neuronal activity, increasing norepinephrine metabolism, and partial action as a presynaptic dopamine antagonist. Studies suggest an indirect effect on benzodiazepine gamma-aminobutyric acid (GABA)–chloride receptor complex or GABA receptors, or on other neurotransmitter systems.

Buspirone is not pharmacologically related to benzodiazepines, barbiturates, or other sedative and anxiolytic agents. It exhibits both a nontraditional clinical profile and is uniquely anxiolytic. It has no anticonvulsant or muscle relaxant activity and does not appear to cause physical dependence or significant sedation.

Pharmacokinetics

- *Absorption:* Drug is absorbed rapidly and completely after oral administration, but extensive first-pass metabolism limits absolute bioavailability to 1% to 13% of the oral dose. Food slows absorption but increases the amount of unchanged drug in systemic circulation.
- *Distribution:* Drug is 95% protein-bound; it does not displace other highly protein-bound medications such as warfarin. Onset of therapeutic effect may require 1 to 2 weeks.
- *Metabolism:* Drug is metabolized in the liver by hydroxylation and oxidation, resulting in at least one pharmacologically active metabolite—1, pyrimidinylpiperazine (1-PP).
- *Excretion:* 29% to 63% is excreted in urine in 24 hours, primarily as metabolites; 18% to 38% is excreted in feces.

Contraindications and precautions

Contraindicated in patients hypersensitive to drug or within 14 days of therapy with an MAO inhibitor.

Use cautiously in patients with renal or hepatic impairment.

Interactions

When used concomitantly with *MAO inhibitors*, buspirone may elevate blood pressure; avoid this combination.

Buspirone may displace *digoxin* from serum-binding sites when the drugs are used concomitantly.

Use cautiously with *alcohol* or other *CNS depressants* because sedation may result, especially with doses greater than 30 mg/day. Buspirone does not increase alcohol-induced impairment of mental and motor performance; however, CNS effects in individuals are not predictable. Serum *haloperidol* levels may increase.

Effects on diagnostic tests

None reported.

Adverse reactions

CNS: *dizziness, drowsiness,* nervousness, insomnia, headache, light-headedness, fatigue, numbness.
EENT: blurred vision.
GI: dry mouth, nausea, diarrhea, abdominal distress.

Overdose and treatment

Signs of overdose include severe dizziness, drowsiness, unusual constriction of pupils, and stomach upset, including nausea and vomiting.

Treatment of overdose is symptomatic and supportive; empty stomach with immediate gastric lavage. Monitor respiration, pulse, and blood pressure. No specific antidote is known. Effect of dialysis is unknown.

☑ Special considerations

- Patients who have been treated with benzodiazepines previously may not show good clinical response to this agent.
- Although buspirone does not appear to cause tolerance or physical or psychological dependence, the possibility exists that patients prone to drug abuse may experience these effects.
- Buspirone does not block the withdrawal syndrome associated with benzodiazepines or other common sedative and hypnotic agents; therefore, these agents should be withdrawn gradually before replacement with buspirone therapy.
- Monitor hepatic and renal function; hepatic and renal impairment impedes metabolism and excretion of drug and may lead to toxic accumulation; dosage reduction may be necessary.

Patient education

- Advise patient to take drug exactly as prescribed; explain that therapeutic effect may not occur for 2 weeks or more. Warn patient not to double the dose if one is missed, but to take a missed dose as soon as possible, unless it is almost time for next dose.
- Caution patient to avoid hazardous tasks requiring alertness until drug's effects are known. The effects of alcohol and other CNS depressants (such as antihistamines, sedatives, tranquilizers, sleeping aids, prescription pain medication, barbiturates, seizure medicine, muscle relaxants, anesthetics, and medicines for colds, coughs, hay fever, or allergies) may be enhanced by additive sedation and drowsiness caused by buspirone.
- Tell patient to store drug away from heat and light and out of children's reach.
- Explain importance of regular follow-up visits to check progress. Urge patient to report adverse reactions immediately.
- Inform patient that results may not be seen in 3 to 4 weeks; however, an improvement may be noted within 7 to 10 days.

Breast-feeding

- Reports of animal studies show that buspirone and its metabolites are excreted in the breast milk of rats; however, the extent of excretion in human milk is unknown. Buspirone should be avoided in breast-feeding women.

busulfan

Myleran

Pharmacologic classification: alkylating agent (cell cycle–phase nonspecific)
Therapeutic classification: antineoplastic
Pregnancy risk category D

How supplied

Available by prescription only
Tablets (scored): 2 mg

Indications, route, and dosage

Dosage and indications may vary. Check current literature for recommended protocol.

Chronic myelogenous leukemia

Adults: For remission induction, usual dosage is 4 to 8 mg P.O. daily; however, may range from 1 to 12 mg P.O. daily (0.06 mg/kg or 1.8 mg/m^2). For maintenance therapy, 1 to 3 mg P.O. daily.
Children: 0.06 to 0.12 mg/kg or 1.8 to 4.6 mg/m^2 P.O. daily. Dosage should be titrated to maintain WBC count of about 20,000/mm^3.

◊ ***Myelofibrosis***

Adults: 2 to 4 mg P.O. two to three times weekly.

Pharmacodynamics

Antineoplastic action: Busulfan is an alkylating agent that exerts its cytotoxic activity by interfering with DNA replication and RNA transcription, causing a disruption of nucleic acid function.

Pharmacokinetics

- *Absorption:* Busulfan is well absorbed from the GI tract.
- *Distribution:* Distribution into the brain and CSF is unknown.
- *Metabolism:* Drug is metabolized in the liver.
- *Excretion:* Busulfan is cleared rapidly from the plasma. Drug and its metabolites are excreted in urine.

Contraindications and precautions
Contraindicated in patients whose chronic myelogenous leukemia has demonstrated prior resistance to drug. Also contraindicated in patients with chronic lymphocytic leukemia or acute leukemia and in those in "blastic" crisis of chronic myelogenous leukemia.

Use cautiously in patients recently given other myelosuppressants or radiation treatment; in those with depressed neutrophil or platelet counts, head trauma, and seizures; or in patients taking other medications that reduce seizure threshold.

Interactions
None reported.

Effects on diagnostic tests
Drug-induced cellular dysplasia may interfere with interpretation of cytologic studies.

Busulfan therapy may increase blood and urine levels of uric acid as a result of increased purine catabolism that accompanies cell destruction.

Adverse reactions
CNS: unusual tiredness or weakness, fatigue.
GI: cheilosis, dry mouth, anorexia.
Hematologic: leukopenia (WBC count decreasing after about 10 days and continuing to decrease for 2 weeks after stopping drug), ***thrombocytopenia, anemia, severe pancytopenia.***
Respiratory: ***irreversible pulmonary fibrosis (commonly called "busulfan lung").***
Skin: alopecia, *transient hyperpigmentation,* rash, urticaria, anhidrosis.
Other: gynecomastia, Addison-like wasting syndrome, profound hyperuricemia caused by increased cell lysis, cataracts, jaundice.

Overdose and treatment
Clinical manifestations of overdose include hematologic manifestations, such as leukopenia and thrombocytopenia.

Treatment is supportive and includes transfusion of blood components and antibiotics for infections that may develop.

☑ Special considerations
- Avoid all I.M. injections when platelets are less than 100,000/mm³.
- Patient response (increased appetite, sense of well-being, decreased total leukocyte count, reduction in size of spleen) usually begins 1 to 2 weeks after initiating the drug.
- Watch for signs or symptoms of infection (fever, sore throat).
- Pulmonary fibrosis may be delayed for 4 to 6 months.
- Persistent cough and progressive dyspnea with alveolar exudate may result from drug toxicity, not pneumonia. Instruct patient to report symptoms so dose adjustments can be made.
- Monitor uric acid, CBC, and kidney function.
- Minimize hyperuricemia by adequate hydration, alkalinization of urine, and administration of allopurinol.

Patient education
- Advise patient to use caution when taking aspirin-containing products and to promptly report any sign of bleeding.
- Tell patient to take medication at same time each day.
- Emphasize importance of continuing to take medication despite nausea and vomiting.
- Instruct patient about the signs and symptoms of infection and tell him to report them promptly if they occur.
- Advise patient to use contraceptive methods during therapy.

Breast-feeding
- It is not known if drug distributes into breast milk. However, potential for mutagenicity, carcinogenicity, and serious adverse reactions in the infant should be taken into consideration when a decision to breast-feed is made.

butabarbital sodium
Butisol

Pharmacologic classification: barbiturate
Therapeutic classification: sedative-hypnotic
Controlled substance schedule III
Pregnancy risk category D

How supplied
Available by prescription only
Tablets: 15 mg, 30 mg, 50 mg, 100 mg
Elixir: 30 mg/5 ml, 33.3 mg/5 ml

Indications, route, and dosage
Sedation
Adults: 15 to 30 mg P.O. t.i.d. or q.i.d.
Preoperative sedation
Adults: 50 to 100 mg P.O. 60 to 90 minutes before surgery.
Children: 2 to 6 mg/kg; up to a maximum of 100 mg/dose.
Insomnia
Adults: 50 to 100 mg P.O. h.s.

Pharmacodynamics
Sedative-hypnotic action: The exact cellular site and mechanism(s) of action are unknown. Butabarbital acts throughout the CNS as a nonselective depressant with an intermediate onset and duration of action. Particularly sensitive to the drug is the reticular activating system, which controls CNS arousal. Butabarbital decreases both presynaptic and postsynaptic membrane excitability by facilitating the action of gamma-aminobutyric acid.

Pharmacokinetics
- *Absorption.* Butabarbital is well absorbed after oral administration, with peak concentrations occurring in 3 to 4 hours. Onset of action occurs in 45 to 60 minutes. Serum concentrations needed for sedation and hypnosis are 2 to 3 mcg/ml and 25 mcg/ml, respectively.

• *Distribution:* Distributed well throughout body tissues and fluids.
• *Metabolism:* Drug is metabolized extensively in the liver by oxidation. Its duration of action is 6 to 8 hours.
• *Excretion:* Inactive metabolites of butabarbital are excreted in urine. Only 1% to 2% of an oral dose is excreted in urine unchanged. Terminal half-life ranges from 30 to 40 hours.

Contraindications and precautions

Contraindicated in patients with bronchopneumonia, or other severe pulmonary insufficiency, hypersensitivity to barbiturates, or porphyria. Use cautiously in patients with renal or hepatic impairment, acute or chronic pain, or history of drug abuse.

Interactions

Butabarbital may add to or potentiate the CNS and respiratory depressant effects of other *sedative-hypnotics, antihistamines, narcotics, antidepressants, tranquilizers*, and *alcohol*.

Butabarbital enhances the enzymatic degradation of *warfarin* and other *oral anticoagulants*; patients may require increased doses of the *anticoagulants*. Drug also enhances hepatic metabolism of some drugs, including *digitoxin* (not digoxin), *corticosteroids, oral contraceptives* and other *estrogens, theophylline* and other *xanthines*, and *doxycycline*. Butabarbital impairs the effectiveness of *griseofulvin* by decreasing absorption from the GI tract.

Valproic acid, disulfiram, and *MAO inhibitors* decrease the metabolism of butabarbital and can increase its toxicity. *Rifampin* may decrease butabarbital levels by increasing hepatic metabolism.

Effects on diagnostic tests

Butabarbital may cause a false-positive phentolamine test. The physiologic effects of drug may impair the absorption of cyanocobalamin ^{57}Co; it may decrease serum bilirubin concentrations in neonates, epileptic patients, and patients with congenital nonhemolytic unconjugated hyperbilirubinemia. EEG patterns are altered, with a change in low-voltage, fast activity; changes persist for a time after discontinuation of therapy. Barbiturates may increase sulfobromophthalein retention.

Adverse reactions

CNS: *drowsiness, lethargy, hangover,* paradoxical excitement in elderly patients, somnolence.
GI: nausea, vomiting.
Hematologic: exacerbation of porphyria.
Respiratory: ***respiratory depression, apnea.***
Skin: rash, urticaria, ***Stevens-Johnson syndrome.***
Other: ***angioedema,*** physical and psychological dependence.

Overdose and treatment

Clinical manifestations of overdose include unsteady gait, slurred speech, sustained nystagmus, somnolence, confusion, respiratory depression, pulmonary edema, areflexia, and coma. Jaundice, hypothermia followed by fever, oliguria, and typical shock syndrome with tachycardia and hypotension may occur.

To treat, maintain and support ventilation and pulmonary function, as necessary; support cardiac function and circulation with vasopressors and I.V. fluids, as needed. If patient is conscious with a functioning gag reflex and ingestion was recent, induce emesis by administering ipecac syrup. If emesis is contraindicated, perform gastric lavage while a cuffed endotracheal tube is in place, to prevent aspiration. Follow by administering activated charcoal or sodium chloride cathartic. Measure intake and output, vital signs, and laboratory parameters. Maintain body temperature. Alkalinization of urine may be helpful in removing drug from the body; hemodialysis may be useful in severe overdose.

☑ Special considerations

Besides those relevant to all *barbiturates*, consider the following recommendations.
• Tablet may be crushed and mixed with food or fluid if patient has difficulty swallowing. Capsule may be opened and contents mixed with food or fluids to aid in swallowing.
• Assess cardiopulmonary status frequently; monitor vital signs for significant changes.
• Monitor patient for possible allergic reaction resulting from tartrazine sensitivity.
• Periodically evaluate blood counts and renal and hepatic studies for abnormalities and adverse effects.
• Monitor PT carefully when patient on butabarbital starts or ends anticoagulant therapy. Anticoagulant dosage may need to be adjusted.
• Watch for signs of barbiturate toxicity (coma, pupillary constriction, cyanosis, clammy skin, hypotension). Overdose can be fatal.
• Prolonged administration is not recommended; drug has not been shown to be effective after 14 days. A drug-free interval of at least 1 week is advised between dosing periods.

Patient education

• Tell patient to avoid driving and other hazardous activities that require alertness because the drug may cause drowsiness.
• Warn patient that prolonged use can result in physical or psychological dependence.
• Emphasize the dangers of combining drug with alcohol. Excessive depressant effect is possible, even if drug is taken the evening before ingestion of alcohol.

Geriatric use

• Elderly patients are more susceptible to the CNS depressant effects of butabarbital. Confusion, disorientation, and excitability may occur.
• Elderly patients usually require lower doses.

Pediatric use

• Butabarbital may cause paradoxical excitement in children. Dosage is dependent on age and weight of child and degree of sedation required. Use with caution.

Breast-feeding
• Drug passes into breast milk; avoid use in breast-feeding women.

butoconazole nitrate
Femstat

Pharmacologic classification: synthetic imidazole derivative
Therapeutic classification: topical fungistat
Pregnancy risk category C

How supplied
Available by prescription only
Vaginal cream: 2% supplied with applicators

Indications, route, and dosage
Vulvovaginal candidiasis (moniliasis)
Adults (nonpregnant): One applicatorful intravaginally h.s. for 3 days (may be extended to 6 days if necessary).
Adults (pregnant): One applicatorful intravaginally h.s. for 6 days. Use only during second or third trimester.

Pharmacodynamics
Antifungal action: Although the exact mechanism is unknown, it is thought that butoconazole controls or destroys fungi by disrupting the permeability of the cell membrane and reducing its osmotic pressure resistance. Drug is active against many fungi, including dermatophytes and yeasts. It is also active in vitro against some gram-positive bacteria.

Pharmacokinetics
• *Absorption:* Approximately 5.5% of drug is absorbed through the vaginal walls.
• *Distribution:* Unknown.
• *Metabolism:* Systemically absorbed drug appears to be metabolized, probably in the liver.
• *Excretion:* Systemically absorbed drug appears to be excreted in the urine and feces.

Contraindications and precautions
Contraindicated in patients hypersensitive to drug.

Interactions
None reported.

Effects on diagnostic tests
None reported.

Adverse reactions
GU: vulvovaginal burning and itching, soreness, and swelling.
Skin: finger itching.

Overdose and treatment
No information available.

☑ Special considerations
• Ascertain that patient understands directions for use and length of therapy.
• Drug may be used concomitantly with oral contraceptives and antibiotic therapy.

Patient education
• Instruct patient to follow the directions enclosed in the package and to insert the applicator high into the vagina and to wash hands after use.
• Tell patient to complete the full course of therapy, including through menstrual period. However, tell her to avoid using tampons during treatment.
• Advise patient to refrain from sexual contact or to have partner use a condom to avoid reinfection during therapy.
• Tell patient to use a sanitary napkin to prevent staining clothing and to absorb discharge.
• Tell patient to report symptoms that persist after full course of therapy.

Breast-feeding
• Use drug with caution in breast-feeding women because it is unknown if it is distributed into breast milk.

butorphanol tartrate
Stadol, Stadol NS

Pharmacologic classification: narcotic agonist-antagonist; opioid partial agonist
Therapeutic classification: analgesic, adjunct to anesthesia
Pregnancy risk category C

How supplied
Available by prescription only
Injection: 1 mg/ml, 1-ml vials; 2 mg/ml, 1-ml, 2-ml, and 10-ml vials
Nasal spray: 10 mg/ml

Indications, route, and dosage
Moderate to severe pain
Adults: 1 to 4 mg I.M. q 3 to 4 hours p.r.n.; or 0.5 to 2 mg I.V. q 3 to 4 hours p.r.n. or around-the-clock. Alternatively, give 1 mg by nasal spray (1 spray in one nostril). Repeat if pain relief is inadequate after 1 to 1½ hours. Repeat q 3 to 4 hours p.r.n.
Pain during labor
Adults: 1 to 2 mg I.M. or I.V. q 4 hours but not 4 hours before delivery.
Preoperative anesthesia
Adults: 2 mg I.M. 60 to 90 minutes before surgery or 2 mg I.V. shortly before induction.
✦ ***Dosage adjustment.*** Decreased dosages may be necessary in elderly patients.

Pharmacodynamics
Analgesic action: The exact mechanisms of action of butorphanol are unknown. Drug is believed to be a competitive antagonist at some, and an agonist at other, opiate receptors, thus relieving moderate to severe pain. Like narcotic agonists, it causes respiratory depression, sedation, and miosis.

Pharmacokinetics
• *Absorption:* Butorphanol is well absorbed after I.M. administration. Onset of analgesia after par-

enteral administration is less than 10 minutes, with peak analgesic effect at ½ to 1 hour. Onset of analgesia usually occurs within 15 minutes after nasal administration.

- *Distribution:* Drug rapidly crosses the placenta, and neonatal serum concentrations are 0.4 to 1.4 times maternal concentrations.
- *Metabolism:* Metabolized extensively in the liver, primarily by hydroxylation, to inactive metabolites.
- *Excretion:* Duration of effect is 3 to 4 hours after parenteral administration; 4 to 5 hours after nasal administration. Butorphanol is excreted in inactive form, mainly by the kidneys. About 11% to 14% of a parenteral dose is excreted in feces.

Contraindications and precautions

Contraindicated in patients receiving repeated doses of narcotic medications or with narcotic addiction; may precipitate withdrawal syndrome. Also contraindicated in patients with hypersensitivity to drug or to the preservative benzethonium chloride.

Use cautiously in emotionally unstable patients and in those with history of drug abuse, head injuries, increased intracranial pressure, acute MI, ventricular dysfunction, coronary insufficiency, respiratory disease or depression, and renal or hepatic dysfunction.

Interactions

If administered within a few hours of *barbiturate anesthetics* such as *thiopental*, butorphanol may produce additive CNS and respiratory depressant effects and, possibly, apnea. According to some reports, *cimetidine* may potentiate butorphanol toxicity, causing disorientation, respiratory depression, apnea, and seizures. Because data are limited, this combination is not contraindicated; however, be prepared to administer a narcotic antagonist if toxicity occurs.

Reduced doses of butorphanol are usually necessary when drug is used concomitantly with other *CNS depressants* (*narcotic analgesics, antihistamines, phenothiazines, barbiturates, benzodiazepines, sedative-hypnotics, alcohol, tricyclic antidepressants, muscle relaxants*), which may potentiate respiratory and CNS depression, sedation, and hypotensive effects of the drug. Use with *general anesthetics* may also cause severe CV depression.

Drug accumulation and enhanced effects may result if drug is given concomitantly with other drugs that are extensively metabolized in the liver (*rifampin, phenytoin, digitoxin*).

Patients who become physically dependent on opioids may experience acute withdrawal syndrome if given a *narcotic antagonist.* Use with caution and monitor closely.

Concomitant use with *pancuronium* may increase conjunctival changes.

Effects on diagnostic tests

None reported.

Adverse reactions

CNS: *confusion,* nervousness, lethargy, headache, *somnolence, dizziness, insomnia,* anxiety, paresthesia, euphoria, hallucinations, flushing, ***increased intracranial pressure.***
CV: palpitations, vasodilation, hypotension.
EENT: blurred vision, *nasal congestion* (with nasal spray), tinnitus, taste perversion.
GI: *nausea, vomiting, constipation,* anorexia.
Respiratory: ***respiratory depression.***
Skin: rash, hives, *clamminess, excessive diaphoresis.*
Other: sensation of heat.

Overdose and treatment

No information available.

☑ Special considerations

Besides those relevant to all *opioid (narcotic) agonist-antagonists,* consider the following recommendations.

- Patients who are using nasal formulation for severe pain may initiate therapy with 2 mg (one spray in each nostril) provided they remain recumbent. Dosage is not repeated for 3 to 4 hours.
- Drug has the potential to be abused. Closely supervise use in emotionally unstable patients and in those with history of drug abuse when long-term therapy is necessary.
- Mild withdrawal symptoms have been reported with chronic use of the injectable form.

Patient education

- Teach patient how to use nasal spray. Patient should use one spray in one nostril unless otherwise directed.

Geriatric use

- Lower doses are usually indicated for elderly patients because they may be more sensitive to drug's therapeutic and adverse effects. Plasma half-life is increased by 25% in patients over age 65.

Pediatric use

- Safety and efficacy in children under age 18 have not been established.

Breast-feeding

- Use of drug in breast-feeding women is not recommended.

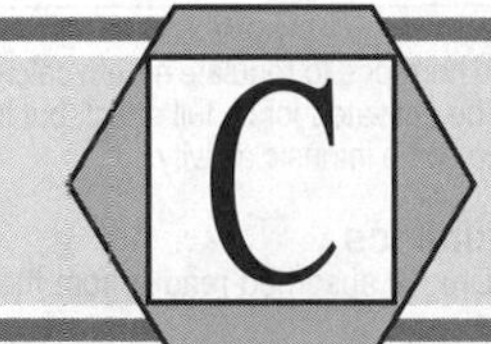

caffeine

Caffedrine, NoDoz, Quick Pep, Vivarin

Pharmacologic classification: methylxanthine
Therapeutic classification: CNS stimulant, analeptic, respiratory stimulant
Pregnancy risk category C

How supplied

Available without a prescription
Tablets: 100 mg, 150 mg, 200 mg

Available by prescription only
Injection: 250 mg/ml, caffeine (121.25 mg/ml) with sodium benzoate (128.75 mg/ml)

Indications, route, and dosage

CNS depression
Adults: 100 to 200 mg P.O. q 3 to 4 hours, p.r.n. For emergencies, 250 to 500 mg I.M. or I.V.
Infants and children: 4 mg/kg I.M., I.V., or S.C. q 4 hours, p.r.n.

Note: This use is strongly discouraged by many clinicians.

◇ ***Neonatal apnea***
Neonates: 5 to 10 mg/kg (base) I.V., I.M., or P.O. as a loading dose, followed by 2.5 to 5 mg/kg I.V., I.M., or P.O. daily. Adjust dosage according to patient tolerance and plasma caffeine levels.

Pharmacodynamics

CNS stimulant action: Caffeine is a xanthine derivative; it increases levels of cAMP by inhibiting phosphodiesterase. Caffeine stimulates all levels of the CNS; it hastens and clarifies thinking and improves arousal and psychomotor coordination.

Respiratory stimulant action: In respiratory depression and in neonatal apnea (unlabeled use), larger doses of caffeine increase respiratory rate. Caffeine increases contractile force and decreases fatigue of skeletal muscle.

Pharmacokinetics

- *Absorption:* Well absorbed from the GI tract; absorption after I.M. injection may be slower.
- *Distribution:* Caffeine is distributed rapidly throughout the body; it crosses the blood-brain barrier and placenta. Approximately 17% protein-bound.
- *Metabolism:* Metabolized by the liver; in neonates, liver metabolism is much less evident and half-life may approach 80 hours. Plasma half-life of caffeine in adults is 3 to 4 hours.
- *Excretion:* Excreted in urine.

Contraindications and precautions

Contraindicated in patients with hypersensitivity to drug. Use cautiously in patients with history of peptic ulcer, symptomatic arrhythmias, or palpitations and after an acute MI.

Interactions

Concomitant use of caffeine with *oral contraceptives, fluoroquinolones* such as *ciprofloxacin* and *enoxacin, cimetidine,* or *disulfiram* inhibits caffeine metabolism and increases its effects; use with other *xanthine derivatives* (*theophylline*) may increase incidence of stimulant-induced adverse reactions, such as tremor, tachycardia, insomnia, and nervousness. Concomitant use of *beta agonists* (*terbutaline, albuterol, metaproterenol*) increases incidence of cardiac effects and tremors. *Smoking* may enhance elimination of caffeine.

Effects on diagnostic tests

Caffeine may increase blood glucose levels and cause false-positive urate levels; it also may cause false-positive test results for pheochromocytoma or neuroblastoma by increasing certain urinary catecholamines.

Adverse reactions

CNS: *insomnia,* restlessness, nervousness, headache, excitement, agitation, muscle tremor, twitching.
CV: *tachycardia, palpitations,* extrasystoles.
GI: nausea, vomiting, diarrhea, stomach pain.
GU: *diuresis.*
Other: abrupt withdrawal symptoms (headache, irritability), tinnitus.

Overdose and treatment

Clinical manifestations of overdose in adults may include insomnia, dyspnea, altered states of consciousness, muscle twitching, seizure, diuresis, arrhythmias, and fever. In infants, symptoms may include alternating hypotonicity and hypertonicity, opisthotonoid posture, tremors, bradycardia, hypotension, and severe acidosis.

Treat overdose symptomatically and supportively; lavage and charcoal may help. Carefully monitor vital signs, ECG, and fluid and electrolyte balance. Seizures may be treated with diazepam or phenobarbital; diazepam can exacerbate respiratory depression.

☑ Special considerations

- Restrict caffeine-containing beverages in patients with arrhythmic symptoms or in those who are taking aminophylline or theophylline.
- Caffeine content in beverages (mg/cup) is the following: cola drinks, 24 to 64; brewed tea, 20 to 110;

instant coffee, 30 to 120; brewed coffee, 40 to 180; decaffeinated coffee, 3 to 5.
- Many OTC pain relievers contain caffeine, but evidence concerning its analgesic effects is conflicting. Caffeine (30%) may be used in a hydrophilic base or hydrocortisone cream to treat atopic dermatitis.
- Caffeine has been used to relieve headache after lumbar puncture and, in topical creams, to treat atopic dermatitis.

Patient education
- Advise patient to avoid excessive caffeine consumption, and therefore CNS stimulation, by learning caffeine content of beverages and foods.
- Warn patient not to exceed recommended dosage, not to substitute caffeine for needed sleep, and to discontinue drug if dizziness or tachycardia occurs.

Geriatric use
- Elderly patients are more sensitive to caffeine and should take lower doses.

Pediatric use
- Unlabeled uses include neonatal apnea. For control of neonatal apnea, maintain plasma caffeine level at 5 to 20 mcg/ml.
- Adverse CNS effects are usually more severe in children.
- In neonates, avoid using caffeine products containing sodium benzoate because they may cause kernicterus.

Breast-feeding
- Caffeine appears in breast milk. Alternative feeding method is recommended during therapy with caffeine.

calcifediol
Calderol

Pharmacologic classification: vitamin D analogue
Therapeutic classification: antihypocalcemic
Pregnancy risk category C

How supplied
Available by prescription only
Capsules: 20 mcg, 50 mcg

Indications, route, and dosage
Management of metabolic bone disease or hypocalcemia in patients on chronic renal dialysis
Adults: Initially, 300 to 350 mcg/week P.O. given daily or every other day. May increase dose at 4-week intervals based on serum levels. Most patients respond to 50 to 100 mcg/day or 100 to 200 mcg every other day.

Pharmacodynamics
Antihypocalcemic action: Calcifediol is a vitamin D analogue (25-hydroxycholecalciferol) that works with parathyroid hormone to regulate serum calcium; drug must be activated for its full effect, but it appears to have some intrinsic activity.

Pharmacokinetics
- *Absorption:* Drug is absorbed readily from the small intestine.
- *Distribution:* Distributed widely and highly protein-bound.
- *Metabolism:* Drug is metabolized in the liver and kidney; half-life is 16 days. It is activated to 1,25 dihydroxycholecalciferol.
- *Excretion:* Excreted in urine and bile.

Contraindications and precautions
Contraindicated in patients with hypercalcemia or vitamin D toxicity.

Interactions
Antacids and *mineral oil* may alter calcifediol absorption. *Barbiturates, phenytoin,* and *primidone* may increase metabolism and reduce activity of calcifediol. The increases in calcium produced by calcifediol may potentiate the effects of *cardiac glycosides. Thiazide diuretics* may result in hypercalcemia. *Corticosteroids* counteract the effects of vitamin D analogues. *Cholestyramine* or *colestipol hydrochloride* may reduce intestinal absorption.

Effects on diagnostic tests
Calcifediol may falsely elevate cholesterol determinations made using the Zlatkis-Zak reaction. Alters concentrations of serum alkaline phosphatase concentrations and may alter electrolytes, such as magnesium, phosphate, and calcium, in the serum and urine.

Adverse reactions
Vitamin D intoxication associated with hypercalcemia:
CNS: headache, somnolence, weakness, irritability, psychosis (rare).
CV: hypertension, ***arrhythmias.***
EENT: conjunctivitis, photosensitivity reactions, rhinorrhea.
GI: constipation, nausea, vomiting, polydipsia, pancreatitis, metallic taste, dry mouth, anorexia, diarrhea.
GU: polyuria, nocturia.
Skin: pruritus.
Other: bone and muscle pain, weight loss, hyperthermia, nephrocalcinosis, decreased libido.

Overdose and treatment
The only clinical manifestation of overdose is hypercalcemia. Treatment involves discontinuing therapy, instituting a low-calcium diet, and increasing fluid intake. Provide supportive measures. Severe overdose has led to death from cardiac and renal failure. Calcitonin administration may be useful in hypercalcemia.

☑ Special considerations
- Before initiating therapy, verify serum phosphate levels are controlled. To avoid ectopic calcification,

serum calcium (mg/dl) times phosphorus (mg/dl) should not be allowed to exceed 70.
• Monitor serum calcium levels several times weekly when initiating therapy.
• There is some evidence that monitoring urine calcium and urine creatinine is very helpful in screening for hypercalciuria. The ratio of urine calcium to urine creatinine should be less than or equal to 0.18. A value above 0.2 suggests hypercalciuria, and the dose should be decreased regardless of serum calcium level.

Patient education
• Explain importance of a calcium-rich diet.

Pediatric use
• Some infants may be hyperreactive to drug.

Breast-feeding
• Very little of drug appears in breast milk; however, the effect of vitamin D levels exceeding the RDA in infants is unknown. Drug should be used cautiously in breast-feeding women.

calcipotriene
Dovonex

Pharmacologic classification: synthetic vitamin D_3 analogue
Therapeutic classification: topical antipsoriatic
Pregnancy risk category C

How supplied
Available by prescription only
Cream, lotion, ointment: 0.005%

Indications, route, and dosage
Moderate plaque psoriasis
Adults: Apply a thin layer to affected skin b.i.d. Rub in gently and completely.

Pharmacodynamics
Antipsoriatic action: Calcipotriene is a synthetic vitamin D_3 analogue that binds to vitamin D_3 receptors in skin cells (keratinocytes), regulating skin cell production and development.

Pharmacokinetics
• *Absorption:* Approximately 6% of the applied dose of calcipotriene is absorbed systemically when the ointment is applied topically to psoriasis plaques or 5% when applied to normal skin.
• *Distribution:* Vitamin D and its metabolites are transported in the blood, bound to specific plasma proteins, to many parts of the body containing keratinocytes. (The scaly red patches of psoriasis are caused by the abnormal growth and production of keratinocytes.)
• *Metabolism:* Drug metabolism after systemic uptake is rapid and occurs via a pathway similar to the natural hormone. The primary metabolites are much less potent than the parent compound.
• *Excretion:* The active form of the vitamin, 1,25-dihydroxy vitamin D_3 (calcitriol), is recycled via the liver and excreted in bile.

Contraindications and precautions
Contraindicated in patients hypersensitive to drug or its components. Also contraindicated in patients with hypercalcemia or evidence of vitamin D toxicity. Use cautiously in breast-feeding patients and in the elderly. Drug should not be used on the face.

Interactions
None reported.

Effects on diagnostic tests
None reported.

Adverse reactions
Skin: *burning, pruritus, irritation,* atrophy, dermatitis, dry skin, erythema, folliculitis, hyperpigmentation, peeling, rash, worsening of psoriasis.
Other: hypercalcemia.

Overdose and treatment
Topically applied calcipotriene can be absorbed in sufficient amounts to produce systemic effects. Serum calcium levels may rise with excessive use.

☑ Special considerations
• Drug is for topical dermatologic use only. It is not intended for ophthalmic, oral, or intravaginal use.
• Clinical studies demonstrate that improvement usually begins after 2 weeks of therapy. Approximately 70% of patients show at least marked improvement after 8 weeks of therapy, but only approximately 10% show complete clearing.
• Know that the safety and effectiveness of topical calcipotriene in dermatoses other than psoriasis have not been established.
• Use of calcipotriene may cause irritation of lesions and surrounding uninvolved skin. If irritation develops, the drug should be discontinued.
• Transient, rapidly reversible elevation of serum calcium has occurred with use of calcipotriene. If the serum calcium level rises outside the normal range, discontinue treatment until normal calcium levels are restored.

Patient education
• Tell patient that drug is for external use only, as directed, and to avoid contact with the face or eyes.
• Instruct patient to wash hands thoroughly after application.
• Advise patient not to use drug for disorders other than that for which it was prescribed.
• Tell patient to report signs of local adverse reactions.

Geriatric use
• Adverse dermatologic effects of topical calcipotriene may be more severe in patients over age 65.

Pediatric use
• Safety and effectiveness in children have not been established.

Breast-feeding

• It is not known if drug is excreted in breast milk. Because many drugs are excreted in human milk, caution should be exercised when calcipotriene ointment is administered to a breast-feeding patient.

calcitonin

Calcimar (salmon), Cibacalcin (human), Miacalcin (salmon)

Pharmacologic classification: thyroid hormone
Therapeutic classification: hypocalcemic
Pregnancy risk category C

How supplied

Available by prescription only
Injection: 200-IU/ml, 2-ml vials (salmon); 0.5 mg/vial (human)
Nasal spray: 200 IU/activation

Indications, route, and dosage

Paget's disease of bone (osteitis deformans)
Adults: Initially, 100 IU calcitonin (salmon) S.C. or I.M. daily or 0.5 mg calcitonin (human) S.C. Maintenance dose is 50 to 100 IU calcitonin (salmon), three times weekly or 0.5 mg calcitonin (human) two or three times weekly or 0.25 mg calcitonin (human) daily.
Hypercalcemia
Adults: 4 IU/kg calcitonin (salmon) I.M. or S.C. q 12 hours; increase by 8 IU/kg q 12 hours.
Postmenopausal osteoporosis
Adults: 100 IU calcitonin (salmon) S.C. or I.M. daily, or 200 IU (one spray) daily in alternating nostril.
◊ ***Osteogenesis imperfecta***
Adults: Give 2 IU/kg calcitonin (salmon) three times weekly.

Pharmacodynamics

Hypocalcemic action: Calcitonin directly inhibits the bone resorption of calcium. This effect is mediated by drug-induced increase of cAMP concentration in bone cells, which alters transport of calcium and phosphate across the plasma membrane of the osteoclast. A secondary effect occurs in the kidneys, where calcitonin directly inhibits tubular resorption of calcium, phosphate, and sodium, thereby increasing their excretion. A clinical effect may not be seen for several months in patients with Paget's disease. Calcitonin salmon and calcitonin human are pharmacologically the same, but calcitonin salmon is more potent and has a longer duration of action.

Pharmacokinetics

• *Absorption:* Drug can be administered parenterally or nasally. Plasma concentrations of 0.1 to 0.4 mg/ml are achieved within 15 minutes of a 200-IU S.C. dose. The maximum effect is seen in 2 to 4 hours; duration of action may be 8 to 24 hours for S.C. or I.M. doses, and ½ to 12 hours for I.V. doses. Peak plasma concentrations appear 31 to 39 minutes after using the nasal form.
• *Distribution:* It is unknown if drug enters the CNS or crosses the placenta.
• *Metabolism:* Rapid metabolism occurs in the kidney, with additional activity in the blood and peripheral tissues. Calcitonin salmon has a longer half-life than calcitonin human, which has a 1-hour half-life.
• *Excretion:* Calcitonin is excreted in urine as inactive metabolites.

Contraindications and precautions

Contraindicated in patients who are hypersensitive to salmon calcitonin. Human calcitonin has no contraindications.

Interactions

None reported.

Effects on diagnostic tests

None reported.

Adverse reactions

CNS: headache, weakness, dizziness, paresthesia.
EENT: eye pain, nasal congestion.
GI: transient *nausea,* unusual taste, diarrhea, anorexia, *vomiting,* epigastric discomfort, abdominal pain.
GU: *increased urinary frequency,* nocturia.
Skin: *facial flushing,* rash, pruritus of ear lobes, *inflammation at injection site.*
Other: hypersensitivity reactions ***(anaphylaxis),*** edema of feet, chills, chest pressure, shortness of breath, tender palms and soles.

Overdose and treatment

Clinical manifestations of overdose include hypocalcemia and hypocalcemic tetany. This usually will occur in patients at higher risk during the first few doses. Parenteral calcium will correct the symptoms and therefore should be readily available.

☑ Special considerations

• Know that S.C. route is the preferred method of administration.
• Before initiating therapy with calcitonin (salmon), a skin test using calcitonin (salmon) should be considered. If patient has allergic reactions to foreign proteins, test for hypersensitivity before therapy. Systemic allergic reactions are possible because hormone is a protein. Epinephrine should be kept readily available.
• Keep parenteral calcium available during the first doses in case of hypocalcemic tetany.
• Periodically monitor serum calcium levels during therapy.
• Observe patient for signs of hypocalcemic tetany during therapy (muscle twitching, tetanic spasms, and convulsions if hypocalcemia is severe).
• Watch for signs of hypercalcemic relapse: bone pain, renal calculi, polyuria, anorexia, nausea, vomiting, thirst, constipation, lethargy, bradycardia, muscle hypotonicity, pathologic fracture, psychosis, and coma. Patients with good initial clinical response to calcitonin who suffer relapse should be evaluated for antibody formation response to the hormone protein.

• Refrigerate solution. Once activated, nasal spray should be stored upright at room temperature.

Patient education

• Instruct patient on self-administration of drug and assist him until proper technique is achieved.

• Tell patient to handle missed doses as follows:

Daily dosing: take as soon as possible; do not double up on doses.

Every other day dosing: take as soon as possible, then restart the alternate days from this dose.

• Stress importance of regular follow-up to assess progress.

• If given for postmenopausal osteoporosis, remind patient to take adequate calcium and vitamin D supplements.

• Instruct patient using the nasal spray to first activate pump.

• Tell patient to call if nasal irritation occurs. Periodic nasal examination should be performed.

Pediatric use

• There are no data to support the use of the nasal spray in pediatric patients.

calcitriol

Calcijex, Rocaltrol

Pharmacologic classification: vitamin D analogue
Therapeutic classification: antihypocalcemic
Pregnancy risk category C

How supplied

Available by prescription only
Capsules: 0.25 mcg, 0.5 mcg
Injection: 1 mcg/ml, 2 mcg/ml

Indications, route, and dosage

Management of hypocalcemia in patients undergoing chronic dialysis

Oral

Adults: Initially, 0.25 mcg P.O. daily. Dosage may be increased by 0.25 mcg daily at 4- to 8-week intervals. Maintenance dose, 0.25 mcg every other day up to 0.5 to 1 mcg daily.

Parenteral

Adults: 0.5 mcg I.V. three times weekly, approximately every other day. Dosage may be increased by 0.25 to 0.5 mcg at 2- to 4-week intervals. Maintenance dose, 0.5 to 3 mcg I.V. three times weekly.

Management of hypoparathyroidism and pseudohypoparathyroidism

Adults and children age 6 and older: Initially, 0.25 mcg P.O. daily in the morning. Dosage may be increased at 2- to 4-week intervals. Maintenance dose, 0.5 to 2 mcg daily.

Children age 1 to 5: (hypoparathyroidism only) 0.25 to 0.75 mcg daily.

◊ ***Psoriasis vulgaris***

Adults: 0.5 mcg/day P.O. for 6 months and topically (0.5 mcg/g petroleum) daily for 8 weeks.

Pharmacodynamics

Antihypocalcemic action: Calcitriol is a vitamin D analogue (1,25 dihydroxycholecalciferol), or activated cholecalciferol. It promotes absorption of calcium from the intestine by forming a calcium-binding protein. It reverses the signs of rickets and osteomalacia in patients who cannot activate or use ergocalciferol or cholecalciferol. In patients with renal failure it reduces bone pain, muscle weakness, and parathyroid serum levels.

Pharmacokinetics

• *Absorption:* Calcitriol is absorbed readily after oral administration.

• *Distribution:* Distributed widely and protein-bound.

• *Metabolism:* Drug is metabolized in the liver and kidney, with a half-life of 3 to 8 hours. No activation step is required.

• *Excretion:* Excreted primarily in the feces.

Contraindications and precautions

Contraindicated in patients with hypercalcemia or vitamin D toxicity. Withhold all preparations containing vitamin D.

Interactions

Antacids, cholestyramine, mineral oil, and *colestipol* may alter calcitriol absorption. *Barbiturates, phenytoin,* and *primidone* may increase metabolism of calcitriol and reduce activity. The increases in calcium may potentiate the effects of *cardiac glycosides. Thiazide diuretics* may result in hypercalcemia. *Corticosteroids* may counteract the effects of vitamin D analogues.

Effects on diagnostic tests

Calcitriol therapy may falsely elevate cholesterol determinations made using the Zlatkis-Zak reaction. It also alters serum alkaline phosphatase concentrations and may alter electrolytes, such as magnesium, phosphate, and calcium in serum and urine.

Adverse reactions

Vitamin D intoxication associated with hypercalcemia:

CNS: headache, somnolence, weakness, irritability, psychosis (rare).
CV: hypertension, ***arrhythmias.***
EENT: conjunctivitis, photophobia, rhinorrhea.
GI: nausea, vomiting, constipation, polydipsia, pancreatitis, metallic taste, dry mouth, anorexia.
GU: polyuria, nocturia.
Skin: pruritus.
Other: bone and muscle pain, weight loss, hyperthermia, nephrocalcinosis, decreased libido.

Overdose and treatment

Clinical manifestation of overdose is hypercalcemia. Treatment requires discontinuation of drug, institution of a low-calcium diet, increased fluid intake, and supportive measures. Calcitonin administration may help reverse hypercalcemia. In severe cases, death has followed CV and renal failure.

☑ Special considerations

- Monitor serum calcium levels several times weekly after initiating therapy.
- There is some evidence that monitoring urine calcium and urine creatinine is very helpful in screening for hypercalciuria. The ratio of urine calcium to urine creatinine should be less than or equal to 0.18. A value above 0.2 suggests hypercalciuria, and the dose should be decreased regardless of serum calcium level. The product of serum calcium times phosphate should not be allowed to exceed 70.
- Protect drug from heat and light.

Patient education

- Instruct patient on the importance of a calcium-rich diet.
- Advise patient to report adverse reactions immediately.
- Tell patient to avoid magnesium-containing antacids and other self-prescribed drugs.

Pediatric use

- Some infants may be hyperreactive to drug.

Breast-feeding

- Very little drug appears in breast milk; however, the effect of vitamin D levels exceeding the RDA in infants is not known. Therefore, large doses should not be administered to breast-feeding women.

calcium polycarbophil

Equalactin, Fiberall, FiberCon, Fiber-Lax, Mitrolan

Pharmacologic classification: hydrophilic
Therapeutic classification: bulk laxative, antidiarrheal
Pregnancy risk category C

How supplied

Available without a prescription
Tablets: 500 mg (FiberCon, Fiber-Lax)
Tablets (chewable): 500 mg (Equalactin, Fiber-Lax, Mitrolan), 1,000 mg (Fiberall)

Indications, route, and dosage

Constipation; acute nonspecific diarrhea associated with irritable bowel syndrome

Adults: 1 g P.O. q.i.d. as required. Maximum dosage, 6 g in 24-hour period.

Children age 6 to 12: 500 mg P.O. one to three times daily as required. Maximum dosage, 3 g in 24-hour period.

Children age 3 to 6: 500 mg P.O. one to two times daily as required. Maximum dosage, 1.5 g in 24-hour period.

Pharmacodynamics

Laxative action: Calcium polycarbophil absorbs water and expands, thereby increasing stool bulk and moisture and promoting normal peristalsis and bowel motility.

Antidiarrheal action: Calcium polycarbophil absorbs intestinal fluid, thereby restoring normal stool consistency and bulk.

Pharmacokinetics

- *Absorption:* None.
- *Distribution:* None.
- *Metabolism:* None.
- *Excretion:* Excreted in feces.

Contraindications and precautions

Contraindicated in patients with GI obstruction because drug may exacerbate this condition.

Interactions

When used concomitantly, calcium polycarbophil may impair *tetracycline* absorption.

Effects on diagnostic tests

None reported.

Adverse reactions

GI: abdominal fullness and increased flatus, intestinal obstruction.
Other: laxative dependence (with long-term or excessive use).

Overdose and treatment

No information available.

☑ Special considerations

- Patient must chew tablets (chewable) before swallowing; administer tablets with 8 oz (240 ml) of fluid. Administer less fluid for antidiarrheal effect.
- When using drug as an antidiarrheal, do not give if patient has high fever.

Patient education

- For chewable tablets: Instruct patient to chew tablets instead of swallowing them whole. If drug is being taken as a laxative, advise patient to drink a full glass (8 oz) of fluid after each tablet; to take less water if he is using drug to treat diarrhea.
- Warn patient not to take more than 12 tablets in 24-hour period (6 tablets for child age 6 to 12; three tablets for child age 3 to 6) and to take for length of time prescribed.
- If patient is taking drug as laxative, advise him to call promptly and discontinue drug if constipation persists after 1 week or if fever, nausea, vomiting, or abdominal pain occurs.
- Instruct patient that dose may be taken every 30 minutes for acute diarrhea, but not to exceed maximum daily dosage.
- Tell patient that if abdominal discomfort or fullness occurs, he may take smaller doses more frequently throughout the day, at regular intervals.

calcium salts

calcium acetate
Phos-Ex, PhosLo

calcium carbonate
Alka-mints, Amitone, Calciday-667, Cal-Plus, Caltrate 600, Chooz, Os-Cal 500, Rolaids, Titralac, Tums, Tums E-X

calcium chloride

calcium citrate
Citracal

calcium glubionate
Neo-Calglucon

calcium gluceptate

calcium gluconate

calcium lactate

calcium phosphate, tribasic
Posture

Pharmacologic classification: calcium supplement
Therapeutic classification: therapeutic agent for electrolyte balance, cardiotonic
Pregnancy risk category C

How supplied
Available by prescription only
calcium chloride
Injection: 10% solution (1 g/10 ml; each ml of solution provides 27.2 mg or 1.36 mEq of calcium) in 10-ml ampules, vials, and syringes
calcium gluceptate
Injection: 1.1 g/5 ml ampules or 50-ml vials for preparation of I.V. admixtures (each ml of solution provides 18 mg or 0.9 mEq of calcium)
calcium gluconate
Injection: 10% solution (1 g/10 ml; each ml of solution provides 9.3 mg or 0.46 mEq of calcium) in 10-ml ampules and vials, or 20-ml vials

Available without a prescription
calcium acetate
Tablets: 250 mg (62.5 mg of calcium), 668 mg (167 mg of calcium), 1,000 mg (250 mg of calcium)
Capsules: 500 mg
calcium carbonate
Tablets: 500 mg, 650 mg, 667 mg, 1.25 g, 1.5 g
Tablets (chewable): 350 mg, 420 mg, 500 mg, 750 mg, 835 mg, 850 mg, 1.25 g
Oral suspension: 1.25 g (500 mg of calcium) per 5 ml
Capsules: 1.25 g (500 mg of calcium), 1.5 g (600 mg of calcium)
Powder: 6.5 g
calcium citrate
Tablets: 950 mg (contains 200 mg of elemental calcium/g)
Tablets (effervescent): 2,376 mg
calcium glubionate
Syrup: 1.8 g/5 ml (contains 115 mg of elemental calcium/g)
calcium gluconate
Tablets: 500 mg, 650 mg, 975 mg, 1 g (contains 90 mg of elemental calcium/g)
calcium lactate
Tablets: 325 mg, 650 mg (contains 130 mg of elemental calcium/g)
calcium phosphate, tribasic
Tablets: 300 mg, 600 mg (contains 400 mg of elemental calcium/g)

Indications, route, and dosage
Emergency treatment of hypocalcemia
calcium chloride
Adults: 500 mg to 1 g I.V. slowly (not to exceed 1 ml/minute).
Children: 0.2 ml/kg I.V. slowly (not to exceed 1 ml/minute).
calcium gluconate
Adults: 7 to 14 mEq I.V. slowly (not to exceed 0.7 to 1.8 mEq/minute).
Children: 1 to 7 mEq I.V. slowly (not to exceed 0.7 to 1.8 mEq/minute).
Repeat above dosage based on clinical laboratory value.
Cardiotonic use
calcium chloride
Adults: 500 mg to 1 g I.V. slowly (not to exceed 1 ml/minute); or 200 to 800 mg intraventricularly as a single dose.
Hyperkalemia
calcium gluconate
Adults: 2.25 to 14 mEq I.V. slowly. Administration must be titrated based on ECG response.
Hypermagnesemia
calcium chloride
Adults: 500 mg I.V. initially, repeated based on clinical response.
calcium gluceptate
Adults: 2 to 5 ml I.M., or 5 to 20 ml I.V.
calcium gluconate
Adults: 4.5 to 9 mEq I.V. slowly.
During exchange transfusions
Adults: 1.35 mEq I.V. concurrently with each 100-ml citrated blood exchange.
Neonates: 0.45 mEq I.V. after every 100 ml of citrated blood exchange.
Hypocalcemia
calcium acetate
Adults: 2 to 4 tablets P.O. with meals.
calcium gluconate
Adults: for hypocalcemic tetany, 4.5 to 16 mEq I.V. until therapeutic response is obtained.
Children: for hypocalcemic tetany, 0.5 to 0.7 mEq/kg I.V. t.i.d. or q.i.d. or until tetany is controlled.
calcium lactate
Adults: 325 mg to 1.3 g P.O. t.i.d. with meals.
Osteoporosis prevention
Adults: 1 to 1.5 g P.O. daily of elemental calcium.
Hyperphosphatemia in end-stage renal failure
calcium acetate
Adults: 2 to 4 tablets with each meal.

Pharmacodynamics

Calcium replacement: Calcium is essential for maintaining the functional integrity of the nervous, muscular, and skeletal systems, and for cell membrane and capillary permeability. Calcium salts are used as a source of calcium cation to treat or prevent calcium depletion in patients in whom dietary measures are inadequate. Conditions associated with hypocalcemia are chronic diarrhea, vitamin D deficiency, steatorrhea, sprue, pregnancy and lactation, menopause, pancreatitis, renal failure, alkalosis, hyperphosphatemia, and hypoparathyroidism.

Pharmacokinetics

- *Absorption:* I.M. and I.V. calcium salts are absorbed directly into the bloodstream. I.V. injection gives an immediate blood level, which will decrease to previous levels in about 30 to 120 minutes. Oral dose is absorbed actively in the duodenum and proximal jejunum and, to a lesser extent, in the distal part of the small intestine. Calcium is absorbed only in the ionized form. Pregnancy and reduction of calcium intake may increase the efficiency of absorption. Vitamin D in its active form is required for calcium absorption.
- *Distribution:* Calcium enters the extracellular fluid and then is incorporated rapidly into skeletal tissue. Bone contains 99% of the total calcium; 1% is distributed equally between the intracellular and extracellular fluids. CSF concentrations are about 50% of serum calcium concentrations.
- *Metabolism:* None significant.
- *Excretion:* Calcium is excreted mainly in the feces as unabsorbed calcium that was secreted via bile and pancreatic juice into the lumen of the GI tract. Most calcium entering the kidney is reabsorbed in the loop of Henle and the proximal and distal convoluted tubules. Only small amounts of calcium are excreted in the urine.

Contraindications and precautions

Contraindicated in patients with ventricular fibrillation, hypercalcemia, hypophosphatemia, or renal calculi. Use cautiously in patients with sarcoidosis, renal or cardiac disease, cor pulmonale, respiratory acidosis, or respiratory failure and in digitalized patients.

Interactions

Concomitant use of calcium salts with *cardiac glycosides* increases *digitalis* toxicity; administer calcium very cautiously, if at all, to digitalized patients.

Calcium may antagonize the therapeutic effects of *calcium channel blocker drugs* (*verapamil*).

Calcium should not be physically mixed with *phosphates, carbonates, sulfates,* or *tartrates*, especially at high concentrations. Calcium competes with *magnesium* and may compete for absorption, thus decreasing the amount of bioavailable *magnesium.* Concurrent administration of oral calcium decreases the therapeutic effect of *tetracycline* as a result of chelation. Concurrent administration with *quinolones* (such as *norfloxacin*), *atenolol*, or *iron salts* may decrease levels of these drugs.

Effects on diagnostic tests

I.V. calcium may produce transient elevation of plasma 11-hydroxycorticosteroid concentrations (Glen-Nelson technique) and false-negative values for serum and urine magnesium as measured by the Titan yellow method.

Adverse reactions

CNS: tingling sensations, sense of oppression or heat waves, headache, irritability, weakness (with I.V. use); syncope (with rapid I.V. injection).
CV: mild fall in blood pressure; vasodilation, bradycardia, ***arrhythmias, cardiac arrest*** (with rapid I.V. injection).
GI: irritation, hemorrhage, *constipation* (with oral use); chalky taste, rebound hyperacidity, *nausea* (with I.V. use); hemorrhage, nausea, vomiting, thirst, abdominal pain (with oral calcium chloride).
GU: hypercalcemia, polyuria, renal calculi.
Skin: local reactions including burning, necrosis, tissue sloughing, cellulitis, soft tissue calcification (with I.M. use).
Other: pain and irritation (with S.C. injection); *vein irritation* (with I.V. use).

Overdose and treatment

Acute hypercalcemia syndrome is characterized by a markedly elevated plasma calcium level, lethargy, weakness, nausea and vomiting, and coma, and may lead to sudden death.

In case of overdose, calcium should be discontinued immediately. After oral ingestion of calcium overdose, treatment includes removal by emesis or gastric lavage followed by supportive therapy, as needed.

☑ Special considerations

- Monitor ECG when giving calcium I.V. Such injections should be given slowly at a rate dependent on salt form used. Stop injection if patient complains of discomfort.
- Calcium chloride should be given I.V. only.
- I.V. route is recommended in children, but not by scalp vein because calcium salts can cause tissue necrosis.
- I.V. calcium should be administered slowly through a small-bore needle into a large vein to avoid extravasation and necrosis.
- After I.V. injection, patient should be recumbent for 15 minutes to prevent orthostasis.
- If perivascular infiltration occurs, discontinue I.V. immediately. Venospasm may be reduced by administering 1% procaine hydrochloride and hyaluronidase to the affected area.
- Use I.M. route only in emergencies when no I.V. route is available. Give I.M. injections in the gluteal region in adults, lateral thigh in infants.
- Monitor serum calcium levels frequently, especially in patients with renal impairment.
- Hypercalcemia may result when large doses are given to patients with chronic renal failure.
- Severe necrosis and sloughing of tissue may occur after extravasation. Calcium gluconate is less irritating to veins and tissue than calcium chloride.
- Assess Chvostek's and Trousseau's signs periodically to check for tetany.

• Crash carts usually contain both gluconate and chloride. Be sure to specify form to be administered.
• If GI upset occurs with oral calcium, give 2 to 3 hours after meals.
• Oxalic acid (found in rhubarb and spinach), phytic acid (in bran and whole-grain cereals), and phosphorus (in milk and dairy products) may interfere with absorption of calcium.
• With oral product, patient may need laxatives or stool softeners to manage constipation.
• Monitor for symptoms of hypercalcemia (nausea, vomiting, headache, mental confusion, anorexia), and report them immediately. Calcium absorption of an oral dose is decreased in patients with certain disease states such as achlorhydria, renal osteodystrophy, steatorrhea, or uremia.

Patient education
• Tell patient not to exceed the manufacturer's recommended dosage of calcium.
• Warn patient not to use bone meal or dolomite as a source of calcium; they may contain lead.
• Advise patient to avoid tobacco and to limit intake of alcohol and caffeine-containing beverages.

Geriatric use
• Calcium absorption (after oral administration) may be decreased in elderly patients.

Pediatric use
• Calcium should be administered cautiously to children by the I.V. route (usually not administered I.M.).

Breast-feeding
• Calcium has been shown to pass into the breast milk, but not in quantities large enough to affect the breast-feeding infant.

cantharidin
Cantharone, Verr-Canth

Pharmacologic classification: cantharide derivative
Therapeutic classification: keratolytic
Pregnancy risk category NR

How supplied
Available by prescription only
Liquid: 0.7% (to be applied by primary health care provider only)

Indications, route, and dosage
Removal of ordinary and periungual warts
Adults and children: No cutting or prior treatment required. Apply directly to lesion and cover completely. Allow to dry, then cover with nonporous adhesive tape. Remove tape in 24 hours (or less if it causes extreme pain) and replace with loose bandage. Reapply, if necessary, in 1 to 2 weeks.
Removal of molluscum contagiosum
Adults and children: Coat each lesion. Repeat in 1 week on new or remaining lesions, this time covering with occlusive tape. Remove tape in 4 to 6 hours.
Removal of plantar warts
Adults and children: Pare away keratin. Apply drug to wart and 1 to 3 mm around the wart. Allow to dry; then cover with nonporous tape. Debride 1 to 2 weeks after treatment. Repeat three times, if necessary, on large lesions.

Pharmacodynamics
Keratolytic action: Cantharidin causes exfoliation of benign epithelial growths as a consequence of acantholytic action. This action does not go beyond the epidermal cells; the basal layer remains intact.

Pharmacokinetics
• *Absorption:* Limited with use.
• *Distribution:* None.
• *Metabolism:* None.
• *Excretion:* None.

Contraindications and precautions
Cantharidin is contraindicated in patients with hypersensitivity to drug. Avoid use near eyes or mucous membranes. Do not use on sensitive areas, such as the face or genitalia, or on moles, birthmarks, or hair-growing warts. Drug should be used with caution in patients with diabetes or impaired peripheral circulation.

Interactions
None reported.

Effects on diagnostic tests
None reported.

Adverse reactions
Skin: irritation, burning, tingling, tenderness at site; may cause annular warts.
Note: Discontinue drug if sensitization develops.

Overdose and treatment
Cantharidin is a strong vesicant. If spillage occurs, follow instructions given under "Special considerations."

☑ Special considerations
• Apply directly to lesion and cover with nonporous tape. Avoid applying to normal skin tissue. Use only on affected area. Be sure to wash hands well after using drug. If spilled on skin, wipe off at once with acetone, alcohol, or tape remover and wash with soap and water.
• Use of mild antibacterial is recommended until tissue re-epithelializes.

Patient education
• Advise patient that drug may cause tingling, itching, or burning a few hours after application and may even cause blistering. The site of application may be extremely tender for 1 week after application.

Breast-feeding
• Safety has not been established; therefore, use of drug in breast-feeding women is not recommended.

capsaicin

Dolorac, Zostrix, Zostrix-HP

Pharmacologic classification: naturally occurring chemical derived from plants of the Solanaceae family
Therapeutic classification: topical analgesic
Pregnancy risk category NR

How supplied

Available without a prescription
Cream: 0.025% (Zostrix), 0.075% (Zostrix-HP), 0.25% (Dolorac)

Indications, route, and dosage

Temporary pain relief from rheumatoid arthritis, osteoarthritis, and certain neuralgias, such as pain associated with shingles (herpes zoster) or diabetic neuropathy
Zostrix
Adults and children over age 2: Apply to affected areas t.i.d. or q.i.d.
Dolorac
Adults and children over age 12: Apply thin film to affected areas b.i.d.

Pharmacodynamics

Analgesic action: Although the precise mechanism of action of capsaicin is not fully understood, current evidence suggests that drug renders skin and joints insensitive to pain by depleting and preventing reaccumulation of substance P in peripheral sensory neurons. Substance P is thought to be the principal chemomediator of pain impulses from the periphery to the CNS. In addition, substance P is released into joint tissues and activates inflammatory mediators involved with the pathogenesis of rheumatoid arthritis.

Pharmacokinetics

- *Absorption:* No information available.
- *Distribution:* No information available.
- *Metabolism:* No information available.
- *Excretion:* No information available.

Contraindications and precautions

Contraindicated in patients hypersensitive to drug.

Interactions

None reported.

Effects on diagnostic tests

None reported.

Adverse reactions

Respiratory: cough, irritation.
Skin: redness, *stinging or burning on application.*

Overdose and treatment

No information available.

☑ Special considerations

- Transient burning or stinging with application is usually evident at initial therapy but will disappear in several days.
- Application schedules of less than three or four times daily may not provide optimum pain relief, and the burning sensation may persist.
- Capsaicin is for external use only. Avoid contact with eyes and broken or irritated skin.
- Do not bandage tightly.

Patient education

- Instruct patient how to apply cream, stressing importance of avoiding the eyes and broken or irritated skin.
- Instruct patient to wash hands after applying cream, avoiding areas where drug was applied.
- Warn patient that transient burning or stinging with application may occur but will disappear with continued use after several days.
- Tell patient not to bandage areas tightly.
- Advise patient to discontinue drug and to call if condition worsens or does not improve after 28 days.

captopril

Capoten

Pharmacologic classification: ACE inhibitor
Therapeutic classification: antihypertensive, adjunctive treatment of heart failure
Pregnancy risk category C (D second and third trimesters)

How supplied

Available by prescription only
Tablets: 12.5 mg, 25 mg, 50 mg, 100 mg

Indications, route, and dosage

Mild to severe hypertension; ◊ idiopathic edema; ◊ Raynaud's phenomenon
Adults: Initially, 25 mg P.O. b.i.d. or t.i.d.; if necessary, dosage may be increased to 50 mg b.i.d. or t.i.d. after 1 to 2 weeks; if control is still inadequate after 1 to 2 weeks more, a diuretic may be added. Dosage may be raised to a maximum of 150 mg t.i.d. (450 mg/day) while continuing the diuretic. Daily dose may be given b.i.d.
Heart failure
Adults: Initially, 25 mg P.O. t.i.d.; may be increased to 50 mg t.i.d., with maximum of 450 mg/day. In patients taking diuretics, initial dosage is 6.25 to 12.5 mg t.i.d.
Prevention of diabetic nephropathy
Adults: 25 mg P.O. t.i.d.
Left ventricular dysfunction after an MI
Adults: Give 6.25 mg P.O. as a single dose 3 days after an MI; then 12.5 mg t.i.d. increasing dose to 25 mg t.i.d. Target dose is 50 mg t.i.d.
✦ ***Dosage adjustment.*** In patients with renal failure and the elderly, use lower initial daily dosages and smaller increments for titration.

Pharmacodynamics

Antihypertensive action: Captopril inhibits ACE, preventing conversion of angiotensin I to angiotensin II, a potent vasoconstrictor. Reduced formation of angiotensin II decreases peripheral arterial resistance, which results in decreased aldosterone secretion, thus reducing sodium and water retention and lowering blood pressure.

Cardiac load-reducing action: Captopril decreases systemic vascular resistance (afterload) and pulmonary capillary wedge pressure (preload), thus increasing cardiac output in patients with heart failure.

Pharmacokinetics

- *Absorption:* 60% to 75% of an oral dose is absorbed through the GI tract; food may reduce absorption by up to 40%. Antihypertensive effect begins in 15 minutes; peak blood levels occur at 1 hour. Maximum therapeutic effect may require several weeks.
- *Distribution:* Distributed into most body tissues except CNS; drug is approximately 25% to 30% protein-bound.
- *Metabolism:* About 50% of drug is metabolized in the liver.
- *Excretion:* Captopril and its metabolites are excreted primarily in urine; small amounts are excreted in feces. Duration of effect is usually 2 to 6 hours; this increases with higher doses. Elimination half-life is less than 3 hours. Duration of action may be increased in patients with renal dysfunction.

Contraindications and precautions

Contraindicated in patients with hypersensitivity to drug or other ACE inhibitors. Use cautiously in patients with impaired renal function, renal artery stenosis, or serious autoimmune diseases (especially lupus erythematosus) and in those taking drugs that affect WBC counts or immune response.

Interactions

Indomethacin, *aspirin*, and *other NSAIDs* may decrease captopril's antihypertensive effect; *antacids* also decrease captopril's effects and should be given at different dose intervals.

Captopril may increase antihypertensive effects of *diuretics* or *other antihypertensive drugs.*

Patients with impaired renal function or heart failure and patients concomitantly receiving drugs that can increase serum potassium levels for example, *potassium-sparing diuretics, potassium supplements*, or *salt substitutes,* may develop hyperkalemia during captopril therapy.

Captopril may increase *lithium* levels, which may lead to *lithium* toxicity. Use together with caution and monitor *lithium* drug levels.

Probenecid may increase plasma levels of captopril and decrease its clearance. Concomitant use with *phenothiazine* may lead to increased pharmacologic effects. Captopril may also increase serum *digoxin* levels.

Effects on diagnostic tests

Captopril may cause false-positive results for urinary acetone; it also may cause hyperkalemia and may transiently elevate liver enzyme levels.

Adverse reactions

CNS: dizziness, fainting, headache, malaise, fatigue.
CV: *tachycardia, hypotension,* angina pectoris.
GI: anorexia, *dysgeusia,* nausea, vomiting, abdominal pain, constipation, dry mouth.
Hematologic: ***leukopenia, agranulocytosis, pancytopenia,*** anemia, ***thrombocytopenia.***
Hepatic: transient increase in hepatic enzymes.
Respiratory: *dry, persistent, tickling, nonproductive cough,* dyspnea.
Skin: *urticarial rash, maculopapular rash,* pruritus, alopecia.
Other: fever, ***angioedema of face and extremities,*** hyperkalemia.

Overdose and treatment

Overdose is manifested primarily by severe hypotension. After acute ingestion, empty stomach by induced emesis or gastric lavage. Follow with activated charcoal to reduce absorption. Subsequent treatment is usually symptomatic and supportive. In severe cases, hemodialysis may be considered.

☑ Special considerations

- Diuretic therapy is usually discontinued 2 to 3 days before beginning ACE inhibitor therapy, to reduce risk of hypotension; if drug does not adequately control blood pressure, diuretics may be reinstated.
- Perform WBC and differential counts before treatment, every 2 weeks for 3 months, and periodically thereafter. Monitor serum potassium levels because potassium retention has been noted.
- Lower drug dosage or reduced dosing frequency is necessary in patients with impaired renal function. Titrate patient to effective levels over a 1- to 2-week interval, then reduce dosage to lowest effective level.
- Several weeks of therapy may be required before the beneficial effects of captopril are seen.
- Proteinuria and nephrotic syndrome may occur in patients.
- Because ACE inhibitors can cause fetal harm or death, drug use should be discontinued as soon as pregnancy is detected.

Patient education

- Tell patient to report feelings of light-headedness, especially in first few days, so dosage can be adjusted; signs of infection, such as sore throat or fever, because drug may decrease WBC count; facial swelling or difficulty breathing, because drug may cause angioedema; and loss of taste, which may necessitate discontinuing drug.
- Instruct patient to take captopril 1 hour before meals to prevent decreased absorption.
- Advise patient to avoid sudden position changes to minimize orthostatic hypotension.

• Warn patient to seek medical approval before taking OTC cold preparations and to call if a persistent, dry cough occurs.
• Instruct patient to call immediately if pregnancy occurs.

Geriatric use
• Elderly patients may need lower doses because of impaired drug clearance. They also may be more sensitive to captopril's hypotensive effects.

Pediatric use
• Safety and efficacy in children have not been established; use only if potential benefit outweighs risk.

Breast-feeding
• Captopril is distributed into breast milk, but its effect on breast-feeding infants is unknown; use drug with caution in breast-feeding women.

carbachol
Carboptic, Isopto Carbachol, Miostat

Pharmacologic classification: cholinergic agonist
Therapeutic classification: miotic
Pregnancy risk category C

How supplied
Available by prescription only
Intraocular injection: 0.01%
Ophthalmic solution: 0.75%, 1.5%, 2.25%, 3%

Indications, route, and dosage
Ocular surgery (to produce pupillary miosis)
Adults: Instill 0.5 ml of 0.01% (intraocular form) gently into the anterior chamber for production of satisfactory miosis. It may be instilled before or after securing sutures.
Open-angle or narrow-angle glaucoma
Adults: Instill 2 drops of 0.75% to 3% solution up to t.i.d.

Pharmacodynamics
Miotic action: Carbachol's cholinergic activity causes contraction of the sphincter muscles of the iris, producing miosis, and contraction of the ciliary muscle, resulting in accommodation. It also acts to deepen the anterior chamber and dilates conjunctival vessels of the outflow tract.

Pharmacokinetics
• *Absorption:* Action begins within 10 to 20 minutes and peaks in less than 4 hours.
• *Distribution:* Unknown.
• *Metabolism:* Unknown.
• *Excretion:* Duration of effect is usually about 8 hours.

Contraindications and precautions
Contraindicated in patients with hypersensitivity to drug or in those in whom cholinergic effects, such as constriction, are undesirable (for example, acute iritis, some forms of secondary glaucoma, pupillary block glaucoma, or acute inflammatory disease of the anterior chamber of the eye).

Use cautiously in patients with acute heart failure, bronchial asthma, peptic ulcer, hyperthyroidism, GI spasm, Parkinson's disease, and urinary tract obstruction.

Interactions
When used concomitantly, *cyclopentolate* or the *ophthalmic belladonna alkaloids* (*atropine, homatropine*) may interfere with the antiglaucoma actions of carbachol.

Effects on diagnostic tests
None reported.

Adverse reactions
CNS: headache, syncope.
CV: ***arrhythmias,*** hypotension.
EENT: spasm of eye accommodation, conjunctival vasodilation, eye and brow pain, transient stinging and burning, corneal clouding, bullous keratopathy, salivation.
GI: abdominal cramps, diarrhea.
GU: urinary urgency.
Respiratory: asthma.
Other: diaphoresis, flushing.

Overdose and treatment
Clinical manifestations of overdose include miosis, flushing, vomiting, bradycardia, bronchospasm, increased bronchial secretion, sweating, tearing, involuntary urination, hypotension, and seizures.

With accidental oral ingestion, vomiting is usually spontaneous; if not, induce emesis and follow with activated charcoal or a cathartic.

Treat dermal exposure by washing the area twice with water. Treat CV or blood pressure responses with epinephrine. Atropine has been suggested as a direct antagonist for toxicity.

☑ Special considerations
• Drug is especially useful in glaucoma patients resistant or allergic to pilocarpine hydrochloride or nitrate.
• Premixed drugs should be used for single-dose intraocular use only.
• Discard unused portions of injectable drug.

Patient education
• Tell patient with glaucoma that long-term use may be necessary. Stress compliance, and explain importance of medical supervision for tonometric readings before and during therapy.
• Instruct patient to apply finger pressure on the lacrimal sac 1 to 2 minutes after topical instillation of the drug.
• Reassure patient that blurred vision usually diminishes with continued use.
• Teach patient how to instill eyedrops correctly and warn him not to touch eye or surrounding area with dropper.
• Warn patient not to drive for 1 or 2 hours after administration until effect on vision is determined.

carbamazepine

Atretol, Carbatrol, Epitol, Tegretol

Pharmacologic classification: iminostilbene derivative; chemically related to tricyclic antidepressants
Therapeutic classification: anticonvulsant, analgesic
Pregnancy risk category D

How supplied

Available by prescription only
Tablets: 200 mg
Tablets (chewable): 100 mg
Capsules (extended-release): 200 mg, 300 mg
Oral suspension: 100 mg/5 ml

Indications, route, and dosage

Generalized tonic-clonic, complex-partial, mixed seizure patterns
Adults and children over age 12: 200 mg P.O. b.i.d. on day 1. May increase by 200 mg/day P.O. at weekly intervals, in divided doses at 6- to 8-hour intervals. Adjust to minimum effective level when control is achieved; do not exceed 1,000 mg/day in children age 12 to 15, or 1,200 mg/day in those over age 15. In rare instances, dosages up to 1,600 mg/day have been used in adults.

For extended-release capsules, initial dose 200 mg P.O. b.i.d. Increase at weekly intervals by up to 200 mg/day until optimal response obtained. Dosage should not exceed 1,000 mg/day in children age 12 to 15 and 1,200 mg/day in patients over 15. Some adult doses may be up to 1,600 mg/day. Maintenance dose usually 800 to 1,200 mg/day.
Children age 6 to 12: Initially, 100 mg P.O. b.i.d. Increase at weekly intervals by adding 100 mg P.O. daily, first using a t.i.d. schedule and then q.i.d. if necessary. Adjust dosage based on patient response. Generally, dose should not exceed 1,000 mg/day. Children taking total daily dosage of immediate-release form of 400 mg or more may be converted to same total daily dosage of extended-release capsules using a b.i.d. regimen.
Oral loading dose for rapid seizure control
Adults and children over age 12: 8 mg/kg of oral suspension.
◊ ***Bipolar affective disorder, intermittent explosive disorder***
Adults: Initially, 200 mg P.O. b.i.d.; increase p.r.n. q 3 to 4 days. Maintenance dosage may range from 600 to 1,600 mg/day.
Trigeminal neuralgia
Adults: 100 mg P.O. b.i.d. with meals on day 1. Increase by 100 mg q 12 hours until pain is relieved. Do not exceed 1.2 g daily. Maintenance dose is 200 to 1,200 mg P.O. daily. For extended-release capsules, 200 mg P.O. day 1. Daily dose may be increased by up to 200 mg/day q 12 hours p.r.n. to achieve freedom from pain. Maintenance dose usually 400 to 800 mg/day.
◊ ***Chorea***
Children: 15 to 25 mg/kg/day.
◊ ***Restless leg syndrome***
Adults: 100 to 300 mg h.s.

Pharmacodynamics

Anticonvulsant action: Carbamazepine is chemically unrelated to other anticonvulsants and its mechanism of action is unknown. The anticonvulsant activity appears principally to involve limitations of seizure propagation by reduction of posttetanic potentiation (PTP) of synaptic transmissions.

Analgesic action: In trigeminal neuralgia, carbamazepine is a specific analgesic through its reduction of synaptic neurotransmission.

Pharmacokinetics

- *Absorption:* Carbamazepine is absorbed slowly from the GI tract; peak plasma concentrations occur at 1.5 hours (suspension), 4 to 6 hours (tablets), and 6 hours (extended-release).
- *Distribution:* Drug is distributed widely throughout body; it crosses the placenta and accumulates in fetal tissue. Approximately 75% is protein-bound. Therapeutic serum levels in adults are 4 to 12 mcg/ml; nystagmus can occur above 4 mcg/ml and ataxia, dizziness, and anorexia at or above 10 mcg/ml. Serum levels may be misleading because an unmeasured active metabolite also can cause toxicity. Carbamazepine levels in breast milk approach 60% of serum levels. There is poor correlation between plasma concentrations and dose in children.
- *Metabolism:* Metabolized by the liver to an active metabolite. It may also induce its own metabolism; over time, higher doses are needed to maintain plasma levels. Half-life is initially 25 to 65 hours and 12 to 17 hours with multiple dosing.
- *Excretion:* Excreted in urine (70%) and feces (30%).

Contraindications and precautions

Contraindicated in patients with history of previous bone marrow suppression or hypersensitivity to drug or tricyclic antidepressants and in patients who have taken an MAO inhibitor within 14 days of therapy. Use cautiously in patients with mixed-type seizure disorders.

Interactions

Concomitant use of carbamazepine with *MAO inhibitors* may cause hypertensive crisis; use with *calcium channel blockers* (*verapamil* and possibly *diltiazem*) may increase serum levels of carbamazepine significantly (therefore, carbamazepine dosage should be decreased by 40% to 50% when given with *verapamil*); concomitant use with *clarithromycin, valproic acid, erythromycin, cimetidine, isoniazid,* or *propoxyphene* also may increase serum carbamazepine levels.

Fluoxetine or *fluvoxamine* may increase carbamazepine levels. Concomitant use with *felbamate* may result in lower serum levels of either agent.

Concomitant use with *phenobarbital, phenytoin,* or *primidone* lowers serum carbamazepine levels. When used with *warfarin, phenytoin, haloperidol, ethosuximide,* or *valproic acid,* carbamazepine may increase the metabolism of these drugs; it may decrease the effectiveness of *theophylline* and *oral contraceptives.*

Effects on diagnostic tests

Carbamazepine may elevate liver enzyme levels; it also may decrease values of thyroid function tests.

Adverse reactions

CNS: *dizziness, vertigo, drowsiness,* fatigue, *ataxia,* ***worsening of seizures*** (usually in patients with mixed-type seizure disorders, including atypical absence seizures), confusion, headache, syncope.
CV: ***heart failure,*** hypertension, hypotension, aggravation of coronary artery disease, ***arrhythmias,*** AV block.
EENT: conjunctivitis, dry mouth and pharynx, blurred vision, diplopia, nystagmus.
GI: *nausea, vomiting,* abdominal pain, diarrhea, anorexia, stomatitis, glossitis.
GU: urinary frequency, urine retention, impotence, albuminuria, glycosuria, elevated BUN.
Hematologic: ***aplastic anemia, agranulocytosis,*** eosinophilia, leukocytosis, ***thrombocytopenia.***
Hepatic: abnormal liver function test results, ***hepatitis.***
Respiratory: pulmonary hypersensitivity.
Skin: rash, urticaria, erythema multiforme, ***Stevens-Johnson syndrome.***
Other: excessive diaphoresis, fever, chills, SIADH.

Overdose and treatment

Symptoms of overdose may include irregular breathing, respiratory depression, tachycardia, blood pressure changes, shock, arrhythmias, impaired consciousness (ranging to deep coma), seizures, restlessness, drowsiness, psychomotor disturbances, nausea, vomiting, anuria, or oliguria.

Treat overdose with repeated gastric lavage, especially if patient ingested alcohol concurrently. Oral charcoal and laxatives may hasten excretion. Carefully monitor vital signs, ECG, and fluid and electrolyte balance. Diazepam may control seizures but can exacerbate respiratory depression.

☑ Special considerations

- Adjust drug dosage based on individual response.
- Drug is structurally similar to tricyclic antidepressants; some risk of activating latent psychosis, confusion, or agitation in elderly patients exists.
- Hematologic toxicity is rare but serious. Routinely monitor hematologic and liver functions.
- Chewable tablets are available for children.
- Unlabeled uses of carbamazepine include hypophyseal diabetes insipidus, certain psychiatric disorders, and management of alcohol withdrawal.
- For administering via a nasogastric tube, mix with an equal volume of diluent (D_5W or 0.9% NaCl solution) and administer; then flush with 100 ml of diluent.

Patient education

- Remind patient to store drug in a cool, dry place, and not in the medicine cabinet. Reduced bioavailability has been reported with use of improperly stored tablets.
- Tell patient that drug may cause GI distress. Patient should take drug with food at equally spaced intervals.
- Warn patient not to stop drug abruptly.
- Encourage patient to promptly report unusual bleeding, bruising, jaundice, dark urine, pale stools, abdominal pain, impotence, fever, chills, sore throat, mouth ulcers, edema, or disturbances in mood, alertness, or coordination.
- Emphasize importance of follow-up laboratory tests and continued medical supervision. Periodic eye examinations are recommended.
- Warn patient that drug may cause drowsiness, dizziness, and blurred vision. Patient should avoid hazardous activities that require alertness, especially during first week of therapy and when dosage is increased.
- Remind patient to shake suspension well before using.
- Tell patient, if necessary, that the Carbatrol capsule can be opened and its contents sprinkled over food (for example, a teaspoon of applesauce), but the capsule or its contents should never be crushed or chewed.

Geriatric use

- Drug may activate latent psychosis, confusion, or agitation in elderly patients; use with caution.

Pediatric use

- Safety and efficacy have not been established for children under age 6.

Breast-feeding

- Significant amounts of drug appear in breast milk; alternative feeding method is recommended during therapy.

carbamide peroxide

Auro Ear Drops, Debrox, Gly-Oxide Liquid, Murine Ear, Orajel, Orajel Perioseptic, Proxigel

Pharmacologic classification: urea hydrogen peroxide
Therapeutic classification: ceruminolytic, topical antiseptic
Pregnancy risk category C

How supplied

Available without a prescription
Otic solution: 6.5% carbamide in glycerin or glycerin and propylene glycol
Oral solution: 10% carbamide with glycerin and propylene glycol; 15% with anhydrous glycerin, methylparaben, and propylene glycol
Oral gel: 10% carbamide in water-free gel base

Indications, route, and dosage

Impacted cerumen
Adults and children age 12 and older: 5 to 10 drops otic solution into ear canal b.i.d. for 3 to 4 days.
Inflammation or irritation of lips, mouth, gums
Adults and children over age 3: Apply several drops of undiluted oral solution to affected area or place 10 drops on tongue (mix with saliva, swish for several minutes and expectorate after 1 to 3 minutes) after meals and h.s.

Children: Apply undiluted gel to affected area (massage into area with finger or swab) q.i.d.

Pharmacodynamics

Ceruminolytic action: Emulsifies and disperses accumulated cerumen.

Antiseptic action: Releases oxygen upon contact with oral mucosa, which results in a cleansing and mild anti-inflammatory action.

Pharmacokinetics

- *Absorption:* No information available.
- *Distribution:* No information available.
- *Metabolism:* No information available.
- *Excretion:* No information available.

Contraindications and precautions

Contraindicated in patients with a perforated eardrum.

Interactions

None reported.

Effects on diagnostic tests

None reported.

Adverse reactions

GI: oral irritation or inflammation.

Overdose and treatment

Clinical manifestations of overdose include mild irritation to mucosal tissue or, if swallowed, irritation, inflammation, and burns in the mouth, throat, esophagus, or stomach. Gastric distention may result from liberation of oxygen. Accidental ocular exposure causes immediate pain and irritation, but severe injury is rare. Irrigate eyes with large amounts of warm water for at least 15 minutes. Accidental dermal exposure bleaches the exposed area. Wash exposed skin twice with soap and water. Treat oral exposure by immediate dilution with water. Spontaneous vomiting may occur.

☑ Special considerations

- Do not use to treat swimmer's ear or itching of the ear canal. Also, do not use if patient has a perforated eardrum.
- Irrigation of ear may be necessary to aid removal of cerumen.
- Tip of dropper should not touch ear or ear canal when using otic preparation.
- Remove cerumen remaining after instillation by using a soft rubber-bulb otic syringe to gently irrigate the ear canal with warm water.

Patient education

- Teach patient correct way to use product.
- Tell patient to call if inflammation or irritation persists.
- Warn patient not to use otic preparation for more than 4 consecutive days and to avoid contact with eyes.
- Instruct patient to keep otic solution in ear for at least 15 minutes by tilting head sideways or putting cotton in ear.
- Tell patient not to rinse mouth or drink for 5 minutes after use.

Pediatric use

- Oral preparations should not be self-administered by children under age 3; otic preparations should not be self-administered by children under 12.

carbenicillin indanyl sodium

Geocillin

Pharmacologic classification: extended-spectrum penicillin, alpha-carboxypenicillin
Therapeutic classification: antibiotic
Pregnancy risk category B

How supplied

Available by prescription only
Tablets: 382 mg

Indications, route, and dosage

Urinary tract infection and prostatitis caused by susceptible organisms

Adults: 382 to 764 mg P.O. q.i.d.

Note: Use drug only in patients whose creatinine clearance is 10 ml/minute or higher to ensure adequate urinary concentrations.

Pharmacodynamics

Antibiotic action: Drug is bactericidal; it adheres to bacterial penicillin-binding proteins, thus inhibiting bacterial cell-wall synthesis. Extended-spectrum penicillins are more resistant to inactivation by certain beta-lactamases, especially those produced by gram-negative organisms, but are still liable to inactivation by certain others.

Drug has an activity spectrum similar to that of carbenicillin disodium, including many gram-negative aerobic and anaerobic bacilli; some gram-positive aerobic and anaerobic bacilli; and many gram-positive and gram-negative aerobic cocci.

Pharmacokinetics

- *Absorption:* Drug is stable in gastric acid, but absorbed incompletely (30% to 40%) from GI tract. Peak plasma concentrations occur at 30 minutes after oral dose; indanyl salt is completely hydrolyzed to carbenicillin in plasma within 90 minutes.
- *Distribution:* Distributed widely after oral administration, but concentrations are insufficient to treat systemic infections. Carbenicillin crosses the placenta and is 30% to 60% protein-bound.
- *Metabolism:* Carbenicillin indanyl sodium is hydrolyzed rapidly in plasma to carbenicillin; carbenicillin is metabolized partially.
- *Excretion:* Drug and its metabolites are excreted primarily (79% to 99%) in urine by renal tubular secretion and glomerular filtration; some drug is excreted in breast milk. Elimination half-life in adults is about 1 hour. In patients with extensive renal impairment, half-life is extended to 9½ to 23 hours; urine concentrations in renal parenchyma and urine in patients with such impairment are insufficient for treating urinary tract infections.

Contraindications and precautions

Contraindicated in patients with hypersensitivity to drug or other penicillins.

Interactions

Concomitant use with *aminoglycoside antibiotics* results in synergistic bactericidal effects against *Pseudomonas aeruginosa, Escherichia coli, Klebsiella, Citrobacter, Enterobacter, Serratia,* and *Proteus mirabilis.* Concomitant use of carbenicillin indanyl sodium (and other extended-spectrum penicillins) with *clavulanic acid* produces synergistic bactericidal effects against certain beta-lactamase–producing bacteria.

Probenecid is used with some penicillins to achieve higher serum concentrations of drug, an undesired effect in urinary tract infection.

Large doses of penicillins may interfere with renal tubular secretion of *methotrexate*, delaying elimination and elevating serum concentration of methotrexate.

Effects on diagnostic tests

Drug alters results of urine glucose tests that use cupric sulfate (Benedict's reagent or Clinitest). Make urine glucose determinations with glucose oxidase methods (Diastix or Chemstrip uG). It causes increased serum uric acid values (cupric sulfate method) and false elevations of urine specific gravity in dehydrated patients with low urine output.

Positive Coombs' tests have been reported after carbenicillin therapy; drug also interferes with some human leukocyte antigen (HLA) tests and could cause inaccurate HLA typing.

Systemic effect of carbenicillin may prolong PTs; it may cause transient elevations in liver function study results and transient reductions in RBC, WBC, and platelet counts.

Carbenicillin may also decrease serum aminoglycoside concentrations.

Adverse reactions

GI: *nausea,* vomiting, *diarrhea, flatulence, abdominal cramps, unpleasant taste,* glossitis, dry mouth, furry tongue.
Hematologic: leukopenia, ***neutropenia,*** eosinophilia, ***hemolytic anemia, thrombocytopenia.***
Other: hypersensitivity reactions (rash, urticaria, pruritus, ***anaphylaxis***), overgrowth of nonsusceptible organisms.

Overdose and treatment

Clinical signs of overdose include neuromuscular hypersensitivity or seizures resulting from CNS irritation by high drug concentrations. No specific treatment is recommended. Treatment is supportive. After recent ingestion (within 4 hours), empty the stomach by induced emesis or gastric lavage. Follow with activated charcoal to reduce absorption. Drug can be removed by hemodialysis.

☑ Special considerations

Besides those relevant to all *penicillins,* consider the following recommendations.

- Administer drug 1 to 2 hours before and 2 to 3 hours after meals with full glass (8 oz) of water to obtain maximum drug levels.
- Because carbenicillin is dialyzable, patients undergoing hemodialysis may need dosage adjustments.

Patient education

- Inform patient of potential adverse reactions.

Geriatric use

- Half-life may be prolonged in elderly patients because of decreased renal function.

Pediatric use

- Safe use in children has not been established. High incidence of nausea, vomiting, and diarrhea has been associated with its use in children.

Breast-feeding

- Drug is distributed into breast milk; use cautiously in breast-feeding women.

carboplatin

Paraplatin

Pharmacologic classification: alkylating agent (cell cycle–phase nonspecific)
Therapeutic classification: antineoplastic
Pregnancy risk category D

How supplied

Available by prescription only
Injection: 50-mg, 150-mg, 450-mg vials

Indications, route, and dosage

Initial and secondary (palliative) treatment of ovarian carcinoma; ◊ retinoblastoma; ◊ advanced bladder cancer; ◊ lung cancer; ◊ head and neck cancer; ◊ Wilms' tumor; ◊ primary brain tumor; ◊ testicular neoplasm

Adults: Initial recommended dose for single-agent therapy is 360 mg/m² I.V. on day 1. Dose is repeated q 4 weeks. In combination therapy (with cyclophosphamide), give 300 mg/m² I.V. on day 1 q 4 weeks for 6 cycles.

✦ ***Dosage adjustment.*** Dosage adjustments are based on the lowest posttreatment platelet or neutrophil value obtained in weekly blood counts.

In patients with impaired renal function, initial recommended dose is 250 mg/m² for creatinine clearance levels between 41 and 59 ml/minute; for creatinine clearance levels between 16 and 40 ml/minute, dose is 200 mg/m².

Lowest platelet count/mm³	Lowest neutrophil count/mm³	Adjusted dose
> 100,000	> 2,000	125%
50,000 to 100,000	500 to 2,000	No adjustment
< 50,000	< 500	75%

Pharmacodynamics
Antitumor action: Carboplatin causes cross-linking of DNA strands.

Pharmacokinetics
• *Absorption:* Drug is administered I.V.
• *Distribution:* Carboplatin's volume of distribution is approximately equal to total body water. Drug is not protein-bound but degraded to platinum-containing products, which are 87% protein-bound at 24 hours.
• *Metabolism:* Drug is hydrolyzed to form hydroxylated and aquated species. Drug's half-life is 2 to 3 hours; terminal half-life for platinum is 4 to 6 days.
• *Excretion:* 65% of drug is excreted by the kidneys within 12 hours, 71% within 24 hours. Enterohepatic recirculation may occur.

Contraindications and precautions
Contraindicated in patients with history of hypersensitivity to cisplatin, platinum-containing compounds, or mannitol or with severe bone marrow suppression or bleeding.

Interactions
Concomitant use with *nephrotoxic agents* produces additive nephrotoxicity of carboplatin.

Effects on diagnostic tests
High doses of carboplatin may cause elevated bilirubin, alkaline phosphatase, AST, serum creatinine, and BUN levels.

Adverse reactions
CNS: dizziness, confusion, peripheral neuropathy, ototoxicity, central neurotoxicity, paresthesia, ***CVA***.
CV: *cardiac failure, embolism.*
EENT: visual disturbances, change in taste.
GI: constipation, diarrhea, *nausea, vomiting.*
Hematologic: **THROMBOCYTOPENIA,** *leukopenia,* **NEUTROPENIA,** *anemia,* **BONE MARROW SUPPRESSION.**
Other: alopecia; hypersensitivity reactions; increased BUN, creatinine, AST, or alkaline phosphatase levels; pain; asthenia; ***anaphylaxis;*** decreased serum electrolyte levels.

Overdose and treatment
Symptoms of overdose result from bone marrow suppression or hepatotoxicity. There is no known antidote for carboplatin overdose.

☑ Special considerations
• Reconstitute with D_5W, 0.9% NaCl solution, or sterile water for injection to make a concentration of 10 mg/ml.
• Drug can be diluted with 0.9% NaCl solution or D_5W.
• Unopened vials should be stored at room temperature. Once reconstituted and diluted as directed, solution is stable at room temperature for 8 hours. Because drug does not contain antibacterial preservatives, unused drug should be discarded after 8 hours.
• Do not use needles or I.V. administration sets containing aluminum because drug may precipitate and lose potency.
• Although drug is promoted as causing less nausea and vomiting than cisplatin, it can cause severe emesis. Administer antiemetic therapy.
• Administration of carboplatin requires the supervision of a physician experienced in the use of chemotherapeutic agents.

Patient education
• Stress importance of adequate fluid intake and increase in urine output, to facilitate uric acid excretion.
• Tell patient to report tinnitus immediately, to prevent permanent hearing loss. Patient should have audiometric testing before initial and subsequent course.
• Advise patient to avoid exposure to people with infections.
• Instruct patient to promptly report unusual bleeding or bruising.
• Advise female patient to use contraception during therapy and to call if pregnancy is suspected.

Geriatric use
• Patients over age 65 are at greater risk for neurotoxicity.

Pediatric use
• Safety has not been established.

Breast-feeding
• It is unknown if drug is distributed in breast milk. However, because of the potential for toxicity to the infant, breast-feeding should be stopped.

carboprost tromethamine
Hemabate

Pharmacologic classification: prostaglandin
Therapeutic classification: oxytocic
Pregnancy risk category C

How supplied
Available by prescription only
Injection: 250 mcg/ml in combination with 83 mcg/ml tromethamine

Indications, route, and dosage
To abort pregnancy between weeks 13 and 20 of gestation
Adults: Initially, administer 250 mcg deep I.M. Administer subsequent doses of 250 mcg at intervals of 1½ to 3½ hours, depending on uterine response. Increments in dosage may be increased to 500 mcg if contractility is inadequate after several 250 mcg doses. Total dose should not exceed 12 mg, and therapy should not continue for more than 2 days.
Postpartum hemorrhage due to uterine atony that has not responded to conventional management
Adults: 250 mcg by deep I.M. injection. May administer repeat doses at 15- to 90-minute intervals. Maximum total dose, 2 mg.

Pharmacodynamics

Oxytocic action: Carboprost tromethamine stimulates myometrial contractions in the gravid uterus similar to the contractions of term labor. Exact mechanism is unknown but effect may be due to one or more of the following: direct stimulation, regulation of cellular calcium transport, or regulation of intracellular concentrations of cAMP. Uterine response increases with the length of the pregnancy. Carboprost tromethamine also facilitates cervical dilation by softening the cervix. The mean abortion time is 16 hours.

Pharmacokinetics

- *Absorption:* Following deep I.M. administration, peak concentrations occur in 15 minutes.
- *Distribution:* Unknown.
- *Metabolism:* The liver appears to be the primary site of oxidation.
- *Excretion:* Drug is excreted primarily as metabolites in urine.

Contraindications and precautions

Contraindicated in patients with hypersensitivity to drug, acute pelvic inflammatory disease, or active cardiac, pulmonary, renal, or hepatic disease. Use cautiously in patients with history of asthma; hypotension or hypertension; CV, renal, or hepatic disease; anemia; jaundice; diabetes; epilepsy; a compromised uterus; or chorioamnionitis.

Interactions

When used concomitantly, drug will enhance the effects of *oxytocin* and other *oxytocics*; however, cervical laceration and trauma have been reported with concomitant use of *oxytocin.*

Effects on diagnostic tests

None reported.

Adverse reactions

CNS: headache, anxiety, hot flashes, paresthesia, syncope, weakness.
CV: chest pain, ***arrhythmias.***
EENT: blurred vision, eye pain.
GI: *vomiting, diarrhea, nausea.*
GU: endometritis, uterine rupture, uterine or vaginal pain.
Respiratory: coughing, wheezing.
Skin: flushing, rash.
Other: *fever,* chills, backache, breast tenderness, diaphoresis, leg cramps.

Overdose and treatment

Clinical manifestations of overdose are extensions of the adverse reactions. Because drug is metabolized rapidly, treatment involves discontinuing drug and providing supportive care.

☑ Special considerations

- Administer only in hospitals with intensive care and surgical facilities available.
- Confirmation of fetal death is imperative before administration when used for missed abortion or intrauterine fetal death.
- Premedicate patient with antiemetic and antidiarrheal agents to minimize GI effects.
- Meperidine may be helpful to reduce abdominal cramps.
- Store drug in refrigerator. (Carboprost is stable at room temperature for 9 days.)
- If fever occurs, differentiate between drug-induced fever and endometritis pyrexia.
- If incomplete abortion occurs, use other measures to ensure complete abortion.

Patient education

- Advise patient of expected adverse reactions.

carisoprodol

Soma

Pharmacologic classification: carbamate derivative
Therapeutic classification: skeletal muscle relaxant
Pregnancy risk category NR

How supplied

Available by prescription only
Tablets: 350 mg

Indications, route, and dosage

Adjunct for relief of discomfort in acute, painful musculoskeletal conditions

Adults and children over age 12: Administer 350 mg P.O. t.i.d. and h.s.

Pharmacodynamics

Skeletal muscle relaxant action: Carisoprodol does not relax skeletal muscle directly but apparently as a result of its sedative effects. However, the exact mechanism of action is unknown. Animal studies suggest that the drug modifies central perception of pain without eliminating peripheral pain reflexes and has slight antipyretic activity.

Pharmacokinetics

- *Absorption:* With usual therapeutic doses, onset of action occurs within 30 minutes and persists 4 to 6 hours.
- *Distribution:* Drug is widely distributed throughout the body.
- *Metabolism:* Metabolized in the liver. Drug may induce microsomal enzymes in the liver; half-life is 8 hours.
- *Excretion:* Excreted in urine mainly as its metabolites; less than 1% of a dose is excreted unchanged. Drug may be removed by hemodialysis or peritoneal dialysis.

Contraindications and precautions

Contraindicated in patients with hypersensitivity to related compounds (for example, meprobamate or tybamate) or intermittent porphyria. Use cautiously in patients with impaired renal or hepatic function.

Interactions
Concomitant use with *other CNS depressants*, including *alcohol*, produces additive CNS depression. When used with other *depressant drugs* (*general anesthetics, opioid analgesics, antipsychotics, tricyclic antidepressants*, or *anxiolytics*), exercise care to avoid overdose. Concurrent use with *MAO inhibitors* or *tricyclic antidepressants* may increase CNS depression, respiratory depression, and hypotensive effects. Dosage adjustments (reduction of one or both) are required.

Effects on diagnostic tests
None reported.

Adverse reactions
CNS: *drowsiness, dizziness,* vertigo, ataxia, tremor, agitation, irritability, headache, depressive reactions, insomnia.
CV: orthostatic hypotension, tachycardia, facial flushing.
GI: nausea, vomiting, hiccups, epigastric distress.
Hematologic: eosinophilia.
Respiratory: asthmatic episodes.
Skin: rash, ***erythema multiforme,*** pruritus.
Other: fever, angioedema, ***anaphylaxis.***

Overdose and treatment
Clinical manifestations of overdose include exaggerated CNS depression, stupor, coma, shock, and respiratory depression.

Treatment of a conscious patient requires emptying the stomach by emesis or gastric lavage; activated charcoal may be used after gastric lavage to adsorb any remaining drug. If patient is comatose, secure endotracheal tube with cuff inflated before gastric lavage. Provide supportive therapy by maintaining adequate airway and assisted ventilation. CNS stimulants and pressor agents should be used cautiously. Monitor vital signs, fluid and electrolyte levels, and neurologic status closely.

Monitor urine output, and avoid overhydration. Forced diuresis using mannitol, peritoneal dialysis, or hemodialysis may be beneficial. Continue to monitor patient for relapse from incomplete gastric emptying and delayed absorption.

☑ Special considerations
- Use with caution with other CNS depressants, because effects may be cumulative.
- Initially, allergic or idiosyncratic reactions may occur (first to the fourth dose). Symptoms usually subside after several hours; treat with supportive and symptomatic measures.
- Psychological dependence may follow long-term use.
- Withdrawal symptoms (abdominal cramps, insomnia, chilliness, headache, and nausea) may occur with abrupt termination of drug after prolonged use of higher-than-recommended doses.
- Commercially available formulations may contain sodium metabisulfite, which may cause an allergic reaction.

Patient education
- Inform patient that drug may cause dizziness and faintness. Symptoms may be controlled by making position changes slowly and in stages. Patient should report persistent symptoms.
- Tell patient to avoid alcoholic beverages and to use cough or cold preparations containing alcohol cautiously while taking this medication. Patient should also avoid other CNS depressants (effects may be additive) unless prescribed.
- Warn patient drug may cause drowsiness. Avoid hazardous activities that require alertness until CNS depressant effects can be determined.
- Advise patient to discontinue drug immediately and to call if rash, diplopia, dizziness, or other unusual signs or symptoms appear.
- Inform patient to store drug away from direct heat and light (not in bathroom medicine cabinet).
- Instruct patient to take missed dose only if remembered within 1 hour. If remembered later, patient should skip that dose and go back to regular schedule. Patient should not double the dose.

Geriatric use
- Elderly patients may be more sensitive to drug's effects.

Pediatric use
- Safety and efficacy have not been established in children under age 12. However, some clinicians suggest a dosage of 25 mg/kg or 750 mg/m² divided q.i.d. for children age 5 and older.

Breast-feeding
- Carisoprodol may be distributed into breast milk at two to four times maternal plasma concentrations.

carmustine (BCNU)
BiCNU, Gliadel

Pharmacologic classification: alkylating agent; nitrosourea (cell cycle–phase nonspecific)
Therapeutic classification: antineoplastic
Pregnancy risk category D

How supplied
Available by prescription only
Injection: 100-mg vial (lyophilized), with a 3-ml vial of absolute alcohol supplied as a diluent
Implant: 7.7 mg wafer

Indications, route, and dosage
Dosage and indications may vary. Check current literature for recommended protocol.
◇ Brain; ◇ breast; ◇ GI tract; ◇ lung; ◇ hepatic cancer; Hodgkin's disease; malignant lymphomas; ◇ malignant melanomas; multiple myeloma
Adults: 75 to 100 mg/m² I.V. by slow infusion daily for 2 consecutive days, repeated q 6 weeks if platelet count is above 100,000/mm³ and WBC count is above 4,000/mm³.

✦ ***Dosage adjustment.*** Reduce dosage p.r.n. using the following guidelines:

Nadir after prior dose		% of prior dose to be given
Leukocytes/ mm^3	Platelets/ mm^3	
> 4,000	> 100,000	100%
3,000 to 3,999	75,000 to 99,999	100%
2,000 to 2,999	25,000 to 74,999	70%
< 2,000	< 25,000	50%

Alternative therapy: 150 to 200 mg/m^2 I.V. slow infusion as a single dose, repeated q 6 to 8 weeks; or 40 mg/m^2 I.V. slow infusion for 5 consecutive days, repeated q 6 weeks.
Recurrent glioblastoma and metastatic brain tumors (adjunct to surgery to prolong survival)
Adults: Implant 8 wafers in the resection cavity if allowed by size and shape of cavity.

Pharmacodynamics
Antineoplastic action: The cytotoxic action of carmustine is mediated through its metabolites, which inhibit several enzymes involved with DNA formation. This agent can also cause cross-linking of DNA. Cross-linking interferes with DNA, RNA, and protein synthesis. Cross-resistance between carmustine and lomustine has been shown to occur.

Pharmacokinetics
• *Absorption:* Drug is not absorbed across the GI tract. Implant wafers are biodegradable in the human brain when implanted into the tumor resection cavity.
• *Distribution:* Drug is cleared rapidly from the plasma. After I.V. administration, carmustine and its metabolites distribute rapidly into the CSF.
• *Metabolism:* Metabolized extensively in the liver.
• *Excretion:* Approximately 60% to 70% of drug and its metabolites are excreted in urine within 96 hours, 6% to 10% is excreted as carbon dioxide by the lungs, and 1% is excreted in feces. Enterohepatic circulation and protein-binding can occur and may cause delayed hematologic toxicity.

Note concerning implant wafer: The absoption, distribution, metabolism and excretion of the copolymer in humans is unknown.

Contraindications and precautions
Contraindicated in patients with hypersensitivity to drug.

Interactions
Concomitant use with *cimetidine* increases the bone marrow toxicity of carmustine. The mechanism of this interaction is unknown. Avoid concomitant use of these drugs. *Phenytoin* serum concentrations may be decreased by a combination chemotherapy regimen including carmustine. *Digoxin* levels may also be decreased.

Effects on diagnostic tests
Carmustine therapy may increase BUN, serum alkaline phosphatase, AST, and bilirubin concentrations.

Adverse reactions
CNS: ataxia, drowsiness.
EENT: ocular toxicities.
GI: *nausea* beginning in 2 to 6 hours (can be severe), *vomiting.*
GU: nephrotoxicity, azotemia, ***renal failure.***
Hematologic: ***cumulative bone marrow suppression*** (delayed 4 to 6 weeks, lasting 1 to 2 weeks); ***leukopenia; thrombocytopenia; acute leukemia, bone marrow dysplasia*** (after long-term use); anemia.
Hepatic: hepatotoxicity.
Respiratory: ***pulmonary fibrosis.***
Skin: facial flushing, hyperpigmentation.
Other: *intense pain at infusion site from venous spasm;* possible hyperuricemia (in lymphoma patients when rapid cell lysis occurs).

Overdose and treatment
Clinical manifestations of overdose include leukopenia, thrombocytopenia, nausea, and vomiting.

Treatment consists of supportive measures, including transfusion of blood components, antibiotics for infections that may develop, and antiemetics.

☑ Special considerations
• Use double gloves and use surgical instruments dedicated to the handling of implant wafers.
• Reconstitute 100-mg vial with the 3 ml of absolute alcohol provided by manufacturer, then dilute further with 27 ml sterile water for injection. Resultant solution contains 3.3 mg carmustine/ml in 10% ethanol. Dilute in 0.9% NaCl or D_5W for I.V. infusion. Give at least 250 ml over 1 to 2 hours. Discard excess drug.
• Wear gloves to administer drug infusion and when changing I.V. tubing. Avoid contact with skin because carmustine will cause a brown stain. If drug comes into contact with skin, wash off thoroughly.
• Solution is unstable in plastic I.V. bags. Administer only in glass containers.
• Carmustine may decompose at temperatures above 80° F (26.6° C).
• If powder liquefies or appears oily, discard it because it is a sign of decomposition.
• Reconstituted solution may be stored in refrigerator for 24 hours.
• Do not mix with other drugs during administration.
• Avoid I.M. injections when platelet count is below 100,000/mm^3.
• To reduce pain on infusion, dilute further or slow infusion rate.
• Intense flushing of the skin may occur during an I.V. infusion, but usually disappears within 2 to 4 hours.
• To reduce nausea, give antiemetic before administering.
• Monitor patient's CBC.
• Know that pulmonary toxicity is more likely in people who smoke.

- At first sign of extravasation, infusion should be discontinued and area infiltrated with liberal injections of 0.5 mEq/ml sodium bicarbonate solution.
- Drug has been applied topically in concentrations of 0.05% to 0.4% to treat mycosis fungoides.
- Prescribe anticoagulants and aspirin products cautiously. Monitor patient closely for signs of bleeding.
- Because drug crosses the blood-brain barrier, it may be used to treat primary brain tumors.

Patient education

- Warn patient to watch for signs of infection and bone marrow toxicity (fever, sore throat, anemia, fatigue, easy bruising, nose or gum bleeds, melena). Patient should take temperature daily.
- Remind patient to return for follow-up blood work weekly, or as needed, and to watch for signs and symptoms of infection.
- Advise patient to avoid exposure to people with infections.
- Tell patient to avoid OTC products containing aspirin because they may precipitate bleeding. Advise patient to report signs of bleeding promptly.
- Advise female patient to avoid becoming pregnant and to call if pregnancy is suspected.

Breast-feeding

- Active metabolites of drug have been found in breast milk. Therefore, it is not advisable for women receiving drug to breast-feed their infants because of risk of serious adverse reactions, mutagenicity, and carcinogenicity in the infant.

carteolol hydrochloride

Cartrol, Ocupress

Pharmacologic classification: beta-adrenergic blocker
Therapeutic classification: antihypertensive
Pregnancy risk category C

How supplied

Available by prescription only
Tablets: 2.5 mg, 5 mg
Ophthalmic solution: 1%

Indications, route, and dosage

Hypertension
Adults: Initially, 2.5 mg as a single daily dose. Gradually increase the dosage as required to 5 mg daily or 10 mg daily as a single dose.

◊ ***Angina***
Adults: 10 mg/day.

✦ ***Dosage adjustment.*** Patients with substantial renal failure should receive the usual dose of carteolol scheduled at longer intervals as shown.

Creatinine clearance (ml/min)	Dosage interval (hr)
> 60	24
20 to 60	48
< 20	72

Open-angle glaucoma
Adults: 1 drop b.i.d. in eye.

Pharmacodynamics

Antihypertensive action: Drug is a nonselective beta-adrenergic blocking agent with intrinsic sympathomimetic activity (ISA). Its antihypertensive effects are probably caused by decreased sympathetic outflow from the brain and decreased cardiac output. Carteolol does not have a consistent effect on renin output.

Pharmacokinetics

- *Absorption.* Rapid, achieving peak plasma levels in 1 to 3 hours. Bioavailability is about 85%.
- *Distribution:* Drug is 20% to 30% bound to plasma proteins.
- *Metabolism:* Only 30% to 50% of drug is metabolized in the liver to 8-hydroxycarteolol, an active metabolite, and the inactive metabolite glucuronoside.
- *Excretion:* Primarily renal. Plasma half-life is about 6 hours.

Contraindications and precautions

Contraindicated in patients hypersensitive to any component of drug and in those with bronchial asthma, severe COPD, sinus bradycardia, second- or third-degree AV block, overt cardiac failure, or cardiogenic shock.

Use cautiously in patients with nonallergic bronchospastic disease, diabetes mellitus, hyperthyroidism, or decreased pulmonary function and in breast-feeding women.

Interactions

The dosage of *insulin* and *oral antidiabetic agents* may have to be adjusted in patients receiving carteolol.

Catecholamine-depleting drugs, such as *reserpine,* may have an additive effect when administered with a beta blocker. Carteolol may potentiate the hypotension produced by *general anesthetics.* Observe carefully for excessive hypotension or bradycardia and for orthostatic hypotension.

Avoid concurrent administration of *oral calcium antagonists* and beta blockers in patients with impaired cardiac function because of the risk of hypotension, left ventricular failure, and AV conduction disturbances. I.V. calcium antagonists should be used with caution.

Effects on diagnostic tests

None reported.

Adverse reactions

CNS: lassitude, fatigue, somnolence, *asthenia, paresthesia.*
CV: *conduction disturbances.*
EENT: transient irritation, conjunctival hyperemia, *edema.*
GI: diarrhea, nausea, abdominal pain.
Other: *muscle cramps,* arthralgia, rash.

Overdose and treatment

No information available. The likely symptoms are bradycardia, bronchospasm, heart failure, and hypotension.

Atropine should be used to treat symptomatic bradycardia. If no response is seen, cautiously use isoproterenol. Bronchospasm should be treated with a $beta_2$ agonist, such as isoproterenol, or theophylline. Cardiac glycosides or diuretics may be useful in treating heart failure. Vasopressors (epinephrine, dopamine, or norepinephrine) should be given to combat hypotension.

☑ Special considerations

Besides those relevant to all *beta-adrenergic blockers,* consider the following recommendations.

- Dosage over 10 mg daily does not produce a greater response; it may actually decrease response.
- Food may slow the rate, but not the extent, of carteolol absorption.
- Steady-state levels are reached rapidly (within 1 to 2 days) in patients with normal renal function.

Patient education

- Advise patient to take drug exactly as prescribed and not to discontinue drug suddenly.
- Advise patient to report shortness of breath or difficulty breathing, unusually fast heartbeat, cough, or fatigue with exertion.
- Inform patient that transient stinging or discomfort may occur with ophthalmic use; if reaction is severe, he should call immediately.

Geriatric use

- No specific age-related recommendations are available.

Pediatric use

- Safety has not been established.

Breast-feeding

- Animal studies indicate that drug may be distributed in breast milk. Use with caution in breast-feeding women.

carvedilol

Coreg

Pharmacologic classification: $alpha_1$-nonselective beta-adrenergic blocker
Therapeutic classification: antihypertensive, adjunct treatment for heart failure
Pregnancy risk category C

How supplied

Available by prescription only
Tablets: 3.125 mg, 6.25 mg, 12.5 mg, 25 mg

Indications, route, and dosage

Hypertension

Adults: Dosage individualized. Initially, 6.25 mg P.O. b.i.d. with food; obtain standing systolic pressure 1 hour after initial dose. If tolerated, continue dose for 7 to 14 days. Can increase to 12.5 mg P.O. b.i.d., repeating monitoring protocol. Maximum dose is 25 mg P.O. b.i.d. as tolerated.

Heart failure

Adults: Dosage individualized and titrated carefully. Stabilize dosing of cardiac glycosides, diuretics, and ACE inhibitors before starting therapy. Initially, 3.125 mg P.O. b.i.d. with food for 2 weeks; if tolerated, can increase to 6.25 mg P.O. b.i.d. for 2 weeks. Dose can be doubled q 2 weeks to highest level tolerated by patient. At initiation of new dose, observe patient for dizziness or light-headedness for 1 hour. Maximum dosing for patients weighing less than 187 lb (85 kg) is 25 mg P.O. b.i.d.; for those weighing over 187 lb, give 50 mg P.O. b.i.d.

Pharmacodynamics

Antihypertensive action: Mechanism not established. Beta blockade shown to reduce cardiac output and tachycardia. Alpha blockade is demonstrated by the attenuated pressor effects of phenylephrine, vasodilation, and decreases in peripheral vascular resistance.

Heart failure: Not fully established. Drug has been shown to decrease systemic blood pressure, pulmonary artery pressure, right atrial pressure, systemic vascular resistance, and heart rate while increasing stroke volume index.

Pharmacokinetics

- *Absorption:* Rapidly and extensively metabolized following oral administration, with absolute bioavailability of 25% to 35% because of significant first-pass metabolism. Mean terminal elimination half-life ranges from 7 to 10 hours.
- *Distribution:* Plasma concentrations are proportional to oral dose administered. Absorption is slowed when administered with food, as evidenced by a delay in the time to reach peak plasma levels with no significant difference in extent of bioavailability.
- *Metabolism:* Extensively metabolized, primarily by aromatic ring oxidation and glucuronidation. The oxidative metabolites are further metabolized by conjugation via glucuronidation and sulfation. Demethylation and hydroxylation at the phenol ring produce three active metabolites with beta-blocking activity.
- *Excretion:* Metabolites are primarily excreted via bile into the feces. Less than 2% of dose is excreted unchanged in urine.

Contraindications and precautions

Contraindicated in patients with New York Heart Association (NYHA) class IV decompensated cardiac failure requiring I.V. inotropic therapy, bronchial asthma or related bronchospastic conditions, second- or third-degree AV block, sick sinus syndrome (unless a permanent pacemaker is in place), cardiogenic shock, severe bradycardia, or hypersensitivity to drug. Drug is not recommended in patients with hepatic impairment.

Use cautiously in hypertensive patients with left ventricular failure, perioperative patients who receive anesthetics that depress myocardial function (for example, ether, cyclopropane, trichloroethylene), or diabetic patients receiving insulin or oral antidiabetic agents and in those subject to spontaneous hypoglycemia. Also use with caution in patients with thyroid disease (may mask hyperthyroidism and drug withdrawal may precipitate thyroid storm or an exacerbation of hyperthyroidism), pheochromocytoma, Prinzmetal's variant angina, or peripheral vascular disease (may precipitate or aggravate symptoms of arterial insufficiency).

Interactions

Although *inhibitors of cytochrome P-2D6 (quinidine, fluoxetine, paroxetine, propafenone)* have not been studied, they would possibly increase carvedilol levels. *Catecholamine-depleting agents* (such as *reserpine, MAO inhibitors)* may cause severe bradycardia or hypotension. *Clonidine* may potentiate blood pressure and heart rate lowering effects. If patient is receiving beta blockers and clonidine, discontinue beta blocker first, then clonidine several days later by titration.

Concentrations of *digoxin* are increased about 15% while on concurrent therapy; because both agents slow AV conduction, monitor digoxin levels. *Rifampin* reduces plasma concentrations of carvedilol by 70%, *cimetidine* increases bioavailability by 30%. *Calcium channel blockers* can cause isolated conduction disturbances; monitor ECG and blood pressure. Concomitant use with *insulin* and *oral antidiabetic agents* may enhance hypoglycemic properties; monitor blood glucose levels.

Effects on diagnostic tests

None reported.

Adverse reactions

CNS: *dizziness, fatigue,* headache, hypesthesia, insomnia, pain, paresthesia, somnolence, vertigo.
CV: aggravated angina pectoris, ***AV block, bradycardia,*** chest pain, fluid overload, hypertension, hypotension, postural hypertension, syncope.
EENT: abnormal vision.
GI: abdominal pain, *diarrhea,* melena, nausea, periodontitis, vomiting.
GU: abnormal renal function, albuminuria, hematuria, urinary tract infection.
Hematologic: decreased PT, purpura, ***thrombocytopenia.***
Hepatic: increased ALT, AST.
Metabolic: dehydration, glycosuria, gout, hypercholesterolemia, *hyperglycemia*, hypertriglyceridemia, hypervolemia, hyperuricemia, hypoglycemia, hyponatremia, weight gain, increased alkaline phosphatase, BUN, or nonprotein nitrogen.
Respiratory: bronchitis, dyspnea, pharyngitis, rhinitis, sinusitis, *upper respiratory tract infection.*
Other: allergy, arthralgia, back pain, edema, fever, hypovolemia, impotence, malaise, myalgia, peripheral edema, ***sudden death***, viral infection.

Overdose and treatment

Overdosage may cause severe hypotension, bradycardia, cardiac insufficiency, cardiogenic shock, and cardiac arrest. Respiratory effects, bronchospasm, vomiting, lapses of consciousness, and generalized seizures may also occur. Place patient in supine position and keep him in intensive care conditions, if needed. Gastric lavage or pharmacologically-induced emesis may be effective shortly after ingestion. May use atropine 2 mg I.V. for bradycardia, glucagon 5 to 10 mg I.V. rapidly over 30 seconds, followed by continuous infusion at 5 mg/hour; sympathomimetics (dobutamine, isoprenaline, adrenaline) at doses based on body weight and effect. If peripheral vasodilation dominates, administer epinephrine or norepinephrine, if necessary, and continuously monitor circulatory conditions. For therapy-resistant bradycardia, perform pacemaker therapy. For bronchospasm, give beta-sympathomimetics by aerosol or I.V. or aminophylline I.V. If seizures occur, slow I.V. injection of diazepam or clonazepam may be effective. If severe intoxication and symptoms of shock occur, continue treatment with antidotes for a sufficiently long period of time consistent with the drug's 7- to 10-hour half-life.

☑ Special considerations

- Mild hepatocellular injury may occur during therapy. At first sign of hepatic dysfunction, perform tests for hepatic injury or jaundice; if present, stop drug.
- Discontinue drug gradually over 1 to 2 weeks. Decrease dosage if heart rate is below 55 beats/minute.
- Monitor heart failure patient for worsened condition, renal dysfunction, or fluid retention; diuretics may need to be increased. Also monitor diabetic patient because hyperglycemia may be worsened.
- Patients on beta blocker therapy with history of severe anaphylactic reaction to several allergens may be more reactive to repeated challenge, either accidental, diagnostic, or therapeutic. They may be unresponsive to the usual doses of epinephrine used to treat allergic reactions.

Patient education

- Tell patient not to interrupt or discontinue drug without medical approval.
- Advise heart failure patient to call if weight gain or shortness of breath occurs.
- Inform patient that he may experience lowered blood pressure when standing. If dizziness and fainting (rare) occur, advise him to sit or lie down.
- Caution patient against performing hazardous tasks during initiation of therapy. If dizziness or fatigue occur, tell him to call for an adjustment in dosage.
- Tell patient to take drug with food.
- Advise diabetic patient to report changes in blood glucose promptly.
- Inform patients who wear contact lenses that decreased lacrimation may occur.

Geriatric use

- Monitor plasma levels carefully; drug occurs about 50% higher in elderly compared with young patients.
- No significant difference was found in adverse effects between older and younger patients; dizziness was slightly more common in the elderly.

Pediatric use

- Safety of drug in patients under age 18 has not been established.

Breast-feeding
• It is unknown if drug is excreted in breast milk. Use drug cautiously.

cascara sagrada

cascara sagrada aromatic fluid extract

Pharmacologic classification: anthraquinone glycoside mixture
Therapeutic classification: laxative
Pregnancy risk category C

How supplied
Available without a prescription
Tablets: 325 mg
Aromatic fluid extract: 1 g/ml with 18% alcohol

Indications, route, and dosage
Acute constipation, preparation for bowel or rectal examination
Adults: 1 tablet P.O. h.s.
Children age 2 to 12: ½ of adult dose.
Children under age 2: ¼ of adult dose.

Pharmacodynamics
Laxative action: Cascara sagrada, obtained from the dried bark of the buckthorn tree *(Rhamnus purshiana),* contains cascarosides A and B (barbaloin glycosides) and cascarosides C and D (chrysaloin glycosides). It exerts a direct irritant action on the colon that promotes peristalsis and bowel motility. It also enhances colonic fluid accumulation, increasing the laxative effect.

Pharmacokinetics
• *Absorption:* Minimal drug absorption occurs in the small intestine. Onset of action usually occurs in about 6 to 12 hours but may not occur for 3 or 4 days.
• *Distribution:* Cascara may be distributed in the bile, saliva, and colonic mucosa.
• *Metabolism:* Metabolized in the liver.
• *Excretion:* Excreted in feces via biliary elimination, in urine, or in both.

Contraindications and precautions
Contraindicated in patients with abdominal pain, nausea, vomiting, or other symptoms of appendicitis or acute surgical abdomen; acute surgical delirium; fecal impaction; and intestinal obstruction or perforation. Use cautiously in patients with rectal bleeding.

Interactions
None reported.

Effects on diagnostic tests
Cascara turns alkaline urine pink to red, red to violet, or red to brown and turns acidic urine yellow to brown in the phenolsulfonphthalein excretion test.

Adverse reactions
GI: *nausea;* vomiting; diarrhea; loss of normal bowel function with excessive use; *abdominal cramps,* especially in severe constipation; malabsorption of nutrients; "cathartic colon" (syndrome resembling ulcerative colitis radiologically and pathologically) with chronic misuse; discoloration of rectal mucosa after long-term use.
Other: hypokalemia, protein enteropathy, electrolyte imbalance (with excessive use), laxative dependence (with long-term or excessive use).

Overdose and treatment
No information available.

☑ Special considerations
• Prescribe doses carefully; fluid extract preparation is five times as potent as aromatic fluid extract.
• Aromatic fluid extract tastes better than fluid extract.
• Drug may color urine reddish pink or brown, depending on urine pH.
• Cascara is a common ingredient in many so-called natural laxatives available without a prescription.
• Bulk-forming or surfactant laxatives are preferred during pregnancy.

Patient education
• Warn patient that drug may turn urine reddish pink or brown.

Geriatric use
• Because many elderly persons use laxatives, they have a particularly high risk of developing laxative dependence. Urge them to use laxatives only for short periods.

Pediatric use
• Use with caution in children.

Breast-feeding
• Cascara may be excreted in breast milk, which may result in increased incidence of diarrhea in infant.

castor oil
Emulsoil, Neoloid, Purge

Pharmacologic classification: glyceride, *Ricinus communis* derivative
Therapeutic classification: stimulant laxative
Pregnancy risk category X

How supplied
Available without a prescription
Liquid: 60 ml, 120 ml
Liquid (95%): 30 ml, 60 ml
Liquid emulsion: 60 ml (95%), 90 ml (67%)

Indications, route, and dosage
Preparation for rectal or bowel examination or surgery; acute constipation (rarely)

Liquid
Adults: 15 to 60 ml (or 30 to 60 ml, 95%) P.O.
Children age 2 to 12: 5 to 15 ml P.O.
Liquid emulsion
Adults: 45 ml (67%) or 15 to 60 ml (95%) mixed with ½ to 1 glass liquid.
Children age 2 to 12: 15 ml (67%) or 5 to 15 ml (95%) mixed with ½ to 1 glass liquid.

Pharmacodynamics

Laxative action: Castor oil acts primarily in the small intestine, where it is metabolized to ricinoleic acid, which stimulates the intestine, promoting peristalsis and bowel motility.

Pharmacokinetics

- *Absorption:* Unknown; action begins in 2 to 6 hours.
- *Distribution:* Castor oil is distributed locally, primarily in the small intestine.
- *Metabolism:* Like other fatty acids, castor oil is metabolized by intestinal enzymes into its active form, ricinoleic acid.
- *Excretion:* Castor oil is excreted in feces.

Contraindications and precautions

Contraindicated in patients with ulcerative bowel lesions; abdominal pain, nausea, vomiting, or other symptoms of appendicitis or acute surgical abdomen; in those with anal or rectal fissures, fecal impaction, or intestinal obstruction or perforation; and during menstruation or pregnancy. Use cautiously in patients with rectal bleeding.

Interactions

Castor oil may decrease absorption of *intestinally absorbed drugs.*

Effects on diagnostic tests

None reported.

Adverse reactions

GI: *nausea;* vomiting; diarrhea; loss of normal bowel function with excessive use; *abdominal cramps,* especially in severe constipation; malabsorption of nutrients; "cathartic colon" (syndrome resembling ulcerative colitis radiologically and pathologically) with chronic misuse; laxative dependence with long-term or excessive use. May cause constipation after catharsis.
Other: hypokalemia, protein-losing enteropathy, other electrolyte imbalances (with excessive use).

Overdose and treatment

No information available.

☑ Special considerations

- Castor oil is not recommended for routine use in constipation; it is commonly used to evacuate the bowels before diagnostic or surgical procedures.
- Do not administer drug at bedtime because of rapid onset of action.
- Drug is most effective when taken on an empty stomach; shake well.
- Observe patient for signs and symptoms of dehydration.
- Flavored preparations are available.

Patient education

- Instruct patient not to take drug at bedtime.
- Recommend that drug be chilled or taken with juice or carbonated beverage for palatability.
- Instruct patient to shake emulsion well.
- Reassure patient that after response to drug he may not need to move bowels again for 1 or 2 days.

Geriatric use

- With chronic use, elderly patients may experience electrolyte depletion, resulting in weakness, incoordination, and orthostatic hypotension.

Breast-feeding

- Breast-feeding women should seek medical approval before using castor oil.

cefaclor

Ceclor, Ceclor CD

Pharmacologic classification: second-generation cephalosporin
Therapeutic classification: antibiotic
Pregnancy risk category B

How supplied

Available by prescription only
Tablets (extended-release): 375 mg, 500 mg
Capsules: 250 mg, 500 mg
Suspension: 125 mg/5 ml, 187 mg/5 ml, 250 mg/5 ml, 375 mg/5 ml

Indications, route, and dosage

Infections of respiratory or urinary tract and skin; otitis media caused by susceptible organisms
Adults: 250 to 500 mg P.O. q 8 hours. Total daily dosage should not exceed 4 g. For extended-release tablets, 375 to 500 mg P.O. q 12 hours for 7 to 10 days.
Children: 20 mg/kg P.O. daily (40 mg/kg for severe infections and otitis media) in divided doses q 8 hours, not to exceed 1 g/day.
◇ ***Acute uncomplicated urinary tract infection***
Adults: Give 2 g as a single dose.
✦ ***Dosage adjustment.*** Because cefaclor is dialyzable, patients who are receiving treatment with hemodialysis or peritoneal dialysis may require dosage adjustment.

Pharmacodynamics

Antibacterial action: Drug is primarily bactericidal; however, it may be bacteriostatic. Activity depends on the organism, tissue penetration, drug dosage, and rate of organism multiplication. It acts by adhering to bacterial penicillin-binding proteins, thereby inhibiting cell-wall synthesis.

Cefaclor has the same bactericidal spectrum as other second-generation cephalosporins, except that it has increased activity against ampicillin- or amoxicillin-resistant *Haemophilus influenzae* and *Branhamella catarrhalis.*

Pharmacokinetics

- *Absorption:* Drug is well absorbed from the GI tract; peak serum levels occur 30 to 60 minutes after an oral dose. Food will delay but not prevent complete GI tract absorption.
- *Distribution:* Cefaclor is distributed widely into most body tissues and fluids; CSF penetration is poor. Cefaclor crosses the placenta; it is 25% protein-bound.
- *Metabolism:* Drug is not metabolized.
- *Excretion:* Excreted primarily in urine by renal tubular secretion and glomerular filtration; small amounts of the drug are excreted in breast milk. Elimination half-life is ½ to 1 hour in patients with normal renal function; end-stage renal disease prolongs half-life to 3 to 5½ hours. Hemodialysis removes cefaclor.

Contraindications and precautions

Contraindicated in patients with hypersensitivity to other cephalosporins. Use cautiously in patients with impaired renal function or penicillin allergy and in breast-feeding women.

Interactions

Probenecid competitively inhibits renal tubular secretion of cephalosporins, resulting in higher, prolonged serum levels of these drugs.

Concomitant use with nephrotoxic agents (*vancomycin, colistin, polymyxin B, aminoglycosides*) or *loop diuretics* may increase the risk of nephrotoxicity.

Concomitant use of cefaclor with bacteriostatic agents (*tetracyclines, erythromycin, chloramphenicol*) may impair its bactericidal activity.

Effects on diagnostic tests

Cefaclor may cause false-positive Coombs' test results. Cefaclor also causes false-positive results in urine glucose tests using cupric sulfate (Benedict's reagent or Clinitest); use glucose oxidase tests (Chemstrip uG, Diastix, or glucose enzymatic test strip) instead.

Cefaclor causes false elevations in serum or urine creatinine levels in tests using Jaffé's reaction.

Adverse reactions

CNS: dizziness, headache, somnolence, malaise.
GI: *nausea,* vomiting, *diarrhea,* anorexia, dyspepsia, abdominal cramps, pseudomembranous colitis, oral candidiasis.
GU: vaginal moniliasis, vaginitis.
Hematologic: transient leukopenia, anemia, eosinophilia, ***thrombocytopenia,*** lymphocytosis.
Skin: *maculopapular rash,* dermatitis, pruritus.
Other: hypersensitivity reactions (serum sickness, ***anaphylaxis***), fever, transient increases in liver enzymes.

Overdose and treatment

Clinical signs of overdose include neuromuscular hypersensitivity; seizure may follow high CNS concentrations. Remove cefaclor by hemodialysis or peritoneal dialysis.

☑ Special considerations

Besides those relevant to all *cephalosporins*, consider the following recommendations.

- To prevent toxic accumulation, reduced dosage may be required if patient's creatinine clearance is below 40 ml/minute.
- Cefaclor may be given with food to minimize GI distress.
- Total daily dosage may be administered b.i.d. rather than t.i.d. with similar therapeutic effect.
- Stock oral suspension is stable for 14 days if refrigerated.

Patient education

- Instruct patient to take extended-release tablets with food and not to cut, crush, or chew them.

Geriatric use

- Dosage reduction may be necessary in patients with reduced renal function.

Pediatric use

- Drug can be used safely in children.

Breast-feeding

- Drug distributes into breast milk and should be used with caution in breast-feeding women.

cefadroxil

Duricef

Pharmacologic classification: first-generation cephalosporin
Therapeutic classification: antibiotic
Pregnancy risk category B

How supplied

Available by prescription only
Tablets: 1 g
Capsules: 500 mg
Suspension: 125 mg/5 ml, 250 mg/5 ml, 500 mg/5 ml

Indications, route, and dosage

Urinary tract, skin, and soft-tissue infections caused by susceptible organisms; pharyngitis; tonsillitis

Adults: 1 to 2 g P.O. daily, depending on the infection treated. Usually given once or twice daily.
Children: 30 mg/kg daily in two divided doses.

✦ ***Dosage adjustment.*** In patients with creatinine clearance below 10 ml/minute, extend dosing interval to q 36 hours; if it ranges between 10 and 25 ml/minute, administer q 24 hours; and if it is between 25 and 50 ml/minute, give q 12 hours.

Because drug is dialyzable, patients who are receiving treatment with hemodialysis may require dosage adjustment.

Pharmacodynamics

Antibacterial action: Cefadroxil is primarily bactericidal; however, it may be bacteriostatic. Activity depends on the organism, tissue penetration, drug dosage, and rate of organism multiplication. It acts by adhering to bacterial penicillin-binding proteins, thereby inhibiting cell-wall synthesis.

Cefadroxil is active against many gram-positive cocci, including penicillinase-producing *Staphylococcus aureus* and *epidermidis; Streptococcus pneumoniae,* group B streptococci, and group A beta-hemolytic streptococci; and susceptible gram-negative organisms, including *Klebsiella pneumoniae, Escherichia coli,* and *Proteus mirabilis.*

Pharmacokinetics

- *Absorption:* Drug is absorbed rapidly and completely from the GI tract after oral administration; peak serum levels occur at 1 to 2 hours.
- *Distribution:* Distributed widely into most body tissues and fluids, including the gallbladder, liver, kidneys, bone, bile, sputum, and pleural and synovial fluids; CSF penetration is poor. Drug crosses the placenta; it is 20% protein-bound.
- *Metabolism:* Cefadroxil is not metabolized.
- *Excretion:* Excreted primarily unchanged in the urine via glomerular filtration and renal tubular secretion; small amounts of drug may be excreted in breast milk. Elimination half-life is about 1 to 2 hours in patients with normal renal function; end-stage renal disease prolongs half-life to 25 hours. Drug can be removed by hemodialysis.

Contraindications and precautions

Contraindicated in patients with hypersensitivity to drug or other cephalosporins. Use cautiously in patients with impaired renal function or penicillin allergy and in breast-feeding women.

Interactions

Probenecid competitively inhibits renal tubular secretion of cephalosporins, resulting in higher, prolonged serum levels of these drugs.

Concomitant use with nephrotoxic agents (*vancomycin, colistin, polymyxin B, aminoglycosides*) or *loop diuretics* may increase the risk of nephrotoxicity.

Concomitant use with bacteriostatic agents (*tetracyclines, erythromycin, chloramphenicol*) may interfere with bactericidal activity.

Effects on diagnostic tests

Cefadroxil causes false-positive results in urine glucose tests utilizing cupric sulfate (Benedict's reagent or Clinitest); use glucose oxidase test (Chemstrip uG, Diastix, or glucose enzymatic test strip) instead. Cefadroxil causes false elevations in serum or urine creatinine levels in tests using Jaffé's reaction.

Positive Coombs' test results occur in about 3% of patients taking cephalosporins.

Adverse reactions

CNS: ***seizures.***
GI: pseudomembranous colitis, *nausea,* vomiting, *diarrhea,* glossitis, abdominal cramps, oral candidiasis.
GU: genital pruritus, moniliasis, vaginitis, renal dysfunction.
Hematologic: transient neutropenia, eosinophilia, leukopenia, anemia, ***agranulocytosis, thrombocytopenia.***
Skin: *maculopapular and erythematous rashes,* urticaria.
Other: hypersensitivity reactions (serum sickness, ***anaphylaxis,*** angioedema), transient increases in liver enzymes, dyspnea, fever.

Overdose and treatment

Clinical signs of overdose include neuromuscular hypersensitivity; seizure may follow high CNS concentrations. Remove cefadroxil by hemodialysis. Other treatment is supportive.

☑ Special considerations

Besides those relevant to all *cephalosporins,* consider the following recommendation.

- Longer half-life of drug permits once- or twice-daily dosing.

Patient education

- Inform patient of potential adverse reactions.

Geriatric use

- Reduce dosage in elderly patients with diminished renal function.

Pediatric use

- Serum half-life is prolonged in neonates and infants under age 1.

Breast-feeding

- Drug distributes into breast milk and should be used with caution in breast-feeding women.

cefamandole nafate

Mandol

Pharmacologic classification: second-generation cephalosporin
Therapeutic classification: antibiotic
Pregnancy risk category B

How supplied

Available by prescription only
Injectable solution: 500 mg, 1 g, 2 g
Pharmacy bulk package: 10 g

Indications, route, and dosage

Serious respiratory, GU, skin and soft-tissue, and bone and joint infections; septicemia; peritonitis from susceptible organisms

Adults: 500 mg to 1 g q 4 to 8 hours. In life-threatening infections, up to 2 g q 4 hours may be required.

Infants and children: 50 to 100 mg/kg daily in equally divided doses q 4 to 8 hours. May be increased to total daily dosage of 150 mg/kg (not to exceed maximum adult dose) for severe infections.

Total daily dosage is same for I.M. or I.V. administration and depends on susceptibility of organism and severity of infection. Drug should be injected deep I.M. into a large muscle mass, such as the gluteus or the lateral aspect of the thigh.

✦ ***Dosage adjustment.*** In patients with impaired renal function, doses or frequency of administration must be modified according to degree of renal impairment, severity of infection, and susceptibility of organism.

DOSAGE IN ADULTS

Creatinine clearance (ml/min/ 1.73 m²)	Severe infections	Life-threatening infections (maximum)
> 80	1 to 2 g q 6 hr	2 g q 4 hr
50 to 80	750 mg to 1.5 g q 6 hr	1.5 g q 4 hr; or 2 g q 6 hr
25 to 50	750 mg to 1.5 g q 8 hr	1.5 g q 6 hr; or 2 g q 8 hr
10 to 25	500 mg to 1 g q 8 hr	1 g q 6 hr; or 1.25 g q 8 hr
2 to 10	500 to 750 mg q 12 hr	670 mg q 8 hr; or 1 g q 12 hr
< 2	250 to 500 mg q 12 hr	500 mg q 8 hr; or 750 mg q 12 hr

Pharmacodynamics

Antibacterial action: Cefamandole is primarily bactericidal; however, it may be bacteriostatic. Activity depends on the organism, tissue penetration, drug dosage, and rate of organism multiplication. It acts by adhering to bacterial penicillin-binding proteins, thereby inhibiting cell-wall synthesis.

Cefamandole is active against *Escherichia coli* and other coliform bacteria, *Staphylococcus aureus* (penicillinase– and nonpenicillinase–producing), *Staphylococcus epidermidis,* group A beta-hemolytic streptococci, *Klebsiella, Haemophilus influenzae, Proteus mirabilis,* and *Enterobacter* as the second-generation drugs. *Bacteroides fragilis* and *Acinetobacter* are resistant.

Pharmacokinetics

- *Absorption:* Cefamandole is not absorbed from the GI tract and must be given parenterally; peak serum levels occur ½ to 2 hours after an I.M. dose.
- *Distribution:* Distributed widely into most body tissues and fluids, including the gallbladder, liver, kidneys, bone, sputum, bile, and pleural and synovial fluids; CSF penetration is poor. Cefamandole crosses the placenta; it is 65% to 75% protein-bound.
- *Metabolism:* Cefamandole is not metabolized.
- *Excretion:* Excreted primarily in urine by renal tubular secretion and glomerular filtration; small amounts of drug are excreted in breast milk. Elimination half-life is about ½ to 2 hours in patients with normal renal function; severe renal disease prolongs half-life to 12 to 18 hours. Hemodialysis removes some cefamandole.

Contraindications and precautions

Contraindicated in patients with hypersensitivity to drug or other cephalosporins. Use cautiously in patients with impaired renal function or penicillin allergy and in breast-feeding women.

Interactions

Probenecid competitively inhibits renal tubular secretion of cephalosporins, resulting in higher, prolonged serum levels of these drugs.

Concomitant use with nephrotoxic agents (*vancomycin, colistin, polymyxin B, aminoglycosides*) or *loop diuretics* may increase the risk of nephrotoxicity. Concomitant use of cefamandole with bacteriostatic agents (*tetracyclines, erythromycin, chloramphenicol*) may impair its bactericidal activity.

Concomitant use with *alcohol* may cause severe disulfiram-like reactions. Concomitant use with *anticoagulants* may increase risk of bleeding.

Effects on diagnostic tests

Cefamandole causes false-positive results in urine glucose tests using cupric sulfate (Benedict's reagent or Clinitest); use glucose oxidase tests (Chemstrip uG, Diastix, or glucose enzymatic test strip) instead. Cefamandole also causes false elevations in serum or urine creatinine levels in tests using Jaffé's reaction.

Drug may cause positive Coombs' test results and may elevate liver function test results or PT.

Adverse reactions

GI: pseudomembranous colitis, nausea, vomiting, *diarrhea,* oral candidiasis.
Hematologic: eosinophilia, coagulation abnormalities.
Skin: *maculopapular and erythematous rashes, urticaria.*
Other: hypersensitivity reactions (serum sickness, ***anaphylaxis***); transient increases in liver enzymes; *pain, induration, sterile abscesses,* temperature elevation, tissue sloughing (at injection site); *phlebitis, thrombophlebitis* (with I.V. injection).

Overdose and treatment

Clinical signs of overdose include neuromuscular hypersensitivity. Seizure may follow high CNS concentrations. Hypoprothrombinemia and bleeding may occur; they may be treated with vitamin K or blood products. Some drug may be removed by hemodialysis.

☑ Special considerations

- For most cephalosporin-sensitive organisms, cefamandole offers little advantage over others; it is less effective than cefoxitin against anaerobic infections. Some clinicians consider it inappropriate for pediatric use, especially for serious infections like *Haemophilus influenzae.*
- For I.V. use, reconstitute 1 g with 10 ml of sterile water for injection, 5% dextrose injection, or 0.9% NaCl injection. Administer slowly, over 3 to 5 minutes, or by intermittent infusion or continuous infusion in compatible solutions. Check package insert.
- Do not mix with I.V. infusions containing magnesium or calcium ions, which are chemically incompatible and may cause irreversible effects.
- Cefamandole injection contains 3.3 mEq of sodium per g of drug.
- For I.M. use, dilute 1 g of cefamandole in 3 ml of sterile water for injection, bacteriostatic water for

injection, 0.9% NaCl solution for injection, or 0.9% bacteriostatic NaCl for injection.

• Administer deeply into large muscle mass to ensure maximum absorption. Rotate injection sites.
• I.M. cefamandole is less painful than cefoxitin injection; it does not require addition of lidocaine.
• After reconstitution, solution remains stable for 24 hours at room temperature or 96 hours under refrigeration. Solution should be light yellow to amber. Do not use solution if it is discolored or contains a precipitate.
• Monitor for signs or symptoms of bleeding. Monitor patient's PT and platelet level. Patient may require prophylactic use of vitamin K to prevent bleeding.
• Bleeding can be reversed by administering vitamin K or blood products.
• Concomitant use with alcohol will lead to disulfiram-like reaction. For patients who drink alcohol, consider alternative drugs if home I.V. antibiotic therapy is necessary.

Patient education

• Inform patient of potential adverse reactions.

Geriatric use

• Dosage reduction may be required in patients with diminished renal function. Hypoprothrombinemia and bleeding have been reported most frequently in elderly, malnourished, and debilitated patients.

Pediatric use

• Safe use in infants under age 1 month has not been established.

Breast-feeding

• Drug distributes into breast milk and should be used with caution in breast-feeding women. Safe use has not been established.

cefazolin sodium

Ancef, Kefzol, Zolicef

Pharmacologic classification: first-generation cephalosporin
Therapeutic classification: antibiotic
Pregnancy risk category B

How supplied

Available by prescription only
Injection (parenteral): 250 mg, 500 mg, 1 g, 5 g, 10 g, 20 g
Infusion: 500 mg/50- or 100-ml vial, 1 g/50- or 100-ml vial, 500-mg or 1-g Redi Vials, Faspaks, or ADD-Vantage vials

Indications, route, and dosage

Serious respiratory, GU, skin and soft-tissue, and bone and joint infections; biliary tract infections; septicemia, endocarditis from susceptible organisms

Adults: 250 mg I.M. or I.V. q 8 hours to 1 g q 8 hours. Maximum dosage is 12 g/day in life-threatening situations.

Children over age 1 month: 50 to 100 mg/kg/day I.M. or I.V. in divided doses q 8 hours.

Total daily dosage is same for I.M. or I.V. administration and depends on the susceptibility of organism and severity of infection. Cefazolin should be injected deep I.M. into a large muscle mass, such as the gluteus or the lateral aspect of the thigh.

✦ ***Dosage adjustment.*** Dose or frequency of administration must be modified according to the degree of renal impairment, severity of infection, susceptibility of organism, and serum levels of drug. Because drug can be removed by hemodialysis, patients undergoing hemodialysis may require dosage adjustment.

Creatinine clearance (ml/min/1.73 m²)	Dosage in adults
≥ 55	Usual adult dose
35 to 54	Full dose q 8 hr or less frequently
11 to 34	½ usual dose q 12 hr
≤ 10	½ usual dose q 18 to 24 hr

Creatinine clearance (ml/min/1.73 m²)	Dosage in children
> 70	Usual pediatric dose
40 to 70	60% of normal daily dose q 12 hr
20 to 40	25% of normal daily dose q 12 hr
5 to 20	10% of normal daily dose q 24 hr

Pharmacodynamics

Antibacterial action: Cefazolin is primarily bactericidal; however, it may be bacteriostatic. Activity depends on the organism, tissue penetration, drug dosage, and rate of organism multiplication. It acts by adhering to bacterial penicillin-binding proteins, thereby inhibiting cell-wall synthesis.

Cefazolin is active against *Escherichia coli, Enterobacteriaceae, Haemophilus influenzae, Klebsiella, Proteus mirabilis, Staphylococcus aureus, Streptococcus pneumoniae,* and group A beta-hemolytic streptococci.

Pharmacokinetics

• *Absorption:* Drug is not well absorbed from the GI tract and must be given parenterally; peak serum levels occur 1 to 2 hours after an I.M. dose.
• *Distribution:* Cefazolin is distributed widely into most body tissues and fluids, including the gallbladder, liver kidneys, bone, sputum, bile, and pleural and synovial fluids; CSF penetration is poor. It crosses the placenta; it is 74% to 86% protein-bound.
• *Metabolism:* Cefazolin is not metabolized.
• *Excretion:* Excreted primarily unchanged in urine by renal tubular secretion and glomerular filtration;

small amounts of drug are excreted in breast milk. Elimination half-life is about 1 to 2 hours in patients with normal renal function; end-stage renal disease prolongs half-life to 12 to 50 hours. Hemodialysis or peritoneal dialysis removes cefazolin.

Contraindications and precautions
Contraindicated in patients with hypersensitivity to other cephalosporins. Use cautiously in patients with impaired renal function or penicillin allergy and in breast-feeding women.

Interactions
Probenecid competitively inhibits renal tubular secretion of cephalosporins, resulting in higher, prolonged serum levels of these drugs.

Concomitant use with nephrotoxic agents (*vancomycin, colistin, polymyxin B, aminoglycosides*) or *loop diuretics* may increase the risk of nephrotoxicity.

Concomitant use with bacteriostatic agents (*tetracyclines, erythromycin, chloramphenicol*) may interfere with bactericidal activity.

Effects on diagnostic tests
Cephalosporins cause false-positive results in urine glucose tests utilizing cupric sulfate (Benedict's reagent or Clinitest); use glucose oxidase tests (Chemstrip uG, Diastix, or glucose enzymatic test strip) instead. Cefazolin causes false elevations in serum or urine creatinine levels in tests using Jaffé's reaction.

Cefazolin also causes positive Coombs' test results and may elevate liver function test results.

Adverse reactions
GI: pseudomembranous colitis, nausea, anorexia, vomiting, *diarrhea,* glossitis, dyspepsia, abdominal cramps, anal pruritus, oral candidiasis.
GU: genital pruritus, candidiasis, vaginitis.
Hematologic: ***neutropenia,*** leukopenia, eosinophilia, ***thrombocytopenia.***
Skin: *maculopapular and erythematous rashes, urticaria, pruritus.*
Other: hypersensitivity reactions (serum sickness, ***anaphylaxis***); transient increases in liver enzymes; Stevens-Johnson syndrome; *pain, induration, sterile abscesses, tissue sloughing* (at injection site); *phlebitis, thrombophlebitis* (with I.V. injection).

Overdose and treatment
Clinical signs of overdose include neuromuscular hypersensitivity; seizure may follow high CNS concentrations. Remove cefazolin by hemodialysis.

☑ Special considerations
Besides those relevant to all *cephalosporins*, consider the following recommendations.
- For patients on sodium restrictions, note that cefazolin injection contains 2 mEq of sodium per gram of drug.
- Because of the long duration of effect, most infections can be treated with a single dose every 8 hours.
- For I.M. use, reconstitute with sterile water, bacteriostatic water, or 0.9% NaCl solution: 2 ml to a 250-mg vial, 2 ml to a 500-mg vial, and 2.5 ml to a 1-g vial produces concentrations of 125 mg/ml, 225 mg/ml, and 330 mg/ml respectively.
- Reconstituted solution is stable for 24 hours at room temperature; for 96 hours if refrigerated.
- I.M. cefazolin injection is less painful than that of other cephalosporins.

Patient education
- Inform patient of potential adverse reactions.

Pediatric use
- Cefazolin has been used in children. However, safety in infants under age 1 month has not been established.

Breast-feeding
- Safety has not been established. Drug should be used with caution in breast-feeding women.

cefdinir
Omnicef

Pharmacologic classification: third-generation cephalosporin
Therapeutic classification: antibiotic
Pregnancy risk category B

How supplied
Available by prescription only
Capsules: 300 mg
Suspension: 125 mg/5 ml

Indications, route, and dosage
Treatment of mild to moderate infections caused by susceptible strains of microorganisms for conditions of community-acquired pneumonia, acute exacerbations of chronic bronchitis, acute maxillary sinusitis, acute bacterial otitis media, and uncomplicated skin and skin structure infections
Adults and adolescents age 13 and older: 300 mg P.O. q 12 hours or 600 mg P.O. q 24 hours for 10 days. (Use q 12-hour dosages for pneumonia and skin infections.)
Children age 6 months to 12 years: 7 mg/kg P.O. q 12 hours or 14 mg/kg P.O. q 24 hours for 10 days, up to maximum dose of 600 mg daily. (Use q 12-hour dosages for skin infections.)
Treatment of pharyngitis and tonsillitis
Adults and adolescents age 13 and older: 300 mg P.O. q 12 hours for 5 to 10 days or 600 mg P.O. q 24 hours for 10 days.
Children 6 months to 12 years: 7 mg/kg P.O. q 12 hours for 5 to 10 days or 14 mg/kg P.O. q 24 hours for 10 days.
✦ ***Dosage adjustment.*** If creatinine clearance is below 30 ml/minute, reduce dosage to 300 mg P.O. once daily for adults and 7 mg/kg P.O. (up to 300 mg) once daily for children.

In patients receiving chronic hemodialysis, 300 mg or 7 mg/kg P.O. at end of each dialysis session and subsequently every other day.

Pharmacodynamics

Antibiotic action: Cefdinir's bactericidal activity results from inhibition of cell wall synthesis. Drug is stable in the presence of some beta-lactamase enzymes, causing some microorganisms resistant to penicillins and cephalosporins to be susceptible to cefdinir. Excluding *Pseudomonas, Enterobacter, Enterococcus,* and methicillin-resistant *Staphylococcus* species, cefdinir's spectrum of activity includes a broad range of gram-positive and gram-negative aerobic microorganisms.

Pharmacokinetics

- *Absorption:* Estimated bioavailability of drug is 21% following administration of a 300-mg capsule dose, 16% following a 600-mg capsule dose, and 25% for the suspension. After administration of capsule or suspension, peak plasma levels occur in 2 to 4 hours; food does not affect absorption.
- *Distribution:* Mean volume of distribution for adults and children is 0.35 and 0.67 L/kg, respectively; distribution to tonsil, sinus, lung, and middle ear tissue and fluid is 15% to 35% of corresponding plasma levels. Drug is 60% to 70% bound to plasma proteins; binding is independent of concentration.
- *Metabolism:* Drug is not metabolized; its activity is due mainly to parent drug.
- *Excretion:* Principally by renal excretion; mean plasma elimination half-life is 1.7 hours. Drug clearance is reduced in patients with renal dysfunction.

Contraindications and precautions

Contraindicated in patients with known allergy to cephalosporins. Use cautiously in patients with known hypersensitivity to penicillin because of risk of cross-sensitivity with other beta-lactam antibiotics and in those with history of colitis.

Interactions

Antacids (magnesium- and aluminum-containing), iron supplements, and *foods fortified with iron (infant formula)* decrease cefdinir's rate of absorption and bioavailability. Administer such preparations 2 hours before or after cefdinir dose. As with other beta-lactam antibiotics, *probenecid* inhibits the renal excretion of cefdinir.

Effects on diagnostic tests

False-positive reactions for ketones (tests using nitroprusside only) and glucose (Clinitest, Benedict's solution, Fehling's solution) in the urine have been reported. Generally, cephalosporins can induce a positive direct Coombs' test.

Adverse reactions

CNS: headache.
GI: abdominal pain, *diarrhea,* nausea, vomiting.
GU: vaginal candidiasis, vaginitis.
Skin: rash.

Overdose and treatment

Information is not available in humans. Toxic signs of overdosage with other beta-lactam antibiotics include nausea, vomiting, epigastric distress, diarrhea, and seizures. Drug is removed by hemodialysis.

Special considerations

- As with many antibiotics, prolonged drug treatment may result in possible emergence and overgrowth of resistant organisms. Alternative therapy should be considered if superinfection occurs.
- Pseudomembranous colitis has been reported with many antibiotics, including cefdinir, and should be considered in diagnosing patients who present with diarrhea subsequent to antibiotic therapy or in those with history of colitis.

Patient education

- Instruct patient to take antacids, iron supplements, and iron-fortified foods 2 hours before or after a dose of cefdinir.
- Inform diabetic patient that each teaspoon of suspension contains 2.86 g of sucrose.
- Tell patient that drug may be taken without regard to meals.
- Advise patient to report severe diarrhea or diarrhea accompanied by abdominal pain.
- Tell patient that mild diarrhea can be treated symptomatically.

Geriatric use

- Cefdinir is well-tolerated in all age groups. Safety and efficacy are comparable in elderly patients and younger patients. Dosage adjustment is not necessary unless patient has renal impairment.

Pediatric use

- Safety and efficacy in infants under age 6 months have not been established. Pharmacokinetic data for pediatric population are comparable to adults.

Breast-feeding

- Drug is not detectable in breast milk following 600-mg doses.

cefepime hydrochloride

Maxipime

Pharmacologic classification: semisynthetic third- or fourth-generation cephalosporin
Therapeutic classification: antibiotic
Pregnancy risk category B

How supplied

Available by prescription only
Injection: 500 mg/15 ml vial, 1 g/100 ml piggyback bottle, 1 g/ADD-Vantage vial, 1 g/15 ml vial, 2 g/100 ml piggyback bottle, 2 g/20 ml vial

Indications, route, and dosage

Mild to moderate urinary tract infections caused by* Escherichia coli, Klebsiella pneumoniae, *or* Proteus mirabilis, *including cases associated with concurrent bacteremia with these microorganisms

Adults and children age 12 and older: 0.5 to 1 g I.M. (use I.M. route only for infections caused by *E. coli*), or I.V. infused over 30 minutes q 12 hours for 7 to 10 days.

***Severe urinary tract infections including pyelonephritis caused by* E. coli *or* K. pneumoniae**
Adults and children age 12 and older: 2 g I.V. infused over 30 minutes q 12 hours for 10 days.
Moderate to severe pneumonia caused by* Streptococcus pneumoniae, Pseudomonas aeruginosa, K. pneumoniae, *or* Enterobacter *species
Adults and children age 12 and older: 1 to 2 g I.V. infused over 30 minutes q 12 hours for 10 days.
***Moderate to severe uncomplicated skin and skin structure infections due to* Staphylococcus aureus *(methicillin-susceptible strains only) or* Streptococcus pyogenes**
Adults and children age 12 and older: 2 g I.V. infused over 30 minutes q 12 hours for 10 days.
✦ ***Dosage adjustment.*** Adjust dosage in patients with impaired renal function.

Pharmacodynamics

Antibiotic action: Cefepime exerts its bactericidal action by inhibition of cell-wall synthesis. It is usually active against gram-positive microorganisms such as *S. pneumoniae, S. aureus,* and *S. pyogenes* and gram-negative microorganisms such as *Enterobacter* species, *E. coli, K. pneumoniae, P. mirabilis,* and *P. aeruginosa.*

Pharmacokinetics

- *Absorption:* Cefepime is completely absorbed after I.M. administration.
- *Distribution:* Drug is widely distributed and is about 20% bound to serum protein.
- *Metabolism:* Cefepime is metabolized rapidly.
- *Excretion:* About 85% is excreted in urine as unchanged drug; less than 1% as the metabolite, 6.8% as the metabolite oxide, and 2.5% as an epimer of cefepime.

Contraindications and precautions

Contraindicated in patients with hypersensitivity to drug, other cephalosporins, penicillins, or other beta-lactam antibiotics. Use cautiously in patients with history of GI disease (especially colitis), impaired renal function, or poor nutritional status and in those receiving a protracted course of antimicrobial therapy.

Interactions

Aminoglycosides may increase risk of nephrotoxicity and ototoxicity. Monitor patient's renal and hearing functions closely. *Potent diuretics* such as *furosemide* may increase risk of nephrotoxicity. Monitor patient's renal function closely.

Effects on diagnostic tests

Cefepime may result in a false-positive reaction for glucose in the urine when using Clinitest tablets. Glucose tests based on enzymatic glucose oxidase reactions (such as Chemstrip uG, Diastix, or glucose enzymatic test strip) should be used instead. A positive direct Coombs' test may occur during treatment with drug.

Adverse reactions

CNS: headache.
GI: colitis, diarrhea, nausea, vomiting, oral moniliasis.
GU: vaginitis.
Skin: rash, pruritus, urticaria.
Other: phlebitis, pain, inflammation, fever.

Overdose and treatment

Overdosage may result in the patient experiencing seizures, encephalopathy, and neuromuscular excitability. Patients who receive an overdose should be carefully observed and given supportive treatment. In the presence of renal insufficiency, hemodialysis, not peritoneal dialysis, is recommended to aid in the removal of cefepime from the body.

☑ Special considerations

Besides those relevant to all *cephalosporins,* consider the following recommendations.

- Obtain culture and sensitivity tests before giving first dose, if appropriate. Therapy may begin pending results.
- For I.V. administration, follow manufacturer guidelines closely when reconstituting drug. Variations occur in constituting drug for administration and depend on concentration of drug required and how drug is packaged (piggyback vial, ADD-Vantage vial, or regular vial). Also know that type of diluent used for constitution varies, depending on product used. Use only solutions recommended by manufacturer. The resulting solution should be administered over 30 minutes.
- Intermittent I.V. infusion with a Y-type administration set can be accomplished with compatible solutions. However, during infusion of a solution containing cefepime, discontinuing the other solution is recommended.
- For I.M. administration, constitute drug using sterile water for injection, 0.9% NaCl solution, 5% dextrose injection, 5% or 1% lidocaine hydrochloride, or bacteriostatic water for injection with parabens or benzyl alcohol. Follow manufacturer guidelines for quantity of diluent to use.
- Inspect solution visually for particulate matter before administration. The powder and its solutions tend to darken depending on storage conditions. However, product potency is not adversely affected when stored as recommended.
- Monitor patient for superinfection. Drug may cause overgrowth of nonsusceptible bacteria or fungi.
- Know that many cephalosporins may cause a fall in prothrombin activity; patients at risk include those with renal or hepatic impairment or poor nutritional status and those receiving prolonged cefepime therapy. Monitor PT in these patients. Administer exogenous vitamin K if necessary.

Patient education

- Warn patient receiving drug I.M. that pain may occur at injection site.
- Instruct patient to report adverse reactions immediately.

Geriatric use

- Use caution when administering cefepime to elderly patients. Dosage adjustment may be necessary in patients with impaired renal function.

Pediatric use
• Safety and effectiveness in children under age 12 have not been established.

Breast-feeding
• Use caution when administering cefepime to breast-feeding women because drug is excreted in breast milk in very low concentrations.

cefixime
Suprax

Pharmacologic classification: third-generation cephalosporin
Therapeutic classification: antibiotic
Pregnancy risk category B

How supplied
Available by prescription only
Tablets: 200 mg, 400 mg
Powder for oral suspension: 100 mg/5 ml

Indications, route, and dosage
Otitis media; acute bronchitis; acute exacerbations of chronic bronchitis, pharyngitis, tonsillitis; uncomplicated urinary tract infections caused by* Escherichia coli *and* Proteus mirabilis; *uncomplicated gonorrhea
Adults: 400 mg P.O. daily in one or two divided doses; for uncomplicated gonorrhea, 400 mg as a single dose.
Children over age 6 months: 8 mg/kg P.O. daily in one or two divided doses.
✦ ***Dosage adjustment.*** In renally impaired patients, doses must be adjusted based on degree of renal impairment, severity of infection, and susceptibility of organism. To prevent toxic accumulation in patients with creatinine clearance below 60 ml/minute/1.73 m^2, reduced dosage may be needed.

Creatinine clearance (ml/min/1.73 m^2)	Dosage in adults
> 60	Usual dose
20 to 60	75% of usual dose
< 20 or patients receiving continuous ambulatory peritoneal dialysis	50% of usual dose

Pharmacodynamics
Antibacterial action: Cefixime is primarily bactericidal; it acts by binding to penicillin-binding proteins in the bacterial cell wall, thereby inhibiting cell-wall synthesis.

It is used in the treatment of otitis media caused by *Haemophilus influenzae* (penicillinase- and non-penicillinase-producing), *Moraxella (Branhamella) catarrhalis* (which is penicillinase-producing), and *Streptococcus pyogenes.* Substantial drug resistance has been noted. Cefixime is also active in the treatment of acute bronchitis and acute exacerbations of chronic bronchitis caused by *S. pneumoniae* and *H. influenzae* (penicillinase- and non-penicillinase-producing), pharyngitis and tonsillitis caused by *S. pyogenes,* and uncomplicated urinary tract infections caused by *E. coli* and *P. mirabilis.*

Pharmacokinetics
• *Absorption:* About 30% to 50% is absorbed following oral administration. The suspension form provides a higher serum level than the tablet form. Absorption is delayed by food, but the total amount absorbed is not affected.
• *Distribution:* Cefixime is widely distributed; about 65% is bound to plasma proteins.
• *Metabolism:* About 50% of drug is metabolized.
• *Excretion:* Cefixime is excreted primarily in the urine. The elimination half-life in patients with normal renal function is 3 to 4 hours. In patients with end-stage renal disease, half-life may be prolonged to 11½ hours

Contraindications and precautions
Contraindicated in patients with hypersensitivity to drug or other cephalosporins. Use cautiously in patients with impaired renal function.

Interactions
Salicylates may increase serum concentration of cefixime.

Effects on diagnostic tests
Cefixime may cause false-positive results in urine glucose tests utilizing cupric sulfate (Benedict's reagent or Clinitest); use glucose oxidase tests (Chemstrip uG, Diastix, or glucose enzymatic test strip) instead. Cefixime may cause false-positive results in tests for urine ketones that utilize nitroprusside (but not nitroferricyanide).

False-positive direct Coombs' test results have been seen with other cephalosporins.

Adverse reactions
CNS: headache, dizziness.
GI: *diarrhea,* loose stools, abdominal pain, nausea, vomiting, dyspepsia, flatulence, pseudomembranous colitis.
GU: genital pruritus, vaginitis, genital candidiasis, transient increases in BUN and serum creatinine levels.
Hematologic: ***thrombocytopenia,*** leukopenia, eosinophilia.
Skin: pruritus, rash, urticaria, erythema multiforme, Stevens-Johnson syndrome.
Other: drug fever, transient increases in liver enzymes, hypersensitivity reactions (serum sickness, ***anaphylaxis***).

Overdose and treatment
No specific antidote available. Gastric lavage and supportive treatment are recommended. Peritoneal dialysis and hemodialysis will remove substantial quantities of drug.

Studies in volunteers revealed no unusual effects after acute ingestion of 2 g of cefixime.

☑ Special considerations

Besides those relevant to all *cephalosporins*, consider the following recommendations.

- Cefixime is the first orally active, third-generation cephalosporin that is effective with once-daily dosage.
- The manufacturer suggests that tablets should not be substituted for suspension when treating otitis media.
- Patients with antibiotic-induced diarrhea should be evaluated for overgrowth of pseudomembranous colitis caused by *Clostridium difficile.* Mild cases usually respond to discontinuation of the drug; moderate to severe cases may require fluid, electrolyte, and protein supplementation. Oral vancomycin is the drug of choice for the treatment of antibiotic-associated *C. difficile* pseudomembranous colitis.
- Acute hypersensitivity reactions should be treated immediately. Emergency measures, such as airway management, pressor amines, epinephrine, oxygen, antihistamines, and corticosteroids, may be required.
- Some cephalosporins may cause seizures, especially in patients with renal failure who receive full therapeutic dosages. If seizures occur, discontinue drug and initiate anticonvulsant therapy.

Patient education

- Instruct patient to report unpleasant effects, such as itching, rash, or severe diarrhea. Note that diarrhea is the most common adverse GI effect.
- Advise patient that oral suspension is stable for 14 days after reconstitution and does not require refrigeration.

Pediatric use

- The incidence of adverse GI effects in children receiving oral suspension is similar to those in adults receiving tablets.

Breast-feeding

- Distribution of drug in breast milk is unknown. The manufacturer recommends that discontinuation of breast-feeding should be considered during cefixime therapy.

cefmetazole sodium

Zefazone

Pharmacologic classification: second-generation cephalosporin
Therapeutic classification: antibiotic
Pregnancy risk category B

How supplied

Available by prescription only
Injection: 1 g, 2 g

Indications, route, and dosage

Serious respiratory, urinary, skin and soft-tissue, abdominal, and ◇ pelvic infections caused by susceptible organisms

Adults: 2 g I.V. q 6 to 12 hours for 5 to 14 days.

Perioperative prophylaxis

Adults: 1 to 2 g I.V. administered 30 to 90 minutes before the procedure. Can repeat dose 8 and 16 hours after first dose for prolonged (over 4 hours) procedures.

✦ ***Dosage adjustment.*** In adult patients with creatinine clearance of 50 to 90 ml/minute, give 1 to 2 g I.V. q 12 hours; if 30 to 49 ml/minute, give 1 to 2 g I.V. q 16 hours; if 10 to 29 ml/minute, 1 to 2 g I.V. q 24 hours; and if it is below 10 ml/minute, give 1 to 2 g I.V. q 48 hours.

Pharmacodynamics

Antibacterial action: Cefmetazole is primarily bactericidal; however, it may be bacteriostatic. Activity depends on the organism, tissue penetration, drug dosage, and rate of organism multiplication. It acts by adhering to bacterial penicillin-binding proteins, thereby inhibiting cell-wall synthesis.

Drug's spectrum of activity resembles that of other second-generation cephalosporins. It is active against many gram-positive organisms and enteric gram-negative bacilli, including *Escherichia coli* and other coliform bacteria, *Staphylococcus aureus* (penicillinase- and nonpenicillinase-producing), *Staphylococcus epidermidis,* streptococci, *Klebsiella, Haemophilus influenzae,* and *Bacteroides* species (including *B. fragilis*). *Enterobacter, Pseudomonas, Acinetobacter, Serratia marcescens, Citrobacter freundii,* and methicillin-resistant *Staphylococcus* are generally resistant to cefmetazole.

Pharmacokinetics

- *Absorption:* Cefmetazole is not absorbed from the GI tract and must be given parenterally. Peak serum levels occur 1½ hours after an I.M. dose.
- *Distribution:* Distributed widely in most body tissues and fluids, including the gallbladder, liver, kidney, bone, sputum, bile, and pleural and synovial fluids. CSF penetration is poor. Cefmetazole is 65% protein-bound.
- *Metabolism:* Only about 15% of a dose is metabolized, probably in the liver.
- *Excretion:* Drug is excreted primarily in the urine by renal tubular secretion and glomerular filtration. Elimination half-life is approximately 1.5 hours in patients with normal renal function. Patients with renal dysfunction require dosage adjustment.

Contraindications and precautions

Contraindicated in patients with hypersensitivity to drug or other cephalosporins. Use cautiously in patients with penicillin allergy and in breast-feeding women.

Interactions

Probenecid competitively inhibits renal tubular secretion of cephalosporins, resulting in higher, prolonged serum levels of these drugs.

Concomitant use of cefmetazole with nephrotoxic agents (*vancomycin, colistin, polymyxin B, aminoglycosides*) or *loop diuretics* may increase the risk of nephrotoxicity. Concomitant use with bacteriostatic agents (*tetracyclines, erythromycin, chloramphenicol*) may impair cefmetazole's bactéricidal activity. Concomitant use with *alcohol* may cause disulfiram-like reactions.

Effects on diagnostic tests

Cefmetazole causes false-positive results of urine glucose tests that use cupric sulfate (Benedict's reagent or Clinitest); use glucose oxidase tests (Chemstrip uG, Diastix, or glucose enzymatic test strip) instead.

Cefmetazole may cause positive Coombs' test results and may elevate liver function test results.

Adverse reactions

CNS: headache, hot flashes.
CV: *shock,* hypotension.
EENT: epistaxis.
GI: nausea, vomiting, *diarrhea,* epigastric pain, pseudomembranous colitis, candidiasis, bleeding.
GU: vaginitis.
Respiratory: pleural effusion, dyspnea, respiratory distress.
Skin: rash, pruritus, generalized erythema.
Other: fever, bacterial or fungal superinfection, hypersensitivity reactions (serum sickness, ***anaphylaxis***), altered color perception, pain at injection site, phlebitis, thrombophlebitis, joint pain and inflammation.

Overdose and treatment

Clinical signs of overdose include neuromuscular hypersensitivity. Seizure may follow high CNS concentrations. Hypoprothrombinemia and bleeding may occur; they may be treated with vitamin K or blood products. Some cefmetazole may be removed by hemodialysis.

☑ Special considerations

- For most cephalosporin-sensitive organisms, cefmetazole offers little advantage over other cephalosporins.
- Concomitant use with alcohol will lead to disulfiram-like reactions. Use cautiously with home I.V. antibiotic patients who drink alcohol, or consider alternative drug therapy.
- Cefmetazole injection contains 2 mEq of sodium per gram of drug.
- Do not use Zefazone I.V. Solution for I.M. administration; I.M. administration is indicated only in treatment of gonorrhea.
- Hypoprothrombinemia may occur. If bleeding occurs or if PT increases, this can be reversed by administering vitamin K.

Patient education

- Inform patient of potential adverse reactions including the possible alteration of color perception.
- Instruct patient to report respiratory problems promptly.

Geriatric use

- Dosage reduction may be required in patients with diminished renal function. Hypoprothrombinemia and bleeding have been reported most frequently in elderly, malnourished, and debilitated patients.

Pediatric use

- Safety and efficacy have not been established.

Breast-feeding

- Trace concentrations have been detected in breast milk. Consider temporarily discontinuing breast-feeding during therapy.

cefonicid sodium

Monocid

Pharmacologic classification: second-generation cephalosporin
Therapeutic classification: antibiotic
Pregnancy risk category B

How supplied

Available by prescription only
Injection: 500 mg, 1 g
Infusion: 1 g
Pharmacy bulk package: 10 g

Indications, route, and dosage

Serious lower respiratory, urinary tract, skin, and skin-structure infections; septicemia; bone and joint infections from susceptible organisms
Adults: Usual dosage is 1 g I.V. or I.M. q 24 hours. In life-threatening infections, 2 g q 24 hours.
Preoperative prophylaxis
Adults: 1 g I.M. or I.V. 1 hour before surgery.
◊ ***Uncomplicated gonorrhea***
Adults: 1 g I.M. as a single dose.

Total daily dosage is same for I.M. or I.V. administration and depends on susceptibility of organism and severity of infection. Cefonicid should be injected deep I.M. into a large muscle mass, such as the gluteus or the lateral aspect of the thigh.

✦ ***Dosage adjustment.*** In patients with impaired renal function, doses or frequency of administration must be modified according to degree of renal impairment, severity of infection, and susceptibility of organism. To prevent toxic accumulation, reduced dosage may be necessary in patients with creatinine clearance below 80 ml/minute (see chart below). Because drug is dialyzable, patients undergoing treatment with hemodialysis may require dosage adjustment.

DOSAGE IN ADULTS

Creatinine clearance (ml/min/1.73 m²)	Mild to moderate infections	Severe infections
≥ 80	Usual adult dose	Usual adult dose
60 to 79	10 mg/kg q 24 hr	25 mg/kg q 24 hr
40 to 59	8 mg/kg q 24 hr	20 mg/kg q 24 hr
20 to 39	4 mg/kg q 24 hr	15 mg/kg q 24 hr

(continued)

DOSAGE IN ADULTS *(continued)*

Creatinine clearance (ml/min/ 1.73 m²)	Mild to moderate infections	Severe infections
10 to 19	4 mg/kg q 48 hr	15 mg/kg q 48 hr
5 to 9	4 mg/kg q 3 to 5 days	15 mg/kg q 3 to 5 days
< 5	3 mg/kg q 3 to 5 days	4 mg/kg q 3 to 5 days

Pharmacodynamics

Antibacterial action: Cefonicid is primarily bactericidal; however, it may be bacteriostatic. Activity depends on the organism, tissue penetration, drug dosage, and rate of organism multiplication. It acts by adhering to bacterial penicillin-binding proteins, thereby inhibiting cell-wall synthesis.

Cefonicid is active against many gram-positive organisms and enteric gram-negative bacilli, including *Streptococcus pneumoniae, Klebsiella pneumoniae, Escherichia coli, Haemophilus influenzae, Proteus mirabilis, Staphylococcus aureus* and *S. epidermidis,* and *Streptococcus pyogenes;* however, *Bacteroides fragilis, Pseudomonas,* and *Acinetobacter* are resistant to cefonicid. Cefonicid is less effective than cefamandole or cefuroxime against gram-positive cocci; it is twice as effective as cefamandole against *H. influenzae* and slightly more active than cefamandole or cefoxitin against gonococci.

Pharmacokinetics

- *Absorption:* Cefonicid is not absorbed from the GI tract and must be given parenterally; peak serum levels occur 1 to 2 hours after an I.M. dose.
- *Distribution:* Distributed widely into most body tissues and fluids, including the gallbladder, liver, kidneys, bone, sputum, bile, and pleural and synovial fluids; CSF penetration is poor. Cefonicid is 90% to 98% protein-bound. Drug crosses the placenta.
- *Metabolism:* Cefonicid is not metabolized.
- *Excretion:* Excreted primarily in urine by renal tubular secretion and glomerular filtration; small amounts of drug are excreted in breast milk. Elimination half-life is about 3½ to 6 hours in patients with normal renal function; 100 hours in patients with severe renal disease. Hemodialysis partially removes cefonicid.

Contraindications and precautions

Contraindicated in patients with hypersensitivity to drug or other cephalosporins. Use cautiously in patients with impaired renal function or penicillin allergy and in breast-feeding women.

Interactions

Probenecid competitively inhibits renal tubular secretion of cephalosporins, resulting in higher, prolonged serum levels of these drugs.

Concomitant use with nephrotoxic agents *(vancomycin, colistin, polymyxin B, aminoglycosides)* or *loop diuretics* may increase the risk of nephrotoxicity.

Concomitant use with bacteriostatic agents *(tetracyclines, erythromycin, chloramphenicol)* may interfere with bactericidal activity.

Effects on diagnostic tests

Cefonicid causes positive Coombs' test results and may elevate liver function test results or PT. Cefonicid also causes false-positive results in urine glucose tests using cupric sulfate (Benedict's reagent or Clinitest); use glucose oxidase tests (Chemstrip uG, Diastix, or glucose enzymatic test strip) instead.

Cefonicid causes false elevations in serum or urine creatinine levels in tests using Jaffé's reaction.

Adverse reactions

CNS: dizziness, headache, malaise, paresthesia.
GI: pseudomembranous colitis, diarrhea.
GU: *acute renal failure,* interstitial nephritis.
Hematologic: neutropenia, leukopenia, eosinophilia, anemia, thrombocytosis, ***thrombocytopenia.***
Skin: *maculopapular and erythematous rashes, urticaria.*
Other: hypersensitivity reactions (serum sickness, ***anaphylaxis***); *pain, induration, sterile abscesses, tissue sloughing* (at injection site); *phlebitis, thrombophlebitis,* fever, myalgia (with I.V. injection).

Overdose and treatment

Clinical signs of overdose include neuromuscular hypersensitivity. Seizure may follow high CNS concentrations. Some cefonicid may be removed by hemodialysis.

☑ Special considerations

Besides those relevant to all *cephalosporins,* consider the following recommendations.

- When used for surgical prophylaxis, administer drug 1 hour before surgery.
- For patients on sodium restrictions, note that cefonicid injection contains 3.7 mEq of sodium per gram of drug.
- Reconstitute I.M. or bolus I.V. dose with sterile water for injection. Shake well to ensure complete drug dissolution. Check for precipitate. Discard solution that contains a precipitate.
- Administer deep I.M. dose into a large muscle mass to decrease pain and local irritation. Rotate injection sites. Apply ice to site after administration to reduce pain. Do not inject more than 1 g into a single I.M. site.
- For I.V. infusion, further dilute drug in 50 to 100 ml of recommended fluid. Administer I.V. bolus slowly over 3 to 5 minutes directly or through I.V. tubing if solution is compatible.
- Reconstituted solution is stable at room temperature for 24 hours; if refrigerated, for 72 hours. Slight yellowing of solution does not indicate loss of potency.

Patient education

- Inform patient of potential adverse reactions.

Geriatric use
- Reduced dosage may be required in patients with diminished renal function.

Pediatric use
- Safety in children has not been established.

Breast-feeding
- Drug distributes into breast milk and should be used with caution in breast-feeding women.

cefoperazone sodium
Cefobid

Pharmacologic classification: third-generation cephalosporin
Therapeutic classification: antibiotic
Pregnancy risk category B

How supplied
Available by prescription only
Parenteral: 1 g, 2 g
Infusion: 1 g, 2 g piggyback

Indications, route, and dosage
Serious respiratory tract, intra-abdominal, gynecologic, skin and structure, urinary tract, and enterococcal infections; bacterial septicemia caused by susceptible organisms
Adults: Usual dosage is 1 to 2 g q 12 hours I.M. or I.V. In severe infections or infections caused by less sensitive organisms, the total daily dosage or frequency may be increased up to 16 g/day in certain situations.

✦ ***Dosage adjustment.*** No dosage adjustment is usually necessary in patients with renal impairment. However, doses of 4 g/day should be given cautiously to patients with hepatic disease. Adults with combined hepatic and renal function impairment should not receive more than 1 g (base) daily without serum determinations. In patients who are receiving hemodialysis treatments, a dose should be scheduled to follow hemodialysis.

Pharmacodynamics
Antibacterial action: Cefoperazone is primarily bactericidal; however, it may be bacteriostatic. Activity depends on the organism, tissue penetration, drug dosage, and rate of organism multiplication. It acts by adhering to bacterial penicillin-binding proteins, thereby inhibiting cell-wall synthesis. Third-generation cephalosporins appear more active against some beta-lactamase–producing gram-negative organisms.

Cefoperazone is active against some gram-positive organisms and many enteric gram-negative bacilli, including *Streptococcus pneumoniae* and *Streptococcus pyogenes, Staphylococcus aureus* (penicillinase- and nonpenicillinase-producing), *Staphylococcus epidermidis, Escherichia coli, Klebsiella, Haemophilus influenzae, Enterobacter, Citrobacter, Proteus,* some *Pseudomonas* species (including *Pseudomonas aeruginosa),* and *Bacteroides fragilis. Acinetobacter* and *Listeria* usually are resistant. Cefoperazone is less effective than moxalactam, cefotaxime, or ceftizoxime against Enterobacteriaceae but is slightly more active than those drugs against *Pseudomonas aeruginosa.*

Pharmacokinetics
- *Absorption:* Cefoperazone is not absorbed from the GI tract and must be given parenterally; peak serum levels occur 1 to 2 hours after an I.M. dose.
- *Distribution:* Drug is distributed widely into most body tissues and fluids, including the gallbladder, liver, kidneys, bone, sputum, bile, and pleural and synovial fluids; CSF penetration is achieved in patients with inflamed meninges. It crosses the placenta. Protein binding is dose-dependent and decreases as serum levels rise; average is 82% to 93%.
- *Metabolism:* Cefoperazone is not substantially metabolized.
- *Excretion:* Excreted primarily in bile; some drug is excreted in urine by renal tubular secretion and glomerular filtration; and small amounts, in breast milk. Elimination half-life is about 1½ to 2½ hours in patients with normal hepatorenal function; biliary obstruction or cirrhosis prolongs half-life to about 3½ to 7 hours. Hemodialysis removes cefoperazone.

Contraindications and precautions
Contraindicated in patients with hypersensitivity to drug or other cephalosporins. Use cautiously in patients with impaired renal or hepatic function or penicillin allergy and in breast-feeding women.

Interactions
Concomitant use with *aminoglycosides* results in synergistic activity against *Pseudomonas aeruginosa* and *Serratia marcescens;* such combined use slightly increases the risk of nephrotoxicity.

Concomitant use with *clavulanic acid* results in synergistic activity against many Enterobacteriaceae, *Bacteroides fragilis, P. aeruginosa,* and *S. aureus.*

Concomitant use with *alcohol* may cause disulfiram-like reactions (flushing, sweating, tachycardia, headache, and abdominal cramping).

Probenecid competitively inhibits renal tubular secretions of cephalosporins, causing prolonged serum levels of these drugs.

Concomitant use with *anticoagulants* may increase risk of bleeding.

Effects on diagnostic tests
Cephalosporins cause false-positive results in urine glucose tests using cupric sulfate (Benedict's reagent or Clinitest); use glucose oxidase (Chemstrip uG, Diastix, or glucose enzymatic test strip) instead.

Cefoperazone may cause positive Coombs' test results, and elevated liver function test results and PT.

Adverse reactions
GI: pseudomembranous colitis, nausea, vomiting, *diarrhea.*
Hematologic: transient neutropenia, *eosinophilia,* anemia, hypoprothrombinemia, bleeding.

Skin: *maculopapular and erythematous rashes, urticaria.*
Other: mildly elevated liver enzymes; hypersensitivity reactions (serum sickness, ***anaphylaxis***); *pain, induration, sterile abscesses, temperature elevation, tissue sloughing* (at injection site); *phlebitis, thrombophlebitis,* drug fever (with I.V. injection).

Overdose and treatment
Clinical signs of overdose include neuromuscular hypersensitivity. Seizure may follow high CNS concentrations. Hypoprothrombinemia and bleeding may occur and may require treatment with vitamin K or blood products. Hemodialysis will remove cefoperazone.

☑ Special considerations
Besides those relevant to all *cephalosporins,* consider the following recommendations.
- Diarrhea may be more common with drug than with other cephalosporins because of high degree of biliary excretion.
- Patients with biliary disease may need lower doses.
- For patients on sodium restriction, note that cefoperazone injection contains 1.5 mEq of sodium per gram of drug.
- To prepare I.M. injection, use the appropriate diluent, including sterile water for injection or bacteriostatic water for injection. Follow manufacturer's recommendations for mixing drug with sterile water for injection and lidocaine 2% injection. Final solution for I.M. injection will contain 0.5% lidocaine and will be less painful upon administration (recommended for concentrations of 250 mg/ml or greater). Cefoperazone should be injected deep I.M. into a large muscle mass, such as the gluteus or the lateral aspect of the thigh.
- Store drug in refrigerator and away from light before reconstituting.
- Allow solution to stand after reconstituting to allow foam to dissipate and solution to clear. Solution can be shaken vigorously to ensure complete drug dissolution.
- After reconstitution, solution is stable for 24 hours at a controlled room temperature or 3 days if refrigerated. Protecting drug from light is unnecessary.
- Because cefoperazone is dialyzable, patients undergoing treatment with hemodialysis may require dosage adjustment.
- Concomitant use with alcohol can lead to disulfiram-like reaction. Use drug cautiously in home antibiotic therapy patients who drink alcohol, or consider alternate drug therapy.

Patient education
- Inform patient of potential adverse reactions.
- Caution patient against the use of alcohol.

Geriatric use
- Hypoprothrombinemia and bleeding have been reported more frequently in elderly patients. Use with caution, and monitor PT and check for signs of abnormal bleeding.

Pediatric use
- Safety and effectiveness in children under age 12 have not been established.

Breast-feeding
- Drug distributes into breast milk and should be used with caution in breast-feeding women.

cefotaxime sodium
Claforan

Pharmacologic classification: third-generation cephalosporin
Therapeutic classification: antibiotic
Pregnancy risk category B

How supplied
Available by prescription only
Injection: 1 g, 2 g
Pharmacy bulk package: 10-g vial
Infusion: 1 g, 2 g

Indications, route, and dosage
Serious lower respiratory, urinary, CNS, bone and joint, intra-abdominal, gynecologic, and skin infections; bacteremia; septicemia caused by susceptible organisms; ◊ pelvic inflammatory disease
Adults and children weighing over 110 lb (50 kg): Usual dosage is 1 g I.V. or I.M. q 6 to 12 hours. Up to 12 g daily can be administered in life-threatening infections.

Total daily dosage is same for I.M. or I.V. administration and depends on susceptibility of organism and severity of infection. Cefotaxime should be injected deep I.M. into a large muscle mass, such as the gluteus or the lateral aspect of the thigh.
Children age 1 month to 12 years weighing under 110 lb (50 kg): 50 to 180 mg/kg/day in four or six equally divided doses. Higher doses are reserved for serious infections (such as meningitis).
Neonates age 1 to 4 weeks: 50 mg/kg I.V. q 8 hours.
Neonates up to 1 week: 50 mg/kg I.V. q 12 hours.
Uncomplicated gonorrhea
Adults and adolescents: 1 g I.M. as a single dose.
Perioperative prophylaxis
Adults: 1 g I.V. or I.M. 30 to 90 minutes before surgery.
◊ Disseminated gonococcal infection
Adults: 1 g I.V. q 8 hours.
◊ Gonococcal ophthalmia; ◊ disseminated gonococcal infection
Neonates and infants: 25 to 50 mg/kg I.V. q 8 to 12 hours for 7 days or 50 to 100 mg/kg I.M. or I.V. q 12 hours for 7 days.
◊ Gonorrheal meningitis or arthritis
Neonates and infants: 25 to 50 mg/kg I.V. q 8 to 12 hours for 10 to 14 days or 50 to 100 mg/kg I.M. or I.V. q 12 hours for 10 to 14 days.
✦ ***Dosage adjustment.*** In patients with impaired renal function, modify dose or frequency of administration based on degree of renal impairment, severity of infection, and susceptibility of organism. To prevent toxic accumulation, reduced dosage

may be required in patients with creatinine clearance below 20 ml/minute.

Pharmacodynamics

Antibacterial action: Cefotaxime is primarily bactericidal; however, it may be bacteriostatic. Activity depends on the organism, tissue penetration, drug dosage, and rate of organism multiplication. It acts by adhering to bacterial penicillin-binding proteins, thereby inhibiting cell-wall synthesis.

Third-generation cephalosporins appear more active against some beta-lactamase producing gram-negative organisms.

Cefotaxime is active against some gram-positive organisms and many enteric gram-negative bacilli, including streptococci (*Streptococcus pneumoniae* and *pyogenes*), *Staphylococcus aureus* (penicillinase- and nonpenicillinase-producing), *Staphylococcus epidermidis, Escherichia coli, Klebsiella* species, *Haemophilus influenzae, Enterobacter* species, *Proteus* species, and *Peptostreptococcus* species, and some strains of *Pseudomonas aeruginosa. Listeria* and *Acinetobacter* are often resistant. The active metabolite of cefotaxime, desacetylcefotaxime, may act synergistically with the parent drug against some bacterial strains.

Pharmacokinetics

• *Absorption:* Drug is not absorbed from the GI tract and must be given parenterally; peak serum levels occur 30 minutes after an I.M. dose.
• *Distribution:* Cefotaxime is distributed widely into most body tissues and fluids, including the gallbladder, liver, kidneys, bone, sputum, bile, and pleural and synovial fluids. Unlike most other cephalosporins, drug has adequate CSF penetration when meninges are inflamed; it crosses the placenta; 13% to 38% is protein-bound.
• *Metabolism:* Cefotaxime is metabolized partially to an active metabolite, desacetylcefotaxime.
• *Excretion:* Drug and its metabolites are excreted primarily in urine by renal tubular secretion; some drug may be excreted in breast milk. About 25% of cefotaxime is excreted in urine as the active metabolite; elimination half-life in normal adults is about 1 to 1½ hours for cefotaxime and about 1½ to 2 hours for desacetylcefotaxime; severe renal impairment prolongs cefotaxime's half-life to 11½ hours and that of the metabolite to as much as 56 hours. Hemodialysis removes both drug and its metabolites.

Contraindications and precautions

Contraindicated in patients with hypersensitivity to drug or other cephalosporins. Use cautiously in patients with impaired renal function or penicillin allergies and in breast-feeding women.

Interactions

Concomitant use with *aminoglycosides* results in apparent synergistic activity against Enterobacteriaceae and some strains of *Pseudomonas aeruginosa* and *Serratia marcescens;* combined use may increase risk of nephrotoxicity.

Probenecid may block renal tubular secretion of cefotaxime and prolong its half-life.

Effects on diagnostic tests

Cephalosporins cause false-positive results in urine glucose tests using cupric sulfate (Benedict's reagent or Clinitest); use glucose oxidase (Chemstrip uG, Diastix, or glucose enzymatic test strip) instead. Cefotaxime also causes false elevations in urine creatinine levels in tests using Jaffé's reaction.

Cefotaxime may cause positive Coombs' tests results and elevations of liver function test results.

Adverse reactions

CNS: headache.
GI: pseudomembranous colitis, nausea, vomiting, *diarrhea.*
GU: vaginitis, moniliasis, interstitial nephritis.
Hematologic: transient neutropenia, eosinophilia, hemolytic anemia, ***thrombocytopenia, agranulocytosis.***
Skin: *maculopapular and erythematous rashes, urticaria.*
Other: hypersensitivity reactions (serum sickness, ***anaphylaxis***); transient increases in liver enzymes; elevated temperature; *pain, induration, sterile abscesses, temperature elevation, tissue sloughing* (at injection site); *phlebitis, thrombophlebitis* (with I.V. injection).

Overdose and treatment

Clinical signs of overdose include neuromuscular hypersensitivity. Seizure may follow high CNS concentrations. Cefotaxime may be removed by hemodialysis.

☑ Special considerations

Besides those relevant to all *cephalosporins,* consider the following recommendations.
• For patients on sodium restriction, note that cefotaxime contains 2.2 mEq of sodium per gram of drug.
• For I.M. injection, add 2 ml, 3 ml, or 5 ml of sterile or bacteriostatic water for injection to each 500-mg, 1-g, or 2-g vial. Shake well to dissolve drug completely. Check solution for particles and discoloration. Color ranges from light yellow to amber.
• Do not inject more than 1 g into a single I.M. site to prevent pain and tissue reaction.
• Do not mix with aminoglycosides or sodium bicarbonate or fluids with a pH above 7.5.
• For I.V. use, reconstitute all strengths of an I.V. dose with 10 ml of sterile water for injection. For infusion bottles, add 50 to 100 ml of 0.9% NaCl solution injection or 5% dextrose injection. May be further reconstituted to 50 to 1,000 ml with fluids recommended by manufacturer.
• Administer drug by direct intermittent I.V. infusion over 3 to 5 minutes. Cefotaxime also may be given more slowly into a flowing I.V. line of compatible solution.
• Solution is stable for 24 hours at room temperature or at least 5 days under refrigeration. Cefotaxime may be stored in disposable glass or plastic syringes.

• Because drug is hemodialyzable, patients undergoing treatment with hemodialysis may require dosage adjustment.

Patient education
• Inform patient of potential adverse reactions.

Geriatric use
• Use with caution in elderly patients with diminished renal function.

Pediatric use
• Cefotaxime may be used in neonates, infants, and children.

Breast-feeding
• Drug distributes into breast milk and should be used with caution in breast-feeding women.

cefotetan disodium
Cefotan

Pharmacologic classification: second-generation cephalosporin, cephamycin
Therapeutic classification: antibiotic
Pregnancy risk category B

How supplied
Available by prescription only
Injection: 1 g, 2 g, 10 g (pharmacy bulk package)
Infusion: 1 g, 2 g piggyback

Indications, route, and dosage
Serious urinary, lower respiratory, gynecologic, skin, intra-abdominal, and bone and joint infections caused by susceptible organisms
Adults: 500 mg to 3 g I.V. or I.M. q 12 hours for 5 to 10 days. Up to 6 g daily in life-threatening infections.
◊ *Children:* 40 to 60 mg/kg daily I.V. divided in equally divided doses q 12 hours.
Preoperative prophylaxis
Adults: 1 to 2 g I.V. 30 to 60 minutes before surgery.
Postcesarean
Adults: 1 to 2 g I.V. as soon as umbilical cord is clamped.

Total daily dosage is same for I.M. or I.V. administration and depends on the susceptibility of the organism and severity of infection. Cefotetan should be injected deep I.M. into a large muscle mass, such as the gluteus or the lateral aspect of the thigh.

✦ ***Dosage adjustment.*** In patients with impaired renal function, doses or frequency of administration must be modified based on degree of renal impairment, severity of infection, and susceptibility of organism. To prevent toxic accumulation, reduced dosage may be necessary in patients with creatinine clearance below 30 ml/minute. Because drug is hemodialyzable, hemodialysis patients may require dosage adjustment.

Creatinine clearance (ml/min/1.73 m²)	Dosage in adults
> 30	Usual adult dose
10 to 30	Usual adult dose q 24 hr; or ½ usual adult dose q 12 hr
< 10	Usual adult dose q 48 hr; or ¼ usual adult dose q 12 hr
Hemodialysis patients	¼ usual adult dose q 24 hr on days between hemodialysis sessions; and ½ usual adult dose on day of hemodialysis

Pharmacodynamics
Antibacterial action: Cefotetan is primarily bactericidal; however, it may be bacteriostatic. Activity depends on the organism, tissue penetration, drug dosage, and rate of organism multiplication. It acts by adhering to bacterial penicillin-binding proteins, thereby inhibiting cell-wall synthesis.

Cefotetan is active against many gram-positive organisms and enteric gram-negative bacilli, including streptococci, *Staphylococcus aureus* (penicillinase- and nonpenicillinase-producing), *Staphylococcus epidermidis, Escherichia coli, Klebsiella* species, *Enterobacter* species, *Proteus* species, *Haemophilus influenzae, Neisseria gonorrhoeae,* and *Bacteroides* species (including some strains of *B. fragilis*); however, some *B. fragilis* strains, *Pseudomonas,* and *Acinetobacter* are resistant to cefotetan. Most Enterobacteriaceae are more susceptible to cefotetan than to other second-generation cephalosporins.

Pharmacokinetics
• *Absorption:* Drug is not absorbed from the GI tract and must be given parenterally; peak serum levels occur 1½ to 3 hours after an I.M. dose.
• *Distribution:* Cefotetan is distributed widely into most body tissues and fluids, including the gallbladder, liver, kidneys, bone, sputum, bile, and pleural and synovial fluids; CSF penetration is poor. Biliary concentration levels of cefotetan can be up to 20 times higher than serum concentrations in patients with good gallbladder function. Cefotetan crosses the placenta; it is 75% to 90% protein-bound.
• *Metabolism:* Drug is not metabolized.
• *Excretion:* Excreted primarily in urine by glomerular filtration and some renal tubular secretion; 20% is excreted in the bile. Small amounts of the drug are excreted in breast milk. Elimination half-life is about 3 to 4½ hours in patients with normal renal function.

Contraindications and precautions
Contraindicated in patients with hypersensitivity to drug or other cephalosporins. Use cautiously in patients with impaired renal function or penicillin allergy and in breast-feeding women.

Interactions
Concomitant use of cefotetan with nephrotoxic agents (*vancomycin, colistin, polymyxin B, aminoglycosides*) or *loop diuretics* may increase the risk of nephrotoxicity.

Concomitant use with *alcohol* may cause disulfiram-like reactions (flushing, sweating, tachycardia, headache, and abdominal cramping).

Concomitant use with *anticoagulants* may increase risk of bleeding.

Effects on diagnostic tests
Cefotetan also causes false-positive results in urine glucose tests using cupric sulfate (Benedict's reagent or Clinitest); use glucose oxidase tests (Chemstrip uG, Diastix, or glucose enzymatic test strip) instead. Cefotetan causes false elevations in serum or urine creatinine levels in tests using Jaffé's reaction. It may cause positive Coombs' test results and may elevate liver function test results and PT.

Adverse reactions
GI: pseudomembranous colitis, nausea, *diarrhea.*
GU: nephrotoxicity.
Hematologic: transient neutropenia, eosinophilia, hemolytic anemia, hypoprothrombinemia, bleeding, thrombocytosis, ***agranulocytosis, thrombocytopenia.***
Skin: *maculopapular and erythematous rashes, urticaria.*
Other: hypersensitivity reactions (serum sickness, ***anaphylaxis***); transient increases in liver enzymes; elevated temperature; *pain, induration, sterile abscesses, tissue sloughing* (at injection site); *phlebitis, thrombophlebitis* (with I.V. injection).

Overdose and treatment
Clinical signs of overdose include neuromuscular hypersensitivity. Seizure may follow high CNS concentrations. Hypoprothrombinemia and bleeding may occur; they may be treated with vitamin K or blood products. Cefotetan may be removed by hemodialysis.

☑ Special considerations
Besides those relevant to all *cephalosporins,* consider the following recommendations.
- For I.V. use, reconstitute with sterile water for injection. Then it may be mixed with 50 to 100 ml D_5W or 0.9% NaCl solution. Infuse intermittently over 30 to 60 minutes.
- For I.M. injection, cefotetan may be reconstituted with sterile water or bacteriostatic water for injection or with 0.9% NaCl or 0.5% or 1% lidocaine hydrochloride. Shake to dissolve and let solution stand until clear.
- Reconstituted solution remains stable for 24 hours at room temperature or for 96 hours when refrigerated.
- Assess for signs and symptoms of overt and occult bleeding. Monitor vital signs. Check CBC with differential, platelet levels, and PT for abnormalities.
- Bleeding can be reversed promptly by administering vitamin K.
- Concomitant use with alcohol may cause severe disulfiram-like reactions.

Patient education
- Inform patient of potential adverse reactions.
- Caution patient against use of alcohol during therapy.
- Instruct patient to promptly report signs of bleeding.

Geriatric use
- Hypoprothrombinemia and bleeding have been reported more frequently in elderly and debilitated patients.

Pediatric use
- Safe use in children has not been established.

Breast-feeding
- Cephalosporins distribute into breast milk and should be used with caution in breast-feeding women. Safe use has not been established.

cefoxitin sodium
Mefoxin

Pharmacologic classification: second-generation cephalosporin, cephamycin
Therapeutic classification: antibiotic
Pregnancy risk category B

How supplied
Available by prescription only
Injection: 1 g, 2 g
Pharmacy bulk package: 10 g
Infusion: 1 g, 2 g in 50-ml containers

Indications, route, and dosage
Serious respiratory, GU, gynecologic, skin, soft-tissue, bone and joint, blood, and intra-abdominal infections caused by susceptible organisms
Adults: 1 to 2 g q 6 to 8 hours for uncomplicated forms of infection. Up to 12 g daily in life-threatening infections.
Children over age 3 months: 80 to 160 mg/kg daily given in four to six equally divided doses.

Total daily dosage is same for I.M. or I.V. administration and depends on susceptibility of organism and severity of infection. Cefoxitin should be injected deep I.M. into a large muscle mass, such as the gluteus or lateral aspect of the thigh.
Preoperative prophylaxis
Adults: 2 g I.V. 30 to 60 minutes before surgery, followed by 2 g I.V. q 6 hours for 24 hours postoperatively.
Children over age 3 months: 30 to 40 mg/kg I.V. 30 to 60 minutes before surgery; then 30 mg/kg I.V. q 6 hours for 24 hours postoperatively.
Uncomplicated gonorrhea
Adults: Give 2 g I.M. as a single dose with 1 g probenecid P.O. at the same time or up to 30 minutes beforehand.
Pelvic inflammatory disease
Adults: 2 g I.V. q 6 hours. (If *Chlamydia trachomatis* is suspected, additional antichlamydial coverage should be given.)

✦ ***Dosage adjustment.*** In patients with impaired renal function, doses or frequency of administration must be modified based on degree of renal impairment, severity of infection, and susceptibility of organism. To prevent toxic accumulation, reduced dosage may be required in patients with creatinine clearance below 50 ml/minute/1.73 m^2.

Creatinine clearance (ml/min/1.73 m^2)	Dosage in adults
> 50	Usual adult dose
30 to 50	1 to 2 g q 8 to 12 hr
10 to 29	1 to 2 g q 12 to 24 hr
5 to 9	500 mg to 1 g q 12 to 24 hr
< 5	500 mg to 1 g q 24 to 48 hr

Pharmacodynamics

Antibacterial action: Cefoxitin is primarily bactericidal; however, it may be bacteriostatic. Activity depends on the organism, tissue penetration, drug dosage, and rate of organism multiplication. It acts by adhering to bacterial penicillin-binding proteins, thereby inhibiting cell-wall synthesis.

Cefoxitin is active against many gram-positive organisms and enteric gram-negative bacilli, including *Escherichia coli* and other coliform bacteria, *Staphylococcus aureus* (penicillinase– and non-penicillinase–producing), *Staphylococcus epidermidis,* streptococci, *Klebsiella, Haemophilus influenzae,* and *Bacteroides* species (including *B. fragilis*). *Enterobacter, Pseudomonas,* and *Acinetobacter* are resistant to cefoxitin.

Pharmacokinetics

- *Absorption:* Cefoxitin is not absorbed from the GI tract and must be given parenterally; peak serum levels occur 20 to 30 minutes after an I.M. dose.
- *Distribution:* Distributed widely into most body tissues and fluids, including the gallbladder, liver, kidneys, bone, sputum, bile, and pleural and synovial fluids; CSF penetration is poor. Cefoxitin crosses the placenta; it is 50% to 80% protein-bound.
- *Metabolism:* About 2% of a cefoxitin dose is metabolized.
- *Excretion:* Excreted primarily in urine by renal tubular secretion and glomerular filtration; small amounts of drug are excreted in breast milk. Elimination half-life is about ½ to 1 hour in patients with normal renal function; half-life is prolonged in patients with severe renal dysfunction to 6½ to 21½ hours. Cefoxitin can be removed by hemodialysis but not by peritoneal dialysis.

Contraindications and precautions

Contraindicated in patients with hypersensitivity to drug or other cephalosporins. Use cautiously in patients with impaired renal function or penicillin allergy and in breast-feeding women.

Interactions

Probenecid competitively inhibits renal tubular secretion of cephalosporins, resulting in higher, prolonged serum levels of these drugs.

Concomitant use of cefoxitin with *nephrotoxic agents* (*vancomycin, colistin, polymixin B, aminoglycosides*) or *loop diuretics* may increase the risk of nephrotoxicity. Concomitant use with bacteriostatic agents (*tetracyclines, erythromycin, chloramphenicol*) may impair cefoxitin's bactericidal activity.

Effects on diagnostic tests

Cefoxitin causes false-positive results in urine glucose tests using cupric sulfate (Benedict's reagent or Clinitest); use glucose oxidase tests (Chemstrip uG, Diastix, or glucose enzymatic test strip) instead. Cefoxitin also causes false elevations in serum or urine creatinine levels in tests using Jaffé's reaction.

Cefoxitin may elevate liver function test results and may cause positive Coombs' test results.

Adverse reactions

CV: hypotension.
GI: pseudomembranous colitis, nausea, vomiting, *diarrhea.*
GU: ***acute renal failure.***
Hematologic: transient neutropenia, eosinophilia, ***hemolytic anemia,*** anemia, ***thrombocytopenia.***
Skin: *maculopapular and erythematous rash, urticaria,* exfoliative dermatitis.
Other: hypersensitivity reactions (serum sickness, ***anaphylaxis***), transient increases in liver enzymes, elevated temperature; *pain, induration, sterile abscesses, tissue sloughing* (at injection site); *phlebitis, thrombophlebitis,* dyspnea (with I.V. injection).

Overdose and treatment

Clinical signs of overdose include neuromuscular hypersensitivity. Seizure may follow high CNS concentrations. Cefoxitin may be removed by hemodialysis.

☑ Special considerations

Besides those relevant to all *cephalosporins,* consider the following recommendations.

- For I.V. use, reconstitute 1 g of cefoxitin with at least 10 ml of sterile water for injection, or 2 g of cefoxitin with 10 to 20 ml. Solutions of dextrose 5% and 0.9% NaCl solution for injection can also be used.
- Cefoxitin has been associated with thrombophlebitis. Assess I.V. site frequently for signs of infiltration or phlebitis. Change I.V. site every 48 to 72 hours.
- For I.M. injection, reconstitute with 0.5% to 1% lidocaine hydrochloride (without epinephrine) to minimize pain at injection site; or with sterile water for injection.
- Administer I.M. dose deep into a large muscle mass. Aspirate before injecting to prevent inadvertent injection into a blood vessel. Rotate injection sites to prevent tissue damage.
- After reconstituting, shake vial and then let stand until clear to ensure complete drug dissolution. So-

lution is stable for 24 hours at room temperature, for 1 week if refrigerated, or 26 weeks if frozen.
• Solution may range from colorless to light amber and may darken during storage. Slight color change does not indicate loss of potency.
• Cefoxitin injection contains 2.3 mEq of sodium per gram of drug.
• Because drug is hemodialyzable, patients undergoing treatment with hemodialysis may require dosage adjustments.

Patient education
• Inform patient of potential adverse reactions.

Geriatric use
• Dosage reduction may be necessary in patients with diminished renal function.

Pediatric use
• Dosage may need to be reduced in infants under age 3 months. Safety has not been established.

Breast-feeding
• Drug distributes into breast milk and should be used with caution in breast-feeding women.

cefpodoxime proxetil
Vantin

Pharmacologic classification: third-generation cephalosporin
Therapeutic classification: antibiotic
Pregnancy risk category B

How supplied
Available by prescription only
Tablets (film-coated): 100 mg, 200 mg
Oral suspension: 50 mg/5 ml, 100 mg/5 ml

Indications, route, and dosage
***Acute, community-acquired pneumonia caused by non-beta-lactamase–producing strains of* Haemophilus influenzae *or* Streptococcus pneumoniae**
Adults: 200 mg P.O. q 12 hours for 14 days.
***Acute bacterial exacerbations of chronic bronchitis caused by non-beta-lactamase–producing strains* of H. influenzae, S. pneumoniae, *or* Moraxella catarrhalis**
Adults: 200 mg P.O. q 12 hours for 10 days.
Uncomplicated gonorrhea in men and women; rectal gonococcal infections in women
Adults: 200 mg P.O. as a single dose. Follow with doxycycline 100 mg P.O. b.i.d. for 7 days.
***Uncomplicated skin and skin structure infections caused by* Staphylococcus aureus *or* Streptococcus pyogenes**
Adults: 400 mg P.O. q 12 hours for 7 to 14 days.
***Acute otitis media caused* by S. pneumoniae, H. influenzae, *or* M. catarrhalis**
Children age 5 months to 12 years: 5 mg/kg (not to exceed 200 mg) P.O. q 12 hours for 10 days.
***Pharyngitis or tonsillitis caused by* S. pyogenes**
Adults: 100 mg P.O. q 12 hours for 7 to 10 days.
Children age 5 months to 12 years: 5 mg/kg (not to exceed 100 mg) P.O. q 12 hours for 10 days.
***Uncomplicated urinary tract infections caused by* Escherichia coli, Klebsiella pneumoniae, Proteus mirabilis, *or* Staphylococcus saprophyticus**
Adults: 100 mg P.O. q 12 hours for 7 days.
✦ ***Dosage adjustment.*** In patients with renal impairment when creatinine clearance is below 30 ml/minute, dosage interval should be increased to q 24 hours. Patients receiving hemodialysis should get drug three times weekly, after dialysis.

Pharmacodynamics
Antibiotic action: A second-generation cephalosporin, cefpodoxime proxetil is a bactericidal agent that inhibits cell-wall synthesis. It is usually active against gram-positive aerobes, such as *S. aureus* (including penicillinase–producing strains), *S. saprophyticus, S. pneumoniae,* and *S. pyogenes,* and gram-negative aerobes, such as *E. coli, H. influenzae* (including beta-lactamase–producing strains), *K. pneumoniae, M. (Branhamella) catarrhalis, Neisseria gonorrhoeae* (including penicillinase–producing strains), and *P. mirabilis.*

Pharmacokinetics
• *Absorption:* Drug is absorbed via the GI tract. Absorption and mean peak plasma concentration levels increase when the drug is administered with food.
• *Distribution:* Cephalosporins are widely distributed to most tissues and fluids. Second-generation cephalosporins do not enter CSF even when the meninges are inflamed, although data on cefpodoxime are not available. Protein-binding ranges from 22% to 33% in serum and from 21% to 29% in plasma.
• *Metabolism:* Cefpodoxime proxetil is de-esterified to its active metabolite, cefpodoxime.
• *Excretion:* Drug is excreted primarily in urine.

Contraindications and precautions
Contraindicated in patients with hypersensitivity to drug or other cephalosporins. Use cautiously in patients with impaired renal function or penicillin allergy and in breast-feeding women.

Interactions
Antacids and *H_2 antagonists* decrease absorption of cefpodoxime proxetil and should not be administered concurrently. *Probenecid* decreases the excretion of cefpodoxime proxetil. Monitor the patient for cefpodoxime toxicity. Although nephrotoxicity has not been noted when cefpodoxime proxetil was given alone in clinical studies, close monitoring of renal function is advised when cefpodoxime proxetil is administered concomitantly with *compounds of known nephrotoxic potential.*

Effects on diagnostic tests
Cefpodoxime proxetil may induce a positive direct Coombs' test.

Adverse reactions
CNS: headache.

GI: *diarrhea,* nausea, vomiting, abdominal pain.
GU: vaginal fungal infections.
Skin: rash.
Other: hypersensitivity reactions ***(anaphylaxis).***

Overdose and treatment

No information on drug overdosage is available. Toxic symptoms after an overdose of beta-lactam antibiotics may include nausea, vomiting, epigastric distress, and diarrhea. In the event of serious toxic reaction from overdosage, hemodialysis or peritoneal dialysis may aid in removing drug from the body, particularly if renal function is compromised.

☑ Special considerations

- Drug is highly stable in presence of beta-lactamase enzymes. As a result, many organisms resistant to penicillins and some cephalosporins, because of presence of beta-lactamases, may be susceptible to cefpodoxime proxetil.
- Cefpodoxime is inactive against most strains of *Pseudomonas, Enterobacter,* and *Enterococcus.*
- As with other antibiotics, prolonged use of cefpodoxime proxetil may result in overgrowth of nonsusceptible organisms. Repeated evaluation of the patient's condition is essential, and appropriate measures should be taken if superinfection occurs during therapy.
- Obtain specimen for culture and sensitivity tests before giving first dose. Therapy may begin pending test results.
- Store suspension in refrigerator (36° to 46° F [2 to 8° C]). Shake well before using. Discard unused portion after 14 days.

Patient education

- Instruct patient to take drug with food to enhance absorption.
- Inform patient that oral suspension of cefpodoxime proxetil should be refrigerated. Instruct patient to shake container well before using and to discard unused portion after 14 days.
- Tell patient to continue taking drug for the prescribed course of therapy, even after feeling better.

Pediatric use

- Safety and efficacy in infants under age 6 months have not been established.

Breast-feeding

- Drug is excreted in breast milk. Because of the potential for serious reactions in breast-fed infants, a decision must be made to discontinue breast-feeding or drug, taking into account the importance of drug to the mother.

cefprozil

Cefzil

Pharmacologic classification: second-generation cephalosporin
Therapeutic classification: antibiotic
Pregnancy risk category B

How supplied

Available by prescription only
Tablets: 250 mg, 500 mg
Oral suspension: 125 mg/5 ml, 250 mg/5 ml

Indications, route, and dosage

***Pharyngitis or tonsillitis caused by* Streptococcus pyogenes**
Adults and children age 13 and older: 500 mg P.O. daily for at least 10 days.
Children age 2 to 12: 7.5 mg/kg q 12 hours for 10 days.
***Otitis media caused by* Streptococcus pneumoniae, Haemophilus influenzae, *and* Moraxella (Branhamella) catarrhalis**
Infants and children age 6 months to 12 years: 15 mg/kg P.O. q 12 hours for 10 days.
***Secondary bacterial infections of acute bronchitis and acute bacterial exacerbation of chronic bronchitis caused by* S. pneumoniae, H. influenzae, *and* M. (B.) catarrhalis**
Adults: 500 mg P.O. q 12 hours for 10 days.
***Uncomplicated skin and skin structure infections caused by* Staphylococcus aureus *and* S. pyogenes**
Adults and children age 13 and older: 250 mg P.O. b.i.d., or 500 mg daily to b.i.d. for 10 days.
Children age 2 to 12: 20 mg/kg q 24 hours for 10 days.
✦ ***Dosage adjustment.*** No adjustments are necessary for patients with creatinine clearance over 30 ml/minute. For patients with creatinine clearance of 30 ml/minute or less, dose should be reduced by 50%; however, dosing interval remains unchanged. Because drug is partially removed by hemodialysis, it should be administered after the hemodialysis session.

Pharmacodynamics

Antibiotic action: Cefprozil interferes with bacterial cell-wall synthesis during cell replication, leading to osmotic instability and cell lysis. Bactericidal or bacteriostatic, depending on concentration.

Pharmacokinetics

Note: Pharmacokinetic data are derived from investigational studies that used an oral capsule formulation which is not commercially available.

- *Absorption:* Cefprozil is approximately 95% absorbed from the GI tract. Peak levels occur within 1½ hours of a dose. Food did not interfere with the capsule formulation; it is unknown if food will interfere with absorption of tablets or oral suspension.
- *Distribution:* Drug is about 36% protein-bound.
- *Metabolism:* Cefprozil is probably metabolized by the liver; plasma half-life increases only slightly in patients with impaired hepatic function.
- *Excretion:* About 60% of a dose is recovered unchanged in the urine. Plasma half-life is 1.3 hours in patients with normal renal function; 2 hours, impaired hepatic function; and 5.2 to 5.9 hours, end-stage renal disease. Drug is removed by hemodialysis.

Contraindications and precautions
Contraindicated in patients with hypersensitivity to drug or other cephalosporins. Use cautiously in patients with impaired renal function or penicillin allergy and in breast-feeding women.

Interactions
Concomitant use with *aminoglycoside* antibiotics may increase the risk of nephrotoxicity of cephalosporins. *Probenecid* may decrease excretion of cefprozil.

Effects on diagnostic tests
Cephalosporins may produce a false-positive test for urine glucose with tests that use copper reduction method (Benedict's test, Fehling's solution, or Clinitest tablets). Instead, use enzymatic methods (such as glucose enzymatic test strip). A false-negative reaction may occur in the ferricyanide test for blood glucose.

Adverse reactions
CNS: dizziness, hyperactivity, headache, nervousness, insomnia, confusion, somnolence.
GI: *diarrhea, nausea,* vomiting, abdominal pain.
GU: elevated BUN level, elevated serum creatinine level, genital pruritus, vaginitis.
Hematologic: decreased leukocyte count, eosinophilia.
Hepatic: elevated liver enzymes, cholestatic jaundice (rare).
Skin: rash, urticaria, diaper rash.
Other: superinfection, hypersensitivity reactions (serum sickness, ***anaphylaxis***).

Overdose and treatment
Because drug is eliminated primarily by the kidneys, the manufacturer states that hemodialysis may aid in removal of drug in cases of extreme overdose, especially in patients with decreased renal function.

☑ Special considerations
Besides those relevant to all *cephalosporins*, consider the following recommendations.
- Pseudomembranous colitis has been reported with nearly all antibacterial agents. Consider this diagnosis in patients who develop diarrhea secondary to antibiotic therapy. Although most patients respond to withdrawal of drug therapy alone, it may be necessary to institute treatment with an antibacterial agent effective against *Clostridium difficile,* an organism linked to this disorder.
- Obtain specimen for culture and sensitivity tests before giving first dose. Therapy may begin pending test results.
- Drug may cause overgrowth of nonsusceptible bacteria or fungi. Monitor for signs and symptoms of superinfection.
- Advise patients with phenylketonuria that oral suspension contains 28 mg/5 ml phenylalanine.

Patient education
- Tell patient to take all of drug as prescribed, even if he feels better.

Geriatric use
- Elderly volunteers (age 65 and over) exhibited a higher area under the plasma-concentration-versus-time curve and lower renal clearance compared with younger subjects.

Pediatric use
- Oral suspensions contain drug in a bubble gum flavored vehicle to improve palatability and compliance in children. Reconstituted suspension should be stored in the refrigerator, and unused drug should be discarded after 14 days. Shake suspension well before measuring dose.

Breast-feeding
- It is unknown if drug is excreted in breast milk. Use with caution in breast-feeding women.

ceftazidime
Ceptaz, Fortaz, Tazicef, Tazidime

Pharmacologic classification: third-generation cephalosporin
Therapeutic classification: antibiotic
Pregnancy risk category B

How supplied
Available by prescription only
Injection: 500 mg, 1 g, 2 g
Pharmacy bulk package: 6 g, 10 g
Infusion: 1 g, 2 g in 20-, 50-, and 100-ml vials and bags

Indications, route, and dosage
Bacteremia, septicemia, and serious respiratory, urinary, gynecologic, bone and joint, intra-abdominal, CNS, and skin infections from susceptible organisms
Adults: 1 g I.V. or I.M. q 8 to 12 hours; up to 6 g daily in life-threatening infections.
Children age 1 month to 12 years: 30 to 50 mg/kg I.V. q 8 hours to a maximum of 6 g/day (Fortaz, Tazicef, and Tazidime only).
Neonates up to 4 weeks: 30 mg/kg I.V. q 12 hours (Fortaz, Tazicef, and Tazidime only).

Total daily dosage is the same for I.M. or I.V. administration and depends on susceptibility of organism and severity of infection. Ceftazidime should be injected deep I.M. into a large muscle mass, such as the gluteus or lateral aspect of the thigh.

✦ ***Dosage adjustment.*** In patients with impaired renal function, doses or frequency of administration must be modified according to the degree of renal impairment, severity of infection, and susceptibility of organism. To prevent toxic accumulation, reduced dosage may be required in patients with creatinine clearance below 50 ml/minute/1.73 m^2.

Creatinine clearance (ml/min/1.73 m²)	Dosage in adults
> 50	Usual adult dose
31 to 50	1 g q 12 hr
16 to 30	1 g q 24 hr
6 to 15	500 mg q 24 hr
≤ 5	500 mg q 48 hr
Hemodialysis patients	1 g after each hemodialysis period
Peritoneal dialysis patients	500 mg q 24 hr

Pharmacodynamics

Antibacterial action: Ceftazidime is primarily bactericidal; however, it may be bacteriostatic. Activity depends on the organism, tissue penetration, drug dosage, and rate of organism multiplication. It acts by adhering to bacterial penicillin-binding proteins, thereby inhibiting cell-wall synthesis. Third-generation cephalosporins appear more active against some beta-lactamase–producing gram-negative organisms.

Ceftazidime is active against some gram-positive organisms and many enteric gram-negative bacilli, as well as streptococci (*Streptococcus pneumoniae* and *S. pyogenes*); *Staphylococcus aureus* (penicillinase- and nonpenicillinaseproducing); *Escherichia coli; Klebsiella* species; *Proteus* species; *Enterobacter species; Haemophilus influenzae; Pseudomonas* species; and some strains of *Bacteroides* species. It is more effective than any cephalosporin or penicillin derivative against *Pseudomonas.* Some other third-generation cephalosporins are more active against gram-positive organisms and anaerobes.

Pharmacokinetics

- *Absorption:* Drug is not absorbed from the GI tract and must be given parenterally; peak serum levels occur 1 hour after an I.M. dose.
- *Distribution:* Drug is distributed widely into most body tissues and fluids, including the gallbladder, liver, kidneys, bone, sputum, bile, and pleural and synovial fluids; unlike most other cephalosporins, ceftazidime has good CSF penetration; it crosses the placenta. Ceftazidime is 5% to 24% protein-bound.
- *Metabolism:* Ceftazidime is not metabolized.
- *Excretion:* Excreted primarily in urine by glomerular filtration; small amounts of drug are excreted in breast milk. Elimination half-life is about 1½ to 2 hours in patients with normal renal function; up to 35 hours in patients with severe renal disease. Hemodialysis or peritoneal dialysis removes ceftazidime.

Contraindications and precautions

Contraindicated in patients with hypersensitivity to drug or other cephalosporins. Use cautiously in breast-feeding women and in patients with impaired renal function or penicillin allergy.

Interactions

Concomitant use with *aminoglycosides* results in synergistic activity against *Pseudomonas aeruginosa* and some strains of enterobacteriaceae; such combined use may slightly increase the risk of nephrotoxicity.

Concomitant use with *clavulanic acid* results in synergistic activity against some strains of *Bacteroides fragilis.*

Effects on diagnostic tests

Ceftazidime causes false-positive results in urine glucose tests using cupric sulfate (Benedict's reagent or Clinitest); use glucose oxidase (Chemstrip uG, Diastix, or glucose enzymatic test strip) instead. Ceftazidime also causes false elevations in urine creatinine levels in tests using Jaffé's reaction.

Ceftazidime may cause positive Coombs' test results and elevated liver function test results.

Adverse reactions

CNS: headache, dizziness, paresthesia, ***seizures.***
GI: pseudomembranous colitis, nausea, vomiting, diarrhea, candidiasis, abdominal cramps.
GU: vaginitis.
Hematologic: eosinophilia, thrombocytosis, leukopenia, hemolytic anemia, ***agranulocytosis, thrombocytopenia.***
Skin: *maculopapular and erythematous rash, urticaria.*
Other: hypersensitivity reactions (serum sickness, ***anaphylaxis***), transient elevation in liver enzymes; *pain, induration, sterile abscesses, tissue sloughing* (at injection site); *phlebitis, thrombophlebitis* (with I.V. injection).

Overdose and treatment

Clinical signs of overdose include neuromuscular hypersensitivity. Seizure may follow high CNS concentrations. Drug may be removed by hemodialysis or peritoneal dialysis.

☑ Special considerations

Besides those relevant to all *cephalosporins,* consider the following recommendations.

- For patients on sodium restriction, note that ceftazidime contains 2.3 mEq of sodium per gram of drug.
- Ceftazidime powders (excluding Ceptaz) for injection contain 118 mg sodium carbonate per gram of drug; ceftazidime sodium is more water-soluble and is formed in situ upon reconstitution.
- Vials are supplied under reduced pressure. When the antibiotic is dissolved, carbon dioxide is released and a positive pressure develops. Each brand of ceftazidime includes specific instructions for reconstitution. Read and follow these instructions carefully.
- Because drug is hemodialyzable, patients undergoing treatments with hemodialysis or peritoneal dialysis may require dosage adjustment.
- Separate I.V. sites should be used for aminoglycosides and ceftazidime.

Patient education
• Inform patient of potential adverse reactions.

Geriatric use
• Reduced dosage may be necessary in elderly patients with diminished renal function.

Pediatric use
• Only Fortaz, Tazicef, and Tazidime may be used in infants and children. Ceptaz should not be used in children under age 12 because of the arginine component in this product.

Breast-feeding
• Drug is distributed into breast milk and should be used with caution in breast-feeding women. Safe use has not been established.

ceftibuten
Cedax

Pharmacologic classification: third-generation cephalosporin
Therapeutic classification: antibiotic
Pregnancy risk category B

How supplied
Available by prescription only
Capsules: 400 mg
Oral suspension: 90 mg/5 ml, 180 mg/5 ml

Indications, route, and dosage
***Acute bacterial exacerbations of chronic bronchitis due to* Haemophilus influenzae, Moraxella catarrhalis, *or* Streptococcus pneumoniae**
Adults and children age 12 and over: 400 mg P.O. daily for 10 days.
***Pharyngitis and tonsillitis due to* S. pyogenes; *acute bacterial otitis media due to* H. influenzae, M. catarrhalis, *or* S. pyogenes**
Adults and children age 12 and older: 400 mg P.O. daily for 10 days.
Children under age 12: 9 mg/kg P.O. daily for 10 days. Children weighing over 99 lb (45 kg) should receive the maximum daily dose of 400 mg.
✦ ***Dosage adjustment.*** No adjustments are necessary for patients with creatinine clearance over 50 ml/minute. Give 4.5 mg/kg (or 200 mg) daily to patients with creatinine clearance between 30 and 49 ml/minute and 2.25 mg/kg (or 100 mg) daily for those with creatinine clearance of 5 to 29 ml/minute. For patients undergoing hemodialysis two or three times weekly, give a single 400-mg dose (capsule form) or administer a single dose of 9 mg/kg (maximum dose, 400 mg) using oral suspension at the end of each hemodialysis session.

Pharmacodynamics
Antibiotic action: Ceftibuten exerts its bactericidal action by binding to essential target proteins of the bacterial cell wall. This binding leads to inhibition of cell-wall synthesis. It is usually active against gram-positive aerobes (*S. pneumoniae, S. pyogenes*) and gram-negative aerobes (*H. influenzae, M. catarrhalis*).

Pharmacokinetics
• *Absorption:* Ceftibuten is rapidly absorbed from GI tract. Food decreases the bioavailabiity of drug.
• *Distribution:* Drug is 65% bound to plasma proteins.
• *Metabolism:* Ceftibuten is metabolized to its predominant component, cis-ceftibuten. About 10% of ceftibuten is converted to the transisomer.
• *Excretion:* Drug is excreted in urine and feces.

Contraindications and precautions
Contraindicated in patients with hypersensitivity to the cephalosporin group of antibiotics. Use cautiously if administering to patients with history of hypersensitivity to penicillin because up to 10% of these patients will exhibit cross-sensitivity to a cephalosporin. Also use cautiously in patients with impaired renal function and GI disease (especially colitis).

Interactions
None reported.

Effects on diagnostic tests
Although ceftibuten has not been known to affect the direct Coombs' test to date, other cephalosporins have caused a false-positive direct Coombs' test. Therefore, it should be recognized that a positive Coombs' test could be due to drug.

Adverse reactions
CNS: headache, dizziness, fatigue, paresthesia, somnolence, taste perversion, agitation, hyperkinesia, insomnia, irritability, rigors.
EENT: nasal congestion.
GI: nausea, dyspepsia, abdominal pain, vomiting, anorexia, constipation, dry mouth, eructation, flatulence, loose stools.
GU: dysuria, hematuria, elevated BUN and serum creatinine level, vaginitis.
Hepatic: elevated levels of liver enzymes, bilirubin, and alkaline phosphatase.
Hematologic: elevated amount of eosinophils, decreased hemoglobin level, altered platelet count, decreased leukocyte count.
Respiratory: dyspnea
Skin: rash, pruritus, diaper dermatitis, urticaria.
Other: candidiasis, dehydration, fever.

Overdose and treatment
Overdosage of cephalosporins can cause cerebral irritation leading to seizures. Ceftibuten is readily dialyzable and significant quantities (65% of plasma concentrations) can be removed from the circulation by a single hemodialysis session. Information does not exist with regard to removal of ceftibuten by peritoneal dialysis.

☑ Special considerations
Besides those relevant to all *cephalosporins*, consider the following recommendations.
• Pseudomembranous colitis has been reported with nearly all antibacterial agents; consider this diagnosis in patients who develop diarrhea secondary to antibiotic therapy. Although most patients respond to withdrawal of drug therapy alone, it may

be necessary to institute treatment with an antibacterial agent effective against *Clostridium difficile,* an organism linked to this disorder.
• Obtain specimen for culture and sensitivity tests before giving first dose. Therapy may begin pending test results.
• When preparing oral suspension, first tap the bottle to loosen powder. Follow chart supplied by manufacturer for amount of water to add to powder when mixing oral suspension form. Add water in two portions, shaking well after each aliquot. After mixing, the suspension may be kept for 14 days and must be stored in the refrigerator.
• Drug may cause overgrowth of nonsusceptible bacteria or fungi. Monitor patient for signs and symptoms of superinfection.

Patient education
• Tell patient to take all of drug as prescribed, even if feeling better.
• Instruct patient using oral suspension to take it at least 2 hours before or 1 hour after a meal.
• Inform diabetic patient that oral suspension contains 1 g of sucrose per teaspoon of suspension.
• Instruct patient using oral suspension to shake bottle well before measuring dose.
• Tell patient to keep oral suspension in the refrigerator with lid tightly closed and to discard unused drug after 14 days.

Geriatric use
• Use with caution when administering drug to elderly patients. Dosage adjustment may be necessary if patient has impaired renal function.

Pediatric use
• Safety and effectiveness in infants under age 6 months have not been established.

Breast-feeding
• It is not known if drug is excreted in breast milk. Use cautiously in breast-feeding women.

ceftizoxime sodium
Cefizox

Pharmacologic classification: third-generation cephalosporin
Therapeutic classification: antibiotic
Pregnancy risk category B

How supplied
Available by prescription only
Injection: 500 mg, 1 g, 2 g, 10 g
Infusion: 1 g, 2 g in 100-ml vials; 50 ml in D_5W

Indications, route, and dosage
Bacteremia, septicemia, meningitis, pelvic inflammatory disease, and serious respiratory, urinary, gynecologic, intra-abdominal, bone and joint, and skin infections from susceptible organisms
Adults: Usual dosage is 500 mg to 2 g I.V. or I.M. q 8 to 12 hours. In life-threatening infections, 3 to 4 g I.V. q 8 hours.
Children age 6 months and older: 50 mg/kg q 6 to 8 hours.

Total daily dosage is same for I.M. or I.V. administration and depends on susceptibility of organism and severity of infection. Ceftizoxime should be injected deep I.M. into a large muscle mass, such as the gluteus or lateral aspect of the thigh.
Uncomplicated gonorrhea
Adults: 1 g I.M. given as a single dose.
✦ ***Dosage adjustment.*** In patients with impaired renal function, modify doses or frequency of administration according to degree of renal impairment, severity of infection, and susceptibility of organism. To prevent toxic accumulation, reduced dosage may be required in patients with creatinine clearance below dosage 80 ml/minute.

DOSAGE IN ADULTS

Creatinine clearance (ml/min/ 1.73 m²)	Less severe infections	Life-threatening infections
≥ 80	Usual adult dose	Usual adult dose
50 to 79	500 mg q 8 hr	750 mg to 1.5 g q 8 hr
5 to 49	250 to 500 mg q 12 hr	500 mg to 1 g q 12 hr
≤ 4	500 mg q 48 hr; or 250 mg q 24 hr	500 mg to 1 g q 48 hr; or 500 mg q 24 hr

Pharmacodynamics
Antibacterial action: Ceftizoxime is primarily bactericidal; however, it may be bacteriostatic. Activity depends on the organism, tissue penetration, drug dosage, and rate of organism multiplication. It acts by adhering to bacterial penicillin-binding proteins, thereby inhibiting cell-wall synthesis. Third-generation cephalosporins appear more active against some beta-lactamase-producing gram-negative organisms.

Drug is active against some gram-positive organisms and many enteric gram-negative bacilli, as well as streptococci (*Streptococcus pneumoniae* and *pyogenes*); *Staphylococcus aureus* (penicillinase- and non-penicillinase-producing); *Staphylococcus epidermidis; Escherichia coli; Klebsiella* species; *Haemophilus influenzae; Enterobacter* species; *Proteus* species; *Bacteroides* species (including *Bacteroides fragilis*); *Peptostreptococcus* species; some strains of *Pseudomonas* and *Acinetobacter.* Cefotaxime and moxalactam are slightly more active than ceftizoxime against gram-positive organisms but are less active against gram-negative organisms.

Pharmacokinetics
• *Absorption:* Ceftizoxime is not absorbed from the GI tract and must be given parenterally; peak serum levels occur at ½ to 1½ hours after an I.M. dose.

• *Distribution:* Distributed widely into most body tissues and fluids, including the gallbladder, liver, kidneys, bone, sputum, bile, and pleural and synovial fluids; unlike most other cephalosporins, ceftizoxime has good CSF penetration and achieves adequate concentration in inflamed meninges; ceftizoxime crosses the placenta. Ceftizoxime is 30% protein-bound.
• *Metabolism:* Drug is not metabolized.
• *Excretion:* Excreted primarily in urine by renal tubular secretion and glomerular filtration; small amounts of drug are excreted in breast milk. Elimination half-life is about 1½ to 2 hours in patients with normal renal function; severe renal disease prolongs half-life up to 30 hours. Hemodialysis or peritoneal dialysis removes minimal amounts of ceftizoxime.

Contraindications and precautions
Contraindicated in patients with hypersensitivity to ceftizoxime or other cephalosporins. Use cautiously in breast-feeding women and in patients with impaired renal function or penicillin allergy.

Interactions
Probenecid competitively inhibits renal tubular secretion of cephalosporins, causing higher, prolonged serum levels.

Concomitant use with *aminoglycosides* may slightly increase the risk of nephrotoxicity.

Effects on diagnostic tests
Ceftizoxime causes false-positive results in urine glucose tests utilizing cupric sulfate (Benedict's reagent or Clinitest); use glucose oxidase (Chemstrip uG, Diastix, or glucose enzymatic test strip) instead. Ceftizoxime also causes false elevations in urine creatinine levels using Jaffé's reaction.

Ceftizoxime may cause positive Coombs' test results and elevated liver function test results.

Adverse reactions
GI: pseudomembranous colitis, nausea, anorexia, vomiting, *diarrhea.*
GU: vaginitis.
Hematologic: transient neutropenia, eosinophilia, hemolytic anemia, thrombocytosis, anemia, ***thrombocytopenia.***
Skin: *maculopapular and erythematous rash, urticaria.*
Other: hypersensitivity reactions (serum sickness, ***anaphylaxis***), dyspnea, elevated temperature; *pain, induration, sterile abscesses, tissue sloughing* (at injected site); *phlebitis, thrombophlebitis,* transient elevation in liver enzymes (with I.V. injection).

Overdose and treatment
Clinical signs of overdose include neuromuscular hypersensitivity. Seizure may follow high CNS concentrations. Ceftizoxime may be removed by hemodialysis.

☑ Special considerations
Besides those relevant to all *cephalosporins,* consider these recommendations.

• For patients on sodium restriction, note that ceftizoxime contains 2.6 mEq of sodium per gram of drug.
• Drug may be supplied as frozen, sterile solution in plastic containers. Thaw at room temperature. Thawed solution is stable for 24 hours at room temperature or for 10 days if refrigerated. Do not refreeze.
• For I.M. use, reconstitute with sterile water for injection. Shake vial well to ensure complete dissolution of drug. To administer a dose that exceeds 1 g, divide the dose and inject it into separate sites to prevent tissue injury.
• For I.V. use, reconstitute I.V. dose with sterile water for injection. Solution should clear after shaking well and range in color from yellow to amber. If particles are visible, discard solution. Reconstituted solution is stable for 24 hours at room temperature or 96 hours if refrigerated.
• Administer I.V. as a direct injection slowly over 3 to 5 minutes directly or through tubing of compatible infusion fluid. If given as intermittent infusion, dilute reconstituted drug in 50 to 100 ml of compatible fluid. Check package insert.

Patient education
• Inform patient of potential adverse reactions.

Geriatric use
• Reduced dosage may be necessary in elderly patients with diminished renal function.

Pediatric use
• Safely and efficacy have not been established in infants under age 6 months.

Breast-feeding
• Drug is distributed into breast milk and should be used with caution in breast-feeding women. Safe use has not been established.

ceftriaxone sodium
Rocephin

Pharmacologic classification: third-generation cephalosporin
Therapeutic classification: antibiotic
Pregnancy risk category B

How supplied
Available by prescription only
Injection: 250 mg, 500 mg, 1 g, 2 g
Pharmacy bulk package: 10 g
Infusion: 1 g, 2 g

Indications, route, and dosage
Bacteremia, septicemia, and serious respiratory, bone, joint, urinary, gynecologic, intra-abdominal, and skin infections from susceptible organisms
Adults: 1 to 2 g I.M. or I.V. once daily or in equally divided doses b.i.d. Total daily dosage should not exceed 4 g.
Children: Total daily dose is 50 to 75 mg/kg, given in divided doses q 12 hours.

Gonococcal meningitis, endocarditis
Adults: 1 to 2 g I.V. q 12 hours for 10 to 14 days for meningitis and 3 to 4 weeks for endocarditis.
Children: 50 to 100 mg/kg (maximum daily dose, 4 g) as a single dose or divided q 12 hours for 7 to 14 days for meningitis and 28 days for endocarditis.

May give an initial dose of 100 mg/kg (not to exceed 4 g) to initiate therapy. Total daily dosage is same for I.M. or I.V. administration and depends on susceptibility of organism and severity of infection. Ceftriaxone should be injected deep I.M. into a large muscle mass, such as the gluteus or lateral aspect of the thigh.

Preoperative prophylaxis
Adults: 1 g I.M. or I.V. 30 minutes to 2 hours before surgery.

Uncomplicated gonorrhea
Adults: 125 to 250 mg I.M. given as a single dose; ◊ 1 to 2 g I.M. or I.V. daily until improvement occurs.

◊ **Haemophilus ducreyi *infection***
Adults: 250 mg I.M. as a single dose.

◊ ***Sexually transmitted epididymitis, pelvic inflammatory disease***
Adults: 250 mg I.M. as a single dose; follow up with other antibiotics.

◊ ***Anti-infectives for sexual assault victims***
Adults: 125 mg I.M. as a single dose in conjunction with other antibiotics.

◊ ***Lyme disease***
Adults: 1 to 2 g I.M. or I.V. q 12 to 24 hours.

✦ ***Dosage adjustment.*** In patients with impaired hepatic and renal function, dosage should not exceed 2 g/day without monitoring serum drug levels.

Pharmacodynamics

Antibacterial action: Ceftriaxone is primarily bactericidal; however, it may be bacteriostatic. Activity depends on organism, tissue penetration, and drug dosage and on rate of organism multiplication. It acts by adhering to bacterial penicillin-binding proteins, thereby inhibiting cell-wall synthesis. Third-generation cephalosporins appear more active against some beta-lactamase-producing gram-negative organisms.

Ceftriaxone is active against some gram-positive organisms and many enteric gram-negative bacilli, as well as streptococci; *Streptococcus pneumoniae* and *pyogenes; Staphylococcus aureus* (penicillinase and non-penicillinase producing); *Staphylococcus epidermidis; Escherichia coli; Klebsiella* species; *Haemophilus influenzae, Enterobacter; Proteus;* some strains of *Pseudomonas* and *Peptostreptococcus* and spirochetes such as *Borrelia burgdorferi* (the causative organism of Lyme disease). Most strains of *Listeria, Pseudomonas,* and *Acinetobacter* are resistant. Generally, ceftriaxone's activity is most like that of cefotaxime and ceftizoxime.

Pharmacokinetics

- *Absorption:* Drug is not absorbed from the GI tract and must be given parenterally; peak serum levels occur at 2 to 3 hours after an I.M. dose.
- *Distribution:* Ceftriaxone is distributed widely into most body tissues and fluids, including the gallbladder, liver, kidneys, bone, sputum, bile, and pleural and synovial fluids; unlike most other cephalosporins, ceftriaxone has good CSF penetration. Ceftriaxone crosses the placenta. Protein binding is dose-dependent and decreases as serum levels rise; average is 84% to 96%.
- *Metabolism:* Ceftriaxone is partially metabolized.
- *Excretion:* Excreted principally in urine; some drug is excreted in bile by biliary mechanisms, and small amounts are excreted in breast milk. Elimination half-life is 5½ to 11 hours in adults with normal renal function; severe renal disease prolongs half-life only moderately. Neither hemodialysis nor peritoneal dialysis will remove ceftriaxone.

Contraindications and precautions

Contraindicated in patients with hypersensitivity to ceftriaxone or other cephalosporins. Use cautiously in breast-feeding women and in patients with penicillin allergy.

Interactions

Concomitant use with *aminoglycosides* produces synergistic antimicrobial activity against *Pseudomonas aeruginosa* and some strains of *enterobacteriaceae.* High doses of *probenecid* may increase clearance by blocking biliary secretion and displacement of ceftriaxone from plasma proteins.

Effects on diagnostic tests

Ceftriaxone causes false-positive results in urine glucose tests utilizing cupric sulfate (Benedict's reagent or Clinitest); use glucose oxidase (Chemstrip uG, Diastix, or glucose enzymatic test strip) instead. Ceftriaxone also causes false elevations in urine creatinine levels in tests using Jaffé's reaction.

Ceftriaxone may cause positive Coombs' test results and elevations in liver function test results.

Adverse reactions

CNS: headache, dizziness.
GI: pseudomembranous colitis, nausea, vomiting, diarrhea, urolithiasis.
GU: genital pruritus, moniliasis, elevated BUN levels.
Hematologic: eosinophilia, thrombocytosis, leukopenia.
Skin: pain, induration, tenderness (at injection site); phlebitis; *rash;* pruritus.
Other: hypersensitivity reactions (serum sickness, ***anaphylaxis***), elevated temperature, chills, jaundice.

Overdose and treatment

Clinical signs of overdose include neuromuscular hypersensitivity. Seizure may follow high CNS concentrations. Treatment is supportive.

☑ Special considerations

Besides those relevant to all *cephalosporins,* consider the following recommendations.

- For patients on sodium restriction, note that ceftriaxone injection contains 3.6 mEq of sodium per gram of drug.
- Ceftriaxone is used commonly in home care programs for management of serious infections, such as osteomyelitis.

• Dosage adjustment usually is not necessary in patients with renal insufficiency because of partial biliary excretion.

Patient education
• Inform patient of potential adverse reactions.

Pediatric use
• Ceftriaxone may be used in neonates and children. Use cautiously in hyperbilirubinemic neonates due to drug's ability to displace bilirubin.

Breast-feeding
• Drug is distributed into breast milk. Use with caution in breast-feeding women.

cefuroxime axetil
Ceftin

cefuroxime sodium
Kefurox, Zinacef

Pharmacologic classification: second-generation cephalosporin
Therapeutic classification: antibiotic
Pregnancy risk category B

How supplied
Available by prescription only
cefuroxime axetil
Tablets: 125 mg, 250 mg, 500 mg
Suspension: 125 mg/5 ml
cefuroxime sodium
Injection: 750 mg, 1.5 g
Infusion: 750 mg, 1.5-g infusion packets, 7.5-g bulk packets

Indications, route, and dosage
Serious lower respiratory, urinary tract, skin and skin-structure infections; septicemia; meningitis caused by susceptible organisms
Adults: Usual dosage is 750 mg to 1.5 g I.M. or I.V. q 8 hours, usually for 5 to 10 days. For life-threatening infections and infections caused by less susceptible organisms, 1.5 g I.M. or I.V. q 6 hours; for bacterial meningitis, up to 3 g I.V. q 8 hours.
Children and infants over age 3 months: 50 to 100 mg/kg/day I.M. or I.V. in divided doses q 6 to 8 hours. Some clinicians give 100 to 150 mg/kg/day. For meningitis, the usual starting dose is 200 to 240 mg/kg/day I.V. in divided doses q 6 to 8 hours, reduced to 100 mg/kg/day when clinical improvement is seen. However, some clinicians prefer other agents for meningitis.

Total daily dosage is same for I.M. or I.V. administration and depends on susceptibility of organism and severity of infection. Cefuroxime should be injected deep I.M. into a large muscle mass, such as the gluteus or lateral aspect of the thigh.
Pharyngitis, tonsillitis, lower respiratory infection, urinary tract infection
Adults and children over age 12: 125 to 500 mg P.O. b.i.d. for 10 days.
Children under age 12 who can swallow pills: 125 to 250 mg P.O. b.i.d. (tablets) for 10 days.
Children age 3 months to 12 years: 20 mg/kg/day in divided doses b.i.d. (oral suspension) to maximum dose of 500 mg for 10 days.
Otitis media, impetigo
Children age 3 months to 12 years: 30 mg/kg/day P.O. oral suspension divided into two doses (maximum dose, 1 g) for 10 days.
Children who can swallow pills: 250 mg P.O. b.i.d. for 10 days.

Note: Compliance may be a problem when treating otitis media in children. Order suspension form if child is unable to swallow pills.
Preoperative prophylaxis
Adults: 1.5 g I.V. 30 to 60 minutes before surgery; then 750 mg I.M. or I.V. q 8 hours intraoperatively for a prolonged procedure.
◊ ***Gonorrhea (uretheral, endocervical,*** ◊ ***rectal)***
Adults: 1.5 g I.M. given as a single dose, alone or with other antibiotics.
***Lyme disease (erythema migrans) caused by* Borrelia burgdoferi**
Adults and children age 13 and older: 500 mg P.O. b.i.d. for 20 days.
✦ ***Dosage adjustment.*** Safety of drug in renal patients has not been established. In patients with impaired renal function, dose or frequency of administration must be modified based on degree of renal impairment, severity of infection, and susceptibility of organism. To prevent toxic accumulation, reduced I.M. or I.V. dosage may be required in patients with creatinine clearance below 20 ml/minute/1.73 m².

Creatinine clearance (ml/min/1.73 m²)	Dosage in adults
> 20	750 mg to 1.5 g q 8 hr
10 to 20	750 mg q 12 hr
< 10	750 mg q 24 hr
Hemodialysis patients	750 mg at end of each dialysis period in addition to regular dose

Pharmacodynamics
Antibacterial action: Cefuroxime is primarily bactericidal; however, it may be bacteriostatic. Activity depends on the organism, tissue penetration, drug dosage, and rate of organism multiplication. It acts by adhering to bacterial penicillin-binding proteins, thereby inhibiting cell-wall synthesis.

Cefuroxime is active against many gram-positive organisms and enteric gram-negative bacilli, including *Streptococcus pneumoniae* and *S. pyogenes, Haemophilus influenzae, Klebsiella* species, *Staphylococcus aureus, Escherichia coli, Enterobacter,* and *Neisseria gonorrhoeae;* its spectrum is similar to that of cefamandole, but it is more stable against beta-lactamases. *Bacteroides fragilis, Pseudomonas,* and *Acinetobacter* are resistant to cefuroxime.

Pharmacokinetics
• *Absorption:* Cefuroxime sodium is not well absorbed from the GI tract and must be given par-

enterally; peak serum levels occur 15 to 60 minutes after an I.M. dose.

Cefuroxime axetil is better absorbed orally, with between 37% to 52% of an oral dose reaching the systemic circulation. Peak serum levels after oral administration occur in about 2 hours. Food appears to enhance absorption. Tablets and suspension are not bioequivalent.

• *Distribution:* Drug is distributed widely into most body tissues and fluids, including the gallbladder, liver, kidneys, bone, bile, and pleural and synovial fluids; CSF penetration is greater than that of most first- and second-generation cephalosporins and achieves adequate therapeutic levels in inflamed meninges. Cefuroxime crosses the placenta; it is 33% to 50% protein-bound.

• *Metabolism:* Cefuroxime is not metabolized.

• *Excretion:* Drug is primarily excreted in urine by renal tubular secretion and glomerular filtration; elimination half-life is 1 to 2 hours in patients with normal renal function; end-stage renal disease prolongs half-life 15 to 22 hours. Some drug is excreted in breast milk. Hemodialysis removes cefuroxime.

Contraindications and precautions

Contraindicated in patients with hypersensitivity to cefuroxime or other cephalosporins. Use cautiously in breast-feeding women and in those with impaired renal function or penicillin allergy.

Interactions

Probenecid competitively inhibits renal tubular secretion of cephalosporins, resulting in higher, prolonged serum levels of these drugs.

Concomitant use of cefuroxime with *nephrotoxic agents* (*vancomycin, colistin, polymixin B*, or *aminoglycosides*) or *loop diuretics* may increase the risk of nephrotoxicity.

Effects on diagnostic tests

Drug causes false-positive results in urine glucose tests using cupric sulfate (Benedict's reagent or Clinitest); use glucose oxidase tests (Chemstrip uG, Diastix, or glucose enzymatic test strip) instead. Cefuroxime also causes false elevations in serum or urine creatinine levels in tests using Jaffé's reaction.

Cefuroxime may elevate liver function test results and may cause positive Coombs' test results.

Adverse reactions

GI: pseudomembranous colitis, nausea, anorexia, vomiting, *diarrhea.*

Hematologic: transient neutropenia, eosinophilia, ***hemolytic anemia, thrombocytopenia,*** decreased hemoglobin and hematocrit levels.

Skin: *maculopapular and erythematous rash, urticaria.*

Other: transient increases in liver enzymes, hypersensitivity reactions (serum sickness, ***anaphylaxis***); *pain, induration, sterile abscesses, temperature elevation, tissue sloughing* (at injection site); *phlebitis, thrombophlebitis* (with I.V. injection).

Overdose and treatment

Clinical signs of overdose include neuromuscular hypersensitivity. Seizure may follow high CNS concentrations. Hemodialysis or peritoneal dialysis will remove cefuroxime.

☑ Special considerations

Besides those relevant to all *cephalosporins*, consider the following recommendations.

• Cefuroxime is a second-generation cephalosporin similar to cefamandole. However, cefuroxime has not been associated with prothrombin deficiency and bleeding. It offers the advantage of effectiveness in treating meningitis.

• Tablets and suspension are not bioequivalent and cannot be substituted on a mg/mg basis.

• For patients on sodium restriction, note that cefuroxime sodium contains 2.4 mEq of sodium per gram of drug.

• Check solutions for particulate matter and discoloration. Solution may range in color from light yellow to amber without affecting potency.

• Shake I.M. solution gently before administration to ensure complete drug dissolution. Administer deep I.M. in a large muscle mass, preferably the gluteus area. Aspirate before injecting to prevent inadvertent injection into a blood vessel. Rotate injection sites to prevent tissue damage. Apply ice to injection site to relieve pain.

• For direct intermittent I.V., inject solution slowly into vein over 3 to 5 minutes or slowly through tubing of free-running, compatible I.V. solution.

• Reconstituted solution retains potency for 24 hours at room temperature or for 48 hours if refrigerated.

• Because drug is hemodialyzable, patients undergoing treatment with hemodialysis or peritoneal dialysis may require dosage adjustments.

• Reconstituted suspension can be stored at room temperature or in refrigerator. Unused portion should be discarded after 10 days. Shake well before each dose.

Patient education

• Inform patient of potential adverse reactions.

Geriatric use

• Use with caution in elderly patients.

Pediatric use

• Safe use in infants under age 3 months has not been established.

Breast-feeding

• Drug distributes into breast milk and should be used with caution in breast-feeding women.

cephalexin hydrochloride

Keftab

cephalexin monohydrate

Biocef, C-Lexin*, Keflex, Novo-Lexin*

Pharmacologic classification: first-generation cephalosporin
Therapeutic classification: antibiotic
Pregnancy risk category B

How supplied

Available by prescription only
cephalexin hydrochloride
Tablets: 500 mg
cephalexin monohydrate
Tablets: 250 mg, 500 mg, 1 g
Capsules: 250 mg, 500 mg
Suspension: 125 mg/5 ml, 250 mg/5 ml

Indications, route, and dosage

Respiratory, GU, skin and soft-tissue, or bone and joint infections caused by susceptible organisms
Adults: 250 mg to 1 g P.O. q 6 hours.
Children: 25 to 50 mg/kg/day divided into four doses. In patients over age 1 with streptococcal pharyngitis or skin and structure infections, dose may be administered q 12 hours.
Otitis media
Adults: 250 mg to 1 g P.O. q 6 hours.
Children: 75 to 100 mg/kg/day divided into four doses.
✦ ***Dosage adjustment.*** To prevent toxic accumulation in patients with impaired renal function with creatinine clearance below 40 ml/minute, give reduced dosage. If creatinine clearance is below 5 ml/minute, give 250 mg q 12 to 24 hours; if it ranges between 5 and 10 ml/minute, give 250 mg q 12 hours; and if it is 11 to 40 ml/minute, give 500 mg q 8 to 12 hours.

Pharmacodynamics

Antibacterial action: Cephalexin is primarily bactericidal; however, it may be bacteriostatic. Activity depends on the organism, tissue penetration, drug dosage, and rate of organism multiplication. It acts by adhering to bacterial penicillin-binding proteins, thereby inhibiting cell-wall synthesis.

Cephalexin is active against a number of gram-positive organisms, including penicillinase-producing *Staphylococcus aureus* and *S. epidermidis, Streptococcus pneumoniae,* group B streptococci, and group A beta-hemolytic streptococci; susceptible gram-negative organisms include *Klebsiella pneumoniae, Escherichia coli, Proteus mirabilis,* and *Shigella.*

Pharmacokinetics

• *Absorption:* Drug is absorbed rapidly and completely from the GI tract after oral administration; peak serum levels occur within 1 hour. The base monohydrate is probably converted to the hydrochloride in the stomach before absorption. Food delays but does not prevent complete absorption.
• *Distribution:* Distributed widely into most body tissues and fluids, including the gallbladder, liver, kidneys, bone, sputum, bile, and pleural and synovial fluids; CSF penetration is poor. Cephalexin crosses the placenta; it is 6% to 15% protein-bound.
• *Metabolism:* Cephalexin is not metabolized.
• *Excretion:* Excreted primarily unchanged in urine by glomerular filtration and renal tubular secretion; small amounts of drug may be excreted in breast milk. Elimination half-life is about ½ to 1 hour in patients with normal renal function; 7½ to 14 hours in patients with severe renal impairment. Hemodialysis or peritoneal dialysis removes cephalexin.

Contraindications and precautions

Contraindicated in patients with hypersensitivity to cephalosporins. Use cautiously in patients with impaired renal function or penicillin allergy and in breast-feeding women.

Interactions

Probenecid competitively inhibits renal tubular secretion of cephalosporins, resulting in higher, prolonged serum levels of these drugs.

Concomitant use with *nephrotoxic agents* (*vancomycin, colistin, polymixin B, aminoglycosides*) or *loop diuretics* may increase the risk of nephrotoxicity.

Effects on diagnostic tests

Drug causes false-positive results in urine glucose tests utilizing cupric sulfate (Benedict's reagent or Clinitest); use glucose oxidase test (Chemstrip uG, Diastix, or glucose enzymatic test strip) instead. Cephalexin also causes false elevations in serum or urine creatinine levels in tests using Jaffé's reaction.

Positive Coombs' test results occur in about 3% of patients taking cephalexin.

Adverse reactions

CNS: dizziness, headache, fatigue, agitation, confusion, hallucinations.
GI: pseudomembranous colitis, *nausea, anorexia,* vomiting, *diarrhea,* gastritis, glossitis, dyspepsia, abdominal pain, anal pruritus, tenesmus, oral candidiasis.
GU: genital pruritus and candidiasis, vaginitis, interstitial nephritis.
Hematologic: ***neutropenia,*** eosinophilia, anemia, ***thrombocytopenia.***
Skin: *maculopapular and erythematous rash, urticaria.*
Other: transient increases in liver enzymes, hypersensitivity reactions (serum sickness, **anaphylaxis**), arthritis, arthralgia, joint pain.

Overdose and treatment

Clinical signs of overdose include neuromuscular hypersensitivity; seizure may follow high CNS concentrations. Remove cephalexin by hemodialysis or peritoneal dialysis. Other treatment is supportive.

☑ Special considerations

Besides those relevant to all *cephalosporins,* consider the following recommendations.
• To prepare the oral suspension, add the required amount of water to the powder in two portions. Shake well after each addition. After mixing, store in refrigerator. Suspension is stable for 14 days without significant loss of potency. Store mixture in tightly closed container. Shake well before using.
• Because cephalexin is dialyzable, patients undergoing treatment with hemodialysis or peritoneal dialysis may require dosage adjustment.

Patient education

• Inform patient of potential adverse reactions.

Geriatric use

• Reduce dosage in elderly patients with diminished renal function.

Pediatric use

• Serum half-life is prolonged in neonates and in infants under age 1. Safety and effectiveness in children have not been established.

Breast-feeding

• Drug distributes into breast milk and should be used with caution in breast-feeding women.

cephalothin sodium

Keflin

Pharmacologic classification: first-generation cephalosporin
Therapeutic classification: antibiotic
Pregnancy risk category B

How supplied

Available by prescription only
Injection: 1 g, 2 g, 4 g
Infusion: 1 g/50 ml, 2 g/50 ml, 1 g/dl, 2 g/dl
Pharmacy bulk package: 20 g

Indications, route, and dosage

Serious respiratory, GU, GI, skin and soft-tissue, bone and joint infections; septicemia; endocarditis; meningitis
Adults: 500 mg to 1 g I.M. or I.V. (or intraperitoneally) q 4 to 6 hours; in life-threatening infections, up to 2 g q 4 hours.
Children: 80 to 160 mg/kg/day in divided doses I.V. q 6 hours; dosage should be proportionately reduced based on age, weight, and severity of infection.

Cephalothin should be injected deep I.M. into a large muscle mass, such as the gluteus or lateral aspect of the thigh. I.V. route is preferable in severe or life-threatening infections.

Preoperative prophylaxis
Adults: 1 to 2 g I.V. 30 to 60 minutes before surgery; then 1 to 2 g I.M. or I.V. q 6 hours postoperatively.
Children: 20 to 30 mg/kg I.V. 30 to 60 minutes before surgery; then 20 to 30 mg/kg I.M. or I.V. q 6 hours postoperatively. Discontinue within 24 hours of surgery.

◊ ***Ventriculitis***
Children: 15 to 100 mg/day intraventricularly.

✦ **Dosage adjustment.** Dosage schedule is determined by degree of renal impairment, severity of infection, and susceptibility of causative organism. To prevent toxic accumulation, reduced dosage may be required in patients with creatinine clearance below 50 ml/minute.

Because cephalothin is dialyzable, patients undergoing treatment with hemodialysis or peritoneal dialysis may require dosage adjustments.

Creatinine clearance (ml/min/1.73 m^2)	Dosage in adults
> 80	Usual adult dose
50 to 80	Up to 2 g q 6 hr
25 to 50	Up to 1.5 g q 6 hr
10 to 25	Up to 1 g q 6 hr
2 to 10	Up to 500 mg q 6 hr
< 2	Up to 500 mg q 8 hr

Pharmacodynamics

Antibacterial action: Cephalothin is primarily bactericidal; however, it may be bacteriostatic. Activity depends on the organism, tissue penetration, drug dosage, and rate of organism multiplication. It acts by adhering to bacterial penicillin-binding proteins, thereby inhibiting cell-wall synthesis.

Like other first-generation cephalosporins, cephalothin is active mainly against gram-positive organisms and some gram-negative organisms. Susceptible organisms include some strains of *Escherichia coli* and other coliform bacteria, group A beta-hemolytic streptococci, *Haemophilus influenzae, Klebsiella, Proteus mirabilis, Salmonella, Staphylococcus aureus, Shigella, Streptococcus pneumoniae,* staphylococci, and *Streptococcus viridans.*

Pharmacokinetics

• *Absorption:* Cephalothin is not absorbed from the GI tract and must be given parenterally; peak serum levels occur 30 minutes after an I.M. dose.
• *Distribution:* Drug is distributed widely into most body tissues and fluids, including the gallbladder, liver, kidneys, bone, sputum, bile, and pleural and synovial fluids; CSF penetration is poor. Cephalothin crosses the placenta; it is 65% to 79% protein-bound.
• *Metabolism:* Metabolized partially by the liver and kidneys.
• *Excretion:* Excreted primarily in urine by renal tubular secretion and glomerular filtration. Small amounts of drug are excreted in breast milk. Elimination half-life is ½ to 1 hour in patients with normal renal function; 19 hours in patients with severe renal disease. Hemodialysis or peritoneal dialysis removes drug.

Contraindications and precautions

Contraindicated in patients with hypersensitivity to cephalothin or other cephalosporins. Use cautiously in patients with impaired renal function or penicillin allergy and in breast-feeding women.

Interactions

Probenecid competitively inhibits renal tubular secretion of cephalosporins, resulting in higher, prolonged serum levels of these drugs.

Concomitant use with *nephrotoxic agents* (*vancomycin, colistin, polymixin B, aminoglycosides*) or *loop diuretics* may increase risk of nephrotoxicity.

Effects on diagnostic tests

Cephalothin causes false-positive results in urine glucose tests utilizing cupric sulfate (Benedict's reagent or Clinitest); use glucose oxidase tests (Chemstrip uG, Diastix, or glucose enzymatic test strip) instead. Cephalothin also causes false elevations in serum or urine creatinine levels in tests using Jaffé's reaction.

Drug may cause positive Coombs' test results or elevate liver function test results.

Adverse reactions

CNS: headache, malaise, paresthesia, dizziness.
GI: pseudomembranous colitis, nausea, anorexia, vomiting, *diarrhea,* dyspepsia, abdominal cramps.
GU: nephrotoxicity, genital pruritus, candidiasis.
Hematologic: transient neutropenia, eosinophilia, ***hemolytic anemia, thrombocytopenia.***
Skin: *maculopapular and erythematous rash, urticaria.*
Other: transient increases in liver enzymes, hypersensitivity reactions (serum sickness, ***anaphylaxis***); *pain, induration, sterile abscesses, tissue sloughing* (at injection site); *phlebitis, thrombophlebitis* (with I.V. injection).

Overdose and treatment

Clinical signs of overdose include neuromuscular hypersensitivity; seizure may follow high CNS concentrations. Remove drug by hemodialysis or peritoneal dialysis.

☑ Special considerations

Besides those relevant to all *cephalosporins,* consider the following recommendations.

- Avoid I.M. injection if possible because it is painful. Inject I.M. dose deeply into a large muscle mass to reduce pain. Apply ice to injection site. Rotate injection sites to prevent tissue irritation.
- For I.M. administration, reconstitute each gram of cephalothin with 4 ml of sterile water for injection, providing 500 mg in each 2.2 ml. If contents do not dissolve completely, add an additional 0.2 to 0.4 ml of diluent, and warm contents slightly.
- For intermittent I.V. infusion, dissolve 4 g cephalothin in 40 ml of sterile water for injection, 5% dextrose, or 0.9% NaCl injection. Discontinue other infusion during administration. For continuous infusion, dissolve 1 or 2 g of drug in at least 10 ml sterile water for injection and add to one of the following I.V. solutions: lactated Ringer's injection, dextrose 5% injection, dextrose 5% in lactated Ringer's injection, Ionosol B in D_5W, Normosol-M in D_5W, acetated Ringer's injection, or 0.9% NaCl injection. Choose solution and fluid volume according to patient's fluid and electrolyte status.
- Administer reconstituted I.M. and I.V. solutions within 12 hours. Solutions for continuous infusion should start within 12 hours and be completed within 24 hours.
- Reconstituted solutions are stable for 96 hours under refrigeration. Low temperature may cause solution to precipitate. Warm to room temperature with gentle agitation before using.
- Discoloration in solution stored at room temperature does not indicate loss of potency.
- Do not freeze drug in plastic syringes.
- Solutions reconstituted in original container and frozen immediately are stable for as long as 12 weeks at – 4° F (–20° C). Do not thaw solution until ready to use. Do not heat to thaw or refreeze once thawed

Patient education

- Inform patient of potential adverse reactions.

Geriatric use

- Dosage reduction may be required in patients with diminished renal function.

Breast-feeding

- Drug distributes into breast milk; use with caution in breast-feeding women.

cephradine

Velosef

Pharmacologic classification: first-generation cephalosporin
Therapeutic classification: antibiotic
Pregnancy risk category B

How supplied

Available by prescription only
Capsules: 250 mg, 500 mg
Suspension: 125 mg/5 ml, 250 mg/5 ml
Injection: 250 mg, 500 mg, 1 g, 2 g

Indications, route, and dosage

Serious respiratory, GU, skin and soft-tissue, bone and joint infections; septicemia; endocarditis; and otitis media

Adults: 250 to 500 mg P.O. q 6 hours. Severe or chronic infections may require larger or more frequent doses (up to 1 g P.O. q 6 hours). Alternatively, 500 mg to 1 g I.M. or I.V. q 6 hours.

Children over age 9 months: 25 to 100 mg/kg P.O. daily in equally divided doses q 6 to 12 hours. Alternatively, 12.5 to 25 mg/kg I.M. or I.V. q 6 hours.

Larger doses (up to 1 g q.i.d.) may be given for severe or chronic infections in all patients regardless of age and weight.

✦ ***Dosage adjustment.*** To prevent toxic accumulation, reduced dosage may be required in patients with creatinine clearance below 20 ml/minute as follows:

Creatinine clearance (ml/min/1.73 m²)	Dosage in adults
> 20	500 mg q 6 hr
5 to 20	250 mg q 6 hr
< 5	250 mg q 12 hr

For patients on chronic intermittent dialysis, give 250 mg initially; repeat in 12 hours and after 36 to 48 hours. Children may require dose modifications proportional to weight and severity of infection.

Pharmacodynamics

Antibacterial action: Drug is primarily bactericidal; however, it may be bacteriostatic. Activity depends on the organism, tissue penetration, drug dosage, and rate of organism multiplication. It acts by adhering to bacterial penicillin-binding proteins, thereby inhibiting cell-wall synthesis.

Like other first-generation cephalosporins, cephradine is active against many gram-positive organisms and some gram-negative organisms. Susceptible organisms include *Escherichia coli* and other coliform bacteria, group A beta-hemolytic streptococci, *Hemophilus influenzae, Klebsiella, Proteus mirabilis, Staphylococcus aureus, Streptococcus pneumoniae,* staphylococci, and *Streptococcus viridans.*

Pharmacokinetics

- *Absorption:* Cephradine is well absorbed from the GI tract; peak serum levels occur within 1 hour after an oral dose.
- *Distribution:* Drug is distributed widely into most body tissues and fluids, including the gallbladder, liver, kidneys, bone, sputum, bile, and pleural and synovial fluids; CSF penetration is poor. Cephradine crosses the placenta; it is 6% to 20% protein-bound.
- *Metabolism:* Cephradine is not metabolized.
- *Excretion:* Drug is excreted primarily in urine by renal tubular and glomerular filtration; small amounts of drug are excreted in breast milk. Elimination half-life is about ½ to 2 hours in normal renal function; end-stage renal disease prolongs half-life to 8 to 15 hours. Hemodialysis or peritoneal dialysis removes drug.

Contraindications and precautions

Contraindicated in patients with hypersensitivity to drug and other cephalosporins. Use cautiously in patients with impaired renal function or penicillin allergy and in breast-feeding women.

Interactions

Probenecid competitively inhibits renal tubular secretion of cephalosporins, resulting in higher, prolonged serum levels of these drugs.

Concomitant use with *nephrotoxic agents* (*vancomycin, colistin, polymixin B,* or *aminoglycosides*) or *loop diuretics* may increase the risk of nephrotoxicity.

Concomitant use with *bacteriostatic agents* (*tetracyclines, erythromycin,* or *chloramphenicol*) may interfere with bactericidal activity.

Effects on diagnostic tests

Drug causes false-positive results in urine glucose tests utilizing cupric sulfate (Benedict's reagent or Clinitest); use glucose oxidase tests (Chemstrip uG, Diastix, or glucose enzymatic test strip) instead. Cephradine also causes false elevations in serum or urine creatinine levels in tests using Jaffé's reaction.

Cephradine may cause positive Coombs' test results or elevate liver function test results.

Adverse reactions

CNS: dizziness, headache, malaise, paresthesia.
GI: pseudomembranous colitis, *nausea, anorexia,* vomiting, heartburn, abdominal cramps, *diarrhea,* oral candidiasis.
GU: genital pruritus and candidiasis, vaginitis.
Hematologic: transient neutropenia, eosinophilia, ***thrombocytopenia.***
Skin: *maculopapular and erythematous rash, urticaria.*
Other: transient increases in liver enzymes, hypersensitivity reactions (serum sickness, ***anaphylaxis***).

Overdose and treatment

Clinical signs of overdose include neuromuscular hypersensitivity; seizure may follow high CNS concentrations. Remove cephradine by hemodialysis.

☑ Special considerations

Besides those relevant to all *cephalosporins,* consider the following recommendations.

- Reconstituted oral suspension may be stored for 7 days at room temperature or for 14 days in the refrigerator.
- Because drug is dialyzable, patients undergoing treatment with hemodialysis may require dosage adjustments.

Patient education

- Inform patient of potential adverse reactions.

Geriatric use

- Reduced dosage may be required in patients with reduced renal function. Use with caution.

Pediatric use

- Serum half-life is prolonged in neonates and infants under age 1. Safe use has not been established.

Breast-feeding

- Drug distributes into breast milk; use with caution in breast-feeding women. Safe use has not been established.

cerivastatin sodium

Baycol

Pharmacologic classification: 3-hydroxy-3-methylglutaryl-coenzyme A (HMG-CoA) reductase inhibitor
Therapeutic classification: antilipidemic
Pregnancy risk category X

How supplied

Available by prescription only
Tablets: 0.2 mg, 0.3 mg

Indications, route, and dosage

Adjunct to diet for reducing elevated total and low-density lipoprotein (LDL) cholesterol levels in patients with primary hypercholesterolemia and mixed dyslipidemia when diet

and other nonpharmacologic measures have been inadequate
Adults: 0.3mg, P.O., once daily in the evening.
✦ ***Dosage adjustment.*** In patients with significant renal impairment (creatinine clearance 60 ml/minute/1.73 m^2 or less), 0.2 mg P.O. once daily in the evening.

Pharmacodynamics

Antilipidemic action: Competitive inhibitor of HMG-CoA reductase that is responsible for conversion of HMG-CoA to mevalonate, a precursor of sterols including cholesterol. Reducing the level of cholesterol in hepatic cells stimulates synthesis of LDL receptors, leading to an increase in uptake of LDL particles.

Pharmacokinetics

- *Absorption:* Absorbed in the active form. Mean absolute bioavailability of 0.2-mg tablet is 60%, with peak concentrations occurring about 2.5 hours after a dose. Absorption is similar if taken with an evening meal or 4 hours after an evening meal.
- *Distribution:* Mean volume of distribution is 0.3 L/kg. Over 99% of circulating drug is bound to plasma proteins (80% bound to albumin).
- *Metabolism:* Extensively metabolized to two active metabolites, M1 and M23. A demethylation reaction forms M1, and a hydroxylation reaction forms M23. The relative potencies of M1 and M23 are 50% and 80% of the active compound, respectively. Relative concentrations of these metabolites in comparison to the parent compound are significantly less. Therefore, cholesterol-lowering effect of cerivastatin is due primarily to parent compound.
- *Excretion:* Drug does not occur in urine or feces; M1 and M23 are the major metabolites excreted by these routes. Following an oral dose of 0.4 mg ^{14}C-cerivastatin to healthy volunteers, excretion of radioactivity is about 24% in the urine and 70% in the feces. The parent compound, cerivastatin accounts for less than 2% of total radioactivity excreted.

Contraindications and precautions

Contraindicated in patients with active liver disease, unexplained persistent elevations of serum transaminases, or known hypersensititivy to drug. Also contraindicated during pregnancy and in breast-feeding patients. Avoid use in women of childbearing age unless patient is highly unlikely to conceive because of potential for fetal harm. If patient becomes pregnant during therapy, discontinue drug. Use cautiously in patients with history of liver disease or chronic alcohol ingestion.

Interactions:

Cholestyramine given within 4 hours of drug results in decreased absorption and decreased peak plasma levels of cerivastatin. However, administration of cerivastatin at bedtime and cholestyramine 1 hour before the evening meal does not result in a significant decrease in the clinical effect of cerivastatin. *Azole antifungals, cyclosporine, erythromycin, fibric acid derivatives* and *niacin* may increase the risk of myopathy. *Erythromycin* decreases hepatic metabolism of drug and increases serum concentrations of cerivastatin up to 50%.

Effects on diagnostic tests

Drug therapy may elevate transaminases, CK, alkaline phosphatase, gamma glutamyl transpeptidase, and bilirubin. Thyroid function abnormalities have been reported.

Adverse reactions

CNS: asthenia, dizziness, *headache*, insomnia.
CV: chest pain, peripheral edema.
EENT: *pharyngitis, rhinitis,* sinusitis.
GI: abdominal pain, constipation, diarrhea, dyspepsia, flatulence, nausea.
GU: urinary tract infection.
Musculoskeletal: arthralgia, back or leg pain, myalgia.
Respiratory: increased cough.
Skin: rash.
Other: flu syndrome.

Overdose and treatment

There are no specific recommendations regarding the treatment of overdose. If overdose occurs, treat symptomatically and provide supportive measures. Because of extensive drug binding to plasma proteins, hemodialysis may not enhance drug clearance.

☑ Special considerations

- Withhold drug temporarily in patients with acute or serious conditions predisposing them to renal failure secondary to rhabdomyolysis; these include trauma; major surgery; severe metabolic, endocrine and electrolyte disorders; severe acute infection; hypotension; and uncontrolled seizures. Rare cases of rhabdomyolysis have been reported with other HMG-CoA reductase inhibitors.
- Therapy with lipid-lowering drugs should be a component of multiple risk factor intervention program and attempts should be made to control cholesterol with appropriate diet, exercise, and weight reduction before initiating therapy with lipid-lowering drugs.
- Before initiating treatment, exclude secondary causes for hypercholesterolemia and perform a baseline lipid profile. Periodic liver function tests and lipid levels should be done before starting treatment, at 6 and 12 weeks after initiation, or after an increase in dosage and periodically thereafter.
- Because maximal effect of drug is seen within 4 weeks, lipid determinations should be performed at this time.
- Drug may be taken with or without food.
- Drug should be given to women of childbearing age only if conception is highly unlikely and they have been warned of potential risks to fetus.

Patient education

- Teach patient proper dietary management, weight control, and exercise.
- Explain importance in controlling elevated serum lipid levels.
- Tell patient to take drug in the evening with or without food.
- Warn patient to avoid alcohol.

• Inform patient that it may take up to 4 weeks for full therapeutic effect to occur.
• Caution female patient that drug may cause fetal damage. Advise her to call immediately if pregnancy occurs or is suspected.
• Tell patient to immediately report unexplained muscle pain, tenderness, or weakness, especially if accompanied by fever or malaise.

Geriatric use
• Plasma drug levels are similar in healthy elderly male patients over age 65 and in young male patients below age 40.

Pediatric use
• Safety and efficacy have not been established.

Breast-feeding
• Because of potential for adverse reactions in breast-fed infants, women taking cerivastatin should not breast-feed.

cetirizine hydrochloride
Zyrtec

Pharmacologic classification: selective H_1-receptor antagonist
Therapeutic classification: antihistamine
Pregnancy risk category B

How supplied
Available by prescription only
Tablets: 5 mg, 10 mg
Syrup: 5 mg/ml

Indications, route, and dosage
Seasonal allergic rhinitis, perennial allergic rhinitis, chronic urticaria
Adults and children age 6 and older: 5 or 10 mg P.O. daily.
✦ ***Dosage adjustment.*** In hemodialysis patients or those with hepatic impairment or creatinine clearance below 31 ml/minute, 5 mg P.O. daily.

Pharmacodynamics
Antihistaminic action: Cetirizine's principal effects are mediated via selective inhibition of peripheral H_1 receptors.

Pharmacokinetics
• *Absorption:* Cetirizine is rapidly absorbed.
• *Distribution:* Drug is about 93% bound to plasma protein.
• *Metabolism:* Cetirizine is metabolized to a very limited extent by oxidative O-dealkylation to a metabolite with negligible antihistaminic activity.
• *Excretion:* Primarily excreted in urine with 50% as unchanged drug. A small amount is excreted in feces.

Contraindications and precautions
Contraindicated in patients with hypersensitivity to drug or hydroxyzine. Use cautiously in patients with impaired renal function.

Interactions
Ethanol and other *CNS depressants* may cause a possible additive effect. Avoid concomitant use. *Theophylline* may cause decreased clearance of cetirizine. Monitor patient closely.

Effects on diagnostic tests
None reported.

Adverse reactions
CNS: somnolence, fatigue, dizziness.
GI: dry mouth.
Other: pharyngitis.

Overdose and treatment
Overdosage may result in somnolence. If overdosage occurs, treatment should be symptomatic or supportive. There is no known specific antidote for cetirizine and the drug is not effectively removed by dialysis.

☑ Special considerations
• There is no information to indicate that abuse or dependency occurs with cetirizine use.

Patient education
• Caution patient not to perform hazardous activities if somnolence occurs with drug use.
• Instruct patient not to consume alcohol or other CNS depressants while taking drug because of additive effect.

Pediatric use
• Safety and effectiveness in children under age 6 have not been established.

Breast-feeding
• Drug has been reported to be excreted in breast milk. Avoid use of drug in breast-feeding women.

chloral hydrate
Aquachloral Supprettes, Noctec, Novo-Chlorhydrate*

Pharmacologic classification: general CNS depressant
Therapeutic classification: sedative-hypnotic
Controlled substance schedule IV
Pregnancy risk category C

How supplied
Available by prescription only
Capsules: 250 mg, 500 mg
Syrup: 250 mg/5 ml, 500 mg/5 ml
Suppositories: 325 mg, 500 mg, 650 mg

Indications, route, and dosage
Sedation
Adults: 250 mg P.O. t.i.d. after meals.
Children: 8 mg/kg P.O. t.i.d. Maximum dosage, 500 mg t.i.d.
Management of alcohol withdrawal symptoms
Adults: 500 to 1,000 mg; may repeat q 6 hours p.r.n.

Insomnia
Adults: 500 mg to 1 g P.O. or P.R. 15 to 30 minutes before bedtime.
Children: 50 mg/kg P.O. single dose. Maximum dose, 1 g.
Premedication for EEG
Children: 20 to 25 mg/kg P.O. single dose. Maximum dose, 1 g.
Hypnosis
Children: 50 mg/kg P.O. or 1.5 g/m^2 as a single dose. Maximum dose, 1 g.
✦ ***Dosage adjustment.*** Decrease dosage in elderly patients.

Pharmacodynamics
Sedative-hypnotic action: Chloral hydrate has CNS depressant activities similar to those of the barbiturates. Nonspecific CNS depression occurs at hypnotic doses; however, respiratory drive is only slightly affected. Drug's primary site of action is the reticular activating system, which controls arousal. The cellular site(s) of action are not known.

Pharmacokinetics
- *Absorption:* Chloral hydrate is absorbed well after oral and rectal administration. Sleep occurs 30 to 60 minutes after a 500-mg to 1-g dose.
- *Distribution:* Drug and its active metabolite, trichloroethanol, are distributed throughout the body tissue and fluids. Trichloroethanol is 35% to 41% protein-bound.
- *Metabolism:* Metabolized rapidly and nearly completely in the liver and erythrocytes to the active metabolite trichloroethanol. It is further metabolized in the liver and kidneys to trichloroacetic acid and other inactive metabolites.
- *Excretion:* Inactive metabolites of drug hydrate are excreted primarily in urine. Minor amounts are excreted in bile. Half-life of trichloroethanol is 8 to 10 hours.

Contraindications and precautions
Contraindicated in patients with impaired hepatic or renal function, severe cardiac disease, or hypersensitivity to drug. Oral administration contraindicated in patients with gastric disorders. Use with extreme caution in patients with mental depression, suicidal tendencies, or history of drug abuse.

Interactions
Concomitant use with *alcohol, sedative-hypnotics, narcotics, antihistamines, tranquilizers, tricyclic antidepressants*, or other *CNS depressants* will add to or potentiate their effects. Concomitant use with *alcohol* may cause vasodilation, tachycardia, sweating, and flushing in some patients.

Administration of drug followed by I.V. *furosemide* may cause a hypermetabolic state by displacing thyroid hormone from binding sites, resulting in sweating, hot flashes, tachycardia, and variable blood pressure.

Chloral hydrate may displace *oral anticoagulants* such as *warfarin* from protein-binding sites, causing increased hypoprothrombinemic effects.

Elimination of *phenytoin* may be increased.

Effects on diagnostic tests
Drug therapy may produce false-positive results for urine glucose with tests using cupric sulfate, such as Benedict's reagent and possibly Clinitest. It does not interfere with Chemstrip uG, Diastix, or glucose enzymatic test strip results. It will interfere with fluorometric tests for urine catecholamines; do not use drug for 48 hours before the test. Drug may also interfere with Reddy-Jenkins-Thorn test for urinary 17-hydroxycorticosteroids. It also may cause a false-positive phentolamine test.

Adverse reactions
CNS: drowsiness, nightmares, dizziness, ataxia, paradoxical excitement, hangover, somnolence, disorientation, delirium, light-headedness, hallucinations, confusion, vertigo, malaise.
GI: *nausea, vomiting, diarrhea,* flatulence.
Hematologic: eosinophilia, leukopenia.
Skin: hypersensitivity reactions (rash, urticaria).
Other: physical and psychological dependence.

Overdose and treatment
Clinical manifestations of overdose include stupor, coma, respiratory depression, pinpoint pupils, hypotension, and hypothermia. Esophageal stricture may follow gastric necrosis and perforation. GI hemorrhage has also been reported. Hepatic damage and jaundice may occur.

Treatment is supportive of respiration (including mechanical ventilation if needed), blood pressure, and body temperature. If patient is conscious, empty stomach by emesis or gastric lavage. Hemodialysis will remove drug and its metabolite. Peritoneal dialysis may be effective.

☑ Special considerations
- Chloral hydrate is not a first-line drug because of potential for adverse or toxic adverse effects.
- Know that some brands contain tartrazine, which may cause allergic reactions in susceptible individuals.
- Assess level of consciousness before administering drug to ensure appropriate baseline level.
- Give drug capsules with a full glass (8 oz [240 ml]) of water to lessen GI upset; dilute syrup in a half glass of water or juice before administration to improve taste.
- Monitor vital signs frequently.
- Store in dark container away from heat and moisture to prevent breakdown of medicine. Store suppositories in refrigerator.

Patient education
- Advise patient to take drug with a full glass (8 oz) of water and to dilute syrup with juice or water before use.
- Instruct patient in proper administration of drug form prescribed.
- Warn patient not to attempt tasks that require mental alertness or physical coordination until the CNS effects of drug are known.
- Tell patient to avoid alcohol and other CNS depressants.
- Instruct patient to call before using OTC allergy or cold preparations.

• Warn patient not to increase dose or stop drug except as prescribed.

Geriatric use
• Elderly patients may be more susceptible to drug's CNS depressant effects because of decreased elimination. Lower doses are indicated.

Pediatric use
• Drug is safe and effective as a premedication for EEG and other procedures.

Breast-feeding
• Small amounts pass into the breast milk and may cause drowsiness in breast-fed infants of mothers taking drug; avoid use in breast-feeding women.

chlorambucil
Leukeran

Pharmacologic classification: alkylating agent (cell cycle–phase nonspecific)
Therapeutic classification: antineoplastic
Pregnancy risk category D

How supplied
Available by prescription only
Tablets (sugar-coated): 2 mg

Indications, route, and dosage
Dosage and indications may vary. Check current literature for recommended protocol.

Chronic lymphocytic leukemia, malignant lymphomas including lymphosarcoma, giant follicular lymphomas, Hodgkin's disease, ◊ autoimmune hemolytic anemias, ◊ nephrotic syndrome, ◊ polycythemia vera, ◊ macroglobulinemia, ◊ ovarian neoplasms
Adults: 100 to 200 mcg/kg P.O. daily or 3 to 6 mg/m^2 P.O. daily as a single dose or in divided doses; for 3 to 6 weeks. Usual dose is 4 to 10 mg daily. Reduce dose if within 4 weeks of a full course of radiation therapy.

◊ Macroglobulinemia
Adults: 2 to 10 mg P.O. daily.

◊ Metastatic trophoblastic neoplasia
Adults: 6 to 10 mg P.O. daily for 5 days; repeat q 1 to 2 weeks.

◊ Idiopathic uveitis
Adults: 6 to 12 mg P.O. daily for 1 year.

◊ Rheumatoid arthritis
Adults: 0.1 to 0.3 mg/kg P.O. daily.

Pharmacodynamics
Antineoplastic action: Drug exerts its cytotoxic activity by cross-linking strands of cellular DNA and RNA, disrupting normal nucleic acid function.

Pharmacokinetics
• *Absorption:* Chlorambucil is well absorbed from the GI tract.
• *Distribution:* Not well understood. However, drug and its metabolites have been shown to be highly bound to plasma and tissue proteins.
• *Metabolism:* Drug is metabolized in the liver. Its primary metabolite, phenylacetic acid mustard, also possesses cytotoxic activity.
• *Excretion:* Drug's metabolites are excreted in urine. Half-life of parent compound is 2 hours; the phenylacetic acid metabolite, 2½ hours. Drug is probably not dialyzable.

Contraindications and precautions
Contraindicated in patients with hypersensitivity or resistance to previous therapy. Patients hypersensitive to other alkylating agents also may be hypersensitive to drug. Use cautiously in patients with history of head trauma or seizures and in those receiving other drugs that lower seizure threshold.

Interactions
None reported.

Effects on diagnostic tests
Drug therapy may increase concentrations of serum alkaline phosphatase, AST, and blood and urine uric acid.

Adverse reactions
CNS: ***seizures,*** peripheral neuropathy, tremor, muscle twitching, confusion, agitation, ataxia, flaccid paresis.
GI: *nausea, vomiting, stomatitis,* diarrhea.
GU: *azoospermia, infertility.*
Hematologic: ***neutropenia,*** delayed up to 3 weeks, lasting up to 10 days after last dose; ***bone marrow suppression; thrombocytopenia; anemia.***
Hepatic: hepatotoxicity.
Respiratory: interstitial pneumonitis, ***pulmonary fibrosis*** (rare).
Skin: rash, hypersensitivity.
Other: allergic febrile reaction.

Overdose and treatment
Clinical manifestations of overdose include reversible pancytopenia in adults and vomiting, ataxia, abdominal pain, muscle twitching, and major motor seizures in children. Treatment is usually supportive with transfusion of blood components if necessary and appropriate anticonvulsant therapy if seizures occur. Induction of emesis, activated charcoal, and gastric lavage may be useful in removing unabsorbed drug.

☑ Special considerations
• Oral suspension can be prepared in the pharmacy by crushing tablets and mixing powder with a suspending agent and simple syrup.
• Avoid all I.M. injections when platelets are below 100,000/mm^3.
• Anticoagulants and aspirin products should be used cautiously. Watch closely for signs of bleeding.
• Drug-induced pancytopenia generally lasts 1 to 2 weeks but may persist for 3 to 4 weeks. It is reversible up to a cumulative dose of 6.5 mg/kg in a single course.
• To prevent hyperuricemia with resulting uric acid nephropathy, allopurinol may be used with adequate hydration. Monitor uric acid.

• Store tablets in a tightly closed, light-resistant container.

Patient education

• Emphasize importance of continuing medication despite nausea and vomiting, and of keeping appointments for periodic blood work.
• Advise patient to call if vomiting occurs shortly after taking dose or if symptoms of infection or bleeding are present.
• Tell patient to avoid exposure to people with infections.
• Instruct patient to avoid OTC products containing aspirin.
• Advise patient to use contraceptive measures during therapy.

Pediatric use

• Safety and efficacy in children have not been established. The potential benefits versus risks must be evaluated.

Breast-feeding

• It is unknown if drug distributes into breast milk. The risk of potential serious adverse reactions, mutagenicity, and carcinogenicity in breast-feeding infants and the mother's need for the medication should be considered in deciding whether to discontinue drug or breast-feed.

chloramphenicol

Chloromycetin, Chloroptic, Econochlor, Fenicol*, Ophthochlor, Pentamycetin*

chloramphenicol sodium succinate

Chloromycetin Sodium Succinate, Pentamycetin*

Pharmacologic classification: dichloroacetic acid derivative
Therapeutic classification: antibiotic
Pregnancy risk category C

How supplied

Available by prescription only
Powder for solution: 25 mg/vial
Injection: 1-g, 10-g vial
Ophthalmic solution: 0.5%
Ophthalmic ointment: 1%
Otic solution: 0.5%, 4.5%*

Indications, route, and dosage

Severe meningitis, brain abscesses, bacteremia, or other serious infections
Adults and children: 50 to 100 mg/kg I.V. daily, divided q 6 hours. Maximum dose, 100 mg/kg daily.
Premature infants and neonates weighing less than 4.4 lb (2 kg) or age under 7 days: 25 mg/kg I.V. daily.
Neonates weighing more than 4.4 lb and age 7 days or older: 25 mg/kg I.V. q 12 hours. I.V. route must be used to treat meningitis.
Superficial infections of the skin caused by susceptible bacteria
Adults and children: Rub into affected area b.i.d. or t.i.d.
External ear canal infection
Adults and children: Instill 2 to 3 drops into ear canal t.i.d or q.i.d.
Surface bacterial infection involving conjunctiva or cornea
Adults and children: Instill 2 drops of solution in eye q hour until condition improves, or instill q.i.d., depending on severity of infection. Apply small amount of ointment to lower conjunctival sac at bedtime as supplement to drops. To use ointment alone, apply small amount to lower conjunctival sac q 3 to 6 hours or more frequently if necessary. Continue with treatment up to 48 hours after condition improves.

Pharmacodynamics

Antibacterial action: Chloramphenicol palmitate and chloramphenicol sodium succinate must be hydrolyzed to chloramphenicol before antimicrobial activity can take place. The active compound then inhibits bacterial protein synthesis by binding to the ribosome's 50S subunit, thus inhibiting peptide bond formation.

Drug usually produces bacteriostatic effects on susceptible bacteria, including *Rickettsia, Chlamydia, Mycoplasma,* and certain *Salmonella* strains, as well as most gram-positive and gram-negative organisms. Chloramphenicol is used to treat *Haemophilus influenzae,* Rocky Mountain spotted fever, meningitis, lymphogranuloma, psittacosis, severe meningitis, and bacteremia.

Pharmacokinetics

• *Absorption:* With I.V. administration, serum concentrations vary greatly, depending on patient's metabolism.
• *Distribution:* Drug is distributed widely to most body tissues and fluids, including CSF, liver, and kidneys; it readily crosses the placenta. Approximately 50% to 60% of drug binds to plasma proteins.
• *Metabolism:* Parent drug is metabolized primarily by hepatic glucuronyl transferase to inactive metabolites.
• *Excretion:* About 8% to 12% of dose is excreted by the kidneys as unchanged drug; the remainder is excreted as inactive metabolites. (However, some drug may be excreted in breast milk.) Plasma half-life ranges from about 1½ to 4½ hours in adults with normal hepatic and renal function. Plasma half-life of parent drug is prolonged in patients with hepatic dysfunction. Peritoneal hemodialysis does not remove significant drug amounts. Plasma chloramphenicol levels may be elevated in patients with renal impairment after I.V. chloramphenicol administration.

Contraindications and precautions

Contraindicated in patients with hypersensitivity to chloramphenicol.

Use cautiously in patients with impaired renal or hepatic function, acute intermittent porphyria, or

G6PD deficiency and in those taking drugs that suppress bone marrow function.

Interactions

When used concomitantly, chloramphenicol inhibits hepatic metabolism of *phenytoin, dicumarol, tolbutamide, chlorpropamide, phenobarbital*, and *cyclophosphamide* (by inhibiting microsomal enzyme activity); that leads to prolonged plasma half-life of these drugs and possible toxicity from increased serum drug concentrations. When used concomitantly, chloramphenicol may antagonize *penicillin*'s bactericidal activity.

Concomitant use with *acetaminophen* causes an elevated serum chloramphenicol level (by an unknown mechanism), possibly resulting in an enhanced pharmacologic effect. Concomitant use with *iron salts, folic acid*, and *vitamin B_2* reduces the hematologic response to these substances.

Effects on diagnostic tests

False elevation of urinary para-aminobenzoic acid (PABA) levels will result if chloramphenicol is administered during a bentiromide test for pancreatic function. Drug therapy will cause false-positive results on tests for urine glucose level using cupric sulfate (Clinitest). Erythrocyte, platelet, and leukocyte counts in the blood and possibly the bone marrow may decrease during drug therapy (from reversible or irreversible bone marrow depression). Hemoglobinuria or lactic acidosis may also occur with chloramphenicol treatment.

Adverse reactions

CNS: headache, mild depression, confusion, delirium, peripheral neuropathy with prolonged therapy.
EENT: optic neuritis (in patients with cystic fibrosis), glossitis, decreased visual acuity, optic atrophy in children, stinging or burning of eye after instillation, blurred vision (with ointment).
GI: nausea, vomiting, stomatitis, diarrhea, enterocolitis.
Hematologic: ***aplastic anemia, hypoplastic anemia, agranulocytosis, thrombocytopenia.***
Skin: possible contact sensitivity; burning, urticaria, pruritus, angioedema in hypersensitive patients.
Other: hypersensitivity reactions (fever, rash, urticaria, ***anaphylaxis***), jaundice, ***gray syndrome in neonates (abdominal distention, gray cyanosis, vasomotor collapse, respiratory distress, death within a few hours of onset of symptoms).***

Overdose and treatment

Clinical effects of parenterally administered overdose include anemia and metabolic acidosis followed by hypotension, hypothermia, abdominal distention, and possible death.

Initial treatment is symptomatic and supportive. Drug may be removed by charcoal hemoperfusion.

☑ Special considerations

- Culture and sensitivity tests may be done concurrently with first dose and repeated as needed.
- Use drug only when clearly indicated for severe infection. Because of drug's potential for severe toxicity, it should be reserved for potentially life-threatening infections.
- Refrigerate ophthalmic solution.
- If administering drug concomitantly with penicillin, give penicillin 1 hour or more before chloramphenicol to avoid reduction in penicillin's bactericidal activity.
- For I.V. administration, reconstitute 1-g vial of powder for injection with 10 ml of sterile water for injection; concentration will be 100 mg/ml. Solution remains stable for 30 days at room temperature; however, refrigeration is recommended. Do not use cloudy solutions. Administer I.V. infusion slowly, over at least 1 minute. Check injection site daily for phlebitis and irritation.
- Therapeutic range is 10 to 20 mcg/ml for peak levels and 5 to 10 mcg/ml for trough levels.
- Monitor CBC, platelet count, reticulocyte count, and serum iron level before therapy begins and every 2 days during therapy. Discontinue immediately if test results indicate anemia, reticulocytopenia, leukopenia, or thrombocytopenia.
- Observe patient for signs and symptoms of superinfection by nonsusceptible organisms.

Patient education

- Instruct patient to report adverse reactions, especially nausea, vomiting, diarrhea, bleeding, fever, confusion, sore throat, or mouth sores.
- Tell patient to take drug for prescribed period and to take it exactly as directed, even after he feels better.
- Instruct patient to wash hands before and after applying topical ointment or solution.
- Warn patient using otic solution not to touch ear with dropper.
- Caution patient using topical cream to avoid sharing washcloths and towels with family members.
- Tell patient using ophthalmic drug to clean eye area of excess exudate before applying drug, and show him how to instill drug in eye. Warn him not to touch applicator tip to eye or surrounding tissue. Instruct him to observe for signs and symptoms of sensitivity, such as itchy eyelids or constant burning, and to discontinue drug and call immediately should any occur.

Geriatric use

- Administer drug cautiously to elderly patients with impaired liver function.

Pediatric use

- Use drug cautiously in children under age 2 because of risk of gray syndrome (although most cases occur in first 48 hours after birth). Drug has prolonged half-life in neonates, necessitating special dose.

Breast-feeding

- Drug is excreted in breast milk in low concentrations, posing risk of bone marrow depression and slight risk of gray syndrome. Alternative feeding method is recommended during treatment with chloramphenicol.

chlordiazepoxide
Libritabs

chlordiazepoxide hydrochloride
Librium, Mitran, Reposans-10

Pharmacologic classification: benzodiazepine
Therapeutic classification: antianxiety, anticonvulsant, sedative-hypnotic
Controlled substance schedule IV
Pregnancy risk category D

How supplied
Available by prescription only
Tablets: 5 mg, 10 mg, 25 mg
Capsules: 5 mg, 10 mg, 25 mg
Powder for injection: 100 mg/ampule

Indications, route, and dosage
Mild to moderate anxiety and tension
Adults: 5 to 10 mg t.i.d. or q.i.d.
Children over age 6 and elderly or debilitated patients: 5 mg P.O. b.i.d. to q.i.d. Maximum dosage, 10 mg P.O. b.i.d. or t.i.d.
Severe anxiety and tension
Adults: 20 to 25 mg P.O. t.i.d. or q.i.d.
Withdrawal symptoms of acute alcoholism
Adults: 50 to 100 mg P.O., I.M., or I.V. Maximum dosage, 300 mg/day.
Preoperative apprehension and anxiety
Adults: 5 to 10 mg P.O. t.i.d. or q.i.d. on day before surgery; or 50 to 100 mg I.M. 1 hour before surgery.

Note: Parenteral form is not recommended in children under age 12.

Pharmacodynamics
Anxiolytic action: Chlordiazepoxide depresses the CNS at the limbic and subcortical levels of the brain. It produces an antianxiety effect by influencing the effect of the neurotransmitter gamma-aminobutyric acid (GABA) on its receptor in the ascending reticular activating system, which increases inhibition and blocks both cortical and limbic arousal after stimulation of the reticular formation.

Anticonvulsant action: Drug suppresses the spread of seizure activity produced by the epileptogenic foci in the cortex, thalamus, and limbic structures by enhancing presynaptic inhibition.

Pharmacokinetics
- *Absorption:* When given orally, drug is absorbed well through the GI tract. Action begins within 30 to 45 minutes, with peak action in 1 to 3 hours. I.M. administration results in erratic absorption of drug; onset of action usually occurs in 15 to 30 minutes. After I.V. administration, rapid onset of action occurs in 1 to 5 minutes after injection.
- *Distribution:* Drug is distributed widely throughout the body; 90% to 98% is protein-bound.
- *Metabolism:* Chlordiazepoxide is metabolized in the liver to several active metabolites.
- *Excretion:* Most metabolites are excreted in urine as glucuronide conjugates. Half-life of drug is 5 to 30 hours.

Contraindications and precautions
Contraindicated in patients hypersensitive to drug. Use cautiously in patients with impaired renal or hepatic function, mental depression, or porphyria.

Interactions
Chlordiazepoxide potentiates the CNS depressant effects of *phenothiazines, narcotics, barbiturates, alcohol, antihistamines, MAO inhibitors, general anesthetics,* and *antidepressants.* Concomitant use with *cimetidine* and possibly *disulfiram* diminishes hepatic metabolism of chlordiazepoxide, which increases its plasma concentration. *Heavy smoking* accelerates chlordiazepoxide's metabolism, thus lowering clinical effectiveness. *Oral contraceptives* may impair the metabolism of chlordiazepoxide.

Antacids may delay the absorption of chlordiazepoxide. Concomitant use with *levodopa* may decrease the therapeutic effects of levodopa. Benzodiazepines may decrease serum levels of *haloperidol. Phenytoin* and *digoxin* levels may be increased.

Effects on diagnostic tests
Drug therapy may elevate results of liver function tests. Minor changes in EEG patterns, usually low-voltage, fast activity, may occur during and after chlordiazepoxide therapy. Chlordiazepoxide may cause a false-positive pregnancy test, depending on method used. It may also alter urinary 17-ketosteroids (Zimmerman reaction), urine alkaloid determination (Frings thin-layer chromatography method), and urinary glucose determinations (with Chemstrip uG and Diastix, but not glucose enzymatic test strip).

Adverse reactions
CNS: *drowsiness, lethargy,* ataxia, confusion, extrapyramidal symptoms, EEG changes.
GI: nausea, constipation.
GU: increased or decreased libido, menstrual irregularities.
Hematologic: ***agranulocytosis.***
Hepatic: jaundice.
Skin: *swelling, pain at injection site,* skin eruptions, edema.

Overdose and treatment
Clinical manifestations of overdose include somnolence, confusion, coma, hypoactive reflexes, dyspnea, labored breathing, hypotension, bradycardia, slurred speech, and unsteady gait or impaired coordination.

Support blood pressure and respiration until drug effects subside; monitor vital signs. Flumazenil, a specific benzodiazepine antagonist, may be useful. Mechanical ventilatory assistance via endotracheal tube may be required to maintain a patent airway and support adequate oxygenation. Use I.V. fluids and vasopressors, such as dopamine and phenylephrine, to treat hypotension as needed. Use gastric lavage if ingestion was recent, but only if an endotracheal tube is in place to prevent aspiration. Induce emesis if the patient is conscious. After emesis or lavage, administer activated charcoal with a cathartic as a single dose. Do not administer barbiturates if excitation occurs. Dialysis is of limited value.

☑ Special considerations

Besides those relevant to all *benzodiazepines*, consider the following recommendations.

- I.M. administration is not recommended because of erratic and slow absorption. However, if I.M. route is used, reconstitute with special diluent only. Do not use diluent if hazy. Discard unused portion. Inject I.M. deep into large muscle mass.
- For I.V. administration, drug should be reconstituted with sterile water or 0.9% NaCl solution and infused slowly, directly into a large vein, at a rate not exceeding 50 mg/minute for adults. Do not infuse chlordiazepoxide into small veins. Avoid extravasation into subcutaneous tissue. Observe infusion site for phlebitis. Keep resuscitation equipment nearby in case of an emergency.
- Prepare solutions for I.V. or I.M. use immediately before administration. Discard unused portions.
- Patients should remain in bed under observation for at least 3 hours after parenteral administration of chlordiazepoxide.
- Lower doses are effective in patients with renal or hepatic dysfunction. Closely monitor renal and hepatic studies for signs of dysfunction.

Patient education

- Warn patient that sudden changes in position may cause dizziness. Advise patient to dangle legs a few minutes before getting out of bed to prevent falls and injury.
- Advise patient to avoid driving or performing other tasks that require alertness because drug may cause drowsiness.
- Tell patient to avoid alcohol consumption.

Geriatric use

- Elderly patients demonstrate a greater sensitivity to the CNS depressant effects of drug. Some may require supervision with ambulation and activities of daily living during initiation of therapy or after an increase in dose.
- Lower doses are usually effective in elderly patients because of decreased elimination.
- Parenteral administration of drug is more likely to cause apnea, hypotension, and bradycardia in elderly patients.

Pediatric use

- Safety of oral form has not been established in children under age 6. Safety of parenteral form has not been established in children under age 12.

Breast-feeding

- The breast-fed infant of a mother who uses chlordiazepoxide may become sedated, have feeding difficulties, or lose weight. Do not administer drug to breast-feeding women.

chloroquine hydrochloride
Aralen Hydrochloride

chloroquine phosphate
Aralen Phosphate

Pharmacologic classification: 4-aminoquinoline
Therapeutic classification: antimalarial, amebicide, anti-inflammatory
Pregnancy risk category C

How supplied

Available by prescription only
chloroquine hydrochloride
Injection: 50 mg/ml (40 mg/ml base)
chloroquine phosphate
Tablets: 250 mg (150-mg base), 500 mg (300-mg base)

Indications, route, and dosage

Suppressive prophylaxis
Adults: Give 500 mg (300-mg base) P.O. on same day once weekly beginning 2 weeks before exposure.
Children: 5 mg (base)/kg P.O. on same day once weekly (not to exceed adult dosage) beginning 2 weeks before exposure.

Treatment of acute attacks of malaria
Adults: 1 g (600-mg base) P.O. followed by 500 mg (300-mg base) P.O. after 6 to 8 hours; then a single dose of 500 mg (300-mg base) P.O. for next 2 days or 4 to 5 ml (160- to 200-mg base) I.M. and repeated in 6 hours if needed; change to P.O. as soon as possible.
Children: Initial dose is 10 mg (base)/kg P.O.; then 5 mg (base)/kg after 6 hours. Third dose is 5 mg (base)/kg 18 hours after second dose; fourth dose is 5 mg (base)/kg 24 hours after third dose; or 5 mg (base)/kg I.M. May repeat in 6 hours and change to P.O. as soon as possible.

Extraintestinal amebiasis
Adults: 1 g (600-mg base) daily for 2 days, then 500 mg (300-mg base) daily for 2 to 3 weeks or 4 to 5 ml (160- to 200-mg base) I.M. for 10 to 12 days; change to P.O. as soon as possible.

◊ ***Rheumatoid arthritis***
Adults: 250 mg daily (chloroquine phosphate) with evening meal.

◊ ***Lupus erythematosus***
Adults: 250 mg daily (chloroquine phosphate) with evening meal; reduce dosage gradually over several months when lesions regress.

Pharmacodynamics

Antimalarial action: Chloroquine binds to DNA, interfering with protein synthesis. It also inhibits both DNA and RNA polymerases.

Amebicidal action: Mechanism of action is unknown.

Anti-inflammatory action: Mechanism of action is unknown. Drug may antagonize histamine and serotonin and inhibit prostaglandin effects by inhibiting conversion of arachidonic acid to prostaglandin F_2; it also may inhibit chemotaxis of polymorphonuclear leukocytes, macrophages, and eosinophils.

Chloroquine's spectrum of activity includes the asexual erythrocytic forms of *Plasmodium malariae, P. ovale, P. vivax*, many strains of *P. falciparum*, and *Entamoeba histolytica*.

Pharmacokinetics

- *Absorption:* Chloroquine is absorbed readily and almost completely, with peak plasma concentrations occurring at 1 to 2 hours.
- *Distribution:* Drug is 55% bound to plasma proteins. It concentrates in erythrocytes, liver, spleen, kidneys, heart, and brain and is strongly bound in melanin-containing cells.
- *Metabolism:* About 30% of an administered dose is metabolized by the liver to monodesethylchloroquine and bidesethylchloroquine.
- *Excretion:* About 70% of an administered dose is excreted unchanged in urine; unabsorbed drug is excreted in feces. Small amounts of the drug may be present in urine for months after the drug is discontinued. Renal excretion is enhanced by urinary acidification. It is excreted in breast milk.

Contraindications and precautions

Contraindicated in patients with hypersensitivity to drug and in those with retinal or visual field changes or porphyria. Use cautiously in patients with GI, neurologic, or blood disorders.

Interactions

Concomitant administration of *kaolin* or *magnesium trisilicate* may decrease absorption of chloroquine. Chloroquine may interfere with antibody response to *intradermal human diploid cell rabies vaccine*. *Cimetidine* may reduce oral clearance and metabolism.

Effects on diagnostic tests

Drug may cause inversion or depression of the T wave or widening of the QRS complex on ECG. Rarely it may cause decreased WBC, RBC, or platelet counts.

Adverse reactions

CNS: mild and transient headache, psychic stimulation, ***seizures,*** dizziness, neuropathy.
CV: hypotension, ECG changes.
EENT: visual disturbances (blurred vision; difficulty in focusing; reversible corneal changes; typically irreversible, sometimes progressive or delayed retinal changes, such as narrowing of arterioles; macular lesions; pallor of optic disk; optic atrophy; patchy retinal pigmentation, typically leading to blindness); ototoxicity (nerve deafness, vertigo, tinnitus).
GI: anorexia, abdominal cramps, diarrhea, nausea, vomiting, stomatitis.
Hematologic: *agranulocytosis, aplastic anemia,* hemolytic anemia, ***thrombocytopenia.***
Skin: pruritus, lichen planus eruptions, skin and mucosal pigmentary changes, pleomorphic skin eruptions.

Overdose and treatment

Symptoms of drug overdose may appear within 30 minutes after ingestion and may include headache, drowsiness, visual changes, CV collapse, and seizures followed by respiratory and cardiac arrest.

Treatment is symptomatic. Empty stomach by emesis or lavage. After lavage, activated charcoal in an amount at least five times the estimated amount of drug ingested may be helpful if given within 30 minutes of ingestion.

Ultra-short-acting barbiturates may help control seizures. Intubation may become necessary. Peritoneal dialysis and exchange transfusions also may be useful. Forced fluids and acidification of the urine are helpful after the acute phase.

☑ Special considerations

- Baseline and periodic ophthalmologic examinations are necessary in prolonged or high-dosage therapy.
- Give immediately before or after meals on the same day each week to minimize gastric distress. Patients who cannot tolerate drug because of GI distress may tolerate hydroxychloroquine.
- Resistance of *P. falciparum* to chloroquine has spread to most areas with malaria except the Dominican Republic, Haiti, Central America west of the Panama Canal, the Middle East, and Egypt.
- It may also be advisable to provide travelers with sulfadoxine and pyrimethamine (Fansidar) to be taken with them. Patients should be instructed to take drug if a febrile illness occurs and professional medical care is not available. (The recommended prescriptive dose for adults is 1,500 mg sulfadoxine and 75 mg pyrimethamine, or three tablets.) Emphasize that such self-treatment is a temporary measure, and that they must seek medical care as soon as possible. They should continue prophylaxis after the treatment dose of Fansidar.

Patient education

- Tell patient to report blurred vision, increased sensitivity to light, hearing loss, pronounced GI disturbances, or muscle weakness promptly.
- Warn patient to avoid excessive exposure to the sun to prevent drug-induced dermatoses.

Pediatric use

- Children are extremely susceptible to toxicity; monitor closely for adverse effects.

Breast-feeding

- Safety has not been established. Use with caution in breast-feeding women.

chlorotrianisene

Tace

Pharmacologic classification: estrogen
Therapeutic classfication: estrogen replacement, antineoplastic
Pregnancy risk category X

How supplied
Available by prescription only
Capsules: 12 mg, 25 mg

Indications, route, and dosage
Prostatic cancer
Adults: 12 to 25 mg P.O. daily.
Menopausal symptoms or management of atrophic vaginitis or kraurosis vulvae
Adults: 12 to 25 mg P.O. daily in 30-day cycles (3 weeks on, 1 week off).
Female hypogonadism
Adults: 12 to 25 mg P.O. for 21 days, followed by one dose of progesterone 100 mg I.M. or 5 days of oral progestogen given concurrently with last 5 days of chlorotrianisene (that is, medroxyprogesterone 5 to 10 mg). Begin on day 5 of menstrual cycle.
Inoperable prostate carcinoma
Adults: 12 to 25 mg P.O. daily.

Pharmacodynamics
Estrogenic action: Drug mimics the action of endogenous estrogen in treating menopausal symptoms and atrophic vaginitis. It inhibits growth of hormone-sensitive tissue in advanced, inoperable prostatic cancer.

Pharmacokinetics
Very little pharmacokinetic data are available. Chlorotrianisene appears to have a longer duration of action than the naturally occurring estrogens, possibly as a result of extensive distribution into, and subsequent release from, fatty tissue.

Contraindications and precautions
Contraindicated in patients with thrombophlebitis or thromboembolic disorders; in those with breast, reproductive organ, or genital cancer; in those with undiagnosed abnormal genital bleeding; and during pregnancy.

Use cautiously in patients with cerebrovascular or coronary artery disease; asthma; bone disease; migraine; seizures; cardiac, renal, or hepatic dysfunction; hypercalcemia caused by metastatic breast disease; or in those with a family history of breast or genital tract cancer, breast nodules, fibrocystic disease, or an abnormal mammogram.

Interactions
Concomitant administration of drugs that induce hepatic metabolism, such as *rifampin, barbiturates, primidone, carbamazepine,* and *phenytoin* may decrease estrogenic effects from a given dose. These drugs are known to accelerate the rate of metabolism of certain other agents.

Estrogen may decrease the action of *oral anticoagulants* and may enhance the anti-inflammatory effect of *hydrocortisone.*

Effects on diagnostic tests
In patients with diabetes, chlorotrianisene may increase blood glucose levels, necessitating dosage adjustment of insulin or oral hypoglycemic drugs.

Adverse reactions
CNS: headache, dizziness, chorea, migraine, depression, ***seizures.***
CV: thrombophlebitis; ***thromboembolism;*** hypertension; edema; ***increased risk of CVA, pulmonary embolism, MI.***
EENT: worsening of myopia or astigmatism, intolerance of contact lenses.
GI: *nausea,* vomiting, abdominal cramps, bloating, colitis, acute pancreatitis, anorexia, increased appetite, excessive thirst, weight changes.
GU: in women, breakthrough bleeding, altered menstrual flow, dysmenorrhea, ***increased risk of endometrial cancer, possibility of increased risk of breast cancer,*** amenorrhea, cervical erosion or abnormal secretions, enlargement of uterine fibromas, vaginal candidiasis; in men, *gynecomastia, testicular atrophy, impotence.*
Hepatic: cholestatic jaundice, ***hepatic adenoma.***
Skin: melasma, urticaria, hirsutism or hair loss, erythema nodosum, dermatitis.
Other: breast changes (tenderness, enlargement, secretion), hypercalcemia, gallbladder disease.

Overdose and treatment
Specific recommendations are unavailable. Drug overdose may cause nausea. Treatment should be supportive.

☑ Special considerations
Besides those relevant to all *estrogens,* consider the following recommendations.
- Because of its prolonged duration of action, drug is not recommended for correcting menstrual disorders.
- Chlorotrianisene contains tartrazine dye, which can cause an allergic reaction.

Patient education
- Warn patient to report immediately abdominal pain, numbness, or stiffness in legs or buttocks; pressure or pain in chest; shortness of breath; severe headaches; visual disturbances, such as blind spots, flashing lights, or blurriness; vaginal bleeding or discharge; breast lumps; swelling of hands or feet; yellow skin and sclera; dark urine; and light-colored stools.

Geriatric use
- Because of potential for numerous adverse effects, use with caution in elderly patients. Administration of estrogens to postmenopausal women may be associated with increased incidence of endometrial or breast cancer.

Breast-feeding
- Drug is contraindicated in breast-feeding women.

chlorpheniramine maleate

Aller-Chlor, Chlo-Amine, Chlor-100, Chlor-Pro, Chlorspan-12, Chlortab-4, Chlortab-8, Chlor-Trimeton, Chlor-Tripolon*, Novo-Pheniram*, Pfeiffer's Allergy, Phenetron, Teldrin, Trymegen

Pharmacologic classification: propylamine-derivative antihistamine
Therapeutic classification: antihistamine (H_1-receptor antagonist)
Pregnancy risk category B

How supplied

Available with or without a prescription
Tablets: 4 mg, 8 mg, 12 mg
Tablets (chewable): 2 mg
Tablets (timed-release): 8 mg, 12 mg
Capsules (timed-release): 8 mg, 12 mg
Syrup: 2 mg/5 ml
Injection: 10 mg/ml, 100 mg/ml

Indications, route, and dosage

Rhinitis, allergy symptoms

Adults and children age 12 or older: 4 mg of tablets or syrup q 4 to 6 hours; or 8 to 12 mg of timed-release tablets b.i.d. or t.i.d. Maximum dosage, 24 mg/day; 10 to 20 mg S.C., I.V., or I.M. also may be used.

Children age 6 to 11: 2 mg of tablets or syrup q 4 to 6 hours; or one 8-mg timed-release tablet in 24 hours. Maximum dosage, 12 mg/day.

Children age 2 to 5: 1 mg of syrup q 4 to 6 hours. Maximum dosage, 6 mg/day.

Pharmacodynamics

Antihistamine action: Antihistamines compete with histamine for histamine H_1-receptor sites on smooth muscle of the bronchi, GI tract, uterus, and large blood vessels; they bind to cellular receptors, preventing access of histamine, thereby suppressing histamine-induced allergic symptoms. They do not directly alter histamine or its release.

Pharmacokinetics

- *Absorption:* Drug is well absorbed from the GI tract; action begins within 30 to 60 minutes, and peaks in 2 to 6 hours. Food in the stomach delays absorption but does not affect bioavailability.
- *Distribution:* Chlorpheniramine is distributed extensively into the body; drug is about 72% protein-bound.
- *Metabolism:* Drug is metabolized largely in GI mucosal cells and liver (first-pass effect).
- *Excretion:* Half-life is 12 to 43 hours in adults and 10 to 13 hours in children; drug and metabolites are excreted in urine.

Contraindications and precautions

Contraindicated in patients having acute asthmatic attacks. Antihistamines are not recommended for breast-feeding women because small amounts of drug are excreted in breast milk.

Use cautiously in the elderly and in patients with increased intraocular pressure, hyperthyroidism, CV or renal disease, hypertension, bronchial asthma, urine retention, prostatic hyperplasia, bladder neck obstruction, or stenosing peptic ulcers.

Interactions

MAO inhibitors interfere with the detoxification of chlorpheniramine and thus prolong and intensify its central depressant and anticholinergic effects; additive sedation may occur when antihistamines are given concomitantly with other *CNS depressants,* such as *alcohol, barbiturates, tranquilizers, sleeping aids* or *antianxiety agents.*

Chlorpheniramine enhances the effects of *epinephrine* and may diminish the effects of *sulfonylureas,* and partially counteract the anticoagulant action of *heparin.*

Effects on diagnostic tests

Discontinue drug 4 days before diagnostic skin tests; antihistamines can prevent, reduce, or mask positive skin test response.

Adverse reactions

CNS: *stimulation,* sedation, *drowsiness,* excitability (in children).
CV: hypotension, palpitations.
GI: epigastric distress, *dry mouth.*
GU: urine retention.
Respiratory: thick bronchial secretions.
Skin: rash, urticaria.
Other: local stinging, burning sensation (after parenteral administration), pallor, weak pulse, transient hypotension.

Overdose and treatment

Clinical manifestations of overdose may include either CNS depression (sedation, reduced mental alertness, apnea, and CV collapse) or CNS stimulation (insomnia, hallucinations, tremors, and seizures). Atropine-like symptoms, such as dry mouth, flushed skin, fixed and dilated pupils, and GI symptoms, are common, especially in children.

Treat overdose by inducing emesis with ipecac syrup (in conscious patient), followed by activated charcoal to reduce further drug absorption. Use gastric lavage if patient is unconscious or ipecac fails. Treat hypotension with vasopressors, and control seizures with diazepam or phenytoin. *Do not give stimulants.* Administering ammonium chloride or vitamin C to acidify urine will promote drug excretion.

☑ Special considerations

Besides those relevant to all *antihistamines,* consider the following recommendations.

- Give 100 mg/ml of injectable form S.C. or I.M. *only.* Do not give I.V.; I.V. preparation contains preservatives.
- Do not use parenteral solutions intradermally.
- Administer I.V. solution slowly, over 1 minute.

Patient education

- Instruct patient to swallow sustained-release tablets whole; they should not be crushed or chewed.

• Inform patient to store syrup and parenteral solution away from light.

Geriatric use

• Elderly patients are usually more sensitive to adverse effects of antihistamines and are especially likely to experience a greater degree of dizziness, sedation, hyperexcitability, dry mouth, and urine retention than younger patients. Symptoms usually respond to a decrease in medication dosage.

Pediatric use

• Drug is not indicated for use in premature or newborn infants.
• Children, especially those under age 6, may experience paradoxical hyperexcitability.

Breast-feeding

• Antihistamines such as chlorpheniramine should not be used during breast-feeding. Many of these drugs are secreted in breast milk, exposing the infant to risks of unusual excitability; premature infants are at particular risk for seizures.

chlorpromazine hydrochloride

Chlorpromanyl-5*, Chlorpromanyl-20*, Largactil*, Novo-Chlorpromazine*, Ormazine, Thorazine, Thor-Prom

Pharmacologic classification: aliphatic phenothiazine
Therapeutic classification: antipsychotic, antiemetic
Pregnancy risk category C

How supplied

Available by prescription only
Tablets: 10 mg, 25 mg, 50 mg, 100 mg, 200 mg
Capsules (sustained-release): 30 mg, 75 mg, 150 mg, 200 mg, 300 mg
Syrup: 10 mg/5 ml
Oral concentrate: 30 mg/ml, 100 mg/ml
Suppositories: 25 mg, 100 mg
Injection: 25 mg/ml

Indications, route, and dosage

Psychosis
Adults: 30 to 75 mg P.O. daily in two to four divided doses. Dosage may be increased twice weekly by 20 to 50 mg until symptoms are controlled. Most patients respond to 200 mg daily, but doses up to 800 mg may be necessary.
Children age 6 months or more: 0.5 to 1 mg/kg P.O. q 4 to 6 hours; or 0.25 mg/lb I.M. q 6 to 8 hours; or 0.5 mg/lb P.R. q 6 to 8 hours. Maximum dosage is 40 mg in children under age 5, and 75 mg in children age 5 to 12.
Acute management of psychosis in severely agitated patients
Adults: 25 mg I.M.; may be repeated with 25 to 50 of 400 mg q 4 to 6 hours.
Nausea, vomiting
Adults: 10 to 25 mg P.O. or 25 mg I.M. q 4 to 6 hours, p.r.n.; or 100 mg rectally q 6 to 8 hours, p.r.n.
Children and infants: 0.25 mg/lb P.O. q 4 to 6 hours; or 0.25 mg/lb I.M. q 6 to 8 hours; or 0.5 mg/lb P.R. q 6 to 8 hours.
Intractable hiccups
Adults: 25 to 50 mg P.O. or I.M t.i.d. or q.i.d.
Mild alcohol withdrawal, acute intermittent porphyria, tetanus
Adults: 25 mg to 50 mg I.M. t.i.d. or q.i.d.

Pharmacodynamics

Antipsychotic action: Drug is thought to exert its antipsychotic effects by postsynaptic blockade of CNS dopamine receptors, thereby inhibiting dopamine-mediated effects; antiemetic effects are attributed to dopamine receptor blockade in the medullary chemoreceptor trigger zone (CTZ). Drug has many other central and peripheral effects; it produces both alpha and ganglionic blockade and counteracts histamine- and serotonin-mediated activity. Its most prominent adverse reactions are antimuscarinic and sedative.

Pharmacokinetics

• *Absorption:* Rate and extent of absorption vary with route of administration. Oral tablet absorption is erratic and variable, with onset ranging from ½ to 1 hour; peak effects occur at 2 to 4 hours and duration of action is 4 to 6 hours. Sustained-release preparations have similar absorption, but action lasts for 10 to 12 hours. Suppositories act in 60 minutes and last 3 to 4 hours. Oral concentrates and syrups are much more predictable; I.M. drug is absorbed rapidly.
• *Distribution:* Distributed widely into the body, including breast milk; concentration is usually higher in CNS than plasma. Steady-state serum level is achieved within 4 to 7 days. Drug is 91% to 99% protein-bound.
• *Metabolism:* Drug is metabolized extensively by the liver and forms 10 to 12 metabolites; some are pharmacologically active.
• *Excretion:* Mostly excreted as metabolites in urine; some is excreted in feces via the biliary tract. It may undergo enterohepatic circulation.

Contraindications and precautions

Contraindicated in patients with hypersensitivity to drug or in patients experiencing CNS depression, bone marrow suppression, subcortical damage, and coma.

Use cautiously in acutely ill or dehydrated children; elderly or debilitated patients; and in patients with impaired renal or hepatic function, severe CV disease, glaucoma, prostatic hyperplasia, respiratory or seizure disorders, hypocalcemia, reaction to insulin or electroconvulsive therapy, or exposure to heat, cold, or organophosphate insecticides.

Interactions

Concomitant use of chlorpromazine with *sympathomimetics*, including *epinephrine, phenylephrine, phenylpropanolamine*, and *ephedrine* (often found in *nasal sprays*), and *appetite suppressants* may decrease their stimulatory and pressor effects. Chlorpromazine may cause *epinephrine* reversal: the beta-adrenergic agonist activity of *epinephrine* is evident whereas its alpha effects are blocked, leading to decreased diastolic and increased systolic pressures and tachycardia.

Chlorpromazine may inhibit blood pressure response to *centrally acting antihypertensive drugs* such as *guanethidine, guanabenz, guanadrel, clonidine, methyldopa*, and *reserpine*. Additive effects are likely after concomitant use of chlorpromazine and *CNS depressants* (*including alcohol, analgesics, barbiturates, narcotics, tranquilizers*, and *general, spinal*, or *epidural anesthetics*), or *parenteral magnesium sulfate* (oversedation, respiratory depression, and hypotension); *antiarrhythmic agents, quinidine, disopyramide*, and *procainamide* (increased incidence of arrhythmias and conduction defects); *atropine* and other *anticholinergic drugs*, including *antidepressants, MAO inhibitors* in risk of seizures).

Beta-blocking agents may inhibit chlorpromazine metabolism, increasing plasma levels and toxicity.

Concomitant use with *propylthiouracil* increases risk of agranulocytosis; concomitant use with *lithium* may cause severe neurologic toxicity with an encephalitis-like syndrome, and a decreased therapeutic response to chlorpromazine.

Pharmacokinetic alterations and subsequent decreased therapeutic response to chlorpromazine may follow concomitant use with *phenobarbital* (enhanced renal excretion), *aluminum- and magnesium-containing antacids* and *antidiarrheals* (decreased absorption), *caffeine*, and with *heavy smoking* (increased metabolism).

Chlorpromazine may antagonize the therapeutic effect of *bromocriptine* on prolactin secretion; it also may decrease the vasoconstricting effects of high-dose *dopamine* and may decrease effectiveness and increase toxicity of *levodopa* (by dopamine blockade). Chlorpromazine may inhibit metabolism and increase toxicity of *phenytoin*.

Effects on diagnostic tests

Drug causes false-positive test results for urinary porphyrins, urobilinogen, amylase, and 5-hydroxyindoleacetic acid because of darkening of urine by metabolites; it also causes false-positive results in urine pregnancy tests using human chorionic gonadotropin.

Chlorpromazine elevates tests for liver function and protein-bound iodine and causes quinidine-like ECG effects.

Adverse reactions

CNS: *extrapyramidal reactions*, drowsiness, *sedation*, ***seizures***, *tardive dyskinesia*, pseudoparkinsonism, dizziness.
CV: *orthostatic hypotension*, tachycardia, ECG changes.
EENT: ocular changes, blurred vision, nasal congestion.
GI: *dry mouth, constipation*, nausea.
GU: *urine retention*, menstrual irregularities, gynecomastia, inhibited ejaculation, priapism.
Hematologic: leukopenia, ***agranulocytosis***, eosinophilia, hemolytic anemia, ***aplastic anemia, thrombocytopenia.***
Hepatic: jaundice, abnormal liver function test results.
Skin: *mild photosensitivity*, allergic reactions, *pain at I.M. injection site*, sterile abscess, skin pigmentation.
Other: ***neuroleptic malignant syndrome.***

After abrupt withdrawal of long-term therapy: gastritis, nausea, vomiting, dizziness, tremor.

Overdose and treatment

CNS depression is characterized by deep, unarousable sleep and possible coma, hypotension or hypertension, extrapyramidal symptoms, abnormal involuntary muscle movements, agitation, seizures, arrhythmias, ECG changes, hypothermia or hyperthermia, and autonomic nervous system dysfunction.

Treatment is symptomatic and supportive, including maintaining vital signs, airway, stable body temperature, and fluid and electrolyte balance.

Do not induce vomiting: drug inhibits cough reflex, and aspiration may occur. Use gastric lavage, then activated charcoal and sodium chloride cathartics; dialysis does not help. Regulate body temperature as needed. Treat hypotension with I.V. fluids: *do not give epinephrine*. Treat seizures with parenteral diazepam or barbiturates; arrhythmias with parenteral phenytoin (1 mg/kg with rate titrated to blood pressure); extrapyramidal reactions with benztropine 1 to 2 mg or parenteral diphenhydramine 10 to 50 mg.

☑ Special considerations

Besides those relevant to all *phenothiazines*, consider the following recommendations.

- A pink-brown discoloration of urine may be observed.
- Chlorpromazine has a high incidence of sedation, orthostatic hypotension, and photosensitivity reactions (3%). Patient should avoid exposure to sunlight or heat lamps.
- Sustained-release preparations should not be crushed or opened, but swallowed whole.
- Oral formulations may cause stomach upset and may be administered with food or fluid.
- Dilute concentrate in 2 to 4 oz (60 to 120 ml) of liquid, preferably water, carbonated drinks, fruit juice, tomato juice, milk, puddings, or applesauce.
- Store suppository form in a cool place.
- If tissue irritation occurs, chlorpromazine injection may be diluted with 0.9% NaCl solution or 2% procaine.
- I.V. form should be used only during surgery or for severe hiccups. Dilute injection to 1 mg/ml with 0.9% NaCl solution and administer at a rate of 1 mg/2 minutes for children and 1 mg/minute for adults.
- I.M. injection should be given deep in the upper outer quadrant of the buttocks. Injection is usually painful; massaging the area after administration may prevent abscess formation.
- Liquid and injectable forms may cause a rash if skin contact occurs.
- Solution for injection may be slightly discolored. Do not use if drug is excessively discolored or if a

precipitate is evident. Monitor blood pressure before and after parenteral administration.

Patient education

- Explain risks of dystonic reactions and tardive dyskinesia, and tell patient to report abnormal body movements.
- Tell patient to avoid sun exposure and to wear sunscreen when going outdoors, to prevent photosensitivity reactions. (Note that sunlamps and tanning beds also may cause burning of the skin or skin discoloration.)
- Warn patient to avoid extremely hot or cold baths or exposure to temperature extremes, sunlamps, or tanning beds. Drug may cause thermoregulatory changes.
- Tell patient not to spill the liquid preparation on the skin because rash and irritation may result.
- Instruct patient to take drug exactly as prescribed and not to double dose to compensate for missed ones.
- Explain that many drug interactions are possible. Patient should seek medical approval before taking *any* self-prescribed medications.
- Tell patient not to stop taking drug suddenly.
- Encourage patient to report difficulty urinating, sore throat, dizziness, or fainting.
- Advise patient to avoid hazardous activities that require alertness until drug's effect is established. Excessive sedative effects tend to subside after several weeks.
- Tell patient to avoid alcohol and medications that may cause excessive sedation.
- Explain what fluids are appropriate for diluting the concentrate and the dropper technique for measuring dose. Teach patient how to use suppository form.
- Inform patient that sugarless chewing gum or hard candy, ice chips, or artificial saliva may help to alleviate dry mouth.

Geriatric use

- Older patients tend to require lower doses, titrated individually. They also are more likely to develop adverse reactions, especially tardive dyskinesia and other extrapyramidal effects.

Pediatric use

- Drug is not recommended for patients under age 6 months. Sudden infant death syndrome has been reported to occur in children under age 1 receiving drug.

Breast-feeding

- Drug enters into the breast milk. Potential benefits to the mother should outweigh the potential harm to the infant.

chlorpropamide

Diabinese, Novo-Propamide*

Pharmacologic classification: sulfonylurea
Therapeutic classification: antidiabetic
Pregnancy risk category C

How supplied

Available by prescription only
Tablets: 100 mg, 250 mg

Indications, route, and dosage

Adjunct to diet to lower blood glucose levels in patients with non-insulin-dependent diabetes mellitus (type 2)

Adults: 250 mg P.O. daily with breakfast or in divided doses if GI disturbances occur. First dosage increase may be made after 5 to 7 days because of extended duration of action, then dose may be increased q 3 to 5 days by 50 to 125 mg, if needed, to a maximum of 750 mg daily.

✦ ***Dosage adjustment.*** In adults over age 65, initial dosage should be 100 to 125 mg daily.

To change from insulin to oral therapy

Adults: If insulin dosage is less than 40 U daily, insulin may be stopped and oral therapy started as above. If insulin dosage is 40 U or more daily, start oral therapy as above, with insulin dose reduced 50% the first few days. Further insulin reductions should be made based on patient response.

Pharmacodynamics

Antidiabetic action: Chlorpropamide lowers blood glucose levels by stimulating insulin release from beta cells in the pancreas. After prolonged administration, it produces hypoglycemic effects through extrapancreatic mechanisms, including reduced basal hepatic glucose production and enhanced peripheral sensitivity to insulin; the latter may result either from an increased number of insulin receptors or from changes in events that follow insulin binding.

Antidiuretic action: Drug appears to potentiate the effects of minimal levels of antidiuretic hormone.

Pharmacokinetics

- *Absorption:* Chlorpropamide is absorbed readily from the GI tract. Onset of action occurs within 1 hour, with a maximum decrease in serum glucose levels at 3 to 6 hours.
- *Distribution:* Not fully understood, but is probably similar to that of the other sulfonylureas. It is highly protein-bound.
- *Metabolism:* Approximately 80% of drug is metabolized by the liver. Whether the metabolites have hypoglycemic activity is unknown.
- *Excretion:* Drug and its metabolites are excreted in urine. Rate of excretion depends on urinary pH; it increases in alkaline urine and decreases in acidic urine. Duration of action is up to 60 hours; half-life is 36 hours.

Contraindications and precautions

Contraindicated for treating type 1 diabetes (insulin-dependent) or diabetes that can be adequately controlled by diet. Also contraindicated in patients with type 2 diabetes complicated by ketosis, acidosis, diabetic coma, major surgery, severe infections, severe trauma, during pregnancy or breast-feeding as well as those with hypersensitivity to drug.

Use cautiously in elderly, debilitated, or malnourished patients and those with porphyria or impaired renal or hepatic function.

Interactions

Concomitant use of chlorpropamide with *alcohol* may produce a disulfiram-like reaction consisting of nausea, vomiting, abdominal cramps, and headaches. Concomitant use with *anticoagulants* may increase plasma levels of both drugs and, after continued therapy, may reduce plasma levels and anticoagulant effects.

Concomitant use with *chloramphenicol, guanethidine, insulin, MAO inhibitors, probenecid, salicylates,* or *sulfonamides* may enhance hypoglycemic effects by displacing chlorpropamide from its protein-binding sites.

Concomitant use with nonspecific *beta-adrenergic blocking agents,* including *ophthalmics,* may increase the risk of hypoglycemia by masking its symptoms, such as rising pulse rate and blood pressure. Use with drugs that may increase blood glucose levels (*acetazolamide, adrenocorticoids, glucocorticoids, amphetamines, baclofen, corticotropin, epinephrine, estrogens, ethacrynic acid, furosemide, oral contraceptives, phenytoin, thiazide diuretics, triamterene, thyroid hormones*) may require dosage adjustments. Chlorpropamide appears to potentiate the effects of minimal levels of antidiuretic hormone.

Because *smoking* increases corticosteroid release, patients who smoke may require higher dosages of chlorpropamide.

Effects on diagnostic tests

Drug therapy alters cholesterol, alkaline phosphatase, bilirubin, urine phenyl ketone, porphyrins, and protein levels, and cephalin flocculation (thymol turbidity).

Adverse reactions

CNS: paresthesia, fatigue, dizziness, vertigo, malaise, headache.
EENT: tinnitis.
GI: nausea, heartburn, epigastric distress.
GU: tea-colored urine.
Hematologic: leukopenia, ***thrombocytopenia, aplastic anemia, agranulocytosis,*** hemolytic anemia.
Skin: rash, pruritus, erythema, urticaria.
Other: ***hypersensitivity reactions, prolonged hypoglycemia, dilutional hyponatremia.***

Overdose and treatment

Clinical manifestations of overdose include low blood glucose levels, tingling of lips and tongue, hunger, nausea, decreased cerebral function (lethargy, yawning, confusion, agitation, and nervousness), increased sympathetic activity (tachycardia, sweating, and tremor), and ultimately seizures, stupor, and coma.

Mild hypoglycemia (without loss of consciousness or neurologic findings) can be treated with oral glucose and dosage adjustments. If patient loses consciousness or experiences neurologic symptoms, he should receive rapid injection of dextrose 50%, followed by a continuous infusion of dextrose 10% at a rate to maintain blood glucose levels greater than 100 mg/dl. Because of chlorpropamide's long half-life, monitor patient for 3 to 5 days.

☑ Special considerations

Besides those relevant to all *sulfonylureas,* consider the following recommendations.

- To avoid GI intolerance in those patients who require dosages of 250 mg/day or more and to improve control of hyperglycemia, divided doses are recommended. These are given before the morning and evening meals.
- Elderly, debilitated, or malnourished patients and those with impaired renal or hepatic function usually require a lower initial dosage.
- Patients switching from chlorpropamide to another sulfonylurea should be monitored closely for 1 week because of chlorpropamide's prolonged retention in the body.
- Because of drug's long duration of action, adverse reactions, especially hypoglycemia, may be more frequent or severe than with some other sulfonylureas.
- Patients with severe diabetes who do not respond to 500 mg usually will not respond to higher doses.
- Drug may accumulate in patients with renal insufficiency. Watch for such signs as dysuria, anuria, and hematuria.
- Chlorpropamide may potentiate antidiuretic effects of vasopressin. Watch for drowsiness, muscle cramps, seizures, unconsciousness, water retention, and weakness.
- Oral hypoglycemic agents have been associated with an increased risk of CV mortality compared with diet or diet and insulin treatments.

Patient education

- Emphasize importance of following prescribed diet, as well as the exercise and medical regimen.
- Instruct patient to take medication at the same time each day. If a dose is missed, it should be taken immediately, unless it's almost time for the next dose. Patient should never take double doses.
- Tell patient to avoid alcohol, and remind him that many foods and OTC medications contain alcohol. Alcohol may cause a disulfiram-like reaction.
- Encourage patient to wear a medical identification bracelet or necklace.
- Instruct patient to take drug with food if it causes GI upset.
- Teach patient how to monitor blood glucose, urine glucose, and ketone levels, as needed.
- Teach patient to recognize the signs and symptoms of hypoglycemia and hyperglycemia and what to do if they occur.
- Reassure patient that skin reactions are transient and usually subside with continuation of therapy.

Geriatric use

- Elderly patients may be more sensitive to the effects of drug because of reduced metabolism and elimination. They are more likely to develop neurologic symptoms of hypoglycemia.
- Avoid drug in elderly patients because of its longer duration of action.
- Elderly patients usually require a lower initial dosage.

Pediatric use
• Drug is ineffective in insulin-dependent (type 1, juvenile-onset) diabetes.

Breast-feeding
• Drug is excreted in breast milk and should not be used in breast-feeding women.

chlorthalidone
Apo-Chlorthalidone*, Hygroton, Novo-Thalidone*, Thalitone, Uridon*

Pharmacologic classification: thiazide-like diuretic
Therapeutic classification: diuretic, antihypertensive
Pregnancy risk category B

How supplied
Available by prescription only
Tablets: 15 mg, 25 mg, 50 mg, 100 mg

Indications, route, and dosage
Edema
Adults: 50 to 100 mg (Thalitone, 30 to 60 mg) P.O. daily or 100 mg (Thalitone, 60 mg) P.O. every other day.
Children: 2 mg/kg P.O. three times weekly.
Hypertension
Adults: 25 to 100 mg (Thalitone, 15 to 50 mg) P.O. daily.
Children: 2 mg/kg P.O. three times weekly.

Pharmacodynamics
Diuretic action: Chlorthalidone increases urinary excretion of sodium and water by inhibiting sodium reabsorption in the cortical diluting tubule of the nephron, thus relieving edema.

Antihypertensive action: The exact mechanism of drug hypotensive effect is unknown. This effect may partially result from direct arteriolar vasodilation and a decrease in total peripheral resistance.

Pharmacokinetics
• *Absorption:* Drug is absorbed from the GI tract; extent of absorption is unknown.
• *Distribution:* Chlorthalidone is 90% bound to erythrocytes.
• *Metabolism:* Data are limited.
• *Excretion:* Between 30% and 60% of a given dose of chlorthalidone is excreted unchanged in urine; half-life is 54 hours. Duration of action is 24 to 72 hours.

Contraindications and precautions
Contraindicated in patients with anuria or hypersensitivity to thiazides or other sulfonamide-derived drugs. Use cautiously in patients with impaired renal or hepatic function.

Interactions
Chlorthalidone potentiates the hypotensive effects of most other *antihypertensive drugs*; this may be used to therapeutic advantage.

Chlorthalidone may potentiate hyperglycemic, hypotensive, and hyperuricemic effects of *diazoxide*, and its hyperglycemic effect may increase *insulin* or *sulfonylurea* requirements in diabetic patients. Chlorthalidone may reduce renal clearance of *lithium*, elevating serum lithium levels, and may necessitate reduction in lithium dosage by 50%.

Chlorthalidone turns urine slightly more alkaline and may decrease urinary excretion of some *amines*, such as *amphetamine* and *quinidine*; alkaline urine also may decrease therapeutic efficacy of *methenamine compounds* such as *methenamine mandelate*.

Cholestyramine and *colestipol* may bind to chlorthalidone, preventing its absorption; give drugs 1 hour apart. Chlorthalidone may increase the risk of *NSAID*-induced renal failure.

Effects on diagnostic tests
Drug therapy may alter serum electrolyte levels and may increase serum urate, glucose, cholesterol, and triglyceride levels.

Chlorthalidone may interfere with tests for parathyroid function and should be discontinued before such tests.

Adverse reactions
CNS: dizziness, vertigo, headache, paresthesia, weakness, restlessness.
CV: volume depletion and dehydration, vasculitis.
GI: anorexia, nausea, pancreatitis, vomiting, abdominal pain, diarrhea, constipation.
GU: impotence.
Hematologic: ***aplastic anemia, agranulocytosis,*** leukopenia, ***thrombocytopenia.***
Hepatic: jaundice.
Skin: dermatitis, photosensitivity, rash, purpura, urticaria.
Other: hypersensitivity reactions; hypokalemia; asymptomatic hyperuricemia; hyperglycemia and impairment of glucose tolerance; fluid and electrolyte imbalances, including dilutional hyponatremia and hypochloremia, metabolic alkalosis, hypercalcemia; gout.

Overdose and treatment
Clinical signs of overdose include GI irritation and hypermotility, diuresis, and lethargy, which may progress to coma.

Treatment is mainly supportive; monitor and assist respiratory, CV, and renal function as indicated. Monitor fluid and electrolyte balance. Induce vomiting with ipecac in conscious patient; otherwise, use gastric lavage to avoid aspiration. Do not give cathartics; these promote additional loss of fluids and electrolytes.

☑ Special considerations
Recommendations for use of chlorthalidone and for care and teaching of the patient during therapy are the same as those for all *thiazide* and *thiazide-like diuretics*.

Geriatric use
• Elderly and debilitated patients require close observation and may require reduced dosages. They

are more sensitive to excess diuresis because of age-related changes in CV and renal function. Excess diuresis promotes orthostatic hypotension, dehydration, hypovolemia, hyponatremia, hypomagnesemia, and hypokalemia.

Breast-feeding

• Drug is distributed in breast milk; its safety and effectiveness in breast-feeding women have not been established.

chlorzoxazone

Paraflex, Parafon Forte DSC, Remular-S

Pharmacologic classification: benzoxazole derivative
Therapeutic classification: skeletal muscle relaxant
Pregnancy risk category C

How supplied

Available by prescription only
Tablets: 250 mg, 500 mg
Caplets (film-coated): 250 mg, 500 mg

Indications, route, and dosage

Adjunct in acute, painful musculoskeletal conditions

Adults: 250, 500, or 750 mg P.O. t.i.d. or q.i.d. Reduce to lowest effective dose after response is obtained.
Children: 20 mg/kg or 600 mg/m^2 P.O. daily divided t.i.d. or q.i.d., or 125 to 500 mg t.i.d. or q.i.d., depending on age and weight.

Pharmacodynamics

Skeletal muscle relaxant action: Chlorzoxazone does not relax skeletal muscle directly, but apparently as a result of its sedative effects. However, exact mechanism of action is unknown. Animal studies suggest that drug modifies central perception of pain without eliminating peripheral pain reflexes.

Pharmacokinetics

• *Absorption:* Drug is rapidly and completely absorbed from the GI tract. Onset of action occurs within 1 hour; duration of action is 3 to 4 hours.
• *Distribution:* Widely distributed in the body.
• *Metabolism:* Drug is metabolized in the liver to inactive metabolites. The half-life of chlorzoxazone is 66 minutes.
• *Excretion:* Excreted in urine as glucuronide metabolite.

Contraindications and precautions

Contraindicated in patients with hypersensitivity to drug or impaired hepatic function.

Interactions

Concomitant use with other *CNS depressants*, including *alcohol*, produces further CNS depression. When used with other *depressant drugs* (*general anesthetics, opioid analgesics, antipsychotics, anxiolytics, tricyclic antidepressants*), exercise care to avoid overdose. Concurrent use with *MAO inhibitors* or *tricyclic antidepressants* may result in increased CNS depression, respiratory depression, and hypotensive effects. Reduce dosage of one or both agents.

Effects on diagnostic tests

None reported.

Adverse reactions

CNS: *drowsiness, dizziness, light-headedness,* malaise, headache, overstimulation, tremor.
GI: anorexia, nausea, vomiting, heartburn, abdominal distress, constipation, diarrhea.
GU: urine discoloration (orange or purple-red).
Hepatic: hepatic dysfunction.
Skin: urticaria, redness, pruritus, petechiae, bruising, angioneurotic edema, ***anaphylaxis.***

Overdose and treatment

Clinical manifestations of overdose include nausea, vomiting, diarrhea, drowsiness, dizziness, lightheadedness, headache, malaise, or sluggishness, followed by loss of muscle tone, decreased or absent deep tendon reflexes, respiratory depression, and hypotension.

To treat overdose, induce emesis or perform gastric lavage followed by activated charcoal. Closely monitor vital signs and neurologic status. Provide general supportive measures, including maintenance of adequate airway and assisted ventilation. Use caution if administering pressor agents.

☑ Special considerations

• Drug may cause drowsiness.
• Urine may turn orange or reddish purple.
• Know if patient is taking other CNS depressant drugs because of cumulative effects.
• Monitor liver function tests in patients receiving long-term therapy.

Patient education

• Caution patient to avoid hazardous activities that require alertness or physical coordination until CNS depression is determined.
• Warn patient to avoid alcoholic beverages and to use caution when taking cough and cold preparations because they may contain alcohol.
• Advise patient to store drug away from direct heat or light (not in bathroom medicine cabinet, where heat and humidity cause deterioriation of drug).
• Tell patient to take missed dose only if remembered within 1 hour of scheduled time. If beyond 1 hour, patient should skip dose and go back to regular schedule. Patient should not double-dose.
• Inform patient not to stop taking drug without calling for specific instructions.
• Tell patient urine may turn orange or reddish purple, but this is a harmless effect.
• Warn athletic patient that skeletal muscle relaxants are banned in competition sponsored by the U.S. Olympics Committee and the National Collegiate Athletic Association. Use can lead to disqualification.

Geriatric use
- Elderly patients may be more sensitive to drug's effects.

Pediatric use
- Tablets may be crushed and mixed with food, milk, or fruit juice to aid dosing in children.

Breast-feeding
- It is unknown if drug is excreted in breast milk. No clinical problems have been reported.

cholera vaccine

Pharmacologic classification: vaccine
Therapeutic classification: cholera prophylaxis
Pregnancy risk category C

How supplied
Available by prescription only
Injection: suspension of killed *Vibrio cholerae* (each milliliter contains 8 U of Inaba and Ogawa serotypes) in 1.5-ml and 20-ml vials

Indications, route, and dosage
Primary immunization
Adults and children over age 10: 2 doses of 0.5 ml I.M. or S.C., 1 week to 1 month apart, before traveling in cholera area. Booster dosage is 0.5 ml q 6 months for as long as protection is needed.
Children age 5 to 10: 0.3 ml I.M. or S.C. Boosters of same dose should be given q 6 months for as long as protection is needed.
Children age 6 months to 4 years: 0.2 ml I.M. or S.C. Boosters of same dose should be given q 6 months for as long as protection is needed.

Pharmacodynamics
Cholera prophylaxis: Vaccine promotes active immunity to cholera in approximately 50% of those immunized.

Pharmacokinetics
- *Absorption:* No information available.
- *Distribution:* No information available. Virus-induced immunity begins to taper off within 3 to 6 months.
- *Metabolism:* No information available.
- *Excretion:* No information available.

Contraindications and precautions
Contraindicated in patients with acute illness or history of severe systemic reaction or allergic response to vaccine.

Interactions
Concomitant use of cholera vaccine with *corticosteroids* or *immunosuppressants* may impair the immune response to cholera vaccine and therefore should be avoided.

The simultaneous administration of cholera vaccine with *yellow fever vaccine* may decrease the response to both.

Effects on diagnostic tests
None reported.

Adverse reactions
CNS: headache.
Other: *erythema, swelling, pain, induration (at injection site);* malaise, fever.

Overdose and treatment
No information available.

☑ Special considerations
- Obtain a thorough history of allergies and reactions to immunizations.
- Epinephrine solution 1:1,000 should be available to treat allergic reactions.
- When possible, cholera and yellow fever vaccines should be administered at least 3 weeks apart; however, they may be administered simultaneously if time constraints make this necessary.
- Cholera vaccine may be given intradermally (0.2 ml) in persons over age 5, but higher levels of antibody may be achieved in children under age 5 by the S.C. or I.M. route.
- Shake vial well before removing a dose.
- Administer I.M. in deltoid muscle in adults and children over age 3 and in the anterolateral thigh in children under age 3.
- Do not use I.M. route in patients with thrombocytopenia or other coagulation disorders that would contraindicate I.M. injection. Cholera vaccine should not be administered I.V. Aspirate before S.C. or I.M. injection.
- Store vaccine at 36° to 46° F (2° to 8° C). Do not freeze.

Patient education
- Tell patient to report skin changes, difficulty breathing, fever, or joint pain.
- Inform patient that acetaminophen may be taken to relieve minor adverse effects, such as pain and tenderness at injection site.
- Tell patient that use of vaccine does not prevent infection.
- Advise patient to avoid consumption of contaminated food or water.

Pediatric use
- Drug is not recommended for infants under age 6 months.

Breast-feeding
- It is not known if cholera vaccine is distributed into breast milk or if transmission of cholera vaccine to a breast-fed infant presents any unusual risk.

cholestyramine
Questran, Questran Light

Pharmacologic classification: anion exchange resin
Therapeutic classification: antilipemic, bile acid sequestrant
Pregnancy risk category C

How supplied
Available by prescription only
Powder: 378-g cans, 9-g single-dose packets (Questran). 5-g single dose packets (Questran Light). Each scoop of powder or single-dose packet contains 4 g of cholestyramine resin.

Indications, route, and dosage
Primary hyperlipidemia and hypercholesterolemia unresponsive to dietary measures alone; to reduce the risks of atherosclerotic coronary artery disease and MI; to relieve pruritus associated with partial biliary obstruction; ◊ cardiac glycoside toxicity
Adults: 4 g before meals and h.s. not to exceed 32 g daily. Can be given in one to six divided doses.
Children age 6 to 12: 80 mg/kg, or 2.35 g/m^2 t.i.d. Safe dosage has not been established for children under age 6.

Pharmacodynamics
Antilipemic action: Bile is normally excreted into the intestine to facilitate absorption of fat and other lipid materials. Cholestyramine binds with bile acid, forming an insoluble compound that is excreted in feces. With less bile available in the digestive system, less fat and lipid materials in food are absorbed, more cholesterol is used by the liver to replace its supply of bile acids, and the serum cholesterol level decreases. In partial biliary obstruction, excess bile acids accumulate in dermal tissue, resulting in pruritus; by reducing levels of dermal bile acids, cholestyramine combats pruritus.

Drug can also act as an antidiarrheal in postoperative diarrhea caused by bile acids in the colon.

Pharmacokinetics
- *Absorption:* Drug is not absorbed. Cholesterol levels may begin to decrease 24 to 48 hours after the start of therapy and may continue to fall for up to 12 months. In some patients, the initial decrease is followed by a return to or above baseline cholesterol levels on continued therapy. Relief of pruritus associated with cholestasis occurs 1 to 3 weeks after initiation of therapy. Diarrhea associated with bile acids may cease in 24 hours.
- *Distribution:* None.
- *Metabolism:* None.
- *Excretion:* Insoluble cholestyramine with bile acid complex is excreted in feces.

Contraindications and precautions
Contraindicated in patients with hypersensitivity to bile-acid sequestering resins and in those with complete biliary obstruction. Use cautiously in patients with coronary artery disease or a predisposition to constipation.

Interactions
Cholestyramine may reduce absorption of other oral medications, such as *acetaminophen, corticosteroids, thiazide diuretics, thyroid preparations,* and *cardiac glycosides,* thus decreasing their therapeutic effects. Its binding potential may also decrease anticoagulant effects of *warfarin;* concurrent depletion of *vitamin K* may either negate this effect or increase anticoagulant activity; careful monitoring of PT is mandatory.

Dosage of *oral medications* may require adjustment to compensate for possible binding with cholestyramine; give other drugs at least 1 hour before or 4 to 6 hours after cholestyramine (longer if possible); readjustment must also be made when cholestyramine is withdrawn, to prevent high-dose toxicity.

Effects on diagnostic tests
Drug therapy alters serum concentrations of ALT, AST, chloride, phosphorus, potassium, calcium, and sodium. Impaired calcium absorption may lead to osteoporosis.

Cholecystography using iopanoic acid will yield abnormal results because iopanoic acid is also bound by cholestyramine.

Adverse reactions
CNS: headache, anxiety, vertigo, dizziness, insomnia, fatigue, syncope, tinnitus.
GI: *constipation,* ***fecal impaction,*** hemorrhoids, *abdominal discomfort,* flatulence, *nausea,* vomiting, steatorrhea, GI bleeding, diarrhea, anorexia.
GU: hematuria, dysuria.
Skin: *rash;* irritation of skin, tongue, and perianal area.
Other: *vitamin A, D, E, and K deficiencies from decreased absorption;* hyperchloremic acidosis (with long-term use or very high doses); anemia; ecchymoses; backache; muscle and joint pain; bleeding tendencies; osteoporosis.

Overdose and treatment
Drug overdose has not been reported. Chief potential risk is intestinal obstruction; treatment would depend on location and degree of obstruction and on amount of gut motility.

☑ Special considerations
- To mix, sprinkle powder on surface of preferred beverage or wet food, let stand a few minutes and stir to obtain uniform suspension; avoid excess foaming by using large glass and mixing slowly. Use at least 90 ml of water or other fluid, soups, milk, or pulpy fruit; rinse container and have patient drink this liquid to be sure he ingests entire dose.
- Drug has been used to treat cardiac glycoside overdose because it binds these agents and prevents enterohepatic recycling. When used as an adjunct to hyperlipidemia, monitor levels of cardiac glycosides and other drugs to ensure appropriate dosage during and after therapy with cholestyramine.
- Determine serum cholesterol level frequently during first few months of therapy and periodically thereafter.
- Monitor bowel function. Treat constipation promptly by decreasing dosage, adding a stool softener, or discontinuing drug.
- Monitor for signs of vitamin A, D, or K deficiency.
- Questran Light contains aspartame and provides 1.6 calories per packet or scoop.

Patient education
- Explain disease process and rationale for therapy, and encourage patient to comply with continued blood testing and special diet; although therapy is not curative, it helps control serum cholesterol level.
- Encourage patient to control weight and to stop smoking as part of attempt to increase awareness of other cardiac risk factors.
- Tell patient not to take the powder in dry form; teach him to mix drug with fluids or pulpy fruits.

Geriatric use
- Patients over age 60 are more likely to experience adverse GI effects as well as adverse nutritional effects.

Pediatric use
- Children may be at greater risk of hyperchloremic acidosis during cholestyramine therapy.

Breast-feeding
- Safety in breast-feeding women has not been established.

choline magnesium trisalicylates
Tricosal, Trilisate

choline salicylate
Arthropan

Pharmacologic classification: salicylate
Therapeutic classification: nonnarcotic analgesic, antipyretic, anti-inflammatory
Pregnancy risk category C

How supplied
Available by prescription only
Tablets: 500 mg, 750 mg, 1,000 mg of salicylate (as choline and magnesium salicylate)
Solution: 500 mg of salicylate/5 ml (as choline and magnesium salicylate); 870 mg/5 ml (as choline salicylate)

Indications, route, and dosage
Rheumatoid arthritis, osteoarthritis
Adults: 1,500 mg P.O. b.i.d. or 3,000 mg h.s.
✦ ***Dosage adjustment.*** In elderly patients, give 750 mg t.i.d.
Arthritis, mild; antipyresis
Adults: 2,000 to 3,000 mg P.O. daily in divided doses b.i.d.
Mild-to-moderate pain and fever
Children: Based on weight, and the doses should be divided b.i.d.
Children weighing 26 to 28.5 lb (12 to 13 kg): 500 mg P.O. daily.
Children weighing 30 to 37.5 lb (14 to 17 kg): 750 mg P.O. daily.
Children weighing 39 to 48.5 lb (18 to 22 kg): 1,000 mg P.O. daily.
Children weighing 50 to 59.5 lb (23 to 27 kg): 1,250 mg P.O. daily.
Children weighing 61 to 70.5 lb (28 to 32 kg): 1,500 mg P.O. daily.
Children weighing 73 to 81.5 lb (33 to 37 kg): 1,750 mg P.O. daily.

Pharmacodynamics
Analgesic action: Choline salicylates produce analgesia by an ill-defined effect on the hypothalamus (central action) and by blocking generation of pain impulses (peripheral action). The peripheral action may involve inhibition of prostaglandin synthesis.

Anti-inflammatory action: These drugs exert their anti-inflammatory effect by inhibiting prostaglandin synthesis; they may also inhibit the synthesis or action of other inflammation mediators.

Antipyretic action: Choline salicylates relieve fever by acting on the hypothalamic heat-regulating center to produce peripheral vasodilation. This increases peripheral blood supply and promotes sweating, which leads to loss of heat and to cooling by evaporation. These drugs do not affect platelet aggregation and should not be used to prevent thrombosis.

Pharmacokinetics
- *Absorption:* These salicylate salts are absorbed rapidly and completely from the GI tract. Peak therapeutic effect occurs in 2 hours.
- *Distribution:* Protein binding depends on concentration and ranges from 75% to 90%, decreasing as serum concentration increases. Severe toxic effects may occur at serum concentrations greater than 400 mcg/ml.
- *Metabolism:* Drug is hydrolyzed to salicylate in the liver.
- *Excretion:* Metabolites are excreted in urine.

Contraindications and precautions
Contraindicated in patients hypersensitive to drug. Also contraindicated in patients with hemophilia, bleeding ulcers, hemorrhagic states, and for patients who consume 3 or more alcoholic beverages per day. Use cautiously in patients with impaired renal or hepatic function, peptic ulcer disease, or gastritis. Do not give to children or teenagers with chickenpox or influenza-like illnesses.

Interactions
Concomitant use of choline salicylates with drugs that are highly protein-bound (*phenytoin, sulfonylureas, warfarin*) may cause displacement of either drug, and adverse effects. Monitor therapy closely for both drugs. Concomitant use with *methotrexate* may cause displacement of bound methotrexate and inhibition of renal excretion. The adverse GI effects of choline salicylates may be potentiated by concomitant use of other *GI-irritant drugs* (such as *steroids, antibiotics, other NSAIDs*). Use together with caution. Choline salicylates decrease renal clearance of *lithium carbonate,* thus increasing serum lithium levels and the risk of adverse effects. *Ammonium chloride* and *other urine acidifiers* increase choline salicylate blood levels; monitor for choline salicylate blood levels and thus toxicity. *Antacids* in high doses, and other *urine al-*

kalizers, decrease choline salicylate blood levels; monitor for decreased salicylate effect. *Corticosteroids* enhance salicylate elimination; monitor for decreased effect. *Food* and *antacids* delay and decrease absorption of choline salicylates. Salicylates enhance the hypoprothrombinemic effects of *warfarin.* The hypoglycemic effects of *sulfonylureas* may be enhanced by salicylates.

Effects on diagnostic tests
Choline salicylates may interfere with urinary glucose analysis performed via Chemstrip uG, Diastix, glucose enzymatic test strip, Clinitest, and Benedict's solution. These drugs also interfere with urinary 5-hydroxyindole acetic acid and vanillylmandelic acid. Free T_4 levels may be elevated.

Adverse reactions
EENT: tinnitus, hearing loss.
GI: GI distress, nausea, vomiting.
Skin: rash.
Other: hypersensitivity reactions ***(anaphylaxis), Reye's syndrome, acute tubular necrosis with renal failure.***

Overdose and treatment
Clinical manifestations of overdose include metabolic acidosis with respiratory alkalosis, hyperpnea, and tachypnea from increased carbon dioxide production and direct stimulation of the respiratory center.

To treat overdose of choline salicylates, empty stomach immediately by inducing emesis with ipecac syrup, if patient is conscious, or by gastric lavage. Administer activated charcoal via nasogastric tube. Provide symptomatic and supportive measures (respiratory support and correction of fluid and electrolyte imbalances). Monitor laboratory parameters and vital signs closely. Hemodialysis is effective in removing choline salicylates but is used only in severe poisoning. Forced diuresis with alkalinizing agent accelerates salicylate excretion.

☑ Special considerations
Besides those relevant to all *salicylates,* consider the following recommendations.
- Do not mix choline salicylates with antacids.
- Administer oral solution of choline salicylate mixed with fruit juice. Follow with a full 8-oz (240 ml) glass of water to ensure passage into stomach.
- Monitor serum magnesium levels to prevent possible magnesium toxicity.
- Use of choline salicylates should be avoided in the third trimester of pregnancy.

Geriatric use
- Patients over age 60 may be more susceptible to the toxic effects of these drugs.

Pediatric use
- Safety of long-term drug use in children under age 14 has not been established.
- Because of epidemiologic association with Reye's syndrome, the Centers for Disease Control and Prevention recommend that children with chickenpox or flulike symptoms should not be given salicylates.
- Febrile, dehydrated children can develop toxicity rapidly. Usually, they should not receive more than five doses in 24 hours.

Breast-feeding
- Salicylates are distributed into breast milk. Avoid use in breast-feeding women.

chorionic gonadotropin, human (HCG)
A.P.L., Chorex 5, Chorex 10, Choron 10, Gonic, Pregnyl, Profasi, Profasi HP*

Pharmacologic classification: gonadotropin
Therapeutic classification: ovulation stimulant, spermatogenesis stimulant
Pregnancy risk category X

How supplied
Available by prescription only
Injection: 500 USP U/ml, 1,000 USP U/ml, 2,000 USP U/ml

Indications, route, and dosage
To induce ovulation and pregnancy
Adults: 5,000 to 10,000 USP U I.M. 1 day after last dose of menotropins.
Hypogonadotropic hypogonadism
Adults: 500 to 1,000 USP U I.M. three times weekly for 3 weeks, then twice weekly for 3 weeks; or 4,000 USP U I.M. three times weekly for 6 to 9 months, then 2,000 USP U three times weekly for 3 more months.
Nonobstructive prepubertal cryptorchidism
Children age 4 to 9: 5,000 USP U I.M. every other day for four doses; or 4,000 USP U I.M. three times weekly for 3 weeks; or 15 doses of 500 to 1,000 USP U I.M. given over 6 weeks; or 500 USP U three times weekly for 4 to 6 weeks, which may be repeated if unsuccessful in 1 month, giving 1,000 USP U per injection.

Pharmacodynamics
Ovulation stimulant action: HCG mimics the action of luteinizing hormone in stimulating the ovulation of a mature ovarian follicle.

Spermatogenesis stimulant action: HCG stimulates androgen production in Leydig's cells of the testis and causes maturation of the cells lining the seminiferous tubules of the testes.

Pharmacokinetics
- *Absorption:* HCG must be administered I.M. Peak blood concentrations occur within 6 hours.
- *Distribution:* HCG is distributed primarily into the testes and the ovaries.
- *Metabolism:* Initial half-life of HCG is 11 hours with a terminal phase of 23 hours.
- *Excretion:* HCG is excreted in urine.

Contraindications and precautions
Contraindicated in patients with precocious puberty or androgen-responsive cancer (prostatic, testicular, male breast) because it stimulates androgen production, and in patients with known hypersensitivity to HCG.

Use only by clinicians experienced in treating infertility disorders. Use with caution in patients with asthma, seizure disorders, migraines, or cardiac or renal diseases because it may exacerbate these conditions.

Interactions
None reported.

Effects on diagnostic tests
May interfere with radioimmunoassays for gonadotropins.

Adverse reactions
CNS: headache, fatigue, irritability, restlessness, depression.
GU: early puberty (growth of testes, penis, pubic and axillary hair; voice change; down on upper lip; growth of body hair), hyperstimulation (ovarian enlargement), ***rupture of ovarian cysts*** (after use of gonadotropins).
Skin: pain (at injection site).
Other: gynecomastia, edema.

☑ Special considerations
- Young male patients receiving HCG must be observed carefully for the development of precocious puberty.
- Carefully monitor patients with disorders that may be aggravated by fluid retention.
- Pregnancies that occur after stimulation of ovulation with gonadotropins show a relatively high incidence of multiple births.
- HCG is usually used only after failure of clomiphene in anovulatory patients.
- In infertility, encourage daily intercourse from day before HCG is given until ovulation occurs.
- Be alert to symptoms of ectopic pregnancy, usually evident between 8 and 12 weeks' gestation.

Patient education
- Teach patient and family how to assess for edema and to report it promptly.
- Advise patient and family to report signs of precocious puberty promptly.
- Inform patient receiving HCG for infertility that multiple births are possible.

Geriatric use
- Drug is not indicated for use in the elderly.

Pediatric use
- Treating prepubertal cryptorchidism with HCG can help predict future need for orchidopexy. Induction of androgen secretion may induce precocious puberty in patients treated for cryptorchidism. Instruct parent to report the following: axillary, facial, or pubic hair; penile growth; acne; and deepening of voice.

chymopapain
Chymodiactin

Pharmacologic classification: proteolytic enzyme
Therapeutic classification: chemonucleolytic agent
Pregnancy risk category C

How supplied
Available by prescription only
Powder for injection: 4,000 or 10,000 pKat unit vials

Indications, route, and dosage
Herniated lumbar intervertebral disk
Adults: 2,000 to 4,000 pKat U per disk injected intradiskally. Maximum dose in a patient with multiple disk herniation is 8,000 pKat U.

Pharmacodynamics
Chemonucleolytic action: Mechanism of action has not been clearly established in humans; in animals, chymopapain hydrolyzes the noncollagenous polypeptides or proteins that maintain the chondromucoprotein structure of the nucleus pulposus. Hydrolysis of chondromucoprotein decreases intradiskal osmotic pressure and fluid accumulation, thereby reducing symptoms of compression. Drug has no effect on collagen.

Pharmacokinetics
- *Absorption:* Drug is available only for intradiskal administration. It acts directly at the site of injection.
- *Distribution:* After intradiskal injection, chymopapain and its immunologically reactive fragments (CIP) are detectable in serum.
- *Metabolism:* Chymopapain serum levels are low, and drug is inactivated rapidly by plasma alpha-2 macroglobulin; extradiskal activity is unlikely.
- *Excretion:* Chymopapain and CIP serum levels remain steady for 24 hours and then decline. Only small amounts of CIP occur in urine.

Contraindications and precautions
Contraindicated in patients with history of allergy to drug, papaya, or papaya derivatives (such as meat tenderizers); in patients who have previously received an injection of chymopapain; and in those with severe spondylolisthesis in addition to spinal stenosis, severe progressing paralysis, or evidence of spinal cord tumor or a cauda equina lesion.

Interactions
Concomitant use with *radiographic contrast media* increases risk of neurotoxicity.

Effects on diagnostic tests
None reported.

Adverse reactions
CNS: ***seizures, subarachnoid and intracerebral hemorrhage,*** headache, dizziness.
GI: nausea, various GI disturbances.

Skin: erythema, rash, pruritic urticaria.
Other: ***anaphylaxis, anaphylactoid reaction; paraplegia, acute transverse myelitis,*** leg weakness, paresthesia, numbness of legs and toes, *back pain, stiffness, back spasm, soreness,* conjunctivitis, vasomotor rhinitis, angioedema.

Overdose and treatment
Doses of over 100 times the recommended amount have been given *without* toxic effects; toxic effects after overdosage would probably be extreme manifestations of adverse reactions. Treat symptomatically.

☑ Special considerations
- Administer drug in the health care facility by clinicians experienced and trained in diagnosis of lumbar disk disease.
- Before treatment, question patient about allergy to papaya or its derivatives.
- Monitor patient for at least 1 hour after injection for hypersensitivity reaction; hypotension and bronchospasm can rapidly lead to anaphylaxis and death. Maintain an open I.V. line to permit rapid management of anaphylaxis, and keep resuscitative measures available.
- Anaphylaxis occurs in 0.4% to 1% of patients and may occur immediately or up to 1 hour after injection; risk of anaphylaxis is greater in women with elevated erythrocyte sedimentation rate and in patients undergoing general anesthesia.
- One in 18,000 patients develops acute transverse myelitis or myelopathy, manifested by acute onset of severe back pain, weakness, and sensory changes at the thoracic level that progress to paraplegia or paraparesis over 4 to 48 hours; patients with injection of two or more disks after diskography have an increased risk.
- A skin test (ChymoFAST) may detect hypersensitivity.
- Pretreatment of the patient with histamine-receptor antagonists (H_1 and H_2) is recommended to decrease the severity of chymopapain-induced allergic reactions.
- Patient should be well hydrated before the procedure because of the abrupt decrease in intravascular volume during anaphylaxis.

Patient education
- Warn patient to call at once if a delayed allergic reaction of rash, itching, or urticaria develops (up to 15 days postinjection) or if sudden, severe pain, muscle weakness, or sensory changes in the back develops.
- Tell patient that back pain, stiffness, and soreness may occur; back spasm may also occur after treatment. Reassure patient this is temporary but may last for several days.

Geriatric use
- Drug should be used with caution in elderly patients.

ciclopirox olamine
Loprox

Pharmacologic classification: N-hydroxypyridinone derivative
Therapeutic classification: topical antifungal
Pregnancy risk category B

How supplied
Available by prescription only
Cream: 1%
Lotion: 1%

Indications, route, and dosage
Tinea pedis, tinea cruris, and tinea corporis; cutaneous candidiasis; tinea versicolor
Adults and children over age 10: Massage gently into the affected and surrounding areas b.i.d., in the morning and evening.

Pharmacodynamics
Antifungal and antibacterial activity: Although the exact mechanism of action is unknown, ciclopirox appears to act by causing intracellular depletion of essential cellular components or ions. The drug is active against many fungi, including dermatophytes and yeast, as well as against some gram-positive and gram-negative bacteria.

Pharmacokinetics
- *Absorption:* Rapid but minimal percutaneous absorption.
- *Distribution:* Minimal.
- *Metabolism:* After percutaneous absorption, ciclopirox has an elimination half-life of about 2 hours.
- *Excretion:* After percutaneous absorption, ciclopirox and its metabolites are excreted rapidly in the urine.

Contraindications and precautions
Contraindicated in patients hypersensitive to drug.

Effects on diagnostic tests
None reported.

Interactions
None reported.

Adverse reactions
Skin: pruritus, burning, irritation, redness.

Overdose and treatment
No information available.

☑ Special considerations
- Drug is for topical use only; avoid contact with eyes.
- Do not apply occlusive dressings.

Patient education
- Instruct patient to use drug for full treatment period even if symptoms have improved. He should call if no improvement occurs in 4 weeks.
- Tell patient to avoid occlusive wrapping or dressing.

- Advise patient to wash hands thoroughly after applying drug, to avoid contacting eyes with drug.
- Tell patient to discontinue drug and call promptly if sensitivity or chemical irritation occurs.
- Inform patient with tinea versicolor that hypopigmentation from the disease will not resolve immediately.

Pediatric use
- Safety and efficacy in children under age 10 have not been established.

Breast-feeding
- It is unknown if drug is excreted in breast milk; use with caution in breast-feeding women.

cidofovir
Vistide

Pharmacologic classification: nucleotide analogue
Therapeutic classification: antiviral
Pregnancy risk category C

How supplied
Available by prescription only
Injection: 75 mg/ml

Indications, route, and dosage
Cytomegalovirus (CMV) retinitis in patients with AIDS
Adults: Give 5 mg/kg I.V infused over 1 hour once weekly for 2 consecutive weeks followed by a maintenance dosage of 5 mg/kg I.V. infused over 1 hour once q 2 weeks. Probenecid must be administered concomitantly.

✦ ***Dosage adjustment.*** For patients with creatinine clearance of 41 to 55 ml/minute, induction and maintenance dosages should be reduced to 2 mg/kg; if creatinine clearance is 30 to 40 ml/minute, induction and maintenance doses should be reduced to 1.5 mg/kg; if creatinine clearance is 20 to 29 ml/minute, induction and maintenance doses should be reduced to 1 mg/kg; and if creatinine clearance is 19 ml/minute or less, induction and maintenance doses should be reduced to 0.5 mg/kg.

Pharmacodynamics
Antiviral action: Cidofovir suppresses CMV replication by selective inhibition of viral DNA synthesis.

Pharmacokinetics
- *Absorption:* Cidofovir is administered only I.V.
- *Distribution:* Unknown.
- *Metabolism:* Not metabolized.
- *Excretion:* 80% to 100% of cidofovir is excreted unchanged in urine.

Contraindications and precautions
Contraindicated in patients with hypersensitivity to drug or history of clinically severe hypersensitivity to probenecid or other sulfa-containing medications. Do not administer as a direct intraocular injection (direct injection may be associated with significant decreases in intraocular pressure and vision impairment). Use cautiously in patients with impaired renal function.

Interactions
Avoid concomitant administration of cidofovir and agents with nephrotoxic potential, such as *amphotericin B, aminoglycosides, foscarnet,* and *I.V. pentamidine.*

Effects on diagnostic tests
None reported.

Adverse reactions
CNS: *asthenia, headache,* amnesia, anxiety, confusion, ***seizure,*** depression, dizziness, abnormal gait, hallucinations, insomnia, neuropathy, paresthesia, somnolence, vasodilation.
CV: hypotension, postural hypotension, pallor, syncope, tachycardia.
EENT: amblyopia, conjunctivitis, eye disorders, ocular hypotony, iritis, retinal detachment, taste perversion, uveitis, abnormal vision, pharyngitis, rhinitis, sinusitis.
GI: *nausea, vomiting, diarrhea, anorexia, abdominal pain,* dry mouth, colitis, constipation, tongue discoloration, dyspepsia, dysphagia, flatulence, gastritis, melena, oral candidiasis, rectal disorders, stomatitis, aphthous stomatitis, mouth ulceration.
GU: *elevated creatinine levels, nephrotoxicity, proteinuria,* decreased creatinine clearance levels, glycosuria, hematuria, urinary incontinence, urinary tract infection.
Hematologic: NEUTROPENIA, *anemia,* ***thrombocytopenia.***
Hepatic: hepatomegaly, abnormal liver function tests, increased alkaline phosphatase levels.
Metabolic: fluid imbalances, hyperglycemia, hyperlipemia, hypocalcemia, hypokalemia, weight loss.
Musculoskeletal: arthralgia, myasthenia, myalgia.
Respiratory: asthma, bronchitis, coughing, dyspnea, hiccups, increased sputum, lung disorders, pneumonia.
Skin: *rash, alopecia,* acne, skin discoloration, dry skin, herpes simplex, pruritus, sweating, urticaria.
Other: *fever; infections; chills;* allergic reactions; facial edema; malaise; pain in back, chest, or neck; ***sarcoma, sepsis.***

Overdose and treatment
No information on drug overdose is available. However, hemodialysis and hydration may reduce drug plasma concentrations in patients who receive an overdosage of the drug. Probenecid may reduce the potential for nephrotoxicity in patients who receive a drug overdose through reduction of active tubular secretion.

☑ Special considerations
- Renal impairment is the major toxicity of cidofovir. To minimize possible nephrotoxicity, use I.V. prehydration with 0.9% NaCl and administer probenecid with each cidofovir infusion.
- Administer 1 L of 0.9% NaCl solution over a 1- to 2-hour period immediately before each cidofovir infusion. Administer a second liter in patients who can tolerate the additional fluid load. If the second

liter is given, administer either at the start of the cidofovir infusion or immediately afterward, and infuse it over a 1- to 3-hour period.
• Administer 2 g of probenecid P.O. 3 hours before the cidofovir dose and 1 g at 2 hours, and again at 8 hours after completion of the 1-hour infusion (total 4 g).
• Because of the potential for increased nephrotoxicity, doses exceeding the recommended dose should not be administered and the frequency or rate of administration should not be exceeded.
• To prepare infusion, extract the appropriate amount of cidofovir from the vial with a syringe and transfer the dose to an infusion bag containing 100 ml 0.9% NaCl solution. Infuse the entire volume I.V. into the patient at a constant rate over a 1-hour period. Use a standard infusion pump for administration.
• Because of the mutagenic properties of cidofovir, drug should be prepared in a class II laminar flow biological safety cabinet. Personnel preparing drug should wear surgical gloves and a closed front surgical-type gown with knit cuffs.
• If drug contacts the skin, wash membranes and flush thoroughly with water. Excess drug and all other materials used in the admixture preparation and administration should be placed in a leak-proof, puncture-proof container. The recommended method of disposal is high temperature incineration.
• Cidofovir infusion admixtures should be administered within 24 hours of preparation; refrigerator or freezer storage should not be used to extend this 24-hour period. If admixtures are not to be used immediately, they may be refrigerated at 36° to 46° F (2° to 8° C) for no more than 24 hours. Refrigerated admixtures should be allowed to equilibrate to room temperature before use.
• No other drug and supplements should be added to the cidofovir admixture for concurrent administration. Compatibility with Ringer's solution, lactated Ringer's solution, or bacteriostatic infusion fluids has not been evaluated.
• WBC counts with differential should be monitored before each dose.
• Renal function (serum creatinine and urine protein) should be monitored before each dose of the drug and the dosage modified for changes in renal function.
• Granulocytopenia has been observed in association with cidofovir treatment; monitor neutrophil counts during therapy.
• Intraocular pressure, visual acuity, and ocular symptoms should be monitored periodically.
• Drug is indicated only for the treatment of CMV retinitis in patients with AIDS. Safety and efficacy of drug have not been established for treating other CMV infections, congenital or neonatal CMV disease, and CMV disease in patients not infected with the human immunodeficiency virus.
• In animal studies, cidofovir was carcinogenic and teratogenic and caused hypospermia.
• Drug should not be initiated in patients with baseline serum creatinine exceeding 1.5 mg/dl or calculated creatinine clearances of 55 ml/minute or less unless the potential benefits exceed the potential risks.
• Fanconi's syndrome and decreased serum bicarbonate levels associated with evidence of renal tubular damage have been reported in patients receiving cidofovir. Monitor patient closely.
• Discontinue zidovudine therapy or reduce dosage by 50% in patients receiving zidovudine on the days cidofovir is administered, because probenecid reduces metabolic clearance of zidovudine.

Patient education
• Inform patient that drug is not a cure for CMV retinitis and that regular ophthalmologic follow-up examinations are necessary.
• Alert patients on zidovudine therapy that they will need to obtain dosage guidelines on days that cidofovir is administered.
• Tell patient that close monitoring of renal function will be needed during cidofovir therapy and that an abnormality may require a change in cidofovir therapy.
• Stress importance of completing a full course of probenecid with each cidofovir dose. Tell patient to take probenecid after a meal to decrease nausea.
• Advise patient that cidofovir is considered a potential carcinogen in humans.
• Instruct women of childbearing potential to use effective contraception during and for 1 month after treatment with cidofovir. Tell men to practice barrier contraceptive methods during and for 3 months after drug treatment.

Geriatric use
• Use with caution when administering cidofovir to elderly patients. Dosage adjustment will be necessary if patient is renally impaired.

Pediatric use
• Safety and effectiveness in children have not been established.

Breast-feeding
• It is not known if drug is excreted in breast milk. Do not administer to breast-feeding women.

cimetidine
Tagamet, Tagamet HB

Pharmacologic classification: H_2-receptor antagonist
Therapeutic classification: antiulcer
Pregnancy risk category B

How supplied
Available by prescription only
Tablets: 200 mg, 300 mg, 400 mg, 800 mg
Injection: 150 mg/ml, 300 mg/50 ml (premixed)
Liquid: 300 mg/5 ml

Available without a prescription
Tablets: 100 mg

Indications, route, and dosage
Duodenal ulcer (short-term treatment)
Adults: 800 mg h.s. for maximum of 8 weeks. Alternatively, give 400 mg P.O. b.i.d. or 300 mg P.O.

q.i.d. with meals and h.s. When healing occurs, stop treatment or give h.s. dose only to control nocturnal hypersecretion.

Parenteral

300 mg diluted to 20 ml with 0.9% NaCl solution or other compatible I.V. solution by I.V. push over 5 minutes q 6 hours. Or 300 mg diluted in 50 ml dextrose 5% solution or other compatible I.V. solution by I.V. infusion over 15 to 20 minutes q 6 to 8 hours. Or 300 mg I.M. q 6 to 8 hours (no dilution necessary). To increase dose, give more frequently to maximum daily dose of 2,400 mg.

Duodenal ulcer prophylaxis

Adults: 400 mg h.s.

Active benign gastric ulcer

Adults: 800 mg h.s., or 300 mg q.i.d. with meals and h.s. for up to 8 weeks.

Pathologic hypersecretory conditions (such as Zollinger-Ellison syndrome, systemic mastocytosis, and multiple endocrine adenomas); ◇ short-bowel syndrome

Adults: 300 mg P.O. q.i.d. with meals and h.s.; adjust to patient needs. Maximum daily dose, 2,400 mg.

Parenteral

300 mg diluted to 20 ml with 0.9% NaCl solution or other compatible I.V. solution by I.V. push over 5 minutes q 6 to 8 hours. Or 300 mg diluted in 50 ml dextrose 5% solution or other compatible I.V. solution by I.V. infusion over 15 to 20 minutes q 6 to 8 hours. To increase dose, give 300 mg doses more frequently to maximum daily dose of 2,400 mg.

Symptomatic relief of gastroesophageal reflux

Adults: 800 mg P.O. b.i.d. or 400 mg q.i.d., before meals and h.s.

◇ Active upper GI bleeding, peptic esophagitis, stress ulcer

Adults: 1 to 2 g I.V. or P.O. daily, in four divided doses.

Children: 20 to 40 mg/kg daily in divided doses.

Continuous infusion for patients unable to tolerate oral medication

Adults: 37.5 mg/hour (900 mg/day) by continuous I.V. infusion. Use an infusion pump if total volume is below 250 ml/day.

Heartburn, acid indigestion, sour stomach

Adults: 200 mg P.O. up to a maximum of b.i.d. (400 mg).

✦ ***Dosage adjustment.*** In patients with renal failure, recommended dose is 300 mg P.O. or I.V. q 8 to 12 hours at end of dialysis. Dosage may be decreased further if hepatic failure is also present.

Pharmacodynamics

Antiulcer action: Cimetidine competitively inhibits histamine's action at H_2 receptors in gastric parietal cells, inhibiting basal and nocturnal gastric acid secretion (such as from stimulation by food, caffeine, insulin, histamine, betazole, or pentagastrin). Cimetidine may also enhance gastromucosal defense and healing.

A 300-mg oral or parenteral dose inhibits about 80% of gastric acid secretion for 4 to 5 hours.

Pharmacokinetics

- *Absorption:* Approximately 60% to 75% of oral dose is absorbed. Absorption rate (but not extent) may be affected by food.
- *Distribution:* Drug is distributed to many body tissues. About 15% to 20% of drug is protein-bound. Cimetidine apparently crosses the placenta and is distributed in breast milk.
- *Metabolism:* Approximately 30% to 40% of dose is metabolized in the liver. Drug has a half-life of 2 hours in patients with normal renal function; half-life increases with decreasing renal function.
- *Excretion:* Excreted primarily in urine (48% of oral dose, 75% of parenteral dose); 10% of oral dose is excreted in feces. Some drug is excreted in breast milk.

Contraindications and precautions

Contraindicated in patients hypersensitive to drug. Use with caution in elderly or debilitated patients.

Interactions

Cimetidine decreases the metabolism of the following drugs, thus increasing potential toxicity and possibly necessitating dosage reduction: *beta-adrenergic blockers* (such as *propranolol*), *phenytoin, lidocaine, procainamide, quinidine, benzodiazepines, disulfiram, metronidazole, xanthines, tricyclic antidepressants, oral contraceptives, isoniazid, warfarin, carmustine,* and *triamterene.* It also may affect the absorption of *ketoconazole, ferrous salts, indomethacin,* and *tetracyclines* by altering gastric pH. Serum *digoxin* concentrations may be reduced. Concomitant administration with *flecainide* may increase pharmacologic effects: serum concentrations of *flecainide* may be increased.

Effects on diagnostic tests

Cimetidine may antagonize pentagastrin's effect during gastric acid secretion tests; it may cause false-negative results in skin tests using allergen extracts.

Cimetidine therapy increases prolactin levels, serum alkaline phosphatase levels, and serum creatinine levels.

FD and C blue dye #2 used in Tagamet tablets may impair interpretation of Hemoccult and Gastroccult tests on gastric content aspirate. Be sure to wait at least 15 minutes after tablet administration before drawing the sample, and follow test manufacturer's instructions closely.

Adverse reactions

CNS: confusion, dizziness, headache, peripheral neuropathy, somnolence, hallucinations.
GI: *mild and transient diarrhea.*
GU: transient elevations in serum creatinine levels, impotence, mild gynecomastia if used for over 1 month.
Hematologic: ***agranulocytosis*** (rare), ***neutropenia, thrombocytopenia*** (rare), ***aplastic anemia*** (rare).
Hepatic: jaundice (rare).
Other: hypersensitivity reactions, muscle pain, arthralgia.

Overdose and treatment

Clinical effects of overdose include respiratory failure and tachycardia. Overdose is rare; intake of up to 10 g has caused no untoward effects.

Support respiration and maintain a patent airway. Induce emesis or use gastric lavage; follow with activated charcoal to prevent further absorption. Treat tachycardia with propranolol if necessary.

☑ Special considerations

Besides those relevant to all *H_2-receptor antagonists,* consider the following recommendations.

- For I.V. use, cimetidine must be diluted prior to administration. Do not dilute drug with sterile water for injection; use 0.9% NaCl solution, D_5W or $D_{10}W$ injection, lactated Ringer's solution, or 5% sodium bicarbonate injection to a total volume of 20 ml. I.M. administration may be painful.
- After administration of the liquid via nasogastric tube, tube should be flushed to clear it and ensure drug's passage to stomach.
- Hemodialysis removes drug; schedule dose after dialysis session.
- Other unlabeled uses of drug include pancreatic insufficiency, hives, and hirsutism.

Patient education

- Warn patient to take drug as directed and to continue taking it even after pain subsides, to allow for adequate healing. Urge patient to avoid smoking, because it may increase gastric acid secretion and worsen disease.

Geriatric use

- Use caution when administering cimetidine to elderly patients because of the potential for adverse reactions affecting the CNS.

Breast-feeding

- Drug is excreted in breast milk. Avoid use in breast-feeding women.

ciprofloxacin (systemic)

Cipro

Pharmacologic classification: fluoroquinolone antibiotic
Therapeutic classification: antibiotic
Pregnancy risk category C

How supplied

Available by prescription only
Tablets: 250 mg, 500 mg, 750 mg
Injection: 200 mg/20-ml vial; 400 mg/40-ml vial; 200 mg in 100 ml D_5W; 400 mg in 200 ml D_5W

Indications, route, and dosage

Mild to moderate urinary tract infection caused by susceptible bacteria
Adults: 250 mg P.O. or 200 mg I.V. q 12 hours.
Infectious diarrhea, mild to moderate respiratory tract infections, bone and joint infections, severe or complicated urinary tract infections
Adults: 500 mg P.O. q 12 hours or 400 mg I.V. q 12 hours.
Severe or complicated infections of the respiratory tract, bones, joints, skin, or skin structures; ◊ mycobacterial infections
Adults: 750 mg P.O. q 12 hours or 400 mg I.V. q 12 hours.
Typhoid fever
Adults: 500 mg P.O. q 12 hours.
Intra-abdominal infections (in combination with metronidazole)
Adults: 500 mg P.O. q 12 hours
◊ Uncomplicated gonorrhea
Adults: 250 mg P.O. as a single dose
◊ Neisseria meningitidis in nasal passages
Adults: 500 to 750 mg P.O. as a single dose, or 250 mg P.O. b.i.d. for 2 days, or 500 mg P.O. b.i.d. for 5 days.
✦ ***Dosage adjustment.*** For patients with renal failure, refer to following chart.

ORAL CIPROFLOXACIN

Creatinine clearance (ml/min)	Dose
> 50	No adjustment
30 to 50	250 to 500 mg q 12 hr
5 to 29	250 to 500 mg q 18 hr
Patients on hemodialysis or peritoneal dialysis	250 to 500 mg q 24 hr (after dialysis)

I.V. CIPROFLOXACIN

Creatinine clearance (ml/min)	Dose
> 30	No adjustment
5 to 29	200 to 400 mg I.V. q 18 to 24 hr

Pharmacodynamics

Antibiotic action: Ciprofloxacin inhibits DNA gyrase, preventing bacterial DNA replication. The following organisms have been reported to be susceptible (in-vitro) to ciprofloxacin: *Campylobacter jejuni, Citrobacter diversus, Citrobacter freundii, Enterobacter cloacae, Escherichia coli* (including enterotoxigenic strains), *Haemophilus parainfluenzae, Klebsiella pneumoniae, Morganella morganii, Proteus mirabilis, Proteus vulgaris, Providencia stuartii, Providencia rettgeri, Pseudomonas aeruginosa, Serratia marcescens, Shigella flexneri, Shigella sonnei, Staphylococcus aureus* (penicillinase– and non-penicillinase–producing strains), *Staphylococcus epidermidis, Streptococcus faecalis,* and *Streptococcus pyogenes.*

Pharmacokinetics

- *Absorption:* About 70% is absorbed after oral administration. Food delays rate of absorption but not extent.
- *Distribution:* Peak serum levels occur within 1 to 2 hours after oral dosing. Drug is 20% to 40% pro-

tein-bound; CSF levels are only about 10% of plasma levels.
• *Metabolism:* Probably hepatic. Four metabolites have been identified; each has less antimicrobial activity than the parent compound.
• *Excretion:* Primarily renal. Serum half-life is about 4 hours in adults with normal renal function.

Contraindications and precautions
Contraindicated in patients sensitive to fluoroquinolone antibiotics. Use cautiously in patients with CNS disorders or those at risk for seizures.

Interactions
Aluminum-, *calcium-*, and *magnesium-containing antacid supplements* may interfere with ciprofloxacin absorption. Antacids may be safely administered 2 hours prior to 6 hours after ciprofloxacin. Concomitant use with *probenecid* interferes with renal tubular secretion and results in higher plasma levels of ciprofloxacin; use with *sucralfate* reduces absorption of ciprofloxacin by 50%. Ciprofloxacin may attenuate elimination of *theophylline*, increasing the risk of *theophylline* toxicity. Ciprofloxacin also prolongs elimination half-life of *caffeine*.

Synergistic effects have occurred with concurrent use of *beta-lactams* and *aminoglycosides*. PT has increased with use of ciprofloxin and *warfarin*. *Vitamins, minerals*, and *iron* may interfere with absorption of ciprofloxacin.

Effects on diagnostic tests
None reported.

Adverse reactions
CNS: headache, restlessness, tremor, dizziness, fatigue, drowsiness, insomnia, depression, lightheadedness, confusion, hallucinations, ***seizures,*** paresthesia.
GI: *nausea, diarrhea,* vomiting, abdominal pain or discomfort, oral candidiasis, pseudomembranous colitis, dyspepsia, flatulence, constipation.
GU: crystalluria, increased serum creatinine and BUN levels, interstitial nephritis.
Musculoskeletal: arthralgia, joint or back pain, joint inflammation, joint stiffness, aching, neck or chest pain.
Skin: *rash,* photosensitivity, toxic epidermal necrolysis, exfoliative dermatitis.
Other: photosensitivity, elevated liver enzymes, Stevens-Johnson syndrome, hypersensitivity; thrombophlebitis, burning, pruritus, erythema, edema (with I.V. administration).

Overdose and treatment
To treat drug overdose, empty the stomach by induced vomiting or lavage. Provide general supportive measures and maintain hydration. Peritoneal dialysis or hemodialysis may be helpful, particularly if patient's renal function is compromised.

☑ Special considerations
• Duration of therapy depends on type and severity of infection. Therapy should continue for 2 days after symptoms have abated. Most infections are well controlled in 1 to 2 weeks, but bone or joint infections may require therapy for 4 weeks or longer.
• Closer monitoring of theophylline levels may be necessary because of increased risk of theophylline toxicity in patient receiving ciprofloxacin.

Patient education
• Tell patient that drug may be taken without regard to meals. The preferred time is 2 hours after a meal.
• Advise patient to avoid taking drug with antacids, iron, or calcium and to drink plenty of fluids during therapy.
• Inform patient that, because dizziness, lightheadedness, or drowsiness may occur, he should avoid hazardous activities that require mental alertness until CNS effects of drug are determined.

Pediatric use
• Avoid use in children.

Breast-feeding
• Drug may be secreted in breast milk. Consider discontinuing breast-feeding or drug therapy to avoid serious toxicity in the infant.

ciprofloxacin hydrochloride (ophthalmic)
Ciloxan

Pharmacologic classification: fluoroquinolone
Therapeutic classification: antibacterial
Pregnancy risk category C

How supplied
Available by prescription only
Ophthalmic solution: 0.3% in 2.5- and 5-ml containers

Indications, route, and dosage
***Corneal ulcers caused by* Pseudomonas aeruginosa, Staphylococcus aureus, Staphylococcus epidermidis, Streptococcus pneumoniae, *and* possibly Serratia marcescens *and* Streptococcus viridans**
Adults and children over age 12: Instill 2 drops in the affected eye q 15 minutes for first 6 hours, then 2 drops q 30 minutes for remainder of first day. On day 2, instill 2 drops hourly. On days 3 to 14, instill 2 drops q 4 hours.
***Bacterial conjunctivitis caused by* S. aureus *and* S. epidermidis *and possibly* S. pneumoniae**
Adults and children over age 12: Instill 1 or 2 drops into the conjunctival sac of affected eye q 2 hours while awake, for first 2 days. Then 1 or 2 drops q 4 hours while awake, for next 5 days.

Pharmacodynamics
Antibacterial action: Inhibits bacterial DNA gyrase, an enzyme necessary for bacterial replication. Bacteriostatic or bactericidal, depending on concentration.

Pharmacokinetics

- *Absorption:* Systemic absorption is limited. One study in which the drug was administered in each eye every 2 hours while awake for 2 days, followed by every 4 hours while awake for an additional 5 days, showed that the maximum plasma concentration was below 5 ng/ml, and the mean plasma concentration was usually below 2.5 ng/ml.
- *Distribution:* Unknown.
- *Metabolism:* Unknown.
- *Excretion:* Unknown.

Contraindications and precautions

Contraindicated in patients with history of hypersensitivity to drug or other fluoroquinolone antibiotics. Use with caution in breast-feeding women.

Interactions

None reported.

Effects on diagnostic tests

None reported.

Adverse reactions

EENT: *local burning or discomfort, white crystalline precipitate* (in the superficial portion of the corneal defect in patients with corneal ulcers), *margin crusting, crystals or scales, foreign body sensation, itching, conjunctival hyperemia,* bad or bitter taste in mouth, corneal staining, allergic reactions, keratopathy, lid edema, tearing, photophobia, decreased vision.
GI: nausea.

Overdose and treatment

A topical overdose of drug may be flushed from the eye with warm tap water.

☑ Special considerations

- If corneal epithelium is still compromised after 14 days of treatment, continue therapy.

Patient education

- Teach patient how to instill drug correctly. Remind him not to touch the tip of the bottle with his hands and to avoid contact of the tip with the eye or surrounding tissue.
- Remind patient not to share washcloths or towels with other family members to avoid spreading infection.
- Advise patient to wash hands before and after instilling solution.

Pediatric use

- Safety and efficacy in children under age 12 have not been established.

Breast-feeding

- It is unknown if drug is excreted in breast milk after application to the eye; however, systemically administered ciprofloxacin has been detected in breast milk. Use caution.

cisapride

Propulsid

Pharmacologic classification: serotonin-4 receptor agonist
Therapeutic classification: GI prokinetic
Pregnancy risk category C

How supplied

Available by prescription only
Tablets: 10 mg, 20 mg
Suspension: [illegible] mg/ml

Indications, route, and dosage

Symptomatic treatment of nocturnal heartburn due to gastroesophageal reflux disease that does not respond adequately to lifestyle modifications, antacids, and gastric acid–reducing agents
Adults: 10 mg P.O. q.i.d. at least 15 minutes before meals and h.s. Dosage may be increased to 20 mg q.i.d., if needed.

Pharmacodynamics

GI prokinetic action: Cisapride is thought to enhance release of acetylcholine at the myenteric plexus, increasing GI motility. Cisapride does not induce muscarinic or nicotinic receptor stimulation, nor does it inhibit acetylcholinesterase activity. It also does not increase or decrease basal- or pentagastrin-induced gastric acid secretion.

Pharmacokinetics

- *Absorption:* Cisapride is rapidly absorbed; onset of action is approximately 30 to 60 minutes after oral administration. Peak plasma concentrations are reached 1 to 1½ hours after administration.
- *Distribution:* Extensively distributed (the volume of distribution is about 180 L). About 97.5% to 98% binds to plasma proteins, mainly to albumin.
- *Metabolism:* Cisapride is extensively metabolized in the liver. Norcisapride, formed by N-dealkylation, is the principal metabolite in plasma, feces, and urine.
- *Excretion:* Drug is excreted in urine and feces. Unchanged drug accounts for less than 10% of urinary and fecal recovery after oral administration. The mean terminal half-life ranges from 6 to 12 hours.

Contraindications and precautions

Contraindicated in patients hypersensitive to drug. Also contraindicated in patients in whom increased GI motility may be harmful, such as those with mechanical obstruction, hemorrhage, or perforation of the GI tract.

Concurrent use with macrolides, antifungals, protease inhibitors, and nefazodine is contraindicated. Also contraindicated in patients with history of prolonged QT intervals, ventricular arrhythmias, ischemic heart disease, uncorrected electrolyte disorders (such as hypokalemia, hypomagnesemia), and heart, renal, or respiratory failure. Use cautiously in breast-feeding women.

Interactions

Anticholinergic agents may decrease cisapride's therapeutic effects. Cisapride may affect the absorption of other drugs by accelerating gastric emptying. Patients receiving narrow therapeutic ratio drugs or other drugs that require careful titration should be monitored closely and plasma levels reassessed.

Administration of cisapride during *anticoagulant* therapy has led to increased coagulation times. It is advisable to check coagulation time 1 week after the start and discontinuation of cisapride therapy, with an appropriate adjustment of the anticoagulant dose, if necessary.

Cimetidine coadministration leads to an increased peak plasma concentration of cisapride. GI absorption of *cimetidine* and *ranitidine* is accelerated when they are coadministered with cisapride.

Cisapride may increase the absorption of *digoxin.* Concurrent administration with *clarithromycin, erythromycin, fluconazole, indinavir, itraconazole, ketoconazole, miconazole, nefazodone, ritonavir, troleandomycin,* and *agents that inhibit cytochrome P-450 IIIA4* is contraindicated because of the increased risk of prolonged QT intervals and arrhythmias.

Effects on diagnostic tests

None reported.

Adverse reactions

CNS: *headache,* insomnia, anxiety, nervousness.
EENT: abnormal vision, rhinitis, sinusitis.
GI: *diarrhea, abdominal pain,* nausea, constipation, flatulence, dyspepsia.
GU: frequency, urinary tract infection, vaginitis.
Respiratory: cough, upper respiratory tract infections.
Skin: rash, pruritus.
Other: pain, fever, viral infections, arthralgia.

Overdose and treatment

Symptoms of overdose may include retching, borborygmi, flatulence, and increased stool and urinary frequency. Treatment should include gastric lavage or activated charcoal, close observation, and general supportive measures.

☑ Special considerations

- Be aware that cisapride may accelerate the sedative effects of benzodiazepines and alcohol.

Patient education

- Instruct patient to take cisapride at least 15 minutes before meals and at bedtime.
- Warn patient that drug may accelerate the sedative effects of benzodiazepines and alcohol.
- Caution patient against use of oral fluconazole, ketoconazole, itraconazole, miconazole, erythromycin, clarithromycin, indinavir, nefazodone, ritonavir, troleandomycin because of potential for serious adverse reactions.

Geriatric use

- Steady-state plasma levels of cisapride are generally higher in older patients than in younger ones because of a moderately prolonged elimination half-life. Therapeutic doses, however, are similar to those used in younger adults.

Pediatric use

- Safety and effectiveness in children have not been established.

Breast-feeding

- Drug is excreted in breast milk at concentrations approximately one-twentieth of those observed in plasma. Use caution when administering cisapride to breast-feeding patients.

cisatracurium besylate

Nimbex

Pharmacologic classification: nondepolarizing neuromuscular blocker
Therapeutic classification: skeletal muscle relaxant
Pregnancy risk category B

How supplied

Available by prescription only
Injection: 2 mg/ml, 10 mg/ml

Indications, route, and dosage

Adjunct to general anesthesia, to facilitate tracheal intubation, and to provide skeletal muscle relaxation during surgery or mechanical ventilation in the intensive care unit

Adults and children age 12 and older: Initially, 0.15 or 0.20 mg/kg I.V.; then 0.03 mg/kg I.V. q 40 to 50 minutes after an initial dose of 0.15 mg/kg and q 50 to 60 minutes following an initial dose of 0.20 mg/kg for maintenance in prolonged surgical procedures. Alternatively, administer 3 mcg/kg/minute maintenance infusion after initial dose and then decrease to 1 to 2 mcg/kg/minute p.r.n.

Children age 2 to 12: 0.1 mg/kg I.V. over 5 to 10 seconds. Administer 3 mcg/kg/minute maintenance I.V. infusion after initial dose and then decrease to 1 to 2 mcg/kg/minute p.r.n. in prolonged surgical procedures.

Maintenance of neuromuscular blockade in intensive care unit

Adults: 3 mcg/kg/minute I.V. infusion.

Note: There may be wide variability among patients in dosage requirements and these may increase or decrease over time.

Pharmacodynamics

Skeletal muscle relaxation action: Cisatracurium binds competitively to cholinergic receptors on the motor end-plate to antagonize the action of acetylcholine, resulting in blockage of neuromuscular transmission.

Pharmacokinetics

- *Absorption:* Drug is only administered I.V.

• *Distribution:* Volume of distribution is limited by its large molecular weight and high polarity. Drug binding to plasma proteins has not been successfully studied because of its rapid degradation at physiologic pH.
• *Metabolism:* The degradation of cisatracurium is largely independent of liver metabolism. It is believed that drug undergoes Hofmann elimination (a pH- and temperature-dependent chemical process) to form laudanosine and the monoquaternary acrylate metabolite.
• *Excretion:* The metabolites of cisatracurium are excreted primarily in urine and feces. Elimination half-life is between 22 and 29 minutes.

Contraindications and precautions

Contraindicated in patients with hypersensitivity to drug, other bis-benzylisoquinolinium agents, or benzyl alcohol. Use cautiously in pregnant patients.

Interactions

Aminoglycosides, bacitracin, clindamycin, colistin, lincomycin, lithium, local anesthetics, magnesium salts, polymyxins, procainamide, quinidine, tetracyclines, and *colistimethate sodium* may enhance the neuromuscular blocking action of cisatracurium. Use together cautiously. *Carbamazepine* and *phenytoin* may cause slightly shorter duration of neuromuscular blockage requiring higher infusion rate requirements. Monitor patient closely. *Isoflurane* or *enflurane* administered with *nitrous oxide* or *oxygen* may prolong the clinically effective duration of action of initial and maintenance doses of cisatracurium. In long surgical procedures, less frequent maintenance dosing, lower maintenance doses, or reduced infusion rates of cisatracurium may be needed.

Effects on diagnostic tests

None reported.

Adverse reactions

CV: bradycardia, hypotension.
Respiratory: ***bronchospasm.***
Skin: flushing, rash.

Overdose and treatment

Overdosage with neuromuscular blocking agents may result in neuromuscular block beyond the time needed for surgery and anesthesia. The primary treatment is maintenance of a patent airway and controlled ventilation until recovery of normal neuromuscular function is assured. Once recovery from neuromuscular block begins, further recovery may be facilitated by administration of an anticholinesterase agent (neostigmine, edrophonium) and an appropriate anticholinergic agent.

☑ Special considerations

• Drug is not recommended for rapid sequence endotracheal intubation because of its intermediate onset of action.
• Cisatracurium has no known effect on consciousness, pain threshold, or cerebration. To avoid patient distress, neuromuscular block should not be induced before patient is unconscious.
• For I.V. use 20-ml vial is intended for use in the intensive care unit only. Drug is not compatible with propofol injection or ketorolac injection for Y-site administration. Drug is acidic and may also not be compatible with an alkaline solution having a pH greater than 8.5 such as barbiturate solutions for Y-site administration. Drug should not be diluted in lactated Ringer's injection USP because of chemical instability.
• Drug is a colorless to slightly yellow or greenish-yellow solution. Inspect vial visually for particulate matter and discoloration before administration. Solutions that are not clear or contain visible particulates should not be used.
• Monitor neuromuscular function during drug administration with a nerve stimulator. Additional doses of drug should not be given before there is a definite response to nerve stimulation. If no response occurs, infusion should be discontinued until a response returns.
• To avoid inaccurate dosing, neuromuscular monitoring should be performed on a nonparetic limb in patients with hemiparesis or paraparesis.
• In patients with neuromuscular disease (myasthenia gravis and myasthenic syndrome), prolonged neuromuscular block may occur. The use of a peripheral nerve stimulator and a dose not exceeding 0.02 mg/kg is recommended to assess the level of neuromuscular block and to monitor dosage requirements.
• Because patients with burns have been shown to develop resistance to nondepolarizing neuromuscular blocking agents, these patients may require increased dosing requirements and exhibit shortened duration of action. Monitor closely.
• Monitor patient's acid-base balance and electrolyte levels. Acid-base or serum electrolyte abnormalities may potentiate or antagonize the action of cisatracurium.
• Monitor patient for malignant hyperthermia.
• Administer pain medication, if necessary, regularly as patient will feel pain but not be able to exhibit signs of its presence.

Patient education

• Inform patient and family of need for drug and how it is administered.
• Reassure patient and family that patient will be monitored continuously throughout drug use.

Geriatric use

• Use with caution when administering cisatracurium to elderly patients. The time to maximum block is about 1 minute slower in elderly patients.

Pediatric use

• Safety and effectiveness in children under age 2 have not been established.

Breast-feeding

• Use caution when administering cisatracurium to breast-feeding women because it is not known if drug is excreted in breast milk.

cisplatin (cis-platinum)
Platinol, Platinol AQ

Pharmacologic classification: alkylating agent (cell cycle–phase nonspecific)
Therapeutic classification: antineoplastic
Pregnancy risk category D

How supplied
Available by prescription only
Injection: 10-mg, 50-mg vials (lyophilized); 50-mg, 100-mg vials (aqueous)

Indications, route, and dosage
Dosage and indications may vary. Check current literature for recommended protocol.
Adjunctive therapy in metastatic testicular cancer
Adults: 20 mg/m² I.V. daily for 5 days. Repeat q 3 weeks for three cycles or more. Usually used in therapeutic regimen with bleomycin and vinblastine.
Adjunctive therapy in metastatic ovarian cancer
Adults: 75 to 100 mg/m² I.V. Repeat q 4 weeks or 50 mg/m² I.V. q 3 weeks with concurrent doxorubicin hydrochloride therapy.
Treatment of advanced bladder cancer
Adults: 50 to 70 mg/m² I.V. once q 3 to 4 weeks. Patients who have received other antineoplastics or radiation therapy should receive 50 mg/m² q 4 weeks.
◊ ***Head and neck cancer***
Adults: 80 to 120 mg/m² I.V. once q 3 weeks.
◊ ***Cervical cancer***
Adults: 50 mg/m² I.V. once q 3 weeks.
◊ ***Non-small-cell lung cancer***
Adults: 70 to 120 mg/m² I.V. once q 3 to 6 weeks.
◊ ***Brain tumor***
Children: 60 mg/m² I.V. for 2 days q 3 to 4 weeks.
◊ ***Osteogenic sarcoma or neuroblastoma***
Children: 90 mg/m² I.V. q 3 weeks.

Note: Prehydration and mannitol diuresis may significantly reduce renal toxicity and ototoxicity.

Pharmacodynamics
Antineoplastic action: Cisplatin exerts its cytotoxic effects by binding with DNA and inhibiting DNA synthesis and, to a lesser extent, by inhibition of protein and RNA synthesis. Cisplatin also acts as a bifunctional alkylating agent, causing intrastrand and interstrand cross-links of DNA. Interstrand cross-linking appears to correlate well with the cytotoxicity of drug.

Pharmacokinetics
• *Absorption:* Drug is not administered orally or intramuscularly.
• *Distribution:* Cisplatin distributes widely into tissues, with the highest concentrations found in the kidneys, liver, and prostate. Drug can accumulate in body tissues, with drug being detected up to 6 months after the last dose. Cisplatin does not readily cross the blood-brain barrier. Drug is extensively and irreversibly bound to plasma proteins and tissue proteins.
• *Metabolism:* Metabolic fate of cisplatin is unclear.
• *Excretion:* Excreted primarily unchanged in urine. In patients with normal renal function, the half-life of the initial elimination phase is 25 to 79 minutes and the terminal phase 58 to 78 hours. The terminal half-life of total cisplatin is up to 10 days.

Contraindications and precautions
Contraindicated in patients with hypersensitivity to drug or to other platinum-containing compounds and in those with severe renal disease, hearing impairment, or myelosuppression.

Interactions
Concomitant use with *aminoglycosides* potentiates the cumulative nephrotoxicity caused by cisplatin; additive toxicity is the mechanism for this interaction. Therefore, aminoglycosides should not be used within 2 weeks of cisplatin therapy. Concomitant use with *loop diuretics* increases the risk of ototoxicity; closely monitor patient's audiologic status. Concomitant use with *phenytoin* may decrease serum concentration of *phenytoin.*

Effects on diagnostic tests
Cisplatin therapy may increase BUN, serum creatinine, and serum uric acid levels. It may decrease creatinine clearance, serum calcium, magnesium, phosphate, and potassium levels, indicating nephrotoxicity.

Adverse reactions
CNS: *peripheral neuritis,* loss of taste, ***seizures.***
EENT: *tinnitus, hearing loss, ototoxicity,* vestibular toxicity.
GI: *nausea, vomiting* (beginning 1 to 4 hours after dose and lasting 24 hours).
GU: more prolonged and SEVERE RENAL TOXICITY with repeated courses of therapy.
Hematologic: MYELOSUPPRESSION; ***leukopenia, thrombocytopenia; anemia;*** nadirs in circulating platelet and WBC counts on days 18 to 23, with recovery by day 39.
Other: ***anaphylactoid reaction,*** *hypomagnesemia,* hypokalemia, hypocalcemia, hyponatremia, hypophosphatemia, hyperuricemia.

Overdose and treatment
Clinical manifestations of overdose include leukopenia, thrombocytopenia, nausea, and vomiting.

Treatment is generally supportive and includes transfusion of blood components, antibiotics for possible infections, and antiemetics. Cisplatin can be removed by dialysis, but only within 3 hours after administration.

☑ Special considerations
• Review hematologic status and creatinine clearance before therapy.
• Reconstitute 10-mg vial with 10 ml and 50-mg vial with 50 ml of sterile water for injection to yield a concentration of 1 mg/ml. The drug may be diluted further in a sodium chloride-containing solution for I.V. infusion.

• Do not use aluminum needles for reconstitution or administration of cisplatin; a black precipitate may form. Use stainless steel needles.
• Drug is stable for 24 hours in 0.9% NaCl solution at room temperature. Do not refrigerate because precipitation may occur. Discard solution containing precipitate.
• Infusions are most stable in chloride-containing solutions, such as 0.9% NaCl, 0.45% NaCl, or 0.225% NaCl.
• Mannitol may be given as a 12.5-g I.V. bolus before starting cisplatin infusion. Follow by infusion of mannitol at rate of up to 10 g/hour, as necessary, to maintain urine output during cisplatin infusion and for 6 to 24 hours after infusion.
• I.V. sodium thiosulfate may be administered with cisplatin infusion to decrease risk of nephrotoxicity.
• Hydrate patient with 0.9% NaCl solution before giving drug. Maintain urine output of 100 ml/hour for 4 consecutive hours before and for 24 hours after infusion.
• Hydrate patient by encouraging oral fluid intake when possible.
• Avoid all I.M. injections when platelets are low.
• Nausea and vomiting may be severe and protracted (up to 24 hours). Antiemetics can be started 24 hours before therapy. Monitor fluid intake and output. Continue I.V. hydration until patient can tolerate adequate oral intake.
• High-dose metoclopramide (2 mg/kg I.V.) has been used to prevent and treat nausea and vomiting. Dexamethasone 10 to 20 mg has been given I.V. with metoclopramide to help alleviate nausea and vomiting. Many patients respond favorably to treatment with ondansetron (Zofran). Pretreatment with this 5-HT_3 antagonist should begin 30 minutes before cisplatin therapy.
• Treat extravasation with local injections of a 1/6 M sodium thiosulfate solution (prepared by mixing 4 ml of sodium thiosulfate 10% and 6 ml of sterile water for injection).
• Monitor CBC, platelet count, and renal function studies before initial and subsequent doses. Do not repeat dose unless platelet count is over 100,000/mm^3, WBC count is over 4,000/mm^3, serum creatinine level is under 1.5 mg/dl, or BUN level is under 25 mg/dl.
• Renal toxicity becomes more severe with repeated doses. Renal function must return to normal before next dose can be given.
• Monitor electrolytes extensively; aggressive supplementation is often required after a course of therapy.
• Anaphylactoid reaction usually responds to immediate treatment with epinephrine, corticosteroids, or antihistamines.
• Avoid contact with skin. If contact occurs, wash drug off immediately with soap and water.

Patient education
• Stress importance of adequate fluid intake and increase in urine output, to facilitate uric acid excretion.
• Tell patient to report tinnitus immediately, to prevent permanent hearing loss. Patient should have audiometric tests before initial and subsequent courses.
• Advise patient to avoid exposure to people with infections.
• Inform patient to promptly report unusual bleeding or bruising.

Pediatric use
• Pediatric dosage of cisplatin has not been fully established. Unlabeled uses of cisplatin include osteogenic sarcoma and neuroblastoma.
• Ototoxicity appears to be more severe in children.

Breast-feeding
• It is unknown if drug distributes into breast milk. However, because of risk to infant of serious adverse reactions, mutagenicity, and carcinogenicity, breast-feeding is not recommended.

cladribine
Leustatin

Pharmacologic classification: purine nucleoside analogue
Therapeutic classification: antineoplastic
Pregnancy risk category D

How supplied
Available by prescription only
Injection: 1 mg/ml

Indications, route, and dosage
Active hairy cell leukemia
Adults: 0.09 mg/kg daily by continuous I.V. infusion for 7 days.
◊ ***Advanced cutaneous T-cell lymphomas, chronic lymphocytic leukemia, malignant lymphomas, acute myeloid leukemias, autoimmune hemolytic anemia, mycosis fungoides, or Sézary syndrome***
Adults: Usually 0.1 mg/kg/day by continuous I.V. infusion for 7 days.

Pharmacodynamics
Antineoplastic action: Cladribine enters tumor cells, where it is phosphorylated by deoxycytidine kinase and subsequently converted into an active triphosphate deoxynucleotide. This metabolite impairs synthesis of new DNA, inhibits repair of existing DNA, and disrupts cellular metabolism.

Pharmacokinetics
• *Absorption:* Drug is not administered P.O. or I.M.
• *Distribution:* Approximately 20% of cladribine is bound to plasma proteins.
• *Metabolism:* Information not available.
• *Excretion:* For patients with normal renal function, the mean terminal half-life of cladribine is 5.4 hours.

Contraindications and precautions
Contraindicated in patients hypersensitive to drug. Use cautiously in patients with impaired renal or hepatic function.

Interactions
There are no known drug interactions with cladribine. However, *amphotericin B* may increase the risk of nephrotoxiciy, hypotension and bronchospasm. Also, caution should be exercised when administering cladribine after or in conjunction with *other drugs known to cause myelosuppression.*

Effects on diagnostic tests
Cladribine frequently alters hematologic studies because of its suppressive effect on bone marrow. It may increase blood and urine concentrations of uric acid.

Adverse reactions
CNS: *headache, fatigue,* dizziness, insomnia, asthenia.
CV: tachycardia, edema.
EENT: epistaxis.
GI: *nausea, decreased appetite, vomiting, diarrhea,* constipation, abdominal pain.
GU: acute renal insufficiency.
Hematologic: NEUTROPENIA, ***anemia, thrombocytopenia.***
Respiratory: *abnormal breath or chest sounds, cough,* shortness of breath.
Skin: *rash, pruritus, erythema, purpura,* petechiae.
Other: *fever,* INFECTION, *local reaction at the injection site, chills, diaphoresis, malaise, trunk pain, myalgia, arthralgia,* hyperuricemia.

Overdose and treatment
High doses of cladribine have been associated with irreversible neurologic toxicity (paraparesis/quadriparesis), acute nephrotoxicity, and severe bone marrow suppression that results in neutropenia, anemia, and thrombocytopenia. No antidote specific to cladribine overdose is known. Besides discontinuation of cladribine, treatment consists of careful observation and appropriate supportive measures. It is not known if drug can be removed from the circulation by dialysis or hemofiltration.

☑ Special considerations
• Cladribine is a toxic drug, and some toxicity is expected during treatment. Monitor hematologic function closely, especially during the first 4 to 8 weeks of therapy. Severe bone marrow suppression, including neutropenia, anemia, and thrombocytopenia, commonly has been observed in patients treated with drug; many patients also have preexisting hematologic impairment from their disease.
• Fever is commonly observed during the first month of therapy and frequently requires antibiotic therapy.
• Because of risk of hyperuricemia from tumor lysis, allopurinol should be administered during therapy.
• For a 24-hour infusion, add the calculated dose to a 500-ml infusion bag of 0.9% NaCl solution injection. Once diluted, administer promptly or store in the refrigerator for no more than 8 hours before administration. Do not use solutions that contain dextrose because studies have shown increased degradation of drug. Because the product does not contain bacteriostatic agents, use strict aseptic technique to prepare the admixture. Solutions containing cladribine should not be mixed with other I.V. drugs or infused simultaneously via a common I.V. line.
• Alternatively, prepare a 7-day infusion solution, using bacteriostatic sodium chloride injection, which contains 0.9% benzyl alcohol. First, pass the calculated amount of drug through a disposable 0.22-micron hydrophilic syringe filter into a sterile infusion reservoir. Next, add sufficent bacteriostatic sodium chloride injection to bring the total volume to 100 ml. Clamp off the line; then disconnect and discard the filter. If necessary, aseptically aspirate air bubbles from the reservoir, using a new filter or sterile vent filter assembly.
• Studies have shown acceptable physical and chemical stability using Pharmacia Deltec medication cassettes.
• Refrigerate unopened vials at 36° to 46° F (2° to 8° C), and protect from light. Although freezing does not adversely affect the drug, a precipitate may form; this will disappear if the drug is allowed to warm to room temperature gradually and the vial is vigorously shaken. Do not heat, microwave, or refreeze.

Patient education
• Tell female patient of childbearing age to avoid pregnancy during drug therapy because of risk of fetal malformations.

Pediatric use
• Safety and effectiveness in children have not been established.

Breast-feeding
• It is not known if drug is excreted in breast milk. A decision should be made whether to discontinue breast-feeding or drug, taking into account the importance of drug to the mother.

clarithromycin
Biaxin

Pharmacologic classification: macrolide
Therapeutic classification: antibiotic
Pregnancy risk category C

How supplied
Available by prescription only
Tablets: 250 mg, 500 mg
Suspension: 125 mg/5 ml, 250 mg/5 ml

Indications, route, and dosage
***Pharyngitis or tonsillitis caused by* Streptococcus pyogenes**
Adults: 250 mg P.O. q 12 hours for 10 days.
Children: 15 mg/kg/day divided q 12 hours for 10 days.
***Acute maxillary sinusitis caused by* Streptococcus pneumoniae, Haemophilus influenzae, *or* Moraxella catarrhalis**
Adults: 500 mg P.O. q 12 hours for 14 days.

Children: 15 mg/kg/day divided q 12 hours for 10 days.
***Acute exacerbations of chronic bronchitis caused by* M. (Branhamella) catarrhalis *or* S. pneumoniae; *pneumonia caused by* S. pneumoniae *or* Mycoplasma pneumoniae**
Adults: 250 mg P.O. q 12 hours for 7 to 14 days.
***Acute exacerbations of chronic bronchitis caused by* H. influenzae**
Adults: 500 mg P.O. q 12 hours for 7 to 14 days.
***Uncomplicated skin and skin structure infections caused by* Staphylococcus aureus *or* S. pyogenes**
Adults: 250 mg P.O. q 12 hours for 7 to 14 days.
***Prophylaxis and treatment of disseminated infection due to* Mycobacterium avium complex**
Adults: 500 mg P.O. b.i.d.
Children: 7.5 mg/kg b.i.d. up to 500 mg b.i.d.
***Acute otitis media caused by* H. influenzae, M. catarrhalis, *or* S. pneumoniae**
Children: 7.5 mg/kg b.i.d. up to 500 mg b.i.d.
✦ ***Dosage adjustment.*** In patients with creatinine clearance of less than 30 ml/minute, dose should be halved or frequency interval doubled.

Pharmacodynamics

Antibiotic action: Clarithromycin, a macrolide antibiotic that is a derivative of erythromycin, binds to the 50S subunit of bacterial ribosomes, blocking protein synthesis. It is bacteriostatic or bactericidal, depending on the concentration.

Pharmacokinetics

- *Absorption:* Drug is rapidly absorbed from the GI tract; absolute bioavailability is about 50%. Peak serum levels are achieved within 2 hours of dosing. Although food slightly delays onset of absorption and formation of the active metabolite, clarithromycin may be taken without regard to meals because food doesn't alter the total amount of drug absorbed.
- *Distribution:* Drug is widely distributed; because it readily penetrates cells, tissue concentrations are higher than plasma levels. Plasma half-life is dose-dependent; half-life is 3 to 4 hours at doses of 250 mg q 12 hours and increases to 5 to 7 hours at doses of 500 mg q 12 hours.
- *Metabolism:* Clarithromycin's major metabolite, 14-hydroxy clarithromycin, has significant antimicrobial activity. It is about twice as active against *H. influenzae* as the parent drug.
- *Excretion:* In patients taking 250 mg q 12 hours, about 20% is eliminated in the urine unchanged; this increases to 30% in patients taking 500 mg q 12 hours. The major metabolite accounts for about 15% of drug in the urine. Elimination half-life of the active metabolite is dose-dependent: 5 to 6 hours with 250 mg q 12 hours; 7 hours with 500 mg q 12 hours.

Contraindications and precautions

Contraindicated in patients with hypersensitivity to erythromycin or other macrolides and in those receiving astemizole who have preexisting cardiac abnormalities or electrolyte disturbances. Use cautiously in patients with impaired renal or hepatic function.

Interactions

Preliminary studies indicate that clarithromycin may increase serum levels of *theophylline* and *carbamazepine.* Monitor plasma levels of these agents carefully. Other macrolides have been associated with various drug interactions, including increased PT in patients taking *warfarin*; increased *digoxin* levels in patients receiving *digoxin*; acute *ergot* toxicity in patients receiving *ergotamine* or *dihydroergotamine*; and decreased metabolism of *cyclosporine, triazolam,* or *phenytoin.*

Effects on diagnostic tests

None reported.

Adverse reactions

CNS: headache.
GI: *diarrhea, nausea, abnormal taste,* dyspepsia, abdominal pain or discomfort.
Hematologic: increased PT; decreased WBC; elevated liver function test results, BUN, creatinine.

Overdose and treatment

No information available.

☑ Special considerations

- Obtain specimen for culture and sensitivity tests before giving first dose. Therapy may begin pending test results.
- Drug may be taken without regard to meals.
- Drug may cause overgrowth of nonsusceptible bacteria or fungi. Monitor for signs and symptoms of superinfection.
- Reconstituted suspension should not be refrigerated; discard any unused portion after 14 days.

Patient education

- Tell patient to take all of drug as prescribed, even if he feels better.
- Inform patient that he may take drug without regard to meals.
- Instruct patient to shake suspension well before use; do not refrigerate.

Pediatric use

- Safety and efficacy in children under age 12 have not been established.

Breast-feeding

- It is unknown if drug is excreted in breast milk; however, other macrolides have been found in breast milk. Use with caution.

clemastine fumarate

Tavist, Tavist-1

Pharmacologic classification: ethanolamine-derivative antihistamine
Therapeutic classification: antihistamine (H_1-receptor antagonist)
Pregnancy risk category C

How supplied

Available without a prescription

Tablets: 1.34 mg (Tavist-1), 2.68 mg (Tavist)

Syrup: 0.67 mg/5 ml (equivalent to 0.5 mg base/5 ml)

Indications, route, and dosage

Rhinitis, allergy symptoms

Adults and children age 12 or older: 1.34 to 2.68 mg P.O. b.i.d. or t.i.d. Maximum recommended daily dose: 8.04 mg.

Children age 6 to 11: 0.67 mg b.i.d.; not to exceed 4.02 mg/day.

Allergic skin manifestation of urticaria and angioedema

Adults and children age 12 or older: 2.68 mg up to t.i.d. maximum.

Children age 6 to 11: 1.34 mg b.i.d.; not to exceed 4.02 mg/day.

Pharmacodynamics

Antihistamine action: Antihistamines compete with histamine for histamine H_1-receptor sites on the smooth muscle of the bronchi, GI tract, uterus, and large blood vessels; by binding to cellular receptors, they prevent access of histamine and suppress histamine-induced allergic symptoms, even though they do not prevent its release.

Pharmacokinetics

- *Absorption:* Clemastine is absorbed readily from the GI tract; action begins in 15 to 30 minutes and peaks in 2 to 7 hours.
- *Distribution:* Unknown.
- *Metabolism:* Clemastine is extensively metabolized.
- *Excretion:* Drug is excreted in urine.

Contraindications and precautions

Contraindicated in patients with hypersensitivity to drug or other antihistamines of similar chemical structure; in those with acute asthma; in neonates or premature infants; and in breast-feeding patients.

Use cautiously in the elderly and in patients with increased intraocular pressure, glaucoma, hyperthyroidism, CV or renal disease, hypertension, bronchial asthma, pyloroduodenal obstruction, prostatic hyperplasia, bladder neck obstruction, and stenosing peptic ulcers.

Interactions

MAO inhibitors interfere with the detoxification of clemastine and thus prolong and intensify their central depressant and anticholinergic effects. Additive CNS depression may occur when clemastine is given concomitantly with other *CNS depressants,* such as *alcohol, barbiturates, tranquilizers, sleeping aids,* or *antianxiety agents.*

Clemastine may diminish the effects of *sulfonylureas* and may partially counteract the anticoagulant effects of *heparin.*

Effects on diagnostic tests

Discontinue clemastine 4 days before diagnostic skin tests; antihistamines can prevent, reduce, or mask positive skin test response.

Adverse reactions

CNS: *sedation, drowsiness,* ***seizures,*** nervousness, tremor, confusion, restlessness, vertigo, headache, *sleepiness, dizziness, incoordination,* fatigue.

CV: hypotension, palpitations, tachycardia.

GI: *epigastric distress,* anorexia, diarrhea, nausea, vomiting, constipation, *dry mouth.*

GU: urine retention, urinary frequency.

Hematologic: hemolytic anemia, ***thrombocytopenia, agranulocytosis.***

Respiratory: *thick bronchial secretions.*

Skin: rash, urticaria, photosensitivity, diaphoresis.

Other: ***anaphylactic shock.***

Overdose and treatment

Clinical manifestations of overdose may include either CNS depression, sedation, reduced mental alertness, apnea, and CV collapse) or CNS stimulation (insomnia, hallucinations, tremors, or seizures). Anticholinergic symptoms, such as dry mouth, flushed skin, fixed and dilated pupils, and GI symptoms, are common, especially in children.

Treat overdose by inducing emesis with ipecac syrup (in conscious patient), followed by activated charcoal to reduce further drug absorption. Use gastric lavage if patient is unconscious or if ipecac fails. Treat hypotension with vasopressors, and control seizures with diazepam or phenytoin. *Do not give stimulants.*

☑ Special considerations

Besides those relevant to all *antihistamines,* consider the following recommendation.

- Drug is indicated for treatment of urticaria only at dosages of 2.68 mg up to t.i.d.

Patient education

- Inform patient of potential adverse reactions.

Geriatric use

- Elderly patients are more susceptible to the sedative effect of drug. Instruct the older patient to change positions slowly and gradually. Elderly people may experience dizziness or hypotension more readily than younger people.

Pediatric use

- Drug is not indicated for use in premature infants or neonates. Children, especially those under age 6, may experience paradoxical hyperexcitability.

Breast-feeding

- Drug should not be used during breast-feeding because it is secreted in breast milk, exposing infant to risks of unusual excitability; premature infants are at particular risk for seizures.

clindamycin hydrochloride
Cleocin

clindamycin palmitate hydrochloride
Cleocin Pediatric

clindamycin phosphate
Cleocin Phosphate, Cleocin T

Pharmacologic classification: lincomycin derivative
Therapeutic classification: antibiotic
Pregnancy risk category NR (B vaginal and topical creams)

How supplied
Available by prescription only
Capsules: 75 mg, 150 mg, 300 mg
Solution: 75 mg/5 ml
Injection: 150 mg/ml
Infusion for I.V. use: 300 mg, 600 mg, 900 mg
Gel, lotion, topical solution: 1%

Indications, route, and dosage
Infections caused by sensitive organisms
Adults: 150 to 450 mg P.O. q 6 hours; or 600 to 2,700 mg/day I.M. or I.V. divided into two to four equal doses.
Children over age 1 month: 8 to 20 mg/kg/day P.O. or 20 to 40 mg/kg/day I.V. divided into three or four equal doses.
Children under age 1 month: 15 to 20 mg/kg/day I.V. divided into three or four equal doses.
Bacterial vaginosis
Adults: 100 mg intravaginally h.s. for 7 days.
Acne vulgaris
Adults: Apply thin film of topical solution to affected areas b.i.d.
◇ ***Toxoplasmosis (cerebral or ocular) in immunocompromised patients***
Adults: 1,200 to 4,800 mg/day I.V. or P.O. Also administered with pyrimethamine in doses up to 75 mg/day P.O. and with folinic acid in a dose of 10 mg/day P.O.
◇ **Pneumocystis carinii *pneumonia***
Adults: 600 mg I.V. q 6 hours or 300 to 450 mg P.O. q.i.d. With primaquine, give 15 to 30 mg P.O. daily.

Pharmacodynamics
Antibacterial action: Drug inhibits bacterial protein synthesis by binding to ribosome's 50S subunit. Clindamycin may produce bacteriostatic or bactericidal effects on susceptible bacteria, including most aerobic gram-positive cocci and anaerobic gram-negative and gram-positive organisms. It is considered a first-line drug in the treatment of *Bacteroides fragilis* and most other gram-positive and gram-negative anaerobes. It is also effective against *Mycoplasma pneumoniae, Leptotrichia buccalis,* and some gram-positive cocci and bacilli.

Pharmacokinetics
- *Absorption:* When administered orally, drug is absorbed rapidly and almost completely from the GI tract, regardless of formulation. Peak concentrations of 1.9 to 3.9 mcg/ml occur in 45 to 60 minutes. Drug may also be given I.M. with good absorption. Peak concentrations occur in about 3 hours. With 300-mg dose, peak concentrations are about 6 mcg/ml; with 600-mg dose, about 10 mcg/ml.
- *Distribution:* Distributed widely to most body tissues and fluids (except CSF) and crosses the placenta. Approximately 93% of drug is bound to plasma proteins.
- *Metabolism:* Clindamycin is metabolized partially to inactive metabolites.
- *Excretion:* About 10% of dose is excreted unchanged in urine; rest is excreted as inactive metabolites (with some drug excreted in breast milk). Plasma half-life is 2½ to 3 hours in patients with normal renal function; 3½ to 5 hours in anephric patients; and 7 to 14 hours in patients with hepatic disease. Peritoneal dialysis and hemodialysis do not remove drug.

Contraindications and precautions
Contraindicated in patients with hypersensitivity to the antibiotic congener lincomycin; in those with a history of ulcerative colitis, regional enteritis, or antibiotic-associated colitis; and in those with a history of atopic reactions.

Use cautiously in patients with asthma, impaired renal or hepatic function, or history of GI diseases or significant allergies.

Interactions
When used concomitantly, clindamycin may potentiate the action of *neuromuscular blocking agents* (such as *tubocurarine* and *pancuronium*). Concomitant use with *kaolin products* may reduce GI absorption of clindamycin. Concomitant use with such *antidiarrheals* as *diphenoxylate* and *opiates* may prolong or worsen clindamycin-induced diarrhea by reducing excretion of bacterial toxins. When used concomitantly, *erythromycin* may act as an antagonist blocking clindamycin from reaching its site of action. When used concurrently with other *acne preparations* (such as *benzoyl peroxide* or *tretinoin*), topical clindamycin may cause a cumulative irritant or drying effect. Reportedly, clindamycin inactivates *aminoglycosides* in vitro.

Effects on diagnostic tests
Liver function test results may become abnormal in some patients during clindamycin therapy.

Adverse reactions
GI: *nausea,* vomiting, abdominal pain, ***diarrhea, pseudomembranous colitis.***
GU: *cervicitis, vaginitis, Candida albicans* overgrowth, *vulvar irritation.*
Hematologic: transient leukopenia, eosinophilia, ***thrombocytopenia.***
Skin: maculopapular rash, urticaria, dryness, *redness,* pruritus, swelling, irritation, contact dermatitis, burning.
Other: ***anaphylaxis,*** jaundice, abnormal liver function test results.

Overdose and treatment
No information available.

☑ Special considerations
• Culture and sensitivity tests should be done before treatment starts and should be repeated as needed.
• Do not refrigerate reconstituted oral solution, because it will thicken. Drug remains stable for 2 weeks at room temperature.
• I.M. preparation should be given deep I.M. Rotate sites. Doses exceeding 600 mg are not recommended.
• I.M. injection may increase creatinine phosphokinase levels because of muscle irritation.
• For I.V. infusion, dilute each 300 mg in 50 ml of dextrose 5%, 0.9% NaCl, or lactated Ringer's solution and give no faster than 30 mg/minute. Do not administer more than 1.2 g/hour.
• Topical form may produce adverse systemic effects.
• Monitor renal, hepatic, and hematopoietic functions during prolonged therapy.
• Do not administer diphenoxylate compound (Lomotil) to treat drug-induced diarrhea because this may worsen and prolong diarrhea.

Patient education
• Warn patient that I.M. injection may be painful.
• Instruct patient to report adverse effects, especially diarrhea. Warn patient not to self-treat diarrhea.
• Advise patient to take capsules with full glass (8 oz [240 ml]) of water to prevent dysphagia.
• Instruct patient using topical solution to wash, rinse, and dry affected areas before application. Warn patient not to use topical solution near eyes, nose, mouth, or other mucous membranes, and caution about sharing washcloths and towels with family members.

Geriatric use
• Elderly patients may tolerate drug-induced diarrhea poorly. Monitor closely for change in bowel frequency.

Pediatric use
• Administer drug cautiously, if at all, to neonates and infants. Monitor closely, especially for diarrhea.

Breast-feeding
• Drug is excreted in breast milk. Alternative feeding method is recommended during clindamycin therapy.

clobetasol propionate
Dermovate*, Temovate

Pharmacologic classification: topical adrenocorticoid
Therapeutic classification: anti-inflammatory
Pregnancy risk category C

How supplied
Available by prescription only
Cream: 0.05%
Lotion: 0.05%
Ointment: 0.05%

Indications, route, and dosage
Inflammation of corticosteroid-responsive dermatoses
Adults: Apply a thin layer to affected skin areas b.i.d., once in the morning and once at night. Limit treatment to 14 days, with no more than 50 g of the cream or ointment or 50 ml of lotion (25 mg total) weekly.

Pharmacodynamics
Anti-inflammatory action: Drug is effective because of anti-inflammatory, antipruritic, and vasoconstrictive actions; however, the exact mechanism of its actions is unknown. Clobetasol is a high-potency group I fluorinated corticosteroid that is usually reserved for the management of severe dermatoses that have not responded satisfactorily to a less potent formulation.

Pharmacokinetics
• *Absorption:* Amount absorbed depends on the potency of the preparation, the amount applied, and the nature of the skin at the application site. It ranges from about 1% in areas with a thick stratum corneum (such as the palms, soles, elbows, and knees) to as high as 36% in areas with a thin stratum corneum (face, eyelids, and genitals). Absorption increases in areas of skin damage, inflammation, or occlusion. Some systemic absorption of topical steroids occurs, especially through the oral mucosa.
• *Distribution:* After topical application, clobetasol is distributed throughout the local skin. Any drug absorbed into the circulation is rapidly removed from the blood and distributed into muscle, liver, skin, intestines, and kidneys.
• *Metabolism:* After topical administration, drug is metabolized primarily in the skin. The small amount absorbed into systemic circulation is metabolized primarily in the liver to inactive compounds.
• *Excretion:* Inactive metabolites are excreted by the kidneys, primarily as glucuronides and sulfates, but also as unconjugated products. Small amounts of the metabolites are also excreted in feces.

Contraindications and precautions
Contraindicated in patients hypersensitive to corticosteroids.

Interactions
None reported.

Effects on diagnostic tests
None reported.

Adverse reactions
Skin: burning, pruritus, irritation, dryness, erythema, folliculitis, perioral dermatitis, allergic contact dermatitis, hypopigmentation, hypertrichosis, acneiform eruptions.

Other: ***hypothalamic-pituitary-adrenal (HPA) axis suppression,*** Cushing's syndrome, hyperglycemia, glucosuria.

Overdose and treatment
No information available.

☑ Special considerations
Besides those relevant to all *topical adrenocorticoids,* consider the following recommendations.
- Clobetasol should not be used with occlusive dressings. Advise patient not to cover affected area or use occlusive dressings. Apply sparingly in light film.
- "Pulse" therapy is sometimes used with topical steroids of this potency, that is, b.i.d. for 3 days, then none for 3 days. Intermittent use prevents cumulative effects. Drug suppresses HPA axis at doses as low as 2 g/day.

Patient education
- Inform patient of potential adverse reactions.
- Advise patient to avoid contact with eyes.

Pediatric use
- Drug treatment is not recommended in patients under age 12.

clocortolone pivalate
Cloderm

Pharmacologic classification: topical adrenocorticoid
Therapeutic classification: anti-inflammatory
Pregnancy risk category C

How supplied
Available by prescription only
Cream: 0.1%

Indications, route, and dosage
Inflammation of corticosteroid-responsive dermatoses
Adults and children: Apply cream sparingly and gently rub into affected area daily to q.i.d.

Pharmacodynamics
Anti-inflammatory action: Clocortolone is effective because of anti-inflammatory, antipruritic, and vasoconstrictive actions; however, the exact mechanism of its actions is unknown. Clocortolone cream is a group III fluorinated glucocorticoid with a potency similar to that of betamethasone valerate cream 0.01%, flurandrenolide cream 0.025%, and hydrocortisone valerate cream and ointment 0.2%.

Pharmacokinetics
- *Absorption:* Amount absorbed depends on the amount applied and on the nature of the skin at the application site. It ranges from about 1% in areas with a thick stratum corneum (such as the palms, soles, knees, and elbows) to as much as 36% in areas of the thinnest stratum corneum (face, eyelids, and genitals). Absorption increases in areas of skin damage, inflammation, or occlusion. Some systemic absorption of topical steroids occurs, especially through the oral mucosa.
- *Distribution:* After topical application, clocortolone is distributed throughout the local skin. Any drug that is absorbed into circulation is removed rapidly from the blood and distributed into muscle, liver, skin, intestines, and kidneys.
- *Metabolism:* After topical administration, drug is metabolized primarily in the skin. The small amount that is absorbed into systemic circulation is metabolized primarily in the liver to inactive compounds.
- *Excretion:* Inactive metabolites are excreted by the kidneys, primarily as glucuronides and sulfates, but also as unconjugated products. Small amounts of the metabolites are also excreted in feces.

Contraindications and precautions
Contraindicated in patients hypersensitive to drug.

Interactions
None significant.

Effects on diagnostic tests
None reported.

Adverse reactions
Skin: burning, pruritus, irritation, dryness, erythema, folliculitis, striae, acneiform eruptions, perioral dermatitis, hypertrichosis, hypopigmentation, allergic contact dermatitis; ***secondary infection, maceration, atrophy, striae, miliaria*** (with occlusive dressings).
Other: ***hypothalamic-pituitary-adrenal axis suppression,*** Cushing's syndrome, hyperglycemia, glucosuria.

Overdose and treatment
No information available.

☑ Special considerations
Recommendations for use of clocortolone, for care and teaching of patients during therapy, and for use in elderly patients, children, and breast-feeding women are the same as those for all *topical adrenocorticoids.*
- Occlusive dressing may be used for severe or resistant dermatoses.

Patient education
- Inform patient of potential adverse reactions.

clofazimine
Lamprene

Pharmacologic classification: substituted iminophenazine dye
Therapeutic classification: leprostatic
Pregnancy risk category C

How supplied
Available by prescription only
Capsules: 50 mg, 100 mg

Indications, route, and dosage

Dapsone-sensitive multibacillary leprosy

Adults: Combination therapy with two other drugs for at least 2 years until skin smears are negative, followed by monotherapy.

Dapsone-resistant leprosy

Adults: 100 mg P.O. once daily; usually given in combination with one or more other antileprosy drugs for at least 3 years followed by monotherapy of 100 mg Lamprene daily.

Erythema nodosum leprosum

Adults: 100 to 200 mg P.O. daily for up to 3 months. Taper dosage to 100 mg daily as soon as possible. Dosages above 200 mg daily are not recommended.

◇ ***Atypical mycobacterial infections***

Adults: 100 mg P.O. q 8 hours. Usually given with several other antitubercular agents.

Pharmacodynamics

Leprostatic action: Clofazimine is a bright red iminophenazine dye, a relative of aniline dyes. It exerts a slow bactericidal effect on *Mycobacterium leprae* (Hansen's bacillus). Clinical benefit is usually noted in 1 to 3 months, with clearing observed by 6 months. Administration with dapsone produces a more rapid effect on leprosy lesions. No cross-resistance with dapsone or rifampin has been reported. Clofazimine inhibits mycobacterial growth and preferentially binds to mycobacterial DNA. Although the precise mechanism is unknown, drug also exhibits anti-inflammatory properties in controlling erythema nodosum leprosum reactions.

Clofazimine also appears to have an important role in the treatment of atypical mycobacterial infections, such as *Mycobacterium avium* infections, which have become prominent recently in patients with AIDS. Some efficacy has been demonstrated when used in combination with ansamycin, ethionamide, or ethambutol. Further clinical information is required.

Pharmacokinetics

- *Absorption:* Absorption is variable (45% to 62%) after oral administration.
- *Distribution:* Highly lipophilic, drug is distributed widely into fatty tissues and is taken up by macrophages into the reticuloendothelial system. Little, if any, crosses the blood-brain barrier or enters the CNS.
- *Metabolism:* Drug's metabolism has not been completely defined; however, some evidence exists of enterohepatic cycling. Serum half-lives of up to 70 days have been noted.
- *Excretion:* Mostly excreted in feces; some in sputum, sebum, and sweat; very little in urine. Drug occurs in breast milk.

Contraindications and precautions

No known contraindications. Use cautiously in patients with GI dysfunction, such as abdominal pain or diarrhea.

Interactions

Dapsone may inhibit the anti-inflammatory activity of clofazimine, but this is unconfirmed; continued treatment with both drugs is still advisable.

Coadministration with *isoniazid* may increase plasma and urinary concentrations of clofazamine and decrease levels in the skin.

Effects on diagnostic tests

Clofazinine therapy can elevate blood sugar, albumin, serum bilirubin, and AST and can cause hypokalemia and eosinophilia.

Adverse reactions

EENT: *conjunctival and corneal pigmentation, dryness, burning, itching, irritation.*
GI: *epigastric pain, diarrhea, nausea, vomiting, GI intolerance,* ***bowel obstruction, GI bleeding.***
Skin: *pink to brownish-black pigmentation, ichthyosis, dryness,* rash, pruritus.
Other: ***splenic infarction,*** discolored body fluids and excrement.

Overdose and treatment

No specific information on signs and symptoms is available. In case of overdose, empty the stomach by inducing vomiting or by gastric lavage. Treatment includes usual supportive measures.

☑ Special considerations

- Administer with meals. Use clofazimine in combination with other antileprosy drugs.
- Severe GI symptoms may necessitate withdrawal of drug if dosage reduction does not relieve symptoms.
- Pink to brownish-black pigmentation of skin occurs in 75% to 100% of patients.
- Observe patient for signs of depression.

Patient education

- Tell patient to take drug with meals to minimize GI problems.
- Advise patient to store drug away from heat and light and out of children's reach.
- Explain that pink to brownish-black pigmentation of skin may occur. Although reversible, it may take several months or years to disappear after drug is stopped. Also explain that discoloration of eyes, urine, feces, sputum, sweat, and tears also may occur.
- Tell patient not to expect benefits for 1 to 3 months; observable benefits may take up to 6 months.
- Recommend use of skin oil or cream to help relieve dryness or ichthyosis.

Breast-feeding

- Drug is excreted in breast milk; it should not be used in breast-feeding women unless potential benefit to mother exceeds risk to infant.

clofibrate

Atromid-S

Pharmacologic classification: fibric acid derivative
Therapeutic classification: antilipemic
Pregnancy risk category C

How supplied

Available by prescription only
Capsules: 500 mg

Indications, route, and dosage

Hyperlipidemia and xanthoma tuberosum; type III hyperlipidemia that does not respond adequately to diet
Adults: 2 g P.O. daily in two to four divided doses. Some patients may respond to lower doses as assessed by serum lipid monitoring.
◊ ***Diabetes insipidus***
Adults: 1.5 to 2 g P.O. daily in divided doses.

Clofibrate should not be used in children.

Pharmacodynamics

Antilipemic action: Clofibrate may lower serum triglyceride levels by accelerating catabolism of very low-density lipoproteins; drug lowers serum cholesterol levels (to a lesser degree) by inhibiting cholesterol biosynthesis. Both mechanisms are unknown. Drug is closely related to gemfibrozil.

Pharmacokinetics

- *Absorption:* Drug is absorbed slowly but completely from GI tract. Peak plasma concentration occurs 2 to 6 hours after a single dose. Serum triglyceride levels decrease in 2 to 5 days, with peak clinical effect at 21 days.
- *Distribution:* Clofibrate is distributed into extracellular space as its active form, clofibric acid, which is up to 98% protein-bound. Animal studies suggest that fetal concentration levels may exceed maternal concentration levels.
- *Metabolism:* Clofibrate is hydrolyzed by serum enzymes to clofibric acid, which is metabolized by the liver.
- *Excretion:* 20% of clofibric acid is excreted unchanged in urine; 70% is eliminated in urine as conjugated metabolite. Plasma half-life after a single dose ranges from 6 to 25 hours; in patients with renal impairment and cirrhosis, half-life can be as long as 113 hours.

Contraindications and precautions

Contraindicated in patients with significant hepatic or renal dysfunction, primary biliary cirrhosis, or hypersensitivity to drug and in pregnant or breast-feeding women. Use cautiously in patients with peptic ulcer or history of gallbladder disease.

Interactions

Clofibrate potentiates the effects of *oral anticoagulants,* which may cause fatal hemorrhage; if such a combination is necessary, reduce *oral anticoagulant* dosage by 50%, and evaluate PT frequently.

Clofibrate may also enhance the effects of *sulfonylureas,* causing hypoglycemia; a dosage adjustment may be needed.

Concomitant use with *furosemide* may cause increased diuresis as both drugs compete for albumin binding sites; use cautiously.

Concomitant administration with *cholestyramine* decreases absorption rate of clofibrate.

Effects on diagnostic tests

Clofibrate therapy may increase serum levels of CK, serum transaminase, serum amylase, ALT, and AST. Drug may decrease plasma beta-lipoprotein and plasma fibrinogen concentrations.

Adverse reactions

CNS: fatigue, weakness, drowsiness, dizziness, headache.
CV: ***arrhythmias,*** angina, ***thromboembolic events,*** intermittent claudication.
GI: *nausea, diarrhea, vomiting,* stomatitis, *dyspepsia,* flatulence, ***cholelithiasis, cholecystitis.***
GU: impotence and decreased libido, renal dysfunction (dysuria, hematuria, proteinuria, decreased urine output)
Hematologic: leukopenia, anemia, eosinophilia.
Hepatic: gallstones, *transient and reversible elevations of liver function test results,* hepatomegaly.
Skin: rash, urticaria, pruritus, dry skin and hair.
Other: myalgia and arthralgia, resembling a flulike syndrome; *weight gain; polyphagia.*

Overdose and treatment

No information available.

☑ Special considerations

- Clofibrate should not be used indiscriminately; it may pose an increased risk of gallstones, heart disease, and cancer.
- Monitor serum cholesterol and triglyceride levels regularly during clofibrate therapy.
- Observe patient for following serious adverse reactions: thrombophlebitis, pulmonary embolism, angina, and dysrhythmias; monitor renal and hepatic function, blood counts, and serum electrolyte and blood glucose levels.
- Studies suggest clofibrate may increase risk of death from cancer, postcholecystectomy complications, and pancreatitis.

Patient education

- Warn patient to report flulike symptoms immediately.
- Stress importance of close medical supervision and of reporting adverse reactions; encourage patient to comply with prescribed regimen and diet.
- Warn patient not to exceed prescribed dose.
- Advise patient to take drug with food to minimize GI discomfort.
- Emphasize that drug therapy will not replace diet, exercise, and weight reduction for the control of hyperlipidemia.

Pediatric use

- Safety and efficacy have not been established in children under age 14.

Breast-feeding
• Available data suggest clofibrate may enter breast milk; alternative feeding method is recommended during therapy.

clomiphene citrate
Clomid, Milophene, Serophene

Pharmacologic classification: chlorotrianisene derivative
Therapeutic classification: ovulation stimulant
Pregnancy risk category X

How supplied
Available by prescription only
Tablets: 50 mg

Indications, route, and dosage
To induce ovulation
Adults: 50 mg P.O. daily for 5 days, starting any time in patients who have had no recent uterine bleeding; or 50 mg P.O. daily starting on day 5 of menstrual cycle (first day of menstrual flow is day 1). Dose may be increased to 100 mg if ovulation does not occur. Repeat the 5-day course each ovulatory cycle until conception occurs or until 3 courses of therapy are completed.
◊ ***Male infertility***
Adults: 50 to 400 mg P.O. daily for 2 to 12 months.

Pharmacodynamics
Ovulation stimulant action: The precise mechanism of action for inducing ovulation in anovulatory females has not been determined. The drug appears to stimulate the release of the pituitary gonadotropin, follicle-stimulating hormone (FSH), and luteinizing hormone (LH), which results in development and maturation of the ovarian follicle, ovulation, and subsequent development and function of the corpus luteum.

Pharmacokinetics
• *Absorption:* Clomiphene citrate is absorbed readily from the GI tract.
• *Distribution:* Drug may undergo enterohepatic recirculation or may be stored in body fat.
• *Metabolism:* Clomiphene citrate is metabolized by the liver.
• *Excretion:* Half-life is approximately 5 days. Drug is excreted principally in the feces via biliary elimination.

Contraindications and precautions
Contraindicated during pregnancy and in patients with undiagnosed abnormal genital bleeding, ovarian cyst not due to polycystic ovarian syndrome, hepatic disease or dysfunction, uncontrolled thyroid or adrenal dysfunction, or presence of organic intracranial lesion (such as a pituitary tumor).

Interactions
None reported.

Effects on diagnostic tests
Drug therapy may increase levels of serum thyronine, thyroxine-binding globulin, and sex hormone-binding globulin. It may also increase sulfobromophthalein retention and FSH and LH secretion.

Adverse reactions
CNS: headache, restlessness, insomnia, dizziness, light-headedness, depression, fatigue, aggressive behavior.
EENT: blurred vision, diplopia, scotoma, photophobia.
GI: nausea, vomiting, bloating, distention, weight gain.
GU: urinary frequency and polyuria; abnormal uterine bleeding; *ovarian enlargement* and cyst formation, which regress spontaneously when drug is stopped.
Hematologic: ***thrombocytopenia,*** leukopenia, anemia.
Respiratory: pharyngitis, rhinitis, sinusitus, coughing, epistaxis, dyspnea.
Skin: alopecia, urticaria, rash, dermatitis.
Other: *hot flashes,* reversible *breast discomfort.*

Overdose and treatment
No information available.

☑ Special considerations
• Human chorionic gonadotropin (5,000 to 10,000 U) may be administered 5 to 7 days after the last dose of drug to stimulate ovulation.

Patient education
• Instruct patient on all aspects of infertility testing and therapy.
• Tell patient to report visual disturbances immediately.
• Advise patient of possibility of multiple births, which increases with higher doses.
• Teach patient to take basal body temperature every morning (starting on day 1 of menstrual period) and chart on a graph to detect ovulation.
• Instruct patient on importance of properly timed coitus.
• Advise patient to discontinue drug immediately if abdominal symptoms, weight gain, edema, or bloating occur, because these may indicate ovarian enlargement or ovarian cysts.
• Warn patient to avoid hazardous tasks until response to drug is known because dizziness or visual disturbances may occur.
• Advise patient to discontinue drug and call immediately if she suspects she is pregnant because drug may have teratogenic effects.

clomipramine hydrochloride
Anafranil

Pharmacologic classification: tricyclic antidepressant (TCA)
Therapeutic classification: antiobsessional
Pregnancy risk category C

How supplied

Available by prescription only
Capsules: 25 mg, 50 mg, 75 mg

Indications, route, and dosage

Treatment of obsessive-compulsive disorder (OCD)
Adults: Initially, 25 mg P.O. daily, gradually increasing to 100 mg P.O. daily (in divided doses, with meals) during the first 2 weeks. Maximum dosage, 250 mg daily. After titration, entire daily dose may be given h.s.
Children and adolescents: Initially, 25 mg P.O. daily, gradually increased to a maximum of 3 mg/kg or 100 mg P.O. daily, whichever is smaller (in divided doses, with meals) over the first 2 weeks. Maximum daily dosage is 3 mg/kg or 200 mg, whichever is smaller. After titration, entire daily dose may be given h.s.

Pharmacodynamics

Antiobsessional action: A selective inhibitor of serotonin (5-HT) reuptake into neurons within the CNS. It may also have some blocking activity at postsynaptic dopamine receptors. The exact mechanism by which clomipramine treats OCD is unknown.

Pharmacokinetics

- *Absorption:* Clomipramine is well absorbed from GI tract, but extensive first-pass metabolism limits bioavailablity to about 50%.
- *Distribution:* Drug distributes well into lipophilic tissues; the volume of distribution is about 12 L/kg; 98% is bound to plasma proteins.
- *Metabolism:* Primarily hepatic. Several metabolites have been identified; desmethylclomipramine is the primary active metabolite.
- *Excretion:* About 66% is excreted in the urine and the remainder in the feces. Mean elimination half-life of the parent compound is about 36 hours; the elimination half-life of desmethylclomipramine has a mean of 69 hours. After multiple dosing, the half-life may increase.

Contraindications and precautions

Contraindicated in patients with hypersensitivity to drug or other TCAs; in those who have taken MAO inhibitors within the previous 14 days; and in patients during acute recovery period after MI.

Use cautiously in patients with urine retention, suicidal tendencies, glaucoma, increased intraocular pressure, brain damage, or seizure disorders and in those taking medications that may lower the seizure threshold. Also use cautiously in patients with impaired renal or hepatic function, hyperthyroidism, or tumors of the adrenal medulla and in those undergoing elective surgery or receiving thyroid medication or electroconvulsive treatment.

Interactions

Concomitant administration of *MAO inhibitors* with TCAs may cause hyperpyretic crisis, seizures, coma, and death.

Concurrent use of *barbiturates* increases the activity of hepatic microsomal enzymes with repeated doses and may decrease TCA blood levels. Monitor for decreased effectiveness. *Barbiturates, alcohol* and other *CNS depressants* may cause an exaggerated depressant effect when used concomitantly with TCAs.

Methylphenidate may increase TCA blood levels. *Epinephrine* and *norepinephrine* may produce an increased hypertensive effect in patients taking TCAs.

Effects on diagnostic tests

None reported.

Adverse reactions

CNS: *somnolence, tremor, dizziness, headache, insomnia, nervousness, myoclonus, fatigue,* EEG changes, ***seizures.***
CV: postural hypotension, palpitations, tachycardia.
EENT: *pharyngitis, rhinitis, visual changes.*
GI: *dry mouth, constipation, nausea, dyspepsia, increased appetite,* diarrhea, *anorexia, abdominal pain.*
GU: *urinary hesitancy,* urinary tract infection, *dysmenorrhea, ejaculation failure, impotence.*
Hematologic: purpura, anemia.
Skin: *diaphoresis,* rash, pruritus, dry skin.
Other: *myalgia, weight gain, altered libido.*

Overdose and treatment

Signs and symptoms of clomipramine overdose are similar to those of other TCAs and have included sinus tachycardia, intraventricular block, hypotension, irritability, fixed and dilated pupils, drowsiness, delirium, stupor, hyperreflexia, and hyperpyrexia.

Treatment should include gastric lavage with large quantities of fluid. Lavage should be continued for 12 hours because the anticholinergic effects of the drug slow gastric emptying. Hemodialysis, peritoneal dialysis, and forced diuresis are ineffective because of the high degree of plasma protein binding. Support respirations and monitor cardiac function. Treat shock with plasma expanders or corticosteroids; treat seizures with diazepam.

☑ Special considerations

- To minimize risk of overdose, dispense drug in small quantities.
- Monitor for urine retention and constipation. Suggest stool softener or high-fiber diet, as needed, and encourage adequate fluid intake.
- Do not withdraw drug abruptly.
- Activation of mania or hypomania may occur with clomipramine therapy.

Patient education

- Warn patient to avoid hazardous activities that require alertness or good psychomotor coordination until adverse CNS effects are known. This is especially important during initial titration period when daytime sedation and dizziness may occur.
- Instruct patient to avoid alcohol and other depressants.
- Suggest that dry mouth may be relieved with saliva substitutes or sugarless candy or gum.

• Tell patient adverse GI effects can be minimized by taking drug with meals during the titration period. Later, the entire daily dose may be taken at bedtime to limit daytime drowsiness.
• Inform patient to avoid using OTC medications, particularly antihistamines and decongestants, unless recommended by primary health care provider or pharmacist.
• Encourage patient to continue therapy, even if adverse reactions are troublesome.

Breast-feeding
• It is not known if drug is excreted in breast milk. Use with caution in breast-feeding women.

clonazepam
Klonopin, Rivotril*

Pharmacologic classification: benzodiazepine
Therapeutic classification: anticonvulsant
Controlled substance schedule IV
Pregnancy risk category C

How supplied
Available by prescription only
Tablets: 0.5 mg, 1 mg, 2 mg

Indications, route, and dosage
Absence and atypical absence seizures; akinetic and myoclonic seizures; ◊ generalized tonic-clonic seizures
Adults: Initial dosage should not exceed 1.5 mg P.O. daily, divided into three doses. May be increased by 0.5 to 1 mg q 3 days until seizures are controlled. Maximum recommended daily dosage, 20 mg.
Children up to age 10 or weighing 66 lb (30 kg) or less: 0.01 to 0.03 mg/kg P.O. daily (not to exceed 0.05 mg/kg daily), divided q 8 hours. Increase dosage by 0.25 to 0.5 mg q third day to a maximum maintenance dosage of 0.1 to 0.2 mg/kg daily.
◊ Leg movements during sleep; ◊ adjunct treatment in schizophrenia
Adults: 0.5 to 2 mg P.O. h.s.
◊ Parkinsonian dysarthria
Adults: 0.25 to 0.5 mg P.O. daily.
◊ Acute manic episodes
Adults: 0.75 to 16 mg P.O. daily.
◊ Multifocal tic disorders
Adults: 1.5 to 12 mg P.O. daily.
◊ Neuralgia
Adults: 2 to 4 mg P.O. daily.

Pharmacodynamics
Anticonvulsant action: Mechanism of anticonvulsant activity is unknown; drug appears to act in the limbic system, thalamus, and hypothalamus.

Drug is used to treat myoclonic, atonic, and absence seizures resistant to other anticonvulsants and to suppress or eliminate attacks of sleep-related nocturnal myoclonus (restless legs syndrome).

Pharmacokinetics
• *Absorption:* Clonazepam is well absorbed from the GI tract; action begins in 20 to 60 minutes and persists for 6 to 8 hours in infants and children and up to 12 hours in adults.
• *Distribution:* Drug is distributed widely throughout the body; it is approximately 85% protein-bound.
• *Metabolism:* Clonazepam is metabolized by the liver to several metabolites. The half-life of drug is 18 to 39 hours.
• *Excretion:* Excreted in urine.

Contraindications and precautions
Contraindicated in patients with significant hepatic disease; in those with sensitivity to benzodiazepines; and in patients with acute angle-closure glaucoma. Use cautiously in children and in patients with mixed-type seizures, respiratory disease, or glaucoma.

Interactions
Concomitant use of clonazepam with other *CNS depressants* (*alcohol, narcotics, tranquilizers, anxiolytics, barbiturates*) and other *anticonvulsants* will produce additive CNS depressant effects. Concomitant use with *valproic acid* may induce absence seizures. Concomitant use of clonazepam with *ritonavir* may significantly increase levels of clonazepam.

Effects on diagnostic tests
Clonazepam may elevate phenytoin levels and liver function test values.

Adverse reactions
CNS: ***drowsiness, ataxia, behavioral disturbances*** (especially in children), slurred speech, tremor, confusion, psychosis, agitation.
CV: palpitations.
EENT: nystagmus, abnormal eye movements, sore gums.
GI: constipation, gastritis, change in appetite, nausea, anorexia, diarrhea.
GU: dysuria, enuresis, nocturia, urine retention.
Hematologic: leukopenia, ***thrombocytopenia,*** eosinophilia.
Respiratory: ***respiratory depression,*** chest congestion, shortness of breath.
Skin: rash.

Overdose and treatment
Symptoms of overdose may include ataxia, confusion, coma, decreased reflexes, and hypotension. Treat overdose with gastric lavage and supportive therapy. Flumazenil, a specific benzodiazepine antagonist, may be useful. Vasopressors should be used to treat hypotension. Carefully monitor vital signs, ECG, and fluid and electrolyte balance. Clonazepam is not dialyzable.

☑ Special considerations
• Abrupt withdrawal may precipitate status epilepticus; after long-term use, lower dosage gradually.
• Concomitant use with barbiturates or other CNS depressants may impair ability to perform tasks re-

quiring mental alertness, such as driving a car. Warn patient to avoid such combined use.
- Monitor CBC and liver function tests periodically.
- Monitor for oversedation, especially in elderly patients.

Patient education
- Explain rationale for therapy and risks and benefits that may be anticipated.
- Teach patient signs and symptoms of adverse reactions and need to report them promptly.
- Tell patient to avoid alcohol and other sedatives to prevent added CNS depression.
- Warn patient not to discontinue drug or change dosage unless prescribed.
- Advise patient to avoid tasks that require mental alertness until degree of sedative effect is determined.

Geriatric use
- Elderly patients may require lower doses because of diminished renal function; such patients also are at greater risk for oversedation from CNS depressants.

Pediatric use
- Long-term safety in children has not been established.

Breast-feeding
- Alternative feeding method is recommended during clonazepam therapy.

clonidine hydrochloride
Catapres, Catapres-TTS, Dixarit*

Pharmacologic classification: centrally acting alpha-adrenergic agonist antiadrenergic
Therapeutic classification: antihypertensive
Pregnancy risk category C

How supplied
Available by prescription only
Tablets: 0.1 mg, 0.2 mg, 0.3 mg
Transdermal: TTS-1 (releases 0.1 mg/24 hours), TTS-2 (releases 0.2 mg/24 hours), TTS-3 (releases 0.3 mg/24 hours)

Indications, route, and dosage
Hypertension
Adults: Initially, 0.1 mg P.O. b.i.d.; then increased by 0.1 to 0.2 mg daily or every few days until desired response is achieved. Usual dosage range is 0.2 to 0.6 mg daily in divided doses. Maximum effective dosage is 2.4 mg/day. If transdermal patch is used, apply to area of hairless intact skin once q 7 days.
Children: No dosing recommendations for children.
◊ ***Adjunctive therapy in nicotine withdrawal***
Adults: Initially, 0.15 mg P.O. daily, gradually increased to 0.4 mg P.O. daily as tolerated. Alternatively, apply transdermal patch (0.2 mg/24 hours) and replace weekly for the first 2 or 3 weeks after smoking cessation.
◊ ***Prophylaxis for vascular headache***
Adults: 0.025 mg P.O. b.i.d. to q.i.d. up to 0.15 mg P.O. daily in divided doses.
◊ ***Adjunctive treatment of menopausal symptoms***
Adults: 0.025 to 0.075 mg P.O. b.i.d.
◊ ***Adjunctive therapy in opiate withdrawal***
Adults: 5 to 17 mcg/kg P.O. daily in divided doses for up to 10 days. Adjust dosage to avoid hypotension and excessive sedation, and slowly withdraw drug.
◊ ***Ulcerative colitis***
Adults: 0.3 mg P.O. t.i.d.
◊ ***Neuralgia***
Adults: 0.2 mg P.O. daily.
◊ ***Tourette syndrome***
Adults: 0.15 to 0.2 mg P.O. daily.
◊ ***Diabetic diarrhea***
Adults: 0.15 to 1.2 mg/day P.O. or 1 to 2 patches/week (0.3 mg/24 hours).
◊ ***Growth delay in children***
Children: 0.0375 to 0.15 mg/m^2 P.O. daily.
◊ ***To diagnose pheochromocytoma***
Adults: 0.3 mg given once.

Pharmacodynamics
Antihypertensive action: Clonidine decreases peripheral vascular resistance by stimulating central alpha-adrenergic receptors, thus decreasing cerebral sympathetic outflow; drug may also inhibit renin release. Initially, clonidine may stimulate peripheral alpha-adrenergic receptors, producing transient vasoconstriction.

Pharmacokinetics
- *Absorption:* Clonidine is absorbed well from the GI tract when administered orally; after oral administration, blood pressure begins to decline in 30 to 60 minutes, with maximal effect occurring in 2 to 4 hours. Clonidine is absorbed well percutaneously after transdermal topical administration; transdermal therapeutic plasma levels are achieved 2 to 3 days after initial application.
- *Distribution:* Clonidine is distributed widely into the body.
- *Metabolism:* Drug is metabolized in the liver, where nearly 50% is transformed to inactive metabolites.
- *Excretion:* Approximately 65% of a given dose is excreted in urine; 20% is excreted in feces. Half-life of clonidine ranges from 6 to 20 hours in patients with normal renal function. After oral administration, the antihypertensive effect lasts up to 8 hours; after transdermal application, the antihypertensive effect persists for up to 7 days.

Contraindications and precautions
Contraindicated in patients with hypersensitivity to drug. Transdermal form is contraindicated in patients with hypersensitivity to any component of the adhesive layer of the transdermal system. Use cautiously in patients with severe coronary disease, recent MI, cerebrovascular disease, and impaired hepatic or renal function.

* Canada only

◊ Unlabeled clinical use

Interactions
Clonidine may increase CNS depressant effects of *alcohol, barbiturates*, and other *sedatives*.

Tricyclic antidepressants, MAO inhibitors, and *tolazoline* may inhibit the antihypertensive effects of clonidine; use with *propranolol* or *other beta blockers* may have an additive effect, producing bradycardia. This may increase rebound hypertension upon withdrawal.

Effects on diagnostic tests
Clonidine may decrease urinary excretion of vanillylmandelic acid and catecholamines; it may slightly increase blood or serum glucose levels and may cause a weakly positive Coombs' test.

Adverse reactions
CNS: *drowsiness, dizziness*, fatigue, *sedation, weakness*, malaise, agitation, depression.
CV: orthostatic hypotension, bradycardia, ***severe rebound hypertension.***
GI: *constipation, dry mouth*, nausea, vomiting, anorexia.
GU: urine retention, impotence, loss of libido.
Skin: *pruritus, dermatitis* (with transdermal patch), rash.
Other: weight gain.

Overdose and treatment
Clinical signs of overdose include bradycardia, CNS depression, respiratory depression, hypothermia, apnea, seizures, lethargy, agitation, irritability, diarrhea, and hypotension; hypertension has also been reported.

After overdose with oral clonidine, *do not induce emesis*, because rapid onset of CNS depression can lead to aspiration. After adequate airway is assured, empty stomach by gastric lavage followed by administration of activated charcoal. If overdose occurs in patients receiving transdermal therapy, remove transdermal patch. Further treatment is usually symptomatic and supportive.

☑ Special considerations
- Monitor pulse and blood pressure frequently; dosage is usually adjusted to patient's response and tolerance.
- Do not discontinue abruptly; reduce dosage gradually over 2 to 4 days to prevent severe rebound hypertension.
- Patients with renal impairment may respond to smaller doses of drug.
- Give 4 to 6 hours before scheduled surgery.
- Clonidine may be used to lower blood pressure quickly in some hypertensive emergencies.
- Monitor weight daily during initiation of therapy, to monitor fluid retention.
- Therapeutic plasma levels are achieved 2 or 3 days after applying transdermal form. Patient may need oral antihypertensive therapy during this interim period.
- Transdermal systems should be removed when attempting defibrillation or synchronized cardioversion because of electrical conductivity.

Patient education
- Explain disease and rationale for therapy; emphasize importance of follow-up visits in establishing therapeutic regimen.
- Teach patient signs and symptoms of adverse effects and need to report them; patient should also report excessive weight gain (more than 5 lb [2.27 kg] weekly).
- Warn patient to avoid hazardous activities that require mental alertness until tolerance develops to sedation, drowsiness, and other CNS effects.
- Advise patient to avoid sudden position changes to minimize orthostatic hypotension.
- Inform patient that ice chips, hard candy, or gum will relieve dry mouth.
- Warn patient to call for specific instructions before taking OTC cold preparations.
- Advise taking last dose at bedtime to ensure nighttime blood pressure control.
- Tell patient not to discontinue drug suddenly; rebound hypertension may develop.

Geriatric use
- Elderly patients may require lower doses because they may be more sensitive to clonidine's hypotensive effects.

Pediatric use
- Efficacy and safety in children have not been established; use drug only if potential benefit outweighs risk.

Breast-feeding
- Clonidine is distributed into breast milk. An alternate feeding method is recommended during treatment.

clopidogrel bisulfate
Plavix

Pharmacologic classification: inhibitor of ADP-induced platelet aggregation
Therapeutic classification: antiplatelet agent
Pregnancy risk category B

How supplied
Available by prescription only
Tablets: 75 mg

Indications, route, and dosage
To reduce atherosclerotic events (MI, CVA, vascular death) in patients with atherosclerosis documented by recent CVA, MI, or peripheral arterial disease
Adults: 75 mg P.O. once daily with or without food.

Pharmacodynamics
Antiplatelet action: Inhibits the binding of adenosine diphosphate (ADP) to its platelet receptor and the subsequent ADP-mediated activation of glycoprotein IIb/IIIa complex, thereby inhibiting platelet aggregation. Because clopidogrel acts by irreversibly modifying the platelet ADP receptor, platelets exposed to the drug are affected for their lifespan.

Dose-dependent inhibition of platelet aggregation can be seen 2 hours after single doses, and becomes maximal after 3 to 7 days of repeated dosing. Following discontinuation of drug, platelet aggregation and bleeding time return to baseline after treatment is discontinued, in approximately 5 days.

Pharmacokinetics

• *Absorption:* After repeated oral doses, plasma concentrations of parent compound, which has no platelet-inhibiting effect, are very low and generally below quantification limit. Pharmacokinetic evaluations are generally stated in terms of the main circulating metabolite. Rapidly absorbed after oral dosing with peak plasma levels of the main circulating metabolite occurring about 1 hour after dosing. Following oral administration, approximately 50% of dose is absorbed.
• *Distribution:* Clopidogrel and main circulating metabolite binds reversibly to human plasma proteins (98% and 94%, respectively).
• *Metabolism:* Extensively metabolized by the liver. Main circulating metabolite is the carboxylic acid derivative that has no effect on platelet aggregation. It represents about 85% of circulating drug. Elimination half-life of main circulating metabolite is 8 hours after single and repeated doses.
• *Excretion:* Following oral administration, about 50% is excreted in the urine and 46% in the feces.

Contraindications and precautions

Contraindicated in patients with pathologic bleeding, such as peptic ulcer or intracranial hemorrhage, and in those with known hypersensitivity to drug or its components.

Use with caution in patients at risk for increased bleeding from trauma, surgery, or other pathologic conditions and in those with hepatic impairment or severe hepatic disease.

Interactions

Aspirin may increase risk for GI bleeding; it does not modify the clopidogrel-mediated inhibition of ADP-induced platelet aggregation.

Safe use with *heparin* or *warfarin* has not been established. Use together cautiously. Clopidogrel did not alter the heparin dose or the effect of heparin on coagulation. Coadministration of heparin had no effect on inhibition of platelet aggregation induced by clopidogrel.

Coadministration with *NSAIDs* is associated with an increased occult GI blood loss. Use with caution.

Effects on diagnostic tests

None reported.

Adverse reactions

CNS: asthenia, depression, dizziness, fatigue, headache, paresthesia, syncope.
CV: chest pain, edema, hypertension, palpitation.
EENT: epistaxis, rhinitis.
GI: abdominal pain, constipation, diarrhea, dyspepsia, gastritis, hemorrhage, nausea, vomiting.
GU: urinary tract infection.
Hematologic: purpura.
Respiratory: bronchitis, coughing, dyspnea, upper respiratory infection.
Skin: rash, pruritus.
Other: arthralgia, flu symptoms, pain.

Overdose and treatment

No adverse effects were reported after single oral administration of 600 mg (equivalent to eight standard 75-mg tablets). The bleeding time was prolonged by a factor of 1.7, which is similar to that observed with the therapeutic dose of 75 mg daily. Symptoms of acute toxicity in animal studies included vomiting, prostration, GI hemorrhage, and difficulty breathing.

Based on biological plausibility, platelet transfusion may be appropriate to reverse the pharmacologic effects of clopidogrel if quick reversal is required.

☑ Special considerations

• Drug is usually used in patients who are hypersensitive or intolerant to aspirin.
• If patient is to undergo surgery and an antiplatelet effect is not desired, drug should be stopped 7 days before surgery.

Patient education

• Inform patient it may take longer than usual to stop bleeding; therefore, advise him to refrain from activities in which trauma and bleeding may occur. Encourage use of seat belts.
• Instruct patient to report unusual bleeding or bruising.
• Tell patient to inform primary health care provider or dentist of clopidogrel use before scheduling surgery or taking new drugs.
• Inform patient that drug may be taken without regard to meals.

Pediatric use

• Safety and efficacy have not been established.

Breast-feeding

• It is not known if drug or its metabolite occur in breast milk. A decision to discontinue breast-feeding or drug should be made.

---

clorazepate dipotassium

Novoclopate*, Tranxene*, Tranxene-SD, Tranxene-SD Half Strength

Pharmacologic classification: benzodiazepine
Therapeutic classification: antianxiety agent; anticonvulsant; sedative-hypnotic
Controlled substance schedule IV
Pregnancy risk category NR

How supplied

Available by prescription only
Tablets: 3.75 mg, 7.5 mg, 11.25 mg, 15 mg, 22.5 mg
Capsules: 3.75 mg, 7.5 mg, 15 mg

Indications, route, and dosage

Acute alcohol withdrawal

Adults: Day 1—initially, 30 mg P.O., followed by 30 to 60 mg P.O. in divided doses; day 2—45 to 90 mg P.O. in divided doses; day 3—22.5 to 45 mg P.O. in divided doses; day 4—15 to 30 mg P.O. in divided doses; gradually reduce daily dose to 7.5 to 15 mg.

Anxiety

Adults: 15 to 60 mg P.O. daily.

As an adjunct in treatment of partial seizures

Adults and children over age 12: Maximum recommended initial dosage is 7.5 mg P.O. t.i.d. Dosage increases should not exceed 7.5 mg/week. Maximum daily dosage should not exceed 90 mg.

Children age 9 and 12: Maximum recommended initial dosage is 7.5 mg P.O. b.i.d. Dosage increases should not exceed 7.5 mg/week. Maximum daily dosage should not exceed 60 mg.

Pharmacodynamics

Anxiolytic and sedative actions: Clorazepate depresses the CNS at the limbic and subcortical levels of the brain. It produces an antianxiety effect by enhancing the effect of the neurotransmitter gamma-aminobutyric acid (GABA) on its receptor in the ascending reticular activating system, which increases inhibition and blocks both cortical and limbic arousal.

Anticonvulsant action: Drug suppresses spread of seizure activity produced by epileptogenic foci in the cortex, thalamus, and limbic structures by enhancing presynaptic inhibition.

Pharmacokinetics

- *Absorption:* After oral administration, clorazepate is hydrolyzed in the stomach to desmethyldiazepam, which is absorbed completely and rapidly. Peak serum levels occur at 1 to 2 hours.
- *Distribution:* Drug is distributed widely throughout the body. Approximately 80% to 95% of an administered dose is bound to plasma protein.
- *Metabolism:* Desmethyldiazepam is metabolized in the liver to conjugated oxazepam.
- *Excretion:* Inactive glucuronide metabolites are excreted in urine. The half-life of desmethyldiazepam ranges from 30 to 100 hours.

Contraindications and precautions

Contraindicated in patients with hypersensitivity to drug or other benzodiazepines and acute angle-closure glaucoma. Avoid use in pregnant patients, especially during the first trimester.

Use cautiously in patients with impaired renal or hepatic function, suicidal tendencies, or history of drug abuse.

Interactions

Clorazepate potentiates the CNS depressant effects of *phenothiazines, narcotics, barbiturates, alcohol, antihistamines, MAO inhibitors, general anesthetics,* and *antidepressants.* Concomitant use with *cimetidine* and possibly *disulfiram* causes diminished hepatic metabolism of clorazepate, which increases its plasma concentration.

Heavy smoking accelerates clorazepate's metabolism, thus lowering clinical effectiveness. *Antacids* delay drug's absorption and reduce the total amount absorbed.

Benzodiazepines may reduce serum levels of *haloperidol.* Clorazepate may decrease the therapeutic effectiveness of *levodopa.*

Effects on diagnostic tests

Drug therapy may elevate liver function test results. Minor changes in EEG patterns, usually low-voltage, fast activity, may occur during and after clorazepate therapy.

Adverse reactions

CNS: *drowsiness,* dizziness, nervousness, confusion, headache, insomnia, depression, irritability, tremor.
CV: hypotension.
EENT: blurred vision, diplopia.
GI: nausea, vomiting, abdominal discomfort, dry mouth.
GU: urine retention, incontinence.
Skin: rash.

Overdose and treatment

Clinical manifestations of overdose include somnolence, confusion, coma, hypoactive reflexes, dyspnea, labored breathing, hypotension, bradycardia, slurred speech, and unsteady gait or impaired coordination.

Support blood pressure and respiration until drug effects subside; monitor vital signs. Flumazenil, a specific benzodiazepine antagonist, may be useful. Mechanical ventilatory assistance via endotracheal tube may be required to maintain a patent airway and support adequate oxygenation. Treat hypotension with I.V. fluids and vasopressors such as dopamine and phenylephrine as needed. Induce emesis if patient is conscious. Use gastric lavage if ingestion was recent, but only if an endotracheal tube is present to prevent aspiration. After emesis or lavage, administer activated charcoal with a cathartic as a single dose. Dialysis is of limited value. Do not use barbiturates because they may worsen CNS adverse effects.

☑ Special considerations

Besides those relevant to all *benzodiazepines,* consider the following recommendations.

- Lower doses are effective in elderly patients and patients with renal or hepatic dysfunction.
- Store in a cool, dry place away from direct light.

Patient education

- Advise patient of potential for physical and psychological dependence with chronic use of clorazepate.
- Instruct patient not to alter drug regimen without medical approval.
- Warn patient that sudden position changes may cause dizziness. Advise patient to dangle legs for a few minutes before getting out of bed to prevent falls and injury.
- Advise patient to take antacids 1 hour before or after clorazepate.
- Inform patient not to suddenly stop taking drug.

Geriatric use

- Lower doses are usually effective in elderly patients because of decreased elimination. Use with caution.
- Elderly patients who receive this drug require supervision with ambulation and activities of daily living during initiation of therapy or after an increase in dose.

Pediatric use

- Safety has not been established in children under age 9.

Breast-feeding

- The breast-fed infant of a mother who uses clorazepate may become sedated, have feeding difficulties, or lose weight. Avoid use in breast-feeding women.

clotrimazole

FemCare, Gyne-Lotrimin, Lotrimin, Lotrimin AF, Mycelex, Mycelex-G, Mycelex OTC, Mycelex-7

Pharmacologic classification: synthetic imidazole derivative
Therapeutic classification: topical antifungal
Pregnancy risk category B (C, oral form)

How supplied

Available by prescription only
Vaginal tablets: 500 mg
Topical cream: 1%
Topical lotion: 1%
Topical solution: 1%
Lozenges: 10 mg

Available without a prescription
Vaginal tablets: 100 mg
Vaginal cream: 1%
Combination pack: Vaginal tablets 500 mg/topical cream 1%

Indications, route, and dosage

Tinea pedis, tinea cruris, tinea versicolor, tinea corporis, cutaneous candidiasis

Adults and children: Apply thinly and massage into cleansed affected and surrounding area, morning and evening, for prescribed period (usually 1 to 4 weeks; however, therapy may take up to 8 weeks).

Vulvovaginal candidiasis

Adults: Insert one tablet intravaginally h.s. for 7 consecutive days. If vaginal cream is used, insert one applicatorful intravaginally, h.s. for 7 to 14 consecutive days.

Oropharyngeal candidiasis

Adults and children: Administer orally and dissolve slowly (15 to 30 minutes) in mouth; usual dosage is one lozenge five times daily for 14 consecutive days.

◇ ***Keratitis***

Adults: 1% ointment in sterile peanut oil q 2 to 4 hours for up to 6 weeks.

Pharmacodynamics

Antifungal action: Clotrimazole alters cell membrane permeability by binding with phospholipids in the fungal cell membrane. Clotrimazole inhibits or kills many fungi, including yeast and dermatophytes, and also is active against some gram-positive bacteria.

Pharmacokinetics

- *Absorption:* Absorption is limited with topical administration. Absorption following dissolution of a lozenge in the mouth not determined.
- *Distribution:* Minimal with local application.
- *Metabolism:* Unknown.
- *Excretion:* Unknown.

Contraindications and precautions

Contraindicated in patients hypersensitive to drug. Also contraindicated for ophthalmic use.

Interactions

None reported.

Effects on diagnostic tests

Abnormal liver function test results have been reported in patients receiving clotrimazole lozenges.

Adverse reactions

GI: nausea, vomiting (with lozenges); lower abdominal cramps.
GU: *mild vaginal burning or irritation* (with vaginal use), cramping, urinary frequency.
Skin: blistering, *erythema,* edema, blistering, pruritus, burning, stinging, peeling, urticaria, skin fissures, general irritation.

Overdose and treatment

Discontinue therapy.

☑ Special considerations

- Patients treated with clotrimazole lozenges, especially those who have preexisting liver dysfunction, should have periodic liver function tests.

Patient education

- Advise patient that lozenges must dissolve slowly in the mouth to achieve maximum effect. Tell patient not to chew lozenges.
- Instruct patients using intravaginal application to insert drug high into the vagina and to refrain from sexual contact during treatment period to avoid reinfection. Also tell patient to use a sanitary napkin to prevent staining of clothing and to absorb discharge.
- Tell patient to complete the full course of therapy. Improvement usually will be noted within 1 week. Patient should call if no improvement occurs in 4 weeks or if condition worsens.
- Advise patient to watch for and report irritation or sensitivity and, if this occurs, to discontinue use.

Pediatric use

- Drug is not recommended for use in children under age 3.

Breast-feeding
• It is unknown if drug is excreted in breast milk. Drug should be used with caution in breast-feeding women.

cloxacillin sodium
Cloxapen, Tegopen

Pharmacologic classification: penicillinase-resistant penicillin
Therapeutic classification: antibiotic
Pregnancy risk category B

How supplied
Available by prescription only
Capsules: 250 mg, 500 mg
Oral solution: 125 mg/5 ml (after reconstitution)

Indications, route, and dosage
Systemic infections caused by penicillinase-producing staphylococci organisms
Adults: 250 to 500 mg q 6 hours.
Children: 50 to 100 mg/kg P.O. daily, divided into doses given q 6 hours.

Pharmacodynamics
Antibiotic action: Cloxacillin is bactericidal; it adheres to bacterial penicillin-binding proteins, thereby inhibiting bacterial cell-wall synthesis.

Cloxacillin resists the effects of penicillinases—enzymes that inactivate penicillin—and therefore is active against many strains of penicillinase-producing bacteria; this activity is most pronounced against penicillinase-producing staphylococci; some strains may remain resistant. Cloxacillin is also active against gram-positive aerobic and anaerobic bacilli but has no significant effect on gram-negative bacilli.

Pharmacokinetics
• *Absorption:* Absorbed rapidly but incompletely (37% to 60%) from the GI tract; it is relatively acid stable. Peak plasma concentrations occur ½ to 2 hours after an oral dose. Food may decrease both rate and extent of absorption.
• *Distribution:* Cloxacillin is distributed widely. CSF penetration is poor but enhanced in meningeal inflammation. Cloxacillin crosses the placenta; it is 90% to 96% protein-bound.
• *Metabolism:* Drug is only partially metabolized.
• *Excretion:* Cloxacillin and metabolites are excreted in urine by renal tubular secretion and glomerular filtration; they are also excreted in breast milk. Elimination half-life in adults is ½ to 1 hour, extended minimally to 2½ hours in patients with renal impairment.

Contraindications and precautions
Contraindicated in patients with hypersensitivity to drug or other penicillins.

Interactions
Concomitant use with *aminoglycosides* produces synergistic bactericidal effects against *Staphylococcus aureus.* However, the drugs are physically and chemically incompatible and are inactivated when mixed or given together. In vivo inactivation has been reported when *aminoglycosides* and penicillins are used concomitantly.

Probenecid blocks renal tubular secretion of carbenicillin, raising its serum concentrations.

Effects on diagnostic tests
Cloxacillin alters test results for urine and serum proteins; it produces false-positive or elevated results in turbidimetric urine and serum protein tests using sulfosalicylic acid or trichloroacetic acid; it also reportedly produces false results on the Bradshaw screening test for Bence Jones protein.

Cloxacillin may cause transient elevations in liver function study results and transient reductions in RBC, WBC, and platelet counts.

Elevated liver function test results may indicate drug-induced cholestasis or hepatitis.

Cloxacillin may falsely decrease serum aminoglycoside concentrations.

Adverse reactions
CNS: lethargy, hallucinations, ***seizures,*** anxiety, confusion, agitation, depression, dizziness, fatigue.
GI: *nausea,* vomiting, *epigastric distress, diarrhea,* enterocolitis, pseudomembranous colitis, black "hairy" tongue, abdominal pain.
GU: interstitial nephritis, nephropathy.
Hematologic: eosinophilia, anemia, ***thrombocytopenia,*** leukopenia, hemolytic anemia, ***agranulocytosis.***
Other: hypersensitivity reactions (rash, urticaria, chills, fever, sneezing, wheezing, ***anaphylaxis***), intrahepatic cholestasis, overgrowth of nonsusceptible organisms.

Overdose and treatment
Clinical signs of overdose include neuromuscular irritability or seizures. No specific recommendation is available. Treatment is symptomatic. After recent ingestion (within 4 hours), empty the stomach by induced emesis or gastric lavage; follow with activated charcoal to reduce absorption. Cloxacillin is not appreciably removed by hemodialysis or peritoneal dialysis.

☑ Special considerations
Besides those relevant to all *penicillins,* consider the following recommendations.
• Give drug with water only; acid in fruit juice or carbonated beverage may inactivate drug.
• Give dose on empty stomach; food decreases absorption.
• Refrigerate oral suspension and discard any unused medication after 14 days. Unrefrigerated suspension is stable for 3 days.

Patient education
• Inform patient of potential adverse reactions.
• Instruct patient to take on an empty stomach and take with water only.
• Tell patient to refrigerate oral suspension and to discard any unused suspension after the course of treatment.

Pediatric use
• Elimination of cloxacillin is reduced in neonates; safe use of drug in neonates has not been established.

Breast-feeding
• Drug is excreted into breast milk; use cautiously in breast-feeding women.

clozapine
Clozaril

Pharmacologic classification: tricyclic dibenzodiazepine derivative
Therapeutic classification: antipsychotic
Pregnancy risk category B

How supplied
Available by prescription only
Tablets: 25 mg, 100 mg

Indications, route, and dosage
Treatment of schizophrenia in severely ill patients unresponsive to other therapies
Adults: Initially, 12.5 mg P.O. once or twice daily, titrated upward at 25 to 50 mg daily (if tolerated) to a daily dosage of 300 to 450 mg by end of 2 weeks. Individual dosage is based on clinical response, patient tolerance, and adverse reactions. Subsequent increases of dosage should occur no more than once or twice weekly and should not exceed 100 mg. Many patients respond to dosages of 300 to 600 mg daily, but some patients require as much as 900 mg daily. Do not exceed 900 mg/day.

Pharmacodynamics
Antipsychotic action: Clozapine binds to dopamine receptors (D-1, D-2, D-3, D-4, and D-5) within the limbic system of the CNS. It also may interfere with adrenergic, cholinergic, histaminergic, and serotoninergic receptors.

Pharmacokinetics
• *Absorption:* Peak levels occur about 2½ hours after oral administration. Food does not appear to interfere with bioavailability. Only 27% to 50% of the dose reaches systemic circulation.
• *Distribution:* Drug is about 95% bound to serum proteins.
• *Metabolism:* Nearly complete; very little unchanged drug appears in the urine.
• *Excretion:* Approximately 50% of drug appears in the urine and 30% in the feces, mostly as metabolites. Elimination half-life appears proportional to dose and may range from 4 to 66 hours.

Contraindications and precautions
Contraindicated in patients with uncontrolled epilepsy or history of clozapine-induced agranulocytosis; in patients with a WBC count below 3,500/mm³; in patients with severe CNS depression or coma; in patients taking other drugs that suppress bone marrow function; and in those with myelosuppressive disorders.

Use cautiously in patients with renal, hepatic, or cardiac disease, prostatic hyperplasia, or angle-closure glaucoma and in those receiving general anesthesia.

Interactions
Clozapine may potentiate the hypotensive effects of *antihypertensives. Anticholinergics* may potentiate the anticholinergic effects of clozapine.

Administration of clozapine to a patient taking a *benzodiazepine* may pose a risk of respiratory arrest and severe hypotension. Avoid concomitant use.

Increased serum levels of *warfarin, digoxin,* and *other highly protein-bound drugs* may occur. Monitor closely for adverse reactions.

Potentially increased bone marrow toxicity may follow concomitant use with *drugs that suppress bone marrow function.* Use together with *other CNS-active drugs* cautiously because of the potential for additive effects.

Clozapine may decrease *phenytoin* levels. It also may lower the seizure threshold; therefore, avoid use with other drugs that have the same effect.

Use cautiously with other *drugs metabolized by cytochrome P450 2D6,* including *antidepressants, phenothiazines, carbamazepine,* and *type IC antiarrhythmics* (*propafenone, flecainide, encainide*) or *drugs that inhibit this enzyme,* such as *quinidine.*

Effects on diagnostic tests
Toxic drug effects may be evidenced by depressed blood counts.

Adverse reactions
CNS: *drowsiness, sedation,* ***seizures,*** dizziness, syncope, vertigo, headache, tremor, disturbed sleep or nightmares, restlessness, hypokinesia or akinesia, agitation, rigidity, akathisia, confusion, fatigue, insomnia, hyperkinesia, weakness, lethargy, ataxia, slurred speech, depression, myoclonus, anxiety, neuroleptic malignant syndrome.
CV: *tachycardia, hypotension,* hypertension, chest pain, ECG changes, orthostatic hypotension.
GI: *dry mouth, constipation,* nausea, vomiting, *excessive salivation,* heartburn, constipation, diarrhea.
GU: urinary abnormalities (urinary frequency or urgency, urine retention), incontinence, abnormal ejaculation.
Hematologic: ***leukopenia, agranulocytosis.***
Skin: rash.
Other: fever, muscle pain or spasm, muscle weakness, weight gain, visual disturbances, diaphoresis.

After abrupt withdrawal of long-term therapy: possible abrupt recurrence of psychotic symptoms. Monitor patient closely.

Overdose and treatment
Fatalities have occurred at doses exceeding 2.5 g. Symptoms include drowsiness, delirium, coma, hypotension, hypersalivation, tachycardia, respiratory depression, and, rarely, seizures.

Treat symptomatically. Establish an airway and ensure adequate ventilation. Gastric lavage with activated charcoal and sorbitol may be effective. Monitor vital signs. Avoid epinephrine (and derivatives), quinidine, and procainamide when treating hypotension and arrhythmias.

☑ Special considerations

- Clozapine therapy must be given with a monitoring program that ensures weekly testing of WBC counts. Blood tests must be performed weekly, and no more than a 1-week supply of drug can be distributed.
- To discontinue clozapine therapy, withdraw drug gradually (over a 1- to 2-week period). However, changes in the patient's clinical status (including the development of leukopenia) may require abrupt discontinuation of the drug. If so, monitor closely for recurrence of psychotic symptoms.
- To reinstate therapy in patients withdrawn from drug, follow usual guidelines for dosage buildup. However, reexposure of the patient may increase the risk and severity of adverse reactions. If therapy was terminated for WBC counts below 2,000/mm³ or granulocyte counts below 1,000/mm³, drug should not be continued.
- Some patients experience transient fevers (temperature above 100.4° F [38° C]), especially in the first 3 weeks of therapy. Monitor patients closely.
- Assess patient periodically for abnormal body movement.

Patient education

- Warn patient about risk of developing agranulocytosis. He should know that safe use of drug requires weekly blood tests to monitor for agranulocytosis. Advise patient to promptly report flulike symptoms, fever, sore throat, lethargy, malaise, or other signs of infection.
- Advise patient to call before taking OTC drugs or alcohol.
- Tell patient that ice chips or sugarless candy or gum may help to relieve dry mouth.
- Warn patient to rise slowly to upright position to avoid orthostatic hypotension.

Pediatric use

- Safe use in children has not been established.

Breast-feeding

- Animal studies have shown that drug is excreted in breast milk. Women taking clozapine should not breast-feed.

codeine phosphate

codeine sulfate

Pharmacologic classification: opioid
Therapeutic classification: analgesic, antitussive
Controlled substance schedule II
Pregnancy risk category C

How supplied

Available by prescription only
Tablets: 15 mg, 30 mg, 60 mg; 15 mg, 30 mg, 60 mg (soluble)
Oral solution: 15 mg/5 ml codeine phosphate
Injection: 15 mg/ml, 30 mg/ml, 60 mg/ml codeine phosphate

Indications, route, and dosage

Mild to moderate pain
Adults: 15 to 60 mg P.O. or 15 to 60 mg (phosphate) S.C. or I.M. q 4 to 6 hours, p.r.n., or around-the-clock.
Children: 0.5 mg/kg (or 15 mg/m²) q 4 to 6 hours. (Do not use I.V.)
Nonproductive cough
Adults and children age 12 and older: 10 to 20 mg P.O. q 4 to 6 hours. Maximum dosage is 120 mg/24 hours.
Children age 6 to 11: 5 to 10 mg q 4 to 6 hours, not to exceed 60 mg daily.
Children age 2 to 6: 1 mg/kg daily divided into four equal doses, administered q 4 to 6 hours, not to exceed 30 mg in 24 hours.

Pharmacodynamics

Analgesic action: Codeine (methylmorphine) has analgesic properties that result from its agonist activity at the opiate receptors.

Antitussive action: Codeine has a direct suppressant action on the cough reflex center.

Pharmacokinetics

- *Absorption:* Codeine is well absorbed after oral or parenteral administration. It is about two thirds as potent orally as parenterally. After oral or subcutaneous administration, action occurs in less than 30 minutes. Peak analgesic effect is seen at ½ to 1 hour, and the duration of action is 4 to 6 hours.
- *Distribution:* Distributed widely throughout the body; it crosses the placenta and enters breast milk.
- *Metabolism:* Codeine is metabolized mainly in the liver, by demethylation, or conjugation with glucuronic acid.
- *Excretion:* Excreted mainly in the urine as norcodeine and free and conjugated morphine.

Contraindications and precautions

Contraindicated in patients with hypersensitivity to drug. Use cautiously in patients with impaired renal or hepatic function, head injuries, increased intracranial pressure, increased CSF pressure, hypothyroidism, Addison's disease, acute alcoholism, CNS depression, bronchial asthma, COPD, respiratory depression, or shock, and in elderly or debilitated patients.

Interactions

Concomitant use with other *CNS depressants* (*narcotic analgesics, general anesthetics, antihistamines, phenothiazines, barbiturates, benzodiazepines, sedative-hypnotics, tricyclic antidepressants, MAO inhibitors, alcohol, muscle relaxants*) potentiates drug's respiratory and CNS depression, sedation, and hypotensive effects. Concomitant use with *cimetidine* may also increase respiratory and CNS depression, causing confusion, disorientation, apnea, or seizures.

Drug accumulation and enhanced effects may result from concomitant use with other drugs that are extensively metabolized in the liver (*rifampin, phenytoin, digitoxin*); combined use with *anticholinergics* may cause paralytic ileus. Use with drugs which induce P450 enzymes results in increased clearance and decreased effect of codeine.

Patients who become physically dependent on drug may experience acute withdrawal syndrome if given a *narcotic antagonist*.

Severe CV depression may result from concomitant use with *general anesthetics*.

Effects on diagnostic tests

Drug may increase plasma amylase and lipase levels, delay gastric emptying, increase biliary tract pressure resulting from contraction of the sphincter of Oddi, and may interfere with hepatobiliary imaging studies.

Adverse reactions

CNS: *sedation, clouded sensorium, euphoria, dizziness, light-headedness.*
CV: *hypotension,* bradycardia.
GI: *nausea, vomiting, constipation, dry mouth,* ileus.
GU: *urine retention.*
Respiratory: ***respiratory depression.***
Skin: pruritus, flushing, *diaphoresis.*
Other: physical dependence.

Overdose and treatment

The most common signs and symptoms of overdose are CNS depression, respiratory depression, and miosis (pinpoint pupils). Other acute toxic effects include hypotension, bradycardia, hypothermia, shock, apnea, cardiopulmonary arrest, circulatory collapse, pulmonary edema, and seizures.

To treat acute overdose, first establish adequate respiratory exchange via a patent airway and ventilation as needed; administer narcotic antagonist (naloxone) to reverse respiratory depression. (Because the duration of action of codeine is longer than that of naloxone, repeated naloxone dosing is necessary.) Naloxone should not be given unless the patient has clinically significant respiratory or CV depression. Monitor vital signs closely.

If patient presents within 2 hours of ingestion of an oral overdose, empty the stomach immediately by inducing emesis (ipecac syrup) or using gastric lavage. Use caution to avoid risk of aspiration. Administer activated charcoal via nasogastric tube for further removal of drug in an oral overdose.

Provide symptomatic and supportive treatment (continued respiratory support, correction of fluid or electrolyte imbalance). Monitor laboratory parameters, vital signs, and neurologic status closely.

☑ Special considerations

Besides those relevant to all *opioids,* consider the following recommendations.
- Codeine and aspirin have additive analgesic effects. Give together for maximum pain relief.
- Codeine has much less abuse potential than morphine.

Patient education

- Inform patient that codeine may cause drowsiness, dizziness, or blurring of vision; tell him to use caution while driving or performing tasks that require mental alertness.
- Advise patient to avoid consumption of alcohol and other CNS depressants and to take drug with food if GI upset occurs.

Geriatric use

- Lower doses are usually indicated for elderly patients, who may be more sensitive to the therapeutic and adverse effects of drug.

Pediatric use

- Administer cautiously to children. Codeine-containing cough preparations may be hazardous in young children. Use a calibrated measuring device and do not exceed the recommended daily dose.

Breast-feeding

- Drug is excreted in breast milk; assess risk to benefit ratio before administering.

colchicine

Pharmacologic classification: Colchicum autumnale alkaloid
Therapeutic classification: antigout
Pregnancy risk category C (oral), D (parenteral)

How supplied

Available by prescription only
Injection: 1 mg (1/60 grain)/2-ml ampule
Tablets: 0.6 mg (1/100 grain), 0.5 mg (1/120 grain) as sugar-coated granules

Indications, route, and dosage

To prevent acute attacks of gout as prophylactic or maintenance therapy
Adults: 0.5 or 0.6 mg P.O. one to four times weekly.
To prevent attacks of gout in patients undergoing surgery
Adults: 0.5 to 0.6 mg P.O. t.i.d. 3 days before and 3 days after surgery.
Acute gout, acute gouty arthritis
Adults: Initially, 0.5 to 1.3 mg P.O., followed by 0.5 to 0.65 mg P.O. q 1 to 2 hours or 1 to 1.3 mg P.O. q 2 hours; total daily dose is usually 4 to 8 mg P.O.; give until pain is relieved or until nausea, vomiting, or diarrhea ensues. Or 2 mg I.V. followed by 0.5 mg I.V. q 6 hours if necessary. Total I.V. dose over 24 hours (one course of treatment) not to exceed 4 mg.
◊ ***Familial Mediterranean fever***
Colchicine has been used effectively to treat familial Mediterranean fever (hereditary disorder characterized by acute episodes of fever, peritonitis, and pleuritis).
Adults: 1 to 2 mg/day in divided doses.
◊ ***Amyloidosis suppressant***
Adults: 500 to 600 mcg P.O. once daily to b.i.d.
◊ ***Dermatitis herpetiformis suppressant***
Adults: 600 mcg P.O. b.i.d. or t.i.d.
◊ ***Hepatic cirrhosis***
Adults: 1 mg 5 days weekly.

◇ ***Primary biliary cirrhosis***
Adults: 0.6 mg b.i.d.

Pharmacodynamics
Antigout action: Colchicine's exact mechanism of action is unknown, but it is involved in leukocyte migration inhibition; reduction of lactic acid production by leukocytes, resulting in decreased deposits of uric acid; and interference with kinin formation.

Anti-inflammatory action: Colchicine reduces the inflammatory response to deposited uric acid crystals and diminishes phagocytosis.

Pharmacokinetics
- *Absorption:* When administered P.O., colchicine is rapidly absorbed from the GI tract. Unchanged drug may be reabsorbed from the intestine by biliary processes.
- *Distribution:* Colchicine is distributed rapidly into various tissues after reabsorption from the intestine. It is concentrated in leukocytes and distributed into the kidneys, liver, spleen, and intestinal tract, but is absent in the heart, skeletal muscle, and brain.
- *Metabolism:* Drug is metabolized partially in the liver and also slowly metabolized in other tissues.
- *Excretion:* Drug and its metabolites are excreted primarily in the feces, with lesser amounts excreted in urine.

Contraindications and precautions
Contraindicated in patients with hypersensitivity to drug; blood dyscrasias; or serious CV, renal, or GI disease. Use cautiously in elderly or debilitated patients and in those with early signs of CV, renal, or GI disease.

Interactions
Colchicine induces reversible malabsorption of *vitamin B_{12}*, may increase sensitivity to *CNS depressants*, and may enhance the response to *sympathomimetic agents*. Colchicine is inhibited by *acidifying agents* and by *alcohol consumption*; its actions are increased by *alkalinizing* agents. Concomitant use with cyclosporine may cause GI dysfunction, hepatonephropathy, and neuromyopathy.

Effects on diagnostic tests
Colchicine therapy may increase alkaline phosphatase, AST, and ALT levels and may decrease serum carotene, cholesterol, and thrombocyte values.

Colchicine may cause false-positive results of urine tests for RBCs or hemoglobin.

Adverse reactions
CNS: peripheral neuritis.
GI: *nausea, vomiting, abdominal pain, diarrhea.*
Hematologic: ***aplastic anemia, thrombocytopenia, and agranulocytosis*** (with long-term use); nonthrombocytopenic purpura.
Skin: alopecia, urticaria, dermatitis, hypersensitivity reactions.
Other: severe local irritation if extravasation occurs, myopathy, reversible azoospermia.

Overdose and treatment
Clinical manifestations of overdose include nausea, vomiting, abdominal pain, and diarrhea. Diarrhea may be severe and bloody from hemorrhagic gastroenteritis. Burning sensations in the throat, stomach, and skin also may occur. Extensive vascular damage may result in shock, hematuria, and oliguria, indicating kidney damage. Patient develops severe dehydration, hypotension, and muscle weakness with an ascending paralysis of the CNS. Patient usually remains conscious, but delirium and convulsions may occur. Death may result from respiratory depression.

There is no known specific antidote. Treatment begins with gastric lavage and preventive measures for shock. Recent studies support the use of hemodialysis and peritoneal dialysis; atropine and morphine may relieve abdominal pain; paregoric usually is administered to control diarrhea and cramps. Respiratory assistance may be needed.

☑ Special considerations
- To avoid cumulative toxicity, a course of oral colchicine should not be repeated for at least 3 days; a course of I.V. colchicine should not be repeated for several weeks.
- Do not administer I.M. or S.C.; severe local irritation occurs.
- Obtain baseline laboratory studies, including CBC, before initiating therapy and periodically thereafter.
- Give I.V. by slow I.V. push over 2 to 5 minutes by direct I.V. injection or into tubing of a free-flowing I.V. with compatible I.V. fluid. Avoid extravasation. Do not dilute colchicine injection with bacteriostatic 0.9% NaCl solution, dextrose 5% injection, or any other fluid that might change pH of colchicine solution. If lower concentration of colchicine injection is needed, dilute with sterile water or 0.9% NaCl solution. However, if diluted solution becomes turbid, do not inject.
- Discontinue drug if weakness, anorexia, nausea, vomiting, or diarrhea appears. First sign of acute overdosage may be GI symptoms, followed by vascular damage, muscle weakness, and ascending paralysis. Delirium and convulsions may occur without loss of consciousness.
- Store drug in a tightly closed, light-resistant container, away from moisture and high temperatures.

Patient education
- Advise patient to report rash, sore throat, fever, unusual bleeding, bruising, tiredness, weakness, numbness, or tingling.
- Tell patient to discontinue drug as soon as gout pain is relieved or at the first sign of nausea, vomiting, stomach pain, or diarrhea. Advise patient to report persistent symptoms.
- Instruct patient to avoid alcohol during drug therapy, because alcohol may inhibit drug action.

Geriatric use
- Administer with caution to elderly or debilitated patients, especially those with renal, GI, or heart disease or hematologic disorders. Reduce dosage if weakness, anorexia, nausea, vomiting, or diarrhea appears.

Pediatric use
- Safety and efficacy in children have not been established.

Breast-feeding
- Safe use has not been established. It is not known if drug is excreted in breast milk.

colestipol hydrochloride
Colestid

Pharmacologic classification: anion exchange resin
Therapeutic classification: antilipemic
Pregnancy risk category C

How supplied
Available by prescription only
Tablets: 1 g
Granules: 300-g and 500-g multidose bottles, 5-g packets

Indications, route, and dosage
Primary hypercholesterolemia and xanthomas
Adults: **Tablets:** Initially, 2 g P.O. once daily or b.i.d., then increase in 2-g increments at 1- to 2-month intervals. Usual dose is 2 to 16 g P.O. daily given as a single dose or in divided doses.
Granules: Initially, 5 g P.O. once daily or b.i.d., then increase in 5-g increments at 1- to 2-month intervals. Usual dose is 5 to 30 g P.O. daily given as a single dose or in divided doses.
◊ *Children:* 10 to 20 g or 500 mg/kg daily in two to four divided doses (lower dosages of 125 to 250 mg/kg used when serum cholesterol levels were 15% to 20% above normal after only dietary management).
◊ ***Digitoxin overdose***
Adults: Initially, 10 g P.O. followed by 5 g P.O. q 6 to 8 hours.

Pharmacodynamics
Antilipemic action: Bile is normally excreted into the intestine to facilitate absorption of fat and other lipid materials. Colestipol binds with bile acid, forming an insoluble compound that is excreted in feces. With less bile available in the digestive system, less fat and lipid materials in food are absorbed, more cholesterol is used by the liver to replace its supply of bile acids, and the serum cholesterol level decreases.

Pharmacokinetics
- *Absorption:* Colestipol is not absorbed. Cholesterol levels may decrease in 24 to 48 hours, with peak effect occurring at 1 month. In some patients, the initial decrease is followed by a return to or above baseline cholesterol levels on continued therapy.
- *Distribution:* None.
- *Metabolism:* None.
- *Excretion:* Drug is excreted in feces; cholesterol levels return to baseline within 1 month after therapy stops.

Contraindications and precautions
Contraindicated in patients with hypersensitivity reactions to bile-acid sequestering resins. Use cautiously in patients prone to constipation and in those with conditions aggravated by constipation, such as symptomatic coronary artery disease.

Interactions
Colestipol impairs absorption of *cardiac glycosides* (including *digoxin* and *digitoxin*), *tetracycline, penicillin G, chenodiol, thiazide diuretics,* thus decreasing their therapeutic effect.

Dosage of any *oral medication* may require adjustment to compensate for possible binding with colestipol; give other drugs at least 1 hour before or 4 to 6 hours after colestipol (longer if possible); readjustment must also be made when colestipol is withdrawn to prevent high-dose toxicity.

Colestipol may interfere with *oral phosphate supplements.* The drug also may decrease GI absorption of *propranolol.*

Effects on diagnostic tests
Drug alters serum levels of alkaline phosphatase, ALT, AST, chloride, phosphorus, potassium, and sodium.

Adverse reactions
CNS: headache, dizziness, anxiety, vertigo, insomnia, fatigue, syncope, tinnitus.
GI: *constipation, **fecal impaction,*** hemorrhoids, abdominal discomfort, flatulence, nausea, vomiting, steatorrhea, ***GI bleeding,*** diarrhea, anorexia.
GU: dysuria, hematuria.
Skin: rash; irritation of tongue and perianal area.
Other: vitamin A, D, E, and K deficiencies from decreased absorption; hyperchloremic acidosis with long-term use or high dosage; anemia; ecchymoses; bleeding tendencies; backache; muscle and joint pain; osteoporosis.

Overdose and treatment
Overdose of colestipol has not been reported. Chief potential risk is intestinal obstruction; treatment would depend on location and degree of obstruction and on amount of gut motility.

☑ Special considerations
- To mix, sprinkle granules on surface of preferred beverage or wet food, let stand a few minutes, and stir to obtain uniform suspension; avoid excess foaming by using large glass and mixing slowly. Use at least 90 ml of water or other fluid, soups, milk, or pulpy fruit; rinse container and have patient drink this to be sure he ingests entire dose. Tablets should be swallowed whole.
- Monitor levels of cardiac glycosides and other drugs to ensure appropriate dosage during and after therapy with colestipol.
- Determine serum cholesterol level frequently during first few months of therapy and periodically thereafter.
- Drug effects are most successful if used concomitantly with a diet and exercise program.

• Monitor bowel habits; treat constipation promptly by decreasing dosage, increasing fluid intake, adding a stool softener, or discontinuing drug.
• Monitor for signs of vitamin A, D, or K deficiency.

Patient education
• Explain disease process and rationale for therapy and encourage patient to comply with continued blood testing and special diet; although therapy is not curative, it helps control serum cholesterol level.
• Teach patient how to administer drug. Other medications should be taken at least 1 hour before or 4 hours after colestipol.

Geriatric use
• Elderly patients are more likely to experience adverse GI effects, as well as adverse nutritional effects.

Pediatric use
• Safety in children has not been established; drug is not usually recommended; however, it has been used in a limited number of children with hypercholesteremia.

Breast-feeding
• Safety in breast-feeding women has not been established.

colfosceril palmitate
Exosurf Neonatal

Pharmacologic classification: phospholipid
Therapeutic classification: lung surfactant
Pregnancy risk category NR

How supplied
Available by prescription only
Intratracheal suspension: 108 mg/10-ml vial (13.5 mg/ml when reconstituted with 8 ml sterile water for injection provided)

Indications, route, and dosage
Prevention and treatment (rescue) of respiratory distress syndrome (RDS) in premature infants
Prophylaxis: 5 ml/kg of body weight intratracheally for the first dose, administered as soon as possible after birth; second and third doses should be administered approximately 12 and 24 hours later to all infants remaining on mechanical ventilation at those times.
Rescue: Initially, give 5 ml/kg of body weight intratracheally, administer as soon as possible after diagnosis of RDS is confirmed; second dose of 5 ml/kg, approximately 12 hours after the first, provided the infant remains on mechanical ventilation.
Administer using endotracheal tube adapter supplied by manufacturer. Infant should be suctioned before administration; however, suction should not be performed for 2 hours after administration except when necessary.

Pharmacodynamics
Surfactant action: Endogenous pulmonary surfactant lowers surface tension on alveolar surfaces during respiration and stabilizes alveoli against collapse at rest in transpulmonary pressures. Colfosceril replenishes surfactant and restores surface activity to the lungs.

Pharmacokinetics
• *Absorption:* Colfosceril is administered directly to the target organ, where biophysical effects occur at the alveolar surface. Most of the dose becomes lung-associated within hours of administration.
• *Distribution:* Distributed into lung tissue.
• *Metabolism:* Catabolized in lung tissue and reutilized for further phospholipid synthesis and secretion.
• *Excretion:* Unknown.

Contraindications and precautions
No known contraindications.

Interactions
None reported.

Effects on diagnostic tests
Abnormal laboratory values are common in critically ill, mechanically ventilated patients. No higher incidence was seen in drug-treated patients.

Adverse reactions
CNS: ***seizures.***
CV: ***intraventricular hemorrhage,*** patent ductus arteriosus, hypotension.
Hematologic: ***thrombocytopenia.***
Respiratory: **PULMONARY HEMORRHAGE, APNEA,** *pulmonary air leak, pneumonia.*
Other: *hyperbilirubinemia, sepsis,* meningitis, ***death from sepsis.***

Overdose and treatment
Overdose may result in acute airway obstruction. Treatment should be symptomatic and supportive.

☑ Special considerations
• Five different-sized endotracheal tube adapters are supplied; select size based on inside diameter of endotracheal tube.
• To prepare, reconstitute immediately before use with 8 ml of sterile water for injection (supplied). Fill a 10- or 12-ml syringe with 8 ml of sterile water using an 18G or 19G needle. Allow vacuum to draw water into vial. Aspirate as much as possible of the 8 ml out of the vial into the syringe while maintaining the vacuum; then, suddenly release the syringe plunger. The last step should be repeated three or four times to ensure adequate mixing. If vacuum is not present, do not use vial.
• The appropriate volume for the entire dose should be drawn into the syringe from below the froth of the vial. Reconstituted suspension will be milky white. Each ml contains 13.5 mg colfosceril, 1.5 mg cetyl alcohol, 1 mg tyloxapol, and NaCl to provide a 0.1 normal concentration.
• Continuous ECG and transcutaneous oxygen saturation monitoring is recommended. During dos-

ing, heart rate, color, chest expansion, facial expressions, oximeter, and endotracheal tube patency and position should be monitored.
- A videotape is available from the manufacturer demonstrating techniques for safe administration and should be viewed by the health care professional who will administer drug.

Patient education
- Inform patient of potential adverse reactions.

coral snake, North American (*Micrurus fulvius*), antivenin

Pharmacologic classification: antivenin
Therapeutic classification: snake antivenin
Pregnancy risk category C

How supplied
Available by prescription only
Injection: Combination package—1 vial antivenin and 1 vial diluent (10 ml bacteriostatic water for injection)

Indications, route, and dosage
Eastern and Texas coral snake bite
Adults and children: 3 to 5 vials slow I.V. through running I.V. of 0.9% NaCl solution. Give first 1 to 2 ml over 3 to 5 minutes and watch for signs of allergic reaction. If no signs develop, continue injection. Up to 15 vials may be needed. Not effective for Sonoran or Arizona coral snake bites.

Pharmacodynamics
Antivenin action: This product neutralizes and binds venom.

Pharmacokinetics
- *Absorption:* I.V. effect is rapid. I.M. absorption may not peak until the second day.
- *Distribution:* No information available.
- *Metabolism:* No information available.
- *Excretion:* Mean half-life is under 15 days.

Contraindications and precautions
Use with caution in persons with sensitivity to horse serum-derived preparations.

Interactions
None reported.

Effects on diagnostic tests
None reported.

Adverse reactions
Other: ***hypersensitivity, anaphylaxis.***
Note: Discontinue drug if severe systemic reactions occur.

Overdose and treatment
No information available.

☑ Special considerations
- If possible, hospitalize patient for observation.
- Splint bitten limb to prevent spread of venom.
- Obtain a thorough patient history of allergies, especially to horses and horse immune serum, and of previous reactions to immunizations.
- Before administering antivenin, a skin test for sensitivity to equine serum should be performed, because this product is derived from horses immunized with Eastern coral snake venom. For an intradermal test, use a 1:10 dilution of the antivenin serum in 0.9% NaCl solution.
- Epinephrine solution 1:1,000 should be available to treat allergic reactions.
- Ask patient when he received his last tetanus immunization; a booster may be appropriate at this time.
- Venom is neurotoxic and may rapidly cause respiratory paralysis and death. Monitor patient carefully for 24 hours. Be ready to take supportive measures, such as mechanical ventilation.
- Avoid use of narcotic analgesics and other drugs that produce sedation or respiratory depression.
- Monitor patient closely over the next 24 hours for reactions to both the snake bite and the antivenin.
- Refrigerate antivenin at 36° to 46° F (2° to 8° C).

Patient education
- Tell patient that product is derived from an animal source (that is, horses) and that he may experience allergic reactions, such as rash, joint swelling or pain, or difficulty breathing.

Pediatric use
- Amount of antivenin given to a child is not based on weight. Children receive the same dosage as adults.

Breast-feeding
- Patient should discontinue breast-feeding until venom's effects have subsided and if symptoms of serum sickness develop.

corticotropin (adrenocorticotropic hormone, ACTH)

ACTH, Acthar, Cortrophin-Zinc, H.P. Acthar Gel

Pharmacologic classification: anterior pituitary hormone
Therapeutic classification: diagnostic aid, replacement hormone, multiple sclerosis, and nonsuppurative thyroiditis treatment
Pregnancy risk category C

How supplied
Available by prescription only
Injection: 25 U/vial, 40 U/vial
Repository injection: 40 U/ml, 80 U/ml

Indications, route, and dosage
Diagnostic test of adrenocortical function
Adults: Up to 80 U I.M. or S.C. in divided doses; or a single dose of repository form; or 10 to 25 U

(aqueous form) in 500 ml of D_5W I.V. over 8 hours, between blood samplings.

Individual dosages vary with adrenal glands' sensitivity to stimulation and with the specific disease. Infants and younger children require larger doses per kilogram than do older children and adults.

Replacement hormone
Adults: 20 U S.C. or I.M. q.i.d.

Exacerbations of multiple sclerosis
Adults: 80 to 120 U I.M. daily for 2 to 3 weeks.

Severe allergic reactions, collagen disorders, dermatologic disorders, inflammation
Adults: 40 to 80 U/day I.M. or S.C. Adjust dosage based upon patient response.

Infantile spasms
Infants: 20 to 40 U I.M. (of repository injection) daily or 80 U I.M. every other day for 3 months or 1 month after spasm ceases.

Pharmacodynamics

Diagnostic action: Corticotropin is used to test adrenocortical function. Corticotropin binds with a specific receptor in the adrenal cell plasma membrane, stimulating the synthesis of the entire spectrum of adrenal steroids, one of which is cortisol. The effect of corticotropin is measured by analyzing plasma cortisol before and after drug administration. In patients with primary adrenocortical insufficiency, corticotropin does not increase plasma cortisol concentrations significantly.

Anti-inflammatory action: In nonsuppurative thyroiditis and acute exacerbations of multiple sclerosis, corticotropin stimulates release of adrenal cortex hormones, which combat tissue responses to inflammatory processes.

Pharmacokinetics

- *Absorption:* Drug is absorbed rapidly after I.M. administration; absorption occurs over 8 to 16 hours after I.M. administration of zinc or repository form. Maximum stimulation occurs after infusing 1 to 6 U of corticotropin over 8 hours. Peak cortisol levels are achieved within 1 hour of I.M. or rapid I.V. administration of corticotropin. Peak 17-hydroxycorticosteroid levels are achieved within 7 to 24 hours with zinc and 3 to 12 hours with the repository form.
- *Distribution:* Exact distribution of corticotropin is unknown, but it is removed rapidly from plasma by many tissues.
- *Metabolism:* Unknown.
- *Excretion:* Probably excreted by the kidneys. Drug's duration of action is about 2 hours with zinc form and up to 3 days with the repository form. Half-life is about 15 minutes.

Contraindications and precautions

Contraindicated in patients with peptic ulcer, scleroderma, osteoporosis, systemic fungal infections, ocular herpes simplex, peptic ulceration, heart failure, hypertension, sensitivity to pork and pork products, adrenocortical hyperfunction or primary insufficiency, or Cushing's syndrome. Also contraindicated in those who have had surgery recently.

Use cautiously in pregnant patients and in women of childbearing age. Also use cautiously in patients being immunized and in those with latent tuberculosis, hypothyroidism, cirrhosis, acute gouty arthritis, psychotic tendencies, renal insufficiency, diverticulitis, ulcerative colitis, thromboembolic disorders, seizures, uncontrolled hypertension, or myasthenia gravis.

Use with caution if surgery or emergency treatment is required.

Interactions

Concomitant use of corticotropin with *diuretics* may accentuate the electrolyte loss associated with *diuretic* therapy; use with *amphotericin B* or *carbonic anhydrase inhibitors* may cause severe hypokalemia. *Amphotericin B* also decreases adrenal responsiveness to corticotropin. Concurrent use with *insulin* or *oral antidiabetic agents* may require increased dosage of the *antidiabetic agent*; use with *hepatic enzyme-inducing agents* may increase corticotropin metabolism resulting from induction of hepatic microsomal enzymes; use with *cardiac glycosides* may increase the risk of arrhythmias or *digitalis* toxicity associated with hypokalemia; and use with *cortisone, hydrocortisone*, or *estrogens* may elevate plasma cortisol levels abnormally.

Because of ulcerogenic effects, drug should be used cautiously with *salicylates, NSAIDs*, and *indomethacin*.

Effects on diagnostic tests

Corticotropin therapy alters blood and urinary glucose levels; sodium and potassium levels; protein-bound iodine levels; radioactive iodine (^{131}I) uptake and T_3 uptake; total protein values; serum amylase, urine amino acid, serotonin, uric acid, calcium, and 17-ketosteroid levels; and leukocyte counts.

High plasma cortisol concentrations may be reported erroneously in patients receiving spironolactone, cortisone, or hydrocortisone when fluorometric analysis is used. This does not occur with the radioimmunoassay or competitive protein-binding method. However, therapy can be maintained with prednisone, dexamethasone, or betamethasone because they are not detectable by the fluorometric method.

Adverse reactions

CNS: ***seizures,*** *dizziness,* vertigo, ***increased intracranial pressure with papilledema,*** pseudotumor cerebri.
CV: hypertension, ***heart failure,*** necrotizing vasculitis, ***shock.***
EENT: cataracts, glaucoma.
GI: ***peptic ulceration with perforation and hemorrhage,*** pancreatitis, abdominal distention, ulcerative esophagitis, nausea, vomiting.
Skin: impaired wound healing; thin, fragile skin; petechiae; ecchymoses; facial erythema; diaphoresis; acne; hyperpigmentation; allergic reactions; hirsutism.
Other: muscle weakness, steroid myopathy, loss of muscle mass, osteoporosis, vertebral compression fractures, pneumonia, abscess and septic infection, cushingoid symptoms, suppression of growth in children, activation of latent diabetes mellitus, progressive increase in antibodies, loss of corticotropin stimulatory effect, hypersensitivity reac-

tions (rash, ***bronchospasm***), *sodium and fluid retention,* calcium and potassium loss, hypokalemic alkalosis, negative nitrogen balance, menstrual irregularities.

Overdose and treatment
Specific information unavailable. Treatment is supportive, as appropriate.

☑ Special considerations
• Cosyntropin is less antigenic and less likely to cause allergic reactions than corticotropin. However, allergic reactions occur rarely with corticotropin.
• In patient with suspected sensitivity to porcine proteins, skin testing should be performed. To decrease the risk of anaphylactic reaction in patient with limited adrenal reserves, 1 mg of dexamethasone may be given at midnight before the corticotropin test and 0.5 mg at start of test.
• Observe neonates of corticotropin-treated women for signs of hypoadrenalism.
• Counteract edema by low-sodium, high-potassium intake; nitrogen loss by high-protein diet; and psychotic symptoms by reducing corticotropin dosage or administering sedatives.
• Drug may mask signs of chronic disease and decrease host resistance and ability to localize infection.
• Insulin or oral antidiabetic dosages may need to be increased during corticotropin therapy.
• Monitor weight, fluid exchange, and resting blood pressure levels until minimal effective dosage is achieved.
• Refrigerate reconstituted product and use within 24 hours.
• If administering gel, warm it to room temperature, draw into large needle, and give slowly, deep I.M. with a 22G needle.
• Do not discontinue drug abruptly, especially after prolonged therapy. An Addisonian crisis may occur.

Patient education
• Warn patient that injection is painful.
• Tell patient to report marked fluid retention, muscle weakness, abdominal pain, seizures, or headache.
• Instruct patient not to be vaccinated during corticotropin therapy.
• Teach patient how to monitor for edema, and tell him about the need for fluid and salt restriction as appropriate.
• Warn patient not to stop drug except as prescribed. Tell him that abrupt discontinuation may provoke severe adverse reactions.

Geriatric use
• Use with caution in elderly patients because they are more likely to develop osteoporosis.

Pediatric use
• Use with caution because prolonged use of drug will inhibit skeletal growth. Intermittent administration is recommended.

Breast-feeding
• Safety has not been established. Because the potential for severe adverse reactions exists, benefits and risks must be weighed.

cortisone acetate
Cortone

Pharmacologic classification: glucocorticoid, mineralocorticoid
Therapeutic classification: anti-inflammatory, replacement therapy
Pregnancy risk category NR

How supplied
Available by prescription only
Tablets: 5 mg, 10 mg, 25 mg
Injection (I.M. use): 50 mg/ml suspension

Indications, route, and dosage
Adrenal insufficiency, allergy, inflammation
Adults: 25 to 300 mg P.O. or 20 to 300 mg I.M. daily or on alternate days. Doses highly individualized, depending on severity of disease.
Children: 20 to 300 mg/m² P.O. daily in four divided doses or 7 to 37.5 mg/m² I.M. once or twice daily. Dosage must be highly individualized.

Pharmacodynamics
Adrenocorticoid replacement: Cortisone acetate is an adrenocorticoid with both glucocorticoid and mineralocorticoid properties. A weak anti-inflammatory agent, drug has only about 80% of the anti-inflammatory activity of an equal weight of hydrocortisone. It is a potent mineralocorticoid, however, having twice the potency of prednisone. Cortisone (or hydrocortisone) is usually the drug of choice for replacement therapy in patients with adrenal insufficiency. It is usually not used for inflammatory or immunosuppressant activity because of the extremely large doses that must be used and because of the unwanted mineralocorticoid effects. Injectable form has a slow onset but a long duration of action. It is usually used only when the oral dosage form cannot be used.

Pharmacokinetics
• *Absorption:* Cortisone is absorbed readily after oral administration, with peak effects in about 1 to 2 hours. The suspension for injection has a variable onset of 24 to 48 hours.
• *Distribution:* Drug is distributed rapidly to muscle, liver, skin, intestines, and kidneys. Cortisone is extensively bound to plasma proteins (transcortin and albumin). Only the unbound portion is active. Cortisone is distributed into breast milk and through the placenta.
• *Metabolism:* Drug is metabolized in the liver to the active metabolite hydrocortisone, which in turn is metabolized to inactive glucuronide and sulfate metabolites. Duration of hypothalamic-pituitary-adrenal (HPA) axis suppression is 1.25 to 1.5 days.
• *Excretion:* Inactive metabolites and small amounts of unmetabolized drug are excreted by the kidneys. Insignificant quantities of the drug are also excret-

ed in feces. Biological half-life of cortisone is 8 to 12 hours.

Contraindications and precautions
Contraindicated in patients with hypersensitivity to drug or its ingredients or systemic fungal infections. Use cautiously in patients with renal disease, recent MI, GI ulcer, hypertension, osteoporosis, diabetes mellitus, hypothyroidism, cirrhosis, diverticulitis, ulcerative colitis, recent intestinal anastamosis, thromboembolic disorders, seizures, myasthenia gravis, heart failure, tuberculosis, ocular herpes, emotional instability, or psychotic tendencies.

Interactions
When used concomitantly, cortisone may decrease the effects of *oral anticoagulants* by unknown mechanisms (rarely); increase the metabolism of *isoniazid* and *salicylates*; and cause hyperglycemia, requiring dosage adjustment of *insulin* or *oral antidiabetic agents* in diabetic patients.

Use with *barbiturates, phenytoin,* or *rifampin* may cause decreased corticosteroid effects because of increased hepatic metabolism. Use with *cholestyramine, colestipol,* or *antacids* decreases cortisone's effect by adsorbing the corticosteroid, decreasing the amount absorbed.

Cortisone may enhance hypokalemia associated with *diuretic* or *amphotericin B* therapy. The hypokalemia may increase the risk of toxicity in patients concurrently receiving *cardiac glycosides.*

Concomitant use with *estrogens* may reduce the metabolism of cortisone by increasing the concentration of transcortin. The half-life of cortisone is then prolonged because of increased protein binding. Concomitant administration of *ulcerogenic drugs,* such as the *NSAIDs,* may increase the risk of GI ulceration.

Cortisone may have a diminished response to *toxoids* or inactivated vaccines.

Effects on diagnostic tests
Drug therapy suppresses reactions to skin tests; causes false-negative results in the nitroblue tetrazolium test for systemic bacterial infections; and decreases ^{131}I uptake and protein-bound iodine concentrations in thyroid function tests.

It may increase glucose and cholesterol levels; decrease serum potassium, calcium, thyroxine, and triiodothyronine levels; and increase urine glucose and calcium levels.

Adverse reactions
Most adverse reactions to corticosteroids are dose- or duration-dependent.
CNS: euphoria, insomnia, psychotic behavior, pseudotumor cerebri, vertigo, headache, paresthesia, ***seizures.***
CV: ***heart failure,*** hypertension, edema, ***arrhythmias,*** thrombophlebitis, ***thromboembolism.***
EENT: cataracts, glaucoma.
Endocrine: menstrual irregularities, cushingoid symptoms (moonface, buffalo hump, central obesity).
GI: *peptic ulcer,* GI irritation, increased appetite, pancreatitis, nausea, vomiting.
Skin: delayed wound healing, acne, various skin eruptions, atrophy at I.M. injection sites.
Other: muscle weakness, osteoporosis, hirsutism, susceptibility to infections; possible hypokalemia, hyperglycemia, and carbohydrate intolerance; growth suppression in children; ***acute adrenal insufficiency may follow increased stress (infection, surgery, trauma) or abrupt withdrawal after long-term therapy.***

After abrupt withdrawal: rebound inflammation, fatigue, weakness, arthralgia, fever, dizziness, lethargy, depression, fainting, orthostatic hypotension, dyspnea, anorexia, hypoglycemia. ***After prolonged use, sudden withdrawal may be fatal.***

Overdose and treatment
Acute ingestion, even in massive doses, is rarely a clinical problem. Toxic signs and symptoms rarely occur if the drug is used for less than 3 weeks, even at large dosage ranges. However, chronic use causes adverse physiologic effects, including suppression of the HPA axis, cushingoid appearance, muscle weakness, and osteoporosis.

☑ Special considerations
Recommendations for use of cortisone and for care and teaching of patients during therapy are the same as those for all *systemic adrenocorticoids.*

Patient education
- Inform patient of potential adverse reactions.

Pediatric use
- Chronic use of cortisone in children and adolescents may delay growth and maturation.

cosyntropin
Cortrosyn

Pharmacologic classification: anterior pituitary hormone
Therapeutic classification: diagnostic
Pregnancy risk category C

How supplied
Available by prescription only
Injection: 0.25 mg/vial

Indications, route, and dosage
Diagnostic test of adrenocortical function
Adults and children age 2 and older: 0.25 to 0.75 mg I.M. or I.V. (unless label prohibits I.V. administration) between blood samplings. To administer as I.V. infusion, dilute 0.25 mg in D_5W or 0.9% NaCl solution, and infuse over 6 hours (40 mcg/hour).
Children under age 2: 0.125 mg I.M. or I.V.

Pharmacodynamics
Diagnostic action: Cosyntropin is used to test adrenal function. Drug binds with a specific receptor in the adrenal cell plasma membrane to initiate synthesis of its entire spectrum of hormones, one of which is cortisol. In patients with primary adrenocortical insufficiency, cosyntropin does not increase plasma cortisol levels significantly.

Pharmacokinetics

- *Absorption:* Drug is inactivated by the proteolytic enzymes in the GI tract. After I.M. administration, cosyntropin is absorbed rapidly. After rapid I.V. administration in patients with normal adrenocortical function, plasma cortisol levels begin to rise within 5 minutes and double within 15 to 30 minutes. Peak levels occur within 1 hour after I.M. or rapid I.V. administration and begin to decrease in 2 to 4 hours.
- *Distribution:* Not fully understood, but drug is removed rapidly from plasma by many tissues.
- *Metabolism:* Unknown.
- *Excretion:* Probably excreted by the kidneys.

Contraindications and precautions

Contraindicated in patients with hypersensitivity to drug.

Interactions

Concomitant use of cosyntropin with *cortisone, hydrocortisone*, or *estrogens* may cause abnormally elevated plasma cortisol levels. High plasma cortisol levels may be reported erroneously in patients receiving *spironolactone, cortisone*, or *hydrocortisone* when fluorometric analysis is used. This does not occur with the radioimmunoassay or competitive protein-binding method. However, therapy can be maintained with *prednisone, dexamethasone*, or *betamethasone* because these are not detectable by the fluorometric method.

Effects on diagnostic tests

Drug therapy alters blood glucose levels.

Adverse reactions

CNS: ***seizures,*** dizziness, vertigo, ***increased intracranial pressure with papilledema,*** pseudotumor cerebri.
EENT: cataracts, glaucoma.
GI: peptic ulcer, ***pancreatitis,*** abdominal distension, ulcerative esophagitis, nausea, vomiting.
Skin: pruritus; impaired wound healing; thin, fragile skin; petechiae; ecchymoses; facial erythema; diaphoresis; acne; hyperpigmentation; hirsutism.
Other: flushing, hypersensitivity reactions, muscle weakness, steroid myopathy, loss of muscle mass, osteoporosis, vertebral compression, fractures, cushingoid symptoms, menstrual irregularities.

Overdose and treatment

Acute overdose probably requires no therapy other than symptomatic treatment and supportive care, as appropriate.

☑ Special considerations

- More cortisol is secreted if dosage is given slowly, not rapidly I.V.
- Cosyntropin is less antigenic than corticotropin and less likely to produce allergic reactions.
- For rapid screening, plasma cortisol levels are determined prior to and 30 minutes after administration of 0.25 mg I.M. or I.V. injection over 2 minutes. Some clinicians prefer plasma cortisol concentration determinations at 60 minutes after injection of cosyntropin.
- Determine if patient is taking medications containing spironolactone, cortisone, hydrocortisone, or estrogen.
- Reconstitute powder by adding 1 ml of 0.9% NaCl solution to 0.25-mg vial to yield a solution containing 0.25 mg/ml.
- Reconstituted solution remains stable at room temperature for 24 hours or for 21 days at 36° to 46° F (2° to 8° C).
- A normal response to cosyntropin includes morning control plasma cortisol level exceeding 5 mcg/100 ml plasma; 30 minutes after the injection, cortisol levels rise by 7 mcg/100 ml above control; 30 minute cortisol levels exceed 18 mcg/100 ml.

Patient education

- Inform patient taking spironolactone, cortisone, hydrocortisone, or estrogen that these medications may interfere with test results.

---

co-trimoxazole (trimethoprim-sulfamethoxazole)

Apo-Sulfatrim*, Bactrim, Bactrim DS, Bactrim I.V., Cotrim, Cotrim D.S., Novo-Trimel*, Roubac*, Septra, Septra DS, Septra I.V., SMZ-TMP, Sulfatrim

Pharmacologic classification: sulfonamide and folate antagonist
Therapeutic classification: antibiotic
Pregnancy risk category C

How supplied

Available by prescription only
Tablets: trimethoprim 80 mg and sulfamethoxazole 400 mg; trimethoprim 160 mg and sulfamethoxazole 800 mg
Suspension: trimethoprim 40 mg and sulfamethoxazole 200 mg/5 ml
Injectable: trimethoprim 80 mg and sulfamethoxazole 400 mg/5 ml

Indications, route, and dosage

Urinary tract infections and shigellosis
Adults: 1 double-strength or 2 regular-strength tablets P.O. q 12 hours for 10 to 14 days or 5 days for shigellosis. Or, 8 to 10 mg/kg (based on trimethoprim) I.V. daily given in 2 to 4 equally divided doses for up to 14 days (5 days for shigellosis). Maximum daily dose, 960 mg.
Children over age 2 months: 8 mg/kg trimethoprim and 40 mg/kg sulfamethoxazole P.O. daily in two divided doses q 12 hours (10 days for urinary tract infections; 5 days for shigellosis).
Otitis media
Children over age 2 months: 8 mg/kg trimethoprim and 40 mg/kg sulfamethoxazole P.O. daily, in two divided doses q 12 hours for 10 days.
Pneumocystis carnii *pneumonitis*
Adults and children over age 2 months: 15 to 20 mg/kg trimethoprim and 75 to 100 mg/kg sulfamethoxazole P.O. daily, in equally divided doses, q 6 to 8 hours for 14 to 21 days.

Chronic bronchitis
Adults: 1 double-strength or 2 regular-strength tablets q 12 hours for 14 days.
Traveler's diarrhea
Adults: 1 double-strength or 2 regular-strength tablets q 12 hours for 5 days.

Note: For the following unlabeled uses, dosages refer to oral trimethoprim (as co-trimoxazole).

◊ ***Septic agranulocytosis***
Adults: 2.5 mg/kg I.V. q.i.d.; for prophylaxis, 80 to 160 mg b.i.d.
◊ ***Nocardia infection***
Adults: 640 mg P.O. daily for 7 months.
◊ ***Pharyngeal gonococcal infections***
Adults: 720 mg P.O. daily for 5 days.
◊ ***Chancroid***
Adults: 160 mg P.O. b.i.d for 7 days.
◊ ***Pertussis***
Adults: 320 mg P.O. daily in two divided doses.
Children: 40 mg/kg/day P.O. in two divided doses.
◊ ***Cholera***
Adults: 160 mg P.O. b.i.d for 3 days.
Children: 5 mg/kg P.O. b.i.d for 3 days.
◊ ***Isosporiasis***
Adults: 160 mg P.O. q.i.d. for 10 days, followed by 160 mg b.i.d. for 3 weeks.

✦ ***Dosage adjustment.*** In patients with impaired renal function, adjust dose or frequency of administration of parenteral form according to degree of renal impairment, severity of infection, and susceptibility of organism.

Creatinine clearance (ml/min/1.73 m²)	Dosage
> 30	Usual regimen
15 to 30	½ usual regimen
< 15	Use is not recommended

Pharmacodynamics

Antibacterial action: Co-trimoxazole is generally bactericidal; it acts by sequential blockade of folic acid enzymes in the synthesis pathway. The sulfamethoxazole component inhibits formation of dihydrofolic acid from para-aminobenzoic (PABA), whereas trimethoprim inhibits dihydrofolate reductase. Both drugs block folic acid synthesis, preventing bacterial cell synthesis of essential nucleic acids.

Co-trimoxazole is effective against *Escherichia coli, Klebsiella, Enterobacter, Proteus mirabilis, Haemophilus influenzae, Streptococcus pneumoniae, Staphylococcus aureus, Acinetobacter, Salmonella, Shigella,* and *Pneumocystis carinii.*

Pharmacokinetics

- *Absorption:* Co-trimoxazole is well absorbed from the GI tract after oral administration; peak serum levels occur at 1 to 4 hours.
- *Distribution:* Co-trimoxazole is distributed widely into body tissues and fluids, including middle ear fluid, prostatic fluid, bile, aqueous humor, and CSF. Protein binding is 44% for trimethoprim, 70% for sulfamethoxazole. Co-trimoxazole crosses the placenta.
- *Metabolism:* Co-trimoxazole is metabolized by the liver.
- *Excretion:* Both components of co-trimoxazole are excreted primarily in urine by glomerular filtration and renal tubular secretion; some drug is excreted in breast milk. Trimethoprim's plasma half-life in patients with normal renal function is 8 to 11 hours, extended to 26 hours in severe renal dysfunction; sulfamethoxazole's plasma half-life is normally 10 to 13 hours, extended to 30 to 40 hours in severe renal dysfunction. Hemodialysis removes some co-trimoxazole.

Contraindications and precautions

Contraindicated in patients with hypersensitivity to trimethoprim or sulfonamides, severe renal impairment (creatinine clearance below 15 ml/minute), or porphyria; in those with megaloblastic anemia caused by folate deficiency; in pregnant women at term; in breast-feeding women; and in children under 2 months.

Use cautiously in patients with impaired renal or hepatic function, severe allergies, severe bronchial asthma, G6PD deficiency, or blood dyscrasia.

Interactions

Co-trimoxazole may inhibit hepatic metabolism of *oral anticoagulants*, displacing them from binding sites and enhancing anticoagulant effects. Concomitant use of co-trimoxazole with *PABA* antagonizes sulfonamide effects. Concomitant use with *oral sulfonylureas* enhances their hypoglycemic effects, probably by displacement of *sulfonylureas* from protein-binding sites.

Phenytoin's hepatic clearance may be decreased (27%) and the half-life prolonged (39%). Concomitant use with *methotrexate* can displace it from plasma-binding sites and increase concentrations. Serum levels of *zidovudine* may be increased due to reduced renal clearance. A decreased therapeutic effect of *cyclosporine* and an increased risk of nephrotoxicity have occurred.

Effects on diagnostic tests

Trimethoprim can interfere with serum methotrexate assay as determined by the competitive binding protein technique. No inteference occurs if radioimmunoassay is used.

Co-trimoxazole may elevate liver function test results; it may decrease serum concentration levels of erythrocytes, platelets, or leukocytes.

The effects of cyclosporine may be decreased and nephrotoxicity may be increased.

Adverse reactions

CNS: headache, mental depression, aseptic meningitis, tinnitus, apathy, ***seizures,*** hallucinations, ataxia, nervousness, fatigue, muscle weakness, vertigo, insomnia.
GI: *nausea, vomiting, diarrhea,* abdominal pain, anorexia, stomatitis, ***pancreatitis,*** pseudomembranous colitis.
GU: *toxic nephrosis with oliguria and anuria,* crystalluria, hematuria, interstitial nephritis.

Hematologic: ***agranulocytosis, aplastic anemia,*** megaloblastic anemia, ***thrombocytopenia,*** leukopenia, ***hemolytic anemia.***
Hepatic: jaundice, ***hepatic necrosis.***
Respiratory: pulmonary infiltrates.
Skin: ***erythema multiforme (Stevens-Johnson syndrome),*** *generalized skin eruptions,* ***epidermal necrolysis, exfoliative dermatitis,*** photosensitivity, urticaria, pruritus.
Other: hypersensitivity reactions (*serum sickness, drug fever,* ***anaphylaxis***), thrombophlebitis, arthralgia, myalgia.

Overdose and treatment

Clinical signs of overdose include mental depression, drowsiness, anorexia, jaundice, confusion, headache, nausea, vomiting, diarrhea, facial swelling, slight elevations in liver function test results, and bone marrow depression.

Treat by emesis or gastric lavage, followed by supportive care (correction of acidosis, forced oral fluid, and I.V. fluids). Treatment of renal failure may be required; transfuse appropriate blood products in severe hematologic toxicity; use folinic acid to rescue bone marrow. Hemodialysis has limited ability to remove co-trimoxazole. Peritoneal dialysis is not effective.

☑ Special considerations

Besides those relevant to all *sulfonamides,* consider the following recommendations.

- Co-trimoxazole has been used effectively to treat chronic bacterial prostatitis and as prophylaxis against recurrent urinary tract infection in women and traveler's diarrhea.
- For I.V. use, dilute infusion in D_5W. Do not mix with other drugs. Do not administer by rapid infusion or bolus injection. Infuse slowly over 60 to 90 minutes. Change infusion site every 48 to 72 hours.
- I.V. infusion must be diluted before use. Each 5 ml should be added to 125 ml D_5W. Do not refrigerate solution; diluted solutions must be used within 6 hours. A dilution of 5 ml per 75 ml D_5W may be prepared for patients requiring fluid restriction, but these solutions should be used within 2 hours.
- Check solution carefully for precipitate before starting infusion. Do not use solution containing a precipitate.
- Assess I.V. site for signs of phlebitis or infiltration.
- Shake oral suspension thoroughly before administering.
- Note that DS means double-strength.

Patient education

- Inform patient of potential adverse reactions.

Pediatric use

- Drug is not recommended for infants under age 2 months.

Geriatric use

- In elderly patients, diminished renal function may prolong half-life. Such patients also have an increased risk of adverse reactions.

Breast-feeding

- Drug is not recommended in breast-feeding women.

cromolyn sodium

Gastrocrom, Intal Aerosol Spray, Intal Nebulizer Solution, Nasalcrom, Opticrom

Pharmacologic classification: chromone derivative
Therapeutic classification: mast cell stabilizer, antiasthmatic
Pregnancy risk category B

How supplied

Available by prescription only
Capsules: 100 mg
Aerosol: 800 mcg/metered spray
Solution: 20 mg/2 ml for nebulization
Ophthalmic solution: 4%
Nasal solution: 5.2 mg/metered spray (40 mg/ml)
Powder for inhalation: 20 mg (in capsules)

Indications, route, and dosage

Adjunct in treatment of severe perennial bronchial asthma
Adults and children over age 5: 2 inhalations q.i.d. at regular intervals; aqueous solution administered through a nebulizer, 1 ampule q.i.d; or, 1 capsule (20 mg) of powder for inhalation q.i.d.
Prevention and treatment of allergic rhinitis
Adults and children age 6 and over: 1 spray (5.2 mg) of nasal solution in each nostril t.i.d or q.i.d. May give up to six times daily.
Prevention of exercise-induced bronchospasm
Adults and children over age 5: 2 metered sprays using inhaler, or 1 capsule (20 mg) of powder for inhalation no more than 1 hour before anticipated exercise.

Inhalation of 20 mg of oral inhalation solution may be used in adults or children age 2 and over. Repeat inhalation as required for protection during long exercise.
Allergic ocular disorders (giant papillary conjunctivitis, vernal keratoconjunctivitis, vernal keratitis, allergic keratoconjunctivitis)
Adults and children over age 4: Instill 1 to 2 drops in each eye four to six times daily at regular intervals. One drop contains approximately 1.6 mg cromolyn sodium.
Systemic mastocytosis
Adults: 200 mg P.O. q.i.d.
Children age 2 to 12: 100 mg P.O. q.i.d.
Children under age 2: 20 mg/kg daily P.O. divided in four equal doses.
◇ ***Food allergy, inflammatory bowel disease***
Adults: 200 mg P.O. q.i.d. 15 to 20 minutes before meals.

Pharmacodynamics

Antiasthmatic action: Cromolyn prevents release of the mediators of Type I allergic reactions, including histamine and slow-reacting substance of anaphylaxis (SRS-A), from sensitized mast cells after the antigen-antibody union has taken place. Cromolyn does not inhibit the binding of the IgE to the mast cell nor the interaction between the cell-bound IgE and the specific antigen. It does inhibit the release of substances (such as histamine and SRS-A) in response to the IgE binding to the mast cell. The main site of action occurs locally on the lung mucosa, nasal mucosa, and eyes.

Bronchodilating action: Besides the mast cell stabilization, recent evidence suggests that drug may have a bronchodilating effect by an unknown mechanism. Comparative studies have shown cromolyn and theophylline to be equally efficacious but less effective than orally inhaled $beta_2$-adrenergic agonists in preventing this bronchospasm.

Ocular antiallergy action: Cromolyn inhibits the degranulation of sensitized mast cells that occurs after exposure to specific antigens, preventing the release of histamine and SRS-A.

Cromolyn has no direct anti-inflammatory, vasoconstrictor, antihistamine, antiserotonin, or corticosteroid-like properties.

Cromolyn dissolved in water and given orally has been found to be effective in managing food allergy, inflammatory bowel disease (Crohn's disease, ulcerative colitis), and systemic mastocytosis.

Pharmacokinetics

- *Absorption:* Only 0.5% to 2% of an oral dose is absorbed. The amount reaching the lungs depends on patient's ability to use inhaler correctly, amount of bronchoconstriction, and size or presence of mucous plugs. The degree of absorption depends on method of administration; most absorption occurs with the aerosol via metered-dose inhaler, and least occurs with the administration of the solution via power-operated nebulizer. Less than 7% of an intranasal dose of cromolyn as a solution is absorbed systemically. Only minimal absorption (0.03%) of an ophthalmic dose occurs after instillation into the eye. Absorption half-life from the lung is 1 hour. A plasma concentration of 9 ng/ml can be achieved 15 minutes after following a 20-mg dose.
- *Distribution:* Cromolyn does not cross most biological membranes because it is ionized and lipid-insoluble at the body's pH. Less than 0.1% of a cromolyn dose crosses to the placenta; it is not known if drug is distributed into breast milk.
- *Metabolism:* None significant.
- *Excretion:* Excreted unchanged in urine (50%) and bile (approximately 50%). Small amounts may be excreted in the feces or exhaled. Elimination half-life is 81 minutes.

Contraindications and precautions

Contraindicated in patients experiencing acute asthma attacks or status asthmaticus and in patients with hypersensitivity to drug. Use inhalation form cautiously in patients with cardiac disease or arrhythmias.

Interactions

Animal studies have shown adverse fetal effects when administered parenterally in high doses with high-dose *isoproterenol.*

Effects on diagnostic tests

None reported.

Adverse reactions

CNS: dizziness, headache.
EENT: *irritated throat and trachea,* nasal congestion, pharyngeal irritation, *sneezing,* nasal burning and irritation, epistaxis.
GI: nausea, esophagitis, abdominal pain.
GU: dysuria, urinary frequency.
Respiratory: ***bronchospasm*** (after inhalation of dry powder), *cough,* wheezing, *eosinophilic pneumonia.*
Skin: rash, urticaria.
Other: joint swelling and pain, lacrimation, swollen parotid gland, ***angioedema,*** bad taste in mouth.

Overdose and treatment

No information available.

☑ Special considerations

- Monitor pulmonary status before and immediately after therapy.
- Bronchospasm or cough occasionally occur after inhalation and may require stopping therapy. Prior bronchodilation may help but it may still be necessary to stop the cromolyn therapy.
- Asthma symptoms may recur if cromolyn dosage is reduced below the recommended dosage.
- Use reduced dosage in patients with impaired renal or hepatic function.
- Eosinophilic pneumonia or pulmonary infiltrates with eosinophilia requires stopping drug.
- Nasal solution may cause nasal stinging or sneezing immediately after instillation of drug but this reaction rarely requires discontinuation of drug.
- Watch for recurrence of asthmatic symptoms when corticosteroids are also used. Use only when acute episode has been controlled, airway is cleared, and patient is able to inhale.
- Perform pulmonary function tests to confirm significant bronchodilator-reversible component of airway obstruction in patients considered for cromolyn therapy.
- Protect oral solution and ophthalmic solution from direct sunlight.
- Therapeutic effects may not be seen for 2 to 4 weeks after initiating therapy.

Patient education

- Teach correct use of metered-dose inhaler: exhale completely before placing mouthpiece between lips, then inhale deeply and slowly with steady, even breath; remove inhaler from mouth, hold breath for 5 to 10 seconds, and exhale.
- Urge patient to call if drug causes wheezing or coughing.
- Instruct patient with asthma or seasonal or perennial allergic rhinitis to administer drug at regular intervals to ensure clinical effectiveness.
- Advise patient that gargling and rinsing mouth after administration can help reduce mouth dryness.
- Tell patient taking prescribed adrenocorticoids to continue taking them during therapy, if appropriate.

• Instruct patient who uses a bronchodilator inhaler to administer dose about 5 minutes before taking cromolyn (unless otherwise indicated); explain that this step helps reduce adverse reactions.

Pediatric use
• Cromolyn use in children under age 5 is limited to the inhalation route of administration. The safety of the nebulizer solution in children under age 2 has not been established. Safety of nasal solution in children under age 6 has not been established.

crotaline (Crotalidae) antivenin, polyvalent

Pharmacologic classification: antivenin
Therapeutic classification: snake antivenin
Pregnancy risk category C

How supplied
Available by prescription only
Injection: combination package—one vial of lyophilized serum, one vial of diluent (10 ml bacteriostatic water for injection), and one 1-ml vial of normal horse serum (diluted 1:10) for sensitivity testing

Indications, route, and dosage
Crotalid (pit viper) bites, including those from rattlesnakes, copperheads, and cotton-mouth moccasins
Adults and children: The following initial doses (given I.M. or I.V.) are recommended (based on level of envenomation): minimal—2 to 4 vials; moderate—5 to 9 vials; severe—10 to 15 or more vials. Administer I.M. into large muscle mass—preferably in gluteal area. Never inject into finger or toe.

Subsequent dosages are based on the patient's response. The smaller the patient, the larger the initial dose. The amount of antivenin given to a child is not based on weight. Children may require a larger dose than adults.

Note: I.V. route is preferred and is mandatory if shock is present.

Pharmacodynamics
Antivenin action: Crotaline antivenin neutralizes and binds venom.

Pharmacokinetics
• *Absorption:* When given I.M., crotaline antivenin may not reach maximum blood levels until about 8 hours after administration.
• *Distribution:* No information available.
• *Metabolism:* No information available.
• *Excretion:* No information available.

Contraindications and precautions
Contraindicated in patients hypersensitive to drug and in those with history of allergy to horses.

Interactions
Concomitant use of crotaline antivenin with *corticosteroids* may mask the severity of hypovolemia in moderate to severe envenomation and may have little, if any, effect on the local tissue response to snake venoms. However, *corticosteroids* may be administered, if necessary, to treat immediate or delayed allergic reactions to antivenin.

Effects on diagnostic tests
None reported.

Adverse reactions
Systemic: *hypersensitivity reactions,* ***anaphylaxis****, serum sickness,* lymphadenopathy, arthralgia, fever.
Other: pain, erythema, urticaria.

Overdose and treatment
No information available.

☑ Special considerations
• Immobilize patient immediately. Splint the bitten extremity.
• Obtain a thorough patient history of allergies, especially to horses and horse immune serum, and previous reactions to immunizations.
• Early use of antivenin (within 4 hours of the bite) is recommended for best results.
• Product is derived from horses immunized with *Crotalidae* venom. Therefore, test patient for sensitivity (against a control of 0.9% NaCl solution in opposing extremity) before giving it. Give 0.02 to 0.03 ml of the 1:10 dilution of horse serum (provided) intradermally. Read results after 5 to 30 minutes.
Positive reaction: wheal with or without pseudopodia and surrounding erythema. If sensitivity test is positive, follow desensitization schedule.
• Epinephrine solution 1:1,000 should be available to treat allergic reactions.
• Pregnancy is not a contraindication to use of crotaline antivenin when indicated.
• Monitor circumference of bitten area before and after antivenin administration.
• Find out when patient received last tetanus immunization; a booster may be indicated.
• Type and crossmatch as soon as possible because hemolysis from venom prevents accurate crossmatching.
• Monitor fluid intake and urine output.
• Watch patient carefully for delayed allergic reactions or relapse.
• This painful snakebite requires supportive, symptomatic, and pharmacologic management.
• Monitor vital signs at frequent intervals (every 30 minutes) until symptoms subside (usually in 1 to 3 hours). Also monitor hemoglobin and hematocrit levels, CBC with differential, platelets, coagulation studies (PT and partial thromboplastin time), bleeding time, chemistry panel, and urinalysis.
• Antibiotic therapy may be necessary for wound infection.
• Store at room temperature. Do not freeze. Use dilutions within 12 hours and reconstituted solutions within 48 hours.

Patient education

- Tell patient that he may experience allergic reactions (such as rash, joint swelling or pain, fever, or difficulty breathing) because this product is derived from an animal source, namely horses. Explain that he will be monitored closely and given medication, as needed, to ease such effects.
- Warn patient that delayed reactions to antivenin may occur up to 24 days after its administration. Have patient call if he experiences such symptoms as fever, general malaise, swollen lymph nodes, edema, nausea and vomiting, or joint and muscle pain.

Breast-feeding

- Patient should discontinue breast-feeding until effects of venom have subsided and if symptoms of serum sickness develop.

crotamiton

Eurax

Pharmacologic classification: synthetic chloroformate salt
Therapeutic classification: scabicide, antipruritic
Pregnancy risk category C

How supplied

Available by prescription only
Cream: 10%
Lotion: 10% (emollient base)

Indications, route, and dosage

Scabicide
Adults: Wash thoroughly and scrub away loose scales, then towel dry; massage drug onto skin of the entire body from the neck to the toes (with special attention to skin folds, creases, and interdigital spaces). Repeat application in 24 hours. Take a cleansing bath 48 hours after the final application. Repeat if necessary.
Antipruritic
Adults: Massage gently into affected areas until medication is completely absorbed. Repeat p.r.n.

Pharmacodynamics

Scabicidal/antipruritic action: Mechanisms of drug action are unknown. Crotamiton is toxic to the parasitic mite *Sarcoptes scabiei.*

Pharmacokinetics

Absorption, distribution, metabolism, and excretion of crotamiton have not been reported.

Contraindications and precautions

Contraindicated when skin is raw or inflamed and in patients hypersensitive to drug.

Interactions

None reported.

Effects on diagnostic test

None reported.

Adverse reactions

Skin: *irritation.*

Overdose and treatment

Discontinue therapy.

☑ Special considerations

- Avoid applying crotamiton to the face, eyes, mucous membranes, or urethral meatus.
- Patients may require isolation and special care of linens until treatment is complete.
- If primary irritation or hypersensitivity occurs, discontinue treatment and remove drug with soap and water.
- Treatment may be repeated 7 to 10 days after a successful course if new lesions appear.

Patient education

- Inform patient to machine wash all clothing and bed linen used by him in hot water and dry in hot dryer or dry-clean.
- Tell patient to reapply drug if accidentally washed off; avoid overuse.
- Advise patient that pruritus may persist after treatment.

Pediatric use

- Safety and effectiveness have not been established in children.

cyanocobalamin (vitamin B_{12})

Bedoz,* Cobex, Crystamine, Cyanoject, Cyomin, Rubesol-1000, Rubramin PC, Vibal

hydroxocobalamin (vitamin B_{12})

Hydrobexan, Hydro-Cobex, LA-12

Pharmacologic classification: water-soluble vitamin
Therapeutic classification: vitamin, nutrition supplement
Pregnancy risk category C (parenteral)

How supplied

Available by prescription only
Injection: 30-ml vials (30 mcg/ml, 100 mcg/ml, 120 mcg/ml with benzyl alcohol, 1,000 mcg/ml, 1,000 mcg/ml with benzyl alcohol), 10-ml vials (100 mcg/ml, 100 mcg/ml with benzyl alcohol, 1,000 mcg/ml, 1,000 mcg/ml with benzyl alcohol, 1,000 mcg/ml with methyl and propyl parabens), 5-ml vials (1,000 mcg/ml with benzyl alcohol), 1-ml vials (1,000 mcg/ml with benzyl alcohol), 1-ml unimatic (1,000 mcg/ml with benzyl alcohol)
Tablets: 25 mcg, 50 mcg, 100 mcg, 250 mcg, 500 mcg, 1,000 mcg

Indications, route, and dosage

Vitamin B_{12} deficiency from any cause except malabsorption related to pernicious anemia or other GI disease
Adults: 25 mcg P.O. daily as dietary supplement, or 30 to 100 mcg S.C. or I.M. daily for 5 to 10 days,

depending on severity of deficiency. (I.M. route recommended for pernicious anemia.)

Maintenance dosage is 100 to 200 mcg I.M. monthly. For subsequent prophylaxis, advise adequate nutrition and daily RDA vitamin B_{12} supplements.

Children: 100 mcg I.M. or S.C. over the course of 2 or more weeks to maximum dose of 1-5 mg. Maintenance dose, 60 mcg/month I.M. or S.C.

Diagnostic test for vitamin B_{12} deficiency without concealing folate deficiency in patients with megaloblastic anemias

Adults and children: 1 mcg I.M. daily for 10 days with diet low in vitamin B_{12} and folate. Reticulocytosis between days 3 and 10 confirms diagnosis of vitamin B_{12} deficiency.

Schilling test flushing dose

Adults and children: 1,000 mcg I.M. in a single dose.

Pharmacodynamics

Nutritional action: Vitamin B_{12} can be converted to coenzyme B_{12} in tissues and, as such, is essential for conversion of methyl-malonate to succinate and synthesis of methionine from homocystine, a reaction that also requires folate. Without coenzyme B_{12}, folate deficiency occurs. Vitamin B_{12} is also associated with fat and carbohydrate metabolism and protein synthesis. Cells characterized by rapid division (epithelial cells, bone marrow, and myeloid cells) appear to have the greatest requirement for vitamin B_{12}.

Vitamin B_{12} deficiency may cause megaloblastic anemia, GI lesions, and neurologic damage; it begins with an inability to produce myelin followed by gradual degeneration of the axon and nerve. Parenteral administration of vitamin B_{12} completely reverses the megaloblastic anemia and GI symptoms of vitamin B_{12} deficiency.

Pharmacokinetics

- *Absorption:* After oral administration, vitamin B_{12} is absorbed irregularly from the distal small intestine. Vitamin B_{12} is protein-bound, and this bond must be split by proteolysis and gastric acid before absorption. Absorption depends on sufficient intrinsic factor and calcium. Vitamin B_{12} is inadequate in malabsorptive states and in pernicious anemia. Vitamin B_{12} is absorbed rapidly from I.M. and S.C. injection sites; the plasma level peaks within 1 hour. After oral administration of doses below 3 mcg, peak plasma levels are not reached for 8 to 12 hours.
- *Distribution:* Vitamin B_{12} is distributed into the liver, bone marrow, and other tissues, including the placenta. At birth, the vitamin B_{12} concentration in neonates is three to five times that in the mother. Vitamin B_{12} is distributed into breast milk in concentrations approximately equal to the maternal vitamin B_{12} concentration. Unlike cyanocobalamin, hydroxocobalamin is absorbed more slowly parenterally and may be taken up by the liver in larger quantities; it also produces a greater increase in serum cobalamin levels and less urinary excretion.
- *Metabolism:* Cyanocobalamin and hydroxocobalamin are metabolized in the liver.
- *Excretion:* In healthy persons receiving only dietary vitamin B_{12}, approximately 3 to 8 mcg of the vitamin is secreted into the GI tract daily, mainly from bile, and all but about 1 mcg is reabsorbed; less than 0.25 mcg is usually excreted in the urine daily. When vitamin B_{12} is administered in amounts that exceed the binding capacity of plasma, the liver, and other tissues, it is free in the blood for urinary excretion.

Contraindications and precautions

Contraindicated in patients hypersensitive to vitamin B_{12} or cobalt and in patients with early Leber's disease. Use cautiously in anemic patients with coexisting cardiac, pulmonary, or hypertensive disease and in those with severe vitamin B_{12}–dependent deficiencies.

Interactions

Concomitant use of the following drugs decreases vitamin B_{12} absorption from the GI tract: *aminoglycosides, colchicine, extended-release potassium preparations, aminosalicylic acid and its salts, anticonvulsants, cobalt irradiation* of the small bowel, and *excessive alcohol intake.* Concurrent administration of *colchicine* may increase *neomycin*-induced malabsorption of vitamin B_{12}. Large amounts of *ascorbic acid* should not be administered within 1 hour of taking vitamin B_{12} because *ascorbic acid* may destroy vitamin B_{12}. In patients with pernicious anemia, vitamin B_{12} absorption and intrinsic factor secretion may be increased. Vitamin B_{12} and *chloramphenicol* should not be given concurrently because of an antagonized hematopoietic response. Careful monitoring of the hematologic response and alternate therapy is necessary.

Effects on diagnostic tests

Vitamin B_{12} therapy may cause false-positive results for intrinsic factor antibodies, which are present in the blood of half of all patients with pernicious anemia.

Methotrexate, pyrimethamine, and most anti-infectives invalidate diagnostic blood assays for vitamin B_{12}.

Adverse reactions

CV: peripheral vascular thrombosis, pulmonary edema, heart failure.

GI: transient diarrhea.

Skin: itching, transitory exanthema, urticaria.

Other: ***anaphylaxis, anaphylactoid reactions*** (with parenteral administration); pain, burning (at S.C. or I.M. injection sites).

Overdose and treatment

Not applicable. Even in large doses, vitamin B_{12} is usually nontoxic.

☑ Special considerations

- Recommended RDA for vitamin B_{12} is 0.3 mcg in infants to 2 mcg in adults, as follows:

Infants up to age 6 months: 0.3 mcg
Children age 6 months to 1 year: 0.5 mcg
Children age 1 to 3: 0.7 mcg
Children age 4 to 6: 1 mcg

Children age 7 to 10: 1.4 mcg
Children age 11 to adult: 2 mcg
Pregnant women: 2.2 mcg
Breast-feeding women: 2.6 mcg

- Determine patient's diet and drug history, including patterns of alcohol use, to identify poor nutritional habits.
- Oral solution should be administered promptly after mixing with fruit juice. Ascorbic acid causes instability of vitamin B_{12}.
- Administer oral vitamin B_{12} with meals to increase absorption.
- Monitor bowel function because regularity is essential for consistent absorption of oral preparations.
- Do not mix the parenteral form with dextrose solutions, alkaline or strongly acidic solutions, or oxidizing and reducing agents, because anaphylactic reactions may occur with I.V. use. Check compatibility with pharmacist.
- Parenteral therapy is preferred for patients with pernicious anemia because oral administration may be unreliable. In patients with neurologic complications, prolonged inadequate oral therapy may lead to permanent spinal cord damage. Oral therapy is appropriate for mild conditions without neurologic signs and for those patients who refuse or are sensitive to the parenteral form.
- Monitor vital signs in patients with cardiac disease and those receiving parenteral vitamin B_{12}. Watch for symptoms of pulmonary edema, which tend to develop early in therapy.
- Patients with a history of sensitivities and those suspected of being sensitive to vitamin B_{12} should receive an intradermal test dose before therapy begins. Sensitization to vitamin B_{12} may develop after as many as 8 years of treatment.
- Expect therapeutic response to occur within 48 hours; it is measured by laboratory values and effect on fatigue, GI symptoms, anorexia, pallid or yellow complexion, glossitis, distaste for meat, dyspnea on exertion, palpitation, neurologic degeneration (paresthesia, loss of vibratory and position sense and deep reflexes, incoordination), psychotic behavior, anosmia, and visual disturbances.
- Therapeutic response to vitamin B_{12} may be impaired by concurrent infection, uremia, folic acid or iron deficiency, or drugs having bone marrow suppressant effects. Large doses of vitamin B_{12} may improve folate-deficient megaloblastic anemia.
- Expect reticulocyte concentration to rise in 3 to 4 days, peak in 5 to 8 days, and then gradually decline as erythrocyte count and hemoglobin rise to normal levels (in 4 to 6 weeks).
- Monitor potassium levels during the first 48 hours, especially in patients with pernicious anemia or megaloblastic anemia. Potassium supplements may be required. Conversion to normal erythropoiesis increases erythrocyte potassium requirement and can result in fatal hypokalemia in these patients.
- Patients with mild peripheral neurologic defects may respond to concomitant physical therapy. Usually, neurologic damage that does not improve after 12 to 18 months of therapy is considered irreversible. Severe vitamin B_{12} deficiency that persists for 3 months or longer may cause permanent spinal cord degeneration.
- Continue periodic hematologic evaluations throughout patient's lifetime.

Patient education

- Emphasize importance of a well-balanced diet. To prevent progression of subacute combined degeneration, do not use folic acid instead of vitamin B_{12} to prevent anemia.
- Tell patient to avoid smoking, which appears to increase requirement for vitamin B_{12}.
- Instruct patient to report infection or disease in case his condition requires increased dosage of vitamin B_{12}.
- Tell patient with pernicious anemia that he must have lifelong treatment with vitamin B_{12} to prevent recurring symptoms and the risk of incapacitating and irreversible spinal cord damage.
- Inform patient to store tablets in a tightly closed container at room temperature.

Pediatric use

- Safety and efficacy of vitamin B_{12} for use in children have not been established. Intake for children should be 0.5 to 2 mcg daily, as recommended by the Food and Nutrition Board of the National Academy of Sciences—National Research Council.
- Some of these products contain benzyl alcohol, which has been associated with a fatal "gasping syndrome" in premature infants.

Breast-feeding

- Vitamin B_{12} is excreted in breast milk in concentrations that approximate the maternal vitamin B_{12} level. The Food and Nutrition Board of the National Academy of Sciences—National Research Council recommends that breast-feeding women consume 2.6 mcg/day of vitamin B_{12}.

cyclizine hydrochloride
Marezine

cyclizine lactate
Marezine, Marzine*

Pharmacologic classification: piperazine-derivative antihistamine
Therapeutic classification: antiemetic, antivertigo
Pregnancy risk category B

How supplied
Available with or without a prescription
cyclizine hydrochloride
Tablets: 50 mg
cyclizine lactate
Injection: 50 mg/ml

Indications, route, and dosage
Motion sickness (prophylaxis and treatment)
Adults and children over age 12: 50 mg P.O. (hydrochloride) 30 minutes before travel, then q 4 to 6 hours, p.r.n., to maximum of 200 mg daily; or 50 mg I.M. (lactate) q 4 to 6 hours, p.r.n.

Children age 6 to 12: 25 mg P.O. up to t.i.d. under medical supervision.

Pharmacodynamics

Antiemetic action: Cyclizine probably inhibits nausea and vomiting by centrally depressing sensitivity of the labyrinth apparatus that relays stimuli to the chemoreceptor trigger zone and thus stimulates the vomiting center in the brain.

Antivertigo action: Drug depresses conduction in vestibular-cerebellar pathways and reduces labyrinth excitability.

Pharmacokinetics

• *Absorption:* Not well characterized; onset of action is between 30 and 60 minutes.
• *Distribution:* Drug is well distributed throughout the body.
• *Metabolism:* Cyclizine is metabolized in the liver.
• *Excretion:* Unknown; drug effect lasts 4 to 6 hours.

Contraindications and precautions

Contraindicated in patients hypersensitive to drug. Use cautiously in patients with heart failure and who have recently had surgery.

Interactions

Additive sedative and CNS depressant effects may occur when cyclizine is used concomitantly with other *CNS depressants*, such as *alcohol, barbiturates, tranquilizers, sleeping agents*, or *antianxiety agents*; drug should not be given to patients taking *ototoxic medications*, such as *aminoglycosides, salicylates, vancomycin, loop diuretics*, and *cisplatin*, because it may mask signs of ototoxicity.

Effects on diagnostic tests

Discontinue cyclizine 4 days before diagnostic skin testing, to avoid preventing, reducing, or masking test response.

Adverse reactions

CNS: *drowsiness,* auditory and visual hallucinations, restlessness, excitation, nervousness.
CV: hypotension, palpitations, tachycardia.
EENT: blurred vision, diplopia, tinnitus, dry nose and throat.
GI: constipation, dry mouth, anorexia, nausea, vomiting, diarrhea, cholestatic jaundice.
GU: urine retention, urinary frequency.
Skin: urticaria, rash.

Overdose and treatment

Overdose and treatment for cyclizine is not documented; however, symptoms may be anticipated to approximate those of other antihistamine H_1-receptor antagonists. Clinical manifestations of overdose may include either CNS depression (sedation, reduced mental alertness, apnea, and CV collapse) or CNS stimulation (insomnia, hallucinations, tremors, or seizures). Anticholinergic symptoms, such as dry mouth, flushed skin, fixed and dilated pupils, and GI symptoms, are common, especially in children.

Treat overdose with gastric lava[ge] stomach contents; inducing emesis [...] syrup may be ineffective. Treat hypotension with vasopressors and control seizures with diazepam or phenytoin. *Do not give stimulants.*

☑ Special considerations

Besides those relevant to all *antihistamines*, consider the following recommendations.
• Injectable cyclizine is for I.M. use only. When giving I.M., aspirate and check carefully for blood return; inadvertent I.V. administration can cause anaphylactic reaction.
• Injectable solution is incompatible with many drugs; check compatibility before mixing in same syringe.
• Store in a cool place; at room temperature, injection may turn slightly yellow but does not indicate loss of potency.

Patient education

• Instruct patient to position himself in places of minimal motion (such as in the middle, not front or back, of ship), to avoid excessive intake of food or drink, and not to read while in motion.
• Tell patient to avoid hazardous activities requiring mental alertness until CNS reaction is determined.

Geriatric use

• Elderly patients are usually more sensitive to adverse effects of antihistamines and are especially likely to experience a greater degree of dizziness, sedation, hyperexcitability, dry mouth, and urine retention than younger patients.

Pediatric use

• Drug is not indicated for use in children under age 6; they may experience paradoxical hyperexcitability. The manufacturer states that the safety and efficacy of I.M. administration in children have not been established and, therefore, is not recommended.

Breast-feeding

• Antihistamines such as cyclizine should not be used during breast-feeding. Most are secreted in breast milk, exposing the infant to risks of unusual excitability; premature infants are at particular risk for seizures. Cyclizine also may inhibit lactation.

cyclobenzaprine hydrochloride

Flexeril

Pharmacologic classification: tricyclic antidepressant derivative
Therapeutic classification: skeletal muscle relaxant
Pregnancy risk category B

How supplied

Available by prescription only
Tablets: 10 mg

Indications, route, and dosage

Adjunct in acute, painful musculoskeletal conditions

Adults: 20 to 40 mg P.O. divided b.i.d. to q.i.d.; maximum dosage, 60 mg daily. Drug should not be administered for more than 2 weeks.

◇ ***Fibrositis***

Adults: 10 to 40 mg P.O. daily.

Pharmacodynamics

Skeletal muscle relaxant action: Cyclobenzaprine relaxes skeletal muscles through an unknown mechanism of action. Cyclobenzaprine is a CNS depressant.

Drug also potentiates the effects of norepinephrine and exhibits anticholinergic effects similar to those of tricyclic antidepressants, including central and peripheral antimuscarinic actions, sedation, and in increase in heart rate.

Pharmacokinetics

- *Absorption:* Drug is almost completely absorbed during first pass through GI tract. Onset of action occurs within 1 hour, with peak concentrations in 3 to 8 hours. Duration of action is 12 to 24 hours.
- *Distribution:* About 93% is plasma protein-bound.
- *Metabolism:* During first pass through GI tract and liver, drug and metabolites undergo enterohepatic recycling. The half-life of cyclobenzaprine is 1 to 3 days.
- *Excretion:* Excreted primarily in urine as conjugated metabolites; also in feces via bile as unchanged drug.

Contraindications and precautions

Contraindicated in patients who have received MAO inhibitors within 14 days; during acute recovery phase of MI; and in patients with hyperthyroidism, hypersensitivity to drug, heart block, arrhythmias, conduction disturbances, or heart failure. Use cautiously in elderly or debilitated patients and in those with increased intraocular pressure, glaucoma, or urine retention.

Interactions

Concomitant use with *CNS depressant drugs*, including *alcohol, narcotics, anxiolytics, antipsychotics, tricyclic antidepressants*, and *parenteral magnesium salts*, may potentiate the CNS depressant's effects.

Antimuscarinic effects may be potentiated when cyclobenzaprine is used with *antidyskinetics* or *antimuscarinics* (especially *atropine and related compounds).*

Cyclobenzaprine may decrease or block the antihypertensive effects of *guanadrel* or *guanethidine*. Concurrent use with *MAO inhibitors* is not recommended for outpatients.

Hyperpyretic crisis, severe seizures, and death have resulted from the tricyclic antidepressant-like effect of cyclobenzaprine. Allow 14 days to elapse after discontinuance of *MAO inhibitor* therapy before starting cyclobenzaprine, and 5 to 7 days after discontinuance of cyclobenzaprine therapy and start of MAO inhibitor.

Effects on diagnostic tests

None reported.

Adverse reactions

CNS: *drowsiness,* headache, insomnia, fatigue, asthenia, nervousness, confusion, paresthesia, *dizziness,* depression, visual disturbances, ***seizures.***
CV: tachycardia, syncope, ***arrhythmias,*** palpitations, hypotension, vasodilation.
EENT: blurred vision, *dry mouth.*
GI: dyspepsia, abnormal taste, constipation, nausea.
GU: urine retention, urinary frequency.
Skin: rash, urticaria, pruritus.
Other: with high doses, watch for adverse reactions similar to those of other tricyclic antidepressants.

Overdose and treatment

Clinical manifestations of overdose include severe drowsiness, troubled breathing, syncope, seizures, tachycardia, arrhythmias, hallucinations, increase or decrease in body temperature, and vomiting.

To treat overdose, induce emesis or perform gastric lavage. As ordered, give 20 to 30 g activated charcoal every 4 to 6 hours for 24 to 48 hours. Take ECG and monitor cardiac functions for arrhythmias. Monitor vital signs, especially body temperature and ECG. Maintain adequate airway and fluid intake. If needed, 1 to 3 mg I.V. physostigmine may be given to combat severe life-threatening antimuscarinic effects. Provide supportive therapy for arrhythmias, cardiac failure, circulatory shock, seizures, and metabolic acidosis as necessary.

☑ Special considerations

- Drug may cause effects and adverse reactions similar to those of tricyclic antidepressants.
- Note that drug's antimuscarinic effect may inhibit salivary flow, resulting in development of dental caries, periodontal disease, oral candidiasis, and mouth discomfort.
- Allow 14 days to elapse after discontinuance of MAO inhibitors before starting cyclobenzaprine; 5 to 7 days after discontinuing cyclobenzaprine before starting MAO inhibitors.
- Monitor patient for GI problems.
- Drug is intended for short-term (2 or 3 weeks) treatment, because risk-benefit ratio associated with prolonged use is not known. Additionally, muscle spasm accompanying acute musculoskeletal conditions is usually transient.
- Spasmolytic effect usually begins within 1 or 2 days and may be manifested by lessening of pain and tenderness and an increase in range of motion and ability to perform activities of daily living.

Patient education

- Warn patient about possible drowsiness and dizziness. Tell him to avoid hazardous activities that require alertness until reaction to drug is known.
- Instruct patient to avoid alcohol and other CNS depressants (unless prescribed), because combined use with drug will cause additive effects.

• Advise patient to relieve dry mouth (anticholinergic effect) with frequent clear water rinses, extra fluid intake, or with sugarless gum or candy.
• Tell patient to report discomfort immediately.
• Inform patient to use cough and cold preparations cautiously because some products contain alcohol.
• Instruct patient to check with dentist to minimize risk of dental disease (tooth decay, fungal infections, or gum disease) if treatment lasts longer than 2 weeks.

Geriatric use
• Elderly patients are more sensitive to drug's effects.

Pediatric use
• Drug is not recommended for children under age 15.

cyclopentolate hydrochloride
AK-Pentolate, Cyclogyl, I-Pentolate, Minims Cyclopentolate*, Pentolair

Pharmacologic classification: anticholinergic
Therapeutic classification: cycloplegic, mydriatic
Pregnancy risk category C

How supplied
Available by prescription only
Ophthalmic solution: 0.5%, 1%, 2%

Indications, route, and dosage
Diagnostic procedures requiring mydriasis and cycloplegia
Adults: Instill 1 drop of 1% solution in eye, followed by another drop in 5 minutes, 40 to 50 minutes before procedure. Use 2% solution in heavily pigmented irises.
Children: Instill 1 drop of 0.5%, 1%, or 2% solution in each eye, followed by 1 drop of 0.5% or 1% solution in 5 minutes, if necessary, 40 to 50 minutes before procedure.

Pharmacodynamics
Cycloplegic and mydriatic action: Anticholinergic action prevents the sphincter muscle of the iris and the muscle of the ciliary body from responding to cholinergic stimulation. This results in unopposed adrenergic influence, producing pupillary dilation (mydriasis) and paralysis of accommodation (cycloplegia).

Pharmacokinetics
• *Absorption:* Peak mydriatic effect occurs within 15 to 60 minutes and cycloplegic effect within 15 to 60 minutes.
• *Distribution:* Unknown.
• *Metabolism:* Unknown.
• *Excretion:* Recovery from mydriasis usually occurs in about 24 hours; recovery from cycloplegia may occur in 6 to 24 hours.

Contraindications and precautions
Contraindicated in patients with glaucoma, hypersensitivity to drug or belladonna alkaloids, or adhesions between the iris and lens. Use cautiously in children, the elderly, and in patients with increased intraocular pressure.

Interactions
Cyclopentolate may interfere with the antiglaucoma action of *pilocarpine, carbachol,* or *cholinesterase inhibitors.*

Effects on diagnostic tests
None reported.

Adverse reactions
CNS: irritability, confusion, somnolence, hallucinations, ataxia, ***seizures,*** behavioral disturbances in children.
CV: tachycardia
EENT: eye burning on instillation, blurred vision, eye dryness, *photophobia,* ocular congestion, contact dermatitis in eye, conjunctivitis, increased intraocular pressure, transient stinging and burning, irritation, hyperemia.
GU: urine retention.
Skin: dryness.

Overdose and treatment
Clinical manifestations of overdose include flushing, warm dry skin, dry mouth, dilated pupils, delirium, hallucinations, tachycardia, bladder distention, ataxia, hypotension, respiratory depression, coma, and death. Induce emesis or give activated charcoal. Use physostigmine to antagonize cyclopentolate's anticholinergic activity, and in severe toxicity; propranolol may be used to treat symptomatic tachyarrhythmias unresponsive to physostigmine.

☑ Special considerations
• Superior to homatropine hydrobromide, cyclopentolate has a shorter duration of action.
• Recovery usually occurs within 24 hours; however, 1 to 2 drops of a 1% or 2% pilocarpine solution instilled into the eye may reduce recovery time to 3 to 6 hours.
• To minimize systemic absorption, primary health care provider should apply light finger-pressure to lacrimal sac during and for 1 to 2 minutes following topical instillation especially in children and when the 2% solution is used.

Patient education
• Warn patient that drug will cause burning sensation when instilled.
• Advise patient to protect eyes from bright illumination; dark glasses may reduce sensitivity.
• Tell patient to use care to avoid contamination of the dropper tip.

Geriatric use
• Drug should be used with caution in elderly patients because undiagnosed narrow-angle glaucoma may be present.

Pediatric use

- Avoid getting preparation in child's mouth while administering.
- Infants and young children may experience an increased sensitivity to the cardiopulmonary and CNS effects of drug.
- Young infants should not be given solution more concentrated than 0.5%.

Breast-feeding

- No data are available; however, use drug with extreme caution in breast-feeding women because of potential for CNS and cardiopulmonary effects in infants.

cyclophosphamide

Cytoxan, Neosar

Pharmacologic classification: alkylating agent (cell cycle–phase nonspecific)
Therapeutic classification: antineoplastic
Pregnancy risk category D

How supplied

Available by prescription only
Tablets: 25 mg, 50 mg
Injection: 100-mg, 200-mg, 500-mg, 1-g, 2-g vials

Indications, route, and dosage

Dosage and indications may vary. Check literature for recommended protocols.

Breast, head, neck, lung, and ovarian carcinoma; Hodgkin's disease; chronic lymphocytic or myelocytic and acute lymphoblastic leukemia; neuroblastoma; retinoblastoma; malignant lymphomas; multiple myeloma; mycosis fungoides; sarcomas; severe rheumatoid disorders; glomerular and nephrotic syndrome (in children); immunosuppression after transplants

Adults: 40 to 50 mg/kg I.V. in divided doses over 2 to 5 days. Oral dosing for initial and maintenance dosage is 1 to 5 mg/kg P.O. daily.

◊ ***Polymyositis***

Adults: 1 to 2 mg/kg P.O. daily.

◊ ***Rheumatoid arthritis***

Adults: 1.5 to 3 mg/kg P.O. daily.

◊ ***Wegener's granulomatosis***

Adults: 1 to 2 mg/kg P.O. daily (usually administered with prednisone).

◊ ***Nephrotic syndrome in children***

Children: 2.5 to 3 mg/kg P.O. daily for 60 to 90 days.

✦ ***Dosage adjustment.*** Adjust dosage of cyclophosphamide in patients with renal impairment.

Pharmacodynamics

Antineoplastic action: Cytotoxic action of cyclophosphamide is mediated by its two active metabolites. These metabolites function as alkylating agents, preventing cell division by cross-linking DNA strands. This results in an imbalance of growth within the cell, leading to cell death. Cyclophosphamide also has significant immunosuppressive activity.

Pharmacokinetics

- *Absorption:* Almost completely absorbed from the GI tract at doses of 100 mg or less. Higher doses (300 mg) are approximately 75% absorbed.
- *Distribution:* Drug is distributed throughout the body, although only minimal amounts have been found in saliva, sweat, and synovial fluid. The concentration in the CSF is too low for treatment of meningeal leukemia. The active metabolites are approximately 50% bound to plasma proteins.
- *Metabolism:* Metabolized to its active form by hepatic microsomal enzymes. The activity of these metabolites is terminated by metabolism to inactive forms.
- *Excretion:* Drug and its metabolites are eliminated primarily in urine, with 15% to 30% excreted as unchanged drug. The elimination half-life ranges from 3 to 12 hours.

Contraindications and precautions

Contraindicated in patients with hypersensitivity to drug or with severe bone marrow suppression. Use cautiously in patients with impaired renal or hepatic function, leukopenia, thrombocytopenia, or malignant cell infiltration of bone marrow and in those who have recently undergone radiation therapy or chemotherapy.

Interactions

Concomitant use of cyclophosphamide with *barbiturates, phenytoin*, or *chloral hydrate* increases the rate of metabolism of cyclophosphamide. These agents are known to be inducers of hepatic microsomal enzymes.

Corticosteroids are known to initially inhibit the metabolism of cyclophosphamide, reducing its effect. Eventual reduction of dose or discontinuation of steroids may increase metabolism of cyclophosphamide to a toxic level. Other drugs that may inhibit cyclophosphamide metabolism include *allopurinol, chloramphenicol, chloroquine, imipramine, phenothiazines, potassium iodide*, and *vitamin A*.

Patients on cyclophosphamide therapy who receive *succinylcholine* as an adjunct to anesthesia may experience prolonged respiratory distress and apnea. This may occur up to several days after the discontinuation of cyclophosphamide. The mechanism of this interaction is that cyclophosphamide depresses the activity of pseudocholinesterases, the enzyme responsible for the inactivation of *succinylcholine*. Use *succinylcholine* with caution or not at all.

Concomitant use of cyclophosphamide may potentiate the cardiotoxic effects of *doxorubicin*.

Effects on diagnostic tests

Drug may suppress positive reaction to *Candida*, mumps, tricophyton, and tuberculin TB skin tests. A false-positive result for the Papanicolaou test may occur. Drug therapy may also increase serum uric acid levels and decrease serum pseudocholinesterase concentrations.

Adverse reactions

CV: *cardiotoxicity* (with very high doses and with doxorubicin).
GI: anorexia, *nausea, vomiting* (within 6 hours); abdominal pain; stomatitis; mucositis.
GU: HEMORRHAGIC CYSTITIS, fertility impairment.
Hematologic: *leukopenia,* nadir between days 8 to 15, recovery in 17 to 28 days; ***thrombocytopenia; anemia.***
Respiratory: ***pulmonary fibrosis*** (with high doses).
Other: *reversible alopecia,* ***secondary malignant disease, anaphylaxis,*** hypersensitivity reactions, ***hepatotoxicity.***

Overdose and treatment

Clinical manifestations of overdose include myelosuppression, alopecia, nausea, vomiting, and anorexia. Treatment is generally supportive and includes transfusion of blood components and antiemetics. Drug is dialyzable.

☑ Special considerations

- Follow institutional guidelines for safe preparation, administration, and disposal of chemotherapeutic drugs.
- Reconstitute vials with appropriate volume of bacteriostatic or sterile water for injection to give a concentration of 20 mg/ml.
- Reconstituted solution is stable 6 days if refrigerated or 24 hours at room temperature.
- Drug can be given by direct I.V. push into a running I.V. line or by infusion in 0.9% NaCl solution or D_5W.
- Avoid all I.M. injections when platelet counts are low.
- Oral medication should be taken with or after a meal. Higher oral doses (400 mg) may be tolerated better if divided into smaller doses.
- Administration with cold foods such as ice cream may improve toleration of oral dose.
- Push fluid (3 L daily) to prevent hemorrhagic cystitis. Some clinicians use uroprotectant agents such as mesna. Drug should not be given at bedtime, because voiding afterward is too infrequent to avoid cystitis. If hemorrhagic cystitis occurs, discontinue drug. Cystitis can occur months after therapy has been discontinued.
- Reduce drug dosage if patient is also receiving corticosteroid therapy and develops viral or bacterial infections.
- Monitor for cyclophosphamide toxicity if patient's corticosteroid therapy is discontinued.
- Monitor uric acid, CBC, and renal and hepatic functions.
- Observe for hematuria and ask patient if he has dysuria.
- Nausea and vomiting are most common with high doses of I.V. cyclophosphamide.
- Drug has been used successfully to treat many nonmalignant conditions, for example, multiple sclerosis, because of its immunosuppressive activity.

Patient education

- Advise both male and female patients to practice contraception while taking drug and for 4 months after because drug has teratogenic properties.
- Emphasize importance of continuing medication despite nausea and vomiting.
- Advise patient to report vomiting that occurs shortly after an oral dose.
- Warn patient that alopecia is likely to occur, but that it is reversible.
- Encourage adequate fluid intake to prevent hemorrhagic cystitis and to facilitate uric acid excretion.
- Tell patient to promptly report unusual bleeding or bruising.
- Advise patient to avoid individuals with infections and to call immediately if fever, chills, or signs of infection occur.

Breast-feeding

- Drug is excreted into breast milk; therefore, breast-feeding should be discontinued because of risk of serious adverse reactions, mutagenicity, and carcinogenicity in the infant.

cycloserine

Seromycin

Pharmacologic classification: isoxizolidone, d-alanine analogue
Therapeutic classification: antitubercular
Pregnancy risk category C

How supplied

Available by prescription only
Capsules: 250 mg

Indications, route, and dosage

Adjunctive treatment in pulmonary or extrapulmonary tuberculosis
Adults: Initially, 250 mg P.O. q 12 hours for 2 weeks; then, if blood levels are below 25 to 30 mcg/ml and there are no clinical signs of toxicity, dosage is increased to 250 mg P.O. q 8 hours for 2 weeks. If optimum blood levels are still not achieved, and there are no signs of clinical toxicity, then dosage is increased to 250 mg P.O. q 6 hours. Maximum dosage is 1 g/day. If CNS toxicity occurs, drug is discontinued for 1 week, then resumed at 250 mg/day for 2 weeks. If no serious toxic effects occur, dose is increased by 250-mg increments q 10 days until blood levels reach 25 to 30 mcg/ml.
◊ *Children:* 10 to 20 mg/kg (maximum, 750 to 1,000 mg) daily administered in two equally divided doses.
Urinary tract infections
Adults: 250 mg P.O. q 12 hours for 2 weeks.

Pharmacodynamics

Antibiotic action: Cycloserine inhibits bacterial cell utilization of amino acids, thereby inhibiting cell-wall synthesis. Its action is bacteriostatic or bactericidal, depending on organism susceptibility and drug concentration at infection site. Cycloserine is active against *Mycobacterium tuberculosis, My-*

cobactrium bovis, and some strains of *Mycobacterium kansasii, Mycobacterium marinum, Mycobacterium ulcerans, Mycobacterium avium, Mycobacterium smegmatis,* and *Mycobacterium intracellulare.* It is also active against some gram-negative and gram-positive bacteria, including *Staphylococcus aureus, Enterobacter,* and *Escherichia coli.* Cycloserine is considered adjunctive therapy in tuberculosis and is combined with other antituberculosis agents to prevent or delay development of drug resistance by *Mycobacterium tuberculosis.*

Pharmacokinetics

• *Absorption:* About 80% of oral dose is absorbed from the GI tract; peak serum concentrations occur 3 to 4 hours after ingestion.
• *Distribution:* Distributed widely into body tissues and fluids, including CSF. Drug crosses the placenta; it does not bind to plasma proteins.
• *Metabolism:* Cycloserine may be metabolized partially.
• *Excretion:* Excreted primarily in urine by glomerular filtration. Small amounts of drug are excreted in feces and breast milk. Elimination plasma half-life in adults is 10 hours. Drug is hemodialyzable.

Contraindications and precautions

Contraindicated in patients with hypersensitivity to drug and in those with seizure disorders, depression or severe anxiety, psychosis, severe renal insufficiency, or excessive concurrent use of alcohol. Use cautiously in patients with impaired renal function.

Interactions

Concomitant use with *isoniazid* or *ethionamide* increases hazard of CNS toxicity, drowsiness, and dizziness; concomitant use with *alcohol* may increase incidence of seizures.

Cycloserine may inhibit metabolism of *phenytoin,* producing toxic blood levels of *phenytoin.* Dosage adjustment may be required.

Effects on diagnostic tests

Cycloserine may elevate serum transaminase levels, especially in patients with preexisting hepatic disease.

Adverse reactions

CNS: ***seizures***, drowsiness, somnolence, headache, tremor, dysarthria, vertigo, confusion, loss of memory, ***possible suicidal tendencies,*** psychosis, hyperirritability, character changes, aggression, paresthesia, paresis, hyperreflexia, ***coma.***
CV: ***sudden-onset heart failure.***
Other: hypersensitivity reactions (allergic dermatitis), skin rash, elevated transaminase level.

Overdose and treatment

Signs of overdose include CNS depression accompanied by dizziness, hyperreflexia, confusion, or seizures.

Treat with gastric lavage and supportive care, including oxygen, I.V. fluids, pressor agents (for circulatory shock), and body temperature stabilization. Treat seizures with anticonvulsants and pyridoxine.

☑ Special considerations

• Give drug after meals to avoid gastric irritation.
• Obtain specimens for culture and sensitivity testing before giving first dose, but therapy can begin before test results are complete; repeat periodically to detect drug resistance.
• Monitor hematologic, renal, and liver function studies before and periodically during therapy to minimize toxicity; toxic reactions may occur at blood levels in excess of 30 mcg/ml.
• Assess level of consciousness and neurologic function; monitor for personality changes and other early signs of CNS toxicity.
• Pyrodoxine (200 to 300 mg daily) may be used to treat or prevent neurotoxic effects.
• Anticonvulsants, tranquilizers, or sedatives may be prescribed to relieve adverse reactions.

Patient education

• Explain disease process and rationale for long-term therapy.
• Teach signs and symptoms of hypersensitivity and other adverse reactions, and emphasize need to report *any* unusual effects and rash promptly.
• Warn patient to avoid hazardous tasks that require mental alertness because drug may cause patient to become drowsy or dizzy.
• Warn patient not to use alcohol; explain hazard of serious CNS toxicity.
• Advise patient to take drug after meals to avoid gastric irritation.
• Urge patient to complete entire prescribed regimen, to comply with instructions for around-the-clock dosage, and not to discontinue drug without medical approval.
• Explain importance of follow-up appointments.

Geriatric use

• Because elderly patients commonly have renal impairment, which decreases excretion of drugs, use drug with caution.

Breast-feeding

• Drug is excreted in breast milk; use cautiously in breast-feeding women.

cyclosporine

Neoral, Sandimmune

Pharmacologic classification: polypeptide antibiotic
Therapeutic classification: immunosuppressant
Pregnancy risk category C

How supplied

Available by prescription only
Capsules: 25 mg, 50 mg, 100 mg
Oral solution: 100 mg/ml
Capsules for microemulsion: 25 mg, 100 mg
Injection: 50 mg/ml

Indications, route, and dosage

Prophylaxis of organ rejection in kidney, liver, heart, bone marrow, ◇ pancreas, ◇ cornea transplants

Adults and children: 15 mg/kg P.O. daily 4 to 12 hours before transplantation. Continue daily dose postoperatively for 1 to 2 weeks. Then, gradually reduce dosage by 5% weekly to maintenance level of 5 to 10 mg/kg/day. Alternatively, administer an I.V. concentrate of 5 to 6 mg/kg 4 to 12 hours before transplantation.

Postoperatively, administer 5 to 6 mg/kg daily as an I.V. dilute solution infusion (50 mg per 20 to 100 ml infused over 2 to 6 hours) until patient can tolerate oral forms.

Note: Sandimmune and Neoral are not bioequivalent and cannot be used interchangeably without primary health care provider's supervision. When converting to Neoral from Sandimmune, start with same daily dose (1:1) and follow serum trough levels frequently.

Pharmacodynamics

Immunosuppressant action: Exact mechanism is unknown; purportedly, its action is related to the inhibition of induction of interleukin II, which plays a role in both cellular and humoral immune responses.

Pharmacokinetics

- *Absorption:* Absorption after oral administration varies widely between patients and in the same individual. Only 30% of an oral dose reaches systemic circulation; peak levels occur at 3 to 4 hours. Neoral has a greater bioavailability than Sandimmune.
- *Distribution:* Drug is distributed widely outside the blood volume. About 33% to 47% is found in plasma; 4% to 9%, in leukocytes; 5% to 12%, in granulocytes; and 41% to 58%, in erythrocytes. In plasma, approximately 90% is bound to proteins, primarily lipoproteins. Cyclosporine crosses the placenta; cord blood levels are about 60% those of maternal blood. Cyclosporine enters breast milk.
- *Metabolism:* Drug is metabolized extensively in the liver.
- *Excretion:* Primarily excreted in the feces (biliary excretion) with only 6% of drug found in urine.

Contraindications and precautions

Contraindicated in patients hypersensitive to drug or to polyoxyethylated castor oil (found in injectable form).

Interactions

Concomitant use with *amphotericin B* or *aminoglycosides* is likely to increase nephrotoxicity because both drugs are nephrotoxic, and *amphotericin* may increase cyclosporine blood levels.

Except for *corticosteroids*, cyclosporine should not be used concomitantly with *immunosuppressive agents* because of the increased risk of malignancy (lymphoma) and susceptibility to infection.

Erythromycin, ketoconazole, diltiazem, verapamil, fluconazole, itraconazole, and possibly *corticosteroids* impair hepatic enzyme metabolism and increase plasma cyclosporine levels; reduced dosage of cyclosporine may be necessary. *Phenytoin, rifampin, phenobarbital,* and *co-trimoxazole* increase hepatic metabolism and may lower plasma levels of cyclosporine.

Concomitant administration of Neoral with *food* decreases the area under the curve and maximum concentration of cyclosporine. Administration with *grapefruit juice* can increase trough concentrations.

Effects on diagnostic tests

Cyclosporine therapy may alter CBC and differential blood tests and may increase serum lipid levels; drug elevation of serum BUN and creatinine and liver function tests may signal nephrotoxicity or hepatotoxicity.

Adverse reactions

CNS: *tremor, headache,* ***seizures,*** confusion, paresthesia.
CV: *hypertension.*
EENT: *gum hyperplasia,* oral candidiasis, sinusitis.
GI: *nausea, vomiting,* diarrhea, abdominal discomfort.
GU: NEPHROTOXICITY.
Hematologic: anemia, ***leukopenia, thrombocytopenia,*** hemolytic anemia.
Hepatic: ***hepatotoxicity.***
Skin: acne, flushing.
Other: increased low-density lipoprotein levels, ***infections,*** hirsutism, ***anaphylaxis,*** gynecomastia.

Overdose and treatment

Clinical manifestations of overdose include extensions of common adverse effects. Hepatotoxicity and nephrotoxicity often accompany nausea and vomiting; tremor and seizures may occur. Up to 2 hours after ingestion, empty stomach by induced emesis or lavage; thereafter, treat supportively. Monitor vital signs and fluid and electrolyte levels closely. Drug is not removed by hemodialysis or charcoal hemoperfusion.

☑ Special considerations

- Cyclosporine usually is prescribed with corticosteroids.
- Possible kidney rejection should be considered before discontinuation of drug for suspected nephrotoxicity.
- Monitor hepatic and renal function tests routinely; hepatotoxicity may occur in first month after transplantation, but renal toxicity may be delayed for 2 to 3 months.
- Dose should be given at same time each day. Oral solution should be measured carefully in oral syringe and mixed with plain or chocolate milk or fruit juice to increase palatability; it should be served in a glass to minimize drug adherence to container walls. Drug can be taken with food to minimize nausea.
- Neoral capsules and oral solution are bioequivalent. Sandimmune capsules and oral solution have decreased bioavailability compared with Neoral.

Patient education

- Teach patient about rationale for therapy; explain possible adverse effects and importance of reporting them, especially fever, sore throat, mouth sores, abdominal pain, unusual bleeding or bruising, pale stools, or dark urine.
- Encourage compliance with therapy and follow-up visits.
- Teach patient how and when to take medication for optimal benefit and minimal discomfort; caution against discontinuing drug without medical approval.
- Advise patient to make oral solution more palatable by diluting with room temperature milk, chocolate milk, or orange juice. Do not use grapefruit juice or food when taking Neoral.
- Tell patient not to rinse syringe with water.

Pediatric use

- Safety and efficacy have not been established; however, drug has been used in children as young as 6 months. Use with caution.

Breast-feeding

- Safety has not been established; breast-feeding women should avoid drug.

cyproheptadine hydrochloride

Periactin

Pharmacologic classification: piperidine-derivative antihistamine
Therapeutic classification: antihistamine (H_1-receptor antagonist), antipruritic
Pregnancy risk category B

How supplied

Available by prescription only
Tablets: 4 mg
Syrup: 2 mg/5 ml

Indications, route, and dosage

Allergy symptoms, pruritus, cold urticaria, allergic conjunctivitis, appetite stimulant, vascular cluster headaches
Adults: 4 mg P.O. t.i.d. or q.i.d. Maximum dosage, 0.5 mg/kg daily.
Children age 7 to 14: 4 mg P.O. b.i.d. or t.i.d. Maximum dosage, 16 mg daily.
Children age 2 to 6: 2 mg P.O. b.i.d. or t.i.d. Maximum dosage, 12 mg daily.
◊ ***Cushing's syndrome***
Adults: 8 to 24 mg P.O. daily in divided doses.

Pharmacodynamics

Antihistamine action: Antihistamines compete with histamine for histamine H_1-receptor sites on smooth muscle of the bronchi, GI tract, uterus, and large blood vessels; they bind to cellular receptors, preventing access of histamine, thereby suppressing histamine-induced allergic symptoms. They do not directly alter histamine or its release.

Drug also displays significant anticholinergic and antiserotonin activity.

Pharmacokinetics

- *Absorption:* Well absorbed from the GI tract; peak action occurs in 6 to 9 hours.
- *Distribution:* Unknown.
- *Metabolism:* Drug appears to be almost completely metabolized in the liver.
- *Excretion:* Drug's metabolites are excreted primarily in urine; unchanged drug is not excreted in urine. Small amounts of unchanged cyproheptadine and metabolites are excreted in feces.

Contraindications and precautions

Contraindicated in patients with hypersensitivity to drug or other drugs of similar chemical structure; in those with acute asthma, angle-closure glaucoma, stenosing peptic ulcer, symptomatic prostatic hyperplasia, bladder neck obstruction, and pyloroduodenal obstruction; in concurrent therapy with MAO inhibitors; in neonates or premature infants; in elderly or debilitated patients, and in breast-feeding patients.

Use cautiously in patients with increased intraocular pressure, hyperthyroidism, CV disease, hypertension, or bronchial asthma.

Interactions

MAO inhibitors interfere with the detoxification of antihistamines and thus prolong and intensify their central depressant and anticholinergic effects; additive sedative effects result when cyproheptadine is used concomitantly with *alcohol* or other *CNS depressants*, such as *barbiturates, tranquilizers, sleeping aids*, and *antianxiety agents.*

Serum amylase and prolactin concentrations may be increased when these drugs are administered with *thyrotropin-releasing hormone.*

Effects on diagnostic tests

Discontinue drug 4 days before diagnostic skin tests. Antihistamines can prevent, reduce, or mask positive skin test response.

Adverse reactions

CNS: *drowsiness,* dizziness, headache, fatigue, sedation, sleepiness, incoordination, confusion, restlessness, insomnia, nervousness, tremor, ***seizures.***
CV: hypotension, palpitations, tachycardia.
GI: nausea, vomiting, epigastric distress, *dry mouth,* diarrhea, constipation.
GU: urine retention, urinary frequency.
Hematologic: hemolytic anemia, leukopenia, ***agranulocytosis, thrombocytopenia.***
Skin: rash, urticaria, photosensitivity.
Other: weight gain, ***anaphylactic shock.***

Overdose and treatment

Clinical manifestations of overdose may include either CNS depression (sedation, reduced mental alertness, apnea, and CV collapse) or CNS stimulation (insomnia, hallucinations, tremors, or seizures). Anticholinergic symptoms, such as dry mouth, flushed skin, fixed and dilated pupils, and GI symptoms, are common, especially in children.

Treat overdose by inducing emesis with ipecac syrup (in conscious patient), followed by activated charcoal to reduce further drug absorption. Use gastric lavage if patient is unconscious or ipecac fails. Treat hypotension with vasopressors, and control seizures with diazepam or phenytoin. *Do not give stimulants.*

☑ Special considerations

Besides those relevant to all *antihistamines,* consider the following recommendations.

- Drug can cause weight gain. Monitor weight.
- Drug also has been used experimentally to stimulate appetite and increase weight gain in children.
- In some patients, sedative effect disappears within 3 or 4 days.

Patient education

- Inform patient about potential adverse reactions.

Geriatric use

- Elderly patients are more susceptible to the sedative effect of drug. Instruct patient to change positions slowly and gradually. Elderly patients may experience dizziness or hypotension more readily than younger patients.

Pediatric use

- CNS stimulation (agitation, confusion, tremors, hallucinations) is more common in children and may require dosage reduction. Drug is not indicated for use in newborn or premature infants.

Breast-feeding

- Antihistamines such as cyproheptadine should not be used during breast-feeding. Many of these drugs are secreted in breast milk, exposing the infant to risks of unusual excitability; premature infants are at particular risk for seizures.

cytarabine (ara-C, cytosine arabinoside)

Cytosar-U

Pharmacologic classification: antimetabolite (cell cycle–phase specific, S phase)
Therapeutic classification: antineoplastic
Pregnancy risk category D

How supplied

Available by prescription only
Injection: 100-mg, 500-mg, 1-g, 2-g vials

Indications, route, and dosage

Dosage and indications may vary. Check literature for recommended protocols.

Acute myelocytic and other acute leukemias
Adults and children: 100 mg/m^2 I.V. once daily or q 12 hours by continuous I.V. infusion or rapid I.V. injection in divided doses for 5 days at 2-week intervals for remission induction; or 30 mg/m^2 intrathecally (range, 5 to 75 mg/m^2) q 4 days until CSF findings are normal, then followed by one additional dose. Dosages up to 3 g/m^2 q 12 hours for up to 12 doses have been given by continuous infusion for refractory acute leukemias.

Pharmacodynamics

Antineoplastic action: Cytarabine requires conversion to its active metabolite within the cell. This metabolite acts as a competitive inhibitor of the enzyme DNA polymerase, disrupting the normal synthesis of DNA.

Pharmacokinetics

- *Absorption:* Poorly absorbed (less than 20%) across the GI tract because of rapid deactivation in the gut lumen. After I.M. or subcutaneous administration, peak plasma levels are less than after I.V. administration.
- *Distribution:* Cytarabine rapidly distributes widely through the body. Approximately 13% of the drug is bound to plasma proteins. Drug penetrates the blood-brain barrier only slightly after a rapid I.V. dose; however, when administered by continuous I.V. infusion, CSF levels achieve a concentration 40% to 60% of that of plasma levels.
- *Metabolism:* Cytarabine is metabolized primarily in the liver but also in the kidneys, GI mucosa, and granulocytes.
- *Excretion:* Biphasic elimination of drug, with an initial half-life of 8 minutes and a terminal phase half-life of 1 to 3 hours. Cytarabine and its metabolites are excreted in urine. Less than 10% of a dose is excreted as unchanged drug in urine.

Contraindications and precautions

Contraindicated in patients hypersensitive to drug. Use cautiously in patients with impaired hepatic function.

Interactions

When used concomitantly, cytarabine decreases the cellular uptake of *methotrexate,* reducing its effectiveness.

Cytarabine may antagonize the activity of *gentamicin.*

Combination chemotherapy (including cytarabine) may decrease *digoxin* absorption even several days after stopping chemotherapy. *Digoxin* capsules and *digitoxin* do not appear to be affected.

Effects on diagnostic tests

Cytarabine therapy may increase blood and urine levels of uric acid. It may also increase serum alkaline phosphatase, AST, and bilirubin concentrations, which indicate drug-induced hepatotoxicity.

Adverse reactions

CNS: neurotoxicity, malaise, dizziness, headache.
EENT: conjunctivitis.
GI: *nausea; vomiting;* diarrhea; anorexia; anal ulcer; abdominal pain; oral ulcers in 5 to 10 days; high dose given rapidly I.V. may cause projectile vomiting.
Hematologic: ***leukopenia,*** with initial WBC count nadir 7 to 9 days after drug is stopped and a second (more severe) nadir 15 to 24 days after drug is stopped; anemia; reticulocytopenia; ***thrombocytopenia,*** with platelet count nadir occurring between days 12 to 15; *megaloblastosis.*
Hepatic: hepatotoxicity (usually mild and reversible), jaundice.

Skin: rash, pruritus.
Other: flulike syndrome, hyperuricemia, infection, fever, thrombophlebitis, myalgia, bone pain, ***anaphylaxis,*** renal dysfunction, edema.

Overdose and treatment

Clinical manifestations of overdose include myelosuppression, nausea, vomiting, and megaloblastosis.

Treatment is usually supportive and includes transfusion of blood components and antiemetics.

☑ Special considerations

- To reconstitute the 100-mg vial for I.V. administration use 5 ml bacteriostatic water for injection (20 mg/ml) and for the 500-mg vial with 10 ml bacteriostatic water for injection (50 mg/ml).
- Drug may be further diluted with D_5W or 0.9% NaCl solution for continuous I.V. infusion.
- For intrathecal injection, dilute drug in 5 to 15 ml of lactated Ringer's solution, Elliot's B solution, or 0.9% NaCl solution with no preservative, and administer after withdrawing an equivalent volume of CSF.
- Do not reconstitute drug with bacteriostatic diluent for intrathecal administration because the preservative, benzyl alcohol, has been associated with a higher incidence of neurologic toxicity.
- Reconstituted solutions are stable for 48 hours at room temperature. Infusion solutions up to a concentration of 5 mg/ml are stable for 7 days at room temperature. Discard cloudy reconstituted solution.
- Dose modification may be required in thrombocytopenia, leukopenia, renal or hepatic disease, and after other chemotherapy or radiation therapy.
- Watch for signs of infection (cough, fever, sore throat). Monitor CBC.
- Excellent mouth care can help prevent adverse oral reactions.
- Nausea and vomiting are more frequent when large doses are administered rapidly by I.V. push. These reactions are less frequent with infusion. To reduce nausea, give antiemetic before administering.
- Monitor intake and output carefully. Maintain high fluid intake and give allopurinol, if ordered, to avoid urate nephropathy in leukemia induction therapy. Monitor uric acid and plasma digoxin levels.
- Monitor hepatic function.
- Monitor patients receiving high doses for cerebellar dysfunction.
- Prescribe steroid eyedrops (dexamethasone) to prevent drug-induced keratitis.
- Avoid I.M. injections of any drugs in patients with severely depressed platelet count (thrombocytopenia) to prevent bleeding.
- Pyridoxine supplements may be administered to prevent neuropathies; reportedly, however, prophylactic use of pyridoxine does not prevent cytarabine neurotoxicity.

Patient education

- Encourage adequate fluid intake to increase urine output and facilitate excretion of uric acid.
- Advise patient to avoid exposure to people with infections. Tell him to call immediately if signs of infection or unusual bleeding occurs.

Breast-feeding

- It is not known if drug distributes into breast milk. However, because of the risk of serious adverse reactions, mutagenicity, and carcinogenicity in the infant, breast-feeding is not recommended.

cytomegalovirus immune globulin intravenous, human (CMV-IGIV)

CytoGam

Pharmacologic classification: immune globulin
Therapeutic classification: immune serum
Pregnancy risk category C

How supplied

Available by prescription only
Injection: 2.5 g as lyophilized powder with 50 ml sterile water (diluent supplied)

Indications, route, and dosage

To attenuate primary cytomegalovirus (CMV) disease in seronegative kidney transplant recipients who receive a kidney from a CMV-seropositive donor

Adults: Maximum total dosage per infusion is 150 mg/kg I.V. administered as follows:
Within 72 hours of transplant: 150 mg/kg
2 weeks posttransplant: 100 mg/kg
4 weeks posttransplant: 100 mg/kg
6 weeks posttransplant: 100 mg/kg
8 weeks posttransplant: 100 mg/kg
12 weeks posttransplant: 50 mg/kg
16 weeks posttransplant: 50 mg/kg.

Administer initial dose I.V. at a rate of 15 mg/kg/hour. If no adverse reactions occur after 30 minutes, increase the rate to 30 mg/kg/hour. If no adverse reactions occur after a subsequent 30 minutes, the infusion may be increased to 60 mg/kg/hour. Volume should not exceed 75 ml/hour. Subsequent doses may be administered at 15 mg/kg/hour for 15 minutes, increasing as with initial dose at 15-minute intervals, if no adverse reactions occur to a maximum rate of 60 mg/kg/hour.

Pharmacodynamics

Immune action: CMV immune globulin contains a relatively high concentration of immunoglobulin G (IgG) antibodies against CMV and can raise relevant antibodies in CMV-exposed patients to levels sufficient to attenuate or reduce the incidence of serious CMV disease.

Pharmacokinetics

- *Absorption:* CMV immune globulin is administered I.V.
- *Distribution:* Unknown; other immune globulins distribute between the intravascular and extravascular spaces.

- *Metabolism:* Unknown.
- *Excretion:* Unknown.

Contraindications and precautions
Contraindicated in patients with sensitivity to other human immunoglobulin preparations or with selective immunoglobulin A (IgA) deficiency.

Interactions
Vaccination with *live-virus vaccines* should be deferred for at least 3 months after CMV immune globulin administration because of the potential for interference with the immune response to *live virus vaccines.*

Adverse reactions
CV: hypotension.
GI: nausea, vomiting.
Other: ***anaphylaxis,*** wheezing, flushing, chills, muscle cramps, back pain, fever.

Overdose and treatment
Little data are available. Presumed major manifestations would be related to volume overload.

If anaphylaxis or drop in blood pressure occurs, discontinue infusion and administer supportive therapy, including drugs such as diphenhydramine and epinephrine.

☑ Special considerations
- Monitor patient closely during each change or infusion rate.
- Infusion should begin within 6 hours and finish within 12 hours of reconstitution.
- Administer through a separate I.V. line using a constant infusion pump. Filters are not necessary.
- If unable to administer through separate line, piggyback into preexisting line of NaCl injection or one of the following dextrose solutions with or without NaCl: $D_{2.5}W$, D_5W, $D_{10}W$, or $D_{20}W$. Do not dilute more than 1:2 with any of the above solutions.
- Monitor vital signs before infusion, midway through infusion, after the infusion, and before increase in infusion rate.
- Reconstitute drug as follows. Remove tab portion of vial cap and clean rubber stopper with 70% alcohol or equivalent. Add 50 ml sterile water for injection. *Do not shake vial; avoid foaming.* After adding water, release residual vacuum in vial to hasten the dissolving process. Rotate vial gently to wet all undissolved powder. Allow 30 minutes for powder to dissolve before administration. Inspect vial for clarity and particles.
- Store drug in refrigerator at 35.6° to 46.4° F (2° to 8° C).
- CMV immune globulin provides passive immunity.

Patient education
- Inform patient of the potential adverse reactions.

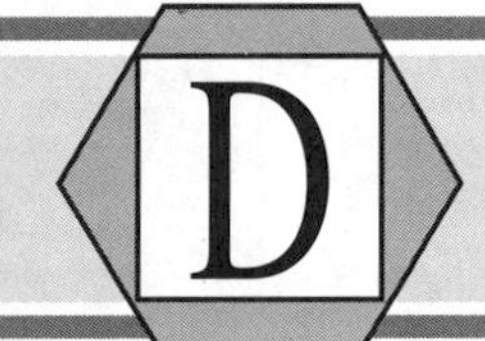

dacarbazine (DTIC)

DTIC-Dome

Pharmacologic classification: alkylating agent (cell cycle–phase nonspecific)
Therapeutic classification: antineoplastic
Pregnancy risk category C

How supplied

Available by prescription only
Injection: 100 mg, 200 mg

Indications, route, and dosage

Dosage and indications may vary. Check current literature for recommended protocols.

Metastatic malignant melanoma

Adults: 2 to 4.5 mg/kg I.V. daily for 10 days, then repeat q 4 weeks as tolerated; or 250 mg/m^2 I.V. daily for 5 days, repeated at 3-week intervals.

Hodgkin's disease

Adults: 150 mg/m^2 I.V. (in combination with other agents) for 5 days, repeat q 4 weeks; or 375 mg/m^2 on day 1 of a combination regimen, repeated q 15 days.

✦ ***Dosage adjustment.*** Reduce dosage when giving repeated doses to patients with severely impaired renal function. Use lower dose if renal function or bone marrow is impaired.

Pharmacodynamics

Antineoplastic action: Three mechanisms have been proposed to explain the cytotoxicity of dacarbazine: alkylation, in which DNA and RNA synthesis are inhibited; antimetabolite activity as a false precursor for purine synthesis; and binding with protein sulfhydryl groups.

Pharmacokinetics

- *Absorption:* Because of poor absorption from the GI tract, dacarbazine is not administered orally.
- *Distribution:* Drug is believed to localize in body tissues, especially the liver. It crosses the blood-brain barrier to a limited extent and is minimally bound to plasma proteins.
- *Metabolism:* Dacarbazine is rapidly metabolized in the liver to several compounds, some of which may be active.
- *Excretion:* Drug elimination occurs in a biphasic manner, with an initial phase half-life of 19 minutes and terminal phase of 5 hours in patients with normal renal and hepatic function. Approximately 30% to 45% of a dose is excreted unchanged in urine.

Contraindications and precautions

Contraindicated in patients hypersensitive to drug. Use cautiously in patients with impaired bone marrow function.

Interactions

Drug may increase risk of nephrotoxicity when used in combination with *amphotericin B*; may potentiate the activity of *allopurinol* by inhibiting xanthine oxidase, *phenobarbitol* and *phenytoin* may increase the metabolism of dacarbazine.

Effects on diagnostic tests

Dacarbazine therapy causes transient increases in serum BUN, ALT, AST, and alkaline phosphatase levels.

Adverse reactions

GI: *severe nausea and vomiting, anorexia*, diarrhea (rare).
Hematologic: ***leukopenia, thrombocytopenia.***
Hepatic: transient increase in liver enzyme levels, ***hepatotoxicity*** (rare).
Skin: phototoxicity, rash, facial flushing.
Other: *flulike syndrome* (fever, malaise; myalgia, beginning 7 days after treatment ends and lasting possibly 7 to 21 days), alopecia, ***anaphylaxis;*** severe pain (if I.V. solution infiltrates or if solution is too concentrated); tissue damage; facial paresthesia.

Overdose and treatment

Clinical manifestations of overdose include myelosuppression and diarrhea. Treatment is usually supportive and includes transfusion of blood components and monitoring of hematologic parameters.

☑ Special considerations

- To reconstitute drug for I.V. administration, use a volume of sterile water for injection that gives a concentration of 10 mg/ml (9.9 ml for 100-mg vial, 19.7 ml for 200-mg vial).
- Drug may be diluted further with D_5W or 0.9% NaCl to a volume of 100 to 200 ml for I.V. infusion over 30 minutes. Increase volume or slow the rate of infusion to decrease pain at infusion site.
- Drug may be administered I.V. push over 1 to 2 minutes.
- A change in solution color from ivory to pink indicates *some* drug degradation. During infusion, protect solution from light to avoid possible drug breakdown.
- Treatment of extravasation with application of hot packs may relieve burning sensation, local pain, and irritation.
- Discard refrigerated solution after 72 hours; room temperature solution after 8 hours.

• Nausea and vomiting may be minimized by administering dacarbazine by I.V. infusion and by hydrating patient 4 to 6 hours before therapy.
• Monitor uric acid levels.
• Stop drug if WBC count falls to 3,000/mm³ or platelet count drops to 100,000/mm³. Monitor CBC.
• Monitor daily temperature. Observe for signs of infection.
• Avoid all I.M. injections when platelet count is below 100,000/mm³.
• Anticoagulants and aspirin products should be used cautiously. Watch closely for signs of bleeding.

Patient education
• Advise patient to avoid sunlight and sunlamps for first 2 days after treatment.
• Instruct patient to avoid contact with people who have infections and to report signs of infection or unusual bleeding immediately.
• Reassure patient that growth of hair should return 4 to 8 weeks after treatment has ended, but hair is usually of a different texture and color will be lost as therapy continues.
• Reassure patient that flulike syndrome may be treated with mild antipyretics such as acetaminophen.
• Tell patient to avoid aspirin and aspirin-containing products. Teach him the signs and symptoms of bleeding, and urge him to report them promptly.

Breast-feeding
• It is not known if drug is distributed into breast milk. However, because of the risk of serious adverse reactions, mutagenicity, and carcinogenicity in the infant, breast-feeding is not recommended.

daclizumab
Zenapax

Pharmacologic classification: humanized immunoglobulin G1 monoclonal antibody
Therapeutic classification: immunosuppressive agent
Pregnancy risk category C

How supplied
Available by prescription only
Injection (for I.V. use): 25 mg/5 ml

Indications, route, and dosage
Prophylaxis of acute organ rejection in patients receiving renal transplants
Adults: 1.0 mg/kg in 50 ml 0.9% NaCl I.V. given over 15 minutes via a central or peripheral line. The standard course of therapy is five doses. Administer first dose no more than 24 hours before transplantation; remaining four doses are given at 14-day intervals.

Drug is used as part of an immunosuppressive regimen that includes corticosteroids and cyclosporine.

Pharmacodynamics
Immunosuppressive action: An interleukin(IL)-2 receptor antagonist that binds to the 1-alpha Tac subunit of the IL-2 receptor complex and inhibits IL-2 binding. This effect prevents IL-2 mediated activation of lymphocytes, a critical pathway in the cellular immune response against allografts. Once in circulation, drug impairs the response of the immune system to antigenic challenges. Following drug administration, the Tac subunit of the IL-2 receptor is saturated for approximately 120 days posttransplant.

Pharmacokinetics
• *Absorption:* Serum concentrations increase between first and fifth doses.
• *Distribution:* Unknown.
• *Metabolism:* Unknown, but given a known relationship between body weight and systemic clearance, dosing is based on mg/kg.
• *Excretion:* Estimated terminal elimination half-life is 20 days (480 hours).

Contraindications and precautions
Contraindicated in patients with a known hypersensitivity to drug or any of its components.

It is not known if drug has a long-term effect on the immune response to antigens first encountered during therapy. Readministration of drug after initial course of treatment has not been studied. The possible risks of prolonged immunosuppression, anaphylaxis, or anaphylactoid reactions have not been identified.

Interactions
None reported.

Effect on diagnostic tests
None reported.

Adverse reactions
CNS: *tremor, headache, dizziness, insomnia,* generalized weakness, prickly sensation, *fever, pain, fatigue,* depression, anxiety.
CV: tachycardia, hypertension, ***pulmonary edema,*** hypotension, aggravated hypertension, *edema,* fluid overload, chest pain.
EENT: blurred vision, pharyngitis, rhinitis.
GI: constipation, nausea, diarrhea, vomiting, abdominal pain, dyspepsia, pyrosis, abdominal distention, epigastric pain, flatulance, gastritis, hemorrhoids.
GU: ***oliguria,*** *dysuria,* ***renal tubular necrosis, renal damage,*** urinary retention, hydronephrosis, urinary tract bleeding, urinary tract disorder, ***renal insufficiency.***
Hematologic: *lymphocele.*
Metabolic: diabetes mellitus, dehydration.
Musculoskeletal: *musculoskeletal or back pain,* arthralgia, myalgia, leg cramps.
Respiratory: *dyspnea, coughing,* atelectasis, congestion, ***hypoxia,*** rales, abnormal breath sounds, pleural effusion.
Skin: *acne, impaired wound healing without infection,* pruritis, hirsutism, rash, night sweats, increased sweating.
Other: *posttraumatic pain,* shivering, extremity edema.

Overdose and treatment
No information available. Maximum tolerated dosage has not been determined. Doses up to 1.5 mg/kg have been administered to bone marrow transplant recipients without associated adverse effects.

☑ Special considerations
• Only clinicians experienced in immunosuppressive therapy, management, and follow up of organ transplant patients should use drug. Patients receiving drug should be managed in facilities equipped and staffed with adequate laboratory and supportive medical care.
• Incidence of lipoproliferative disorders and opportunistic infections was no greater when compared with placebo in clinical trials. However, patients undergoing immunosuppressive therapy are at increased risk; monitor them carefully.
• Drug is not for direct injection.
• Other drugs should not be added or infused simultaneously through the same I.V. line.

Patient education
• Tell patient to consult primary health care provider before taking other medications during drug therapy.
• Advise patient to practice infection prevention precautions.
• Inform patient that neither he nor any household member should receive vaccinations unless medically approved.
• Tell patient to report wounds that fail to heal, unusual bruising or bleeding, or fever immediately.
• Advise patient to drink plenty of fluids during drug therapy, and to report painful urination, blood in the urine, or decrease in urine amount.

Geriatric use
• Use drug cautiously in elderly patients.

Pediatric use
• No adequate or well-controlled clinical trial exists involving children. The immune response to vaccines, infection, or other antigenic stimuli during or after therapy is not known.

Breast-feeding
• It is not known if drug is excreted in breast milk. Because of the potential risks, either the drug or breast-feeding should be discontinued.

---

dactinomycin (actinomycin D)
Cosmegen

Pharmacologic classification: antibiotic antineoplastic (cell cycle–phase nonspecific)
Therapeutic classification: antineoplastic
Pregnancy risk category C

How supplied
Available by prescription only
Injectable: 500-mcg vial

Indications, route, and dosage
Dosage and indications may vary. Check current literature for recommended protocols.
Uterine cancer, testicular cancer, Wilms' tumor, rhabdomyosarcoma, Ewing's sarcoma, sarcoma botryoides, ◊ Kaposi's sarcoma, ◊ acute organ (kidney or heart) rejection, ◊ malignant melanoma, ◊ acute lymphocytic leukemia, ◊ advanced tumors of breast or ovary, ◊ Paget's disease of bone
Adults: 500 mcg (0.5 mg) I.V. daily for a maximum of 5 days. Maximum dosage is 15 mcg/kg/day or 400 to 600 mcg/m²/day for 5 days. After bone marrow recovery, course may be repeated.
Children: 15 mcg/kg (0.015 mg/kg) I.V. daily for a maximum of 5 days. Alternatively, give a total dosage of 2,500 mcg/m² I.V. over a 1-week period. Maximum dosage is 15 mcg/kg/day or 400 to 600 mcg/m²/day. After bone marrow recovery, course may be repeated.

For isolation-perfusion, use 50 mcg/kg for lower extremity or pelvis; 35 mcg/kg for upper extremity.

Dose should be based on body surface area in obese or edematous patients.

Pharmacodynamics
Antineoplastic action: Dactinomycin exerts its cytotoxic activity by intercalating between DNA base pairs and uncoiling the DNA helix. The result is inhibition of DNA synthesis and DNA-dependent RNA synthesis.

Pharmacokinetics
• *Absorption:* Due to its vesicant properties, dactinomycin must be administered I.V.
• *Distribution:* Widely distributed into body tissues, with highest levels found in the bone marrow and nucleated cells. Drug does not cross the blood-brain barrier to a significant extent.
• *Metabolism:* Dactinomycin is only minimally metabolized in the liver.
• *Excretion:* Drug and its metabolites are excreted in the urine and bile. Plasma elimination half-life of drug is 36 hours.

Contraindications and precautions
Contraindicated in patients with chickenpox or herpes zoster.

Interactions
In combination with *amphotericin B* may increase risk of nephrotoxicity; may increase serum uric acid levels when used in combination with *antigout* medications.

Effects on diagnostic tests
Drug therapy may increase blood and urine concentrations of uric acid.

Adverse reactions
GI: *anorexia, nausea, vomiting,* abdominal pain, diarrhea, *stomatitis,* ulceration, proctitis.
Hematologic: ***anemia, leukopenia, thrombocytopenia, pancytopenia, aplastic anemia, agranulocytosis.***
Hepatic: ***hepatotoxicity.***

Skin: *erythema;* desquamation; *hyperpigmentation of skin, especially in previously irradiated areas; acnelike eruptions* (reversible).
Other: phlebitis and severe damage to soft tissue at injection site, reversible alopecia, malaise, fatigue, lethargy, fever, myalgia, hypocalcemia, ***death.***

Overdose and treatment

Clinical manifestations of overdose include myelosuppression, nausea, vomiting, glossitis, and oral ulceration.

Treatment is generally supportive and includes antiemetics and transfusion of blood components.

☑ Special considerations

- To reconstitute for I.V. administration, add 1.1 ml of preservative-free sterile water for injection to drug to give a concentration of 0.5 mg/ml. Do not use a preserved diluent, as precipitation may occur.
- Use gloves when preparing and administering this drug.
- Drug may be diluted further with D_5W or 0.9% NaCl for administration by I.V. infusion.
- Discard unused solution because it doesn't contain preservatives.
- May administer by I.V. push injection into the tubing of a freely flowing I.V. infusion. Do *not* administer through an in-line I.V. filter.
- Use body surface area calculation in obese or edematous patients.
- Treatment of extravasation includes topical administration of dimethyl sulfoxide and cold compresses.
- To reduce nausea, give antiemetic before administering. Nausea usually occurs within 30 minutes of a dose.
- Monitor CBC daily and platelet counts every third day. Leukocyte and platelet nadirs usually occur 14 to 21 days after completion of course of therapy. Observe for signs of bleeding.
- Monitor renal and hepatic functions.
- Patients who have received other cytotoxic drugs or radiation within 6 weeks of dactinomycin may exhibit erythema, followed by hyperpigmentation or edema, or both; desquamation; vesiculation; and, rarely, necrosis.

Patient education

- Advise patient to avoid exposure to people with infections.
- Warn patient that alopecia may occur but is usually reversible.
- Tell patient to promptly report sore throat, fever, or signs of bleeding.

Pediatric use

- Restrict use of drug in infants age 6 months or older; adverse reactions are more frequent in infants under age 6 months.

Breast-feeding

- Distribution of drug in breast milk is unknown. However, because of risks of serious adverse reactions, mutagenicity, and carcinogenicity in infants, breast-feeding is not recommended.

dalteparin sodium

Fragmin

Pharmacologic classification: low-molecular-weight heparin derivative
Therapeutic classification: anticoagulant
Pregnancy risk category B

How supplied

Available by prescription only
Injection: 2,500 anti-factor Xa IU/0.2 ml, 5,000 anti-factor Xa IU/0.2 ml

Indications, route, and dosage

Prophylaxis against deep vein thrombosis (DVT) in patients undergoing abdominal surgery who are at risk for thromboembolic complications (including those who are over age 40, obese, undergoing general anesthesia lasting longer than 30 minutes, and with history of DVT or pulmonary embolism)
Adults: 2,500 IU S.C. daily, starting 1 to 2 hours before surgery and repeated once daily for 5 to 10 days postoperatively.

Pharmacodynamics

Anticoagulant action: Drug acts by enhancing the inhibition of factor Xa and thrombin by antithrombin.

Pharmacokinetics

- *Absorption:* Drug's absolute bioavailability measured in anti-factor Xa activity is about 87%.
- *Distribution:* Volume of distribution for dalteparin anti-factor Xa activity is 40 to 60 ml/kg.
- *Metabolism:* Unknown.
- *Excretion:* Unknown.

Contraindications and precautions

Contraindicated in patients with hypersensitivity to drug, heparin, or pork products; active major bleeding; or thrombocytopenia associated with positive in vitro tests for antiplatelet antibody in the presence of drug.

Use with extreme caution in patients with history of heparin-induced thrombocytopenia or in those with increased risk of hemorrhage, such as those with severe uncontrolled hypertension, bacterial endocarditis, congenital or acquired bleeding disorders, active ulceration and angiodysplastic GI disease, hemorrhagic stroke, or shortly after brain, spinal, or ophthalmic surgery. Use cautiously in patients with bleeding diathesis, thrombocytopenia, or platelet defects; severe liver or kidney insufficiency; hypertensive or diabetic retinopathy; and recent GI bleeding.

Interactions

Oral anticoagulants or *platelet inhibitors* may increase risk of bleeding. Use together with caution.

Effects on diagnostic tests

Dalteparin may falsely elevate AST and ALT levels; these increases are fully reversible.

Adverse reactions
Hematologic: ***thrombocytopenia.***
Skin: pruritus, rash; *hematoma,* pain or skin necrosis (rare) (at injection site).
Other: hemorrhage, ecchymoses, bleeding complications, fever, ***anaphylactoid reactions*** (rare).

Overdose and treatment
Overdosage may cause hemorrhagic complications. These may generally be stopped by the slow I.V. injection of protamine sulfate (1% solution), at a dose of 1 mg protamine for every 100 anti-factor Xa IU of dalteparin given. A second infusion of 0.5 mg protamine sulfate per 100 anti-factor Xa IU of dalteparin may be administered if the activated partial thromboplastin time (APTT) measured 2 to 4 hours after the first infusion remains prolonged. Even with these additional doses of protamine sulfate, the APTT may remain more prolonged than would usually be found following administration of conventional heparin.

☑ Special considerations
- Patient should assume a sitting or lying down position when drug is administered. Dalteparin should be injected S.C. deeply. Injection sites include a U-shaped area around the navel, the upper outer side of the thigh, or the upper outer quadrangle of the buttock. Sites should be rotated daily. When the area around the navel or the thigh is used, the thumb and forefinger should be used to lift up a fold of skin while the injection is being given. The entire length of the needle should be inserted at a 45- to 90-degree angle.
- Dalteparin should never be administered I.M.
- Do not mix drug with other injections or infusions unless specific compatibility data are available that support such mixing.
- Drug is not interchangeable (unit for unit) with unfractionated heparin or other low-molecular-weight heparins.
- Periodic routine CBC, including platelet count, and stool occult blood tests are recommended in patients receiving treatment with dalteparin. Patients do not require regular monitoring of PT or APTT.
- Monitor patient closely for thrombocytopenia.
- Discontinue drug if a thromboembolic event occurs despite dalteparin prophylaxis.

Patient education
- Instruct patient and his family to watch for signs of bleeding and report them immediately.
- Tell patient to avoid OTC medications containing aspirin or other salicylates.

Pediatric use
- Safety and effectiveness in children have not been established.

Breast-feeding
- It is not known if drug occurs in breast milk; use with caution in breast-feeding women.

danaparoid sodium
Orgaran Injection

Pharmacologic classification: glycosaminoglycuronan
Therapeutic classification: antithrombotic
Pregnancy risk category B

How supplied
Available by prescription only
Ampule: 750 anti-Xa units/0.6 ml
Syringe: 750 anti-Xa units/0.6 ml

Indications, route, and dosage
Prophylaxis against postoperative deep vein thrombosis (DVT) which may lead to pulmonary embolism in patients undergoing elective hip replacement surgery
Adults: 750 anti-Xa units S.C. b.i.d. beginning 1 to 4 hours preoperatively; then no sooner than 2 hours after surgery. Continue treatment for 7 to 10 days postoperatively or until risk of DVT has diminished.

Pharmacodynamics
Antithrombotic action: Prevents fibrin formation by inhibiting generation of thrombin by anti-Xa and anti-IIa. Because of its predominant anti-Xa activity, danaparoid injection has little effect on clotting assays such as PT and partial thromboplastin time (PTT). Drug has only minor effect on platelet function and platelet aggregability.

Pharmacokinetics
Drug pharmacokinetics have been described by monitoring its biologic activity (plasma anti-Xa activity) because no specific chemical assay methods are currently available.
- *Absorption:* S.C. administration is approximately 100% bioavailable, compared with same dose administered I.V. Onset and duration are unknown. Peak anti-Xa activity occurs in 2 to 5 hours.
- *Distribution:* Not reported.
- *Metabolism:* Not reported.
- *Excretion:* Drug is mainly eliminated through the kidneys. Mean value for the terminal half-life is about 24 hours. In patients with severely impaired renal function, elimination half-life of plasma anti-Xa activity may be prolonged.

Contraindications and precautions
Contraindicated in patients with hypersensitivity to drug or to pork products, severe hemorrhagic diathesis (such as hemophilia or idiopathic thrombocytopenic purpura), active major bleeding (including hemorrhagic stroke in the acute phase), or type II thrombocytopenia associated with positive in vitro tests for antiplatelet antibody in the presence of the drug.

Use with extreme caution in patients at increased risk of hemorrhage, such as in severe uncontrolled hypertension, acute bacterial endocarditis, congenital or acquired bleeding disorders, active ulcerative and angiodysplastic GI disease, nonhemorrhagic stroke, postoperative use of indwelling epidural catheter, or shortly after brain, spinal, or ophthalmic surgery.

Use cautiously in patients with impaired renal function and in those receiving oral anticoagulants or platelet inhibitors.

Interactions
Oral anticoagulants or *platelet inhibitors* may increase the risk of bleeding; use together cautiously.

Effects on diagnostic tests
Monitoring of anticoagulant activity of oral anticoagulants by PT and Thrombotest is unreliable within 5 hours after danaparoid administration.

Adverse reactions
CNS: insomnia, headache, asthenia, dizziness.
CV: peripheral edema, ***hemorrhage.***
GI: *nausea, constipation,* vomiting.
GU: urinary tract infection, urine retention.
Hematologic: anemia.
Musculoskeletal: joint disorder, pain.
Skin: rash, pruritis.
Other: *fever,* pain at injection site, infection, edema.

Overdose and treatment
Overdosage of danaparoid injection may lead to bleeding complications. The effects of danaparoid on anti-Xa activity cannot be currently antagonized with other known agents. Although protamine sulfate partially neutralizes the anti-Xa activity of danaparoid and can be safely coadministered, there is no evidence that protamine sulfate is capable of reducing severe nonsurgical bleeding during treatment with danaparoid. If serious bleeding occurs, stop drug and administer blood or blood products as needed.

Symptoms of acute toxicity after I.V. dosing were respiratory depression, prostration, and twitching.

☑ Special considerations
- Drug contains sodium sulfite, which may cause allergic-type reactions, including anaphylactic symptoms and life-threatening or less severe asthmatic episodes in certain patients. The overall prevalence of sulfite allergy in the general population is unknown and probably low. Sulfite sensitivity is seen more frequently in asthmatic than in nonasthmatic patients.
- Risks and benefits of danaparoid injection should be carefully considered before use in patients with severely impaired renal function or hemorrhagic disorders.
- Do not give drug I.M. To administer drug, have patient lie down. Give S.C. injection deeply, using a 25G to 26G needle. Alternate injection sites between the left and right anterolateral and posterolateral abdominal wall. Gently pull up a skin fold with thumb and forefinger and insert entire length of the needle into tissue. Do not rub or pinch afterward.
- Know that drug is not interchangeable (unit for unit) with heparin or low-molecular-weight heparin.
- Periodic, routine CBCs (including platelet count) and fecal occult blood tests are recommended during therapy. Patients do not require regular monitoring of PT and PTT.
- Drug has little effect on PT, PTT, fibrinolytic activity, and bleeding time.
- Monitor patient's hematocrit and blood pressure closely; a decrease in either may signal hemorrhage. If serious bleeding occurs, stop drug and transfuse blood products if needed.
- Monitor patient with severely impaired renal function carefully.
- Carefully monitor patients with serum creatinine level of 2 mg/dl or more.

Patient education
- Instruct patient and family to watch for and report signs of bleeding.
- Tell patient to avoid OTC drugs containing aspirin or other salicylates.

Pediatric use
- Safety and effectiveness in pediatric patients have not been established.

Breast-feeding
- It is not known if drug is excreted in breast milk; use cautiously in breast-feeding patients.

danazol
Cyclomen*, Danocrine

Pharmacologic classification: androgen
Therapeutic classification: antiestrogen, androgen
Pregnancy risk category X

How supplied
Available by prescription only
Capsules: 50 mg, 100 mg, 200 mg

Indications, route, and dosage
Mild endometriosis
Adults: Initially, 100 to 200 mg P.O. b.i.d. uninterrupted for 3 to 6 months; may continue for 9 months. Subsequent dosage based on patient response.
Moderate to severe endometriosis
Adults: 400 mg P.O. b.i.d. uninterrupted for 3 to 6 months; may continue for 9 months.
Fibrocystic breast disease
Adults: 100 to 400 mg P.O. daily in two divided doses uninterrupted for 2 to 6 months.
Prevention of hereditary angioedema
Adults: 200 mg P.O. b.i.d. or t.i.d., continued until favorable response is achieved. Then, dosage should be decreased by half at 1- to 3-month intervals.

Pharmacodynamics
Antiestrogenic action: Danazol's antiestrogenic actions cause regression and atrophy of normal and ectopic endometrial tissue. Drug also decreases the rate of growth and nodularity of abnormal breast tissue in fibrocystic breast disease.

Androgenic action: Danazol's androgenic effects increase levels of the C1 and C4 components of complement, which reduces the frequency and severity of attacks associated with hereditary angioedema.

Pharmacokinetics

- *Absorption:* Amount of danazol absorbed by the body is not proportional to the administered dose; doubling drug dose produces an increase of only 35% to 40% in drug absorption.
- *Distribution:* Unknown.
- *Metabolism:* Drug is metabolized to 2-hydroxymethylethisterone.
- *Excretion:* Unknown.

Contraindications and precautions

Contraindicated in patients with undiagnosed abnormal genital bleeding; porphyria; or impaired renal, cardiac, or hepatic function; during pregnancy; and in breast-feeding patients.

Use cautiously in patients with seizure disorders or migraine headaches.

Interactions

In patients with diabetes, danazol may cause decreases in blood glucose levels, which may require adjustment of *insulin* or *oral antidiabetic drugs.* Danazol may potentiate the action of *warfarin-type anticoagulants,* prolonging PT. It may increase the plasma concentrations of *carbamazepine* in patients taking both drugs.

Effects on diagnostic tests

Glucose tolerance test results may be abnormal. Total serum T_4 may be decreased; T_3 may be increased. PT (especially in patients on anticoagulant therapy) may be prolonged.

Adverse reactions

CNS: dizziness, headache, sleep disorders, fatigue, tremor, irritability, excitation, lethargy, mental depression, chills, paresthesia.
CV: elevated blood pressure.
EENT: visual disturbances.
GI: gastric irritation, nausea, vomiting, diarrhea, constipation, change in appetite.
GU: hematuria, *hypoestrogenic effects (flushing, diaphoresis, vaginitis [including itching, dryness,* and *burning]; vaginal bleeding, nervousness, emotional lability, menstrual irregularities).*
Hepatic: reversible jaundice, elevated liver enzyme levels, hepatic dysfunction.
Other: muscle cramps or spasms; androgenic effects in women *(weight gain, hirsutism,* hoarseness, clitoral enlargement, *decreased breast size,* acne, edema, changes in libido, *oily skin or hair,* voice deepening).

Overdose and treatment

No information available. Empty stomach by induced emesis or gastric lavage; follow with activated charcoal to reduce absorption. Treatment is supportive.

☑ Special considerations

Besides those relevant to all *androgens,* consider the following recommendations.

- Because drug may cause hepatic dysfunction, periodic liver function studies should be performed.
- To treat endometriosis and fibrocystic breast disease, danazol therapy should begin during menstruation.
- Tests should rule out pregnancy before therapy with danazol. Urge female patient to use effective barrier methods of contraception during danazol therapy.
- Danazol provides alternative therapy for patients who cannot tolerate or fail to respond to other means of therapy. (It is *not* indicated in cases in which surgery is the best choice.)

Patient education

- Tell patient desiring birth control to use a nonhormonal contraceptive; during danazol treatment, ovulation may not be suppressed by hormonal contraceptives.
- Advise patient to report voice changes or other signs of virilization promptly. Some androgenic effects such as deepening of the voice may not be reversible on discontinuation of drug.
- Instruct patient to immediately report nausea, vomiting, headache, and visual disturbances, which may suggest pseudotumor cerebri.
- Advise patient who is taking danazol for fibrocystic disease to examine breasts regularly. If breast nodule enlarges during treatment, she should call immediately.
- Advise female patient that amenorrhea usually occurs after 6 to 8 weeks of therapy.
- Advise male patient that periodic evaluation of semen may be indicated.

Geriatric use

- Use with caution. Observe elderly male patients for the development of prostatic hypertrophy; symptomatic prostatic hypertrophy or prostatic carcinoma mandates discontinuation of danazol.

Pediatric use

- Use with caution because of possible androgenic effects. Use danazol with extreme caution in children to avoid precocious puberty and premature closure of the epiphyses. Conduct X-ray examinations every 6 months to assess skeletal maturation.

Breast-feeding

- Because of the potential for serious adverse reactions in the infant, a decision should be made to discontinue breast-feeding or the drug, depending on drug's importance to patient.

dantrolene sodium

Dantrium

Pharmacologic classification: hydantoin derivative
Therapeutic classification: skeletal muscle relaxant
Pregnancy risk category C

How supplied

Available by prescription only
Capsules: 25 mg, 50 mg, 100 mg
Injection: 20 mg parenteral (contains 3 g mannitol)

Indications, route, and dosage

Spasticity resulting from upper motor neuron disorders

Adults: 25 mg P.O. daily, increased gradually in increments of 25 mg at 4- to 7-day intervals, up to 100 mg b.i.d. to q.i.d., to maximum of 400 mg daily.
Children over age 5: 0.5 mg/kg P.O. b.i.d., increased to t.i.d., then q.i.d. Increase dosage further p.r.n. by 0.5 mg/kg up to 3 mg/kg b.i.d. to q.i.d. Maximum dosage is 100 mg q.i.d.

Prevention of malignant hyperthermia in susceptible patients who require surgery

Adults: 4 to 8 mg/kg/day P.O. given in three to four divided doses for 1 to 2 days before procedure; administer last dose 3 to 4 hours before procedure. Alternatively, give 2.5 mg/kg I.V. over 1 hour approximately 75 minutes before anesthesia.

Management of malignant hyperthermia crisis

Adults and children: Initially, 1 mg/kg I.V.; then continue until symptoms subside or maximum cumulative dose of 10 mg/kg has been reached.

Prevention of recurrence of malignant hyperthermia after crisis

Adults: 4 to 8 mg/kg/day P.O. given in four divided doses for up to 3 days after crisis. Alternatively, give 1 mg/kg or more I.V. based on clinical situation.

◊ ***To reduce succinylcholine-induced muscle fasciculations and postoperative muscle pain***

Adults under 99 lb (45 kg): 100 mg P.O. 2 hours before succinylcholine.
Adults over 99 lb: 150 mg P.O. 2 hours before succinylcholine.

Pharmacodynamics

Skeletal muscle relaxant action: A hydantoin derivative, dantrolene is chemically and pharmacologically unrelated to other skeletal muscle relaxants. It directly affects skeletal muscle, reducing muscle tension. It interferes with the release of calcium ions from the sarcoplasmic reticulum, resulting in decreased muscle contraction. This mechanism is of particular importance in malignant hyperthermia when increased myoplasmic calcium ion concentrations activate acute catabolism in the skeletal muscle cell. Dantrolene prevents or reduces the increase in myoplasmic calcium concentrations associated with malignant hyperthermia crises.

Pharmacokinetics

- *Absorption:* 35% of oral dose is absorbed through GI tract, with serum half-life reached within 8 to 9 hours after oral administration, and 5 hours after I.V. administration. Therapeutic effect in patients with upper motor neuron disorders may take 1 week or more.
- *Distribution:* Dantrolene is substantially plasma protein-bound, mainly to albumin.
- *Metabolism:* Drug is metabolized in the liver to its less active 5-hydroxy derivatives, and to its amino derivative by reductive pathways.
- *Excretion:* Excreted in urine as metabolites.

Contraindications and precautions

Contraindicated in patients when spasticity is used to maintain motor function in those with upper motor neuron disorders, for spasms in rheumatic disorders, in patients with active hepatic disease, and in breast-feeding patients. Contraindicated in combination with verapamil in management of malignant hyperthermia. Use cautiously in women (especially those taking estrogen), in patients over age 35, and in patients with severely impaired cardiac or pulmonary function or preexisting hepatic disease.

Interactions

Concomitant use with other *CNS depressant drugs,* including *alcohol, narcotics, anxiolytics, antipsychotics,* and *tricyclic antidepressants,* may increase CNS depression. Reduce dosage of one or both if used concurrently. Use of dantrolene in women over age 35 who are also receiving *estrogen* therapy may increase incidence of hepatotoxicity. Concomitant administration with *verapamil* has resulted in rare reports of cardiac collapse.

Effects on diagnostic tests

Dantrolene therapy alters liver function test results (increased ALT, AST, alkaline phosphatase, and LD), BUN levels, and total serum bilirubin.

Adverse reactions

CNS: *muscle weakness, drowsiness, dizziness, light-headedness, malaise, fatigue, headache, confusion, nervousness, insomnia,* ***seizures.***
CV: tachycardia, blood pressure changes.
EENT: excessive lacrimation, speech disturbance, altered taste, diplopia, visual disturbances.
GI: anorexia, constipation, cramping, dysphagia, metallic taste, severe diarrhea, GI bleeding.
GU: urinary frequency, hematuria, incontinence, nocturia, dysuria, crystalluria, difficult erection, urine retention.
Hepatic: ***hepatitis.***
Respiratory: pleural effusion with pericarditis.
Skin: eczematous eruption, pruritus, urticaria.
Other: abnormal hair growth, diaphoresis, myalgia, chills, fever, back pain.

Overdose and treatment

Clinical manifestations of overdose include exaggeration of adverse reactions, particularly CNS depression, and nausea and vomiting.

Treatment includes supportive measures, gastric lavage, and observation of symptoms. Maintain adequate airway, have emergency ventilation equipment on hand, monitor ECG, and administer large quantities of I.V. solutions to prevent crystalluria. Monitor vital signs closely. The benefit of dialysis is not known.

☑ Special considerations

- To prepare suspension for single oral dose, dissolve contents of appropriate number of capsules in fruit juice or other suitable liquid.
- Before therapy begins, check patient's baseline neuromuscular functions—posture, gait, coordination, range of motion, muscle strength and tone, presence of abnormal muscle movements, and reflexes—for later comparisons.
- Drug may cause muscle weakness and impaired walking ability. Use with caution and carefully su-

pervise patients receiving drug for prophylactic treatment for malignant hyperthermia.
• Walking should be supervised until patient's reaction to drug is known. With relief of spasticity, patient may lose ability to maintain balance.
• Improvement may require 1 week or more of drug therapy.
• Because of the risk of hepatic injury, discontinue drug if improvement is not evident within 45 days.
• Perform baseline and regularly scheduled liver function tests (alkaline phosphatase, ALT, AST, and total bilirubin), blood cell counts, and renal function tests.
• Risk of hepatotoxicity may be greater in women, patients over age 35, and in those taking other medications (especially estrogen) or high dantrolene doses (400 mg or more daily) for prolonged periods.
• Clinical signs of malignant hyperthermia include skeletal muscle rigidity (often the first sign), sudden tachycardia, arrhythmias, cyanosis, tachypnea, severe hypercarbia, unstable blood pressure, rapidly rising temperature, acidosis, and shock.
• In malignant hyperthermia crisis, drug should be given by rapid I.V. injection as soon as reaction is recognized.
• To reconstitute, add 60 ml sterile water for injection to 20-mg vial. Do not use bacteriostatic water, D_5W, or 0.9% NaCl for injection. Reconstituted solution should be stored away from direct sunlight at room temperature, and should be discarded after 6 hours.
• Treating malignant hyperthermia requires continual monitoring of body temperature, management of fever, correction of acidosis, maintenance of fluid and electrolyte balance, monitoring of intake and output, adequate oxygenation, and seizure precautions.

Patient education
• Instruct patient to report promptly the onset of jaundice: yellow skin or sclerae, dark urine, clay-colored stools, itching, and abdominal discomfort. Hepatotoxicity occurs more frequently between the third and twelfth month of therapy.
• Advise patient susceptible to malignant hyperthermia to wear medical identification (for example, Medic Alert) indicating diagnosis, primary health care provider's name and telephone number, drug causing reaction, and treatment used.
• Because hepatotoxicity occurs more commonly after concurrent use of other drugs with dantrolene, warn patient to avoid OTC medications, alcoholic beverages, and other CNS depressants except as prescribed.
• Advise patient to avoid excessive or unnecessary exposure to sunlight and to use protective clothing and a sunscreen agent because photosensitivity reactions may occur.
• Warn patient to avoid hazardous activities that require alertness until CNS depressant effects are determined. Drug may cause drowsiness.
• Advise patient to report adverse reactions immediately.
• Tell patient to store drug away from heat and direct light (not in bathroom medicine cabinet). Keep out of reach of children.
• If patient misses a dose, tell him to take it within 1 hour; otherwise, he should omit the dose and return to regular dosing schedule. Tell him not to double doses.

Geriatric use
• Administer drug with extreme caution to elderly patients.

Pediatric use
• Drug is not recommended for long-term use in children under age 5.

Breast-feeding
• Contraindicated for use by breast-feeding women.

dapsone
Avlosulfon*

Pharmacologic classification: synthetic sulfone
Therapeutic classification: antileprotic, antimalarial
Pregnancy risk category C

How supplied
Available by prescription only
Tablets: 25 mg, 100 mg

Indications, route, and dosage
All forms of leprosy (Hansen's disease) except for cases of proven dapsone resistance
Adults: 100 mg P.O. daily for at least 2 years, plus rifampin 600 mg daily for 6 months.
Children: 1 to 1.5 mg/kg P.O. daily.
Prophylaxis for leprosy patient's close contacts
Adults and children age 12 and older: 50 mg P.O. daily.
Children age 6 to 12: 25 mg P.O. daily.
Children age 2 to 5: 25 mg P.O. three times weekly.
Infants age 6 to 23 months: 12 mg P.O. three times weekly.
Infants under age 6 months: 6 mg P.O. three times weekly.
Dermatitis herpetiformis
Adults: Initially, 50 mg P.O. daily; may increase dose p.r.n. to obtain full control.
✦ ***Dosage adjustment.*** Dapsone levels are influenced by acetylation rates. Patients with high acetylation rates may require dose adjustments.
◇ ***Malaria suppression or prophylaxis***
Adults: 100 mg P.O. weekly, with pyrimethamine 12.5 mg P.O. weekly.
Children: 2 mg/kg P.O. weekly, with pyrimethamine 0.25 mg/kg weekly.
Continue prophylaxis throughout exposure and 6 months postexposure.
◇ ***Treatment of* Pneumocystis carinii *pneumonia***
Adults: 100 mg P.O. daily. Usually administered with trimethoprim, 20 mg/kg daily, for 21 days.

Pharmacodynamics

Antibiotic action: Drug is bacteriostatic and bactericidal; like sulfonamides, it is thought to act principally by inhibition of folic acid. It acts against *Mycobacterium leprae* and *M. tuberculosis* and has some activity against *P. carinii* and *Plasmodium*.

Pharmacokinetics

• *Absorption:* When given orally, drug is rapidly and almost completely absorbed. Peak serum levels occur 2 to 8 hours after ingestion.
• *Distribution:* Distributed widely into most body tissues and fluids; 50% to 90% is protein-bound.
• *Metabolism:* Drug undergoes acetylation by liver enzymes; rate varies and is genetically determined. Almost 50% of Blacks and Whites are slow acetylators, whereas over 80% of Chinese, Japanese, and Eskimos are fast acetylators.
• *Excretion:* Drug and metabolites are excreted primarily in urine; small amounts of drug are excreted in feces; and substantial amounts in breast milk. Dapsone undergoes enterohepatic circulation; half-life in adults ranges between 10 and 50 hours (average 28 hours). Orally administered charcoal may enhance excretion. Dapsone is dialyzable.

Contraindications and precautions

Contraindicated in patients with hypersensitivity to drug. Use cautiously in patients with impaired renal, hepatic, or CV disease; refractory types of anemia; and G6PD deficiency.

Interactions

Activated charcoal may decrease dapsone's GI absorption and enterohepatic recycling; monitor closely. Use with *didanosine* may produce a possible therapeutic failure of dapsone, leading to an increase in infection. Avoid concomitant use.

Use with *folic acid antagonists* such as *methotrexate* is associated with increased risk of adverse hematologic reactions. Avoid concomitant use.

PABA may antagonize the effect of dapsone by interfering with the primary mechanism of action. Monitor for lack of efficacy. *Probenecid* reduces urinary excretion of dapsone metabolites, increasing plasma concentrations. Monitor closely.

Use with *rifampin* or barbiturates is associated with increased hepatic metabolism of dapsone. Monitor for lack of efficacy. Increased serum levels of both dapsone and *trimethoprim* may occur when they are used together, possibly increasing the pharmacologic and toxic effects of each drug. Monitor closely.

Effects on diagnostic tests

None reported.

Adverse reactions

CNS: insomnia, psychosis, headache, paresthesia, peripheral neuropathy, vertigo.
EENT: tinnitus, blurred vision.
GI: anorexia, abdominal pain, nausea, vomiting.
GU: albuminuria, nephrotic syndrome, renal papillary necrosis.
Hematologic: ***hemolytic anemia*** (dose-related), ***agranulocytosis, aplastic anemia.***
Skin: lupus erythematosus, phototoxity, ***exfoliative dermatitis, toxic erythema, erythema multiforme, toxic epidermal necrolysis, morbiliform and scarlatiniform reactions***, urticaria, ***erythema nodosum.***
Other: fever, tachycardia, ***pancreatitis,*** male infertility, pulmonary eosinophilia, infectious mononucleosis-like syndrome, ***sulfone syndrome (fever, malaise, jaundice*** [with hepatic necrosis], ***exfoliative dermatitis, lymphadenopathy, methemoglobinemia, hemolytic anemia).***

Leprosy reactional states

When treating leprosy with dapsone, it is essential to recognize two types of leprosy reactional states that are related to effectiveness of dapsone treatment.

Type I, reversal reaction, includes erythema, followed by swelling of skin and nerve lesions in tuberculoid patients; skin lesions may ulcerate and multiply, and acute neuritis may cause neural dysfunction. Severe cases require hospitalization, analgesics, corticosteroids, and nerve trunk decompression while dapsone therapy is continued.

Type II, erythema nodosum leprosum, occurs primarily in lepromatous leprosy, with an incidence of about 50% during the first year of therapy. Signs and symptoms include tender erythematous skin nodules, fever, malaise, orchitis, neuritis, albuminuria, iritis, joint swelling, epistaxis, and depression; skin lesions may ulcerate. Treatment includes corticosteroids and analgesics while dapsone is continued.

Additional treatment guidelines are available from National Hansen's Disease Center, (800) 642-7771.

Overdose and treatment

Signs of overdose include nausea, vomiting, and hyperexcitability, occurring within minutes or up to 24 hours after ingestion; methemoglobin-induced depression, cyanosis, and seizures may occur. Hemolysis is a late complication (up to 14 days after ingestion).

Treatment is by gastric lavage, followed by activated charcoal; dapsone-induced methemoglobinemia (in patients without G6PD-deficiency) can be treated with methylene blue. Hemodialysis may also be used to enhance elimination.

☑ Special considerations

• Give drug with or after meals to avoid gastric irritation. Ensure adequate fluid intake.
• Obtain specimens for culture and sensitivity testing before giving first dose, but therapy may begin before test results are complete; repeat periodically to detect drug resistance.
• Observe patient for adverse effects and monitor hematologic and liver function studies to minimize toxicity.
• Monitor dapsone serum concentrations periodically to maintain effective levels. Levels of 0.1 to 7 mcg/ml (average 2.3 mcg/ml) are usually effective and safe.

- Observe skin and mucous membranes for early signs of allergic reactions or leprosy reactional states.
- Isolation of patient with inactive leprosy is not required; however, surfaces in contact with discharge from nose or skin lesions should be disinfected.
- Therapeutic effect on leprosy may not be evident until 3 to 6 months after start of therapy.
- Monitor vital signs frequently during early weeks of drug therapy. Frequent or high fever may require reduced dosage or discontinuation of drug.
- Because drug is dialyzable, patients undergoing hemodialysis may require dosage adjustments.

Patient education

- Explain disease process and rationale for long-term therapy to patient and family; emphasize that improvement may not occur for 3 to 6 months, and that treatment must contimue for at least 1 to 2 years.
- Teach signs and symptoms of hypersensitivity and other adverse reactions, and emphasize need to report these promptly; explain possibility of cumulative effects; urge patient to report *any* unusual effects or reactions and to report loss of appetite, nausea, or vomiting promptly.
- Teach patient how to take drug and the need to comply with prescribed regimen. Encourage patient to report no improvement or worsening of symptoms after 3 months of drug treatment. Urge patient not to discontinue drug without medical approval.
- Explain importance of follow-up visits and need to monitor close contacts at 6- to 12-month intervals for 10 years.
- Teach sanitary disposal of secretions from nose or skin lesions.
- Assure patient and family that inactive leprosy is no barrier to employment or school attendance.
- New mothers need not be separated from infant during therapy; teach signs of cyanosis and methemoglobinemia.
- Tell patient to avoid prolonged exposure to sunlight.

Geriatric use

- Elderly patients often have decreased renal function, which decreases drug excretion. Use with caution in elderly patients.

Pediatric use

- Use drug with caution in children.

Breast-feeding

- Dapsone is excreted in breast milk and is tumorigenic in animals. An alternative feeding method is recommended during therapy with dapsone.

---

daunorubicin hydrochloride

Cerubidine

Pharmacologic classification: antibiotic antineoplastic (cell cycle–phase nonspecific)
Therapeutic classification: antineoplastic
Pregnancy risk category D

How supplied

Available by prescription only
Injection: 20-mg vials (with 100 mg of mannitol)

Indications, route, and dosage

Dosage and indications may vary. Check current literature for recommended protocols.

Remission induction in acute nonlymphocytic leukemia (myelogenous, monocytic, erythroid)
Adults under age 60: 45 mg/m² I.V. daily on days 1 to 3 of first course and on days 1 and 2 of subsequent courses. Give all courses in combination with cytosine arabinoside infusions
Adults age 60 and over: 30 mg/m² I.V. daily on days 1 to 3 of first course and on days 1 and 2 of subsequent courses. Give all courses in combination with cytosine arabinoside infusions

Remission induction in acute lymphocytic leukemia
Adults: 45 mg/m²/day I.V. on days 1 to 3; give in combination with vincristine, prednisone, and l-asparaginase
Children age 2 and over: 25 mg/m² I.V. on day 1 weekly for up to 6 weeks, if needed; give in combination with vincristine and prednisone.
Children under age 2 or with a body surface area of under 0.5 m²: Dose should be calculated based on body weight (1 mg/kg), rather than body surface area.

✦ ***Dosage adjustment.*** Use reduced dosage if patient has hepatic or renal impairement. In patients with serum bilirubin of 1.2 to 3 mg/dl, reduce dose by 25%; with serum bilirubin or creatinine levels over 3 mg/dl, reduce dose by 50%.

Pharmacodynamics

Antineoplastic action: Drug exerts its cytotoxic activity by intercalating between DNA base pairs and uncoiling the DNA helix. The result is inhibition of DNA synthesis and DNA-dependent RNA synthesis. Drug may also inhibit polymerase activity.

Pharmacokinetics

- *Absorption:* Owing to its vesicant nature, drug must be given I.V.
- *Distribution:* Drug is widely distributed into body tissues, with the highest concentrations found in the spleen, kidneys, liver, lungs, and heart. It does not cross the blood-brain barrier.
- *Metabolism:* Drug is extensively metabolized in the liver by microsomal enzymes. One of the metabolites has cytotoxic activity.
- *Excretion:* Drug and its metabolites are primarily excreted in bile, with a small portion excreted in urine. Plasma elimination has been described as biphasic, with an initial phase half-life of 45 minutes and a terminal phase half-life of 18½ hours.

Contraindications and precautions

No known contraindications. Use cautiously in patients with myelosuppression or impaired cardiac, renal, or hepatic function.

Interactions

When used concomitantly, other *hepatotoxic drugs* may increase the risk of hepatotoxicity with daunorubicin.

Do not mix daunorubicin with either *heparin sodium* or *dexamethasone phosphate*. Admixture of these agents results in the formation of a precipitate.

Effects on diagnostic tests
Daunorubicin therapy may increase blood and urine concentrations of uric acid. Drug therapy may also cause an increase in serum alkaline phosphatase, AST, and bilirubin levels, indicating drug-induced hepatotoxicity.

Adverse reactions
CV: *irreversible cardiomyopathy* (dose-related), ECG changes.
GI: *nausea, vomiting,* diarrhea, *mucositis* (may occur 3 to 7 days after administration).
GU: red urine (transient).
Hematologic: ***bone marrow suppression*** (lowest blood counts 10 to 14 days after administration).
Hepatic: ***hepatotoxicity.***
Skin: rash.
Other: *severe cellulitis, tissue sloughing* (if drug extravasates); *alopecia,* fever, chills, hyperuricemia.

Overdose and treatment
Clinical manifestations of overdose include myelosuppression, nausea, vomiting, and stomatitis.

Treatment is usually supportive and includes transfusion of blood components and antiemetics.

☑ Special considerations
- To reconstitute drug for I.V. administration, add 4 ml of sterile water for injection to a 20-mg vial to give a concentration of 5 mg/ml.
- Drug may be diluted further into 100 ml of D_5W or 0.9% NaCl solution and infused over 30 to 45 minutes.
- For I.V. push administration, withdraw reconstituted drug into syringe containing 10 to 15 ml of 0.9% NaCl or D_5W and inject over 2 to 3 minutes into the tubing of a freely flowing I.V. infusion. Reconstituted solution is stable for 24 hours at room temperature and 48 hours in refrigeration.
- Reddish color of drug looks similar to that of doxorubicin (Adriamycin). Do not confuse the two drugs.
- Erythematous streaking along the vein or flushing in the face indicate that the drug is being administered too rapidly.
- Extravasation may be treated with topical application of dimethyl sulfoxide and ice packs to the site.
- Antiemetics may be used to prevent or treat nausea and vomiting.
- Darkening or redness of the skin may occur in prior radiation fields.
- ECG monitoring or monitoring of systolic injection fraction may help to identify early changes associated with drug-induced cardiomyopathy. An ECG or determination of systolic injection fraction should be performed before each course of therapy.
- To prevent cardiomyopathy, limit cumulative dose in adults to 500 to 600 mg/m^2 (400 to 450 mg/m^2 when patient has been receiving other cardiotoxic agents, such as cyclophosphamide, or radiation therapy that encompasses the heart).
- Monitor CBC and hepatic function.
- Note if resting pulse rate is high (a sign of cardiac adverse reactions).
- Do not use a scalp tourniquet or apply ice to prevent alopecia, because this may compromise effectiveness of drug.
- Nausea and vomiting may be very severe and last 24 to 48 hours.

Patient education
- Warn patient that urine may be red for 1 to 2 days and that this is a drug effect, not bleeding.
- Advise patient that alopecia may occur, but that it is usually reversible.
- Tell patient to avoid exposure to people with infections.
- Encourage adequate fluid intake to increase urine output and facilitate excretion of uric acid.
- Warn patient that nausea and vomiting may be severe and may last for 24 to 48 hours.
- Instruct patient to call if a sore throat, fever, or signs of bleeding occur.

Geriatric use
- Elderly patients have an increased incidence of drug-induced cardiotoxicity.
- Monitor for hematologic toxicity because some elderly patients have poor bone marrow reserve.

Pediatric use
- Children have an increased incidence of drug-induced cardiotoxicity, which may occur at lower doses. Total lifetime dosage for children over age 2 is 300 mg/m^2; for children under age 2, 10 mg/kg.

Breast-feeding
- It is not known if drug occurs in breast milk. However, because of the potential for serious adverse reactions, mutagenicity, and carcinogenicity in the infant, breast-feeding is not recommended.

deferoxamine mesylate
Desferal

Pharmacologic classification: chelating agent
Therapeutic classification: heavy metal antagonist
Pregnancy risk category C

How supplied
Available by prescription only
Injectable powder for injection: 500-mg vial

Indications, route, and dosage
Acute iron intoxication
Adults and children: 1 g I.M. or I.V. (I.M. injection is preferred route for all patients in shock), followed by 500 mg I.M. or I.V. q 4 hours for two doses; then 500 mg I.M. or I.V. q 4 to 12 hours if needed. I.V. infusion rate should not exceed 15 mg/kg/hour. Do not exceed 6 g in 24 hours. (I.V. infusion should be reserved for patients in CV collapse.)

Chronic iron overload resulting from multiple transfusions
Adults and children: 500 mg to 1 g I.M. daily and 2 g slow I.V. infusion in separate solution along with each unit of blood transfused. I.V. infusion rate should not exceed 15 mg/kg/hour. Alternatively, give 1 to 2 g via a S.C. infusion pump over 8 to 24 hours.

Pharmacodynamics
Chelating action: Deferoxamine chelates iron by binding ferric ions to the 3 hydroxamic groups of the molecule, preventing it from entering into further chemical reactions. It also chelates aluminum to a lesser extent.

Pharmacokinetics
- *Absorption:* Drug is absorbed poorly after oral administration; however, absorption may occur in patients with acute iron toxicity.
- *Distribution:* Distributes widely into the body after parenteral administration.
- *Metabolism:* Small amounts of drug are metabolized by plasma enzymes.
- *Excretion:* Drug is excreted in urine as unchanged drug or as ferrioxamine, the deferoxamine-iron complex.

Contraindications and precautions
Contraindicated in patients with severe renal disease or anuria. Use cautiously in patients with impaired renal function.

Interactions
None reported.

Effects on diagnostic tests
None reported.

Adverse reactions
CV: tachycardia (with long-term use).
EENT: blurred vision, cataracts, hearing loss.
GI: diarrhea, abdominal discomfort (with long-term use).
GU: dysuria (with long-term use.)
Other: hypersensitivity reactions (cutaneous wheal formation, pruritus, rash, ***anaphylaxis***); pain and induration at injection site; leg cramps; fever; *erythema, urticaria, hypotension,* ***shock*** (after too-rapid I.V. administration).

Overdose and treatment
Acute intoxication is anticipated to include extension and exacerbation of adverse reactions. Treat symptomatically. Drug can be removed by hemodialysis.

☑ Special considerations
- Observe closely and be prepared to treat hypersensitivity reactions; monitor renal, vision, and hearing function throughout therapy.
- Use I.M. route for acute iron intoxication, if patient is not in shock. If patient is in shock, administer I.V. *slowly;* avoid S.C. route.
- Drug has been used to treat iron overload from congenital anemias and in the diagnosis and treatment of primary hemochromatosis. It also has been applied topically to remove corneal rust rings and has been used I.V. or intraperitoneally to promote aluminum excretion or removal.
- Drug has also been used experimentally as a chelator to reduce aluminum levels in bones of patients with renal failure and in patients presenting with dialysis-induced encephalopathy. It has also been shown to slow cognitive deterioration by 50% in long-term clinical trials.

Patient education
- Advise patient that ophthalmic and, possibly, audiometric examinations are needed every 3 to 6 months during continuous therapy; stress importance of reporting changes in vision or hearing.
- Explain that drug may turn urine red.

Geriatric use
- Drug should be used with caution, because elderly patients are more likely to have visual or hearing impairment and renal dysfunction than younger patients.

Pediatric use
- Drug is safe and effective in children over age 3.

delavirdine mesylate
Rescriptor

Pharmacologic classification: non-nucleoside reverse-transcriptase inhibitor of HIV-1
Therapeutic classification: antiviral
Pregnancy risk category C

How supplied
Available by prescription only
Tablets: 100 mg

Indications, route, and dosage
HIV infection
Adults: 400 mg P.O. t.i.d.; use with other antiretroviral agents as appropriate.

Pharmacodynamics
Antiviral action: Delavirdine is a non-nucleoside reverse transcriptase (RT) inhibitor of HIV-1. It binds directly to RT and blocks RNA-dependent and DNA-dependent DNA polymerase activities.

Pharmacokinetics
- *Absorption:* Rapidly absorbed following oral administration with peak occurring at approximately 1 hour.
- *Distribution:* 98% bound to plasma proteins, primarily albumin. Distribution into CSF, saliva, and semen is approximately 0.4%, 6%, and 2%, respectively, of the corresponding plasma concentrations.
- *Metabolism:* Converted to several inactive metabolites; primarily metabolized in liver by cytochrome P-450 3A (CYP3A) enzyme system. However, in vitro data also suggest that CYP2D6 may also be involved. Delavirdine can reduce CYP3A activity

and can inhibit its own metabolism; this is usually reversed within 1 week after discontinuation of the drug. In vitro data also suggest that CYP2C9 and CYP2C19 activity are also reduced by delavirdine.

• *Excretion:* After multiple doses, 44% of the dose was recovered in feces and 51% was excreted in urine. Less than 5% of the dose was recovered unchanged in urine. Mean elimination half-life was 5.8 hours.

Contraindications and precautions

Contraindicated in patients with hypersensitivity to drug's formulation. Use caution when administering to patients with impaired hepatic function. Nonnucleoside RT inhibitors, when used alone or in combination, may confer cross-resistance to other drugs in that class.

Interactions

Use caution when coadministering delaviridine to patients receiving *enzyme-inducing or inhibiting agents* such as *rifampin* and *phenobarbitol.*

Coadministration of delaviridine *with nonsedating antihistamines, indinavir, saquinavir, clarithromycin, dapsone, rifabutin, benzodiazepines, sedative hypnotics, quinidine, warfarin, calcium channel blockers, ergot alkaloid preparations, amphetamines,* and *cisapride* may result in increased plasma concentrations of these drugs. Higher plasma concentration of these drugs could increase or prolong both therapeutic and adverse effects; therefore, dose reduction of the agents may be necessary. *Ketoconazole, clarithromycin,* and *fluoxetine* caused a 50% increase in delavirdine bioavailability.

Carbamazepine, phenobarbital, phenytoin, rifabutin, and *rifampin* decrease plasma delavirdine levels; use with caution. Because the absorption of delavirdine is reduced when coadministered with *antacids,* separate doses by at least 1 hour. *H_2-receptor antagonists* increase gastric pH and may reduce the absorption of delavirdine. Although the effects of these drugs on delavirdine absorption has not been evaluated, chronic use of these drugs with delaviridne is not recommended, Coadministration with *didanosine* should be separated by at least 1 hour because bioavailability of both drugs is reduced by 20%. Due to an increase in *indinavir* plasma concentrations (preliminary results) a lower dose of indinavir should be considered when coadministered with delavirdine. Concurrent use of *saquinavir* resulted in a five-fold increase in bioavailability. In a small, preliminary study, increased liver enzymes occurred in 13% of patients. Monitor AST and ALT levels frequently when used together.

Effects on diagnostic tests

None reported.

Adverse reactions

CNS: headache, abnormal coordination, agitation, amnesia, anxiety, change in dreams, cognitive impairment, confusion, depression, disorientation, emotional lability, hallucinations, hyperesthesia, hyperreflexia, hypesthesia, impaired concentration, insomnia, manic symptoms, muscle cramps, nervousness, neuropathy, nightmares, nystagmus, paralysis, paranoid symptoms, paresthesia, restlessness, somnolence, tingling, tremor, vertigo, weakness, pallor.
CV: bradycardia, palpitation, postural hypotension, syncope, tachycardia, vasodilation, chest pain.
EENT: blepharitis, conjunctivitis, diplopia, dry eyes, ear pain, epistaxis, pharyngitis, rhinitis, sinusitis, photophobia, taste perversion, tinnitus.
GI: *nausea,* vomiting, diarrhea, anorexia, aphthous stomatitis, bloody stools, colitis, constipation, decreased appetite, diverticulitis, duodenitis, dry mouth, dyspepsia, dysphagia, enteritis, esophagitis, fecal incontinence, flatulence, gagging, gastritis, gastroesophageal reflux, ***GI bleeding,*** gingivitis, gum hemorrhage, increased thirst and appetite, increased saliva, mouth ulcer, nonspecific hepatitis, ***pancreatitis,*** sialadenitis, stomatitis, tongue edema or ulceration, abdominal cramps, distention, pain (generalized or localized).
GU: breast enlargement, renal calculi, epididymitis, hematuria, hemospermia, impotence, renal pain, metrorrhagia, nocturia, polyuria, proteinuria, vaginal moniliasis.
Hematologic: ***anemia,*** ecchymosis, eosinophilia, ***granulocytosis, neutropenia, pancytopenia,*** petechia, prolonged PTT, purpura, spleen disorder, ***thrombocytopenia.***
Hepatic: *increased ALT and AST levels.*
Metabolic: alcohol intolerance; bilirubinemia; hyperkalemia; hyperuricemia; hypocalcemia; hyponatremia; hypophosphatemia; increased gamma-glutamyl transferase, lipase, serum alkaline phosphatase, serum amylase, and serum CK; peripheral edema, weight gain or loss.
Respiratory: upper respiratory infection, bronchitis, chest congestion, cough, dyspnea, laryngismus.
Skin: *rash, pruritus,* ***angioedema,*** dermal leukocytoblastic vasculitis, dermatitis, desquamation, diaphoresis, dry skin, erythema multiforme, folliculitis, fungal dermatitis, alopecia, nail disorder, petechial rash, seborrhea, skin nodule, ***Stevens-Johnson syndrome,*** urticaria.
Other: bruise, *fatigue,* allergic reaction, asthenia, back pain, chills, edema (generalized or localized), epidermal cyst, fever, flank pain, flu syndrome, lethargy, lip edema, malaise, neck rigidity, pain (generalized or localized), sebaceous cyst, trauma, arthralgia or arthritis of single and multiple joints, bone pain, leg cramps, muscular weakness, myalgia, tendon disorder, tenosynovitis, tetany, decreased libido.

Overdose and treatment

Although no information is available, provide supportive treatment. Remove drug by gastric lavage or emesis if needed. Dialysis is unlikely to be effective because drug is highly protein-bound.

☑ Special considerations

• Drug-induced rash—typically diffuse, maculopapular, erythematous and often pruritic—occurs commonly; its incidence does not appear to be significantly reduced by titrated drug doses.

• Rash is more common in patients with lower CD4+ cell counts and usually occurs within the first 3 weeks of treatment. Severe rash occurred in 3.6% of patients. In most cases, rash lasted less than 2 weeks and did not require dose reduction or drug discontinuation. Most patients were able to resume therapy after treatment interruption caused by rash.
• Rash occurred mainly on the upper body and proximal arms, with decreasing lesion intensity on the neck and face and less on the rest of the trunk and limbs. Erythema multiforme and Stevens-Johnson syndrome were rarely seen, and resolved after drug was stopped. Occurrence of drug-related rash after 1 month of therapy is uncommon unless prolonged interruption of drug treatment occurs.
• Neutropenia (absolute neutrophil count below 750/mm^3), anemia (hemoglobin less than 7 g/dl), thrombocytopenia (platelet count under 50,000/mm^3), ALT and AST (over five times upper limit of normal), bilirubin (over 2½ times upper limit of normal) and amylase (over twice upper limit of normal) may occur while on delavirdine. Monitor patient carefully.
• Symptomatic relief may been obtained by using diphenhydramine, hydroxyzine, or topical corticosteroids.
• Monitor patients with hepatic or renal impairment because effect of drug has not been studied.
• Drug has not been shown to reduce risk of transmission of HIV-1.

Patient education
• Instruct patient to discontinue drug and call if severe rash or symptoms such as fever, blistering, oral lesions, conjunctivitis, swelling, or muscle or joint aches occur.
• Tell patient that drug is not a cure for HIV-1 infection. He may continue to acquire illnesses associated with HIV-1 infection, including opportunistic infections. Therapy has not been shown to reduce the incidence or frequency of such illnesses.
• Advise patient to remain under medical supervision when taking drug because long-term effects are not known.
• Inform patient to take drug as prescribed and not to alter doses without medical approval. If a dose is missed, tell him to take the next dose as soon as possible; he should not double the next dose.
• Inform patient that drug may be dispersed in water before ingestion. Add tablets to at least 3 oz (90 ml) of water, allow to stand for a few minutes, and stir until a uniform dispersion occurs. Tell patient to drink dispersion promptly, rinse glass, and swallow the rinse to ensure that entire dose is consumed.
• Tell patient that drug may be taken with or without food.
• Advise patient with achlorhydria to take drug with an acidic beverage such as orange or cranberry juice.
• Instruct patient to take drug and antacids at least 1 hour apart.
• Advise patient to report the use of other prescription or OTC medications.

Geriatric use
• Safety and effectiveness have not been studied in patients over age 65.

Pediatric use
• Safety and effectiveness have not been studied in patients under age 16.

Breast-feeding
• Women infected with HIV are advised not to breast-feed.

demeclocycline hydrochloride
Declomycin

Pharmacologic classification: tetracycline antibiotic
Therapeutic classification: antibiotic
Pregnancy risk category D

How supplied
Available by prescription only
Tablets: 150 mg, 300 mg
Capsules: 150 mg

Indications, route, and dosage
Infections caused by susceptible organisms
Adults: 150 mg P.O. q 6 hours, or 300 mg P.O. q 12 hours.
Children over age 8: 6.6 to 13.2 mg/kg P.O. daily, divided q 6 to 12 hours.
Gonorrhea
Adults: 600 mg P.O. initially, then 300 mg P.O. q 12 hours for 4 days (total, 3 g).
◊ ***SIADH secretion (a hyposmolar state)***
Adults: 600 to 1,200 mg P.O. daily in three or four divided doses.

Pharmacodynamics
Antibacterial action: Demeclocycline is bacteriostatic. Tetracyclines bind reversibly to ribosomal subunits, thereby inhibiting bacterial protein synthesis. Demeclocycline is active against many gram-negative and gram-positive organisms, *Mycoplasma, Rickettsia, Chlamydia,* and spirochetes.

Pharmacokinetics
• *Absorption:* About 60% to 80% is absorbed from the GI tract after oral administration; peak serum levels occur at 3 to 4 hours. Food or milk reduces absorption by 50%; antacids chelate with tetracyclines and further reduce absorption. Drug has the greatest affinity of all tetracyclines for calcium ions.
• *Distribution:* Distributed widely into body tissues and fluids, including synovial, pleural, prostatic, and seminal fluids; bronchial secretions; saliva; and aqueous humor; CSF penetration is poor. Drug crosses the placenta; about 36% to 91% is protein-bound.
• *Metabolism:* Drug is not metabolized.
• *Excretion:* Excreted primarily unchanged in urine by glomerular filtration; some drug may be excreted in breast milk. Plasma half-life is 10 to 17 hours in adults with normal renal function. Hemodialysis

and peritoneal dialysis remove only minimal amounts of demeclocycline.

Contraindications and precautions
Contraindicated in patients with hypersensitivity to drug or other tetracyclines. Use cautiously in women during second half of pregnancy, in children under age 8, and in patients with impaired renal or hepatic function.

Interactions
Oral absorption of tetracyclines is impaired by concomitant use with *antacids containing aluminum, calcium, or magnesium* or *laxatives containing magnesium* because of chelation; absorption of tetracyclines is also impaired by *food, milk* and *other dairy products, iron products,* and *sodium bicarbonate.*

Tetracyclines may antagonize bactericidal effects of *penicillin,* inhibiting cell growth because of bacteriostatic action; administer penicillin 2 to 3 hours before tetracycline.

Concomitant use of tetracyclines increases the risk of nephrotoxicity from *methoxyflurane.* When used concomitantly with *oral anticoagulants,* it necessitates lowered dosages of oral anticoagulants because of enhanced effects; and when used with *digoxin,* lowered dosages of *digoxin* because of increased bioavailability.

Concurrent use of tetracyclines with *oral contraceptives* may render oral contraceptives less effective. Breakthrough bleeding has been reported.

Effects on diagnostic tests
Drug causes false-negative results in urine tests using glucose oxidase reagent (Diastix, Chemstrip uG, or glucose enzymatic test strip). It also causes false elevations in fluorometric tests for urinary catecholamines.

Demeclocycline may elevate serum BUN levels in patients with decreased renal function.

Adverse reactions
CNS: ***intracranial hypertension (pseudotumor cerebri)***, dizziness.
CV: pericarditis.
EENT: dysphagia, glossitis, tinnitus, visual disturbances.
GI: anorexia, *nausea, vomiting, diarrhea,* enterocolitis, anogenital inflammation, ***pancreatitis.***
Hematologic: neutropenia, eosinophilia, ***thrombocytopenia, hemolytic anemia.***
Skin: *maculopapular and erythematous rash, photosensitivity, increased pigmentation, urticaria.*
Other: hypersensitivity reactions ***(anaphylaxis),*** elevated liver enzymes, *increased BUN level,* diabetes insipidus syndrome (polyuria, polydipsia, weakness), permanent tooth discoloration or bone growth retardation if used in children under age 8.

Overdose and treatment
Clinical signs of overdose are usually limited to the GI tract. Treatment may include antacids or gastric lavage if ingestion occurred within the preceding 4 hours.

☑ Special considerations
Besides those relevant to all *tetracyclines,* consider the following recommendations.
- As an anti-infective, drug is usually reserved for patients intolerant of other antibiotics.
- A reversible diabetes insipidus syndrome has been reported with long-term use of demeclocycline; monitor patient for this disorder (weakness, polyuria, polydipsia).

Patient education
- Advise patient to take drug at least 1 hour before or 2 hours after meals. Drug should not be taken with dairy products.
- Tell patient to avoid prolonged exposure to sunlight.
- Advise female patient taking oral contraceptives to use barrier contraceptives for duration of drug treatment.

Pediatric use
- Avoid use in children under age 8.

Breast-feeding
- Avoid use of drug in breast-feeding women.

desipramine hydrochloride
Norpramin

Pharmacologic classification: dibenzazepine tricyclic antidepressant
Therapeutic classification: antidepressant
Pregnancy risk category NR

How supplied
Available by prescription only
Tablets: 10 mg, 25 mg, 50 mg, 75 mg, 100 mg, 150 mg

Indications, route, and dosage
Depression
Adults: 100 to 200 mg P.O. daily in divided doses, increasing to maximum of 300 mg daily. Alternatively, the entire dosage can be given once daily, usually h.s.
Elderly patients and adolescents: 25 to 100 mg P.O. daily, increasing gradually to a maximum of 100 mg daily (maximum 150 mg/daily only for the severely ill in these age groups).

Pharmacodynamics
Antidepressant action: Drug is thought to exert its antidepressant effects by inhibiting reuptake of norepinephrine and serotonin in CNS nerve terminals (presynaptic neurons), which results in increased concentrations and enhanced activity of these neurotransmitters in the synaptic cleft. Desipramine more strongly inhibits reuptake of norepinephrine than serotonin; it has a lesser incidence of sedative effects and less anticholinergic and hypotensive activity than its parent compound, imipramine.

Pharmacokinetics
- *Absorption:* Drug is absorbed rapidly from the GI tract after oral administration.

• *Distribution:* Distributed widely into the body, including the CNS and breast milk. Drug is 90% protein-bound. Peak effect occurs in 4 to 6 hours; steady state, within 2 to 11 days, with full therapeutic effect in 2 to 4 weeks. Proposed therapeutic plasma levels (parent drug and metabolite) range from 125 to 300 ng/ml.
• *Metabolism:* Desipramine is metabolized by the liver; a significant first-pass effect may explain variability of serum concentrations in different patients taking the same dosage.
• *Excretion:* Drug is excreted primarily in urine.

Contraindications and precautions

Contraindicated in patients with hypersensitivity to drug, in those who have taken MAO inhibitors within the previous 14 days, and in patients during acute recovery phase of MI. Use with extreme caution in patients with history of seizure disorders or urine retention, CV or thyroid disease, or glaucoma and in those taking thyroid medication.

Interactions

Concomitant use of desipramine with sympathomimetics, including *epinephrine, phenylephrine, phenylpropanolamine,* and *ephedrine* (often found in nasal sprays) may increase blood pressure; use with *warfarin* may increase PT and cause bleeding.

Concomitant use with *thyroid medication, pimozide,* or *antiarrhythmic agents* (*quinidine, disopyramide, procainamide*) may increase incidence of arrhythmias and conduction defects.

Desipramine may decrease hypotensive effects of *centrally acting antihypertensive drugs,* such as *guanethidine, guanabenz, guanadrel, clonidine, methyldopa,* and *reserpine.* Concomitant use with *disulfiram* or *ethchlorvynol* may cause delirium and tachycardia. Additive effects are likely after concomitant use of desipramine and *CNS depressants,* including *alcohol, analgesics, barbiturates, narcotics, tranquilizers,* and *anesthetics* (oversedation); *atropine* and *other anticholinergic drugs,* including *phenothiazines, antihistamines, meperidine,* and *antiparkinsonian agents* (oversedation, paralytic ileus, visual changes, and severe constipation); and *metrizamide* (increased risk of seizures).

Barbiturates and *heavy smoking* induce desipramine metabolism and decrease therapeutic efficacy; *phenothiazines* and *haloperidol* decrease its metabolism, decreasing therapeutic efficacy. *Methylphenidate, cimetidine, oral contraceptives, propoxyphene,* and *beta blockers* may inhibit desipramine metabolism, increasing plasma levels and toxicity.

Use caution when using desipramine with *selective serotonin-uptake inhibiting agents* because patient may become toxic to tricyclic antidepressant at much lower dosages.

Effects on diagnostic tests

Drug may prolong conduction time (elongation of QT and PR intervals, flattened T waves on ECG); it also may elevate liver function test results, decrease WBC counts, and decrease or increase serum glucose levels.

Adverse reactions

CNS: *drowsiness, dizziness,* excitation, tremor, weakness, confusion, anxiety, restlessness, agitation, headache, nervousness, EEG changes, ***seizures,*** extrapyramidal reactions.
CV: orthostatic hypotension, *tachycardia, ECG changes,* hypertension, **sudden death.**
EENT: *blurred vision,* tinnitus, mydriasis.
GI: *dry mouth, constipation,* nausea, vomiting, anorexia, paralytic ileus.
GU: *urine retention.*
Skin: rash, urticaria, photosensitivity.
Other: *diaphoresis,* hypersensitivity reaction, ***sudden death*** (in children).

After abrupt withdrawal of long-term therapy: nausea, headache, malaise (does not indicate addiction).

Overdose and treatment

The first 12 hours after acute ingestion are a stimulatory phase characterized by excessive anticholinergic activity (agitation, irritation, confusion, hallucinations, parkinsonian symptoms, hyperthermia, seizures, urine retention, dry mucous membranes, pupillary dilatation, constipation, and ileus). This is followed by CNS depressant effects, including hypothermia, decreased or absent reflexes, sedation, hypotension, cyanosis, and cardiac irregularities, including tachycardia, conduction disturbances, and quinidine-like effects on the ECG.

Severity of overdose is best indicated by widening of the QRS complex, which usually represents a serum level in excess of 1,000 ng/ml; serum levels are generally not helpful. Metabolic acidosis may follow hypotension, hypoventilation, and seizures.

Treatment is symptomatic and supportive, including maintaining airway, stable body temperature, and fluid and electrolyte balance. Induce emesis with ipecac if patient is conscious; follow with gastric lavage and activated charcoal to prevent further absorption. Dialysis is of little use. Physostigmine may be used with caution to reverse CV abnormalities or coma; too rapid administration may cause seizures. Treat seizures with parenteral diazepam or phenytoin; arrhythmias, with parenteral phenytoin or lidocaine; and acidosis, with sodium bicarbonate. *Do not give barbiturates;* these may enhance CNS and respiratory depressant effects.

☑ Special considerations

Besides those relevant to all *tricyclic antidepressants,* consider the following recommendations.
• Dispense drug in the smallest possible quantities to depressed outpatients, as suicide has been accomplished with drug.
• Check standing and sitting blood pressure to assess orthostasis before administering desipramine.
• Drug has a lesser incidence of sedative effects and fewer anticholinergic and hypotensive effects than its parent compound imipramine.
• The full dose may be given at bedtime to help offset daytime sedation.
• Tolerance usually develops to the sedative effects of drug during initial weeks of therapy.

• Do not withdraw drug abruptly; taper gradually over 3 to 6 weeks.
• Discontinue drug at least 48 hours before surgical procedures.
• Drug therapy in patients with biploar illness may induce a hypomanic state.

Patient education
• Tell patient to take the full dose at bedtime to alleviate daytime sedation.
• Explain that full effects of drug may not become apparent for 4 weeks or more after initiation of therapy.
• Tell patient to take the medication exactly as prescribed and not to double dose for missed ones.
• To prevent dizziness, advise patient to lie down for about 30 minutes after each dose at start of therapy and to avoid sudden postural changes, especially when rising to upright position.
• Warn patient not to stop taking drug suddenly.
• Encourage patient to report unusual or troublesome effects, especially confusion, movement disorders, rapid heartbeat, dizziness, fainting, or difficulty urinating.
• Tell patient sugarless chewing gum or hard candy or ice may alleviate dry mouth.
• Stress importance of regular dental hygiene to avoid caries.
• Warn patient to avoid alcohol and prolonged sunlight while taking this medication.
• Tell patient to store drug safely away from children.

Geriatric use
• Elderly patients may be more susceptible to adverse cardiac reactions.

Pediatric use
• Avoid use in children under age 12.

Breast-feeding
• Drug is excreted in breast milk in concentrations equal to those in maternal serum. The potential benefit to the mother should outweigh the possible adverse reactions in the infant.

desmopressin acetate
DDAVP, Stimate

Pharmacologic classification: posterior pituitary hormone
Therapeutic classification: antidiuretic, hemostatic
Pregnancy risk category B

How supplied
Available by prescription only
Tablets: 0.1 mg, 0.2 mg
Nasal solution: 0.1 mg/ml, 1.5 mg/ml
Injection: 4 mcg/ml in 1-ml single-dose ampules and 10-ml multiple-dose vials; 15 mcg/ml in 1-ml and 2-ml ampules

Indications, route, and dosage
Central cranial diabetes insipidus, temporary polyuria, polydipsia associated with pituitary trauma
Adults: 0.1 to 0.4 ml (10 to 40 mcg) intranasally in one to three divided doses daily. Adjust morning and evening doses separately for adequate diurnal rhythm of water turnover.

Alternatively, 0.05 mg P.O. b.i.d. initially. Adjust individual dosage in increments of 0.1 mg to 1.2 mg daily, divided into two or three doses. Optimal dosage range is 0.1 to 0.8 mg daily in divided doses. Or give 0.5 ml (2 mcg) to 1 ml (4 mcg) I.V. or S.C. daily, usually in two divided doses
Children age 3 months to 12 years: 0.05 to 0.3 ml (5 to 30 mcg) intranasally daily in one or two doses.
Hemophilia A, von Willebrand's disease
Adults and children: 0.3 mcg/kg diluted in 0.9% NaCl solution and infused I.V. slowly over 15 to 30 minutes. May repeat dosage, if necessary, as indicated by laboratory response and patient's condition. Alternatively, give one spray per nostril.
Primary nocturnal enuresis
Children age 6 and older: 20 mcg (two to four metered sprays), intranasally h.s. Dosage adjusted according to response. Maximum recommended dose is 40 mcg daily.

Pharmacodynamics
Antidiuretic action: Drug is used to control or prevent signs and complications of neurogenic diabetes insipidus. The site of action is primarily at the renal tubular level. Desmopressin increases water permeability at the renal tubule and collecting duct, resulting in increased urine osmolality and decreased urinary flow rate.

Hemostatic action: Desmopressin increases factor VIII activity by releasing endogenous factor VIII from plasma storage sites.

Pharmacokinetics
• *Absorption:* Drug is destroyed in the GI tract. After intranasal administration, 10% to 20% of dose is absorbed through nasal mucosa; antidiuretic action occurs within 1 hour and peaks in 1 to 5 hours. After I.V. infusion, plasma factor VIII activity increases within 15 to 30 minutes and peaks between 1½ and 3 hours.
• *Distribution:* Not fully understood.
• *Metabolism:* Unknown.
• *Excretion:* Plasma levels decline in two phases: the half-life of the fast phase is about 8 minutes; the slow phase, 75 minutes. Duration of action after intranasal administration is 8 to 20 hours; after I.V. administration, it is 12 to 24 hours for mild hemophilia and approximately 3 hours for von Willebrand's disease.

Contraindications and precautions
Contraindicated in patients hypersensitive to drug and in patients with type IIB von Willebrand's disease.

Use cautiously in patients with coronary artery insufficiency or hypertensive CV disease, or in those with conditions associated with fluid and electrolyte imbalances such as cystic fibrosis, because these patients are prone to hyponatremia.

Interactions
Concomitant use of desmopressin with *carbamazepine, chlorpropamide, or clofibrate* may potentiate desmopressin's antidiuretic action. Concomitant use with *lithium, epinephrine, norepinephrine, demeclocycline, heparin,* or *alcohol* may decrease the antidiuretic effect.

Effects on diagnostic tests
None reported.

Adverse reactions
CNS: headache.
CV: slight rise in blood pressure (at high dosage).
EENT: rhinitis, epistaxis, sore throat, cough.
GI: nausea, abdominal cramps.
GU: vulval pain.
Other: flushing, local erythema, swelling, burning (after injection).

Overdose and treatment
Clinical manifestations of overdose include drowsiness, listlessness, headache, confusion, anuria, and weight gain (water intoxication). Treatment requires water restriction and temporary withdrawal of desmopressin until polyuria occurs. Severe water intoxication may require osmotic diuresis with mannitol, hypertonic dextrose, or urea—alone or with furosemide.

☑ Special considerations
Besides those relevant to all *posterior pituitary hormones,* consider the following recommendations.
- Desmopressin may be administered intranasally through a flexible catheter called a rhinyle. A measured quantity is drawn up into the catheter, one end is inserted into patient's nose, and patient blows on the other end to deposit drug into nasal cavity. Alternatively, drug is newly available in nasal spray, which may be easier for some patients.
- Patients may be switched from intranasal to S.C. desmopressin (for example, during episodes of rhinorrhea). They should receive 1/10 of their usual dosage parenterally.
- Observe for early signs of water intoxication—drowsiness, listlessness, headache, confusion, anuria, and weight gain—to prevent seizures, coma, and death.
- Adjust patient's fluid intake to reduce risk of water intoxication and of sodium depletion, especially in young or elderly patients.
- Weigh patient daily and observe for edema.
- Desmopressin is not indicated for hemophilia A patients with factor VIII levels up to 5% or in patients with severe von Willebrand's disease.
- Drug therapy may enable some patients to avoid the hazards of contaminated blood products.
- Check expiration date of drug.

Patient education
- Teach patient correct administration technique, then evaluate his proficiency at drug administration and accurate measurement on return visits; some may have difficulty measuring and inhaling drug into nostrils.
- Emphasize that patient should not increase or decrease dosage unless it is prescribed.
- Review with patient fluid intake measurement and methods for measuring fluid output.
- Assist patient in planning a schedule for fluid intake if oral fluids must be reduced to decrease the possibility of water intoxification and hyponatremia. A diuretic may be administered if excessive fluid retention occurs.
- Instruct patient to call if signs of water intoxication (drowsiness, listlessness, headache, or shortness of breath) occur.
- Tell patient to store drug away from heat and direct light, not in bathroom, where heat and moisture can cause drug to deteriorate.

Geriatric use
- Elderly patients have an increased risk of hyponatremia and water intoxication; therefore, restriction of their fluid intake is recommended.
- Because elderly patients are more sensitive to drug's effects, they may need a lower dosage.

Pediatric use
- Drug is not recommended in infants under age 3 months because of their increased tendency to develop fluid imbalance.
- Use with caution in infants because of risk of hyponatremia and water intoxication.
- Safety and efficacy of parenteral desmopressin have not been established for management of diabetes insipidus in children under age 12.

desonide
DesOwen, Tridesilon

Pharmacologic classification: topical adrenocorticoid
Therapeutic classification: anti-inflammatory
Pregnancy risk category C

How supplied
Available by prescription only
Cream, lotion, ointment: 0.05%

Indications, route, and dosage
Adjunctive therapy for inflammation in acute and chronic corticosteroid-responsive dermatoses
Adults and children: Apply sparingly to affected area b.i.d. to q.i.d.

Pharmacodynamics
Anti-inflammatory action: Desonide stimulates the synthesis of enzymes needed to decrease the inflammatory response. Desonide is a group IV nonfluorinated glucocorticoid with a potency similar to that of alclometasone dipropionate 0.05% and fluocinolone acetonide 0.01%.

Pharmacokinetics

• *Absorption:* Amount of drug absorbed depends on the amount applied and on the nature of the skin at the application site. It ranges from about 1% in areas with a thick stratum corneum (such as the palms, soles, elbows, and knees) to as much as 36% in areas of the thinnest stratum corneum (face, eyelids, and genitals). Absorption increases in areas of skin damage, inflammation, or occlusion. Some systemic absorption of topical steroids occurs, especially through the oral mucosa.
• *Distribution:* After topical application, desonide is distributed throughout the local skin layer. Any drug that is absorbed into circulation is removed rapidly from the blood and distributed into muscle, liver, skin, intestines, and kidneys.
• *Metabolism:* After topical administration, drug is metabolized primarily in the skin. The small amount that is absorbed into systemic circulation is metabolized primarily in the liver to inactive compounds.
• *Excretion:* Inactive metabolites are excreted by the kidneys, primarily as glucuronides and sulfates, but also as unconjugated products. Small amounts of the metabolites are also excreted in feces.

Contraindications and precautions

Contraindicated in patients hypersensitive to drug.

Interactions

None significant.

Effects on diagnostic tests

None reported.

Adverse reactions

Skin: burning, pruritus, irritation, dryness, erythema, folliculitis, perioral dermatitis, allergic contact dermatitis, hypertrichosis, hypopigmentation, acneiform eruptions; *maceration of skin, secondary infection, atrophy, striae, miliaria* (with occlusive dressings).
Other: ***hypothalamic-pituitary-adrenal axis suppression,*** Cushing's syndrome, hyperglycemia, glucosuria.

Overdose and treatment

No information available.

☑ Special considerations

Recommendations for use of desonide, for care and teaching of patients during therapy, and for use in elderly patients, children, and breast-feeding women are the same as those for all *topical adrenocorticoids.*

desoximetasone

Topicort

Pharmacologic classification: topical adrenocorticoid
Therapeutic classification: anti-inflammatory
Pregnancy risk category C

How supplied

Available by prescription only
Cream: 0.05%, 0.25%
Gel: 0.05%
Ointment: 0.25%

Indications, route, and dosage

Inflammation and pruritus of corticosteroid-responsive dermatoses
Adults and children: Apply sparingly in a very thin film and rub in gently to the affected area b.i.d.

Pharmacodynamics

Anti-inflammatory action: Desoximetasone stimulates the synthesis of enzymes needed to decrease the inflammatory response. Desoximetasone is a synthetic fluorinated corticosteroid. The 0.05% cream has a potency of group III; the 0.25% cream and ointment and the 0.05% gel have a potency of group II.

Pharmacokinetics

• *Absorption:* The amount of drug absorbed depends on the strength of the preparation, the amount applied, and the nature of the skin at the application site. It ranges from about 1% in areas with a thick stratum corneum (such as the palms, soles, elbows, and knees) to as much as 36% in areas of the thinnest stratum corneum (face, eyelids, and genitals). Absorption increases in areas of skin damage, inflammation, or occlusion. Some systemic absorption of topical steroids, especially through the oral mucosa, may occur.
• *Distribution:* After topical application, drug is distributed throughout the local skin. Any drug that is absorbed into circulation is removed rapidly from the blood and distributed into muscle, liver, skin, intestines, and kidneys.
• *Metabolism:* After topical administration, drug is metabolized primarily in the skin. The small amount that is absorbed into systemic circulation is metabolized primarily in the liver to inactive compounds.
• *Excretion:* Inactive metabolites are excreted by the kidneys, primarily as glucuronides and sulfates, but also as unconjugated products. Small amounts of the metabolites are also excreted in feces.

Contraindications and precautions

Contraindicated in patients hypersensitive to drug.

Interactions

None significant.

Effects on diagnostic tests

None reported.

Adverse reactions

Skin: burning, pruritus, irritation, dryness, erythema, folliculitis, hypertrichosis, acneiform eruptions, perioral dermatitis, hypopigmentation, allergic contact dermatitis; *maceration, secondary infection, atrophy, striae, miliaria* (with occlusive dressings).
Other: ***hypothalamic-pituitary-adrenal axis suppression,*** Cushing's syndrome, hyperglycemia, glucosuria.

Overdose and treatment
No information available.

☑ Special considerations
Recommendations for use of desoximetasone, for care and teaching of patients during therapy, and for use in elderly patients, children, and breast-feeding women are the same as those for all *topical adrenocorticoids.*

dexamethasone (ophthalmic suspension)
Maxidex

dexamethasone sodium phosphate
AK-Dex, Decadron, Dexair, I-Methasone, Ocu-Dex

Pharmacologic classification: corticosteroid
Therapeutic classification: ophthalmic anti-inflammatory
Pregnancy risk category C

How supplied
Available by prescription only
dexamethasone
Ophthalmic suspension: 0.1%
dexamethasone sodium phosphate
Ophthalmic ointment: 0.05%
Ophthalmic solution: 0.1%

Indications, route, and dosage
Uveitis; iridocyclitis; inflammation of eyelids, conjunctiva, cornea, anterior segment of globe; corneal injury from burns or penetration by foreign bodies; allergic conjunctivitis; suppression of graft rejection after keratoplasty
Adults and children: Instill 1 to 2 drops of suspension or solution or apply 1.25 to 2.5 cm of ointment into conjunctival sac. For initial therapy of severe cases, instill the solution or suspension into the conjunctival sac every hour, gradually discontinue dose as patient's condition improves. In mild condition, use drops up to four to six times daily or apply ointment t.i.d. or q.i.d. As patient's condition improves, taper dose to b.i.d. then once daily. Treatment may extend from a few days to several weeks.

Pharmacodynamics
Anti-inflammatory action: Corticosteroids stimulate the synthesis of enzymes needed to decrease the inflammatory response. Dexamethasone, a long-acting fluorinated synthetic adrenocorticoid with strong anti-inflammatory activity and minimal mineralocorticoid activity, is 25 to 30 times more potent than an equal weight of hydrocortisone.

Drug is poorly soluble and therefore has a slower onset of action but a longer duration of action when applied in a liquid suspension. The sodium phosphate salt is highly soluble and has a rapid onset but short duration of action.

Pharmacokinetics
- *Absorption:* After ophthalmic administration, drug is absorbed through the aqueous humor. Because only low doses are administered, little if any systemic absorption occurs.
- *Distribution:* Drug is distributed throughout the local tissue layers. Drug absorbed into circulation is rapidly removed from the blood and distributed into muscle, liver, skin, intestines, and kidneys.
- *Metabolism:* Dexamethasone is primarily metabolized locally. The small amount that is absorbed into systemic circulation is metabolized primarily in the liver to inactive compounds.
- *Excretion:* Inactive metabolites are excreted by the kidneys, primarily as glucuronides and sulfates, but also as unconjugated products. Small amounts of the metabolites are also excreted in feces.

Contraindications and precautions
Contraindicated in patients with acute superficial herpes simplex (dendritic keratitis), vaccinia, varicella, or other fungal or viral diseases of cornea and conjunctiva; ocular tuberculosis; or acute, purulent, untreated infections of the eye.

Use cautiously in patients with corneal abrasions that may be infected (especially with herpes). Also use cautiously in patients with glaucoma because intraocular pressure may increase. Glaucoma medications may need to be increased to compensate.

Interactions
None reported.

Effects on diagnostic tests
None reported.

Adverse reactions
EENT: increased intraocular pressure; thinning of cornea, interference with corneal wound healing, increased susceptibility to viral or fungal corneal infection, corneal ulceration; glaucoma exacerbation, cataracts, defects in visual acuity and visual field, optic nerve damage; mild blurred vision; burning, stinging, or redness of eyes; watery eyes, discharge, discomfort, ocular pain, foreign body sensation (with excessive or long-term use).
Other: systemic effects and adrenal suppression (with excessive or long-term use).

Overdose and treatment
No information available.

☑ Special considerations
- Watch for corneal ulceration; may require stopping drug.
- Shake suspension well before use.
- Drug is not recommended for long-term use.

dexamethasone (systemic)

Decadron, Deronil*, Dexasone*, Dexone, Hexadrol

dexamethasone acetate

Dalalone D.P., Decadron-L.A., Decaject-L.A., Dexasone-L.A., Dexone L.A., Solurex L.A.

dexamethasone sodium phosphate

AK-Dex, Dalalone, Decadrol, Decadron, Decaject, Dexameth, Dexasone, Dexone, Hexadrol Phosphate, Oradexon*, Solurex

Pharmacologic classification: glucocorticoid
Therapeutic classification: anti-inflammatory, immunosuppressant
Pregnancy risk category NR

How supplied

Available by prescription only
dexamethasone
Tablets: 0.25 mg, 0.5 mg, 0.75 mg, 1 mg, 1.5 mg, 2 mg, 4 mg, 6 mg
Elixir: 0.5 mg/5 ml
Oral solution: 0.5 mg/0.5 ml, 0.5 mg/5 ml
dexamethasone acetate
Injection: 8 mg/ml, 16 mg/ml suspension
dexamethasone sodium phosphate
Injection: 4 mg/ml, 10 mg/ml, 20 mg/ml, 24 mg/ml

Indications, route, and dosage

Cerebral edema
dexamethasone sodium phosphate
Adults: Initially, 10 mg I.V., then 4 mg I.M. q 6 hours for 2 to 4 days, then taper over 5 to 7 days.
Inflammatory conditions, allergic reactions, neoplasias
Adults: 0.75 to 9 mg P.O. daily divided b.i.d., t.i.d., or q.i.d.
Children: 0.024 to 0.34 mg/kg P.O. daily in four divided doses.
dexamethasone acetate
Adults: 4 to 16 mg intra-articularly or into soft tissue q 1 to 3 weeks; 0.8 to 1.6 mg into lesions q 1 to 3 weeks; or 8 to 16 mg I.M. q 1 to 3 weeks p.r.n.
dexamethasone sodium phosphate
Adults: 0.2 to 6 mg intra-articularly, intralesionally, or into soft tissue; or 0.5 to 9 mg I.M.
Shock (other than adrenal crisis)
dexamethasone sodium phosphate
Adults: 1 to 6 mg/kg I.V. daily as a single dose; or 40 mg I.V. q 2 to 6 hours p.r.n.
Dexamethasone suppression test
Adults: 0.5 mg P.O. q 6 hours for 48 hours.
Adrenal insufficiency
Adults: 0.75 to 9 mg P.O. daily in divided doses.
Children: 0.024 to 0.34 mg/kg P.O. daily in four divided doses.
dexamethasone sodium phosphate
Adults: 0.5 to 9 mg I.M. or I.V. daily.
Children: 0.235 to 1.25 mg/m^2 I.M. or I.V. once daily or b.i.d.
◊ ***Prevention of hyaline membrane disease in premature infants***
Adults: 5 mg (phosphate) I.M. t.i.d. to mother for 2 days before delivery.
◊ ***Prevention of cancer chemotherapy-induced nausea and vomiting***
Adults: 10 to 20 mg I.V. before administration of chemotherapy. Additional doses (individualized for each patient and usually lower than initial dose) may be administered I.V. or P.O. for 24 to 72 hours following cancer chemotherapy, if needed.

Pharmacodynamics

Anti-inflammatory action: Dexamethasone stimulates the synthesis of enzymes needed to decrease the inflammatory response. It causes suppression of the immune system by reducing activity and volume of the lymphatic system, producing lymphocytopenia (primarily T-lymphocytes), decreasing passage of immune complexes through basement membranes and possibly by depressing reactivity of tissue to antigen-antibody interactions.

Drug is a long-acting synthetic adrenocorticoid with strong anti-inflammatory activity and minimal mineralocorticoid properties. It is 25 to 30 times more potent than an equal weight of hydrocortisone.

The acetate salt is a suspension and should not be used I.V. It is particularly useful as an anti-inflammatory agent in intra-articular, intradermal, and intralesional injections.

The sodium phosphate salt is highly soluble and has a more rapid onset and a shorter duration of action than does the acetate salt. It is most commonly used for cerebral edema and unresponsive shock. It can also be used in intra-articular, intralesional, or soft tissue inflammation. Other uses for dexamethasone are symptomatic treatment of bronchial asthma, chemotherapy-induced nausea, and as a diagnostic test for Cushing's syndrome.

Pharmacokinetics

- *Absorption:* After oral administration, drug is absorbed readily, and peak effects occur in about 1 to 2 hours. The suspension for injection has a variable onset and duration of action (ranging from 2 days to 3 weeks), depending on whether it is injected into an intra-articular space, a muscle, or the blood supply to the muscle. After I.V. injection, dexamethosone is rapidly and completely absorbed into the tissues.
- *Distribution:* Drug is removed rapidly from the blood and distributed to muscle, liver, skin, intestines, and kidneys. Dexamethasone is bound weakly to plasma proteins (transcortin and albumin). Only the unbound portion is active. Adrenocorticoids are distributed into breast milk and through the placenta.
- *Metabolism:* Metabolized in the liver to inactive glucuronide and sulfate metabolites.
- *Excretion:* The inactive metabolites and small amounts of unmetabolized drug are excreted by the kidneys. Insignificant quantities of drug are also excreted in feces; biologic half-life is 36 to 54 hours.

Contraindications and precautions

Contraindicated in patients hypersensitive to any component of drug and in those with systemic fungal infections.

Use cautiously in patients with recent MI, GI ulcer, renal disease, hypertension, osteoporosis, diabetes mellitus, hypothyroidism, cirrhosis, diverticulitis, nonspecific ulcerative colitis, recent intestinal anastomoses, thromboembolic disorders, seizures, myasthenia gravis, heart failure, tuberculosis, ocular herpes simplex, emotional instability, and psychotic tendencies. Because some formulations contain sulfite preservatives, also use cautiously in patients sensitive to sulfites.

Interactions

When used concomitantly, dexamethasone may in rare cases decrease the effects of *oral anticoagulants* by unknown mechanisms.

Dexamethasone increases the metabolism of *isoniazid* and *salicylates*; causes hyperglycemia, requiring dosage adjustment of *insulin* or *oral antidiabetic agents* in diabetic patients; and may enhance hypokalemia associated with *diuretic* or *amphotericin B* therapy. The hypokalemia may increase the risk of toxicity in patients concurrently receiving *cardiac glycosides*.

Concomitant use of *barbiturates*, *phenytoin*, and *rifampin* may cause decreased corticosteroid effects because of increased hepatic metabolism. *Cholestyramine, colestipol*, and *antacids* decrease the corticosteroid effect by adsorbing the corticosteroid, decreasing the amount absorbed.

Concomitant use with *estrogens* may reduce the metabolism of dexamethasone by increasing the concentration of transcortin. The half-life of the corticosteroid is then prolonged because of increased protein-binding. Concomitant administration of *ulcerogenic drugs*, such as *NSAIDs*, may increase the risk of GI ulceration.

Effects on diagnostic tests

Dexamethasone suppresses reactions to skin tests; causes false-negative results in the nitroblue tetrazolium test for systemic bacterial infections; and decreases ^{131}I uptake and protein-bound iodine concentrations in thyroid function tests.

Dexamethasone may increase glucose and cholesterol levels; may decrease levels of serum potassium, calcium, thyroxine, and triiodothyronine; and may increase urine glucose and calcium levels.

Adverse reactions

Most adverse reactions to corticosteroids are dose-dependent or duration-dependent.

CNS: *euphoria, insomnia,* psychotic behavior, pseudotumor cerebri, vertigo, headache, paresthesia, ***seizures.***

CV: ***heart failure,*** hypertension, edema, ***arrhythmias,*** thrombophlebitis, ***thromboembolism.***

EENT: cataracts, glaucoma.

Endocrine: menstrual irregularities, cushingoid state (moonface, buffalo hump, central obesity).

GI: *peptic ulceration,* GI irritation, increased appetite, pancreatitis, nausea, vomiting.

Skin: delayed wound healing, acne, various skin eruptions; atrophy (at I.M. injection sites).

Other: muscle weakness, osteoporosis, hirsutism, susceptibility to infections; hypokalemia, hyperglycemia, and carbohydrate intolerance; growth suppression in children; ***acute adrenal insufficiency may follow increased stress (infection, surgery, or trauma) or abrupt withdrawal after long-term therapy.***

After abrupt withdrawal: rebound inflammation, fatigue, weakness, arthralgia, fever, dizziness, lethargy, depression, fainting, orthostatic hypotension, dyspnea, anorexia, hypoglycemia. ***After prolonged use, sudden withdrawal may be fatal.***

Overdose and treatment

Acute ingestion, even in massive doses, rarely poses a clinical problem. Toxic signs and symptoms rarely occur if drug is used for less than 3 weeks, even at large dosage ranges. However, chronic use causes adverse physiologic effects, including suppression of the hypothalamic-pituitary-adrenal axis, cushingoid appearance, muscle weakness, and osteoporosis.

☑ Special considerations

Recommendations for use of dexamethasone, for care and teaching of patients during therapy, and for use in elderly patients and breast-feeding women are the same as those for all *systemic adrenocorticoids.*

- Drug is being used investigationally to prevent hyaline membrane disease (respiratory distress syndrome) in premature infants. The suspension (phosphate salt) is administered I.M. to the mother two or three times daily for 2 days before delivery.

Pediatric use

- Chronic use of drug in children and adolescents may delay growth and maturation.

dexamethasone (topical)

Aeroseb-Dex, Decaspray

dexamethasone sodium phosphate

Decadron Phosphate

Pharmacologic classification: corticosteroid
Therapeutic classification: anti-inflammatory
Pregnancy risk category C

How supplied

Available by prescription only
dexamethasone
Aerosol: 0.01%, 0.04%
Gel: 0.1%
dexamethasone sodium phosphate
Cream: 0.1%

Indications, route, and dosage

Inflammation of corticosteroid-responsive dermatoses

Adults and children: Apply sparingly t.i.d. or q.i.d. For aerosol use on scalp, shake can well and apply to dry scalp after shampooing. Hold can upright. Slide applicator tube under hair so that it touches scalp. Spray while moving tube to all affected areas, keeping tube under hair and in contact with scalp throughout spraying, which should take about 2 seconds. Inadequately covered areas may be spot sprayed. Slide applicator tube through hair to touch scalp, press and immediately release spray button. Do not massage medication into scalp or spray forehead or eyes.

Pharmacodynamics

Anti-inflammatory action: Dexamethasone is a synthetic fluorinated corticosteroid. It is usually classed as a group VII potency anti-inflammatory agent. Occlusive dressings may be used in severe cases. The aerosol spray is usually used for dermatologic conditions of the scalp.

Pharmacokinetics

- *Absorption:* Drug absorption depends on the potency of the preparation, the amount applied, the vehicle used, and the nature of the skin at the application site. It ranges from about 1% in areas with a thick stratum corneum (such as the palms, soles, elbows, and knees) to 25% in areas of the thinnest stratum corneum (face, eyelids, and genitals). Inflamed or damaged skin may absorb more than 33%. Absorption increases in areas of skin damage, inflammation, or occlusion. Some systemic absorption occurs, especially through the oral mucosa.
- *Distribution:* After topical applications, dexamethasone is distributed throughout the local skin layer. If absorbed into circulation, the drug is distributed rapidly into muscle, liver, skin, intestines, and kidneys.
- *Metabolism:* After topical administration, dexamethasone is metabolized primarily in the skin. The small amount that is absorbed into systemic circulation is primarily metabolized in the liver to inactive compounds.
- *Excretion:* Inactive metabolites are excreted by the kidneys, primarily as glucuronides and sulfates, but also as unconjugated products. Small amounts of the metabolites are also excreted in feces.

Contraindications and precautions

Contraindicated in patients hypersensitive to drug.

Interactions

None significant.

Effects on diagnostic tests

None reported.

Adverse reactions

Skin: burning, pruritus, irritation, dryness, erythema, folliculitis, hypertrichosis, acneiform eruptions, perioral dermatitis, hypopigmentation, allergic contact dermatitis; *maceration, secondary infection, atrophy, striae, miliaria* (with occlusive dressings).

Other: ***hypothalamic-pituitary-adrenal axis suppression,*** Cushing's syndrome, hyperglycemia, glucosuria.

Overdose and treatment

Topical corticosteroids can be absorbed in sufficient amounts to produce systemic effects.

☑ Special considerations

Recommendations for use of dexamethasone, for care and teaching of patients during therapy, and for use in elderly patients, children, and breast-feeding women are the same as those for all *topical adrenocorticoids.*

dexamethasone sodium phosphate

Nasal inhalant
Dexacort Phosphate Turbinaire

Oral inhalant
Dexacort Phosphate in Respihaler

Pharmacologic classification: glucocorticoid
Therapeutic classification: anti-inflammatory, antiasthmatic
Pregnancy risk category NR

How supplied

Available by prescription only
Nasal aerosol: 100 mcg of dexamethasone sodium phosphate/metered spray, (equivalent to 84 mcg of dexamethasone); 170 doses/canister
Oral inhalation aerosol: 100 mcg of dexamethasone sodium phosphate/metered spray, (equivalent to 84 mcg of dexamethasone); 170 doses/canister

Indications, route, and dosage

Control of bronchial asthma in patients with steroid-dependent asthma

Oral inhaler

Adults: 3 inhalations t.i.d. or q.i.d., to a maximum dosage of 12 inhalations daily.
Children: 2 inhalations t.i.d. or q.i.d., to a maximum dosage of 8 inhalations daily.

Allergic or inflammatory conditions, nasal polyps (excluding polyps originating within the sinuses)

Nasal inhaler

Adults: 2 sprays (168 mcg) into each nostril b.i.d. or t.i.d. Maximum dosage of 12 sprays daily (1,008 mcg).
Children age 6 to 12: 1 or 2 sprays (84 to 168 mcg) into each nostril b.i.d. Maximum dosage is 8 sprays daily (672 mcg).

Pharmacodynamics

Anti-inflammatory action: Dexamethasone stimulates the synthesis of enzymes needed to decrease the inflammatory response.

Antiasthmatic action: Used as a nasal inhalant for the symptomatic treatment of seasonal or perennial rhinitis and nasal polyposis. It is used as an oral inhalant to treat bronchial asthma in patients who require corticosteroids to control symptoms.

Pharmacokinetics

• *Absorption:* Approximately 30% to 50% of an orally inhaled dose is systemically absorbed. Onset of action usually occurs within a few days, but may take as long as 7 days in some patients.

• *Distribution:* Distribution following intranasal aerosol administration has not been described. After oral aerosol administration, drug is mostly distributed into the mouth and throat; the remainder is distributed through the trachea and bronchial tissue. When absorbed systemically, drug is distributed rapidly to muscle, liver, skin, intestines, and kidneys. Dexamethasone is bound weakly to plasma proteins (transcortin and albumin). Only the unbound portion is active. Dexamethasone transfers across the placenta and is distributed into breast milk.

• *Metabolism:* Drug is metabolized primarily in the liver to inactive glucuronide and sulfate metabolites. Some drug may be metabolized locally in the lung tissue.

• *Excretion:* The inactive metabolites and small amounts of unmetabolized drug are excreted by the kidneys. Insignificant quantities of drug are excreted in feces. The biological half-life of dexamethasone is 36 to 54 hours.

Contraindications and precautions

Oral inhalant is contraindicated in patients hypersensitive to any component of the formulation (fluorocarbons, ethanol) and in those with status asthmaticus, persistent positive sputum cultures for *Candida albicans,* or systemic fungal infections. Use oral inhalant cautiously in patients with ocular herpes simplex, nonspecific ulcerative colitis, diverticulitis, recent intestinal anastomoses, peptic ulcer, renal insufficiency, hypertension, osteoporosis, and myasthenia gravis. Dexamethasone should not be added to therapy if asthma is already controlled by bronchodilators or noncorticosteroids or in those with nonasthmatic bronchial disease.

Nasal inhalant is contraindicated in patients with hypersensitivity to drug or in patients with systemic fungal infections, tuberculosis, viral and fungal nasal conditions, or ocular herpes simplex. Use nasal inhalant cautiously in patients with diabetes mellitus, peptic ulcer, ulcerative colitis, abscess or other pyrogenic infection, diverticulitis, recent intestinal anastomoses, renal insufficiency, hypertension, osteoporosis, and myasthenia gravis.

Interactions

None reported.

Effects on diagnostic tests

None reported.

Adverse reactions

EENT: nasal irritation, dryness, rebound nasal congestion, pharygeal candidiasis (with use of oral inhalant).

Other: hypersensitivity reactions, systemic effects with prolonged use (pituitary-adrenal suppression, sodium retention, ***heart failure,*** hypertension, peptic ulceration, ecchymoses, petechiae, masking of infection).

Overdose and treatment

No information available.

☑ Special considerations

Recommendations for use of inhalant dexamethasone and for care and teaching of the patient during therapy are the same as those for all *inhalant adrenocorticoids.*

Breast-feeding

• Breast-feeding is not recommended because systemically absorbed drug may be excreted in breast milk.

dexpanthenol

Ilopan, Panthoderm

Pharmacologic classification: vitamin B complex analogue
Therapeutic classification: GI stimulant, emollient
Pregnancy risk category C

How supplied

Available by prescription only
Injection: 250 mg/ml in vials, ampules, and prefilled syringes
Topical cream: 2%

Indications, route, and dosage

Emollient and protectant over colostomy area or other surgical sites
Adults and children: Apply thin layer p.r.n.

Itching, wounds, insect bites, poison ivy, poison oak, diaper rash, chafing, mild eczema, decubitus ulcers, dry lesions
Adults and children: Apply thin layer topically p.r.n.

Prevention of postoperative adynamic ileus
Adults: 250 to 500 mg I.M.; repeat in 2 hours. Then give q 6 hours, p.r.n.

Treatment of adynamic ileus
Adults: 500 mg I.M., repeat in 2 hours. Then give q 6 hours, p.r.n.

Pharmacodynamics

Emollient action: By stimulating granulation and epithelialization, dexpanthenol promotes healing and relieves itching.

GI stimulant action: Dexpanthenon is an analogue of pantothenic acid, a precursor of coenzyme A, which serves as a cofactor in the synthesis of acetylcholine. Dexpanthenol stimulates the acetylation of choline to acetylcholine, which increases peristalsis.

Pharmacokinetics

• *Absorption:* Dexpanthenol is absorbed from I.M. sites.

• *Distribution:* After conversion to pantothenic acid, drug is distributed widely, mainly as coenzyme A. Highest concentration occurs in the liver, adrenal glands, heart, and kidneys.

• *Metabolism:* Conversion to pantothenic acid occurs readily.
• *Excretion:* Most metabolites are excreted in urine; remainder in feces.

Contraindications and precautions
Contraindicated in patients with ileus due to obstruction because of potential for severe cramping and worsening of condition and on wounds in patients with hemophilia because of potential for severe bleeding.

Interactions
When dexpanthenol is used concomitantly with *antibiotics* and *barbiturates,* allergic responses to dexpanthenol may occur (very rare). *Succinylcholine's* actions are prolonged in the presence of dexpanthenol; therefore, give these drugs at least 1 hour apart.

Effects on diagnostic tests
None reported.

Adverse reactions
CV: slight decreases in blood pressure.
GI: intestinal colic, vomiting, diarrhea.
Respiratory: breathing difficulties.
Skin: itching, red patches, dermatitis, tingling.
Note: Drug should be discontinued if hypersensitivity reactions occur.

Overdose and treatment
No information available.

☑ Special considerations
• For I.V. administration, dilute in glucose or lactated Ringer's solutions and infuse slowly.
• Be sure to monitor fluid and electrolytes (especially potassium) in patients with adynamic ileus. Anemia, hypoproteinemia, and infection may contribute to the condition.
• Avoid concomitant use with drugs that decrease GI motility.

Patient education
• Advise patient of the adverse reactions.

Geriatric use
• Use cautiously in the elderly; cases of agitation have been reported.

Pediatric use
• Safety of parenteral form has not been established.

dexrazoxane
Zinecard

Pharmacologic classification: intracellular chelating agent
Therapeutic classification: cardioprotective
Pregnancy risk category C

How supplied
Available by prescription only
Injection: 250 mg, 500 mg in single-dose vials

Indications, route, and dosage
Reduction of incidence and severity of doxorubicin-induced cardiomyopathy in women with metastatic breast cancer who have received a cumulative doxorubicin dose of 300 mg/m² but would benefit from continued therapy with doxorubicin
Adults: Dosage ratio of dexrazoxane to doxorubicin must be 10:1 such as 500 mg/m² dexrazoxane:50 mg/m² doxorubicin. After reconstitution, dexrazoxane should be administered by slow I.V. push or rapid drip I.V. infusion. After completion of dexrazoxane administration and before a total elapsed time of 30 minutes from the beginning of the dexrazoxane administration, the I.V. injection of the doxorubicin dose should be given.

Pharmacodynamics
Cardioprotective action: Dexrazoxane's specific mechanism of action is unknown. Drug is a cyclic derivative of EDTA that readily penetrates cell membranes. Studies suggest that drug is converted intracellularly to a ring-opened chelating agent that interferes with iron-mediated free radical generation believed to be responsible, in part, for anthracycline-induced cardiomyopathy.

Pharmacokinetics
• *Absorption:* Dexrazoxane is given I.V.
• *Distribution:* Unknown. Drug is not bound to plasma proteins.
• *Metabolism:* Dexrazoxane is not believed to be metabolized.
• *Excretion:* Drug is primarily excreted in urine.

Contraindications and precautions
Contraindicated in patients who are not receiving doxorubicin as part of the chemotherapy regimen. Use cautiously in all patients because additive effects of immunosuppression may occur from concomitant administration of cytotoxic drugs.

Interactions
None reported.

Effects on diagnostic tests
None reported.

Adverse reactions
The following reactions (except for pain on injection) may be attributed to the FAC regimen (fluorouracil, doxorubicin, cyclophosphamide) given shortly after dexrazoxane.
CNS: *fatigue, malaise, neurotoxicity.*
GI: *nausea, vomiting, anorexia, stomatitis, diarrhea,* esophagitis, dysphagia.
Hematologic: hemorrhage.
Skin: urticaria.
Other: *alopecia, fever, infection, pain on injection, sepsis,* streaking at I.V. insertion site, erythema, phlebitis, extravasation.

Overdose and treatment

There are no known reports of overdosage although myelosuppression is most likely to occur. Because dexrazoxane is not bound to plasma protein, peritoneal dialysis or hemodialysis may be effective in removing drug from body. Suspected overdose should be managed with good supportive care until resolution of myelosuppression and related conditions is complete. Management of overdose should include treatment of infections, fluid regulation, and maintenance of nutritional requirements.

☑ Special considerations

- Doxorubicin should not be given before dexrazoxane. Also, dexrazoxane is not recommended for use with the initiation of doxorubicin therapy but only after an accumulate dosage of doxorubicin of 300 mg/m² has been reached and continuation of doxorubicin is desired.
- Drug must be diluted with the diluent supplied with drug (0.167 M sodium lactate injection) to give a concentration of 10 mg dexrazoxane for each ml of sodium lactate. Reconstituted solution should be given by slow I.V. push or rapid drip I.V. infusion from a bag.
- Reconstituted solution, when transferred to an empty infusion bag, is stable for 6 hours from the time of reconstitution when stored at controlled room temperature (36° to 46° F [2° to 8° C]) or under refrigeration. Discard unused solution.
- Reconstituted drug may be diluted with either 0.9% NaCl solution or D_5W injection to a concentration range of 1.3 to 5.0 mg/ml in I.V. infusion bags. The resultant solution is also stable for 6 hours under the same storage conditions as the diluted drug.
- Dexrazoxane should not be mixed with other drugs because of possible incompatibility.
- Use caution when handling and preparing the reconstituted solution; follow same precautions as handling antineoplastic agents. Be sure to use gloves. If drug powder or solution contacts the skin or mucosa, immediately wash thoroughly with soap and water.
- Monitor CBC closely because drug is always used with other cytotoxic drugs and it may add to the myelosuppressive effects of cytotoxic drugs itself.
- The administration of Zinecard with doxarubicin does not eliminate the possibility of cardiac toxicity. Therefore cardiac function should be carefully monitored.

Patient education

- Inform patient of need for drug during continued doxorubicin therapy.
- Warn patient to watch for signs of infection (fever, sore throat, fatigue) and bleeding (easy bruising, nose bleeds, bleeding gums, melena). Tell patient to take temperature daily and teach him infection control and bleeding precautions.
- Inform patient that alopecia may occur but that it's usually reversible.

Pediatric use

- Safety and effectiveness in children have not been established.

Breast-feeding

- Because of the potential for serious adverse effects in breast-fed infants, breast-feeding is not recommended.

dextran 1

Promit

dextran, low-molecular-weight (dextran 40)

Gentran 40, LMD 10%, Rheomacrodex

dextran, high-molecular-weight (dextran 70, dextran 75)

Gendex 75, Gentran 70, Macrodex

Pharmacologic classification: glucose polymer
Therapeutic classification: plasma volume expander
Pregnancy risk category C

How supplied

Available by prescription only
dextran 1
Injection: 150 mg/ml in 20-ml vials
low-molecular-weight dextran
Injection: 10% dextran 40 in D_5W or 0.9% NaCl
high-molecular-weight dextran
Injection: 6% dextran 70 in 0.9% NaCl or D_5W; 6% dextran 75 in 0.9% NaCl or D_5W

Indications, route, and dosage

Prevention of severe anaphylactic reaction caused by low- or high-molecular-weight dextran
Adults: 20 ml of dextran 1 by rapid I.V. push 1 to 2 minutes before dextran infusion.
Children: 0.3 ml/kg of dextran 1 by rapid I.V. push 1 to 2 minutes before dextran infusion.
Plasma volume expansion
Dosage depends on amount of fluid loss.
Adults: Initially, 500 ml of dextran 40 with central venous pressure (CVP) monitoring. Infuse remaining dose slowly. Total daily dose should not exceed 2 g/kg (20 ml/kg) body weight. If therapy continues past 24 hours, do not exceed 1 g/kg daily. Continue for no longer than 5 days.

Usual dose of dextran 70 or 75 solution is 30 g (500 ml of 6% solution) I.V. In emergencies, may be administered at a rate of 1.2 to 2.4 g/minute (20 to 40 ml/minute). Total dose during the first 24 hours is not to exceed 1.2 g/kg; actual dose depends on the amount of fluid loss and resultant hemoconcentration and must be determined individually. In normovolemic patients, the rate of administration should not exceed 240 mg/minute (4 ml/minute).
Children: Total dosage of dextran 70 or 75 should not exceed 1.2 g/kg (20 ml/kg), with the dose based on the body weight or surface area. If therapy is continued, dosage should not exceed 0.6 g/kg (10 ml/kg) daily.

Priming pump oxygenators
Adults: Dextran 40 can be used as the only priming fluid or as an additive to other primers in pump oxygenators. Dextran 40 is added to the perfusion circuit as the 10% solution in a dose of 1 to 2 g/kg (10 to 20 ml/kg); total dose should not exceed 2 g/kg (20 ml/kg).
Prophylaxis of venous thrombosis and pulmonary embolism
Adults: Dextran 40 therapy should usually be given during the surgical procedure. On the day of surgery, dextran 40 (10% solution) is given at the dose of 50 to 100 g (500 to 1,000 ml or approximately 10 ml/kg). Treatment is continued for 2 to 3 days at a dose of 50 g (500 ml) daily. Then, if needed, 50 g (500 ml) may be given q 2 or 3 days for up to 2 weeks to reduce the risk of thromboembolism (deep venous thrombosis) or pulmonary embolism.

Pharmacodynamics
Plasma-expanding action: Dextran 40 (10%) has an average molecular weight of 40,000, the osmotic equivalent of twice the volume of plasma. Dextran 40 has a duration of action of 2 to 4 hours. Dextran 70 has an average molecular weight of 70,000; the I.V. infusion results in an expansion of the plasma volume slightly in excess of the volume infused. This effect, useful in treating shock, lasts for approximately 12 hours.

Dextran 40, 70, and 75 enhance the blood flow, particularly in the microcirculation. Dextran 40 can be used to prime oxygenator pumps, as the only fluid or in combination with other fluids.

Prophylaxis of venous thrombosis and pulmonary embolism: Dextran 40 inhibits vascular stasis and platelet adhesiveness and alters the structure and lysability of fibrin clots. Dextran 40 increases cardiac output and arterial, venous, and microcirculatory flow and reduces mean transit time, mainly by expanding plasma volume and by reducing blood viscosity through hemodilution and reducing red cell aggregation.

Pharmacokinetics
- *Absorption:* Dextran 40 and 70 are given by I.V. infusion. The plasma concentration depends on the rate of infusion and the rate of disappearance of the drug from the plasma.
- *Distribution:* Dextran is distributed throughout the vascular system.
- *Metabolism:* Dextran molecules with molecular weights above 50,000 are enzymatically degraded by dextranase to glucose at a rate of about 70 to 90 mg/kg/day. This is a variable process.
- *Excretion:* Dextran molecules with molecular weights below 50,000 are eliminated by renal excretion, with 40% of dextran 70 appearing in the urine within 24 hours. Approximately 50% of dextran 40 is excreted in the urine within 3 hours, 60% within 6 hours, and 75% within 24 hours. The remaining 25% is hydrolyzed partially and excreted in urine, excreted partially in feces, and partially oxidized.

Contraindications and precautions
Low-molecular-weight dextran is contraindicated in patients with hypersensitivity to drug and in those with marked hemostatic defects, marked cardiac decompensation, and renal disease with severe oliguria or anuria. High-molecular-weight dextran is also contraindicated in patients with hypervolemic conditions and severe bleeding disorders.

Use low-molecular-weight dextran cautiously in patients with active hemorrhage, thrombocytopenia, or diabetes mellitus. Use high-molecular-weight dextran cautiously in patients with active hemorrhage, thrombocytopenia, impaired renal clearance, chronic liver disease, and abdominal conditions or in those undergoing bowel surgery.

Interactions
Abnormally prolonged bleeding times can occur if either high-molecular weight dextran or low-molecular-weight dextran are given concomitantly with *anticoagulants* or *antiplatelet drugs.*

Effects on diagnostic tests
Falsely elevated blood glucose levels may occur in patients receiving dextran 40 or 70 if the test uses high concentrations of acid. Dextran may cause turbidity, which interferes with bilirubin assays that use alcohol, total protein levels using biuret reagent, and blood glucose levels using the orthotoluidine method.

Blood typing and cross-matching using enzyme techniques may give unreliable readings if the samples are taken after the dextran infusion.

Dextran 40 administration has been associated with abnormal renal and hepatic function test results.

Adverse reactions
GI: nausea, vomiting.
GU: tubular stasis and blocking, increased urine viscosity; oliguria, anuria, increased specific gravity of urine (with high-molecular-weight dextran).
Hematologic: *decreased hemoglobin and hematocrit levels;* increased bleeding time (with higher doses of low-molecular-weight dextran); increased bleeding time and significant suppression of platelet function (with high-molecular-weight dextran in doses of 15 ml/kg body weight).
Hepatic: increased AST and ALT levels.
Other: ***thrombophlebitis,*** hypersensitivity reactions (urticaria, ***anaphylaxis***); fever, arthralgia, nasal congestion (with high-molecular-weight dextran).

Overdose and treatment
No information available.

☑ Special considerations
- Patients with dehydration should be well hydrated before dextran infusions.
- Dextran in NaCl solution is hazardous when given to patients with heart failure, severe renal failure, and clinical states in which edema exists with sodium restriction. (D_5W solution should be used.)
- Dextran works as a plasma expander via colloidal osmotic effect, thereby drawing fluid from interstitial to intravascular space. It provides plasma ex-

pansion slightly greater than volume infused. Observe for circulatory overload or a rise in CVP readings.

- Dextran 1 should be given just before infusing low- or high-molecular-weight dextran. Repeat dosage of dextran 1 if more than 15 minutes elapses during infusion.
- Avoid doses that exceed the recommendations because dose-related increases in the incidence of wound hematoma, wound seroma, wound bleeding, distant bleeding (such as hematuria and melena), and pulmonary edema have been observed.
- Monitor urinary output during administration. If oliguria or anuria occurs or is not reversed by the initial infusion (500 ml), administration should be discontinued.
- Monitor urine or serum osmolarity; urine specific gravity will be increased by urine dextran concentration.
- Monitor CVP when dextran is given by rapid I.V. infusion. A precipitous rise in CVP or other signs of fluid overload indicate the need to stop the infusion.
- Check hemoglobin and hematocrit; do not allow to fall below 30% by volume.
- Observe patient closely during early phase of infusion; check for infiltration, phlebitis, and anaphylactic reactions.
- Dextran may interfere with analysis of blood grouping, cross-matching, bilirubin, blood glucose, and protein.
- Store at constant 77° F (25° C). Solution may precipitate in storage. Discard any solution that is not clear.
- Dextran does not contain a preservative. Discard partially used containers.

Geriatric use
- Use dextran with caution in elderly patients because they may be at increased risk of fluid overload.

Breast-feeding
- It is unknown whether dextran crosses into human milk. A decision should be made to discontinue breast-feeding or use of the drug.

dextranomer
Debrisan

Pharmacologic classification: synthetic polysaccharide
Therapeutic classification: topical debriding agent
Pregnancy risk category NR

How supplied
Available by prescription only
Beads: 4 g, 25 g, 60 g, 120 g
Dressing pad: 3 g
Paste: 10 g

Indications, route, and dosage
Cleaning of exudative wounds
Adults and children: Apply to affected area once or twice daily or more often if drainage is heavy. Apply to at least ¼″ thickness, and cover with sterile gauze.

Pharmacodynamics
Debriding action: Dextranomer cleanses wound surfaces by capillary action, drawing wound exudate, bacteria, and contaminants into the beads and therefore enhancing formation of granulative tissue and promoting wound healing.

Pharmacokinetics
- *Absorption:* Limited with topical use.
- *Distribution:* None.
- *Metabolism:* None.
- *Excretion:* None.

Contraindications and precautions
Contraindicated in deep fistulas, sinus tracts, or any area where complete removal is not assured and in dry wounds because it is ineffective in cleaning them.

Interactions
Dextranomer should not be used concomitantly with *topical antibiotics* or *debriding enzymes.*

Effects on diagnostic tests
None reported.

Adverse reactions
Skin: transient pain at site, bleeding, erythema, contact dermatitis.

Note: Drug should be discontinued if sensitization develops.

Overdose and treatment
No information available.

☑ Special considerations
- Use strict aseptic technique when applying dextranomer.
- Dextranomer is not an enzyme and cannot be used for dry wounds.
- Clean wound before applying, leaving area moist; cover wound to a thickness of at least ¼″, then bandage lightly to hold beads in place. Be sure to leave room for expansion (1 g of beads absorbs 4 ml of exudate).
- When product is saturated and grayish yellow, irrigate wound and remove beads or paste; beads must be removed thoroughly, especially before any surgical treatment, and vigorous irrigation or soaking may be necessary.
- If dressing becomes dry, do not remove it without prior wetting to loosen bandage and beads.
- Stop treatment when area is free of exudate.
- Do not use in areas where complete removal cannot be ensured—for example, in fistulas or sinus tracts.

Patient education
- Teach patient how to perform sterile dressing changes before discharge.
- Advise patient to avoid drug contact with eyes and to wash hands well after application.

Breast-feeding

- Women should avoid breast-feeding if drug is used in breast area.

dextroamphetamine sulfate

Dexedrine, Ferndex

Pharmacologic classification: amphetamine
Therapeutic classification: CNS stimulant, short-term adjunctive anorexigenic agent, sympathomimetic amine
Controlled substance schedule II
Pregnancy risk category C

How supplied

Available by prescription only
Tablets: 5 mg, 10 mg, 20 mg
Capsules (sustained-release): 5 mg, 10 mg, 15 mg
Elixir: 5 mg/5 ml

Indications, route, and dosage

Narcolepsy
Adults: 5 to 60 mg P.O. daily in divided doses. Long-acting dosage forms allow once-daily dosing.
Children over age 12: 10 mg P.O. daily, with 10-mg increments weekly, p.r.n.
Children age 6 to 12: 5 mg P.O. daily, with 5-mg increments weekly, p.r.n.
◇ ***Short-term adjunct in exogenous obesity***
Adults: 5 to 30 mg P.O. daily 30 to 60 minutes before meals in divided doses of 5 to 10 mg. Alternatively, give one 10- or 15-mg sustained-release capsule daily as a single dose in the morning.
Attention deficit hyperactivity disorder
Children age 6 and older: 5 mg once daily or b.i.d., with 5-mg increments weekly, p.r.n. Total daily dose should rarely exceed 40 mg.
Children age 3 to 5: 2.5 mg P.O. daily, with 2.5-mg increments weekly, p.r.n.; not recommended for children under age 3.

Pharmacodynamics

CNS stimulant action: Amphetamines are sympathomimetic amines with CNS stimulant activity; in hyperactive children, they have a paradoxical calming effect.

Anorexigenic action: Anorexigenic effects are thought to occur in the hypothalamus, where decreased smell and taste acuity decreases appetite. They may be tried for short-term control of refractory obesity, with caloric restriction and behavior modification.

The cerebral cortex and reticular activating system appear to be the primary sites of activity; amphetamines release nerve terminal stores of norepinephrine, promoting nerve impulse transmission. At high dosages, effects are mediated by dopamine.

Amphetamines are used to treat narcolepsy and as adjuncts to psychosocial measures in attention deficit disorder in children. Their precise mechanism of action in these conditions is unknown.

Pharmacokinetics

- *Absorption:* Drug is rapidly absorbed from the GI tract; peak serum concentrations occur 2 to 4 hours after oral administration; long-acting capsules are absorbed more slowly and have a longer duration of action.
- *Distribution:* Drug is distributed widely throughout the body.
- *Metabolism:* Unknown.
- *Excretion:* Drug is excreted in urine.

Contraindications and precautions

Contraindicated in patients with hypersensitivity or idiosyncrasy to the sympathomimetic amines, within 14 days of MAO inhibitor therapy, and in those with hyperthyroidism, moderate to severe hypertension, symptomatic CV disease, glaucoma, advanced arteriosclerosis, and history of drug abuse. Use cautiously in patients with motor and phonic tics, Tourette's syndrome, and agitated states.

Interactions

Concomitant use with *MAO inhibitors* (or drugs with MAO-inhibiting activity, such as *furazolidone*) or within 14 days of such therapy may cause hypertensive crisis; use with *antihypertensives* may antagonize antihypertensive effects.

Concomitant use with *antacids, sodium bicarbonate,* or *acetazolamide* enhances reabsorption of dextroamphetamine and prolongs duration of action; use with *ascorbic acid* enhances dextroamphetamine excretion and shortens duration of action.

Concomitant use with *phenothiazines* or *haloperidol* decreases dextroamphetamine effects; *barbiturates* antagonize dextroamphetamine by CNS depression; use with *theophylline, caffeine,* or other *CNS stimulants* produces additive effects.

Dextroamphetamine may alter *insulin* requirements.

Dextroamphetamine given concommitantly with *phenobarbital* or *phenytoin* may produce a synergistic anticonvulsant action.

Effects on diagnostic tests

Drug may elevate plasma corticosteroid levels and may interefere with urinary steroid determinations.

Adverse reactions

CNS: *restlessness,* tremor, *insomnia,* dizziness, headache, chills, overstimulation, dysphoria, euphoria.
CV: *tachycardia, palpitations,* hypertension, ***arrhythmias.***
GI: dry mouth, unpleasant taste, diarrhea, constipation, anorexia, weight loss, other GI disturbances.
GU: impotence.
Skin: urticaria.
Other: altered libido.

Overdose and treatment

Individual responses to overdose vary widely. Toxic symptoms may occur at 15 mg and 30 mg and can cause severe reactions; however, doses of 400 mg or more have not always proved fatal.

Symptoms of overdose include restlessness, tremor, hyperreflexia, tachypnea, confusion, aggressiveness, hallucinations, and panic; fatigue and depression usually follow excitement stage. Other symptoms may include arrhythmias, shock, alterations in blood pressure, nausea, vomiting, diarrhea, and abdominal cramps; death is usually preceded by seizures and coma.

Treat overdose symptomatically and supportively: if ingestion is recent (within 4 hours), use gastric lavage or emesis and sedate with a barbiturate; monitor vital signs and fluid and electrolyte balance. Urinary acidification may enhance excretion. Saline catharsis (magnesium citrate) may hasten GI evacuation of unabsorbed sustained-release drug.

☑ Special considerations

- Administer dextroamphetamine 30 to 60 minutes before meals when using as an anorexigenic agent. To minimize insomnia, avoid giving within 6 hours of bedtime.
- Check vital signs regularly. Observe patient for signs of excessive stimulation.
- When tolerance to anorexigenic effect develops, dosage should be discontinued, not increased.
- Monitor blood and urine glucose levels. Drug may alter daily insulin requirement in patients with diabetes.
- For narcolepsy, patient should take first dose on awakening.

Patient education

- Tell patient to avoid drinks containing caffeine, which increases stimulant effects of the drug.
- Warn patient to avoid hazardous activities that require alertness until CNS response is determined.
- Instruct patient to take drug early in the day to minimize insomnia.
- Tell patient not to crush sustained-release forms or to increase dosage.
- Tell patient to take dose 60 minutes before next meal when drug is used as an appetite suppressant.
- If possible, teach parents to provide drug-free periods for children with attention deficit disorder, especially during periods of reduced stress.

Geriatric use

- Use lower doses in elderly patients.

Pediatric use

- Drug is not recommended for treatment of obesity in children under age 12.

Breast-feeding

- Safety has not been established. Alternative feeding method is recommended during therapy with dextroamphetamine sulfate.

dextromethorphan hydrobromide

Balminil D.M.*, Benylin DM Cough, Broncho-Grippol-DM*, Delsym, DM Syrup*, Hold, Koffex*, Mediquell, Neo-DM*, Robidex*, Sedatuss*, St. Joseph Cough Suppressant for Children, Sucrets Cough Control Formula, Suppress, Trocal, Vicks Formula 44

Pharmacologic classification: levorphanol derivative (dextrorotatory methyl ether)
Therapeutic classification: antitussive (nonnarcotic)
Pregnancy risk category C

How supplied

Available without a prescription
Syrup: 10 mg/5 ml, 15 mg/15 ml
Liquid (sustained-action): 30 mg/5 ml
Liquid: 3.5 mg/5 ml, 7.5 mg/5 ml, 15 mg/5 ml
Lozenges: 2.5 mg, 5 mg, 7.5 mg
Chewable pieces: 15 mg

Indications, route, and dosage

Nonproductive cough (chronic)
Adults and children age 12 and older: 10 to 20 mg q 4 hours, or 30 mg q 6 to 8 hours. Or the controlled-release liquid b.i.d. (60 mg b.i.d.). Maximum dose is 120 mg daily.
Children age 6 to 12: 5 to 10 mg q 4 hours, or 15 mg q 6 to 8 hours. Or the controlled-release liquid b.i.d. (30 mg b.i.d.). Maximum dose is 60 mg daily.
Children age 2 to 6: 2.5 to 5 mg q 4 hours, or 7.5 mg q 6 to 8 hours; or the sustained-action liquid 15 mg b.i.d. Maximum dose is 30 mg daily.

Pharmacodynamics

Antitussive action: Dextromethorphan suppresses the cough reflex by direct action on the cough center in the medulla. Drug is almost equal in antitussive potency to codeine, but causes no analgesia or addiction and little or no CNS depression and has no expectorant action; it also produces fewer subjective and GI adverse effects than codeine. Treatment is intended to relieve cough frequency without abolishing protective cough reflex. In therapeutic doses, drug does not inhibit ciliary activity.

Pharmacokinetics

- *Absorption:* Drug is absorbed readily from the GI tract; action begins within 15 to 30 minutes.
- *Distribution:* Unknown.
- *Metabolism:* Drug is metabolized extensively by the liver. Plasma half-life is approximately 11 hours.
- *Excretion:* Little drug is excreted unchanged: metabolites are excreted primarily in urine; about 7% to 10% is excreted in feces. Antitussive effect persists for 5 to 6 hours.

Contraindications and precautions

Contraindicated in patients currently taking MAO inhibitors or within 2 weeks of discontinuing MAO inhibitors. Use cautiously in atopic children, sedated or debilitated patients, and those confined to the supine position. Also use cautiously in patients with sensitivity to aspirin.

Interactions
Concomitant use with *MAO inhibitors* may cause nausea, hypotension, excitation, hyperpyrexia, and coma; do not give dextromethorphan to patients at any interval less than 2 weeks after MAO inhibitors are discontinued.

Effects on diagnostic tests
None reported.

Adverse reactions
CNS: drowsiness, dizziness.
GI: nausea, vomiting, stomach pain.

Overdose and treatment
Clinical manifestations of overdose may include nausea, vomiting, drowsiness, dizziness, blurred vision, nystagmus, shallow respirations, urine retention, toxic psychosis, stupor, and coma.

Treatment of overdose involves administering activated charcoal to reduce drug absorption and I.V. naloxone to support respiration. Other symptoms are treated supportively.

☑ Special considerations
- Treatment is intended to relieve cough intensity and frequency, without completely abolishing the protective cough reflex.
- Use with percussion and chest vibration.
- Monitor nature and frequency of coughing.

Patient education
- Tell patient to call if cough persists more than 7 days.
- Instruct patient to use sugarless throat lozenges for throat irritation and resulting cough.
- Recommend a humidifier to filter out dust, smoke, and air pollutants.

Pediatric use
- Do not use syrup, tablets, or lozenges in children under age 2. Sustained-action liquid may be used in children under age 2, but dosage must be individualized.

Breast-feeding
- Safety has not been established.

dextrose (d-glucose)
$D_{2.5}W$, D_5W, $D_{10}W$, $D_{20}W$, $D_{25}W$, $D_{30}W$, $D_{38}W$, $D_{40}W$, $D_{50}W$, $D_{60}W$, $D_{70}W$

Pharmacologic classification: carbohydrate
Therapeutic classification: total parenteral nutrition (TPN) component, caloric agent, fluid volume replacement
Pregnancy risk category C

How supplied
Available by prescription only
Injection: 1,000 ml (2.5%, 5%, 10%, 20%, 30%, 40%, 50%, 60%, 70%); 650 ml (38.5%); 500 ml (5%, 10%, 20%, 30%, 40%, 50%, 60%, 70%); 400 ml (5%); 250 ml (5%, 10%); 100 ml (5%); 70-ml pin-top vial (70% for additive use only); 50 ml (5% and 50% available in vial, ampule, and Bristoject); 10 ml (25%); 5-ml ampule (10%); 3-ml ampule (10%)

Indications, route, and dosage
Fluid replacement and caloric supplementation in patients who cannot maintain adequate oral intake or who are restricted from doing so
Adults and children: Dosage depends on fluid and caloric requirements. Use peripheral I.V. infusion of 2.5% or 5% solution, or central I.V. infusion of10% or 20% solution for minimal fluid needs. Use 50% solution to treat insulin-induced hypoglycemia. Solutions from 10% to 70% are used diluted in admixtures, normally with amino acid solutions, and administered via a central vein.

Pharmacodynamics
Metabolic action: Dextrose is a rapidly metabolized source of calories and fluids in patients with inadequate oral intake. While increasing blood glucose concentrations, dextrose may decrease body protein and nitrogen losses, promote glycogen deposition, and decrease or prevent ketosis if sufficient doses are given. Dextrose also may induce diuresis. Parenterally injected doses of dextrose undergo oxidation to carbon dioxide and water. A 5% solution is isotonic and is administered peripherally. Concentrated dextrose infusions provide increased caloric intake with less fluid volume; they may be irritating if given by peripheral infusions. Concentrated solutions (above 10%) should be administered only by central venous catheters.

Pharmacokinetics
- *Absorption:* After oral administration, dextrose (a monosaccharide) is absorbed rapidly by the small intestine, principally by an active mechanism. In patients with hypoglycemia, blood glucose concentrations increase within 10 to 20 minutes after oral administration. Peak blood concentrations may occur 40 minutes after oral administration.
- *Distribution:* As a source of calories and water for hydration, dextrose solutions expand plasma volume.
- *Metabolism:* Dextrose is metabolized to carbon dioxide and water.
- *Excretion:* In some patients, dextrose solutions may produce diuresis.

Contraindications and precautions
Contraindicated in patients in diabetic coma while blood glucose remains excessively high. Use of concentrated solutions contraindicated in patients with intracranial or intraspinal hemorrhage, in dehydrated patients with alcohol withdrawal syndrome, or in patients with severe dehydration, anuria, hepatic coma, or glucose-galactose malabsorption syndrome. Use cautiously in patients with cardiac

or pulmonary disease, hypertension, renal insufficiency, urinary obstruction, or hypovolemia.

Interactions

Dextrose should be administered cautiously, especially if it contains sodium ions, to patients receiving *corticosteroids* or *corticotropin*. Additives must be introduced aseptically, mixed thoroughly, and not stored; incompatibility is possible. Dextrose must not be administered with *blood* through the same infusion set because of possible pseudoagglutination of RBCs.

Dextrose infusions may alter *insulin* or *oral hypoglycemic* drug requirements and may cause vitamin B complex deficiency.

Effects on diagnostic tests

None reported.

Adverse reactions

CNS: confusion, ***unconsciousness in hyperosmolar nonketotic syndrome.***
CV: ***pulmonary edema, exacerbated hypertension, heart failure*** in susceptible patients (with fluid overload); *phlebitis, venous sclerosis,* tissue necrosis (with prolonged or concentrated infusions, especially when administered peripherally).
GU: glycosuria, osmotic diuresis.
Skin: sloughing and tissue necrosis, if extravasation occurs with concentrated solutions.
Other: hyperglycemia, hypervolemia, hypovolemia, dehydration, fever, hyperosmolarity (with rapid infusion of concentrated solution or prolonged infusion); hypoglycemia from rebound hyperinsulinemia, vitamin B complex deficiency (with rapid termination of long-term infusion).

Overdose and treatment

If fluid or solute overload occurs during I.V. therapy, reevaluate patient's condition and institute appropriate corrective treatment. Decrease infusion rate or adjust insulin dosage as needed.

☑ Special considerations

- Monitor infusion rate for maximum dextrose infusion of 0.5 g/kg/hour, using the largest available peripheral vein and a well-placed needle or catheter. However, hypertonic dextrose solutions may cause thrombosis if infused via peripheral vein, therefore, administer via a central venous catheter.
- Avoid rapid administration, which may cause hyperglycemia, hyperosmolar syndrome, or glycosuria.
- Infuse concentrated solutions slowly; rapid infusion can cause hyperglycemia and fluid shifts.
- Hypertonic solutions are more likely than isotonic or hypotonic solutions to cause irritation; they should be administered into larger central veins.
- Injection site should be checked frequently during the day to prevent irritation, tissue sloughing, necrosis, and phlebitis.
- Carefully monitor patient's intake, output, and body weight, especially in patients with renal dysfunction.
- Monitor serum glucose levels during long-term treatment.
- Monitor vital signs for significant changes.
- Depletion of pancreatic insulin production and secretion can occur. To avoid an adverse effect on insulin production, patient may need to have insulin added to infusions.
- Evaluate fluid imbalance or changes in electrolyte concentrations and acid-base balance by periodic laboratory determinations during prolonged therapy. Additional electrolyte supplementation may be required.
- Excessive administration of potassium-free solutions may result in hypokalemia. Potassium should be added to dextrose solutions and administered to fasting patients with good renal function; special precautions should be taken with patients receiving a cardiac glycoside.
- Infuse concentrated solutions via central venous catheter with meticulous aseptic technique, as bacterial contamination thrives in high glucose environments.
- To avoid rebound hypoglycemia, dextrose 5% or 10% solution is advisable upon discontinuation of concentrated dextrose infusions.

Pediatric use

- Use with caution in infants of diabetic women, except as may be indicated in newborn infants who are hypoglycemic.

diazepam

Apo-Diazepam*, Dizac, Novodipam*, Valium, Vivol*, Zetran

Pharmacologic classification: benzodiazepine
Therapeutic classification: antianxiety; skeletal muscle relaxant; amnesic; anticonvulsant; sedative-hypnotic
Controlled substance schedule IV
Pregnancy risk category NR

How supplied

Available by prescription only
Tablets: 2 mg, 5 mg, 10 mg
Capsules (extended-release): 15 mg
Oral solution: 5 mg/ml; 5 mg/5 ml
Oral suspension: 5 mg/5 ml
Injection: 5 mg/ml in 2-ml ampules or 10-ml vials
Disposable syringe: 2-ml Tel-E-Ject

Indications, route, and dosage

Anxiety
Adults: Depending on severity, 2 to 10 mg P.O. b.i.d. to q.i.d. or 15 to 30 mg extended-release capsules P.O. once daily. Alternatively, 2 to 10 mg I.M. or I.V. q 3 to 4 hours p.r.n.
Children age 6 months and older: 1 to 2.5 mg P.O. t.i.d. or q.i.d.; increase dose gradually, as needed and tolerated.
Acute alcohol withdrawal
Adults: 10 mg P.O. t.i.d. or q.i.d. for the first 24 hours; reduce to 5 mg t.i.d. or q.i.d., p.r.n.; or 10 mg I.M. or I.V. initially, followed by 5 to 10 mg q 3 to 4 hours, p.r.n.

Muscle spasm
Adults: 2 to 10 mg P.O. b.i.d. to q.i.d.; or 15 to 30 mg extended-release capsules once daily. Alternatively, 5 to 10 mg I.M. or I.V. q 3 to 4 hours, p.r.n.
Tetanus
Infants over age 30 days to children age 5: 1 to 2 mg I.M. or I.V. slowly, repeated q 3 to 4 hours.
Children age 5 and older: 5 to 10 mg I.M. or I.V. slowly q 3 to 4 hours, p.r.n.
Adjunct to convulsive disorders
Adults: 2 to 10 mg P.O. b.i.d. to q.i.d.
Children age 6 months and older: Initially, 1 to 2.5 mg P.O. t.i.d. or q.i.d.; increase dose as tolerated and needed.
Adjunct to anesthesia; endoscopic procedures
Adults: 5 to 10 mg I.M. before surgery; or administer I.V. slowly just before procedure, titrating dose to effect. Usually, less than 10 mg is used, but up to 20 mg may be given.
Status epilepticus
Adults: 5 to 10 mg I.V. (preferred) or I.M. initially, repeated at 10- to 15-minute intervals up to a maximum dose of 30 mg. Repeat q 2 to 4 hours, p.r.n.
Children age 5 and older: 1 mg I.V. q 2 to 5 minutes up to a maximum dose of 10 mg; repeat in 2 to 4 hours, p.r.n.
Infants over age 30 days to children age 5: 0.2 to 0.5 mg I.V. q 2 to 5 minutes up to a maximum dose of 5 mg.
Cardioversion
Adults: Administer 5 to 15 mg I.V. 5 to 10 minutes before procedure.

Pharmacodynamics
Anxiolytic and sedative-hypnotic actions: Diazepam depresses the CNS at the limbic and subcortical levels of the brain. It produces an anti-anxiety effect by influencing the effect of the neurotransmitter gamma-aminobutyric acid on its receptor in the ascending reticular activating system, which increases inhibition and blocks cortical and limbic arousal.

Anticonvulsant action: Diazepam suppresses the spread of seizure activity produced by epileptogenic foci in the cortex, thalamus, and limbic structures by enhancing presynaptic inhibition.

Amnesic action: The exact mechanism of action is unknown.

Skeletal muscle relaxant action: The exact mechanism is unknown, but it is believed to involve inhibiting polysynaptic afferent pathways.

Pharmacokinetics
- *Absorption:* When administered orally, drug is absorbed through the GI tract. Onset of action occurs within 30 to 60 minutes, with peak action in 1 to 2 hours. I.M. administration results in erratic absorption of the drug; onset of action usually occurs in 15 to 30 minutes. After I.V. administration, rapid onset of action occurs 1 to 5 minutes after injection.
- *Distribution:* Distributed widely throughout the body. Approximately 85% to 95% of an administered dose is bound to plasma protein.
- *Metabolism:* Drug is metabolized in the liver to the active metabolite desmethyldiazepam.
- *Excretion:* Most metabolites of diazepam are excreted in urine, with only small amounts excreted in feces. Half-life of desmethyldiazepam is 30 to 200 hours. Duration of effect is 3 hours; this may be prolonged up to 90 hours in elderly patients and in patients with hepatic or renal dysfunction.

Contraindications and precautions
Contraindicated in patients with hypersensitivity or narrow angle glaucoma; in patients experiencing shock, coma, or acute alcohol intoxication (parenteral form) and in children under age 6 months (oral form). Use cautiously in the elderly, in debilitated patients, and in those with impaired hepatic or renal function, depression, or chronic open-angle glaucoma. Avoid use in pregnant women, especially during the first trimester.

Interactions
Diazepam potentiates the CNS depressant effects of *phenothiazines, narcotics, barbiturates, alcohol, antihistamines, MAO inhibitors, general anesthetics,* and *antidepressants.* Concomitant use with *cimetidine* and possibly *disulfiram* causes diminished hepatic metabolism of diazepam, which increases its plasma concentration.

Antacids may decrease the rate of absorption of diazepam.

Haloperidol may change the seizure patterns of patients treated with diazepam; benzodiazepines also may reduce the serum levels of *haloperidol.*

Diazepam reportedly can decrease *digoxin* clearance; monitor patients for digoxin toxicity.

Patients receiving diazepam and *nondepolarizing neuromuscular blocking agents* such as *pancuronium* and *succinylcholine* have intensified and prolonged respiratory depression.

Heavy smoking accelerates diazepam's metabolism, thus lowering clinical effectiveness.

Oral contraceptives may impair the metabolism of diazepam.

Diazepam may inhibit the therapeutic effect of *levodopa.*

Effects on diagnostic tests
Diazepam therapy may elevate liver function test results. Minor changes in EEG patterns, usually low-voltage, fast activity, may occur during and after diazepam therapy.

Adverse reactions
CNS: *drowsiness,* slurred speech, tremor, transient amnesia, fatigue, ataxia, headache, insomnia, paradoxical anxiety, hallucinations.
CV: hypotension, ***CV collapse,*** bradycardia.
EENT: diplopia, blurred vision, nystagmus.
GI: nausea, constipation.
GU: incontinence, urine retention, altered libido.
Respiratory: ***respiratory depression.***
Skin: rash.
Other: physical or psychological dependence, ***acute withdrawal syndrome*** after sudden discontinuation in physically dependent persons, *pain, phlebitis* (at injection site), *dysarthria, jaundice, neutropenia.*

Overdose and treatment
Clinical manifestations of overdose include somnolence, confusion, coma, hypoactive reflexes, dys-

pnea, labored breathing, hypotension, bradycardia, slurred speech, and unsteady gait or impaired coordination.

Support blood pressure and respiration until drug effects subside; monitor vital signs. Mechanical ventilatory assistance via endotracheal tube may be required to maintain a patent airway and support adequate oxygenation. Flumazenil, a specific benzodiazepine antagonist, may be useful. Use I.V. fluids and vasopressors such as dopamine and phenylephrine to treat hypotension as needed. If the patient is conscious, induce emesis; use gastric lavage if ingestion was recent, but only if an endotracheal tube is present to prevent aspiration. After emesis or lavage, administer activated charcoal with a cathartic as a single dose. Dialysis is of limited value.

☑ Special considerations

Besides those relevant to all *benzodiazepines,* consider the following recommendations.

- Do not discontinue drug suddenly; decrease dosage slowly over 8 to 12 weeks after long-term therapy.
- To enhance taste, oral solution can be mixed with liquids or semisolid foods, such as applesauce or puddings, immediately before administration.
- Extended-release capsule should be swallowed whole; do not let patient crush or chew it.
- Shake oral suspension well before administering.
- When prescribing with opiates for endoscopic procedures, reduce opiate dose by at least one third.
- Parenteral forms of diazepam may be diluted in 0.9% NaCl solution; a slight precipitate may form, but the solution can still be used.
- Diazepam interacts with plastic. Do not store diazepam in plastic syringes or administer it in plastic administration sets, which will decrease availability of the infused drug.
- I.V. route is preferred because of rapid and more uniform absorption.
- For I.V. administration, drug should be infused slowly, directly into a large vein, at a rate not exceeding 5 mg/minute for adults or 0.25 mg/kg of body weight over 3 minutes for children. Do not inject diazepam into small veins to avoid extravasation into subcutaneous tissue. Observe infusion site for phlebitis. If direct I.V. administration is not possible, inject diazepam directly into I.V. tubing at point closest to vein insertion site to prevent extravasation.
- Administration by continuous I.V. infusion is not recommended.
- Inject I.M. dose deep into deltoid muscle. Aspirate for backflow to prevent inadvertent intra-arterial administration. Use I.M. route only if I.V. or oral routes are unavailable.
- Patient should remain in bed under observation for at least 3 hours after parenteral administration of diazepam to prevent potential hazards; keep resuscitation equipment nearby.
- During prolonged therapy, periodically monitor blood counts and liver function studies.
- Lower doses are effective in patients with renal or hepatic dysfunction.
- Assess gag reflex postendoscopy and before resuming oral intake to prevent aspiration.
- Anticipate possible transient increase in frequency or severity of seizures when diazepam is used as adjunctive treatment of convulsive disorders. Impose seizure precautions.
- Do not mix diazepam with other drugs in a syringe or infusion container.

Patient education

- Advise patient of the potential for physical and psychological dependence with chronic use.
- Warn patient that sudden changes of position can cause dizziness. Advise patient to dangle legs for a few minutes before getting out of bed to prevent falls and injury.
- Encourage patient to avoid or limit smoking to prevent increased diazepam metabolism.
- Warn female patient to call immediately if she becomes pregnant.
- Caution patient to avoid alcohol while taking diazepam.
- Advise patient not to suddenly discontinue drug.

Geriatric use

- Elderly patients are more sensitive to the CNS depressant effects of diazepam. Use with caution.
- Lower doses are usually effective in elderly patients because of decreased elimination.
- Elderly patients who receive this drug require assistance with walking and activities of daily living during initiation of therapy or after an increase in dose.
- Parenteral administration of this drug is more likely to cause apnea, hypotension, and bradycardia in elderly patients.

Pediatric use

- Safe use of oral diazepam in infants less than age 6 months has not been established. Safe use of parenteral diazepam in infants under age 30 days has not been established.
- Closely observe neonates of mothers who took diazepam for a prolonged period during pregnancy; the infants may show withdrawal symptoms. Use of diazepam during labor may cause neonatal flaccidity.

Breast-feeding

- Diazepam is distributed into breast milk. The breast-fed infant of a mother who uses diazepam may become sedated, have feeding difficulties, or lose weight. Avoid use of drug in breast-feeding women.

diazoxide

Hyperstat IV, Proglycem

Pharmacologic classification: peripheral vasodilator

Therapeutic classification: antihypertensive, antihypoglycemic

Pregnancy risk category C

How supplied
Available by prescription only
Capsules: 50 mg
Oral suspension: 50 mg/ml in 30-ml bottle
Injection: 300 mg/20 ml ampule

Indications, route, and dosage
Hypertensive crisis
Adults and children: 1 to 3 mg/kg I.V. (up to a maximum of 150 mg) q 5 to 15 minutes until an adequate reduction in blood pressure is achieved.

Note: The use of 300-mg I.V. bolus push is no longer recommended. Switch to therapy with oral antihypertensives as soon as possible.

Hypoglycemia from hyperinsulinism
Adults and children: Usual daily dosage is 3 to 8 mg/kg/day P.O. divided in two or three equal doses.
Infants and newborns: Usual daily dosage is 8 to 15 mg/kg/day P.O. divided in two or three equal doses.

Pharmacodynamics
Antihypertensive action: Diazoxide directly relaxes arteriolar smooth muscle, causing vasodilation and reducing peripheral vascular resistance, thus reducing blood pressure.

Antihypoglycemic action: Diazoxide increases blood glucose levels by inhibiting pancreatic secretion of insulin, by stimulating catecholamine release, or by increasing hepatic release of glucose.

Diazoxide is a nondiuretic congener of thiazide diuretics.

Pharmacokinetics
- *Absorption:* After I.V. administration, blood pressure should decrease promptly, with maximum decrease in under 5 minutes. After oral administration, hyperglycemic effect begins in 1 hour.
- *Distribution:* Drug is distributed throughout the body; highest concentration is found in kidneys, liver, and adrenal glands; diazoxide crosses placenta and blood-brain barrier. Drug is approximately 90% protein-bound.
- *Metabolism:* Metabolized partially in the liver.
- *Excretion:* Drug and its metabolites are excreted slowly by the kidneys. Duration of antihypertensive effect varies widely, ranging from 30 minutes to 72 hours (average 3 to 12 hours) after I.V. administration; after oral administration, antihypoglycemic effect persists for about 8 hours. Antihypertensive and antihypoglycemic effects may be prolonged in patients with renal dysfunction.

Contraindications and precautions
Parenteral form is contraindicated in patients with hypersensitivity to drug, other thiazides, or sulfonamide-derived drugs and in the treatment of compensatory hypertension (such as that associated with coarctation of the aorta or arteriovenous shunt). Oral form is contraindicated in patients with functional hypoglycemia.

Use cautiously in patients with uremia or impaired cerebral or cardiac function.

Interactions
Diazoxide may potentiate antihypertensive effects of other *antihypertensive agents*, especially if I.V. diazoxide is administered within 6 hours after patient has received another antihypertensive agent.

Concomitant use of diazoxide with *phenytoin* may increase metabolism and decrease the plasma protein binding of phenytoin.

Concomitant use of diazoxide with *diuretics* may potentiate antihypoglycemic, hyperuricemic, or antihypertensive effects of diazoxide.

Diazoxide may displace *warfarin,* bilirubin, or other highly protein-bound substances from protein-binding sites.

Concomitant use with other *thiazides* may enhance effects of diazoxide. Diazoxide may alter insulin and oral antidiabetic requirements in previously stable diabetic patients.

Effects on diagnostic tests
Diazoxide inhibits glucose-stimulated insulin release and may cause false-negative insulin response to glucagon. Prolonged use of oral diazoxide may decrease hemoglobin and hematocrit levels.

Adverse reactions
CNS: dizziness, weakness; headache, malaise, anxiety, insomnia, paresthesia (with oral form); headache, ***seizures, paralysis, cerebral ischemia,*** light-headedness, euphoria (with parenteral form).
CV: ***arrhythmias,*** tachycardia, hypotension, hypertension (with oral form); *sodium and water retention, orthostatic hypotension,* diaphoresis, flushing, warmth, angina, myocardial ischemia, ***arrhythmias,*** ECG changes, ***shock, MI*** (with parenteral form).
EENT: diplopia, transient cataracts, blurred vision, lacrimation (with oral administration).
GI: abdominal discomfort, diarrhea; nausea, vomiting, anorexia, taste alteration (with oral form); *nausea, vomiting,* dry mouth, constipation (with parenteral form).
GU: azotemia, reversible nephrotic syndrome, decreased urine output, hematuria, albuminuria (with oral administration).
Hematologic: leukopenia, ***thrombocytopenia,*** anemia, eosinophilia, excessive bleeding (with oral administration).
Skin: rash, pruritus (with oral administration).
Other: *sodium and fluid retention, ketoacidosis and hyperosmolar nonketotic syndrome, hyperuricemia,* hirsutism, fever (with oral administration); inflammation and pain resulting from extravasation, *hyperglycemia:* hyperuricemia, optic nerve infarction (with parenteral form).

Overdose and treatment
Overdose is manifested primarily by hyperglycemia; ketoacidosis and hypotension may occur.

Treat acute overdose supportively and symptomatically. If hyperglycemia develops, give insulin and replace fluid and electrolyte losses; use vasopressors if hypotension fails to respond to conservative treatment. Prolonged monitoring may be necessary because of diazoxide's long half-life.

☑ Special considerations

- Diazoxide is used to treat only hypoglycemia resulting from hyperinsulinism; it is not used to treat functional hypoglycemia. It may be used temporarily to control preoperative or postoperative hypoglycemia in patients with hyperinsulinism.
- I.V. use of diazoxide is seldom necessary for more than 4 or 5 days.
- After I.V. injection, monitor blood pressure every 5 minutes for 15 to 30 minutes, then hourly when patient is stable. Discontinue if severe hypotension develops or if blood pressure continues to fall 30 minutes after drug infusion; keep patient recumbent during this time and have norepinephrine available. Monitor I.V. site for infiltration or extravasation.
- Monitor patient's intake and output carefully. If fluid or sodium retention develops, diuretics may be given 30 to 60 minutes after diazoxide. Keep patient recumbent for 8 to 10 hours after diuretic administration.
- Monitor daily blood glucose and electrolyte levels, watching diabetic patients closely for severe hyperglycemia or hyperglycemic hyperosmolar nonketotic coma; also monitor daily urine glucose and ketone levels, intake and output, and weight. Check serum uric acid levels frequently.
- Protect solutions from light, heat, or freezing; do not administer solutions that have darkened or that contain particulate matter.
- Significant hypotension does not occur after oral administration in doses used to treat hypoglycemia.
- Drug may be given by constant I.V. infusion (7.5 to 30 mg/minute) until adequate blood pressure reduction occurs.

Patient education

- Explain that orthostatic hypotension can be minimized by rising slowly and avoiding sudden position changes.
- Tell patient to report adverse effects immediately, including pain and redness at injection site, which may indicate infiltration.
- Instruct patient to check weight daily and report gains of over 5 lb/week; diazoxide causes sodium and water retention.
- Reassure patient that excessive hair growth is a common reaction that subsides when drug treatment is completed.

Geriatric use

- Elderly patients may have a more pronounced hypotensive response.

Pediatric use

- Use with caution in children.

Breast-feeding

- It is not known if drug occurs in breast milk; an alternative feeding method is recommended during therapy.

dibucaine

Nupercainal

Pharmacologic classification: local anesthetic (amine)
Therapeutic classification: localamide anesthestic
Pregnancy risk category B

How supplied

Available without a prescription
Ointment: 1%
Cream: 0.5%

Indications, route, and dosage

Temporary relief of pain and itching associated with abrasions, sunburn, minor burns, insect bites, and other minor skin conditions
Adults and children: Apply to affected areas, p.r.n. Maximum daily dose of 1% ointment is 30 g for adults and 7.5 g for children.

Temporary relief of pain, itching, and burning caused by hemorrhoids
Adults: Instill 1% ointment into rectum using a rectal applicator each morning and evening and after each bowel movement, p.r.n. Apply additional ointment topically to anal tissues. Maximum daily dose is 30 g.

Pharmacodynamics

Anesthetic action: Dibucaine inhibits conduction of nerve impulses and decreases cell membrane permeability to ions, anesthetizing local nerve endings.

Pharmacokinetics

- *Absorption:* Dibucaine has limited absorption.
- *Distribution:* None.
- *Metabolism:* None.
- *Excretion:* None.

Contraindications and precautions

Contraindicated in patients with known hypersensitivity to drug, sulfites, or other amide-type local anesthetics and for use on large skin areas, on broken skin or mucous membranes, and in eyes.

Interactions

None reported.

Effects on diagnostic tests

None reported.

Adverse reactions

Skin: irritation, inflammation, contact dermatitis, cutaneous lesions.
Other: hypersensitivity reactions (urticaria, edema, burning, stinging, tenderness).

Note: Discontinue drug if sensitization occurs or if condition worsens.

Overdose and treatment

Clean area thoroughly with mild soap and water.

☑ Special considerations

- Use dibucaine topically only, for short periods.

Patient education

- Advise patient to call if condition worsens or if symptoms persist for more than 7 days after use.
- Explain correct use of drug.
- Emphasize need to wash hands thoroughly after use.
- Caution patient to apply drug sparingly to minimize untoward effects.
- Tell patient to keep drug out of reach of children.

Geriatric use

- Dosage should be adjusted to patient's age, size, and physical condition.

Pediatric use

- Dosage should be adjusted to patient's age, size, and physical condition.

Breast-feeding

- Drug should not be used in breast-feeding women.

diclofenac potassium

Cataflam

diclofenac sodium

Voltaren, Voltaren Ophthalmic, Voltaren-XR

Pharmacologic classification: NSAID
Therapeutic classification: antiarthritic, anti-inflammatory
Pregnancy risk category B

How supplied

Available by prescription only
Tablets: 25 mg*, 50 mg
Tablets (enteric-coated): 25 mg, 50 mg, 75 mg, 100 mg
Ophthalmic solution: 0.1%

Indications, route, and dosage

Osteoarthritis
Adults: 50 mg P.O. b.i.d. or t.i.d., or 75 mg P.O. b.i.d. (diclofenac sodium only).
Ankylosing spondylitis
Adults: 25 mg P.O. q.i.d. An additional 25 mg dose may be needed h.s.
Rheumatoid arthritis
Adults: 50 mg P.O. t.i.d. or q.i.d. Alternatively, 75 mg P.O. b.i.d. (diclofenac sodium only).
Analgesia and primary dysmenorrhea
Adults: 50 mg (diclofenac potassium only) P.O. t.i.d. Alternatively, 100 mg (diclofenac potassium only) P.O. initially, followed by 50 mg doses, up to a maximum dose of 200 mg in first 24 hours; subsequent dosing should follow 50 mg t.i.d. regimen.
Postoperative inflammation following cataract removal
Adults: 1 drop in the conjunctival sac q.i.d., beginning 24 hours after surgery and continuing throughout the first 2 weeks of the postoperative period.

Pharmacodynamics

Anti-inflammatory action: Diclofenac exerts its anti-inflammatory and antipyretic actions through an unknown mechanism that may involve inhibition of prostaglandin synthesis.

Pharmacokinetics

- *Absorption:* After oral administration, diclofenac is rapidly and almost completely absorbed, with peak plasma concentrations occurring in 10 to 30 minutes. Absorption is delayed by food, with peak plasma concentrations occurring in 2½ to 12 hours; however, bioavailability is unchanged.
- *Distribution:* Drug is highly (nearly 100%) protein-bound.
- *Metabolism:* Drug undergoes first-pass metabolism, with 60% of unchanged drug reaching systemic circulation. The principal active metabolite, 4′-hydroxydiclofenac, has approximately 3% the activity of the parent compound. Mean terminal half-life is approximately 1.2 to 1.8 hours after an oral dose.
- *Excretion:* Approximately 40% to 60% of diclofenac is excreted in the urine; the balance is excreted in the bile. The 4″-hydroxy metabolite accounts for 20% to 30% of the dose excreted in the urine; the other metabolites account for 10% to 20%; 5% to 10% excreted unchanged in the urine. More than 90% is excreted within 72 hours. Moderate renal impairment does not alter the elimination rate of unchanged diclofenac but may reduce the elimination rate of the metabolites. Hepatic impairment does not appear to affect the pharmacokinetics of diclofenac.

Contraindications and precautions

Oral form is contraindicated in patients with hypersensitivity to drug and in those with hepatic porphyria or a history of asthma, urticaria, or other allergic reactions after taking aspirin or other NSAIDs. Avoid use during late pregnancy or while breast-feeding. Ophthalmic solution is contraindicated in patients with hypersensitivity to any component of the drug and in those wearing soft contact lenses; also avoid use during late pregnancy.

Use oral form cautiously in patients with history of peptic ulcer disease, hepatic or renal dysfunction, cardiac disease, hypertension, or conditions associated with fluid retention.

Use ophthalmic solution cautiously in patients with hypersensitivity to aspirin, phenyl-acetic acid derivatives, and other NSAIDs and in surgical patients with known bleeding tendencies or in those receiving medications that may prolong bleeding time.

Interactions

Concomitant administration of diclofenac and *aspirin* lowers plasma levels of diclofenac and is not recommended. Concomitant use with *warfarin* requires close monitoring of anticoagulant dosage because diclofenac, like other NSAIDs, affects platelet function. Concurrent use with *digoxin, methotrexate,* and *cyclosporine* may increase the toxicity of these drugs; with *lithium* decreases renal clearance of lithium and therefore increases its plasma levels and may lead to lithium toxicity; with *insulin* or *oral antidiabetic agents* may alter the patient's response to these agents. Concurrent use of diclofenac may inhibit the action of *diuretics*; use

* Canada only

with *potassium-sparing diuretics* may increase serum potassium levels.

Effects on diagnostic tests

Diclofenac increases platelet aggregation time but does not affect bleeding time, plasma thrombin clotting time, plasma fibrinogen, or factors V and VII to XII.

Drug increases platelet aggregation time, and may increase ALT and AST levels.

Adverse reactions

Unless otherwise noted, the following adverse reactions refer to oral administration of drug.

CNS: anxiety, depression, dizziness, drowsiness, insomnia, irritability, headache.

CV: ***heart failure,*** hypertension, edema.

EENT: *tinnitus,* laryngeal edema, swelling of the lips and tongue, blurred vision, eye pain, night blindness, epistaxis, taste disorder, reversible hearing loss; *transient stinging and burning, increased intraocular pressure, keratitis,* anterior chamber reaction, ocular allergy (with ophthalmic solution).

GI: *abdominal pain or cramps, constipation, diarrhea, indigestion, nausea,* abdominal distention, flatulence, peptic ulceration, ***bleeding,*** melena, bloody diarrhea, appetite change, colitis.

GU: proteinuria, ***acute renal failure,*** oliguria, interstitial nephritis, papillary necrosis, ***nephrotic syndrome,*** fluid retention.

Hepatic: elevated liver enzymes, jaundice, hepatitis, ***hepatotoxicity.***

Respiratory: asthma.

Skin: rash, pruritus, urticaria, eczema, dermatitis, alopecia, photosensitivity, bullous eruption, ***Stevens-Johnson syndrome*** (rare), allergic purpura.

Other: ***anaphylaxis; anaphylactoid reactions;*** angioedema; back, leg, or joint pain; hypoglycemia; hyperglycemia; vomiting, viral infection (with ophthalmic solution).

Overdose and treatment

No information available. There is no special antidote. Supportive and symptomatic treatment may include induction of vomiting or gastric lavage. Treatment with activated charcoal or dialysis may also be appropriate.

☑ Special considerations

- Concurrent administration with other drugs, such as glucocorticoids, that produce adverse GI effects may aggravate such effects.
- Periodic evaluation of hematopoietic function is recommended because bone marrow abnormalities have occurred. Regular check of hemoglobin level is important to detect toxic effects on the GI tract.
- Because the anti-inflammatory, antipyretic, and analgesic effects of diclofenac may mask the usual signs of infection, monitor carefully for infection.
- Monitor renal function during treatment. Use with caution and at reduced dosage in patients with renal impairment.
- Periodic ophthalmologic examinations are recommended during prolonged therapy.
- Monitor liver function during therapy. Abnormal liver function test results and severe hepatic reactions may occur.

Patient education

- Advise patient to take drug with meals or milk to avoid GI upset.
- Teach patient to restrict salt intake, as diclofenac may cause edema, especially if patient is hypertensive.
- Instruct patient to report symptoms that may be related to GI ulceration, such as epigastric pain and black or tarry stools, as well as other unusual symptoms such as skin rash, pruritis or significant edema or weight gain.

Geriatric use

- Use with caution in elderly patients. Elderly patients may be more susceptible to adverse reactions, especially GI toxicity. Reduce dosage to lowest level that controls symptoms.

Pediatric use

- Drug is not recommended for use in children.

Breast-feeding

- Low levels of diclofenac have been measured in breast milk. Risk-to-benefit ratio must be considered.

dicloxacillin sodium

Dycill, Dynapen, Pathocil

Pharmacologic classification: penicillinase-resistant penicillin
Therapeutic classification: antibiotic
Pregnancy risk category NR

How supplied

Available by prescription only
*Capsules:*125 mg, 250 mg, 500 mg
Oral suspension: 62.5 mg/5 ml (after reconstitution)

Indications, route, and dosage

Systemic infections caused by penicillinase-producing staphylococci

Adults and children weighing 88 lb (40 kg) or more: 125 to 250 mg P.O. q 6 hours.

Infants and children over age 1 month weighing below 88 lb: 12.5 to 50 mg/kg P.O. daily, divided into doses given q 6 hours. Serious infection may require higher dosage (75 to 100 mg/kg/day in divided doses q 6 hours).

Pharmacodynamics

Antibiotic action: Dicloxacillin is bactericidal; it adheres to bacterial penicillin-binding proteins, thus inhibiting bacterial cell wall synthesis. Dicloxacillin resists the effects of penicillinases—enzymes that inactivate penicillin—and is thus active against many strains of penicillinase-producing bacteria; this activity is most important against penicillinase-producing staphylococci; some strains may remain resistant. Dicloxacillin is also active against a few gram-positive aerobic and anaerobic bacilli but has no significant effect on gram-negative bacilli.

Pharmacokinetics

• *Absorption:* Drug is absorbed rapidly but incompletely (35% to 76%) from the GI tract; it is relatively acid stable. Peak plasma levels occur ½ to 2 hours after an oral dose. Food may decrease both rate and extent of absorption.

• *Distribution:* Distributed widely into bone, bile, and pleural and synovial fluids. CSF penetration is poor but is enhanced by meningeal inflammation. Drug crosses the placenta; it is 95% to 99% protein-bound.

• *Metabolism:* Metabolized only partially.

• *Excretion:* Drug and metabolites are excreted in urine by renal tubular secretion and glomerular filtration; also excreted in breast milk. Elimination half-life in adults is ½ to 1 hour, extended minimally to 2.2 hours in patients with renal impairment.

Contraindications and precautions

Contraindicated in patients with hypersensitivity to drug or other penicillins. Use cautiously in patients with other drug allergies, especially to cephalosporins, or in those with mononucleosis.

Interactions

Concomitant use with *aminoglycosides* produces synergistic bactericidal effects against *Staphylococcus aureus.* However, the drugs are physically and chemically incompatible and are inactivated when mixed or given together.

Probenecid blocks renal tubular secretion of dicloxacillin, raising its serum levels.

Effects on diagnostic tests

Dicloxacillin alters test results for urine and serum proteins; it produces false-positive or elevated results in turbidimetric urine and serum protein tests using sulfosalicylic acid or trichloroacetic acid; it also reportedly produces false results on the Bradshaw screening test for Bence Jones protein.

Drug may cause transient elevations in liver function study results and transient reductions in RBC, WBC, and platelet counts. Elevated liver function test results may indicate drug-induced cholestasis or hepatitis.

Dicloxacillin may falsely decrease serum aminoglycoside concentrations.

Adverse reactions

CNS: neuromuscular irritability, ***seizures,*** lethargy, hallucinations, anxiety, confusion, agitation, depression, dizziness, fatigue.
GI: *nausea,* vomiting, *epigastric distress,* flatulence, *diarrhea,* enterocolitis, pseudomembranous colitis, black "hairy" tongue, abdominal pain.
GU: interstitial nephritis, nephropathy.
Hematologic: eosinophilia, anemia, ***thrombocytopenia,*** leukopenia, hemolytic anemia, ***agranulocytosis.***
Other: hypersensitivity reactions (pruritus, urticaria, rash, ***anaphylaxis***), overgrowth of nonsusceptible organisms.

Overdose and treatment

Clinical signs of overdose include neuromuscular irritability or seizures. No specific recommendations. Treatment is supportive. After recent ingestion (4 hours or less), empty the stomach by induced emesis or gastric lavage; follow with activated charcoal to reduce absorption. Drug is not appreciably dialyzable.

☑ Special considerations

Besides those relevant to all *penicillins,* consider the following recommendations.

• Give drug with water only; acid in fruit juice or carbonated beverage may inactivate drug.

• Give dose on empty stomach; food decreases absorption.

• Regularly assess renal, hepatic, and hematopoietic function during prolonged therapy.

Patient education

• Tell patient to report severe diarrhea promptly. He should also report rash or itching.

• Instruct patient to complete full course of treatment.

Geriatric use

• Half-life may be prolonged in elderly patients because of impaired renal function.

Pediatric use

• Elimination of dicloxacillin is reduced in neonates; safe use of drug in neonates has not been established.

Breast-feeding

• Dicloxacillin is excreted into breast milk; drug should be used with caution in breast-feeding women.

dicyclomine hydrochloride

Antispas, A-Spas, Bentyl, Bentylol*, Byclomine, Dibent, Formulex*, Lomine*, Neoquess, Or-Tyl, Spasmoban*, Spasmoject

Pharmacologic classification: anticholinergic
Therapeutic classification: antimuscarinic, GI antispasmodic
Pregnancy risk category B

How supplied

Available by prescription only
Tablets: 20 mg
Capsules: 10 mg, 20 mg
Syrup: 10 mg/5 ml
Injection: 10 mg/ml in 2-ml vials, 10-ml vials, 2-ml ampules

Indications, route, and dosage

Irritable bowel syndrome and other functional GI disorders

Adults: Initially, 20 mg P.O. q.i.d., then increase to 40 mg P.O. q.i.d. during first week of therapy un-

less precluded by adverse reactions. Alternatively, give 20 mg I.M. q 4 to 6 hours.
Children age 2 and older: 10 mg P.O. t.i.d. or q.i.d.
Infants age 6 to 23 months: 5 to 10 mg P.O. t.i.d. or q.i.d.
◇ ***Infant colic***
Infants age 6 months and over: 5 to 10 mg P.O. t.i.d. or q.i.d. Adjust dosage according to patient's needs and response.

Note: High environmental temperatures may induce heatstroke during drug use. If symptoms occur, the drug should be discontinued.

Pharmacodynamics

Antispasmodic action: Dicyclomine exerts a nonspecific, direct spasmolytic action on smooth muscle. It also has some local anesthetic properties that may contribute to spasmolysis in the GI and biliary tracts.

Pharmacokinetics

- *Absorption:* About 67% of an oral dose is absorbed from the GI tract.
- *Distribution:* Largely unknown.
- *Metabolism:* Unknown.
- *Excretion:* After oral administration, 80% of a dose is excreted in urine and 10% in feces.

Contraindications and precautions

Contraindicated in patients with obstructive uropathy, obstructive disease of the GI tract, reflux esophagitis, severe ulcerative colitis, myasthenia gravis, hypersensitivity to anticholinergics, unstable CV status in acute hemorrhage, or glaucoma. Also contraindicated in breast-feeding patients and in children under age 6 months.

Use cautiously in patients with autonomic neuropathy, hyperthyroidism, coronary artery disease, arrhythmias, heart failure, hypertension, hiatal hernia, hepatic or renal disease, prostatic hyperplasia, and ulcerative colitis.

Interactions

Concurrent administration of *antacids* decreases oral absorption of anticholinergics. Administer dicyclomine at least 1 hour before antacids.

Concomitant administration of drugs with *anticholinergic* effects may cause additive toxicity.

Decreased GI absorption of many drugs has been reported after the use of anticholinergics (for example, *levodopa* and *ketoconazole*). Conversely, slowly dissolving *digoxin* tablets may yield higher serum digoxin levels when administered with anticholinergics.

Use cautiously with *oral potassium supplements* (especially *wax-matrix formulations*) because the incidence of potassium-induced GI ulcerations may be increased.

Effects on diagnostic tests

None reported.

Adverse reactions

CNS: *headache; dizziness;* insomnia; light-headedness; drowsiness; nervousness, confusion, excitement (in elderly patients).
CV: *palpitations,* tachycardia.
EENT: blurred vision, increased intraocular pressure, mydriasis.
GI: nausea, vomiting, *constipation, dry mouth,* abdominal distention, heartburn, paralytic ileus.
GU: *urinary hesitancy, urine retention,* impotence.
Skin: urticaria, decreased sweating or possible anhidrosis, other dermal manifestations, local irritation.
Other: fever, allergic reactions.

Dicyclomine is a synthetic tertiary derivative that may have atropine-like adverse reactions.

Overdose and treatment

Clinical signs of overdose include curare-like symptoms, of CNS stimulation followed by depression, and such psychotic symptoms as disorientation, confusion, hallucinations, delusions, anxiety, agitation, and restlessness. Peripheral effects may include dilated, nonreactive pupils; hot, flushed, dry skin; tachycardia; hypertension; and increased respiration.

Treatment is primarily symptomatic and supportive, as necessary. Maintain patent airway. If patient is alert, induce emesis (or use gastric lavage) and follow with a saline cathartic and activated charcoal to prevent further drug absorption. In severe cases, physostigmine may be administered to block dicyclomine's antimuscarinic effects. Give fluids, as needed, to treat shock; diazepam to control psychotic symptoms; and pilocarpine (instilled into the eyes) to relieve mydriasis. If urine retention occurs, catheterization may be necessary.

☑ Special considerations

Besides those relevant to all *anticholinergics,* consider the following recommendation.

- Never give dicyclomine I.V. or S.C.

Patient education

- Tell patient that syrup formulation may be diluted with water.
- Warn patient that high environmental temperatures may induce heatstroke while drug is being used; tell patient to avoid exposure to such temperatures.

Geriatric use

- Drug should be administered cautiously to elderly patients. Lower doses are indicated.

Pediatric use

- Safety and effectiveness in children have not been established. Administer cautiously to infants age 6 months or over; seizures have been reported. Be aware that drug is contraindicated in infants under age 6 months.

Breast-feeding

- Dicyclomine may be excreted in breast milk; it may also decrease milk production. Breast-feeding women should avoid use of drug.

didanosine (ddI)
Videx

Pharmacologic classification: purine analogue
Therapeutic classification: antiviral
Pregnancy risk category B

How supplied
Available by prescription only
Chewable tablets: 25 mg, 50 mg, 100 mg, 150 mg
Powder for solution (buffered): 100 mg/packet, 167 mg/packet, 250 mg/packet, 375 mg/packet
Powder for oral solution (pediatric): 10 mg/ml in 2-g and 4-g bottles

Indications, route, and dosage
Treatment of HIV infection when antiretroviral therapy is warranted
Adults weighing 132 lb (60 kg) and over: 200 mg (tablets) P.O. q 12 hours, or 250 mg buffered powder P.O. q 12 hours.
Adults weighing less than 132 lb: 125 mg (tablets) P.O. q 12 hours, or 167 mg buffered powder P.O. q 12 hours.
Children: 120 mg/m^2 P.O. q 12 hours. Children over age 1 should receive a 2-tablet dose, and children under age 1 should receive a one-tablet dose.
✦ ***Dosage adjustment.*** Patients with renal or hepatic impairment may need their dosage adjusted; however, insufficient data exist to provide specific recommendations.

Pharmacodynamics
Antiviral actions: Didanosine is a synthetic purine analogue of deoxyadenosine. After didanosine enters the cell, it is converted to its active form dideoxyadenosine triphosphate (ddATP), which inhibits replication of HIV by preventing DNA replication. In addition, ddATP inhibits the enzyme HIV-RNA dependent DNA polymerase (reverse transcriptase).

Pharmacokinetics
- *Absorption:* Drug degrades rapidly in gastric acid. Commercially available preparations contain buffers to raise stomach pH. Bioavailability averages about 33%; tablets may exhibit better bioavailability than buffered powder for oral solution. Food can decrease absorption by 50%.
- *Distribution:* Didanosine is widely distributed; drug penetration into the CNS varies, but CSF levels average 46% of concurrent plasma levels.
- *Metabolism:* Not fully understood, but is probably similar to that of endogenous purines.
- *Excretion:* Drug is excreted in urine as allantoin, hypoxanthine, xanthine, and uric acid. Serum half-life averages 0.8 hours.

Contraindications and precautions
Contraindicated in patients with history of hypersensitivity to any component of the formulation.

Use very cautiously in patients with history of pancreatitis. Also use cautiously in patients with peripheral neuropathy, impaired renal or hepatic function, or hyperuricemia.

Interactions
Ketoconazole, dapsone, and other *drugs that require gastric acid for adequate absorption* may be rendered ineffective because of the buffering action of didanosine formulations on gastric acid. Administer such drugs 2 hours before didanosine. *Tetracyclines* and *fluoroquinolones* may show decreased absorption because of buffering agents in didanosine tablets or antacids in pediatric suspension. Concurrently used *antacids* containing magnesium or aluminum hydroxides may produce enhanced adverse effects, such as diarrhea or constipation.

Effects on diagnostic tests
None reported.

Adverse reactions
CNS: *headache,* ***seizures,*** confusion, anxiety, nervousness, abnormal thinking, twitching, depression, *peripheral neuropathy.*
GI: *diarrhea, nausea, vomiting, abdominal pain,* ***pancreatitis,*** dry mouth, anorexia.
Hematologic: *leukopenia,* granulocytosis, ***thrombocytopenia,*** anemia.
Hepatic: ***hepatic failure,*** elevated liver enzymes.
Skin: rash, pruritus.
Other: asthenia, pain, pneumonia, infection, sarcoma, dyspnea, allergic reactions, myopathy, increased serum uric acid levels, *chills, fever.*

Overdose and treatment
No specific information exists regarding the treatment of overdose; however, experience with patients in phase I clinical trials suggest possible effects of overdose. Patients who received doses 10 times greater than the currently recommended dosage developed diarrhea, pancreatitis, peripheral neuropathy, hyperuricemia, and hepatic dysfunction. Treatment is supportive. No specific antidote is known, and it is unknown if drug is dialyzable.

☑ Special considerations
- The major toxicity of drug use is pancreatitis, which must be considered when a patient develops abdominal pain, nausea, and vomiting or biochemical markers are elevated. Discontinue use of drug until pancreatitis is excluded.
- Administer didanosine on an empty stomach, regardless of dosage form used. Studies have shown that administering drug with meals can result in a 50% decrease in absorption.
- Most patients over age 1 should receive two tablets per dose. Tablets contain buffers that raise stomach pH to levels that prevent degradation of the active drug. Tablets should be thoroughly chewed before swallowing, and the patient should drink at least 1 oz water with each dose. If tablets are manually crushed, mix drug in 1 oz (30 ml) water; stir to disperse uniformly, then have patient drink it immediately. Know that single-dose packets containing buffered powder for oral solution are available.
- To administer buffered powder for oral solution, carefully open the packet and pour the contents into 4 oz (120 ml) water. Do not use fruit juice or other acidic beverages. Stir for 2 or 3 minutes until the powder dissolves completely. Administer immediately.

• In early clinical trials, about one third of patients taking buffered powder for oral solution developed diarrhea. Although there is no evidence that other formulations have a lower incidence of diarrhea, consider substituting the chewable tablets if diarrhea occurs.
• When preparing powder or crushing tablets, take care to avoid excessive dispersal of drug particles into the air.
• Pediatric powder for oral solution must be prepared by a pharmacist before dispensing. It must be constituted with water, then diluted with antacid (manufacturer recommends either Mylanta Double Strength Liquid or Maalox TC) to a final concentration of 10 mg/ml. The admixture is stable for 30 days if refrigerated (36° to 46° F [2° to 8° C]). Be sure to shake well before measuring the dose.

Patient education
• Tell patient to take drug on an empty stomach to ensure adequate absorption, to chew tablets thoroughly before swallowing, and to drink at least 1 oz (30 ml) water with each dose.
• Remind patient using buffered powder for oral solution not to use fruit juice or other acidic beverages. Allow 3 minutes for powder to dissolve completely, and take immediately. Be sure he understands how to mix the solution.

Pediatric use
• Retinal depigmentation occurred in some children receiving drug. Children should receive dilated retinal examinations at least every 6 months or if a change in vision occurs.

Breast-feeding
• It is unknown if drug is excreted in breast milk. Because of risk of serious adverse effects in the infant, breast-feeding is not recommended.

dienestrol
Ortho Dienestrol

Pharmacologic classification: estrogen
Therapeutic classification: topical estrogen
Pregnancy risk category X

How supplied
Available by prescription only
Cream: 0.01% dienestrol

Indications, route, and dosage
Atrophic vaginitis and kraurosis vulvae
Postmenopausal adults: One to two intravaginal applications of vaginal cream daily for 1 to 2 weeks; then half that dose for the same period. Maintenance dose of 1 applicatorful one to three times weekly may then be used, if needed.

Pharmacodynamics
Estrogenic action: Drug causes development, cornification, and secretion in atrophic vaginal tissue.

Pharmacokinetics
• *Absorption:* Absorpted significantly when topically applied, particularly when used in large doses. Its pharmacokinetics are not well known.
• *Distribution:* No information available.
• *Metabolism:* No information available.
• *Excretion:* No information available.

Contraindications and precautions
Contraindicated in patients with active thrombophlebitis or thromboembolic disorders associated with estrogen therapy or past history of such events; in those with breast, reproductive organ, or genital cancer; or in those with undiagnosed abnormal genital bleeding. Also contraindicated during pregnancy and in breast-feeding patients.

Use cautiously in patients with cerebrovascular or coronary artery disease, diabetes, hypertension, epilepsy, or migraine and in those with a strong family history of breast cancer or who have breast nodules, fibrocystic disease, or abnormal mammograms. Also use cautiously in patients with cardiac, hepatic, or renal dysfunction; history of depression; or metabolic bone diseases and in young patients in whom bone growth is not complete.

Interactions
None reported.

Effects on diagnostic tests
Dienestrol increases sulfobromophthalein retention, PT and clotting factors VII to X, and norepinephrine-induced platelet aggregability. It decreases antithrombin III concentration. Drug increases thyroid-binding globulin level; thus, total thyroid level (measured by protein-bound iodine or total T_4) increases and free T_3 resin uptake decreases. Serum folate and pyridoxine levels may decrease; triglyceride, glucose, and phospholipid levels may increase. Glucose tolerance may be impaired. Pregnanediol excretion may decrease.

Adverse reactions
GU: vaginal discharge, increased intravaginal discomfort, uterine bleeding (with excessive use), burning sensation.
Other: systemic effects (breast tenderness, peripheral edema).

Overdose and treatment
Serious toxicity has not been reported.

☑ Special considerations
Besides those relevant to all *estrogens,* consider the following recommendations.
• Systemic absorption of drug may occur with intravaginal use, causing systemic reactions.
• After vaginal mucosa has been restored, a maintenance dose of one applicatorful of cream one to three times weekly may be used. Attempts to reduce dosage or discontinue therapy should be made at 3- to 6-month intervals.

Patient education
• Instruct patient to wash vaginal area with soap and water before application and to apply drug at

bedtime to increase its absorption and effectiveness. Patient shouldn't wear tampon while receiving vaginal therapy. She may need to wear sanitary pad to protect clothing.
- Tell patient to remain recumbent for 30 minutes after drug application to prevent drug loss.
- Warn patient not to exceed prescribed dose.
- Withdrawal bleeding may occur if estrogen is stopped suddenly.

Breast-feeding
- Drug is contraindicated in breast-feeding women.

diethylpropion hydrochloride
Tenuate, Tenuate Dospan

Pharmacologic classification: amphetamine
Therapeutic classification: short-term adjunctive anorexigenic, sympathomimetic amine
Controlled substance schedule IV
Pregnancy risk category B

How supplied
Available by prescription only
Tablets: 25 mg
Tablets (controlled-release): 75 mg

Indications, route, and dosage
Short-term adjunct in exogenous obesity
Adults: 25 mg P.O. t.i.d. before meals. An additional 25-mg dose may be added in the evening to control night hunger. Alternatively, give 75 mg controlled-release tablet P.O. at midmorning.
✦ ***Dosage adjustment.*** In elderly patients, lower dosages may be effective because of diminished renal function.

Pharmacodynamics
Anorexigenic action: The precise mechanism of action for appetite control is unknown; anorexigenic effects are thought to occur in the hypothalamus, where decreased smell and taste acuity decreases appetite. The cerebral cortex and reticular activating system appear to be the primary sites of activity; amphetamines release nerve terminal stores of norepinephrine, promoting nerve impulse transmission.

Diethylpropion is used adjunctively with caloric restriction and behavior modification to control appetite in exogenous obesity. Diethylpropion is a sympathomimetic amine and is considered the safest of its class for potential use in patients with mild to moderate hypertension.

Pharmacokinetics
- *Absorption:* Drug is readily absorbed after oral administration; therapeutic effects persist for 4 hours with regular tablets, longer with controlled-release preparation.
- *Distribution:* Widely distributed throughout the body.
- *Metabolism:* Metabolized in the liver.
- *Excretion:* Excreted in urine.

Contraindications and precautions
Contraindicated in patients with hypersensitivity or idiosyncrasy to sympathomimetic amines; within 14 days of MAO inhibitor therapy; in those with hyperthyroidism, severe hypertension, advanced arteriosclerosis, glaucoma, or history of drug abuse; and in agitated patients.

Use cautiously in patients with mild to moderate hypertension, symptomatic CV disease (including arrhythmias), or seizure disorders.

Interactions
Concomitant use with *MAO inhibitors* (or *drugs with MAO-inhibiting effects,* such as *furazolidone*) or within 14 days of such therapy may cause hypertensive crisis.

Diethylpropion may decrease antihypertensive effects of *guanethidine*; it may also decrease *insulin* requirements in diabetic patients as a result of weight loss. Diethylpropion may increase the effects of *antidepressants*; excessive concomitant use of *caffeine* produces additive CNS stimulation. *Barbiturates* antagonize diethylpropion by CNS depression and may decrease its effects.

Effects on diagnostic tests
None reported.

Adverse reactions
CNS: headache, *nervousness,* insomnia, fatigue, anxiety, drowsiness.
CV: *tachycardia, palpitations,* elevated blood pressure, ***pulmonary hypertension,*** ECG changes, ***arrhythmias.***
EENT: blurred vision, mydriasis.
GI: dry mouth, nausea, abdominal cramps, diarrhea, constipation, unpleasant taste, vomiting.
GU: altered libido, changes in menstruation, impotence.
Hematologic: decreased blood glucose levels.
Skin: urticaria, rash.

Overdose and treatment
Symptoms of acute overdose include restlessness, tremor, hyperreflexia, tachypnea, confusion, aggressive behavior, hallucinations, blood pressure changes, arrhythmias, nausea, vomiting, diarrhea, and cramps. Fatigue and depression usually follow initial stimulation; seizures and coma may also occur.

Treat overdose symptomatically and supportively: if ingestion is recent (within 4 hours) use gastric lavage or emesis. Treatment may require administration of a sedative and, if acute hypertension develops, I.V. phentolamine. Monitor vital signs and fluid and electrolyte balance.

☑ Special considerations
- Drug can be used to stop nighttime overeating. Drug rarely causes insomnia.
- Do not crush 75-mg controlled-release tablets.

Patient education
- Tell patient to avoid drinks containing caffeine to prevent overstimulation.

- Tell patient to swallow controlled-release tablet whole and not to chew or crush it.
- Warn patient against exceeding prescribed dosage.
- Tell patient drug may color urine pink to brown. This is not harmful.
- Explain that extreme fatigue and depression may ensue if drug is abruptly discontinued after use for a prolonged period.
- Emphasize importance of careful adherence to the total treatment program, including diet and exercise, if weight control is to be successful. Be sure patient understands dietary restrictions that must accompany drug therapy to obtain maximal benefit.
- Advise patient to avoid foods high in tyromine (including beer, wine, and aged cheese), as hypertensive reactions may occur when combined with drug.

Geriatric use
- Use with caution in elderly patients.

Pediatric use
- Drug is not recommended for weight reduction in children under age 12.

Breast-feeding
- Drug is excreted in breast milk; alternative feeding method is recommended during therapy with drug.

diethylstilbestrol
Stilbestrol*

diethylstilbestrol diphosphate
Honvol*, Stilphostrol

Pharmacologic classification: estrogen
Therapeutic classification: estrogen replacement, antineoplastic, ◇contraceptive (postcoital)
Pregnancy risk category X

How supplied
Available by prescription only
diethylstilbestrol
Tablets: 1 mg, 5 mg
Tablets (enteric-coated): 1 mg, 5 mg
diethystilbestrol diphosphate
Tablets: 50 mg
Injection: 50 mg/ml

Indications, route, and dosage
◇*Postcoital contraception ("morning-after pill")*
Adults: 25 mg P.O. b.i.d. for 5 days, starting not later than 72 hours and preferably within 24 hours after coitus.
Inoperable prostatic cancer
Adults: Initially, 1 to 3 mg P.O. daily; some patients may require higher doses. Subsequent maintenance dose may be decreased to 1 mg daily. Alternatively, give 50 mg P.O. diphosphate t.i.d.; then increase dose up to 200 mg or more t.i.d., p.r.n., or 0.5 g I.V., followed by 1 g daily for 5 or more days, p.r.n. Maintenance dose is 0.25 to 0.5 g I.V. once or twice weekly.
Inoperable breast cancer
Men and postmenopausal women: 15 mg P.O. daily.

Pharmacodynamics
Estrogen replacement action: Diethylstilbestrol mimics the action of endogenous estrogen in treating female hypogonadism, menopausal symptoms, and atrophic vaginitis.

Antineoplastic action: Drug inhibits growth of hormone-sensitive tissue in advanced, inoperable prostatic cancer and in certain carefully selected cases of breast cancer in men and postmenopausal women.

Topical estrogenic action: Drug causes development, cornification, and secretion in atrophic vaginal tissue.

Pharmacokinetics
- *Absorption:* Diethylstilbestrol is well absorbed from the GI tract when administered orally.
- *Distribution:* Very little information is available; drug probably distributes extensively into most body tissues.
- *Metabolism:* Drug undergoes conjugation with glucuronic acid in the liver.
- *Excretion:* Drug appears in both urine and feces, primarily as the glucuronide conjugate.

Contraindications and precautions
Contraindicated in men with known or suspected breast cancer, except in selected patients being treated for metastatic disease; in patients with active thrombophlebitis or thromboembolic disorders, estrogen-dependent neoplasia, undiagnosed abnormal genital bleeding, history of thrombophlebitis, thrombosis, or thromboembolic disorders associated with estrogen use; and during pregnancy.

Use cautiously in patients with hypertension, coronary artery disease, cerebrovascular disease, mental depression, bone disease, migraine, seizures, diabetes mellitus, and cardiac, hepatic, or renal dysfunction.

Interactions
Concomitant administration of diethylstilbestrol with *drugs that induce hepatic metabolism*, such as *rifampin, barbiturates, primidone, carbamazepine*, and *phenytoin*, may result in decreased estrogenic effects from a given dose. These drugs are known to accelerate the rate of metabolism of certain other agents. Concomitant use with *anticoagulants* may decrease the effects of warfarin-type anticoagulants.

Concomitant use with *adrenocorticosteroids* increases the risk of fluid and electrolyte accumulation.

Effects on diagnostic tests
Diethylstilbestrol may cause increases in blood glucose levels, necessitating dosage adjustment of insulin or oral antidiabetic drugs. Diethylstilbestrol increases sulfobromophthalein retention, prothrombin and clotting factors VII to X, and nor-

epinephrine-induced platelet aggregability. Increases in thyroid-binding globulin concentration may occur, resulting in increased total thyroid concentrations (measured by protein-bound iodine or total thyroxine) and decreased uptake of free triiodothyronine resin. Antithrombin III concentrations decrease; serum folate and pyridoxine concentrations and pregnanediol excretion may decrease; triglyceride, glucose, and phospholipid levels may increase. Glucose tolerance may be impaired.

Adverse reactions

CNS: headache, dizziness, chorea, depression, ***seizures.***

CV: thrombophlebitis, ***thromboembolism,*** hypertension, edema, ***increased risk of CVA, pulmonary embolism, MI.***

EENT: worsening of myopia or astigmatism, intolerance of contact lenses.

GI: *nausea,* vomiting, abdominal cramps, bloating, anorexia, increased appetite, excessive thirst, weight changes, pancreatitis.

GU: in women—breakthrough bleeding, altered menstrual flow, dysmenorrhea, amenorrhea, cervical erosion, ***increased risk of endometrial cancer, possibility of increased risk of breast cancer,*** altered cervical secretions, enlargement of uterine fibromas, vaginal candidiasis, loss of libido; in men—gynecomastia, testicular atrophy, impotence.

Hepatic: cholestatic jaundice, ***hepatic adenoma.***

Skin: melasma, urticaria, hirsutism or hair loss, erythema nodosum, dermatitis.

Other: breast tenderness or enlargement, hypercalcemia, gallbladder disease.

Overdose and treatment

Serious toxicity after overdose of this drug has not been reported. Nausea may be expected to occur. Appropriate supportive care should be provided.

☑ Special considerations

Besides those relevant to all *estrogens,* diethylstilbestrol requires the following special considerations.

- Administer diethylstilbestrol diphosphate injection as an I.V. infusion. Dilute the dose in 300 ml of 0.9% NaCl solution or D_5W, and administer no faster than 1 to 2 ml/minute for the first 15 minutes. The flow rate may then be adjusted so that the remainder of the dose is administered over 1 hour.
- To be effective as a postcoital contraceptive ("morning-after pill"), diethylstilbestrol must be taken within 72 hours (preferably within 24 hours) after coitus. Nausea and vomiting are common with this large dose.
- A pregnancy test is advised before starting diethylstilbestrol therapy.
- A higher incidence of CV death has been reported in men taking diethylstilbestrol tablets (5 mg daily) for prostatic cancer over a long time. This effect is not associated with a daily dosage of 1 mg t.i.d.
- According to the U.S. Department of Health and Human Services 1985 DES Task Force, women who used diethylstilbestrol during pregnancy may have a greater risk of breast cancer, but limited data available do not confirm a causal relationship to the drug.
- For women who received diethylstilbestrol during pregnancy, the DES Task Force recommends regular breast examinations according to general National Cancer Institute guidelines, and annual gynecologic examinations.

Patient education

- Warn patient to stop taking drug immediately if she becomes pregnant, because it can adversely affect the fetus.

Geriatric use

- Use with caution in elderly patients. Administering estrogens to postmenopausal women may be associated with increased incidence of endometrial or breast cancer.

Breast-feeding

- Drug is not recommended for use in breast-feeding women.

diflorasone diacetate

Florone, Florone E, Maxiflor, Psorcon

Pharmacologic classification: topical adrenocorticoid
Therapeutic classification: anti-inflammatory
Pregnancy risk category C

How supplied

Available by prescription only
Cream, ointment: 0.05%

Indications, route, and dosage

Inflammation of corticosteroid-responsive dermatoses

Adults and children: Apply sparingly in a thin film once daily to q.i.d., as determined by severity of condition.

Pharmacodynamics

Anti-inflammatory action: Diflorasone stimulates the synthesis of enzymes needed to decrease the inflammatory response. Diflorasone is a group I-II potency anti-inflammatory agent.

Pharmacokinetics

- *Absorption:* The amount of drug absorbed depends on the amount applied and on the nature of the skin at the application site. It ranges from about 1% in areas with a thick stratum corneum (such as the palms, soles, elbows, and knees) to as high as 36% in areas of the thinnest stratum corneum (face, eyelids, and genitals). Absorption increases in areas of skin damage, inflammation, or occlusion. Some systemic absorption of topical steroids occurs, especially through the oral mucosa.
- *Distribution:* After topical application, diflorasone is distributed throughout the local skin. Drug absorbed into the circulation is distributed rapidly into muscle, liver, skin, intestines, and kidneys.

• *Metabolism:* After topical administration, diflorasone is metabolized primarily in the skin. The small amount absorbed into the systemic circulation is metabolized primarily in the liver to inactive compounds.
• *Excretion:* Inactive metabolites are excreted by the kidneys, primarily as glucuronides and sulfates, but also as unconjugated products. Small amounts of the metabolites are also excreted in feces.

Contraindications and precautions
Contraindicated in patients hypersensitive to drug.

Interactions
None significant.

Effects on diagnostic tests
None reported.

Adverse reactions
Skin: burning, pruritus, irritation, dryness, erythema, folliculitis, perioral dermatitis, hypertrichosis, hypopigmentation, acneiform eruptions; *maceration, secondary infection, atrophy, striae, miliaria* (with occlusive dressings).
Other: ***hypothalamic-pituitary-adrenal axis suppression,*** Cushing's syndrome, hyperglycemia, glucosuria.

Overdose and treatment
No information available.

☑ Special considerations
• Recommendations for use of diflorasone, for care and teaching of patients during therapy, and for use in elderly patients, children, and breast-feeding women are the same as those for all *topical adrenocorticoids.*

Patient education
• Tell patient to use drug only as instructed. Use externally only, and keep away from your eyes.
• Advise patient not to use drug other than for what it is prescribed.
• Do not bandage to wrap treated area unless medically approved.
• Tell parents not to put on tight clothes and diapers over treated areas in infants.

diflunisal
Dolobid

Pharmacologic classification: NSAID, salicylic acid derivative
Therapeutic classification: nonnarcotic analgesic, antipyretic, anti-inflammatory
Pregnancy risk category C

How supplied
Available by prescription only
Tablets: 250 mg, 500 mg

Indications, route, and dosage
Mild to moderate pain
Adults: Initiate therapy with 1 g, then 500 mg daily in two or three divided doses, usually q 8 to 12 hours. Maximum dose is 1,500 mg daily.
✦ ***Dosage adjustment.*** In adults over age 65, start with one half the usual adult dose.
Rheumatoid arthritis and osteoarthritis
Adults: 500 to 1,000 mg P.O. daily in two divided doses, usually q 12 hours. Maximum dose is 1,500 mg daily.
✦ ***Dosage adjustment.*** In adults over age 65, start with one half the usual dose.

Pharmacodynamics
Analgesic, antipyretic, and anti-inflammatory actions: Mechanisms of action are unknown, but are probably related to inhibition of prostaglandin synthesis. Diflunisal is a salicylic acid derivative, but is not hydrolyzed to free salicylate in vivo.

Pharmacokinetics
• *Absorption:* Diflunisal is absorbed rapidly and completely via the GI tract. Peak plasma concentrations occur in 2 to 3 hours. Analgesia is achieved within 1 hour and peaks within 2 to 3 hours.
• *Distribution:* Drug is highly protein-bound.
• *Metabolism:* Diflunisal is metabolized in the liver; it is not metabolized to salicylic acid.
• *Excretion:* Drug is excreted in urine. Half-life is 8 to 12 hours.

Contraindications and precautions
Contraindicated in patients with hypersensitivity to the drug or for whom acute asthmatic attacks, urticaria, or rhinitis are precipitated by aspirin or other NSAIDs. Use cautiously in patients with GI bleeding, history of peptic ulcer disease, renal impairment, and compromised cardiac function, hypertension, or other conditions predisposing patient to fluid retention.

Because of the epidemiologic association with Reye's syndrome, the Centers for Disease Control and Prevention recommends not giving salicylates to children and teenagers with chickenpox or influenza-like illness.

Interactions
Concomitant use of diflunisal with *anticoagulants* and *thrombolytic drugs* may potentiate their anticoagulant effects by the platelet-inhibiting effect of diflunisal. Concomitant use of diflunisal with other *highly protein-bound drugs (phenytoin, sulfonylureas, warfarin)* may cause displacement of either drug, and adverse effects. Monitor therapy closely for both drugs. Concomitant use of diflunisal with other *GI-irritating drugs,* such as *alcohol, steroids, antibiotics,* and other *NSAIDs,* may potentiate the adverse GI effects of diflunisal; use together with caution.

Intake of *antacids* and *food* delays and decreases the absorption of diflunisal.

Concurrent use of diflunisal with *hydrochlorothiazide* may increase the plasma concentration of hydrochlorothiazide, but decrease its hyperuricemic, diuretic, antihypertensive, and natriuretic effects. Concomitant use with *furosemide* may decrease furosemide's hyperuricemic effect. Concurrent use with *antihypertensives* may decrease their effect on blood pressure; concurrent use with *diuretics* may increase nephrotoxic potential. Concurrent use with *gold compounds* may increase nephrotoxicity. Concurrent use of diflunisal and *indomethacin* has been associated with decreased renal clearance of indomethacin. Fatal GI hemorrhage has also been reported. Concurrent use with *acetaminophen* may increase serum acetaminophen levels by as much as 50%, leading to potential hepatotoxicity. This interaction may also be nephrotoxic.

Concurrent use with *lithium* may result in increased lithium serum levels. Diflunisal may decrease the renal excretion of *methotrexate, verapamil,* and *nifedipine. Probenecid* may decrease the renal clearance of diflunisal. *Aspirin* may decrease the bioavailibity of diflunisal.

Effects on diagnostic tests

The physiologic effects of drug may prolong bleeding time; increase serum BUN, creatinine, and potassium levels; decrease serum uric acid; and increase liver function tests (serum transaminase, alkaline phosphatase, and LD).

Adverse reactions

CNS: *dizziness,* somnolence, insomnia, *headache,* fatigue.
EENT: *tinnitus, visual disturbances* (rare).
GI: *nausea, dyspepsia, GI pain, diarrhea,* vomiting, constipation, flatulence.
GU: renal impairment, hematuria, interstitial nephritis.
Skin: *rash,* pruritus, sweating, stomatitis, erythema multiforme, ***Stevens-Johnson syndrome.***

Overdose and treatment

Clinical manifestations of overdose include drowsiness, nausea, vomiting, hyperventilation, tachycardia, sweating, tinnitus, disorientation, stupor, and coma.

To treat overdose of diflunisal, empty stomach immediately by inducing emesis with ipecac syrup if patient is conscious, or by gastric lavage. Administer activated charcoal via nasogastric tube. Provide symptomatic and supportive measures (respiratory support and correction of fluid and electrolyte imbalances). Monitor laboratory parameters and vital signs closely. Hemodialysis has little effect.

☑ Special considerations

Besides those relevant to all *NSAIDs,* consider the following recommendations.

- Similar to aspirin, diflunisal is a salicylic acid derivative but is metabolized differently.
- Diflunisal is recommended for twice-daily dosing for added patient convenience and compliance.
- Do not break, crush, or allow patient to chew diflunisal. Patient should swallow medication whole.
- Administer diflunisal with water, milk, or meals to minimize GI upset.
- Do not administer concurrently with aspirin or acetaminophen.
- Monitor results of laboratory tests, especially renal and liver function studies. Assess presence and amount of peripheral edema. Monitor weight frequently.
- Evaluate patient's response to diflunisal therapy as evidenced by a reduction in pain or inflammation. Monitor vital signs frequently, especially temperature.
- Assess patient for signs and symptoms of potential hemorrhage, such as bruising, petechiae, coffee ground emesis, and black, tarry stools.
- Institute safety measures to prevent injury if patient experiences CNS effects.

Patient education

- Instruct patient in diflunisal regimen and need for compliance. Advise him to report adverse reactions.
- Tell patient to take diflunisal with foods to minimize GI upset and to swallow capsule whole.
- Caution patient to avoid activities requiring alertness or concentration, such as driving, until CNS effects are known.
- Instruct patient in safety measures to prevent injury.

Geriatric use

- Patients over age 60 may be more susceptible to the toxic effects (particularly GI toxicity) of these drugs.
- The effects of these drugs on renal prostaglandins may cause fluid retention and edema, a significant drawback for elderly patients, especially those with heart failure or hypertension.

Pediatric use

- Do not use long-term diflunisal therapy in children under age 14; safe use has not been established.

Breast-feeding

- Because drug is distributed into breast milk, breast-feeding is not recommended.

digoxin

Lanoxicaps, Lanoxin, Novodigoxin*

Pharmacologic classification: cardiac glycoside
Therapeutic classification: antiarrhythmic, inotropic
Pregnancy risk category C

How supplied

Available by prescription only
Tablets: 0.125 mg, 0.25 mg, 0.5 mg
Capsules: 0.05 mg, 0.10 mg, 0.20 mg
Elixir: 0.05 mg/ml
Injection: 0.05 mg/ml*, 0.1 mg/ml (pediatric), 0.25 mg/ml

Indications, route, and dosage

Heart failure, atrial fibrillation and flutter, paroxysmal atrial tachycardia

Tablets, elixir

Adults: For rapid digitalization, give 0.75 to 1.25 mg P.O. over 24 hours in two or more divided doses q 6 to 8 hours. For slow digitalization, give 0.125 to 0.5 mg daily for 5 to 7 days. Maintenance dose is 0.125 to 0.5 mg daily.

Children age 10 and older: 10 to 15 mcg/kg P.O. over 24 hours in two or more divided doses q 6 to 8 hours. Maintenance dose is 25% to 35% of total digitalizing dose.

Children age 5 to 10: 20 to 35 mcg/kg P.O. over 24 hours in two or more divided doses q 6 to 8 hours. Maintenance dose is 25% to 35% of total digitalizing dose.

Children age 2 to 5: 30 to 40 mcg/kg P.O. over 24 hours in two or more divided doses q 6 to 8 hours. Maintenance dose is 25% to 35% of total digitalizing dose.

Infants age 1 month to 2 years: 35 to 60 mcg/kg P.O. over 24 hours in two or more divided doses q 6 to 8 hours. Maintenance dose is 25% to 35% of total digitalizing dose.

Neonates: 25 to 35 mcg/kg P.O. over 24 hours in two or more divided doses q 6 to 8 hours. Maintenance dose is 25% to 35% of total digitalizing dose.

Premature infants: 20 to 30 mcg/kg P.O. over 24 hours in two or more divided doses q 6 to 8 hours. Maintenance dose is 20% to 30% of total digitalizing dose.

Capsules

Adults: For rapid digitalization, give 0.4 to 0.6 mg P.O. initially, followed by 0.1 to 0.3 mg q 6 to 8 hours, as needed and tolerated, for 24 hours. For slow digitalization, give 0.05 to 0.35 mg daily in two divided doses for 7 to 22 days p.r.n. until therapeutic serum levels are reached. Maintenance dose is 0.05 to 0.35 mg daily in one or two divided doses.

Children: Digitalizing dose is based on child's age and is administered in three or more divided doses over the first 24 hours. Initial dose should be 50% of the total dose; subsequent doses are given q 4 to 8 hours as needed and tolerated.

Children age 10 and over: For rapid digitalization, give 8 to 12 mcg/kg P.O. over 24 hours, divided as above. Maintenance dose is 25% to 35% of total digitalizing dose, given daily as a single dose.

Children age 5 to 10: For rapid digitalization, give 15 to 30 mcg/kg P.O. over 24 hours, divided as above. Maintenance dose is 25% to 35% of total digitalizing dose, divided and given in two or three equal portions daily.

Children age 2 to 5: For rapid digitalization, give 25 to 35 mcg/kg P.O. over 24 hours, divided as above. Maintenance dose is 25% to 35% of total digitalizing dose, divided and given in two or three equal portions daily.

Injection

Adults: For rapid digitalization, give 0.4 to 0.6 mg I.V. initially, followed by 0.1 to 0.3 mg I.V. q 4 to 8 hours, as needed and tolerated, for 24 hours. For slow digitalization, give appropriate daily maintenance dose for 7 to 22 days as needed until therapeutic serum levels are reached. Maintenance dose is 0.125 to 0.5 mg I.V. daily in one or two divided doses.

Children: Digitalizing dose is based on child's age and is administered in three or more divided doses over the first 24 hours. Initial dose should be 50% of total dose; subsequent doses are given q 4 to 8 hours as needed and tolerated.

Children age 10 and over: For rapid digitalization, give 8 to 12 mcg/kg I.V. over 24 hours, divided as above. Maintenance dose is 25% to 35% of total digitalizing dose, given daily as a single dose.

Children age 5 to 10: For rapid digitalization, give 15 to 30 mcg/kg I.V. over 24 hours, divided as above. Maintenance dose is 25% to 35% of total digitalizing dose, divided and given in two or three equal portions daily.

Children age 2 to 5: For rapid digitalization, give 25 to 35 mcg/kg I.V. over 24 hours, divided as above. Maintenance dose is 25% to 35% of total digitalizing dose, divided and given in two or three equal portions daily.

Infants age 1 month to 2 years: For rapid digitalization, give 30 to 50 mcg/kg I.V. over 24 hours, divided as above. Maintenance dose is 25% to 35% of total digitalizing dose, divided and given in two or three equal portions daily.

Neonates: For rapid digitalization, give 20 to 30 mcg/kg I.V. over 24 hours, divided as above. Maintenance dose is 25% to 35% of the total digitalizing dose, divided and given in two or three equal portions daily.

Premature infants: For rapid digitalization, give 15 to 25 mcg/kg I.V. over 24 hours, divided as above. Maintenance dose is 20% to 30% of the total digitalizing dose, divided and given in two or three equal portions daily.

✦ ***Dosage adjustment.*** Reduce dosage in patients with impaired renal function. Hypothyroid patients are highly sensitive to glycosides; hyperthyroid patients may need larger doses.

Pharmacodynamics

Digoxin is the most widely used cardiac glycoside. Multiple oral forms and a parenteral form are available, facilitating drug's use in both acute and chronic clinical settings.

Inotropic action: Digoxin's effect on the myocardium is dose-related and involves both direct and indirect mechanisms. It directly increases the force and velocity of myocardial contraction, AV node refractory period, and total peripheral resistance; at higher doses, it also increases sympathetic outflow. It indirectly depresses the SA node and prolongs conduction to the AV node. In patients with heart failure, increased contractile force boosts cardiac output, improves systolic emptying, and decreases diastolic heart size. It also reduces ventricular end-diastolic pressure and, consequently, pulmonary and systemic venous pressures. Increased myocardial contractility and cardiac output reflexively reduce sympathetic tone in patients with heart failure. This compensates for drug's direct vasoconstrictive action, thereby reducing total peripheral resistance. It also slows increased heart rate and causes diuresis in edematous patients.

Antiarrhythmic action: Digoxin-induced heart-rate slowing in patients without heart failure is negligible and stems mainly from vagal (cholinergic) and sympatholytic effects on the SA node; however, with toxic doses, heart-rate slowing results from direct depression of SA node automaticity. Therapeutic doses produce little effect on the action potential, but toxic doses increase the automaticity (spontaneous diastolic depolarization) of all cardiac regions except the SA node.

Pharmacokinetics

- *Absorption:* With tablet or elixir administration, 60% to 85% of dose is absorbed. With capsule form, bioavailability increases. About 90% to 100% of a dose is absorbed. With I.M. administration, about 80% of dose is absorbed. With oral administration, onset of action occurs in 30 minutes to 2 hours, with peak effects occurring in 6 to 8 hours. With I.M. administration, onset of action occurs in 30 minutes, with peak effects in 4 to 6 hours. With I.V. administration, action occurs in 5 to 30 minutes, with peak effects in 1 to 5 hours.
- *Distribution:* Digoxin is distributed widely in body tissues; highest concentrations occur in the heart, kidneys, intestine, stomach, liver, and skeletal muscle; lowest concentrations are in the plasma and brain. Digoxin crosses both the blood-brain barrier and the placenta; fetal and maternal digoxin levels are equivalent at birth. About 20% to 30% of drug is bound to plasma proteins. Usual therapeutic range for steady-state serum levels is 0.5 to 2 ng/ml. In treatment of atrial tachyarrhythmias, higher serum levels (such as 2 to 4 ng/ml) may be needed. Because of drug's long half-life, achievement of steady-state levels may take 7 days or longer, depending on patient's renal function. Toxic symptoms may appear within the usual therapeutic range; however, these are more frequent and serious with levels above 2.5 ng/ml.
- *Metabolism:* In most patients, a small amount of digoxin apparently is metabolized in the liver and gut by bacteria. This metabolism varies and may be substantial in some patients. Drug undergoes some enterohepatic recirculation (also variable). Metabolites have minimal cardiac activity.
- *Excretion:* Most of dose is excreted by the kidneys as unchanged drug. Some patients excrete a substantial amount of metabolized or reduced drug. In patients with renal failure, biliary excretion is a more important excretion route. In healthy patients, terminal half-life is 30 to 40 hours. In patients lacking functioning kidneys, half-life increases to at least 4 days.

Contraindications and precautions

Contraindicated in patients with hypersensitivity to drug, digitalis-induced toxicity, ventricular fibrillation, or ventricular tachycardia unless caused by heart failure.

Use very cautiously in the elderly and in patients with acute MI, incomplete AV block, sinus bradycardia, PVCs, chronic constrictive pericarditis, hypertrophic cardiomyopathy, renal insufficiency, severe pulmonary disease, or hypothyroidism.

Interactions

Concomitant use of digoxin with *antacids* containing aluminum or magnesium hydroxide, *magnesium trisilicate, kaolin-pectin, aminosalicylic acid,* and *sulfasalazine* decreases absorption of orally administered digoxin. *Cholestyramine* and *colestipol* may bind digoxin in the GI tract and impair absorption.

Concomitant use with *cytotoxic agents* or *radiation therapy* may decrease digoxin absorption if the intestinal mucosa is damaged. (Use of digoxin elixir or capsules is recommended in this situation.) Concomitant use with *amiodarone, diltiazem, nifedipine, verapamil*, or *quinidine* may cause increased serum digoxin levels, predisposing the patient to toxicity. Concomitant use with cardiac *drugs affecting AV conduction* (such as *procainamide, propranolol*, and *verapamil*) may cause additive cardiac effects. Concomitant use with *sympathomimetics* such as *ephedrine, epinephrine,* and *isoproterenol*) or *rauwolfia alkaloids* may increase the risk of arrhythmias.

When used concomitantly, certain *antibiotics* may interfere with bacterial flora that allow formation of inactive reduction products in the GI tract, possibly causing a significant increase in digoxin bioavailability and, consequently, increased serum digoxin levels.

Concomitant use with I.V. *calcium* preparations may cause synergistic effects that precipitate arrhythmias. Concomitant use with *electrolyte-altering agents* may increase or decrease serum electrolyte concentrations, predisposing the patient to digoxin toxicity. For example, such *diuretics* as *ethacrynic acid, furosemide, bumetanide*, and *thiazides* may cause hypokalemia and hypomagnesemia; thiazides may cause hypercalcemia. Fatal arrhythmias may result. *Amphotericin B, corticosteroids, corticotropin, edetate disodium, laxatives,* and *sodium polystyrene sulfonate* deplete total body potassium, possibly causing digoxin toxicity. *Glucagon, large dextrose doses*, and *dextrose-insulin infusions* reduce extracellular potassium, possibly leading to digitalis toxicity. Concomitant use with *succinylcholine* may precipitate arrhythmias by potentiating digoxin's effects.

Effects on diagnostic tests

None reported.

Adverse reactions

The following signs of toxicity may occur with all cardiac glycosides:

CNS: *fatigue, generalized muscle weakness, agitation, hallucinations,* headache, malaise, dizziness, vertigo, stupor, paresthesia.
CV: ***arrhythmias*** (most commonly, conduction disturbances with or without AV block, PVCs, and supraventricular arrhythmias) that may lead to increased severity of ***heart failure*** and hypotension. ***Toxic effects on the heart may be life-threatening and require immediate attention.***
EENT: *yellow-green halos around visual images, blurred vision,* light flashes, photophobia, diplopia.
GI: *anorexia, nausea,* vomiting, diarrhea.

Overdose and treatment

Clinical effects of overdose are primarily GI, CNS, and cardiac reactions.

Severe intoxication may cause hyperkalemia, which may develop rapidly and result in life-threatening cardiac manifestations. Cardiac signs of digoxin toxicity may occur with or without other toxicity signs and commonly precede other toxic effects. Because toxic cardiac effects also can occur as manifestations of heart disease, determining whether these effects result from underlying heart disease or digoxin toxicity may be difficult. Digoxin has caused almost every kind of arrhythmia; various combinations of arrhythmias may occur in the same patient. Patients with chronic digoxin toxicity commonly have ventricular arrhythmias or AV conduction disturbances. Patients with digoxin-induced ventricular tachycardia have a high mortality because ventricular fibrillation or asystole may result.

If toxicity is suspected, discontinue drug and obtain serum drug level measurements. Usually, drug takes at least 6 hours to distribute between plasma and tissue and reach equilibrium; plasma levels drawn earlier may show higher digoxin levels than those present after drug distributes into the tissues.

Other treatment measures include immediate emesis induction, gastric lavage, and administration of activated charcoal to reduce absorption of drug remaining in the gut. Multiple doses of activated charcoal (such as 50 g q 6 hours) may help reduce further absorption, especially of any drug undergoing enterohepatic recirculation. Some clinicians advocate cholestyramine administration if digoxin was recently ingested; however, it may not be useful if the ingestion is life-threatening. Interacting drugs probably should be discontinued. Ventricular arrhythmias may be treated with I.V. potassium (replacement dose; but not in patients with significant AV block), I.V. phenytoin, I.V. lidocaine, or I.V. propranolol. Refractory ventricular tachyarrhythmias may be controlled with overdrive pacing. Procainamide may be used for ventricular arrhythmias that do not respond to the above treatments. In severe AV block, asystole, and hemodynamically significant sinus bradycardia, atropine restores a normal rate.

Administration of digoxin-specific antibody fragments (digoxin immune Fab [Digibind]) is a treatment for life-threatening digoxin toxicity. Each 40 mg of digoxin immune Fab binds about 0.6 mg of digoxin in the bloodstream. The complex is then excreted in the urine, rapidly decreasing serum levels and therefore cardiac drug concentrations.

☑ Special considerations

- Obtain baseline heart rate and rhythm, blood pressure, and serum electrolyte levels before giving first dose.
- Question patient about use of cardiac glycosides within the previous 2 to 3 weeks before administering a loading dose. Always divide loading dose over first 24 hours unless clinical situation indicates otherwise.
- Adjust dose to patient's clinical condition and renal function; monitor ECG and serum levels of digoxin, calcium, potassium, and magnesium as well as serum creatinine. Therapeutic serum digoxin levels range from 0.5 to 2 ng/ml. Take corrective action before hypokalemia occurs.
- Monitor clinical status. Take apical-radial pulse for a full minute. Watch for significant changes (sudden rate increase or decrease, pulse deficit, irregular beats, and especially regularization of a previously irregular rhythm). Check blood pressure and obtain 12-lead ECG if these changes occur.
- GI absorption may be reduced in patients with heart failure, especially right heart failure.
- Digoxin dosage generally should be reduced and serum level monitoring performed if patient is receiving digoxin concomitantly with amiodarone, diltiazem, nifedipine, verapamil, or quinidine. Also monitor patient closely for signs and symptoms of digoxin toxicity. Obtain serum digoxin levels if you suspect toxicity.
- Because digoxin may predispose patients to postcardioversion asystole, most clinicians withhold digoxin 1 or 2 days before elective cardioversion in patients with atrial fibrillation. (However, consider consequences of increased ventricular response to atrial fibrillation if drug is withheld.)
- Elective cardioversion should be postponed in patients with signs of digoxin toxicity.
- Do not administer calcium rapidly by the I.V. route to patient receiving digoxin. Calcium affects cardiac contractility and excitability in much the same way that digoxin does and may lead to serious arrhythmias.
- Monitor patient's eating patterns. Ask him about nausea, vomiting, anorexia, visual disturbances, and other evidence of toxicity.
- Consider that different brands may not be therapeutically interchangeable.
- Digoxin solution is enclosed in newly available soft capsule (Lanoxicaps). Because these capsules are better absorbed than tablets, dose is usually slightly smaller.

Patient education

- Inform patient and responsible family member about drug action, medication regimen, how to take pulse, reportable signs, and follow-up plans. Patient must understand importance of follow-up laboratory tests, and have access to outpatient lab facilities.
- Instruct patient not to take an "extra" dose of digoxin if dose is missed.
- Tell patient to call if severe nausea, vomiting, or diarrhea occurs because these conditions may make patient more prone to toxicity.
- Advise patient to use the same brand consistently.
- Tell patient to call before using OTC preparations, especially those high in sodium.

Geriatric use

- Digoxin should be used with caution in elderly patients; adjust dosage to prevent systemic accumulation.

Pediatric use

• Pediatric patients have a poorly defined serum concentration range; however, toxicity apparently does not occur at same concentrations considered toxic in adults. Divided daily dosing is recommended for infants and children under age 10; older children require adult doses proportional to body weight.

digoxin immune Fab (ovine)

Digibind

Pharmacologic classification: antibody fragment
Therapeutic classification: cardiac glycoside antidote
Pregnancy risk category C

How supplied

Available by prescription only
Injection: 38-mg vial

Indications, route, and dosage

Potentially life-threatening digoxin or digitoxin intoxication

Adults and children: Administered I.V. over 30 minutes or as a bolus if cardiac arrest is imminent. Dosage varies based on amount of drug to be neutralized; average dose for adults is 6 vials (228 mg). However, if toxicity resulted from acute digoxin ingestion, and neither a serum digoxin level nor an estimated ingestion amount is known, 10 to 20 vials (380 to 760 mg) should be administered. See package insert for complete, specific dosage instructions.

Pharmacodynamics

Cardiac glycoside antidote: Specific antigen-binding fragments bind to free digoxin in extracellular fluid and intravascularly to prevent and reverse pharmacologic and toxic effects of the cardiac glycoside. This binding is preferential for digoxin and digitoxin; preliminary evidence suggests some binding to other digoxin derivatives and cardioactive metabolites.

Once free digoxin is bound and removed from serum, tissue-bound digoxin is released into the serum to maintain efflux-influx balance. As digoxin is released, it, too, is bound and removed by digoxin immune Fab, resulting in a reduction of serum and tissue digoxin. Cardiac glycoside toxicity begins to subside within 30 minutes after completion of a 15- to 30-minute I.V. infusion of digoxin immune Fab. The onset of action and response is variable and appears to depend on rate of infusion, dose administered relative to body load of glycoside, and possibly other, as yet unidentified factors. Reversal of toxicity, including hyperkalemia, is usually complete within 2 to 6 hours after administration of digoxin immune Fab.

Pharmacokinetics

• *Absorption:* Peak serum concentrations occur at the completion of I.V. infusion. Digoxin immune Fab has a serum half-life of 15 to 20 hours. The association reaction between Fab fragments and glycoside molecules appears to occur rapidly; data are limited.

• *Distribution:* Not fully characterized. After I.V. administration, drug appears to distribute rapidly throughout extracellular space, into both plasma and interstitial fluid. It is not known if digoxin immune Fab crosses the placental barrier or is distributed into breast milk.

• *Metabolism:* Unknown.

• *Excretion:* Drug is excreted in urine via glomerular filtration.

Contraindications and precautions

No known contraindications. Use cautiously in patients known to be allergic to ovine proteins. In these high-risk patients, skin testing is recommended because the drug is derived from digoxin-specific antibody fragments obtained from immunized sheep.

Interactions

When used concomitantly, digoxin immune Fab will bind *cardiac glycosides*, including *digoxin, digitoxin, and lanatoside C.* This will also occur if redigitalization is attempted before elimination of digoxin immune Fab is complete (several days with normal renal function; 1 week or longer with renal impairment).

Effects on diagnostic tests

Digoxin immune Fab therapy changes standard cardiac glycoside determinations by radioimmunoassay procedures. Results may be falsely increased or decreased, depending on separation method used. Serum potassium levels may decrease rapidly.

Adverse reactions

CV: ***heart failure,*** rapid ventricular rate (both caused by reversal of cardiac glycoside's therapeutic effects).
Other: hypersensitivity reactions ***(anaphylaxis),*** hypokalemia.

Overdose and treatment

Limited information is available; however, administration of doses larger than needed for neutralizing the cardiac glycoside may subject the patient to increased risk of allergic or febrile reaction or delayed serum sickness. Large doses may also prolong the time span required before redigitalization.

☑ Special considerations

• Give I.V. using a 0.22-micron filter needle over 30 minutes or as a bolus injection when cardiac arrest is imminent. Dose depends on amount of digoxin to be neutralized. Each 38-mg vial binds approximately 0.5 mg of digoxin or digitoxin. Reconstitute vial with 4 ml of sterile water for injection, mix gently, and use immediately. May be stored in refrigerator up to 4 hours.

• To determine appropriate dose, divide the total digitalis body load by 0.5; the resultant number estimates the number of vials required for appropriate dose. Alternatively, in cases of acute ingestion of known quantity of digitalis, multiply the amount of digitalis ingested in milligrams by 0.80 (to account for incomplete absorption).

- Skin testing may be appropriate for high-risk patients. One of two methods may be used:

Intradermal test—dilute 0.1 ml of reconstituted solution in 9.9 ml of sterile saline for injection; then withdraw and inject 0.1 ml of this solution intradermally. Inspect site after 20 minutes for signs of erythema or urticaria.

Scratch test—dilute as for intradermal test. Place one drop of diluted solution on skin and make a ¼" scratch through the drop with a sterile needle. Inspect site after 20 minutes for signs of erythema or urticaria. If results are positive, avoid use of digoxin immune Fab unless necessary. If systemic reaction occurs, treat symptomatically.

- Pretreat patients with sensitivity or allergy to sheep or ovine products, or when skin test results are positive, with an antihistamine such as diphenhydramine and a corticosteroid before administering digoxin immune Fab.
- Keep medications and equipment for cardiopulmonary resuscitation readily available during administration of digoxin immune Fab for patients who respond poorly to withdrawal of digoxin's inotropic effects. Dopamine or dobutamine, or other cardiac load-reducing agents, may be used. Catecholamines may aggravate arrhythmias induced by digitalis toxicity and should be used with caution.
- Measure serum digoxin or digitoxin levels before giving antidote, because serum concentrations may be difficult to interpret after therapy with antidote.
- Closely monitor temperature, blood pressure, ECG, and potassium concentration before, during, and after administration of antidote.
- Potassium levels must be checked repeatedly, because severe digitalis intoxication can cause life-threatening hyperkalemia, and reversal by digoxin immune Fab may lead to rapid hypokalemia.
- Suicidal ingestion often involves more than one medication. Be alert for possible toxic manifestations secondary to these other medications.
- Delay redigitalization until elimination of Fab fragments is complete; may take several days with normal renal function, a week or longer with impaired renal function.

Pediatric use

- Risk-to-benefit ratio must be considered. Use in infants and small children has not produced adverse effects.
- Monitor for volume overload in small children.
- Very small doses may require diluting reconstituted solution with 36 ml of sterile saline for injection to produce a 1 mg/ml solution.
- Infants may require smaller doses; manufacturer recommends reconstituting as directed and administering with a tuberculin syringe.

Breast-feeding

- It is unknown if digoxin immune Fab distributes into breast milk; use with caution in breast-feeding women.

dihydroergotamine mesylate

D.H.E. 45, Migranal

Pharmacologic classification: ergot alkaloid
Therapeutic classification: vasoconstrictor
Pregnancy risk category X

How supplied

Available by prescription only
Injection: 1 mg/ml
Nasal spray: 4 mg/ml

Indications, route, and dosage

To prevent or abort vascular headaches, including migraine headaches

Adults: 1 mg I.M. or I.V., repeated at 1-hour intervals, up to total of 3 mg I.M. or 2 mg I.V. Maximum weekly dose is 6 mg.

To acutely treat migraine headaches with or without aura

Adults: 1 spray (0.5 mg) administered in each nostril, followed by an additional spray in each nostril in 15 minutes for a total of 4 sprays (2 mg).

Pharmacodynamics

Vasoconstrictor action: By stimulating alpha-adrenergic receptors, dihydroergotamine causes peripheral vasoconstriction (if vascular tone is low). However, drug causes vasodilation in hypertonic blood vessels. At high doses, it is a competitive alpha-adrenergic blocker. In therapeutic doses, dihydroergotamine inhibits the reuptake of norepinephrine, which increases its vasoconstricting activity. A weak antagonist of serotonin, drug reduces the increased rate of platelet aggregation caused by serotonin.

In the treatment of vascular headaches, dihydroergotamine probably causes direct vasoconstriction of the dilated carotid artery bed while decreasing the amplitude of pulsations. Its serotoninergic and catecholamine effects also appear to be involved.

Effects on blood pressure are unpredictable but usually minimal. The vasoconstrictor effect is more pronounced on veins and venules than on arteries and arterioles.

Pharmacokinetics

- *Absorption:* Drug is incompletely and irregularly absorbed from the GI tract. Onset of action is probably dependent on how promptly after onset of headache the drug is given. After I.M. injection, onset of action occurs within 15 to 30 minutes, and after I.V. injection, within a few minutes. Duration of action persists 3 to 4 hours after I.M. injection.
- *Distribution:* 90% of a dose is plasma protein-bound.
- *Metabolism:* Drug is extensively metabolized, probably in the liver (extensive first-pass metabolism).
- *Excretion:* 10% of a dose is excreted in urine within 72 hours as metabolites; the rest in feces.

Contraindications and precautions
Contraindicated in patients with hypersensitivity to drug, in pregnant or breast-feeding patients, and in those with peripheral and occlusive vascular disease, coronary artery disease, uncontrolled hypertension, sepsis, hemiplegic or basilar migraine, and severe hepatic or renal dysfunction. Do not use drug within 24 hours of 5-HT_1 agonists, ergotamine-containing or ergot-type medications, or methylsergide. Avoid use in patients with uncontrolled hypertension because it may increase blood pressure.

Interactions
Concomitant use with *antihypertensive* drugs may antagonize their antihypertensive effects. Concomitant use with *erythromycin* may cause ergot toxicity. Concomitant use with *vasodilators* may result in pressor effects and dangerous hypertension.

Effects on diagnostic tests
None reported.

Adverse reactions
CV: numbness and tingling in fingers and toes, transient tachycardia or bradycardia, precordial distress and pain, increased arterial pressure.
GI: *nausea, vomiting.*
Skin: itching.
Other: weakness in legs, muscle pain in extremities, localized edema.

Overdose and treatment
Clinical manifestations of overdose include symptoms of ergot toxicity, including peripheral ischemia, paresthesia, headache, nausea, and vomiting.

Treatment requires prolonged and careful monitoring. Provide respiratory support, treat seizures if necessary, and apply warmth (not direct heat) to ischemic extremities if vasospasm occurs. Administer vasodilator (nitroprusside, prazosin, or tolazoline) if needed.

☑ Special considerations
Besides those relevant to all *ergot alkaloids,* consider the following recommendations.
- Drug is most effective when used at first sign of migraine, or as soon after onset as possible.
- If severe vasospasm occurs, keep extremities warm. Provide supportive treatment to prevent tissue damage. Administer vasodilators (nitroprusside, prazosin, or tolazoline) if needed.
- Protect ampules from heat and light. Do not use if discolored.
- For short-term use only. Do not exceed recommended dose.
- Ergotamine rebound or an increase in frequency or duration of headaches may occur when drug is stopped.
- Drug has also been used to treat postural hypotension as an unlabeled use.

Patient education
- Advise patient to lie down and relax in a quiet, darkened room after dose is administered.
- Urge patient to report immediately feelings of numbness or tingling in fingers and toes, or red or violet blisters on hands or feet.
- Warn patient to avoid alcoholic beverages during drug therapy because alcohol may worsen headaches.
- Caution patient to avoid smoking while on drug therapy because the adverse effects of drug may be increased.
- Tell patient to avoid prolonged exposure to very cold temperatures while taking this medication. Cold may increase adverse reactions.
- Advise patient to report illness or infection, which may increase sensitivity to drug reactions.
- Tell patient that solution in Migranal is for nasal use and should not be injected.
- Instruct patient to prime nasal spray (pump four times) before use.
- Instruct patient to discard nasal spray applicator once it has been prepared together with unused drug after 8 hours.

Geriatric use
- Administer drug cautiously, because elderly patients are more sensitive to drug's reactions. Safety and efficacy in elderly patients have not been established

Breast-feeding
- Breast-feeding is not recommended while patient is receiving drug therapy.

dihydrotachysterol
DHT, DHT Intensol, Hytakerol

Pharmacologic classification: vitamin D analogue
Therapeutic classification: antihypocalcemic
Pregnancy risk category C

How supplied
Available by prescription only
Tablets: 0.125 mg, 0.2 mg, 0.4 mg
Capsules: 0.125 mg
Solution: 0.2 mg/ml (Intensol), 0.2 mg/5 ml (in 4% alcohol), 0.25 mg/ml (in sesame oil)

Indications, route, and dosage
Hypocalcemia associated with hypoparathyroidism and pseudohypoparathyroidism
Adults: Initially, 0.8 to 2.4 mg P.O. daily for several days. Maintenance dose is 0.2 to 1 mg daily, as required for normal serum calcium levels. Average dose is 0.6 mg daily.
Children: Initially, 1 to 5 mg P.O. daily for 4 days, then continue dosage or reduce to one fourth the initial amount. Usual maintenance dosage is 0.5 to 1.5 mg daily, as required for normal serum calcium levels.
Prevention of thyroidectomy-induced hypocalcemia
Adults: 0.25 mg P.O. daily given with calcium supplements until danger of hypocalcemic tetany has passed.

◊ ***Familial hypophosphatemia***
Adults and children: 0.5 to 2 mg P.O. daily (until healing of bones occurs). Maintenance dose is 0.2 to 1.5 mg daily.
◊ ***Renal osteodystrophy in chronic uremia***
Adults: 0.1 to 0.6 mg P.O. daily.
Children: 0.1 to 0.5 mg P.O. daily.
◊ ***Osteoporosis***
Adults: 0.6 mg P.O. daily given with calcium and fluoride.

Pharmacodynamics
Antihypocalcemic action: Once activated to its 25-hydroxy form, dihydrotachysterol works with parathyroid hormone to regulate levels of calcium. It appears to have little activity as the parent compound.

Pharmacokinetics
- *Absorption:* Absorbed readily from the small intestine.
- *Distribution:* Drug is distributed widely; it is largely protein-bound.
- *Metabolism:* Drug is metabolized in the liver, and has a duration of action up to 9 weeks.
- *Excretion:* Excreted in urine and bile.

Contraindications and precautions
Contraindicated in patients with hypercalcemia or vitamin D toxicity. Use cautiously in those with a history of renal calculi.

Interactions
Magnesium-containing *antacids* may alter absorption of dihydrotachysterol. *Barbiturates, phenytoin,* and *primidone* may increase metabolism and therefore reduce activity of dihydrotachysterol. The resulting increases in calcium may potentiate the effects of cardiac glycosides. Excessive use of *mineral oil* may interfere with intestinal absorption of vitamin D analogues. Concurrent use with *cholestyramine* and *colestipol* may result in decreased intestinal absorption of vitamin D analogues.

Effects on diagnostic tests
Drug alters serum alkaline phosphatase concentrations and cholesterol levels and may alter electrolytes, such as magnesium, phosphate, and calcium, in serum and urine.

Adverse reactions
CNS: headache, somnolence, irritability, psychosis (rare).
CV: hypertension, ***arrhythmias.***
EENT: conjunctivitis, photophobia, rhinorrhea.
GI: nausea, vomiting, constipation, polydipsia, pancreatitis, metallic taste, dry mouth, anorexia, diarrhea.
GU: polyuria, nocturia.
Other: weakness, bone and muscle pain, thirst, weight loss, hyperthermia, decreased libido, nephrocalcinosis.

Overdose and treatment
Hypercalcemia is the only clinical manifestation of overdose. Treatment involves discontinuing therapy, instituting a low-calcium diet, increasing fluid intake, and providing supportive measures. In severe cases, death from cardiac and renal failure has occurred. Calcitonin administration may help reverse hypercalcemia.

☑ Special considerations
- Monitor serum and urine calcium levels. Observe patient for signs and symptoms of hypercalcemia.
- There is some evidence that monitoring urine calcium and urine creatinine is very helpful in screening for hypercalcuria. The ratio of urine calcium to urine creatinine should be less than or equal to 0.18. A value of above 0.2 suggests hypercalcuria, and the dose should be decreased regardless of serum calcium.
- Adequate dietary calcium intake is necessary; usually supplemented with 10 to 15 g oral calcium lactate or gluconate daily.
- 1 mg of dihydrotachysterol is equivalent to 120,000 units ergocalciferol (vitamin D_2).
- Store drug in tightly closed, light-resistant containers. Do not refrigerate.

Patient education
- Explain importance of a calcium-rich diet.

Pediatric use
- Some infants may be hyperreactive to drug.

Breast-feeding
- Do not use in breast-feeding women.

diltiazem hydrochloride
Cardizem, Cardizem CD, Cardizem SR, Dilacor XR

Pharmacologic classification: calcium channel blocker
Therapeutic classification: antianginal
Pregnancy risk category C

How supplied
Available by prescription only
Tablets: 30 mg, 60 mg, 90 mg, 120 mg
Capsules (extended-release): 120 mg, 180 mg, 240 mg, 300 mg (Cardizem CD); 120 mg, 180 mg, 240 mg (Dilacor XR)
Capsules (sustained-release): 60 mg, 90 mg, 120 mg (Cardizem SR)
Injection: 5 mg/ml 5-ml vials, Lyo-ject 25 mg syringe

Indications, route, and dosage
Management of Prinzmetal's or variant angina or chronic stable angina pectoris
Adults: 30 mg P.O. q.i.d. before meals and h.s. Increase dose gradually to maximum of 360 mg/day divided into three to four doses, p.r.n. Alternatively, give 120 or 180 mg (extended-release) P.O. once daily. Titrate over a 7- to 14-day period as needed and tolerated up to a maximum dose of 480 mg daily.

Hypertension
Adults: 60 to 120 mg P.O. b.i.d. (sustained-release). Titrate up to maximum recommended dose of 360 mg/day, p.r.n. Alternatively, give 180 to 240 mg (extended-release) P.O. once daily. Adjust dose based on patient response to a maximum dose of 480 mg/day.
Atrial fibrillation or flutter; paroxysmal supraventricular tachycardia
Adults: 0.25 mg/kg I.V. as a bolus injection over 2 minutes. Repeat after 15 minutes if response is not adequate with a dosage of 0.35 mg/kg I.V. over 2 minutes. Follow bolus with continuous I.V. infusion at 5 to 15 mg/hour (for up to 24 hours).

Pharmacodynamics

Antianginal or antihypertensive action: By dilating systemic arteries, diltiazem decreases total peripheral resistance and afterload, slightly reduces blood pressure, and increases cardiac index, when given in high doses (over 200 mg). Afterload reduction, which occurs at rest and with exercise, and the resulting decrease in myocardial oxygen consumption account for diltiazem's effectiveness in controlling chronic stable angina.

Diltiazem also decreases myocardial oxygen demand and cardiac work by reducing heart rate, relieving coronary artery spasm (through coronary artery vasodilation), and dilating peripheral vessels. These effects relieve ischemia and pain. In patients with Prinzmetal's angina, diltiazem inhibits coronary artery spasm, increasing myocardial oxygen delivery.

Antiarrhythmic action: By impeding the slow inward influx of calcium at the AV node, diltiazem decreases conduction velocity and increases refractory period, thereby decreasing the impulses transmitted to the ventricles in atrial fibrillation or flutter. The end result is a decreased ventricular rate.

Pharmacokinetics

- *Absorption:* Approximately 80% of a dose is absorbed rapidly from the GI tract. However, only about 40% of drug enters systemic circulation because of a significant first-pass effect in the liver. Peak serum levels occur in about 2 to 3 hours.
- *Distribution:* About 70% to 85% of circulating drug is bound to plasma proteins.
- *Metabolism:* Diltiazem is metabolized in the liver.
- *Excretion:* About 35% of drug is excreted in the urine and about 65% in the bile as unchanged drug and inactive and active metabolites. Elimination half-life is 3 to 9 hours. Half-life may increase in elderly patients; however, renal dysfunction does not appear to affect half-life.

Contraindications and precautions

Contraindicated in patients with sick sinus syndrome or second- or third-degree AV block in the absence of an artificial pacemaker, in supraventricular tachycardias associated with a bypass tract such as in Wolfe-Parkinson-White syndrome or Lown-Ganong-Levine syndrome, left ventricular failure, hypotension (systolic blood pressure below 90 mm Hg), hypersensitivity to the drug, acute MI, and pulmonary congestion (documented by X-ray).

Use cautiously in the elderly and in patients with heart failure or impaired hepatic or renal function.

Interactions

When used concomitantly, *beta blockers* may cause combined effects that result in heart failure, conduction disturbances, arrhythmias, and hypotension. Concomitant use with *cyclosporine* may cause increased serum cyclosporine levels and subsequent cyclosporine-induced nephrotoxicity. *Cimetidine* may increase diltiazem's plasma level. Patient should be carefully monitored for a change in diltiazem's effects when initiating and discontinuing therapy with cimetidine.

Effects on diagnostic tests

None reported.

Adverse reactions

CNS: *headache,* dizziness, asthenia, somnolence.
CV: *edema,* ***arrhythmias,*** flushing, bradycardia, hypotension, conduction abnormalities, ***heart failure,*** AV block, abnormal ECG.
GI: *nausea, constipation,* abdominal discomfort.
Hepatic: acute hepatic injury.
Skin: *rash.*

Overdose and treatment

Clinical effects of overdose primarily are extensions of drug's adverse reactions. Heart block, asystole, and hypotension are the most serious effects and require immediate attention.

Treatment may involve I.V isoproterenol, norepinephrine, epinephrine, atropine, or calcium gluconate administered in usual doses. Adequate hydration must be ensured. Inotropic agents, including dobutamine and dopamine, may be used, if necessary. If the patient develops severe conduction disturbances (such as heart block and asystole) with hypotension that does not respond to drug therapy, cardiac pacing should be initiated immediately with cardiopulmonary resuscitation measures, as indicated.

☑ Special considerations

Besides those relevant to all *calcium channel blockers,* consider the following recommendations.
- If diltiazem is added to therapy of patient receiving digoxin, monitor serum digoxin levels and observe patient closely for signs of toxicity, especially elderly patients, those with unstable renal function, and those with serum digoxin levels in the upper therapeutic range.
- Sublingual nitroglycerin may be administered concomitantly, as needed, if patient has acute angina symptoms.
- Diltiazem has been used investigationally to prevent reinfarction after nonQ-wave MI; as an adjunct in the treatment of peripheral vascular disorders; and in the treatment of several spastic smooth muscle disorders, including esophageal spasm.

Patient education

- Tell patient that nitrate therapy prescribed during titration of diltiazem dosage may cause dizziness. Urge patient to continue compliance.

- Inform patient of proper use, dose, and adverse effects associated with diltiazem use.
- Instruct patient to continue taking drug even when feeling better.
- Tell patient to report feelings of lightheadedness or dizziness and to avoid sudden position changes.

Geriatric use

- Use drug with caution in elderly patients because the half-life may be prolonged.

Breast-feeding

- Drug is excreted in breast milk; therefore, women should discontinue breast-feeding during diltiazem therapy.

dimenhydrinate

Apo-Dimenhydrinate*, Calm-X, Dimetabs, Dinate, Dommanate, Dramamine, Dramocen, Dramoject, Dymenate, Gravol*, Hydrate, Nauseatol*, Novo-Dimenate*, PMS-Dimenhydrinate*, Travamine*, Wehamine

Pharmacologic classification: ethanolamine-derivative antihistamine
Therapeutic classification: antihistamine (H_1-receptor antagonist), antiemetic, antivertigo
Pregnancy risk category B

How supplied

Available with or without a prescription
Tablets: 50 mg
Capsules: 50 mg
Liquid: 12.5 mg/4 ml, 15 mg/5 ml*
Injection: 50 mg/ml

Indications, route, and dosage

Prophylaxis and treatment of nausea, vomiting, dizziness associated with motion sickness
Adults and children age 12 and older: 50 to 100 mg q 4 to 6 hours P.O., I.V., or I.M. For I.V. administration, dilute each 50-mg dose in 10 ml of 0.9% NaCl solution and inject slowly over 2 minutes.
Children: 1.25 mg/kg/day or 37.5 mg/m²/day P.O. or I.M. q.i.d. not to exceed 300 mg/day, or according to the following schedule:
Children age 6 to 12: 25 to 50 mg P.O. q 6 to 8 hours; maximum dose is 150 mg/day.
Children age 2 to 6: 12.5 to 25 mg P.O. q 6 to 8 hours; maximum dose is 75 mg/day.
◊ ***Ménière's disease***
Adults: 50 mg I.M. for acute attack; maintenance dose is 25 to 50 mg P.O. t.i.d.

Pharmacodynamics

Antiemetic and antivertigo action: Dimenhydrinate probably inhibits nausea and vomiting by centrally depressing sensitivity of the labyrinth apparatus that relays stimuli to the chemoreceptor trigger zone and stimulates the vomiting center in the brain.

Pharmacokinetics

- *Absorption:* Drug is well absorbed. Action begins within 15 to 30 minutes after oral administration, 20 to 30 minutes after I.M. administration, and almost immediately after I.V. administration. Its duration of action is 3 to 6 hours.
- *Distribution:* Drug is well distributed throughout the body and crosses the placenta.
- *Metabolism:* Dimenhydrinate is metabolized in the liver.
- *Excretion:* Metabolites are excreted in urine.

Contraindications and precautions

Contraindicated in patients hypersensitive to drug or its components. I.V. product contains benzyl alcohol, which has been associated with a fatal "gasping syndrome" in premature infants and low birth weight infants.

Use cautiously in patients with seizures, acute angle-closure glaucoma, or enlarged prostate gland and in those receiving ototoxic drugs.

Interactions

Additive CNS sedation and depression may occur when drug is used concomitantly with other *CNS depressants*, such as *alcohol, barbiturates, tranquilizers, sleeping agents,* and *antianxiety agents.*

Dimenhydrinate may mask the signs of ototoxicity caused by known *ototoxic agents*, including the *aminoglycosides, salicylates, vancomycin, loop diuretics,* and *cisplatin.*

Effects on diagnostic tests

Dimenhydrinate may alter or confuse test results for xanthines (caffeine, aminophylline) because of its 8-chlorotheophylline content; discontinue dimenhydrinate 4 days before diagnostic skin tests to avoid preventing, reducing, or masking test response.

Adverse reactions

CNS: *drowsiness,* headache, dizziness, confusion, nervousness, insomnia (especially in children), vertigo, tingling and weakness of hands, lassitude, excitation.
CV: palpitations, hypotension, tachycardia.
EENT: blurred vision, dry respiratory passages, diplopia, nasal congestion.
GI: dry mouth, nausea, vomiting, diarrhea, epigastric distress, constipation, anorexia.
Respiratory: wheezing, thickened bronchial secretions.
Skin: photosensitivity, urticaria, rash.
Other: ***anaphylaxis,*** tightness of chest.

Overdose and treatment

Clinical manifestations of overdose may include either CNS depression (sedation, reduced mental alertness, apnea, and CV collapse) or CNS stimulation (insomnia, hallucinations, tremors, or seizures). Anticholinergic symptoms, such as dry mouth, flushed skin, fixed and dilated pupils, and GI symptoms, are likely to occur, especially in children.

Use gastric lavage to empty stomach contents; emetics may be ineffective. Diazepam or phenytoin may be used to control seizures. Provide supportive treatment.

☑ Special considerations

Besides those relevant to all *antihistamines,* consider the following recommendations.

- Incorrectly administered or undiluted I.V. solution is irritating to veins and may cause sclerosis.
- Parenteral solution is incompatible with many drugs; do not mix other drugs in the same syringe.
- Advise safety measures for all patients; dimenhydrinate has a high incidence of drowsiness. Tolerance to CNS depressant effects usually develops within a few days.
- To prevent motion sickness, patient should take medication 30 minutes before traveling and again before meals and at bedtime.
- Antiemetic effect may diminish with prolonged use.

Patient education

- Tell patient to avoid hazardous activities, such as driving or operating heavy machinery, until adverse CNS effects of drug are known.
- For motion sickness, tell patient to take drug 30 minutes before exposure.

Geriatric use

- Elderly patients are usually more sensitive to adverse effects of antihistamines and are especially likely to experience a greater degree of dizziness, sedation, hyperexcitability, dry mouth, and urine retention than younger patients.

Pediatric use

- Safety in neonates has not been established. Infants and children under age 6 may experience paradoxical hyperexcitability. I.V. dosage for children has not been established.

Breast-feeding

- Avoid use of antihistamines during breast-feeding. Many of these drugs, including dimenhydrinate, are secreted in breast milk, exposing the infant to risks of unusual excitability; premature infants are at particular risk for seizures.

dimercaprol

BAL in Oil

Pharmacologic classification: chelating
Therapeutic classification: heavy metal antagonist
Pregnancy risk category NR

How supplied

Available by prescription only
Injection: 100 mg/ml

Indications, route, and dosage

Severe arsenic or gold poisoning
Adults and children: 3 mg/kg deep I.M. q 4 hours for 2 days, then q.i.d. on day 3; then b.i.d. for 10 days.

Mild arsenic or gold poisoning
Adults and children: 2.5 mg/kg deep I.M. q.i.d. for 2 days, then b.i.d. on day 3; then once daily for 10 days.

Severe gold dermatitis
Adults and children: 2.5 mg/kg deep I.M. q 4 hours for 2 days, then b.i.d. for 7 days.

Gold-induced thrombocytopenia
Adults and children: 100 mg deep I.M. b.i.d. for 15 days.

Mercury poisoning
Adults and children: Initially, 5 mg/kg deep I.M., then 2.5 mg/kg daily or b.i.d. for 10 days.

Acute lead encephalopathy or blood lead level greater than 100 mcg/dl
Adults and children: 4 mg/kg (or 75 to 83 mg/m²) deep I.M. injection, then give simultaneously with edetate calcium disodium (250 mg/m²) q 4 hours for 3 to 5 days. Use separate injection sites.

Pharmacodynamics

Chelating action: The sulfhydryl groups of dimercaprol form heterocyclic ring complexes with heavy metals, particularly arsenic, mercury, and gold, preventing or reversing their binding to body ligands.

Pharmacokinetics

- *Absorption:* Drug is absorbed slowly through the skin. After I.M. injection, peak serum levels occur in 30 to 60 minutes.
- *Distribution:* Distributed to all tissues, mainly the intracellular space, with the highest concentrations of dimercaprol occurring in the liver and kidneys.
- *Metabolism:* Uncomplexed dimercaprol is metabolized rapidly to inactive products.
- *Excretion:* Most dimercaprol-metal complexes and inactive metabolites are excreted in urine and feces.

Contraindications and precautions

Contraindicated in patients with hepatic dysfunction (except postarsenical jaundice). Use cautiously in patients with hypertension or oliguria. Avoid use in pregnant women unless required to treat a life-threatening acute poisoning.

Interactions

Iron, cadmium, selenium, and *uranium* form toxic complexes with dimercaprol. Delay iron therapy for 24 hours after stopping dimercaprol.

Effects on diagnostic tests

Dimercaprol therapy blocks thyroid uptake of ^{131}I, causing decreased values.

Adverse reactions

CNS: pain or tightness in throat, chest, or hands; headache; paresthesia; muscle pain or weakness, anxiety.
CV: *transient increase in blood pressure* (returns to normal in 2 hours), *tachycardia.*
EENT: blepharospasm, conjunctivitis, lacrimation, rhinorrhea, excessive salivation.
GI: *nausea, vomiting; burning sensation in lips, mouth, and throat; abdominal pain.*
Other: *fever* (especially in children).

Overdose and treatment
Clinical signs of overdose include vomiting, seizures, stupor, coma, hypertension, and tachycardia; effects subside in 1 to 6 hours. Support CV and respiratory status; control seizures with diazepam.

☑ Special considerations
- Treat patient as soon as possible after poisoning, for optimal therapeutic effect; administer drug by deep I.M. injection only.
- Monitor vital signs and intake and output during therapy, and keep urine alkaline to prevent renal failure.
- Adverse effects of dimercaprol are usually mild and transitory and occur in about one half of patients who receive an I.M. dose of 5 mg/kg. In patients who receive doses in excess of 5 mg/kg, adverse effects usually occur within 30 minutes after injection and subside in 1 to 6 hours.
- Drug has strong garlic odor.

Patient education
- Advise patient that drug may cause a bad taste in the mouth or bad breath. It also may cause a burning sensation of the lips, mouth, throat, eyes, and penis and pain in the teeth.

Geriatric use
- Drug should be used with caution.

Pediatric use
- Fever is common, usually appearing after the second or third dose, and may persist throughout therapy. Acrodynia in infants and children has been treated with 3 mg/kg of dimercaprol I.M. every 4 hours for 2 days, then every 6 hours for 1 day, followed by every 12 hours for 7 to 8 days.

dinoprostone (prostaglandin E_2)
Cervidil, Prepidil, Prostin E_2

Pharmacologic classification: prostaglandin
Therapeutic classification: oxytocic
Pregnancy risk category C

How supplied
Available by prescription only
Vaginal suppositories: 20 mg
Vaginal gel: 0.5 mg
Vaginal insert: 10 mg

Indications, route, and dosage
Abort second-trimester pregnancy, evacuate uterus in cases of missed abortion, intrauterine fetal deaths up to 28 weeks of gestation, benign hydatidiform mole
Adults: Insert 20-mg suppository high into posterior vaginal fornix. Repeat q 3 to 5 hours until abortion is complete. Do not exceed 240 mg.
Ripening of an unfavorable cervix in pregnant patients at or near term (gel or insert)
Adults: Insert one applicatorful (0.5 mg) of gel into vagina. May repeat the dose in 6 hours if no response. Maximum recommended dose in 24 hours is 1.5 mg. Alternatively, 1-10 mg insert into posterior vaginal fornix. Have patient remain supine for 2 hours. Remove insert upon onset of active labor or 12 hours after insertion.

Pharmacodynamics
Oxytocic action: Dinoprostone stimulates myometrial contractions in the gravid uterus similar to the contractions of term labor. The exact mechanism of action is unknown, but it may result from one or more of the following: direct stimulation, regulation of cellular calcium transport, or regulation of intracellular concentrations of cyclic 3,5-adenosine monophosphate. Reductions in plasma estrogen and progesterone levels play a role in the drug's uterine action, but this effect does not occur consistently. Dinoprostone facilitates cervical dilations by directly softening the cervix.

Pharmacokinetics
- *Absorption:* Following vaginal insertion, dinoprostone is diffused slowly into the maternal blood. There is also some local absorption into the uterus through the cervix or local vascular and lymphatic channels, but this accounts for only a small portion of the dose. Contractions appear within 10 minutes of dosing, with a peak effect in 17 hours. There is no correlation of activity with plasma concentrations.
- *Distribution:* Drug is distributed widely in the mother.
- *Metabolism:* Drug is metabolized in the lungs, liver, kidneys, spleen, and other maternal tissues. There are at least nine inactive metabolites.
- *Excretion:* Drug and metabolites are excreted primarily in urine, with small amounts in feces.

Contraindications and precautions
Gel form is contraindicated where prolonged contractions of the uterus are considered inappropriate and in patients with hypersensitivity to prostaglandins or constituents of the gel. Also contraindicated in patients with placenta previa or unexplained vaginal bleeding during this pregnancy and in whom vaginal delivery is not indicated (that is, because of vasa previa or active herpes genitalia).

Suppository form is contraindicated in patients with hypersensitivity to the drug, acute pelvic inflammatory disease, and active cardiac, pulmonary, renal, or hepatic disease.

Vaginal insert is contraindicated in patients with known hypersensitivity to prostaglandins or when there is clinical suspicion or definite evidence of marked cephalopelvic disproportion or fetal distress where delivery is not imminent. The insert is also contraindicated in patients with unexplained vaginal bleeding during pregnancy, multiparity with six or more previous term pregnancies, and when oxytocic drugs are contraindicated or the patient is already receiving I.V. oxytocic drugs.

Use suppository form cautiously in patients with asthma, seizure disorders, anemia, diabetes, hypertension or hypotension, jaundice, scarred uterus, cervicitis, acute vaginitis, and CV, renal, or hepatic disease. Use gel form cautiously in patients with asthma or history of asthma, glaucoma or raised intraocular pressure, or renal or hepatic dysfunction and in those with ruptured membranes. Insert should be used cautiously in cases of nonvertex presentation and in patients with ruptured membranes or history of previous uterine hypertony, glaucoma, or childhood asthma.

Interactions
Used concomitantly, dinoprostone enhances the effects of *oxytocin* and other *oxytocics*. Cervical laceration and trauma have been reported when oxytocin is used concurrently. When using gel for cervical ripening, concomitant use is not recommended. Rather, allow a dosing interval of 6 to 12 hours before starting oxytocin therapy.

Effects on diagnostic tests
None reported.

Adverse reactions
CNS: *headache, dizziness,* anxiety, hot flashes, paresthesia, weakness, syncope.
CV: chest pain, ***arrhythmias.***
EENT: blurred vision, eye pain.
GI: *nausea, vomiting, diarrhea.*
GU: vaginal pain, vaginitis, endometritis.
Respiratory: coughing, dyspnea.
Skin: rash.
Other: *nocturnal leg cramps, fever, shivering, chills,* backache, breast tenderness, diaphoresis, muscle cramps.

Overdose and treatment
Clinical manifestations of overdose are extensions of adverse reactions. Because the drug is rapidly metabolized, treatment involves discontinuing the drug and providing supportive treatment.

☑ Special considerations
- Store suppositories in the freezer at –4° F (–20° C) and warm to room temperature (in foil) just before use.
- To prevent absorption through the skin, use gloves and keep handling of drug to a minimum.
- Administer drug only in medical facilities where intensive care and surgical facilities are accessible.
- Confirmation of fetal death is imperative before administration when used for missed abortion or intrauterine fetal death.
- Premedicate patient with antiemetic and antidiarrheal agents to minimize GI effects.
- Drug should not be administered P.R.
- Abortion should be complete within 30 hours.
- Drug-induced fever is transient and self-limiting. Sponge baths or increased fluid intake usually corrects this problem.
- After administration, patient should remain supine for 10 minutes.

Patient education
- Advise patient of expected adverse reactions, especially fever, nausea, vomiting (occurs in two-thirds of all patients), or diarrhea (occurs in approximately half of all patients), all of which are self-limiting.
- Instruct patient to remain in prone position for 10 minutes after insertion of drug.

diphenhydramine hydrochloride
Benadryl, Benadryl Allergy, Benylin, Compoz, Diphen AF, Diphen Cough, Diphenadryl, Hydramine, Insomnal*, Nervine Nighttime Sleep-Aid, Nytol with DPH, Sleep-Eze 3, Sominex, Tusstat, Twilite

Pharmacologic classification: ethanolamine-derivative antihistamine
Therapeutic classification: antihistamine (H_1-receptor antagonist), antiemetic, antivertigo, antitussive, sedative-hypnotic, topical anesthetic, antidyskinetic (anticholinergic)
Pregnancy risk category B

How supplied
Available with or without a prescription
Tablets: 25 mg, 50 mg
Capsules: 25 mg, 50 mg
Capsules (chewable): 12.5 mg
Elixir: 12.5 mg/5 ml (14% alcohol)
Syrup: 12.5 mg/5 ml (5% alcohol)
Injection: 50 mg/ml
Cream: 1%, 2%
Gel: 1%, 2%
Spray: 1%, 2%

Indications, route, and dosage
Rhinitis, allergy symptoms, motion sickness, Parkinson's disease
Adults and children age 12 and older: 25 to 50 mg P.O. t.i.d. or q.i.d.; or 10 to 50 mg I.V. or deep I.M. Maximum I.M. or I.V. dose is 400 mg daily.
Children under age 12: 5 mg/kg daily P.O., deep I.M., or I.V. in divided doses q.i.d. Maximum dose is 300 mg daily.
Nonproductive cough
Adults and children age 12 and older: 25 mg P.O. q 4 to 6 hours. Maximum dose is 150 mg daily.
Children age 6 to 12: 12.5 mg P.O. q 4 to 6 hours. Maximum dose is 75 mg daily.
Children age 2 to 6: 6.25 mg P.O. q 4 to 6 hours. Maximum dose is 25 mg daily.
Insomnia
Adults: 50 mg P.O. h.s.
Sedation
Adults: 25 to 50 mg P.O., or deep I.M., p.r.n.

Pharmacodynamics
Antihistamine action: Antihistamines compete for H_1-receptor sites on the smooth muscle of the bronchi, GI tract, uterus, and large blood vessels; by binding to cellular receptors, they prevent access of histamine and suppress histamine-induced allergic symptoms, even though they do not prevent its release.

Antivertigo, antiemetic, and antidyskinetic action: Central antimuscarinic actions of antihistamines probably are responsible for these effects of diphenhydramine.

Antitussive action: Drug suppresses the cough reflex by a direct effect on the cough center.

Sedative action: Mechanism of the CNS depressant effects of diphenhydramine is unknown.

Anesthetic action: Drug is structurally related to local anesthetics, which prevent initiation and transmission of nerve impulses; this is the probable source of its topical and local anesthetic effects.

Pharmacokinetics

- *Absorption:* Well absorbed from the GI tract. Action begins within 15 to 30 minutes and peaks in 1 to 4 hours.
- *Distribution:* Drug is distributed widely throughout the body, including the CNS; drug crosses the placenta and is excreted in breast milk. Drug is approximately 82% protein-bound.
- *Metabolism:* About 50% to 60% of an oral dose of diphenhydramine is metabolized by the liver before reaching the systemic circulation (first-pass effect); virtually all available drug is metabolized by the liver within 24 to 48 hours.
- *Excretion:* Plasma elimination half-life of drug is about 2½ to 9 hours; drug and metabolites are excreted primarily in urine.

Contraindications and precautions

Contraindicated in patients with hypersensitivity to drug, during acute asthmatic attacks, and in newborns, premature neonates, or breast-feeding patients.

Use with extreme caution in patients with angle-closure glaucoma, prostatic hyperplasia, pyloroduodenal and bladder neck obstruction, asthma or COPD, increased intraocular pressure, hyperthyroidism, CV disease, hypertension, and stenosing peptic ulcer.

Interactions

MAO inhibitors interfere with the detoxification of diphenhydramine and thus prolong their central depressant and anticholinergic effects; additive CNS depression may occur when diphenhydramine is given concomitantly with other *CNS depressants,* such as *alcohol, barbiturates, tranquilizers, sleeping aids,* and *antianxiety agents.*

Diphenhydramine may diminish the effects of *sulfonylureas,* enhance the effects of *epinephrine,* and partially counteract the anticoagulant effects of *heparin.*

Effects on diagnostic tests

Discontinue drug 4 days before diagnostic skin tests; antihistamines can prevent, reduce, or mask positive skin test response.

Adverse reactions

CNS: *drowsiness,* confusion, insomnia, headache, vertigo, *sedation, sleepiness, dizziness, incoordination,* fatigue, restlessness, tremor, nervousness, ***seizures.***
CV: palpitations, hypotension, tachycardia.
EENT: diplopia, blurred vision, tinnitus.
GI: *nausea,* vomiting, diarrhea, *dry mouth,* constipation, *epigastric distress,* anorexia.
GU: dysuria, urine retention, urinary frequency.
Hematologic: hemolytic anemia, ***thrombocytopenia, agranulocytosis.***
Respiratory: nasal congestion, *thickening of bronchial secretions.*
Skin: urticaria, photosensitivity, rash.
Other: ***anaphylactic shock.***

Overdose and treatment

Drowsiness is the usual clinical manifestation of overdose. Seizures, coma, and respiratory depression may occur with profound overdose. Anticholinergic symptoms, such as dry mouth, flushed skin, fixed and dilated pupils, and GI symptoms, are common, especially in children.

Treat overdose by inducing emesis with ipecac syrup (in conscious patient), followed by activated charcoal to reduce further drug absorption. Use gastric lavage if patient is unconscious or ipecac fails. Treat hypotension with vasopressors, and control seizures with diazepam or phenytoin. *Do not give stimulants.*

☑ Special considerations

Besides those relevant to all *antihistamines,* consider the following recommendations.

- Diphenhydramine injection is compatible with most I.V. solutions but is *incompatible* with some drugs; check compatibility before mixing in the same I.V. line.
- Alternate injection sites to prevent irritation. Administer deep I.M. into large muscle.
- Drowsiness is the most common adverse effect during initial therapy but usually disappears with continued use of drug.
- Injectable and elixir solutions are light-sensitive; protect them from light.

Patient education

- Advise patient that drowsiness is very common initially, but may be reduced with continued use of drug.
- Warn patient to avoid alcohol during therapy.
- Advise patient undergoing skin testing for allergies to notify primary health care provider of current drug therapy.

Geriatric use

- Elderly patients are usually more sensitive to adverse effects of antihistamines and are especially likely to experience a greater degree of dizziness, sedation, hyperexcitability, dry mouth, and urine retention than younger patients. Symptoms usually respond to a decrease in medication dosage.

Pediatric use

- Drug should not be used in premature infants or neonates. Infants and children, especially those under age 6, may experience paradoxical hyperexcitability.

Breast-feeding

- Avoid use of antihistamines during breast-feeding. Many of these drugs are secreted in breast milk, exposing the infant to risks of unusual excitability; premature infants are at particular risk for seizures.

diphenoxylate hydrochloride with atropine sulfate

Lofene, Logen, Lomanate, Lomotil, Lonox, Lo-Trol, Low-Quel

Pharmacologic classification: opiate
Therapeutic classification: antidiarrheal
Controlled substance schedule V
Pregnancy risk category C

How supplied

Available by prescription only
Tablets: 2.5 mg diphenoxylate hydrochloride and 0.025 mg atropine sulfate per tablet
Liquid: 2.5 mg diphenoxylate hydrochloride and 0.025 mg atropine sulfate/5 ml

Indications, route, and dosage

Acute, nonspecific diarrhea

Adults: 5 mg diphenoxylate component P.O. q.i.d., then adjust p.r.n.
Children age 2 and over: 0.3 to 0.4 mg/kg/day diphenoxylate component in divided doses; or administer according to diphenoxylate component, as follows: *Children age 9 to 12:* 3.5 to 5 ml.
Children age 6 to 8: 2.5 to 5 ml.
Children age 5: 2.5 to 4. 5 ml.
Children age 4: 2 to 4 ml.
Children age 3: 2 to 3 ml.
Children age 2: 1.5 to 3 ml.

Pharmacodynamics

Antidiarrheal action: Diphenoxylate is a meperidine analogue that inhibits GI motility locally and centrally. In high doses, it may produce an opiate effect. Atropine is added in subtherapeutic doses to prevent abuse by deliberate overdose.

Pharmacokinetics

- *Absorption:* About 90% of an oral dose is absorbed. Action begins in 45 to 60 minutes.
- *Distribution:* Drug is distributed in breast milk.
- *Metabolism:* Diphenoxylate is metabolized extensively by the liver.
- *Excretion:* Metabolites are excreted mainly in feces via the biliary tract, with lesser amounts excreted in urine. Duration of effect is 3 to 4 hours.

Contraindications and precautions

Contraindicated in patients with hypersensitivity to diphenoxylate or atropine, acute diarrhea resulting from poison until toxic material is eliminated from GI tract, acute diarrhea caused by organisms that penetrate intestinal mucosa, or diarrhea resulting from antibiotic-induced pseudomembranous enterocolitis or enterotoxin-producing bacteria; also contraindicated in patients with obstructive jaundice and in children under age 2.

Use cautiously in children age 2 and older; in patients with hepatic disease, narcotic dependence, or acute ulcerative colitis; and in pregnant women. Stop therapy immediately if abdominal distention or other signs of toxic megacolon develop.

Interactions

Diphenoxylate may precipitate hypertensive crisis in patients receiving *MAO inhibitors.* Concomitant use with such CNS depressants as *barbiturates, tranquilizers* and *alcohol* may result in an increased depressant effect.

Effects on diagnostic tests

Diphenoxylate may decrease urinary excretion of phenolsulfonphthalein (PSP) during the PSP excretion test; drug may increase serum amylase levels.

Adverse reactions

CNS: *sedation, dizziness,* headache, drowsiness, lethargy, restlessness, depression, euphoria, malaise, confusion, numbness in extremities.
CV: tachycardia.
EENT: mydriasis.
GI: *dry mouth,* nausea, vomiting, abdominal discomfort or distention, ***paralytic ileus,*** anorexia, fluid retention in bowel or megacolon (may mask depletion of extracellular fluid and electrolytes, especially in young children treated for acute gastroenteritis), ***pancreatitis,*** swollen gums, possible physical dependence with long-term use.
GU: urine retention.
Respiratory: ***respiratory depression.***
Skin: pruritus, rash, dry skin.
Other: ***angioedema, anaphylaxis.***

Overdose and treatment

Clinical effects of overdose include drowsiness, low blood pressure, marked seizures, apnea, blurred vision, miosis, flushing, dry mouth and mucous membranes and psychotic episodes.

Treatment is supportive; maintain airway and support vital functions. A narcotic antagonist, such as naloxone may be given. Gastric lavage may be performed. Monitor patient for 48 to 72 hours.

☑ Special considerations

- Monitor vital signs and intake and output; observe patient for adverse reactions, especially CNS reactions.
- Monitor bowel function.
- Drug is usually ineffective in treating antibiotic-induced diarrhea.
- Reduce dosage as soon as symptoms are controlled.

Patient education

- Warn patient to take drug exactly as ordered and not to exceed recommended dose.
- Advise patient to maintain adequate fluid intake during course of diarrhea and teach him about diet and fluid replacement.
- Caution patient to avoid driving during drug therapy because drowsiness and dizziness may occur; warn patient to avoid alcohol while taking drug because additive depressant effect may occur.

• Advise patient to call if drug is not effective within 48 hours.
• Warn patient that prolonged use may result in tolerance and that use of larger-than-recommended doses may result in drug dependence.

Geriatric use
• Elderly patients may be more susceptible to respiratory depression and to exacerbation of preexisting glaucoma.

Pediatric use
• Drug is contraindicated in children under age 2; some children may experience respiratory depression. Children, especially those with Down syndrome, appear to be particularly sensitive to atropine content of drug.

Breast-feeding
• Drug is excreted in breast milk; drug effects have been reported in breast-fed infants of patients taking drug.

diphtheria and tetanus toxoids, adsorbed (Td); DT

Pharmacologic classification: toxoid
Therapeutic classification: diphtheria and tetanus prophylaxis
Pregnancy risk category C

How supplied
Available by prescription only
Available in pediatric (DT) and adult (Td) strengths
Injection: pediatric—6.6 to 15 Lf (limit flocculation) units of inactivated diphtheria and 5 to 10 Lf units of inactivated tetanus per 0.5 ml, in 5-ml vials; adult—2 Lf units of inactivated diphtheria and 2 to 10 Lf units of inactivated tetanus per 0.5 ml, in 5-ml vials

Indications, route, and dosage
Primary immunization
Adults and children age 7 and older: Use adult strength. Give 0.5 ml I.M. 4 to 8 weeks apart for two doses and a third dose 6 to 12 months later. Booster dose is 0.5 ml I.M. q 10 years.
Children age 1 to 7: Use pediatric strength. Give two 0.5-ml doses I.M. 4 to 8 weeks apart. Give a third dose 6 to 12 months after the second injection. If the final immunizing dose is given after the 7th birthday, use the adult strength.
Infants age 6 weeks to 1 year: Use pediatric strength. Give three 0.5-ml doses I.M. 4 to 8 weeks apart. Give a fourth dose 6 to 12 months after third injection.

Pharmacodynamics
Diphtheria and tetanus prophylaxis: Diphtheria and tetanus toxoids promote active immunization to diphtheria and tetanus by inducing production of antitoxins.

Pharmacokinetics
• *Absorption:* No information available.
• *Distribution:* No information available.
• *Metabolism:* No information available.
• *Excretion:* No information available.

Contraindications and precautions
Contraindicated in immunosuppressed patients and in those receiving radiation or corticosteroid therapy. Vaccination should be deferred in patients with respiratory illness and during polio outbreaks; also defer in those with acute illness except during emergency. When polio is a risk, a single antigen is used. In children under age 6, use only when diphtheria, tetanus, and pertussis combination is contraindicated because of pertussis component. DT should not be used in children age 7 or older because of an increased incidence of adverse reactions. Drug also contraindicated in patients with history of adverse reactions to constituents of drug.

Interactions
Concomitant use with *corticosteroids* or *immunosuppressants* may impair the immune response to diphtheria and tetanus toxoids. Avoid elective immunization under these circumstances.

Effects on diagnostic tests
None reported.

Adverse reactions
CV: flushing, tachycardia, hypotension, shock.
Skin: *pain, stinging, edema, erythema, induration at injection site,* urticaria, pruritus.
Other: ***anaphylaxis,*** chills, fever, malaise, headache.

Overdose and treatment
No information available.

☑ Special considerations
• Obtain a thorough history of allergies and reactions to immunizations.
• Epinephrine solution 1:1,000 should be available to treat allergic reactions.
• Diphtheria and tetanus toxoids are used primarily when pertussis vaccine is contraindicated or used separately.
• These toxoids are not used to treat active tetanus or diphtheria infections.
• Teratogenicity has not been reported. Immunization during pregnancy is recommended when needed.
• To prevent sciatic nerve damage, avoid administration in gluteal muscle. During primary immunization, do not inject same site more than once.
• Store toxoids between 36° and 46° F (2° and 8° C). Do not freeze. Shake well before withdrawing each dose.

Patient education
• Inform patient that he may experience discomfort at the injection site and that a nodule may develop there and persist for several weeks after immunization. He also may develop fever, headache, upset stomach, general malaise, or body aches and pains. Tell patient to relieve such effects with acetaminophen.

• Tell patient to report distressing adverse reactions.
• Stress importance of keeping all scheduled appointments for subsequent doses because full immunization requires a series of injections.

diphtheria and tetanus toxoids and pertussis vaccine, adsorbed (DTP)

Acel-Imune, diphtheria and tetanus toxoids and acellular pertussis vaccine adsorbed (DTaP), DTwP, Tri-Immunol, Tripedia

Pharmacologic classification: combination toxoid and vaccine
Therapeutic classification: diphtheria, tetanus, and pertussis prophylaxis
Pregnancy risk category C

How supplied

Available by prescription only
Whole-cell vaccine
Injection: 6.5 Lf (limit flocculation) units inactivated diphtheria, 5 Lf units inactivated tetanus, and 4 protective units pertussis per 0.5 ml, in 2.5-, 5-, and 7.5-ml vials; 10 Lf units inactivated diphtheria, 5.5 Lf units inactivated tetanus, and 4 protective units pertussis per 0.5 ml in 5-ml vials (DTwP); 12.5 Lf units inactivated diphtheria, 5 Lf units inactivated tetanus, and 4 protective units pertussis per 0.5 ml, in 7.5-ml vials (Tri-Immunol)
Acellular vaccine
Injection: 5 Lf units inactivated diphtheria, 5 Lf units inactivated tetanus, and 300 hemagglutinin units of acellular pertussis vaccine per 0.5 ml; 66.7 Lf units inactivated diphtheria, 5 Lf units inactivated tetanus, and 46.8 pertussis antigens per 0.5 ml

Indications, route, and dosage

Primary immunization
Children age 6 weeks to 7 years: Give 0.5 ml I.M. 4 to 8 weeks apart for three doses and a fourth dose 6 to 12 months after the third dose.
Booster immunization
Booster dosage is 0.5 ml I.M. when starting school, at age 4 to 6 unless fourth dose in series was administered after child's fourth birthday; then, a booster is not necessary at time of school entrance. Not advised for adults or for children age 7 or older.

Note: The acellular vaccine may be used only for the fourth or fifth dose in children age 15 months (Tripedia) or 17 months (Acel-Imune) to 7 years who have been immunized with three or four doses of the whole-cell vaccine.

Pharmacodynamics

Diphtheria, tetanus, and pertussis (whooping cough) prophylaxis: Vaccine promotes active immunity to diphtheria, tetanus, and pertussis by inducing production of antitoxin and antibodies.

Pharmacokinetics

• *Absorption:* No information available.
• *Distribution:* No information available.
• *Metabolism:* No information available.
• *Excretion:* No information available.

Contraindications and precautions

Contraindicated in immunosuppressed patients and in those on corticosteroid therapy or with history of seizures. Vaccination should be deferred in patients with acute febrile illness. Children with preexisting neurologic disorders should not receive pertussis component. Also, children who exhibit neurologic signs after injection should not receive pertussis component in any succeeding injections. Diphtheria and tetanus toxoids (called DT) should be given instead.

Interactions

Concomitant use of vaccine with *corticosteroids* or *immunosuppressants* may impair the immune response to the toxoids and vaccine. Avoid elective immunization under these circumstances.

Effects on diagnostic tests

None reported.

Adverse reactions

CNS: ***encephalopathy, seizures.***
Skin: soreness, redness, expected nodule remaining several weeks at injection site.
Other: ***anaphylaxis,*** *fever,* hypersensitivity reactions, peripheral neuropathy, ***shock,*** thrombocytopenic purpura, urticaria.

Overdose and treatment

No information available.

☑ Special considerations

• Obtain history of allergies and reactions to immunizations, especially to pertussis vaccine.
• Epinephrine solution 1:1,000 should be available to treat allergic reactions.
• Vaccine may be given at same time as trivalent oral polio vaccine and, if indicated, when the patient receives vaccines against *Haemophilus influenzae* type b, measles, mumps, and rubella.
• Do not use to treat active tetanus, diphtheria, or pertussis infections.
• Store vaccine between 36° and 46° F (2° and 8° C). Do not freeze. Shake vial well before withdrawing dose.

Patient education

• Explain to parents that child may experience discomfort at the injection site after immunization and that a nodule may develop there and persist for several weeks. Fever, upset stomach, or general malaise may also develop. Recommend acetaminophen liquid to relieve such discomfort.
• Tell parents to report worrisome or intolerable reactions promptly.
• Stress importance of keeping scheduled appointments for subsequent doses. Full immunization requires a series of injections.

diphtheria antitoxin, equine

Pharmacologic classification: antitoxin
Therapeutic classification: diphtheria antitoxin
Pregnancy risk category NR

How supplied

Available by prescription only
Injection: not less than 500 units/ml in 20,000-unit vial

Indications, route, and dosage

Diphtheria prevention
Adults and children: 5,000 to 10,000 units I.M. (dose dependent on length of time since exposure, extent of exposure, and individual's medical condition).

Diphtheria treatment
Adults and children: 20,000 to 120,000 units I.M. or slow I.V. infusion in 0.9% NaCl solution (dose based on extent of disease). A 1:20 dilution of the antitoxin is infused at 1 ml/minute. Additional doses may be given in 24 hours. I.M. route may be used in mild cases. Begin antibiotic therapy.

Pharmacodynamics

Antitoxin action: Diphtheria antitoxin neutralizes and binds toxin.

Pharmacokinetics

- *Absorption:* No information available.
- *Metabolism:* No information available.
- *Distribution:* No information available.
- *Excretion:* No information available.

Contraindications and precautions

Contraindicated in patients hypersensitive to drug. An intradermal or scratch skin test and a conjunctival test for sensitivity to equine serum (against a control of 0.9% NaCl solution) should be performed before administering diphtheria antitoxin. If the sensitivity test is positive, check desensitization schedule.

Interactions

None reported.

Effects on diagnostic tests

None reported.

Adverse reactions

Skin: *pain, erythema.*
Other: ***hypersensitivity reactions (anaphylaxis,*** serum sickness, urticaria, pruritus, fever, malaise, arthralgia) may occur in 7 to 12 days. Discontinue if severe systemic reactions occur.

Overdose and treatment

No information available.

☑ Special considerations

- Obtain a thorough patient history of allergies, especially to horses and horse immune serum; of asthma; and of previous reactions to immunizations.
- Epinephrine solution 1:1,000 should be available to treat allergic reactions.
- All asymptomatic nonimmunized contacts of patients with diphtheria should receive prompt prophylaxis with antibiotic therapy and have cultures taken before and after treatment. The patient should receive diphtheria toxoid and be monitored for 7 days thereafter.
- Therapy should begin immediately, without waiting for culture and sensitivity test results, if patient has clinical symptoms of diphtheria (sore throat, fever, and tonsillar membrane involvement). Continue treatment until all symptoms are controlled.
- Refrigerate antitoxin at 36° to 46° F (2° to 8° C). It may also be warmed to 90° to 93° F (32° to 34° C); higher temperatures will diminish potency.

Patient education

- Tell patient that allergic reactions may occur (rash, joint swelling or pain, or difficulty breathing) but that he will be monitored closely and will receive medication, as needed, to relieve such effects.
- Encourage patient to report all unusual symptoms; delayed effects associated with antitoxin may occur in 7 to 12 days after treatment.

Breast-feeding

- Patient should discontinue breast-feeding until toxin's effects subside or if symptoms of serum sickness develop.

diphtheria toxoid, adsorbed (for pediatric use)

Pharmacologic classification: toxoid
Therapeutic classification: diphtheria prophylaxis
Pregnancy risk category NR

How supplied

Available by prescription only
Injection: suspension of 15 Lf (limit flocculation) units inactivated diphtheria per 0.5 ml, in 5-ml vials or 10-ml vials

Indications, route, and dosage

Diphtheria immunization
Children under age 7: 0.5 ml I.M. 6 to 8 weeks apart for two doses and a third dose 1 year later. Booster dosage is 0.5 ml I.M. at 5- to 10-year intervals. Not advised for adults or for children over age 6; instead, use adult strength of diphtheria toxoid (usually available as diphtheria and tetanus toxoids, adsorbed, combined).

Pharmacodynamics

Diphtheria prophylaxis: Diphtheria toxoid promotes active immunity to diphtheria by inducing production of antitoxin. Protection lasts about 10 years.

Pharmacokinetics

- *Absorption:* No information available.
- *Metabolism:* No information available.
- *Distribution:* No information available.
- *Excretion:* No information available.

Contraindications and precautions
Diphtheria toxoid is contraindicated in patients with febrile illness other than a mild upper respiratory infection or other active infection. Defer elective immunization during these situations and during outbreaks of poliomyelitis.

Defer immunization until age 2 in infants with a history of seizures or CNS damage. (Alternatively, one tenth the recommended initial dosage may be used, followed by standard doses if no untoward effect occurs.)

Diphtheria toxoid is not recommended for adults or for children over age 6. This preparation also is contraindicated in patients with known hypersensitivity to thimerosal, a component of the toxoid, and in immunosuppressed patients (those with congenital immunodeficiencies, cancer, or acquired immunodeficiency syndrome and those undergoing treatment with cortico-steroids, antineoplastic agents, or radiation).

Interactions
Concomitant use of diphtheria toxoid with *corticosteroids* or *immunosuppressants* may impair the immune response to the toxoid. Avoid elective immunization under these circumstances.

Effects on diagnostic tests
None reported.

Adverse reactions
Skin: erythema, pain, and sterile abscess induration at injection site; a nodule may develop and persist for several weeks.
Other: fever, malaise, urticaria, tachycardia, flushing, pruritus, hypotension, myalgia, arthralgia, ***anaphylaxis,*** drowsiness.

Overdose and treatment
No information available.

☑ Special considerations
- Obtain a thorough history of allergies and reactions to immunizations.
- Epinephrine solution 1:1,000 should be available to treat allergic reactions.
- Preparation is used primarily when products containing tetanus toxoid or pertussis vaccine would not be advisable.
- Shake well before using.
- Do not use diphtheria toxoid to treat active diphtheria infections.
- Store drug between 36° and 46° F (2° and 8° C). Do not freeze.

Patient education
- Explain to parents that child may experience discomfort at the injection site after immunization and may develop a nodule there that can persist for several weeks. Fever, general malaise, or body aches and pains may also develop. Recommend acetaminophen liquid to relieve minor discomfort.
- Tell parents to report worrisome or intolerable adverse reactions promptly.
- Emphasize importance of keeping scheduled appointments for subsequent doses. Full immunization requires a series of injections.

dipivefrin hydrochloride
Propine

Pharmacologic classification: sympathomimetic
Therapeutic classification: antiglaucoma
Pregnancy risk category B

How supplied
Available by prescription only
Ophthalmic solution: 0.1%

Indications, route, and dosage
To reduce intraocular pressure in chronic open-angle glaucoma
Adults: For initial glaucoma therapy, 1 drop in eye q 12 hours; then adjust dose based on patient response as determined by tonometric readings.

Pharmacodynamics
Antiglaucoma action: Dipivefrin is a prodrug converted to epinephrine in the eye. It decreases aqueous humor production and enhances outflow. It is often used with a miotic agent.

Pharmacokinetics
- *Absorption:* Action begins in about 30 minutes, with peak effect in 1 hour.
- *Distribution:* Unknown.
- *Metabolism:* Unknown.
- *Excretion:* Unknown.

Contraindications and precautions
Contraindicated in patients with angle-closure glaucoma or hypersensitivity to drug. Use cautiously in patients with asthma, hypersensitivity to epinephrine, and aphakia or CV disease.

Interactions
When used concomitantly, dipivefrin may enhance the lowering of intraocular pressure caused by *miotic agents* and *carbonic anhydrase inhibitors.* Depending on the extent of systemic absorption and the amount present, there may be additive toxic effects with *sympathomimetics*, and an increased risk of arrhythmias with *digoxin, anesthetics,* or *tricyclic antidepressants.*

Effects on diagnostic tests
None reported.

Adverse reactions
CV: tachycardia, hypertension, ***arrhythmias.***
EENT: eye burning or stinging, conjunctival injection, conjunctivitis, mydriasis, allergic reaction, photophobia.

Overdose and treatment
Overdose is quite rare with ophthalmic use but may cause the following effects after accidental ingestion: hypertension with tachycardia or bradycardia,

arrhythmias, precordial pain, anxiety, nervousness, insomnia, muscle tremor, cerebral hemorrhage, seizures, altered mental status, anorexia, nausea and vomiting, and acute renal failure. To treat oral overdose, dilute immediately then initiate emesis followed by activated charcoal and a cathartic, unless the patient is comatose or obtunded. Monitor urinary output. As ordered, treat seizures with I.V. diazepam, and hypertension with nitroprusside; treat arrhythmias appropriately, depending on the type of arrhythmia. Preparations containing sulfites may cause GI or cardiac toxicities and hypotension.

☑ Special considerations

- Drug may cause fewer adverse reactions than with conventional epinephrine therapy; it often is used concomitantly with other antiglaucoma agents.
- Store away from heat and light.

Patient education

- Teach patient the correct way to instill drops and warn him not to touch eye with dropper.
- Teach patient that if also using other eye drops, he should instill dipivefrin first, then wait at least 5 minutes before using the other drops.
- Instruct patient not to blink more than usual and not to close his eyes tightly after instillation.
- Tell patient instillation of drug may cause transient burning or stinging.

Geriatric use

- Drug should be used with caution in elderly patients, to avoid precipitating narrow-angle glaucoma.

dipyridamole

Persantine

Pharmacologic classification: pyrimidine analogue
Therapeutic classification: coronary vasodilator, platelet aggregation inhibitor
Pregnancy risk category B

How supplied

Available by prescription only
Tablets: 25 mg, 50 mg, 75 mg
Injection: 10 mg/ampule

Indications, route, and dosage

Alternative to exercise in thallium myocardial perfusion imaging
Adults: 0.142 mg/kg/minute infused over 4 minutes (0.57 mg/kg total).
Inhibition of platelet adhesion in patients with prosthetic heart valves, in combination with warfarin or aspirin
Adults: 75 to 100 mg P.O. q.i.d.
◊ ***Chronic angina pectoris***
Adults: 50 mg P.O. t.i.d. at least 1 hour before meals; 2 to 3 months of therapy may be required to achieve a clinical response.
◊ ***Prevention of thromboembolic complications in patients with various thromboembolic disorders other than prosthetic heart valves***
Adults: 150 to 400 mg P.O. daily (in combination with warfarin or aspirin).

Pharmacodynamics

Coronary vasodilating action: Dipyridamole increases coronary blood flow by selectively dilating the coronary arteries. Coronary vasodilator effect follows inhibition of serum adenosine deaminase, which allows accumulation of adenosine, a potent vasodilator. Dipyridamole inhibits platelet adhesion by increasing effects of prostacyclin or by inhibiting phosphodiesterase.

Pharmacokinetics

- *Absorption:* Absorption is variable and slow; bioavailability ranges from 27% to 59%. Serum concentrations of dipyridamole peak 45 minutes to 2½ hours after oral administration.
- *Distribution:* Animal studies indicate wide distribution in body tissues; small amounts cross the placenta. Protein binding ranges from 91% to 97%.
- *Metabolism:* Drug is metabolized by the liver.
- *Excretion:* Elimination occurs via biliary excretion of glucuronide conjugates. Some dipyridamole and conjugates may undergo enterohepatic circulation and fecal excretion; a small amount is excreted in urine. Half-life varies from 1 to 12 hours.

Contraindications and precautions

No known contraindications. Use cautiously in patients with hypotension.

Interactions

Aminophylline inhibits the action of dipyridamole. Dipyridimole can enhance the effects of oral anticoagulants and heparin.

Effects on diagnostic tests

Drug's physiologic effects on platelet aggregation will cause an increase in bleeding time. Serum levels of activated PT and activated partial thromboplastin time, as well as platelet count, should remain unchanged.

Adverse reactions

CNS: *headache, dizziness.*
CV: flushing, fainting, *hypotension;* angina, chest pain, *blood pressure lability, hypertension* (with I.V. infusion).
GI: *nausea,* vomiting, diarrhea, abdominal distress.
Skin: rash, irritation (with undiluted injection), pruritus.

Overdose and treatment

Clinical signs of overdose include peripheral vasodilation and hypotension. Maintain blood pressure and treat symptomatically.

☑ Special considerations

- Be alert for adverse reactions, including signs of bleeding and prolonged bleeding time, especially at high doses and during long-term therapy.
- Monitor blood pressure.

• Give drug at least 1 hour before meals.
• When used as a pharmacologic "stress test," total doses beyond 60 mg appear to be unnecessary.
• Dilute I.V. form to at least a 1:2 ratio with 0.45% NaCl injection, 0.9% NaCl injection, or D_5W to a total volume of 20 to 50 ml. Inject thallium within 5 minutes of dipyridamole.

Patient education
• Explain that clinical response may require 2 to 3 months of continuous therapy; encourage patient compliance.
• Discuss adverse reactions and how to manage therapy.

Pediatric use
• Dosage has not been established in children.

Breast-feeding
• Safety in breast-feeding women has not been established.

dirithromycin
Dynabac

Pharmacologic classification: macrolide
Therapeutic classification: antibiotic
Pregnancy risk category C

How supplied
Available by prescription only
Tablets: 250 mg

Indications, route, and dosage
Acute bacterial exacerbations of chronic bronchitis due to* Moraxella catarrhalis *or* Streptococcus pneumoniae*; secondary bacterial infection of acute bronchitis due to* M. catarrhalis *or* S. pneumoniae*; uncomplicated skin and skin structure infections due to* Staphylococcus aureus *(methicillin susceptible)
Adults and children age 12 and older: 500 mg P.O. daily with food for 7 days.
***Community-acquired pneumonia due to* Legionella pneumophila, Mycoplasma pneumoniae, *or* S. pneumoniae**
Adults and children age 12 and older: 500 mg P.O. daily with food for 14 days.
***Pharyngitis or tonsillitis due to* Streptococcus pyogenes**
Adults and children age 12 and older: 500 mg P.O. daily with food for 10 days.

Pharmacodynamics
Antibiotic action: Dirithromycin inhibits bacterial RNA-dependent protein synthesis by binding to the 50S subunit of the ribosome. Its spectrum of activity includes gram-positive aerobes such as *S. aureus* (methicillin-susceptible strains only), *S. pneumoniae, S. pyogenes;* gram-negative aerobes such as *Legionella pneumophila* and *M. catarrhalis;* and other bacteria such as *M. pneumoniae.*

Pharmacokinetics
• *Absorption:* Rapidly absorbed from GI tract and converted by nonenzymatic hydrolysis to the microbiologically active compound erythromycylamine. Food slightly increases bioavailability of drug.
• *Distribution:* Drug is widely distributed throughout the body. The protein binding of erythromycylamine ranges from 15% to 30%.
• *Metabolism:* Dirithromycin undergoes little to no hepatic metabolism.
• *Excretion:* Drug is primarily eliminated in bile or feces with a small amount in urine. Mean half-life of erythromycylamine is about 8 hours.

Contraindications and precautions
Contraindicated in patients with hypersensitivity to dirithromycin, erythromycin, or other macrolide antibiotics.

Use cautiously in patients with hepatic insufficiency and in pregnant women.

Interactions
The absorption of *antacids* and H_2 *antagonists* may be slightly enhanced when dirithromycin is administered immediately after these drugs. Dirithromycin may alter steady-state plasma concentration of *theophylline.* Monitor theophylline plasma concentrations. Dosage adjustments may be needed.

The following drugs have been reported to interact with erythromycin products. It is not known whether these same drug interactions occur with dirithromycin. Until further data are available regarding the potential interaction of dirithromycin with these compounds, caution should be used during coadministration: *alfentanil, anticoagulants, astemizole, bromocriptine, carbamazepine, cyclosporine, digoxin, disopyramide, ergotamine, hexobarbital, lovastatin, phenytoin, triazolam,* and *valproate.*

Effects on diagnostic tests
None reported.

Adverse reactions
CNS: headache, dizziness, vertigo, insomnia.
GI: abdominal pain, nausea, diarrhea, vomiting, dyspepsia, GI disorder, flatulence.
Hematologic: increased platelet, eosinophil, and neutrophil counts.
Respiratory: increased cough, dyspnea.
Skin: rash, pruritus, urticaria.
Other: pain (nonspecific), asthenia, hyperkalemia, decreased bicarbonate levels, increased CK levels.

Overdose and treatment
The symptoms of a macrolide antibiotic overdose may include nausea, vomiting, epigastric distress, and diarrhea.

Treatment should be supportive as forced diuresis, dialysis, or hemoperfusion have not been established to be helpful for an overdose of dirithromycin.

☑ Special considerations
• Obtain culture and sensitivity tests before initiating drug treatment. Therapy may begin pending results.
• Do not use drug in patients with known, suspected, or potential bacteremias because serum levels are inadequate to provide antibacterial coverage of the bloodstream.
• Administer drug with food or within 1 hour of eating.
• Monitor patient for superinfection. Drug may cause overgrowth of nonsusceptible bacteria or fungi.

Patient education
• Tell patient to take all of drug as prescribed, even after he feels better.
• Instruct patient to take drug with food or within 1 hour of having eaten. Tell him not to cut, chew, or crush the tablet.

Pediatric use
• Safety and effectiveness in children under age 12 have not been established.

Breast-feeding
• It is not known if dirithromycin is excreted in breast milk; caution is advised in breast-feeding women.

disopyramide phosphate
Norpace, Norpace CR, Rythmodan*, Rythmodan-LA*

Pharmacologic classification: pyridine derivative antiarrhythmic, group IA antiarrhythmic
Therapeutic classification: ventricular antiarrhythmic, supraventricular antiarrhythmic, atrial antitachyarrhythmic
Pregnancy risk category C

How supplied
Available by prescription only
Capsules: 100 mg, 150 mg
Capsules (extended-release): 100 mg, 150 mg

Indications, route, and dosage
PVCs (unifocal, multifocal, or coupled); ventricular tachycardia; ◇ conversion of atrial fibrillation, atrial flutter, and paroxysmal atrial tachycardia to normal sinus rhythm
Adults: Initially, 200 to 300 mg loading dose. Usual maintenance dosage is 150 mg P.O. q 6 hours or 300 mg (extended-release) P.O. q 12 hours; for patients weighing below 50 kg (110 lb), give 100 mg P.O. q 6 hours or 200 mg (extended-release) P.O. q 12 hours; and for patients with cardiomyopathy or possible cardiac decompensation, give 100 mg P.O. q 6 to 8 hours initially and then adjust p.r.n.
Children age 12 to 18: 6 to 15 mg/kg/day.
Children age 4 to 12: 10 to 15 mg/kg/day.
Children age 1 to 4: 10 to 20 mg/kg/day.
Children under age 1: 10 to 30 mg/kg/day.

All children's doses should be divided into equal amounts and given q 6 hours. Extended-release capsules not recommended for use in children.

✦ ***Dosage adjustment.*** Elderly patients may need dosage reduction. Adults with hepatic insufficiency or moderately impaired renal function should receive 100 mg P.O. q 6 hours or 200 mg (extended-release) q 12 hours. Patients with severe impaired renal function should receive only 100 mg (regular-release) at the following intervals:

Creatinine clearance (ml/min)	Dosage interval
30 to 40	q 8 hr
15 to 30	q 12 hr
< 15	q 24 hr

Pharmacodynamics
A class IA antiarrhythmic agent, disopyramide depresses phase O of the action potential. It is considered a myocardial depressant because it decreases myocardial excitability and conduction velocity and may depress myocardial contractility. It also possesses anticholinergic activity that may modify the drug's direct myocardial effects. In therapeutic doses, disopyramide reduces conduction velocity in the atria, ventricles, and His-Purkinje system. By prolonging the effective refractory period (ERP), it helps control atrial tachyarrhythmias (however, this indication is unapproved in the United States). Its anticholinergic action, which is much greater than quinidine's, may increase AV node conductivity.

Disopyramide also has a greater myocardial depressant (negative inotropic) effect than quinidine. It helps manage premature ventricular beats by suppressing automaticity in the His-Purkinje system and ectopic pacemakers. At therapeutic doses, it usually does not prolong the QRS segment duration and PR interval but may prolong the QT interval.

Pharmacokinetics
• *Absorption:* Disopyramide is rapidly and well absorbed from the GI tract; about 60% to 80% of drug reaches systemic circulation. Onset of action usually occurs in 30 minutes; peak blood levels occur approximately 2 hours after administration of conventional capsules and 5 hours after administration of extended-release capsules.
• *Distribution:* Drug is well distributed throughout extracellular fluid but is not extensively bound to tissues. Plasma protein binding varies, depending on drug concentration levels, but generally ranges from about 50% to 65%. Usual therapeutic serum level ranges from 2 to 4 mcg/ml, although some patients may require up to 7 mcg/ml. Levels above 9 mcg/ml generally are considered toxic.
• *Metabolism:* Metabolized in the liver to one major metabolite that possesses little antiarrhythmic activity but greater anticholinergic activity than the parent compound.
• *Excretion:* About 90% of an orally administered dose is excreted in the urine as unchanged drug and metabolites; 40% to 60% is excreted as unchanged drug. Usual elimination half-life is about

7 hours but lengthens in patients with renal or hepatic insufficiency. Duration of effect is usually 6 to 7 hours.

Contraindications and precautions
Contraindicated in patients with hypersensitivity to drug, cardiogenic shock, or second- or third-degree heart block in the absence of an artificial pacemaker.

Use very cautiously and avoid, if possible, in patients with heart failure. Use cautiously in patients with underlying conduction abnormalities, urinary tract diseases (especially prostatic hyperplasia), hepatic or renal impairment, myasthenia gravis, or acute angle-closure glaucoma.

Interactions
When used concomitantly, *other antiarrhythmic agents* may cause additive or antagonistic cardiac effects and additive toxicity. Concomitant use with *enzyme inducers*, such as *rifampin*, may impair disopyramide's antiarrhythmic activity. Concomitant use with *anticholinergic agents* may cause additive anticholinergic effects. Concomitant use with *warfarin* may potentiate anticoagulant effects. *Oral antidiabetic agents* or *insulin* may cause additive hypoglycemia. *Erythromycin* may increase disopyramide levels causing arrhythmias and increased QT intervals.

Effects on diagnostic tests
The physiologic effects of disopyramide may cause a decrease in blood glucose concentrations.

Adverse reactions
CNS: dizziness, agitation, depression, fatigue, muscle weakness, syncope.
CV: *hypotension, **heart failure,** heart block,* edema, weight gain, ***arrhythmias,*** shortness of breath, chest pain.
EENT: *blurred vision, dry eyes or nose.*
GI: nausea, vomiting, anorexia, bloating, abdominal pain, diarrhea.
Hepatic: cholestatic jaundice.
Skin: rash, pruritus, dermatosis.
Other: aches, pain, muscle weakness, hypoglycemia (rare).

Overdose and treatment
Clinical manifestations of overdose include anticholinergic effects, severe hypotension, widening of QRS complex and QT interval, ventricular arrhythmias, cardiac conduction disturbances, bradycardia, heart failure, asystole, loss of consciousness, seizures, apnea episodes, and respiratory arrest.

Treatment involves general supportive measures (including respiratory and CV support) and hemodynamic and ECG monitoring. If ingestion was recent, gastric lavage, emesis induction, and administration of activated charcoal may decrease absorption. Isoproterenol or dopamine may be administered to correct hypotension, after adequate hydration has been ensured. Digoxin and diuretics may be administered to treat heart failure. Hemodialysis and charcoal hemoperfusion may effectively remove disopyramide. Some patients may require intra-aortic balloon counterpulsation, mechanically assisted respiration, or endocardial pacing.

☑ Special considerations
- Correct underlying electrolyte abnormalities, especially hypokalemia, before administering drug, because disopyramide may be ineffective in patients with these problems.
- Do not give sustained-release capsules for rapid control of ventricular arrhythmias if therapeutic blood drug levels must be attained rapidly, or if patient has cardiomyopathy, possible cardiac decompensation, or severe renal impairment.
- Watch for signs of developing heart block, such as QRS complex widening by more than 25% or QT interval lengthening by more than 25% above baseline.
- Drug may cause hypoglycemia in some patients; monitor serum glucose levels in patients with altered serum glucose regulatory mechanisms.
- If drug causes constipation, administer laxatives and ensure proper diet.
- Drug is commonly prescribed for patients who cannot tolerate quinidine or procainamide.
- Patients with atrial flutter or fibrillation should be digitalized prior to disopyramide administration to ensure that enhanced AV conduction does not lead to ventricular tachycardia.
- Pharmacist may prepare disopyramide suspension; 100-mg capsules are used with cherry syrup to prepare suspension (this may be best form for young children).
- Drug is removed by hemodialysis. Dosage adjustments may be necessary in patients undergoing dialysis.

Patient education
- When changing from immediate-release to sustained-release capsules, advise patient to begin taking sustained-release capsule 6 hours after last immediate-release capsule.
- Teach patient importance of taking drug on time, exactly as prescribed. To do this, he may have to use an alarm clock for night doses.
- Advise patient to use sugarless gum or hard candy to relieve dry mouth.

Geriatric use
- Monitor closely for toxicity signs; also monitor serum electrolyte and drug levels.

Pediatric use
- Although drug's safety and effectiveness in children has not been established, current recommendations call for total daily dosage given in equally divided doses every 6 hours or at intervals based on individual requirements.
- Monitor pediatric patients during initial titration period; dose titration should begin at lower end of recommended ranges. Monitor serum drug levels and therapeutic response carefully.

Breast-feeding
- Drug is distributed into breast milk; recommend alternate infant feeding methods during drug therapy.

disulfiram
Antabuse

Pharmacologic classification: aldehyde dehydrogenase inhibitor
Therapeutic classification: alcoholic deterrent
Pregnancy risk category NR

How supplied
Available by prescription only
Tablets: 250 mg, 500 mg

Indications, route, and dosage
Adjunct in management of chronic alcoholism
Adults: Give maximum dose of 500 mg P.O. as a single dose in the morning for 1 to 2 weeks. Can be taken in evening if drowsiness occurs. Maintenance dosage is 125 to 500 mg daily (average dose 250 mg) until permanent self-control is established. Treatment may continue for months or years.

Pharmacodynamics
Antialcoholic action: Disulfiram irreversibly inhibits aldehyde dehydrogenase, which prevents the oxidation of alcohol after the acetaldehyde stage. It interacts with ingested alcohol to produce acetaldehyde levels five to ten times higher than are produced by normal alcohol metabolism. Excess acetaldehyde produces a highly unpleasant reaction (nausea and vomiting) to even a small quantity of alcohol. Tolerance to disulfiram does not occur; rather, sensitivity to alcohol increases with longer duration of therapy.

Pharmacokinetics
- *Absorption:* Disulfiram is absorbed completely after oral administration, but 3 to 12 hours may be required before effects occur. Toxic reactions to alcohol may occur up to 2 weeks after the last dose of disulfiram.
- *Distribution:* Drug is highly lipid-soluble and is initially localized in adipose tissue.
- *Metabolism:* Mostly oxidized in the liver and excreted in urine as free drug and metabolites (for example, diethyldithiocarbamate, diethylamine, and carbon disulfide).
- *Excretion:* 5% to 20% is unabsorbed and is eliminated in feces. A small amount is eliminated through the lungs, but most is excreted in the urine. Several days may be required for total elimination of drug.

Contraindications and precautions
Contraindicated in patients intoxicated by alcohol and within 12 hours of alcohol ingestion; in those with psychoses, myocardial disease, coronary occlusion, or hypersensitivity to disulfiram or to other thiuram derivatives used in pesticides and rubber vulcanization; and in patients receiving metronidazole, paraldehyde, alcohol, or alcohol-containing preparations.

Use with extreme caution in patients with diabetes mellitus, hypothyroidism, seizure disorder, cerebral damage, or nephritis or hepatic cirrhosis or insufficiency and with concurrent phenytoin therapy. Drug should not be administered during pregnancy.

Interactions
Disulfiram interferes with the metabolism of *alcohol, diazepam, chlordiazepoxide, barbiturates, coumarin anticoagulants, paraldehyde,* and *phenytoin;* therefore, it may increase the blood concentration of these drugs.

Disulfiram inhibits the metabolism of *caffeine,* greatly increasing its half-life. Exaggerated or prolonged effects of caffeine may occur.

Concomitant use of disulfiram with *metronidazole* can produce psychosis or confusion and should be avoided. Use with *isoniazid* may produce ataxia, unsteady gait, or marked behavioral changes and should be avoided.

Disulfiram has been reported to produce a synergistic CNS stimulation when used with *marijuana.*

Effects on diagnostic tests
Disulfiram may decrease urinary vanillylmandelic acid excretion and increase urinary concentrations of homovanillic acid. Decrease of ^{131}I; uptake or protein-bound iodine levels may occur rarely. Serum cholesterol levels may be elevated.

Adverse reactions
CNS: drowsiness, headache, fatigue, delirium, depression, neuritis, peripheral neuritis, polyneuritis, restlessness, psychotic reactions.
EENT: optic neuritis.
GI: metallic or garlic aftertaste.
GU: impotence.
Skin: acneiform or allergic dermatitis, occasional eruptions.
Other: disulfiram reaction (precipitated by ethanol use), which may include flushing, throbbing headache, dyspnea, nausea, copious vomiting, diaphoresis, thirst, chest pain, palpitations, hyperventilation, hypotension, syncope, anxiety, weakness, blurred vision, confusion, arthropathy. ***In severe reactions—respiratory depression, CV collapse, arrhythmias, MI, acute heart failure, seizures, unconsciousness, or death.***

Overdose and treatment
Overdose symptoms include GI upset and vomiting, abnormal EEG findings, drowsiness, altered consciousness, hallucinations, speech impairment, incoordination, and coma. Treat overdose or accidental over-ingestion by gastric aspiration or lavage along with supportive therapy.

Treatment of alcohol-induced disulfiram reaction is supportive and symptomatic. These reactions are not usually life-threatening. Emergency equipment and drugs should be available, because arrhythmias and severe hypotension may occur. Treat severe reactions like shock by administering plasma or electrolyte solutions as needed. Large I.V. doses of ascorbic acid, iron, and antihistamines have been used but are of questionable value. Hypokalemia has been reported; it requires careful monitoring and potassium supplements.

☑ Special considerations

- Drug use requires close medical supervision. Patients should clearly understand consequences of disulfiram therapy and give informed consent before use.
- Use drug only in patients who are cooperative and well motivated, and are receiving supportive psychiatric therapy.
- Complete physical examination and laboratory studies (CBC, electrolytes, transaminases) should precede therapy and be repeated regularly.
- Disulfiram should *not* be administered for at least 12 hours after the last alcohol ingestion.

Patient education

- Explain that although disulfiram can help discourage use of alcohol, it is not a cure for alcoholism.
- Inform patient of seriousness of disulfiram-alcohol reaction and the consequences of alcohol use.
- Warn patient to avoid all sources of alcohol: sauces or soups made with sherry or other wines or alcohol (even "cooking alcohol") and cough syrups. External applications of after-shave lotion, liniments, or other topical preparations may cause disulfiram reaction (because of the products' alcohol content).
- Tell patient that alcohol reaction may occur for up to 2 weeks after a single dose of disulfiram. The longer the disulfiram therapy, the more sensitive patient will be to alcohol.
- Warn patient that drug may cause drowsiness.
- Instruct patient to carry identification card stating that disulfiram is being used and including the phone number of the primary health care provider or clinic to contact if a reaction occurs.

dobutamine hydrochloride

Dobutrex

Pharmacologic classification: adrenergic, $beta_1$ agonist
Therapeutic classification: inotropic
Pregnancy risk category B

How supplied

Available by prescription only
Injection: 12.5 mg/ml in 20-ml vials (parenteral)

Indications, route, and dosage

To increase cardiac output in short-term treatment of cardiac decompensation caused by depressed contractility
Adults: 2.5 to 15 mcg/kg/minute as an I.V. infusion. Rarely, infusion rates up to 40 mcg/kg/minute may be needed. Titrate dosage carefully to patient response.

✦ ***Dosage adjustment.*** Elderly patients require lower doses because they may be more sensitive to drug's effects.

Pharmacodynamics

Inotropic action: Dobutamine selectively stimulates $beta_1$-adrenergic receptors to increase myocardial contractility and stroke volume, resulting in increased cardiac output (a positive inotropic effect in patients with normal hearts or in heart failure). At therapeutic doses, dobutamine decreases peripheral resistance (afterload), reduces ventricular filling pressure (preload), and may facilitate AV node conduction. Systolic blood pressure and pulse pressure may remain unchanged or increased from increased cardiac output. Increased myocardial contractility results in increased coronary blood flow and myocardial oxygen consumption. Heart rate usually remains unchanged; however, excessive doses do have chronotropic effects. Dobutamine does not appear to affect dopaminergic receptors, nor does it cause renal or mesenteric vasodilation; however, urine flow may increase because of increased cardiac output.

Pharmacokinetics

- *Absorption:* After I.V. administration, onset of action occurs within 2 minutes, with peak concentrations achieved within 10 minutes. Effects persist a few minutes after I.V. is discontinued.
- *Distribution:* Drug is widely distributed throughout the body.
- *Metabolism:* Dobutamine is metabolized by the liver and by conjugation to inactive metabolites.
- *Excretion:* Drug is excreted mainly in urine, with minor amounts in feces, as its metabolites and conjugates.

Contraindications and precautions

Contraindicated in patients with hypersensitivity to drug or its formulation and in those with idiopathic hypertrophic subaortic stenosis. Use cautiously in patients with a history of hypertension or after recent myocardial infarction. Drug may precipitate an exaggerated pressor response.

Interactions

Concomitant use with *inhalation hydrocarbon anesthetics*, especially *halothane* and *cyclopropane*, may trigger ventricular arrhythmias. *Beta-adrenergic blockers* may antagonize the cardiac effects of dobutamine, resulting in increased peripheral resistance and predominance of alpha-adrenergic effects.

Dobutamine may decrease the hypotensive effects of *guanadrel* and *guanethidine*; however, these agents may potentiate the pressor effects of dobutamine, possibly resulting in hypertension and arrhythmias. Concomitant use with *nitroprusside* may cause higher cardiac output and lower pulmonary wedge pressure. Theoretically, *rauwolfia alkaloids* may prolong the actions of dobutamine (a denervation supersensitivity response).

Effects on diagnostic tests

None reported.

Adverse reactions
CNS: headache.
CV: *increased heart rate,* ***hypertension, PVCs,*** angina, nonspecific chest pain, palpitations, hypotension.
GI: nausea, vomiting.
Respiratory: shortness of breath, ***asthmatic episodes.***
Other: phlebitis, hypersensitivity reactions ***(anaphylaxis).***

Overdose and treatment
Clinical manifestations of overdose include nervousness and fatigue. No treatment is necessary beyond dosage reduction or withdrawal of drug.

☑ Special considerations
Besides those relevant to all *adrenergics,* consider the following recommendations.
- Before administration of dobutamine, correct hypovolemia with appropriate plasma volume expanders.
- Monitor ECG, blood pressure, cardiac output, and pulmonary wedge pressure.
- Before giving dobutamine, administer a cardiac glycoside if patient has atrial fibrillation (dobutamine increases AV conduction).
- Most patients experience an increase of 10 to 20 mm Hg in systolic blood pressure; some show an increase of 50 mm Hg or more. Most also experience an increase in heart rate of 5 to 15 beats/minute; some show increases of 30 or more beats/minute. Premature ventricular arrhythmias may also occur in about 5% of patients. Dosage reduction may be necessary when these occur.
- Dose should be adjusted to meet individual needs and achieve desired clinical response. Drug must be administered by I.V. infusion using an infusion pump or other device to control flow rate.
- Concentration of infusion solution should not exceed 5,000 mcg/ml; the solution should be used within 24 hours. Rate and duration of infusion depend on patient response.
- Pink discoloration of solution indicates slight oxidation but no significant loss of potency.
- Dobutamine is incompatible with alkaline solution (sodium bicarbonate). Also, do not mix with or give through same I.V. line as heparin, hydrocortisone, cefazolin, cefamandole, or penicillin.

Patient education
- Advise patient to report adverse reactions.
- Inform patient that he'll need frequent monitoring of vital signs.

Geriatric use
- Use with caution in elderly patients.

Pediatric use
- Drug is not recommended for use in children. Safety and efficacy have not been established.

Breast-feeding
- It is unknown if dobutamine is excreted in breast milk. Administer cautiously to breast-feeding women.

docetaxel
Taxotere

Pharmacologic classification: taxoid
Therapeutic classification: antineoplastic
Pregnancy risk category D

How supplied
Available by prescription only
Injection: 20 mg, 80 mg

Indications, route, and dosage
Treatment of patients with locally advanced or metastatic breast cancer who have progressed during anthracycline-based therapy or have relapsed during anthracycline-based adjuvant therapy
Adults: 60 to 100 mg/m^2 I.V. over 1 hour q 3 weeks.

Pharmacodynamics
Antineoplastic action: Docetaxel acts by disrupting the microtubular network in cells that is essential for mitotic and interphase cellular functions.

Pharmacokinetics
- *Absorption:* Docetaxel is administered I.V.
- *Distribution:* Docetaxel is about 94% protein-bound.
- *Metabolism:* Docetaxel undergoes oxidative metabolism.
- *Excretion:* Docetaxel is eliminated primarily in feces with a small amount being eliminated in urine.

Contraindications and precautions
Contraindicated in patients with history of severe hypersensitivity to drug or other drugs formulated with polysorbate 80. Docetaxel should not be used in patients with neutrophil counts below 1,500 cells/mm^3.

Interactions
The metabolism of docetaxel may be modified by the concomitant administration of *compounds that induce, inhibit, or are metabolized by cytochrome P-450 3A4,* such as *cyclosporine, ketoconazole, erythromycin,* and *troleandomycin.* Use caution when administering these agents concomitantly with docetaxel.

Effects on diagnostic tests
None reported.

Adverse reactions
CNS: paresthesia, dysesthesia, pain (including burning sensation), weakness.
CV: fluid retention, hypotension.
GI: *stomatitis,* nausea, vomiting, diarrhea.
Hematologic: *anemia,* **NEUTROPENIA, FEBRILE NEUTROPENIA,** ***myelosuppression*** (dose-limiting), **LEUKOPENIA,** ***thrombocytopenia.***
Skin: *alopecia,* macropapular eruptions, desquamation, nail pigmentation alteration, onycholysis, nail pain, flushing, rash.
Other: hypersensitivity reactions, *infections,* chest tightness, back pain, dyspnea, drug fever, chills.

Overdose and treatment

Clinical manifestations of overdose may include bone marrow suppression, peripheral neurotoxicity, and mucositis. There is no known antidote for docetaxel. Patient should be kept in a specialized unit where vital functions can be closely monitored.

☑ Special considerations

- Patients with bilirubin values greater than the upper limits of normal (ULN) should generally not receive docetaxel. Also, patients with ALT or AST that exceeds 1.5 times ULN concomitant with alkaline phosphatase greater than 2.5 times ULN should generally not receive drug.
- All patients should be premedicated with oral corticosteroids such as dexamethasone 16 mg daily for 5 days starting 1 day before docetaxel administration to reduce the incidence and severity of fluid retention and hypersensitivity reactions.
- Docetaxel requires dilution before administration using the diluent supplied with drug. Allow drug and diluent to stand at room temperature for about 5 minutes before mixing. After adding the entire contents of diluent to the vial of docetaxel, gently rotate the vial for about 15 seconds. Then allow solution to stand for a few minutes to allow any foam that appeared to dissipate. It is not required that all foam dissipate before continuing the preparation process.
- To prepare the docetaxel infusion solution, aseptically withdraw the required amount of premix solution from the vial and inject into a 250-ml infusion bag or bottle of 0.9% NaCl solution or D_5W solution to produce a final concentration of 0.3 to 0.9 mg/ml. Doses exceeding 240 mg require a larger volume of infusion solution so that a concentration of 0.9 mg/ml of docetaxel is not exceeded. Thoroughly mix the infusion by manual rotation.
- Caution should be used during preparation and administration of docetaxel. Use of gloves is recommended. If solution contacts skin, wash skin immediately and thoroughly with soap and water. If docetaxel contacts mucous membranes, the membranes should be flushed thoroughly with water. Mark all waste materials with CHEMOTHERAPY HAZARD labels.
- Contact of the undiluted concentrate with plasticized polyvinyl chloride equipment or devices used to prepare solutions for infusion is not recommended. Prepare and store infusion solutions in bottles (glass, polypropylene) or plastic bags (polypropylene, polyolefin) and administer through polyethylene-lined administration sets.
- Patients who are dosed initially at 100 mg/m^2 and who experience either febrile neutropenia, a neutrophil count under 500 cells/mm^3 for more than 1 week, severe or cumulative cutaneous reactions, or severe peripheral neuropathy during docetaxel therapy should have dosage adjusted from 100 to 75 mg/m^2. If the patient continues to experience these reactions, dosage should either be decreased from 75 to 55 mg/m^2 or the treatment discontinued.
- Patients who are dosed initially at 60 mg/m^2 and who do not experience febrile neutropenia, a neutrophil count below 500 cells/mm^3 for more than 1 week, severe or cumulative cutaneous reactions, or severe peripheral neuropathy during docetaxel therapy may tolerate higher doses.
- Bone marrow toxicity is the most frequent and dose-limiting toxicity. Frequent blood count monitoring is necessary during therapy.
- Monitor patient closely for hypersensitivity reactions, especially during the first and second infusions. If minor reactions such as flushing or localized skin reactions occur, interruption of therapy is not required. More severe reactions require the immediate discontinuation of docetaxel and aggressive treatment.

Patient education

- Advise patient of childbearing age to avoid becoming pregnant during therapy with docetaxel because of the potential harm to the fetus.
- Warn patient that alopecia occurs in almost 80% of all patients.
- Tell patient to promptly report a sore throat or fever or unusual bruising or bleeding.

Pediatric use

- Safety and effectiveness in children under age 16 have not been established.

Breast-feeding

- Because of potential for serious adverse reactions in breast-fed infants, it is recommended that breast-feeding be discontinued during docetaxel therapy.

---

docusate calcium
Pro-Cal-Sof, Surfak

docusate potassium
Dialose, Diocto-K, Kasof

docusate sodium
Colace, Diocto, Dioeze, Diosuccin, Disonate, DOK, DOS, Doxinate, D-S-S, Duosol, Modane Soft, Pro-Sof, Regulax SS, Regulex*, Regutol, Theravac-SB

Pharmacologic classification: surfactant
Therapeutic classification: emollient laxative
Pregnancy risk category C

How supplied

Available without a prescription
Tablets: 50 mg, 100 mg
Capsules: 50 mg, 60 mg, 100 mg, 120 mg, 240 mg, 250 mg, 300 mg
Syrup: 50 mg/15 ml, 60 mg/15 ml
Liquid: 150 mg/15 ml
Solution: 50 mg/ml

Indications, route, and dosage

Stool softener
docusate sodium
Adults and children age 12 and older: 50 to 200 mg P.O. daily until bowel movements are normal. Alternatively, add 50 to 100 mg to saline or oil retention enema to treat fecal impaction.
Children age 6 to 12: 40 to 120 mg P.O. daily.

Children age 3 to 6: 20 to 60 mg P.O. daily.
Children under age 3: 10 to 40 mg P.O. daily.
docusate calcium or potassium
Adults: 240 mg (calcium) or 100 to 300 mg (potassium) P.O. daily until bowel movements are normal. Higher doses are for initial therapy. Adjust dose to individual response.
Children age 6 and older: 50 to 150 mg (calcium) or 100 mg (potassium) P.O. daily.

Pharmacodynamics
Laxative action: Docusate salts act as detergents in the intestine, reducing surface tension of interfacing liquids; this promotes incorporation of fat and additional liquid, softening the stool.

Pharmacokinetics
- *Absorption:* Docusate salts are absorbed minimally in the duodenum and jejunum; drug acts in 1 to 3 days.
- *Distribution:* Docusate salts are distributed primarily locally, in the gut.
- *Metabolism:* None.
- *Excretion:* Docusate salts are excreted in feces.

Contraindications and precautions
Contraindicated in patients hypersensitive to drug and in those with intestinal obstruction, undiagnosed abdominal pain, vomiting or other signs of appendicitis, fecal impaction, or acute surgical abdomen.

Interactions
Docusate salts may increase absorption of *mineral oil.*

Effects on diagnostic tests
None reported.

Adverse reactions
GI: bitter taste, mild abdominal cramping, diarrhea, laxative dependence (with long-term or excessive use).

Overdose and treatment
No information available.

☑ Special considerations
- Liquid or syrup must be given in 6 to 8 oz (180 to 240 ml) of milk or fruit juice or in infant's formula to prevent throat irritation.
- After administration of liquid through nasogastric tube, tube should be flushed afterward to clear it and ensure dispersion into stomach.
- Avoid using docusate sodium in sodium-restricted patients.
- Docusate salts are available in combination with casanthranol (Peri-Colace), senna (Senokot, Gentlax), and phenolphthalein (Ex-Lax, Feen-a-Mint, Correctol).
- Docusate salts are the preferred laxative for most patients who must avoid straining at stool, such as those recovering from MI or rectal surgery. They also are used commonly to treat patients with postpartum constipation.
- Docusate salts are less likely than other laxatives to cause laxative dependence; however, their effectiveness may decrease with long-term use.

Patient education
- Docusate salts lose their effectiveness over time; advise patient to report failure of medication.

Geriatric use
- Docusate salts are good choices for elderly patients because they rarely cause laxative dependence and cause fewer adverse effects and are gentler than some other laxatives.

Breast-feeding
- Because absorption of docusate salts is minimal, they presumably pose no risk to breast-feeding infants.

dolasetron mesylate
Anzemet

Pharmacologic classification: selective serotonin 5-HT_3 receptor antagonist
Therapeutic classification: antinauseant, antiemetic
Pregnancy risk category B

How supplied
Available by prescription only
Tablets: 50 mg, 100 mg
Injection: 20 mg/ml as 12.5 mg/0.625 ml ampules or 100 mg/5 ml vials

Indications, route, and dosage
Prevention of nausea and vomiting associated with cancer chemotherapy
Adults: 100 mg P.O. given as a single dose 1 hour before chemotherapy, or 1.8 mg/kg as a single I.V. dose given 30 minutes before chemotherapy, or a fixed dose of 100 mg I.V. given 30 minutes before chemotherapy.
Children age 2 to 16: 1.8 mg/kg P.O. given 1 hour before chemotherapy, or 1.8 mg/kg as a single I.V. dose given 30 minutes before chemotherapy. Injectable form can be mixed with apple or apple-grape juice and administered P.O. 1 hour before chemotherapy. Maximum daily dose of 100 mg.
Prevention of postoperative nausea and vomiting
Adults: 100 mg P.O. within 2 hours before surgery; 12.5 mg as a single I.V. dose approximately 15 minutes before cessation of anesthesia.
Children age 2 to 16: 1.2 mg/kg P.O. given within 2 hours before surgery, up to maximum of 100 mg; or 0.35 mg/kg (up to 12.5 mg) given as a single I.V. dose approximately 15 minutes before the cessation of anesthesia. Injectable form (1.2 mg/kg up to 100-mg dose) can be mixed with apple or apple-grape juice and administered P.O. 2 hours before surgery.
Treatment of postoperative nausea and vomiting (I.V. form only)
Adults: 12.5 mg as a single I.V. dose as soon as nausea or vomiting presents.

Children age 2 to 16: 0.35 mg/kg, up to a maximum dose of 12.5 mg, given as a single I.V. dose as soon as nausea or vomiting occurs.

Pharmacodynamics

Antinauseant and antiemetic action: A selective serotonin 5-HT_3 receptor antagonist that blocks the action of serotonin. 5HT_3 receptors are located on the nerve terminals of the vagus nerve in the periphery and in the central chemoreceptor trigger zone. Blocking the activity of the serotonin receptors prevents serotonin from stimulating the vomiting reflex.

Pharmacokinetics

- *Absorption:* Orally administered dolasetron, injection, the I.V. solution, and tablets are bioequivalent. Oral dolasetron is well absorbed, although parent drug is rarely detected in plasma due to rapid and complete metabolism to the most clinically relevant metabolite, hydrodolasetron.
- *Distribution:* Widely distributed in the body, with a mean apparent volume of distribution of 5.8 L/kg; 69% to 77% of hydrodolasetron is bound to plasma protein.
- *Metabolism:* A ubiquitous enzyme, carbonyl reductase, mediates the reduction of dolasetron to hydrodolasetron. Cytochrome P-450 (CYP)2D6 and CYP3A are responsible for subsequent hydroxylation and N-oxidation of hydrodolasetron, respectively.
- *Excretion:* Two-thirds of dose is excreted in the urine and one third in the feces. Mean elimination half-life of hydrodolasetron is 8.1 hours.

Contraindications and precautions

Contraindicated in patients hypersensitive to drug.

Use drug cautiously in patients with or at risk for developing prolonged cardiac conduction intervals, particularly QTc. These include patients taking antiarrhythmic drugs or other drugs which lead to QT prolongation; hypokalemia or hypomagnesemia; a potential for electrolyte abnormalities, including those receiving diuretics; congenital QT syndrome; and those who have received cumulative high-dose anthracycline therapy.

Interactions

Administration with *drugs that prolong ECG intervals* (such as *antiarrhythmic drugs*) can increase the risk of arrhythmias. Monitor patient closely.

Drugs that *inhibit the P-450 enzymes* (such as *cimetidine*) can increase hydrodolasetron levels. Monitor patient for adverse effects.

Drugs that *induce the P-450 enzymes* (such as *rifampin*) may decrease hydrodolasetron levels. Monitor patient for decreased efficacy of antiemetic.

Effects on diagnostic tests

None reported.

Adverse reactions

CNS: *headache*, dizziness, drowsiness, fatigue.
CV: ***arrhythmia,*** ECG changes, hypotension, hypertension, tachycardia, bradycardia.
GI: *diarrhea*, dyspepsia, abdominal pain, constipation, anorexia.
GU: oliguria, urinary retention.
Skin: pruritus, rash.
Other: fever, elevation of liver function tests, chills, pain at injection site.

Overdose and treatment

There is no specific antidote for dolasetron overdose; provide supportive care. It is not known if drug is removed by hemodialysis or peritoneal dialysis.

☑ Special considerations

- Safety and efficacy of multiple drug doses have not been evaluated. Efficacy studies have all been conducted with single doses of drug.
- **I.V. use:** Injection can be infused as rapidly as 100 mg/30 seconds or diluted in 50 ml compatible solution and infused over 15 minutes.
- Injection for oral administration is stable in apple or apple-grape juice for 2 hours at room temperature.

Patient education

- Inform patient that oral doses of drug must be taken 1 to 2 hours before surgery or 1 hour before chemotherapy to be effective.
- Teach patient about potential adverse effects.
- Instruct patient not to mix injection in juice for oral administration until just before dosing.
- Tell patient to report if nausea or vomiting occurs.

Geriatric use

- Dosage adjustment is not needed in patients over age 65.
- Effectiveness in prevention on nausea and vomiting in elderly patients was no different that in younger age groups.

Pediatric use

- There is no experience in pediatric patients under 2 years of age.
- Efficacy information in pediatric patients age 2 to 17 receiving cancer chemotherapy are consistent with those obtained in adults.
- No efficacy information was collected in the pediatric postoperative nausea and vomiting studies.

Breast-feeding

- It is not known if drug is excreted in breast milk. Use caution when administering drug to breast-feeding patient.

donepezil hydrochloride

Aricept

Pharmacologic classification: acetylcholinesterase inhibitor
Therapeutic classification: cholinomimetic
Pregnancy risk category C

How supplied

Available by prescription only
Tablets: 5 mg, 10 mg

Indications, route, and dosage

Mild to moderate dementia of the Alzheimer's type

Adults: Initially, 5 mg P.O. daily h.s. After 4 to 6 weeks, dosage may be increased to 10 mg daily.

Pharmacodynamics

Anticholinesterase action: Drug is believed to inhibit the enzyme acetylcholinesterase in the CNS, increasing the concentration of acetylcholine and temporarily improving cognitive function in patients with Alzheimer's disease. Drug does not alter the course of the underlying disease process.

Pharmacokinetics

- *Absorption:* Donepezil is well absorbed with a relative bioavailability of 100% and reaches peak plasma concentrations in 3 to 4 hours. Steady state is reached within 15 days.
- *Distribution:* Steady state volume of distribution is 12 L/kg. Donepezil is approximately 96% bound to plasma proteins, mainly to albumins (about 75%) and alpha$_1$-acid glycoprotein (about 21%) over the concentration range of 2 to 1,000 ng/ml.
- *Metabolism:* Extensively metabolized to four major metabolites (two are known to be active) and several minor metabolites (not all have been identified). Donepezil is metabolized by CYP 450 isoenzymes 2D6 and 3A4 and undergoes glucuronidation.
- *Excretion:* Drug is both excreted in the urine intact and extensively metabolized by the liver. Elimination half-life is about 70 hours and mean apparent plasma clearance is 0.13 L/hour/kg. About 17% of drug is eliminated by the kidneys as unchanged drug.

Contraindications and precautions

Contraindicated in patients with known hypersensitivity to drug or to piperidine derivatives. Use very cautiously in patients with "sick sinus syndrome" or other supraventricular cardiac conduction conditions because drug may cause bradycardia. Use cautiously in patients with CV disease, asthma, or history of ulcer disease and in those taking NSAIDs.

Interactions

Concurrent use with *anticholinergics* may interfere with anticholinergic activity. *Carbamazepine, dexamethasone, rifampin, phenytoin,* and *phenobarbital* may increase rate of elimination of donepezil. Monitor patient.

Cholinomimetics and *cholinesterase inhibitors* may produce synergistic effect. Monitor patient closely. Concomitant use with *succinylcholine* or *bethanechol* may produce additive effects. Monitor patient closely.

Effects on diagnostic tests

None reported.

Adverse reactions

CNS: abnormal dreams or crying, aggression, aphasia, ataxia, dizziness, depression, *headache, insomnia,* irritability, nervousness, paresthesia, restlessness, somnolence, seizures, tremor, vertigo.
CV: atrial fibrillation, chest pain, hypertension, vasodilation, hypotension, syncope.
EENT: blurred vision, cataract, eye irritation.
GI: anorexia, bloating, *diarrhea,* epigastric pain, fecal incontinence, GI bleeding, *nausea,* vomiting.
GU: frequent urination, hot flashes, nocturia.
Hematologic: ecchymosis.
Musculoskeletal: arthritis, bone fracture, muscle cramps, toothache.
Respiratory: bronchitis, dyspnea, sore throat.
Skin: diaphoresis, pruritus, urticaria.
Other: accident, dehydration, fatigue, increased libido, influenza, pain, weight loss.

Overdose and treatment

Overdosage can result in cholinergic crisis characterized by severe nausea, vomiting, salivation, sweating, bradycardia, hypotension, respiratory depression, collapse, and seizures. Increasing muscle weakness may also occur and may result in death if respiratory muscles are involved. Tertiary anticholinergics such as atropine may be used as an antidote for drug overdosage. I.V. atropine sulfate titrated to effect is recommended; give an initial dose of 1 to 2 mg I.V. and base subsequent doses on response. Atypical responses in blood pressure and heart rate have been reported with other cholinomimetics when co-administered with quaternary anticholinergics such as glycopyrrolate. It is not known if donepezil or its metabolites can be removed by dialysis.

☑ Special considerations

- Syncopal episodes have been reported with drug use.
- Drug may increase gastric acid secretion owing to increased cholinergic activity. Closely monitor patients at increased risk for developing ulcers (such as those with history of ulcer disease or those receiving NSAIDs) for symptoms of active or occult GI bleeding.
- Diarrhea, nausea, and vomiting occur more frequently with the 10-mg dose than with the 5-mg dose. These effects are mostly mild and transient, sometimes lasting 1 to 3 weeks, and resolve during continued drug therapy.
- Although not observed in clinical trials, drug may cause bladder outflow obstruction.
- Cholinomimetics have potential to cause generalized seizures. However, seizure activity also may be due to Alzheimer's disease.

Patient education

- Explain to patient and caregiver that drug does not alter disease but can alleviate symptoms. Effects of therapy depend on drug administration at regular intervals.
- Tell caregiver to give drug in the evening, just before bedtime.
- Advise patient and caregiver to immediately report significant adverse effects or changes in overall health status.
- Tell patient and caregiver to inform healthcare team that patient takes drug before he receives anesthesia.

Geriatric use

• Mean plasma drug levels of elderly patients with Alzheimer's disease are comparable with those observed in young healthy volunteers.

Pediatric use

• Safety and efficacy in children have not been established.

Breast-feeding

• It is not known whether donepezil is excreted in breast milk. Avoid use of donepezil in breast-feeding patients.

dopamine hydrochloride

Intropin

Pharmacologic classification: adrenergic
Therapeutic classification: inotropic, vasopressor
Pregnancy risk category C

How supplied

Available by prescription only
Injection: 40 mg/ml, 80 mg/ml, and 160 mg/ml parenteral concentrate for injection for I.V. infusion; 0.8 mg/ml (200 or 400 mg) in D_5W 1.6 mg/ml (400 or 800 mg) in D_5W, and 3.2 mg/ml (800 mg) in D_5W parenteral injection for I.V. infusion

Indications, route, and dosage

Adjunct in shock to increase cardiac output, blood pressure, and urine flow
Adults: 1 to 5 mcg/kg/minute I.V. infusion, up to 20 - 50 mcg/kg/minute. Infusion rate may be increased by 1 to 4 mcg/kg/minute at 10- to 30-minute intervals until optimum response is achieved. In severely ill patient, infusion may begin at 5 mcg/kg/minute and gradually increase by increments of 5 to 10 mcg/kg/minute until optimum response is achieved.
Short-term treatment of severe, refractory, chronic heart failure
Adults: Initially, 0.5 to 2 mcg/kg/minute I.V. infusion. Dosage may be increased until desired renal response occurs. Average dosage, 1 to 3 mcg/kg/minute.

Pharmacodynamics

Vasopressor action: An immediate precursor of norepinephrine, dopamine stimulates dopaminergic, beta-adrenergic, and alpha-adrenergic receptors of the sympathetic nervous system. The main effects produced are dose-dependent. It has a direct stimulating effect on $beta_1$ receptors (in I.V. doses of 2 to 10 mcg/kg/minute) and little or no effect on $beta_2$ receptors. In I.V. doses of 0.5 to 2 mcg/kg/minute it acts on dopaminergic receptors, causing vasodilation in the renal, mesenteric, coronary, and intracerebral vascular beds; in I.V. doses above 10 mcg/kg/minute, it stimulates alpha receptors.

Low to moderate doses result in cardiac stimulation (positive inotropic effects) and renal and mesenteric vasodilation (dopaminergic response). High doses result in increased peripheral resistance and renal vasoconstriction.

Pharmacokinetics

• *Absorption:* Onset of action after I.V. administration occurs within 5 minutes and persists for less than 10 minutes.
• *Distribution:* Drug is widely distributed throughout the body; however, it does not cross the blood-brain barrier.
• *Metabolism:* Dopamine is metabolized to inactive compounds in the liver, kidneys, and plasma by MAO and catechol-O-methyltransferase. About 25% is metabolized to norepinephrine within adrenergic nerve terminals.
• *Excretion:* Drug is excreted in urine, mainly as its metabolites.

Contraindications and precautions

Contraindicated in patients with uncorrected tachyarrhythmias, pheochromocytoma, or ventricular fibrillation. Use cautiously in patients with occlusive vascular disease, cold injuries, diabetic endarteritis, and arterial embolism; in those taking MAO inhibitors; and in pregnant women.

Interactions

Concomitant use with *MAO inhibitors* may prolong and intensify the effects of dopamine. Use with *beta blockers* antagonizes the cardiac effects of dopamine; use with *alpha blockers* may antagonize the peripheral vasoconstriction caused by high doses of dopamine.

Combined use with *general anesthetics,* especially *halothane* and *cyclopropane,* may cause ventricular arrhythmias and hypertension. Use with I.V. *phenytoin* may cause hypotension and bradycardia; use with *diuretics* increases diuretic effects of both agents. Use with *oxytocics* may cause advanced vasoconstriction. Dosage adjustments may be needed.

Effects on diagnostic tests

Dopamine may cause elevated urinary catecholamine levels. Drug may also cause increased serum glucose levels although level usually doesn't rise above normal limits.

Adverse reactions

CNS: headache.
CV: ectopic beats, tachycardia, anginal pain, palpitations, *hypotension;* bradycardia, conduction disturbances, hypertension, vasoconstriction, widening of QRS complex (less frequently).
GI: nausea, vomiting.
Other: necrosis and tissue sloughing with extravasation, piloerection, dyspnea, ***anaphylactic reactions, asthmatic episodes,*** azotemia.

Overdose and treatment

Clinical manifestations of overdose include excessive, severe hypertension. No treatment is necessary beyond dosage reduction or withdrawal of drug. If that fails to lower blood pressure, a short-acting alpha-adrenergic blocking agent may be helpful.

☑ Special considerations

Besides those relevant to all *adrenergics*, consider the following recommendations.

- Hypovolemia should be corrected with appropriate plasma volume expanders before administration of dopamine.
- Dopamine is administered by I.V. infusion using an infusion device to control rate of flow.
- Administer drug into a large vein to prevent the possibility of extravasation. If necessary to administer in hand or ankle veins, change injection site to larger vein as soon as possible. Monitor continuously for free flow. Central venous access is recommended.
- Adjust dose to meet individual needs of patient and to achieve desired clinical response. If dose required to obtain desired systolic blood pressure exceeds optimum rate of renal response, reduce dose as soon as hemodynamic condition is stabilized.
- Severe hypotension may result with abrupt withdrawal of infusion; therefore, reduce dose gradually.
- If extravasation occurs, stop infusion and infiltrate site promptly with 10 to 15 ml NaCl injection containing 5 to 10 mg of phentolamine. Use syringe with a fine needle, and infiltrate area liberally with phentolamine solution.
- Do not mix other drugs in dopamine solutions. Discard solutions after 24 hours.
- Monitor blood pressure, cardiac output, ECG, and intake and output during infusion, especially if dose exceeds 20 mcg/kg/minute. Watch for cold extremities.

Patient education

- Advise patient to report adverse reactions.
- Inform patient of need for frequent monitoring of his vital signs and condition.

Geriatric use

- Lower doses are indicated because elderly patients may be more sensitive to drug's effects.

dornase alfa

Pulmozyme

Pharmacologic classification: recombinant human deoxyribonuclease I, a mucolytic enzyme
Therapeutic classification: respiratory inhalant
Pregnancy risk category B

How supplied

Available by prescription only
Inhalation solution: 2.5 ml ampule containing 1 mg/ml dornase alfa

Indications, route, and dosage

To improve pulmonary function and reduce the frequency of moderate to severe respiratory infections in patients with cystic fibrosis (CF)

Adults and children age 5 and over: One ampule (2.5 mg/2.5 ml) inhaled once daily. Treatment usually takes 10 to 15 minutes. Use drug only with an approved nebulizer. Patients over age 21 and those with a baseline forced vital capacity greater than 85% may require twice-daily dosing.

Pharmacodynamics

Respiratory inhalant action: Dornase alfa is a purified solution of recombinant human deoxyribonuclease I, an enzyme that selectively breaks down DNA. Patients with CF retain thick, purulent pulmonary secretions rich in extracellular DNA. Dornase alfa hydrolyzes the excess DNA, reducing sputum viscosity.

Pharmacokinetics

- *Absorption:* After inhalation, drug achieves a mean sputum concentration of 3 mcg/ml within 15 minutes, declining to an average of 0.6 mcg/ml within 2 hours.
- *Distribution:* No information available.
- *Metabolism:* No information available.
- *Excretion:* No information available.

Contraindications and precautions

Contraindicated in patients hypersensitive to drug or Chinese hamster ovary cell-derived products.

Interactions

None reported.

Effects on diagnostic tests

None reported.

Adverse reactions

EENT: *pharyngitis, voice alteration,* laryngitis, conjunctivitis.
Skin: *rash,* urticaria.
Other: *chest pain.*

Overdose and treatment

CF patients have received up to 20 mg twice daily for up to 6 days and 10 mg twice daily intermittently (2 weeks on, 2 weeks off) for 168 days. These doses were well tolerated.

☑ Special considerations

- Mixing dornase alfa with other drugs in the nebulizer could cause adverse changes in one or both drugs.
- Drug should be used in conjunction with standard therapies prescribed for CF.
- Safety and efficacy of daily administration have not been demonstrated in patients with forced vital capacity less than 40% of the predicted value or for longer than 12 months.

Patient education

- Inform patient to store drug in refrigerator at 36° to 46° F (2° to 8° C) and protect it from strong light. It should be refrigerated during transport and should not be exposed to room temperatures for a total time of 24 hours.
- Tell patient to discard solution if it is cloudy or discolored.

- Inform patient that drug contains no preservative and, once opened, the entire ampule must be used or discarded.
- Instruct patient in the proper use and maintenance of the nebulizer and compressor system used in its delivery.

Pediatric use
- Safety and efficacy of daily administration have not been demonstrated in patients under age 5.

Breast-feeding
- It is not known if drug occurs in breast milk. Use cautiously when administering drug to breast-feeding women.

dorzolamide hydrochloride
Trusopt

Pharmacologic classification: sulfonamide
Therapeutic classification: antiglaucoma
Pregnancy risk category C

How supplied
Available by prescription only
Ophthalmic solution: 2%

Indications, route, and dosage
Treatment of increased intraocular pressure in patients with ocular hypertension or open-angle glaucoma
Adults: Instill 1 drop in the conjunctival sac of affected eye t.i.d.

Pharmacodynamics
Antiglaucoma action: Dorzolamide inhibits carbonic anhydrase in the ciliary processes of the eye, which decreases aqueous humor secretion, presumably by slowing the formation of bicarbonate ions with subsequent reduction in sodium and fluid transport. The result is a reduction in intraocular pressure.

Pharmacokinetics
- *Absorption:* Dorzolamide reaches the systemic circulation when applied topically.
- *Distribution:* Drug accumulates in RBCs during chronic dosing as a result of binding to carbonic anhydrase II.
- *Metabolism:* Unknown.
- *Excretion:* Drug is primarily excreted unchanged in urine.

Contraindications and precautions
Contraindicated in patients with hypersensitivity to any component of drug or in those with impaired renal function. Use cautiously in patients with impaired hepatic function.

Interactions
Oral carbonic anhydrase inhibitors pose the potential for additive effects. Do not administer concomitantly.

Effects on diagnostic tests
None reported.

Adverse reactions
EENT: *ocular burning, stinging, discomfort; superficial punctate keratitis; ocular allergic reactions; blurred vision; lacrimation; dryness; photophobia;* iridocyclitis.
Other: *bitter taste,* headache, nausea, asthenia, fatigue, rash, urolithiasis.

Overdose and treatment
Overdosage may result in electrolyte imbalance, acidosis, and possible CNS effects. Serum electrolyte levels (especially potassium) and blood pH levels should be monitored. Treatment is supportive.

☑ Special considerations
- Because dorzolamide is a sulfonamide and is absorbed systemically, the same types of adverse reactions that are attributable to sulfonamides may occur with topical administration of dorzolamide.
- If signs of serious adverse reactions or hypersensitivity occur, drug should be discontinued.

Patient education
- Instruct patient that if more than one topical ophthalmic drug is being used, they should be administered at least 10 minutes apart.
- Teach patient how to instill drops. Advise him to wash hands before and after instilling solution, and warn him not to touch dropper or tip to eye or surrounding tissue.
- Advise patient to apply light finger pressure on lacrimal sac for 1 minute after instillation to minimize systemic absorption of drug.
- Tell patient that the same types of adverse reactions that are attributable to sulfonamides may occur with topical administration. If signs of serious adverse reactions or hypersensitivity occur, tell patient to discontinue the drug and call immediately.
- Inform patient to report ocular reactions, particularly conjunctivitis and lid reactions, and discontinue drug.
- Tell patient not to wear soft contact lenses while using drug.
- Stress importance of compliance with recommended therapy.

Geriatric use
- Use with caution because greater sensitivity to drug may occur in older adults.

Pediatric use
- Safety and effectiveness in children have not been established.

Breast-feeding
- It is not known if drug is excreted into breast milk. Because of the risk for serious adverse reactions to the breast-fed infant, its use in breast-feeding women is not recommended.

doxacurium chloride

Nuromax

Pharmacologic classification: nondepolarizing neuromuscular blocker
Therapeutic classification: skeletal muscle relaxant
Pregnancy risk category C

How supplied

Available by prescription only
Injection: 1 mg/ml

Indications, route, and dosage

To provide skeletal muscle relaxation for endotracheal intubation and during surgery as an adjunct to general anesthesia

Adults: Dosage is highly individualized; 0.05 mg/kg rapid I.V. produces adequate conditions for endotracheal intubation in 5 minutes in about 90% of patients when used as part of a thiopental-narcotic induction technique. Lower doses may require longer delay before intubation is possible. Neuromuscular blockade at this dose lasts an average of 100 minutes.

Children over age 2: Dosage is highly individualized; an initial dose of 0.03 mg/kg I.V. administered during halothane anesthesia produces effective blockade in 7 minutes and has a duration of 30 minutes. Under the same conditions, 0.05 mg/kg produces a blockade in 4 minutes and lasts 45 minutes.

Maintenance of neuromuscular blockade during long procedures

Adults and children over age 2: After initial dose of 0.05 mg/kg I.V., maintenance dosages of 0.005 and 0.01 mg/kg will prolong neuromuscular blockade for an average of 30 minutes and 45 minutes, respectively. Children usually require more frequent administration of maintenance dosages.

✦ ***Dosage adjustment.*** Adjust dosage to ideal body weight in obese patients (patients whose weight is 30% or more above their ideal weight) to avoid prolonged neuromuscular blockade.

Pharmacodynamics

Skeletal muscle relaxant action: Doxacurium binds competitively to cholinergic receptors on the motor end-plate to antagonize the action of acetylcholine, resulting in a block of neuromuscular transmission.

Pharmacokinetics

- *Absorption:* First signs of neuromuscular blockade occur within about 2 minutes following I.V. administration. Maximum effects occur in about 3 to 6 minutes.
- *Distribution:* Plasma protein binding of drug is approximately 30% in human plasma.
- *Metabolism:* Doxacurium is thought not to be metabolized.
- *Excretion:* Drug is primarily eliminated as unchanged drug in urine and bile.

Contraindications and precautions

Contraindicated in patients with hypersensitivity to drug and in neonates. Drug contains benzyl ethanol, which has been associated with death in newborns.

Use cautiously, perhaps at a reduced dose, in debilitated patients; in patients with metastatic cancer, severe electrolyte disturbances, or neuromuscular diseases; and in those in whom potentiation or difficulty in reversal of neuromuscular blockade is anticipated. Patients with myasthenia gravis or myasthenic syndrome (Eaton-Lambert syndrome) are particularly sensitive to the effects of nondepolarizing relaxants. Shorter-acting agents are recommended for use in such patients.

Interactions

Isoflurane, enflurane, and *halothane* decrease the ED_{50} (the effective dose required to produce a 50% suppression of the response to ulnar nerve stimulation) of doxacurium by 30% to 45%. These agents also may prolong the clinically effective duration of action of doxacurium by up to 25%.

The neuromuscular blocking action of doxacurium may be enhanced by certain *antibiotics* (such as *aminoglycosides, tetracyclines, bacitracin, polymyxins, lincomycin, clindamycin, colistin,* and *colistimethate sodium), magnesium salts, lithium, local anesthetics, procainamide,* and *quinidine.*

Phenytoin and *carbamazepine* delay onset of neuromuscular blockade induced by doxacurium and shorten its duration.

Effects on diagnostic tests

None reported.

Adverse reactions

Respiratory: dyspnea, respiratory depression, ***respiratory insufficiency or apnea.***
Other: prolonged muscle weakness.

Overdose and treatment

Overdosage with neuromuscular blocking agents such as doxacurium may result in neuromuscular block beyond the time needed for surgery and anesthesia. The primary treatment is maintenance of a patent airway and controlled ventilation until recovery of normal neuromuscular function is assured. Once initial evidence of recovery is observed, further recovery may be facilitated by administration of an anticholinesterase agent (such as neostigmine or edrophonium) in conjunction with an appropriate anticholinergic agent.

☑ Special considerations

- All times of onset and duration of neuromuscular blockade are averages; considerable individual variation in dosages is normal.
- As with other nondepolarizing neuromuscular blocking agents, a reduction in dosage of doxacurium must be considered in cachectic or debilitated patients; in patients with neuromuscular diseases, severe electrolyte abnormalities, or carcinomatosis; and in other patients in whom potentiation of neuromuscular block or difficulty with reversal is anticipated. Increased doses of doxacurium may be required in burn patients.

• Drug has no effect on consciousness or pain threshold. To avoid distress to the patient, it should not be administered until patient's consciousness is obtunded by general anesthetic.
• Drug may prolong neuromuscular block in patients undergoing renal transplantation, and onset and duration of the block may vary with patients undergoing liver transplantation.
• Use drug only under direct medical supervision by personnel familiar with the use of neuromuscular blocking agents and techniques involved in maintaining a patent airway. Do not use unless facilities and equipment for mechanical ventilation, oxygen therapy, and intubation and an antagonist are within reach.
• Use of a peripheral nerve stimulator will permit the most advantageous use of doxacurium, minimize the possibility of overdosage or underdosage, and assist in the evaluation of recovery.
• Doxacurium is acidic (pH 3.9 to 5.0) and may not be compatible with alkaline solutions having a pH above 8.5 (for example, barbiturate solutions).
• Doxacurium diluted up to 1:10 in D_5W injection, USP or 0.9% NaCl injection, USP, has been shown to be physically and chemically stable when stored in polypropylene syringes at 41° to 77° F (5° to 25° C) for up to 24 hours. Because dilution diminishes the preservative effectiveness of benzyl alcohol, aseptic techniques should be used to prepare the diluted product. Immediate use of the diluted product is preferred, and any unused portion should be discarded after 8 hours.

Geriatric use
• Elderly patients may be more sensitive to the drug's effects. They may experience a slower onset of the blockade and a longer duration.

Pediatric use
• Drug use has not been studied in children younger than age 2.

Breast-feeding
• It is not known if drug is excreted in breast milk. Because many drugs are excreted in breast milk, use with caution when administering to breast-feeding patients.

doxapram hydrochloride
Dopram

Pharmacologic classification: analeptic
Therapeutic classification: CNS and respiratory stimulant
Pregnancy risk category B

How supplied
Available by prescription only
Injection: 20 mg/ml (benzyl alcohol 0.9%)

Indications, route, and dosage
Postanesthesia respiratory stimulation
Adults: 0.5 to 1 mg/kg of body weight as a single I.V. injection (not to exceed 1.5 mg/kg) or as multiple injections q 5 minutes, not to exceed 2 mg/kg total dosage. Alternatively, 250 mg in 250 ml of 0.9% NaCl solution or D_5W infused at an initial rate of 5 mg/minute I.V. until a satisfactory response is achieved. Maintain at 1 to 3 mg/minute. Recommended total dosage for infusion should not exceed 4 mg/kg.
Drug-induced CNS depression
Adults: For injection, priming dose of 2 mg/kg I.V. repeated in 5 minutes and again q 1 to 2 hours until patient awakens (and if relapse occurs). Maximum daily dosage is 3 g.

For infusion, priming dose of 2 mg/kg I.V., repeated in 5 minutes and again in 1 to 2 hours if needed. If response occurs, give I.V. infusion (1 mg/ml) at 1 to 3 mg/minute until patient awakens. Do not infuse for longer than 2 hours or administer more than 3 g/day. May resume I.V. infusion after a rest period of 30 minutes to 2 hours, if needed.
Chronic pulmonary disease associated with acute hypercapnia
Adults: Infusion of 1 to 2 mg/minute (using 2 mg/ml solution). Maximum dosage is 3 mg/minute for a maximum duration of 2 hours. *Do not use drug with mechanical ventilation.* Use infusion pump to regulate rate.

Pharmacodynamics
Respiratory stimulant action: Doxapram increases respiratory rate by direct stimulation of the medullary respiratory center and possibly by indirect action on chemoreceptors in the carotid artery and aortic arch. Doxapram causes increased release of catecholamines.

Pharmacokinetics
• *Absorption:* After I.V. administration, action begins within 20 to 40 seconds; peak effect occurs in 1 to 2 minutes. Pharmacologic action persists for 5 to 12 minutes.
• *Distribution:* Distributed throughout the body.
• *Metabolism:* Drug is 99% metabolized by the liver.
• *Excretion:* Metabolites are excreted in urine.

Contraindications and precautions
Contraindicated in patients with seizure disorders; head injury; CV disorders; frank, uncompensated heart failure; severe hypertension; CVA; respiratory failure or incompetence secondary to neuromuscular disorders, muscle paresis, flail chest, obstructed airway, pulmonary embolism, pneumothorax, restrictive respiratory disease, acute bronchial asthma, or extreme dyspnea; or hypoxia not associated with hypercapnia. Drug also contraindicated in newborns because product contains benzyl alcohol.

Use cautiously in patients with bronchial asthma, severe tachycardia or arrhythmias, cerebral edema or increased CSF pressure, hyperthyroidism, pheochromocytoma, or metabolic disorders.

Interactions
Concomitant use with *MAO inhibitors* or *sympathomimetic drugs* may produce added pressor effects.

Discontinue *anesthetics*, such as *halothane, cyclopropane*, and *enflurane*, at least 10 minutes before giving doxapram; these agents sensitize the myocardium to catecholamines.

Doxapram temporarily may mask residual effects of *neuromuscular blockers* used after anesthesia.

Effects on diagnostic tests

Doxapram may cause T-wave depression on ECG, decreased erythrocyte and leukocyte counts, reduced hemoglobin and hematocrit levels, increased BUN levels, and albuminuria.

Adverse reactions

CNS: ***seizures,*** *headache,* dizziness, apprehension, disorientation, hyperactivity, bilateral Babinski's signs, paresthesia.
CV: *chest pain and tightness, variations in heart rate, hypertension,* lowered T waves, ***arrhythmias.***
EENT: sneezing, ***laryngospasm.***
GI: nausea, vomiting, diarrhea.
GU: urine retention, bladder stimulation with incontinence.
Respiratory: cough, ***bronchospasm,*** dyspnea.
Skin: pruritus.
Other: hiccups, rebound hypoventilation, muscle spasms, diaphoresis, flushing.

Overdose and treatment

Signs of overdose include hypertension, tachycardia, arrhythmias, skeletal muscle hyperactivity, and dyspnea.

Treatment is supportive. Keep oxygen and resuscitative equipment available, but use oxygen with caution because rapid increase in partial pressure of oxygen can suppress carotid chemoreceptor activity. Keep I.V. anticonvulsants available to treat seizures.

☑ Special considerations

- Doxapram's use as an analeptic is strongly discouraged; drug should be used only in surgery or emergency room.
- Establish adequate airway before administering drug; prevent aspiration of vomitus by placing patient on his side.
- Monitor blood pressure, heart rate, deep tendon reflexes, and arterial blood gas (ABG) levels before giving drug and every 30 minutes afterward. Discontinue drug if ABG levels deteriorate or mechanical ventilation is started.
- For I.V. infusion, dilute to 1 mg/ml. Do not infuse doxapram faster than recommended rate because hemolysis may occur. Drug should be used only on an intermittent basis; maximum infusion period is 2 hours.
- Avoid repeated injections in the site for long periods because of risk of thrombophlebitis or local skin irritation.
- Do not combine doxapram, which is acidic, with alkaline solutions, such as thiopental sodium; solution is compatible with D_5W or $D_{10}W$ and 0.9% NaCl.
- Give concomitant oxygen cautiously to patients with COPD who are narcotized or those who have just undergone surgery; doxapram-stimulated respiration increases oxygen demand.
- Monitor patient for signs of toxicity—tachycardia, muscle tremor, spasticity, and hyperactive reflexes—and blood pressure changes, especially hypertensive patients.

Geriatric use

- No specific recommendations exist for drug use in elderly patients. However, elderly patients may be predisposed to one of several illnesses that preclude its use.

Pediatric use

- Safety in children under age 12 has not been established.

Breast-feeding

- Safe use in breast-feeding has not been established. Distribution into breast milk is unknown.

doxazosin mesylate

Cardura

Pharmacologic classification: alpha-adrenergic blocker
Therapeutic classification: antihypertensive
Pregnancy risk category C

How supplied

Available by prescription only
Tablets: 1 mg, 2 mg, 4 mg, 8 mg

Indications, route, and dosage

Essential hypertension

Adult: Dosage must be individualized. Initially, administer 1 mg P.O. daily and determine effect on standing and supine blood pressure at 2 to 6 hours and 24 hours after dosing. If necessary, increase dose to 2 mg daily. To minimize adverse reactions, titrate dose slowly (dosage typically increased only q 2 weeks). If necessary, increase dose to 4 mg daily, then 8 mg. Maximum daily dose is 16 mg, but doses exceeding 4 mg daily are associated with a greater incidence of adverse reactions.

Benign prostatic hyperplasia

Adults: initially, 1 mg P.O. once daily in the morning or evening; increase to 2 mg and, thereafter, to 4 mg and 8 mg once daily. Recommended titration interval is 1 to 2 weeks.

Pharmacodynamics

Hypotensive action: Doxazosin selectively blocks postsynaptic $alpha_1$-adrenergic receptors, dilating both resistance (arterioles) and capacitance (veins) vessels. It lowers both supine and standing blood pressure, producing more pronounced effects on diastolic pressure. Maximum reductions occur 2 to 6 hours after dosing and are associated with a small increase in standing heart rate. Doxazosin has a greater effect on blood pressure and heart rate in the standing position.

Benign prostatic hyperplasia: Doxazosin improves urine flow related to relaxation of smooth muscles produced by blockade of alpha adrenoreceptors in the bladder neck and prostate.

Pharmacokinetics

• *Absorption:* Readily absorbed from the GI tract after oral administration. Peak plasma levels are obtained in 2 to 3 hours.
• *Distribution:* Drug is 98% protein-bound. It is distributed in breast milk in concentrations about 20 times greater than in maternal plasma.
• *Metabolism:* Extensively metabolized in the liver by *O*-demethylation or hydroxylation. Secondary peaking of plasma levels suggests enterohepatic recycling.
• *Excretion:* 63% is excreted in bile and feces (4.8% as unchanged drug); 9% is excreted in urine.

Contraindications and precautions

Contraindicated in patients with hypersensitivity to drug and quinazoline derivatives (including prazosin and terazosin). Use cautiously in patients with impaired hepatic function.

Interactions

Antihypertensive effects of *clonidine* may be decreased.

Effects on diagnostic tests

Mean WBC and neutrophil counts may be decreased.

Adverse reactions

CNS: *dizziness,* vertigo, somnolence, drowsiness, *asthenia, headache.*
CV: *orthostatic hypotension,* hypotension, edema, palpitations, ***arrhythmias,*** tachycardia.
GI: nausea, vomiting, diarrhea, constipation.
Skin: rash, pruritus.
Other: rhinitis, arthralgia, myalgia, pain, dyspnea, pharyngitis, abnormal vision.

Overdose and treatment

Keep patient supine to restore blood pressure and heart rate. If necessary, treat shock with volume expanders. Administer vasopressors and monitor and support renal function.

☑ Special considerations

• Postural effects are most likely to occur 2 to 6 hours after dose. Monitor blood pressure during this time after the first dose and after subsequent increases in dosage. Daily doses above 4 mg increase the potential of excessive postural effects.
• Tolerance to doxazosin's antihypertensive effects has not been observed.
• No apparent differences exist in the hypotensive response of whites and blacks or of elderly patients.
• First-dose effect (orthostatic hypotension) occurs with doxazosin but is less pronounced than with prazosin or terazosin.

Patient education

• Tell patient that orthostatic hypotension and syncope may occur, especially after first few doses and with dosage changes. Patient should arise slowly to prevent orthostatic hypertension.
• Caution patient that drug may cause drowsiness and somnolence. Patient should avoid driving and other hazardous tasks that require alertness for 12 to 24 hours after first dose, after dosage increases, and after resumption of interrupted therapy.
• Tell patient to report bothersome palpitations or dizziness.
• Tell patient drug may be taken with food if nausea occurs. Inform patient that nausea should improve as therapy continues.

Pediatric use

• Safety and efficacy have not been established.

Breast-feeding

• Drug accumulates in breast milk in concentrations about 20 times greater than in maternal plasma concentrations.

doxepin hydrochloride

Adapin, Sinequan, Triadapin*

Pharmacologic classification: tricyclic antidepressant
Therapeutic classification: antidepressant
Pregnancy risk category NR

How supplied

Available by prescription only
Capsules: 10 mg, 25 mg, 50 mg, 75 mg, 100 mg, 150 mg
Oral concentrate: 10 mg/ml

Indications, route, and dosage

Depression or anxiety
Adults: Initially, 25 to 75 mg P.O. daily in divided doses, to a maximum of 300 mg daily. Alternatively, give entire maintenance dosage once daily with a maximum dose of 150 mg P.O.
✦ ***Dosage adjustment.*** Reduce dosage in the elderly, debilitated or adolescent patients, and in those receiving other medications (especially anticholinergics).

Pharmacodynamics

Antidepressant action: Doxepin is thought to exert its antidepressant effects by inhibiting reuptake of norepinephrine and serotonin in CNS nerve terminals (presynaptic neurons), which results in increased levels and enhanced activity of these neurotransmitters in the synaptic cleft. Doxepin more actively inhibits reuptake of serotonin than norepinephrine. Anxiolytic effects of this drug usually precede antidepressant effects. Doxepin also may be used as an anxiolytic. Doxepin has the greatest sedative effect of all tricyclic antidepressants; tolerance to this effect usually develops in a few weeks.

Pharmacokinetics

• *Absorption:* Drug is absorbed rapidly from the GI tract after oral administration.
• *Distribution:* Doxepin is distributed widely into the body, including the CNS and breast milk. Drug is 90% protein-bound. Peak effect occurs in 2 to 4

hours; steady state is achieved within 7 days. Therapeutic concentrations (parent drug and metabolite) are thought to range from 150 to 250 ng/ml.
• *Metabolism:* Drug is metabolized by the liver to the active metabolite desmethyldoxepin. A significant first-pass effect may explain variability of serum concentrations in different patients taking the same dosage.
• *Excretion:* Mostly excreted in urine.

Contraindications and precautions
Contraindicated in patients with hypersensitivity to drug, glaucoma, or tendency to retain urine.

Interactions
Concomitant use of doxepin with *sympathomimetics*, including *epinephrine, phenylephrine, phenylpropanolamine*, and *ephedrine* (often found in nasal sprays), may increase blood pressure; use with *warfarin* may increase PT and cause bleeding.

Concomitant use with *thyroid medication, pimozide*, and *antiarrhythmic agents (quinidine, disopyramide, procainamide)* may increase incidence of arrhythmias and conduction defects.

Doxepin may decrease hypotensive effects of *centrally acting antihypertensive drugs*, such as *guanethidine, guanabenz, guanadrel, clonidine, methyldopa*, and *reserpine*. Concomitant use with *disulfiram* or *ethchlorvynol* may cause delirium and tachycardia. Additive effects are likely after concomitant use of doxepin with CNS depressants, including *alcohol, analgesics, barbiturates, narcotics, tranquilizers*, and *anesthetics* (oversedation); *atropine* and other *anticholinergic drugs*, including *phenothiazines, antihistamines, meperidine*, and *antiparkinsonian agents* (oversedation, paralytic ileus, visual changes, and severe constipation); and *metrizamide* (increased risk of seizures).

Barbiturates and *heavy smoking* induce doxepin metabolism and decrease therapeutic efficacy; *phenothiazines* and *haloperidol* decrease its metabolism, decreasing therapeutic efficacy; *methylphenidate, cimetidine, oral contraceptives, propoxyphene*, and *beta blockers* may inhibit doxepin metabolism, increasing plasma levels and toxicity.

Effects on diagnostic tests
Doxepin may prolong conduction time (elongation of QT and PR intervals, flattened T waves on ECG); it also may elevate liver function test results, decrease WBC counts, and decrease or increase serum glucose levels.

Adverse reactions
CNS: *drowsiness, dizziness*, confusion, numbness, hallucinations, paresthesia, ataxia, weakness, headache, ***seizures***, extrapyramidal reactions.
CV: *orthostatic hypotension, tachycardia.*
EENT: *blurred vision*, tinnitus.
GI: *dry mouth, constipation*, nausea, vomiting, anorexia.
GU: urine retention.
Hematologic: ***eosinophilia, bone marrow depression.***
Skin: rash, urticaria, photosensitivity.
Other: *diaphoresis*, hypersensitivity reaction.

After abrupt withdrawal of long-term therapy: nausea, headache, malaise (does not indicate addiction).

Overdose and treatment
The first 12 hours after acute ingestion are a stimulatory phase characterized by excessive anticholinergic activity (agitation, irritation, confusion, hallucinations, hyperthermia, parkinsonian symptoms, seizures, urine retention, dry mucous membranes, pupillary dilatation, constipation, and ileus). This is followed by CNS depressant effects, including hypothermia, decreased or absent reflexes, sedation, hypotension, cyanosis, and cardiac irregularities, including tachycardia, conduction disturbances, and quinidine-like effects on the ECG.

Severity of overdose is best indicated by widening of QRS complex. Usually, this represents a serum concentration in excess of 1,000 ng/ml. Serum concentrations are usually not helpful. Metabolic acidosis may follow hypotension, hypoventilation, and seizures.

Treatment is symptomatic and supportive, including maintaining airway, stable body temperature, and fluid and electrolyte balance. Induce emesis with ipecac if patient is conscious; follow with gastric lavage and activated charcoal to prevent further absorption. Dialysis is of little use. Physostigmine may be cautiously used to reverse central anticholinergic effects. Treat seizures with parenteral diazepam or phenytoin; arrhythmias with parenteral phenytoin or lidocaine; and acidosis with sodium bicarbonate. *Do not give barbiturates:* these may enhance CNS and respiratory depressant effects.

☑ Special considerations
Recommendations for administration of doxepin, care of patients during therapy, and use in pediatric patients are the same as those for all *tricyclic antidepressants.*

Patient education
• Teach patient to dilute oral concentrate with 120 ml water, milk, or juice (grapefruit, orange, pineapple, prune, or tomato). Drug is incompatible with carbonated beverages.
• Tell patient to use ice chips, sugarless gum or hard candy, or saliva substitutes to treat dry mouth.
• Advise patient to avoid alcohol or other sedative drugs while taking doxepin. Drug has a strong sedative effect and such combinations can cause excessive sedation.
• Warn patient to avoid taking other drugs while taking doxepin unless they have been prescribed.
• Instruct patient to take full dose at bedtime.
• Tell patient to store drug safely away from children.

Geriatric use
• Elderly patients are more likely to develop adverse CNS reactions.

Pediatric use
• Doxepin is rarely used for the treatment of anxiety in pediatric patients.

Breast-feeding

• Drug is excreted in breast milk. Avoid use of drug in breast-feeding patients, especially if high doses are used.

doxorubicin hydrochloride

Adriamycin PFS, Adriamycin RDF, Rubex

Pharmacologic classification: antineoplastic antibiotic (cell cycle–phase nonspecific)
Therapeutic classification: antineoplastic
Pregnancy risk category D

How supplied

Available by prescription only
Injection: 10 mg, 20 mg, 50 mg, 100 mg, 150 mg vials
Injection (preservative-free): 2 mg/ml

Indications, route, and dosage

Dosage and indications may vary. Check current literature for recommended protocol or for information on liposomal doxorubicin.

Bladder, breast, lung, ovarian, stomach, and thyroid cancers; Hodgkin's disease; acute lymphoblastic and myeloblastic leukemia; Wilms' tumor; neuroblastoma; lymphoma; sarcoma
Adults: 60 to 75 mg/m^2 I.V. as a single dose q 21 days; or 25 to 30 mg/m^2 I.V. as a single daily dose on days 1 to 3 of 4-week cycle. Alternatively, 20 mg/m^2 I.V. once weekly. Maximum cumulative dosage is 550 mg/m^2 (450 mg/m^2 in patients who have received chest irradiation).

Pharmacodynamics

Antineoplastic action: Doxorubicin exerts its cytotoxic activity by intercalating between DNA base pairs and uncoiling the DNA helix. The result is inhibition of DNA synthesis and DNA-dependent RNA synthesis. Doxorubicin also inhibits protein synthesis.

Pharmacokinetics

• *Absorption:* Because of its vesicant effects, doxorubicin must be administered I.V.
• *Distribution:* Drug distributes widely into body tissues, with the highest concentrations found in the liver, heart, and kidneys. It does not cross the blood-brain barrier.
• *Metabolism:* Extensively metabolized by hepatic microsomal enzymes to several metabolites, one of which possesses cytotoxic activity.
• *Excretion:* Drug and its metabolites are excreted primarily in bile. A minute amount is eliminated in urine. The plasma elimination of doxorubicin is described as biphasic with a half-life of about 15 to 30 minutes in the initial phase and 16½ hours in the terminal phase.

Contraindications and precautions

Contraindicated in patients with marked myelosuppression induced by previous treatment with other antitumor agents or by radiotherapy and in those who have received lifetime cumulative dosage of 550 mg/m^2.

Interactions

Concomitant use with *streptozocin* may increase the plasma half-life of doxorubicin by an unknown mechanism, increasing the activity of doxorubicin. Concomitant use of *daunorubicin* or *cyclophosphamide* may potentiate the cardiotoxicity of doxorubicin through additive effects on the heart. Doxorubicin should not be mixed with *heparin sodium, fluorouracil, aminophylline, cephalosporins, dexamethasone phosphate,* or *hydrocortisone sodium phosphate* because it will result in a precipitate. Serum *digoxin* levels may be decreased if used concomitantly with doxorubicin. Doxorubicin may worsen *cyclophosphamide*-induced hemorrhagic cystitis and *mercaptopurine*-induced hepatotoxicity.

Effects on diagnostic tests

Doxorubicin therapy may increase blood and urine concentrations of uric acid.

Adverse reactions

CV: cardiac depression, seen in such ECG changes as sinus tachycardia, T-wave flattening, ST-segment depression, voltage reduction; ***arrhythmias; acute left ventricular failure; irreversible cardiomyopathy.***
EENT: conjunctivitis.
GI: *nausea, vomiting,* diarrhea, *stomatitis,* esophagitis, anorexia.
GU: red urine (transient).
Hematologic: *leukopenia* during days 10 to 15 with recovery by day 21; ***thrombocytopenia;* MYELOSUPPRESSION.**
Skin: urticaria, facial flushing.
Other: *severe cellulitis or tissue sloughing* (if drug extravasates); hyperuricemia; *complete alopecia within 3 to 4 weeks* (hair may regrow 2 to 5 months after drug is stopped); fever; chills; ***anaphylaxis.***

Overdose and treatment

Clinical manifestations of overdose include myelosuppression, nausea, vomiting, mucositis, and irreversible myocardial toxicity.

Treatment is usually supportive and includes transfusion of blood components, antiemetics, antibiotics for infections which may develop, symptomatic treatment of mucositis, and cardiac glycoside preparations.

☑ Special considerations

• To reconstitute, add 5 ml of 0.9% NaCl injection, USP, to the 10 mg vial, 10 ml to the 20 mg vial, and 25 ml to the 50 mg vial, to yield a concentration of 2 mg/ml.
• Drug may be further diluted with 0.9% NaCl solution or D_5W and administered by I.V. infusion.
• Drug may be administered by I.V. push injection over 5 to 10 minutes into the tubing of a freely flowing I.V. infusion.
• The alternative dosage schedule (once-weekly dosing) has been found to cause a lower incidence of cardiomyopathy.

• If cumulative dose exceeds 550 mg/m^2 body surface area, 30% of patients develop cardiac adverse reactions, which begin 2 weeks to 6 months after stopping drug. With high doses of adriamycin, consider concommitant dosing with the cardioprotective agent dexrazoxane.
• The occurrence of streaking along a vein or facial flushing indicates that drug is being administered too rapidly.
• Applying a scalp tourniquet or ice may decrease alopecia. However, *do not* use these if treating leukemias or other neoplasms where tumor stem cells may be present in scalp.
• Drug should be discontinued or rate of infusion slowed if tachycardia develops. Treat extravasation with topical application of dimethyl sulfoxide and ice packs.
• Monitor CBC and hepatic function.
• Decrease dosage as follows if serum bilirubin level increases: 50% of dose when bilirubin level is 1.2 to 3 mg/100 ml; 25% of dose when bilirubin level exceeds 3 mg/100 ml.
• Esophagitis is very common in patients who have also received radiation therapy.

Patient education
• Encourage adequate fluid intake to increase urine output and facilitate excretion of uric acid.
• Advise patient to avoid exposure to people with infections.
• Warn patient that alopecia will occur. Explain that hair growth should resume 2 to 5 months after drug is stopped.
• Advise patient that urine will appear red for 1 to 2 days after the dose and does not indicate bleeding. The urine may stain clothes.
• Instruct patient not to receive immunizations during therapy and for several weeks after. Other members of the patient's household should also not receive immunizations during the same period.
• Tell patient to call if unusual bruising or bleeding or signs of an infection occur.

Geriatric use
• Patients over age 70 have an increased incidence of drug-induced cardiotoxicity. Caution should be taken in elderly patients with low bone marrow reserve to prevent serious hematologic toxicity.

Pediatric use
• Children under age 2 have a higher incidence of drug-induced cardiotoxicity.

Breast-feeding
• It is not known whether doxorubicin distributes into breast milk. However, because of the risk of serious adverse reactions, mutagenicity, and carcinogenicity in the infant, breast-feeding is not recommended.

doxycycline
Vibramycin

doxycycline calcium
Vibramycin

doxycycline hyclate
Doryx, Doxy-100, Doxy-200, Doxy-Caps, Vibramycin, Vibra-Tabs

doxycycline monohydrate
Monodox, Vibramycin

Pharmacologic classification: tetracycline
Therapeutic classification: antibiotic
Pregnancy risk category D

How supplied
Available by prescription only
doxycycline
Oral suspension: 25 mg/5 ml
doxycycline calcium
Oral suspension: 50 mg/5 ml
doxycycline hyclate
Tablets: 100 mg
Capsules: 50 mg, 100 mg
Injection: 100 mg, 200 mg
doxycycline monohydrate
Capsules: 50 mg, 100 mg
Oral suspension: 25 mg/5 ml

Indications, route, and dosage
Infections caused by sensitive organisms
Adults and children weighing 99 lb (45 kg) and over: 100 mg P.O. q 12 hours on day 1, then 100 mg P.O. daily; or 200 mg I.V. on day 1 in one or two infusions, then 100 to 200 mg I.V. daily.
Children over age 8 weighing less than 99 lb: 4.4 mg/kg P.O. or I.V. daily, divided q 12 hours day 1, then 2.2 to 4.4 mg/kg daily.

Give I.V. infusion slowly (minimum 1 hour). Infusion must be completed within 12 hours (within 6 hours in lactated Ringer's solution or D_5W in lactated Ringer's solution).
Gonorrhea in patients allergic to penicillin
Adults: 100 mg P.O. b.i.d. for 7 days; or 300 mg P.O. initially and repeat dose in 1 hour.
◇ ***Syphilis in patients allergic to penicillin***
Adults: 100 mg P.O. b.i.d. for 2 weeks (early detection) or 4 weeks (if more than 1 year's duration).
Chlamydia trachomatis, *nongonococcal urethritis, and uncomplicated urethral, endocervical, or rectal infections*
Adults: 100 mg P.O. b.i.d. for at least 7 days.
Acute pelvic inflammatory disease (PID)
Adults: 250 mg I.M. ceftriaxone, followed by 100 mg doxycycline P.O. b.i.d. for 10 to 14 days.
***Acute epididymoorchitis caused by* C. trachomatis *or* Neisseria gonorrhoeae**
Adults: 100 mg P.O. b.i.d for at least 10 days.
◇ ***To prevent traveler's diarrhea commonly caused by enterotoxigenic* Escherichia coli**
Adults: 100 mg P.O. daily for up to 3 days.
◇ ***Prophylaxis for rape victims***
Adults and adolescents: 100 mg P.O. b.i.d. for 7

days after a single 2-g oral dose of metronidazole is given in conjunction with a single 125-mg I.M. dose of ceftriaxone.

Chemoprophylaxis for malaria in travelers to areas where chloroquine-resistant* Plasmodium falciparum *is endemic and mefloquine is contraindicated

Adults: 100 mg P.O. once daily. Begin prophylaxis 1 to 2 days before travel to malarious areas; continue daily while in affected area, and continue for 4 weeks after return from malarious area.

Children over age 8: Give 2 mg/kg P.O. daily as a single dose; do not exceed 100 mg daily. Use the same dosage schedule as for adults.

◇ ***Lyme disease***

Adults and children age 9 and older: 100 mg P.O. b.i.d. or t.i.d. for 10 to 30 days.

◇ ***Pleural effusions associated with cancer***

Adults: 500 mg of doxycycline diluted in 250 ml of 0.9% saline and instilled into pleural space via a chest tube.

Pharmacodynamics

Antibacterial action: Doxycycline is bacteriostatic; it binds reversibly to ribosomal units, thereby inhibiting bacterial protein synthesis.

Drug's spectrum of activity includes many gram-negative and gram-positive organisms, *Mycoplasma, Rickettsia, Chlamydia,* and spirochetes.

Pharmacokinetics

- *Absorption:* About 90% to 100% is absorbed after oral administration; peak serum levels occur at 1½ to 4 hours. Doxycycline has the least affinity for calcium of all tetracyclines; its absorption is insignificantly altered by milk or other dairy products.
- *Distribution:* Drug is distributed widely into body tissues and fluids, including synovial, pleural, prostatic, and seminal fluids; bronchial secretions; saliva; and aqueous humor. CSF penetration is poor. Doxycycline readily crosses the placenta; it is 25% to 93% protein-bound.
- *Metabolism:* Doxycycline is insignificantly metabolized; some hepatic degradation occurs.
- *Excretion:* Drug is excreted primarily unchanged in urine by glomerular filtration; some may be excreted in breast milk. Plasma half-life is 22 to 24 hours after multiple dosing in adults with normal renal function; 20 to 30 hours in patients with severe renal impairment. Some drug is excreted in feces.

Contraindications and precautions

Contraindicated in patients with hypersensitivity to drug or other tetracyclines. Use cautiously in patients with impaired renal or hepatic function. Use during last half of pregnancy and in children under age 8 may cause permanent discoloration of teeth, enamel defects, and bone growth retardation.

Interactions

Concomitant use of doxycycline with *antacids containing aluminum, calcium,* or *magnesium* or *laxatives* containing magnesium decreases oral absorption of doxycycline because of chelation. *oral iron products* and *sodium bicarbonate* also impair absorption of tetracyclines.

Doxycycline may antagonize bactericidal effects of *penicillin*, inhibiting cell growth because of bacteriostatic action; administer penicillin 2 to 3 hours before tetracycline.

Concomitant use of doxycycline with *oral anticoagulants* necessitates lowered dosage of oral anticoagulants because of enhanced effects; when used with *digoxin*, lowered dosages of digoxin because of increased bioavailability.

Effects on diagnostic tests

Doxycycline causes false-negative results in urine tests using glucose oxidase reagent (Diastix, Chemstrip uG, or glucose enzymatic test strip); parenteral dosage form may cause false-negative Clinitest results.

Doxycycline also causes false elevations in fluorometric tests for urinary catecholamines.

Adverse reactions

CNS: ***intracranial hypertension (pseudotumor cerebri).***

CV: pericarditis.

EENT: glossitis, dysphagia.

GI: anorexia, *epigastric distress, nausea,* vomiting, *diarrhea,* oral candidiasis, enterocolitis, anogenital inflammation.

Hematologic: ***neutropenia,*** eosinophilia, ***thrombocytopenia,*** hemolytic anemia.

Skin: *maculopapular and erythematous rashes, photosensitivity, increased pigmentation, urticaria.*

Other: hypersensitivity reactions ***(anaphylaxis);*** elevated liver enzymes; permanent discoloration of teeth, enamel defects, bone growth retardation if used in children under age 8; superinfection; thrombophlebitis.

Overdose and treatment

Clinical signs of overdose are usually limited to the GI tract; give antacids or empty stomach by gastric lavage if ingestion occurred within the preceding 4 hours.

☑ Special considerations

Besides those relevant to all *tetracyclines,* consider the following recommendations.

- Reconstitute powder for injection with sterile water for injection. Use 10 ml in a 100-mg vial and 20 ml in a 200-mg vial. Dilute solution to 100 to 1,000 ml for I.V. infusion. Do not infuse solutions more concentrated than 1 mg/ml.
- Reconstituted solution is stable for 72 hours if refrigerated and protected from light.
- Do not inject S.C. or I.M.
- Drug may be used in patients with impaired renal function; it does not accumulate or cause a significant rise in BUN levels.

Pediatric use

- Avoid use of drug in children under age 9.

Breast-feeding

- Avoid use in breast-feeding women.

dronabinol

Marinol

Pharmacologic classification: cannabinoid
Therapeutic classification: antiemetic/ appetite stimulant
Controlled substance schedule II
Pregnancy risk category C

How supplied

Available by prescription only
Capsules: 2.5 mg, 5 mg, 10 mg

Indications, route, and dosage

Nausea and vomiting associated with cancer chemotherapy
Adults and children: 5 mg/m² P.O. 1 to 3 hours before administration of chemotherapy; then same dose q 2 to 4 hours after chemotherapy for a total of 4 to 6 doses daily. Dose may be increased in increments of 2.5 mg/m² to a maximum of 15 mg/m² per dose.
Appetite stimulation in the treatment of anorexia associated with AIDS-related weight loss
Adults: 2.5 mg P.O. b.i.d. before lunch and supper; increased, if necessary, to a maximum of 20 mg daily.

Pharmacodynamics

Antiemetic action: Dronabinol is a synthetic cannabinoid that inhibits vomiting centers in the brain and possibly in the chemoreceptor trigger zone and other sites.

Pharmacokinetics

- *Absorption:* Almost 90% to 95% of dose is absorbed; action begins in 30 to 60 minutes, with peak action in 1 to 3 hours.
- *Distribution:* Distributed rapidly into many tissue sites. Drug is 97% to 99% protein-bound.
- *Metabolism:* Drug undergoes extensive metabolism in the liver. Metabolite activity is unknown.
- *Excretion:* Excreted primarily in feces, via the biliary tract. Drug effect may persist for several days after treatment ends; duration varies considerably among patients.

Contraindications and precautions

Contraindicated in patients hypersensitive to sesame oil or cannabinoids. Use cautiously in elderly, pregnant, or breast-feeding patients and in those with heart disease, psychiatric illness, or a history of drug abuse.

Interactions

When used concomitantly with *alcohol* or other *sedatives* or *psychotomimetic drugs*, dronabinol may have an additive sedative effect. Dronabinol may alter *ethanol* elimination, increasing it in some patients and decreasing it in others. Concomitant use with *anticholinergics* may cause tachycardia.

Effects on diagnostic tests

None reported.

Adverse reactions

CNS: *dizziness, drowsiness, euphoria, ataxia,* depersonalization, hallucinations, somnolence, headache, muddled thinking, asthenia, amnesia, confusion, *paranoia.*
CV: tachycardia, orthostatic hypotension, palpitations, vasodilation.
GI: *dry mouth, nausea, vomiting,* diarrhea.
Other: visual disturbances.

Overdose and treatment

Treat overdose with symptomatic and supportive therapy. Observe patient in a quiet environment and provide supportive measures.

☑ Special considerations

- Drug is used only in patients with nausea and vomiting resulting from cancer chemotherapy who do not respond to other treatment; drug should be given before chemotherapy infusion.
- Monitor frequency and degree of vomiting.
- Monitor pulse, blood pressure, and fluid intake and output to help prevent dehydration; observe for signs of confusion.
- Drug is the major active ingredient of *Cannabis sativa* (marijuana) and therefore has a potential for abuse.

Patient education

- Warn patient to avoid driving and other activities requiring sound judgment until extent of CNS depressant effects are known.
- Urge family to ensure that patient is supervised by a responsible person during and immediately after treatment.
- Caution patient and family to anticipate drug's mood-altering effects.

Geriatric use

- Elderly patients may be more susceptible to adverse reactions.

Breast-feeding

- Drug is concentrated and excreted in breast milk and is absorbed by breast-feeding infants.

droperidol

Inapsine

Pharmacologic classification: butyrophenone derivative
Therapeutic classification: tranquilizer
Pregnancy risk category C

How supplied

Available by prescription only
Injection: 2.5 mg/ml

Indications, route, and dosage

Anesthetic premedication
Adults: 2.5 to 10 mg I.M. 30 to 60 minutes before induction of general anesthesia.
Children age 2 to 12: 0.088 to 0.165 mg/kg I.V. or I.M.

Adjunct for induction of general anesthesia
Adults: 0.22 to 0.275 mg/kg I.V. (preferably) or I.M. concomitantly with an analgesic or general anesthetic.
Children: 0.088 to 0.165 mg/kg I.V. or I.M.
Adjunct for maintenance of general anesthesia
Adults: 1.25 to 2.5 mg I.V.
For use without a general anesthetic during diagnostic procedures
Adults: 2.5 to 10 mg I.M. 30 to 60 minutes before the procedure. Additional doses of 1.25 to 2.5 mg I.V. are given p.r.n.
Adjunct to regional anesthesia
Adults: 2.5 to 5 mg I.M. or slow I.V. injection.
◊ ***Antiemetic in conjunction with cancer chemotherapy***
Adults: 6.25 mg I.M. or by slow I.V. injection.

Pharmacodynamics

Tranquilizer action: Droperidol produces marked sedation by directly blocking subcortical receptors. Droperidol also blocks CNS receptors at the chemoreceptor trigger zone, producing an antiemetic effect.

Pharmacokinetics

- *Absorption:* Drug is well absorbed after I.M. injection. Sedation begins in 3 to 10 minutes, peaks at 30 minutes, and lasts for 2 to 4 hours; some alteration of consciousness may persist for 12 hours.
- *Distribution:* Not well understood; drug crosses the blood-brain barrier and is distributed in the CSF. It also crosses the placenta.
- *Metabolism:* Droperidol is metabolized by the liver to *p*-fluoro-phenylacetic acid and *p*-hydroxypiperidine.
- *Excretion:* Drug and its metabolites are excreted in urine and feces.

Contraindications and precautions

Contraindicated in patients with known hypersensitivity or intolerance to drug. Use cautiously in patients with hypotension and other CV disease because of its vasodilatory effects, in patients with hepatic or renal disease in whom drug clearance may be impaired, and in patients taking other CNS depressants, including alcohol, opiates, and sedatives, because droperidol may potentiate the effects of these drugs.

Interactions

Droperidol potentiates the CNS depressant effects of *opiate* or other *analgesics* and has an additive or potentiating effect when used concomitantly with other *CNS depressants*, such as *alcohol, barbiturates, tranquilizers*, and *sedative-hypnotics*. When used concurrently, the dosage of both drugs should be reduced.

Effects on diagnostic tests

Drug temporarily alters the EEG pattern, which returns slowly to normal after administration of the drug. Droperidol may decrease pulmonary artery pressure.

Adverse reactions

CNS: *sedation*, altered consciousness, respiratory depression, postoperative hallucinations, extrapyramidal reactions (dystonia [extended tongue, stiff rotated neck, upward rotation of eyes], akathisia [restlessness], fine tremors of limbs).
CV: *hypotension* with rebound tachycardia, bradycardia (occasional), hypertension when combined with fentanyl or other parenteral analgesics (rare).

Note: Discontinue drug if patient shows signs of ***hypersensitivity, severe persistent hypotension, respiratory depression, paradoxical hypertension, or dystonia.***

Overdose and treatment

Clinical signs of overdose include extension of the drug's pharmacologic actions. Treat overdose symptomatically and supportively.

☑ Special considerations

- Monitor vital signs and watch carefully for extrapyramidal reactions. Droperidol is related to haloperidol and is more likely than other antipsychotics to cause extrapyramidal symptoms.
- If opiates are required during recovery from anesthesia to prevent potentiation of respiratory depression, they should be used initially in reduced dosages (as low as one fourth to one third of the usual recommended dosage).
- Droperidol has been used for its antiemetic effects in preventing or treating cancer chemotherapy-induced nausea and vomiting, especially that produced by cisplatin.
- Observe patient for postoperative hallucinations or emergence delirium and drowsiness.
- Be prepared to treat severe hypotension.

Patient education

- Advise patient of possible postoperative effects.

Geriatric use

- Drug should be used with caution.

Pediatric use

- Safety and efficacy in children under age 2 have not been established.

Breast-feeding

- It is unknown if droperidol occurs in breast milk.

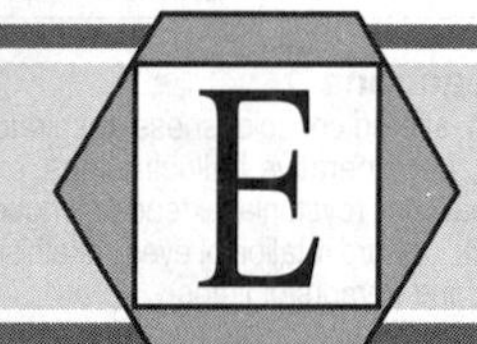

echothiophate iodide
Phospholine Iodide

Pharmacologic classification: cholinesterase inhibitor
Therapeutic classification: miotic
Pregnancy risk category NR

How supplied
Available by prescription only
Ophthalmic: powder for reconstitution to make 0.03%, 0.06%, 0.125%, 0.25% solutions

Indications, route, and dosage
Open-angle glaucoma, conditions obstructing aqueous outflow
Adults and children: Instill 1 drop of 0.03% to 0.125% solution into conjunctival sac daily. Maximum dosage is 1 drop b.i.d. Use lowest possible dosage to continuously control intraocular pressure.
Diagnosis of convergent strabismus
Adults: Instill 1 drop of 0.125% solution daily h.s. for 2 to 3 weeks.
Treatment of convergent strabismus
Adults: Instill 1 drop of 0.03% to 0.125% solution daily or every other day h.s. Alternatively, instill 1 drop of 0.06% solution daily.

Pharmacodynamics
Miotic action: Echothiophate inhibits the enzymatic destruction of acetylcholine by inactivating cholinesterase. Acetylcholine acts on the effector cells of the iridic sphincter and ciliary muscles, causing pupillary constriction and accommodation spasm.

Pharmacokinetics
- *Absorption:* Unknown.
- *Distribution:* Unknown.
- *Metabolism:* Unknown.
- *Excretion:* Duration of effect can be up to 1 week or longer.

Contraindications and precautions
Contraindicated in patients with hypersensitivity to drug or iodine, acute angle-closure glaucoma before iridectomy, and other forms of glaucoma (except for primary open-angle glaucoma). Use with extreme caution, if at all, in patients with seizure disorders, vasomotor instability, parkinsonism, bronchial asthma, spastic GI conditions, urinary tract obstruction, peptic ulcer, severe bradycardia or hypotension, vascular hypertension, MI, or history or risk of retinal detachment. Use cautiously in patients with corneal abrasion.

Interactions
When used concomitantly, echothiophate may increase the neuromuscular-blocking effects of *succinylcholine,* antagonize the antiglaucoma effect of *cyclopentolate* and the *belladonna alkaloids,* increase the toxicity of *carbonate organophosphate insecticides* and *cholinesterase inhibitors,* and add to effects of *systemic anticholinesterase agents used for myasthenia gravis.*

Effects on diagnostic tests
Drug therapy decreases plasma cholinesterase activity.

Adverse reactions
CNS: fatigue, muscle weakness, paresthesia, headache.
CV: bradycardia, hypotension.
EENT: ciliary spasm or spasm of eye accommodation, ciliary or circumcorneal injection, nonreversible cataract formation (time- and dose-related), reversible iris cysts, pupillary block, blurred or dimmed vision, eye or brow pain, twitching of eyelids, hyperemia, photophobia, lens opacities, lacrimation, retinal detachment.
GI: diarrhea, nausea, vomiting, abdominal pain, intestinal cramps, salivation.
GU: frequent urination.
Respiratory: ***bronchoconstriction.***
Other: diaphoresis, flushing.

Overdose and treatment
Clinical manifestations of overdose include tremor, syncope, headache, bradycardia, hypotension, arrhythmias, diarrhea, nausea, vomiting, abdominal pain, excessive salivation, urinary incontinence, and dyspnea. Toxicity can be cumulative, with symptoms appearing weeks to months after initiating therapy.

To treat accidental overdose after ingestion, employ general measures, such as emesis, cathartics, or lavage to remove drug from the GI tract. Treat dermal exposure by washing the area twice with soap and water. The extent of echothiophate's potential toxicity is not well known; observe patient closely for signs and symptoms, and treat symptomatically and supportively. Atropine sulfate (S.C., I.M., or I.V.) has been suggested as the antidote of choice.

☑ Special considerations
- Reconstitute powder carefully to avoid contamination; use only diluent provided. Discard refrigerated, reconstituted solution after 6 months; discard solution at room temperature after 1 month.
- Discontinue drug at least 2 weeks preoperatively if succinylcholine is to be used in surgery. Inform anesthesiologist.

• Echothiophate iodide is a potent, long-acting, irreversible drug.

Patient education
• Warn patient that transient brow ache or dimmed or blurred vision is common at first but usually disappears within 5 to 10 days; advise instillation at bedtime to minimize effects of blurred vision.
• Tell patient or family to inform primary health care provider or anesthesiologist about use of drug before general anesthesia is administered.
• Teach patient correct use, storage, and reconstitution of product.

Geriatric use
• Elderly patients may be at increased risk for adverse reactions.

Pediatric use
• Safety and efficacy have not been established; iris cysts have been reported, but these generally resolve spontaneously when drug is discontinued. Many ophthalmologists avoid using drug in children because of reports of lens opacities in adults.

econazole nitrate
Spectazole

Pharmacologic classification: synthetic imidazole derivative
Therapeutic classification: antifungal
Pregnancy risk category C

How supplied
Available by prescription only
Cream: 1% (water-soluble base)

Indications, route, and dosage
Cutaneous candidiasis
Adults and children: Gently rub sufficient quantity into affected areas b.i.d. in the morning and evening.
Tinea pedis, tinea cruris, tinea corporis, and tinea versicolor
Adults and children: Gently rub into affected area once daily.

Pharmacodynamics
Antifungal action: Although exact mechanism of action is unknown, drug is thought to exert its effects by altering cellular membranes and interfering with intracellular enzymes. Econazole is active against many fungi, including dermatophytes and yeasts, as well as some gram-positive bacteria.

Pharmacokinetics
• *Absorption:* Minimal but rapid percutaneous absorption.
• *Distribution:* Minimal.
• *Metabolism:* Unknown.
• *Excretion:* Unknown.

Contraindications and precautions
Contraindicated in patients hypersensitive to drug.

Interactions
None reported.

Effects on diagnostic tests
None reported.

Adverse reactions
Skin: burning, pruritus, stinging, erythema.

Overdose and treatment
Overdose in humans has not been reported. If a reaction suggesting sensitivity or chemical irritation occurs, discontinue therapy.

☑ Special considerations
• Wash affected area with soap and water, and dry thoroughly before applying drug.
• Do not apply drug to the eye or administer intravaginally.

Patient education
• Instruct patient to wash hands well after application.
• Advise patient to use medication for entire treatment period even though symptoms lessen. Relief of symptoms usually occurs within 1 to 2 weeks of therapy.
• Inform patient with tinea pedis (athlete's foot) to wear well-fitting, well-ventilated shoes and to change shoes and all-cotton socks daily.

Breast-feeding
• Use with caution in breast-feeding women because it is unknown whether drug occurs in breast milk.

edetate calcium disodium (calcium EDTA)
Calcium Disodium Versenate

Pharmacologic classification: chelating agent
Therapeutic classification: heavy metal antagonist
Pregnancy risk category NR

How supplied
Available by prescription only
Injection: 200 mg/ml

Indications, route, and dosage
Acute lead encephalopathy or blood lead levels above 70 mcg/dl
Adults and children: 1.5 g/m² I.V. or I.M. daily in divided doses at 12-hour intervals for 3 to 5 days, usually in conjunction with dimercaprol. Administer second course in 5 to 7 days if necessary.
Lead poisoning without encephalopathy or asymptomatic with blood levels below 70 mcg/dl
Children: 1 g/m² I.V. or I.M. daily in divided doses.
◊ ***Other heavy metal poisonings***
Adults: 1 g in 500 ml of D_5W or 0.9% NaCl injection infused I.V. over a 5-hour period once daily for 3 days.

Pharmacodynamics

Chelating action: Calcium in edetate calcium disodium is displaced by divalent and trivalent heavy metals, forming a soluble complex, which is then excreted in urine, removing the heavy metal.

Pharmacokinetics

- *Absorption:* Well absorbed after I.M. or S.C. injection. After I.V. administration, chelated lead appears in urine within 1 hour; peak excretion of lead occurs in 24 to 48 hours.
- *Distribution:* Drug is distributed primarily in extracellular fluid.
- *Metabolism:* None.
- *Excretion:* Excreted rapidly in urine. After I.V. administration, 50% of drug is excreted in urine unchanged or as a metal chelate in 1 hour; 95% of drug is excreted in 24 hours.

Contraindications and precautions

Contraindicated in patients with anuria, hepatitis, and acute renal disease. Use with extreme caution in patients with mild renal disease.

Interactions

None reported.

Effects on diagnostic tests

None reported.

Adverse reactions

CNS: tremor, headache, numbness, tingling.
CV: hypotension, cardiac rhythm irregularities.
GI: cheilosis, nausea, vomiting, anorexia, thirst.
GU: proteinuria, hematuria; ***nephrotoxicity with renal tubular necrosis leading to fatal nephrosis.***
Hematologic: transient bone marrow depression.
Hepatic: *mild increases in ALT and AST.*
Other: pain (at I.M. injection site), fever, chills, malaise, fatigue, myalgia, arthralgia.

Overdose and treatment

Clinical signs of overdose include acute renal failure with anuria and altered consciousness consistent with increased intracranial pressure, in patients with lead encephalopathy. Reduce intracranial pressure with hyperventilation and furosemide or mannitol; monitor vital signs and ECG closely. Barbiturate infusion may be needed in severe cases; hemodialysis may be needed in acute renal failure.

☑ Special considerations

- Add 1% procaine or lidocaine to solution before I.M. injection to decrease pain at site.
- Avoid rapid I.V. infusion and infusions of large fluid volumes in patients with lead encephalopathy.
- Hydrate patient before giving drug, to ensure adequate urine flow; monitor renal status frequently.
- Monitor intake and output, urinalysis, BUN levels, and ECG throughout therapy.
- Parenterally administered edetate calcium disodium has been used in poisoning by radioactive and nuclear fusion products and other heavy metals except mercury, gold, or arsenic poisoning. It has also been used to aid diagnosis of lead poisoning.
- For I.V. infusion, dilute drug with D_5W solution or 0.9% NaCl; administer one half the daily dose over at least a 1-hour period in asymptomatic patients, 2 hours in symptomatic patients. The second daily infusion should be given 6 or more hours after the first infusion. If administered as a single dose, infuse over 12 to 24 hours.
- If drug is administered as a continuous I.V. infusion, interrupt infusion for at least 1 hour before a blood lead concentration to avoid a falsely elevated value.

Patient education

- As appropriate, explain measures to avoid future heavy metal poisoning.

Pediatric use

- I.M. route is recommended for children.

edetate disodium (EDTA)

Disotate, Endrate, Meritate

Pharmacologic classification: chelating agent
Therapeutic classification: heavy metal antagonist
Pregnancy risk category NR

How supplied

Available by prescription only
Injection: 150 mg/ml

Indications, route, and dosage

Hypercalcemia

Adults: 50 mg/kg daily by slow I.V. infusion to a maximum of 3 g in 24 hours. Dilute in 500 ml of D_5W or 0.9% NaCl. Give over 3 or more hours.
Children: 40 mg/kg by slow I.V. infusion, diluted to a maximum concentration of 30 mg/ml in D_5W or 0.9% NaCl solution administered over 3 or more hours. Maximum daily dose is 70 mg/kg.

Cardiac glycoside–induced ventricular arrhythmias

Adults and children: I.V. infusion of 15 mg/kg/hour; maximum dose is 60 mg/kg daily. Dilute in D_5W.

Pharmacodynamics

Chelating agent: Edetate disodium binds many divalent and trivalent ions but has the strongest affinity for calcium, with which it forms a stable complex readily excreted by the kidneys.

Edetate disodium also chelates magnesium, zinc, and other trace metals, increasing their excretion in urine; it does not decrease CSF calcium concentrations.

Pharmacokinetics

- *Absorption:* Drug is absorbed poorly from the GI tract.
- *Distribution:* Drug does not enter the CSF in significant amounts but distributes widely throughout the rest of the body.
- *Metabolism:* None.

• *Excretion:* After I.V. administration, drug is excreted rapidly in urine; 95% of dose is excreted within 24 hours.

Contraindications and precautions
Contraindicated in patients with hypersensitivity to drug, anuria, known or suspected hypocalcemia, significant renal disease, active or healed tubercular lesions, or history of seizures or intracranial lesions.

Use cautiously in patients with limited cardiac reserve, heart failure, or hypokalemia.

Interactions
Edetate disodium interferes with the cardiac effects of *cardiac glycosides* indirectly by decreasing intracellular calcium by both chelation and urinary excretion of extracellular calcium.

Drug may decrease *insulin requirements* in diabetic patients by chelation of zinc in exogenous insulin.

Effects on diagnostic tests
Edetate disodium lowers serum calcium concentrations when measured by oxalate or other precipitation methods and by colorimetry. The drug also lowers blood glucose concentration in diabetic patients. Edetate disodium–induced hypomagnesemia decreases serum alkaline phosphatase levels.

Adverse reactions
CNS: circumoral paresthesia, numbness, headache, seizures.
CV: hypotension.
EENT: erythema.
GI: nausea, vomiting, diarrhea.
GU: nephrotoxicity with urinary urgency, nocturia, dysuria, polyuria, proteinuria, renal insufficiency, ***acute renal failure, acute tubular necrosis*** (in excessive doses).
Skin: exfoliative dermatitis.
Other: ***severe hypocalcemia,*** decreased magnesium, pain at site of infusion, thrombophlebitis, extravasation.

Overdose and treatment
Clinical signs of overdose may include hypotension, arrhythmias, and cardiac arrest. Treat hypotension with fluids, if necessary. Treat arrhythmias with lidocaine and seizures and tetany with calcium replacement; use I.V. diazepam for refractory seizures. Replace magnesium and potassium, as needed.

☑ Special considerations
• Monitor infusion site closely. Extravasation severely irritates tissue; rotate infusion sites with multiple doses or chronic therapy.
• Do not exceed recommended rate of infusion or dosage; rapid infusion or high concentrations of edetate disodium may precipitously decrease serum calcium levels, causing seizures and death. Therefore, have I.V. calcium replacement readily available whenever drug is administered.
• Monitor calcium levels, and observe patient for seizures or altered vital signs and ECG during infusion. Administer infusion over at least 3 hours; have patient remain supine for 20 to 30 minutes after infusion because of possible postural hypotension. Drug also exerts a negative inotropic effect on the heart.
• Edetate disodium also has been used topically or by iontophoresis to treat corneal calcium deposits.
• Although once considered useful in treating cardiac glycoside–induced arrhythmias, edetate disodium has been replaced by digoxin immune fab as drug of choice for digoxin toxicity.

Patient education
• Explain possible adverse reactions; stress importance of reporting signs and symptoms of adverse reactions promptly.
• Tell diabetic patients that insulin dosage may need adjustment.

Geriatric use
• Elderly patients with renal or cardiac failure are at increased risk; lower doses are recommended.

Pediatric use
• Give recommended dose slowly, over at least 3 hours.

edrophonium chloride
Enlon, Reversol, Tensilon

Pharmacologic classification: cholinesterase inhibitor
Therapeutic classification: cholinergic agonist, diagnostic
Pregnancy risk category NR

How supplied
Available by prescription only
Injection: 10 mg/ml in 1-ml ampule, 10-ml vial, 15-ml vial

Indications, route, and dosage
Curare antagonist (to reverse neuromuscular blocking action)
Adults: 10 mg I.V. given over 30 to 45 seconds, repeated p.r.n. to 40 mg maximum dose. Larger doses may potentiate rather than antagonize effect of curare.
Diagnostic aid in myasthenia gravis
Adults: 2 mg I.V. within 15 to 30 seconds, then 8 mg if no response (increase in muscular strength) occurs. Alternatively, 10 mg I.M. If cholinergic reaction occurs, 2 mg I.M. 30 minutes later to rule out false-negative response.
Children weighing over 75 lb (34 kg): 2 mg I.V. If no response within 45 seconds, give 1 mg q 45 seconds to maximum dose of 10 mg; alternatively, 5 mg I.M.
Children weighing 75 lb or less: 1 mg I.V. If no response within 45 seconds, give 1 mg q 45 seconds to maximum dose of 5 mg; alternatively, 2 mg I.M.
Infants: 0.5 mg I.V.

To differentiate myasthenic crisis from cholinergic crisis
Adults: 1 mg I.V. If no response occurs in 1 minute, repeat dose once. Increased muscular strength confirms myasthenic crisis; no increase or exaggerated weakness confirms cholinergic crisis.
Tensilon test for evaluating treatment requirements in myasthenia gravis
Adults: 1 to 2 mg I.V. administered 1 hour after oral intake of drug being used in treatment. Response will be myasthenic in the undertreated patient, adequate in the controlled patient, and cholinergic in the overtreated patient.
◊ ***To terminate paroxysmal atrial tachycardia or as an aid in diagnosing supraventricular tachyarrhythmias and evaluating the function of demand pacemakers***
Adults: 10 mg I.V. over 5 minutes.
✦ ***Dosage adjustment.*** In elderly or digitalized adults, 5 to 7 mg I.V. over 5 minutes.
To slow supraventricular tachyarrhythmias unresponsive to a cardiac glycoside
Adults: 2 mg/minute I.V test dose, followed by 2 mg q minute until a total dose of 10 mg is given. If heart rate decreases in response to this dose, infusion of 0.25 mg/minute may be started; rate of infusion may be increased to 2 mg/minute if necessary.

Pharmacodynamics
Cholinergic action: Edrophonium blocks acetylcholine's hydrolysis by cholinesterase, resulting in acetylcholine accumulation at cholinergic synapses. That leads to increased cholinergic receptor stimulation at the neuromuscular junction and vagal sites. Edrophonium is a short-acting agent, which makes it particularly useful for the diagnosis of myasthenia gravis.

Pharmacokinetics
- *Absorption:* Action begins 30 to 60 seconds after I.V. administration and 2 to 10 minutes after I.M. administration.
- *Distribution:* Not clearly identified.
- *Metabolism:* Exact metabolic fate is unknown; drug is not hydrolyzed by cholinesterases. Duration of effect ranges from 5 to 10 minutes after I.V. administration and 5 to 30 minutes after I.M. administration.
- *Excretion:* Exact excretion mode is unknown.

Contraindications and precautions
Contraindicated in patients with hypersensitivity to anticholinesterase agents and in those with mechanical obstruction of the intestine or urinary tract. Use cautiously in patients with bronchial asthma or arrhythmias.

Interactions
Concomitant use with *procainamide* or *quinidine* may reverse edrophonium's cholinergic effect on muscle. Use with *corticosteroids* may decrease edrophonium's cholinergic effects; when corticosteroids are stopped, however, cholinergic effects may increase, possibly affecting muscle strength.

Concomitant use with *succinylcholine* may cause prolonged respiratory depression from plasma esterase inhibition, leading to delayed succinylcholine hydrolysis. Concomitant use with *ganglionic blockers,* such as *mecamylamine,* may lead to a critical blood pressure decrease, usually preceded by abdominal symptoms.

Magnesium administration has a direct depressant effect on skeletal muscle and concomitant administration may antagonize edrophonium's anticholinesterase effect.

Concomitant use with *other cholinergic drugs* may lead to additive toxicity.

Effects on diagnostic tests
None reported.

Adverse reactions
CNS: ***seizures,*** weakness, dysarthria, dysphagia.
CV: hypotension, bradycardia, AV block.
EENT: excessive lacrimation, diplopia, miosis, conjunctival hyperemia.
GI: nausea, vomiting, *diarrhea, abdominal cramps,* excessive salivation.
GU: urinary frequency, incontinence.
Respiratory: ***paralysis of muscles of respiration, central respiratory paralysis, bronchospasm, laryngospasm,*** increased bronchial secretions.
Other: muscle cramps, muscle fasciculation, diaphoresis.

Overdose and treatment
Clinical signs of overdose include muscle weakness, nausea, vomiting, diarrhea, blurred vision, miosis, excessive tearing, bronchospasm, increased bronchial secretions, hypotension, incoordination, excessive sweating, cramps, fasciculations, paralysis, bradycardia or tachycardia, excessive salivation, and restlessness or agitation. Muscles first weakened by overdose include neck, jaw, and pharyngeal muscles, followed by muscle weakening of the shoulder, upper extremities, pelvis, outer eye, and legs.

Discontinue drug immediately. Support respiration; bronchial suctioning may be performed. Atropine may be given to block edrophonium's muscarinic effects but will not counter the drug's paralytic effects on skeletal muscle. Avoid atropine overdose, because it may lead to bronchial plug formation.

☑ Special considerations
- Of all cholinergics, edrophonium has the most rapid onset of action but the shortest duration of effect; consequently, it is not used to treat myasthenia gravis.
- When giving edrophonium to differentiate myasthenic crisis from cholinergic crisis, evaluate patient's muscle strength closely.
- For easier administration, use a tuberculin syringe with an I.V. needle.
- Atropine sulfate injection should always be readily available as an antagonist for the muscarinic effects of edrophonium.

Patient education

• Tell patient drug's adverse effects will be transient because of its short duration of effect.

Geriatric use

• Elderly patients may be more sensitive to effects of this drug. Use with caution.

Pediatric use

• Children may require I.M. administration; with this route, drug effects may be delayed for 2 to 10 minutes.

Breast-feeding

• Safety has not been established. Breast-feeding women should avoid edrophonium.

eflornithine hydrochloride (DFMO)

Ornidyl

Pharmacologic classification: ornithine decarboxylase inhibitor
Therapeutic classification: antiprotozoal
Pregnancy risk category C

How supplied

Available by prescription only
Injection: 200 mg/ml in 100-ml vials (concentrated)

Indications, route, and dosage

Treatment of meningoencephalitic stage of* Trypanosoma brucei gambiense *infection (sleeping sickness); treatment of* Pneumocystis carinii *pneumonia in patients with AIDS

Adults: 100 mg/kg (46 mg/lb) q 6 hours administered by I.V. infusion over a minimum of 45 minutes daily for 14 days.

✦ ***Dosage adjustment.*** In patients with renal failure, excretion of drug parallels creatinine clearance. Estimate creatinine clearance from serum creatinine as follows:

Males:

$$\text{Creatinine clearance} = \frac{\text{weight (kg)} \times (140 - \text{age})}{72 \times \text{serum creatinine (mg/dl)}}$$

Females: 0.85 × male value.

Pharmacodynamics

Antiprotozoal action: Eflornithine is a selective, enzyme-activated, irreversible inhibitor of ornithine decarboxylase, blocking the conversion of ornithine to putrescine—the first and rate-limiting step in the biosynthesis of polyamine—which is thought to play an important role in cell differentiation and division.

Pharmacokinetics

• *Absorption:* Not applicable; administered by I.V. infusion.
• *Distribution:* Drug is not significantly bound to plasma proteins. It does cross the blood-brain barrier, diffusing into the CNS in CSF at levels up to 51% of corresponding serum concentrations.
• *Metabolism:* Not significant.
• *Excretion:* 80% of I.V. dose is excreted unchanged in the urine within 24 hours. Terminal plasma elimination half-life is 3 to 4 hours.

Contraindications and precautions

Contraindicated in patients with hypersensitivity to drug. Use cautiously in patients with impaired renal function because most (about 80%) of drug is excreted unchanged in the urine.

Interactions

None reported.

Effects on diagnostic tests

None reported.

Adverse reactions

CNS: ***seizures,*** hearing impairment, dizziness, headache, asthenia.
GI: diarrhea, vomiting, abdominal pain, anorexia.
Hematologic: *anemia, leukopenia,* ***thrombocytopenia, myelosupression,*** eosinophilia.
Other: facial edema, alopecia.

Overdose and treatment

No information available.

☑ Special considerations

• Because drug is a myelosuppressant, careful monitoring of hematologic status is necessary for safe and effective use. Some degree of myelosuppression may be unavoidable; in most patients, problems resolve after discontinuation of drug.
• Eflornithine concentrate is hypertonic and must be diluted with sterile water for injection before use. Diluted drug must be used within 24 hours of preparation and stored at 39° F (4° C) to minimize risk of microbial proliferation.
• Other drugs should not be administered I.V. simultaneously during eflornithine administration.
• Perform CBC and platelet counts before therapy, twice weekly during therapy, and weekly after completion of therapy until hematologic values return to baseline.
• Monitor patient for at least 24 months to ensure further therapy in the event of relapse.
• To prepare solutions within 10% of plasma tonicity, use strict aseptic technique; withdraw the entire contents of each 100-ml vial of eflornithine and inject 25 ml into each of four diluent bags (100 ml of sterile water for injection per bag). Concentration will be 40 mg/ml (5,000 mg of eflornithine in 125 ml final volume).
• Serial audiograms are recommended to monitor degree of hearing impairment.

Patient education

• Inform patient of need for frequent blood tests.
• Advise patient that audiograms will be done to monitor for hearing problems.

Geriatric use

• Use cautiously because elderly patients may develop some degree of renal impairment.

Pediatric use
- Safety and efficacy have not been established.

Breast-feeding
- It is unknown if drug is excreted in breast milk. Consider potential for serious adverse reactions in breast-fed infants against importance of drug to mother.

enalaprilat
Vasotec I.V.

enalapril maleate
Vasotec

Pharmacologic classification: ACE inhibitor
Therapeutic classification: antihypertensive
Pregnancy risk category C (D in second and third trimesters)

How supplied
Available by prescription only
Tablets: 2.5 mg, 5 mg, 10 mg, 20 mg
Injection: 1.25 mg/ml in 2-ml vials

Indications, route, and dosage
Hypertension
Adults: For patient not receiving diuretics, initially 5 mg P.O. once daily, then adjusted according to response. Usual dosage range is 10 to 40 mg daily as a single dose or two divided doses. Alternatively, 1.25 mg I.V. infusion q 6 hours over 5 minutes. For patient on diuretics, initially 2.5 mg P.O. once daily. Alternatively, administer 0.625 mg I.V. over 5 minutes, repeat in 1 hour if needed, then follow by 1.25 mg I.V. q 6 hours.
To convert from I.V. therapy to oral therapy
Adults: If patient was not treated with diuretics and was receiving 1.25 mg q 6 hours, then initially, 5 mg P.O. once daily. If patient is being treated with diuretics and was receiving 0.625 mg I.V. q 6 hours, then 2.5 mg P.O. once daily. Adjust dose according to response.
To convert from oral therapy to I.V. therapy
Adults: 1.25 mg I.V. over 5 minutes q 6 hours. Higher doses have not demonstrated greater efficacy.
✦ ***Dosage adjustment.*** In hypertensive patients with renal failure who have a creatinine clearance below 30 ml/minute, begin therapy at 2.5 mg/day. Gradually titrate dosage according to response. Patients undergoing hemodialysis should receive a supplemental dose of 2.5 mg on days of dialysis.
Heart failure
Adults: Initially, 2.5 mg P.O. Recommended dosing range is 2.5 to 20 mg b.i.d. Titrate dosage upward, as tolerated, over a period of a few days or weeks. Maximum daily dose is 40 mg P.O. daily in divided doses.
Asymptomatic left ventricular dysfunction
Adults: Initially, 2.5 mg P.O. b.i.d.; titrate dosage to targeted daily dose of 20 mg (in divided doses) as tolerated.
✦ ***Dosage adjustment.*** In patients with heart failure and renal impairment or hyponatremia (serum sodium less than 130 mEq/L or serum creatinine above 1.6 mg/dl), begin therapy with 2.5 mg P.O. daily. Increase dosage to 2.5 mg b.i.d., then 5 mg b.i.d. and higher p.r.n., usually at intervals of 4 days or more.

Pharmacodynamics
Antihypertensive action: Enalapril inhibits ACE, preventing conversion of angiotensin I to angiotensin II, a potent vasoconstrictor. Reduced angiotensin II levels decrease peripheral arterial resistance, lowering blood pressure, and decrease aldosterone secretion, thus reducing sodium and water retention.

Pharmacokinetics
- *Absorption:* Approximately 60% of a given dose of enalapril is absorbed from the GI tract; blood pressure decreases within 1 hour, with peak antihypertensive effect at 4 to 6 hours.
- *Distribution:* Full distribution pattern of enalapril is unknown; drug does not appear to cross the blood-brain barrier.
- *Metabolism:* Enalapril is metabolized extensively to the active metabolite enalaprilat.
- *Excretion:* About 94% of a dose of enalapril is excreted in urine and feces as enalaprilat and enalapril.

Contraindications and precautions
Contraindicated in patients with hypersensitivity to drug or history of angioedema related to previous treatment with an ACE inhibitor. Use cautiously in patients with impaired renal function.

Interactions
Indomethacin and *aspirin* may decrease enalapril's antihypertensive effect; enalapril may increase antihypertensive effects of *diuretics, phenothiazines,* or *other antihypertensive drugs.*

Enalapril may enhance effects of *potassium-sparing diuretics, potassium supplements,* and *salt substitutes,* thereby causing hyperkalemia; such products should be used cautiously.

Enalapril may decrease the renal clearance of *lithium* and may decrease pharmacologic effects of *rifampin.*

Enalapril, similar to other ACE-inhibitors, may cause a dry hacking cough.

Effects on diagnostic tests
Enalapril may elevate BUN and serum creatinine levels and, less commonly, liver enzyme and bilirubin levels; it may slightly decrease hemoglobin and hematocrit levels. Rare cases of neutropenia, thrombocytopenia, and bone marrow depression have been reported.

Adverse reactions
CNS: *headache, dizziness, fatigue,* vertigo, asthenia, syncope.
CV: *hypotension,* chest pain.
GI: diarrhea, nausea, abdominal pain, vomiting.
GU: decreased renal function (in patients with bilateral renal artery stenosis or heart failure).

Hematologic: ***neutropenia, agranulocytosis.***
Respiratory: *dry, persistent, tickling, nonproductive cough;* dyspnea.
Skin: rash.
Other: ***angioedema.***

Overdose and treatment

Little clinical data are available. The most likely manifestation would be hypotension. After acute ingestion, empty stomach by induced emesis or gastric lavage. Follow with activated charcoal to reduce absorption. Consider hemodialysis in severe cases. Subsequent treatment is usually symptomatic and supportive.

☑ Special considerations

- Discontinue diuretic therapy 2 to 3 days before beginning enalapril therapy, to reduce risk of hypotension; if drug does not adequately control blood pressure, diuretics should be reinstated.
- Perform WBC and differential counts before treatment, every 2 weeks for 3 months, and periodically thereafter.
- Proteinuria and nephrotic syndrome may occur in patients who are on enalapril therapy.
- Give drug before, during, or after meals because food does not appear to affect absorption.

Patient education

- Tell patient to report feelings of light-headedness, especially in first few days, so dosage can be adjusted; signs of infection, such as sore throat and fever, because drug may decrease WBC count; facial swelling or difficulty breathing, because drug may cause angioedema; and loss of taste, which may necessitate discontinuing drug.
- Advise patient not to change position suddenly to minimize orthostatic hypotension.
- Warn patient to seek medical approval before taking OTC cold preparations particularly cough medications.

Geriatric use

- Elderly patients may need lower doses because of impaired drug clearance.

Pediatric use

- Safety and efficacy of enalapril in children have not been established; use only if potential benefit outweighs risk.

Breast-feeding

- It is unknown if drug occurs in breast milk; an alternative feeding method is recommended during therapy.

enoxacin

Penetrex

Pharmacologic classification: fluoroquinolone antibacterial
Therapeutic classification: antibiotic
Pregnancy risk category C

How supplied

Available by prescription only
Tablets (film-coated): 200 mg, 400 mg

Indications, route, and dosage

Uncomplicated urinary tract infections (cystitis) caused by **Escherichia coli, Staphylococcus epidermidis, *or* Staphylococcus saprophyticus**
Adults: 200 mg P.O. q 12 hours for 7 days.
Complicated urinary tract infections caused by **E. coli, Klebsiella pneumoniae, Proteus mirabilis, Pseudomonas aeruginosa, Staphylococcus epidermidis, *or* Enterobacter cloacae**
Adults: 400 mg P.O. q 12 hours for 14 days.
Uncomplicated urethral or endocervical gonorrhea caused by **Neisseria gonorrhoeae**
Adults: 400 mg P.O. as a single dose.
✦ ***Dosage adjustment.*** In patients with renal impairment, if creatinine clearance is 30 ml/minute/1.73 m^2 or less, start therapy with the usual initial dose. Decrease subsequent doses by 50%.

Note*:* Discontinue therapy if hypersensitivity or phototoxicity occurs.

Pharmacodynamics

Antibiotic action: Enoxacin, a bactericidal agent, inhibits the bacterial enzyme DNA gyrase, which is necessary for DNA replication. The drug is active against most strains of gram-positive aerobes, such as *Staphylococcus epidermidis* and *Staphylococcus saprophyticus,* and against many gram-negative aerobes, such as *Enterobacter cloacae, Escherichia coli, Klebsiella pneumoniae, Neisseria gonorrhoeae, Proteus mirabilis,* and *Pseudomonas aeruginosa.*

Pharmacokinetics

- *Absorption:* Following oral administration, peak plasma concentrations may be achieved within 1 to 3 hours. Absolute oral bioavailability is about 90%.
- *Distribution:* Drug is approximately 40% bound to plasma proteins in healthy individuals and 14% bound to plasma proteins in patients with impaired renal function.
- *Metabolism:* Five metabolites of enoxacin have been identified in human urine; they account for 15% to 20% of the administered dose.
- *Excretion:* Excreted primarily by the kidneys. Drug's plasma half-life is 3 to 6 hours.

Contraindications and precautions

Contraindicated in patients with hypersensitivity to drug or other fluoroquinolone antibiotics.

Use cautiously in patients with CNS disorders, such as severe cerebral arteriosclerosis or seizure disorders, and in those at increased risk for seizures. Enoxacin may cause CNS stimulation. Use with caution and with dosage adjustments in patients with impaired renal or hepatic function.

Interactions

Enoxacin interferes with the metabolism of *theophylline,* resulting in a dose-related decrease in theophylline clearance. Elevated serum theophylline concentrations may increase the risk of theophylline-related adverse reactions. Enoxacin also interferes with the metabolism of *caffeine*, resulting in a decrease in caffeine clearance of up to 80%. This effect increases caffeine-related adverse effects. Instruct patient not to consume caffeine products while taking enoxacin.

Bismuth subsalicylate, given within 60 minutes after enoxacin, decreases enoxacin bioavailability by approximately 25%. Concomitant administration should be avoided.

Elevated cyclosporine levels have been reported with concomitant use of *cyclosporine* and *members of the quinolone class*. Monitor patients receiving cyclosporine and enoxacin concurrently.

Enoxacin may raise serum *digoxin* levels in some patients. If signs and symptoms of digoxin toxicity occur, obtain serum digoxin levels and adjust digoxin doses appropriately.

Quinolones form chelates with metal cations. Therefore, administration of quinolones with *antacids containing calcium, magnesium, or aluminum;* with *sucralfate;* with *divalent or trivalent cations*, such as *iron*; or with *multivitamins containing zinc* may substantially interfere with drug absorption and result in insufficient plasma and tissue quinolone concentrations. These agents should not be taken for 8 hours before or for 2 hours after enoxacin administration.

Oral bioavailability of enoxacin is reduced by 60% with coadministration of *ranitidine*. Thus, ranitidine should not be administered for 8 hours before or for 2 hours after enoxacin.

Effects on diagnostic tests
None reported.

Adverse reactions
CNS: headache, restlessness, tremor, light-headedness, confusion, hallucinations, ***seizures.***
GI: *nausea, diarrhea*, vomiting, abdominal pain or discomfort, oral candidiasis.
GU: crystalluria.
Musculoskeletal: tendon pain, tendon rupture.
Skin: *rash*, pruritus, photosensitivity.
Other: eosinophilia, dyspnea, cough, elevated liver enzymes, hypersensitivity.

Overdose and treatment
In the event of acute overdosage, the stomach should be emptied by inducing vomiting or by gastric lavage and the patient carefully observed and given supportive treatment. Enoxacin is poorly removed (less than 5% over 4 hours) by hemodialysis.

☑ Special considerations
- Obtain specimen for culture and sensitivity tests before giving first dose. Therapy may begin pending results.
- Safety and efficacy of enoxacin in pregnant women have not been established.
- Pseudomembranous colitis has been reported with enoxacin and may range in severity from mild to life-threatening. This diagnosis should be considered in patients who present with diarrhea after enoxacin administration.
- Moderate-to-severe phototoxicity reactions have been observed in patients exposed to direct sunlight while receiving enoxacin.

Patient education
- Advise patient to avoid excessive sunlight and to take other precautions as necessary to prevent phototoxicity.
- Instruct patient to call immediately if pregnancy is suspected.
- Tell patient not to take magnesium-, aluminum-, or calcium-containing antacids; bismuth subsalicylate; iron-containing products; or multivitamins that contain zinc for 8 hours before enoxacin administration.
- Instruct patient to drink fluid liberally but to avoid consumption of caffeine-containing products during enoxacin therapy.
- Caution patient that enoxacin may cause dizziness and light-headedness; advise him not to operate an automobile or other hazardous machinery or to engage in activities requiring mental alertness and coordination until response to therapy is known.
- Advise patient that enoxacin may be associated with hypersensitivity reaction, even after the first dose. Tell him to discontinue drug and call at the first sign of rash or other allergic reactions.
- Instruct patient to take enoxacin at least 1 hour before or at least 2 hours after a meal.

Pediatric use
- Safety and effectiveness of enoxacin in children have not been established.

Breast-feeding
- Safety and effectiveness of enoxacin in breast-feeding patients have not been established.

enoxaparin sodium
Lovenox

Pharmacologic classification: low-molecular-weight heparin
Therapeutic classification: anticoagulant
Pregnancy risk category B

How supplied
Available by prescription only
Ampules: 30 mg/0.3 ml
Syringes (prefilled): 30 mg/0.3 ml; 40 mg/0.4 ml
Syringes (graduated prefilled): 60 mg/0.6 ml; 80 mg/0.8 ml; 100 mg/1 ml

Indications, route, and dosage
Prevention of deep vein thrombosis (DVT), which may lead to pulmonary embolism, following hip or knee replacement surgery
Adults: 30 mg S.C. q 12 hours for 7 to 10 days. Give initial dose between 12 and 24 hours postoperatively provided hemostasis has been established.
Prevention of DVT, which may lead to pulmonary embolism, following abdominal surgery
Adults: 40 mg S.C. once daily for 7 to 10 days. Give initial dose 2 hours hours prior to surgery.

Prevention of ischemic complications of unstable angina and non-Q-wave MI, when concurrently administered with aspirin
Adults: 1 mg/kg S.C. q 12 hours for 2 to 8 days in conjunction with oral aspirin therapy (100 to 325 mg once daily).

Note: To minimize risk of bleeding following vascular instrumentation during the treatment of unstable angina, adhere precisely to the intervals recommended between enoxaparin doses.

Pharmacodynamics
Anticoagulant action: Enoxaparin is a low-molecular-weight heparin that accelerates formation of antithrombin III-thrombin complex and deactivates thrombin, preventing conversion of fibrinogen to fibrin. It has a higher anti-factor Xa to anti-factor IIa activity than unfractionated heparin.

Pharmacokinetics
- *Absorption:* Maximum anti-factor Xa and antifactor IIa (antithrombin) activities occur 3 to 5 hours after S.C. injection of enoxaparin.
- *Distribution:* Volume of distribution of antifactor Xa activity is approximately 6 L.
- *Metabolism:* Information not available.
- *Excretion:* Elimination half-life based on antifactor Xa activity is about 4.5 hours after S.C. administration.

Contraindications and precautions
Contraindicated in patients with hypersensitivity to drug or heparin or pork products; in patients with active, major bleeding or thrombocytopenia; and in those who demonstrate antiplatelet antibodies in the presence of drug.

Use with extreme caution in patients with history of heparin-induced thrombocytopenia. Use cautiously in patients with conditions that put them at increased risk for hemorrhage, such as bacterial endocarditis; congenital or acquired bleeding disorders; ulcer disease; angiodysplastic GI disease; hemorrhagic stroke; or recent spinal, eye, or brain surgery; or in those treated concomitantly with NSAIDs, platelet inhibitors, or other anticoagulants that affect hemostasis. Also use cautiously in patients with a bleeding diathesis, uncontrolled arterial hypertension, or history of recent GI ulceration, diabetic retinopathy, and hemorrhage. Use with care in the elderly and patients with renal insufficiency who may show delayed elimination of enoxaparin.

Use with extreme caution in patients with postoperative indwelling epidural catheters. Cases of epidural or spinal hematomas have been reported with the use of enoxaparin and spinal or epidural anesthesia or spinal puncture resulting in long-term or permanent paralysis.

Interactions
Concomitant use of enoxaparin with other *anticoagulants* or *antiplatelet agents* increases the risk of bleeding.

Effects on diagnostic tests
Enoxaparin therapy may decrease patient's platelet count and may increase AST and ALT levels.

Adverse reactions
CNS: confusion.
CV: edema, peripheral edema.
GI: nausea.
Hematologic: hypochromic anemia, ***thrombocytopenia.***
Other: irritation, pain, hematoma, erythema (at injection site); fever; pain; ***hemorrhage;*** ecchymoses; bleeding complications.

Overdose and treatment
Accidental overdose after drug administration may lead to hemorrhagic complications. This may be largely neutralized by the slow I.V. injection of protamine sulfate (1%) solution. The dose of protamine sulfate should be equal to the dose of enoxaparin injection (1 mg of protamine neutralizes 1 mg of enoxaparin).

☑ Special considerations
- Enoxaparin is not intended for I.M. administration.
- Drug cannot be used interchangeably (unit for unit) with unfractionated heparin or other low-molecular-weight heparins.
- Do not mix drug with other injections or infusions.
- Screen all patients before prophylactic administration of enoxaparin to rule out a bleeding disorder.
- There is usually no need for daily monitoring of the effect of enoxaparin in patients with normal presurgical coagulation parameters.
- Administer drug by deep S.C. injection with patient lying down. The full length of the needle should be introduced into a skin fold held between the thumb and forefinger, and the skin fold should be held throughout the injection. Alternate administration sites exist between the left and right anterolateral and left and right posterolateral abdominal wall.
- Do not expel air bubble from syringe before injection because drug may be lost.
- If thromboembolic events occur despite enoxaparin prophylaxis, discontinue drug and initiate appropriate therapy.
- Consider the potential benefit versus risk before neuraxial intervention in patients anticoagulated or to be anticoagulated for thromboprophylaxis. When epidural or spinal anesthesia or spinal puncture is employed, patients anticoagulated with enoxaparin are at risk of developing an epidural or spinal hematoma. Patients should be frequently monitored for signs and symptoms of neurological impairment. If neurologic compromise is noted, urgent treatment is necessary.

Pediatric use
- Safety and effectiveness of enoxaparin in children have not been established.

Breast-feeding
- It is not known if drug is excreted in breast milk. Therefore, use with caution when administering to breast-feeding patients.

ephedrine

ephedrine hydrochloride

ephedrine sulfate

Ephedrine Sulphate Capsules,
Ephedrine Sulfate Injection

Pharmacologic classification: adrenergic
Therapeutic classification: bronchodilator, vasopressor (parenteral form), nasal decongestant
Pregnancy risk category C

How supplied

Available with and without a prescription
Capsules: 25 mg, 50 mg
Nasal preparations: 1% jelly; 0.25% spray; 0.5% drops
Injection: 25 mg/ml, 50 mg/ml (parenteral)

Indications, route, and dosage

To correct hypotensive states
Adults: 25 to 50 mg I.M. or S.C., or 10 to 25 mg slow I.V. bolus. If necessary, a second I.M. dose of 50 mg or I.V. dose of 25 mg may be administered. Additional I.V. doses may be given in 5 to 10 minutes. Maximum dosage is 150 mg daily.
Children: 3 mg/kg or 100 mg/m^2 S.C. or I.V. daily, divided into four to six doses.
Orthostatic hypotension
Adults: 25 mg P.O. once daily to q.i.d.
Children: 3 mg/kg P.O. daily, divided into four to six doses.
Bronchodilator or nasal decongestant
Adults: 25 to 50 mg q 3 to 4 hours p.r.n.; 12.5 to 25 mg I.M., I.V., or S.C. repeated based on patient response.
As nasal decongestant, 2 to 3 drops instilled into each nostril or on a nasal pack. Instill no more often than q 4 hours.
Children age 2 and older: 2 to 3 mg/kg or 100 mg/m^2 P.O. daily in four to six divided doses.
Severe, acute bronchospasm
Adults: 12.5 to 25 mg I.M., S.C., or I.V.
Enuresis
Adults: 25 to 50 mg P.O. h.s.
Myasthenia gravis
Adults: 25 mg t.i.d. to q.i.d.

Pharmacodynamics

Ephedrine is both a direct- and indirect-acting sympathomimetic that stimulates alpha- and beta-adrenergic receptors. Release of norepinephrine from its storage sites is one of its indirect effects. In therapeutic doses, ephedrine relaxes bronchial smooth muscle and produces cardiac stimulation with increased systolic and diastolic blood pressure when norepinephrine stores are not depleted.

Bronchodilator action: Ephedrine relaxes bronchial smooth muscle by stimulating beta$_2$-adrenergic receptors, resulting in increased vital capacity, relief of mild bronchospasm, improved air exchange, and decreased residual volume.

Vasopressor action: Drug produces positive inotropic effects with low doses by action on beta$_1$-receptors in the heart. Vasodilation results from its effect on beta$_2$-adrenergic receptors; vasoconstriction from its alpha-adrenergic effects. Pressor effects may result from vasoconstriction or cardiac stimulation; however, when peripheral vascular resistance is decreased, blood pressure elevation results from increased cardiac output.

Nasal decongestant action: Ephedrine stimulates alpha-adrenergic receptors in blood vessels of nasal mucosa, producing vasoconstriction and nasal decongestion.

Pharmacokinetics

- *Absorption:* Rapidly and completely absorbed after oral, S.C., or I.M. administration. After oral administration, onset of action occurs within 15 to 60 minutes and persists 2 to 4 hours. Pressor and cardiac effects last 1 hour after I.V. dose of 10 to 25 mg or I.M. or S.C. dose of 25 to 50 mg; they last up to 4 hours after oral dose of 15 to 50 mg.
- *Distribution:* Drug is widely distributed throughout the body.
- *Metabolism:* Ephedrine is slowly metabolized in the liver by oxidative deamination, demethylation, aromatic hydroxylation, and conjugation.
- *Excretion:* Dose is mostly excreted unchanged in urine; rate of excretion depends on urine pH.

Contraindications and precautions

Contraindicated in patients with hypersensitivity to drug and other sympathomimetics; in those with porphyria, severe coronary artery disease, arrhythmias, angle-closure glaucoma, psychoneurosis, angina pectoris, substantial organic heart disease, and CV disease; and in those taking MAO inhibitors.

Nasal solution is contraindicated in patients with angle-closure glaucoma, psychoneurosis, angina pectoris, substantial organic heart disease, CV disease, and hypersensitivity to drug or other sympathomimetics.

Use with extreme caution in elderly men and in those with hypertension, hyperthyroidism, nervous or excitable states, diabetes, and prostatic hyperplasia. Use nasal solution cautiously in patients with hyperthyroidism, hypertension, diabetes mellitus, or prostatic hyperplasia.

Interactions

Use with *other sympathomimetic agents* may add to their effects and toxicity. Use with *alpha-adrenergic blocking agents* may decrease vasopressor effects of ephedrine. Concomitant *beta-adrenergic blocking agents* may block CV and bronchodilating effects of ephedrine. Use with *general anesthetics* (especially *cyclopropane, halothane)* and *cardiac glycosides* may sensitize myocardium to effects of ephedrine, causing arrhythmias.

MAO inhibitors may potentiate the pressor effects of ephedrine, possibly resulting in hypertensive crisis. Allow 14 days to lapse after withdrawal of MAO inhibitor before using ephedrine. *Reserpine, guanethidine, methyldopa,* and *diuretics* may decrease ephedrine's pressor effects.

Concomitant use with *atropine* blocks reflex bradycardia and enhances pressor effects. Administration with a *theophylline derivative* such as *aminophylline* reportedly produces a greater incidence of adverse reactions than either drug when used alone.

Effects on diagnostic tests
None reported.

Adverse reactions
CNS: *insomnia, nervousness,* dizziness, headache, muscle weakness, diaphoresis, euphoria, confusion, delirium; nervousness, excitation (with nasal solution).
CV: *palpitations,* tachycardia, hypertension, precordial pain; *tachycardia* (with nasal solution).
EENT: dry nose and throat; rebound nasal congestion with long-term or excessive use, mucosal irritation (with nasal solution).
GI: nausea, vomiting, anorexia.
GU: urine retention, painful urination due to visceral sphincter spasm.

Overdose and treatment
Clinical manifestations of overdose include exaggeration of common adverse reactions, especially arrhythmias, extreme tremor or seizures, nausea and vomiting, fever, and CNS and respiratory depression.

Treatment requires supportive and symptomatic measures. If patient is conscious, induce emesis with ipecac followed by activated charcoal. If patient is depressed or hyperactive, perform gastric lavage. Maintain airway and blood pressure. Do not administer vasopressors. Monitor vital signs closely.

A beta blocker (such as propranolol) may be used to treat arrhythmias. A cardioselective beta blocker is recommended in asthmatic patients. Phentolamine may be used for hypertension, paraldehyde or diazepam for seizures, and dexamethasone for pyrexia.

☑ Special considerations
Besides those relevant to all *adrenergics,* consider the following recommendations.
- As a pressor agent, ephedrine is not a substitute for blood, plasma, fluids, or electrolytes. Correct fluid volume depletion before administration.
- Tolerance may develop after prolonged or excessive use. Increased dose may be needed. Also, if drug is discontinued for a few days and readministered, effectiveness may be restored.
- To prevent insomnia, last dose should be taken at least 2 hours before bedtime.
- With parenteral dosing, monitor vital signs closely during infusion. Tachycardia is common.

Patient education
- Tell patient using OTC product to follow directions on label, to take last dose a few hours before bedtime to reduce possibility of insomnia, to take only as directed, and not to increase dose or frequency.
- Advise patient to store drug away from heat and light (not in bathroom medicine cabinet) and to keep out of reach of children.
- Instruct patient who misses a dose to take it as soon as remembered if within 1 hour. If beyond 1 hour, patient should skip dose and return to regular schedule.
- Teach patient to be aware of palpitations and significant pulse rate changes.
- Instruct patient to clear nose before instillation of nasal solutions.

Geriatric use
- Administer cautiously, because elderly patients may be more sensitive to drug's effects. Lower dose may be recommended.

Pediatric use
- Use cautiously in children.

Breast-feeding
- Avoid breast-feeding during treatment with ephedrine.

epinephrine
Bronkaid Mist, Bronkaid Mistometer*, EpiPen, EpiPen Jr., Primatene Mist, Sus-Phrine

epinephrine bitartrate
AsthmaHaler

epinephrine hydrochloride
Adrenalin Chloride, AsthmaNefrin, Epifrin, Glaucon, microNefrin, Vaponefrin

epinephryl borate
Epinal

Pharmacologic classification: adrenergic
Therapeutic classification: bronchodilator, vasopressor, cardiac stimulant, local anesthetic (adjunct), topical antihemorrhagic, antiglaucoma
Pregnancy risk category C

How supplied
Available by prescription only
Injection: 0.01 mg/ml (1:100,000), 0.1 mg/ml (1:10,000), 0.5 mg/ml (1:2,000), 1 mg/ml (1:1,000) parenteral; 5 mg/ml (1:200) parenteral suspension
Ophthalmic: 0.1%, 0.25%, 0.5%, 1%, 2% solution

Available without a prescription
Nebulizer inhaler: 1% (1:100), 1.25%, 2.25%
Aerosol inhaler: 160 mcg, 200 mcg, 250 mcg/metered spray
Nasal solution: 0.1%

Indications, route, and dosage
Bronchospasm, hypersensitivity reactions, anaphylaxis
Adults: Initially, 0.1 to 0.5 mg (0.1 to 0.5 ml of a 1:1,000 solution) S.C. or I.M.; may be repeated at 10- to 15-minute intervals p.r.n. Alternatively, 0.1 to 0.25 mg (1 to 2.5 ml of a 1:10,000 solution) I.V. slowly over 5 to 10 minutes. May be repeated q 5

to 15 minutes if needed or followed by a 1 to 4 mcg/minute I.V. infusion.

Children: 0.01 mg/kg (0.01 ml/kg of a 1:1,000 solution) or 0.3 mg/m² (0.3 ml/m² of a 1:1,000 solution) S.C. Dose not to exceed 0.5 mg. May be repeated at 20-minute to 4-hour intervals, p.r.n. Alternatively, 0.02 to 0.025 mg/kg (0.004 to 0.005 ml/kg) or 0.625 mg/m² (0.125 ml/m²) of a 1:200 solution. May be repeated but not more often than q 6 hours. Alternatively, 0.1 mg (10 ml of a 1:100,000 dilution) I.V. slowly over 5 to 10 minutes followed by a 0.1 to 1.5 mcg/kg/minute I.V. infusion.

Bronchodilator

Adults and children: 1 inhalation via metered aerosol, repeated once if needed after 1 minute; subsequent doses should not be repeated for at least 3 hours. Alternatively, 1 or 2 deep inhalations via hand-bulb nebulizer of a 1% (1:100) solution; may be repeated at 1- to 2-minute intervals. Alternatively, 0.03 ml (0.3 mg) of a 1% solution via intermittent positive pressure breathing.

To restore cardiac rhythm in cardiac arrest

Adults: Initially, 0.5 to 1 mg (range, 0.1 to 1 mg to 10 ml of a 1:10,000 solution) I.V. bolus; may be repeated q 3 to 5 minutes p.r.n. Alternatively, initial dose followed by 0.3 mg S.C. or 1 to 4 mcg/minute I.V. infusion. Alternatively, 1 mg (10 ml of a 1:10,000 solution) intratracheally, or 0.1 to 1 mg (1 to 10 ml of a 1:10,000 solution) by intracardiac injection.

Children: Initially, 0.01 mg/kg (0.1 ml/kg of a 1:10,000 solution) I.V. bolus or intratracheally; may be repeated q 5 minutes p.r.n.

Alternatively, initially, 0.1 mcg/kg/minute; may increase in increments of 0.1 mcg/kg/minute to a maximum of 1 mcg/kg/minute. Alternatively, 0.005 to 0.01 mg/kg (0.05 to 0.1 ml/kg of a 1:10,000 solution) by intracardiac injection.

Infants: Initially, 0.01 to 0.03 mg/kg (0.1 to 0.3 ml/kg of a 1:10,000 solution) I.V. bolus or by intratracheal injection. May be repeated q 5 minutes p.r.n.

Hemostatic use

Adults: 1:50,000 to 1:1,000, applied topically.

To prolong local anesthetic effect

Adults and children: 1:500,000 to 1:50,000 mixed with local anesthetic.

Open-angle glaucoma

Adults: 1 or 2 drops of 1% to 2% solution instilled daily or b.i.d.

Nasal congestion, local superficial bleeding

Adults and children: Instill 1 or 2 drops of solution.

Pharmacodynamics

Epinephrine acts directly by stimulating alpha- and beta-adrenergic receptors in the sympathetic nervous system. Its main therapeutic effects include relaxation of bronchial smooth muscle, cardiac stimulation, and dilation of skeletal muscle vasculature.

Bronchodilator action: Epinephrine relaxes bronchial smooth muscle by stimulating $beta_2$-adrenergic receptors. Epinephrine constricts bronchial arterioles by stimulating alpha-adrenergic receptors, resulting in relief of bronchospasm, reduced congestion and edema, and increased tidal volume and vital capacity. By inhibiting histamine release, it may reverse bronchiolar constriction, vasodilation, and edema.

CV and vasopressor actions: As a cardiac stimulant, epinephrine produces positive chronotropic and inotropic effects by action on $beta_1$-receptors in the heart, increasing cardiac output, myocardial oxygen consumption, and force of contraction and decreasing cardiac efficiency. Vasodilation results from its effect on $beta_2$-receptors; vasoconstriction results from alpha-adrenergic effects.

Local anesthetic (adjunct) action: Epinephrine acts on alpha receptors in skin, mucous membranes, and viscera; it produces vasoconstriction, which reduces absorption of local anesthetic, thus prolonging its duration of action, localizing anesthesia, and decreasing risk of anesthetic's toxicity.

Local vasoconstriction action: Epinephrine's effect results from action on alpha receptors in skin, mucous membranes, and viscera, which produces vasoconstriction and hemostasis in small vessels.

Antiglaucoma action: Epinephrine's exact mechanism of lowering intraocular pressure is unknown. When applied topically to the conjunctiva or injected into the interior chamber of the eye, epinephrine constricts conjunctival blood vessels, contracts the dilator muscle of the pupil, and may dilate the pupil.

Pharmacokinetics

- *Absorption:* Well absorbed after S.C. or I.M. injection, epinephrine has a rapid onset of action and short duration of action. Bronchodilation occurs within 5 to 10 minutes and peaks in 20 minutes after S.C. injection; onset after oral inhalation is within 1 minute.

Topical administration or intraocular injection usually produces local vasoconstriction within 5 minutes and lasts less than 1 hour. After topical application to the conjunctiva, reduction of intraocular pressure occurs within 1 hour, peaks in 4 to 8 hours, and persists up to 24 hours.

- *Distribution:* Epinephrine is distributed widely throughout the body.
- *Metabolism:* Drug is metabolized at sympathetic nerve endings, liver, and other tissues to inactive metabolites.
- *Excretion:* Epinephrine is excreted in urine, mainly as its metabolites and conjugates.

Contraindications and precautions

Contraindicated in patients with angle-closure glaucoma, shock (other than anaphylactic shock), organic brain damage, cardiac dilation, arrhythmias, coronary insufficiency, or cerebral arteriosclerosis. Also contraindicated in patients during general anesthesia with halogenated hydrocarbons or cyclopropane and in patients in labor (may delay second stage).

Some commercial products contain sulfites; contraindicated in patients with sulfite allergies except when epinephrine is being used for treatment of serious allergic reactions or other emergencies.

In conjunction with local anesthetics, epinephrine is contraindicated for use in fingers, toes, ears, nose, or genitalia.

Ophthalmic preparation is contraindicated in patients with angle-closure glaucoma or when nature of the glaucoma has not been established and in patients with hypersensitivity to the drug, organic mental syndrome, or cardiac dilation and coronary insufficiency. Nasal solution is contraindicated in patients with hypersensitivity to drug.

Use with extreme caution in patients with long-standing bronchial asthma and emphysema who have developed degenerative heart disease. Also use cautiously in elderly patients and in those with hyperthyroidism, CV disease, hypertension, psychoneurosis, and diabetes.

Use ophthalmic preparation cautiously in the elderly and in patients with diabetes, hypertension, Parkinson's disease, hyperthyroidism, aphakia (eye without lens), cardiac disease, cerebral arteriosclerosis, or bronchial asthma.

Interactions

Concomitant use with other *sympathomimetics* may produce additive effects and toxicity. *Beta-adrenergic blockers* antagonize cardiac and bronchodilating effects of epinephrine; *alpha-adrenergic blockers* antagonize vasoconstriction and hypertension. Use with *general anesthetics* (especially *cyclopropane, halothane)* and *cardiac glycosides* may sensitize the myocardium to epinephrine's effects, causing arrhythmias. Use with *tricyclic antidepressants, antihistamines,* and *thyroid hormones* may potentiate adverse cardiac effects of epinephrine. Concomitant use with *oxytocics* or *ergot alkaloids* may cause severe hypertension.

Because *phenothiazines* may cause reversal of its pressor effects, epinephrine should not be used to treat circulatory collapse or hypotension caused by phenothiazines; such use may cause further lowering of blood pressure.

Use with *guanethidine* may decrease its hypotensive effects while potentiating epinephrine's effects, resulting in hypertension and arrhythmias.

Concomitant use with *antidiabetic agents* may decrease their effects. Dosage adjustments may be necessary.

Concomitant use of ophthalmic epinephrine with *topical miotics, topical beta-adrenergic blocking agents, osmotic agents,* and *carbonic anhydrase inhibitors* may cause additive lowering of intraocular pressure. Concomitant use with *miotics* offers the advantage of reducing the ciliary spasm, mydriasis, blurred vision, and increased intraocular pressure that may occur with miotics or epinephrine alone.

Effects on diagnostic tests

Epinephrine therapy alters blood glucose and serum lactic acid levels (both may be increased), increases BUN levels, and interferes with tests for urinary catecholamines.

Adverse reactions

CNS: *nervousness, tremor,* vertigo, *headache,* disorientation, agitation, *drowsiness,* fear, pallor, dizziness, weakness, ***cerebral hemorrhage, CVA.*** In patients with Parkinson's disease, drug increases rigidity, tremor; browache, headache, light-headedness (with ophthalmic preparation); nervousness, excitation (with nasal solution).

CV: *palpitations;* widened pulse pressure; ***hypertension; tachycardia; ventricular fibrillation; shock;*** anginal pain; ECG changes, including a decreased T-wave amplitude; palpitations, tachycardia, ***arrhythmias,*** hypertension (with ophthalmic preparation); *tachycardia (with nasal solution).*

EENT: corneal or conjunctival pigmentation or corneal edema in long-term use, follicular hypertrophy, chemosis, conjunctivitis, iritis, hyperemic conjunctiva, maculopapular rash, eye pain, allergic lid reaction, ocular irritation, eye stinging, burning, and tearing on instillation (with ophthalmic preparation); rebound nasal congestion, slight sting upon application (with nasal solution).

GI: *nausea, vomiting.*

Respiratory: dyspnea.

Skin: urticaria, pain, hemorrhage (at injection site).

Overdose and treatment

Clinical manifestations of overdose may include a sharp increase in systolic and diastolic blood pressure, rise in venous pressure, severe anxiety, irregular heartbeat, severe nausea or vomiting, severe respiratory distress, unusually large pupils, unusual paleness and coldness of skin, pulmonary edema, renal failure, and metabolic acidosis.

Treatment includes symptomatic and supportive measures, because epinephrine is rapidly inactivated in the body. Monitor vital signs closely. Trimethaphan or phentolamine may be needed for hypotension; beta blockers (such as propranolol) for arrhythmias.

☑ Special considerations

Besides those relevant to all *adrenergics,* consider the following recommendations.

- After S.C. or I.M. injection, massaging the site may hasten absorption.
- Epinephrine is destroyed by oxidizing agents, alkalies (including sodium bicarbonate), halogens, permanganates, chromates, nitrates, and salts of easily reducible metals such as iron, copper, and zinc.
- A tuberculin syringe may assure greater accuracy in measurement of parenteral doses.
- To avoid hazardous medication errors, check carefully type of solution prescribed, concentration, dosage, and route before administration. Do not mix with alkali.
- Before withdrawing epinephrine suspension into syringe, shake vial or ampule thoroughly to disperse particles; then inject promptly. Do not use if preparation is discolored or contains a precipitate.
- Repeated injections may cause tissue necrosis from vascular constriction. Rotate injection sites, and observe for signs of blanching.
- Avoid I.M. injection into buttocks. Epinephrine-induced vasoconstriction favors growth of the anaerobe *Clostridium perfringens.*
- Monitor blood pressure, pulse, respirations, and urine output, and observe patient closely. Epinephrine may widen pulse pressure. If arrhythmias occur, discontinue epinephrine immediately. Watch for changes in intake and output ratio.

• Patients receiving I.V. epinephrine should be on cardiac monitor. Keep resuscitation equipment available.
• When drug is administered I.V., check patient's blood pressure repeatedly during first 5 minutes, then every 3 to 5 minutes until patient is stable.
• Intracardiac administration requires external cardiac massage to move drug into coronary circulation.
• Drying effect on bronchial secretions may make mucus plugs more difficult to dislodge. Bronchial hygiene program, including postural drainage, breathing exercises, and adequate hydration, may be necessary.
• Epinephrine may increase blood glucose levels. Closely observe patients with diabetes for loss of diabetes control.
• Monitor amount, consistency, and color of sputum.

Inhalation
• Treatment should start with first symptoms of bronchospasm. Patient should use the fewest number of inhalations that provide relief. To prevent excessive dosage, at least 1 or 2 minutes should elapse before taking additional inhalations of epinephrine. Dosage requirements vary. Warn patient that overuse or too-frequent use can cause severe adverse reactions.

Nasal
• Instill nose drops with patient's head in lateral, head-low position to prevent entry of drug into throat.

Ophthalmic
• Ophthalmic preparation may cause mydriasis with blurred vision and sensitivity to light in some patients being treated for glaucoma. Drug is usually administered at bedtime or after prescribed miotic to minimize these symptoms.
• Patients, especially elderly patients, should have regular tonometer readings during continuous therapy.
• When using separate solutions of epinephrine and a topical miotic, instill the miotic 2 to 10 minutes before epinephrine.

Patient education

• Urge patient to report diminishing effect. Repeated or prolonged use of epinephrine can cause tolerance to drug's effects. Continuing to take epinephrine despite tolerance can be hazardous. Interrupting drug therapy for 12 hours to several days may restore responsiveness to drug.

Inhalation
• Instruct patient in correct use of inhaler.
• Tell patient to avoid contact with eyes and to take no more than 2 inhalations at a time with 1- to 2-minute intervals between them.
• Instruct patient to rinse mouth and throat with water immediately after inhalation to avoid swallowing residual drug (the propellant in the aerosol preparation may cause epigastric pain and systemic effects) and to prevent dryness of oropharyngeal membranes.
• Tell patient to save applicator; refills may be available.
• Advise patient to call immediately if he receives no relief within 20 minutes or if condition worsens.

Nasal
• Tell patient to call if symptoms are not relieved in 20 minutes or if they become worse and to report bronchial irritation, nervousness, or sleeplessness, which require reduction of dosage.
• Warn patient that intranasal applications may sting slightly and cause rebound congestion or drug-induced rhinitis after prolonged use. Nose drops should be used for 3 or 4 days only. Encourage patient to use drug exactly as prescribed.
• Tell patient to rinse nose dropper or spray tip with hot water after each use to avoid contaminating the solution.
• Instruct patient to gently press finger against nasolacrimal duct for at least 1 or 2 minutes immediately after drug instillation to avoid excessive systemic absorption.

Ophthalmic
• To minimize systemic absorption, tell patient to press finger to lacrimal sac during and for 1 to 2 minutes after instillation of eyedrops.
• To prevent contamination, tell patient not to touch applicator tip to any surface; keep container tightly closed.
• Tell patient not to use if epinephrine solution is discolored or contains a precipitate.
• Advise patient to remove soft contact lenses before instilling eyedrops to avoid staining or damaging them.
• Tell patient to apply a missed dose as soon as possible. If too close to time for next dose, the patient should wait and apply at regularly scheduled time.
• Tell patient to store drug away from heat and light (not in bathroom medicine cabinet where heat and moisture can cause drug to deteriorate) and out of children's reach.

Geriatric use

• Elderly patients may be more sensitive to effects of epinephrine, so lower doses are indicated.

Pediatric use

• Safety and efficacy of ophthalmic epinephrine in children have not been established. Use with caution.

Breast-feeding

• Drug is excreted in breast milk. Patient should avoid breast-feeding during therapy with epinephrine.

epoetin alfa (erythropoietin)

Epogen, Procrit

Pharmacologic classification: glycoprotein
Therapeutic classification: antianemic
Pregnancy risk category C

How supplied

Available by prescription only
Injection: 2,000 units, 3,000 units, 4,000 units, 10,000 units, 20,000 units

Indications, route, and dosage

Anemia associated with chronic renal failure

Adults: Initiate therapy at 50 to 100 units/kg three times weekly. Patients receiving dialysis should receive drug I.V.; chronic renal failure patients not on dialysis may receive drug S.C. or I.V.

Reduce dosage when target hematocrit is reached or if hematocrit rises more than four points within a 2-week period. Increase dosage if hematocrit does not rise by five to six points after 8 weeks of therapy and hematocrit is below target range. Maintenance dosage is highly individualized.

Anemia related to zidovudine therapy in patients infected with HIV

Adults: Before therapy, determine endogenous serum epoetin alfa levels. Patients with levels of 500 milliunits/ml or more are unlikely to respond to therapy.

Initial dose for patients with levels of under 500 milliunits/ml who are receiving 4,200 mg weekly or less of zidovudine less is 100 units/kg I.V. or S.C. three times weekly for 8 weeks. If response is inadequate after 8 weeks, increase dose by increments of 50 to 100 units/kg three times weekly and reevaluate response q 4 to 8 weeks. Individualize maintenance dose to maintain response, which may be influenced by zidovudine dose or infection or inflammation.

Anemia secondary to cancer chemotherapy

Adults: 150 units/kg S.C. three times weekly for 8 weeks or until target hemoglobin level is reached. If response is not satisfactory after 8 weeks, increase dose up to 300 units/kg S.C. three times weekly.

Reduction of need for allogeneic blood transfusion in anemic patients scheduled to undergo elective, noncardiac, nonvascular surgery

Adults: 300 units/kg/day S.C. daily for 10 days before surgery, on day of surgery, and for 4 days after surgery. Alternatively, 600 units/kg S.C. in once-weekly doses (21, 14, and 7 days before surgery), plus a fourth dose on day of surgery. Before initiating treatment, establish that hemoglobin is above 10 g/dl and less than or equal to 13 g/dl.

Pharmacodynamics

Antianemic action: Epoetin alfa is a glycoprotein consisting of 165 amino acids synthesized using recombinant DNA technology. It mimics naturally occurring erythropoietin, which is produced by the kidneys. It stimulates the division and differentiation of cells within bone marrow to produce RBCs.

Pharmacokinetics

- *Absorption:* Epoetin alfa may be given S.C. or I.V. After S.C. administration, peak serum levels occur within 5 to 24 hours.
- *Distribution:* Unknown.
- *Metabolism:* Unknown.
- *Excretion:* Unknown.

Contraindications and precautions

Contraindicated in patients with uncontrolled hypertension and hypersensitivity to mammalian cell-derived products or albumin (human).

Interactions

None reported.

Effects on diagnostic tests

Moderate increases in BUN, uric acid, creatinine, phosphorus, and potassium levels have been reported.

Adverse reactions

CNS: *headache,* ***seizures,*** *paresthesia, fatigue,* dizziness.
CV: *hypertension, edema.*
GI: *nausea, vomiting, diarrhea.*
Respiratory: *cough, shortness of breath.*
Skin: *rash,* urticaria.
Other: increased clotting of arteriovenous grafts, *pyrexia, arthralgia, cough, injection site reactions, asthenia.*

Overdose and treatment

Maximum safe dose has not been established. Doses up to 1,500 units/kg have been administered three times weekly for 3 weeks without direct toxic effects.

The drug can cause polycythemia; phlebotomy may be used to bring hematocrit within appropriate levels.

☑ Special considerations

- Monitor hematocrit at least twice weekly during initiation of therapy and during any dosage adjustment. Close monitoring of blood pressure is also recommended.
- For HIV-infected patients treated with zidovudine, measure hematocrit once weekly until stabilized and then periodically.
- If a patient fails to respond to epoetin alfa therapy, consider the following possible causes: vitamin deficiency, iron deficiency, underlying infection, occult blood loss, underlying hematologic disease, hemolysis, aluminum intoxication, osteitis fibrosa cystica, or increased dosage of zidovudine.
- Most patients eventually require supplemental iron therapy. Before and during therapy, monitor patient's iron stores, including serum ferritin and transferrin saturation.
- Measure hematocrit twice weekly until it has stabilized and during adjustment to a maintenance dosage in patients with chronic renal failure. An interval of 2 to 6 weeks may elapse before a dosage change is reflected in the hematocrit level.
- Routine monitoring of CBC with differential and platelet counts is recommended.

Patient education

- Explain importance of regularly monitoring blood pressure in light of the potential drug effects.
- Advise patient to adhere to dietary restrictions during therapy. Make sure he understands that drug will not influence disease process.

Pediatric use

- Safety and efficacy in children have not been established.

Breast-feeding
• It is unknown if drug is excreted in breast milk. Use with caution in breast-feeding women.

epoprostenol sodium
Flolan

Pharmacologic classification: naturally occurring prostaglandin
Therapeutic classification: vasodilator, antiplatelet aggregator
Pregnancy risk category B

How supplied
Available by prescription only
Injection: 0.5 mg/17-ml vial, 1.5 mg/17-ml vial

Indications, route, and dosage
Long-term I.V. treatment of primary pulmonary hypertension in New York Heart Association (NYHA) class III and class IV patients
Adults: Initially for acute dose ranging, 2 ng/kg/minute as an I.V. infusion; increase in increments of 2 ng/kg/minute q 15 minutes or longer until dose-limiting pharmacologic effects are elicited. Begin maintenance (chronic) dosing with 4 ng/kg/minute less than the maximum tolerated infusion rate as determined during acute dose ranging. If the maximum tolerated infusion rate is below 5 ng/kg/minute, begin maintenance infusion at one half the maximum tolerated infusion rate. Base subsequent dosage adjustments on persistence, recurrence, or worsening of patient's symptoms of primary pulmonary hypertension and the occurrence of adverse events because of excessive doses of drug. Increases in dose from the initial maintenance dose can generally be expected and are done in increments of 1 to 2 ng/kg/minute at intervals of at least 15 minutes.

Pharmacodynamics
Vasodilator/antiplatelet action: Epoprostenol causes direct vasodilation of pulmonary and systemic arterial vascular beds and inhibits platelet aggregation.

Pharmacokinetics
• *Absorption:* Drug is administered I.V.
• *Distribution:* Unknown.
• *Metabolism:* Epoprostenol is extensively metabolized.
• *Excretion:* Drug is excreted primarily in urine with a small amount excreted in feces.

Contraindications and precautions
Contraindicated in patients with hypersensitivity to drug or structurally related compounds. Chronic use of drug is also contraindicated in patients with heart failure because of severe left ventricular systolic dysfunction or in those who develop pulmonary edema during initial dose ranging.

Interactions
Antihypertensive agents, diuretics, or *other vasodilators* may cause additional reduction in blood pressure. Monitor blood pressure closely. *Anticoagulants* and *antiplatelet agents* may increase risk of bleeding. Monitor closely for bleeding.

Effects on diagnostic tests
None reported.

Adverse reactions
CNS: *headache, anxiety, nervousness, agitation, dizziness, hyperesthesia, paresthesia.*
CV: *tachycardia; hypotension, chest pain,* bradycardia (during initial dose ranging).
GI: *nausea, vomiting;* abdominal pain, dyspepsia (during initial dose ranging); *diarrhea* (during maintenance dosing).
Hematologic: ***thrombocytopenia.***
Respiratory: dyspnea.
Skin: *flushing.*
Other: musculoskeletal pain, back pain, sweating (during initial dose ranging); *jaw pain, flulike symptoms, chills, fever, sepsis, myalgia, nonspecific musculoskeletal pain* (during maintenance dosing).

Overdose and treatment
Overdosage may result in flushing, headache, hypotension, tachycardia, nausea, vomiting, and diarrhea. Treatment usually requires dose reduction of epoprostenol.

☑ Special considerations
• Drug should be used only by staff experienced in the diagnosis and treatment of primary pulmonary hypertension. Determining the appropriate dose for the patient, called dose ranging, must be done in a setting with adequate personnel and equipment for physiologic monitoring and emergency care.
• Reconstitute drug only as directed using sterile diluent for Flolan. Drug must not be reconstituted or mixed with other parenteral medications or solutions before or during administration.
• Follow manufacturer guidelines for reconstituting drug to achieve concentration needed. Be aware that the concentration selected should be compatible with the infusion pump being used with respect to minimum and maximum flow rates, reservoir capacity, and the infusion pump criteria recommended by manufacturer. When used for maintenance infusion, drug should be prepared in a drug delivery reservoir appropriate for the infusion pump with a total reservoir volume of at least 100 ml. Drug should be prepared using two vials of sterile diluent for epoprostenol for use during a 24-hour period.
• Before use, reconstituted solutions of the drug must be protected from light and must be refrigerated at 36° to 46° F (2° to 8° C) if not used immediately. Do not freeze reconstituted solutions of drug. Discard reconstituted solution that has been frozen. Discard reconstituted solution if it has been refrigerated for more than 48 hours.
• Maintenance dosing should be administered by continuous I.V. infusion via a permanent indwelling central venous catheter using an ambulatory infusion pump. During establishment of dosing range, drug may be administered peripherally.

• To facilitate extended use at ambient temperatures exceeding 77° F (25° C), a cold pouch with frozen gel packs can be used. The cold pouches and gel packs used in clinical trials were obtained from Palco Labs, Palo Alto, California. A cold pouch used must be capable of maintaining the temperature of reconstituted drug between 36° and 46° F (2° and 8° C) for 12 hours. If such a cold pouch is used during the infusion, reconstituted solution should be used for no longer than 24 hours.
• Most common dose-limiting pharmacologic effects used to determine maximum dosage during initial dosing have been nausea, vomiting, headache, hypotension, and flushing, but also may include chest pain, anxiety, dizziness, bradycardia, dyspnea, abdominal pain, musculoskeletal pain, and tachycardia.
• Following establishment of a new maintenance infusion rate, observe the patient closely and monitor patient's standing and supine blood pressure and heart rate for several hours to ensure that the new dose is tolerated.
• During maintenance infusion, the occurrence of dose-related pharmacologic events similar to those observed during initial dosing may necessitate a decrease in infusion rate, but the adverse event may occasionally resolve without dosage adjustment.
• Avoid abrupt withdrawal or sudden large reductions in infusion rates. Ensure that patient has access to a backup infusion pump and I.V. infusion sets to avoid potential interruptions in drug delivery. A multilumen catheter should be considered if other I.V. therapies are routinely administered.
• Anticoagulant therapy should be administered during chronic use of drug, unless contraindicated. Monitor PT and INR closely.
• To reduce risk of infection, aseptic technique must be used in the reconstitution and administration of the drug as well as in routine catheter care.

Patient education

• Ensure that patient and family understand before therapy is begun that there is a high likelihood that I.V. therapy with epoprostenol will be needed for prolonged periods, possibly years, and that the patient or family has the ability to accept and care for a permanent I.V. catheter and infusion pump.
• Instruct patient and family how to reconstitute drug and administer drug via infusion pump using sterile technique. Explain how to use infusion pump. Stress importance of maintaining continuous drug therapy. Provide patient and family with instructions on how to switch to a new infusion pump in the event of pump failure. Also instruct patient and family on how to store drug.
• Instruct patient to report adverse reactions regarding drug therapy immediately because dosage adjustments may be necessary.
• Provide patient with telephone number to obtain assistance for 24-hour support.

Geriatric use

• In general, dose selection for an elderly patient should be cautious, reflecting the greater frequency of decreased hepatic, renal, or cardiac function and of concomitant disease or other drug therapy.

Pediatric use

• Safety and effectiveness in children have not been established.

Breast-feeding

• Use drug with caution in breast-feeding patients because it is not known if it occurs in breast milk.

ergocalciferol (vitamin D_2)

Calciferol, Deltalin, Drisdol, Vitamin D

Pharmacologic classification: vitamin
Therapeutic classification: antihypocalcemic
Pregnancy risk category C

How supplied

Available by prescription only
Capsules: 1.25 mg (50,000 units)
Tablets: 1.25 mg (50,000 units)
Injection: 12.5 mg (500,000 units)/ml

Available without a prescription
Liquid: 8,000 units/ml in 60-ml dropper bottle

Indications, route, and dosage

Nutritional rickets or osteomalacia
Adults: 25 to 125 mcg P.O. daily if patient has normal GI absorption. With severe malabsorption, 250 mcg to 7.5 mg P.O. or 250 mcg I.M. daily.
Children: 25 to 125 mcg P.O. daily if patient has normal GI absorption. With malabsorption, 250 to 625 mcg P.O. daily.
Familial hypophosphatemia
Adults: 250 mcg to 1.5 mg P.O. daily with phosphate supplements.
Children: 1 to 2 mg P.O. daily with phosphate supplements. Increase daily dosage in 250- to 500-mcg increments at 3- to 4-month intervals until adequate response is obtained.
Vitamin D-dependent rickets
Adults: 250 mcg to 1.5 mg P.O. daily.
Children: 75 to 125 mcg P.O. daily.
Anticonvulsant-induced rickets and osteomalacia
Adults: 50 mcg to 1.25 mg P.O. daily.
Hypoparathyroidism and pseudohypoparathyroidism
Adults: 625 mcg to 5 mg P.O. daily with calcium supplements.
Children: 1.25 to 5 mg P.O. daily with calcium supplements.
◇ ***Fanconi's syndrome***
Adults: 1.25 to 5 mg. P.O. daily.
Children: 625 mcg to 1.25 mg P.O. daily.
◇ ***Osteoporosis***
Adults: 25 to 250 mcg P.O. daily or 1.25 mg P.O. weekly with calcium and fluoride supplements.

Pharmacodynamics

Antihypocalcemic action: Once activated, ergocalciferol acts to regulate the serum concentrations of calcium by regulating absorption from the GI tract and resorption from bone.

Pharmacokinetics

• *Absorption:* Drug is absorbed readily from the small intestine. Onset of action is 10 to 24 hours.
• *Distribution:* Drug is distributed widely and bound to proteins stored in the liver.
• *Metabolism:* Ergocalciferol is metabolized in the liver and kidneys. It has an average half-life of 24 hours and a duration of up to 6 months.
• *Excretion:* Bile (feces) is the primary excretion route. A small percentage is excreted in urine.

Contraindications and precautions

Contraindicated in patients with hypercalcemia, hypervitaminosis A, or renal osteodystrophy with hyperphosphatemia. Use with extreme caution, if at all, in patients with impaired renal function, heart disease, renal stones, or arteriosclerosis.

Interactions

Concomitant use of ergocalciferol and *cardiac glycosides* may result in arrhythmias. Concomitant use with *thiazide diuretics* may cause hypercalcemia in patients with hypoparathyroidism; with *magnesium-containing antacids* may lead to hypermagnesemia; with *verapamil* may induce recurrence of atrial fibrillation when supplemental calcium and calciferol have induced hypercalcemia. *Corticosteroids* counteract drug's effects. Administration of *phenobarbital* or *phenytoin* may increase drug's metabolism to inactive metabolites. *Cholestyramine, colestipol,* and excessive use of *mineral oil* may interfere with the absorption of ergocalciferol.

Effects on diagnostic tests

Ergocalciferol may falsely increase serum cholesterol levels and may elevate AST and ALT levels.

Adverse reactions

Adverse reactions listed usually occur only in vitamin D toxicity.
CNS: headache, weakness, somnolence, decreased libido, overt psychosis, irritability.
CV: *calcifications of soft tissues, including the heart,* hypertension, ***arrhythmias.***
EENT: rhinorrhea, conjunctivitis (calcific), photophobia.
GI: anorexia, nausea, vomiting, constipation, dry mouth, metallic taste, polydipsia.
GU: polyuria, albuminuria, hypercalciuria, nocturia, ***impaired renal function,*** reversible azotemia.
Skin: pruritus.
Other: bone and muscle pain, bone demineralization, weight loss, ***hypercalcemia,*** hyperthermia.

Overdose and treatment

Clinical manifestations of overdose include hypercalcemia, hypercalciuria, and hyperphosphatemia, which may be treated by stopping therapy, starting a low calcium diet, and increasing fluid intake. A loop diuretic, such as furosemide, may be given with saline I.V. infusion to increase calcium excretion. Supportive measures should be provided. In severe cases, death from cardiac or renal failure may occur. Calcitonin may decrease hypercalcemia.

☑ Special considerations

• I.M. injection of ergocalciferol dispersed in oil is preferable in patients who are unable to absorb the oral form.
• If I.V. route is necessary, use only water-miscible solutions intended for dilution in large-volume parenterals. Use cautiously in cardiac patients, especially if they are receiving cardiotonic glycosides. In such patients, hypercalcemia may precipitate arrhythmias.
• Monitor eating and bowel habits; dry mouth, nausea, vomiting, metallic taste, and constipation can be early signs of toxicity.
• Patients with hyperphosphatemia require dietary phosphate restrictions and binding agents to avoid metastatic calcifications and renal calculi.
• When high therapeutic doses are used, frequent serum and urine calcium, potassium, and urea determinations should be made.
• Malabsorption caused by inadequate bile or hepatic dysfunction may require addition of exogenous bile salts.
• Doses of 60,000 IU daily can cause hypercalcemia.
• Patients taking ergocalciferol should restrict their intake of magnesium-containing antacids.

Patient education

• Explain importance of a calcium-rich diet.
• Caution patient not to increase daily dose on his own initiative. Vitamin D is a fat-soluble vitamin; vitamin D toxicity is thus more likely to occur.
• Tell patient to avoid magnesium-containing antacids and mineral oil.
• Instruct patient to swallow tablets whole without crushing or chewing.

Pediatric use

• Some infants may be hyperreactive to drug.

Breast-feeding

• Very little appears in the breast milk; however, effect on infants of amounts exceeding RDA levels of vitamin D is not known.

ergonovine maleate

Ergotrate Maleate

Pharmacologic classification: ergot alkaloid
Therapeutic classification: oxytocic
Pregnancy risk category NR

How supplied

Available by prescription only
Injection: 0.2 mg/ml ampules

Indications, route, and dosage

Prevent or treat postpartum and postabortion hemorrhage due to uterine atony or subinvolution
Adults: 0.2 mg I.M. q 2 to 4 hours, maximum five doses; or 0.2 mg I.V. (only for severe uterine bleeding or other life-threatening emergency) over 1 minute while blood pressure and uterine contrac-

tions are monitored. I.V. dose may be diluted to 5 ml with 0.9% NaCl injection.

◊ ***To diagnose coronary artery spasm (Prinzmetal's angina)***
Adults: 0.1 to 0.4 mg I.V. for one dose.

Pharmacodynamics

Oxytocic action: Ergonovine maleate stimulates contractions of uterine and vascular smooth muscle. This produces intense uterine contractions, followed by periods of relaxation. The drug produces vasoconstriction of primarily capacitance blood vessels, causing an increased CVP and elevated blood pressure.

The clinical effect is secondary to contraction of the uterine wall around bleeding vessels, producing hemostasis.

Pharmacokinetics

- *Absorption:* Absorption is rapid following I.M. administration. Onset of action is immediate for I.V., 2 to 5 minutes for I.M.
- *Distribution:* Unknown.
- *Metabolism:* Drug is metabolized in the liver.
- *Excretion:* Primarily nonrenal elimination in feces has been suggested.

Contraindications and precautions

Contraindicated in patients sensitive to ergot preparations; in threatened spontaneous abortion, induction of labor, or before delivery of placenta because captivation of placenta may occur; and in those with history of allergic or idiosyncratic reactions to drug.

Because of the potential for adverse CV effects, use cautiously in patients with hypertension, toxemia, sepsis, occlusive vascular disease, and hepatic, renal, and cardiac disease.

Interactions

Ergonovine maleate will enhance the vasoconstrictor potential of *other ergot alkaloids* and *sympathomimetic amines.* Combined use of *local anesthetics with vasoconstrictors (lidocaine with epinephrine)* or *smoking (nicotine)* will enhance vasoconstriction. If patient is not also taking a cardiac glycoside, cautious administration of *calcium gluconate I.V.* may produce desired oxytocic action in calcium-deficient patients.

Effects on diagnostic tests

The concentration of serum prolactin may appear decreased.

Adverse reactions

CNS: headache, confusion, dizziness, ringing in ears.
CV: chest pain, weakness in legs (peripheral vasospasm), hypertension, thrombophlebitis.
GI: nausea, vomiting, diarrhea, cramping.
Respiratory: shortness of breath.
Other: itching; sweating; pain in arms, legs, or lower back; ***hypersensitivity reactions, signs of shock.***

Note: Discontinue drug if hypertension or allergic reactions occur.

Overdose and treatment

Clinical manifestations of overdose include seizures, with nausea, vomiting, diarrhea, dizziness, fluctuations in blood pressure, weak pulse, chest pain, tingling, and numbness and coldness in the extremities. Rarely, gangrene has occurred. Treat seizures with anticonvulsants and hypercoagulability with heparin; give vasodilators to improve blood flow. Gangrene may require amputation.

☑ Special considerations

- Contractions begin immediately after I.V. injection. May continue for 45 minutes after I.V. injection.
- Monitor blood pressure, pulse rate, uterine response, and character and amount of vaginal bleeding. Watch for sudden changes in vital signs and frequent periods of uterine relaxation.
- Hypocalcemia may decrease patient response; I.V. administration of calcium salts is necessary.
- High doses during delivery may cause uterine tetany and possible infant hypoxia or intracranial hemorrhage.
- Store I.V. solutions below 46.4° F (8° C). Daily stock may be kept at cool room temperature for 60 days.
- Drug has been used as a diagnostic agent for angina pectoris.

Patient education

- Tell patient not to smoke while taking drug.
- Advise patient of possible adverse reactions.

Breast-feeding

- Ergot alkaloids inhibit lactation. Drug is excreted in breast milk, and ergotism has been reported in breast-fed infants of mothers treated with other ergot alkaloids. Use with caution.

ergotamine tartrate

Cafergot, Ergomar, Ergostat, Medihaler Ergotamine, Wigraine

Pharmacologic classification: ergot alkaloid
Therapeutic classification: vasoconstrictor
Pregnancy risk category X

How supplied

Available by prescription only
Tablets (S.L.): 2 mg
Tablets: 1 mg* (with or without caffeine 100 mg)
Aerosal inhaler: 360 mcg/metered spray
Suppositories: 2 mg (with caffeine 100 mg)

Indications, route, and dosage

To prevent or abort vascular headache, including migraine and cluster headaches
Adults: Initially, 2 mg S.L. or P.O., then 1 to 2 mg S.L. or P.O. q 30 minutes, to maximum 6 mg per attack or in 24 hours, and 10 mg weekly. Alternatively, initially 1 inhalation; if not relieved in 5 minutes, repeat 1 inhalation. May repeat inhalations at least 5 minutes apart up to maximum of 6 inhalations per 24 hours or 15 inhalations weekly. Patient may also use

rectal suppositories. Initially, 2 mg P.R. at onset of attack; repeat in 1 hour p.r.n. Maximum dosage is 2 suppositories per attack or 5 suppositories weekly.
◊ *Children:* 1 mg S.L. in older children and adolescents; if no improvement, additional 1-mg dose may be given in 30 minutes.

Pharmacodynamics

Vasoconstricting action: By stimulating alpha-adrenergic receptors, ergotamine in therapeutic doses causes peripheral vasoconstriction (if vascular tone is low); however, if vascular tone is high, it produces vasodilation. In high doses, it is a competitive alpha-adrenergic blocker. In therapeutic doses, it inhibits the reuptake of norepinephrine, which increases the vasoconstricting activity of ergotamine. A weaker serotonin antagonist, it reduces the increased rate of platelet aggregation caused by serotonin.

In the treatment of vascular headaches, ergotamine probably causes direct vasoconstriction of dilated carotid artery beds while decreasing the amplitude of pulsations. Its serotoninergic and catecholamine effects also seem to be involved.

Pharmacokinetics

- *Absorption:* Drug is rapidly absorbed after inhalation and variably absorbed after oral administration. Peak concentrations are reached within ½ to 3 hours. Caffeine may increase rate and extent of absorption. Drug undergoes first-pass metabolism after oral administration.
- *Distribution:* Widely distributed throughout the body.
- *Metabolism:* Drug is extensively metabolized in the liver.
- *Excretion:* 4% of a dose is excreted in urine within 96 hours; remainder of a dose presumed to be excreted in feces. Ergotamine is dialyzable. Onset of action depends on how promptly drug is given after onset of headache.

Contraindications and precautions

Contraindicated in patients with peripheral and occlusive vascular diseases, coronary artery disease, hypertension, hepatic or renal dysfunction, severe pruritus, sepsis, or hypersensitivity to ergot alkaloids and during pregnancy.

Interactions

Concomitant use with *propranolol* or other *beta blockers* may intensify ergotamine's vasoconstrictor effects. Use with *troleandomycin* appears to interfere with the detoxification of ergotamine in the liver; use concurrently with caution. Concomitant use with *macrolides* may cause acute ergotism manifested as peripheral ischemia. Concomitant use with *vasodilators* can increase pressor effects, causing dangerous hypertension.

Effects on diagnostic tests

None reported.

Adverse reactions

CV: transient tachycardia or bradycardia, precordial distress and pain, increased arterial pressure, angina pectoris, peripheral vasoconstriction.
GI: nausea, vomiting.
Skin: pruritus, localized edema.
Other: weakness in legs, muscle pain in extremities, numbness and tingling in fingers and toes.

Overdose and treatment

Clinical manifestations of overdose include adverse vasospastic effects, nausea, vomiting, lassitude, impaired mental function, delirium, severe dyspnea, hypotension or hypertension, rapid or weak pulse, unconsciousness, spasms of the limbs, seizures, and shock.

Treatment requires supportive and symptomatic measures, with prolonged and careful monitoring. If patient is conscious and ingestion is recent, empty stomach by emesis or gastric lavage; if comatose, perform gastric lavage after placement of endotracheal tube with cuff inflated. Activated charcoal and a saline (magnesium sulfate) cathartic may be used. Provide respiratory support. Apply warmth (not direct heat) to ischemic extremities if vasospasm occurs. As needed, administer vasodilators (nitroprusside, prazosin, or tolazoline) and, if necessary, I.V. diazepam to treat convulsions. Dialysis may be helpful.

☑ Special considerations

Besides those relevant to all *alpha-adrenergic blocking agents,* consider the following recommendations.

- Drug is most effective when used in prodromal stage of headache or as soon as possible after onset. Provide quiet, low-light environment to relax patient after dose is administered.
- Store drug in light-resistant container.
- Sublingual tablet is preferred during early stage of attack because of its rapid absorption.
- Obtain an accurate dietary history to determine possible relationship between certain foods and onset of headache.
- Rebound headache or an increase in duration or frequency of headache may occur when drug is stopped.
- If patient experiences severe vasoconstriction with tissue necrosis, administer I.V. sodium nitroprusside or intra-arterial tolazoline. I.V. heparin and 10% dextran 40 in D_5W injection also may be administered to prevent vascular stasis and thrombosis.
- Drug is not effective for muscle contraction headaches.

Patient education

- Instruct patient in correct use of inhaler.
- Urge patient to immediately report feelings of numbness or tingling in fingers or toes or red or violet blisters on hands or feet.
- Caution patient to avoid alcoholic beverages, because alcohol may worsen headache, and to avoid smoking, because it may increase adverse effects of drug.
- Warn patient to avoid prolonged exposure to very cold temperatures, which may increase adverse effects of drug.
- Tell patient to promptly report illness or infection, which may increase sensitivity to drug effects.

• Inform patient that the body may need time to adjust after discontinuing the medication depending on the amount used and length of time involved.
• Advise patient who uses an inhaler to call promptly if mouth, throat, or lung infection occurs or if condition worsens. Cough, hoarseness, or throat irritation may occur. He should gargle and rinse mouth after each dose to help prevent hoarseness and irritation.
• Instruct patient to call promptly if persistent numbness or tingling of fingers or toes, and chest, muscle, or abdominal pain occur.
• Advise patient not to exceed recommended dosage.
• Tell patient not to eat, drink, or smoke while sublingual tablet is dissolving.

Geriatric use
• Administer cautiously to elderly patients.

Pediatric use
• Safety and efficacy of ergotamine in children have not been established.

Breast-feeding
• Drug is distributed into breast milk; therefore, it should be used with caution in breast-feeding women. Excessive dosage or prolonged administration of the drug may inhibit lactation.

erythromycin base
E-Base, E-Mycin, Eryc, Eryc Sprinkle*, Ery-Tab, Erythromycin Base/Filmtabs, PCE, Robimycin

erythromycin estolate
Ilosone

erythromycin ethylsuccinate
E.E.S., EryPed, Pediazole

erythromycin gluceptate
Ilotycin Gluceptate

erythromycin lactobionate
Erythrocin Lactobionate

erythromycin stearate
Apo-Erythro-S*, Erythrocin Stearate Filmtab, Novorythro*

erythromycin (topical)
Akne-Mycin, A/T/S, Del-Mycin, Erycette, EryDerm, Erymax, Ery-Sol, Erythra-Derm, Staticin, T-Stat, Theramycin Z

Pharmacologic classification: erythromycin
Therapeutic classification: antibiotic
Pregnancy risk category B

How supplied
Available by prescription only
Oral suspension: 125 mg/5 ml, 200 mg/5 ml, 400 mg/5 ml

erythromycin base
Tablets (enteric-coated): 250 mg, 333 mg, 500 mg
Pellets (enteric-coated): 250 mg
erythromycin estolate
Tablets: 500 mg
Capsules: 250 mg
Suspension: 125 mg/5 ml, 250 mg/5 ml
erythromycin ethylsuccinate
Tablets (chewable): 200 mg
Topical solution: 1.5%, 2%
Topical gel: 2%
Topical ointment: 2%
Oral suspension: 400 mg/5 ml
Powder for oral suspension: 200 mg/5 ml (after reconstitution)
Granules for oral suspension: 400 mg/5 ml (after reconstitution)
Ophthalmic ointment: 5 mg/g
erythromycin gluceptate
Injection: 500-mg, 1-g vials
erythromycin lactobionate
Injection: 500-mg, 1-g vials
erythromycin stearate
Tablets (film-coated): 250 mg, 500 mg

Indications, route, and dosage
***Acute pelvic inflammatory disease caused by* Neisseria gonorrhoeae**
Adults: 500 mg I.V. (gluceptate, lactobionate) q 6 hours for 3 days, then 250 mg (base, estolate, stearate) or 400 mg (ethylsuccinate) P.O. q 6 hours for 7 days.
Endocarditis prophylaxis for dental procedures in patients allergic to penicillin
Adults: Initially, 800 mg (ethylsuccinate) or 1 g (stearate) P.O. 2 hours before procedure; then 400 mg (ethylsuccinate) or 500 mg (stearate) P.O. 6 hours later.
Children: Initially, 20 mg/kg (ethylsuccinate or stearate) P.O. 2 hours before procedure, then 10 mg/kg 6 hours later.
Treatment of intestinal amebiasis in patients who cannot receive metronidazole
Adults: 250 mg (base, estolate, stearate) or 400 mg (ethylsuccinate) P.O. q 6 hours for 10 to 14 days.
Children: 30 to 50 mg/kg (base, estolate, ethylsuccinate, stearate) P.O. daily, divided q 6 hours for 10 to 14 days. (Note: base and stearate forms not available in liquid form).
Mild to moderately severe respiratory tract, skin, and soft-tissue infections caused by susceptible organisms
Adults: 250 to 500 mg (base, estolate, stearate) P.O. q 6 hours; or 400 to 800 mg (ethylsuccinate) P.O. q 6 hours; or 15 to 20 mg/kg (gluceptate, lactobionate) I.V. daily, in divided doses q 6 hours.
Children: 30 mg/kg to 50 mg/kg (oral erythromycin salts) P.O. daily, in divided doses q 6 hours; or 15 to 20 mg/kg I.V. daily, in divided doses q 4 to 6 hours.
Syphilis
Adults: 500 mg (base, estolate, stearate) P.O. q.i.d. for 14 days.
Legionnaire's disease
Adults: 500 mg to 1 g I.V. or P.O. (base, estolate, stearate) or 800 mg to 1,600 mg (ethylsuccinate) P.O. q 6 hours for 21 days.

Uncomplicated urethral, endocervical, or rectal infections when tetracyclines are contraindicated
Adults: 500 mg (base, estolate, stearate) or 800 mg (ethylsuccinate) P.O. q.i.d. for at least 7 days.
Urogenital* Chlamydia trachomatis *infections during pregnancy
Adults: 500 mg (base, estolate, stearate) P.O. q.i.d. for at least 7 days or 250 mg (base, estolate, stearate) or 400 mg (ethylsuccinate) P.O. q.i.d. for at least 14 days.
Conjunctivitis caused by* C. trachomatis *in neonates
Neonates: 50 mg/kg/day P.O. in four divided doses for at least 2 weeks.
***Pneumonia of infancy caused by* C. trachomatis**
Infants: 50 mg/kg/day P.O. in four divided doses for at least 3 weeks.
Topical treatment of acne vulgaris
Adults and children: Apply to the affected area b.i.d.
Prophylaxis of ophthalmia neonatorum
Neonates: Apply 1-cm long ribbon ointment in the lower conjunctival sac of each eye no later than 1 hour after birth. Use new tube for each infant and do not flush after instillation.
Acute and chronic conjunctivitis, trachoma, other eye infections
Adults and children: Apply 1-cm long ribbon ointment directly into infected eye up to six times daily, depending on severity of infection.

Pharmacodynamics

Antibacterial action: Erythromycin inhibits bacterial protein synthesis by binding to the ribosomal 50S subunit. It is used in the treatment of *Haemophilus influenzae, Entamoeba histolytica, Mycoplasma pneumoniae, Corynebacterium diphtheriae* and *Corynebacterium minutissimum, Legionella pneumophila,* and *Bordetella pertussis.* It may be used as an alternative to penicillins or tetracycline in the treatment of *Streptococcus pneumoniae, Streptococcus viridans, Listeria monocytogenes, Staphylococcus aureus, C. trachomatis, Neisseria gonorrhoeae,* and Treponema *pallidium.*

Pharmacokinetics

- *Absorption:* Because base salt is acid-sensitive, it must be buffered or have enteric coating to prevent destruction by gastric acids. Acid salts and esters (estolate, ethylsuccinate, and stearate) are not affected by gastric acidity and therefore are well absorbed. Base and stearate preparations should be given on empty stomach. Absorption of estolate and ethylsuccinate preparations is unaffected or possibly even enhanced by presence of food. When administered topically, erythromycin is absorbed minimally.
- *Distribution:* Erythromycin is distributed widely to most body tissues and fluids except CSF, where it appears only in low concentrations. Drug crosses the placenta. About 80% of base and 96% of erythromycin estolate are protein-bound.
- *Metabolism:* Erythromycin is metabolized partially in the liver to inactive metabolites.
- *Excretion:* Erythromycin is excreted mainly unchanged in bile. Only small drug amounts (less than 5%) are excreted in urine; some drug is excreted in breast milk. In patients with normal renal function, plasma half-life is about 1½ hours. Drug is not dialyzable.

Contraindications and precautions

Contraindicated in patients with hypersensitivity to drug or other macrolides. Erythromycin estolate is contraindicated in patients with hepatic disease. Use erythromycin salts cautiously in patients with impaired hepatic function.

Interactions

Concomitant use of erythromycin may inhibit metabolism of *theophylline* (possibly leading to elevated serum theophylline levels), *warfarin* (causing excessive anticoagulant effect), *carbamazepine* (possibly causing toxicity), and *cyclosporine* (resulting in elevation of serum cyclosporine levels and subsequent nephrotoxicity).

When used concomitantly with *topical desquamating or abrasive acne preparations,* topical erythromycin has a cumulative irritant effect.

Erythromycin preparations should not be administered concurrently with *astemizole* because potentially serious adverse CV effects may occur.

Effects on diagnostic tests

Erythromycin may interfere with fluorometric determination of urinary catecholamines. False elevation of liver function test using calometric assays may occur (rare).

Adverse reactions

EENT: bilateral reversible hearing loss (with high systemic or oral doses in patients with renal or hepatic insufficiency); slowed corneal wound healing, blurred vision (with ophthalmic administration).
GI: *abdominal pain, cramping, nausea, vomiting, diarrhea* (with oral or systemic administration).
Hepatic: cholestatic jaundice (with estolate).
Skin: urticaria, rash, eczema (with oral or systemic administration); urticaria, dermatitis (with ophthalmic administration); sensitivity reactions, erythema, burning, *dryness, pruritus,* irritation, peeling, oily skin (with topical application).
Other: overgrowth of nonsusceptible bacteria or fungi; ***anaphylaxis;*** fever (with oral or systemic administration); *venous irritation, thrombophlebitis* (after I.V. injection); overgrowth of nonsusceptible organisms (with long-term use); hypersensitivity reactions, including itching and burning eyes (with ophthalmic administration).

Overdose and treatment

No information available.

☑ Special considerations

- Perform culture and sensitivity tests before treatment starts and then as needed.
- Administer base and stearate preparations on empty stomach. Absorption of estolate and ethylsuccinate preparations is unaffected or possibly

even enhanced by presence of food. When administered topically, drug is minimally absorbed.
• Erythromycin estolate may cause serious hepatotoxicity (reversible cholestatic jaundice) in adults. Monitor liver function tests for increased serum bilirubin, AST, and alkaline phosphatase levels. Other erythromycin salts can cause less severe hepatotoxicity. (Patients who develop hepatotoxicity from erythromycin estolate may react similarly to any erythromycin preparation.)
• If patient is receiving erythromycin concomitantly with theophylline, monitor serum theophylline levels.
• If patient is receiving erythromycin concomitantly with warfarin, monitor for prolonged PT or INR and abnormal bleeding.
• Reconstitute injectable form (lactobionate) based on manufacturer's instructions and dilute every 250 mg in at least 100 ml of 0.9% NaCl solution. Continuous infusions are preferred, but drug may be given by intermittent infusion at a maximum concentration of 5 mg/ml infused over 20 to 60 minutes.
• Do not administer erythromycin lactobionate with other drugs because of chemical instability. Reconstituted solutions are acidic and should be completely administered within 8 hours of preparation.
• Drug may cause overgrowth of nonsusceptible bacteria or fungi.
• Although drug is bacteriostatic, it may be bactericidal in high concentrations or against highly susceptible organisms.

Patient education
• For best absorption, instruct patient to take oral form with full glass of water 1 hour before or 2 hours after meals. (However, patient receiving enteric-coated tablets may take them with meals). Advise patient not to take drug with fruit juice. If patient is taking chewable tablets, instruct him not to swallow them whole.
• If patient is using topical solution, instruct him to wash, rinse, and dry affected areas before applying it. Warn patient not to apply solution near eyes, nose, mouth, or other mucous membranes. Caution patient to avoid sharing washcloths and towels with family members.
• Instruct patient applying ophthalmic ointment to wash hands before and after applying ointment. Instruct him to cleanse eye area of excess exudate before applying ointment. Warn him not to allow tube to touch the eye or surrounding tissue. Instruct him to promptly report signs of sensitivity, such as itching eyelids and constant burning.
• Tell patient to take drug exactly as directed and to continue taking it for prescribed period, even after he feels better.
• Instruct patient to report adverse reactions at once.

Breast-feeding
• Although drug is excreted in breast milk, no adverse reactions have been reported. Administer cautiously to breast-feeding women.

esmolol hydrochloride
Brevibloc

Pharmacologic classification: beta$_1$-adrenergic blocker
Therapeutic classification: antiarrhythmic
Pregnancy risk category C

How supplied
Available by prescription only
Injection: 10 mg/ml in 10-ml vials; 250 mg/ml in 10-ml ampules

Indications, route, and dosage
Supraventricular tachycardia
Adults: Dosage range is 50 to 200 mcg/kg/minute; average dose is 100 mcg/kg/minute. Individual dosage adjustment requires stepwise titration in which each step consists of a loading dose followed by a maintenance dose.

To begin treatment, administer a loading infusion of 500 mcg/kg/minute for 1 minute followed by a 4-minute maintenance infusion of 50 mcg/kg/minute. If tachycardia does not subside within 5 minutes, repeat loading dose and follow with maintenance infusion increased to 100 mcg/kg/minute. Continue titration, repeating loading infusion and increasing each maintenance infusion by 50 mcg/kg/minute. As patient's heart rate or blood pressure reaches a safety endpoint, omit loading infusion and reduce the increase in maintenance infusion from 50 to 25 mcg/kg/minute or less; also, increase the interval between titration steps from 5 to 10 minutes.

Intraoperative and postoperative tachycardia and hypertension
Adults: For immediate control, 80 mg (approximately 1 mg/kg) I.V. bolus dose over 30 seconds followed by a 150 mcg/kg/minute infusion, if necessary; for gradual control, a loading I.V. infusion of 500 mcg/kg/minute for 1 minute, followed by a 4-minute maintenance infusion of 50 mcg/kg/minute. If an adequate therapeutic effect is not observed within 5 minutes, repeat the same loading dosage and follow with a maintenance infusion increased to 100 mcg/kg/minute (see supraventricular tachycardia, above).

Pharmacodynamics
Antiarrhythmic action: Esmolol, a beta$_1$ blocker with rapid onset and very short duration of action, decreases blood pressure and heart rate in a dose-related, titratable mannner. Its hemodynamic effects are similar to those of propranolol, but it does not increase vascular resistance.

Pharmacokinetics
• *Absorption:* Absorption is immediate after I.V. infusion.
• *Distribution:* Esmolol is distributed rapidly throughout the plasma. Distribution half-life is about 2 minutes. Esmolol is 55% protein-bound.
• *Metabolism:* Drug is hydrolyzed rapidly by plasma esterases.

• *Excretion:* Esmolol is excreted by the kidneys as metabolites. Elimination half-life is about 9 minutes.

Contraindications and precautions

Contraindicated in patients with sinus bradycardia, heart block greater than first-degree, cardiogenic shock, or overt heart failure. Use cautiously in patients with impaired renal function, diabetes, or bronchospasm.

Interactions

Because of esmolol's short duration of action and the short periods of time over which it is used, many of its interactions associated with other beta blockers do not apply. Concurrent use of esmolol with *insulin* or *oral antidiabetic agents* may mask symptoms of developing hypoglycemia, such as rising pulse rate and blood pressure. Use with *nondepolarizing neuromuscular blocking agents such as* succinylcholine, *gallamine, metocurine, pancuronium, or tubocurarine* may potentiate and prolong their action; careful postoperative monitoring of the patient may be necessary after concurrent or sequential use, especially if there is a possibility of incomplete reversal of neuromuscular blockade.

Use with *antihypertensives* may potentiate their hypotensive effects and requires dosage adjustments based on blood pressure measurements.

Concurrent use of esmolol with *I.V. phenytoin* may produce additive cardiac depressant effects. Concurrent use with *reserpine* may result in additive and possibly excessive beta-adrenergic blockade with bradycardia and hypotension. Close observation is recommended.

Concurrent use of esmolol with *sympathomimetic amines having beta-adrenergic stimulant activity* may cause mutual but transient inhibition of therapeutic effects.

Use with *xanthines,* especially *aminophylline or theophylline,* may cause mutual inhibition of therapeutic effects and (except for dyphylline) may decrease theophylline clearance, especially in patients with increased theophylline clearance induced by smoking; concurrent use requires careful monitoring to prevent toxic accumulation of theophylline. Concomitant *I.V. administration with digoxin* may increase digoxin blood levels 10% to 20%; *I.V. administration of morphine* increases esmolol steady-state levels by 46%.

Effects on diagnostic tests

None reported.

Adverse reactions

CNS: dizziness, somnolence, headache, agitation, fatigue, confusion.
CV: HYPOTENSION (sometimes with diaphoresis), peripheral ischemia.
GI: *nausea,* vomiting.
Respiratory: ***bronchospasm,*** wheezing, dyspnea, nasal congestion.
Other: inflammation, induration (at infusion site).

Overdose and treatment

Limited information available. Hypotension would be the most likely symptom.

Symptoms of esmolol overdose usually disappear quickly after esmolol is withdrawn. In addition to immediate discontinuation of esmolol infusion, treatment is supportive and symptomatic.

Glucagon has been reported to effectively combat the CV effects (bradycardia, hypotension) of overdose with beta blockers. An I.V. dose of 2 to 3 mg is administered over 30 seconds and repeated if necessary, followed by infusion at 5 mg/hour until patient's condition has stabilized.

☑ Special considerations

• Dilute drug injection and administer by I.V. infusion. Concentrations exceeding 10 mg of esmolol hydrochloride per ml may produce irritation.
• To prepare esmolol hydrochloride injection for administration by I.V. infusion, aseptically remove 20 ml from a 500-ml bottle of I.V. fluid (D_5W injection USP, 5% dextrose in Ringer's injection, 5% dextrose and 0.45% NaCl injection USP, 5% dextrose and 0.9% NaCl injection USP, lactated Ringer's injection USP, 0.45% NaCl injection USP, or 0.9% NaCl injection USP) and then add 5-g esmolol hydrochloride injection to the bottle to produce a solution containing 10 mg of esmolol hydrochloride per milliliter.
• Drug is not compatible with 5% sodium bicarbonate injection USP.
• Diluted solutions of esmolol hydrochloride are stable for at least 24 hours at room temperature.
• If irritation occurs at infusion site, stop infusion and resume at another site. Do not use butterfly needles for I.V. administration.
• To convert to other antiarrhythmic therapy after control has been achieved with esmolol, reduce infusion rate of esmolol by 50% 30 minutes after administration of first dose of the alternative agent. If after the second dose of the alternative agent a satisfactory response is maintained for 1 hour, then discontinue esmolol.
• Monitor patient's pulse and blood pressure.

Patient education

• Advise patient to report pain at I.V. site.
• Inform patient of need of frequent monitoring of vital signs.

Geriatric use

• Although adequate and well-controlled studies have not been done in the geriatric population, the elderly may be less sensitive to some of the effects of beta blockers. However, reduced metabolic and excretory capabilities in many elderly patients may lead to increased myocardial depression and require dosage reduction of beta blockers. Dosage adjustment should be based on clinical response.

Pediatric use

• Adequate and well-controlled studies have not been done. Safety and efficacy in children have not been established.

Breast-feeding

• It is not known if drug is excreted in breast milk; no problems associated with breast-feeding have been reported.

estazolam

ProSom

Pharmacologic classification: benzodiazepine
Therapeutic classification: hypnotic
Controlled substance schedule IV
Pregnancy risk category X

How supplied

Available by prescription only
Tablets: 1 mg, 2 mg

Indications, route, and dosage

Short-term management of insomnia characterized by difficulty in falling asleep, frequent nocturnal awakenings, or early-morning awakenings

Adults: Initially, 1 mg P.O. h.s.; may increase to 2 mg as needed and tolerated.

✦ ***Dosage adjustment.*** In small or debilitated older adults, initially, 0.5 mg P.O. h.s.; may increase with care to 1 mg if needed.

Pharmacodynamics

Hypnotic action: Estazolam depresses the CNS at the limbic and subcortical levels of the brain. It produces a sedative-hypnotic effect by potentiating the effect of the neurotransmitter gamma-aminobutyric acid on its receptor in the ascending reticular activating system, which increases inhibition and blocks both cortical and limbic arousal.

Pharmacokinetics

- *Absorption:* Estazolam is rapidly and completely absorbed through the GI tract in 1 to 3 hours. Peak levels occur within 2 hours (range is ½ to 6 hours).
- *Distribution:* Estazolam is 93% protein-bound.
- *Metabolism:* Drug is extensively metabolized in the liver.
- *Excretion:* Metabolites are excreted primarily in the urine. Less than 5% is excreted in urine as unchanged drug; 4% of a 2-mg dose is excreted in feces. Elimination half-life ranges from 10 to 24 hours; clearance is accelerated in smokers.

Contraindications and precautions

Contraindicated in pregnant patients or patients with hypersensitivity to drug. Use cautiously in patients with depression, suicidal tendencies, and hepatic, renal, or pulmonary disease.

Interactions

Estazolam potentiates CNS depressant effects of *phenothiazines, narcotics, antihistamines, MAO inhibitors, barbiturates, alcohol, general anesthetics,* and *tricyclic antidepressants.* Concurrent use with *cimetidine, disulfiram, oral contraceptives,* and *isoniazid* may diminish hepatic metabolism, resulting in increased plasma concentrations of estazolam and increased CNS depressant effects. *Heavy smoking* accelerates estazolam's metabolism, resulting in diminished clinical efficacy. Like other benzodiazepines, estazolam increases *phenytoin* and *digoxin* levels, possibly resulting in toxicity. Use with *probenecid* results in more rapid onset and more prolonged benzodiazepine effect. *Theophylline* antagonizes estazolam's pharmacologic effects. *Rifampin* increases clearance and decreases half-life of estazolam.

Effects on diagnostic tests

AST levels may be increased.

Adverse reactions

CNS: fatigue, dizziness, *daytime drowsiness, somnolence, asthenia, hypokinesia, abnormal thinking.*
GI: dyspepsia, abdominal pain.
Other: back pain, stiffness.

Overdose and treatment

Somnolence, confusion with reduced or absent reflexes, respiratory depression, apnea, hypotension, impaired coordination, slurred speech, seizures, or coma can occur from benzodiazepine overdose. If excitation occurs, do not use barbiturates. Remember that multiple agents may have been ingested. Gastric evacuation and lavage should be performed immediately. Monitor respiration, pulse rate, and blood pressure. Use symptomatic and supportive measures. Maintain airway and administer fluids. Flumazenil, a specific benzodiazepine antagonist, may be useful.

☑ Special considerations

Besides those relevant to all *benzodiazepines,* consider the following recommendations.

- Remove all potential safety hazards such as cigarettes from patient's reach.
- Regularly perform blood counts, urinalysis, and blood chemistry analyses.
- Withdraw drug slowly after prolonged use.
- Encourage good sleep habits and regular exercise. Advise the avoidance of caffeine or other stimulants, especially late in the day.

Patient education

- Tell patient to avoid alcohol and other CNS depressants while taking this medication. After taking drug in the evening, patient should avoid alcohol the following day.
- Advise female patient to call immediately if she suspects pregnancy or plans to become pregnant during therapy.
- Tell patient to notify primary health care provider of other medications and of usual alcohol consumption.
- Warn that drug may cause drowsiness. Advise special caution and avoidance of driving or operating hazardous machinery until adverse CNS effects of the drug are known.
- Inform patient that nocturnal sleep may be disturbed for or 2 nights after drug is stopped.
- Caution patient not to discontinue drug abruptly after taking it daily for prolonged period and not to vary dosage or increase dose unless prescribed.
- Advise patient that rebound insomnia may occur after stopping the drug.

Geriatric use

• Elderly patients may be more susceptible to CNS depressant effects of estazolam. Use with caution. Lower dosage may be required. To prevent injury from dizziness and falls, elderly patients should be supervised during daily living activities, especially at the start of treatment and after an increase in dosage.

Pediatric use

• Safety and efficacy have not been established.

Breast-feeding

• Because drug occurs in breast milk, avoid use in breast-feeding patients.

esterified estrogens

Estratab, Menest

Pharmacologic classification: estrogen
Therapeutic classification: estrogen replacement, antineoplastic
Pregnancy risk category X

How supplied

Available by prescription only
Tablets: 0.3 mg, 0.625 mg, 1.25 mg, 2.5 mg

Indications, route, and dosage

Palliative treatment of advanced inoperable prostatic cancer
Adults: 1.25 to 2.5 mg P.O. t.i.d.
Breast cancer
Men and postmenopausal women: 10 mg P.O. t.i.d. for 3 or more months.
Female hypogonadism
Adults: 2.5 mg P.O. daily to t.i.d. in cycles of 20 days on, 10 days off.
Castration, primary ovarian failure
Adults: 2.5 mg daily to t.i.d. in cycles of 3 weeks on, 1 week off.
Vasomotor menopausal symptoms
Adults: 0.3 to 1.25 mg P.O. daily in cycles of 3 weeks on, 1 week off; dosage may be increased to 2.5 or 3.75 mg P.O. daily, if necessary.
Atrophic vaginitis and atrophic urethritis
Adults: 0.3 to 1.25 mg P.O. daily in cycles of 3 weeks on, 1 week off.

Pharmacodynamics

Estrogenic action: Esterified estrogen mimics the action of endogenous estrogen in treating female hypogonadism, menopausal symptoms, and atrophic vaginitis. It inhibits growth of hormone-sensitive tissue in advanced, inoperable prostatic cancer and in certain carefully selected cases of breast cancer in men and postmenopausal women.

Pharmacokinetics

• *Absorption:* After oral administration, esterified estrogens are well absorbed but substantially inactivated by the liver. Therefore, esterified estrogens are usually administered parenterally.
• *Distribution:* Esterified estrogens are approximately 50% to 80% plasma protein-bound, particularly the estradiol-binding globulin. Distribution occurs throughout the body with highest concentrations appearing in fat.
• *Metabolism:* Esterified estrogens are metabolized primarily in the liver, where they are conjugated with sulfate and glucuronide.
• *Excretion:* Most esterified estrogens are eliminated through the kidneys in the form of sulfate or glucuronide conjugates.

Contraindications and precautions

Contraindicated in patients with breast cancer (except metastatic disease), estrogen-dependent neoplasia, active thrombophlebitis or thromboembolic disorders, undiagnosed abnormal genital bleeding, hypersensitivity to drug, history of thromboembolic disease, or during pregnancy.

Use cautiously in patients with history of hypertension, mental depression, liver impairment, or cardiac or renal dysfunction and in those with bone diseases, migraine, seizures, or diabetes mellitus.

Interactions

Concomitant administration of *drugs that induce hepatic metabolism*, such as *rifampin, barbiturates, primidone, carbamazepine,* and *phenytoin,* may result in decreased estrogenic effects from a given dose. These drugs are known to accelerate the rate of metabolism of certain other agents.

In patients with diabetes, esterified estrogens may increase blood glucose levels, necessitating dosage adjustment of *insulin* or *oral antidiabetic agents.*

Concomitant use with *anticoagulants* may decrease the effects of *warfarin-type anticoagulants.* Concomitant use with *adrenocorticosteroids* or *adrenocorticotropic hormone* may cause greater risk of fluid and electrolyte accumulation.

Effects on diagnostic tests

Therapy with esterified estrogens increases sulfobromophthalein retention, PT and clotting factors VII to X, and norepinephrine-induced platelet aggregability. Increases in the thyroid-binding globulin concentration may occur, resulting in increased total thyroid concentrations (measured by protein-bound iodine or total T_4) and decreased uptake of free T_3 resin. Serum folate, pyridoxine, and antithrombin III concentrations may decrease; triglyceride, glucose, and phospholipid levels may increase. Glucose tolerance may be impaired. Pregnanediol excretion may decrease.

Adverse reactions

CNS: headache, dizziness, chorea, depression, ***seizures.***
CV: thrombophlebitis; ***thromboembolism;*** hypertension; edema; ***increased risk of CVA, pulmonary embolism, MI.***
EENT: worsening of myopia or astigmatism, intolerance of contact lenses.
GI: *nausea,* vomiting, abdominal cramps, bloating, anorexia, increased appetite, weight changes, pancreatitis.

GU: in women—breakthrough bleeding, altered menstrual flow, dysmenorrhea, amenorrhea, ***increased risk of endometrial cancer, possibility of increased risk of breast cancer,*** cervical erosion, altered cervical secretions, enlargement of uterine fibromas, vaginal candidiasis; in men—gynecomastia, testicular atrophy, impotence
Hepatic: cholestatic jaundice, ***hepatic adenoma.***
Skin: melasma, rash, hirsutism or hair loss, erythema nodosum, dermatitis.
Other: breast changes (tenderness, enlargement, secretion), gallbladder disease, hypercalcemia.

Overdose and treatment

Serious toxicity after overdose of these drugs has not been reported. Nausea may be expected to occur. Appropriate supportive care should be provided.

☑ Special considerations

Recommendations for administration of esterified estrogens and for care and teaching of the patient during therapy are the same as those for all *estrogens.*

Breast-feeding

- Esterified estrogens are contraindicated in breast-feeding women.

estradiol

Climara, Estrace, Estrace Vaginal Cream, Estraderm, Vivelle

estradiol cypionate

depGynogen, Depo-Estradiol Cypionate, Depogen, Estro-Cyp, Estrofem

estradiol valerate

Delestrogen*, Dioval 40, Dioval XX, Estra-L 40, Gynogen L.A. 20, Gynogen L.A. 20, Valergen-20

polyestradiol phosphate

Estradurin

Pharmacologic classification: estrogen
Therapeutic classification: estrogen replacement, antineoplastic
Pregnancy risk category X

How supplied

Available by prescription only
estradiol
Tablets: 0.5 mg, 1 mg, 2 mg
Vaginal: 0.1 mg/g cream (in nonliquefying base)
Transdermal: 4 mg/10 cm^2 (delivers 0.05 mg/24 hours); 8 mg/20 cm^2 (delivers 0.1 mg/24 hours)
estradiol cypionate
Injection: 5 mg/ml (in oil)
estradiol valerate
Injection: 10 mg/ml, 20 mg/ml, 40 mg/ml (in oil)
polyestradiol phosphate
Injection: 40 mg/2 ml

Indications, route, and dosage

Atrophic vaginitis, atrophic dystrophy of the vulva, vasomotor menopausal symptoms, hypogonadism, female castration, primary ovarian failure
estradiol (tablets)
Adults: 1 to 2 mg P.O. daily, in cycles of 21 days on and 7 days off or cycles of 5 days on and 2 days off; or 0.2 to 1 mg I.M. weekly.
estradiol valerate
Adults: 10 to 20 mg I.M. once monthly.
estradiol (transdermal)
Adults: Place one Estraderm transdermal patch on trunk of the body, preferably the abdomen, twice weekly. Administer on an intermittent cyclic schedule (3 weeks on and 1 week off).
Atrophic vaginitis
estradiol (vaginal cream)
Adults: 2 to 4 g daily for 1 to 2 weeks. When vaginal mucosa is restored, begin maintenance dosage of 1 g one to three times weekly.
Female hypogonadism
estradiol cypionate
Adults: 1.5 to 2 mg I.M. at monthly intervals.
Inoperable breast cancer
estradiol (tablets)
Adults: 10 mg P.O. t.i.d. for 3 months.
Inoperable prostatic cancer
estradiol valerate
Adults: 30 mg I.M. q 1 to 2 weeks.
estradiol (tablets)
Adults: 1 to 2 mg P.O. t.i.d.
polyestradiol phosphate
Adults: 40 mg I.M. q 2 to 4 weeks.

Pharmacodynamics

Estrogenic action: Estradiol mimics the action of endogenous estrogen in treating female hypogonadism, menopausal symptoms, and atrophic vaginitis. It inhibits growth of hormone-sensitive tissue in advanced, inoperable prostatic cancer and in certain carefully selected cases of breast cancer in men and postmenopausal women.

Pharmacokinetics

- *Absorption:* After oral administration, estradiol and the other natural unconjugated estrogens are well absorbed but substantially inactivated by the liver. Therefore, unconjugated estrogens are usually administered parenterally.

After I.M. administration, absorption begins rapidly and continues for days. The cypionate and valerate esters administered in oil have prolonged durations of action because of their slow absorption characteristics.

Topically applied estradiol is absorbed readily into the systemic circulation.
- *Distribution:* Estradiol and the other natural estrogens are approximately 50% to 80% plasma protein-bound, particularly the estradiol-binding globulin. Distribution occurs throughout the body, with highest concentrations appearing in fat.
- *Metabolism:* The steroidal estrogens, including estradiol, are metabolized primarily in the liver, where they are conjugated with sulfate and glucuronide. Because of the rapid rate of metabolism,

nonesterified forms of estrogen, including estradiol, must usually be administered daily.

• *Excretion:* The majority of estrogen elimination occurs through the kidneys in the form of sulfate or glucuronide conjugates.

Contraindications and precautions

Contraindicated in patients with thrombophlebitis or thromboembolic disorders, estrogen-dependent neoplasia, breast or reproductive organ cancer (except for palliative treatment), or undiagnosed abnormal genital bleeding and during pregnancy. Also contraindicated in patients with history of thrombophlebitis or thromboembolic disorders associated with previous estrogen use (except for palliative treatment of breast and prostate cancer).

Use cautiously in patients with cerebrovascular or coronary artery disease, asthma, bone diseases, migraine, seizures, or cardiac, hepatic, or renal dysfunction and in women with a strong family history of breast cancer or who have breast nodules, fibrocystic disease, or abnormal mammographic findings.

Interactions

Concomitant administration of *drugs that induce hepatic metabolism (rifampin, barbiturates, primidone, carbamazepine, phenytoin)* may decrease estrogenic effects from a given dose. These drugs are known to accelerate the rate of metabolism of certain other agents.

In patients with diabetes, estradiol may increase blood glucose levels, necessitating dosage adjustment of *insulin* or *oral antidiabetic agents.*

Concomitant use with *anticoagulants* may decrease the effects of *warfarin-type anticoagulants.*

Use with *adrenocorticosteroids* or *adrenocorticotropic hormone* increases the risk of fluid and electrolyte accumulation.

Use with *hepatotoxic medications (*especially *dantrolene)* increases risk of liver damage.

Effects on diagnostic tests

Estradiol increases sulfobromophthalein retention, prothrombin and clotting factors VII to X, and norepinephrine-induced platelet aggregability. Increases in thyroid-binding globulin concentrations may occur, resulting in increased total thyroid concentrations (measured by protein-bound iodine or total T_4) and decreased uptake of free T_3 resin. Serum folate, pyridoxine, and antithrombin III concentrations may decrease; triglyceride, glucose, and phospholipid levels may increase. Glucose tolerance may be impaired. Pregnanediol excretion may decrease.

Adverse reactions

CNS: headache, dizziness, chorea, depression, ***seizures.***
CV: thrombophlebitis, ***thromboembolism,*** hypertension, edema.
EENT: worsening of myopia or astigmatism, intolerance of contact lenses.
GI: *nausea,* vomiting, abdominal cramps, bloating, increased appetite, weight changes, pancreatitis.
GU: in women—breakthrough bleeding, altered menstrual flow, dysmenorrhea, amenorrhea, ***increased risk of endometrial cancer, possibility of increased risk of breast cancer,*** cervical erosion, altered cervical secretions, enlargement of uterine fibromas, vaginal candidiasis; in men—gynecomastia, testicular atrophy, impotence.
Hepatic: cholestatic jaundice, ***hepatic adenoma.***
Skin: melasma, urticaria, erythema nodosum, dermatitis, hirsutism or hair loss.
Other: breast changes (tenderness, enlargement, secretion), gallbladder disease, hypercalcemia.

Overdose and treatment

Serious toxicity after overdose of drug has not been reported. Nausea may be expected to occur. Provide appropriate supportive care.

☑ Special considerations

Besides those relevant to all *estrogens,* consider the following recommendations.

• Before injection, make sure drug is well dispersed in solution by rolling the reconstituted vial between the palms.
• Administer by deep I.M. injection into large muscles.

Patient education

• Tell patient not to apply patch to her breast areas.
• Remind patient not to use the same skin site for at least 1 week after removal of the transdermal system.

Geriatric use

• Frequent physical examinations are recommended in postmenopausal women taking estrogen.

Breast-feeding

• Drug is contraindicated in breast-feeding women.

estramustine phosphate sodium

Emcyt

Pharmacologic classification: estrogen, alkylating agent
Therapeutic classification: antineoplastic
Pregnancy risk category NR

How supplied

Available by prescription only
Capsules: 140 mg

Indications, route, and dosage

Dosage and indications may vary. Check literature for recommended protocols.

Palliative treatment of metastatic or progressive cancer of the prostate
Adults: 10 to 16 mg/kg P.O. in three or four divided doses. Usual dosage is 14 mg/kg daily. Therapy should continue for up to 3 months and, if successful, be maintained as long as patient responds.

Pharmacodynamics

Antineoplastic action: Exact mechanism of action is unclear. However, the estrogenic portion of the molecule may act as a carrier of the drug to facilitate selective uptake by tumor cells with estradiol hormone receptors, such as those in the prostate gland. At that point, the nitrogen mustard portion of the drug acts as an alkylating agent.

Pharmacokinetics

- *Absorption:* After oral administration, about 75% of a dose is absorbed across the GI tract.
- *Distribution:* Estramustine distributes widely into body tissues.
- *Metabolism:* Extensively metabolized in the liver.
- *Excretion:* Drug and its metabolites are eliminated primarily in feces, with a small amount excreted in urine. Terminal phase of plasma elimination has a half-life of 20 hours.

Contraindications and precautions

Contraindicated in patients hypersensitive to estradiol and nitrogen mustard and in those with active thrombophlebitis or thromboembolic disorders, except when the actual tumor mass is the cause of the thromboembolic phenomenon.

Use cautiously in patients with history of thrombophlebitis or thromboembolic disorders and cerebrovascular or coronary artery disease.

Interactions

Concomitant use of estramustine with *anticoagulants* may decrease the anticoagulant effect by an unknown mechanism and requires increased dosage of anticoagulants.

Effects on diagnostic tests

Drug therapy may increase norepinephrine-induced platelet aggregability. A reduced response to the metyrapone test may occur during therapy with estramustine. Glucose tolerance may be decreased.

Adverse reactions

CNS: lethargy, insomnia, headache, anxiety.
CV: ***MI,*** sodium and fluid retention, thrombophlebitis, ***heart failure, stroke.***
GI: *nausea, vomiting,* diarrhea, anorexia, flatulence, GI bleeding, thirst.
Hematologic: ***leukopenia, thrombocytopenia.***
Respiratory: ***edema, pulmonary embolism,*** dyspnea.
Skin: rash, pruritus, dry skin, flushing.
Other: *painful gynecomastia and breast tenderness,* thinning of hair, leg cramps, chest pain.

Overdose and treatment

Clinical manifestations of overdose include headache, nausea, vomiting, and myelosuppression.

Treatment is usually supportive and includes induction of emesis, gastric lavage, transfusion of blood components, and appropriate symptomatic therapy. Hematologic monitoring should continue for at least 6 weeks after the ingestion.

☑ Special considerations

- Administer drug with meals or antacids to reduce incidence of GI upset. However, milk, milk products, or calcium-rich foods may impair absorption.
- Store capsules in refrigerator.
- Phenothiazines can be used to treat nausea and vomiting.
- Monitor blood pressure at baseline and routinely during therapy. Estramustine may cause hypertension.
- Drug may exaggerate preexisting peripheral edema or heart failure. Weight gain should be monitored regularly in these patients.
- Monitor glucose tolerance periodically during therapy.
- Patient may continue estramustine as long as he's responding favorably. Some patients have taken drug for more than 3 years.

Patient education

- Emphasize importance of continuing medication despite nausea and vomiting.
- Advise patient to call immediately if vomiting occurs shortly after a dose is taken.
- Because of possibility of mutagenic effects, advise patients of childbearing age to use contraceptive measures.

Geriatric use

- Use with caution in elderly patients, who are more likely to have vascular disorders, because the use of estrogen is associated with vascular complications.

estrogen and progestin

Alesse-28, Brevicon, Demulen 1/35, Demulen 1/35-28, Loestrin 21 1/20, Loestrin 21 1.5/30, Loestrin Fe 1/20, Loestrin Fe 1.5/30, Lo/Ovral, Lo/Ovral-28, Modicon 21, Modicon 28, Nordette-21, Nordette-28, Norinyl 1+35 21-Day, Norinyl 1+35 28-Day, Norinyl 1+50 21-Day, Norinyl 1+50 28-Day, Norinyl 1+80 28-Day, Ortho-Novum 1/35 21, Ortho-Novum 1/35 28, Ortho-Novum 1/50 21, Ortho-Novum 1/50 28, Ortho-Novum 7/7/7-21, Ortho-Novum 7/7/7-28, Ortho-Novum 10/11-21, Ortho-Novum 10/11-28, Ovcon-35, Ovcon-50, Ovral, Ovral-28, Tri-Norinyl-21, Tri-Norinyl-28, Triphasil-21, Triphasil-28

Pharmacologic classification: estrogen with progestin
Therapeutic classification: contraceptive (hormonal)
Pregnancy risk category X

How supplied

Available by prescription only
Tablets—monophasic type
Mestranol 0.1 mg and norethynodrel 2.5 mg
Mestranol 0.1 mg and norethindrone 2 mg
Mestranol 0.1 mg and ethynodiol diacetate 1 mg
Mestranol 0.08 mg and norethindrone 1 mg
Mestranol 0.075 mg and norethynodrel 5 mg
Mestranol 0.05 mg and norethindrone 1 mg
Ethinyl estradiol 0.02 mg and levonorgestrel 0.1 mg

Ethinyl estradiol 0.05 mg and norethindrone 1 mg
Ethinyl estradiol 0.05 mg and norethindrone acetate 1 mg
Ethinyl estradiol 0.05 mg and ethynodiol diacetate 1 mg
Ethinyl estradiol 0.05 mg and norethindrone acetate 2.5 mg
Ethinyl estradiol 0.05 mg and norgestrel 0.5 mg
Ethinyl estradiol 0.035 mg and norethindrone 1 mg
Ethinyl estradiol 0.035 mg and norethindrone 0.5 mg
Ethinyl estradiol 0.035 mg and norethindrone 0.4 mg
Ethinyl estradiol 0.035 mg and ethynodiol diacetate 1 mg
Ethinyl estradiol 0.03 mg and norethindrone acetate 1.5 mg
Ethinyl estradiol 0.03 mg and norgestrel 0.3 mg
Ethinyl estradiol 0.03 mg and levonorgestrel 0.15 mg
Ethinyl estradiol 0.02 mg and norethindrone 1 mg

Tablets—biphasic type
10 tablets ethinyl estradiol 0.035 mg and norethindrone 0.5 mg; 11 tablets ethinyl estradiol 0.035 mg and norethindrone 1 mg

Tablets—triphasic type
7 tablets ethinyl estradiol 0.035 mg and norethindrone 0.5 mg; 9 tablets ethinyl estradiol 0.035 mg and norethindrone 1 mg; 5 tablets ethinyl estradiol 0.035 mg and norethindrone 0.5 mg
7 tablets ethinyl estradiol 0.035 mg and norethindrone 0.5 mg; 7 tablets ethinyl estradiol 0.035 mg and norethindrone 0.75 mg; 7 tablets ethinyl estradiol 0.035 mg and norethindrone 1 mg
6 tablets ethinyl estradiol 0.03 and levonorgestrel 0.05 mg; 5 tablets ethinyl estradiol 0.04 mg and levonorgestrel 0.075 mg; 10 tablets ethinyl estradiol 0.03 mg and levonorgestrel 0.125 mg

Indications, route, and dosage

Contraception

Monophasic

Adults: One tablet P.O. daily, beginning on day 5 of menstrual cycle (first day of menstrual flow is day 1), or on the first Sunday after onset of menstruation, or on day 1 of menstrual cycle depending on specific contraceptive. With 20- and 21-tablet packages, new dosing cycle begins 7 days after last tablet taken. With 28-tablet packages, dosage is one tablet daily without interruption; extra tablets are placebos or contain iron. If next menstrual period doesn't begin on schedule, rule out pregnancy before starting new dosing cycle. If menstrual period begins, start new dosing cycle 7 days after last tablet was taken. If all doses have been taken on schedule and one menstrual period is missed, continue dosing cycle. If two consecutive menstrual periods are missed, pregnancy test is required before new dosing cycle is started.

Biphasic

Adults: One color tablet P.O. daily (Ortho-Novum 10/11) for 10 days, then next color tablet for 11 days.

Triphasic

Adults: One tablet P.O. daily (Ortho-Novum 7/7/7, Tri-Norinyl, Triphasil) in the sequence specified by the manufacturer.

Hypermenorrhea

Adults: Use high-dose combinations only. Dosage is same as for contraception.

Endometriosis

Adults: Cyclic therapy: One 10-mg tablet P.O. daily (Ortho-Novum) for 20 days from day 5 to day 24 of menstrual cycle. Suppressive therapy: One 5- or 10-mg tablet P.O. daily (Enovid) for 2 weeks, starting on day 5 of menstrual cycle. Continue without interruption for 6 to 9 months, increasing dose by 5 to 10 mg q 2 weeks, up to 20 mg daily. Up to 40 mg daily may be needed if breakthrough bleeding occurs.

Pharmacodynamics

Contraceptive action: Estrogen components of oral contraceptives inhibit the release of follicle-stimulating hormone, thereby stopping follicular development and suppressing ovulation.

Progestin components of oral contraceptives inhibit the release of luteinizing hormone, preventing ovulation even in the event of incomplete suppression of follicular development. Progestins also change the endometrial environment to inhibit nidation (implantation of the fertilized egg into the endometrium) and cause thickening of the cervical mucus, blocking the upward migration of sperm.

Pharmacokinetics

- *Absorption:* Most components of oral contraceptives are absorbed relatively well from the GI tract. Bioavailabilities range from 40% to 70%; considerable individual variation exists in extent of absorption. Peak concentrations occur from 1 to 2 hours after dosing.
- *Distribution:* Protein binding of the various drugs used in oral contraceptives is high, ranging from 80% to 98%. These agents are distributed extensively into virtually all body tissues.
- *Metabolism:* These drugs undergo metabolic transformation before excretion; their rates of metabolism may thus be affected by agents that induce or inhibit metabolism.
- *Excretion:* Very little, if any, of these drugs is excreted unchanged in urine or feces. They appear primarily as sulfate and glucuronide conjugates.

Contraindications and precautions

Oral contraceptives are contraindicated in patients with thromboembolic disorders, cerebrovascular or coronary artery disease, or MI because of their association with thromboembolic disease; in patients with known or suspected cancer of the breast or reproductive organs or with benign or malignant liver tumors because of their association with tumorigenesis; in patients with undiagnosed abnormal vaginal bleeding; in women known or believed to be pregnant or breast-feeding; in adolescents with incomplete epiphyseal closure; and in women smokers over age 35.

Oral contraceptives should be used cautiously in patients with systemic lupus erythematosus, hypertension, mental depression, migraine, epilepsy, asthma, diabetes mellitus, amenorrhea, scanty or irregular periods, fibrocystic breast disease, family history (mother, grandmother, sister) of breast or genital tract cancer, or renal or gallbladder disease. Development or worsening of any of these conditions should be reported. Prolonged therapy may be inadvisable in women who plan to become pregnant.

Interactions

Concomitant use of certain drugs such as *rifampin, barbiturates, phenylbutazone, phenytoin, primidone, carbamazepine,* and *isoniazid* increases the metabolism of oral contraceptives, resulting in reduced efficacy, breakthrough bleeding, and occasionally contraceptive failure. Similar effects may occur with concomitant use of *neomycin, penicillin V, tetracycline, griseofulvin, chloramphenicol, nitrofurantoin, sulfonamides,* and *antihistamines.*

Oral contraceptive use may require adjustment of dosage of *insulin* or *oral antidiabetic agents.* Oral contraceptives may counteract the effectiveness of *oral warfarin-type anticoagulants* and of *anticonvulsants, antihypertensives,* and *tricyclic antidepressants.*

Effects on diagnostic tests

The following test results may be elevated in users of oral contraceptives: sulfobromophthalein retention, prothrombin and clotting factors VII to X, plasminogen, norepinephrine-induced platelet aggregation, fibrinogen, thyroid-binding globulin, triglycerides, phospholipids, transcortin and corticosteroids, transferrin, prolactin, renin, and vitamin A.

The following test results may be decreased in users of oral contraceptives: antithrombin III, metyrapone, pregnanediol excretion, free T_3 resin uptake, glucose tolerance, zinc, and vitamin B_{12}.

Adverse reactions

CNS: headache, dizziness, depression, libido changes, lethargy, migraine.
CV: ***thromboembolism,*** hypertension, edema.
EENT: worsening of myopia or astigmatism, intolerance of contact lenses, unexplained loss of vision, optic neuritis, diplopia, retinal thrombosis, papilledema.
GI: *nausea, vomiting,* abdominal cramps, bloating, diarrhea, constipation, changes in appetite, weight gain, bowel ischemia.
GU: breakthrough bleeding, granulomatous colitis, dysmenorrhea, amenorrhea, cervical erosion or abnormal secretions, enlargement of uterine fibromas, vaginal candidiasis, urinary tract infections.
Hepatic: gallbladder disease, cholestatic jaundice, liver tumors.
Metabolic: hyperglycemia, hypercalcemia, folic acid deficiency.
Skin: rash, acne, seborrhea, oily skin, erythema multiforme, hyperpigmentation.
Other: breast tenderness, enlargement, or secretion; increase in varicosities; possible increased risk of congenital anomalies.

Adverse effects may be more serious, frequent, and rapid in onset with high-dose than with low-dose combinations.

Note: Discontinue drug if patient becomes hypertensive during therapy.

Overdose and treatment

Serious toxicity after drug overdose has not been reported. Nausea and vomiting may be expected to occur. Withdrawal bleeding may occur.

☑ Special considerations

Besides those relevant to all *estrogens* and *progestins,* oral contraceptives require the following special considerations.

- Astigmatic error and myopic refractive error may be increased twofold to threefold, usually after 6 months of oral contraceptive therapy. Changes in ocular contour and lubricant quality of tears may necessitate change in size and shape of contact lenses.

Patient education

- Warn patient that headache, nausea, dizziness, breast tenderness, spotting, and breakthrough bleeding are common at first. These should diminish after 3 to 6 dosing cycles (months). However, breakthrough bleeding in patients taking high-dose estrogen-progestin combinations for menstrual disorders may necessitate dosage adjustment.
- Advise patient to use an additional method of birth control for the first week of administration in the initial cycle (unless using day-1 start).
- If one menstrual period is missed and tablets have been taken on schedule, tell patient to continue taking them. If two consecutive menstrual periods are missed, tell patient to stop drug and have pregnancy test.
- Teach patient to take drug at the same time each day at 24-hour intervals for efficacy of medication, to keep tablets in original container, and to take them in correct (color-coded) sequence.
- Tell patient that night-time dosing may reduce incidence of nausea and headaches.
- Suggest taking drug with or immediately after food to reduce nausea.
- Stress importance of annual Papanicolaou smears and gynecologic examinations while taking estrogen-progestin combinations.
- Warn patient of possible delay in achieving pregnancy when drug is discontinued.
- Advise patient of increased risks associated with simultaneous use of cigarettes and oral contraceptives, especially the risk of serious cardiovascular side effects. Women who use oral contraceptives should be strongly advised not to smoke.
- Instruct patient to weigh herself at least twice weekly and to report sudden weight gain or edema.
- Warn patient to avoid exposure to ultraviolet light or prolonged exposure to sunlight; chloasma seems to be aggravated by sunlight. With anticipated exposure (as in summer), taking pill at bedtime will reduce daytime levels of circulating hormone.
- Advise patient to avoid pregnancy for 2 months after stopping drug and to seek medical advice about how soon it may be safely attempted after drug is stopped.
- Inform patient that oral contraceptives decrease viscosity of the cervical mucus and increase susceptibility to vaginal infections. Good hygienic practices are essential.

- Instruct patient to use another form of contraception if she is receiving ampicillin, antiepileptics, phenylbutazone, rifampin, or tetracycline, because intermittent bleeding and unwanted pregnancy might result from effect of drug interactions.
- Instruct patient as follows regarding missed doses.

Monophasic or biphasic cycles

For 20-, 21-, or 24-day dosing schedule:

- If one regular dose is missed, take tablet as soon as possible; if remembered on the next day, take two tablets, then continue regular dosing schedule.
- If two consecutive days are missed, take two tablets a day for next 2 days, then resume regular dosing schedule.
- If 3 consecutive days are missed, discontinue drug and substitute other contraceptive method until period begins or pregnancy is ruled out. Then start new cycle of tablets.

For 28-day dosing schedule:

- Follow instructions for 21-day dosing schedule; if 1 of the last 7 tablets is missed, be sure to take first tablet of next month's cycle on regularly scheduled day.

Triphasic cycle

For 21-day dosing schedule:

- If 1 day is missed, take dose as soon as possible; if remembered on the next day, take two tablets, then continue regular dosing schedule while using additional method of contraception for remainder of cycle.
- If 2 consecutive days are missed, take two tablets daily for next 2 days, then continue regular schedule while using additional contraceptive method for remainder of cycle.
- If 3 consecutive days are missed, discontinue drug and use other contraceptive method until period begins or pregnancy is ruled out. Then start new cycle of tablets.

For 28-day dosing schedule:

- Follow instructions for 21-day dosing schedule; if one of the last seven tablets was missed, be sure to take first tablet of next month's cycle on regularly scheduled day.

Pediatric use

- To avoid later fertility and menstrual problems, hormonal contraception is not advised for the adolescent until after at least 2 years of well-established menstrual cycles and completion of physiologic maturation.
- An estrogen-dominant agent is the best choice for the adolescent with scanty menses, moderate or severe acne, or candidiasis. A progestin-dominant agent is the best choice for the adolescent with dysmenorrhea, hypermenorrhea, fibrocystic breast disease, or cyclic premenstrual weight gain.

Breast-feeding

- Oral contraceptives are contraindicated in breast-feeding women.

estrogenic substances, conjugated

Premarin

Pharmacologic classification: estrogen
Therapeutic classification: estrogen replacement, antineoplastic, antiosteoporotic
Pregnancy risk category X

How supplied

Available by prescription only
Tablets: 0.3 mg, 0.625 mg, 0.9 mg, 1.25 mg, 2.5 mg
Injection: 25 mg/5 ml
Vaginal cream: 0.0625%

Indications, route, and dosage

Abnormal uterine bleeding (hormonal imbalance)

Adults: 25 mg I.V. or I.M. Repeat in 6 to 12 hours.

Castration and primary ovarian failure

Adults: 1.25 mg P.O. daily in cycles of 3 weeks on, 1 week off.

Osteoporosis

Adults: 0.625 mg P.O. daily in cycles of 3 weeks on, 1 week off.

Female hypogonadism

Adults: 2.5 to 7.5 mg P.O. daily in divided doses for 20 consecutive days followed by 10 days without drug.

Vasomotor menopausal symptoms

Adults: 1.25 mg P.O. daily in cycles of 3 weeks on, 1 week off.

Atrophic vaginitis or kraurosis vulvae

Adults: 0.3 mg to 1.25 mg or more P.O. daily. Alternatively, 2 to 4 g intravaginally or topically once daily in cycles of 3 weeks on, 1 week off.

Palliative treatment of inoperable prostatic cancer

Adults: 1.25 to 2.5 mg P.O. t.i.d.

Palliative treatment of breast cancer

Adults: 10 mg P.O. t.i.d. for 3 months or more.

Pharmacodynamics

Estrogenic action: Conjugated estrogenic substances mimic the action of endogenous estrogen in treating female hypogonadism, menopausal symptoms, and atrophic vaginitis. They inhibit growth of hormone-sensitive tissue in advanced, inoperable prostatic cancer and in certain carefully selected cases of breast cancer in men and postmenopausal women; they also retard progression of osteoporosis by enhancing calcium and phosphate retention and limiting bone decalcification.

Pharmacokinetics

- *Absorption:* Not well characterized. After I.M. administration, absorption begins rapidly and continues for days.
- *Distribution:* Conjugated estrogens are approximately 50% to 80% plasma protein-bound, particularly the estradiol-binding globulin. Distribution occurs throughout the body, with highest concentrations appearing in fat.

• *Metabolism:* Conjugated estrogens are metabolized primarily in the liver, where they are conjugated with sulfate and glucuronide. Because of the rapid rate of metabolism, nonesterified forms of estrogen, including estradiol, must usually be administered daily.

• *Excretion:* The majority of estrogen elimination occurs through the kidneys, in the form of sulfate or glucuronide conjugates, or both.

Contraindications and precautions

Contraindicated in patients with thrombophlebitis or thromboembolic disorders, estrogen-dependent neoplasia, breast or reproductive organ cancer (except for palliative treatment), or undiagnosed abnormal genital bleeding and during pregnancy.

Use cautiously in patients with cerebrovascular or coronary artery disease, asthma, bone disease, migraine, seizures, or cardiac, hepatic, or renal dysfunction or in women with family history (mother, grandmother, sister) of breast or genital tract cancer or who have breast nodules, fibrocystic disease, or abnormal mammographic findings.

Interactions

Concomitant administration of *drugs that induce hepatic metabolism (rifampin, barbiturates, primidone, carbamazepine, phenytoin)* may decrease estrogenic effects from a given dose. These drugs are known to accelerate the rate of metabolism of certain other agents.

In diabetic patients, estrogens may cause increases in blood glucose levels, requiring dosage adjustment of *insulin* or *oral antidiabetic drugs.*

Use with *anticoagulants* may decrease the effects of warfarin-type anticoagulants. Use with *adrenocorticosteroids* or *adrenocorticotropic hormone* increases the risk of fluid and electrolyte accumulation.

Effects on diagnostic tests

Therapy with estrogens increases sulfobromophthalein retention, prothrombin and clotting factors VII to X, and norepinephrine-induced platelet aggregability. Increases in thyroid-binding globulin level may occur, resulting in increased total thyroid level (measured by protein-bound iodine or total T_4) and decreased uptake of free T_3 resin. Serum folate, pyridoxine, and antithrombin III levels may decrease; triglyceride, glucose, and phospholipid levels may increase. Glucose tolerance may be impaired. Pregnanediol excretion may decrease.

Adverse reactions

CNS: headache, dizziness, chorea, depression, ***seizures.***

CV: thrombophlebitis; ***thromboembolism;*** hypertension; edema; ***increased risk of CVA, pulmonary embolism, MI.***

EENT: worsening of myopia or astigmatism, intolerance of contact lenses.

GI: *nausea,* vomiting, abdominal cramps, bloating, anorexia, increased appetite, weight changes, pancreatitis.

GU: in women—breakthrough bleeding, altered menstrual flow, dysmenorrhea, amenorrhea, ***increased risk of endometrial cancer, possibility of increased risk of breast cancer,*** cervical erosion, altered cervical secretions, enlargement of uterine fibromas, vaginal candidiasis; in men—gynecomastia, testicular atrophy, impotence.

Hepatic: cholestatic jaundice, ***hepatic adenoma.***

Skin: melasma, urticaria, flushing (with rapid I.V. administration), hirsutism or hair loss, erythema nodosum, dermatitis.

Other: breast changes (tenderness, enlargement, secretion), hypercalcemia, gallbladder disease.

Overdose and treatment

Serious toxicity after drug overdose has not been reported. Nausea may be expected to occur. Provide appropriate supportive care.

☑ Special considerations

Besides those relevant to all *estrogens,* consider the following recommendations.

• For the rapid treatment of dysfunctional uterine bleeding or reduction of surgical bleeding, parenteral administration is preferred.

• Refrigerate before reconstitution. After adding diluent, agitate gently until drug is in solution, use within a few hours. Reconstituted drug may be safely stored in refrigeration for up to 60 days.

Geriatric use

• Chronic use for menopausal symptoms may be associated with increased risk of certain cancers. Frequent physical examinations are advised.

Breast-feeding

• Estrogens are contraindicated in breast-feeding women.

estropipate

Ogen, Ortho-Est

Pharmacologic classification: estrogen
Therapeutic classification: estrogen replacement
Pregnancy risk category X

How supplied

Estropipate is available as estrone sodium sulfate. Available by prescription only.
Tablets: 0.625 mg, 1.25 mg, 2.5 mg

Indications, route, and dosage

Atrophic vaginitis, kraurosis vulvae, and vasomotor menopausal symptoms

Adults: 0.625 to 5 mg P.O. daily for 21 days, followed by 7 days off therapy.

Female hypogonadism, primary ovarian failure, or after castration

Adults: 1.25 to 7.5 mg P.O. daily for 3 weeks, followed by 8 to 10 days off therapy. Cycle may be repeated if no withdrawal bleeding occurs within 10 days of discontinuing therapy.

Prevention of osteoporosis

Adults: 0.625 mg P.O. daily for 25 days of a 31-day cycle.

Pharmacodynamics

Estrogenic action: Estropipate mimics the action of endogenous estrogen in treating female hypogonadism, menopausal symptoms, and atrophic vaginitis.

Pharmacokinetics

• *Absorption:* After oral administration, estradiol and the other natural unconjugated estrogens are well absorbed but substantially inactivated by the liver. Therefore, unconjugated estrogens are usually administered parenterally.

After I.M. administration, absorption begins rapidly and continues for days. The cypionate and valerate esters administered in oil have prolonged durations of action because of their slow absorption characteristics.

Topically applied estradiol is absorbed readily into the systemic circulation.

• *Distribution:* Estradiol and the other natural estrogens are approximately 50% to 80% plasma protein-bound, particularly the estradiol-binding globulin. Distribution occurs throughout the body, with highest concentrations appearing in fat.

• *Metabolism:* The steroidal estrogens, including estradiol, are metabolized primarily in the liver, where they are conjugated with sulfate and glucuronide. Because of the rapid rate of metabolism, nonesterified forms of estrogen, including estradiol, must usually be administered daily.

• *Excretion:* Estrogen is mostly eliminated through the kidneys in the form of sulfate or glucuronide conjugates.

Contraindications and precautions

Contraindicated in patients with thrombophlebitis or thromboembolic disorders, estrogen-dependent neoplasia, breast or reproductive organ cancer (except for palliative treatment), or undiagnosed abnormal genital bleeding and during pregnancy.

Use cautiously in patients with cerebrovascular or coronary artery disease, asthma, bone diseases, mental depression, migraine, seizures, or cardiac, hepatic, or renal dysfunction or in women with family history (mother, grandmother, sister) of breast or genital tract cancer or who have breast nodules, fibrocystic disease, or abnormal mammographic findings.

Interactions

Concomitant administration of *drugs that induce hepatic metabolism (rifampin, barbiturates, primidone, carbamazepine, phenytoin)* may decrease estrogenic effects from a given dose. These drugs are known to accelerate the rate of metabolism of certain other agents. Estrogens may decrease elimination rate of *corticosteroids.*

In patients with diabetes, estropipate may cause increases in blood glucose levels, necessitating dosage adjustment of *insulin* or *oral antidiabetic drugs.*

Use with *anticoagulants* may decrease the effects of warfarin-type anticoagulants. Use with *adrenocorticosteroids* or *adrenocorticotropic hormone* increases the risk of fluid and electrolyte accumulation.

Effects on diagnostic tests

Therapy with estrogens increases sulfobromophthalein retention, prothrombin and clotting factors VII to X, and norepinephrine-induced platelet aggregability. Increases in thyroid-binding globulin concentration may occur, resulting in increased total thyroid concentration (measured by protein-bound iodine or total T_4) and decreased uptake of free T_3 resin. Serum folate, pyridoxine, and antithrombin III concentrations may decrease; triglyceride, glucose, and phospholipid levels may increase. Glucose tolerance may be impaired. Pregnanediol excretion may decrease.

Adverse reactions

CNS: headache, dizziness, depression, migraine, ***seizures.***
CV: ***increased risk of CVA, pulmonary embolism, MI, thromboembolism,*** thrombophlebitis, edema.
EENT: worsening of myopia or astigmatism, intolerance of contact lenses.
GI: vomiting, abdominal cramps, bloating, weight changes.
GU: in women—breakthrough bleeding, increased size of uterine fibromas, dysmenorrhea, amenorrhea, vaginal candidiasis, ***increased risk of endometrial cancer, possibility of increased risk of breast cancer,*** altered menstrual flow, cervical erosion, altered cervical secretions; in men—gynecomastia, testicular atrophy; cystitis-like syndrome, condition resembling premenstrual syndrome.
Hepatic: cholestatic jaundice, ***hepatic adenoma.***
Skin: ***erythema multiforme***, erythema nodosum, hair loss, hemorrhagic eruption, hirsutism, melasma.
Other: breast changes (tenderness, enlargement, secretion), hypercalcemia, gallbladder disease, aggravation of porphyria, libido changes.

Overdose and treatment

Serious toxicity after overdose of this drug has not been reported. Nausea may be expected to occur. Provide appropriate supportive care.

☑ Special considerations

Besides those relevant to all *estrogens,* consider the following recommendations.

• When used for progressive, inoperable prostate cancer, remission should be apparent within 3 weeks of therapy.

• When submitting specimens to pathologist for evaluation, be sure to note that patient is taking estrogens.

Geriatric use

• Frequent physical examinations are recommended for postmenopausal women taking estrogens.

Breast-feeding

• Drug is contraindicated in breast-feeding women.

ethacrynate sodium

ethacrynic acid

Edecrin

Pharmacologic classification: loop diuretic
Therapeutic classification: diuretic
Pregnancy risk category B

How supplied

Available by prescription only
Tablets: 25 mg, 50 mg
Injectable: 50 mg (with 62.5 mg of mannitol and 0.1 mg of thimerosal)

Indications, route, and dosage

Acute pulmonary edema
Adults: 50 mg or 0.5 to 1 mg/kg I.V. to a maximum dose of 100 mg of ethacrynate sodium I.V. slowly over several minutes.
Edema
Adults: 50 to 200 mg P.O. daily. Refractory cases may require up to 200 mg b.i.d.
Children: Initially, 25 mg P.O., given cautiously and increased in 25-mg increments daily until desired effect is achieved.
◇ ***Hypertension***
Adults: Initially, 25 mg P.O. daily. Adjust dose p.r.n. Maximum maintenance dosage is 200 mg P.O. daily in two divided doses.

Pharmacodynamics

Diuretic action: Ethacrynic acid inhibits sodium and chloride reabsorption in the proximal part of the ascending loop of Henle, promoting the excretion of sodium, water, chloride, and potassium.

Pharmacokinetics

- *Absorption:* Drug is absorbed rapidly from the GI tract; diuresis occurs in 30 minutes and peaks in 2 hours. After I.V. administration of ethacrynate sodium, diuresis occurs in 5 minutes and peaks in 15 to 30 minutes.
- *Distribution:* In animal studies, ethacrynic acid was found to accumulate in the liver. Ethacrynic acid does not enter the CSF, and its distribution into breast milk or the placenta is unknown.
- *Metabolism:* In animals, drug is metabolized by the liver to a potentially active metabolite.
- *Excretion:* Animal studies show that 30% to 65% of drug is excreted in urine and 35% to 40% is excreted in bile, as the metabolite. Duration of action is 6 to 8 hours after oral administration and about 2 hours after I.V. administration.

Contraindications and precautions

Contraindicated in infants and in patients with anuria or hypersensitivity to drug. Use cautiously in patients with electrolyte abnormalities or impaired hepatic function.

Interactions

Concomitant use of ethacrynic acid with *other diuretics* may enhance the diuretic effect of the other drugs; reduce dosage when adding ethacrynic acid to a diuretic regimen. Concomitant use of *potassium-sparing diuretics (spironolactone, triamterene, amiloride)* may decrease the potassium loss induced by ethacrynic acid and may be a therapeutic advantage; severe potassium loss may occur if ethacrynic acid is administered with other *potassium-depleting drugs*, such as *steroids* and *amphotericin B*. Ethacrynic acid may reduce renal clearance of *lithium*, elevating serum lithium levels; monitor lithium levels and adjust dosage.

Diabetic patients may need increased dosages of *insulin* or *oral antidiabetic agents* when taking ethacrynic acid. Ethacrynic acid may potentiate the hypotensive effect of *antihypertensive agents*; patients may require dosage reduction.

Concomitant administration of ethacrynic acid and *aminoglycosides* or other *ototoxic drugs* may increase the incidence of deafness; avoid use of such combinations.

Effects on diagnostic tests

Drug therapy alters electrolyte balance and liver and renal function tests.

Adverse reactions

CNS: confusion, fatigue, vertigo, headache.
CV: volume depletion and dehydration, orthostatic hypotension.
EENT: transient deafness (with too-rapid I.V. injection), blurred vision, tinnitus, hearing loss.
GI: diarrhea, anorexia, nausea, vomiting, GI bleeding, pancreatitis.
GU: oliguria, hematuria, nocturia, polyuria, frequent urination, azotemia.
Hematologic: ***agranulocytosis, neutropenia, thrombocytopenia***.
Other: hypokalemia; hypochloremic alkalosis; asymptomatic hyperuricemia; fever; chills; malaise; fluid and electrolyte imbalances, including dilutional hyponatremia, hypocalcemia, hypomagnesemia; hyperglycemia; impaired glucose tolerance.

Overdose and treatment

Clinical manifestations of overdose include profound electrolyte and volume depletion, which may precipitate circulatory collapse.

Treatment of ethacrynic acid overdose is primarily supportive; replace fluid and electrolytes as needed.

☑ Special considerations

Besides those relevant to all *loop diuretics*, consider the following recommendations.

- Do not give drug either I.M. or S.C. because it may cause severe local pain and irritation. When giving I.V., check infusion site frequently for infiltration (edema or skin blanching).
- Infuse drug slowly over 20 to 30 minutes, by I.V. infusion or by direct I.V. injection over a period of several minutes; rapid injection may cause hypotension.
- Do not administer drug simultaneously with whole blood or blood products; hemolysis may occur.
- I.V. ethacrynate sodium has been used to treat hypercalcemia and to manage ethylene glycol poisoning and bromide intoxication.

• Periodically assess hearing function in patients receiving high-dose therapy. Ethacrynic acid may potentiate ototoxicity of other medications.

Patient education

• Advise patient receiving I.V. form of drug to report pain or irritation at I.V. site immediately.
• Notify diabetic patient that antidiabetic dosage may need to be increased.

Geriatric use

• Elderly and debilitated patients require close observation because they are more susceptible to drug-induced diuresis. Excessive diuresis promotes rapid dehydration, leading to hypovolemia, hypokalemia, hyponatremia, and circulatory collapse. Reduced dosages may be indicated.

Pediatric use

• Use ethacrynate sodium or ethacrynic acid with caution in neonates. Usual pediatric dosage can be used, but dosage intervals should be extended.

Breast-feeding

• Do not use drug in breast-feeding women.

ethambutol hydrochloride

Myambutol

Pharmacologic classification: semisynthetic antitubercular
Therapeutic classification: antitubercular
Pregnancy risk category NR

How supplied

Available by prescription only
Tablets: 100 mg, 400 mg

Indications, route, and dosage

Adjunctive treatment in pulmonary tuberculosis
Adults and children age 13 and older: Initial treatment for patients who have not received previous antitubercular therapy, 15 mg/kg P.O. daily single dose. Retreatment*:* 25 mg/kg P.O. daily single dose for 60 days with at least one other antitubercular drug; then decrease to 15 mg/kg P.O. daily single dose.

Pharmacodynamics

Antitubercular action: Ethambutol is bacteriostatic; it interferes with mycolic acid incorporation into the mycobacterial cell wall. Ethambutol is active against *Mycobacterium tuberculosis, M. bovis,* and *M.* marinum, some strains of *M. kansasii, M. avium, M. fortuitum,* and *M.* intracellulare, and the combined strain of M. avium and M. intracellulare (MAC). Ethambutol is considered adjunctive therapy in tuberculosis and is combined with other antituberculosis agents to prevent or delay development of drug resistance by *M. tuberculosis.*

Pharmacokinetics

• *Absorption:* Ethambutol is absorbed rapidly from the GI tract; peak serum levels occur 2 to 4 hours after ingestion.
• *Distribution:* Drug is distributed widely into body tissues and fluids, especially into lungs, erythrocytes, saliva, and kidneys; lesser amounts distribute into brain, ascitic, pleural, and CSFs. Ethambutol is 8% to 22% protein-bound.
• *Metabolism:* Ethambutol undergoes partial hepatic metabolism.
• *Excretion:* After 24 hours, about 50% of unchanged ethambutol and 8% to 15% of its metabolites are excreted in urine; 20% to 25% is excreted in feces. Small amounts of drug may be excreted in breast milk. Plasma half-life in adults is about 3¼ hours; half-life is prolonged in decreased renal or hepatic function. Ethambutol can be removed by peritoneal dialysis and to a lesser extent by hemodialysis.

Contraindications and precautions

Contraindicated in children under age 13 and in patients with optic neuritis or hypersensitivity to drug. Use cautiously in patients with impaired renal function, cataracts, recurrent eye inflammations, gout, and diabetic retinopathy.

Interactions

Ethambutol may potentiate adverse effects of *agents that produce neurotoxicity. Aluminum salts* may delay and reduce the absorption of ethambutol. Separate administration times by several hours.

Effects on diagnostic tests

Ethambutol may elevate serum urate levels and liver function test results.

Adverse reactions

CNS: headache, dizziness, mental confusion, possible hallucinations, peripheral neuritis (numbness and tingling of extremities).
EENT: optic neuritis (related to dose and duration of treatment).
GI: anorexia, nausea, vomiting, abdominal pain, GI upset.
Skin: dermatitis, pruritis, toxic epidermal necrolysis.
Other: ***anaphylactoid reactions,*** fever, malaise, bloody sputum, ***thrombocytopenia,*** joint pain, elevated uric acid level, precipitation of acute gout, abnormal liver function tests.

Overdose and treatment

No recommendation available. Treatment is supportive. After recent ingestion (4 hours or less), empty stomach by induced emesis or gastric lavage. Follow with activated charcoal to decrease absorption.

☑ Special considerations

• Give drug with food if necessary to prevent gastric irritation; food does not interfere with absorption.
• Obtain specimens for culture and sensitivity testing before first dose, but therapy can begin before test results are complete; repeat periodically to detect drug resistance.
• Assess visual status before therapy; test visual acuity and color discrimination monthly in patients taking more than 15 mg/kg/day. Visual disturbances are dose-related and reversible if detected in time.

• Monitor blood (including serum uric acid), renal, and liver function studies before and periodically during therapy to minimize toxicity.
• Monitor for change in renal function. Dosage reduction may be necessary.

Patient education
• Explain disease process and rationale for long-term therapy.
• Teach signs and symptoms of hypersensitivity and other adverse reactions, and emphasize need to notify you if these occur; urge patient to report *any* unusual effects, especially blurred vision, red-green color blindness, or changes in urine elimination.
• Assure patient that visual alterations will disappear within several weeks or months after drug is discontinued.
• Urge patient to complete entire prescribed regimen, to comply with instructions for daily dosage, to avoid missing doses, and not to discontinue drug without medical approval. Explain importance of keeping follow-up appointments.

Pediatric use
• Drug is not recommended for use in children under age 13.

Breast-feeding
• Drug is excreted in breast milk; use with caution in breast-feeding women.

ethanolamine oleate
Ethamolin

Pharmacologic classification: oleic acid/2-aminoethanol combination
Therapeutic classification: sclerosing agent
Pregnancy risk category C

How supplied
Available by prescription only
Injection: 5% solution in 2-ml ampules

Indications, route, and dosage
Treatment of bleeding esophageal varices and prevention of recurrent bleeding
Adults: Local injection of 1.5 to 5 ml per varix. Maximum total dose per treatment should not exceed 20 ml or about 0.4 ml/kg. Injections should be performed by staff familiar with sclerotherapy.
✦ ***Dosage adjustment.*** In patients with significant hepatic dysfunction or cardiopulmonary disease, give less than maximum dose.

Pharmacodynamics
Sclerosing action: Ethanolamine oleate is a mild sclerosing agent that initiates a local inflammatory response that leads to scarring, which prevents bleeding. The oleic acid component is responsible for the inflammatory response, and it may also promote local clot formation by initiating the release of tissue factor and activate Hageman factor. However, the ethanolamine component may chelate calcium and inhibit fibrin clot formation *in situ*.

Pharmacokinetics
• *Absorption:* When injected locally, drug is cleared via the portal vein within 5 minutes.
• *Distribution:* Unknown.
• *Metabolism:* Unknown.
• *Excretion:* Unknown.

Contraindications and precautions
Contraindicated in patients hypersensitive to ethanolamine, oleic acid, or ethanolamine oleate. Sclerotherapy is not indicated for patients with esophageal varices that have not bled. It is also not indicated for varicosities of the leg. Use cautiously in elderly or critically ill patients.

Interactions
None reported.

Effects on diagnostic tests
None reported.

Adverse reactions
GI: esophageal ulcer, esophageal stricture, esophagitis, esophageal tearing, local mucosal sloughing or necrosis, *periesophageal abscess and perforation.*
GU: acute renal failure.
Respiratory: *pleural effusion or infiltration,* pneumonia, *aspiration pneumonia.*
Other: pyrexia, retrosternal pain, ***anaphylaxis.***

Overdose and treatment
Overdosage can result in severe esophageal intramural necrosis. Death has resulted from such overdosage. Specific antidotes are not known.

☑ Special considerations
• Be prepared to treat anaphylaxis in patients undergoing sclerotherapy with ethanolamine oleate. Although rare, it has been fatal. Have epinephrine 1:1,000 available, and control allergic reactions with antihistamines.
• Severe injection necrosis may occur. Assess respiratory status.
• Drug will not correct portal hypertension, the cause of esophageal varices. Vascular recanalization and collateral formation may occur, and patients may need further treatment.
• Submucosal injections are not recommended because they are more likely to cause mucosal ulceration.
• Timing of therapy is quite variable with no clear consensus. However, therapy may be initiated at the first bleeding episode, with follow-up sclerotherapy at 1 week, 6 weeks, 3 months, and 6 months, if needed.

Patient education
• Explain technique to patient, and that several follow-up visits will be necessary for successful sclerotherapy.
• Tell patient to report chest pain, shortness of breath, or bleeding immediately.

Pediatric use
• Safe use in children has not been established.

ethinyl estradiol
Estinyl

Pharmacologic classification: estrogen
Therapeutic classification: estrogen replacement, antineoplastic
Pregnancy risk category X

How supplied
Available by prescription only
Tablets: 0.02 mg, 0.05 mg, 0.5 mg

Indications, route, and dosage
Palliative treatment of metastatic breast cancer (at least 5 years after menopause)
Adults: 1 mg P.O. t.i.d. for at least 3 months.
Female hypogonadism
Adults: 0.05 mg daily to t.i.d. for 2 weeks monthly, followed by 2 weeks progesterone therapy; continue for three to six monthly dosing cycles, followed by 2 months off.
Vasomotor menopausal symptoms
Adults: 0.02 to 0.05 mg P.O. daily for cycles of 3 weeks on, 1 week off.
Palliative treatment of metastatic inoperable prostatic cancer
Adults: 0.15 to 2 mg P.O. daily.

Pharmacodynamics
Estrogenic action: Ethinyl estradiol mimics the action of endogenous estrogen in treating female hypogonadism and menopausal symptoms. It inhibits growth of hormone-sensitive tissue in advanced, inoperable prostatic cancer and in certain carefully selected cases of breast cancer in men and postmenopausal women.

Pharmacokinetics
• *Absorption:* After oral administration, estradiol is well absorbed but substantially inactivated by the liver.
• *Distribution:* Estradiol and the other natural estrogens are approximately 50% to 80% plasma protein-bound, particularly the estradiol-binding globulin. Distribution occurs throughout the body, with highest concentrations appearing in fat.
• *Metabolism:* The steroidal estrogens, including estradiol, are metabolized primarily in the liver, where they are conjugated with sulfate and glucuronide. Because of the rapid rate of metabolism, nonesterified forms of estrogen, including estradiol, must usually be administered daily.
• *Excretion:* The majority of estrogen elimination occurs through the kidneys in the form of sulfate or glucuronide conjugates.

Contraindications and precautions
Contraindicated in patients with thrombophlebitis or thromboembolic disorders, estrogen-dependent neoplasia, breast or reproductive organ cancer (except for palliative treatment), or undiagnosed abnormal genital bleeding and during pregnancy.

Use cautiously in patients with cerebrovascular or coronary artery disease, asthma, mental depression, bone disease, or cardiac, hepatic, or renal dysfunction and in women with a family history (mother, grandmother, sister) of breast or genital tract cancer or who have breast nodules, fibrocystic disease, or abnormal mammographic findings.

Interactions
Concomitant administration of *drugs that induce hepatic metabolism (rifampin, barbiturates, primidone, carbamazepine, phenytoin)* may decrease estrogenic effects from a given dose. These drugs are known to accelerate the rate of metabolism of certain other agents. Concomitant use of estrogens with *corticosteroids* may decrease corticosteroid elimination.

In patients with diabetes, ethinyl estradiol may increase blood glucose levels, necessitating dosage adjustment of *insulin* or *oral antidiabetic agents.*

Use with *anticoagulants* may decrease the effects of *warfarin-type anticoagulants.* Use with *adrenocorticosteroids* or *adrenocorticotropic hormone* increases the risk of fluid and electrolyte accumulation.

Effects on diagnostic tests
Therapy with ethinyl estradiol increases sulfobromophthalein retention, prothrombin and clotting factors VII to X, and norepinephrine-induced platelet aggregability. Increases in thyroid-binding globulin concentration may occur, resulting in increased total thyroid concentration (measured by protein-bound iodine or total T_4) and decreased uptake of free T_3 resin. Serum folate, pyridoxine, and antithrombin III concentrations may decrease; triglyceride, glucose, and phospholipid levels may increase. Glucose tolerance may be impaired. Pregnanediol excretion may decrease.

Adverse reactions
CNS: headache, dizziness, chorea, depression, ***seizures.***
CV: thrombophlebitis; ***thromboembolism;*** hypertension; edema, ***increased risk of CVA, pulmonary embolism, MI.***
EENT: worsening of myopia or astigmatism, intolerance to contact lenses.
GI: *nausea,* vomiting, abdominal cramps, bloating, anorexia, increased appetite, weight changes.
GU: in women—breakthrough bleeding, altered menstrual flow, dysmenorrhea, amenorrhea, cervical erosion, ***increased risk of endometrial cancer, possibility of increased risk of breast cancer,*** altered cervical secretions, enlargement of uterine fibromas, vaginal candidiasis; in men—gynecomastia, testicular atrophy, impotence.
Hepatic: cholestatic jaundice, ***hepatic adenoma.***
Skin: melasma, urticaria, acne, seborrhea, oily skin, hirsutism or hair loss, erythema nodosum, dermatitis.
Other: breast changes (tenderness, enlargement, secretion), hypercalcemia, gallbladder disease.

Overdose and treatment
Serious toxicity after overdose of this drug has not been reported. Nausea may be expected to occur. Provide appropriate supportive care.

☑ Special considerations
Recommendations for administration of ethinyl estradiol and for care and teaching of patient during therapy are the same as those for all *estrogens.*

Geriatric use
- Use with caution in patients whose condition may be aggravated by fluid retention.

Breast-feeding
- Drug is contraindicated in breast-feeding women.

ethosuximide
Zarontin

Pharmacologic classification: succinimide derivative
Therapeutic classification: anticonvulsant
Pregnancy risk category NR

How supplied
Available by prescription only
Capsules: 250 mg
Syrup: 250 mg/5 ml

Indications, route, and dosage
Absence seizures
Adults and children age 6 and older: Initially, 250 mg P.O. b.i.d. May increase by 250 mg q 4 to 7 days up to 1.5 g daily.
Children age 3 to 6: 250 mg P.O. daily. Optimal dose is 20 mg/kg/day.

Pharmacodynamics
Anticonvulsant action: Ethosuximide raises the seizure threshold; it suppresses characteristic spike-and-wave pattern by depressing neuronal transmission in the motor cortex and basal ganglia. It is indicated for absence seizures refractory to other drugs.

Pharmacokinetics
- *Absorption:* Ethosuximide is absorbed from the GI tract; steady-state plasma levels occur in 4 to 7 days.
- *Distribution:* Ethosuximide is distributed widely throughout the body; protein binding is minimal.
- *Metabolism:* Drug is metabolized extensively in the liver to several inactive metabolites.
- *Excretion:* Drug is excreted in urine, with small amounts in bile and feces. Plasma half-life is about 60 hours in adults and about 30 hours in children.

Contraindications and precautions
Contraindicated in patients with hypersensitivity to succinimide derivatives. Use with extreme caution in patients with hepatic or renal disease.

Interactions
Concomitant use of ethosuximide and *other CNS depressants (alcohol, narcotics, anxiolytics, antidepressants, antipsychotics, other anticonvulsants)* causes additive CNS depression and sedation.

Effects on diagnostic tests
Ethosuximide may elevate liver enzyme levels and may cause false-positive Coombs' test results. It may also cause abnormal results of renal function tests.

Adverse reactions
CNS: *drowsiness, headache, fatigue, dizziness, ataxia, irritability, hiccups, euphoria, lethargy, depression, psychosis.*
EENT: myopia, tongue swelling, gingival hyperplasia.
GI: *nausea, vomiting, diarrhea, weight loss, cramps, anorexia, epigastric and abdominal pain.*
GU: vaginal bleeding, urinary frequency.
Hematologic: leukopenia, eosinophilia, ***agranulocytosis,*** pancytopenia.
Skin: urticaria, pruritic and erythematous rash, hirsutism, ***Stevens-Johnson syndrome.***

Overdose and treatment
Symptoms of ethosuximide overdose, when used alone or with other anticonvulsants, include CNS depression, ataxia, stupor, and coma. Treatment is symptomatic and supportive. Carefully monitor vital signs and fluid and electrolyte balance.

☑ Special considerations
- Administer ethosuximide with food to minimize GI distress.
- Avoid abrupt discontinuation of drug. This may precipitate petit mal seizures.
- Observe patient for dermatologic reactions, joint pain, unexplained fever, or unusual bruising or bleeding (which may signal hematologic or other severe adverse reactions).
- Perform CBC, liver function tests, and urinalysis periodically.
- Therapeutic plasma concentrations range from 40 to 100 mcg/ml.

Patient education
- Tell patient to take drug with food or milk to prevent GI distress, to avoid use with alcoholic beverages, and to avoid hazardous tasks that require alertness if drug causes drowsiness, dizziness, or blurred vision.
- Warn patient not to discontinue drug abruptly; this may cause seizures.
- Inform patient that drug may color urine pink to reddish-brown.
- Encourage patient to wear a medical identification bracelet or necklace.
- Tell patient to report the following effects: rash, joint pain, fever, sore throat, or unusual bleeding or bruising.
- Advise patient to call immediately if pregnancy is suspected.
- Instruct patient to protect pediatric syrup from freezing.

Geriatric use
- Use with caution in elderly patients.

Pediatric use
• Drug is not recommended for use in children under age 3.

Breast-feeding
• Safe use has not been established. Alternative feeding method is recommended during therapy with ethosuximide.

ethyl chloride (chloroethane)
Ethyl Chloride

Pharmacologic classification: halogenated hydrocarbon
Therapeutic classification: local anesthetic, counterirritant
Pregnancy risk category C

How supplied
Available by prescription only
Topical liquid spray: 3-oz., 3.5-oz. bottles

Indications, route, and dosage
Local anesthetic in minor operative procedures; relief of pain caused by insect stings, burns, bruises, contusions, abrasions, swelling, and minor sprains associated with sports injuries; tinea lesions and creeping eruption
Adults and children: Dosage varies with different procedures. Use smallest dosage needed to produce desired effect. For local anesthesia, use the fine-spray nozzle; hold container about 12 inches (30 cm) from area and spray downward until a light frosting appears.
Infants: Hold a cotton ball saturated with ethyl chloride to area for a few seconds.
Counterirritant to relieve myofascial and visceral pain syndromes
Adults, children, and infants: Dosage varies with use. Use smallest dosage needed to produce desired effect. Use the large-sized nozzle; hold container 24 inches (60 cm) from skin and spray at an acute angle in one direction in a sweeping motion until area has been covered.

Pharmacodynamics
Anesthetic action: Rapid vaporization of ethyl chloride freezes superficial tissues, producing insensitivity of peripheral nerve endings and local anesthesia. Anesthesia lasts for up to 1 minute.

Pharmacokinetics
• *Absorption:* Limited with topical use.
• *Distribution:* None.
• *Metabolism:* None.
• *Excretion:* None.

Contraindications and precautions
Ethyl chloride is contraindicated for use near eyes or on broken skin or mucous membranes; it should not be inhaled. Freezing and thawing process may damage epithelial cells; avoid repeated use over long periods. Ethyl chloride is highly flammable and explosive; it should not be used near open fire and should be stored away from heat or open flame.

Interactions
None reported.

Effects on diagnostic tests
None reported.

Adverse reactions
Skin: skin lesions, rash, urticaria, burning, stinging, tenderness, inflammation, frostbite, tissue necrosis with prolonged use, pain and muscle spasm from excessive cooling.

Note: Discontinue drug if sensitization develops.

Overdose and treatment
Discontinue use and clean area thoroughly.

☑ Special considerations
• Do not apply to broken skin or mucous membranes.
• Protect adjacent skin with petroleum jelly to prevent tissue damage.
• When using ethyl chloride as a counterirritant, avoid frosting the skin because excessive cooling may increase spasms and pain.

Patient education
• Advise patient that drug will produce a temporary numbness.

Pediatric use
• Use smaller amounts of drug.

Breast-feeding
• Clean drug from breast area before breast-feeding.

etidronate disodium
Didronel

Pharmacologic classification: pyrophosphate analogue
Therapeutic classification: antihypercalcemic
Pregnancy risk category C

How supplied
Available by prescription only
Tablets: 200 mg, 400 mg
Injection: 50 mg/ml (300 mg ampule)

Indications, route, and dosage
Symptomatic Paget's disease
Adults: 5 mg/kg P.O. daily as a single dose 2 hours before a meal with water or juice. Patient should not eat, consume milk or milk products, or take antacids or vitamins with mineral supplements for 2 hours after dose. May give up to 10 mg/kg/day in severe cases, not to exceed 6 months. Maximum dosage is 20 mg/kg/day, not to exceed 3 months.
Heterotopic ossification in spinal cord injuries
Adults: 20 mg/kg/day P.O. for 2 weeks, then 10 mg/kg/day for 10 weeks. Total treatment period is 12 weeks.

Heterotopic ossification after total hip replacement
Adults: 20 mg/kg/day P.O. for 1 month before total hip replacement and for 3 months afterward.
Hypercalcemia associated with malignancy
Adults: 7.5 mg/kg I.V. daily for 3 days. May repeat up to 7 days. Then wait 7 days before beginning a second course of treatment.

Pharmacodynamics
Bone-metabolism inhibitor action: Although the exact mechanism is not known, etidronate acts on bone by adsorbing to hydroxyapatite crystals in the bone, thereby inhibiting their growth and dissolution. It also decreases the number of osteoclasts in bone, thereby slowing excessive remodeling of pagetic or heterotopic bone.

Pharmacokinetics
• *Absorption:* Absorption following an oral dose is variable and is decreased in the presence of food. Absorption may also be dose-related.
• *Distribution:* Approximately half of the dose is distributed to bone.
• *Metabolism:* Etidronate is not metabolized.
• *Excretion:* About 50% of drug is excreted within 24 hours in urine.

Contraindications and precautions
Contraindicated in patients with known hypersensitivity to drug or in those with clinically overt osteomalacia. Use cautiously in patients with impaired renal function.

Interactions
None reported.

Effects on diagnostic tests
Drug may elevate serum phosphate levels.

Adverse reactions
GI: occur most frequently at dosage of 20 mg/kg daily—diarrhea, increased frequency of bowel movements, nausea, constipation, stomatitis.
Other: increased or recurrent bone pain, pain at previously asymptomatic sites, increased risk of fracture, *elevated serum phosphate level,* fever, fluid overload, dyspnea, ***seizures,*** abnormal hepatic function, hypersensitivity reactions.

Overdose and treatment
Clinical manifestations of overdose include diarrhea, nausea, and hypocalcemia. Treat with gastric lavage and emesis. Administer calcium if required.

☑ Special considerations
• Drug should be taken in a single dose. However, if nausea occurs, dosage may be divided.
• Monitor drug effect by serum alkaline phosphate and urinary hydroxyproline excretion; both are lowered by effective therapy.

Patient education
• Instruct patient to take drug on an empty stomach with water or juice and to avoid food, milk or milk products, antacids, and vitamins with mineral supplements for 2 hours.
• Remind patient that improvement may take at least 3 months and may continue even after the drug is stopped.

etodolac
Lodine, Lodine XL

Pharmacologic classification: NSAID
Therapeutic classification: antiarthritic
Pregnancy risk category C

How supplied
Available by prescription only
Capsules: 200 mg, 300 mg
Tablets: 400 mg
Tablets (extended-release): 400 mg, 1,000 mg

Indications, route, and dosage
Acute and chronic management of osteoarthritis, rheumatoid arthritis, and pain
Adults: For acute pain, give 200 to 400 mg P.O. q 6 to 8 hours p.r.n., not to exceed 1,200 mg daily. For patients weighing 132 lb (60 kg) or less, total daily dose should not exceed 20 mg/kg.

For osteoarthritis or rheumatoid arthritis, give 800 to 1,200 mg P.O. daily in divided doses initially, followed by adjustments of 600 to 1,200 mg in divided doses: 200 mg P.O. t.i.d. or q.i.d.; 300 mg P.O. b.i.d., t.i.d., or q.i.d.; 400 mg P.O. b.i.d. or t.i.d. Total daily dosage is not to exceed 1,200 mg.

For patients weighing 132 lb or less, total daily dosage should not exceed 20 mg/kg, or 400 to 1,000 mg P.O. daily (extended-release form). Adjust dosage to lowest effective dose based on patient response. Do not exceed maximum dose of 1,000 mg daily.

Pharmacodynamics
Antiarthritic action: Mechanism of action is unknown but is presumed to be associated with inhibition of prostaglandin biosynthesis.

Pharmacokinetics
• *Absorption:* Etodolac is well-absorbed from GI tract, with peak concentrations reached in 1 to 2 hours. Onset of analgesic activity occurs within 30 minutes, lasting 4 to 6 hours. Antacids do not appear to affect absorption of etodolac; however, they can decrease peak concentrations reached by 15% to 20% but have no effect when peak levels are reached.
• *Distribution:* Found in liver, lungs, heart, and kidneys.
• *Metabolism:* Extensively metabolized in the liver.
• *Excretion:* Excreted in urine primarily as metabolites; 16% is excreted in feces.

Contraindications and precautions
Contraindicated in patients with hypersensitivity to drug and in those with history of aspirin- or NSAID-induced asthma, rhinitis, urticaria, or other allergic reactions.

Use cautiously in patients with impaired renal or hepatic function, history of peptic ulcer disease, cardiac disease, hypertension, or conditions associated with fluid retention.

Interactions

Like other NSAIDs, etodolac may cause changes in elimination of *cyclosporine, digoxin, lithium,* and *methotrexate,* resulting in increased levels of these drugs. It may enhance nephrotoxicity associated with cyclosporine. Although the clinical significance is unknown, concurrent use with *aspirin* reduces etodolac's protein-binding without altering its clearance. Use with *warfarin* results in decreased protein-binding of warfarin but does not change its clearance. No dosage adjustment is necessary.

Effects on diagnostic tests

A false-positive test for urinary bilirubin may be caused by phenolic metabolites. Decreased serum uric acid levels and borderline elevations of one or more liver test results may occur.

Adverse reactions

CNS: *asthenia, malaise, dizziness,* depression, drowsiness, nervousness, insomnia.
CV: hypertension, ***heart failure***, syncope, flushing, palpitations, edema, fluid retention.
EENT: blurred vision, tinnitus, photophobia, dry mouth.
GI: *dyspepsia, flatulence, abdominal pain, diarrhea, nausea,* constipation, gastritis, melena, vomiting, anorexia, peptic ulceration with or without ***GI bleeding*** or perforation, ulcerative stomatitis, thirst.
GU: dysuria, urinary frequency, ***renal failure.***
Hematologic: anemia (rare), leukopenia, ***thrombocytopenia,*** hemolytic anemia, ***agranulocytosis.***
Hepatic: hepatitis.
Respiratory: asthma.
Skin: pruritus, rash, ***Stevens-Johnson syndrome.***
Other: chills, fever, weight gain.

Overdose and treatment

Signs of overdose include lethargy, drowsiness, nausea, vomiting, and epigastric pain. Rare symptoms include GI bleeding, coma, renal failure, hypertension, and anaphylaxis. Treatment is symptomatic and supportive, including stomach decontamination.

☑ Special considerations

- Minimal GI blood loss has been reported at doses up to 1,200 mg daily; endoscopy scores are comparable to placebo at doses up to 1,000 mg daily.
- No apparent interaction occurs when administered with diuretics, phenytoin, or glyburide. Use caution with concurrent use of diuretics in patients with cardiac, renal, or hepatic failure.
- Monitor for signs and symptoms of GI ulceration and bleeding.
- Etodolac 1,200 mg was shown to cause less GI bleeding than ibuprofen 2,400 mg daily, indomethacin 200 mg daily, naproxen 750 mg daily, or piroxicam 20 mg daily.
- In chronic conditions, a therapeutic response to therapy is most often seen within 2 weeks.

Patient education

- Instruct patient to report GI effects of drug.
- Caution patient to avoid use during pregnancy.
- Tell patient that drug may be taken with food.

Geriatric use

- Drug is well-tolerated in older and younger adults and generally does not require age-related dosage adjustments. No age-related differences have been reported.

Pediatric use

- Safety and efficacy have not been established in children under age 18.

Breast-feeding

- It is unknown if etodolac is excreted in breast milk. Use with caution.

etomidate

Amidate

Pharmacologic classification: nonbarbiturate hypnotic
Therapeutic classification: I.V. anesthetic, sedative
Pregnancy risk category C

How supplied

Available by prescription only
Injection: 2 mg/ml

Indications, route, and dosage

Induction of general anesthesia
Adults and children over age 10: 0.2 to 0.6 mg/kg I.V. over 30 to 60 seconds.

Pharmacodynamics

Anesthetic and sedative actions: Etomidate, like naturally occurring gamma-aminobutyric acid, decreases the firing rate of neurons within the ascending reticular activating system.

Pharmacokinetics

- *Absorption:* Drug is only given I.V. Onset of action is rapid, usually beginning in 60 seconds; duration of action is usually 3 to 5 minutes.
- *Distribution:* Etomidate distributes widely into body tissue and is highly protein-bound (76%).
- *Metabolism:* Etomidate is metabolized rapidly in the liver.
- *Excretion:* About 75% of a given dose is excreted in urine as an active metabolite; 10% of drug is excreted in bile and 13% in feces.

Contraindications and precautions

Contraindicated in patients allergic to drug. Use cautiously in elderly or debilitated patients with underlying pulmonary disease because of increased respiratory depression. Monitor patients on prolonged use for signs of adrenal insufficiency because etomidate may block adrenal steroid production. It is not recommended for use during labor and delivery because safety has not been established.

Interactions
None significant.

Effects on diagnostic tests
Reduced plasma cortisol levels have been reported, lasting for 6 to 8 hours after induction.

Adverse reactions
CNS: *transient skeletal muscle movements (chiefly myoclonic, some tonic),* averting movements.
CV: hypertension, hypotension, tachycardia, bradycardia, ***arrhythmias.***
GI: postoperative nausea or vomiting after induction of anesthesia.
Local: *transient venous pain on injection.*
Other: hiccups, snoring, transient apnea.

Note: Discontinue drug if patient shows signs of hypersensitivity or adrenal insufficiency or if prolonged apnea occurs.

Overdose and treatment
Clinical signs include CNS depression and respiratory arrest. Treat patient supportively, using mechanical ventilation if necessary, until drug effects subside.

☑ Special considerations
- Drug is compatible with commonly used preanesthetic agents.
- During short procedures in adults, smaller increments of I.V. etomidate may be used to supplement subpotent anesthetics, such as nitrous oxide.
- Transient muscle movements may be reduced by injection of 0.1 mg of fentanyl before giving etomidate, probably by reducing total dose of etomidate.
- Muscle movements are more common in patients with transient venous irritation and pain.
- Drug has a much lower incidence of CV and respiratory effects than thiopental sodium and is therefore used to advantage in high-risk surgical patients.

Geriatric use
- Use cautiously in elderly patients.

Pediatric use
- Use is not recommended in patients under age 10.

Breast-feeding
- It is unknown if drug enters breast milk; therefore, it should be used with caution in breast-feeding women.

etoposide
VePesid

Pharmacologic classification: podophyllotoxin (cell cycle–phase specific, G2 and late S phases)
Therapeutic classification: antineoplastic
Pregnancy risk category D

How supplied
Available by prescription only
Capsules: 50 mg
Injection: 100 mg/5 ml multiple-dose vials

Indications, route, and dosage
Dosage and indications may vary. Check literature for current protocol.

Small-cell carcinoma of the lung
Adults: 70 mg/m²/day P.O. (rounded to the nearest 50 mg) for 4 days; or 100 mg/m² P.O. (rounded to the nearest 50 mg) daily for 5 days. Repeat q 3 to 4 weeks. Alternatively, 35 mg/m² I.V. daily for 4 days or 50 mg/m² I.V. daily for 5 days. Repeat q 3 to 4 weeks.

Testicular carcinoma
Adults: 50 to 100 mg/m² I.V. daily on days 1 to 5; or 100 mg/m²/day on days 1, 3, and 5 of a regimen repeated q 3 or 4 weeks.

✦ ***Dosage adjustment.*** Dosage reduction may be required in patients with impaired renal function.

Pharmacodynamics
Antineoplastic action: Etoposide exerts its cytotoxic action by arresting cells in the metaphase portion of cell division. Drug also inhibits cells from entering mitosis and depresses DNA and RNA synthesis.

Pharmacokinetics
- *Absorption:* Etoposide is only moderately absorbed across the GI tract after oral administration. Bioavailability ranges from 25% to 75%, with an average of 50% of the dose being absorbed.
- *Distribution:* Drug distributes widely into body tissues; the highest concentrations are found in the liver, spleen, kidneys, healthy brain tissue, and brain tumor tissue. It crosses the blood-brain barrier to a limited and variable extent. Etoposide is approximately 94% bound to serum albumin.
- *Metabolism:* Only a small portion of a dose of etoposide is metabolized. Metabolism occurs in the liver.
- *Excretion.* Etoposide is excreted primarily in the urine as unchanged drug. A smaller portion of a dose is excreted in the feces. The plasma elimination of etoposide is described as biphasic, with an initial phase half-life of about ½ to 2 hours and a terminal phase of about 5¼ to 11 hours.

Contraindications and precautions
Contraindicated in patients hypersensitive to drug. Use cautiously in patients who have had cytotoxic or radiation therapy.

Interactions
Concomitant use of etoposide increases the cytotoxicity of *cisplatin* against certain tumors. The mechanism of this synergistic cytotoxic activity is unknown. Concomitant administration with *warfarin* may cause elongation of PT.

Effects on diagnostic tests
None reported.

Adverse reactions
CNS: peripheral neuropathy.

CV: hypotension (from too-rapid infusion).
GI: *nausea and vomiting, anorexia, diarrhea,* abdominal pain, *stomatitis.*
Hematologic: *anemia,* ***myelosuppression*** (dose-limiting), LEUKOPENIA, THROMBOCYTOPENIA.
Other: *reversible alopecia,* ***anaphylaxis*** (rare), phlebitis at injection site (infrequent).

Overdose and treatment

Clinical manifestations of overdose include myelosuppression, nausea, and vomiting.

Treatment is usually supportive and includes transfusion of blood components, antiemetics, and appropriate symptomatic therapy.

☑ Special considerations

- To prepare solution, dilute prescribed dose to a concentration of 0.2 to 0.4 mg/ml with 0.9% NaCl solution or D_5W. Higher concentrations may crystallize. Discard solution if cloudy.
- Solutions diluted to 0.2 mg/ml are stable for 96 hours at room temperature in plastic or glass unprotected from light; solutions diluted to 0.4 mg/ml are stable for 48 hours under the same conditions.
- Administer infusion over 30 to 60 minutes to avoid hypotensive reactions.
- Treatment of extravasation includes local injections of hyaluronidase, which aids in systemic reabsorption of etoposide.
- Pretreatment with antiemetics may reduce frequency and duration of nausea and vomiting.
- GI toxicity occurs more frequently after oral administration.
- At doses below 200 mg, extent of absorption after oral administration is not affected by food.
- Intrapleural and intrathecal administration of drug is contraindicated due to severe toxicity.
- Store capsules in refrigerator.
- Have diphenhydramine, hydrocortisone, epinephrine, and airway available in case of an anaphylactic reaction.
- Monitor blood pressure before infusion and at 30-minute intervals during infusion. If systolic blood pressure falls below 90 mm Hg, stop infusion.
- Monitor CBC. Observe patient for signs of bone marrow depression. Withhold drug if platelet count is below 50,000/mm^3 or absolute neutrophil count is below 500/mm^3 until blood counts have sufficiently recovered.
- Etoposide has produced complete remissions in small-cell lung cancer and testicular cancer.

Patient education

- Emphasize importance of continuing medication despite nausea and vomiting.
- Tell patient to call immediately if vomiting occurs shortly after dose is taken.
- Advise patient to avoid exposure to people with infections.
- Tell patient not to receive immunizations during therapy with etoposide; other family members also should not receive immunizations during duration of therapy.
- Instruct patient to promptly report a sore throat or fever or unusual bruising or bleeding.
- Reassure patient that hair should grow back after treatment has ended.
- Advise patient to use contraceptive measures during therapy.

Geriatric use

- Elderly patients may be particularly susceptible to the hypotensive effects of etoposide.

Pediatric use

- Safety and effectiveness in children have not been established.

Breast-feeding

- Because drug is excreted into breast milk, its use in breast-feeding patients is not recommended.

etoposide phosphate

Etopophos

Pharmacologic classification: semi-synthetic derivative of podophyllotoxin
Therapeutic classification: antineoplastic
Pregnancy risk category D

How supplied

Available by prescription only
Injection: Single-dose vial containing etoposide phosphate that is equivalent to 100 mg etoposide (20 mg etoposide = 22.7 mg etoposide phosphate)

Indications, route, and dosage

Adjunct treatment of refractory testicular cancer
Adults: Etoposide phosphate doses that are equivalent to 50 to 100 mg/m^2/day of etoposide I.V. on days 1 through 5 of each cycle and given in conjunction with other approved chemotherapeutic agents. Cycle is repeated when adequate recovery from drug toxicity has occurred (usually at 3- to 4-week intervals). Alternatively, etoposide phosphate doses that are equivalent to 100 mg/m^2/day of etoposide I.V. on days 1, 3, and 5 of each cycle and given in conjunction with other approved chemotherapeutic agents. Cycle is repeated at 3- to 4-week intervals if adequate recovery from drug toxicity has occurred. Infusion rate may range from 5 minutes to 210 minutes.
Adjunct treatment of small-cell lung cancer
Adults: Dosage is individualized but may range from etoposide phosphate doses that are equivalent to 35 mg/m^2/day etoposide I.V. for 4 days to etoposide phosphate doses that are equivalent to 50 mg/m^2/day etoposide I.V. for 5 days and given in conjunction with other approved chemotherapeutic agents. Cycle is repeated when adequate recovery from drug toxicity has occurred (usually at 3- to 4-week intervals). Infusion rate may range from 5 minutes to 210 minutes.
✦ ***Dosage adjustment.*** In patients with renal failure with creatinine clearance above 50 ml/minute, give usual dosage; for creatinine clearance between 15 and 50 ml/minute, give 75% of usual dosage.

Pharmacodynamics

Antineoplastic action: Althought action is unknown, it is believed to exert its cytotoxic action by arresting cells in the metaphase portion of cell division. Drug may also inhibit cells from entering mitosis and depressing DNA and RNA synthesis.

Pharmacokinetics

- *Absorption:* Drug is only administered as an I.V. infusion.
- *Distribution:* Distribution is believed to be similiar to etoposide. Etoposide crosses the blood-brain barrier to a limited and variable extent and is about 97% bound to serum albumin.
- *Metabolism:* Drug is rapidly and completely converted to etoposide in plasma.
- *Excretion:* After etoposide phosphate is converted to etoposide, etoposide is excreted primarily in the urine as unchanged drug. A smaller portion of a dose is excreted in the feces. The plasma elimination of etoposide is described as biphasic, with an initial phase half-life of about ½ to 2 hours and a terminal phase of about 5¼ to 11 hours.

Contraindications and precautions

Contraindicated in patients with history of hypersensitivity to etoposide phosphate, etoposide, or other components of the formulation.

Interactions

Caution should be used when administering etoposide phosphate with *drugs that are known to inhibit phosphatase activities* (such as *levamisole hydrochloride*). *High-dose cyclosporine* may increase the toxic effects of etoposide phosphate because of delayed excretion of the drug.

Effects on diagnostic tests

None reported.

Adverse reactions

CNS: *asthenia, malaise,* dizziness, peripheral neurotoxicity.
CV: hypertension, hypotension.
GI: *nausea, vomiting, anorexia, mucositis,* constipation, abdominal pain, diarrhea, taste alteration.
Hematologic: *anemia,* ***myelosuppression*** (dose-limiting), **LEUKOPENIA, THROMBOCYTOPENIA, NEUTROPENIA.**
Skin: facial flushing, rash.
Other: *reversible alopecia, chills, fever,* phlebitis, ***anaphylaxis.***

Overdose and treatment

Because etoposide phosphate is rapidly converted to etoposide, clinical manifestations of overdose would be expected to be similiar. Clinical manifestations of overdose of etoposide include myelosuppression, nausea, and vomiting. Treatment is usually supportive and includes transfusion of blood components, antiemetics, and appropriate symptomatic therapy.

☑ Special considerations

- To prepare solution, reconstitute each vial with either 5 or 10 ml sterile water for injection, D_5W, 0.9% NaCl solution, bacteriostatic water for injection with benzyl alcohol, or bacteriostatic NaCl for injection with benzyl alcohol to a concentration equivalent to 20 mg/ml or 10 mg/ml etoposide (22.7 mg/ml or 11.4 mg/ml etoposide phosphate), respectively.
- Use of gloves is recommended when handling etoposide phosphate. If etoposide phosphate solution comes into contact with the skin or mucosa, immediately and thoroughly wash the skin with soap and water and flush the mucosa with water.
- After reconstitution, solution may be administered without further dilution or it can be further diluted to concentrations as low as 0.1 mg/ml etoposide with either D_5W injection or 0.9% NaCl solution.
- Unopened vials of etoposide phosphate are stable until the date indicated on the package when stored under refrigeration in the original package. When reconstituted or diluted as directed, etoposide phosphate can be stored in glass or plastic containers at room temperature or under refrigeration for 24 hours. Refrigerated solutions should be used immediately upon return to room temperature.
- I.V. infusions may be administered at rates from 5 to 210 minutes.
- Modify dosage to take into account the myelosuppressive effect of other drugs in the combination therapy or the effects of previous radiation or chemotherapy.
- Monitor CBC. Observe patient for signs of bone marrow depression. Withhold drug if platelet count is below 50,000/mm³ or absolute neutrophil count is below 500/mm³ until the blood counts have sufficiently recovered.
- If an anaphylactic reaction occurs, terminate infusion immediately and administer pressor agents, corticosteroids, antihistamines, or volume expanders as needed.
- Patients with low serum albumin may be at an increased risk for etoposide-associated toxicities.

Patient education

- Warn women of childbearing age to avoid becoming pregnant. If pregnancy is suspected, tell patient to promptly report it.
- Advise patient to avoid exposure to people with infections.
- Tell patient to promptly report a sore throat or fever or unusual bruising or bleeding.
- Reassure patient that hair should grow back after treatment has ended.

Pediatric use

- Safety and effectiveness in children have not been established. Anaphylactic reactions have been reported in pediatric patients who received etoposide.

Breast-feeding

- It is unknown if drug is excreted in breast milk. Therefore, because of the potential risk of serious adverse reactions, mutagenicity, and carcinogenicity in the infant, breast-feeding is not recommended.

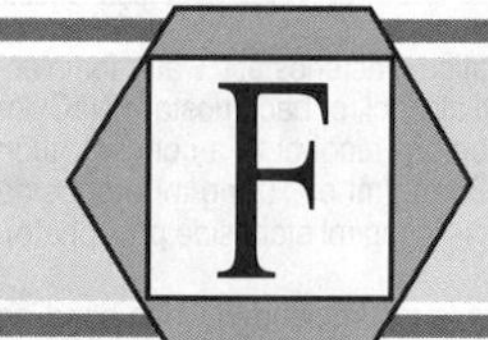

factor IX complex
Konyne 80, Profilnine SD, Proplex T

factor IX (human)
AlphaNine SD, Mononine

factor IX (recombinant)
BeneFix

Pharmacologic classification: blood derivative
Therapeutic classification: systemic hemostatic
Pregnancy risk category C

How supplied
Available by prescription only
Injection: Vials, with diluents. Units specified on label.

Indications, route, and dosage
Factor IX deficiency (hemophilia B or Christmas disease), anticoagulant overdose
factor IX complex and factor IX (human)
Adults and children: Determine units required by multiplying 0.8 to 1 by body weight (in kg), then by percent of desired factor IX level increase; administer by slow I.V. infusion or I.V. push. Dosage is highly individualized, depending on degree of deficiency, desired level of factor IX, body weight, and severity of bleeding.

Factor IX complex can also be used to reverse Coumadin anticoagulation when emergencies such as surgery preclude less hazardous therapy.
Factor IX deficiency (hemophilia B or Christmas disease)
BeneFix only
Adults and children: Determine units required by multiplying 1.2 by body weight (in kg) multiplied by the percent of factor IX increase desired. Administer I.V. over several minutes . Repeat q 12 to 24 hours titrating dose to clinical response.
Hemostasis in patients with factor VIII inhibitors
factor IX complex
Adults and children: Usual dose is 75 IU/kg I.V. Repeat q 12 hours p.r.n.
Hemostasis in factor VII deficiency
Proplex T only
Adults and children: Determine units required by multiplying 0.5 by body weight (kg) multiplied by percent of factor VII increase desired. Administer I.V. and repeat q 4 to 6 hours.

Pharmacodynamics
Hemostatic action: Factor IX complex directly replaces deficient clotting factor.

Pharmacokinetics
- *Absorption:* Factor IX complex must be given parenterally for systemic effect.
- *Distribution:* Equilibration within extravascular space takes 4 to 6 hours.
- *Metabolism:* Factor IX complex is rapidly cleared by plasma.
- *Excretion:* Half-life is approximately 24 hours.

Contraindications and precautions
Contraindicated in patients with hepatic disease in whom there is any suspicion of intravascular coagulation or fibrinolysis. Mononine is contraindicated in patients with hypersensitivity to murine (mouse) protein. BeneFix is produced in a Chinese hamster ovary cell line so it is contraindicated in patients with a known sensitivity to hamster protein. Use cautiously in infants.

Interactions
Concurrent administration with *aminocaproic acid* increases the risk of thrombosis.

Effects on diagnostic tests
Increases coagulation assays (PT, INR).

Adverse reactions
CNS: headache.
CV: ***thromboembolic reactions, MI, DIC, pulmonary embolism,*** changes in blood pressure.
GI: nausea, vomiting.
Skin: urticaria.
Other: *transient fever, chills, flushing, tingling.*

Overdose and treatment
Clinical manifestations of overdose include a risk of DIC on repeated use because of increased levels of factors II, IX, and X.

☑ Special considerations
- Refrigerate vials until needed; before reconstituting, warm to room temperature. Use 20 ml sterile water for injection of each vial of lyophilized drug. To mix, gently roll vial between hands; do not shake or mix with other I.V. solutions. Keep product away from heat (but do not refrigerate, because this may cause precipitation of active ingredient), and use within 3 hours.
- BeneFix only*:* Refrigerate vials until needed; before reconstituting, warm to room temperature. Reconstitute per package instructions using sterile double-ended needle and filter spike provided. Administer within 3 hours.
- Adverse reactions are usually related to too-rapid infusion. Take baseline pulse rate before I.V. administration; if pulse rate increases significantly during infusion, reduce flow rate or stop drug. If pa-

tient complains of tingling sensation, fever, chills, or headache, decrease flow rate. A rate of 100 units/minute is usually well-tolerated; do not give drug faster than 3 ml/minute.

- Monitor coagulation studies before and during therapy; monitor vital signs regularly, and be alert for allergic reactions.
- Human derivative forms of drug may contain the causative agents of hepatitis and other viral diseases (human immunodeficiency virus). The risk of infection with use of these agents cannot be totally eliminated. The DNA-recombinant form of factor IX is inheritantly free from the risk of blood-borne pathogens, but is only indicated for the treatment of Factor IX deficiency.
- Immunize patient with hepatitis B vaccine to decrease risk of transmission of hepatitis.

Patient education

- Teach or review proper storage, preparation, and injection technique for the specific product that the patient uses.

Pediatric use

- Administer human forms of this medication cautiously to neonates and other infants because of increased risk of hepatitis; only heat-treated products are now available, thus decreasing the risk. The DNA-recombinant form is the treatment of choice in the pediatric population.

famciclovir

Famvir

Pharmacologic classification: synthetic acyclic guanine derivative
Therapeutic classification: antiviral
Pregnancy risk category B

How supplied

Available by prescription only
Tablets: 125 mg, 250 mg, 500 mg

Indications, route, and dosage

Management of acute herpes zoster
Adults: 500 mg P.O. q 8 hours for 7 days
✦ ***Dosage adjustment.*** Dosage in adult patients with reduced renal function.

Creatinine clearance (ml/min)	Dosage regimen
≥ 60	500 mg q 8 hr
40 to 59	500 mg q 12 hr
20 to 39	500 mg q 24 hr
< 20	250 mg q 48 hr

Recurrent genital herpes
Adults: 125 mg P.O. b.i.d. for 5 days.
✦ ***Dosage adjustment.*** Dosage in adult patients with reduced renal function.

Creatinine clearance (ml/min)	Dosage regimen
≥ 40	125 mg q 12 hr
20 to 39	125 mg q 24 hr
< 20	125 mg q 48 hr

Pharmacodynamics

Antiviral action: Famciclovir is a prodrug that undergoes rapid biotransformation to the active antiviral compound penciclovir. It enters viral cells (herpes simplex types 1 and 2, varicella zoster), where it inhibits DNA polymerase, viral DNA synthesis, and, therefore, viral replication.

Pharmacokinetics

- *Absorption:* Absolute bioavailability of famciclovir is 77%. Because bioavailability is not affected by food intake, the drug can be taken without regard to meals.
- *Distribution:* Famciclovir is less than 20% bound to plasma proteins.
- *Metabolism:* Drug is extensively metabolized in the liver to the active drug penciclovir (98.5%) and other inactive metabolites.
- *Excretion:* Penciclovir is primarily eliminated in the urine.

Contraindications and precautions

Contraindicated in patients with hypersensitivity to drug. Use cautiously in patients with impaired renal or hepatic function.

Interactions

Concurrent use of famciclovir with *probenecid* or *other drugs significantly eliminated by active renal tubular secretion* may result in increased plasma concentrations of penciclovir. Monitor patient for increased adverse effects.

Effects on diagnostic tests

None reported.

Adverse reactions

CNS: *headache,* fatigue, dizziness, paresthesia, somnolence.
EENT: pharyngitis, sinusitis.
GI: diarrhea, *nausea,* vomiting, constipation, anorexia, abdominal pain.
Musculoskeletal: back pain, arthralgia.
Skin: pruritus; zoster-related signs, symptoms, and complications.
Other: fever, injury, pain, rigors.

Overdose and treatment

No acute overdosage has been reported. Appropriate symptomatic and supportive therapy should be given. It is not known if hemodialysis removes famciclovir from the blood. However, hemodialysis does enhance the elimination of acyclovir, a related nucleoside analogue.

☑ Special considerations
- Information is based on current literature and may change with further clinical experience.

Patient education
- Inform patient that drug may be taken without regard to meals.
- Teach patient to recognize early symptoms of herpes zoster infection, such as tingling, itching, and pain. Explain that treatment is more effective when started within 48 hours of rash onset.

Pediatric use
- Safety and effectiveness have not been established in children under age 18.

Breast-feeding
- It is not known if drug is excreted in breast milk. A decision should be made whether to discontinue breast-feeding or the drug, taking into account the importance of the drug to the mother.

famotidine
Pepcid, Pepcid AC

Pharmacologic classification: H_2-receptor antagonist
Therapeutic classification: antiulcer
Pregnancy risk category B

How supplied
Available by prescription only
Tablets: 20 mg, 40 mg
Injection: 10 mg/ml
Injection, premixed: 20 mg/50 ml 0.9% NaCl solution
Suspension: 40 mg/5 ml

Available without a prescription
Tablets: 10 mg

Indications, route, and dosage
Duodenal and gastric ulcer
Adults: For acute therapy, 40 mg P.O. h.s. for 4 to 8 weeks; for maintenance therapy, 20 mg P.O. h.s.
Pathologic hypersecretory conditions (such as Zollinger-Ellison syndrome)
Adults: 20 mg P.O. q 6 hours. As much as 160 mg q 6 hours may be administered.
Short-term treatment of gastroesophageal reflux disease (GERD)
Adults: 20 to 40 mg P.O. b.i.d. for up to 12 weeks.
Hospitalized patients with intractable ulcers or hypersecretory conditions or patients who cannot take oral medication; ◊ patients with GI bleeding; ◊ to control gastric pH in critically ill patients
Adults: 20 mg I.V. q 12 hours.
Prevention or treatment of heartburn
Pepcid AC
Adults: 10 mg P.O. when symptoms occur; or 10 mg P.O. 1 hour before meals for prevention of symptoms. Drug can be used b.i.d. if necessary.
✦ ***Dosage adjustment.*** In patients with severe renal insufficiency (creatinine clearance below 10 ml/minute), dosage may be reduced to 20 mg h.s. or the dosing interval may be prolonged to 36 to 48 hours to avoid excess accumulation of drug.

Pharmacodynamics
Antiulcer action: Famotidine competitively inhibits histamine's action at H_2-receptors in gastric parietal cells. This inhibits basal and nocturnal gastric acid secretion resulting from stimulation by such factors as caffeine, food, and pentagastrin.

Pharmacokinetics
- *Absorption:* When administered orally, approximately 40% to 45% of dose is absorbed; onset of action occurs in 1 hour, with peak action in 1 to 3 hours. After parenteral administration, peak action occurs in 30 minutes.
- *Distribution:* Drug is distributed widely to many body tissues.
- *Metabolism:* About 30% to 35% of an administered dose is metabolized by the liver (minimal first-pass metabolism).
- *Excretion:* Most drug is excreted unchanged in urine. Famotidine has a longer duration of effect than its 2½- to 4-hour half-life suggests.

Contraindications and precautions
Contraindicated in patients hypersensitive to drug.

Interactions
Famotidine may cause *enteric coatings* to dissolve too rapidly because of increased gastric pH. It may decrease *ketoconazole's* absorption, requiring an increased dose of ketoconazole.

Effects on diagnostic tests
Drug may antagonize pentagastrin during gastric acid secretion tests. Famotidine may elevate hepatic enzyme levels. In skin tests using allergen extracts, drug may cause false-negative results.

Adverse reactions
CNS: *headache,* dizziness, vertigo, malaise, paresthesia.
EENT: tinnitus, taste disorder, orbital edema.
GI: diarrhea, constipation, anorexia, dry mouth.
GU: increased BUN and creatinine levels.
Skin: acne, dry skin, flushing.
Other: transient irritation (at I.V. site), musculoskeletal pain, palpitations, fever.

Overdose and treatment
Overdose has not been reported. Treatment should include gastric lavage or induced emesis, followed by activated charcoal to prevent further absorption and supportive and symptomatic therapy. Hemodialysis does not remove famotidine.

☑ Special considerations
Besides those relevant to all *H_2-receptor antagonists*, consider the following recommendations.
- Drug is not recommended for use longer than 8 weeks in patients with uncomplicated duodenal ulcer.

• After administration via nasogastric tube, tube should be flushed to clear it and ensure drug's passage to stomach.
• For I.V. push administration, dilute with 0.9% NaCl solution to total volume of 5 to 10 ml; administer over period exceeding 2 minutes. For I.V. infusion, dilute in 100 ml of D_5W, administer over 15 to 30 minutes. Drug is stable at room temperature for 48 hours. Do not use drug if it is discolored or contains precipitate.
• Antacids may be administered concurrently.
• Drug appears to cause fewer adverse reactions and drug interactions than cimetidine.

Patient education
• Caution patient to take drug only as directed and to continue taking doses even after pain subsides, to ensure adequate healing.
• Instruct patient to take dose at bedtime.

Geriatric use
• Use drug cautiously in elderly patients because of increased risk of adverse reactions, particularly those affecting the CNS.

Breast-feeding
• Drug may be excreted in breast milk. Use with caution in breast-feeding women.

fat emulsions
Intralipid 10%, Intralipid 20%, Intralipid 30%, Liposyn II 10%, Liposyn II 20%, Liposyn III 10% and 20%

Pharmacologic classification: lipid
Therapeutic classification: total parenteral nutrition (TPN)
Pregnancy risk category C

How supplied
Available by prescription only
Injection: 50 ml (10%, 20%), 100 ml (10%, 20%, 30%), 200 ml (10%, 20%), 250 ml (10%, 20%), 500 ml (10%, 20%)

Indications, route, and dosage
Source of calories adjunctive to TPN
Intralipid
Adults: 1 ml/minute I.V. for 15 to 30 minutes (10% emulsion); or 0.5 ml/minute I.V. for 15 to 30 minutes (20% emulsion). If no adverse reactions occur, increase rate to deliver 500 ml over 4 to 8 hours. Total daily dose should not exceed 2.5 g/kg (10% emulsion) and 3 g/kg (20% emulsion).
Children: 0.1 ml/minute for 10 to 15 minutes (10% emulsion); or 0.05 ml/minute I.V. for 10 to 15 minutes (20% emulsion). If no adverse reactions occur, increase rate to deliver 1 g/kg over 4 hours. Daily dose should not exceed 4 g/kg, which equals 60% of daily caloric intake. Protein-carbohydrate TPN should supply remaining 40%.
Fatty acid deficiency
Intralipid
Adults and children: 8% to 10% of total caloric intake I.V.

Pharmacodynamics
Metabolic action: I.V. fat emulsions are prepared from soybean or safflower oil and provide a mixture of neutral triglycerides, predominantly fatty acids. Besides the major component, fatty acids (linoleic, oleic, palmitic, stearic, and linolenic), these preparations also contain 1.2% egg yolk phospholipids (an emulsifier) and glycerol (to adjust tonicity). I.V. fat emulsions are isotonic and may be given centrally or peripherally.

Linoleic, linolenic, and arachidonic acids are essential in humans. Clinical manifestations of essential fatty acid deficiency (EFAD) include scaly dermatitis, alopecia, growth retardation, poor wound healing, thrombocytopenia, and fatty liver. I.V. fat emulsions prevent or reverse the biochemical and clinical manifestations of EFAD and provide 1.1 kcal/ml (10%) or 2 kcal/ml (20%).

Pharmacokinetics
• *Absorption:* These products are administered as an I.V. infusion, through either a peripheral or a central vein.
• *Distribution:* Fat emulsions distribute through the plasma compartment.
• *Metabolism:* Fat emulsions are metabolized and used as an energy source, causing increased heat production, decreased respiratory quotient, and increased oxygen consumption.
• *Excretion:* The infused fat particles are cleared from the bloodstream in a manner similar to chylomicrons.

Contraindications and precautions
Contraindicated in patients with hyperlipidemia, lipid nephrosis, acute pancreatitis accompanied by hyperlipidemia, or severe egg allergies. Use cautiously in patients with severe hepatic disease, pulmonary disease, anemia, or blood coagulation disorders (especially thrombocytopenia) and in those at risk for fat embolism.

Interactions
None reported.

Effects on diagnostic tests
Abnormally high mean corpuscular hemoglobin and mean corpuscular hemoglobin concentration values may be found in blood samples drawn during or shortly after fat emulsion infusion. Fat emulsions may cause transient abnormalities in liver function tests and may alter results of serum bilirubin tests (especially in infants).

Adverse reactions
Early reactions to fat overload:
CNS: headache, sleepiness, dizziness.
EENT: pressure over eyes.
GI: nausea, vomiting.
Hematologic: ***hypercoagulability, thrombocytopenia in neonates*** (rare).
Respiratory: dyspnea, cyanosis.
Skin: flushing, diaphoresis.
Other: hyperlipidemia, fever, chest and back pain, hypersensitivity reactions, irritation (at infusion site).

Delayed reactions:
CNS: ***focal seizures.***
Hematologic: ***thrombocytopenia,*** leukopenia, leukocytosis.
Hepatic: transient increases in liver function test values, hepatomegaly.
Other: fever, splenomegaly.

Overdose and treatment

Clinical manifestations of overdose or "overloading syndrome" include focal seizures, splenomegaly, leukocytosis, fever, and shock. The infusion should be discontinued until visual inspection of the plasma, determination of triglyceride concentrations, or nephelometric measurement of plasma light-scattering activity confirms clearance of the lipid. Reevaluate the patient and institute appropriate corrective measures.

☑ Special considerations

- Some brands of fat emulsion can be mixed with amino acid solution and dextrose in the same I.V. container. The order of mixing is important; see package insert for further information.
- Do not use an in-line filter when administering this drug because the fat particles (0.5 mcg) are larger than the 0.22 mcg cellulose filter.
- Fat emulsions may extract small amounts of plasticizers from I.V. administration sets made of polyvinyl chloride. Nonphthalate administration sets are available; however, phthalate extraction can be minimized from regular I.V. tubing by not storing primed administration sets.
- Discard the fat emulsion if it separates or becomes oily.
- Change all I.V. tubing at each infusion because lipids support bacterial growth.
- Avoid rapid infusion by using an infusion pump to regulate the rate.
- Check injection site daily for signs of inflammation or infection.
- Watch closely for adverse effects, especially during the first half hour of infusion.
- Monitor serum lipid levels closely when patient is receiving fat emulsion therapy. Lipemia must clear between dosing.
- Monitor hepatic function carefully in long-term use.
- Do not store contents of partly used containers for later use.
- Store Intralipid 10% and Liposyn 10% at room temperature (77° F [25° C]) or below. Do not freeze.

Pediatric use

- Premature and small-for-gestational-age infants have poor clearance of I.V. fat emulsions, so lower doses are necessary to decrease the likelihood of fat overload.
- Because free fatty acids displace bilirubin bound to albumin, caution must be observed when administering fat emulsions to jaundiced or premature infants. Deaths in preterm infants have been reported from intravascular fat accumulation in the lungs.
- Monitor infant's ability to eliminate the infused fat (triglycerides or plasma free fatty acids) daily.
- Check platelet count frequently in neonates receiving fat emulsions I.V. because they tend to develop thrombocytopenia.

felodipine

Plendil

Pharmacologic classification: calcium channel blocker
Therapeutic classification: antihypertensive
Pregnancy risk category C

How supplied

Available by prescription only
Tablets (extended-release): 2.5 mg, 5 mg, 10 mg

Indications, route, and dosage

Hypertension

Adults: 5 mg P.O. daily. Adjust dosage based on patient response, generally at intervals not less than 2 weeks. Usual dose is 2.5 to 10 mg daily; doses exceeding 10 mg daily increase rate of peripheral edema and vasodilatory adverse effects.
✦ ***Dosage adjustment.*** Elderly patients or patients with impaired hepatic function should receive a starting dose of 2.5 mg daily. Doses above 10 mg should not be considered.

Pharmacodynamics

Antihypertensive action: A dihydropyridine-derivative calcium channel blocker, felodipine blocks the entry of calcium ions into vascular smooth muscle and cardiac cells. This type of calcium channel blocker shows some selectivity for smooth muscle as compared with cardiac muscle. Effects on vascular smooth muscle is relaxation; vasodilation.

Pharmacokinetics

- *Absorption:* Felodipine is almost completely absorbed, but extensive first-pass metabolism reduces absolute bioavailability to about 20%. Plasma levels peak within 2½ to 5 hours after a dose.
- *Distribution:* Drug is over 99% bound to plasma proteins.
- *Metabolism:* Metabolism of felodipine is probably hepatic; at least six inactive metabolites have been identified.
- *Excretion:* Over 70% of a dose appears in urine, and 10% appears in feces as metabolites.

Contraindications and precautions

Contraindicated in patients hypersensitive to drug. Use cautiously in patients with impaired hepatic function or heart failure, especially those receiving beta-adrenergic blockers.

Interactions

Felodipine may alter the pharmacokinetics of *metoprolol.* No dosage adjustment appears necessary; however, monitor for adverse effects. *Cimetidine* decreases the clearance of felodipine. Lower doses of felodipine should be used. In clinical trials, felodipine decreased peak serum levels of *digox-*

in, but total absorbed drug was unchanged. Clinical significance is unknown.

Effects on diagnostic tests
None reported.

Adverse reactions
CNS: *headache,* dizziness, paresthesia, asthenia.
CV: *peripheral edema,* chest pain, palpitations.
EENT: rhinorrhea, pharyngitis.
GI: abdominal pain, nausea, constipation, diarrhea.
Respiratory: upper respiratory infection, cough.
Skin: rash, *flushing.*
Other: muscle cramps, back pain, gingival hyperplasia.

Overdose and treatment
Expected symptoms would be peripheral vasodilation, bradycardia, and hypotension. Provide supportive care. I.V. fluids or sympathomimetics may be useful in treating hypotension, and atropine (0.5 to 1 mg I.V.) may treat bradycardia. It is not known if the drug may be removed by dialysis.

☑ Special considerations
Besides those relevant to all *calcium channel blockers,* consider the following recommendations.
- Peripheral edema appears to be both dose- and age-dependent. It's more common in patients taking higher doses, especially those age 60 and over.
- Drug may be administered without regard to meals. However, a small study reported a more than twofold increase of bioavailability when drug was taken with doubly concentrated grapefruit juice compared with water or orange juice.

Patient education
- Tell patient to observe good oral hygiene and to see a dentist regularly because drug has been associated with mild gingival hyperplasia.
- Remind patient to swallow tablet whole and not to crush or chew it.
- Inform patient that he should continue taking drug, even when feeling better. He should watch his diet and call before taking other medications, including OTC drugs.

Geriatric use
- Higher blood levels of drug are seen in elderly patients. Mean clearance of drug from elderly hypertensive patients (average age 74) was less than half of that observed in young patients (average age 26). Check blood pressures closely during dosage adjustment. Maximum daily dose is 10 mg.

Pediatric use
- Safety and efficacy in children have not been established.

Breast-feeding
- It is unknown if drug is excreted in breast milk. Because of risk of serious adverse effects to the infant, breast-feeding is not recommended.

fenofibrate
Tricor

Pharmacologic classification: fibric acid derivative
Therapeutic classification: antihyperlipidemic
Pregnancy risk category C

How supplied
Available by prescription only
Capsules (micronized): 67 mg

Indications, route, and dosage
Adjunct to diet for treatment of patients with very high serum triglyceride levels (type IV and V hyperlipidemia) who are at high risk of pancreatitis and who do not respond adequately to diet alone
Adults: Initiate therapy with one (67-mg) capsule P.O. once daily. Based on response, increase dose if necessary following repeat triglyceride levels at 4- to 8-week intervals to maximum dose of three capsules daily (201 mg).
✦ ***Dosage adjustment.*** Minimize dose in renally impaired patients. Initiate therapy at dose of 67 mg/day and increase only after effects on renal function and triglyceride levels have been evaluated at this dose.

Pharmacodynamics
Antihyperlipidemic action: Exact mechanism of action is not known; drug is thought to lower triglyceride levels by inhibiting triglyceride synthesis, resulting in a decrease in the amount of very-low-density lipoprotein released into the circulation. Fenofibrate may stimulate the breakdown of triglyceride-rich protein.

Pharmacokinetics
- *Absorption:* Drug is well absorbed. Peak plasma concentrations occur within 6 to 8 hours after administration. Food increases the absorption of drug by 35%.
- *Distribution:* Steady-state plasma concentrations are achieved within 5 days after initiation of therapy. Drug is almost entirely bound to plasma protein.
- *Metabolism:* Drug is rapidly hydrolyzed by esterases to fenofibric acid, an active metabolite. Fenofibric acid is primarily conjugated with glucruonic acid and excreted in urine.
- *Excretion:* Drug is primarily excreted in the urine; 25% is excreted in the feces; elimination half-life is 20 hours.

Contraindications and precautions
Contraindicated in patients with preexisting gallbladder disease, hepatic dysfunction (including primary biliary cirrhosis), severe renal dysfunction, unexplained persistent liver function abnormalities, or hypersensitivity to drug.

Interactions

Use extreme caution when administering drug with *coumarin-type anticoagulants* due to protein binding displacement of the anticoagulant and potentiation of its effects. Reduce dose of anticoagulant to maintain PT within desired range.

No data are available on the concomitant use with *HMG-CoA inhibitors (statins)* with fenofibrate; however, because of risk of myopathy, rhabdomyolosis, and acute renal failure reported with the combination use of statins with gemfibrozil (another fibrate derivative), these drugs should not be given together.

Bile acid resins may bind and inhibit absorption of fenofibrate. Therefore, fenofibrate should be taken 1 hour before or 4 to 6 hours after taking these agents.

Cyclosporine-induced renal dysfunction may compromise the elimination of fenofibrate; therefore use cyclosporine and fenofibrate together cautiously.

Effect on diagnostic tests

ALT or AST levels may be increased. Creatinine and BUN levels are increased and hemoglobin and uric acid levels are decreased.

Adverse reactions

CNS: dizziness, miscellaneous pain, asthenia, fatigue, paresthesia, insomnia, increased appetite, headache, decreased libido.
CV: ***arrhythmia.***
EENT: eye irritation, eye floaters, earache, conjunctivitis, blurred vision, rhinitis, sinusitis.
GI: dyspepsia, eructation, flatulence, nausea, vomiting, abdominal pain, constipation, diarrhea.
GU*:* polyuria, vaginitis.
Musculoskeletal: arthralgia.
Respiratory: cough.
Skin: urticaria, pruritis, rash.
Other: *infections,* flu syndrome.

Overdose and treatment:

No cases of overdose have been reported. If overdose dose occur, initiate supportive measures. Because drug is highly protein bound, hemodialysis is unlikely to be of value.

☑ Special considerations

- Withdraw therapy in patients who do not achieve an adequate response after 2 months of treatment with the maximum daily dosage.
- Fenofibrate lowers serum uric acid levels in normal patients as well as hyperuricemic patients by increasing uric acid excretion.
- Drug should not be used for primary or secondary prevention of coronary artery disease.
- If possible, change or discontinue the use of beta-adrenergic blocking agents, estrogens, and thiazide diuretics because they may increase plasma triglyceride levels.
- Drug may cause excretion of cholesterol into the bile leading to cholelithiasis. If suspected, perform appropriate tests and discontinue drug.
- Mild to moderate decreases in hemoglobin, hematocrit, and WBC count may occur on initiation of therapy but stabilize on long-term administration.
- Pancreatitis may occur in patients receiving fenofibrate; myositis and rhabdomyolysis may occur in those with renal failure. Assess CK levels in patients with myalgia, muscle tenderness, or weakness.

Patient education

- Advise patient to promptly report symptoms of unexplained muscle weakness, pain, or tenderness, especially if it is accompanied by malaise or fever.
- Instruct patient to follow a triglyceride-lowering diet during treatment.
- Inform patient to take drug with meals to optimize drug absorption.
- Advise patient to continue weight-control measures, including diet and exercise, as to reduce alcohol intake before starting drug therapy.

Geriatric use

- Drug acts similarly in the elderly (age 77 to 87) as in young adults; similar dosing regimens can be used.

Pediatric use

- Drug is not indicated for use in the pediatric population. Safety and efficacy have not been established.

Breast-feeding

- Do not use drug in breast-feeding patients; either the drug or breast-feeding should be discontinued.

fenoldopam mesylate

Corlopam

Pharmacologic classification: dopamine D_1-like receptor agonist
Therapeutic classification: antihypertensive
Pregnancy risk category B

How supplied

Available by prescription only
Ampules: 10 mg/ml in single-dose 1-ml, 2-ml, 5-ml ampules

Indications, route, and dosage

Short-term (up to 48 hours) in-hospital management of severe hypertension when rapid but quickly reversible reduction of blood pressure is indicated, including malignant hypertension with deteriorating end-organ function
Adults: Administer by continuous I.V. infusion. Infusion rate is initiated at 0.025 to 0.3 mcg/kg/minute and titrated upward or downward at a frequency not exceeding q 15 minutes to achieve desired blood pressure. Recommended increments for titration are 0.05 to 0.1 mcg/kg/minute.

Pharmacodynamics

Antihypertensive action: Rapid-acting vasodilator. Fenoldopam is an agonist for D_1-like dopamine receptors and binds with moderate affinity to alpha$_2$-adrenoceptors. No significant affinity for D_2-like receptors, alpha$_1$ or beta adrenoreceptors, 5HT, 5HT$_2$, or muscarinic receptors has been noted. In addition, fenoldopam has no effect on ACE activity, although it may increase norepinephrine plasma concentrations.

Pharmacokinetics

- *Absorption:* Not reported. Drug is given by I.V. infusion only.
- *Distribution:* Not reported. Steady-state plasma concentrations of 3.2 to 4 ng/ml were reported with infusion rates of 0.1 mcg/kg/minute.
- *Metabolism:* Principle routes of conjugation are methylation, glucuronidation, and sulfation.
- *Excretion:* Elimination is largely by conjugation, without participation of cytochrome P-450 enzymes. Elimination half-life is reported to be about 5 minutes. Following I.V. administration, 90% of drug is excreted in urine and 10% in the feces. Only 4% of drug is excreted unchanged.

Contraindications and precautions

No known contraindications. Use cautiously because drug is a rapid-acting, potent vasodilator that may precipitate severe hypotension.

Use with caution in patients with glaucoma or ocular hypertension because dose-dependent increases in intraocular pressure may occur. Drug may cause symptomatic hypotension; use particular caution when administering to patients who have sustained an acute cerebral infarction or hemorrhage.

Fenoldopam contains sodium metabisulfite, which may cause allergic-type reactions (including anaphylactic symptoms and severe asthmatic episodes in certain susceptible individuals). Sulfite sensitivity is more frequent in asthmatic than in nonasthmatic people.

Interactions

Beta blockers were prohibited in clinical trials. Caution should be exercised because unexpected hypotension could result from beta-blocker inhibition of the reflex response to fenoldopam. Avoid concurrent use.

Effects on diagnostic tests

None reported.

Adverse reactions

CNS: dizziness, headache, insomnia.
CV: hypotension, orthostatic hypotension, palpitations, bradycardia, tachycardia, angina, ***MI, heart failure,*** T-wave inversion, flushing.
EENT: nasal congestion.
GI: nausea, vomiting, abdominal pain, constipation, diarrhea.
GU: oliguria, urinary tract infection
Hematologic: leukocytosis, bleeding.
Metabolic: increased creatinine and BUN, serum glucose, LD, transaminases; hypokalemia.
Musculoskeletal: limb cramp, back pain.
Respiratory dyspnea.
Other: pyrexia, nonspecific chest pain, injection site reaction.

Overdose and treatment

Intentional overdosage has not been reported. The most likely reaction would be excessive hypotension, which should be treated with drug discontinuation and appropriate supportive measures.

☑ Special considerations

- Use during pregnancy only if clearly needed.
- Drug causes a dose-related tachycardia, which diminishes over time but remains substantial at higher doses.
- Follow manufacturer's instructions for diluting drug before I.V. use. Diluted solution is stable at room temperature for at least 24 hours.
- Infuse drug with a calibrated mechanical infusion pump.

Do *not* use a bolus dose.

- Drug may be abruptly discontinued or infusion gradually tapered. Oral antihypertensive agents can be added once blood pressure is stable during infusion or after its discontinuation.
- Monitor blood pressure frequently during infusions. Check blood pressure and heart rate every 15 minutes until patient is stable.
- Monitor serum electrolytes and watch for hypokalemia.

Patient education

- Tell patient that drug causes dose-related decreases in blood pressure and increases in heart rate. Advise patient to change positions slowly to avoid orthostatic symptoms.
- Inform patient that drug must be given by controlled infusion, which should last no more than 48 hours.
- Encourage patient to report adverse reactions promptly.

Pediatric use

- Safety and effectiveness in children have not been established.

Breast-feeding

- Drug may be excreted in milk; use caution in administering to breast-feeding women.

fenoprofen calcium

Nalfon

Pharmacologic classification: NSAID
Therapeutic classification: nonnarcotic analgesic, antipyretic, anti-inflammatory
Pregnancy risk category NR

How supplied

Available by prescription only
Tablets: 600 mg
Capsules: 200 mg, 300 mg

Indications, route, and dosage

Rheumatoid arthritis and osteoarthritis
Adults: 300 to 600 mg P.O. t.i.d. to q.i.d. Maximum dosage is 3.2 g daily.
Mild to moderate pain
Adults: 200 mg P.O. q 4 to 6 hours, p.r.n.
◇ ***Fever***
Adults: Single oral doses up to 400 mg.
◇ ***Acute gouty arthritis***
Adults: 200 mg P.O. q 6 hours; decrease dose based on patient response.

Pharmacodynamics

Analgesic, anti-inflammatory, and antipyretic actions: Mechanisms of action unknown, but drug is thought to inhibit prostaglandin synthesis. Fenoprofen decreases platelet aggregation and may prolong bleeding time.

Pharmacokinetics

- *Absorption:* Drug is absorbed rapidly and completely from the GI tract. The onset of analgesic activity occurs within 15 to 30 minutes, with peak plasma levels achieved in 2 hours. Duration of action is approximately 4 to 6 hours.
- *Distribution:* Fenoprofen is about 99% protein-bound.
- *Metabolism:* Fenoprofen is metabolized in the liver.
- *Excretion:* Drug is excreted chiefly in urine with a serum half-life of 2½ to 3 hours. A small amount is excreted in feces.

Contraindications and precautions

Contraindicated during pregnancy and in patients with hypersensitivity to drug, significantly impaired renal function, or history of aspirin- or NSAID-induced asthma, rhinitis, or urticaria.

Use cautiously in the elderly and in patients with history of GI events, peptic ulcer disease, compromised cardiac function, or hypertension.

Interactions

Concomitant use of fenoprofen with *anticoagulants* and *thrombolytic drugs (coumarin derivatives, heparin, streptokinase, urokinase)* may potentiate anticoagulant effects. Bleeding problems may occur if fenoprofen is used with *other drugs that inhibit platelet aggregation,* such as *dextran, dipyridamole, mezlocillin, piperacillin, sulfinpyrazone, ticarcillin, valproic acid,* or with *cefamandole, cefoperazone, plicamycin, aspirin, salicylates,* or *other anti-inflammatory agents.* Concomitant use with *salicylates, anti-inflammatory agents, alcohol, corticotropin,* or *steroids* may cause increased GI adverse reactions, including ulceration and hemorrhage. *Aspirin* may decrease the bioavailability of fenoprofen.

Because of the influence of prostaglandins on glucose metabolism, concomitant use with *insulin* or *oral antidiabetic agents* may potentiate hypoglycemic effects. Fenoprofen may displace *highly protein-bound drugs* from binding sites. Toxicity may occur with *coumarin derivatives, phenytoin, verapamil,* or *nifedipine.* Increased nephrotoxicity may occur with *gold compounds, other anti-inflammatory agents,* or *acetaminophen.* Fenoprofen may decrease the renal clearance of *methotrexate* and *lithium.*

Fenoprofen may decrease the effectiveness of *antihypertensives* or *diuretics.* Concomitant use with *diuretics* may increase nephrotoxic potential.

Effects on diagnostic tests

The physiologic effects of drug may increase bleeding time, BUN, serum creatinine, potassium, alkaline phosphatase, LD, and transaminase concentrations. Drug may also cause false elevations in both free and total serum T_3, but thyroid-stimulating hormone and T_4 are unaffected.

Adverse reactions

CNS: *headache,* dizziness, *somnolence,* fatigue, nervousness, asthenia, tremor, confusion.
CV: peripheral edema, palpitations.
EENT: tinnitus, blurred vision, decreased hearing.
GI: *epigastric distress, nausea,* ***GI bleeding,*** vomiting, occult blood loss, peptic ulceration, constipation, anorexia, *dyspepsia,* flatulence.
GU: oliguria, interstitial nephritis, proteinuria, reversible renal failure, papillary necrosis, cystitis, hematuria.
Hematologic: prolonged bleeding time, anemia, ***aplastic anemia, agranulocytosis, thrombocytopenia, hemorrhage,*** bruising, hemolytic anemia.
Hepatic: elevated enzymes, hepatitis.
Respiratory: dyspnea, upper respiratory tract infections, nasopharyngitis.
Skin: *pruritus,* rash, urticaria, increased diaphoresis.
Other: ***anaphylaxis,*** angioedema.

Overdose and treatment

Little is known about the acute toxicity of fenoprofen. Nonoliguric renal failure, tachycardia, and hypotension have been observed. Other symptoms include drowsiness, dizziness, confusion and lethargy, nausea, vomiting, headache, tinnitus, and blurred vision. Elevations in serum creatinine and BUN levels have been reported. To treat an overdose of fenoprofen, empty stomach immediately by inducing emesis with ipecac syrup or by gastric lavage. Administer activated charcoal via nasogastric tube. Provide symptomatic and supportive measures (respiratory support and correction of fluid and electrolyte imbalances). Monitor laboratory parameters and vital signs closely. Dialysis is of little value.

☑ Special considerations

Besides those relevant to all *NSAIDs,* consider the following recommendations.

- Fenoprofen has been used to treat fever, acute gouty arthritis, and juvenile arthritis.
- Monitor for potential CNS effects. Institute safety measures to prevent injury.
- Monitor renal, hepatic, and auditory function in patients on long-term therapy. Stop drug if abnormalities occur.

Patient education

- Tell patient to avoid activities that require alertness or concentration until CNS effects of drug are known.
- Instruct patient in safety measures to prevent injury.
- Advise patient to call for specific instruction before taking OTC analgesics.

Geriatric use

- Patients over age 60 may be more susceptible to the toxic effects of fenoprofen, especially adverse GI reactions. Use with caution.
- The effects of drug on renal prostaglandins may cause fluid retention and edema, a significant drawback for elderly patients and those with heart failure.

Pediatric use

- Safe use of fenoprofen in children has not been established. Drug is not recommended for use in children under age 14.

Breast-feeding

- Because drug occurs in breast milk, avoid use in breast-feeding women.

fentanyl citrate
Sublimaze

fentanyl transdermal system
Duragesic-25, Duragesic-50, Duragesic-75, Duragesic-100

fentanyl transmucosal
Fentanyl Oralet

Pharmacologic classification: opioid agonist
Therapeutic classification: analgesic, adjunct to anesthesia, anesthetic
Controlled substance schedule II
Pregnancy risk category C

How supplied

Available by prescription only
Injection: 50 mcg/ml
Transdermal system: patches designed to release 25 mcg, 50 mcg, 75 mcg, or 100 mcg of fentanyl/hour.
Transmucosal: 200 mcg, 300 mcg, 400 mcg

Indications, route, and dosage

Preoperatively
Adults: 50 to 100 mcg I.M. 30 to 60 minutes before surgery. Alternatively, one oralet unit consisting of 200 mcg, 300 mcg, or 400 mcg P.O. for patient to suck until dissolved, 20 to 40 minutes before surgery.
Adjunct to general anesthetic
Low-dose regimen for minor procedures
Adults: 2 mcg/kg I.V.
Moderate-dose regimen for major procedures
Adults: Initial dose is 2 to 20 mcg/kg I.V.; may give additional doses of 25 to 100 mcg I.V. or I.M. p.r.n.
High-dose regimen for complicated procedures
Adults: Initial dose is 20 to 50 mcg/kg; additional doses of 25 mcg to one half the initial dose may be administered p.r.n.
Adjunct to regional anesthesia
Adults: 50 to 100 mcg I.M. or slow I.V. over 1 to 2 minutes.
Induction and maintenance of anesthesia
Children age 2 to 12: Reduced dose as low as 2 to 3 mcg/kg.
Postoperative analgesic
Adults: 50 to 100 mcg I.M. q 1 to 2 hours, p.r.n.
Management of chronic pain in patients who cannot be managed by lesser means
Adults: Apply one transdermal system to a portion of the upper torso on an area of skin that is not irritated and has not been irradiated. Initiate therapy with the 25-mcg/hour system; adjust dosage as needed and tolerated. Each system may be worn for 72 hours.
✦ ***Dosage adjustment.*** Lower doses are usually indicated for elderly patients because they may be more sensitive to drug's therapeutic and adverse effects.

Pharmacodynamics

Analgesic action: Fentanyl binds to the opiate receptors as an agonist to alter the patient's perception of painful stimuli, thus providing analgesia for moderate to severe pain. Its CNS and respiratory depressant effects are similar to those of morphine. Drug has little hypnotic activity and rarely causes histamine release.

Pharmacokinetics

- *Absorption:* Onset of action after I.V. administration is immediate; within 7 to 8 minutes of I.M. injection; within 5 to 15 minutes of transmucosal use; onset after transdermal use may take several hours as it is absorbed through the skin. Peak effect after I.V. use occurs in 3 to 5 minutes; after I.M. or transmucosal use, 20 to 30 minutes; after transdermal use, 1 to 3 days.
- *Distribution:* Redistribution has been suggested as the main cause of the brief analgesic effect of fentanyl.
- *Metabolism:* Drug is metabolized in the liver.
- *Excretion:* Fentanyl is excreted in the urine as metabolites and unchanged drug. Elimination half-life is about 7 hours after parenteral use, 5 to 15 hours after transmucosal use, and 18 hours after transdermal use.

Contraindications and precautions

Contraindicated in patients with known intolerance of drug. Use cautiously in elderly or debilitated patients and in those with head injuries, increased CSF pressure, COPD, decreased respiratory reserve, compromised respirations, arrhythmias, or hepatic, renal, or cardiac disease.

Interactions

Concomitant use with *other CNS depressants (narcotic analgesics, general anesthetics, antihistamines, phenothiazines, barbiturates, benzodiazepines, sedative-hypnotics, tricyclic antidepres-*

sants, alcohol, muscle relaxants) potentiates drug's respiratory and CNS depression, sedation, and hypotensive effects. Concomitant use with *cimetidine* may also increase respiratory and CNS depression, causing confusion, disorientation, apnea, or seizures; such use requires that dosage of fentanyl be reduced by one quarter to one third.

Drug accumulation and enhanced effects may result from concomitant use with other *drugs that are extensively metabolized in the liver (rifampin, phenytoin, digitoxin*); combined use with *anticholinergics* may cause paralytic ileus.

Patients who become physically dependent on drug may experience acute withdrawal syndrome if given a *narcotic antagonist*.

Severe CV depression may result from concomitant use with *general anesthetics; diazepam* may produce CV depression when given with high doses of fentanyl.

When used to supplement conduction anesthesia, such as *spinal anesthesia* and some *peridural anesthetics*, fentanyl can alter respiration by blocking intercostal nerves.

When used with fentanyl, *droperidol* may cause hypotension and a decrease in pulmonary artery pressure. (A droperidol-fentanyl combination, Innovar, is available.) The manufacturer warns that fentanyl should not be given to a patient who has received *MAO inhibitors* within the past 14 days.

Effects on diagnostic tests

Drug increases plasma amylase and lipase levels.

Adverse reactions

CNS: *sedation, somnolence, clouded sensorium, euphoria,* dizziness, headache, *confusion, asthenia,* nervousness, hallucinations, anxiety, depression.
CV: *hypotension,* hypertension, ***arrhythmias,*** chest pain.
GI: *nausea, vomiting, constipation,* ileus, abdominal pain, *dry mouth,* anorexia, diarrhea, dyspepsia.
GU: *urine retention.*
Respiratory: ***respiratory depression,*** hypoventilation, dyspnea, apnea.
Skin: reaction at application site (erythema, papules, edema), *pruritus, diaphoresis.*
Other: physical dependence.

Overdose and treatment

The most common signs and symptoms of fentanyl overdose are an extension of its actions. They include CNS depression, respiratory depression, and miosis (pinpoint pupils). Other acute toxic effects include hypotension, bradycardia, hypothermia, shock, apnea, cardiopulmonary arrest, circulatory collapse, pulmonary edema, and seizures.

To treat acute overdose, first establish adequate respiratory exchange via a patent airway and ventilation as needed; administer a narcotic antagonist (naloxone) to reverse respiratory depression. (Because the duration of action of fentanyl is longer than that of naloxone, repeated dosing is necessary.) Naloxone should not be given unless the patient has clinically significant respiratory or CV depression. Monitor vital signs closely.

Provide symptomatic and supportive treatment (continued respiratory support, correction of fluid or electrolyte imbalance). Monitor laboratory parameters, vital signs, and neurologic status closely.

☑ Special considerations

Besides those relevant to all *opioid (narcotic) agonists,* consider the following recommendations.

- Observe patient for delayed onset of respiratory depression. The high lipid solubility of fentanyl may contribute to this potential adverse effect.
- Monitor patient's heart rate. Fentanyl may cause bradycardia. Pretreatment with an anticholinergic (such as atropine or glycopyrrolate) may minimize this effect.
- High doses can produce muscle rigidity. This effect can be reversed by naloxone.
- Many anesthesiologists use epidural and intrathecal fentanyl as a potent adjunct to epidural anesthesia.

Transdermal form

- Transdermal fentanyl is not recommended for postoperative pain.
- Dosage equivalent charts are available to calculate the fentanyl transdermal dose based on daily morphine intake—for example, for every 90 mg of oral morphine or 15 mg of I.M. morphine per 24 hours, 25 mcg/hour of transdermal fentanyl is required. Some patients will require alternative means of opiate administration when the dose exceeds 300 mcg/hour.
- Dosage adjustments in patients using the transdermal system should be made gradually. Reaching steady-state levels of a new dose may take up to 6 days; delay dose adjustment until after at least two applications.
- Monitor patients who develop adverse reactions to the transdermal system for at least 12 hours after removal. Serum levels of fentanyl drop very gradually and may take as long as 17 hours to decline by 50%.
- Most patients experience good control of pain for 3 days while wearing the transdermal system, although a few may need a new application after 48 hours. Because serum fentanyl concentration rises for the first 24 hours after application, analgesic effect cannot be evaluated for the first day. Be sure the patient has adequate supplemental analgesic to prevent breakthrough pain.
- When reducing opiate therapy or switching to a different analgesic, withdraw the transdermal system gradually. Because fentanyl's serum level drops very gradually after removal, give half of the equianalgesic dose of the new analgesic 12 to 18 hours after removal.

Patient education

- Teach patient proper application of the transdermal patch. Clip hair at the application site, but do not use a razor, which may irritate the skin. Wash area with clear water if necessary, but not with soaps, oils, lotions, alcohol, or other substances that may irritate the skin or prevent adhesion. Dry area completely before application.

• Tell patient to remove the transdermal system from the package just before applying. Hold in place for 10 to 20 seconds, and be sure the edges of the patch adhere to the patient's skin.
• Teach patient to dispose of the transdermal patch by folding so the adhesive side adheres to itself and then flushing it down the toilet.
• If another patch is needed after 72 hours, tell patient to apply to a new site.

Geriatric use
• Use with caution in elderly patients.

Pediatric use
• Safe use in children under age 2 has not been established for parenteral use and children of all ages for transdermal system.

Breast-feeding
• Drug occurs in breast milk; administer cautiously to breast-feeding women.

ferrous fumarate
Femiron, Feostat, Fumasorb, Fumerin, Hemocyte, Ircon, Ircon-FA, Neo-Fer*, Nephro-Fer, Novofumar*, Palafer*, Span-FF

Pharmacologic classification: oral iron supplement
Therapeutic classification: hematinic
Pregnancy risk category A

How supplied
Available without a prescription. Ferrous fumarate is 33% elemental iron.
Tablets: 63 mg, 195 mg, 200 mg, 324 mg, 325 mg, 350 mg
Tablets (chewable): 100 mg
Capsules (extended-release): 325 mg
Suspension: 100 mg/5 ml
Drops: 45 mg/0.6 ml

Indications, route, and dosage
Iron-deficiency states
Adults: 50 to 100 mg P.O. of elemental iron. t.i.d. Adjust dose gradually, as needed and as tolerated.
Children: 4 to 6 mg/kg P.O. daily divided into three doses.
✦ ***Dosage adjustment.*** Elderly patients may need higher doses because reduced gastric secretions and achlorhydria may lower capacity for iron absorption.

Pharmacodynamics
Hematinic action: Ferrous fumarate replaces iron, an essential component in the formation of hemoglobin.

Pharmacokinetics
• *Absorption:* Iron is absorbed from the entire length of the GI tract, but primary absorption sites are the duodenum and proximal jejunum. Up to 10% of iron is absorbed by healthy individuals; patients with iron-deficiency anemia may absorb up to 60%. Enteric coating and some extended-release formulas have decreased absorption because they are designed to release iron past the points of highest absorption; food may decrease absorption by 33% to 50%.
• *Distribution:* Iron is transported through GI mucosal cells directly into the blood, where it is immediately bound to a carrier protein, transferrin, and transported to the bone marrow for incorporation into hemoglobin. Iron is highly protein-bound.
• *Metabolism:* Iron is liberated by the destruction of hemoglobin, but is conserved and reused by the body.
• *Excretion:* Healthy individuals lose only small amounts of iron each day. Men and postmenopausal women lose about 1 mg/day, and premenopausal women about 1.5 mg/day. The loss usually occurs in nails, hair, feces, and urine; trace amounts are lost in bile and sweat.

Contraindications and precautions
Contraindicated in patients with primary hemochromatosis or hemosiderosis, hemolytic anemia unless iron deficiency anemia is also present, peptic ulcer disease, regional enteritis, or ulcerative colitis and in those receiving repeated blood transfusions. Use cautiously on long-term basis.

Interactions
Ascorbic acid (vitamin C) increases ferrous fumarate absorption. *Antacids, cholestyramine, pancreatic extracts,* and *vitamin E* decrease ferrous fumarate absorption (separate doses by 1- to 2-hour intervals); *doxycycline* may interfere with ferrous fumarate absorption even when doses are separated; *chloramphenicol* delays response to iron therapy. Concomitant use of ferrous fumarate and *tetracycline* inhibits absorption of both drugs; give tetracycline 3 hours after or 2 hours before iron supplement.

Ferrous fumarate decreases *penicillamine* absorption; separate doses by at least 2 hours. Drug may decrease absorption of *quinolones.*

Effects on diagnostic tests
Ferrous fumarate blackens feces and may interfere with tests for occult blood in the stool; the guaiac test and orthotoluidine test may yield false-positive results, but the benzidine test is usually not affected.

Iron overload may decrease uptake of technetium 99m and thus interfere with skeletal imaging.

Adverse reactions
GI: *nausea,* epigastric pain, vomiting, *constipation,* diarrhea, black stools, anorexia.
Other: temporary staining of teeth (with suspension and drops).

Overdose and treatment
The lethal dose of iron is between 200 to 250 mg/kg; fatalities have occurred with lower doses. Symptoms may follow ingestion of 20 to 60 mg/kg. Clinical signs of acute overdose may occur as follows.

Between 30 minutes and 8 hours after ingestion, patient may experience lethargy, nausea and vomiting, green then tarry stools, weak and rapid pulse, hypotension, dehydration, acidosis, and coma. If death does not immediately ensue, symptoms may clear for about 24 hours.

At 12 to 48 hours, symptoms may return, accompanied by diffuse vascular congestion, pulmonary edema, shock, seizures, anuria, and hyperthermia. Death may follow.

Treatment requires immediate support of airway, respiration, and circulation. In conscious patient with intact gag reflex, induce emesis with ipecac; if not, empty stomach by gastric lavage. Follow emesis with lavage, using a 1% sodium bicarbonate solution, to convert iron to less irritating, poorly absorbed form. (Phosphate solutions have been used, but carry hazard of other adverse effects.) X-ray abdomen to determine continued presence of excess iron; if serum iron levels exceed 350 mg/dl, deferoxamine may be used for systemic chelation.

Survivors are likely to sustain organ damage, including pyloric or antral stenosis, hepatic cirrhosis, CNS damage, and intestinal obstruction.

☑ Special considerations

- Drug may cause dark-colored stools.
- Drug may stain teeth.

Patient education

- Instruct patient to take tablets with orange juice or water, but not with milk or antacids.
- Tell patient to take suspension with straw and place drops at back of throat.

Geriatric use

- Iron-induced constipation is common in elderly patients; stress proper diet to these patients.

Pediatric use

- Iron overdose may be fatal; treat *immediately.*

Breast-feeding

- Iron supplements are often recommended for breast-feeding women; no adverse effects of such use have been documented.

ferrous gluconate

Apo-Ferrous Gluconate*, Fergon, Ferralet, Fertinic*, Novoferrogluc*, Simron

Pharmacologic classification: oral iron supplement
Therapeutic classification: hematinic
Pregnancy risk category A

How supplied

Available without a prescription. Ferrous gluconate is 11.6% elemental iron.
Tablets: 300 mg (contains 35 mg Fe^{+}), 320 mg, 325 mg (320-mg tablet contains 37 mg Fe^{+})
Capsules: 86 mg (contains 10 mg Fe^{+}), 325 mg (contains 38 mg Fe^{+})
Elixir: 300 mg/5 ml (contains 35 mg Fe^{+})

Indications, route, and dosage

Iron deficiency

Adults: 325 mg P.O. q.i.d., dosage increased as needed and tolerated, up to 650 mg q.i.d.
Children age 2 to 12: 3 mg/kg/day P.O. in three or four divided doses.
Children age 6 months to 2 years: Up to 6 mg/kg/day in three or four divided doses.
Infants: 10 to 25 mg/day P.O. divided into three or four doses.

✦ ***Dosage adjustment.*** Elderly patients may need higher doses because reduced gastric secretions and achlorhydria may lower capacity for iron absorption.

Pharmacodynamics

Hematinic action: Ferrous gluconate replaces iron, an essential component in the formation of hemoglobin.

Pharmacokinetics

- *Absorption:* Iron is absorbed from the entire length of the GI tract, but primary absorption sites are the duodenum and proximal jejunum. Up to 10% of iron is absorbed by healthy individuals; patients with iron-deficiency anemia may absorb up to 60%. Food may decrease absorption by 33% to 50%.
- *Distribution:* Iron is transported through GI mucosal cells directly into the blood, where it is immediately bound to a carrier protein, transferrin, and transported to the bone marrow for incorporation into hemoglobin. Iron is highly protein-bound.
- *Metabolism:* Iron is liberated by the destruction of hemoglobin, but is conserved and reused by the body.
- *Excretion:* Healthy individuals lose only small amounts of iron each day. Men and postmenopausal women lose about 1 mg/day, premenopausal women about 1.5 mg/day. Loss usually occurs in nails, hair, feces, and urine; trace amounts are lost in bile and sweat.

Contraindications and precautions

Contraindicated in patients with peptic ulceration, regional enteritis, ulcerative colitis, hemosiderosis, primary hemochromatosis, or hemolytic anemia unless iron deficiency anemia is also present and in those receiving repeated blood transfusions. Use cautiously on long-term basis.

Interactions

Ascorbic acid (vitamin C) increases ferrous gluconate absorption. *Antacids, cholestyramine, pancreatic extracts,* and *vitamin E* decrease ferrous gluconate absorption (separate doses by 1- to 2-hour intervals); *doxycycline* may interfere with ferrous gluconate absorption even when doses are separated; *chloramphenicol* delays response to iron therapy. Concomitant use of ferrous gluconate and *tetracycline* inhibits absorption of both drugs; give tetracycline 3 hours after or 2 hours before iron supplement.

Ferrous gluconate decreases *penicillamine* absorption; separate doses by at least 2 hours. Drug may decrease absorption of *quinolones*.

Effects on diagnostic tests

Ferrous gluconate blackens feces and may interfere with test for occult blood in the stools; the guaiac test and orthotoluidine test may yield false-positive results, but the benzidine test is usually not affected.

Iron overload may decrease uptake of technetium 99m and thus interfere with skeletal imaging.

Adverse reactions

GI: *nausea*, epigastric pain, vomiting, *constipation*, diarrhea, *black stools*, anorexia.
Other: temporary staining of teeth (with elixir).

Overdose and treatment

The lethal dose of iron is between 200 to 250 mg/kg; fatalities have occurred with lower doses. Symptoms may follow ingestion of 20 to 60 mg/kg. Clinical signs of acute overdose may occur as follows.

Between 30 minutes and 8 hours after ingestion, patient may experience lethargy, nausea and vomiting, green then tarry stools, weak and rapid pulse, hypotension, dehydration, acidosis, and coma. If death does not immediately ensue, symptoms may clear for about 24 hours.

At 12 to 48 hours, symptoms may return, accompanied by diffuse vascular congestion, pulmonary edema, shock, seizures, anuria, and hyperthermia. Death may follow.

Treatment requires immediate support of airway, respiration, and circulation. In conscious patient with intact gag reflex, induce emesis with ipecac; if not, empty stomach by gastric lavage. Follow emesis with lavage, using a 1% sodium bicarbonate solution, to convert iron to less irritating, poorly absorbed form. (Phosphate solutions have been used, but carry hazard of other adverse effects.) Take abdominal X-ray to determine continued presence of excess iron; if serum iron levels exceed 350 mg/dl, deferoxamine may be used for systemic chelation.

Survivors are likely to sustain organ damage, including pyloric or antral stenosis, hepatic cirrhosis, CNS damage, and intestinal obstruction.

☑ Special considerations

- Drug can be given between meals or with some food, but absorption may be decreased.

Geriatric use

- Iron-induced constipation is common in elderly patients; stress proper diet to these patients.

Pediatric use

- Overdose may be fatal; treat *immediately.*

Breast-feeding

- Iron supplements are often recommended for breast-feeding women; no adverse effects of such use have been documented.

ferrous sulfate

Apo-Ferrous Sulfate*, Feosol, Feratab, Fer-In-Sol, Fer-Iron, Fero-Grad-500*, Fero-Gradumet, Ferospace, Ferralyn Lanacaps, Ferra-TD, Mol-Iron, Novoferrosulfa*, PMS Ferrous Sulfate*, Slow FE

Pharmacologic classification: oral iron supplement
Therapeutic classification: hematinic
Pregnancy risk category A

How supplied

Available without a prescription. Ferrous sulfate is 20% elemental iron; dried and powdered (exsiccated), it is about 32% elemental iron.
Tablets: 195 mg, 300 mg, 324 mg, 325 mg; 200 mg (exsiccated); 160 mg (exsiccated, extended-release); 525 mg (timed-release)
Capsules: 150 mg, 190 mg, 250 mg
Capsules (extended-release): 150 mg, 159 mg, 250 mg
Syrup: 90 mg/5 ml
Elixir: 220 mg/5 ml
Liquid: 75 mg/0.6 ml, 125 mg/ml

Indications, route, and dosage

Iron deficiency
Adults: 300 mg P.O. b.i.d.; dosage gradually increased to 300 mg q.i.d. as needed and tolerated. For extended-release capsule, 150 to 250 mg P.O. once or twice daily; for extended-release tablets, 160 to 525 mg once or twice daily.
Children age 2 to 12: 3 mg/kg/day P.O. in three or four divided doses.
Children age 6 months to 2 years: Up to 6 mg/kg/day P.O. in three or four divided doses.
Infants: 10 to 25 mg/day P.O. in three or four divided doses.

✦ ***Dosage adjustment.*** Elderly patients may need higher doses because reduced gastric secretions and achlorhydria may lower capacity for iron absorption.

Pharmacodynamics

Hematinic action: Ferrous sulfate replaces iron, an essential component in the formation of hemoglobin.

Pharmacokinetics

- *Absorption:* Iron is absorbed from the entire length of the GI tract, but primary absorption sites are the duodenum and proximal jejunum. Up to 10% of iron is absorbed by healthy individuals; patients with iron-deficiency anemia may absorb up to 60%. Enteric coating and some extended-release formulas have decreased absorption because they are designed to release iron past the points of highest absorption; food may decrease absorption by 33% to 50%.
- *Distribution:* Iron is transported through GI mucosal cells directly into the blood, where it is immediately bound to a carrier protein, transferrin,

and transported to the bone marrow for incorporation into hemoglobin. Iron is highly protein-bound.
• *Metabolism:* Iron is liberated by the destruction of hemoglobin, but is conserved and reused by the body.
• *Excretion:* Healthy individuals lose very little iron each day. Men and postmenopausal women lose about 1 mg/day, and premenopausal women about 1.5 mg/day. The loss usually occurs in nails, hair, feces, and urine; trace amounts are lost in bile and sweat.

Contraindications and precautions

Contraindicated in patients with hemosiderosis, primary hemochromatosis, hemolytic anemia unless iron deficiency anemia is also present, peptic ulceration, ulcerative colitis, or regional enteritis and in those receiving repeated blood transfusions. Use cautiously on long-term basis.

Interactions

Ascorbic acid (vitamin C) increases ferrous sulfate absorption. *Antacids, cholestyramine, pancreatic extracts*, and *vitamin E* decrease ferrous sulfate absorption (separate doses by 1- to 2-hour intervals); *doxycycline* may interfere with ferrous sulfate absorption even when doses are separated; *chloramphenicol* delays response to iron therapy. Concomitant use of ferrous sulfate and *tetracycline* inhibits absorption of both drugs; give tetracycline 3 hours after or 2 hours before iron supplement.

Ferrous sulfate decreases *penicillamine* absorption; separate doses by at least 2 hours. Drug may decrease the absorption of *quinolones*.

Effects on diagnostic tests

Ferrous sulfate blackens feces and may interfere with tests for occult blood in the stool; the guaiac test and orthotoluidine test may yield false-positive results, but the benzidine test is usually not affected.

Iron overload may decrease uptake of technetium 99m and thus interfere with skeletal imaging.

Adverse reactions

GI: *nausea*, epigastric pain, vomiting, *constipation, black stools*, diarrhea, anorexia.
Other: temporary staining of teeth (with liquid forms).

Overdose and treatment

The lethal dose of iron is 200 to 250 mg/kg; fatalities have occurred with lower doses. Symptoms may follow ingestion of 20 to 60 mg/kg. Clinical signs of acute overdose may occur as follows.

Between 30 minutes to 8 hours after ingestion, patient may experience lethargy, nausea and vomiting, green then tarry stools, weak and rapid pulse, hypotension, dehydration, acidosis, and coma. If death does not immediately ensue, symptoms may clear for about 24 hours.

At 12 to 48 hours, symptoms may return, accompanied by diffuse vascular congestion, pulmonary edema, shock, seizures, anuria, and hyperthermia. Death may follow.

Treatment requires immediate support of airway, respiration, and circulation. In conscious patient with intact gag reflex, induce emesis with ipecac; if not, empty stomach by gastric lavage. Follow emesis with lavage, using a 1% sodium bicarbonate solution, to convert iron to less irritating, poorly absorbed form. (Phosphate solutions have been used, but carry hazard of other adverse effects.) Take abdominal X-ray to determine continued presence of excess iron; if serum iron levels exceed 350 mg/dl, deferoxamine may be used for systemic chelation.

Survivors are likely to sustain organ damage, including pyloric or antral stenosis, hepatic cirrhosis, CNS damage, and intestinal obstruction.

☑ Special considerations

• Drug may cause dark-colored stools.
• Drug may stain teeth.

Patient education

• Instruct patient not to crush or chew extended-release forms.
• Inform parents that three or four tablets can cause serious iron poisoning in children.

Geriatric use

• Iron-induced constipation is common in elderly patients; stress proper diet to minimize this adverse effect.

Pediatric use

• Iron extended-release capsules or tablets are usually not recommended for children. Overdose may be fatal; *treat immediately*.

Breast-feeding

• Iron supplements often are recommended for breast-feeding women; no adverse effects have been documented.

fexofenadine hydrochloride

Allegra

Pharmacologic classification: H_1-receptor antagonist
Therapeutic classification: antihistaminic
Pregnancy risk category C

How supplied

Available by prescription only
Capsules: 60 mg

Indications, route, and dosage

Seasonal allergic rhinitis
Adults and children age 12 and older: 60 mg P.O. b.i.d.
✦ ***Dosage adjustment.*** In patients with impaired renal function, 60 mg P.O. once daily.

Pharmacodynamics

Antihistaminic action: Fexofenadine's principal effects are mediated through a selective inhibition of peripheral H_1 receptors.

Pharmacokinetics
- *Absorption:* Drug is rapidly absorbed.
- *Distribution:* Fexofenadine is 60% to 70% bound to plasma protein.
- *Metabolism:* About 5% of drug is metabolized.
- *Excretion:* Mainly excreted in feces; less so in urine. Mean elimination half-life of drug is 14.4 hours.

Contraindications and precautions
Contraindicated in patients with hypersensitivity to drug or its components. Use cautiously in patients with impaired renal function.

Interactions
None reported.

Effects on diagnostic tests
None reported.

Adverse reactions
CNS: fatigue, drowsiness.
GI: nausea, dyspepsia.
Other: viral infection, dysmenorrhea.

Overdose and treatment
Overdose of up to 800 mg did not result in significant clinical adverse reactions. If overdosage occurs, treatment should be symptomatic or supportive. Fexofenadine is not effectively removed by hemodialysis.

☑ Special considerations
- There is no information to indicate that abuse or dependency occurs with fexofenadine use.

Patient education
- Caution patient not to perform hazardous activities if drowsiness occurs with drug use.
- Instruct patient not to exceed prescribed dosage and to take drug only when needed.

Pediatric use
- Safety and effectiveness in children under age 12 have not been established.

Breast-feeding
- It is not known if drug is excreted in breast milk. Caution is recommended when administering fexofenadine to breast-feeding women.

fibrinolysin and deoxyribonuclease, combined (bovine)
Elase

Pharmacologic classification: proteolytic enzyme
Therapeutic classification: topical debriding
Pregnancy risk category C

How supplied
Available by prescription only
Dry powder: 25 units fibrinolysin and 15,000 units deoxyribonuclease in a 30-ml vial
Ointment: 1 unit/g fibrinolysin and 666.6 units/g deoxyribonuclease in 10-g and 30-g tubes

Indications, route, and dosage
Topical debridement of inflamed and infected skin lesions and wounds
Adults and children: Apply ointment or solution as a spray at intervals for as long as enzyme action is desired, usually at least once daily, but b.i.d. or t.i.d. may be preferred; apply solution as a wet dressing t.i.d. or q.i.d.
Intravaginal treatment of cervicitis and vaginitis
Adults: Using applicator, insert 5 ml of ointment (or 10 ml of solution) high into the vagina once daily h.s. for 5 days, or as prescribed. After 1 or 2 minutes, insert tampon if using solution. Remove tampon before next treatment.
Irrigating agent for the treatment of abscesses, empyema cavities, fistulae, sinus tracts, or subcutaneous hematomas
Adults: Irrigate and replace solution q 6 to 10 hours.

Pharmacodynamics
Debriding action: Digests necrotic tissues by proteolytic action; fibrinolysis is directed toward denatured proteins in devitalized tissues. Produces clear surfaces and facilitates wound healing.

Pharmacokinetics
- *Absorption:* Limited with topical use.
- *Distribution:* None.
- *Metabolism:* None.
- *Excretion:* None.

Contraindications and precautions
Contraindicated in patients with hypersensitivity to drug or to bovine products; not for parenteral use (fibrinolysin may be antigenic).

Interactions
None reported.

Effects on diagnostic tests
None reported.

Adverse reactions
Other: hyperemia (with high doses), hypersensitivity reactions.

Overdose and treatment
No information available.

☑ Special considerations
- Use solution promptly after preparation; do not use after 24 hours.
- Enzyme must be in constant contact with substrate surface for optimal activity. Therefore, remove dense, dry skin before applying drug.
- To apply ointment, clean wound and skin area carefully with 0.9% NaCl solution, hydrogen peroxide, or water; moisten thoroughly, then gently dry area. Apply a thin layer of ointment to the affected area, and cover with loose-fitting, nonadhering or pertrolatum gauze dressing.

• Change dressing at least once daily; flush away enzyme and debris before reapplication.
• Solution may be applied topically as a spray or as a wet dressing. As a spray, apply using an atomizer; as a wet dressing, saturate gauze dressing with solution and pack affected area.
• Avoid using spray near eyes or mucous membranes.

Patient education
• Be sure patient understands how to use product; teach correct application.

Breast-feeding
• Clean breast area thoroughly before breast-feeding.

filgrastim (granulocyte colony stimulating factor, G-CSF)
Neupogen

Pharmacologic classification: biologic response modifier
Therapeutic classification: colony stimulating factor
Pregnancy risk category C

How supplied
Available by prescription only
Injection: 300 mcg/ml in 1-ml and 1.6-ml single-dose vials

Indications, route, and dosage
To decrease incidence of infection after cancer chemotherapy for nonmyeloid malignancies, chronic severe neutropenia, after bone marrow transplantation in cancer patients; to treat ◊ agranulocytosis, ◊ pancytopenia with colchicine overdose, ◊ acute leukemia, ◊ myelodysplastic syndrome, ◊ hematologic toxicity with zidovudine antiviral therapy
Adults: Initially, 5 mcg/kg S.C. or I.V. as a single daily dose; may increase dose incrementally by 5 mcg/kg for each course of chemotherapy according to duration and severity of absolute neutrophil count (ANC) nadir.

Do not administer earlier than 24 hours after or within 24 hours before chemotherapy.

Filgrastim should be given daily for up to 2 weeks until ANC nadir reaches 10,000/mm^3 after the anticipated chemoinduced ANC nadir. Duration of treatment depends on the myelosuppressive potential of the chemotherapy used. Discontinue if ANC nadir surpasses 10,000/mm^3.
◊ AIDS
Adults: 0.3 to 3.6 mcg/kg/day S.C. or I.V.
◊ Aplastic anemia
Adults: 800 to 1,200 mcg/m^2/day S.C. or I.V.
◊ Hairy cell leukemia, myelodysplasia
Adults: 15 to 500 mcg/m^2/day S.C. or I.V.

Pharmacodynamics
Immunostimulant action: Filgrastim is a naturally occurring cytokine glycoprotein that stimulates proliferation, differentiation, and functional activity of neutrophils, causing a rapid rise in WBC counts within 2 to 3 days in patients with normal bone marrow function or 7 to 14 days in patients with bone marrow suppression. Blood counts return to pretreatment levels, usually within 1 week after therapy ends.

Pharmacokinetics
• *Absorption:* After S.C. bolus dose, blood levels suggest rapid absorption with peak levels in 2 to 8 hours.
• *Distribution:* Unknown.
• *Metabolism:* Unknown.
• *Excretion:* Elimination half-life is approximately 3½ hours.

Contraindications and precautions
Contraindicated in patients hypersensitive to proteins derived from *Escherichia coli* or to drug or its components.

Interactions
None reported.

Effects on diagnostic tests
WBC counts may be increased to 100,000/mm^3 or more. Transient increases in neutrophils, as well as reversible elevations in uric acid, LD, and alkaline phosphatase levels, have been reported. Transient decreases in blood pressure and increases in serum creatinine and aminotransferase levels were also reported.

Adverse reactions
CNS: headache, weakness.
CV: ***MI, arrhythmias,*** chest pain.
GI: *nausea, vomiting, diarrhea, mucositis,* stomatitis, constipation.
Hematologic: ***thrombocytopenia,*** leukocytosis.
Respiratory: dyspnea, cough.
Skin: *alopecia,* rash, cutaneous vasculitis.
Other: *skeletal pain, fever, fatigue, hypersensitivity reactions.*

Overdose and treatment
Maximum tolerated dose has not been determined. There have been no reports of overdose.

☑ Special considerations
• Store drug in refrigerator; do not freeze. Avoid shaking. Before injection, allow to reach room temperature for a maximum of 24 hours. Discard after 24 hours. Use only one dose per vial; do not reenter vial.
• Obtain CBC and platelet counts before and twice weekly during therapy.
• Filgrastim is not compatible with 0.9% NaCl.
• Regular monitoring of hematocrit and platelet counts is recommended.
• Adult respiratory distress syndrome may occur in septic patients because of the influx of neutrophils at the site of inflammation.
• MI and arrhythmias have occurred; closely monitor patients with preexisting cardiac conditions.

• Bone pain is the most frequent adverse reaction and may be controlled with nonnarcotic analgesics if mild to moderate or may require narcotic analgesics if severe.

Patient education
• Review "Information for Patients" section of package insert with patient. Thorough instruction is essential if home use is prescribed.
• When drug can be safely and effectively self-administered, instruct patient in proper dosage and administration techniques.
• Manufacturer has reimbursement hotline to answer questions about insurance reimbursement procedures. Hotline operates from Monday through Friday 9 a.m. to 5 p.m. Eastern Standard Time: 1-800-272-9376; in Washington, D.C., 1-202-637-6698.

Geriatric use
• No age-related problems have been reported.

Pediatric use
• Although efficacy is not established, there is no evidence of greater toxicity occurring in children than in adults.

Breast-feeding
• It is unknown if drug occurs in breast milk. Risk-to-benefit ratio must be assessed.

finasteride
Propecia, Proscar

Pharmacologic classification: steroid (synthetic 4-azasteroid) derivative
Therapeutic classification: androgen synthesis inhibitor
Pregnancy risk category X

How supplied
Available by prescription only
Tablets: 1 mg, 5 mg

Indications, route and dosage
Symptomatic benign prostatic hyperplasia (BPH), ◊ adjuvant therapy after radical prostatectomy, ◊ first-stage prostate cancer, ◊ acne, ◊ hirsutism
Adults: 5 mg P.O. daily, usually for 6 to 12 months.
Male pattern baldness (androgenetic alopecia)
Adults: 1 mg P.O. daily, usually for 3 months or more. Continued use is recommended to sustain benefit. Withdrawal of treatment leads to reversal of effect within 12 months.

Pharmacodynamics
Androgen synthesis inhibition action: Finasteride competitively inhibits steroid 5µ-reductase, an enzyme responsible for formation of the potent androgen 5µ-dihydrotestosterone (DHT) from testosterone. Because DHT influences development of the prostate gland, decreasing levels of this hormone in adult males should relieve the symptoms associated with BPH. In men with male pattern baldness, the balding scalp contains miniaturized hair follicles and increased amounts of DHT. Finasteride decreases scalp and serum DHT concentrations in these men.

Pharmacokinetics
• *Absorption:* Average bioavailability was 63% in one study. Maximum plasma concentrations are reached within 2 hours of a dose.
• *Distribution:* Finasteride is about 90% bound to plasma proteins. Drug crosses the blood-brain barrier.
• *Metabolism:* Drug is extensively metabolized by the liver; at least 2 metabolites have been identified. Metabolites are responsible for less than 20% of the drug's total activity.
• *Excretion:* 39% of an oral dose is excreted in urine as metabolites; 57%, in feces. No unchanged drug is found in urine.

Contraindications and precautions
Contraindicated in patients hypersensitive to drug. Although drug is not used in women, manufacturer indicates pregnancy as a contraindication.

Interactions
Small, clinically insignificant increases in *theophylline* clearance and decreased half-life (10%) have been observed.

Effects on diagnostic tests
Finasteride will decrease levels of prostate-specific antigen (PSA) even in prostate cancer. This does not indicate a beneficial effect.

Adverse reactions
GU: impotence, decreased volume of ejaculate.
Other: decreased libido.

Overdose and treatment
Experience with overdose is limited. Patients have received single doses of 400 mg and multiple doses of up to 80 mg daily for 3 months without adverse effects.

☑ Special considerations
• Closely evaluate patient for conditions that might mimic BPH before therapy, including hypotonic bladder, prostate cancer, infection, stricture, or other neurologic conditions.
• Because it is not possible to identify prospectively which patients will respond to finasteride, a minimum of 6 months of therapy may be necessary.
• Patients who have large residual urine volumes or severely diminished urine flows should be monitored carefully. Not all patients respond to drug, and these patients may not be candidates for finasteride therapy.
• Long-term effects of drug on the complications of BPH, including acute urinary obstruction, or the incidence of surgery are not known.
• No dosage adjustments are necessary in patients with renal impairment. Decreased urinary excretion of metabolites is associated with an increased excretion of metabolites in the feces.

• Sustained increases in serum PSA should be carefully evaluated. In patients receiving finasteride therapy, this could indicate noncompliance to therapy.
• Current investigations aim to determine drug's effectiveness as adjuvant therapy after radical prostatectomy; as adjunctive treatment of prostate cancer; acne, and hirsutism.

Patient education
• Advise female patient who is or may become pregnant not to handle crushed tablets because of risk of adverse effects on a male fetus.
• Instruct male patient whose sexual partner is or may become pregnant to avoid exposing her to his semen or to discontinue drug.
• Explain to male patients that drug may decrease the volume of ejaculate but does not appear to impair normal sexual function. However, impotence and decreased libido have occurred in less than 4% of patients treated with drug.
• Inform patient that Propecia is indicated for the treatment of male pattern hair loss in men only. It is not indicated for use in women

Geriatric use
• Although drug's elimination rate is decreased in elderly patients, dosage adjustments are not necessary.

Pediatric use
• Drug is not indicated for use in children.

Breast-feeding
• It is unknown if drug is excreted in breast milk; however, it is not indicated for use in women.

flavoxate hydrochloride
Urispas

Pharmacologic classification: flavone derivative
Therapeutic classification: urinary tract spasmolytic
Pregnancy risk category B

How supplied
Available by prescription only
Tablets (film-coated): 100 mg

Indications, route, and dosage
Symptomatic relief of dysuria, frequency, urgency, nocturia, incontinence, and suprapubic pain associated with urologic disorders
Adults and children over age 12: 100 to 200 mg P.O. t.i.d. or q.i.d.

Pharmacodynamics
Spasmolytic action: Flavoxate exerts a direct spasmolytic effect on smooth muscle, primarily in the urinary tract. Acting on the detrusor muscle, this agent increases bladder capacity in patients with bladder spasticity; by cholinergic blockade, drug also has local anesthetic and analgesic effects.

Pharmacokinetics
• *Absorption:* Drug is absorbed well from the GI tract; peak levels occur in approximately 2 hours.
• *Distribution:* Unknown.
• *Metabolism:* Unknown.
• *Excretion:* Drug is excreted in the urine; 10% to 30% appears in the urine within 6 hours.

Contraindications and precautions
Contraindicated in patients with pyloric or duodenal obstruction, obstructive intestinal lesions or ileus, achalasia, GI hemorrhage, or obstructive uropathies of lower urinary tract. Use cautiously in patients with or suspected of having glaucoma.

Interactions
Flavoxate may potentiate the effects of *CNS depressants.*

Effects on diagnostic tests
None reported.

Adverse reactions
CNS: *confusion* (especially in elderly patients), nervousness, dizziness, headache, drowsiness.
CV: tachycardia, palpitations.
EENT: *blurred vision,* disturbed eye accommodation, increased ocular tension.
GI: dry mouth, nausea, vomiting.
GU: dysuria.
Hematologic: eosinophila, leukopenia.
Skin: urticaria, dermatoses.
Other: fever.

Overdose and treatment
Clinical manifestations of overdose include clumsiness, dizziness, drowsiness, fever, flushing, hallucinations, shortness of breath, nervousness, restlessness, or irritability. Treatment begins with gastric lavage or emesis and may include physostigmine rarely in cases of otherwise refractory life-threatening emergencies.

☑ Special considerations
• Dosage may be reduced with improvement of symptoms.

Patient education
• Warn patient to avoid driving or other hazardous activities that require alertness because of potential for drowsiness, blurred vision, and confusion.

Geriatric use
• Warn family members that elderly patients are more likely to become confused.

Pediatric use
• Safety has not been established in children under age 12.

Breast-feeding
• It is unknown if drug is distributed into breast milk. Use cautiously in breast-feeding women.

flecainide acetate

Tambocor

Pharmacologic classification: benzamide derivative local anesthetic (amide)
Therapeutic classification: ventricular antiarrhythmic
Pregnancy risk category C

How supplied

Available by prescription only
Tablets: 50 mg, 100 mg, 150 mg

Indications, route, and dosage

Life-threatening ventricular tachycardia and PVCs

Adults: 100 mg P.O. q 12 hours; may increase in increments of 50 mg b.i.d. q 4 days until efficacy is achieved. Maximum dosage is 400 mg daily.

Paroxysmal supraventricular tachycardia, paroxysmal atrial fibrillation or flutter in patients without structural heart disease

Adults: 50 mg P.O. q 12 hours; may increase in increments of 50 mg b.i.d. q 4 days until efficacy is achieved. Maximum dosage is 300 mg/day.

✦ ***Dosage adjustment.*** Reduce dosage in patients with renal impairment (creatinine clearance below 35 ml/minute/1.73 m^2) beginning at 100 mg/day (50 mg b.i.d.); increase dosage cautiously at intervals longer than 4 days. For patients with less severe renal failure, initial dose is 100 mg q 12 hours, increasing cautiously at intervals longer than 4 days.

Pharmacodynamics

Antiarrhythmic action: A class IC antiarrhythmic agent, flecainide suppresses SA node automaticity and prolongs conduction in the atria, AV node, ventricles, accessory pathways, and His-Purkinje system. It has the most pronounced effect on the His-Purkinje system, as shown by QRS complex widening; this leads to a prolonged QT interval. The drug has relatively little effect on action potential duration except in Purkinje's fibers, where it shortens it. A proarrhythmic (arrhythmogenic) effect may result from the drug's potent effects on the conduction system. Effects on the sinus node are strongest in patients with sinus node disease (sick sinus syndrome). Flecainide also exerts a moderate negative inotropic effect.

Pharmacokinetics

- *Absorption:* Flecainide is rapidly and almost completely absorbed from the GI tract; bioavailability of commercially available tablets is 85% to 90%. Peak plasma levels usually occur within 2 to 3 hours.
- *Distribution:* Drug is apparently well distributed throughout the body. Only about 40% binds to plasma proteins. Trough serum levels ranging from 0.2 to 1 mcg/ml provide the greatest therapeutic benefit. Trough serum levels higher than 0.7 mcg/ml have been associated with increased adverse effects.
- *Metabolism:* Flecainide is metabolized in the liver to inactive metabolites. About 30% of an orally administered dose escapes metabolism and is excreted in the urine unchanged.
- *Excretion:* Elimination half-life averages about 20 hours. Plasma half-life may be prolonged in patients with heart failure and renal disease.

Contraindications and precautions

Contraindicated in patients with hypersensitivity to drug or cardiogenic shock and in those with preexisting second- or third-degree AV block or right bundle branch block when associated with a left hemiblock (in the absence of an artificial pacemaker).

Use cautiously in patients with heart failure, cardiomyopathy, severe renal or hepatic disease, prolonged QT interval, sick sinus syndrome, or blood dyscrasia.

Tambocor has demonstrated proarrythmic effects in patients with atrial fibrillation or flutter; therefore it is not recommended for use in these patients.

Interactions

Concomitant use with *digoxin* may cause increased serum digoxin levels; concomitant use with *beta-adrenergic blockers* (such as *propranolol*) may cause additive negative inotropic effects. When used concomitantly, *other antiarrhythmic drugs* may cause additive, synergistic, or antagonistic cardiac effects and may cause additive adverse effects. For example, *amiodarone* may increase serum flecainide levels; *disopyramide* may cause an additive negative inotropic effect; *verapamil* also may have an additive negative inotropic effect and may exacerbate AV nodal dysfunction.

Concomitant use with *acidifying and alkalizing agents* changes urinary pH, which in turn alters flecainide elimination; alkalization decreases renal flecainide excretion, and acidification increases it. When drugs that can markedly affect urine acidity (such as *ammonium chloride*) or alkalinity (such as *high-dose antacids, carbonic anhydrase inhibitors, sodium bicarbonate*) are given, monitor for possible subtherapeutic or toxic levels and effects. *Cimetidine* may decrease both the renal and nonrenal clearance of flecainide.

Effects on diagnostic tests

None reported.

Adverse reactions

CNS: *dizziness, headache,* fatigue, tremor, anxiety, insomnia, depression, malaise, paresthesia, ataxia, vertigo, *light-headedness, syncope,* asthenia.
CV: ***new or worsened arrhythmias,*** chest pain, flushing, edema, ***heart failure, cardiac arrest,*** palpitations.
EENT: *blurred vision and other visual disturbances.*
GI: nausea, constipation, abdominal pain, dyspepsia, vomiting, diarrhea, anorexia.
Skin: rash.
Other: *dyspnea,* fever.

Overdose and treatment

Clinical effects of overdose include increased PR and QT intervals, increased QRS complex duration, decreased myocardial contractility, conduction disturbances, and hypotension.

Treatment generally involves symptomatic and supportive measures along with ECG, blood pressure, and respiratory monitoring. Inotropic agents, including dopamine and dobutamine, may be used. Hemodynamic support, including use of an intra-aortic balloon pump and transvenous pacing, may be needed. Because of drug's long half-life, supportive measures may need to be continued for extended periods. Hemodialysis is ineffective in reducing serum drug levels.

☑ Special considerations

- Tambocor has been associated with excessive mortality or nonfatal cardiac arrest rate in national multicenter trials. Its use should be restricted to those patients in which the benefits outweigh the risks.
- Tambocor is a strong negative inotrope and may cause or worsen heart failure, especially in those with cardiomyopathy, preexisting heart failure, or low ejection fraction.
- Hypokalemia or hyperkalemia may alter drug effects and should be corrected before drug therapy begins.
- Initiation of therapy should be done in the hospital with careful monitoring of patients with symptomatic heart failure, sinus node dysfunction, sustained ventricular tachycardia, or underlying structural heart disease and in patients changing from another antiarrhythmic in whom discontinuation of current antiarrhythmic is likely to cause life-threatening arrhythmias.
- Loading doses may exacerbate arrhythmias and therefore are not recommended. Dosage adjustments should be made at intervals of at least 4 days because of drug's long half-life.
- Most patients can be adequately maintained on an every-12-hour dosage schedule, but some need to receive drug every 8 hours.
- Twice-daily dosing improves patient compliance.
- Drug's full therapeutic effect may take 3 to 5 days. I.V. lidocaine may be administered while awaiting full effect.
- Flecainide is a first class IC antiarrhythmic. Incidence of adverse effects increases when trough serum drug levels exceed 0.7 mcg/ml. Periodically monitor blood levels, especially in patients with renal failure or heart failure. Therapeutic levels range from 0.2 to 1.0 mcg/mL.
- Drug may increase acute and chronic endocardial pacing thresholds and may suppress ventricular escape rhythms. Pacing threshold should be determined before drug is administered, after 1 week of therapy, and regularly thereafter. It should not be given to patients with preexisting poor thresholds or nonprogrammable artificial pacemakers unless pacing rescue is available.
- In heart failure and myocardial dysfunction, initial dosage should not exceed 100 mg every 12 hours; common initial dosage is 50 mg every 12 hours.
- Use in hepatic impairment has not been fully evaluated; however, because flecainide is metabolized extensively (probably in the liver) it should be used in patients with significant hepatic impairment only when benefits clearly outweigh risks. Dosage reduction may be necessary and patients should be monitored carefully for signs of toxicity. Serum levels also must be monitored.

Geriatric use

- Elderly patients are more susceptible to adverse effects. Monitor patient carefully.

Pediatric use

- Safety and efficacy have not been established in children under age 18. Limited data suggest usefulness in management of paroxysmal reentrant supraventricular tachycardia.

Breast-feeding

- Limited data indicate that drug is excreted in breast milk. Breast-feeding is not recommended during flecainide therapy because of the risk of adverse effects on the infant.

floxuridine

FUDR

Pharmacologic classification: anti-metabolite (cell cycle–phase specific, S phase)
Therapeutic classification: antineoplastic
Pregnancy risk category D

How supplied

Available by prescription only
Injection: 500-mg vials

Indications, route, and dosage

Dosage and indications may vary. Check current literature for recommended protocol.

Palliative management of GI adenocarcinoma metastatic to the liver; brain, head, neck, gallbladder, bile duct cancer
Adults: 0.1 to 0.6 mg/kg daily by intra-arterial infusion; or 0.4 to 0.6 mg/kg daily into hepatic artery.

◊ ***Solid tumors***
Adults: 0.5 to 1 mg/kg daily by I.V. infusion for 6 to 15 days or until toxicity occurs; or 30 mg/kg daily by single injection for 5 days, then 15 mg/kg every other day for up to 11 days or until toxicity occurs.

Pharmacodynamics

Antineoplastic action: Floxuridine exerts its cytotoxic activity after conversion to its active form, by competitively inhibiting the enzyme thymidylate synthetase; this halts DNA synthesis and leads to cell death.

Pharmacokinetics

- *Absorption:* Drug is not administered orally.
- *Distribution:* Floxuridine crosses the blood-brain barrier to a limited extent.
- *Metabolism:* Floxuridine is metabolized to fluorouracil in the liver after intra-arterial infusions and rapid I.V. injections.
- *Excretion:* Approximately 60% of a dose is excreted through the lungs as carbon dioxide. A small

amount is excreted by the kidneys as unchanged drug and metabolites.

Contraindications and precautions

Contraindicated in patients with poor nutritional state, bone marrow suppression, or serious infection. Use cautiously in patients following high-dose pelvic radiation therapy or use of alkalating agents and in those with impaired renal or hepatic function.

Interactions

None significant.

Effects on diagnostic tests

Floxuridine therapy may increase serum concentrations of ALT, AST, alkaline phosphatase, bilirubin, and LD; these increases indicate drug-induced hepatotoxicity.

Adverse reactions

CNS: cerebellar ataxia, malaise, weakness, headache, lethargy, disorientation, confusion, euphoria.
CV: myocardial ischemia, angina.
EENT: blurred vision, nystagmus, photophobia, epistaxis.
GI: *anorexia, stomatitis, nausea, vomiting, diarrhea, bleeding, enteritis,* GI ulceration.
Hematologic: ***leukopenia, anemia, thrombocytopenia, agranulocytosis.***
Skin: *erythema,* dermatitis, pruritus, rash, alopecia, photosensitivity.
Other: thrombophlebitis, ***anaphylaxis,*** fever.

Overdose and treatment

Clinical manifestations of overdose include myelosuppression, diarrhea, alopecia, dermatitis, and hyperpigmentation.

Treatment is usually supportive and includes transfusion of blood components and antidiarrheal agents.

☑ Special considerations

- To reconstitute, use 5 ml sterile water for injection to give a concentration of 100 mg/ml.
- Dilute to appropriate volume for infusion device with D_5W or 0.9% NaCl solution.
- Administration by infusion pump maintains a continuous, uniform rate. Reconstituted drug solutions are stable for 14 days when refrigerated.
- Observe arterial perfused area. Check line for bleeding, blockage, displacement, or leakage.
- Drug is often administered via hepatic arterial infusion in treating hepatic metastases.
- Discontinue drug if severe skin and GI adverse reactions occur.
- Monitor patient's intake and output, CBC, and renal and hepatic function.
- Therapeutic effect may be delayed 1 to 6 weeks. Make sure patient is aware of time required for improvement.
- To prevent bleeding, avoid I.M. injections of drugs in patients with thrombocytopenia.

Patient education

- Advise patient to report nausea, vomiting, stomach pain, signs of infection, or unusual bruising or bleeding.
- Inform patient that excellent mouth care can help prevent oral adverse reactions.

Breast-feeding

- It is not known if drug occurs in breast milk. However, because of risk of serious adverse reactions, mutagenicity, and carcinogenicity in the infant, breast-feeding is not recommended.

fluconazole

Diflucan

Pharmacologic classification: bis-triazole derivative
Therapeutic classification: antifungal
Pregnancy risk category C

How supplied

Available by prescription only
Tablets: 50 mg, 100 mg, 150 mg, 200 mg
Injection: 200 mg/100 ml, 400 mg/200 ml
Suspension: 350 mg/35 ml, 1,400 mg/35 ml

Indications, route, and dosage

Oropharyngeal and esophageal candidiasis
Adults: 200 mg P.O. or I.V. on day 1 followed by 100 mg P.O. or I.V. once daily. As much as 400 mg daily has been used for esophageal disease. Treatment should continue for at least 2 weeks after resolution of symptoms.
Children: 6 mg/kg on day 1, followed by 3 mg/kg for at least 2 weeks.
Systemic candidiasis
Adults: Up to 400 mg P.O. or I.V. once daily. Treatment should be continued for at least 2 weeks after resolution of symptoms.
Cryptococcal meningitis
Adults: 400 mg I.V. or P.O. on day 1, followed by 200 mg once daily. Continue treatment for 10 to 12 weeks after CSF culture becomes negative. For suppression of relapse in patients with AIDS, give 200 mg once daily.
Vaginal candidiasis
Adults: 150 mg P.O. as a single dose.
Urinary tract infection or peritonitis
Adults: 50 to 200 mg P.O. or I.V. daily.
Prophylaxis in patients undergoing bone marrow transplantation
Adults: 400 mg P.O. or I.V. daily for several days before transplantation and 7 days after neutrophil count rises above 1,000 cells/mm^3.
◇ ***Candidal infection, long-term suppression in patients with HIV infection***
Adults: 100 to 200 mg P.O. or I.V. daily.
◇ ***Prophylaxis against mucocutaneous candidiasis, cryptococcosis, coccidioidomycosis, or histoplasmosis in patients with HIV infection***
Adults: 200 to 400 mg P.O. or I.V. daily.
Children and infants: 2 to 8 mg/kg P.O. daily.

✦ ***Dosage adjustment.*** Patients receiving hemodialysis should receive one full dose after each session.

Creatinine clearance (ml/min)	Percentage of usual adult dose
> 50	100
21 to 49	50
11 to 20	25

Pharmacodynamics
Antifungal action: Fluconazole exerts its fungistatic effects by inhibiting fungal cytochrome P-450 and interfering with sterols in the fungal cell. The spectrum of activity includes *Cryptococcus neoformans, Candida* sp. (including systemic *C. albicans), Aspergillus flavus, A. fumigatus, Coccidioides immitis,* and *Histoplasma capsulatum.*

Pharmacokinetics
- *Absorption:* After oral administration, absorption is rapid and complete. Peak plasma concentration after an oral dose occurs in 1 to 2 hours.
- *Distribution:* Fluconazole is well distributed to various sites, including CNS, saliva, sputum, blister fluid, urine, normal skin, nails, and blister skin. CNS concentrations approach 50% to 90% of that of serum. Fluconazole is 12% protein-bound.
- *Metabolism:* Fluconazole is partially metabolized.
- *Elimination:* Drug is primarily excreted via the kidneys. Over 80% of an administered dose is excreted unchanged in the urine. Excretion rate diminishes as renal function decreases.

Contraindications and precautions
Contraindicated in patients with hypersensitivity to drug and other drugs in the same classification.

Interactions
Concomitant use with *cimetidine* may reduce fluconazole's serum concentrations; use with *phenytoin* may significantly increase phenytoin serum levels. Fluconazole has been shown to increase the hypoglycemic effects of the *sulfonylureas tolbutamide, glyburide,* and *glipizide.* Fluconazole therapy may increase *cyclosporine* levels and may enhance the hypoprothrombinemic effects of *warfarin.*

Rifampin can lower fluconazole levels; *hydrochlorothiazide* has decreased fluconazole's clearance, raising the drug's serum levels. The incidence of elevated hepatic transaminase levels is higher in patients taking *rifampin, isoniazid sulfonylureas, phenytoin,* or *valproic acid.*

Fluconazole may interact with *cisapride,* and *astemizole* causing prolongation of the QT interval resulting in arrhythmias and serious CV effects.

Effects on diagnostic tests
Increased liver transaminase serum levels may occur with fluconazole.

Adverse reactions
CNS: headache.
GI: *nausea,* vomiting, abdominal pain, diarrhea.
Hepatic: ***hepatotoxicity*** (rare), elevated liver enzymes.
Skin: rash, ***Stevens-Johnson syndrome*** (rare).
Other: ***anaphylaxis.***

Overdose and treatment
Treatment is largely supportive.

☑ Special considerations
- Adjust dose in patients with renal dysfunction.
- Fluconazole is not compatible with other I.V. medications.
- Bioavailability of oral drug is comparable to I.V. dosing. Administer drug via oral route whenever possible.
- Adverse reactions (including transaminase elevations) are more frequent and more severe in patients with severe underlying illness (including AIDS and malignancies).

Breast-feeding
- Drug is excreted in breast milk at concentrations similar to those of plasma. Therefore, its use in breast-feeding women is not recommended.

flucytosine (5-FC)
Ancobon

Pharmacologic classification: fluorinated pyrimidine
Therapeutic classification: antifungal
Pregnancy risk category C

How supplied
Available by prescription only
Capsules: 250 mg, 500 mg

Indications, route, and dosage
***Severe fungal infections caused by susceptible strains of* Candida *and* Cryptococcus**
Adults and children weighing over 110 lb (50 kg): 50 to 150 mg/kg/day P.O., administered in divided doses q 6 hours.
Adults and children weighing below 110 lb: 1.5 to 4.5 g/m^2/day in four divided doses P.O.
◇ ***Chromomycosis***
Adults: 150 mg/kg P.O. daily.
✦ ***Dosage adjustment.*** In patients with renal failure who have a creatinine clearance of 50 ml/minute or less, reduce dosage by 20% to 80%. Alternatively, in patients with creatinine clearance of 20 to 40 ml/minute, increase dosage interval to q 12 hours; creatinine clearance of 10 to 20 ml/minute, increase dosage interval to q 24 hours; and for those with creatinine clearance below 10 ml/minute, increase dosage interval to q 24 to 48 hours. Serum levels should be monitored. Flucytosine is removed by hemodialysis and peritoneal dialysis.

Dosage of 20 to 50 mg/kg P.O. immediately after hemodialysis q 2 to 3 days ensures therapeutic blood levels.

Pharmacodynamics

Antifungal action: Flucytosine penetrates fungal cells, where it is converted to fluorouracil, which interferes with pyrimidine metabolism; it also may be converted to fluorodeoxyuredylic acid, which interferes with DNA synthesis. Because human cells lack the enzymes needed to convert drug to these toxic metabolites, flucytosine is selectively toxic to fungal, not host cells. It is active against some strains of *Cryptococcus* and *Candida*.

Pharmacokinetics

• *Absorption:* About 75% to 90% of an oral dose is absorbed. Peak serum concentrations occur at 2 to 6 hours after a dose. Food decreases rate of absorption.
• *Distribution:* Drug is distributed widely into the liver, kidneys, spleen, heart, bronchial secretions, joints, peritoneal fluid, and aqueous humor. CSF levels vary from 60% to 100% of serum levels. It is 2% to 4% bound to plasma proteins.
• *Metabolism:* Only small amounts of flucytosine are metabolized.
• *Excretion:* About 75% to 95% of a dose is excreted unchanged in urine; less than 10% is excreted unchanged in feces. Serum half-life is 2½ to 6 hours with normal renal function; as long as 1,160 hours with creatinine clearance below 2 ml/minute.

Contraindications and precautions

Contraindicated in patients with hypersensitivity to drug. Use cautiously in patients with impaired renal or hepatic function and bone marrow suppression.

Interactions

Flucytosine potentiates the efficacy and toxicity of *amphotericin B*.

Effects on diagnostic tests

Flucytosine causes falsely elevated creatinine values on iminohydrolase enzymatic assay.

Drug may increase alkaline phosphatase, AST, ALT, BUN, and serum creatinine levels and may decrease WBC, RBC, and platelet counts.

Adverse reactions

CNS: headache, vertigo, sedation, fatigue, weakness, confusion, hallucinations, psychosis, ataxia, hearing loss, paresthesia, parkinsonism, peripheral neuropathy.
CV: ***cardiac arrest.***
GI: nausea, vomiting, diarrhea, abdominal pain, emesis, dry mouth, duodenal ulcer, ***hemorrhage,*** ulcerative colitis.
GU: azotemia, elevated creatinine and BUN levels, crystalluria, ***renal failure.***
Hematologic: anemia, ***leukopenia, bone marrow suppression, thrombocytopenia,*** eosinophilia, ***agranulocytosis, aplastic anemia.***
Hepatic: elevated liver enzymes, elevated serum alkaline phosphatase, jaundice.
Respiratory: ***respiratory arrest,*** chest pain, dyspnea.
Skin: occasional rash, pruritus, urticaria, photosensitivity.
Other: hypoglycemia, hypokalemia.

Overdose and treatment

Flucytosine overdose may affect CV and pulmonary function. Treatment is largely supportive. Induced emesis or lavage may be useful within 4 hours after ingestion. Activated charcoal and osmotic cathartics also may be helpful. Flucytosine is readily removed by either hemodialysis or peritoneal dialysis.

☑ Special considerations

• Hematologic studies and renal and hepatic function studies should also precede therapy and should be repeated frequently thereafter, to evaluate dosage and monitor for adverse effects.
• Give capsules over a 15-minute period to reduce nausea, vomiting, and GI distress.
• Monitor intake and output to ensure adequate renal function.
• Flucytosine is usually given concomitantly with amphotericin B because they are synergistic.
• Protect drug from light.
• Because drug is removed by hemodialysis, adjust dosage in patients undergoing hemodialysis.
• Prolonged serum concentrations in excess of 100 mcg/ml may be associated with toxicity; monitor serum levels, especially in patients with renal insufficiency.

Patient education

• Teach patient the signs and symptoms of adverse reactions and the need to report them.
• Tell patient to call promptly if urine output decreases or signs of bleeding or bruising occur.
• Explain that adequate response may require several weeks or months of therapy. Advise patient to adhere to medical regimen and to return as instructed for follow-up visits.

Breast-feeding

• Safety has not been established.

fludarabine phosphate

Fludara

Pharmacologic classification: antimetabolite
Therapeutic classification: antineoplastic
Pregnancy risk category D

How supplied

Available by prescription only
Injection: 50 mg as lyophilized powder

Indications, route, and dosage

Treatment of B-cell chronic lymphocytic leukemia (CLL) in patients who have not responded or responded inadequately to at least one standard alkylating agent regimen, ◇ mycosis fungoides, ◇ hairy-cell leukemia, ◇ Hodgkin's and malignant lymphoma
Adults: Usually, 25 mg/m² I.V. over 30 minutes (◇ rapid I.V. injection or continuous I.V. infusion) for

* Canada only ◇ Unlabeled clinical use

5 consecutive days q 28 days. Therapy based on patient response and tolerance.

◊ ***Chronic lymphocytic leukemia***
Adults: Usually, 18 to 30 mg/m² I.V. over 30 minutes (◊ rapid I.V. injection or continuous I.V. infusion) for 5 consecutive days q 28 days. Therapy based on patient response and tolerance.

Pharmacodynamics

Antineoplastic action: After rapid conversion of fludarabine to its active metabolite, the metabolite appears to inhibit DNA synthesis by inhibiting DNA polymerase alpha, ribonucleotide reductase, and DNA primase. The exact mechanism of action is not fully established.

Pharmacokinetics

- *Absorption:* Drug is administered I.V.
- *Distribution:* Widely distributed with a volume of distribution of 96 to 98 L/m² at steady state.
- *Metabolism:* Drug is rapidly dephosphorylated and then phosphorylated intracellularly to its active metabolite.
- *Excretion:* 23% is excreted in urine as unchanged active metabolite. Half-life is approximately 10 hours.

Contraindications and precautions

Contraindicated in patients hypersensitive to drug or its components. Use cautiously in patients with renal insufficiency.

Interactions

Concomitant use with other *myelosuppressive agents* may cause additive toxicity.

Effects on diagnostic tests

None reported.

Adverse reactions

CNS: *fatigue, malaise, weakness, paresthesia,* peripheral neuropathy, headache, sleep disorder, depression, cerebellar syndrome, ***CVA***, agitation, *confusion,* ***coma.***
CV: *edema,* angina, transient ischemic attack, phlebitis, ***arrhythmias, heart failure,*** supraventricular tachycardia, deep venous thrombosis, ***aneurysm,*** hemorrhage.
EENT: *visual disturbances,* hearing loss, delayed blindness (with high doses), sinusitis, pharyngitis, epistaxis.
GI: *nausea, vomiting, diarrhea,* constipation, *anorexia,* stomatitis, *GI bleeding,* esophagitis, mucositis.
GU: dysuria, *urinary infection* or hesitancy, proteinuria, hematuria, ***renal failure.***
Hematologic: ***myelosuppression.***
Hepatic: liver failure, cholelithiasis.
Respiratory: *cough, pneumonia, dyspnea, upper respiratory tract infection,* allergic pneumonitis, hemoptysis, hypoxia, bronchitis.
Skin: *rash,* pruritus, seborrhea.
Other: *fever, chills, infection, pain, myalgia,* tumor lysis syndrome, alopecia, ***anaphylaxis, death*** (with very high doses), diaphoresis, hypocalcemia, hyperkalemia, hyperglycemia, dehydration, hyperuricemia, hyperphosphatemia.

Overdose and treatment

Irreversible CNS toxicity characterized by delayed blindness, coma, and death is associated with high doses. Severe thrombocytopenia and neutropenia secondary to bone marrow suppression also occur. There is no specific antidote, and treatment consists of discontinuing therapy and taking supportive measures.

☑ Special considerations

- Drug has been used investigationally in the treatment of malignant lymphoma, macroglobulinemic lymphoma, prolymphocytic leukemia or prolymphocytoid variant of CLL, mycosis fungoides, hairy cell leukemia, and Hodgkin's disease.
- Drug should be administered under the direct supervision of a physician experienced in antineoplastic therapy.
- Careful hematologic monitoring is required, especially of neutrophil and platelet counts.
- Tumor lysis syndrome (hyperuricemia, hyperphosphatemia, hypocalcemia, metabolic acidosis, hyperkalemia, hematuria, urate crystalluria, and renal failure) has occurred in CLL patients with large tumors.
- Severe neurologic effects, including blindness, are seen when high doses are used to treat acute leukemia.
- Advanced age, renal insufficiency, and bone marrow impairment may predispose patient to severe toxicity; toxic effects are dose-dependent.
- Optimal duration of therapy has not been established; three additional cycles after achieving maximal response are recommended before discontinuing drug.
- To prepare, add 2 ml of sterile water for injection to the solid cake of fludarabine. Dissolution should occur within 15 seconds and each ml will contain 25 mg of drug, 25 mg of mannitol, and sodium hydroxide. Use within 8 hours of reconstitution. Fludarabine has been further diluted in 100 ml or 125 ml of D_5W or 0.9% NaCl.
- Follow institutional protocol and guidelines for proper handling and disposal of chemotherapeutic agents.
- Store drug in refrigerator at 35.6° to 46.4° F (2° to 8° C).

Patient education

- Tell patient to avoid contact with infected persons and report signs of infection or unusual bleeding immediately.

Geriatric use

- Advanced age may increase toxicity potential.

Pediatric use

- Safety and efficacy have not been established.

Breast-feeding

- It is unknown if drug is excreted in breast milk. Risk-benefit ratio must be determined.

fludrocortisone acetate

Florinef

Pharmacologic classification: mineralocorticoid, glucocorticoid
Therapeutic classification: mineralocorticoid replacement therapy
Pregnancy risk category C

How supplied

Available by prescription only
Tablets: 0.1 mg

Indications, route, and dosage

Adrenal insufficiency (partial replacement), salt-losing adrenogenital syndrome
Adults: 0.1 to 0.2 mg P.O. daily.
Children: 0.05 to 0.1 mg P.O. daily.
Postural hypotension in diabetic patients, ◊ orthostatic hypotension
Adults: 0.1 to 0.4 mg P.O. daily.
Postural hypotension due to levodopa therapy
Adults: 0.05 to 0.2 mg P.O. daily.

Pharmacodynamics

Adrenal hormone replacement: Fludrocortisone, a synthetic glucocorticoid with potent mineralocorticoid activity, is used for partial replacement of steroid hormones in adrenocortical insufficiency and in salt-losing forms of congenital adrenogenital syndrome. In treating adrenocortical insufficiency, an exogenous glucocorticoid must also be administered for adequate control. (Cortisone or hydrocortisone are usually the drugs of choice for replacement because they produce both mineralocorticoid and glucocorticoid activity.) Fludrocortisone is administered on a variable schedule ranging from three times weekly to twice daily, depending on individual requirements.

Pharmacokinetics

- *Absorption:* Fludrocortisone is absorbed readily from the GI tract.
- *Distribution:* Removed rapidly from blood and distributed to muscle, liver, skin, intestines, and kidneys. It has a plasma half-life of about 30 minutes. It is extensively bound to plasma proteins (transcortin and albumin). Only the unbound portion is active. Adrenocorticoids are distributed into breast milk and through the placenta.
- *Metabolism:* Drug is metabolized in the liver to inactive glucuronide and sulfate metabolites.
- *Excretion:* Inactive metabolites and small amounts of unmetabolized drug are excreted by the kidneys. Insignificant quantities of drug are also excreted in feces. Biological half-life is 18 to 36 hours; plasma half-life is 3½ hours or more.

Contraindications and precautions

Contraindicated in patients with systemic fungal infections or hypersensitivity to drug.

Use cautiously in patients with hypothyroidism, cirrhosis, ocular herpes simplex, emotional instability, psychotic tendencies, nonspecific ulcerative colitis, diverticulitis, fresh intestinal anastamoses, peptic ulcer, renal insufficiency, hypertension, osteoporosis, and myasthenia gravis.

Interactions

Concomitant use with *barbiturates, phenytoin,* or *rifampin* may cause decreased corticosteroid effects because of increased hepatic metabolism. Fludrocortisone may enhance hypokalemia associated with *diuretic* or *amphotericin B* therapy. The hypokalemia may increase the risk of toxicity in patients concurrently receiving *cardiac glycosides.* Fludrocortisone may increase the metabolism of *isoniazid* and *salicylates.*

Effects on diagnostic tests

Drug therapy increases serum sodium levels and decreases serum potassium levels. Glucose tolerance tests should be performed only if necessary, because addisonian patients tend to develop severe hypoglycemia within 3 hours of the test.

Adverse reactions

CV: *sodium and water retention,* hypertension, cardiac hypertrophy, edema, ***heart failure.***
Skin: bruising, diaphoresis, urticaria, allergic rash.
Other: hypokalemia.

Overdose and treatment

Acute toxicity is manifested as an extension of the therapeutic effect, such as disturbances in fluid and electrolyte balance, hypokalemia, edema, hypertension, and cardiac insufficiency. In acute toxicity, administer symptomatic treatment and correct fluid and electrolyte imbalance.

☑ Special considerations

Besides those relevant to all *systemic adrenocorticoids,* consider the following recommendations.
- Use only with other supplemental measures, such as glucocorticoids, control of electrolytes, and control of infection.
- Supplemental dosages may be required in times of physiologic stress from serious illness, trauma, or surgery.
- Monitor for significant patient weight gain, edema, hypertension, or severe headaches.

Patient education

- Teach patient to recognize signs of electrolyte imbalance: muscle weakness, paresthesia, numbness, fatigue, anorexia, nausea, altered mental status, increased urination, altered heart rhythm, severe or continuing headaches, unusual weight gain, or swelling of the feet.
- Tell patient to take missed doses as soon as possible, unless it is almost time for the next dose, and not to double dose.

Pediatric use

- Chronic use in children and adolescents may delay growth and maturation.

flumazenil
Romazicon

Pharmacologic classification: benzodiazepine antagonist
Therapeutic classification: antidote
Pregnancy risk category C

How supplied
Available by prescription only
Injection: 0.1 mg/ml in 5-ml and 10-ml multiple-dose vials

Indications, route, and dosage
Complete or partial reversal of the sedative effects of benzodiazepines after anesthesia or short diagnostic procedures (conscious sedation)
Adults: Initially, 0.2 mg I.V. over 15 seconds. If patient does not reach desired level of consciousness after 45 seconds, repeat dose. Repeat at 1-minute intervals until a cumulative dose of 1 mg has been given (initial dose plus four additional doses). Most patients respond after 0.6 to 1 mg of drug. If resedation occurs, dosage may be repeated after 20 minutes, but no more than 1 mg should be given at one time, and patient should not receive more than 3 mg/hour.
Management of suspected benzodiazepine overdose
Adults: Initially, 0.2 mg I.V. over 30 seconds. If patient does not reach desired level of consciousness after 30 seconds, administer 0.3 mg over 30 seconds. If patient still does not respond adequately, give 0.5 mg over 30 seconds; then repeat 0.5-mg doses at 1-minute intervals until cumulative dose of 3 mg has been given. Most patients with benzodiazepine overdose respond to cumulative doses between 1 and 3 mg; rarely, patients who respond partially after 3 mg may require additional doses. Do not give more than 5 mg over 5 minutes initially; sedation that persists after this dosage is unlikely to be caused by benzodiazepines. If resedation occurs, may repeat dosage after 20 minutes, but give no more than 1 mg at one time; patient should not receive more than 3 mg/hour.

Pharmacodynamics
Antidote action: Drug competitively inhibits the actions of benzodiazepines on the gamma-aminobutyric acid-benzodiazepine receptor complex.

Pharmacokinetics
- *Absorption:* After I.V. administration, onset of action is within 1 to 2 minutes; peak effect occurs at 6 to 10 minutes.
- *Distribution:* After administration, drug redistributes rapidly (initial distribution half-life is 7 to 15 minutes). It is about 50% bound to plasma proteins.
- *Metabolism:* Drug is rapidly extracted from the blood and metabolized by the liver. Metabolites that have been identified are inactive. Ingestion of food during an I.V. infusion enhances extraction of drug from plasma, probably by increasing hepatic blood flow.
- *Excretion:* About 90% to 95% appears in the urine as metabolites; rest is excreted in the feces. Plasma half-life is about 54 minutes.

Contraindications and precautions
Contraindicated in patients hypersensitive to drug or benzodiazepines; in patients who show evidence of serious tricyclic antidepressant overdose; and in those who received a benzodiazepine to treat a potentially life-threatening condition (such as status epilepticus).

Use cautiously in alcohol-dependent or psychiatric patients, in those at high risk for developing seizures, or in those with head injuries, signs of seizures, or recent high intake of benzodiazepines (such as patients in the intensive care unit).

Interactions
Flumazenil should not be used in *mixed overdose* because it can obscure symptoms of poisoning by *drugs that can cause seizures or arrhythmias,* such as *antidepressants.* Seizures or arrhythmias can develop after flumazenil removes the effects of the *benzodiazepine overdose.*

Effects on diagnostic tests
None reported.

Adverse reactions
CNS: *dizziness, abnormal or blurred vision, headache,* ***seizures,*** agitation, emotional lability, tremor, insomnia.
CV: ***arrhythmias,*** cutaneous vasodilation, palpitations.
GI: nausea, vomiting.
Respiratory: dyspnea, hyperventilation.
Other: *diaphoresis, pain* (at injection site).

Overdose and treatment
In clinical trials, large doses of flumazenil were administered I.V. to volunteers in the absence of a benzodiazepine agonist. No serious adverse reactions, clinical signs or symptoms, or altered laboratory tests were noted.

In patients with benzodiazepine overdosage, large doses of flumazenil may produce agitation or anxiety, hyperesthesia, increased muscle tone, or seizures. Seizures may be treated with barbiturates, phenytoin, or benzodiazepines.

☑ Special considerations
- Onset of action is usually evident within 1 to 2 minutes of injection, and peak effect occurs within 6 to 10 minutes. Because duration of action of flumazenil is shorter than that of benzodiazepines, monitor patient carefully and administer additional drug as needed. Duration and degree of effect depend on plasma levels of the sedating benzodiazepine and the dose of flumazenil.
- To minimize pain at injection site, drug should be given through a freely flowing I.V. solution running into a large vein. Compatible solutions include D_5W, lactated Ringer's injection, or 0.9% NaCl solution.
- Resedation may occur after reversal of benzodiazepine effect because flumazenil has a shorter duration of action than that of benzodiazepines. Pa-

tients should be monitored for resedation according to duration of drug being reversed: monitor closely after long-acting benzodiazepines (such as diazepam) or after high doses of shorter-acting benzodiazepines (such as 10 mg of midazolam). Usually, serious resedation is unlikely in patients who fail to show signs of resedation 2 hours after a 1-mg dose of flumazenil.

• Do not expect patients to recall information from the postprocedure period because drug does not reverse the amnesiac effects of benzodiazepines. Therefore, give important instructions to the family or caregiver or in writing to the patient.

• Flumazenil can be administered by direct injection or diluted with a compatible solution. Discard unused drug that has been drawn into a syringe or diluted within 24 hours.

Patient education

• Because of risk of resedation, advise patient to avoid hazardous activities (such as driving a car), alcohol, CNS depressants, and OTC drugs within 24 hours of the procedure.

Pediatric use

• Because clinical trials have not been performed to identify flumazenil's clinical risks, benefits, or dosage range, manufacturer does not recommend its use in children.

Breast-feeding

• It is unknown if drug is excreted in breast milk. Use with caution.

flunisolide

Nasal inhalant
Nasalide

Oral inhalant
AeroBid, AeroBid-M

Pharmacologic classification: glucocorticoid
Therapeutic classification: anti-inflammatory, antiasthmatic
Pregnancy risk category C

How supplied

Available by prescription only
Nasal inhalant: 25 mcg/metered spray; 200 doses/bottle
Oral inhalant: 250 mcg/metered spray; at least 100 doses/inhaler

Indications, route, and dosage

Steroid-dependent asthma
Adults: Two inhalations b.i.d. for a total daily dose of 1 mg. Do not exceed 8 inhalations (2 mg)/day.
Children age 6 and older: Two inhalations b.i.d. Do not exceed four inhalations daily.

Seasonal or perennial rhinitis
Adults: 2 sprays (50 mcg) in each nostril b.i.d. (total dose 200 mcg/day). If needed, increase to 2 sprays in each nostril t.i.d. (total dose 300 mcg/day).
Children age 6 to 14: 1 spray (25 mcg) in each nostril t.i.d. or 2 sprays (50 mcg) in each nostril b.i.d. (total dose 150 to 200 mcg/day).

Pharmacodynamics

Anti-inflammatory action: Flunisolide stimulates the synthesis of enzymes needed to decrease the inflammatory response. The anti-inflammatory and vasoconstrictor potency of topically applied flunisolide is several hundred times greater than that of hydrocortisone and about equal to that of an equal weight of triamcinolone; the metabolite, 6-beta-hydroxyflunisolide, has about three times the activity of hydrocortisone.

Antiasthmatic action: The nasal inhalant form is used in the symptomatic treatment of seasonal or perennial rhinitis. In patients who require corticosteroids to control symptoms, the oral inhalant form is used to treat bronchial asthma.

Pharmacokinetics

• *Absorption:* Approximately 50% of a nasally inhaled dose is absorbed systemically; peak plasma concentrations occur within 10 to 30 minutes. After oral inhalation, about 40% of dose is absorbed from the lungs and GI tract; only about 20% of an orally inhaled dose reaches systemic circulation unmetabolized because of extensive metabolism in the liver. Onset of action usually occurs in a few days but may take as long as 4 weeks.

• *Distribution:* Distribution following intranasal administration or oral inhalation has not been described. No evidence exists of tissue storage of flunisolide or its metabolites.

• *Metabolism:* Flunisolide that is swallowed undergoes rapid metabolism in the liver or GI tract to several metabolites, one of which has glucocorticoid activity. Flunisolide and its 6-beta-hydroxy metabolite are eventually conjugated in the liver, by glucuronic acid or surface sulfate, to inactive metabolites.

• *Excretion:* Unknown when drug is administered by inhalation; however, when it is given systemically, metabolites are excreted in approximately equal portions in feces and urine. Biologic half-life of drug averages about 2 hours.

Contraindications and precautions

Contraindicated in patients hypersensitive to drug. Use of nasal inhalant is contraindicated in the presence of untreated localized infection involving nasal mucosa; oral inhalant should not be used in patients with status asthmaticus or respiratory infections.

Use nasal inhalant cautiously in patients with tuberculosis; untreated fungal, bacterial, or systemic viral or ocular herpes simplex infections; or septal ulcers, trauma, surgery in the nasal region. Oral inhalant is not recommended for patients with asthma controlled by bronchodilators or other noncorticosteroids alone or those with nonasthma bronchial diseases.

Interactions

None reported.

Effects on diagnostic tests
None reported.

Adverse reactions
CNS: headache (with nasal inhalant); dizziness, irritability, nervousness (with oral inhalant).
EENT: nasopharyngeal fungal infection; *mild, transient nasal burning and stinging,* stinging, dryness, sneezing, epistaxis, watery eyes (with nasal inhalant).
GI: nausea, vomiting (with nasal inhalant); dry mouth, abdominal pain, decreased appetite, *nausea, vomiting, diarrhea, upset stomach (with oral inhalant).*
Other: *upper respiratory tract infection, cold symptoms, flu,* edema, fever, chest pain, rash, pruritus (with oral inhalant).

Overdose and treatment
No information available.

☑ Special considerations
Recommendations for use of flunisolide and for care and teaching of the patient during therapy are the same as those for all *inhalant adrenocorticoids.*

fluocinolone acetonide
Derma-Smoothe/FS, Fluoderm*, Fluolar*, Fluonid, Fluonide*, Flurosyn, FS Shampoo, Synalar, Synalar-HP, Synamol*, Synemol

Pharmacologic classification: topical adrenocorticoid
Therapeutic classification: anti-inflammatory
Pregnancy risk category C

How supplied
Available by prescription only
Cream: 0.01%, 0.025%, 0.2%
Oil: 0.01%
Ointment: 0.025%
Shampoo: 0.01%
Solution: 0.01%

Indications, route, and dosage
Inflammation of corticosteroid-responsive dermatoses
Adults and children over age 2: Apply cream, ointment, or solution sparingly b.i.d. to q.i.d. Treat multiple or extensive lesions sequentially, applying to only small areas at one time. Occlusive dressings may be used for severe or resistant dermatoses.

Pharmacodynamics
Anti-inflammatory action: Fluocinolone stimulates the synthesis of enzymes needed to decrease the inflammatory response. It is a high-potency fluorinated glucocorticoid. Preparations of 0.01% potency are in group VI; 0.025% potency in group III or IV; and 0.2% potency in group IV.

Pharmacokinetics
• *Absorption:* Absorbed amount depends on strength of preparation, amount applied, and nature of skin at application site. It ranges from about 1% in areas with a thick stratum corneum (such as the palms, soles, elbows, and heels) to as high as 36% in areas of the thinnest stratum corneum (face, eyelids, and genitals). Absorption increases in areas of skin damage, inflammation, or occlusion. Some systemic absorption of topical steroids occurs, especially through the oral mucosa.
• *Distribution:* After topical application, drug is distributed throughout the local skin. Any drug absorbed into the circulation is distributed rapidly into muscle, liver, skin, intestines, and kidneys.
• *Metabolism:* After topical administration, drug is metabolized primarily in the skin. The small amount absorbed into systemic circulation is metabolized primarily in the liver to inactive compounds.
• *Excretion:* Inactive metabolites are excreted by the kidneys, primarily as glucuronides and sulfates, but also as unconjugated products. Small amounts of the metabolites are also excreted in feces.

Contraindications and precautions
Contraindicated in patients hypersensitive to drug.

Interactions
None significant.

Effects on diagnostic tests
None reported.

Adverse reactions
Skin: burning, pruritus, irritation, dryness, erythema, folliculitis, hypertrichosis, hypopigmentation, acneiform eruptions, perioral dermatitis, allergic contact dermatitis; *maceration, secondary infection, atrophy, striae, miliaria* (with occlusive dressings).
Other: ***hypothalamic-pituitary-adrenal axis suppression,*** Cushing's syndrome, hyperglycemia, glucosuria.

Overdose and treatment
No information available.

☑ Special considerations
Recommendations for use of fluocinolone, for care and teaching of patients during therapy, and for use in elderly patients, children, and breast-feeding women are the same as those for all *topical adrenocorticoids.*

fluocinonide
Lidemol*, Lidex, Lidex-E, Lyderm*

Pharmacologic classification: topical adrenocorticoid
Therapeutic classification: anti-inflammatory
Pregnancy risk category C

How supplied
Available by prescription only
Cream, gel, ointment, solution: 0.05%

Indications, route, and dosage

Inflammation of corticosteroid-responsive dermatoses

Adults and children: Apply sparingly b.i.d. or t.i.d. Occlusive dressings may be used for severe or resistant dermatoses.

Pharmacodynamics

Anti-inflammatory action: Fluocinonide stimulates the synthesis of enzymes needed to decrease the inflammatory response. Fluocinonide is a high-potency fluorinated glucocorticoid categorized as a group II topical steroid.

Pharmacokinetics

- *Absorption:* Amount absorbed depends on amount applied and on nature of skin at application site. It ranges from about 1% in areas of thick stratum corneum (such as the palms, soles, elbows, and knees) to as high as 36% in areas of thin stratum corneum (face, eyelids, and genitals). Absorption increases in areas of skin damage, inflammation, or occlusion. Some systemic absorption of steroids occurs, especially through the oral mucosa.
- *Distribution:* After topical application, drug is distributed throughout the local skin. Any drug absorbed into circulation is removed rapidly from the blood and distributed into muscle, liver, skin, intestines, and kidneys.
- *Metabolism:* After topical administration, fluocinonide is metabolized primarily in the skin. The small amount absorbed into systemic circulation is metabolized primarily in the liver to inactive compounds.
- *Excretion:* Inactive metabolites are excreted by the kidneys, primarily as glucuronides and sulfates, but also as unconjugated products. Small amounts of the metabolites are excreted in feces.

Contraindications and precautions

Contraindicated in patients hypersensitive to drug.

Interactions

None significant.

Effects on diagnostic tests

None reported.

Adverse reactions

Skin: burning, pruritus, irritation, dryness, erythema, folliculitis, hypertrichosis, hypopigmentation, acneiform eruptions, perioral dermatitis, allergic contact dermatitis; *maceration, secondary infection, atrophy, striae, miliaria* (with occlusive dressings).

Other: ***hypothalamic-pituitary-adrenal axis suppression,*** Cushing's syndrome, hyperglycemia, glucosuria.

Overdose and treatment

No information available.

☑ Special considerations

Recommendations for use of fluocinonide, for care and teaching of patients during therapy, and for use in elderly patients, children and breast-feeding women are the same as those for all *topical adrenocorticoids.*

fluorescein sodium

AK-Fluor, Fluorescite, Fluorets, Fluor-I-Strip, Fluor-I-Strip-A.T., Ful-Glo, Ophthifluor

Pharmacologic classification: dye
Therapeutic classification: diagnostic aid
Pregnancy risk category C

How supplied

Available by prescription only
Parenteral injection: 10%, 25%
Ophthalmic solution: 2%
Ophthalmic strips: 9 mg

Available without a prescription
Ophthalmic strips: 0.6 mg, 1 mg

Indications, route, and dosage

Diagnostic aid in corneal abrasions and foreign bodies, fitting hard contact lenses; lacrimal patency; fundus photography; applanation tonometry

Adults and children: For topical solution, instill 1 drop of 2% solution followed by irrigation, or moisten strip with sterile water. Touch conjunctiva or fornix with moistened tip. Flush eye with irrigating solution. Patient should blink several times after application.

Retinal angiography

Adults: 5 ml of 10% solution (500 mg) or 3 ml of 25% solution (750 mg) injected rapidly into antecubital vein by primary health care provider or a specially trained nurse.

Children: 7.5 mg/kg injected rapidly into antecubital vein by primary health care provider.

Pharmacodynamics

Diagnostic adjunct: Fluorescein stains abraded or ulcerated areas of the cornea fluorescent green under normal light and bright yellow if viewed under cobalt blue light. Foreign bodies appear surrounded by a green fluorescent ring, and lesions of the conjunctiva appear orange-yellow.

Pharmacokinetics

- *Absorption:* Unknown.
- *Distribution:* Unknown.
- *Metabolism:* Unknown.
- *Excretion:* Drug is excreted in urine. Urine attains a bright yellow color that fades in 24 to 36 hours.

Contraindications and precautions

Contraindicated in patients with hypersensitivity to drug. Also avoid use in patients wearing soft contact lenses (lenses may become discolored). Use cautiously in patients with history of allergy or bronchial asthma.

Interactions

None reported.

Effects on diagnostic tests
Bright yellow discoloration of urine may interfere with routine urinalysis.

Adverse reactions
Topical use:
EENT: eye stinging or burning, yellow tears.
I.V. use:
CNS: headache, dizziness, syncope, ***seizures.***
CV: hypotension, ***shock, cardiac arrest, thrombophlebitis.***
GI: nausea, vomiting, GI distress.
GU: bright yellow urine (persists for 24 to 36 hours).
Respiratory: transient dyspnea, ***bronchospasm.***
Skin: yellow skin discoloration (fades in 6 to 12 hours), urticaria, pruritus.
Other: hypersensitivity reactions, including urticaria and ***anaphylaxis;*** extravasation at injection site; fever; angioedema.

Overdose and treatment
The 2% solution of fluorescein sodium alone is considered nontoxic; however, some preparations may contain boric acid. In other cases, as little as 5 g in infants or 20 g in adults has been fatal. Clinical manifestations of overdose include hypotension, shock, restlessness, weakness, seizures, nausea, vomiting, diarrhea, oliguria, hypothermia, hyperthermia, and erythematous rash.

Use emesis followed by a cathartic for substantial accidental ingestion unless the patient is comatose or obtunded. Treat hypotension with fluids and Trendelenburg's positioning. Treat seizures with I.V. diazepam.

☑ Special considerations
- Never instill drug in eye of patient wearing soft contact lens; this will cause permanent discoloration of lens.
- Topical anesthetic may be used before instillation to partially relieve burning and irritation.
- Use strict aseptic technique; preparation is contaminated easily by *Pseudomonas.*
- Fluorescein is water-soluble. Do not freeze; store below 80° F (26.7° C).
- After I.V. injection, yellow skin discoloration may last 6 to 12 hours; urine will be bright yellow for 24 to 36 hours, and routine urinalysis of sample taken within 1 hour will be abnormal.
- Keep emergency supplies and medications on hand to manage or treat respiratory and cardiac arrest.
- Intermittent nausea lasting 1 to 4 minutes follows I.V. injection in 5% to 10% of patients; assist patient as necessary.

Patient education
- Inform patient that fluorescein may discolor soft contact lenses; he should remove the lenses before drug use. After using fluorescein, patient should flush eyes with 0.9% NaCl solution and allow at least 1 hour before replacing lenses.
- Explain that yellow skin discoloration may persist for 6 to 12 hours and that urine will be bright yellow for 24 to 36 hours after I.V. injection; reassure patient that this is not harmful.
- Tell patient that, although uncommon, mild nausea may occur; reassure patient that it will subside in a few minutes.

fluorometholone
Fluor-Op Ophthalmic, FML Forte, FML Liquifilm Ophthalmic, FML S.O.P.

Pharmacologic classification: corticosteroid
Therapeutic classification: ophthalmic anti-inflammatory
Pregnancy risk category C

How supplied
Available by prescription only
Ophthalmic ointment: 0.1%
Ophthalmic suspension: 0.1%, 0.25%

Indications, route, and dosage
Inflammatory and allergic conditions of cornea, conjunctiva, sclera, anterior uvea
Adults and children: In severe cases, instill 2 drops of suspension in conjunctival sac q 1 to 2 hours or ½" ointment q 4 hours during the first 1 to 2 days of therapy. In mild to moderate cases, 1 to 2 drops of suspension may be used b.i.d. to q.i.d. or ½" ointment daily to t.i.d.

Pharmacodynamics
Anti-inflammatory action: Fluorometholone stimulates the synthesis of enzymes needed to decrease the inflammatory response. Fluorometholone is a synthetic fluorinated corticosteroid that is less likely than hydrocortisone, prednisolone, or dexamethasone to cause intraocular hypertension.

Pharmacokinetics
- *Absorption:* After ophthalmic administration, drug is absorbed mainly into the aqueous humor. Slight systemic absorption typically occurs.
- *Distribution:* Drug is distributed throughout the local tissue layers. Any drug absorbed into circulation is removed rapidly from the blood and distributed into muscle, liver, skin, intestines, and kidneys.
- *Metabolism:* Primarily metabolized locally. The small amount absorbed into systemic circulation is metabolized primarily in liver to inactive compounds.
- *Excretion:* Inactive metabolites are excreted by the kidneys, primarily as glucuronides and sulfates, but also as unconjugated products. Small amounts of the metabolites are also excreted in the feces.

Contraindications and precautions
Contraindicated in patients with vaccinia, varicella, acute superficial herpes simplex (dendritic keratitis), or other fungal or viral eye diseases; ocular tuberculosis; or any acute, purulent, untreated eye infection.

Use cautiously in patients with corneal abrasions that may be contaminated (especially with herpes).

Interactions
None reported.

Effects on diagnostic tests
None reported.

Adverse reactions
EENT: increased intraocular pressure, thinning of cornea, interference with corneal wound healing, corneal ulceration, increased susceptibility to viral or fungal corneal infections; with excessive or long-term use, glaucoma exacerbation, discharge, discomfort, ocular pain, foreign body sensation, cataracts, decreased visual acuity, diminished visual field, optic nerve damage.
Other: systemic effects and adrenal suppression in excessive or long-term use.

Overdose and treatment
No information available.

☑ Special considerations
- Be aware that drug is less likely to cause increased intraocular pressure with long-term use than other ophthalamic anti-inflammatory drugs (except medrysone).

Pediatric use
- Safety and efficacy in children under age 2 have not been established.

fluorouracil (5-FU)
Adrucil, Efudex

Pharmacologic classification: antimetabolite (cell cycle–phase specific, S phase)
Therapeutic classification: antineoplastic
Pregnancy risk category D (injection), X (cream)

How supplied
Available by prescription only
Injection: 50 mg/ml in 10-ml, 20-ml, 50-ml, 100-ml vials
Cream: 1%, 5%
Topical solution: 1%, 2%, 5%

Indications, route, and dosage
Dosage and indications may vary. Check current literature for recommended protocol.
Palliative management of colon, rectal, breast, ◊ ovarian, ◊ cervical, gastric, ◊ bladder, ◊ liver, pancreatic cancers
Adults and children: 12 mg/kg I.V. for 4 days, then if no toxicity occurs, give 6 mg/kg I.V. on days 6, 8, 10, and 12. Maintanence therapy is a repeated course q 30 days. Do not exceed 800 mg/day (400 mg/day in severely ill patients).
Actinic or solar keratoses
Adults: Sufficient cream or lotion to cover lesions b.i.d. for 2 to 4 weeks. Usually, 1% preparations are used on head, neck, and chest, 2% and 5% on hands.
Superficial basal cell carcinomas
Adults: 5% solution or cream in a sufficient amount to cover lesion b.i.d. for 3 to 6 weeks, up to 12 weeks.

Pharmacodynamics
Antineoplastic action: Fluorouracil exerts its cytotoxic activity by acting as an antimetabolite, competing for the enzyme that is important in the synthesis of thymidine, an essential substrate for DNA synthesis. Therefore, DNA synthesis is inhibited. Drug also inhibits RNA synthesis to a lesser extent.

Pharmacokinetics
- *Absorption:* Drug is given parenterally because it is absorbed poorly after oral administration.
- *Distribution:* Distributes widely into all areas of body water and tissues, including tumors, bone marrow, liver, and intestinal mucosa. Fluorouracil crosses the blood-brain barrier to a significant extent.
- *Metabolism:* A small amount is converted in the tissues to the active metabolite, with most of drug degraded in the liver.
- *Excretion:* Metabolites of fluorouracil are primarily excreted through the lungs as carbon dioxide. A small portion of a dose is excreted in urine as unchanged drug.

Contraindications and precautions
Contraindicated in patients hypersensitive to drug; patients who are in a poor nutritional state; patients with bone marrow suppression (WBC counts of 5,000/mm³ or less or platelet counts of 100,000/mm³ or less); patients with potentially serious infections; and in those who have had major surgery within the previous month.

Use cautiously in patients after high-dose pelvic radiation therapy or use of alkylating agents. Also use with caution in patients with widespread neoplastic infiltration of bone marrow and impaired renal or hepatic function.

Interactions
Leucovorin calcium may enhance the toxicity of fluorouracil.

Effects on diagnostic tests
Fluorouracil may decrease plasma albumin concentration because of drug-induced protein malabsorption.

Adverse reactions
CNS: acute cerebellar syndrome, confusion, disorientation, euphoria, ataxia, headache, nystagmus, *weakness, malaise.*
CV: myocardial ischemia, angina.
GI: *stomatitis, GI ulcer* (may precede leukopenia), *nausea, vomiting, diarrhea, anorexia,* GI bleeding.
Hematologic: ***leukopenia, thrombocytopenia, agranulocytosis,*** anemia; WBC count nadir 9 to 14 days after first dose; platelet count nadir in 7 to 14 days.
Skin: *dermatitis; erythema; scaling; pruritus;* nail changes; pigmented palmar creases; erythematous, contact dermatitis; desquamative rash of hands and feet with long-term use ("hand-foot syndrome").

Other: *reversible alopecia, pain, burning,* soreness, suppuration, swelling (with topical use), ***anaphylaxis,*** thrombophlebitis.

Overdose and treatment

Clinical manifestations of overdose include myelosuppression, diarrhea, alopecia, dermatitis, hyperpigmentation, nausea, and vomiting. Treatment is usually supportive and includes transfusion of blood components, antiemetics, and antidiarrheals.

☑ Special considerations

- Drug may be administered I.V. push over 1 to 2 minutes.
- Drug may be further diluted in D_5W or 0.9% NaCl solution for infusions up to 24 hours in duration.
- Use plastic I.V. containers for administering continuous infusions. Solution is more stable in plastic I.V. bags than in glass bottles.
- Do not use cloudy solution. If crystals form, redissolve by warming at a temperature of 140° F (60° C) with vigorous shaking. Allow solution to cool to body temperature before using.
- Use new vein site for each dose.
- Give antiemetic before administering to decrease nausea.
- If extravasation occurs, treat as a chemical phlebitis with warm compresses.
- Do not refrigerate fluorouracil.
- Drug can be diluted in 120 ml of water and administered orally; however this is not an FDA-approved method of adminstration, and absorption is erratic.
- General photosensitivity occurs for 2 to 3 months after a dose.
- Ingestion and systemic absorption may cause leukopenia, thrombocytopenia, stomatitis, diarrhea or GI ulceration, bleeding, and hemorrhage. A topical local anesthetic may be used to soothe mouth lesions. Encourage good and frequent mouth care.
- Monitor intake and output, CBC, and renal and hepatic function.
- Avoid I.M. injections in patients with low platelet counts.
- Apply topical drug while using plastic gloves. Wash hands immediately after handling medication. Avoid topical use with occlusive dressings.
- Apply topical solution with caution near eyes, nose, and mouth.
- Topical application to larger ulcerated areas may cause systemic toxicity.
- For superficial basal cell carcinoma confirmed by biopsy, use 5% strength. Apply 1% concentration on the face. Reserve higher concentrations for thicker-skinned areas or resistant lesions. Occlusion may be required.
- Do not continue to treat lesions resistant to fluorouracil; they should be biopsied.

Patient education

- Warn patient to avoid strong sunlight or ultraviolet light because it will intensify the skin reaction. Encourage use of sunscreens.
- Tell patient to avoid exposure to people with infections. Advise patient to promptly report signs of infection or unusual bleeding.
- Reassure patient that hair should grow back after treatment is discontinued.
- Tell patient to apply topical fluorouracil with gloves and wash hands thoroughly after application.
- Warn patient that treated area may be unsightly during therapy and for several weeks after therapy is stopped. Complete healing may not occur until 1 or 2 months after treatment is stopped.
- Advise female patient of childbearing age to avoid becoming pregnant during therapy.

Breast-feeding

- It is not known if drug occurs in breast milk. However, because of potential for serious adverse reactions, mutagenicity, and carcinogenicity in the infant, breast-feeding is not recommended.

fluoxetine

Prozac, Prozac Pulvules

Pharmacologic classification: selective serotonin reuptake inhibitor (SSRI)
Therapeutic classification: antidepressant
Pregnancy risk category B

How supplied

Available by prescription only
Capsules: 10 mg, 20 mg
Oral solution: 20 mg/5 ml

Indications, route, and dosage

Depression, ◊ panic disorder; ◊ bipolar disorder; ◊ alcohol dependence; ◊ cataplexy; ◊ myoclonus
Adults: 20 mg P.O. daily in the morning. Increase dosage p.r.n. after several weeks to 40 mg daily with a dose in the morning and midday. Do not exceed 80 mg daily.
Obsessive-compulsive disorder
Adults: Initially, 20 mg P.O. daily. Gradually increase dosage as needed and tolerated to 60 to 80 mg daily.
◊ ***Obesity***
Adults: 20 to 60 mg P.O. daily.
◊ ***Eating disorders***
Adults: 60 to 80 mg P.O. daily.

Pharmacodynamics

Antidepressant action: The antidepressant action of fluoxetine is purportedly related to its inhibition of CNS neuronal uptake of serotonin. Fluoxetine blocks uptake of serotonin, but not of norepinephrine, into human platelets. Animal studies suggest it is a much more potent uptake inhibitor of serotonin than of norepinephrine.

Pharmacokinetics

- *Absorption:* Well absorbed after oral administration. Its absorption is not altered by food.
- *Distribution:* Drug is apparently highly protein-bound (about 95%).
- *Metabolism:* Metabolized primarily in the liver to active metabolites.

• *Excretion:* Drug is excreted by the kidneys. Elimination half-life is 2 to 3 days. Norfluoxetine (the primary active metabolite) has an elimination half-life of 7 to 9 days.

Contraindications and precautions

Contraindicated in patients hypersensitive to drug and in patients taking MAO inhibitors within 14 days of starting therapy. Use cautiously in patients at high risk of suicide or in those with a history of seizures, diabetes mellitus, or renal, hepatic, or CV disease.

Interactions

Concomitant use with *diazepam* may prolong half-life of diazepam. Concomitant use with *tryptophan* may lead to increased adverse CNS effects (agitation, restlessness) and GI distress. Avoid concomitant administration with other highly *protein-bound drugs* (such as *warfarin*). Avoid concomitant administration with other *psychoactive drugs (MAO inhibitors, antipsychotics).*

Effects on diagnostic tests

None reported.

Adverse reactions

CNS: *nervousness, anxiety, insomnia, headache, drowsiness, tremor, dizziness, asthenia,* fatigue.
CV: palpitations, hot flashes.
EENT: nasal congestion, pharyngitis, cough, sinusitis.
GI: *nausea, diarrhea, dry mouth, anorexia, dyspepsia,* constipation, abdominal pain, vomiting, flatulence, increased appetite.
GU: sexual dysfunction.
Respiratory: upper respiratory infection, respiratory distress.
Skin: *rash, pruritus,* diaphoresis.
Other: flulike syndrome, muscle pain, *weight loss,* fever.

Overdose and treatment

Symptoms of overdose include agitation, restlessness, hypomania, and other signs of CNS excitation; and, in patients who took higher doses of fluoxetine, nausea and vomiting. Among approximately 38 reports of acute overdose with fluoxetine, two fatalities involved plasma concentrations of 4.57 mg/L and 1.93 mg/L. One involved 1.8 g of fluoxetine with an undetermined amount of maprotiline; another death involved combined ingestion of fluoxetine, codeine, and temazepam. One other patient developed two tonic-clonic seizures after taking 3 g of fluoxetine; these seizures remitted spontaneously and did not require treatment with anticonvulsants.

To treat fluoxetine overdose, establish and maintain an airway; ensure adequate oxygenation and ventilation. Activated charcoal, which may be used with sorbitol, may be as effective as emesis or lavage.

Monitor cardiac and vital signs, and provide usual supportive measures. Fluoxetine-induced seizures that do not subside spontaneously may respond to diazepam. Forced diuresis, dialysis, hemoperfusion, and exchange transfusion are unlikely to be of benefit.

☑ Special considerations

• Consider the inherent risk of suicide until significant improvement of depressive state occurs. High-risk patients should have close supervision during initial drug therapy. To reduce risk of suicidal overdose, prescribe the smallest quantity of pulvules consistent with good management.
• Full antidepressant effect may be delayed until 4 weeks of treatment or longer.
• Treatment of acute depression usually requires at least several months of continuous drug therapy; optimal duration of therapy has not been established.
• Because of its long elimination half-life, changes in fluoxetine dosage will not be reflected in plasma for several weeks, affecting titration to final dose and withdrawal from treatment.
• Fluoxetine therapy may activate mania or hypomania.
• Impaired hepatic function can delay the elimination of fluoxetine and its metabolite norfluoxetine, prolonging the drug's elimination half-life. Therefore, use fluoxetine with caution in patients with liver disease.
• In patients with severely impaired renal function, chronic administration of fluoxetine is associated with significant accumulation of this drug or its metabolites.
• Prescribe lower or less frequent dosages in patients with renal or hepatic impairment. Also consider lower or less frequent dosages in elderly patients and others with concurrent disease or multiple drug therapy.

Patient education

• Inform patient drug may cause dizziness or drowsiness. Patient should avoid hazardous tasks that require alertness until CNS response to drug is established.
• Caution patient to avoid ingestion of alcohol and to seek medical approval before taking other drugs.
• Tell patient to promptly report rash or hives, anxiety, nervousness, anorexia (especially in underweight patients), suspicion of pregnancy, or intent to become pregnant.

fluoxymesterone

Halotestin

Pharmacologic classification: androgen
Therapeutic classification: androgen replacement, antineoplastic
Controlled substance schedule III
Pregnancy risk category X

How supplied

Available by prescription only
Tablets: 2 mg, 5 mg, 10 mg

Indications, route, and dosage

Male hypogonadism
Adults: 5 to 20 mg P.O. daily, in a single dose or in three or four divided doses.

Palliation of breast cancer in women
Adults: 10 to 40 mg P.O. daily in three or four divided doses.
Postpartum breast engorgement
Adults: 2.5 mg P.O. shortly after parturition followed by 5 to 10 mg daily for 4 to 5 days in divided doses.
Vasomotor symptoms associated with menopause
Adults: 1 to 2 mg P.O. b.i.d. combined with ethinyl estradiol 0.02 or 0.04 mg P.O. b.i.d. for 21 days; then 7 days without drug. Repeat regimen when necessary.
Treatment of delayed puberty
Males: 2.5 to 20 mg daily. Most patients respond to dosages of 2.5 to 10 mg daily.

Pharmacodynamics

Androgenic action: Fluoxymesterone mimics the action of the endogenous androgen testosterone by stimulating receptors in androgen-responsive organs and tissues. It exerts inhibitory, anti-estrogenic effects on hormone-responsive breast tumors and metastases.

Antianemic action: Drug enhances the production of erythropoietic stimulating factors, thereby increasing the production of RBCs.

Pharmacokinetics

Fluoxymesterone is eliminated primarily by hepatic metabolism. Its pharmacokinetics are otherwise poorly described.

Contraindications and precautions

Contraindicated in patients with hypersensitivity to drug, in males with breast cancer or prostate cancer, in those with cardiac, hepatic, or renal decompensation; during pregnancy; and in breast-feeding patients.

Use cautiously in prepubertal males and patients with benign prostatic hyperplasia or aspirin sensitivity.

Interactions

In patients with diabetes, decreased blood glucose levels may require adjustment of *insulin* or *oral antidiabetic drug* dosage.

Fluoxymesterone may potentiate the action of *anticoagulants*, resulting in increased PT.

Effects on diagnostic tests

Fluoxymesterone may cause abnormal results of the glucose tolerance test. Thyroid function test results (protein-bound iodine, ^{131}I uptake, thyroid-binding capacity) may decrease. PT (especially in patients on anticoagulant therapy) may be prolonged. Abnormal liver function test results may occur. Because of drug's anabolic activity, serum sodium, potassium, calcium, phosphate, and cholesterol levels may all rise.

Adverse reactions

CNS: headache, anxiety, depression, paresthesia, sleep apnea syndrome.
CV: edema.
GI: nausea.
GU: *hypoestrogenic effects in women (flushing; diaphoresis; vaginitis, including itching, dryness, and burning; vaginal bleeding; nervousness; emotional lability; menstrual irregularities); excessive hormonal effects in men* (prepubertal—*premature epiphyseal closure,* acne, *priapism, growth of body and facial hair,* phallic enlargement; postpubertal—testicular atrophy, oligospermia, decreased ejaculatory volume, impotence, gynecomastia, epididymitis).
Hematologic: polycythemia, elevated serum lipid levels, suppression of clotting factors.
Hepatic: reversible jaundice, peliosis hepatis, elevated liver enzyme levels, ***liver cell tumors.***
Other: hypercalcemia; hypersensitivity skin manifestations; androgenic effects in women (acne, edema, *weight gain, hirsutism,* hoarseness, clitoral enlargement, deepening voice, *decreased breast size,* changes in libido, male-pattern baldness, *oily skin or hair).*

Overdose and treatment

No information available.

☑ Special considerations

Besides those relevant to all *androgens,* consider the following recommendations.
- Observe female patient carefully for signs of excessive virilization. If possible, discontinue drug at first sign of virilization because some adverse effects (deepening of the voice, clitoral enlargement) are not reversible.
- Patients with metastatic breast cancer should have regular determinations of serum calcium levels to identify potential for serious hypercalcemia.
- When drug is used in breast cancer, subjective effects may not appear for about 1 month; objective improvement not for 3 months.
- Watch for symptoms of hypoglycemia in patients with diabetes. Dosage of antidiabetic drug may need adjustment.
- If patient is receiving anticoagulants concurrently with fluoxymesterone, monitor for ecchymoses, petechiae, and other signs of bleeding.
- Halotestin contains tartrazine. Observe for signs of allergic reactions in patients sensitive to aspirin or tartrazine.
- Women with an intact uterus receiving drug in combination with ethinyl estradiol must be monitored closely for endometrial carcinoma. Rule out malignancy if recurrent vaginal bleeding occurs.

Patient education

- Explain to patient taking drug for palliation of breast cancer that virilization usually occurs at dosage used. Tell patient to report androgenic effects immediately. Stopping drug will prevent further androgenic changes but probably will not reverse those already present.
- Tell female patient to report menstrual irregularities and to discontinue therapy pending etiologic determination.
- Advise male patient to report overly frequent or persistent penile erections.
- Advise patient to report persistent GI distress, diarrhea, or the onset of jaundice.

Geriatric use
- Use with caution. Observe elderly male patients for the development of prostatic hypertrophy. Development of symptomatic prostatic hypertrophy or prostatic cancer mandates discontinuing drug.

Pediatric use
- Use with extreme caution in pediatric patients to avoid precocious puberty and premature closure of the epiphyses. X-ray examinations every 6 months are recommended to assess skeletal maturation.

Breast-feeding
- Because of potential adverse effects on the infant, a decision should be made to discontinue breast-feeding or to discontinue drug, depending on patient's need for drug.

fluphenazine decanoate
Modecate Decanoate*, Prolixin Decanoate

fluphenazine enanthate
Moditen Enanthate*, Prolixin Enanthate

fluphenazine hydrochloride
Permitil Hydrochloride, Prolixin Hydrochloride

Pharmacologic classification: phenothiazine (piperazine derivative)
Therapeutic classification: antipsychotic
Pregnancy risk category NR

How supplied
Available by prescription only
fluphenazine decanoate
Depot injection: 25 mg/ml
fluphenazine enanthate
Depot injection: 25 mg/ml
fluphenazine hydrochloride
Tablets: 1 mg, 2.5 mg, 5 mg, 10 mg
Oral concentrate: 5 mg/ml (Prolixin contains 14% alcohol and Permitil contains 1% alcohol)
Elixir: 2.5 mg/5 ml (with 14% alcohol)
I.M. injection: 2.5 mg/ml

Indications, route, and dosage
Psychotic disorders
Adults: Initially, 0.5 to 10 mg fluphenazine hydrochloride P.O. daily in divided doses q 6 to 8 hours; may increase cautiously to 20 mg. Maintenance dosage is 1 to 5 mg P.O. daily. I.M. doses are one third to one half that of oral doses (starting dose is 1.25 mg I.M.).
✦ ***Dosage adjustment.*** Use lower doses for geriatric patients (1 to 2.5 mg daily).

Pharmacodynamics
Antipsychotic action: Fluphenazine is thought to exert its antipsychotic effects by postsynaptic blockade of CNS dopamine receptors, thereby inhibiting dopamine-mediated effects.

Fluphenazine has many other central and peripheral effects; it produces both alpha and ganglionic blockade and counteracts histamine- and serotonin-mediated activity. Its most prominent adverse reactions are extrapyramidal.

Pharmacokinetics
- *Absorption:* Rate and extent of absorption vary with route of administration; oral tablet absorption is erratic and variable. Oral and I.M. dosages have an onset of action of within 1 hour. Long-acting decanoate and enanthate salts act within 24 to 72 hours.
- *Distribution:* Drug is distributed widely into the body, including breast milk. CNS concentrations are usually higher than those in plasma. Drug is 91% to 99% protein-bound. Peak effects of oral dose usually occur at 2 hours; steady-state serum levels are achieved within 4 to 7 days.
- *Metabolism:* Fluphenazine is metabolized extensively by the liver, but no active metabolites are formed; duration of action is about 6 to 8 hours after oral administration; 1 to 6 weeks (average, 2 weeks) after I.M. depot administration.
- *Excretion:* Drug is mostly excreted in urine via the kidneys; some is excreted in feces via the biliary tract.

Contraindications and precautions
Contraindicated in patients with hypersensitivity or in patients experiencing coma, CNS depression, bone marrow suppression or other blood dyscrasia, subcortical damage, or liver damage.

Use cautiously in elderly or debilitated patients and in those with pheochromocytoma, severe CV disease, peptic ulcer disease, exposure to extreme hot or cold (including antipyretic therapy), phosphorus insecticides, respiratory or seizure disorders, hypocalcemia, severe reaction to insulin or electroconvulsive therapy, mitral insufficiency, glaucoma, or prostatic hyperplasia. Use parenteral form cautiously in patients with asthma and those allergic to sulfites.

Interactions
Concomitant use of fluphenazine with *sympathomimetics,* including *epinephrine, phenylephrine, phenylpropanolamine,* and *ephedrine* (often found in *nasal sprays*), and *appetite suppressants* may decrease their stimulatory and pressor effects.

Fluphenazine may inhibit blood pressure response to *centrally acting antihypertensive drugs* such as *guanethidine, guanabenz, guanadrel, clonidine, methyldopa,* and *reserpine.* Additive effects are likely after concomitant use of fluphenazine with *CNS depressants,* including *alcohol, analgesics, barbiturates, narcotics, tranquilizers,* and *general, spinal, or epidural anesthetics,* or *parenteral magnesium sulfate* (oversedation, respiratory depression, and hypotension); *antiarrhythmic agents, quinidine, disopyramide,* and *procainamide* (increased incidence of arrhythmias and conduction defects); *atropine* or other *anticholinergic drugs,* including *antidepressants, MAO inhibitors, phenothiazines, antihistamines, meperidine,* and *antiparkinsonian agents* (oversedation, paralytic ileus, visual changes, and severe constipation); *nitrates* (hypotension); and *metrizamide* (increased risk of seizures).

Beta-blocking agents may inhibit fluphenazine metabolism, increasing plasma levels and toxicity.

Concomitant use with *propylthiouracil* increases risk of agranulocytosis; concomitant use with *lithium* may result in severe neurologic toxicity with an encephalitis-like syndrome, and a decreased therapeutic response to fluphenazine.

Pharmacokinetic alterations and subsequent decreased therapeutic response to fluphenazine may follow concomitant use with *phenobarbital* (enhanced renal excretion), *aluminum-* and *magnesium-containing antacids* and *antidiarrheals* (decreased absorption), or *caffeine*, and with *heavy smoking* (increased metabolism).

Fluphenazine may antagonize therapeutic effect of *bromocriptine* on prolactin secretion; it also may decrease the vasoconstricting effects of high-dose *dopamine*, and may decrease effectiveness and increase toxicity of *levodopa* (by dopamine blockade). Fluphenazine may inhibit metabolism and increase toxicity of *phenytoin* and *tricyclic antidepressants*.

Effects on diagnostic tests

Fluphenazine causes false-positive test results for urinary porphyrins, urobilinogen, amylase, and 5-hydroxyindoleacetic acid, because of darkening of urine by metabolites; it also causes false-positive urine pregnancy test results using human chorionic gonadotropin.

Fluphenazine elevates test results for liver enzymes and protein-bound iodine, and causes quinidine-like ECG effects.

Adverse reactions

CNS: *extrapyramidal reactions, tardive dyskinesia, sedation, pseudoparkinsonism, EEG changes, drowsiness,* ***seizures,*** dizziness.

CV: *orthostatic hypotension,* tachycardia, ECG changes.

EENT: ocular changes, *blurred vision,* nasal congestion.

GI: *dry mouth, constipation.*

GU: *urine retention,* dark urine, menstrual irregularities, gynecomastia, inhibited ejaculation.

Hematologic: leukopenia, ***agranulocytosis,*** eosinophilia, hemolytic anemia, ***aplastic anemia,*** thrombocytopenia.

Hepatic: cholestatic jaundice, abnormal liver function test results.

Skin: *mild photosensitivity,* allergic reactions.

Other: weight gain; increased appetite; rarely, ***neuroleptic malignant syndrome.***

After abrupt withdrawal of long-term therapy: gastritis, nausea, vomiting, dizziness, tremor, feeling of warmth or cold, diaphoresis, tachycardia, headache, insomnia.

Overdose and treatment

CNS depression is characterized by deep, unarousable sleep and possible coma, hypotension or hypertension, extrapyramidal symptoms, dystonia, abnormal involuntary muscle movements, agitation, seizures, arrhythmias, ECG changes, hypothermia or hyperthermia, and autonomic nervous system dysfunction.

Treatment is symptomatic and supportive, including maintaining vital signs, airway, stable body temperature, and fluid and electrolyte balance.

Do not induce vomiting: drug inhibits cough reflex, and aspiration may occur. Use gastric lavage, then activated charcoal and saline cathartics; dialysis does not help. Regulate body temperature as needed. Treat hypotension with I.V. fluids: *do not give epinephrine.* Treat seizures with parenteral diazepam or barbiturates; arrhythmias with parenteral phenytoin (1 mg/kg with rate titrated to blood pressure); extrapyramidal reactions with benztropine 1 to 2 mg or parenteral diphenhydramine at 10 to 50 mg.

☑ Special considerations

Besides those relevant to all *phenothiazines,* consider the following recommendations.

- Note that depot injection (25 mg/ml) and I.M. injection (2.5 mg/ml) are not interchangeable.
- Depot injection is not recommended for patients who are not stabilized on a phenothiazine. This form has a prolonged elimination; its action could not be terminated in case of adverse reactions.

Patient education

- Inform patient that drug may cause dizziness or drowsiness. Patient should avoid hazardous tasks that require alertness until CNS response to drug is established.
- Tell patient to avoid ingestion of alcohol and to seek medical approval before taking other drugs.
- Instruct patient to promptly report rash or hives, anxiety, nervousness, anorexia (especially in underweight patients), suspicion of pregnancy, or intent to become pregnant.

Pediatric use

- Safety and efficacy in children below age 12 have not been established.

Breast-feeding

- Drug enters breast milk. Use with caution; potential benefits to the mother should outweigh the potential harm to the infant.

flurandrenolide

Cordran, Cordran SP, Drenison*

Pharmacologic classification: topical adrenocorticoid
Therapeutic classification: anti-inflammatory
Pregnancy risk category C

How supplied

Available by prescription only
Cream: 0.025%, 0.05%
Lotion: 0.05%
Ointment: 0.025%, 0.05%
Tape: 4 mcg/cm^2

Indications, route, and dosage

Inflammation of corticosteroid-responsive dermatoses

Adults and children: Apply cream, lotion, or ointment sparingly daily to q.i.d. Apply tape q 12 hours.

Occlusive dressings may be used for severe or resistant dermatoses. The tape is usually applied as an occlusive dressing to clean, dry affected areas.

Pharmacodynamics

Anti-inflammatory action: Flurandrenolide stimulates the synthesis of enzymes needed to decrease the inflammatory response. Flurandrenolide is a group III (0.05%, 0.025%) fluorinated glucocorticoid.

Pharmacokinetics

- *Absorption:* Amount absorbed depends on strength of preparation, amount applied, and nature of skin at application site. It ranges from about 1% in areas with a thick stratum corneum (such as the palms, soles, elbows, and knees) to as high as 36% in areas of the thinnest stratum corneum (face, eyelids, and genitals). Absorption increases in areas of skin damage, inflammation, or occlusion. Some systemic absorption may occur, especially through the oral mucosa.
- *Distribution:* After topical application, drug is distributed throughout the local skin. Any drug that is absorbed into circulation is removed rapidly from the blood and distributed into muscle, liver, skin, intestines, and kidneys.
- *Metabolism:* After topical administration, drug is metabolized primarily in the skin. The small amount that is absorbed into systemic circulation is metabolized primarily in the liver to inactive compounds.
- *Excretion:* Inactive metabolites are excreted by the kidneys, primarily as glucuronides and sulfates, but also as unconjugated products. Small amounts of the metabolites are also excreted in feces.

Contraindications and precautions

Contraindicated in patients hypersensitive to drug.

Interactions

None significant.

Effects on diagnostic tests

None reported.

Adverse reactions

Skin: burning, pruritus, irritation, dryness, erythema, folliculitis, hypertrichosis, hypopigmentation, acneiform eruptions, allergic contact dermatitis; *maceration, secondary infection, atrophy, striae, miliaria* (with occlusive dressings); purpura, stripping of epidermis, furunculosis (with tape).

Other: ***hypothalamic-pituitary-adrenal axis suppression,*** Cushing's syndrome, hyperglycemia, glucosuria.

Overdose and treatment

No information available.

☑ Special considerations

Recommendations for use of flurandrenolide, for care and teaching of patients during therapy, and for use in elderly patients, children, and breast-feeding women are the same as those for all *topical adrenocorticoids.*

flurazepam hydrochloride

Apo-Flurazepam*, Dalmane, Novoflupam*

Pharmacologic classification: benzodiazepine
Therapeutic classification: sedative-hypnotic
Controlled substance schedule IV
Pregnancy risk category X

How supplied

Available by prescription only
Capsules: 15 mg, 30 mg

Indications, route, and dosage

Insomnia

Adults: 15 to 30 mg P.O. h.s.

✦ ***Dosage adjustment.*** In patients over age 65, 15 mg P.O. h.s.

Pharmacodynamics

Sedative action: Flurazepam depresses the CNS at the limbic and subcortical levels of the brain. It produces a sedative effect by potentiating the effect of the neurotransmitter gamma-aminobutyric acid on its receptor in the ascending reticular activating system, which increases inhibition and blocks both cortical and limbic arousal.

Pharmacokinetics

- *Absorption:* When administered orally, flurazepam is absorbed rapidly through the GI tract. Onset of action occurs within 20 minutes, with peak action in 1 to 2 hours. Duration of action is 7 to 10 hours.
- *Distribution.* Distributed widely throughout the body. Approximately 97% of an administered dose is bound to plasma protein.
- *Metabolism.* Drug is metabolized in the liver to the active metabolite desalkylflurazepam.
- *Excretion.* Desalkylflurazepam is excreted in urine; half-life is 50 to 100 hours.

Contraindications and precautions

Contraindicated in patients with hypersensitivity to drug and during pregnancy. Use cautiously in patients with impaired renal or hepatic function, chronic pulmonary insufficiency, mental depression, suicidal tendencies, or history of drug abuse.

Interactions

Flurazepam potentiates the CNS depressant effects of *phenothiazines, narcotics, barbiturates, alcohol, antihistamines, MAO inhibitors, general anesthetics,* and *antidepressants.*

Concomitant use with *cimetidine, ritonavir,* and possibly *disulfiram* causes diminished hepatic metabolism of flurazepam, which increases its plasma concentration.

Heavy smoking accelerates flurazepam's metabolism, thus lowering clinical effectiveness.

Benzodiazepines may decrease plasma levels of *haloperidol*. Flurazepam may decrease the therapeutic effects of *levodopa*.

Effects on diagnostic tests

Flurazepam therapy may elevate liver function test results. Minor changes in EEG patterns, usually low-voltage, fast activity, may occur during and after flurazepam therapy.

Adverse reactions

CNS: *daytime sedation, dizziness, drowsiness, disturbed coordination,* lethargy, confusion, *headache,* light-headedness, nervousness, hallucinations, staggering, ataxia, disorientation, ***coma.***
GI: nausea, vomiting, heartburn, diarrhea, abdominal pain.
Hepatic: elevated liver enzymes.
Other: physical or psychological dependence.

Overdose and treatment

Clinical manifestations of overdose include somnolence, confusion, hypoactive reflexes, dyspnea, labored breathing, hypotension, bradycardia, slurred speech, unsteady gait or impaired coordination and, eventually, coma.

Support blood pressure and respiration until drug effects subside; monitor vital signs. Mechanical ventilatory assistance via endotracheal (ET) tube may be required to maintain a patent airway and support adequate oxygenation. Use I.V. fluids to promote diuresis and vasopressors such as dopamine and phenylephrine to treat hypotension, as needed. Flumazenil, a specific benzodiazepine antagonist, may be useful as an adjunct to supportive therapy.

If patient is conscious, induce emesis. Use gastric lavage if ingestion was recent, but only if an ET tube is present to prevent aspiration. After emesis or lavage, administer activated charcoal with a cathartic as a single dose. Dialysis is of limited value. Do not use barbiturates if excitation occurs to avoid exacerbation of excitatory state or potentiation of CNS depressant effects.

☑ Special considerations

Besides those relevant to all *benzodiazepines,* consider the following recommendations.

- Studies have demonstrated a "carryover effect." Drug is most effective after 3 or 4 nights of use because of long half-life. Do not increase dose more frequently than every 5 days.
- Monitor hepatic function, and AST, ALT, bilirubin, and alkaline phosphatase levels for changes.
- Drug is useful for patients who have trouble falling asleep and who awaken frequently at night and early in the morning.
- Although prolonged use is not recommended, this drug has proven effective for up to 4 weeks of continuous use.
- Rapid withdrawal after prolonged use can cause withdrawal symptoms.
- Lower doses are effective in patients with renal or hepatic dysfunction.
- Store in a cool, dry place, away from light.

Patient education

- Warn patient to avoid alcohol while taking drug.
- Advise female patient not to take drug if she is pregnant. Tell her to call immediately if she suspects pregnancy.
- Emphasize the potential for excessive CNS depression if drug is taken with alcohol, even if it is taken the evening before ingestion of alcohol.
- Advise patient that rebound insomnia may occur after stopping drug.
- Warn patient not to discontinue medication abruptly after prolonged therapy.
- Advise patient not to exceed prescribed dosage.

Geriatric use

- Elderly patients are more susceptible to CNS depressant effects of flurazepam. They may require assistance and supervision with walking and daily activities during initiation of therapy or after an increase in dose.
- Lower doses usually are effective in elderly patients because of decreased elimination.

Pediatric use

- Closely observe a neonate for withdrawal symptoms if the mother took flurazepam during pregnancy. Use of flurazepam during labor may cause neonatal flaccidity.
- Drug is not for use in children under age 15.
- Neonates are more sensitive to flurazepam because of slower metabolism. The possibility of toxicity is greatly increased.

Breast-feeding

- Drug is excreted in breast milk. A breast-fed infant may become sedated, have feeding difficulties, or lose weight. Avoid use in breast-feeding women.

flurbiprofen

Ansaid

Pharmacologic classification: NSAID, phenylalkanoic acid derivative
Therapeutic classification: antiarthritic
Pregnancy risk category B

How supplied

Available by prescription only
Tablets: 50 mg, 100 mg

Indications, route, and dosage

Rheumatoid arthritis and osteoarthritis
Adults: 200 to 300 mg P.O. daily, divided b.i.d., t.i.d., or q.i.d.

✦ ***Dosage adjustment.*** Patients with end-stage renal disease may exhibit accumulation of flurbiprofen metabolites, but half-life of parent compound is unchanged. Monitor patient closely and adjust dosage accordingly.

Pharmacodynamics
Anti-inflammatory action: An NSAID, flurbiprofen interferes with the synthesis of prostaglandins.

Pharmacokinetics
• *Absorption:* Well absorbed after oral administration, with peak levels occurring in about 1½ hours. Administering with food alters rate, but not extent, of absorption.
• *Distribution:* Flurbiprofen is highly bound (more than 99%) to plasma proteins.
• *Metabolism:* Primarily in the liver. The major metabolite shows little anti-inflammatory activity.
• *Excretion:* Primarily in the urine. Average elimination half-life is 6 to 10 hours.

Contraindications and precautions
Contraindicated in patients with hypersensitivity to drug, or history of aspirin- or NSAID-induced asthma, urticaria, or other allergic-type reactions. Use cautiously in elderly or debilitated patients and those with history of peptic ulcer disease, herpes simplex keratitis, impaired renal or hepatic function, cardiac disease, or conditions associated with fluid retention.

Interactions
Patients taking *oral anticoagulants* may exhibit increased bleeding tendencies. Monitor closely. *Aspirin* may decrease flurbiprofen levels. Concomitant use is not recommended.

Drug may decrease the effectiveness of *diuretics.* Monitor patient closely. *Antacids* and *food* may decrease the rate, but not the extent, of absorption.

Effects on diagnostic tests
None reported.

Adverse reactions
CNS: *headache,* anxiety, insomnia, dizziness, increased reflexes, tremors, amnesia, asthenia, drowsiness, malaise, depression.
CV: *edema,* ***heart failure,*** hypertension, vasodilation.
EENT: rhinitis, tinnitus, visual changes, epistaxis.
GI: *dyspepsia, diarrhea, abdominal pain, nausea,* constipation, ***bleeding,*** flatulence, vomiting.
GU: *symptoms suggesting urinary tract infection,* hematuria, interstitial nephritis, ***renal failure.***
Hematologic: ***thrombocytopenia,*** neutropenia, anemia, ***aplastic anemia.***
Hepatic: *elevated liver enzymes, jaundice.*
Respiratory: asthma.
Skin: rash, photosensitivity, urticaria, angioedema.
Other: weight changes.

Overdose and treatment
Overdosage has resulted in lethargy, coma, respiratory depression, epigastric pain and distress.

Treatment should be supportive. Emptying the stomach by emesis or lavage would be of little use if the ingestion took place more than an hour before treatment, but is still recommended.

☑ Special considerations
Besides those relevant to all *NSAIDs*, consider the following recommendations.
• Closely monitor patient with impaired hepatic or renal function and elderly or debilitated patients; they may need lower doses. These patients may be at risk for renal toxicity. Periodically monitor renal function.
• Patients receiving long-term therapy should have periodic liver function studies, ophthalmologic and auditory examinations, and hematocrit determinations.

Patient education
• Teach patient the signs and symptoms of GI bleeding, and tell him to discontinue the drug and call promptly if these occur.
• Tell patient to take drug with food, milk, or antacid to minimize GI upset.
• Advise patient to avoid hazardous activities that require alertness until the adverse CNS effects of the drug are known.
• Tell patient to immediately report edema, substantial weight gain, black stools, rash, itching, or visual disturbances.

Pediatric use
• Safe use in children has not been established.

Breast-feeding
• A breast-feeding woman taking 200 mg of flurbiprofen daily could deliver as much as 0.1 mg to the infant daily. Breast-feeding is not recommended during therapy with flurbiprofen.

flurbiprofen sodium
Ocufen Liquifilm

Pharmacologic classification: NSAID
Therapeutic classification: ophthalmic anti-inflammatory, antimiotic
Pregnancy risk category C

How supplied
Available by prescription only
Ophthalmic solution: 0.03%

Indications, route, and dosage
Inhibition of intraoperative miosis
Adults: Instill 1 drop into the eye(s) undergoing surgery approximately q 30 minutes, beginning 2 hours before surgery. Give a total of 4 drops.

Pharmacodynamics
Anti-inflammatory action: Flurbiprofen acts by inhibiting the cyclo-oxygenase enzyme that is essential in converting arachidonic acid to prostaglandin. When applied topically, it inhibits prostaglandin synthesis in the iris, ciliary body, and conjunctiva. It does not affect intraocular pressure or tonographic aqueous outflow resistance.

Antimiotic action: Drug inhibits or reduces miosis and possibly some manifestations of ocular inflammation induced by ocular trauma. When administered prophylactically, topical flurbiprofen inhibits intraoperative trauma-induced miosis. However, drug has little, if any, effect, if administered after trauma-induced miosis is present. Flurbiprofen does not inhibit or reduce light-induced miosis.

Pharmacokinetics

- *Absorption:* No information is available concerning absorption after ophthalmic administration.
- *Distribution:* Flurbiprofen is at least 99% bound to plasma proteins. Whether flurbiprofen crosses the placenta or is distributed into breast milk is unknown.
- *Metabolism:* After ophthalmic administration, flurbiprofen is absorbed systemically and is metabolized primarily in the liver where it is converted mainly to inactive glucuronide and sulfate compounds.
- *Excretion:* Inactive metabolites are excreted by the kidneys, primarily as glucuronides and sulfates. Biologic half-life of orally administered flurbiprofen is 6 to 10 hours.

Contraindications and precautions

Contraindicated in patients with hypersensitivity to drug. Use cautiously in patients with history of herpes simplex keratitis, aspirin or NSAID allergy, bleeding tendencies, and those receiving medications that may prolong clotting times.

Interactions

None reported.

Effects on diagnostic tests

None reported.

Adverse reactions

EENT: transient burning and stinging on instillation, ocular irritation.

Overdose and treatment

Overdosage ordinarily will not cause acute complications. After accidental ingestion, fluids are recommended to dilute the drug.

☑ Special considerations

- Store away from heat in a dark, tightly closed container; protect drug from freezing.

Patient education

- Teach patient not to touch eye dropper to eye.
- Remind patient to keep drug container closed tightly.
- Advise patient not to use more drug than the amount prescribed or to use flurbiprofen for other eye problems unless prescribed.
- Instruct patient to discard drug when outdated or no longer needed.

Pediatric use

- Safety and efficacy in children have not been established.

flutamide

Eulexin

Pharmacologic classification: nonsteroidal antiandrogen
Therapeutic classification: antineoplastic
Pregnancy risk category D

How supplied

Available by prescription only
Capsules: 125 mg

Indication, route, and dosage

Treatment of metastatic prostatic carcinoma (stage D2) in combination with leutinizing hormone-releasing hormone analogues, such as leuprolide acetate
Adults: 250 mg P.O. q 8 hours.

Pharmacodynamics

Antitumor action: Flutamide inhibits androgen uptake or prevents binding of androgens in nucleus of cells within target tissues. Prostatic carcinoma is known to be androgen-sensitive.

Pharmacokinetics

- *Absorption:* Rapid and complete absorption occurs after oral administration.
- *Distribution:* Studies in animals show that drug concentrates in the prostate. Drug and its active metabolite is about 95% protein bound.
- *Metabolism:* Rapid, with at least six metabolites identified. More than 97% of the drug is metabolized within 1 hour of administration.
- *Excretion:* More than 95% in the urine.

Contraindications and precautions

Contraindicated in patients hypersensitive to drug.

Interactions

None reported.

Effects on diagnostic tests

Elevation of plasma testosterone and estradiol levels has been reported. Serum ALT, AST, bilirubin, and creatinine levels may be increased.

Adverse reactions

CNS: *drowsiness, confusion, depression, anxiety, nervousness.*
CV: *peripheral edema, hypertension.*
GI: *diarrhea, nausea, vomiting.*
GU: *impotence, loss of libido.*
Hematologic: anemia, leukopenia, ***thrombocytopenia,*** hemolytic anemia.
Hepatic: elevated liver enzyme levels, hepatitis.
Skin: rash, photosensitivity.
Other: *hot flashes,* gynecomastia.

Overdose and treatment

No experience with overdose in humans has been reported. Dosage as high as 1,500 mg daily for 36 weeks has been reported without serious adverse effects.

☑ Special considerations

• Flutamide must be taken continuously with the agent used for medical castration (such as leuprolide acetate) to produce full benefit of therapy. Leuprolide suppresses testosterone production, while flutamide inhibits testosterone action at the cellular level. Together they can impair the growth of androgen-responsive tumors.

Patient education

• Tell patient not to discontinue either leuprolide or flutamide without medical approval.
• Explain that some symptoms may worsen initially before they improve.

Pediatric use

• Safe use in children has not been established.

Breast-feeding

• It is unknown if drug is excreted in breast milk. Avoid use in breast-feeding women.

---

fluticasone propionate

Cutivate, Flonase, Flovent

Pharmacologic classification: corticosteroid
Therapeutic classification: topical/inhalation anti-inflammatory
Pregnancy risk category C

How supplied

Available by prescription only
Cream: 0.05%
Ointment: 0.005%
Metered nasal spray: 50 mcg/actuation
Inhalation aerosol: 44 mcg/actuation, 110 mcg/actuation, 220 mcg/actuation
Inhalation powder: 50-mcg, 100-mcg, 250-mcg rotadisk

Indications, route, and dosage

Relief of inflammation and pruritus of corticosteroid-responsive dermatoses
Adults: Apply sparingly to affected area b.i.d. and rub in gently and completely.
Allergic rhinitis
Adults: 2 sprays in each nostril once daily or 1 spray b.i.d.
Children age 12 or older: 1 spray in each nostril daily. May increase dosage to 2 sprays in each nostril for severe symptoms; depending on patient's response, dosage may be decreased again to 1 spray.
Maintenance treatment of asthma as prophylactic therapy
Adults and children 12 and older: 88 to 220 mcg inhalation aerosol b.i.d., titrating to maximum 440 mcg inhalation aerosol b.i.d.
Adults and adolescents: 100 mcg inhalation powder b.i.d., titrating to maximum 500 mcg inhalation powder b.i.d.
Children age 4 to 11: 50 mcg inhalation powder b.i.d., titrating to maximum 100 mcg inhalation powder b.i.d.

See also package insert for dosing considerations in combination with oral corticosteroids.

Pharmacodynamics

Anti-inflammatory action: Fluticasone stimulates synthesis of enzymes needed to decrease inflammation.

Pharmacokinetics

• *Absorption:* Amount of fluticasone absorbed depends on the amount applied, application site, vehicle used, use of occlusive dressing, and integrity of epidermal barrier. Some systemic absorption does occur.
• *Distribution:* Drug is distributed throughout the local skin.
• *Metabolism:* Fluticasone is metabolized primarily by the skin. Absorbed drug is extensively metabolized by the liver.
• *Excretion:* Less than 5% is excreted in urine as metabolites; rest is excreted in feces as parent drug and metabolites.

Contraindications and precautions

Contraindicated in patients hypersensitive to drug or its components and in patients with viral, fungal, herpetic, or tubercular skin lesions.

Flovent inhalation aerosol and powder are contraindicated as the primary treatment in status asthmaticus or other acute episodes of asthma where intensive measures are required.

Use care when transferring patients from systemically active corticosteroids to Flovent inhalation aerosol or powder because deaths have occurred in asthmatic patients during and after transfer from systemic corticosteroids to less systemically available inhalation corticosteroids. During periods of stress or severe asthma attack, patients who have been withdrawn from systemic corticosteroids should be instructed to resume oral corticosteroids in large doses immediately and contact their primary health care providers for further assistance.

Interactions

None significant.

Effects on diagnostic tests

None reported.

Adverse reactions

CNS: dizziness, giddiness.
GU: dysmenorrhea.
Musculoskeletal: pain in joints, sprain or strain aches and pains, pain in limbs.
Respiratory: bronchitis, chest congestion.
Skin: stinging, burning, pruritus, irritation, dryness, erythema, folliculitis, skin atrophy, leukoderma, vesicles, numbness of fingers, rash, hypertrichosis, acneiform eruptions, hypopigmentation, perioral dermatitis, allergic contact dermatitis, secondary infection, striae, miliaria.
Other: ***hypothalamic-pituitary-adrenal axis suppression,*** Cushing's syndrome, hyperglycemia, glucosuria, fever.

☑ Special considerations

- Do not use for treatment of rosacea, perioral dermatitis, or acne.
- Mixing with other bases or vehicles may affect potency far beyond expectations.
- Risk of adverse reactions may be minimized by changing to a less potent agent.
- During withdrawal from oral corticosteroids, some patients may experience symptoms of systemically active corticosteroid withdrawal, such as joint or musculoskeletal pain, malaise, and depression, despite maintenance or improvement of respiratory function.
- Because of the possibility of systemic absorption of inhalation steroids, patients treated with these drugs should be observed carefully for any evidence of sytemic corticosteroid effects. Special care should be taken during periods of stress or postoperatively for adrenal insufficiency.
- Flovent inhalation aerosol and powder are not indicated for the relief of acute bronchospasm.

Patient education

- Inform patient to apply agent sparingly and rub in lightly. Washing the area before application may increase drug penetration.
- Instruct patient to report burning, irritation, or persistent or worsened condition.
- Tell patient to avoid prolonged use, contact with eyes, or use around genital area, rectal area, on face, and in skin creases.
- Inform patient to rinse mouth well after steroid inhalation.
- Teach patient on inhalation steroids to avoid exposure to chickenpox or measles, and if they are exposed, to consult their primary health care provider immediately.

Pediatric use

- Safety and efficacy of topical form have not been established in children. Safety and efficacy of nasal form have not been established in children under age 12; use of drug is not recommended in these patients.
- A reduction of growth velocity in children or teenagers may occur as a result of the use of corticosteroids for treatment or from inadequate control of chronic disease such as asthma. The benefits of asthma control from corticosteroid therapy must be weighed against the possibilty of growth suppression in these patients.

Breast-feeding

- Use with caution in breast-feeding women because it is unknown if topical or inhalation corticosteroids undergo sufficient absorption to produce systemic effects in the infant.

fluvastatin sodium

Lescol

Pharmacologic classification: hydroxymethylglutaryl-coenzyme A (HMG-CoA) reductase inhibitor
Therapeutic classification: cholesterol-lowering antilipemic
Pregnancy risk category X

How supplied

Available by prescription only
Capsules: 20 mg, 40 mg

Indications, route, and dosage

Reduction of low-density lipoprotein and total cholesterol levels in patients with primary hypercholesterolemia (types IIa and IIb) when response to diet and other nonpharmacologic measures has been inadequate

Adults: Initially, 20 mg P.O. h.s. Increase dosage p.r.n. to a maximum of 40 mg daily.

✦ ***Dosage adjustment.*** With a persistent increase in ALT or AST levels of at least three times the upper limit of normal, withdrawal of fluvastatin is recommended. Because fluvastatin is cleared hepatically, with less than 5% of the dose excreted into urine, dosage adjustments for mild to moderate renal impairment are not necessary. Exercise caution with severe impairment.

Pharmacodynamics

Antilipemic action: Fluvastatin is a competitive inhibitor of HMG-CoA reductase, which is responsible for the conversion of HMG-CoA to mevalonate, a precursor of sterols, including cholesterol. This enzyme is an early (and rate-limiting) step in the synthetic pathway of cholesterol. Fluvastatin increases high-density lipoproteins and decreases low-density lipoproteins, very-low-density lipoproteins, and plasma triglycerides.

Pharmacokinetics

- *Absorption:* Drug is absorbed rapidly and virtually completely (98%) after oral administration on an empty stomach.
- *Distribution:* Over 98% of circulating drug is bound to plama proteins.
- *Metabolism:* Fluvastatin is completely metabolized in the liver. It has no active metabolites.
- *Excretion:* Approximately 5% of fluvastatin is excreted in urine and 90% in feces.

Contraindications and precautions

Contraindicated in patients with hypersensitivity to drug; in those with active liver disease or conditions associated with unexplained persistent elevations of serum transaminase levels; in pregnant and breast-feeding women; and in women of childbearing age unless there is no risk of pregnancy.

Use cautiously in patients with impaired renal function and history of hepatic disease or heavy alcohol consumption.

Interactions
Cholestyramine or *colestipol* may bind fluvastatin in the GI tract and decrease absorption. Administer fluvastatin at bedtime, at least 2 hours after the resin, to avoid significant interaction from the drug binding to the resin. *Cimetidine, omeprazole,* and *ranitidine* decrease fluvastatin metabolism. The patient should be monitored closely. *Cyclosporine* and other *immunosuppressants, erythromycin, gemfibrozil,* and *niacin* increase the risk of polymyositis and rhabdomyolysis when administered concomitantly with fluvastatin; therefore, concomitant use should be avoided. Fluvastatin may alter *digoxin* pharmacokinetics. Monitor the patient's serum digoxin levels carefully. *Rifampin* enhances fluvastatin metabolism and decreases plasma levels. Monitor the patient closely for lack of effect.

Effects on diagnostic tests
Fluvastatin may elevate serum ALT, AST, CK, alkaline phosphatase, and bilirubin levels. Thyroid function test abnormalities also can occur.

Adverse reactions
CNS: headache, fatigue, dizziness, insomnia.
GI: dyspepsia, diarrhea, nausea, vomiting, abdominal pain, constipation, flatulence, tooth disorder.
Hematologic: thrombocytopenia, leukopenia, ***hemolytic anemia.***
Respiratory: sinusitis, *upper respiratory infection,* rhinitis, cough, pharyngitis, bronchitis.
Other: arthropathy, muscle pain, hypersensitivity reactions (rash, pruritus), increased liver enzyme levels.

Overdose and treatment
No information available. If an accidental overdose occurs, treat symptomatically and institute supportive measures as required. The dialyzability of fluvastatin and its metabolites in humans is unknown.

☑ Special considerations
• Institute fluvastatin only after diet and other nonpharmacologic therapies have proven ineffective. Maintain patient on a standard low-cholesterol diet during therapy.
• Drug may be taken without regard to meals; however, efficacy is enhanced if drug is taken in the evening.
• Monitor patient closely for signs of myositis.
• Liver function tests should be performed at the start of therapy, every 4 to 6 weeks during the first 3 months of therapy, every 6 to 12 weeks during the next 12 months, and at 6-month intervals thereafter.

Patient education
• Tell patient to take fluvastatin at bedtime to enhance effectiveness.
• Instruct patient on a standard low-cholesterol diet and emphasize importance of dietary compliance as part of therapy. Also stress importance of weight control and exercise in controlling elevated serum lipid levels.
• Warn patient to restrict alcohol intake because of potentially serious adverse effects.
• Tell patient to report adverse reactions, particularly muscle aches and pains.

Pediatric use
• Safety and effectiveness in patients under age 18 have not been established. Use in pediatric patients is not recommended.

Breast-feeding
• Preclinical data suggest that drug occurs in breast milk in a 2:1 ratio (milk:plasma). The potential for serious adverse reactions in nursing infants indicates that breast-feeding women should not take fluvastatin.

fluvoxamine maleate
Luvox

Pharmacologic classification: selective serotonin reuptake inhibitor (SSRI)
Therapeutic classification: anticompulsive
Pregnancy risk category C

How supplied
Available by prescription only
Tablets: 50 mg, 100 mg

Indications, route, and dosage
Obsessive-compulsive disorder
Adults: Initially, 50 mg P.O. daily h.s. Increase in 50-mg increments q 4 to 7 days until maximum benefit is achieved. Maximum daily dosage is 300 mg. Total daily dosages exceeding 100 mg should be given in two divided doses.
✦ ***Dosage adjustment.*** Because the elderly and patients with hepatic impairment have been observed to have decreased clearance of fluvoxamine maleate, dose titration may be appropriate.

Pharmacodynamics
Anticompulsive action: The exact mechanism of action is unknown. Fluvoxamine is a potent selective inhibitor of the neuronal uptake of serotonin, which is thought to improve obsessive-compulsive behavior.

Pharmacokinetics
• *Absorption:* Absolute bioavailablility of drug is 53%.
• *Distribution:* Mean apparent volume of distribution is about 25 L/kg. About 80% of drug is bound to plasma protein (mostly albumin).
• *Metabolism:* Drug is extensively metabolized in the liver mostly by oxidative demethylation and deamination.
• *Excretion:* Fluvoxamine's metabolites are primarily excreted in urine.

Contraindications and precautions
Contraindicated in patients with hypersensitivity to drug or to other phenylpiperazine antidepressants and within 14 days of MAO inhibitor therapy. Use

cautiously in patients with hepatic dysfunction, concomitant conditions that may affect hemodynamic responses or metabolism, or history of mania or seizures.

Interactions

Astemizole may cause decreased metabolism leading to increased levels of the antihistamine and cardiotoxicity. Avoid concomitant use. Fluvoxamine causes reduced clearance of *benzodiazepines, theophylline*, and *warfarin;* use together cautiously. However, *diazepam* should not be coadministered with fluvoxamine. An adjustment in diazepam dosage may be necessary.

Drug may cause elevated serum levels of *carbamazepine, clozapine, methadone, metoprolol, propranolol*, and *tricyclic antidepressants*. Use together with caution and monitor patient closely for adverse reactions. Dosage adjustments may be necessary. *Diltiazem* may cause bradycardia; therefore, monitor patient's heart rate.

Because *lithium* and *tryptophan* may enhance fluvoxamine's effects, use together cautiously. *MAO inhibitors* may cause severe excitation, hyperpyrexia, myoclonus, delirium, and coma. Avoid concomitant use.

Effects on diagnostic tests

None reported.

Adverse reactions

CNS: headache, asthenia, somnolence, insomnia, nervousness, dizziness, tremor, anxiety, vasodilation, hypertonia, agitation, depression, CNS stimulation, taste perversion.
CV: palpitations, vasodilation.
EENT: amblyopia.
GI: *nausea, diarrhea, constipation, dyspepsia,* anorexia, *vomiting,* flatulence, tooth disorder, dysphagia, *dry mouth.*
GU: decreased libido, abnormal ejaculation, urinary frequency, impotence, anorgasmia, urine retention.
Respiratory: upper respiratory infection, dyspnea, yawning.
Skin: sweating.
Other: flulike syndrome, chills.

Overdose and treatment

Common signs and symptoms of fluvoxamine overdosage include drowsiness, vomiting, diarrhea, and dizziness; coma, tachycardia, bradycardia, hypotension, ECG abnormalities, liver function abnormalities, and seizures may also occur. Symptoms such as aspiration pneumonitis, respiratory difficulties, or hypokalemia may occur because of loss of consciousness or vomiting.

Treatment is supportive. Besides maintaining an open airway and monitoring vital signs and ECG, administration of activated charcoal may be as effective as emesis or lavage. Because absorption with overdose may be delayed, measures to minimize absorption may be necessary for up to 24 hours postingestion. Dialysis is not believed to be beneficial.

☑ Special considerations

- At least 14 days should be allowed after stopping fluvoxamine before patient is started on an MAO inhibitor. Also, at least 14 days should be allowed before patient may start fluvoxamine after MAO inhibitor therapy has been discontinued.
- Record mood changes. Monitor patient for suicidal tendencies, and allow a minimum supply of drug.

Patient education

- Warn patient not to engage in hazardous activity until CNS effects are known.
- Advise patient to avoid alcoholic beverages while taking fluvoxamine.
- Alert patient that smoking may decrease the effectiveness of drug.
- Instruct female patient to call immediately if pregnancy is suspected or if she intends to become pregnant during therapy.
- Tell patient to report rash, hives, or a related allergic reaction.
- Inform patient that several weeks of therapy may be required to obtain the full antidepressant effect. Once improvement is seen, advise patient not to discontinue the drug until directed by primary health care provider.
- Advise patient to call before taking OTC drugs because of possible drug interactions.

Geriatric use

- Drug clearance is decreased by about 50% in elderly patients compared with younger patients. Administer drug cautiously in this age group and dosage titrated slowly during initiation of therapy.

Pediatric use

- Safety and effectiveness in children under age 18 have not been established.

Breast-feeding

- Drug is excreted in breast milk and should not be given to breast-feeding women.

folic acid

Folvite

Pharmacologic classification: folic acid derivative
Therapeutic classification: vitamin supplement
Pregnancy risk category A

How supplied

Available by prescription only
Tablets: 1 mg
Injection: 10-ml vials (folic acid 5 mg/ml contains 1.5% benzyl alcohol and EDTA; Folvite 5 mg/ml contains 1.5% benzyl alcohol)

Available without a prescription
Tablets: 0.4 mg, 0.8 mg

Indications, route, and dosage

Megaloblastic or macrocytic anemia secondary to folic acid deficiency, hepatic disease, alcoholism, intestinal obstruction, excessive hemolysis

Pregnant and breast-feeding women: 0.8 mg P.O., S.C., or I.M. daily.

Adults and children age 4 and older: 0.4 mg P.O., S.C., or I.M. daily for 4 to 5 days. After anemia secondary to folic acid deficiency is corrected, proper diet and RDA supplements are necessary to prevent recurrence.

Children under age 4: Up to 0.3 mg P.O., S.C., or I.M. daily.

Prevention of megaloblastic anemia of pregnancy and fetal damage

Adults: 1 mg P.O., S.C., or I.M. daily during pregnancy.

Nutritional supplement

Adults: Give 0.15 to 0.2 mg P.O., S.C., or I.M. daily for males; 0.15 to 0.18 mg P.O., S.C., or I.M. daily for females.

Children: 0.05 mg P.O. daily.

Tropical sprue

Adults: 3 to 15 mg P.O. daily.

Pharmacodynamics

Nutritional action: Exogenous folate is required to maintain normal erythropoiesis and to perform nucleoprotein synthesis. Folic acid stimulates production of RBCs, WBCs, and platelets in certain megaloblastic anemias.

Dietary folic acid is present in foods, primarily as reduced folate polyglutamate. This vitamin may be absorbed only after hydrolysis, reduction, and methylation occur in the GI tract. Conversion to active tetrahydrofolate may require vitamin B_{12}.

Oral synthetic form of folic acid is a monoglutamate and is absorbed completely after administration, even in malabsorption syndromes.

Pharmacokinetics

- *Absorption:* Folic acid is absorbed rapidly from the GI tract, mainly from the proximal part of the small intestine. Peak folate activity in blood occurs within 30 to 60 minutes after oral administration. Normal serum folate concentrations range from 0.005 to 0.015 mcg/ml. Usually, serum levels below 0.005 mcg/ml indicate folate deficiency; those below 0.002 mcg/ml usually result in megaloblastic anemia.
- *Distribution:* The active tetrahydrofolic acid and its derivatives are distributed into all body tissues; the liver contains about half of the total body folate stores. Folate is actively concentrated in the CSF. Folic acid is distributed into breast milk.
- *Metabolism:* Folic acid is metabolized in the liver to *N*-methyltetrahydrofolic acid, the main form of folate storage and transport.
- *Excretion:* A single 0.1-mg to 0.2-mg dose of folic acid usually results in only a trace amount of drug in the urine. After administering large doses, excessive folate is excreted unchanged in urine. Small amounts of folic acid have been recovered in feces. About 0.05 mg/day of normal body folate stores is lost by a combination of urinary and fecal excretion and oxidative cleavage of the molecule.

Contraindications and precautions

Contraindicated in patients with undiagnosed anemia because it may mask pernicious anemia. Also contraindicated in those with vitamin B_{12} deficiency.

Interactions

Concomitant use of folic acid (15 to 20 mg/day) decreases serum *phenytoin* levels to subtherapeutic concentrations, possibly with increased frequency of seizures. Folic acid appears to increase the metabolic clearance of phenytoin and cause redistribution of phenytoin in the CSF and brain.

Conversely, phenytoin and *primidone* may decrease serum folate levels and produce symptoms of folic acid deficiency in long-term therapy. *Para-aminosalicylic acid* and *sulfasalazine* may cause a similar deficiency. Although *oral contraceptives* may also impair folate metabolism and produce folate depletion, they are unlikely to induce anemia or megaloblastic changes.

Folic acid may interfere with the antimicrobial actions of *pyrimethamine* against toxoplasmosis.

Folic acid antagonists, pyrimethamine, trimethoprim, or *triamterene* may cause dihydrofolate reductase deficiency, which may interfere with folic acid utilization.

Effects on diagnostic tests

Folic acid therapy alters serum and erythrocyte folate concentrations; falsely low serum and erythrocyte folate levels may occur with the *Lactobacillus casei* assay in patients receiving anti-infectives, such as tetracycline, which suppress the growth of this organism.

Adverse reactions

Respiratory: ***bronchospasm.***
Skin: allergic reactions (rash, pruritus, erythema).
Other: general malaise.

Overdose and treatment

Folic acid is relatively nontoxic. Adverse GI and CNS effects have been reported rarely in patients receiving 15 mg of folic acid daily for 1 month.

☑ Special considerations

- The RDA for folic acid is 25 to 200 mcg in children and 180 to 200 mcg in adults; 100 mcg/day is considered an adequate oral supplement. Pregnant women require 400 mcg daily. During the first 6 months of breast-feeding, women require 280 mcg daily; during the second 6 months, this requirement decreases to 260 mcg daily.
- The preferred route of administration for folic acid is P.O. The manufacturer recommends deep I.M., S.C. or I.V. only when P.O. treatment is not feasible or when malabsorption is suspected.
- Many drugs, such as oral contraceptives and alcohol, can cause folate deficiencies.
- Ensure that patients do not also have vitamin B_{12} deficiency; folic acid can improve hematologic measurements while allowing progression of neurologic

damage. Do not use as sole treatment of pernicious anemia.
- Patients undergoing renal dialysis are at risk for folate deficiency.
- Monitor CBC to measure effectiveness of drug treatment.
- Protect folic acid injections from light.

Patient education
- Teach patient about dietary sources of folic acid, such as yeast, whole grains, leafy vegetables, beans, nuts, and fruit.
- Tell patient that folate is destroyed by overcooking and canning.
- Stress importance of administering folic acid only under medical supervision.

Breast-feeding
- Folic acid is excreted in breast milk. Daily doses of 0.8 mg are sufficient to maintain a normoblastic bone marrow after clinical symptoms have subsided and blood components have returned to normal.

foscarnet sodium (phosphonoformic acid)
Foscavir

Pharmacologic classification: pyrophosphate analogue
Therapeutic classification: antiviral
Pregnancy risk category C

How supplied
Injection: 24 mg/ml in 250-ml and 500-ml vials

Indications, route, and dosage
Cytomegalovirus (CMV) retinitis in patients with AIDS
Adults: Initially, 60 mg/kg I.V. as an induction treatment in patients with normal renal function. Administer as an I.V. infusion over 1 hour q 8 hours for 2 or 3 weeks, depending on response. Follow with a maintenance infusion of 90 mg/kg daily administered over 2 hours; increase as needed and tolerated to 120 mg/kg daily if disease shows signs of progression.

Mucocutaneous acyclovir-resistant herpes simplex virus (HSV) infection
Adults: 40 mg/kg I.V. Administer as an I.V. infusion over 1 hour q 8 to 12 hours for 2 or 3 weeks, depending on response.

◊ ***Varicella zoster infection***
Adults: mg/kg I.V. q 8 hours for 10 to 21 days.

✦ **Dosage adjustment.** For adult patients with renal failure, calculate patient's weight-adjusted creatinine clearance (ml/minute/kg) from this equation:
for male patients:

$$\text{creatinine clearance} = \frac{(140 - \text{age})}{(\text{serum creatinine} \times 72)};$$

for female patients: multiply the above value by 0.85.

Administer according to the following tables.

Induction dose

Creatinine clearance (ml/min/kg)	Dose to be administered q 8 hr (mg/kg)
≥1.6	60
1.5	57
1.4	53
1.3	49
1.2	46
1.1	42
1	39
0.9	35
0.8	32
0.7	28
0.6	25
0.5	21
0.4	18

Maintenance dose

Creatinine clearance (ml/min/kg)	Equivalent to 90 mg/kg daily	Equivalent to 120 mg/kg daily
≥1.4	90	120
1.2 to 1.4	78	104
1 to 1.2	75	100
0.8 to 1	71	94
0.6 to 0.8	63	84
0.4 to 0.6	57	76

Pharmacodynamics
Antiviral action: An organic analogue of pyrophosphate, a compound used in many enzymatic reactions, foscarnet inhibits all known herpes viruses in vitro by blocking the pyrophosphate binding site on DNA polymerases and reverse transcriptases.

Pharmacokinetics
- *Absorption:* Unknown.
- *Distribution:* Foscarnet is about 14% to 17% bound to plasma proteins. Animal studies indicate that the drug is deposited in bone.
- *Metabolism:* Unknown.
- *Excretion:* About 80% to 90% of drug appears in the urine unchanged. Drug clearance is dependent on renal function. Plasma half-life is about 3 hours.

Contraindications and precautions
Contraindicated in patients with hypersensitivity to drug. Use with extreme caution in patients with impaired renal function.

Interactions
Nephrotoxic drugs, such as *amphotericin B* and *aminoglycosides*, may increase risk of nephrotoxicity. Avoid concomitant use.

Pentamidine may increase the risk of nephrotoxicity; severe hypocalcemia has also been reported. Don't use together. *Zidovudine* may increase the incidence or severity of anemia. Monitor blood counts.

Adverse reactions

CNS: *headache, **seizures,*** fatigue, malaise, asthenia, paresthesia, dizziness, hypoesthesia, neuropathy, tremor, ataxia, generalized spasms, dementia, stupor, sensory disturbances, meningitis, aphasia, abnormal coordination, EEG abnormalities, depression, confusion, anxiety, insomnia, somnolence, nervousness, amnesia, agitation, aggressive reaction, hallucinations.
CV: *hypertension, palpitations, ECG abnormalities, sinus tachycardia,* cerebrovascular disorder, *first-degree atrioventricular block, hypotension, flushing,* edema.
EENT: visual disturbances, taste perversion, eye pain, conjunctivitis.
GI: *nausea, diarrhea, vomiting, abdominal pain, anorexia,* constipation, dysphagia, rectal hemorrhage, dry mouth, dyspepsia, melena, flatulence, ulcerative stomatitis, ***pancreatitis.***
GU: *abnormal renal function, decreased creatinine clearance and increased serum creatinine levels, albuminuria, dysuria, polyuria, urethral disorder, urine retention, urinary tract infections, **acute renal failure,*** moniliasis.
Hematologic: ***anemia, granulocytopenia, leukopenia, bone marrow suppression, thrombocytopenia,*** platelet abnormalities, thrombocytosis, WBC count abnormalities, lymphadenopathy.
Respiratory: *cough, dyspnea,* pneumonitis, sinusitis, pharyngitis, rhinitis, respiratory insufficiency, pulmonary infiltration, stridor, pneumothorax, ***bronchospasm,*** hemoptysis, flulike symptoms.
Skin: *rash, increased sweating,* pruritus, skin ulceration, erythematous rash, seborrhea, skin discoloration, facial edema.
Other: ***death,** fever,* pain, infection, sepsis, hypokalemia, hypomagnesemia, hypophosphatemia or hyperphosphatemia, hypocalcemia, leg cramps, rigors, inflammation and pain at infusion site, lymphoma-like disorder, sarcoma, back or chest pain, abnormal hepatic function, bacterial or fungal infections, abscess, increased liver enzymes, arthralgia, myalgia.

☑ Special considerations

- Anemia is common (up to 33% of patients treated with drug) and may be severe enough to require transfusions.
- Do not exceed the recommended dosage, infusion rate, or frequency of administration. Know that all doses must be individualized according to patient's renal function.
- An infusion pump must be used to administer foscarnet.
- Unlike ganciclovir, foscarnet does not require cellular activation by thymidine kinase or other kinases. Foscarnet may be active against certain CMV strains resistant to ganciclovir.

Patient education

- Make sure patient understands that adverse reactions to drug are common and that he should report for all laboratory studies and follow-up appointments to check his progress.
- Advise patient to report perioral tingling, numbness in the extremities, and paresthesia.

Geriatric use

- It is unknown if age alters drug response. However, elderly patients are likely to have preexisting renal function impairment, which requires alterations in dosage.

Pediatric use

- Safety and efficacy in children have not been established. Postmortem studies in animals show that up to 40% of a dose is deposited in the teeth and bones. It is likely that similar deposition may be seen in growing children.

Breast-feeding

- It is unknown if drug is excreted in breast milk; however, animal studies indicate that drug may concentrate in breast milk when administered at high doses. Use with caution.

fosfomycin tromethamine
Monurol

Pharmacologic classification: phosphonic acid derivative
Therapeutic classification: antibiotic
Pregnancy risk category B

How supplied

Available by prescription only
Single-dose sachet: 3 g

Indications, route, and dosage

***Uncomplicated urinary tract infections (acute cystitis) in women caused by susceptible strains of* Escherichia coli *and* Enterococcus faecalis**
Women over age 18: 1 sachet P.O. mixed with 3 to 4 oz (½ cup) of cold water just before ingestion.

Pharmacodynamics

Bactericidal action: Drug inhibits bacterial cell wall synthesis. It is effective in the urinary tract because it reduces adherence of bacteria to uroepithelial cells.

Pharmacokinetics

- *Absorption:* Drug is rapidly absorbed following oral administration and converted to free acid, fosfomycin. Peak concentration when taken on an empty stomach occurs within 2 hours; when drug is taken with food, peak concentrations occur within 4 hours.
- *Distribution:* Mean apparent steady-state volume of distribution is 136 L following oral administration of fosfomycin. Fosfomycin is not bound to plasma proteins; it is distributed to the kidneys, bladder wall, prostate, and seminal vesicles. Drug crosses the placenta.

• *Metabolism:* Not reported
• *Excretion:* Drug is excreted unchanged in both urine and feces.

Contraindications and precautions
Contraindicated in patients with known hypersensitivity to drug. Use cautiously in patients with renal impairment.

Interactions
Metoclopramide lowers serum concentration and urinary excretion of fosfomycin. Avoid concomitant use. *Other drugs that increase GI motility* may produce similar effects.

Effects on diagnostic tests
None reported.

Adverse reactions
CNS: asthenia, dizziness, *headache.*
EENT: pharyngitis, rhinitis.
GI: abdominal pain, *diarrhea,* dyspepsia, nausea.
GU: dysmenorrhea, vaginitis.
Skin: rash.
Other: back pain.

Overdose and treatment
There have been no reported cases of overdosage. If overdosage occurs, provide symptomatic and supportive treatment.

☑ Special considerations
• Obtain urine specimens for culture and sensitivity before and after therapy has been completed.
• Know that using more than one single-dose sachet to treat a single episode of acute cystitis will not improve clinical success and may cause adverse reactions.

Patient education
• Instruct patient how to properly take drug. Drug should not be taken in its dry form. The entire contents of a single-dose sachet should be mixed with 3 to 4 oz (½ cup) cold water. Stir to dissolve, and drink immediately.
• Tell patient to call if symptoms do not improve in 2 to 3 days.
• Inform patient that drug may be taken without regard to food.

Geriatric use
• There were no clinically significant differences in the effectiveness or safety of drug therapy in women age 65 or less compared with those over age 65.

Pediatric use
• Safety and effectiveness in children age 12 and under have not been established.

Breast-feeding
• It is not known if drug is excreted in breast milk. Because many drugs are excreted in breast milk, a decision should be made whether to stop breast-feeding or taking the drug.

fosinopril sodium
Monopril

Pharmacologic classification: ACE inhibitor
Therapeutic classification: antihypertensive
Pregnancy risk category C (D second and third trimesters)

How supplied
Available by prescription only
Tablets: 10 mg, 20 mg, 40 mg

Indications, route, and dosage
Treatment of hypertension
Adults: Initially, 10 mg P.O. daily; adjust dose based on blood pressure response at peak and trough levels. Usual dose: 20 to 40 mg daily; maximum up to 80 mg daily. Dose may be divided.
Treatment of heart failure
Adults: Initially, 10 mg P.O. daily; maximum dose up to 40 mg daily. Doses may be divided.

Pharmacodynamics
Antihypertensive action: Fosinopril is believed to lower blood pressure primarily by suppressing the renin-angiotensin-aldosterone system, although it has also been effective in patients with low-renin hypertension.

Pharmacokinetics
• *Absorption:* Absorbed slowly through GI tract, primarily via proximal small intestine.
• *Distribution:* Over 95% is protein-bound; peak concentrations are achieved in about 3 hours.
• *Metabolism:* Hydrolyzed primarily in the liver and gut wall by esterases.
• *Excretion:* 50% of drug is excreted in urine; rest in feces.

Contraindications and precautions
Contraindicated in patients with hypersensitivity to drug or other ACE inhibitors and in breast-feeding patients. Use cautiously in patients with impaired renal or hepatic function.

Interactions
Excessive hypotension may occur with concurrent use of *diuretics,* especially if patient is volume depleted. Effect may be minimized by stopping diuretic. Concurrent use of *potassium supplements* or *potassium-sparing diuretics* may result in hyperkalemia; monitor potassium levels. When used with *lithium,* increased serum lithium levels and symptoms of lithium toxicity may occur; monitor lithium levels frequently. Risk is increased if *diuretic* is also used.

Antacids may impair absorption of fosinopril; separate administration by at least 2 hours.

Effects on diagnostic tests
False low measurements of digoxin levels may result with the DIGI TAB radioimmunoassay kit for digoxin; other kits may be used. Transient eleva-

tions of BUN and serum creatinine levels and liver function tests and decreases in hematocrit or hemoglobin may also occur.

Adverse reactions

CNS: headache, dizziness, fatigue, syncope, paresthesia, sleep disturbance, ***CVA.***
CV: chest pain, angina, ***MI, hypertensive crisis,*** rhythm disturbances, palpitations, hypotension, orthostatic hypotension.
EENT: tinnitus, sinusitis.
GI: nausea, vomiting, diarrhea, pancreatitis, hepatitis, dry mouth, abdominal distention, abdominal pain, constipation.
GU: sexual dysfunction, decreased libido, renal insufficiency.
Respiratory: *dry, persistent, tickling, nonproductive cough; bronchospasm.*
Skin: urticaria, rash, photosensitivity, pruritus.
Other: *angioedema,* arthralgia, musculoskeletal pain, myalgia, gout, hyperkalemia.

Overdose and treatment

Human overdose has never been reported; however, the most common manifestation of overdose is likely to be hypotension. Treat with infusion of 0.9% NaCl. Hemodialysis and peritoneal dialysis are not effective in removing the drug.

☑ Special considerations

- Diuretic therapy is usually discontinued 2 to 3 days before start of ACE inhibitor therapy to reduce risk of hypotension. If fosinopril does not adequately control blood pressure, diuretic may be reinstituted with care. Monitor potassium levels.
- Perform CBC with differential counts before therapy, then every 2 weeks for 3 months and periodically thereafter.
- Incidence of postural hypotension is low.
- Blood pressure is lowered within 1 hour of a single dose of 10 to 40 mg, with peak reductions occurring 2 to 6 hours after dose. The antihypertensive effect lasts 24 hours.
- Effectiveness of fosinopril is unaffected by age, sex, or weight.

Patient education

- Tell patient to take dose 1 hour before or 2 hours after food or antacids.
- Tell patient to report light-headedness in the first few days of therapy and signs of infection such as fever or sore throat. He should also call if the following occur and discontinue drug immediately: swelling of tongue, lips, face, mucous membranes, eyes, lips, or extremities; difficulty swallowing or breathing; or hoarseness.
- Advise that patient maintain the same salt intake as before therapy, because salt restriction can lead to precipitous drop in blood pressure with initial doses of this drug. Large reductions in blood pressure may also occur with excessive perspiration and dehydration.
- Warn patient to avoid sudden position changes until effect of drug is known; however, postural hypotension is infrequent.
- Instruct female patient of childbearing age to call immediately if pregnancy is suspected.

Geriatric use

- No age-related differences have been observed.

Pediatric use

- Safety and efficacy have not been established.

Breast-feeding

- Avoid use of drug; significant levels have been detected in breast milk.

fosphenytoin sodium

Cerebyx

Pharmacologic classification: hydantoin derivative
Therapeutic classification: anticonvulsant
Pregnancy risk category D

How supplied

Available by prescription only
Injection: 2 ml (150 mg fosphenytoin sodium equivalent to 100 mg phenytoin sodium), 10 ml (750 mg fosphenytoin sodium equivalent to 500 mg phenytoin sodium)

Indications, route, and dosage

Status epilepticus
Adults: Give 15 to 20 mg phenytoin sodium equivalent (PE)/kg I.V. at 100 to 150 PE/minute as a loading dose and then, 4 to 6 mg PE/kg/day I.V. as a maintenance dose. (Phenytoin may be used instead of fosphenytoin as maintenance using the appropriate dose.)
Prevention and treatment of seizures during neurosurgery
Adults: Administer 10 to 20 mg PE/kg I.M. or I.V. at an I.V. infusion rate not exceeding 150 mg PE/minute as a loading dose. Maintenance dose is 4 to 6 mg PE/kg/day I.V.
Short-term substitution for oral phenytoin therapy
Adults: Same total daily dosage as oral phenytoin sodium therapy given as a single daily dose I.M. or I.V. at an I.V. infusion rate not exceeding 150 mg PE/minute. (Some patients may require more frequent dosing.)

Pharmacodynamics

Anticonvulsant action: Fosphenytoin is a prodrug of phenytoin and therefore, its anticonvulsant action is that of phenytoin. Phenytoin stabilizes neuronal membranes and limits seizure activity by modulation of voltage-dependent sodium channels of neurons, inhibition of calcium flux across neuronal membranes, modulation of voltage-dependent calcium channels of neurons, and enhancement of sodium-potassium adenosine triphosphatase activity of neurons and glial cells.

Pharmacokinetics

• *Absorption:* Peak plasma concentrations of fosphenytoin occur about 30 minutes after I.M. administration or at end of the I.V. infusion.
• *Distribution:* About 95% to 99% is bound to plasma proteins, primarily albumin. Volume of distribution increases with dose and rate and ranges from 4.3 to 10.8 L.
• *Metabolism:* Conversion half-life of fosphenytoin to phenytoin is about 15 minutes. Phosphatases are believed to play a major role in the conversion.
• *Excretion:* Unknown, although it is not excreted in urine.

Contraindications and precautions

Contraindicated in patients with hypersensitivity to the drug or its components, phenytoin, or other hydantoins. Also contraindicated in patients with sinus bradycardia, SA block, second- and third-degree AV block, and Adams-Stokes syndrome because of the effect of parenteral phenytoin on ventricular automaticity.

Use cautiously in patients with hypotension, severe myocardial insufficiency, impaired renal or hepatic function, hypoalbuminemia, porphyria, diabetes mellitus, and history of hypersensitivity to similiarly structured drugs, such as barbiturates and succinimides.

Interactions

Most significant drug interactions expected to occur are those that are commonly seen with phenytoin.

Drugs that may increase plasma phenytoin concentrations (and thus its therapeutic effects) include *acute alcohol intake, amiodarone, chloramphenicol, chlordiazepoxide, cimetidine, diazepam, dicumarol, disulfiram, estrogens, ethosuximide, fluoxetine, H_2-antagonists, halothane, isoniazid, methylphenidate, phenothiazines, phenylbutazone, salicylates, succinimides, sulfonamides, tolbutamide,* and *trazodone.*

Plasma phenytoin levels may be decreased by *carbamazepine, chronic alcohol abuse,* or *reserpine.*

Drugs that may increase or decrease plasma phenytoin levels include *phenobarbital, valproic acid,* and *sodium valproate.* Similarly, the effects of phenytoin on the concentrations of these drugs is unpredictable.

Drugs whose efficacy may be decreased by phenytoin due to increased hepatic metabolism include *coumarin, digitoxin, doxycycline, estrogens, furosemide, oral contraceptives, rifampin, quinidine, theophylline,* and *vitamin D.*

Tricyclic antidepressants may lower seizure threshold and may require adjustments in phenytoin dosage.

Effects on diagnostic tests

Fosphenytoin may decrease serum concentrations of T_4. It may also produce artificially low results in dexamethasone or metyrapone tests. Phenytoin may also cause increased serum concentrations of glucose, alkaline phosphatase, and gamma glutamyl transpeptidase.

Adverse reactions

CNS: increased reflexes, speech disorder, dysarthria, intracranial hypertension, thinking abnormality, nervousness, hypesthesia, confusion, twitching, positive Babinski's sign, circumoral paresthesia, hemiplegia, hypotonia, seizure, extrapyramidal syndrome, insomnia, meningitis, depersonalization, CNS depression, hypokinesia, hyperkinesia, brain edema, paralysis, psychosis, aphasia, emotional lability, ***coma,*** hyperesthesia, myoclonus, personality disorder, acute brain syndrome, encephalitis, subdural hematoma, encephalopathy, hostility, akathisia, amnesia, neurosis, migraine, syncope, cerebral infarct, asthenia, headache, *nystagmus, dizziness, somnolence, ataxia,* stupor, incoordination, paresthesia, tremor, agitation, vertigo.
CV: hypertension, ***cardiac arrest, cerebral hemorrhage,*** palpitation, sinus bradycardia, atrial flutter, ***bundle branch block,*** cardiomegaly, orthostatic hypotension, ***pulmonary embolus,*** QT interval prolongation, thrombophlebitis, ventricular extrasystoles, ***heart failure,*** vasodilation, tachycardia, hypotension.
EENT: taste perversion, deafness, visual field defect, eye pain, conjunctivitis, photophobia, hyperacusis, mydriasis, parosmia, ear pain, taste loss, tinnitus, diplopia, amblyopia.
Endocrine: diabetes insipidus.
GI: constipation, dyspepsia, diarrhea, anorexia, GI hemorrhage, increased salivation, abnormal liver function tests, tenesmus, tongue edema, dysphagia, flatulence, gastritis, ileus, nausea, dry mouth, vomiting.
GU: urine retention, oliguria, dysuria, vaginitis, albuminuria, genital edema, kidney failure, polyuria, urethral pain, urinary incontinence, vaginal moniliasis.
Hematologic: ***thrombocytopenia,*** anemia, leukocytosis, hypochromic anemia, leukopenia, ecchymosis.
Musculoskeletal: myasthenia, myopathy, leg cramps, arthralgia, myalgia.
Respiratory: cyanosis, pneumonia, pharyngitis, sinusitis, hyperventilation, rhinitis, apnea, aspiration pneumonia, asthma, dyspnea, atelectasis, increased cough, increased sputum, epistaxis, hypoxia, pneumothorax, hemoptysis, bronchitis.
Skin: petechia, rash, maculopapular rash, urticaria, sweating, skin discoloration, contact dermatitis, pustular rash, skin nodule, *pruritus.*
Other: lymphadenopathy, hypokalemia, hyperglycemia, hypophosphatemia, alkalosis, acidosis, dehydration, hyperkalemia, ketosis, pelvic pain, back pain.

Overdose and treatment

There have been no reports of fosphenytoin overdosage. However because it is a prodrug of phenytoin, overdosage may be similiar. Early signs of phenytoin overdose may include drowsiness, nausea, vomiting, nystagmus, ataxia, dysarthria, tremor, and slurred speech; hypotension, respiratory depression, and coma may follow. Death is caused by respiratory and circulatory depression. Estimated lethal dose of phenytoin in adults is 2 to 5 g.

Formate and phosphate are metabolites of fosphenytoin and therefore may contribute to signs of toxicity following overdosage. Signs of formate toxicity are similar to those of methanol toxicity and are associated with severe anion-gap metabolic acidosis. Large amounts of phosphate, delivered rapidly, could potentially cause hypocalcemia with paresthesia, muscle spasms, and seizures. Ionized free calcium levels can be measured and, if low, used to guide treatment.

Treatment is with gastric lavage or emesis and followed by supportive treatment. Monitor vital signs and fluid and elecytrolyte balance. Forced diuresis is of little or no value. Hemodialysis or peritoneal dialysis may be helpful.

☑ Special considerations

- Fosphenytoin should always be prescribed and dispensed in phenytoin sodium equivalent units (PE). Do not, therefore, make adjustments in the recommended doses when substituting fosphenytoin for phenytoin and vice versa.
- Before I.V. infusion, dilute fosphenytoin in D_5W or 0.9% saline solution for injection to a concentration ranging from 1.5 to 25 mg PE/ml. Do not administer at a rate exceeding 150 mg PE/minute.
- Dose of I.V. fosphenytoin used to treat status epilepticus should be administered at a maximum rate of 150 mg PE/minute. The typical infusion of drug administered to a 50-kg patient takes 5 to 7 minutes whereas that of an identical molar dose of phenytoin cannot be accomplished in less than 15 to 20 minutes because of the untoward CV effects that accompany the direct I.V. administration of phenytoin at rates above 50 mg/minute. Do not use I.M. fosphenytoin because therapeutic phenytoin concentrations may not be reached as rapidly as with I.V. administration.
- If rapid phenytoin loading is a primary goal, I.V. administration of fosphenytoin is preferred because the time to achieve therapeutic plasma phenytoin concentrations is greater following I.M. than that following I.V. administration.
- Monitor patient's ECG, blood pressure, and respiration continuously throughout the period where maximal serum phenytoin concentrations occur, about 10 to 20 minutes after the end of fosphenytoin infusions. Severe CV complications are most commonly encountered in elderly or gravely ill patients. Reduction in rate of administration or discontinuation of dosing may be needed.
- Patients receiving fosphenytoin at doses of 20 mg PE/kg at 150 mg PE/minute are expected to experience some sensory discomfort, with the groin being the most common location. The occurrence and intensity of the discomfort can be lessened by slowing or temporarily stopping the infusion.
- The phosphate load provided by fosphenytoin (0.0037 mmol phosphate/mg PE fosphenytoin) must be taken into consideration when treating patients who require phosphate restriction, such as those with severe renal impairment.
- Discontinue drug if rash appears. If rash is exfoliative, purpuric, or bullous or if lupus erythematosus, Stevens-Johnson syndrome, or toxic epidermal necrolysis is suspected, do not resume use of drug, and seek alternative therapy. If the rash is mild (measleslike or scarlatiniform), therapy may be resumed after it has completely disappeared. If the rash recurs on reinstitution of therapy, further fosphenytoin or phenytoin administration is contraindicated.
- Discontinue drug in patients with acute hepatotoxicity and do not readminister to these patients.
- I.M. drug administration generates systemic phenytoin concentrations that are similar enough to oral phenytoin sodium to allow essentially interchangeable use.
- A dose of 15 to 20 mg PE/kg of fosphenytoin infused I.V. at 100 to 150 mg PE/minute yields plasma-free phenytoin concentrations over time that approximate those achieved when an equivalent dose of phenytoin sodium (such as parenteral dilantin) is administered at 50 mg/minute I.V.
- Following drug administration, it is recommended that phenytoin concentrations not be monitored until conversion to phenytoin is essentially complete; about 2 hours after the end of an I.V. infusion or 4 hours after I.M. administration.
- Interpretation of total phenytoin plasma concentrations should be made cautiously in patients with renal or hepatic disease or hypoalbuminemia due to an increased fraction in unbound phenytoin. Unbound phenytoin concentrations may be more useful in these patients. Also, these patients are at increased risk for both the frequency and severity of adverse reactions when fosphenytoin is administered I.V.
- Abrupt withdrawal of drug may precipitate status epilepticus.

Patient education

- Warn patient that sensory disturbances may occur with I.V. drug administration.
- Tell patient to report adverse reactions, especially rash, immediately.

Geriatric use

- Elderly patients metabolize and excrete phenytoin slowly; therefore, fosphenytoin should be administered cautiously to older adults.

Pediatric use

- Safety and effectiveness in children have not been established

Breast-feeding

- Because it is not known if fosphenytoin is excreted in breast milk, breast-feeding is not recommended.

furosemide

Apo-Furosemide*, Lasix, Lasix Special*, Novosemide*, Uritol*

Pharmacologic classification: loop diuretic
Therapeutic classification: diuretic, antihypertensive
Pregnancy risk category C

How supplied

Available by prescription only
Tablets: 20 mg, 40 mg, 80 mg

* Canada only ◊ Unlabeled clinical use

Solution: 10 mg/ml, 40 mg/5 ml
Injection: 10 mg/ml

Indications, route, and dosage

Acute pulmonary edema
Adults: 40 mg I.V. injected slowly; then 80 mg I.V. within 1 hour p.r.n.
Infants and children: 1 mg/kg I.M. or I.V. q 2 hours until response is achieved; maximum dosage is 6 mg/kg.
Edema
Adults: 20 to 80 mg P.O. daily in morning, with second dose given in 6 to 8 hours, carefully titrated up to 600 mg daily p.r.n.; or 20 to 40 mg I.M. or I.V. Increase by 20 mg q 2 hours until desired response is achieved. I.V. dosage should be given slowly over 1 to 2 minutes.
Infants and children: 2 mg/kg/day P.O., increased by 1 to 2 mg/kg in 6 to 8 hours p.r.n., carefully titrated not to exceed 6 mg/kg/day.
Hypertension
Adults: 40 mg P.O. b.i.d. Adjust dosage according to response.
◊ ***Hypercalcemia***
Adults: 80 to 100 mg I.V. q 1 to 2 hours; or 120 mg P.O. daily.
✦ ***Dosage adjustment.*** Reduced dosages may be indicated in elderly patients.

Pharmacodynamics

Diuretic action: Loop diuretics inhibit sodium and chloride reabsorption in the proximal part of the ascending loop of Henle, promoting the excretion of sodium, water, chloride, and potassium.

Antihypertensive action: This drug effect may be the result of renal and peripheral vasodilatation and a temporary increase in glomerular filtration rate and a decrease in peripheral vascular resistance.

Pharmacokinetics

- *Absorption:* About 60% of a given furosemide dose is absorbed from the GI tract after oral administration. Food delays oral absorption but does not alter diuretic response. Diuresis begins in 30 to 60 minutes; peak diuresis occurs 1 to 2 hours after oral administration. Diuresis follows I.V. administration within 5 minutes and peaks in 20 to 60 minutes.
- *Distribution:* About 95% of drug is plasma protein-bound. It crosses the placenta and distributes into breast milk.
- *Metabolism:* Drug is metabolized minimally by the liver.
- *Excretion:* About 50% to 80% of a dose is excreted in urine; plasma half-life is about 30 minutes. Duration of action is 6 to 8 hours after oral administration and about 2 hours after I.V. administration.

Contraindications and precautions

Contraindicated in patients with anuria or history of hypersensitivity to drug. Use cautiously in patients with hepatic cirrhosis and during pregnancy.

Interactions

Furosemide potentiates the hypotensive effect of *most other antihypertensive agents* and of other *diuretics*; both actions are used to therapeutic advantage.

Concomitant use with *potassium-sparing diuretics (spironolactone, triamterene, amiloride)* may decrease furosemide-induced potassium loss; use with other potassium-depleting drugs, such as *steroids* and *amphotericin B*, may cause severe potassium loss.

Furosemide may reduce renal clearance of *lithium* and increase lithium levels; lithium dosage may require adjustment.

Indomethacin and *probenecid* may reduce furosemide's diuretic effect; their combined use is not recommended. However, if there is no therapeutic alternative, an increased furosemide dosage may be required.

Concomitant administration of furosemide with *ototoxic or nephrotoxic drugs* may result in enhanced toxicity. Furosemide could prolong neuromuscular blockade by *muscle relaxants*.

Patients receiving I.V. furosemide within 24 hours of a dose of *chloral hydrate* have experienced sweating, flushing, and blood pressure fluctuations; if possible, use an alternative sedative in patients receiving I.V. furosemide.

Effects on diagnostic tests

Drug therapy alters electrolyte balance and liver and renal function tests.

Adverse reactions

CNS: vertigo, headache, dizziness, paresthesia, restlessness.
CV: volume depletion and dehydration, orthostatic hypotension.
EENT: transient deafness with too rapid I.V. injection, blurred vision.
GI: abdominal discomfort and pain, diarrhea, anorexia, nausea, vomiting, constipation, pancreatitis.
GU: nocturia, polyuria, frequent urination, oliguria.
Hematologic: ***agranulocytosis,*** leukopenia, ***thrombocytopenia,*** azotemia, anemia, ***aplastic anemia.***
Skin: dermatitis, purpura.
Other: hypokalemia; hypochloremic alkalosis; asymptomatic hyperuricemia; fever; muscle spasm; weakness; fluid and electrolyte imbalances, including dilutional hyponatremia, hypocalcemia, hypomagnesemia; hyperglycemia and impaired glucose tolerance; transient pain (at I.M. injection site); thrombophlebitis (with I.V. administration).

Overdose and treatment

Clinical manifestations of overdose include profound electrolyte and volume depletion, which may precipitate circulatory collapse. Treatment is chiefly supportive; replace fluids and electrolytes.

☑ Special considerations

Besides those relevant to all *loop diuretics*, consider the following recommendations.

• Give I.V. furosemide slowly, over 1 to 2 minutes; for I.V. infusion, dilute furosemide in D_5W, 0.9% NaCl solution, or lactated Ringer's solution, and use within 24 hours. If high-dose furosemide therapy is needed, administer as a controlled infusion not exceeding 4 mg/minute.

Patient education

• Warn patient that photosensitivity reaction may occur. Explain that reaction is a photoallergy in which ultraviolet radiation alters drug structure, causing allergic reactions in some individuals.
• Tell patient that photosensitivity reactions occur 10 days to 2 weeks after initial sun exposure.

Geriatric use

• Elderly and debilitated patients require close observation because they are more susceptible to drug-induced diuresis. Excessive diuresis promotes rapid dehydration, leading to hypovolemia, hypokalemia, hyponatremia, and circulatory collapse.

Pediatric use

• Use drug with caution in neonates. The usual pediatric dosage can be used, but dosing intervals should be extended. Sorbitol content of oral preparations may cause diarrhea, especially at high dosages.

Breast-feeding

• Drug should not be used by breast-feeding women.

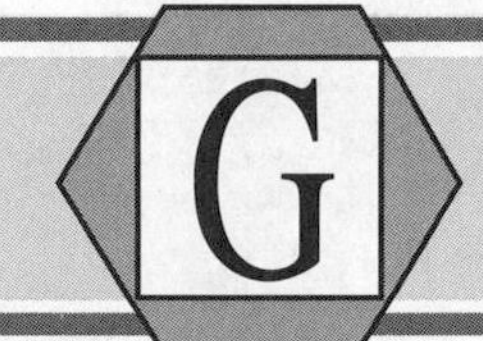

gabapentin
Neurontin

Pharmacologic classification: 1-aminomethyl cyclohexoneacetic acid
Therapeutic classification: anticonvulsant
Pregnancy risk category C

How supplied
Available by prescription only
Capsules: 100 mg, 300 mg, 400 mg

Indications, route, and dosage
Adjunctive treatment of partial seizures with and without secondary generalization
Adults: 300 mg P.O. on day 1, 300 mg P.O. b.i.d. on day 2, and 300 mg P.O. t.i.d. on day 3. Increase dosage as needed and tolerated to 1,800 mg daily, in three divided doses. Usual dosage is 300 to 600 mg P.O. t.i.d., although dosages up to 3,600 mg/day have been well tolerated.

✦ ***Dosage adjustment.*** In adult patients with renal failure, if creatinine clearance is above 60 ml/minute, give 400 mg P.O. t.i.d.; if creatinine clearance is between 30 and 60 ml/minute, give 300 mg P.O. b.i.d.; if creatinine clearance is between 15 and 30 ml/minute, give 300 mg P.O. daily; and if creatinine clearance is less than 15 ml/minute, give 300 mg P.O. every other day. Patients on hemodialysis should receive a loading dose of 300 to 400 mg P.O.; then 200 mg to 300 mg P.O. q 4 hours after hemodialysis.

Pharmacodynamics
Anticonvulsant action: Gabapentin's mechanism of action is unknown. Although it is structurally related to gamma-aminobutyric acid (GABA), the drug does not interact with GABA receptors, is not converted metabolically into GABA or a GABA agonist, and does not inhibit GABA uptake or degradation. Gabapentin does not exhibit affinity for other common receptor sites.

Pharmacokinetics
- *Absorption:* Drug bioavailability is not dose proportional. A 400-mg dose, for example, is about 25% less bioavailable than a 100-mg dose. Over the recommended dose range of 300 to 600 mg t.i.d., however, differences in bioavailability are not large and bioavailability is about 60%. Food has no effect on the rate or extent of absorption.
- *Distribution:* Gabapentin circulates largely unbound (less than 3%) to plasma protein. Drug crosses the blood-brain barrier with approximately 20% of the corresponding plasma concentrations found in CSF.
- *Metabolism:* Drug is not appreciably metabolized in humans.
- *Excretion:* Gabapentin is eliminated from the systemic circulation by renal excretion as unchanged drug. Its elimination half-life is 5 to 7 hours. Drug can be removed from plasma by hemodialysis.

Contraindications and precautions
Contraindicated in patients hypersensitive to drug.

Interactions
Antacids decrease the absorption of gabapentin. Administration of the two drugs should be separated by at least 2 hours.

Effects on diagnostic tests
Gabapentin causes false-postive results with the Ames N-Multistix SG dipstick test for urinary protein when added to other antiepileptic drugs. The more specific sulfosalicylic acid precipitation procedure is recommended to determine the presence of urine protein.

Adverse reactions
CNS: *fatigue, somnolence, dizziness, ataxia, nystagmus, tremor,* nervousness, dysarthria, amnesia, depression, abnormal thinking, twitching, incoordination.
CV: peripheral edema, vasodilation.
EENT: *diplopia, rhinitis,* pharyngitis, dry throat, coughing, *amblyopia.*
GI: nausea, vomiting, dyspepsia, dry mouth, constipation.
GU: impotence.
Hematologic: leukopenia, decreased WBC count.
Skin: pruritus, abrasion.
Other: dental abnormalities, increased appetite, weight gain, back pain, myalgia, fractures.

Overdose and treatment
Acute overdose of gabapentin may cause double vision, slurred speech, drowsiness, lethargy, and diarrhea. Supportive care is recommended. In addition, gabapentin can be removed by hemodialysis and may be indicated by the patient's clinical state or in patients with significant renal impairment.

☑ Special considerations
- Discontinue drug therapy or substitute alternative medication gradually over at least 1 week to minimize risk of precipitating seizures. Do not suddenly withdraw other anticonvulsant drugs in patients starting gabapentin therapy.
- Routine monitoring of plasma drug levels is not necessary. Drug does not appear to alter plasma levels of other anticonvulsants.

• Do not use Ames N-Multistix SG dipstick to test for urine protein; false-positive results can occur.

Patient education

• Warn patient to avoid driving or operating heavy machinery until adverse CNS effects of drug are known.
• Instruct patient to take first dose of drug at bedtime to minimize drowsiness, dizziness, fatigue, and ataxia.
• Inform patient that drug can be taken without regard to meals.

Pediatric use

• Safety and effectiveness in children under age 12 have not been established.

Breast-feeding

• It is not known if drug is excreted in breast milk. Use in breast-feeding patients only if the benefits clearly outweigh the risks.

gallium nitrate

Ganite

Pharmacologic classification: heavy metal
Therapeutic classification: antihypercalcemic
Pregnancy risk category C

How supplied

Available by prescription only
Injection: 500 mg in 20-ml single-dose vial (25 mg/ml)

Indications, route, and dosage

Treatment of cancer-related hypercalcemia after hydration
Adults. Usually, 200 mg/m² I.V. daily for 5 consecutive days. In patients who are hypercalcemic with few symptoms, 100 mg/m² I.V. for 5 days may be used. Dilute in 1,000 ml of 0.9% NaCl solution or D_5W and administer by I.V. infusion over 24 hours. Maintain adequate hydration throughout treatment. If serum calcium levels return to within normal limits in less than 5 days, discontinue therapy.

Pharmacodynamics

Hypocalcemic action: Gallium inhibits calcium resorption from bone by reducing increased bone turnover, but the precise mechanism for inhibiting calcium resorption is unknown.

Pharmacokinetics

• *Absorption:* Plasma half-life is dependent on dosage.
• *Distribution:* Steady-state levels are achieved in 24 to 48 hours.
• *Metabolism:* Drug is not metabolized by liver or kidneys.
• *Excretion:* Excreted by the kidneys; hydration and diuresis do not affect renal clearance of gallium.

Contraindications and precautions

Contraindicated in patients with severe renal impairment. Use cautiously in patients with reduced CV function.

Interactions

Concurrent use with other potentially *nephrotoxic drugs*, such as *aminoglycosides* and *amphotericin B*, may increase risk of renal insufficiency.

Effects on diagnostic tests

During gallium citrate Ga 67 scintigraphy for tumor or abscess localization, gallium nitrate competes with gallium citrate Ga 67 for plasma protein binding sites, resulting in reduced tumor or abscess uptake, increased skeletal uptake, increased renal excretion, and reduced liver uptake of gallium citrate Ga 67.

Adverse reactions

CNS: lethargy, confusion, paresthesia.
CV: tachycardia, lower extremity edema, decreased mean systolic and diastolic blood pressures.
EENT: visual or hearing impairment, acute optic neuritis.
GI: nausea and vomiting, diarrhea, constipation.
GU: *acute renal failure, increased BUN and creatinine levels.*
Hematologic: anemia, leukopenia.
Respiratory: dyspnea, crackles, rhonchi, pulmonary infiltrates, pleural effusion.
Skin: rash.
Other: *hypophosphatemia, hypocalcemia, decreased serum bicarbonate,* fever, hypothermia.

Overdose and treatment

Nausea, vomiting, and renal insufficiency may follow rapid I.V. infusion of gallium or use of doses higher than 200 mg/m². Treat by discontinuing drug and by vigorous hydration with or without diuretics. Monitor serum calcium levels, renal function, and urine output. Balance intake and output levels.

☑ Special considerations

• Store undiluted solution at room temperature. After further dilution, solution may be stored at room temperature for 48 hours or in refrigerator for 7 days. Discard unused portion because product contains no preservatives.
• Gallium is nontoxic to bone cells and its use does not interfere with subsequent chemotherapy.
• Gallium is significantly more effective than calcitonin in reaching normocalcemia (75% versus 27%) and superior in maintaining normocalcemia. Median duration of normocalcemia and hypocalcemia after therapy is 7.5 days.
• Monitor serum creatinine levels; elevated BUN and serum creatinine levels have been observed.
• Adequate hydration of patient is essential. Use extreme care to avoid fluid overload in cardiac-compromised patients.

Geriatric use

• No age-specific data available.

Pediatric use
- Safety and efficacy have not been established.

Breast-feeding
- It is unknown if gallium is excreted in breast milk; risk-benefit ratio must be assessed.

ganciclovir (DHPG)
Cytovene

Pharmacologic classification: synthetic nucleoside
Therapeutic classification: antiviral
Pregnancy risk category C

How supplied
Available by prescription only
Injection: 500-mg vial
Capsules: 250 mg

Indications, route, and dosage
Treatment of cytomegalovirus (CMV) retinitis
Adults: Initially, 5 mg/kg I.V. (given at a constant rate over 1 hour) q 12 hours for 14 to 21 days; followed by a maintenance dose of 5 mg/kg I.V. once daily for 7 days weekly; or 6 mg/kg I.V. once daily for 5 days weekly. These I.V. infusions should be given at a constant rate over 1 hour. Alternately, a maintenance dose of 1,000 mg P.O. t.i.d. or 500 mg P.O. q 3 hours while awake (six times daily) may be used.
Prevention of CMV in transplant recipients
Adults: 5 mg/kg I.V. over 1 hour q 12 hours for 7 to 14 days, followed by a maintenance dose of 5 mg/kg once daily for 7 days weekly or 6 mg/kg once daily for 5 days weekly.
◊ ***Other CMV infections***
Adults: 5 mg/kg I.V. over 1 hour q 12 hours for 14 to 21 days; or 2.5 mg/kg I.V. q 8 hours for 14 to 21 days.
✦ ***Dosage adjustment.*** Adjust dosage in patients with renal failure. A dosage reduction should also be considered for patients with neutropenia, anemia, or thrombocytopenia.

Creatinine clearance (ml/min)	Dosage
I.V. induction dose	
≥ 70	5 mg/kg I.V. q 12 hr
50 to 69	2.5 mg/kg I.V. q 12 hr
25 to 49	2.5 mg/kg I.V. q 24 hr
10 to 24	1.25 mg/kg I.V. q 24 hr
< 10	1.25 mg/kg I.V. three times weekly following hemodialysis

Creatinine clearance (ml/min)	Dosage
P.O. dose	
≥ 70	1,000 mg P.O. t.i.d. or 500 mg q 3 hr, 6 times daily
50 to 69	1,500 mg P.O. daily or 500 mg P.O. t.i.d.
25 to 49	1,000 mg P.O. daily or 500 mg P.O. b.i.d.
10 to 24	500 mg P.O. daily
< 10	500 mg P.O. three times weekly following hemodialysis

Pharmacodynamics
Antiviral action: Ganciclovir is a synthetic nucleoside analogue of 2′-deoxyguanosine. It competitively inhibits viral DNA polymerase, and may be incorporated within viral DNA to cause early termination of DNA replication. It has shown activity against CMV, herpes simplex virus type 1 and type 2 (HSV-1 and HSV-2), varicella zoster virus, Epstein-Barr virus, and hepatitis B virus.

Pharmacokinetics
- *Absorption:* Administered I.V. because less than 7% is absorbed after oral administration.
- *Distribution:* Drug is only 2% to 3% protein-bound. It preferentially concentrates within CMV-infected cells because of action of cellular kinases that convert it to ganciclovir triphosphate.
- *Metabolism:* Mostly (over 90%) excreted unchanged.
- *Excretion:* Elimination half-life is about 3 hours in patients with normal renal function; it can be as long as 30 hours in patients with severe renal failure. The primary route of excretion is through the kidneys by glomerular filtration and some renal tubular secretion.

Contraindications and precautions
Contraindicated in patients with hypersensitivity to drug and with an absolute neutrophil count below 500 mm^3 or a platelet count below 25,000 mm^3. Use cautiously in patients with impaired renal function.

Interactions
There may be a higher incidence of neutropenia in patients also receiving *zidovudine*. Use with *cytotoxic drugs* may result in additive toxicity (bone marrow depression, stomatitis, alopecia). Use with *probenecid* may decrease the renal clearance of ganciclovir. Concomitant use of *imipenem-cilastatin* may increase the risk of seizures.

Effects on diagnostic tests
None reported.

Adverse reactions

CNS: altered dreams, confusion, ataxia, headache, ***seizures, coma,*** dizziness, somnolence, tremor, abnormal thinking, agitation, amnesia, anxiety, neuropathy, paresthesia, asthenia.
EENT: retinal detachment (in CMV retinitis patients).
GI: *nausea, vomiting, diarrhea, anorexia, abdominal pain,* flatulence, dyspepsia, dry mouth.
Hematologic: *granulocytopenia,* ***thrombocytopenia,*** *leukopenia, anemia.*
Hepatic: abnormal liver function tests, increased serum creatinine levels.
Respiratory: pneumonia.
Skin: *rash; sweating;* pruritus, inflammation, pain (at injection site).
Other: phlebitis, chills, sepsis, *fever,* infection.

Overdose and treatment

Overdose may result in emesis, neutropenia, or GI disturbances. Treatment should be symptomatic and supportive. Hemodialysis may be useful. Hydrate the patient to reduce plasma levels.

☑ Special considerations

- Administer drug over 1 hour; do not administer as a rapid I.V. bolus. Do not give I.M. or S.C.
- Reconstitute with sterile water for injection. Do not reconstitute with bacteriostatic water for injection because this may lead to the formation of a precipitate.
- Reconstituted solutions are stable for 12 hours. Do not refrigerate.
- Monitor CBC to detect neutropenia, which may occur in as many as 40% of patients. It usually appears after about 10 days of therapy, and may be associated with a higher dosage (15 mg/kg/day). Neutropenia is reversible, but may necessitate discontinuation of therapy. Patients may resume drug therapy when blood counts return to normal.
- Patients with renal failure will probably need dosage adjustments to prevent toxicity.

Patient education

- Tell patient that maintenance infusions are necessary to prevent recurrence of disease.
- Instruct patients to have regular opthalmic examinations to monitor retinitis.
- Advise patient to immediately report signs or symptoms of infection (fever, sore throat) or easy bruising or bleeding.
- Inform patient to take oral dose with food.

Geriatric use

- Use cautiously in elderly patients with compromised renal function.

Pediatric use

- There has been very little experience with drug in children under age 12. Use with extreme caution, keeping in mind the possible potential for carcinogenic and reproductive toxicity.

Breast-feeding

- Do not use drug in breast-feeding patients. Instruct patient to discontinue breast-feeding until at least 72 hours after last treatment.

gemcitabine hydrochloride

Gemzar

Pharmacologic classification: nucleoside analogue
Therapeutic classification: antitumor
Pregnancy risk category D

How supplied

Available by prescription only
Powder for injection: 200-mg/10 ml, 1-g/50 ml vials

Indications, route, and dosage

Locally advanced (nonresectable stage II or stage III) or metastatic pancreatic adenocarcinoma (stage IV) and in patients previously treated with fluorouracil
Adults: 1,000 mg/m^2 I.V. over 30 minutes once weekly for up to 7 weeks or until toxicity necessitates reducing or holding a dose. Monitor patient's CBC (including differential) and platelet count before each dose. Treatment course of 7 weeks is followed by 1 week rest. Subsequent dosage cycles consist of one infusion weekly for 3 out of 4 consecutive weeks.

✦ ***Dosage adjustment.*** Adjust dosage if bone marrow suppression is detected. Full dose should be given if absolute granulocyte count (AGC) is 1,000/mm^3 or more and platelet count is 100,000/mm^3 or more. If AGC is 500/mm^3 to 999/mm^3, or if platelet count is 50,000/mm^3 to 99,000/mm^3, give 75% of dose. Hold dose if AGC is below 500/mm^3 or platelet count is below 50,000/mm^3. Adjust dosage for subsequent cycles based on AGC and platelet count nadirs and degree of nonhematologic toxicity.

Pharmacodynamics

Cytotoxic action: Drug is cell-phase specific; it inhibits DNA synthesis and blocks progression of cells through G1/S-phase boundary.

Pharmacokinetics

- *Absorption:* Not reported.
- *Distribution:* The volume of distribution (V_d) increases with increased infusion time. Following an infusion lasting under 70 minutes, V_d was 50 L/m^2, suggesting that drug is not extensively distributed. The V_d rose to 370 L/m^2 for longer infusions, reflecting slow equilibration of gemcitabine with the tissue compartment. Plasma protein-binding is negligible. Longer infusion time results in longer drug half-life.
- *Metabolism:* Drug is metabolized to an inactive uracil metabolite.
- *Excretion:* Drug clearance decreases with increasing age; it is also less in women than men. This results in an increased half-life with increased age and in women. In studies, 92% to 98% of drug was recovered almost entirely in the urine.

Contraindications and precautions

Contraindicated in patients with hypersensitivity to drug.

Interactions
None reported.

Effects on diagnostic tests
None reported.

Adverse reactions
CNS: *paresthesia, somnolence.*
GI: *constipation, diarrhea, nausea, stomatitis, vomiting.*
GU: *elevated BUN* and creatinine, *hematuria, proteinuria.*
Hematologic: *anemia*, **LEUKOPENIA, NEUTROPENIA, THROMBOCYTOPENIA.**
Hepatic: *elevated liver enzymes.*
Respiratory: bronchospasm, *dyspnea.*
Other: *alopecia, edema, fever, flulike symptoms,* **HEMORRHAGE, INFECTION,** *pain, peripheral edema, rash.*

Overdose and treatment
There is no known antidote for drug overdosage. If overdose is suspected, monitor patient with appropriate blood counts and provide supportive therapy.

☑ Special considerations
- Perform renal and hepatic function tests before treatment and periodically thereafter.
- Prolongation of infusion time beyond 60 minutes and more frequently than weekly dosing have been shown to increase drug toxicity.
- Monitor CBC, differential, and platelet count before giving each dose. Drug can suppress bone marrow function as manifested by leukopenia, thrombocytopenia, and anemia.
- Follow institutional policy to reduce risks. Preparation and administration of parenteral form of drug is associated with mutagenic, teratogenic, and carcinogenic risks for personnel.
- Age, gender, and renal impairment may predispose patient to toxicity.

Patient education
- Advise patient to watch for signs of infection (fever, sore throat, fatigue) and bleeding (easy bruising, nosebleeds, bleeding gums, melena). Also, tell patient to take temperature daily.
- Advise women of childbearing age to avoid pregnancy or breast-feeding during therapy.

Geriatric use
- Drug clearance is affected by age. There is no evidence, however, that unusual dose adjustments, other than those already recommended, are necessary. Grade 3 to 4 thrombocytopenia was more common in the elderly.

Pediatric use
- Drug has not been studied in pediatric patients.

Breast-feeding
- It is not known if drug is excreted in breast milk. Use with caution.

gemfibrozil
Lopid

Pharmacologic classification: fibric acid derivative
Therapeutic classification: antilipemic
Pregnancy risk category C

How supplied
Available by prescription only
Tablets: 600 mg

Indications, route, and dosage
Type IV hyperlipidemia (hypertriglyceridemia) and severe hypercholesterolemia unresponsive to diet and other drugs; reducing risk of cardiac disease, only in type IIb patients without history of disease
Adults: 1,200 mg P.O. administered in two divided doses 30 minutes before morning and evening meals.

Pharmacodynamics
Antilipemic action: Gemfibrozil decreases serum triglyceride levels and very-low-density lipoprotein (VLDL) cholesterol while increasing serum high-density lipoprotein cholesterol, inhibits lipolysis in adipose tissue, and reduces hepatic triglyceride synthesis; drug is closely related to clofibrate pharmacologically.

Pharmacokinetics
- *Absorption:* Drug is well absorbed from the GI tract; peak plasma concentrations occur 1 to 2 hours after an oral dose. Plasma levels of VLDL decrease in 2 to 5 days; peak clinical effect occurs in 4 weeks. Further decreases in plasma VLDL levels occur over several months.
- *Distribution:* Drug is 95% protein-bound.
- *Metabolism:* Gemfibrozil is metabolized by the liver.
- *Excretion:* Drug is eliminated mostly in urine but some is excreted in feces. After a single dose, half-life is 1½ hours; after multiple doses, half-life decreases to about 1¼ hours.

Contraindications and precautions
Contraindicated in patients with hypersensitivity to drug, hepatic or severe renal dysfunction (including primary biliary cirrhosis), and preexisting gallbladder disease.

Interactions
Gemfibrozil enhances effect of *oral anticoagulants*, increasing risk of hemorrhage; adjust anticoagulant dose to maintain the desired PT, and monitor frequently. Myopathy with rhabdomyolysis can occur with use of gemfibrozil and *lovastatin*, as well as with similar *cholesterol-lowering drugs* (such as *simvastatin* and *pravastatin*). Avoid concomitant use.

Effects on diagnostic tests
Drug therapy may elevate serum levels of CK, ALT, AST, alkaline phosphatase, and LD; it may also decrease serum potassium, hematocrit, hemoglobin, and WBC counts.

Adverse reactions

CNS: headache, fatigue, vertigo.
CV: atrial fibrillation.
GI: abdominal and epigastric pain, diarrhea, nausea, vomiting, *dyspepsia,* constipation, acute appendicitis.
Hematologic: anemia, leukopenia, eosinophilia, ***thrombocytopenia.***
Hepatic: bile duct obstruction, elevated liver enzymes.
Skin: rash, dermatitis, pruritus, eczema.

Overdose and treatment

No information available.

☑ Special considerations

- Because drug is pharmacologically related to clofibrate, adverse reactions associated with clofibrate may also occur with gemfibrozil. Some studies suggest clofibrate increases risk of death from cancer, postcholecystectomy complications, and pancreatitis. These hazards have not been studied in gemfibrozil but should be kept in mind.

Patient education

- Stress importance of close medical supervision and tell patient to report adverse reactions promptly; encourage him to comply with prescribed regimen, diet, and exercise.
- Warn patient not to exceed prescribed dose.
- Advise patient to take drug with food to minimize GI discomfort.

Pediatric use

- Safety and efficacy in children under age 18 have not been established.

Breast-feeding

- Safety in breast-feeding women has not been established.

gentamicin sulfate

Cidomycin*, Garamycin, Genoptic, Genoptic S.O.P., Gentacidin, Gentak, Jenamicin

Pharmacologic classification: aminoglycoside
Therapeutic classification: antibiotic
Pregnancy risk category NR

How supplied

Available by prescription only
Injection: 40 mg/ml (adult), 10 mg/ml (pediatric), 2 mg/ml (intrathecal)
Ophthalmic ointment: 3 mg/g
Ophthalmic solution: 3 mg/ml
Topical cream or ointment: 0.1%

Indications, route, and dosage

Serious infections caused by susceptible organisms
Adults with normal renal function: 3 mg/kg/day I.M. or I.V. infusion (in 50 to 100 ml of 0.9% NaCl solution or D_5W infused over 30 minutes to 2 hours) daily in divided doses q 8 hours. May be given by direct I.V. push if necessary. For life-threatening infections, patient may receive up to 5 mg/kg/day in three to four divided doses.
Children with normal renal function: 2 to 2.5 mg/kg I.M. or I.V. infusion q 8 hours.
Infants and neonates over age 1 week with normal renal function: 2.5 mg/kg I.M. or I.V. infusion q 8 hours.
Neonates under age 1 week: 2.5 mg/kg I.M. or I.V. infusion q 12 hours. For I.V. infusion, dilute in 0.9% NaCl solution or D_5W and infuse over 30 minutes to 2 hours.
Meningitis
Adults: Systemic therapy as above; may also use 4 to 8 mg intrathecally daily.
Children: Systemic therapy as above; may also use 1 to 2 mg intrathecally daily.
Endocarditis prophylaxis for GI or GU procedure or surgery
Adults: 1.5 mg/kg I.M. or I.V. 30 to 60 minutes before procedure or surgery and q 8 hours after, for two doses. Given separately with aqueous penicillin g or ampicillin.
Children: 2 mg/kg I.M. or I.V. 30 to 60 minutes before procedure or surgery and q 8 hours after, for two doses. Given separately with aqueous penicillin g or ampicillin.
External ocular infections caused by susceptible organisms
Adults and children: Instill 1 to 2 drops in eye q 4 hours. In severe infections, may use up to 2 drops q hour. Apply ointment to lower conjunctival sac b.i.d. or t.i.d.
Primary and secondary bacterial infections; superficial burns; skin ulcers; and infected lacerations, abrasions, insect bites, or minor surgical wounds
Adults and children over age 1: Rub in small amount gently t.i.d. or q.i.d., with or without gauze dressing.
Pelvic inflammatory disease
Adults: Initially 2 mg/kg I.M. or I.V; then 1.5 mg/kg q 8 hours.
✦ ***Dosage adjustment.*** In patients with renal failure, initial dose is same as for those with normal renal function. Subsequent doses and frequency determined by renal function studies and blood concentrations; keep peak serum concentrations between 4 and 10 mcg/ml, and trough serum levels; between 1 and 2 mcg/ml. One method is to administer 1 mg/kg doses and adjust the dosing interval based on steady-state serum creatinine, using this formula:

$$\text{creatinine (mg/100 ml)} \times 8 = \text{dosing interval (hours)}$$

Posthemodialysis to maintain therapeutic blood levels
Adults: 1 to 1.7 mg/kg I.M. or I.V. infusion after each dialysis.
Children: 2 to 2.5 mg/kg I.M. or I.V. infusion after each dialysis.

Pharmacodynamics

Antibiotic action: Gentamicin is bactericidal; it binds directly to the 30S ribosomal subunit, thus inhibiting bacterial protein synthesis. Its spectrum of activity includes many aerobic gram-negative organisms (including most strains of *Pseudomonas aeruginosa*) and some aerobic gram-positive organisms. Gentamicin may act against some bacterial strains resistant to other aminoglycosides; bacterial strains resistant to gentamicin may be susceptible to tobramycin, netilmicin, or amikacin.

Pharmacokinetics

- *Absorption:* Absorbed poorly after oral administration and is given parenterally; after I.M. administration, peak serum concentrations occur at 30 to 90 minutes.
- *Distribution:* Drug is distributed widely after parenteral administration; intraocular penetration is poor. CSF penetration is low even in patients with inflamed meninges. Intraventricular administration produces high concentrations throughout the CNS. Protein-binding is minimal. Gentamicin crosses the placenta.
- *Metabolism:* Not metabolized.
- *Excretion:* Excreted primarily in urine by glomerular filtration; small amounts may be excreted in bile and breast milk. Elimination half-life in adults is 2 to 3 hours. In patients with severe renal damage, half-life may extend to 24 to 60 hours.

Contraindications and precautions

Contraindicated in patients hypersensitive to drug or in those who may exhibit cross-sensitivity with other aminoglycosides, such as neomycin. Use systemic treatment cautiously in neonates, infants, the elderly, or in patients with renal or neuromuscular disorders.

Interactions

Concomitant use with the following drugs may increase the hazard of nephrotoxicity, ototoxicity, or neurotoxicity: *methoxyflurane, polymyxin B, vancomycin, capreomycin, cisplatin, cephalosporins, amphotericin B,* and other *aminoglycosides*; hazard of ototoxicity is also increased during use with *ethacrynic acid, furosemide, bumetanide, urea,* or *mannitol. Dimenhydrinate* and other *antiemetic* and *antivertigo drugs* may mask gentamicin-induced ototoxicity.

Concomitant use with a *penicillin* results in synergistic bactericidal effect against *Pseudomonas aeruginosa, Escherichia coli, Klebsiella, Citrobacter, Enterobacter, Serratia,* and *Proteus mirabilis*; however, the drugs are physically and chemically incompatible and are inactivated when mixed or given together.

Gentamicin may potentiate neuromuscular blockade produced by *general anesthetics* or *neuromuscular blocking agents* such as *succinylcholine* and *tubocurarine.*

Effects on diagnostic tests

Gentamicin-induced nephrotoxicity may elevate BUN, nonprotein nitrogen, and serum creatinine levels, and increase urinary excretion of casts.

Adverse reactions

CNS: headache, lethargy, encephalopathy, confusion, dizziness, ***seizures***, numbness, peripheral neuropathy (with injected form).
CV: hypotension (with injected form).
EENT: *ototoxicity,* blurred vision (with injected form); burning, stinging, blurred vision (with ophthalmic ointment), transient irritation (with ophthalmic solution), conjunctival hyperemia (with ophthalmic form).
GI: vomiting, nausea (with injected form).
GU: *nephrotoxicity (with injected form).*
Hematologic: anemia, eosinophilia, leukopenia, ***thrombocytopenia,*** granulocytopenia (with injected form).
Respiratory: ***apnea*** (with injected form).
Skin: rash, urticaria, pruritus, tingling (with injected form); minor skin irritation, possible photosensitivity, allergic contact dermatitis (with topical administration).
Other: fever, muscle twitching, myasthenia gravis-like syndrome, ***anaphylaxis,*** pain at injection site (with injected form); hypersensitivity reactions, overgrowth of nonsusceptible organisms (with ophthalmic form and long-term use).

Note: Systemic absorption from excessive use may cause systemic toxicities.

Overdose and treatment

Clinical signs of overdose include ototoxicity, nephrotoxicity, and neuromuscular toxicity. Drug can be removed by hemodialysis or peritoneal dialysis. Treatment with calcium salts or anticholinesterases reverses neuromuscular blockade.

☑ Special considerations

Besides those relevant to all *aminoglycosides,* consider the following recommendations.

- Increased risk of toxicity is associated with prolonged peak serum concentration above 10 mcg/ml and trough serum concentration above 2 mcg/ml.
- For local application to skin infections, remove crusts by gently soaking with warm water and soap or wet compresses before applying ointment or cream; cover with protective gauze.
- Because drug is dialyzable, patients undergoing hemodialysis may need dosage adjustments.

Patient education

- Teach patient proper topical application of drug; emphasize need to call promptly if lesions worsen or skin irritation occurs.

---

glatiramer acetate (formerly copolymer-1)

Copaxone

Pharmacologic classification: the acetate salts of synthetic peptides containing four naturally occurring amino acids (L-alanine; L-glutamic acid; L-lysine; L-tyrosine)
Therapeutic classification: immune response modifier
Pregnancy risk category B

How supplied

Available by prescription only

Injection for S.C. use: sterile lyophilized material containing 20 mg glatiramer acetate and 40 mg mannitol, USP, in a single-use 2-ml vial (amber glass); 1-ml vials of sterile water for injection (in clear glass) are included for reconstitution

Indications, route, and dosage

To reduce frequency of relapses in patients with relapsing-remitting multiple sclerosis

Adults: 20 mg S.C. daily.

Pharmacodynamics

Immune response modifier action: Mechanism of action in patients with multiple sclerosis is unknown. It is thought to act by modifying immune processes responsible for the pathogenesis of multiple sclerosis.

Pharmacokinetics

Studies in humans not done; pharmacokinetics in patients with impaired renal function are not known.

- *Absorption:* Based on animal data, a substantial fraction of dose injected S.C. may be hydrolyzed locally. Some is presumed to enter the lymphatic circulation, and thus regional lymph nodes, and some may enter the systemic circulation.
- *Distribution:* Not reported.
- *Metabolism:* Not reported.
- *Excretion:* Not reported.

Contraindications and precautions

Contraindicated in patients with known hypersensitivity to drug or mannitol.

Interactions

Interactions between glatiramer acetate and other drugs have not been fully evaluated. Results from clinical trials do not suggest significant interactions with other therapies commonly used in patients with multiple sclerosis (including concurrent use of *corticosteroids* for up to 28 days). Interactions between drug and *interferon beta* have not been studied; however, 10 patients who switched to glatiramer acetate reported no serious or unexpected adverse effects related to treatment.

Effects on diagnostic tests

None reported.

Adverse reactions

CNS: abnormal dreams, agitation, *anxiety, asthenia,* confusion, emotional lability, foot drop, *hypertonia,* migraine, nervousness, nystagmus, speech disorder, stupor, tremor, vertigo.
CV: *chest pain,* hypertension, *palpitations, vasodilatation,* syncope, tachycardia.
EENT: ear pain, eye disorder, *rhinitis.*
GI: anorexia, *diarrhea,* gastroenteritis, GI disorder, *nausea,* oral moniliasis, salivary gland enlargement, tooth caries, ulcerative stomatitis, vomiting.
GU: amenorrhea, bowel urgency, dysmenorrhea, hematuria, impotence, menorrhagia, suspicious Papanicalaou smear, *urinary urgency,* vaginal moniliasis, vaginal hemorrhage.
Hematologic: ecchymosis, *lymphadenopathy.*
Metabolic: edema, peripheral edema, weight gain.
Respiratory: bronchitis, *dyspnea,* hyperventilation, laryngismus.
Skin: eczema, erythema, herpes simplex and zoster, *pruritus, rash,* skin atrophy, skin nodule, *sweating,* urticaria, warts.
Other: arthralgia, *back pain,* bacterial infection, chills, cyst, facial edema, fever, *flulike syndrome, infection, injection site reaction* or hemorrhage, neck pain, *pain.*

Overdose and treatment

No information available.

☑ Special considerations

- Administer drug by S.C. injection only.
- Store drug in the freezer (– 4° to 14° F [–20° to –10° C]); diluent can be kept at room temperature.
- Use immediately after reconstitution because drug does not contain preservatives. Discard unused drug.
- Immediate postinjection reactions have occurred in 10% of patients with multiple sclerosis; symptoms include flushing; chest pain, palpitations, anxiety, dyspnea, constriction of the throat, and urticaria. These reactions were transient, self-limited, and did not require specific treatment. Onset may occur several months after initiation of treatment and patients may have more than one episode.
- Approximately 26% of patients experienced at least one episode of transient chest pain which usually began at least 1 month after treatment began; it was not accompanied by other symptoms and appeared not to be clinically important.
- Because drug can modify immune response, it could interfere with useful immune function. Although evidence is lacking, there has been no evaluation of this risk.
- Drug is an antigenic material and may lead to induction of untoward host responses. Systemic study of these effects has not been done.

Patient education

- Instruct patient how to reconstitute and self-inject drug. Supervise first self-injection.
- Explain need for aseptic self-injection techniques and warn patient against reuse of needles and syringes. Periodically review proper disposal of needles and syringes.
- Instruct patient to call if pregnancy occurs, is suspected, or if pregnancy is being planned.
- Tell patient to call if she is breast-feeding.
- Advise patient not to change drug or dosing schedule or to stop drug without medical approval.
- Inform patient to call immediately if dizziness, hives, sweating, chest pain, difficulty breathing, or severe pain occurs following drug injection.

Geriatric use

- Drug has not been studied specifically in elderly patients.

Pediatric use

- Safety and efficacy have not been established in children under age 18.

Breast-feeding
- It is not known if drug is excreted in breast milk.

glimepiride
Amaryl

Pharmacologic classification: sulfonylurea
Therapeutic classification: antidiabetic
Pregnancy risk category C

How supplied
Available by prescription only
Tablets: 1 mg, 2 mg, 4 mg

Indications, route, and dosage
Adjunct to diet and exercise to lower blood glucose in patients with non-insulin-dependent diabetes mellitus whose hyperglycemia cannot be managed by diet and exercise alone
Adults: Initially, 1 to 2 mg P.O. once daily with first main meal of the day; usual maintenance dosage is 1 to 4 mg P.O. once daily. Maximum recommended dosage is 8 mg once daily. After dose of 2 mg is reached, increases in dosage should be made in increments not exceeding 2 mg at 1- to 2-week intervals based on patient's blood glucose response.
Adjunct to insulin therapy in patients with non-insulin-dependent diabetes mellitus whose hyperglycemia cannot be managed by diet and exercise in conjunction with an oral hypoglycemic agent
Adults: 8 mg P.O. once daily with first main meal of the day in combination with low-dose insulin. Upward adjustments of insulin should be done weekly as needed and guided by patient's blood glucose response.
✦ ***Dosage adjustment.*** Patients with renal impairment require cautious dosing. Give 1 mg P.O. once daily with first main meal of the day, followed by appropriate dose titration p.r.n.

Pharmacodynamics
Antidiabetic action: Exact mechanism of glimepiride to lower blood glucose appears to depend on stimulating the release of insulin from functioning pancreatic beta cells. Also, drug can lead to increased sensitivity of peripheral tissues to insulin.

Pharmacokinetics
- *Absorption:* Drug is completely absorbed from the GI tract. Significant absorption occurs within 1 hour after administration and peak drug levels occur at 2 to 3 hours.
- *Distribution:* Glimepiride's protein binding is greater than 99.5%.
- *Metabolism:* Drug is completely metabolized by oxidative biotransformation.
- *Excretion:* Glimepiride's metabolites are excreted in urine (about 60%) and feces (about 40%).

Contraindications and precautions
Contraindicated in patients with hypersensitivity to drug and in those with diabetic ketoacidosis (with or without coma) because this condition should be treated with insulin. Use cautiously in debilitated or malnourished patients and in those with adrenal, pituitary, hepatic, or renal insufficiency because these patients are more susceptible to the hypoglycemic action of glucose-lowering drugs.

Interactions
NSAIDs and other *drugs that are highly protein-bound* (such as *salicylates, sulfonamides, chloramphenicol, coumarins, probenecid, MAO inhibitors,* and *beta-adrenergic blocking agents*) may potentiate the hypoglycemic action of sulfonylureas such as glimepiride.

Concomitant use of *drugs that tend to produce hyperglycemia,* such as *thiazides* and *other diuretics, estrogens, oral contraceptives, corticosteroids, phenothiazines, thyroid products, phenytoin, nicotinic acid, sympathomimetics,* and *isoniazid,* may require dosage adjustments.

Concomitant use with *beta-adrenergeric blocking agents* may mask symptoms of hypoglycemia.

Effects on diagnostic tests
None reported.

Adverse reactions
CNS: dizziness, asthenia, headache.
EENT: changes in accommodation, blurred vision.
GI: vomiting, abdominal pain, nausea, diarrhea.
Hematologic: leukopenia, hemolytic anemia, agranulocytosis, ***thrombocytopenia, aplastic anemia, pancytopenia.***
Hepatic: cholestatic jaundice.
Skin: allergic skin reactions (pruritus, erythema, urticaria, morbilliform or maculopapular eruptions).
Other: hypoglycemia, elevated transaminase levels.

Overdose and treatment
Overdosage of sulfonylureas can produce hypoglycemia. Mild hypoglycemic symptoms without loss of consciousness or neurologic findings should be treated aggressively with oral glucose and adjustments in drug dosage and meal patterns. Monitor patient closely until he is out of danger. Severe hypoglycemic reactions with coma, seizure, or other neurologic impairment occur infrequently but constitute medical emergencies requiring immediate hospitalization. If hypoglycemic coma occurs or is suspected, give a rapid I.V. injection of concentrated (50%) glucose solution followed by continuous infusion of a more dilute (10%) glucose solution at a rate that will maintain the blood glucose at a level above 100 mg/dl. Patient should be closely monitored for at least 24 to 48 hours because hypoglycemia may recur after apparent clinical recovery.

☑ Special considerations
Besides those relevant to all *sulfonylureas,* consider the following recommendations.
- In elderly, debilitated, or malnourished patients or in patients with renal or hepatic insufficiency, the initial dosing, dose increments, and maintenance dosage should be conservative to avoid hypoglycemic reactions.

• During maintenance therapy, glimepiride should be discontinued if satisfactory lowering of blood glucose is no longer achieved. Secondary failures to glimepiride monotherapy can be treated with glimepiride-insulin combination therapy.
• Fasting blood glucose should be monitored periodically to determine therapeutic response. Glycosylated hemoglobin should also be monitored, usually every 3 to 6 months, to more precisely assess long-term glycemic control.
• Oral hypoglycemic agents have been associated with an increased risk of CV mortality compared with diet or diet and insulin therapy.

Patient education
• Instruct patient to take drug with first meal of the day.
• Make sure patient understands that therapy relieves symptoms but doesn't cure disease.
• Stress importance of adhering to specific diet, weight reduction, exercise, and personal hygiene programs. Explain how and when to perform self-monitoring of blood glucose level.
• Teach patient how to recognize and manage the signs and symptoms of hyperglycemia and hypoglycemia.
• Advise patient to carry medical identification regarding diabetic status.

Geriatric use
• Elderly patients may be more sensitive to the effects of drug because of reduced metabolism and elimination.

Pediatric use
• Safety and effectiveness in pediatric patients have not been established.

Breast-feeding
• It is not known if drug is excreted in breast milk. Because of the potential for hypoglycemia in nursing infants, it should not be administered to breast-feeding women.

glipizide
Glucotrol, Glucotrol XL

Pharmacologic classification: sulfonylurea
Therapeutic classification: antidiabetic
Pregnancy risk category C

How supplied
Available by prescription only
Tablets: 5 mg, 10 mg
Tablets (extended-release): 5 mg, 10 mg

Indications, route, and dosage
Adjunct to diet to lower blood glucose levels in patients with non-insulin-dependent diabetes mellitus
Adults: Initially, 5 mg P.O. daily 30 minutes before breakfast; dose should be adjusted in increments of 2.5 to 5 mg. Usual maintenance dosage is 10 to 15 mg. Maximum recommended daily dose is 40 mg. Total daily doses above 15 mg should be divided except when using extended-release tablets.
✦ ***Dosage adjustment.*** Initial dosage in elderly patients or those with hepatic disease may be 2.5 mg
Extended-release tablets
Adults: Initially, 5 mg P.O. daily. Titrate in 5-mg increments q 3 months based on level of glycemic control. Maximum daily dose is 20 mg.
To replace insulin therapy
Adults: If insulin dosage is more than 20 units daily, patient may be started at usual dosage of glipizide besides 50% of insulin dosage. If insulin dosage is below 20 units, insulin may be discontinued.

Pharmacodynamics
Antidiabetic action: Glipizide lowers blood glucose levels by stimulating insulin release from functioning beta cells in the pancreas. After prolonged administration the drug's hypoglycemic effects appear to reflect extrapancreatic effects, possibly including reduction of basal hepatic glucose production and enhanced peripheral sensitivity to insulin. The latter may result either from an increase in the number of insulin receptors or from changes in events subsequent to insulin binding.

Pharmacokinetics
• *Absorption:* Drug is absorbed rapidly and completely from the GI tract. Onset of action occurs within 15 to 30 minutes, with maximum hypoglycemic effects within 2 to 3 hours.
• *Distribution:* Glipizide probably is distributed within the extracellular fluid. It is approximately 92% to 99% protein-bound.
• *Metabolism:* Drug is metabolized almost completely by the liver to inactive metabolites.
• *Excretion.* Drug and its metabolites are excreted primarily in urine; small amounts in feces. Renal clearance of unchanged glipizide increases with increasing urinary pH. Duration of action is 10 to 24 hours; half-life is 2 to 4 hours.

Contraindications and precautions
Contraindicated in patients with hypersensitivity to drug, diabetic ketoacidosis with or without coma, and during pregnancy or breast-feeding. Use cautiously in patients with impaired renal or hepatic function and in elderly, malnourished, or debilitated patients.

Interactions
Concomitant use of glipizide with *alcohol* may produce a disulfiram-like reaction consisting of nausea, vomiting, abdominal cramps, and headaches. Use with *anticoagulants* may increase plasma levels of both drugs and, after continued therapy, may reduce plasma levels and effectiveness of the anticoagulant. Concomitant use with *chloramphenicol, guanethidine, insulin, MAO inhibitors, probenecid, salicylates,* or *sulfonamides* may enhance the hypoglycemic effect by displacing glipizide from its protein-binding sites. *Cimetidine* may potentiate the hypoglycemic effects by preventing hepatic metabolism.

Concomitant use with *beta-adrenergic blocking agents* (including *ophthalmics*) may mask symptoms of hypoglycemia, such as rising pulse rate and blood pressure, and may prolong hypoglycemia by blocking gluconeogenesis. Use with *drugs that may increase blood glucose levels (adrenocorticoids, glucocorticoids, amphetamines, baclofen, corticotropin, epinephrine, estrogens, ethacrynic acid, furosemide, oral contraceptives, phenytoin, thiazide diuretics, triamterene,* and *thyroid hormones*) may require dosage adjustments.

Because *smoking* increases corticosteroid release, patients who smoke may require higher dosages of glipizide.

Effects on diagnostic tests
Glipizide therapy alters cholesterol, alkaline phosphatase, AST, LD, and BUN levels.

Adverse reactions
CNS: dizziness, drowsiness, headache.
GI: nausea, constipation, diarrhea.
Hematologic: leukopenia, hemolytic anemia, ***agranulocytosis, thrombocytopenia, aplastic anemia.***
Hepatic: cholestatic jaundice.
Skin: rash, pruritus.
Other: ***hypoglycemia.***

Overdose and treatment
Clinical manifestations of overdose include low blood glucose levels, tingling of lips and tongue, hunger, nausea, decreased cerebral function (lethargy, yawning, confusion, agitation, and nervousness), increased sympathetic activity (tachycardia, sweating, and tremor), and ultimately seizures, stupor, and coma.

Mild hypoglycemia (without loss of consciousness or neurologic findings) responds to treatment with oral glucose and dosage adjustments. If the patient loses consciousness or experiences other neurologic changes, he should receive a rapid injection of dextrose 50%, followed by continuous infusion of dextrose 10% at a rate to maintain blood glucose levels more than 100 mg/dl. Monitor for 24 to 48 hours.

☑ Special considerations
Besides those relevant to all *sulfonylureas,* consider the following recommendations.
- To improve glucose control in patients who receive 15 mg/day or more, divided doses, usually given 30 minutes before the morning and evening meals, are recommended.
- Some patients taking glipizide can be controlled effectively on a once-daily regimen; others show better response with divided dosing.
- Glipizide is a second-generation sulfonylurea oral hypoglycemic. It appears to cause fewer adverse reactions than first-generation sulfonylureas.
- Drug has a mild diuretic effect that may be useful in patients with heart failure or cirrhosis.
- When substituting glipizide for chlorpropamide, monitor patient carefully during the first week because of the prolonged retention of chlorpropamide.
- Patients who may be more sensitive to drug, such as elderly, debilitated, or malnourished individuals, should begin therapy with lower dosage (2.5 mg once daily).
- Use in pregnancy is usually not recommended. If glipizide must be used, manufacturer recommends that drug be discontinued at least 1 month before expected delivery to prevent neonatal hypoglycemia.
- Oral antidiabetic agents have been associated with an increased risk of CV mortality as compared with diet or diet and insulin therapy.

Patient education
- Emphasize importance of following prescribed diet, exercise, and medical regimen.
- Instruct patient to take the medication at the same time each day.
- Tell patient that, if a dose is missed, it should be taken immediately, unless it's almost time to take the next dose. He should not take double doses.
- Advise patient to avoid alcohol when taking glipizide. Remind him that many foods and OTC medications contain alcohol.
- Encourage patient to wear a medical identification bracelet or necklace.
- If glipizide causes GI upset, suggest that the drug be taken with food.
- Teach patient how to monitor blood glucose, urine glucose, and ketone levels, as prescribed.
- Teach patient how to recognize and manage the signs and symptoms of hyperglycemia and hypoglycemia.

Geriatric use
- Elderly patients may be more sensitive to the effects of drug.
- Hypoglycemia causes more neurologic symptoms in elderly patients.

Pediatric use
- Glipizide is ineffective in insulin-dependent diabetes. Safety and effectiveness in children have not been established.

glucagon
Pharmacologic classification: antihypoglycemic
Therapeutic classification: antihypoglycemic, diagnostic
Pregnancy risk category B

How supplied
Available by prescription only
Powder for injection: 1 mg (1 unit)/vial, 10 mg (10 units)/vial

Indications, route, and dosage
Coma of insulin-shock therapy
Adults: 0.5 to 1 mg S.C., I.M., or I.V. 1 hour after coma develops; may repeat within 25 minutes, if necessary. In deep coma, give glucose 10% to 50% I.V. for faster response. When patient responds, give additional carbohydrate immediately.

Severe insulin-induced hypoglycemia during diabetic therapy
Adults: 0.5 to 1 mg S.C., I.M., or I.V.; may repeat q 20 minutes for two doses, if necessary.
Children: 0.025 mg/kg S.C., I.M., or I.V. 1 hour after coma develops; may repeat within 25 minutes, if necessary. In deep coma, 10% to 50% glucose I.V. for faster response. When patient responds, give additional carbohydrate immediately.
Diagnostic aid for radiologic examination
Adults: 0.25 to 2 mg I.V. or I.M. before initiation of radiologic procedure.

Pharmacodynamics

Antihypoglycemic action: Glucagon increases plasma glucose levels and causes smooth muscle relaxation and an inotropic myocardial effect because of the stimulation of adenylate cyclase to produce cAMP. cAMP initiates a series of reactions that leads to the degradation of glycogen to glucose. Hepatic stores of glycogen are necessary for glucagon to exert an antihypoglycemic effect.

Diagnostic action: The mechanism by which glucagon relaxes the smooth muscles of the stomach, esophagus, duodenum, small bowel, and colon has not been fully defined.

Pharmacokinetics

- *Absorption:* Glucagon is destroyed in the GI tract; therefore, it must be given parenterally. After I.V. administration, hyperglycemic activity peaks within 30 minutes; relaxation of the GI smooth muscle occurs within 1 minute. After I.M. administration, relaxation of the GI smooth muscle occurs within 10 minutes. Administration to comatose hypoglycemic patients (with normal liver glycogen stores) usually produces a return to consciousness within 20 minutes.
- *Distribution:* Distribution is not fully understood.
- *Metabolism:* Glucagon is degraded extensively by the liver, in the kidneys and plasma, and at its tissue receptor sites in plasma membranes.
- *Excretion:* Metabolic products are excreted by the kidneys. Half-life is about 3 to 10 minutes. Duration after I.M. administration is up to 32 minutes; after I.V. administration, up to 25 minutes.

Contraindications and precautions

Contraindicated in patients with pheochromocytoma or hypersensitivity to drug. Use cautiously in patients with insulinoma.

Interactions

Concomitant use of glucagon with *epinephrine* increases and prolongs the hyperglycemic effect. *Phenytoin* appears to inhibit glucagon-induced insulin release. Use with caution as a diagnostic agent in patients with diabetes mellitus.

Effects on diagnostic tests

Glucagon lowers serum potassium levels.

Adverse reactions

CV: hypotension.
GI: nausea, vomiting.
Respiratory: respiratory distress.
Other: hypersensitivity reactions (***bronchospasm,*** rash, dizziness, light-headedness).

Overdose and treatment

Clinical manifestations of overdose include nausea, vomiting, and hypokalemia. Treat symptomatically.

☑ Special considerations

- Glucagon should be used only under direct medical supervision.
- If patient experiences nausea and vomiting from glucagon administration and cannot retain some form of sugar for 1 hour, consider administration of I.V. dextrose
- For I.V. drip infusion, glucagon is compatible with dextrose solution but forms a precipitate in chloride solutions.
- Glucagon has a positive inotropic and chronotropic action on the heart and may be used to treat overdose of beta-adrenergic blockers.
- Glucagon may be used as a diagnostic aid in radiologic examination of the stomach, duodenum, small intestine, and colon when a hypotonic state is desirable.
- Mixed solutions with diluent are stable for 48 hours when stored at 41° F (5° C). Following reconstitution with sterile water, use immediately.

Patient education

- Teach patient how to mix and inject the medication properly, using an appropriate-sized syringe and injecting at a 90-degree angle. *Instructions for mixing injection:* For 2 mg or less, must use manufacturer's diluent; for doses over 2 mg, use sterile water for injection rather than manufacturer's diluent.
- Instruct patient and family members how to administer glucagon and how to recognize hypoglycemia. Urge them to call immediately in emergencies.
- Tell patient to expect response usually within 20 minutes after injection and that injection may be repeated if no response occurs. Patient should seek medical assistance if second injection is needed.

Pediatric use

- Drug should not be used to treat newborn asphyxia or hypoglycemia in premature infants or in infants who have had intrauterine growth retardation.

Breast-feeding

- No information is available about the occurrence of drug in breast milk. However, because glucagon is destroyed in the GI tract and because of its short-term use, it is unlikely to cause problems in a breast-fed infant.

glyburide

DiaBeta, Glynase PresTab, Micronase

Pharmacologic classification: sulfonylurea
Therapeutic classification: antidiabetic
Pregnancy risk category C

How supplied

Available by prescription only
Tablets: 1.25 mg, 2.5 mg, 5 mg
Tablets (micronized): 1.5 mg, 3 mg, 6 mg

Indications, route, and dosage

Adjunct to diet to lower blood glucose levels in patients with non-insulin-dependent diabetes mellitus

Adults: Initially, 2.5 to 5 mg P.O. daily with breakfast. Patients who are more sensitive to hypoglycemic drugs should be started at 1.25 mg daily. Usual maintenance dosage is 1.25 to 20 mg daily, either as a single dose or in divided doses.

For micronized tablets, initially give 1.5 to 3 mg P.O. with breakfast. Usual maintenance dosage is 0.75 to 12 mg P.O. daily.

✦ ***Dosage adjustment.*** In elderly, debilitated, or malnourished patients or those with renal or liver dysfunction, start therapy with 1.25 mg once daily.

To replace insulin therapy

Adults: If insulin dosage is more than 40 units/day, patient may be started on 5 mg of glyburide daily besides 50% of the insulin dose. Patients maintained on less than 20 units/day should receive 2.5 to 5 mg/day; those maintained on 20 to 40 units/day should receive 5 mg/day. In all patients, glyburide is substituted and insulin discontinued abruptly.

For micronized tablets, if insulin dosage is more than 40 units/day, give 3 mg P.O. with a 50% reduction in insulin. Patients maintained on 20 to 40 units/day should receive 3 mg P.O. as a single daily dose; those maintained on less than 20 units/day should receive 1.5 to 3 mg/day as a single dose.

Pharmacodynamics

Antidiabetic action: Glyburide lowers blood glucose levels by stimulating insulin release from functioning beta cells in the pancreas. After prolonged administration, the drug's hypoglycemic effects appear to be related to extrapancreatic effects, possibly including reduction of basal hepatic glucose production and enhanced peripheral sensitivity to insulin. The latter may result either from an increase in the number of insulin receptors or from changes in events subsequent to insulin binding.

Pharmacokinetics

- *Absorption:* Almost completely absorbed from GI tract. Onset of action occurs within 2 hours; hypoglycemic effects peak within 3 to 4 hours. A micronized tablet results in significant absorption: a 3-mg miconized tablet provides blood levels similar to a 5-mg conventional tablet.
- *Distribution:* Glyburide is 99% protein-bound. Its distribution is not fully understood.
- *Metabolism:* Drug is metabolized completely by the liver to inactive metabolites.
- *Excretion:* Drug is excreted as metabolites in urine and feces in equal proportions. Its duration of action is 24 hours; its half-life is 10 hours.

Contraindications and precautions

Contraindicated in patients with hypersensitivity to drug or diabetic ketoacidosis with or without coma, and during pregnancy or breast-feeding. Use cautiously in patients with impaired renal or hepatic function and in elderly, malnourished, or debilitated patients.

Interactions

Concomitant use of glyburide with *alcohol* may produce a disulfiram-like reaction consisting of nausea, vomiting, abdominal cramps, and headaches. Use with anticoagulants may increase plasma levels of both drugs and, after continued therapy, may reduce plasma levels and anticoagulant effect. Use with *chloramphenicol, guanethidine, insulin, MAO inhibitors, probenecid, salicylates,* or *sulfonamides* may enhance the hypoglycemic effect by displacing glyburide from its protein-binding sites.

Concomitant use of glyburide with *beta-adrenergic blocking agents* (including *ophthalmics*) may increase the risk of hypoglycemia, mask its symptoms (increased pulse rate and blood pressure), and prolong its effects by blocking gluconeogenesis. Use with drugs that may increase blood glucose levels *(adrenocorticoids, diazoxide, glucocorticoids, amphetamines, baclofen, corticotropin, epinephrine, ethacrynic acid, furosemide, phenytoin,* thiazide diuretics, triamterene, and thyroid hormones) may require dosage adjustments.

Because *smoking* increases corticosteroid release, smokers may require higher dosages of glyburide.

Effects on diagnostic tests

Glyburide therapy alters cholesterol, alkaline phosphatase, and BUN levels.

Adverse reactions

EENT: changes in accommodation or blurred vision.
GI: nausea, epigastric fullness, heartburn.
Hematologic: leukopenia, hemolytic anemia, ***agranulocytosis, thrombocytopenia, aplastic anemia.***
Hepatic: cholestatic jaundice, hepatitis, abnormal liver function.
Skin: rash, pruritus, other allergic reactions.
Other: ***hypoglycemia,*** arthralgia, myalgia, angioedema.

Overdose and treatment

Clinical manifestations of overdose include low blood glucose levels, tingling of lips and tongue, hunger, nausea, decreased cerebral function (lethargy, yawning, confusion, agitation, and nervousness), increased sympathetic activity (tachycardia, sweating, and tremor) and ultimately seizures, stupor, and coma.

Mild hypoglycemia, without loss of consciousness or neurologic findings, responds to treatment with oral glucose and dosage adjustments. The patient with severe hypoglycemia should be hospitalized immediately. If hypoglycemic coma is suspected, the patient should receive rapid injection of dextrose 50%, followed by a continuous infusion of dextrose 10% at a rate to maintain blood glucose levels greater than 100 mg/dl. Monitor for 24 to 48 hours.

☑ Special considerations

Besides those relevant to all *sulfonylureas,* consider the following recommendations.

- To improve control in patients receiving 10 mg/day or more, divided doses, usually given before the morning and evening meals, are recommended.
- Some patients taking glyburide may be controlled effectively on a once-daily regimen, whereas others show better response with divided dosing.
- Glyburide is a second-generation sulfonylurea oral antidiabetic agent. It appears to cause fewer adverse reactions than first-generation drugs.
- Drug has a mild diuretic effect that may be useful in patients who have chronic heart failure or cirrhosis.
- When substituting glyburide for chlorpropamide, monitor patient closely during the first week because of the prolonged retention of chlorpropamide in the body.
- Oral antidiabetic agents have been associated with an increased risk of CV mortality compared with diet or diet and insulin therapy.

Patient education

- Emphasize importance of following prescribed diet, exercise, and medical regimen.
- Tell patient to take drug at the same time each day. If a dose is missed, it should be taken immediately, unless it's almost time to take the next dose. Instruct patient not to take double doses.
- Advise patient to avoid alcohol while taking glyburide. Remind him that many foods and OTC medications contain alcohol.
- Encourage patient to wear a medical identification bracelet or necklace.
- Suggest drug be taken with food if GI upset occurs.
- Teach patient how to monitor blood glucose and urine glucose and ketone levels as prescribed.
- Teach patient how to recognize the signs and symptoms of hyperglycemia and hypoglycemia and what to do if they occur.

Geriatric use

- Elderly patients may be more sensitive to drug's effects because of reduced metabolism and elimination.
- Hypoglycemia causes more neurologic symptoms in elderly patients.

Pediatric use

- Glyburide is ineffective in insulin-dependent (type 1, juvenile-onset) diabetes. Safety and effectiveness in children have not been established.

glycerin (glycerol)

Fleet Babylax, Ophthalgan, Osmoglyn, Sani-Supp

Pharmacologic classification: trihydric alcohol, ophthalmic osmotic vehicle
Therapeutic classification: laxative (osmotic), ophthalmic osmotic, adjunct in treating glaucoma, lubricant
Pregnancy risk category C

How supplied

Available by prescription only
Ophthalmic solution: 7.5-ml containers
Oral solution: 50% (0.6 g/ml), 75% (0.94 g/ml)

Available without a prescription
Suppository: 1.5 g (for infants), 3 g (adults)
Rectal solution: 4 ml/applicator

Indications, route, and dosage

Constipation
Adults and children age 6 and older: 3 g as a suppository or 5 to 15 ml as an enema.
Children under age 6: 1 to 1.5 g as a suppository or 2 to 5 ml as an enema.

Reduction of intraocular pressure
Adults: 1 to 2 g/kg P.O. 60 to 90 minutes preoperatively.

Drug is useful in acute angle-closure glaucoma; before iridectomy (with carbonic anhydrase inhibitors or topical miotics); in trauma or disease, such as congenital glaucoma and some secondary glaucoma forms; and before or after surgery, such as retinal detachment surgery, cataract extraction, or keratoplasty.

Reduction of corneal edema
Adults: 1 to 2 drops of ophthalmic solution topically before eye examination; 1 to 2 drops q 3 to 4 hours for corneal edema.

Drug is used to facilitate ophthalmoscopic and gonioscopic examination and to differentiate superficial edema and deep corneal edema.

To act as an osmotic diuretic
Adults: 1 to 2 g/kg P.O. 1 to 1½ hours before surgery.

Pharmacodynamics

Laxative action: Glycerin suppositories produce laxative action by causing rectal distention, thereby stimulating the urge to defecate; by causing local rectal irritation; and by triggering a hyperosmolar mechanism that draws water into the colon.

Antiglaucoma action: Orally administered glycerin helps reduce intraocular pressure by increasing plasma osmotic pressure, thereby drawing water into the blood from extravascular spaces. It also reduces intraocular fluid volume independently of routine flow mechanisms, decreasing intraocular pressure; it may cause tissue dehydration and decreased CSF pressure.

Topically applied glycerin produces a hygroscopic (moisture-retaining) effect that reduces edema and improves visualization in ophthalmoscopy or gonioscopy. Glycerin reduces fluid in the cornea via its osmotic action and clears corneal haze.

Pharmacokinetics

Rectal form

- *Absorption:* Glycerin suppositories are absorbed poorly; after rectal administration, laxative effect occurs in 15 to 30 minutes.
- *Distribution:* When administered by suppository, glycerin is distributed locally.
- *Metabolism:* Not reported.
- *Excretion:* Drug is excreted in the feces.

Oral form

- *Absorption:* Absorbed rapidly from GI tract, with peak serum levels occurring in 60 to 90 minutes with oral administration; intraocular pressure decreases in 10 to 30 minutes. Peak action occurs in 30 minutes to 2 hours, with effects persisting for 4 to 8 hours. Intracranial pressure (ICP) decreases in 10 to 60 minutes; this effect persists for 2 to 3 hours.
- *Distribution:* Distributed throughout the blood but does not enter ocular fluid; drug may enter breast milk.
- *Metabolism:* After oral administration, about 80% of dose is metabolized in the liver, 10% to 20% in the kidneys.
- *Excretion:* Drug is excreted in feces and urine.

Contraindications and precautions

Contraindicated in patients hypersensitive to drug. Rectal administration of drug is contraindicated in those with intestinal obstruction, undiagnosed abdominal pain, vomiting or other signs of appendicitis, fecal impaction, or acute surgical abdomen.

Use oral form cautiously in elderly or dehydrated patients and in those with diabetes or cardiac, renal, or hepatic disease.

Interactions

Concomitant use with *diuretics* may result in additive effects.

Effects on diagnostic tests

None reported.

Adverse reactions

CNS: mild headache, dizziness (with oral administration).
EENT: eye pain, irritation.
GI: cramping pain, thirst, nausea, vomiting, diarrhea (with oral administration); rectal discomfort, hyperemia of rectal mucosa (with rectal administration).
Other: mild hyperglycemia, mild glycosuria.

Note: Drug should be discontinued if symptoms of hypersensitivity occur.

Overdose and treatment

If excess glycerin is administered into eye, irrigate conjunctiva with sterile 0.9% NaCl solution or water. Systemic effects are not expected.

☑ Special considerations

- When administering glycerin orally, do not give hypotonic fluids to relieve thirst and headache from glycerin-induced dehydration because these will counteract drug's osmotic effects.
- Use topical tetracaine hydrochloride or proparacaine before ophthalmic instillation to prevent discomfort.
- Don't touch tip of dropper to eye, surrounding tissues, or tear-film; glycerin will absorb moisture.
- To prevent or relieve headache, have patient remain supine during and after oral administration.
- Monitor diabetic patients for possible alteration of serum and urine glucose levels; dosage adjustment may be necessary.
- Commercially available solutions may be poured over ice and sipped through a straw.
- Hyperosmolar laxatives are used most commonly to help laxative-dependent patients reestablish normal bowel habits.
- Other uses include reducing ICP in patients with CVA, meningitis, encephalitis, Reye's syndrome, or CNS trauma or tumors and reducing brain volume during neurosurgical procedures through oral or I.V. administration, or both.
- Store drug in tightly closed original container.

Patient education

- Instruct patient to call if he experiences severe headache from oral dose.
- Teach patient correct way to instill drops and warn him not to touch eye with the dropper.
- Tell patient to lie down during and after administration of glycerin to prevent or relieve headache.

Geriatric use

- Dehydrated elderly patients may experience seizures and disorientation.

Pediatric use

- Safety and effectiveness of ophthalmic glycerin solutions in children have not been established.

Breast-feeding

- Safety in breast-feeding women has not been established; possible risks must be weighed against benefits.

glycopyrrolate

Robinul, Robinul Forte

Pharmacologic classification: anticholinergic
Therapeutic classification: antimuscarinic, GI antispasmodic
Pregnancy risk category B

How supplied

Available by prescription only
Tablets: 1 mg, 2 mg

Injection: 0.2 mg/ml in 1-ml, 2-ml, 5-ml, 20-ml vials

Indications, route, and dosage

Blockade of cholinergic effects of anticholinesterase drugs used to reverse neuromuscular blockade

Adults and children: 0.2 mg I.V. for each 1 mg neostigmine or 5 mg of pyridostigmine. May be given I.V. without dilution or may be added to dextrose injection and given by infusion.

Preoperatively to diminish secretions and block cardiac vagal reflexes

Adults: 0.0044 mg/kg of body weight given I.M. 30 to 60 minutes before anesthesia.

Adjunctive therapy in peptic ulcers and other GI disorders

Adults: 1 to 2 mg P.O. t.i.d. or 0.1 mg I.M. t.i.d. or q.i.d. Dosage should be individualized.

Pharmacodynamics

Anticholinergic action: Glycopyrrolate inhibits acetylcholine's muscarinic actions on autonomic effectors innervated by postganglionic cholinergic nerves. That action blocks adverse muscarinic effects associated with anticholinesterase agents used to reverse curariform-induced neuromuscular blockade. Glycopyrrolate decreases secretions and GI motility by the same mechanism. Glycopyrrolate blocks cardiac vagal reflexes by blocking vagal inhibition of the SA node.

Pharmacokinetics

- *Absorption:* Poorly absorbed from GI tract (10% to 25%) after oral administration. Glycopyrrolate is rapidly absorbed when given I.M.; serum concentrations peak in 30 to 45 minutes. Action begins in 1 minute after I.V. and 15 to 30 minutes after I.M. or S.C. administration.
- *Distribution:* Drug is rapidly distributed. Because it is a quaternary amine, it does not cross the blood-brain barrier or enter the CNS.
- *Metabolism:* Exact metabolic fate is unknown. Duration of effect is up to 7 hours when given parenterally and up to 12 hours when given orally.
- *Excretion:* Small amount of drug is eliminated in the urine as unchanged drug and metabolites. Drug is mostly excreted unchanged in feces or bile.

Contraindications and precautions

Contraindicated in patients with hypersensitivity to drug and in those with glaucoma, obstructive uropathy, obstructive disease of the GI tract, myasthenia gravis, paralytic ileus, intestinal atony, unstable CV status in acute hemorrhage, severe ulcerative colitis, or toxic megacolon.

Use cautiously in patients with autonomic neuropathy, hyperthyroidism, coronary artery disease, arrhythmias, heart failure, hypertension, hiatal hernia, hepatic or renal disease, and ulcerative colitis. Also use with caution in hot or humid conditions where drug-induced heat stroke may occur.

Interactions

Concurrent administration of *antacids* decreases oral absorption of anticholinergics. Administer glycopyrrolate at least 1 hour before antacids.

Concomitant administration of *drugs with anticholinergic effects* may cause additive toxicity.

Decreased GI absorption of many drugs has been reported after the use of anticholinergics (for example, *levodopa* and *ketoconazole*). Conversely, slowly dissolving *digoxin* tablets may yield higher serum digoxin levels when administered with anticholinergics.

Use cautiously with *oral potassium supplements* (especially *wax-matrix formulations*) because the incidence of potassium-induced GI ulcerations may be increased.

Effects on diagnostic tests

None reported.

Adverse reactions

CNS: weakness, nervousness, insomnia, drowsiness, dizziness, headache, confusion or excitement (in elderly patients).
CV: palpitations, tachycardia.
EENT: *dilated pupils, blurred vision,* photophobia, increased intraocular pressure.
GI: *constipation, dry mouth,* nausea, loss of taste, abdominal distension, vomiting, epigastric distress.
GU: *urinary hesitancy, urine retention,* impotence.
Skin: urticaria, decreased sweating or anhidrosis, other dermal manifestations.
Other: allergic reactions ***(anaphylaxis),*** fever.

Overdose and treatment

Clinical effects of overdose include such peripheral effects as dilated, nonreactive pupils; blurred vision; flushed, hot, dry skin; dryness of mucous membranes; dysphagia; decreased or absent bowel sounds; urine retention; hyperthermia; tachycardia; hypertension; and increased respiration.

Treatment is primarily symptomatic and supportive, as needed. If patient is alert, induce emesis (or use gastric lavage) and follow with a saline cathartic and activated charcoal to prevent further drug absorption. In severe life-threatening cases, physostigmine may be administered to block glycopyrrolate's antimuscarinic effects. Give fluids, as needed, to treat shock. If urine retention occurs, catheterization may be necessary.

☑ Special considerations

Besides those relevant to all *anticholinergics,* consider the following recommendations.

- Check all dosages carefully. Even a slight overdose can lead to toxic effects.
- For immediate treatment of bradycardia, some clinicians prefer atropine over glycopyrrolate.
- Do not mix glycopyrrolate with I.V. solutions containing sodium chloride or bicarbonate.
- Drug may be administered with neostigmine or physostigmine in same syringe.
- Drug is incompatible with thiopental, methohexital, secobarbital, pentobarbital, chloramphenicol, dimenhydrinate, and diazepam.

Geriatric use
• Administer glycopyrrolate cautiously to elderly patients. However, glycopyrrolate may be the preferred anticholinergic in elderly patients.

Pediatric use
• Drug is not recommended for children under age 12 for managing peptic ulcer.

Breast-feeding
• Drug may be excreted in breast milk, possibly resulting in infant toxicity. Breast-feeding women should avoid this drug. Glycopyrrolate may decrease milk production.

gold sodium thiomalate
Aurolate, Myochrysine

Pharmacologic classification: gold salt
Therapeutic classification: antiarthritic
Pregnancy risk category C

How supplied
Available by prescription only
Injection: 25 mg/ml, 50 mg/ml with benzyl alcohol

Indications, route, and dosage
Rheumatoid arthritis, ◊ ***psoriatic arthritis,*** ◊ ***Felty's syndrome***
Adults: Initially, 10 mg I.M.; then 25 mg in second week and continue for a third dose the following week. Continue until 1 g (cumulative) has been given, unless toxicity occurs. If improvement occurs without toxicity before initial 1-g dose, a maintanence dose of 25 to 50 mg every other week for 2 to 20 weeks may be started. Then continue to every third then every fourth week indefinitely. Weekly injections may be restarted anytime, if necessary. If patient does not respond after reaching inital 1-g dose, then discontinue therapy, or give 25 to 50 mg I.M. for an additional 10 weeks, or increase dose by 10 mg q 1 to 4 weeks (maximum dose per injection is 100 mg).
Children: Initiate therapy with 10-mg test dose, then give 1 mg/kg weekly. Continue dosage and administration as listed for adults. Maximum single dose for children under age 12 is 50 mg.
◊ ***Palindromic rheumatism***
Adults: Initially, 10 to 15 mg I.M. weekly until dose of 1 g is reached.
◊ ***Pemphigus***
Adults: Initially, 10 mg I.M.; then 25 mg I.M. for second week, then 50 mg I.M. weekly. When patient is off corticosteroid therapy, maintenance dose of 25 to 50 mg I.M. q 2 weeks may be given.

Pharmacodynamics
Antiarthritic action: Gold sodium thiomalate is thought to be effective against rheumatoid arthritis by altering the immune system to reduce inflammation. Although the exact mechanism of action remains unknown, these compounds have reduced serum concentrations of immunoglobulins and rheumatoid factors in patients with arthritis.

Pharmacokinetics
• *Absorption:* Absorption of gold sodium thiomalate is rapid, with peak levels occurring within 3 to 6 hours.
• *Distribution:* Higher tissue concentrations occur with parenteral gold salts, with a mean steady-state plasma level of 1 to 5 mcg/ml. Drug is distributed widely throughout the body in lymph nodes, bone marrow, kidneys, liver, spleen, and tissues. About 85% to 90% is protein-bound.
• *Metabolism:* Drug is not broken down into its elemental form. The half-life with cumulative dosing is 14 to 40 days.
• *Excretion:* About 70% of drug is excreted in the urine, 30% in feces.

Contraindications and precautions
Contraindicated in patients with hypersensitivity to drug; in those with history of severe toxicity from previous exposure to gold or heavy metals, hepatitis, or exfoliative dermatitis; and in patients with severe uncontrollable diabetes, renal disease, hepatic dysfunction, uncontrolled heart failure, systemic lupus erythematosus, colitis, or Sjögren's syndrome. Also contraindicated in patients with urticaria, eczema, hemorrhagic conditions, or severe hematologic disorders and in those who have recently received radiation therapy.

Use with extreme caution in patients with rash, marked hypertension, compromised cerebral or CV function, or history of renal or hepatic disease, drug allergies, or blood dyscrasias.

Interactions
Concomitant use with *other drugs known to cause blood dyscrasias* causes an additive risk of hematologic toxicity.

Effects on diagnostic tests
Serum protein-bound iodine test, especially when done by the chloric acid digestion method, gives false readings during and for several weeks after gold therapy.

Adverse reactions
Adverse reactions to gold are considered severe and potentially life-threatening.
CNS: confusion, hallucinations, ***seizures.***
CV: bradycardia, hypotension.
EENT: corneal gold deposition, corneal ulcers.
GI: *metallic taste, stomatitis, diarrhea,* anorexia, abdominal cramps, nausea, vomiting, ulcerative enterocolitis.
GU: albuminuria, proteinuria, ***nephrotic syndrome,*** nephritis, acute tubular necrosis, hematuria, ***acute renal failure.***
Hematologic: ***thrombocytopenia*** (with or without purpura), ***aplastic anemia, agranulocytosis,*** leukopenia, eosinophilia, anemia.
Hepatic: hepatitis, jaundice, elevated liver function tests.
Skin: photosensitivity, *rash, dermatitis,* erythema, exfoliative dermatitis.
Other: ***anaphylaxis, angioedema,*** diaphoresis.

Overdose and treatment

When severe reactions to gold occur, corticosteroids, dimercaprol (a chelating agent), or penicillamine may be given to aid in the recovery. Prednisone 40 to 100 mg/day in divided doses is recommended to manage severe renal, hematologic, pulmonary, or enterocolitic reactions to gold. Dimercaprol may be used concurrently with steroids to facilitate the removal of the gold when the steroid treatment alone is ineffective.

☑ Special considerations

- Gold salts should be administered only under close medical supervision.
- Most adverse reactions are readily reversible if drug is discontinued immediately.
- Vasomotor adverse effects are more common with gold sodium thiomalate than with other gold salts.
- Administer all gold salts I.M., preferably intragluteally. Normal color of drug is pale yellow; do not use if it darkens.
- Observe patient for 30 minutes after administration because of possible anaphylactic reaction.
- When administering drug, advise patient to lie down and to remain recumbent for 10 to 20 minutes after injection.
- Obtain patient's urine for analysis for protein and sediment changes before each injection.
- Monitor patient's CBC and platelet count monthly or before every other injection.
- If adverse reactions are mild, some rheumatologists order resumption of gold therapy after 2 to 3 weeks' rest.

Patient education

- Urge patient to have scheduled monthly platelet counts. Drug should be stopped if platelet count falls below 100,000/mm³.
- Reassure patient that beneficial drug effect may be delayed for 3 months. However, if response is inadequate after 6 months, gold sodium thiomalate will probably be discontinued.
- Explain that vasomotor adverse reactions—faintness, weakness, dizziness, flushing, nausea, vomiting, diaphoresis—may occur immediately after injection. Advise patient to lie down until symptoms subside.
- Instruct patient to continue taking drug if he experiences mild diarrhea; however, if diarrhea persists, or if he notes blood in his stool, he should call immediately.
- Tell patient that stomatitis is often preceded by a metallic taste. Advise him to report this symptom immediately.
- Advise patient to report rash or other skin problems immediately.
- Encourage patient to take the drug exactly as prescribed.
- Tell patient to continue taking concomitant drug therapy, such as NSAIDs, as prescribed.
- Tell patient that drug may increase sensitivity to sunlight and tanning beds. He should avoid exposure to excessive sunlight, wear protective clothing, and use a sunscreen.

Geriatric use

- Administer usual adult dose. Use cautiously in patients with decreased renal function.

Pediatric use

- Use in children under age 6 is not recommended.

Breast-feeding

- Drug is not recommended for use in breast-feeding women.

gonadorelin acetate

Lutrepulse

Pharmacologic classification: gonadotropin-releasing hormone (GnRH)
Therapeutic classification: fertility
Pregnancy risk category B

How supplied

Available by prescription only
Injection: 0.8 mg/10 ml, 3.2 mg/10 ml, in 10-ml vials
Supplied as a kit with I.V. supplies and portable infusion pump.

Indications, route, and dosage

To induce ovulation in women with primary hypothalamic amenorrhea

Adults: 5 mcg I.V. q 90 minutes (using a Lutrepulse pump, 0.8 mg solution at 50 microliters/pulse) for 21 days. If no response after three treatment intervals, dosage may be increased. Usual dose is 1 to 20 mcg.

Pharmacodynamics

Ovulation-stimulating action: Mimics the action of GnRH, which results in the synthesis and release of luteinizing hormone (LH) from the anterior pituitary. LH subsequently acts on the reproductive organs to regulate hormone synthesis.

Pharmacokinetics

- *Absorption:* Drug is administered I.V. using a portable pump designed to administer the drug in a pulsatile fashion to mimic the endogenous hormone.
- *Distribution:* Drug has a low plasma volume of distribution (10 to 15 L) and a high rate of clearance from plasma.
- *Metabolism:* Rapidly metabolized. Several biologically inactive peptide fragments have been identified.
- *Excretion:* Excreted primarily in the urine. The high initial clearance rate (half-life of 2 to 10 minutes) is followed by a somewhat slower terminal half-life of 10 to 40 minutes.

Contraindications and precautions

Contraindicated in patients hypersensitive to drug, in women with conditions that could be complicated by pregnancy (such as prolactinoma), in those who are anovulatory from any cause other than a hypothalamic disorder, and in those with ovarian cysts.

Interactions
Concomitant use of *ovarian-stimulating drugs* should be avoided to decrease the risk of ovarian hyperstimulation.

Effects on diagnostic tests
None reported.

Adverse reactions
Skin: hematoma, local infection, inflammation, mild phlebitis.
Other: multiple pregnancy, ovarian hyperstimulation.

Overdose and treatment
No harmful effects are expected if the pump were to malfunction and deliver the entire contents of the highest concentration vial (3.2 mg). Bolus doses of up to 3,000 mcg have not proven harmful in clinical trials. However, continuous exposure (nonpulsatile administration) to gonadorelin might temporarily reduce pituitary responsiveness.

☑ Special considerations
- Patients usually require pelvic ultrasound on days 7 and 14 after establishment of a baseline scan, although the interval between scans may be shortened.
- To mimic the action of the naturally occurring hormone, gonadorelin requires a pulsatile administration with the special portable infusion pump. The pulse period is set at 1 minute (drug is infused over 1 minute); pulse interval is set at 90 minutes.
- To administer 2.5 mcg/pulse, reconstitute the 0.8-mg vial with 8 ml of supplied diluent, and set the pump to deliver 25 microliters/pulse. To administer 5 mcg/pulse, use the same dosage strength and dilution but set the pump to deliver 50 microliters/pulse.
- Some patients may require higher doses. To administer 10 mcg/pulse, reconstitute the 3.2-mg vial with 8 ml of supplied diluent, and set the pump to deliver 25 microliters/pulse. To administer 20 mcg/pulse, use this dosage strength and dilution but set the pump to deliver 50 microliters/pulse.

Patient education
- Because similar drugs have caused anaphylaxis, teach patient the signs and symptoms of hypersensitivity reactions (hives, wheezing, difficulty breathing) and instruct her to report them immediately.
- Make sure patient understands that a multiple pregnancy is possible (incidence about 12%). Close monitoring of dosage and ultrasonography of the ovaries are necessary to monitor drug response.
- Encourage patient to adhere to the close monitoring schedule required by the therapy. Regular pelvic examinations, midluteal phase serum progesterone determinations, and multiple ovarian ultrasound scans are necessary. Inspect the I.V. site at each visit.
- Instruct patient about proper aseptic technique and I.V. site care. Provide available written instructions. The catheter and I.V. site should be monitored and changed at appropriate intervals for the type of catheter used.

Pediatric use
- Safety and efficacy in children under age 18 have not been established.

Breast-feeding
- It is not known if drug is excreted in breast milk; however, there is no reason to administer drug to a breast-feeding woman.

goserelin acetate
Zoladex, Zoladex 3-month

Pharmacologic classification: synthetic decapeptide
Therapeutic classification: luteinizing hormone-releasing hormone (LHRH; GnRH) analogue
Pregnancy risk category X (10.8-mg implant); D (3.6-mg implant)

How supplied
Available by prescription only
Implant: 3.6 mg, 10.8 mg

Indications, route, and dosage
Palliative treatment of advanced carcinoma of the prostate, endometriosis, advanced breast carcinoma
Adults: 1 (3.6 mg) implant S.C. q 28 days into the upper abdominal wall for 6 months. Treatment of endometriosis should not exceed 6 months.
Palliative treatment of advanced carcinoma of the prostate
Adult males: 1 (10.8 mg) implant S.C. q 12 weeks into the upper abdominal wall.

Pharmacodynamics
Hormonal action: Chronic administration of goserelin, an LHRH, acts on the pituitary to decrease the release of follicle-stimulating hormone (FSH) and luteinizing hormone. In males, the result is dramatically lowered serum levels of testosterone.

Pharmacokinetics
- *Absorption:* Goserelin is slowly absorbed from implant site. Drug levels peak in 12 to 15 days.
- *Distribution:* Administration of the implant results in measurable concentrations of drug in serum throughout the dosing period.
- *Metabolism:* Clearance of goserelin following S.C. administration of the drug is rapid and occurs via a combination of hepatic metabolism and urinary excretion.
- *Excretion:* Elimination half-life is about 4.2 hours in patients with normal renal function. Substantial renal impairment prolongs half-life, but this does not appear to increase the incidence of adverse effects.

Contraindications and precautions
Contraindicated in patients with hypersensitivity to LHRH, LHRH agonist analogues, or to goserelin

acetate. Also contraindicated during pregnancy or breast-feeding. The 10.8-mg implant is contraindicated for use in women.

Use cautiously in patients at risk for osteoporosis, chronic alcohol or tobacco abuse, or use of anticonvulsants or corticosteriods.

Interactions
None reported.

Effects on diagnostic tests
Serum testosterone levels increase during the first week of therapy and then decrease. Serum acid phosphatase may increase initially and wil decrease by week 4.

Adverse reactions
CNS: lethargy, pain (worsened in the first 30 days), dizziness, *insomnia,* anxiety, *depression, headache,* chills, *emotional lability.*
CV: edema, ***heart failure, arrhythmias,*** *peripheral edema,* ***CVA,*** hypertension, ***MI,*** peripheral vascular disorder, chest pain.
GI: nausea, vomiting, diarrhea, constipation, ulcer, anorexia, abdominal pain.
GU: *impotence, sexual dysfunction, lower urinary tract symptoms,* renal insufficiency, urinary obstruction, *vaginitis,* urinary tract infection, amenorrhea.
Hematologic: anemia.
Respiratory: COPD, upper respiratory infection.
Skin: rash, *diaphoresis, acne, seborrhea,* hirsutism.
Other: *hot flashes,* gout, hyperglycemia, weight increase, breast swelling and tenderness, *changes in breast size, pain, changes in libido, asthenia, infection,* breast pain, back pain.

Overdose and treatment
No information is available regarding accidental or intentional overdosage in humans. In animal studies, doses up to 1 mg/kg/day did not produce nonendocrine-related symptoms.

☑ Special considerations
- The implant comes in a preloaded syringe. If the package is damaged, do not use the syringe. Make sure that the drug is visible in the translucent chamber of the syringe.
- Drug should be given every 28 days for the 3.6-mg implant and every 12 weeks for the 10.8-mg implant, always under direct medical supervision. Local anesthesia may be used before injection.
- In the unlikely event of the need to surgically remove goserelin, it may be localized by ultrasound.
- Administer drug in the upper abdominal wall using aseptic technique. After cleaning the area with an alcohol swab (and injecting a local anesthetic), stretch the patient's skin with one hand while grasping the barrel of the syringe with the other. Insert the needle into the S.C. fat, then change the needle direction to parallel the abdominal wall. Push the needle in until the hub touches the patient's skin, then withdraw it about 1 cm (this creates a gap for the drug to be injected) before depressing the plunger completely.
- After inserting the needle, do not aspirate because blood will be seen instantly in the chamber if a large vessel is penetrated (a new syringe and injection site will be needed).
- Store drug at room temperature, not to exceed 77° F (25° C).

Patient education
- Advise patient to report every 28 days or 12 weeks, as appropriate, for a new implant. However, a delay of a couple of days is permissible.

Pediatric use
- Safety and efficacy in children under age 18 have not been established.

Breast-feeding
- It is not known if drug is excreted in breast milk.

granisetron hydrochloride
Kytril

Pharmacologic classification: selective 5-hydroxytryptamine (5-HT_3) receptor antagonist
Therapeutic classification: antiemetic, antinausea
Pregnancy risk category B

How supplied
Available by prescription only
Tablets: 1 mg
Injection: 1 mg/ml

Indications, route, and dosage
Prevention of nausea and vomiting associated with emetogenic cancer chemotherapy
Adults and children age 2 to 16: 10 mcg/kg I.V. infused over 5 minutes. Begin infusion within 30 minutes before administration of chemotherapy.
Oral form
Adults: 1 mg P.O. b.i.d. Give the first 1-mg tablet 1 hour before chemotherapy administration and the second tablet 12 hours after the first. Give only on days when chemotherapy is given. Continued treatment while not on chemotherapy has not been found to be useful.

Pharmacodynamics
Antiemetic action: Granisetron as a selective 5-hydroxytryptamine (5-HT_3) receptor antagonist is thought to bind to serotonin receptors of the 5-HT_3 type located peripherally on vagal nerve terminals and centrally in the chemoreceptor trigger zone of the area postrema. This binding blocks serotonin stimulation and subsequent vomiting after emetogenic stimuli, such as cisplatin.

Pharmacokinetics
- *Absorption:* Not determined.
- *Distribution:* Drug is distributed freely between plasma and RBCs. Plasma protein binding is approximately 65%.

• *Metabolism:* Drug is metabolized by the liver, possibly mediated by the cytochrome P-450 3A subfamily.
• *Excretion:* Approximately 12% of drug is eliminated unchanged in the urine in 48 hours; rest is excreted as metabolites, 48% in the urine and 38% in the feces.

Contraindications and precautions
Contraindicated in patients hypersensitive to drug.

Interactions
None significant.

Effects on diagnostic tests
None reported.

Adverse reactions
CNS: *headache, asthenia,* somnolence, dizziness, anxiety.
CV: hypertension.
GI: diarrhea, *constipation,* abdominal pain, *nausea,* vomiting, decreased appetite.
Hematologic: *leukopenia,* anemia, ***thrombocytopenia.***
Other: fever, alopecia, elevated liver function tests.

Overdose and treatment
No antidote for overdosage exists. Symptomatic treatment should be given. Overdosage of up to 38.5 mg of granisetron has been reported without symptoms or only the occurrence of a slight headache.

☑ Special considerations
• Dilute drug with 0.9% NaCl injection or D_5W to a volume of 20 to 50 ml. Infuse I.V. over 5 minutes. Diluted solutions are stable for 24 hours at room temperature.
• Do not mix with other drugs; information about compatibility is limited.
• Although clearance is slower and half-life is prolonged in elderly patients and in patients with hepatic disease, dosage adjustments aren't necessary.
• No dosage adjustment is recommended in patients with renal impairment.

Patient education
• Tell patient to watch for signs of an anaphylactoid reaction—local or generalized hives, chest tightness, wheezing, and dizziness or weakness—and to report them immediately.

Pediatric use
• Safety and effectiveness in children under age 2 have not been established. Safety and effectiveness in children have not been established for the oral form.

Breast-feeding
• It is not known if drug is excreted in breast milk. Use with caution in breast-feeding women.

grepafloxacin hydrochloride
Raxar

Pharmacologic classification: fluoroquinolone antibiotic
Therapeutic classification: antibiotic
Pregnancy risk category C

How supplied
Available by prescription only
Tablets: 200 mg (base)

Indications, route, and dosage
***Acute bacterial exacerbations of chronic bronchitis caused by susceptible strains of* Haemophilus influenzae, Streptococcus pneumoniae, *or* Moraxella catarrhalis**
Adults: 400 or 600 mg P.O. once daily for 10 days with or without food.
***Community-acquired pneumonia caused by susceptible strains of* H. influenzae, S. pneumoniae, M. catarrhalis, *or* Mycoplasma pneumoniae**
Adults: 600 mg P.O. once daily for 10 days.
***Uncomplicated gonorrhea (urethral in males and endocervical and rectal in females) caused by* Neisseria gonorrhoeae**
Adults: 400 mg P.O. as a single dose.
***Nongonococcal urethritis and cervicitis caused by* Chlamydia trachomatis**
Adults: 400 mg P.O. once daily for 7 days.

Pharmacodynamics
Antibiotic action: Exact mechanism is unknown, but bactericidal effects may result from drug inhibiting bacterial DNA gyrase and preventing replication in susceptible bacteria. Drug has *in-vitro* activity against a wide range of gram-positive and gram-negative aerobic microorganisms, as well as some atypical microorganisms.

Pharmacokinetics
• *Absorption:* Rapidly and extensively absorbed following oral administration; absolute bioavailability is approximately 70%. Peak plasma concentrates are achieved within 2 to 3 hours.
• *Distribution:* Apparent volume of distribution after oral administration of grepafloxacin is 5.1 L/kg, suggesting wide distribution into extravascular spaces. Binding to human plasma proteins is low (approximately 50%).
• *Metabolism:* Eliminated primarily through hepatic metabolism and biliary excretion. Metabolites include glucuronide (major metabolite) and sulfate conjugates and oxidative metabolites. Metabolites have little or no antimicrobial activity. Plasma elimination half-life at steady state is about 16 hours.
• *Excretion:* Less than 10% of an oral dose is excreted unchanged in the urine. Fecal elimination (50% of an oral dose) has been observed. Dose adjustment is not required in renal impairment.

Contraindications and precautions
Contraindicated in patients with hypersensitivity to drug or other quinolones, hepatic failure, or a known

QT prolongation, and in those receiving concomitant therapy with medications known to produce an increase in the QT interval or torsade de pointes.

Use cautiously in patients with known or suspected CNS disorders that predispose patient to seizures. Drug is not recommended for patients with proarrhythmic conditions.

Interactions

Antacids containing aluminum, magnesium, or calcium; iron; sucralfate; and *multiple vitamins containing zinc* substantially interfere with absorption of grepafloxacin. These agents should not be taken within 4 hours before or after grepafloxacin administration.

Administration with *antidiabetic agents* may cause disturbances of blood glucose, including hyperglycemia and hypoglycemia. Monitor serum glucose level closely.

Grepafloxacin has the potential to affect the metabolism of CYP 3A4 substrates, such as *astemizole, cyclosporine, cisapride, midazolam, triazolam* and *other quinolone drugs.* Clinical relevance of this possible interaction is unknown. Monitor patient if given concurrently.

Concomitant administration of *NSAIDs* with grepafloxacin may increase risk of CNS stimulation and seizures. Use with caution.

Serum theophylline concentrations increase when grepafloxacin is initiated in patients maintained on *theophylline.* When initiating a multiday course of grepafloxacin in patients maintained on theophylline, half the maintenance dose of theophylline for the period of concurrent therapy. Monitor theophylline serum concentrations.

Grepafloxacin may enhance effects of *warfarin.* Monitor INR.

Drug interferes with metabolism of *caffeine* and *theobromines* and may enhance their effects. Use together cautiously. *Dairy products* can decrease absorption of grepafloxacin. Do not give drug with dairy products.

Photosensitivity reactions may *occur with sun exposure.* Take precautions. Stop drug if reactions occur.

Effects on diagnostic tests

Eosinophilia, leukocytosis, lymphocytosis, hyperuricemia, hyperglycemia, hypoglycemia, hyperlipidemia, hypernatremia, increased alkaline phosphatase, increased BUN, increased creatinine, increased gamma glutamyl transpeptidase, and increased AST and ALT have been reported.

Adverse reactions

CNS: asthenia, dizziness, headache, insomnia, pain, nervousness, somnolence.
EENT: dry mouth.
GI: *nausea,* abdominal pain, anorexia, constipation, diarrhea, dyspepsia, *taste perversion,* vomiting.
GU: leukorrhea, vaginitis.
Skin: pruritus, photosensitivity reactions, rash.
Other: infection.

Overdose and treatment

If acute overdosage occurs, the stomach should be emptied by induced vomiting or gastric lavage. Observe patient carefully and provide supportive treatment. Because of the possibility of prolongation of the QTc interval and complications including arrhythmias, ECG monitoring is recommended after overdosage. It is unknown if hemodialysis or peritoneal dialysis can efficiently remove grepafloxacin.

☑ Special considerations

- Serious and sometimes fatal events of uncertain etiology have been reported in patients receiving therapy with quinolones.
- Discontinue drug if allergic reaction or signs of hypersensitivity occur.
- Drug therapy may start pending results of culture and sensitivity tests.
- Pseudomembranous colitis, which may range in severity from mild to life-threatening, has been reported in patients receiving quinolones.
- Test patients treated for gonorrhea should also be tested for syphillis at time of diagnosis and 3 months after treatment with grepafloxacin.
- Achilles and other tendon ruptures that require surgical repair have been reported in patients receiving quinolone antibiotics. Grepafloxacin should be discontinued if patient experiences pain, inflammation or rupture of a tendon.
- Phototoxicity reactions have been observed in patients who were exposed to direct sunlight or tanning booths. Excessive sunlight should be avoided. Therapy should be discontinued if phototoxicity occurs.
- No dose adjustment is necessary in patients with renal impairment.

Patient education

- Inform patient that drug may be taken with or without meals.
- Instruct patient to drink plenty of fluids.
- Tell patient that drug may increase the effects of caffeine.
- Instruct patient to inform health care provider if he begins taking theophylline.
- Advise patient of possible hypersensitivity reactions. Tell him to stop drug at first sign of rash, hives, or other skin reactions, rapid heartbeat, or difficulty breathing or swallowing.
- Warn patient to avoid hazardous activities, such as driving or operating heavy equipment, until the effects of drug are known, as grepafloxacin may cause dizziness or light-headedness.
- Tell patient to avoid excessive sunlight or artificial ultraviolet light during drug therapy and to discontinue therapy if sunburn or skin eruptions occur.
- Inform patient to stop drug, sit and rest, and notify primary health care provider immediately if pain, inflammation, or rupture of tendon occurs.
- Advise patient not to take antacids, multivitamins, or sucralfate within 4 hours before or after taking drug.

Geriatric use
- There is no apparent difference in the frequency, type, or severity of adverse effects in elderly adults compared with other adults.

Pediatric use
- Safety and efficacy in children and adolescents (below age 18) have not been established. Related quinolone-class drugs produce erosions of cartilage of weight-bearing joints and other signs of arthropathy in immature animals of various species.

Breast-feeding
- Safety in breast-feeding patients has not been established.
- Drug is excreted in breast milk; therefore a decision should be made to discontinue breast-feeding or the drug, based on importance of drug to the mother.

---

griseofulvin microsize
Fulvicin-U/F, Grifulvin V, Grisactin

griseofulvin ultramicrosize
Fulvicin P/G, Grisactin Ultra, Gris-PEG

Pharmacologic classification: penicillium antibiotic
Therapeutic classification: antifungal
Pregnancy risk category C

How supplied
Available by prescription only
Microsize
Capsules: 250 mg
Tablets: 250 mg, 500 mg
Oral suspension: 125 mg/5 ml
Ultramicrosize
Tablets: 125 mg, 165 mg, 250 mg, 330 mg
Tablets (film-coated): 125 mg, 250 mg

Indications, route, and dosage
Tinea corporis, tinea capitis, tinea barbae, or tinea cruris infections
Adults: 330 mg ultramicrosize P.O. daily, or 500 mg microsize P.O. daily.
Children over age 2: 3.3 mg/lb ultramicrosize P.O. daily; or 125 to 250 mg microsize P.O. daily for children weighing 30 to 50 lb (14 to 23 kg) or 250 to 500 mg microsize P.O. daily for children weighing over 50 lb.
Tinea pedis or tinea unguium infections
Adults: 660 mg ultramicrosize P.O. daily or 1 g microsize P.O. daily.
Children over age 2: 3.3 mg/lb ultramicrosize P.O. daily; or 125 to 250 mg microsize P.O. daily for children weighing 30 to 50 lb, or 250 to 500 mg microsize P.O. daily for children weighing over 50 lb.

Pharmacodynamics
Antifungal action: Griseofulvin disrupts the fungal cell's mitotic spindle, interfering with cell division; it also may inhibit DNA replication. Drug is also deposited in keratin precursor cells, inhibiting fungal invasion. It is active against *Trichophyton, Microsporum,* and *Epidermophyton.*

Pharmacokinetics
- *Absorption:* Absorbed primarily in the duodenum and varies among individuals. Ultramicrosize preparations are absorbed almost completely; microsize absorption ranges from 25% to 70% and may be increased by giving with a high-fat meal. Peak concentrations occur at 4 to 8 hours.
- *Distribution:* Drug concentrates in skin, hair, nails, fat, liver, and skeletal muscle; it is tightly bound to new keratin.
- *Metabolism:* Griseofulvin is oxidatively demethylated and conjugated with glucuronic acid to inactive metabolites in the liver.
- *Excretion:* About 50% of drug and its metabolites is excreted in urine and 33% in feces within 5 days. Less than 1% of a dose appears unchanged in urine. Griseofulvin is also excreted in perspiration. Elimination half-life is 9 to 24 hours.

Contraindications and precautions
Contraindicated in those with hypersensitivity to drug and in those with porphyria or hepatocellular failure. Also contraindicated in pregnant patients or women who intend to become pregnant during therapy. Use cautiously in penicillin-sensitive patients.

Interactions
Griseofulvin may potentiate the effects of *alcohol,* producing tachycardia and flushing; it may decrease PT in patients taking *warfarin,* by enzyme induction; and it may decrease the efficacy of *oral contraceptives.*

Concomitant use of *barbiturates* may impair absorption of griseofulvin and increase dosage requirements.

Effects on diagnostic tests
Griseofulvin can cause proteinuria; it also may decrease granulocyte counts.

Adverse reactions
CNS: headache (in early stages of treatment), transient decrease in hearing, fatigue with large doses, occasional mental confusion, impaired performance of routine activities, psychotic symptoms, dizziness, insomnia, paresthesia of the hands and feet after extended therapy.
GI: nausea, vomiting, flatulence, diarrhea, epigastric distress, *bleeding.*
GU: proteinuria.
Hematologic: leukopenia, ***granulocytopenia*** (requires discontinuation of drug), porphyria.
Hepatic: ***hepatic toxicity.***
Skin: *rash, urticaria,* photosensitivity, angioneurotic edema.
Other: oral thrush, hypersensitivity reactions (rash), menstrual irregularities, lupus erythematosus.

Overdose and treatment
Symptoms of overdose include headache, lethargy, confusion, vertigo, blurred vision, nausea, vomiting, and diarrhea. Treatment is supportive. After recent ingestion (within 4 hours), empty stomach

by induced emesis or gastric lavage. Follow with activated charcoal to decrease absorption. A cathartic may also be helpful.

☑ Special considerations

- Commercial formulation of drug has changed, decreasing the dosage required for an equivalent therapeutic effect. Dosages equivalent to the original formulation (before 1971) for 1 g of griseofulvin are 250 mg ultramicrosize or 500 mg microsize. Dosages may vary slightly depending on the manufacturer.
- Identification of organism should be confirmed before therapy begins.
- Give drug with or after meals consisting of a high-fat content (if allowed), to minimize GI distress.
- Assess nutrition and monitor food intake; drug may alter taste sensation, suppressing appetite.
- Check CBCs regularly for possible adverse effects; monitor renal and liver function studies periodically.
- Treatment of tinea pedis may require combined oral and topical therapy.
- Ultramicrosize griseofulvin is absorbed more rapidly and completely than microsize and is effective at one half to two thirds the usual dose.

Patient education

- Encourage patient to maintain adequate nutritional intake; offer suggestions to improve taste of food.
- Stress importance of completing prescribed regimen to prevent relapse even though symptoms may abate quickly.
- Teach signs and symptoms of adverse effects and hypersensitivity, and tell patient to report them immediately.
- Advise patient to avoid exposure to intense indoor light and sunlight to reduce the risk of photosensitivity reactions.
- Explain that drug may potentiate alcohol effects, and advise patient to avoid alcohol during therapy.
- Teach correct personal hygiene and skin care.

Pediatric use

- Safety in children under age 2 has not been established.

Breast-feeding

- Safety has not been established.

guaifenesin

Amonidrin, Anti-Tuss, Balminil Expectorant*, Breonesin, Fenesin, Gee-Gee, Genatuss, GG-Cen, Glyate, Glycotuss, Glytuss, Guiatuss, Halotussin, Humibid L.A., Humibid Sprinkle, Hytuss, Hytuss 2X, Malotuss, Mytussin, Naldecon Senior EX, Neo-Spec*, Organidin NR, Resyl*, Robitussin, Scot-tussin, Uni-tussin

Pharmacologic classification: propanediol derivative
Therapeutic classification: expectorant
Pregnancy risk category C

How supplied

Available without a prescription
Tablets: 100 mg, 200 mg
Tablets (extended-release): 600 mg
Capsules: 200 mg
Capsules (extended-release): 300 mg
Syrup: 100 mg/5 ml, 200 mg/5 ml

Indications, route, and dosage

As expectorant

Adults and children age 12 and older: 100 to 400 mg q 4 hours; maximum dosage is 2.4 g/day.
Children age 6 to 11: 100 to 200 mg q 4 hours; maximum dosage is 1.2 g/day.
Children age 2 to 5: 50 to 100 mg q 4 hours; maximum dosage is 600 mg/day.
Children under age 2: Individualize dosage.

Extended-release

Adults and children over age 12: 600 to 1,200 mg q 12 hours, not to exceed 2,400 mg in 24 hours.
Children age 6 to 12: 600 mg q 12 hours, not to exceed 1,200 mg in 24 hours.
Children age 2 to 6: 300 mg q 12 hours, not to exceed 600 mg in 24 hours.

For self medication, recommended dosage is half the usual dosage.

Pharmacodynamics

Expectorant action: Guaifenesin increases respiratory tract fluid by reducing adhesiveness and surface tension, decreasing viscosity of the secretions and thereby facilitating their removal.

Pharmacokinetics

- *Absorption:* No information available.
- *Distribution:* No information available.
- *Metabolism:* No information available.
- *Excretion:* No information available.

Contraindications and precautions

Contraindicated in patients hypersensitive to drug.

Interactions

None significant.

Effects on diagnostic tests

Drug may cause color interference with tests for 5-hydroxyindoleacetic acid and vanillylmandelic acid.

Adverse reactions

CNS: dizziness, headache.
GI: vomiting and nausea (with large doses).
Skin: rash.

Overdose and treatment

No information available.

☑ Special considerations

- Efficacy of drug as an expectorant has not been established.
- Drug should be taken with a glass of water.

Patient education

- Instruct patient to call if cough persists for more than 1 week, if cough recurs, or if cough is accompanied by fever, rash, or persistent headache.

- Advise patient to use sugarless throat lozenges to decrease throat irritation and associated cough and to report cough that persists longer than 7 days.
- Recommend patient uses a humidifier to filter out dust, smoke, and air pollutants.
- Encourage patient to perform deep-breathing exercises.

Geriatric use
- No specific recommendations are available. Note that most liquid preparations contain alcohol (3.5% to 10%).

Pediatric use
- Individualize dosage for children under age 2.

Breast-feeding
- Distribution into breast milk is unknown. Safe use in breast-feeding has not been established.

guanabenz acetate
Wytensin

Pharmacologic classification: centrally acting antiadrenergic
Therapeutic classification: antihypertensive
Pregnancy risk category C

How supplied
Available by prescription only
Tablets: 4 mg, 8 mg

Indications, route, and dosage
Hypertension (generally considered a step 2 agent)
Adults: Initially, 2 to 4 mg P.O. b.i.d. Dosage may be increased in increments of 4 to 8 mg/day q 1 to 2 weeks. The usual maintenance dosage ranges from 8 to 16 mg daily. Maximum dosage is 32 mg b.i.d.
Children age 12 and older: Initially, 0.5 to 4 mg daily; maintenance dosage ranges from 4 to 24 mg daily, administered in two divided doses.
◊ ***Management of opiate withdrawal***
Adults: 4 mg P.O. b.i.d. to q.i.d.

Pharmacodynamics
Antihypertensive action: Guanabenz lowers blood pressure by stimulating central $alpha_2$-adrenergic receptors, decreasing cerebral sympathetic outflow and thus decreasing peripheral vascular resistance. Guanabenz may also antagonize antidiuretic hormone (ADH) secretion and ADH activity in the kidney.

Pharmacokinetics
- *Absorption:* After oral administration, 70% to 80% of guanabenz is absorbed from the GI tract; antihypertensive effect occurs within 60 minutes, peaking at 2 to 4 hours.
- *Distribution:* Appears to be distributed widely into the body; drug is about 90% protein-bound.
- *Metabolism:* Drug is metabolized extensively in the liver; several metabolites are formed.
- *Excretion:* Guanabenz and its metabolites are excreted primarily in urine; remaining drug is excreted in feces. Duration of antihypertensive effect varies from 6 to 12 hours.

Contraindications and precautions
Contraindicated in patients with hypersensitivity to drug. Use cautiously in the elderly and in patients with impaired renal or hepatic function, severe coronary insufficiency, recent MI, and cerebrovascular disease.

Interactions
Guanabenz may increase CNS depressant effects of *alcohol, phenothiazines, benzodiazepines, barbiturates*, and other *sedatives; tricyclic antidepressants* may inhibit antihypertensive effects of guanabenz.

Effects on diagnostic tests
Guanabenz may reduce serum cholesterol and total triglyceride levels slightly, but it does not alter high-density lipoprotein fraction; drug may cause nonprogressive elevations in liver enzyme levels.

Chronic use of guanabenz decreases plasma norepinephrine, dopamine, beta-hydroxylase, and plasma renin activity.

Adverse reactions
CNS: *drowsiness, sedation, dizziness, weakness,* headache.
CV: *rebound hypertension.*
GI: *dry mouth.*

Overdose and treatment
Clinical signs of overdose include bradycardia, CNS depression, respiratory depression, hypothermia, apnea, seizures, lethargy, agitation, irritability, diarrhea, and hypotension.

Do not induce emesis; CNS depression occurs rapidly. After adequate respiration is assured, empty stomach by gastric lavage; then give activated charcoal and a saline cathartic to decrease absorption. Follow with symptomatic and supportive care.

☑ Special considerations
- To ensure overnight blood pressure control and minimize daytime drowsiness, give last dose at bedtime.
- Investigational uses include managing opiate withdrawal and adjunctive therapy in patients with chronic pain.
- Abrupt discontinuation of guanabenz will cause severe rebound hypertension; reduce dosage gradually over 2 to 4 days.
- Reduced dosages may be required in patients with hepatic impairment.

Patient education
- Explain signs and symptoms of adverse effects and importance of reporting them.
- Warn patient to avoid hazardous activities that require mental alertness and to avoid alcohol and other CNS depressants.

• Suggest taking drug at bedtime until tolerance develops to sedation, drowsiness, and other CNS effects.
• Advise patient to avoid sudden position changes to minimize orthostatic hypotension, and to relieve dry mouth with ice chips or sugarless gum.
• Warn patient to seek medical approval before taking OTC cold preparations.
• Advise patient not to discontinue drug suddenly; severe rebound hypertension may occur.

Geriatric use
• Elderly patients may be more sensitive to the antihypertensive and sedative effects of guanabenz.

Pediatric use
• Drug has been used to treat hypertension in a limited number of children over age 12; its safety and efficacy in younger children have not been established.

Breast-feeding
• It is not known if guanabenz is distributed into breast milk; an alternative feeding method is recommended during therapy.

guanadrel sulfate
Hylorel

Pharmacologic classification: adrenergic neuron blocker
Therapeutic classification: antihypertensive
Pregnancy risk category B

How supplied
Available by prescription only
Tablets: 10 mg, 25 mg

Indications, route, and dosage
Hypertension
Adults: Initially, 5 mg P.O. b.i.d.; adjust dosage until blood pressure is controlled. Most patients require 20 to 75 mg daily, usually given b.i.d. (400 mg daily is rarely used).
✦ ***Dosage adjustment.*** In patient with renal impairment, if creatinine clearance is 30 to 60 ml/minute, reduce dose to 5 mg q 24 hours; if creatinine clearance is below 30 ml/minute, increase dosing interval to q 48 hours.

Pharmacodynamics
Antihypertensive action: Guanadrel reduces blood pressure by peripheral inhibition of norepinephrine release in adrenergic nerve endings, thus decreasing arteriolar vasoconstriction.

Pharmacokinetics
• *Absorption:* Guanadrel is absorbed rapidly and almost completely from the GI tract. Antihypertensive effect usually occurs at ½ to 2 hours; peak effect occurs at 4 to 6 hours.
• *Distribution:* Drug is distributed widely into the body; drug is about 20% protein-bound; it does not enter the CNS.
• *Metabolism:* Approximately 40% to 50% of a given dose is metabolized by the liver.
• *Excretion:* Drug and its metabolites are eliminated primarily in urine. Antihypertensive activity persists for 4 to 14 hours. Plasma half-life is about 10 hours but varies considerably with each individual.

Contraindications and precautions
Contraindicated in patients with hypersensitivity to drug, known or suspected pheochromocytoma, or frank heart failure. Also contraindicated in patients receiving MAO inhibitors or within 1 week of discontinuing MAO inhibitor therapy.

Use cautiously in patients with regional vascular disease, bronchial asthma, or peptic ulcer disease.

Interactions
Guanadrel may potentiate antihypertensive effects of other *antihypertensive agents* and pressor effects of such agents as *norepinephrine* and *metaraminol. MAO inhibitors, ephedrine, norepinephrine, methylphenidate, tricyclic antidepressants, phenothiazines,* or *amphetamines* may antagonize antihypertensive effects of guanadrel; concomitant use of *alcohol* may increase risk of guanadrel-induced orthostatic hypotension. Concomitant use of *diuretics* or other *antihypertensive agents* increases the antihypertensive effects of guanadrel.

Effects on diagnostic tests
None reported.

Adverse reactions
CNS: *fatigue, drowsiness, faintness, headache, confusion, paresthesia.*
CV: *palpitations, chest pain, peripheral edema, orthostatic hypotension.*
EENT: *glossitis.*
GI: *diarrhea,* dry mouth, *indigestion,* constipation, anorexia, nausea, vomiting, abdominal pain.
GU: impotence, *ejaculation disturbances, nocturia, urination frequency.*
Respiratory: *shortness of breath, cough.*
Other: *weight gain, aching limbs, leg cramps, visual disturbances.*

Overdose and treatment
Signs of overdose include hypotension, dizziness, blurred vision, and syncope.

After acute ingestion, empty stomach by induced emesis or gastric lavage. The effect of activated charcoal in absorbing guanadrel has not been determined. Further treatment is usually symptomatic and supportive.

☑ Special considerations
• Monitor supine and standing blood pressure, especially during periods of dosage adjustment.
• Assess for signs and symptoms of edema.
• Discontinue guanadrel 48 to 72 hours before surgery, to minimize risk of vascular collapse during anesthesia.
• Separate use of guanadrel and MAO inhibitors by at least 1 week.

Patient education

- Teach patient signs and symptoms of adverse effects and importance of reporting them; patient should also report excessive weight gain (more than 5 lb [2.25 kg] weekly).
- Explain that orthostatic hypotension can be minimized by rising slowly from a supine position and avoiding sudden position changes; it may be aggravated by fever, hot weather, hot showers, prolonged standing, exercise, and alcohol.
- Warn patient to avoid hazardous activities that require mental alertness and to take drug at bedtime until tolerance develops to sedation, drowsiness, and other CNS effects.
- Advise patient to use ice chips or sugarless hard candy or gum to relieve dry mouth.
- Warn patient to seek medical approval before taking OTC cold preparations.

Geriatric use

- Elderly patients may be more sensitive to orthostatic hypotension.

Pediatric use

- Safety and efficacy in children have not been established; use drug only if potential benefit outweighs risk.

Breast-feeding

- It is not known if drug occurs in breast milk. An alternative feeding method is recommended during therapy.

guanethidine monosulfate

Ismelin

Pharmacologic classification: adrenergic neuron blocker
Therapeutic classification: antihypertensive
Pregnancy risk category C

How supplied

Available by prescription only
Tablets: 10 mg, 25 mg

Indications, route, and dosage

Moderate to severe hypertension,* ◊ *signs and symptoms of thyrotoxicosis

Adults: Initially, 10 mg P.O. once daily; increase by 10 mg at weekly to monthly intervals, p.r.n. Usual dosage is 25 to 50 mg once daily; some patients may require up to 300 mg.

Pharmacodynamics

Antihypertensive action: Guanethidine acts peripherally; it decreases arteriolar vasoconstriction and reduces blood pressure by inhibiting norepinephrine release and depleting norepinephrine stores in adrenergic nerve endings.

Pharmacokinetics

- *Absorption:* Drug is absorbed incompletely from the GI tract. Maximal antihypertensive effects usually are not evident for 1 to 3 weeks.
- *Distribution:* Distributed throughout the body; it is not protein-bound but demonstrates extensive tissue binding.
- *Metabolism:* Guanethidine undergoes partial hepatic metabolism to pharmacologically less-active metabolites.
- *Excretion:* Drug and metabolites are excreted primarily in urine; small amounts are excreted in feces. Elimination half-life after chronic administration is biphasic.

Contraindications and precautions

Contraindicated in patients with pheochromocytoma, frank heart failure, or hypersensitivity to drug and in those receiving MAO inhibitors. Use cautiously in patients with severe cardiac disease, recent MI, cerebrovascular disease, peptic ulcer, impaired renal function, or bronchial asthma and in those taking other antihypertensive agents.

Interactions

Concomitant use of guanethidine with *diuretics, other antihypertensive agents, levodopa,* or *alcohol* may potentiate guanethidine's antihypertensive effect; guanethidine potentiates pressor effects of such agents as *norepinephrine, metaraminol,* and *oral sympathomimetic nasal decongestants.*

Concomitant use with *cardiac glycosides* may result in additive bradycardia; use with *rauwolfia alkaloids* may cause excessive postural hypotension, bradycardia, and mental depression.

Concomitant administration with *MAO inhibitors, tricyclic antidepressants,* or *oral contraceptives* may antagonize the antihypertensive effect of guanethidine.

Effects on diagnostic tests

None reported.

Adverse reactions

CNS: *syncope, fatigue, headache, drowsiness, paresthesia, confusion.*
CV: *palpitations, chest pain, orthostatic hypotension, peripheral edema.*
EENT: *visual disturbances,* glossitis.
GI: *diarrhea, indigestion, constipation, anorexia,* nausea, vomiting.
GU: *nocturia, urination frequency, ejaculation disturbances,* impotence.
Respiratory: shortness of breath, cough.
Other: *weight gain, aching limbs, leg cramps.*

Overdose and treatment

Signs of overdose include hypotension, blurred vision, syncope, bradycardia, and severe diarrhea.

After acute ingestion, empty stomach by induced emesis or gastric lavage and give activated charcoal to reduce absorption. Further treatment is usually symptomatic and supportive.

☑ Special considerations

- Dosage requirements may be reduced in the presence of fever.
- If diarrhea develops, atropine or paregoric may be prescribed.

• Discontinue drug 2 to 3 weeks before elective surgery to reduce risk of CV collapse during anesthesia.
• When drug is replacing MAO inhibitors, wait at least 1 week before initiating guanethidine; if replacing ganglionic blocking agents, withdraw them slowly to prevent a spiking blood pressure response during the transfer period.
• Guanethidine has been used topically as a 5% ophthalmic solution to treat chronic open-angle glaucoma or endocrine ophthalmopathy.

Patient education
• Teach patient signs and symptoms of adverse effects and importance of reporting them; tell patient to also report persistent diarrhea and excessive weight gain (5 lb [2.25 kg] weekly). Advise him not to discontinue the drug but to call for further instructions if adverse reactions occur.
• Warn patient to avoid hazardous activities that require mental alertness and to take drug at bedtime until tolerance develops to sedation, drowsiness, and other CNS effects.
• Advise patient to avoid sudden position changes, strenuous exercise, heat, and hot showers, to minimize orthostatic hypotension; and to relieve dry mouth with ice chips, hard candy, or gum.
• Tell patient not to double next scheduled dose if he misses one; he should take only the next scheduled dose.
• Advise patient to seek medical approval before taking OTC cold preparations.

Geriatric use
• Elderly patients may be more sensitive to drug's antihypertensive effects.

Pediatric use
• Safety and efficacy have not been established.

Breast-feeding
• Small amounts of drug occur in breast milk; an alternative feeding method is recommended during therapy.

guanfacine hydrochloride
Tenex

Pharmacologic classification: centrally acting antiadrenergic
Therapeutic classification: antihypertensive
Pregnancy risk category B

How supplied
Available by prescription only
Tablets: 1 mg, 2 mg

Indications, route, and dosage
Mild to moderate hypertension
Adults: Initially, 0.5 to 1 mg P.O. daily h.s. Average dose is 1 to 3 mg daily.
◊ ***Heroin withdrawal***
Adults: 0.03 to 1.5 mg P.O. daily.
◊ ***Migraine***
Adults: 1 mg P.O. daily for 12 weeks.

Pharmacodynamics
Antihypertensive action: Guanfacine is a centrally acting $alpha_2$-adrenoreceptor agonist whose mechanism of action is not clearly understood. It appears to stimulate central $alpha_2$-adrenergic receptors that decrease peripheral release of norepinephrine, thus decreasing peripheral vascular resistance and lowering blood pressure. Drug reduces heart rate by reducing sympathetic nerve impulses from the vasomotor center to the heart. Systolic and diastolic blood pressure are both decreased; cardiac output is not altered.

Elevated plasma renin activity and plasma catecholamine levels are lowered; however, there is no correlation with individual blood pressure. Single doses of guanfacine stimulate growth hormone secretion, but long-term use has no effect on growth hormone levels.

Pharmacokinetics
• *Absorption:* Guanfacine is absorbed well and completely after oral administration and is approximately 80% bioavailable. Peak plasma concentrations occur in 1 to 4 hours.
• *Distribution:* Approximately 70% is protein-bound; high distribution to tissues is suggested.
• *Metabolism:* Drug is metabolized in the liver.
• *Excretion:* About 50% is eliminated in urine as unchanged drug, rest as conjugates of metabolites.

Contraindications and precautions
Contraindicated in patients with hypersensitivity to drug. Use cautiously in patients with renal or hepatic insufficiency, severe coronary insufficiency, recent MI, or cerebrovascular disease.

Interactions
Guanfacine may enhance the depressant effects of *alcohol* and other *CNS depressants*, such as *phenothiazines, barbiturates,* and *benzodiazepines.*

Concurrent use with other *antihypertensive agents* or *diuretic* combinations may potentiate the antihypertensive effects; this often is used to therapeutic advantage.

NSAIDs (especially *indomethacin*), *estrogens,* and *sympathomimetics* may reduce the antihypertensive effects of guanfacine. *Indomethacin* and other *NSAIDs* may inhibit renal prostaglandin synthesis or cause sodium and fluid retention, thus antagonizing the antihypertensive activity of guanfacine. Blood pressure may be increased by *estrogen*-induced fluid retention; monitor patient carefully.

Effects on diagnostic tests
Drug therapy alters urinary catecholamine concentrations and urinary vanillylmandelic acid excretion (may be decreased during therapy but may increase on abrupt withdrawal). Plasma growth hormone levels may be increased after a single dose; chronic elevation does not follow long-term use.

Adverse reactions

CNS: *dizziness,* fatigue, headache, insomnia, *somnolence,* asthenia.
CV: bradycardia.
GI: *constipation,* diarrhea, nausea, *dry mouth.*
Skin: dermatitis, pruritus.

Overdose and treatment

Clinical manifestations of overdose include difficult breathing, extreme dizziness, faintness, slow heartbeat, severe or unusual tiredness or weakness.

Treat symptomatically, with careful cardiac monitoring. Perform gastric lavage and infuse isoproterenol as appropriate. Drug is dialyzed poorly.

☑ Special considerations

- Give drug at bedtime to reduce daytime drowsiness.
- Withdrawal syndrome may occur if guanfacine is stopped abruptly or discontinued before surgery; therefore, anesthesiologist must be informed if drug was withdrawn more than 2 days before surgery, or if drug has not been withdrawn.
- Dry mouth may contribute to development of dental caries, periodontal disease, oral candidiasis, and discomfort.
- Monitor blood pressure at regular intervals.

Patient education

- Stress importance of diet and the possible need for sodium restriction and weight reduction.
- Tell patient to take medication as directed even if feeling well and to take daily dose at bedtime to minimize daytime drowsiness.
- Advise patient that medication may cause drowsiness or dizziness. Urge patient to avoid use of alcohol and other CNS depressants, which may add to this effect. Tell patient to avoid driving or performing other tasks that require alertness until effects of drug are known.
- Inform patient to take a missed dose as soon as possible; if taking more than one dose per day and it is almost time for next dose, skip the missed dose and return to regular schedule.
- Store drug away from heat and light, and out of children's reach.
- Tell patient to advise new primary health care provider that he is taking this medication before having surgery, including dental surgery, or emergency treatment.
- Advise chewing sugarless gum, candy, ice, or saliva substitute for treatment of dry mouth. If condition continues longer than 2 weeks, patient should call for further recommendations.
- Instruct patient not to take other medications unless they have been prescribed. This is particularly important with medications for cough, cold, asthma, hay fever, or sinus.
- Tell patient not to stop taking medication abruptly; rebound hypertension may occur.

Geriatric use

- Dizziness, drowsiness, hypotension, or faintness occur more frequently in elderly patients, who may be more sensitive to effects of guanfacine.

Breast-feeding

- It is not known if drug is excreted in breast milk. Exercise caution when administering drug to breast-feeding patients.

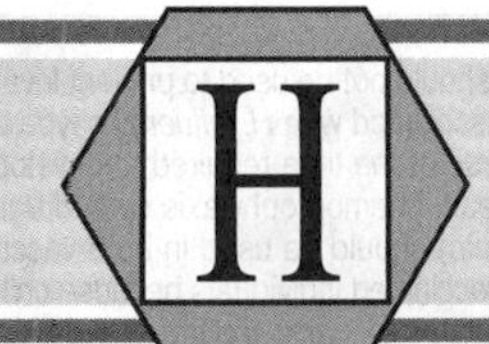

Haemophilus b vaccines

Haemophilus b conjugate vaccine, diphtheria CRM_{197} protein conjugate (HbOC)
HibTITER

Haemophilus b conjugate vaccine, diphtheria toxoid conjugate (PRP-D)
ProHIBiT

Haemophilus b conjugate vaccine, meningococcal protein conjugate (PRP-OMP)
PedvaxHIB

Haemophilus b polysaccharide conjugate vaccine, tetanus toxoid
ActHIB, OmniHIB

Pharmacologic classification: vaccine
Therapeutic classification: bacterial vaccine
Pregnancy risk category C

How supplied
Available by prescription only
Conjugate vaccine, diphtheria CRM_{197} protein conjugate
Injection: 10 mcg of purified *Haemophilus* b saccharide and approximately 25 mcg CRM_{197} protein per 0.5 ml
Conjugate vaccine, diphtheria toxoid conjugate
Injection: 25 mcg of *Haemophilus influenzae* type B (Hib) capsular polysaccharide and 18 mcg of diphtheria toxoid protein per 0.5 ml
Conjugate vaccine, meningococcal protein conjugate
Powder for injection: 15 mcg *Haemophilus* b polysaccharide, 250 mcg *Neisseria meningitidis* OMPC per dose
Conjugate vaccine, tetanus toxoid
Powder for injection: 10 mcg *Haemophilus* b purified capsular polysaccharide, 24 mcg of tetanus toxoid, and 8.5% sucrose

Indications, route, and dosage
Routine immunization
***Haemophilus* b conjugate vaccine, diphtheria CRM_{197} protein conjugate**
Children age 2 to 6 months: 0.5 ml I.M.; repeat in 2 months and again in 4 months (for total of three doses). A booster dose is required at age 15 months.
Previously unvaccinated children age 7 to 11 months: 0.5 ml I.M.; repeat in 2 months (for total of two doses before age 15 months). A booster dose is required at age 15 months (but no sooner than 2 months after last vaccination).
Previously unvaccinated children age 12 to 14 months: 0.5 ml I.M. A booster dose is required at age 15 months (but no sooner than 2 months after last vaccination).
Previously unvaccinated children age 15 to 60 months: 0.5 ml I.M.
***Haemophilus* b conjugate vaccine, diphtheria toxoid conjugate**
Children age 15 to 60 months: 0.5 ml I.M.
***Haemophilus* b conjugate vaccine, meningococcal protein conjugate**
Previously unvaccinated infants age 2 to 10 months: 0.5 ml I.M. ideally at 2 months. Repeat 2 months later (or as soon as possible thereafter). A booster dose of 0.5 ml I.M. should be administered at 12 to 15 months (but no sooner than 2 months after last vaccination).
Previously unvaccinated children age 11 to 14 months: 0.5 ml I.M.; repeat in 2 months.
Previously unvaccinated children age 15 to 71 months: 0.5 ml I.M.
***Haemophilus* b polysaccharide conjugate vaccine, tetanus toxoid**
Previously unvaccinated children age 2 to 6 months: Three 0.5-ml I.M. doses, at 8-week intervals followed by a booster dose at age 15 to 18 months.
Previously unvaccinated children age 7 to 11 months: Two 0.5-ml I.M. doses at 8-week intervals, followed by a booster dose at age 15 to 18 months.
Previously unvaccinated children age 12 to 14 months: 0.5 ml I.M., followed by a booster dose at age 15 to 18 months. Administer no earlier than 2 months after previous dose.
Previously unvaccinated children age 15 to 60 months: 0.5 ml I.M.

Pharmacodynamics
H. influenzae *type b prophylaxis:* Vaccine promotes active immunity to *H. influenzae* type b.

Pharmacokinetics
• *Absorption:* After I.M. or S.C. administration, increases in *H. influenzae* type b capsular antibody levels in serum are detectable in about 2 weeks and peak within 3 weeks.
• *Distribution:* Limited data indicate that antibodies to *H. influenzae* type b can be detected in fetal blood and in breast milk after administration of the vaccine to pregnant and breast-feeding women.

• *Metabolism:* No information available.
• *Excretion:* The vaccine polysaccharide has been detected in urine for up to 11 days after administration to children.

Contraindications and precautions

Contraindicated in patients with acute illness or hypersensitivity to any component of vaccine, including thimerosal. Do not administer to patients less than 10 days before or during treatment with immunosuppressive drugs or irradiation.

Interactions

Concomitant use of *Haemophilus* b vaccine with *corticosteroids* or *immunosuppressants* may impair the immune response to the vaccine. Avoid vaccination under these circumstances.

Effects on diagnostic tests

None reported.

Adverse reactions

GI: diarrhea, vomiting.
Other: ***anaphylaxis,*** fever, *erythema, pain at injection site,* irritability.

Overdose and treatment

No information available.

☑ Special considerations

• Obtain a thorough history of allergies and reactions to immunizations.
• Epinephrine solution 1:1,000 should be available to treat allergic reactions.
• Do not administer intradermally or I.V.
• Vaccine may be given simultaneously with diphtheria, tetanus, and pertussis (DTP) vaccine; measles, mumps, and rubella (MMR) vaccine; poliovirus vaccine, inactivated (IPV); meningococcal vaccine; or pneumococcal vaccine, but should be administered at different sites. It may also be given concomitantly with oral poliovirus vaccine (OPV). It is generally not recommended in pregnancy.
• Store vaccine in the refrigerator and protect it from light. Do not freeze. Hib conjugate vaccine is produced by covalent bonding of the capsular polysaccharide of *H. influenzae* type b to a protein antigen. This produces an antigen resulting in both an enhanced antibody response and an immunologic memory.
• The ACIP currently recommends that beginning at age 2 months children receive one of the conjugate vaccines licensed for this age-group (*Haemophilus* b conjugate vaccine, diphtheria CRM_{197} protein conjugate [HibTITER] or *Haemophilus* b conjugate vaccine, meningococcal protein conjugate [PedvaxHIB], or *Haemophilus* b conjugate vaccine, tetanus toxoid conjugate). Check the package insert to see if the vaccine is licensed for use in specific age-groups.
• Administer same vaccine throughout the vaccination series; no data are available to support the interchangeability of the vaccines.
• Children under age 24 months who develop invasive *H. influenzae* type b disease should be vaccinated because natural immunity may not develop.
• Vaccination should not be used to prevent invasive disease associated with *H. influenzae* type b disease because of the time required to develop immunity. Instead, chemoprophylaxis (with drugs such as rifampin) should be used in both vaccinated and unvaccinated individuals because children with immunity may carry and transmit the organism. However, if every child in a household or day-care group has been fully vaccinated, chemoprophylaxis is not necessary.
• Note that a conjugate vaccine containing meningococcal proteins will not prevent meningococcal disease; one containing diphtheria proteins will not produce immunity against diphtheria; and one containing the tetanus toxoid conjugate will not produce immunity against tetanus toxoid. DTP vaccine should be administered according to the recommended schedule.

Patient education

• *H. influenzae* type b is a cause of meningitis in infants and preschool children. Explain to parents that this vaccine will protect children only against meningitis caused by this organism.
• Tell parents that child may experience swelling and inflammation at injection site and fever. Recommend acetaminophen liquid for fever.
• Tell parents to report worrisome or persistent adverse reactions promptly.

Pediatric use

• These vaccines are indicated only in children between age 2 months and 5 years.
• Check package insert for age limitations.

halcinonide

Halog, Halog-E

Pharmacologic classification: topical adrenocorticoid
Therapeutic classification: anti-inflammatory
Pregnancy risk category C

How supplied

Available by prescription only
Cream: 0.025%, 0.1%
Ointment: 0.1%
Topical solution: 0.1%

Indications, route, and dosage

Inflammation of acute and chronic corticosteroid-responsive dermatoses
Adults and children: Apply cream, ointment, or solution sparingly b.i.d. or t.i.d.; for Halog-E, apply daily to t.i.d. Occlusive dressing may be used for severe or resistant dermatoses.

Pharmacodynamics

Anti-inflammatory action: Halcinonide stimulates the synthesis of enzymes needed to decrease the inflammatory response. Depending on its strength, halcinonide is a group II (0.1%) or group III (0.025%) fluorinated corticosteroid.

Pharmacokinetics

• *Absorption:* Amount absorbed depends on strength of preparation, amount applied, and nature of skin at application site. It ranges from about 1% in skin with a thick stratum corneum (such as the palms, soles, elbows, and knees) to as high as 36% in areas of the thinnest stratum corneum (face, eyelids, and genitals). Absorption increases in areas of skin damage, inflammation, or occlusion. Some systemic absorption of topical steroids may occur, especially through the oral mucosa.
• *Distribution:* After topical application, halcinonide is distributed throughout the local skin. Any drug absorbed into the circulation is distributed into muscle, liver, skin, intestines, and kidneys.
• *Metabolism:* After topical administration, drug is metabolized primarily in the skin. The small amount absorbed into systemic circulation is metabolized primarily in the liver to inactive compounds.
• *Excretion:* Inactive metabolites are excreted by the kidneys, primarily as glucuronides and sulfates, but also as unconjugated products. Small amounts of the metabolites are also excreted in feces.

Contraindications and precautions

Contraindicated in patients hypersensitive to drug, as monotherapy in primary bacterial infections, or for ophthalmic use.

Interactions

None significant.

Effects on diagnostic tests

None reported.

Adverse reactions

Skin: burning, pruritus, irritation, dryness, erythema, folliculitis, hypertrichosis, hypopigmentation, acneiform eruptions, allergic contact dermatitis; *maceration, secondary infection, atrophy, striae, miliaria* (with occlusive dressings).
Other: ***hypothalamic-pituitary-adrenal axis suppression,*** Cushing's syndrome, hyperglycemia, glucosuria.

Overdose and treatment

No information available.

☑ Special considerations

Recommendations for use of halcinonide, for care and teaching of patient during therapy, and for use in elderly patients, children, and breast-feeding women are the same as those for all *topical adrenocorticoids.*

halobetasol propionate

Ultravate

Pharmacologic classification: corticosteroid
Therapeutic classification: topical anti-inflammatory
Pregnancy risk category C

How supplied

Available by prescription only
Cream: 0.05%
Ointment: 0.05%

Indications, route, and dosage

Relief of inflammation and pruritus of corticosteroid-responsive dermatoses

Adults: Apply sparingly to affected areas daily to b.i.d. and rub in gently and completely. Treatment beyond 2 consecutive weeks is not recommended; total dosage should not exceed 50 g weekly. Do not use an occlusive dressing.

Pharmacodynamics

Anti-inflammatory action: Halobetasol is classified as a "super high potency" (group I) corticosteroid. Its anti-inflammatory response results from stimulation of the synthesis of enzymes needed to decrease inflammation.

Pharmacokinetics

• *Absorption:* Amount absorbed depends on amount applied, application site, vehicle, use of occlusive dressing, and integrity of skin. Some systemic absorption occurs.
• *Distribution:* Throughout the local skin.
• *Metabolism:* Metabolized primarily by the skin.
• *Excretion:* Information not available.

Contraindications and precautions

Contraindicated in patients hypersensitive to drug or its components; not for use as monotherapy in primary bacterial infections or ophthalmic use.

Interactions

None significant.

Effects on diagnostic tests

None reported.

Adverse reactions

Skin: stinging, burning, pruritus, irritation, dryness, erythema, folliculitis, skin atrophy, leukoderma, vesicles, rash, hypertrichosis, acneiform eruptions, hypopigmentation, perioral dermatitis, allergic contact dermatitis, secondary infection, striae, miliaria.
Other: ***hypothalamic-pituitary-adrenal (HPA) axis suppression,*** Cushing's syndrome, hyperglycemia, glucosuria, fluid retention.

Overdose and treatment

Sufficient amounts can be absorbed to produce systemic effects—specifically, suppression of the HPA axis, Cushing's syndrome, hyperglycemia, and glucosuria—which are reversible after discontinuation of therapy.

☑ Special considerations

• The corticotropin-stimulation test, morning plasma cortisol, and urinary cortisol levels are useful in determining the extent of HPA axis suppression.
• Treatment should be limited to 2 weeks in dosage below 50 g weekly.
• Do not use occlusive dressings.

• Do not use to treat rosacea or perioral dermatitis. Discontinue drug if infection occurs.
• If HPA axis suppression occurs, discontinue drug or reduce frequency of application or substitute a less potent corticosteroid.
• Do not use on face, groin, or axilla.

Patient education
• Warn patient to use externally and only as directed and to avoid contact with eyes.
• Tell patient not to cover, bandage, or wrap treated area unless instructed.
• Tell patient to report signs of stinging, burning, or irritation.
• Caution patient to use drug exactly as prescribed.

Pediatric use
• Safety and effectiveness have not been established. Use with caution, because children are more susceptible to systemic absorption and effects because of higher ratio of skin surface area to body mass.

Breast-feeding
• It is unknown if topically applied corticosteroids appear in breast milk; however, caution is advised because systemically administered corticosteroids appear in breast milk and could suppress the infant's growth.

haloperidol
Apo-Haloperidol*, Haldol, Novo-Peridol*, Peridol*

haloperidol decanoate
Haldol Decanoate, Haldol Decanoate 100, Haldol LA*

haloperidol lactate
Haldol, Haldol Concentrate, Haloperidol Intensol

Pharmacologic classification: butyrophenone
Therapeutic classification: antipsychotic
Pregnancy risk category C

How supplied
Available by prescription only
haloperidol
Tablets: 0.5 mg, 1 mg, 2 mg, 5 mg, 10 mg, 20 mg
haloperidol decanoate
Injection: 50 mg/ml, 100 mg/ml
haloperidol lactate
Oral concentrate: 2 mg/ml
Injection: 5 mg/ml

Indications, route, and dosage
Psychotic disorders, ◊ alcohol dependence
Adults: Dosage varies for each patient and symptomatology. Initial dosage range is 0.5 to 5 mg P.O. b.i.d. or t.i.d.; or 2 to 5 mg I.M. q 4 to 8 hours, increased rapidly if necessary for prompt control. Maximum dosage is 100 mg P.O. daily. Doses over 100 mg have been used for patients with severely resistant conditions.
Chronic psychotic patients who require prolonged therapy
Adults: 100 mg I.M. of haloperidol decanoate q 4 weeks. Experience with doses over 450 mg monthly is limited.
Control of tics, vocal utterances in Tourette syndrome
Adults: 0.5 to 5 mg P.O. b.i.d. or t.i.d., increased p.r.n.
Children age 3 to 12: 0.05 to 0.075 mg/kg/day given b.i.d. or t.i.d.

Pharmacodynamics
Antipsychotic action: Haloperidol is thought to exert its antipsychotic effects by strong postsynaptic blockade of CNS dopamine receptors, thereby inhibiting dopamine-mediated effects; its pharmacologic effects are most similar to those of piperazine antipsychotics. Its mechanism of action in Tourette syndrome is unknown.

Haloperidol has many other central and peripheral effects; it has weak peripheral anticholinergic effects and antiemetic effects, produces both alpha and ganglionic blockade, and counteracts histamine- and serotonin-mediated activity. Its most prominent adverse reactions are extrapyramidal.

Pharmacokinetics
• *Absorption:* Rate and extent of absorption vary with route of administration: oral tablet absorption yields 60% to 70% bioavailability. I.M. dose is 70% absorbed within 30 minutes. Peak plasma levels after oral administration occur at 2 to 6 hours; after I.M. administration, 30 to 45 minutes; and after long-acting I.M. (decanoate) administration, 6 to 7 days.
• *Distribution:* Haloperidol is distributed widely into the body, with high concentrations in adipose tissue. Drug is 90% to 92% protein-bound.
• *Metabolism:* Haloperidol is metabolized extensively by the liver; there may be only one active metabolite that is less active than parent drug.
• *Excretion:* About 40% of a given dose is excreted in urine within 5 days; about 15% is excreted in feces via the biliary tract.

Contraindications and precautions
Contraindicated in patients with hypersensitivity or in those experiencing parkinsonism, coma, or CNS depression.

Use cautiously in elderly or debilitated patients; in patients with history of seizures, EEG abnormalities, CV disorders, allergies, narrow angle glaucoma, or urine retention; and in those receiving anticoagulant, anticonvulsant, antiparkinsonian, or lithium medications.

Interactions
Concomitant use of haloperidol with *sympathomimetics*, including *epinephrine, phenylephrine, phenylpropanolamine,* and *ephedrine* (often found in nasal sprays), and appetite suppressants may decrease their stimulatory and pressor effects.

Haloperidol may inhibit blood pressure response to centrally acting antihypertensive drugs, such as *clonidine, guanabenz, guanadrel, guanethidine, methyldopa,* and *reserpine.* Additive effects are likely after concomitant use of haloperidol with CNS depressants, including *alcohol, analgesics, barbiturates, narcotics, tranquilizers,* and *general, spinal, or epidural anesthetics,* or with *parenteral magnesium sulfate* (oversedation, respiratory depression, and hypotension); *antiarrhythmic agents, disopyramide, procainamide,* or *quinidine* (increased incidence of arrhythmias and conduction defects); *atropine* or other *anticholinergic drugs,* including *antidepressants, antihistamines, MAO inhibitors, meperidine, phenothiazines,* and *antiparkinsonian agents* (oversedation, paralytic ileus, visual changes, and severe constipation); *nitrates* (hypotension); and *metrizamide* (increased risk of seizures).

Beta-blocking agents may inhibit haloperidol metabolism, increasing plasma levels and toxicity.

Concomitant use with *propylthiouracil* increases risk of agranulocytosis; concomitant use with *lithium* may result in severe neurologic toxicity with an encephalitis-like syndrome, and a decreased therapeutic response to haloperidol.

Pharmacokinetic alterations and subsequent decreased therapeutic response to haloperidol may follow concomitant use with *phenobarbital* (enhanced renal excretion); *aluminum- and magnesium-containing antacids* and *antidiarrheals* (decreased absorption); and *heavy smoking* (increased metabolism).

Haloperidol may antagonize therapeutic effect of *bromocriptine* on prolactin secretion; it also may decrease the vasoconstricting effects of high-dose *dopamine,* and may decrease effectiveness and increase toxicity of *levodopa* (by dopamine blockade). Haloperidol may inhibit metabolism and increase toxicity of *phenytoin.*

Effects on diagnostic tests

None reported.

Adverse reactions

CNS: *severe extrapyramidal reactions, tardive dyskinesia,* sedation, drowsiness, lethargy, headache, insomnia, confusion, vertigo, ***seizures.***
CV: tachycardia, hypotension, hypertension, ECG changes.
EENT: *blurred vision.*
GI: dry mouth, anorexia, constipation, diarrhea, nausea, vomiting, dyspepsia.
GU: urine retention, menstrual irregularities, gynecomastia, priapism.
Hematologic: ***leukopenia,*** leukocytosis.
Skin: rash, other skin reactions, diaphoresis.
Other: *neuroleptic malignant syndrome* (rare), altered liver function tests, jaundice.

Overdose and treatment

CNS depression is characterized by deep, unarousable sleep and possible coma, hypotension or hypertension, extrapyramidal symptoms, dystonia, abnormal involuntary muscle movements, agitation, seizures, arrhythmias, ECG changes (may show QT prolongation and torsades de pointes), hypothermia or hyperthermia, and autonomic nervous system dysfunction. Overdose with long-acting decanoate requires prolonged recovery time.

Treatment is symptomatic and supportive, including maintaining vital signs, airway, stable body temperature, and fluid and electrolyte balance. Ipecac may be used to induce vomiting, with due regard for haloperidol's antiemetic properties and hazard of aspiration. Gastric lavage also may be used, followed by activated charcoal and saline cathartics; dialysis does not help.

Regulate body temperature as needed. Treat hypotension with I.V. fluids: do not give epinephrine. Treat seizures with parenteral diazepam or barbiturates; arrhythmias, with parenteral phenytoin (1 mg/kg I.V. with rate titrated to blood pressure not to exceed 50 mg/minute with ECG monitoring; may repeat every 5 minutes up to 10 mg/kg); extrapyramical reactions with benztropine at 1 to 2 mg or parenteral diphenhydramine at 10 to 50 mg.

☑ Special considerations

- Drug has few CV adverse effects and may be preferred in patients with cardiac disease.
- Assess patient periodically for abnormal body movement.
- Tardive dyskinesia may occur after prolonged use. It may not appear until months or years later and may disappear spontaneously or persist for life.
- Protect drug from light. Slight yellowing of injection or concentrate is common; does not affect potency. Discard markedly discolored solutions.
- Do not withdraw drug abruptly unless required by severe adverse reactions.
- Dose of 2 mg is therapeutic equivalent of 100 mg chlorpromazine.
- When changing from tablets to decanoate injection, patient should initially receive 10 to 20 times the oral dose once monthly (maximum, 100 mg).
- Administer drug by deep I.M. injection. Do not administer decanoate form I.V.

Patient education

- Warn patient against activities that require alertness and good psychomotor coordination until CNS response to drug is determined. Drowsiness and dizziness usually subside after a few weeks.
- Tell patient to report adverse effects, such as extrapyramidal reactions.
- Instruct patient to avoid combining with alcohol or other depressants.

Geriatric use

- Especially useful for agitation associated with senile dementia.
- Elderly patients usually require lower initial doses and a more gradual dosage titration.

Pediatric use

- Drug is not recommended for children under age 3. Children are especially prone to extrapyramidal adverse reactions.

heparin sodium

Heparin Lock Flush, Hep-Lock, Hep-Lock U/P, Liquaemin

Pharmacologic classification: anticoagulant
Therapeutic classification: anticoagulant
Pregnancy risk category C

How supplied

Available products are derived from bovine lung or porcine intestinal mucosa. All are injectable and available by prescription only.

heparin sodium
Vials: 1,000 units/ml, 5,000 units/ml, 10,000 units/ml, 20,000 units/ml, 40,000 units/ml
Unit-dose ampules: 1,000 units/ml, 5,000 units/ml, 10,000 units/ml
Disposable syringes: 1,000 units/ml, 2,500 units/ml, 5,000 units/ml, 7,500 units/ml, 10,000 units/ml, 20,000 units/ml
Carpuject: 5,000 units/ml
Premixed I.V. solutions: 1,000 units in 500 ml 0.9% NaCl solution; 2,000 units in 1,000 ml 0.9% NaCl solution; 12,500 units in 250 ml 0.45% NaCl solution; 25,000 units in 250 ml 0.45% NaCl solution; 25,000 units in 500 ml 0.45% NaCl solution; 10,000 units in 100 ml D_5W; 12,500 units in 250 ml D_5W; 25,000 units in 250 ml D_5W; 25,000 units in 500 ml D_5W

heparin sodium flush
Vials: 10 units/ml, 100 units/ml
Disposable syringes: 10 units/ml, 25 units/2.5 ml, 2,500 units/2.5 ml

Indications, route, and dosage

Deep vein thrombosis, pulmonary embolism
Adults: Initially, 5,000 to 10,000 units I.V. push, then adjust dose according to partial thromboplastin time (PTT) results and give dose I.V. q 4 hours (usually 4,000 to 5,000 units); or 5,000 units I.V. bolus, then 20,000 to 40,000 units in 24 hours by I.V. infusion pump. Wait 4 to 6 hours after bolus dose, and adjust hourly rate based on PTT.
Children: Initially, 50 units/kg I.V. bolus. Maintenance dose is 50 to 100 units/kg I.V. drip q 4 hours. Constant infusion: 20,000 units/m^2 daily. Adjust dosage based on PTT.

Embolism prophylaxis, ◊ post MI, ◊ cerebral thrombosis in evolving stroke, ◊ left ventricular thrombi
Adults: 5,000 units S.C. q 8 to 12 hours.

Open-heart surgery
Adults: (total body perfusion) 150 to 400 units/kg continuous I.V infusion.

DIC
Adults: 50 to 100 units/kg I.V. q 4 hours as a single injection or constant infusion. Discontinue if no improvement in 4 to 8 hours.
Children: 25 to 50 units/kg I.V. q 4 hours, as a single injection or constant infusion. Discontinue if no improvement in 4 to 8 hours.

To maintain patency of I.V. indwelling catheters
Adults and children: 10 to 100 units as an I.V. flush (not intended for therapeutic use).

◊ Unstable angina
Adults: Keep PTT 1.5 to 2 times control during first week of anginal pain.

◊ Anticoagulation in blood transfusion and samples
Transfusions and samples: Mix 7,500 units and 100 ml of 0.9% NaCl and add 6 to 8 ml of mixture to each 100 ml of whole blood or 70 to 150 units to each 10 to 20 ml of blood sample.

Note: Heparin dosing is highly individualized, depending on disease state, age, and renal and hepatic status.

Pharmacodynamics

Anticoagulant action: Heparin accelerates formation of antithrombin III-thrombin complex; it inactivates thrombin and prevents conversion of fibrinogen to fibrin.

Pharmacokinetics

- *Absorption:* Drug is not absorbed from the GI tract and must be given parenterally. After I.V. use, onset of action is almost immediate; after S.C. injection, onset of action occurs in 20 to 60 minutes.
- *Distribution:* Drug is extensively bound to lipoprotein, globulins, and fibrinogen; it does not cross the placenta.
- *Metabolism:* Although metabolism is not completely described, drug is thought to be removed by the reticuloendothelial system, with some metabolism occurring in the liver.
- *Excretion:* Little known; a small fraction is excreted in urine as unchanged drug. Drug is not excreted into breast milk. Plasma half-life is 1 to 2 hours.

Contraindications and precautions

Contraindicated in patients with hypersensitivity to drug. Conditionally contraindicated in patients with active bleeding; blood dyscrasia; or bleeding tendencies, such as hemophilia, thrombocytopenia, or hepatic disease with hypoprothrombinemia; suspected intracranial hemorrhage; suppurative thrombophlebitis; inaccessible ulcerative lesions (especially of GI tract) and open ulcerative wounds; extensive denudation of skin; ascorbic acid deficiency and other conditions that cause increased capillary permeability; during or after brain, eye, or spinal cord surgery; during spinal tap or spinal anesthesia; during continuous tube drainage of stomach or small intestine; in subacute bacterial endocarditis; shock; advanced renal disease; threatened abortion; or severe hypertension. Although heparin use is clearly hazardous in these conditions, its risks and its benefits must be evaluated.

Use cautiously in postpartum patients or women during menses; in patients with mild hepatic or renal disease, alcoholism, or history of asthma, allergies, or GI ulcer; or in those with occupations that have a high incidence of accidents.

Interactions

Concomitant use with *oral anticoagulants* and *platelet inhibitors* increases anticoagulant effect; if it is not possible to avoid using these together, monitor INR, PT, and PTT.

Antihistamines, cardiac glycosides, nicotine, or *tetracyclines* may partially counteract the anticoagulant action of heparin.

Effects on diagnostic tests
Heparin therapy prolongs PT, may falsely elevate AST and ALT levels, and may cause false elevations in some tests for serum thyroxine levels.

Adverse reactions
Hematologic: ***hemorrhage*** (with excessive dosage), *overly prolonged clotting time,* thrombocytopenia.
Other: irritation; mild pain; hematoma; ulceration; cutaneous or subcutaneous necrosis; "white clot" syndrome; hypersensitivity reactions (including chills, fever, pruritus, rhinitis, urticaria, anaphylactoid reactions).

Overdose and treatment
The major sign of overdose is hemorrhage. Immediate withdrawal of drug usually allows the hemorrhage to resolve; however, severe hemorrhage may require treatment with protamine sulfate. Usually, 1 mg protamine sulfate will neutralize 90 units of bovine heparin or 115 units of porcine heparin.

Heparin administered by I.V. route disappears rapidly from the blood, so the protamine dose depends on when heparin was administered. Protamine should be given slowly by I.V. injection (over 3 minutes), and not more than 50 mg should be given in any 10-minute period.

Heparin administered by S.C. route is slowly absorbed. Protamine should be given as a 25- to 50-mg loading dose, followed by constant infusion of the remainder of the calculated dose over 8 to 16 hours.

For severe bleeding, transfusions may be required.

☑ Special considerations
- Obtain pretherapy baseline INR, PT, and PTT; measure PTT regularly. Anticoagulation is present when PTT values are 1.5 to 2 times control values; draw blood for PTT 4 to 6 hours after an I.V. bolus dose and 12 to 24 hours after an S.C. dose. Blood may be drawn at any time after 4 to 6 hours of constant I.V. infusion; if I.V. therapy is intermittent, draw blood 30 minutes before next scheduled dose to avoid falsely prolonged PTT. Never draw blood for PTT from the I.V. tubing of the heparin infusion, or from vein of infusion; falsely prolonged PTT will result. Always draw blood from opposite arm.
- I.V. administration is preferred because S.C. and I.M. injections are irregularly absorbed. When possible, administer I.V. heparin by infusion pump for maximum safety.
- When using heparin flush solution, keep intermittent I.V. line patent by flushing it with NaCl solution before and after heparin; many medications are incompatible with heparin, and may form precipitates if they come in contact with heparin.
- For S.C. injection, use one needle to withdraw solution from vial and another to inject drug. Give low-dose S.C. injections sequentially between iliac crests in lower abdomen; give slowly and deep into subcutaneous fat. After inserting needle into skin, do not withdraw plunger to check for blood, to reduce risk of tissue injury and hematoma; leave needle in place for 10 seconds after S.C. injection. Alternate site every 12 hours: right for morning, left for evening. Do not massage after S.C. injection; watch for local bleeding, hematoma, or inflammation. Rotate site
- Check patient regularly for bleeding gums, bruises on arms or legs, petechiae, nosebleeds, melena, tarry stools, hematuria, or hematemesis. Monitor platelet counts regularly.
- Check I.V. infusions regularly, even when pumps are in good working order, to prevent overdose or underdose; do not piggyback other drugs into line while heparin infusion is running, because many antibiotics and other drugs inactivate heparin. Never mix any drug with heparin in syringe when bolus therapy is used.
- Avoid excessive I.M. injection of other drugs to prevent or minimize hematomas. If possible, do not give any I.M. injections.
- Abrupt withdrawal may increase coagulability; heparin is usually followed by prophylactic oral anticoagulant therapy.

Patient education
- Teach injection technique and methods of record-keeping if patient or family will be administering drug.
- Encourage compliance with medication schedule, follow-up appointments, and need for routine monitoring of blood studies; teach patient and family signs of bleeding, and stress importance of calling immediately at first sign of excess bleeding.
- Caution patient not to take double dose if he misses one; tell him to call for further instructions instead.
- Warn patient against use of aspirin and other OTC medications; stress need to seek medical approval before taking new medication, and to inform primary health care provider and dentist about heparin use

Geriatric use
- At least one manufacturer indicates that women over age 60 are at greatest risk of hemorrhage.

hepatitis A vaccine, inactivated
Havrix

Pharmacologic classification: vaccine
Therapeutic classification: viral vaccine
Pregnancy risk category C

How supplied
Available by prescription only
Injection: 360 Elisa units (EL.U.)/0.5 ml, 1,440 EL.U./1 ml

Indications, route, and dosage
Immunization against disease caused by hepatitis A virus
Adults: 1,440 EL.U./1 ml I.M. as a single dose. Give booster dose of 1,440 EL.U./1 ml I.M. anytime be-

tween 6 and 12 months after initial dosage to ensure highest antibody titers.
Children age 2 to 18: Give two doses of 360 EL.U./0.5 ml I.M. 1 month apart and booster dose of 360 EL.U./0.5 ml I.M. anytime between 6 and 12 months after initial dosage to ensure highest antibody titers.

Pharmacodynamics
Immunostimulant action: Hepatitis A vaccine, inactivated, promotes active immunity to hepatitis A virus. Immunity is not permanent or completely predictable.

Pharmacokinetics
- *Absorption:* No information available.
- *Distribution:* No information available.
- *Metabolism:* No information available.
- *Excretion:* No information available.

Contraindications and precautions
Contraindicated in patients with hypersensitivity to any component of vaccine. Use cautiously in patients with thrombocytopenia or bleeding disorders or in those taking anticoagulants because bleeding may occur following I.M. injection in these individuals.

Interactions
None significant.

Effects on diagnostic tests
None reported.

Adverse reactions
CNS: headache, hypertonic episode, insomnia, photophobia, vertigo.
GI: *anorexia, nausea,* abdominal pain, diarrhea, dysgeusia, vomiting.
Hepatic: jaundice, hepatitis.
Musculoskeletal: arthralgia, elevation of CK, myalgia.
Respiratory: pharyngitis, other upper respiratory tract infections.
Skin: pruritus, *rash,* urticara, *induration, redness, swelling,* hematoma.
Other: *fatigue, fever, malaise,* lymphadenopathy.

Overdose and treatment
No information available.

☑ Special considerations
- As with any vaccine, administration of hepatitis A vaccine should be delayed, if possible, in patients with febrile illness.
- Although anaphylaxis is rare, keep epinephrine readily available to treat an anaphylactoid reaction.
- If vaccine is administered to immunosuppressed persons or those receiving immunosuppressive therapy, the expected immune response may not be obtained.
- Persons who should receive the vaccine include people traveling to or living in areas of higher endemicity for hepatitis A (Africa, Asia [except Japan], the Mediterranean basin, Eastern Europe, the Middle East, Central and South America, Mexico, and parts of the Caribbean), military personnel, native people of Alaska and the Americas, persons engaging in high-risk sexual activity, and users of illicit injectable drugs. Also, certain institutional workers, employees of child day-care centers, laboratory workers who handle live hepatitis A virus, and handlers of primate animals may benefit from immunization.
- Shake vial or syringe well before withdrawal and use. With thorough agitation, the vaccine is an opaque white suspension. Discard if it appears otherwise. No dilution or reconstitution is necessary.
- Administer as I.M. injection into the deltoid region in adults. Do not administer in the gluteal region; such injections may result in suboptimal response. Never inject I.V., S.C., or intradermally.
- Hepatitis A vaccine will not prevent infection in persons with unrecognized hepatitis A infection at the time of vaccination.

Patient education
- Inform patient that vaccine will not prevent hepatitis caused by other agents such as hepatitis B virus, hepatitis C virus, hepatitis E virus, or other pathogens known to infect the liver.

Pediatric use
- Vaccine is well tolerated, highly immunogenic, and effective in children age 2 and older.

Breast-feeding
- It is not known if vaccine occurs in breast milk. Because many drugs are excreted in breast milk, administer cautiously in breast-feeding women.

hepatitis B immune globulin, human (HBIG)
H-BIG, Hep-B-Gammagee, HyperHep

Pharmacologic classification: immune serum
Therapeutic classification: hepatitis B prophylaxis
Pregnancy risk category C

How supplied
Available by prescription only
Injection: 1-ml, 4-ml, and 5-ml vials
Prefilled syringe: 0.5 ml

Indications, route, and dosage
Hepatitis B exposure
Adults and children: 0.06 ml/kg I.M. within 7 days after exposure. Repeat 28 days after exposure.
Neonates born to HBsAg-positive women: 0.5 ml I.M. within 12 hours of birth. Initiation of HB vaccination is also indicated.

The American College of Obstetricians and Gynecologists recommends use of HBIG in pregnancy for postexposure prophylaxis. Hepatitis B immune globulin should only be given if clearly needed.

Pharmacodynamics
Postexposure prophylaxis of hepatitis B: HBIG provides passive immunity to hepatitis B.

Pharmacokinetics

• *Absorption:* HBIG is absorbed slowly after I.M. injection. Antibodies to hepatitis B surface antigen (HBsAg) appear in serum within 1 to 6 days, peak within 3 to 11 days, and persist for about 2 to 6 months.
• *Distribution:* Although specific information is not available, HBIG probably crosses the placenta, as do other immunoglobulins. Data on the distribution of HBIG into breast milk are not available.
• *Metabolism:* No information available.
• *Excretion:* Serum half-life for antibodies to HBsAg is reportedly 21 days.

Contraindications and precautions

Contraindicated in patients with history of anaphylactic reactions to immune serum or thimerosal allergy.

Interactions

Concomitant use of HBIG may interfere with immune response to vaccination with *live virus vaccines*, such as *measles, mumps*, and *rubella. Live virus vaccines* should be administered 2 weeks before or 3 months after HBIG whenever possible.

Effects on diagnostic tests

None reported.

Adverse reactions

Other: ***anaphylaxis***, urticaria, angioedema; pain, tenderness (at injection site).

Overdose and treatment

No information available.

☑ Special considerations

• Obtain a thorough history of allergies and reactions to immunizations.
• Epinephrine solution 1:1,000 should be available to treat allergic reactions.
• Administer drug I.M. only. Severe, even fatal, reactions may occur if it is administered I.V.
• Gluteal or deltoid areas are the preferred injection sites.
• HBIG may be given simultaneously, but at different sites, with hepatitis B vaccine.
• Store between 36° and 46° F (2° and 8° C). Do not freeze.
• Hospital staff should receive immunization if exposed to hepatitis B (for example, from a needlestick or direct contact).
• HBIG has not been associated with a higher incidence of AIDS. The immune globulin is devoid of HIV. Immune globulin recipients do not develop antibodies to HIV.

Patient education

• Explain that patient's chances of getting AIDS after receiving HBIG are very small.
• Inform patient that HBIG provides temporary protection against hepatitis B only.
• Tell patient what to expect after vaccination: local pain, swelling, and tenderness at the injection site. Recommend acetaminophen to relieve minor discomfort.
• Encourage patient to promptly report headache, skin changes, or difficulty breathing.

Breast-feeding

• It is not known if HBIG occurs in breast milk.

hepatitis B vaccine, recombinant

Engerix-B, Recombivax HB, Recombivax HB Dialysis Formulation

Pharmacologic classification: vaccine
Therapeutic classification: viral vaccine
Pregnancy risk category C

How supplied

Available by prescription only
Injection: 2.5 mcg hepatitis B surface antigen (HBsAg)/0.5 ml (Recombivax HB pediatric formulation); 5 mcg HBsAg/0.5 ml (Recombivax HB adolescent/high-risk infant formulation); 10 mcg HBsAg/0.5 ml (Engerix-B, pediatric injection); 10 mcg HBsAg/ml (Recombivax HB); 20 mcg HBsAg/ml (Engerix-B); 40 mcg HBsAg/ml (Recombivax HB Dialysis Formulation)

Indications, route, and dosage

Immunization against infection from all known subtypes of hepatitis B; primary preexposure prophylaxis against hepatitis B; postexposure prophylaxis (when given with hepatitis B immune globulin)

Engerix-B

Adults age 20 and older: Initially, give 20 mcg (1-ml adult formulation) I.M., followed by a second dose of 20 mcg I.M. 30 days later. Give a third dose of 20 mcg I.M. 6 months after the initial dose.
Neonates and children up to age 19: Initially, give 10 mcg (0.5-ml pediatric formulation) I.M., followed by a second dose of 10 mcg I.M. 30 days later. Give a third dose of 10 mcg I.M. 6 months after the initial dose.
Adults undergoing dialysis or receiving immunosuppressant therapy: Initially, give 40 mcg I.M. (divided into two 20-mcg doses and administered at different sites). Follow with a second dose of 40 mcg I.M. in 30 days, a third dose after 2 months, and a final dose of 40 mcg I.M. 6 months after the initial dose.

Note: Alternative dosing schedule in certain populations (neonates born to infected mothers, persons recently exposed to the virus, and travelers to high-risk areas) who may receive the initial vaccine dose (20 mcg for adults and children over age 10, and 10 mcg for neonates and children up to age 10 for this dosing schedule) followed by a second dose in 1 month and the third dose after 2 months. For prolonged maintenance of protective antibody titers, a booster dose is recommended 12 months after the initial dose.

Recombivax HB

Adults age 20 and older: Initially, give 10 mcg (1-ml adult formulation) I.M., followed by a second dose of 10 mcg I.M. 30 days later. Give a third dose of 10 mcg I.M. 6 months after the initial dose.

Children age 11 to 19: Initially, give 5 mcg (0.5-ml adolescent/high risk infant formulation) I.M., followed by a second dose of 5 mcg I.M. 30 days later. Give a third dose of 5 mcg I.M. 6 months after the initial dose.
Neonates (born to HBsAg-negative mothers) and children up to age 10: Initially, give 2.5 mcg (0.5-ml pediatric formulation) I.M., followed by a second dose of 2.5 mcg I.M. 30 days later. Give a third dose of 2.5 mcg I.M. 6 months after the initial dose.
Neonates born to HBsAg-positive mothers: Initially, give 5 mcg (0.5-ml adolescent/high-risk infant formulation) I.M. with 0.5 ml hepatitis B immune globulin. Follow with a second dose of 5 mcg I.M. 30 days later. Give a third dose of 5 mcg I.M. 6 months after the initial dose.
Adults undergoing dialysis or receiving immunosuppressant therapy: Initially, give 40 mcg I.M. (1-ml dialysis formulation). Follow with a second dose of 40 mcg I.M. in 30 days, and give a final dose of 40 mcg I.M. 6 months after the initial dose.

Pharmacodynamics
Hepatitis B prophylaxis: Hepatitis B vaccine promotes active immunity to hepatitis B.

Pharmacokinetics
- *Absorption:* After I.M. administration, antibody to HBsAg appears in serum within about 2 weeks, peaks after 6 months, and persists for at least 3 years.
- *Distribution:* No information available.
- *Metabolism:* No information available.
- *Excretion:* No information available.

Contraindications and precautions
Contraindicated in patients hypersensitive to yeast; recombinant vaccines are derived from yeast cultures. Use cautiously in patients with active infections or compromised cardiac and pulmonary status or in those whom a febrile or systemic reaction could pose a risk.

Interactions
When used concomitantly, *corticosteroids* or *immunosuppressants* may impair the immune response to hepatitis B vaccine. Larger-than-usual doses of vaccine may be necessary to develop adequate circulating antibody levels.

Effects on diagnostic tests
None reported.

Adverse reactions
CNS: headache, dizziness, insomnia.
GI: nausea, pharyngitis, anorexia, diarrhea, vomiting.
Other: paresthesia, neuropathy, arthralgia, slight fever, transient malaise, flulike symptoms, myalgia; local inflammation, *soreness* (at injection site).

Overdose and treatment
No information available.

☑ Special considerations
- Obtain a thorough history of allergies and reactions to immunizations.
- Epinephrine solution 1:1,000 should be available to treat allergic reactions.
- The Centers for Disease Control and Prevention reports that response to hepatitis B vaccine is significantly better after injection into the deltoid rather than the gluteal muscle.
- Hepatitis B vaccine may be administered S.C., but only to persons, such as hemophiliacs and patients with thrombocytopenia, who are at risk of hemorrhage from I.M. injection. Do not administer I.V.
- Hepatitis B vaccine may be given simultaneously, but at different sites, with hepatitis B immune globulin, influenza virus vaccine, Haemophilus influenzae type B conjugate vaccine, polyvalent pneumococcal vaccine, or DTP.
- Although not necessary for most patients, serologic testing (to confirm immunity to hepatitis B after the three-dose regimen) is recommended for persons over age 50, those at high risk of needle-stick injury (who might require postexposure prophylaxis), hemodialysis patients, immunocompromised patients, and those who inadvertently received one or more injections into the gluteal muscle.
- Thoroughly agitate vial just before administration to restore a uniform suspension (slightly opaque and white in color).
- Store opened and unopened vial in the refrigerator. Do not freeze.

Patient education
- Tell patient that there is no risk of contracting HIV infection or AIDS from hepatitis B vaccine because it is synthetically derived.
- Explain that hepatitis B vaccine provides protection against hepatitis B only, not against hepatitis A or hepatitis C.
- Tell patient to expect some discomfort at injection site and possible fever, headache, or upset stomach. Recommend acetaminophen to relieve such effects. Encourage patient to report distressing adverse reactions.

Pediatric use
- Routine immunization is now recommended for all neonates, regardless of whether the mother tests positive or negative for HBsAg. It is usually well tolerated and highly immunogenic in children and infants of all ages.

hetastarch (HES, hydroxyethyl starch)
Hespan

Pharmacologic classification: amylopectin derivative
Therapeutic classification: plasma volume expander
Pregnancy risk category C

How supplied

Available by prescription only

Injection: 500 ml (6 g/100 ml in 0.9% NaCl solution)

Indications, route, and dosage

Plasma expander in shock and cardiopulmonary bypass surgery

Adults: 500 to 1,000 ml I.V. dependent on amount of blood lost and resultant hemoconcentration. Total dosage usually should not exceed 20 ml/kg, up to 1,500 ml/day. Up to 20 ml/kg (1.2 g/kg)/hour may be used in hemorrhagic shock; in burns or septic shock, rate should be reduced.

Leukapheresis adjunct

Hetastarch is an adjunct in leukapheresis to improve harvesting and increase the yield of granulocytes.

Adults: Hetastarch 250 to 700 ml is infused at a constant fixed ratio, usually 1:8 to venous whole blood during continous flow centrifugation (CFC) procedures. Up to 2 CFC procedures weekly, with total number of 7 to 10 procedures using hetastarch, have been found safe and effective. Safety of larger numbers of procedures is unknown.

◇Note: Hetastarch can be used as a priming fluid in pump oxygenators for perfusion during extracorporeal circulation or as a cryoprotective agent for long-term storage of whole blood.

Pharmacodynamics

Plasma volume expander: Hetastarch has an average molecular weight of 450,000 and exhibits colloidal properties similar to human albumin. After an I.V. infusion of hetastarch 6%, the plasma volume expands slightly in excess of the volume infused because of the colloidal osmotic effect. Maximum plasma volume expansion occurs in a few minutes and decreases over 24 to 36 hours. Hemodynamic status may improve for 24 hours or longer.

Leukapheresis adjunct: Hetastarch enhances yield of granulocytes by centrifugal means.

Pharmacokinetics

- *Absorption:* After I.V. administration, plasma volume expands within a few minutes.
- *Distribution:* Drug is distributed in the blood plasma.
- *Metabolism:* Hetastarch molecules larger than 50,000 molecular weight are slowly enzymatically degraded to molecules that can be excreted.
- *Excretion:* 40% of hetastarch molecules smaller than 50,000 molecular weight are excreted in urine within 24 hours. Hetastarch molecules that are not hydroxyethylated are slowly degraded to glucose. Approximately 90% of dose is eliminated from the body with an average half-life of 17 days; remainder has a half-life of 48 days.

Contraindications and precautions

Contraindicated in patients with severe bleeding disorders, severe heart failure, or renal failure with oliguria and anuria.

Interactions

None reported.

Effects on diagnostic tests

When added to whole blood, hetastarch increases the erythrocyte sedimentation rate.

Adverse reactions

CNS: headache.
CV: peripheral edema of lower extremities.
EENT: periorbital edema.
GI: nausea, vomiting.
Respiratory: wheezing.
Skin: urticaria.
Other: mild fever, chills, muscle pain.

Overdose and treatment

Clinical manifestations of overdose include the adverse reactions. Stop infusion if an overdose occurs and treat supportively.

☑ Special considerations

- To avoid circulatory overload, carefully monitor patients with impaired renal function and those at high risk of pulmonary edema or heart failure. Hetastarch 6% in 0.9% NaCl contains 77 mEq sodium and chloride per 500 ml.
- Do not administer as a substitute for blood or plasma.
- Discard partially used bottle because it does not contain a preservative.
- Monitor CBC, total leukocyte and platelet counts, leukocyte differential count, hemoglobin, hematocrit, PT, PTT, electrolyte, BUN, and creatinine levels.
- Assess vital signs and cardiopulmonary status to obtain baseline at start of infusion to prevent fluid overload.
- Monitor I.V. site for signs of infiltration and phlebitis.
- Observe patient for edema.

Patient education

- Explain use and administration of drug to patient and family.
- Instruct patient to report adverse reactions promptly.

Geriatric use

- Use hetastarch with caution in elderly patients, who are more prone to fluid overload; a lower dosage may be sufficient to produce desired plasma volume expansion.

Pediatric use

- Safety and efficacy in children have not been established.

Breast-feeding

- Breast-feeding should be temporarily discontinued in women receiving hetastarch.

histrelin acetate

Supprelin

Pharmacologic classification: gonadotropin-releasing hormone
Therapeutic classification: posterior pituitary hormone
Pregnancy risk category X

How supplied

Available by prescription only
Injection: 120 mcg/0.6 ml, 300 mcg/0.6 ml, 600 mcg/0.6 ml

Indications, route, and dosage

Centrally mediated (idiopathic or neurogenic) precocious puberty
Children (girls age 2 to 8; boys age 2 to 9½): 10 mcg/kg S.C. daily as a single injection.

Pharmacodynamics

Hormonal action: Histrelin mimics the effects of gonadotropin-releasing hormone (GnRH; also called luteinizing hormone-releasing hormone, LHRH); however, it is more potent than the naturally occurring hormone. Chronic administration desensitizes the responsiveness of the pituitary gonadotropin, resulting in decreased sex hormone production by the testes or ovaries.

Pharmacokinetics

- *Absorption:* Because histrelin is a peptide, it is broken down in the GI tract when administered orally. Drug is usually administered S.C.
- *Distribution:* No information available. Drug acts within the CNS.
- *Metabolism:* No information available.
- *Excretion:* No information available. Decreases in follicle-stimulating hormone, LH, and sex steroid levels occur within 3 months.

Contraindications and precautions

Contraindicated in patients hypersensitive to any component of drug and in pregnant or breast-feeding patients.

Interactions

None reported.

Effects on diagnostic tests

None reported.

Adverse reactions

CNS: *mood changes, nervousness, dizziness, depression, headache, libido changes, insomnia, anxiety,* paresthesia, cognitive changes, syncope, somnolence, lethargy, impaired consciousness, tremor, hyperkinesia, ***seizures,*** conduct disorder, fatigue.
CV: *vasodilation,* edema, palpitations, pallor, tachycardia, hypertension.
EENT: epistaxis, ear congestion, abnormal pupillary function, otalgia, visual disturbances, hearing loss, polyopia, photophobia, rhinorrhea, sinusitis, nasal infections.
GI: *abdominal pain, nausea, vomiting, diarrhea, flatulence, decreased appetite, dyspepsia,* cramps, constipation, thirst, gastritis, GI distress.
GU: *menstrual changes, vaginal dryness, leukorrhea, hypermenorrhea, vaginal bleeding, vaginitis, dysmenorrhea,* polyuria, incontinence, dysuria, hematuria, hot flashes, nocturia, tenderness of female genitalia, glycosuria.
Hematologic: hyperlipidemia, anemia.
Respiratory: *upper respiratory infection, respiratory congestion, cough,* asthma, breathing disorder, bronchitis, hyperventilation.
Skin: *redness, swelling, acne, rash, diaphoresis,* urticaria, pruritus, alopecia.
Other: *fever, arthralgia, muscle stiffness, muscle cramps, breast pain or edema,* breast discharge, decreased breast size, *weight gain, body pains,* chills, malaise, purpura, acute hypersensitivity reactions ***(anaphylaxis, angioedema).***

Overdose and treatment

There is no experience with human overdosage. Doses up to 200 times the recommended daily dose in humans have been administered to mice with no adverse effects.

☑ Special considerations

- Reevaluate patient if prepubertal levels of sex steroids or GnRH test response are not achieved within 3 months of therapy.
- A complete physical and endocrinologic evaluation is necessary before drug therapy is initiated; several indices should be reexamined at 3 months, then every 6 to 12 months thereafter. Such evaluations should include determinations of height and weight, hand and wrist X-ray for bone age determination, sex steroid (estradiol or testosterone) levels, and GnRH stimulation test. Repeat these tests periodically to determine effectiveness of therapy.
- Additional tests should be performed to rule out other causes of precocious puberty, including beta human chorionic gonadotropin levels (to rule out a chorionic gonadotropin-secreting tumor); pelvic, adrenal, or testicular ultrasound (to rule out steroid-secreting tumor); and computed tomography of the head (to rule out intracranial tumor). Baseline evaluation should document the size of gonads for serial monitoring.

Patient education

- Explain that drug is dispensed as a 7-day kit, which contains a patient information leaflet. Caregivers should read and understand the leaflet.
- Before initiating therapy, both patient and parents should understand importance of strictly adhering to daily administration schedules. To facilitate compliance and ensure adequate dosing, drug should be taken at same time each day.
- Explain importance of rotating injection sites daily. Sites should include upper arms, thighs, and abdomen.
- Tell patient to store drug in its original container, in the refrigerator at 36° to 46° F (2° to 8° C) and protect it from light. Also tell him that each vial should be used only once because drug contains no preser-

vatives and that drug should be allowed to reach room temperature before use.

- Be sure patient and parents understand that they should seek prompt medical attention for signs of immediate hypersensitivity reactions, such as sudden development of rash, difficulty in breathing or swallowing, or rapid heartbeat. They should also report severe or persistent swelling, redness, or irritation at the injection site.
- Be sure patient and parents know the potential risks of therapy and adverse effects. During the first month of treatment, girls commonly experience a slight menstrual flow, which is probably related to decreasing estrogen levels caused by treatment. As estrogen levels drop, menses begins because estrogens support the endometrium.

Pediatric use

- Safety and efficacy in children under age 2 have not been established.

Breast-feeding

- It is unknown if drug is excreted in breast milk. Do not use in breast-feeding women because of risk to the infant.

homatropine hydrobromide

AK-Homatropine, I-Homatrine, Isopto Homatropine, Minims Homatropine*

Pharmacologic classification: anticholinergic

Therapeutic classification: cycloplegic, mydriatic

Pregnancy risk category C

How supplied

Available by prescription only

Ophthalmic solution: 2%, 5%

Indications, route, and dosage

Cycloplegic refraction

Adults: Instill 1 to 2 drops of 2% or 1 drop of 5% solution in eye; repeat in 5 to 10 minutes p.r.n.

Children: Instill 1 drop of 2% solution in the eye; repeat at 10-minute intervals p.r.n.

Uveitis

Adults: Instill 1 to 2 drops of 2% or 5% solution in eye up to q 3 or 4 hours.

Children: Instill 1 drop of 2% solution b.i.d. or t.i.d.

Pharmacodynamics

Cycloplegic and mydriatic action: Anticholinergic action prevents the sphincter muscle of the iris and the muscle of the ciliary body from responding to cholinergic stimulation, resulting in unopposed adrenergic influence and producing pupillary dilation (mydriasis) and paralysis of accommodation (cycloplegia).

Pharmacokinetics

- *Absorption:* Peak effect is reached in 40 to 60 minutes.
- *Distribution:* Unknown.
- *Metabolism:* Unknown.
- *Excretion:* Recovery from cycloplegic and mydriatic effects usually occurs within 1 to 3 days.

Contraindications and precautions

Contraindicated in patients with hypersensitivity to drug or other belladonna alkaloids, such as atropine, and in those with glaucoma or those who have adhesions between the iris and lens. Use cautiously in the elderly and in those with increased ocular pressure.

Interactions

Homatropine may interfere with the antiglaucoma effects of, *carbachol, cholinesterase inhibitors,* or *pilocarpine.*

Effects on diagnostic tests

None reported.

Adverse reactions

CNS: confusion, somnolence, headache.
CV: tachycardia.
EENT: eye irritation, *blurred vision, photophobia,* increased intraocular pressure, transient stinging and burning, conjunctivitis, vascular congestion, edema.
GI: dry mouth.
Skin: dryness, rash.

Overdose and treatment

Clinical manifestations of overdose include flushed dry skin, dry mouth, blurred vision, ataxia, dysarthria, hallucinations, tachycardia, and decreased bowel sounds.

Treat accidental ingestion by emesis or activated charcoal. Use physostigmine to antagonize homatropine's anticholinergic activity in severe toxicity; propranolol may be used to treat symptomatic tachyarrhythmias unresponsive to physostigmine.

☑ Special considerations

- Drug may produce symptoms of atropine sulfate poisoning, such as severe mouth dryness and tachycardia.
- Drug should not be used internally.
- Patient may be photophobic and may benefit from wearing dark glasses to minimize discomfort.

Patient education

- Teach patient how to instill drops and warn him not to touch the eye or surrounding area with dropper.
- Tell patient that vision will be temporarily blurred after instillation, and advise him to use caution when driving or operating machinery.
- Inform patient that drug may produce drowsiness.

Geriatric use

- Use drug cautiously because of risk of undiagnosed glaucoma and increased sensitivity to drug's effects.

Pediatric use

- Use drug cautiously in small children and infants. There is an increased chance of sensitivity in children with Down syndrome, spastic paralysis, or brain damage. Feeding intolerance may result.

hyaluronidase
Wydase

Pharmacologic classification: protein enzyme
Therapeutic classification: adjunctive agent
Pregnancy risk category C

How supplied
Available by prescription only
Injection (lyophilized powder): 150 USP units/vial, 1,500 USP units/vial
Injection (solution): 150 USP units/ml in 1-ml and 10-ml vials

Indications, route, and dosage
Adjunct to increase absorption and dispersion of other injected drugs
Adults and children: Add 150 USP units to solution containing other medication.
Adjunct to increase absorption rate of fluids given by hypodermoclysis
Adults and children: Inject 150 USP units into the rubber tubing close to the needle of the running clysis solution. Generally, 150 USP units will facilitate absorption of 1 L or more of solution, but dosage administration and type of solution should be individualized.
Adjunct in excretory urography
Adults and children: Administer 75 USP units S.C. over each scapula, before administration of the contrast medium.

Pharmacodynamics
Diffusing action: Hyaluronidase is a spreading or diffusing substance that modifies the permeability of connective tissue through the hydrolysis of hyaluronic acid. Drug enhances the diffusion of substances injected subcutaneously provided local interstitial pressure is adequate.

Pharmacokinetics
- *Absorption:* No information available.
- *Distribution:* No information available.
- *Metabolism:* No information available.
- *Excretion:* No information available.

Contraindications and precautions
Contraindicated in patients hypersensitive to drug.

Interactions
Use with *local anesthetics* may increase analgesia, hasten onset, and reduce local swelling but may also increase systemic absorption, increase toxicity, and shorten duration of action.

Effects on diagnostic tests
None reported.

Adverse reactions
Skin: allergic reactions (rare).

Overdose and treatment
Up to 75,000 units have been administered without ill effect; local adverse effects would be anticipated. Treat symptomatically.

☑ Special considerations
- Give skin test for sensitivity before use with an intradermal injection using about 0.02 ml of hyaluronidase solution; a wheal with pseudopods appearing within 5 minutes after injection and lasting for 20 to 30 minutes along with urticaria indicates a positive reaction.
- Avoid contact with eyes; if it occurs, flood with water immediately.
- Drug also may be used to diffuse local anesthetics at injection site, especially in nerve block anesthesia. It also has been used to enhance the diffusion of drugs in management of I.V. extravasation.
- When considering administration of other drugs with hyaluronidase, consult appropriate references for compatibility.

Patient education
- Instruct patient to report unusual and significant adverse effects after injection.

Pediatric use
- If administering drug for hypodermoclysis, take care to avoid overhydration. In children under age 3, clysis should not exceed 200 ml; in premature neonates, clysis should not exceed 25 ml/kg and the rate should not exceed 2 ml/minute.

hydralazine hydrochloride
Apresoline, Novo-Hylazin

Pharmacologic classification: peripheral vasodilator
Therapeutic classification: antihypertensive
Pregnancy risk category C

How supplied
Available by prescription only
Tablets: 10 mg, 25 mg, 50 mg, 100 mg
Injection: 20 mg/ml

Indications, route, and dosage
Moderate to severe hypertension
Adults: Initially, 10 mg P.O. q.i.d. for 2 to 4 days, then increased to 25 mg q.i.d. for remainder of week. If necessary, increase dosage to 50 mg q.i.d. Maximum recommended dosage is 200 mg daily, but some patients may require 300 to 400 mg daily.

For severe hypertension, 10 to 50 mg I.M. or 10 to 20 mg I.V. repeated p.r.n. Switch to oral antihypertensives as soon as possible.

For hypertensive crisis associated with pregnancy, initially 5 mg I.V., followed by 5 to 10 mg I.V. q 20 to 30 minutes until adequate reduction in blood pressure is achieved (usual range, 5 to 20 mg).
Children: Initially, 0.75 mg/kg P.O. daily in four divided doses (25 mg/m^2 daily); may increase gradually to 7.5 mg/kg daily.

I.M. or I.V. drug dosage is 0.4 to 1.2 mg/kg daily or 50 to 100 mg/m^2 daily in four to six divided doses. Initial parenteral dose should not exceed 20 mg.

◊ ***Management of severe heart failure***

Adults: Initially, 50 to 75 mg P.O., then adjusted according to patient response. Most patients respond to 200 to 600 mg daily, divided q 6 to 12 hours, but dosages as high as 3 g daily have been used.

Pharmacodynamics

Antihypertensive action: Hydralazine has a direct vasodilating effect on vascular smooth muscle, thus lowering blood pressure. Hydralazine's effect on resistance vessels (arterioles and arteries) is greater than that on capacitance vessels (venules and veins).

Pharmacokinetics

- *Absorption:* Drug is absorbed rapidly from GI tract after oral administration; peak plasma levels occur in 1 hour; bioavailability is 30% to 50%. Antihypertensive effect occurs 20 to 30 minutes after oral dose, 5 to 20 minutes after I.V. administration, and 10 to 30 minutes after I.M. administration. Food enhances absorption.
- *Distribution:* Distributed widely throughout the body; drug is approximately 88% to 90% protein-bound.
- *Metabolism:* Hydralazine is metabolized extensively in the GI mucosa and the liver. Hydralazine is subject to polymorphic acetylation. Slow acetylators have higher plasma levels, generally requiring lower doses.
- *Excretion:* Mostly excreted in urine, primarily as metabolites; about 10% of an oral dose is excreted in feces. Antihypertensive effect persists 2 to 4 hours after an oral dose and 2 to 6 hours after I.V. or I.M. administration.

Contraindications and precautions

Contraindicated in patients with hypersensitivity to drug, coronary artery disease, or mitral valvular rheumatic heart disease. Use cautiously in patients with suspected cardiac disease, CVA, or severe renal impairment and in those receiving other antihypertensive drugs.

Interactions

Hydralazine may potentiate the effects of *diuretics* and other *antihypertensive medications*; profound hypotension may occur if drug is given with *diazoxide*.

Concomitant administration with *MAO inhibitors* may synergistically decrease blood pressure; hydralazine may decrease the pressor response to *epinephrine*.

Effects on diagnostic tests

Hydralazine may cause positive antinuclear antibody (ANA) titer; positive lupus erythematosus (LE) cell preparation; blood dyscrasias, including leukopenia, agranulocytosis, and purpura; and hematologic abnormalities, including decreased hemoglobin and RBC count.

Adverse reactions

CNS: peripheral neuritis, *headache*, dizziness.
CV: orthostatic hypotension, *tachycardia*, edema, *angina, palpitations.*
GI: *nausea, vomiting, diarrhea, anorexia,* constipation.
Hematologic: ***neutropenia,*** leukopenia, ***agranulocytosis.***
Skin: rash.
Other: *lupus-like syndrome* (especially with high doses).

Overdose and treatment

Clinical signs of overdose include hypotension, tachycardia, headache, and skin flushing; arrhythmias and shock may occur.

After acute ingestion, empty stomach by emesis or gastric lavage and give activated charcoal to reduce absorption. Follow with symptomatic and supportive care.

☑ Special considerations

- CBC, LE cell preparation, and ANA titer determinations should be performed before therapy and at regular intervals during long-term therapy.
- Incidence of drug-induced systemic lupus erythematosus (SLE) syndrome is greatest in patients receiving more than 200 mg/day for prolonged periods.
- Headache and palpitations may occur 2 to 4 hours after first oral dose but should subside spontaneously.
- Advise precautions for postural hypotension.
- Food enhances oral absorption and helps minimize gastric irritation; adhere to consistent schedule.
- Some preparations contain tartrazine, which may precipitate allergic reactions, especially in aspirin-sensitive patients.
- For I.V. use: Monitor blood pressure every 5 minutes until stable, then every 15 minutes; put patient in Trendelenburg's position if he is faint or dizzy. Too-rapid reduction in blood pressure can cause mental changes from cerebral ischemia.
- Inject drug as soon as possible after draining through needle into syringe; drug changes color after contact with metal.
- Remember that patients with renal impairment may respond to lower maintenance doses of hydralazine.
- Sodium retention can occur with long-term use; monitor patient for signs of weight gain and edema.

Patient education

- Teach patient about disease and therapy, and explain why drug should be taken exactly as prescribed, even when he feels well; advise him never to discontinue drug suddenly because severe rebound hypertension may occur.
- Explain adverse effects and advise patient to report unusual effects, especially symptoms of SLE (sore throat, fever, rash, and muscle and joint pain).
- Explain how to minimize impact of adverse effects: to avoid operation of hazardous equipment until tolerance develops to sedation, drowsiness,

and other CNS effects; to avoid sudden position changes, to minimize orthostatic hypotension; to avoid alcohol; and to take drug with meals to enhance absorption and minimize gastric irritation.
• Reassure patient that headaches and palpitations occurring 2 to 4 hours after initial dose usually subside spontaneously; if not, he should report such effects.
• Instruct patient to weigh himself at least weekly. Advise him to report weight gain that exceeds 5 lb (2.3 kg) weekly.
• Warn patient to seek medical approval before taking OTC cold preparations.

Geriatric use
• Elderly patients may be more sensitive to antihypertensive effects. Use with special caution in patients with history of stroke or impaired renal function; patients with renal impairment may respond to lower maintenance dosages.

Pediatric use
• Drug has had limited use in children. Safety and efficacy in children have not been established; use only if potential benefit outweighs risk.

Breast-feeding
• It is not known if drug is excreted into breast milk. An alternative feeding method is recommended during therapy.

hydrochlorothiazide
Apo-Hydro*, Aquazide-H, Diuchlor H*, Esidrix, Hydro-chlor, Hydro-D, HydroDIURIL, Mictrin, Neo-Codema*, Novo-hydrazide*, Oretic, Urozide*

Pharmacologic classification: thiazide diuretic
Therapeutic classification: diuretic, antihypertensive
Pregnancy risk category B

How supplied
Available by prescription only
Tablets: 25 mg, 50 mg, 100 mg
Solution: 50 mg/5 ml, 100 mg/ml

Indications, route, and dosage
Edema
Adults: Initially, 25 to 200 mg P.O. daily for several days or until dry weight is attained. Maintenance dose is 25 to 100 mg P.O. daily or intermittently. A few refractory patients may require up to 200 mg daily.
Children over age 6 months: 1 to 2 mg/kg P.O. daily divided b.i.d.
Children under age 6 months: Up to 3 mg/kg P.O. daily divided b.i.d.
Hypertension
Adults: 25 to 50 mg P.O. once daily or in divided doses. Daily dosage increased or decreased based on blood pressure.

Pharmacodynamics
Diuretic action: Hydrochlorothiazide increases urinary excretion of sodium and water by inhibiting sodium reabsorption in the cortical diluting tubule of the nephron, thus relieving edema.

Antihypertensive action: Exact mechanism of drug's antihypertensive effect is unknown. It may result partially from direct arteriolar vasodilation and a decrease in total peripheral resistance.

Pharmacokinetics
• *Absorption:* Drug is absorbed from the GI tract; rate and extent of absorption vary with different formulations.
• *Distribution:* Unknown.
• *Metabolism:* None.
• *Excretion:* Excreted unchanged in urine, usually within 24 hours; half-life is 5.6 to 14.8 hours.

Contraindications and precautions
Contraindicated in patients with anuria or hypersensitivity to other thiazides or other sulfonamide derivatives. Use cautiously in patients with severely impaired renal or hepatic function or progressive hepatic disease.

Interactions
Hydrochlorothiazide potentiates the hypotensive effects of most other *antihypertensive drugs*; this may be used to therapeutic advantage.

Hydrochlorothiazide may potentiate hyperglycemic, hypotensive, and hyperuricemic effects of *diazoxide*, and its hyperglycemic effect may increase *insulin* or *sulfonylurea* requirements in diabetic patients.

Hydrochlorothiazide may reduce renal clearance of *lithium*, elevating serum lithium levels, and may necessitate reduction in lithium dosage by 50%.

Hydrochlorothiazide turns urine slightly more alkaline and may decrease urinary excretion of some amines, such as *amphetamine* and *quinidine*; alkaline urine also may decrease therapeutic efficacy of methenamine compounds such as *methenamine mandelate*.

Cholestyramine and *colestipol* may bind hydrochlorothiazide, preventing its absorption; give drugs 1 hour apart.

Effects on diagnostic tests
Drug therapy may alter serum electrolyte levels and may increase serum urate, glucose, cholesterol, and triglyceride levels. It also may interfere with tests for parathyroid function and should be discontinued before such tests.

Adverse reactions
CNS: dizziness, vertigo, headache, paresthesia, weakness, restlessness.
CV: volume depletion and dehydration, orthostatic hypotension, allergic myocarditis, vasculitis.
GI: anorexia, nausea, pancreatitis, epigastric distress, vomiting, abdominal pain, diarrhea, constipation.
GU: polyuria, frequent urination, ***renal failure***, interstitial nephritis.

Hematologic: ***aplastic anemia, agranulocytosis***, leukopenia, ***thrombocytopenia***, hemolytic anemia.
Hepatic: jaundice.
Respiratory: respiratory distress, pneumonitis.
Skin: dermatitis, photosensitivity, rash, purpura, alopecia.
Other: hypersensitivity reactions; hypokalemia; asymptomatic hyperuricemia; hyperglycemia and impaired glucose tolerance; fluid and electrolyte imbalances, including dilutional hyponatremia, hypochloremia, metabolic alkalosis, hypercalcemia; gout; muscle cramps; ***anaphylactic reactions.***

Overdose and treatment

Clinical signs of overdose include GI irritation and hypermotility, diuresis, and lethargy, which may progress to coma.

Treatment is mainly supportive; monitor and assist respiratory, CV, and renal function as indicated. Monitor fluid and electrolyte balance. Induce vomiting with ipecac in conscious patient; otherwise, use gastric lavage to avoid aspiration. Do not give cathartics; these promote additional loss of fluids and electrolytes.

☑ Special considerations

Recommendations for preparation and use of hydrochlorothiazide and for care and teaching of the patient during therapy are the same as those for all *thiazide diuretics.*

- Drug may cause glucose intolerance in some people. Monitor blood sugar in diabetics. May require dose adjustment of insulin or oral antidiabetic medication.

Patient education

- Instruct patient to take drug with food to avoid GI upset.
- Tell patient to take drug in morning or early afternoon to avoid nocturia.
- Advise patient to avoid sudden postural changes.
- Encourage patient to use sunblock to avoid photosensitivity reactions.
- Tell patient to consult primary health care provider before taking OTC medications.

Geriatric use

- Elderly and debilitated patients require close observation and may require reduced dosages. They are more sensitive to excess diuresis because of age-related changes in CV and renal function. Excess diuresis promotes orthostatic hypotension, dehydration, hypovolemia, hyponatremia, hypomagnesemia, and hypokalemia.

Breast-feeding

- Drug is distributed in breast milk; safety and effectiveness in breast-feeding women have not been established.

hydrocortisone (systemic)

Cortef, Cortenema, Hycort*, Hydrocortone

hydrocortisone acetate

Cortifoam

hydrocortisone cypionate

Cortef

hydrocortisone sodium phosphate

Hydrocortone Phosphate

hydrocortisone sodium succinate

A-hydroCort, Solu-Cortef

Pharmacologic classification: glucocorticoid, mineralocorticoid
Therapeutic classification: adrenocorticoid replacement
Pregnancy risk category C

How supplied

Available by prescription only
hydrocortisone
Tablets: 5 mg, 10 mg, 20 mg
Injection: 25 mg/ml, 50 mg/ml suspension
Enema: 100 mg/60 ml
hydrocortisone acetate
Injection: 25 mg/ml, 50 mg/ml suspension
Enema: 10% aerosol foam (provides 90 mg/application)
hydrocortisone cypionate
Oral suspension: 10 mg/5 ml
hydrocortisone sodium phosphate
Injection: 50 mg/ml solution
hydrocortisone sodium succinate
Injection: 100 mg/vial, 250 mg/vial, 500 mg/vial, 1,000 mg/vial

Indications, route, and dosage

Severe inflammation, adrenal insufficiency
hydrocortisone
Adults: 5 to 30 mg P.O. b.i.d., t.i.d., or q.i.d. (as much as 80 mg P.O. q.i.d. may be given in acute situations).
Children: 2 to 8 mg/kg or 60 to 240 mg/m² P.O. daily.
hydrocortisone acetate
Adults: 10 to 75 mg into joints or soft tissue at 2- or 3-week intervals. Dose varies with size of joint. In many cases, local anesthetics are injected with dose.
hydrocortisone sodium phosphate
Adults. 15 to 240 mg S.C., I.M., or I.V. daily in divided doses q 12 hours.
hydrocortisone sodium succinate
Adults: Initially, 100 to 500 mg I.M. or I.V., then 50 to 100 mg I.M. as indicated.
Shock (other than adrenal crisis)
hydrocortisone sodium phosphate
Children: 0.16 to 1 mg/kg I.M. daily or b.i.d.

hydrocortisone sodium succinate
Adults: 100 to 500 mg I.M. or I.V. q 2 to 6 hours.
Children: 0.16 to 1 mg/kg or 6 to 30 mg/m² I.M. or I.V. daily to b.i.d.

Life-threatening shock
hydrocortisone sodium succinate
Adults: 0.5 to 2 g I.V. initially, repeated at 2- to 6-hour intervals, p.r.n. High-dose therapy should be continued only until patient's condition has stabilized. Therapy should not be continued beyond 48 to 72 hours.

Adjunctive treatment of ulcerative colitis and proctitis
hydrocortisone
Adults: One enema (100 mg) nightly for 21 days.
hydrocortisone acetate (rectal foam)
Adults: 90 mg (1 applicatorful) once or twice daily for 2 or 3 weeks; decrease frequency to every other day thereafter.

Pharmacodynamics

Adrenocorticoid replacement action: Hydrocortisone is an adrenocorticoid with both glucocorticoid and mineralocorticoid properties. It is a weak anti-inflammatory agent but a potent mineralocorticoid, having potency similar to that of cortisone and twice that of prednisone. Hydrocortisone (or cortisone) is usually drug of choice for replacement therapy in patients with adrenal insufficiency. It is usually not used for immunosuppressant activity because of the extremely large doses necessary and the unwanted mineralocorticoid effects.

Hydrocortisone and hydrocortisone cypionate may be administered orally. Hydrocortisone sodium phosphate may be administered by I.M., S.C., or I.V. injection or by I.V. infusion, usually at 12-hour intervals. Hydrocortisone sodium succinate may be administered by I.M. or I.V. injection or I.V. infusion every 2 to 10 hours, depending on the clinical situation. Hydrocortisone acetate is a suspension that may be administered by intra-articular, intrasynovial, intrabursal, intralesional, or soft tissue injection. It has a slow onset but a long duration of action. Injectable forms are usually used only when the oral dosage forms cannot be used.

Pharmacokinetics

- *Absorption:* Drug is absorbed readily after oral administration. After oral and I.V. administration, peak effects occur in about 1 to 2 hours. The acetate suspension for injection has a variable absorption over 24 to 48 hours, depending on whether it is injected into an intra-articular space or a muscle, and the blood supply to that muscle.
- *Distribution:* Hydrocortisone is removed rapidly from the blood and distributed to muscle, liver, skin, intestines, and kidneys. Hydrocortisone is bound extensively to plasma proteins (transcortin and albumin). Only the unbound portion is active. Adrenocorticoids are distributed into breast milk and through the placenta.
- *Metabolism:* Metabolized in the liver to inactive glucuronide and sulfate metabolites.
- *Excretion:* The inactive metabolites and small amounts of unmetabolized drug are excreted by the kidneys. Insignificant quantities of drug are excreted in feces. Biologic half-life of hydrocortisone is 8 to 12 hours.

Contraindications and precautions

Contraindicated in patients allergic to any component of the formulation, in those with systemic fungal infections, and in premature infants (with hydrocortisone sodium succinate).

Use hydrocortisone sodium phosphate or succinate cautiously in patients with a recent MI, GI ulcer, renal disease, hypertension, osteoporosis, diabetes mellitus, hypothyroidism, cirrhosis, diverticulitis, ulcerative colitis, recent intestinal anastomosis, thromboembolic disorders, seizures, myasthenia gravis, heart failure, tuberculosis, ocular herpes simplex, emotional instability, and psychotic tendencies.

Interactions

When used concomitantly, hydrocortisone may in rare cases decrease the effects of oral anticoagulants by unknown mechanisms. Concomitant use of *barbiturates, phenytoin,* or *rifampin* may decrease corticosteroid effects because of increased hepatic metabolism. *Antacids, cholestyramine,* and *colestipol* decrease corticosteroid effect by adsorbing the corticosteroid, thereby decreasing the amount absorbed.

Hydrocortisone increases the metabolism of *isoniazid* and *salicylates.* It may enhance hypokalemia associated with *diuretic* or *amphotericin B* therapy. The hypokalemia may increase the risk of toxicity in patients receiving *cardiac glycosides.*

Concomitant use of *estrogens* may reduce the metabolism of corticosteroids by increasing the concentration of *transcortin.* The half-life of the corticosteroid is then prolonged from increased protein binding. Concomitant administration of *ulcerogenic drugs,* such as *NSAIDs,* may increase risk of GI ulceration.

Effects on diagnostic tests

Hydrocortisone suppresses reactions to skin tests, causes false-negative results in the nitroblue tetrazolium tests for systemic bacterial infections, and decreases ^{131}I uptake and protein-bound iodine concentrations in thyroid function tests.

Hydrocortisone may increase glucose and cholesterol levels; may decrease serum potassium, calcium, thyroxine, and triiodothyronine levels; and may increase urine glucose and calcium levels.

Adverse reactions

Most adverse reactions to corticosteroids are dose- or duration-dependent.

CNS: *euphoria, insomnia,* psychotic behavior, pseudotumor cerebri, vertigo, headache, paresthesia, ***seizures.***
CV: ***heart failure***, hypertension, edema, ***arrhythmias***, thrombophlebitis, ***thromboembolism.***
EENT: cataracts, glaucoma.
Endocrine: menstrual irregularities, cushingoid state (moonface, buffalo hump, central obesity).
GI: *peptic ulceration,* GI irritation, increased appetite, pancreatitis, nausea, vomiting.
Skin: delayed wound healing, acne, various skin eruptions, easy bruising.

Other: muscle weakness, osteoporosis, hirsutism, susceptibility to infections; possible hypokalemia, hyperglycemia (requiring dosage adjustment in diabetics), carbohydrate intolerance; growth suppression in children; ***acute adrenal insufficiency with increased stress (infection, surgery, trauma) or abrupt withdrawal (after long-term therapy).***

After abrupt withdrawal: rebound inflammation, fatigue, weakness, arthralgia, fever, dizziness, lethargy, depression, fainting, orthostatic hypotension, dyspnea, anorexia, hypoglycemia. ***After prolonged use, sudden withdrawal may be fatal.***

Overdose and treatment

Acute ingestion, even in massive doses, is rarely a clinical problem. Toxic signs and symptoms rarely occur if drug is used for less than 3 weeks, even at large doses. However, chronic use causes adverse physiologic effects, including suppression of the hypothalamic-pituitary-adrenal axis, cushingoid appearance, muscle weakness, and osteoporosis.

☑ Special considerations

Recommendations for use of hydrocortisone and for care and teaching of patients during therapy are the same as those for all *systemic adrenocorticoids.*

Pediatric use

- Chronic use of hydrocortisone in children and adolescents may delay growth and maturation.

hydrocortisone (topical)

Acticort 100, Aeroseb-HC, Ala-Cort, Ala-Scalp, Anusol-HC, Bactine, Barriere-HC*, CaldeCORT, Cetacort, CortaGel, Cortaid, Cortate*, Cort-Dome, Cortizone, Dermacort, DermiCort, Dermolate, Dermtex HC, Emo-Cort*, Hi-Cor, Hydro-Tex, Hytone, LactiCare-HC, Nutracort, Penecort, Rectocort*, S-T Cort, Synacort, Texacort, Unicort*

hydrocortisone acetate

Anusol-HC, CaldeCORT, Cortaid, Cort-Dome, Cortef, Corticaine, Corticreme*, Cortoderm*, Gynecort, Hyderm*, Lanacort, Novohydrocort*, Orabase-HCA, Pharma-Cort, Rhulicort

hydrocortisone buteprate

Pandel

hydrocortisone butyrate

Locoid

hydrocortisone valerate

Westcort

Pharmacologic classification: glucocorticoid
Therapeutic classification: anti-inflammatory
Pregnancy risk category C

How supplied

Available by prescription only
hydrocortisone
Cream: 0.5%, 1%, 2.5%
Ointment: 0.5%, 1%, 2.5%
Lotion: 0.25%, 0.5%, 1%, 2%, 2.5%
Gel: 0.5%, 1%
Solution: 0.5%, 1%, 2.5%
Aerosol: 0.5%, 1%
Pledgets (saturated with solution): 0.5%, 1%
hydrocortisone acetate
Cream: 0.5%, 1%
Ointment: 0.5%, 1%
Lotion: 0.5%
Suppositories: 25 mg
Rectal foam: 10%
Paste: 0.5%
Solution: 1%
hydrocortisone buteprate
Cream: 0.1%
hydrocortisone butyrate
Cream, ointment, solution: 0.1%
hydrocortisone valerate
Cream, ointment: 0.2%

Indications, route, and dosage

Inflammation of corticosteroid-responsive dermatoses, including those on face, groin, armpits, and under breasts; seborrheic dermatitis of scalp

Adults and children: Apply cream, lotion, ointment, foam, or aerosol sparingly once daily to q.i.d.

Aerosol

Shake can well. Direct spray onto affected area from a distance of 60 (15 cm). Apply for only 3 seconds (to avoid freezing tissues). Apply to dry scalp after shampooing; no need to massage or rub medication into scalp after spraying. Apply daily until acute phase is controlled, then reduce dosage to once to three times weekly, p.r.n., to maintain control.

Rectal administration

Shake can well. Apply once daily or b.i.d. for 2 to 3 weeks, then every other day p.r.n.

Dental lesions

Adults and children: Apply paste b.i.d. or t.i.d. and h.s.

Pharmacodynamics

Anti-inflammatory action: Hydrocortisone stimulates the synthesis of enzymes needed to decrease the inflammatory response. Hydrocortisone, a corticosteroid secreted by the adrenal cortex, is about 1.25 times more potent an anti-inflammatory agent than equivalent doses of cortisone, but both have twice the mineralocorticoid activity of the other glucocorticoids. As topical agents, hydrocortisone and hydrocortisone acetate are low-potency group VI glucocorticoids. Hydrocortisone probutate is a medium-potency corticosteroid. Hydrocortisone valerate has group V potency.

Hydrocortisone 0.5%, 1%, and hydrocortisone acetate 0.5% are available without a prescription for the temporary relief of minor skin irritation, itching, and rashes caused by eczema, insect bites, soaps, and detergents.

Hydrocortisone is also administered rectally as a retention enema for the temporary treatment of acute ulcerative colitis. Hydrocortisone acetate suspension is also available as a rectal suppository or aerosol foam suspension for the temporary treatment of inflammatory conditions of the rectum such as hemorrhoids, cryptitis, proctitis, and pruritus ani.

Pharmacokinetics

• *Absorption:* Absorption depends on potency of preparation, amount applied, and nature of skin at application site. It ranges from about 1% in areas with a thick stratum corneum (such as the palms, soles, elbows, and knees) to as high as 36% in areas where the stratum corneum is thinnest (face, eyelids, and genitals). Absorption increases in areas of skin damage, inflammation, or occlusion. Some systemic absorption occurs, especially through the oral mucosa.
• *Distribution:* After topical application, drug is distributed throughout the local skin layers. Any drug absorbed into circulation is removed rapidly from the blood and distributed into muscle, liver, skin, intestines, and kidneys.
• *Metabolism:* After topical administration, hydrocortisone is metabolized primarily in the skin. The small amount that is absorbed into systemic circulation is metabolized primarily in the liver to inactive compounds.
• *Excretion:* Inactive metabolites are excreted by the kidneys, primarily as glucuronides and sulfates, but also as unconjugated products. Small amounts of the metabolites are also excreted in feces.

Contraindications and precautions

Contraindicated in patients hypersensitive to drug.

Interactions

None significant.

Effects on diagnostic tests

None reported.

Adverse reactions

Skin: burning, pruritus, irritation, dryness, erythema, folliculitis, hypertrichosis, hypopigmentation, acneiform eruptions, allergic contact dermatitis; *maceration, secondary infection, atrophy, striae, miliaria* (with occlusive dressings).
Other: ***hypothalamic-pituitary-adrenal axis suppression,*** Cushing's syndrome, hyperglycemia, glucosuria.

Overdose and treatment

No information available.

☑ Special considerations

Recommendations for use of hydrocortisone, for care and teaching of patients during therapy, and for use in elderly patients, children, and breast-feeding women are the same as those for all *topical adrenocorticoids.*

hydromorphone hydrochloride

Dilaudid, Dilaudid-HP, Hydrostat IR

Pharmacologic classification: opioid
Therapeutic classification: analgesic, antitussive
Controlled substance schedule II
Pregnancy risk category C

How supplied

Available by prescription only
Tablets: 1 mg, 2 mg, 3 mg, 4 mg, 8 mg
Oral liquid: 5 mg/5 ml
Injection: 1 mg/ml, 2 mg/ml, 3 mg/ml, 4 mg/ml, 10 mg/ml
Suppository: 3 mg

Indications, route, and dosage

Moderate to severe pain
Adults: 2 to 10 mg P.O. q 3 to 6 hours, p.r.n. or around the clock; or 2 to 4 mg I.M., S.C., or I.V. q 4 to 6 hours, p.r.n. or around the clock (I.V. dose should be given over 3 to 5 minutes); or 3 mg rectal suppository q 6 to 8 hours, p.r.n. or around the clock. (Give 1 to 14 mg Dilaudid-HP S.C. or I.M. q 4 to 6 hours.)

Note: Hydromorphone hydrochloride should be given in the smallest effective dose and as infrequently as possible to minimize the development of tolerance and physical dependence. Dose must be individually adjusted based on patient's severity of pain, age, and size.

Cough
Adults: 1 mg P.O. q 3 to 4 hours, p.r.n.
Children age 6 to 12: 0.5 mg P.O. q 3 to 4 hours, p.r.n.

Pharmacodynamics

Antitussive action: Hydromorphone acts directly on the cough center in the medulla, producing an antitussive effect.

Analgesic action: Hydromorphone has analgesic properties related to opiate receptor affinity, and is recommended for moderate to severe pain. There is no intrinsic limit to the analgesic effect of hydromorphone, unlike the other opioids.

Pharmacokinetics

• *Absorption:* Well absorbed after oral, rectal, or parenteral administration. Onset of action occurs in 15 to 30 minutes, with peak effect at ½ to 1 hour after dosing.
• *Distribution:* Unknown.
• *Metabolism:* Drug is metabolized primarily in the liver, where it undergoes conjugation with glucuronic acid.
• *Excretion:* Excreted primarily in the urine as the glucuronide conjugate. Duration of action is 4 to 5 hours.

Contraindications and precautions

Contraindicated in patients with hypersensitivity to drug, intracranial lesions associated with increased intracranial pressure, and whenever ventilator function is depressed, such as in status asthmaticus,

COPD, cor pulmonale, emphysema, and kyphoscoliosis.

Use cautiously in elderly or debilitated patients and in those with hepatic or renal disease, Addison's disease, hypothyroidism, prostatic hyperplasia, or urethral strictures.

Interactions

Concomitant use with other *CNS depressants* (*narcotic analgesics, general anesthetics, antihistamines, phenothiazines, barbiturates, benzodiazepines, sedative-hypnotics, tricyclic antidepressants, alcohol, muscle relaxants*) potentiates drug's respiratory and CNS depression, sedation, and hypotensive effects. Concomitant use with *cimetidine* may also increase respiratory and CNS depression, causing confusion, disorientation, apnea, or seizures; such use usually requires reduced dosage of *hydromorphone.*

Drug accumulation and enhanced effects may result from concomitant use with other drugs that are extensively metabolized in the liver (*rifampin, phenytoin, digitoxin*); combined use with *anticholinergics* may cause paralytic ileus.

Patients who become physically dependent on drug may experience acute withdrawal syndrome if given a narcotic antagonist.

Severe CV depression may result from concomitant use with *general anesthetics.*

Effects on diagnostic tests

Drug increases plasma amylase and lipase levels. It may also delay gastric emptying; increased biliary tract pressure resulting from contraction of the sphincter of Oddi may interfere with hepatobiliary imaging studies.

Adverse reactions

CNS: *sedation, somnolence, clouded sensorium,* dizziness, *euphoria.*
CV: *hypotension,* bradycardia.
EENT: blurred vision, diplopia, nystagmus.
GI: *nausea, vomiting, constipation,* ileus.
GU: *urine retention.*
Respiratory: ***respiratory depression, bronchospasm.***
Other: induration (with repeated S.C. injections), physical dependence.

Overdose and treatment

The most common signs and symptoms of hydromorphone overdose are CNS depression, respiratory depression, and miosis (pinpoint pupils). Other acute toxic effects include hypotension, bradycardia, hypothermia, shock, apnea, cardiopulmonary arrest, circulatory collapse, pulmonary edema, and seizures.

To treat an acute overdose, first establish adequate respiratory exchange via a patent airway and ventilation as needed; administer a narcotic antagonist (naloxone) to reverse respiratory depression. (Because the duration of action of hydromorphone is longer than that of naxolone, repeated dosing is necessary.) Naloxone should not be given unless patient has clinically significant respiratory or CV depression. Monitor vital signs closely.

If patient presents within 2 hours of ingestion of an oral overdose, empty the stomach immediately by inducing emesis (ipecac syrup) or using gastric lavage. Use caution to avoid risk of aspiration. Administer activated charcoal via nasogastric tube for further removal of an oral overdose.

Provide symptomatic and supportive treatment (continued respiratory support, correction of fluid or electrolyte imbalance). Monitor laboratory parameters, vital signs, and neurologic status closely.

Contact the local or regional poison control center for further information.

☑ Special considerations

Besides those relevant to all *opioids,* consider the following recommendations.

- Before administration, visually inspect all parenteral products for particulate matter and extreme yellow discoloration.
- Oral dosage form is particularly convenient for patients with chronic pain, because tablets are available in several strengths, enabling patient to titrate own dosage precisely.
- Dilaudid-HP, a highly concentrated form (10 mg/ml), may be administered in smaller volumes, preventing discomfort associated with large-volume injections.

Patient education

- Instruct patient to take or ask for drug before pain becomes intense.
- Tell patient to store suppositories in the refrigerator.
- Encourage coughing or deep breathing to avoid atelectasis (postoperatively).
- Instruct patient to avoid hazardous activities that require mental alertness.
- Advise patient to avoid alcohol.

Geriatric use

- Lower doses are usually indicated for elderly patients, because they may be more sensitive to the therapeutic and adverse effects of drug.

Breast-feeding

- It is unknown if drug is excreted in breast milk; use with caution in breast-feeding women.

hydroxychloroquine sulfate

Plaquenil Sulfate

Pharmacologic classification: 4-aminoquinoline
Therapeutic classification: antimalarial, anti-inflammatory
Pregnancy risk category C

How supplied

Available by prescription only
Tablets: 200 mg (155 mg base)

Indications, route, and dosage

Suppressive prophylaxis of malarial attacks
Adults: 400 mg of sulfate (310 mg base) P.O. weekly on exactly the same day each week. (Begin 2

weeks before entering and continue for 8 weeks after leaving the endemic area.)
Infants and children: 5 mg, calculated as base per kilogram of body weight (should not exceed the adult dose regardless of weight) on exactly the same day each week. Start 2 weeks before exposure. If unable, give 10 mg base/kg in two divided doses 6 hours apart.
Treatment of acute attack of malaria
Adults: 800 mg (620 mg base) followed by 400 mg (310 mg base) in 6 to 8 hours and 400 mg (310 mg base) on each of 2 consecutive days.
Infants and children: Initial dose, 10 mg base/kg (but not exceeding a single dose of 620 mg base). Second dose, 5 mg base/kg (but not exceeding a single dose of 310 mg base) 6 hours after first dose. Third dose, 5 mg base/kg 18 hours after second dose. Fourth dose, 5 mg base/kg 24 hours after third dose.
Lupus erythematosus (chronic discoid and systemic)
Adults: 400 mg P.O. daily or b.i.d., continued for several weeks or months, based on response. Prolonged maintenance is 200 to 400 mg P.O. daily.
◇ ***Rheumatoid arthritis***
Adults: Initially, 400 to 600 mg P.O. daily. When good response occurs (usually in 4 to 12 weeks), reduce dosage by half.

Pharmacodynamics

Antimalarial action: Hydroxychloroquine binds to DNA, interfering with protein synthesis. It also inhibits DNA and RNA polymerases. It is active against asexual erythrocytic forms of *Plasmodium malariae, P. ovale, P. vivax,* and many strains of *P. falciparum.*

Amebicidal action: Mechanism of action is unknown.

Anti-inflammatory action: Mechanism of action is unknown. Drug may antagonize histamine and serotonin and inhibit prostaglandin effects by inhibiting conversion of arachidonic acid to prostaglandin F_2; it may also inhibit chemotaxis of polymorphonuclear leukocytes, macrophages, and eosinophils.

Pharmacokinetics

- *Absorption:* Absorbed readily and almost completely, with peak plasma concentrations occurring at 1 to 2 hours.
- *Distribution:* Drug is bound to plasma proteins. It concentrates in the liver, spleen, kidneys, heart, and brain and is strongly bound in melanin-containing cells.
- *Metabolism:* Drug is metabolized by the liver to desethylchloroquine and desethyl hydroxychloroquine.
- *Excretion:* Most of an administered dose is excreted unchanged in urine. Drug and its metabolites are excreted slowly in urine; unabsorbed drug is excreted in feces. Small amounts of drug may be present in urine for months after it is discontinued. Drug is excreted in breast milk.

Contraindications and precautions

Contraindicated in patients with hypersensitivity to drug, in long-term therapy for children, and in patients with retinal or visual field changes or porphyria. Use cautiously in patients with severe GI, neurologic, or blood disorders.

Interactions

Concomitant administration of *kaolin* or *magnesium trisilicate* may decrease absorption of hydroxychloroquine. Use with *digoxin* may increase serum digoxin levels.

Effects on diagnostic tests

Drug may cause inversion or depression of the T wave or widening of the QRS complex on ECG. Rarely, it may cause decreased WBC, RBC, or platelet counts.

Adverse reactions

CNS: irritability, nightmares, ataxia, ***seizures***, psychosis, vertigo, nystagmus, dizziness, hypoactive deep tendon reflexes, ataxia, lassitude, skeletal muscle weakness, headache.
EENT: visual disturbances (blurred vision; difficulty in focusing; reversible corneal changes; typically irreversible, sometimes progressive or delayed retinal changes, such as narrowing of arterioles; macular lesions; pallor of optic disk; optic atrophy; visual field defects; patchy retinal pigmentation, commonly leading to blindness), ototoxicity (irreversible nerve deafness, tinnitus, labyrinthitis).
GI: anorexia, abdominal cramps, diarrhea, nausea, vomiting.
Hematologic: ***agranulocytosis, leukopenia, thrombocytopenia, hemolysis (in patients with G6PD deficiency), aplastic anemia.***
Skin: pruritus, lichen planus eruptions, skin and mucosal pigmentary changes, pleomorphic skin eruptions.
Other: weight loss, alopecia, bleaching of hair.

Overdose and treatment

Symptoms of drug overdose may appear within 30 minutes after ingestion and may include headache, drowsiness, visual changes, CV collapse, and seizures followed by respiratory and cardiac arrest.

Treatment is symptomatic. The stomach should be emptied by emesis or lavage. After lavage, activated charcoal in an amount at least five times the estimated amount of drug ingested may be helpful if given within 30 minutes of ingestion.

Ultra-short-acting barbiturates may help control seizures. Intubation may become necessary. Peritoneal dialysis and exchange transfusions may also be useful. Forced fluids and acidification of the urine are helpful after the acute phase.

☑ Special considerations

- Baseline and periodic ophthalmologic examinations are necessary in prolonged or high-dosage therapy.
- Monitor for blurred vision, increased sensitivity to light, hearing loss, pronounced GI disturbances, or muscle weakness.

• Give drug immediately before or after meals on the same day each week to minimize gastric distress.
• Drug is not effective for chloroquine-resistant strains of *P. falciparum.*

Patient education

• To prevent drug-induced dermatoses, warn patient to avoid excessive exposure to the sun.

Pediatric use

• Children are extremely susceptible to toxicity; monitor closely for adverse effects. Do not use drug for long-term therapy in children and do not exceed recommended dose.

Breast-feeding

• Safety has not been established. Use with caution in breast-feeding women.

---

hydroxyprogesterone caproate

Hy-Gestrone, Hylutin, Hyprogest, Prodrox

Pharmacologic classification: progestin
Therapeutic classification: progestin, antineoplastic
Pregnancy risk category X

How supplied

Available by prescription only
Injection: 125 mg/ml, 250 mg/ml

Indications, route, and dosage

Amenorrhea and uterine bleeding

Adults: 375 mg I.M. May be repeated at 4-week intervals if needed. After 4 days of desquamation or if there is no bleeding within 21 days after administration, begin cyclic therapy with an estrogen.

Endometrial cancer

Adults: 1 g I.M. up to seven times weekly for 12 weeks or as indicated. Therapy is discontinued if relapse occurs or if no objective response is seen after 12 weeks of therapy.

Pharmacodynamics

Progestational action: Drug suppresses ovulation, causes thickening of cervical mucus, and induces sloughing of the endometrium. It inhibits growth progression of progestin-sensitive uterine cancer tissue by an unknown mechanism.

Pharmacokinetics

This compound has a duration of action of 7 to 14 days when used as directed.
• *Absorption:* Hydroxyprogesterone is absorbed slowly after I.M. injection.
• *Distribution:* Unknown.
• *Metabolism:* Primarily hepatic; not well characterized.
• *Excretion:* Primarily renal; not well characterized.

Contraindications and precautions

Contraindicated during pregnancy and in patients with hypersensitivity to drug, thromboembolic disorders, cerebral apoplexy, breast or genital organ cancer, undiagnosed abnormal vaginal bleeding, severe hepatic disease, or missed abortion.

Use cautiously in patients with diabetes mellitus, seizures, migraine, cardiac or renal disease, asthma, mental depression, or impaired liver function.

Interactions

Concomitant use with *bromocriptine* may cause amenorrhea or galactorrhea, thus interfering with the action of *bromocriptine.* Concurrent use of these drugs is not recommended.

Effects on diagnostic tests

Glucose tolerance has been shown to decrease in a small percentage of patients receiving drug. Abnormal thyroid or liver function tests may occur; the metyrapone test may be altered and pregnanediol excretion may decrease.

Adverse reactions

CNS: depression.
CV: thrombophlebitis, ***thromboembolism***, ***CVA, pulmonary embolism***, edema.
EENT: exophthalmos, diplopia.
GU: breakthrough bleeding, dysmenorrhea, amenorrhea, cervical erosion, abnormal secretions.
Hepatic: cholestatic jaundice.
Skin: rash, acne, pruritus, melasma; irritation, pain (at injection site).
Other: breast tenderness, enlargement, or secretion; changes in weight.

Overdose and treatment

No information available.

☑ Special considerations

Besides those relevant to all *progestins,* consider the following recommendations.
• Hydroxyprogesterone caproate is for I.M. administration only. Inject deep into large muscle mass, preferably the gluteal muscle.
• Provide manufacturer's package insert to women receiving drug.
• Monitor diabetic patients during therapy for signs of decreased glucose tolerance.
• Patients receiving drug should have a full physical examination, including a gynecologic examination and a Papanicolaou test, every 6 to 12 months.

Patient education

• Warn patient that edema and weight gain are likely to occur.
• Remind patient that normal menstrual cycles may not resume for 2 to 3 months after discontinuing drug therapy.
• Advise patient of potential risks to the fetus if she becomes pregnant during therapy or is inadvertently exposed to drug during the first 4 months of pregnancy.

Breast-feeding
• Drug use is contraindicated in breast-feeding women.

hydroxyurea
Hydrea

Pharmacologic classification: antimetabolite (cell cycle–phase specific, S phase)
Therapeutic classification: antineoplastic
Pregnancy risk category NR

How supplied
Available by prescription only
Capsules: 500 mg

Indications, route, and dosage
Dosage and indications may vary. Check current literature for recommended protocol.

Solid tumors
Adults: 80 mg/kg P.O. as a single dose q 3 days; or 20 to 30 mg/kg P.O. as a single daily dose.

Head and neck cancer
Adults: 80 mg/kg P.O. as a single dose q 3 days.

Resistant chronic myelocytic leukemia
Adults: 20 to 30 mg/kg P.O. as a single daily dose.

Pharmacodynamics
Antineoplastic action: Exact mechanism of hydroxyurea's cytotoxic action is unclear. Hydroxyurea inhibits DNA synthesis without interfering with RNA or protein synthesis. Drug may act as an antimetabolite, inhibiting the incorporation of thymidine into DNA, and may also damage DNA directly.

Pharmacokinetics
• *Absorption:* Well absorbed after oral administration, with peak serum levels occurring 2 hours after a dose. Higher serum levels are achieved if drug is given as a large, single dose rather than in divided doses.
• *Distribution:* Drug crosses the blood-brain barrier.
• *Metabolism:* Approximately 50% of an oral dose is degraded in the liver.
• *Excretion:* The remaining 50% is excreted in urine as unchanged drug. The metabolites are excreted through the lungs as carbon dioxide and in urine as urea.

Contraindications and precautions
Contraindicated in patients hypersensitive to drug and with marked bone marrow depression (leukopenia [less than 2,500 WBCs/mm^3], thrombocytopenia [less than 100,000 platelets/mm^3], or severe anemia).

Use cautiously in patients with impaired renal function. Do not administer to pregnant women or women of childbearing age who may become pregnant unless potential benefit to patient outweighs possible risk to fetus.

Interactions
Concomitant use of hydroxyurea may decrease the activity of *fluorouracil*. Hydroxyurea appears to inhibit the conversion of *fluorouracil* to its active metabolite. A high incidence of neurotoxicity may occur when these two agents are administered together.

Effects on diagnostic tests
Hydroxyurea therapy elevates BUN, serum creatinine, and serum uric acid levels.

Adverse reactions
CNS: hallucinations, headache, dizziness, disorientation, ***seizures***, malaise.
GI: *anorexia, nausea, vomiting, diarrhea,* stomatitis, constipation.
GU: increased BUN and serum creatinine levels.
Hematologic: *leukopenia, thrombocytopenia,* anemia, *megaloblastosis,* ***bone marrow suppression,*** with rapid recovery (dose-limiting and dose-related).
Skin: rash, alopecia, erythema.
Other: fever, chills.

Overdose and treatment
Clinical manifestations of overdose include myelosuppression, ulceration of buccal and GI mucosa, facial erythema, maculopapular rash, disorientation, hallucinations, and impairment of renal tubular function.

Treatment is usually supportive and includes transfusion of blood components.

☑ Special considerations
• Dose modification may be required following other chemotherapy or radiation therapy.
• Monitor intake and output levels; keep patient hydrated.
• Obtain BUN, uric acid, and serum creatinine levels routinely.
• Drug may exacerbate postirradiation erythema.
• Auditory and visual hallucinations and blood toxicity increase when decreased renal function exists.
• Avoid all I.M. injections when platelet counts are below 100,000/mm^3.
• Store capsules in tight container at room temperature. Avoid exposure to excessive heat.
• Drug is currently under investigation for the treatment of sickle cell anemia. Widespread use of drug for this disease is not recommended because of the potential for toxicity.

Patient education
• Instruct patient to empty contents of capsule in water and drink immediately if capsule cannot be swallowed.
• Emphasize importance of continuing drug therapy despite nausea and vomiting.
• Tell patient to call immediately if vomiting occurs shortly after taking a dose.
• Encourage daily fluid intake of 10 to 12 (8 oz) glasses, to increase urine output and facilitate excretion of uric acid.

• Tell patient to report unusual bruising or bleeding.
• Advise patient to avoid exposure to people with infections and to report signs of infection immediately.

Geriatric use
• Elderly patients may be more sensitive to drug's effects, requiring a lower dosage.

Pediatric use
• Children may be more sensitive to drug's effects, requiring a lower dosage.

Breast-feeding
• It is not known if drug distributes into breast milk. However, because of risk of serious adverse reactions, mutagenicity, and carcinogenicity in the infant, breast-feeding is not recommended.

hydroxyzine hydrochloride
Anxanil, Apo-Hydroxyzine*, Atarax, Hydroxacen, Hyzine-50, Multipax*, Novo-Hydroxyzin*, Quiess, Vistacon-50, Vistazine-50

hydroxyzine pamoate
Vistaril

Pharmacologic classification: antihistamine (piperazine derivative)
Therapeutic classification: antianxiety, sedative, antipruritic, antiemetic, antispasmodic
Pregnancy risk category C

How supplied
Available by prescription only
hydroxyzine hydrochloride
Capsules: 10 mg, 25 mg, 50 mg
Tablets: 10 mg, 25 mg, 50 mg, 100 mg
Syrup: 10 mg/5 ml
Injection: 25 mg/ml, 50 mg/ml
hydroxyzine pamoate
Capsules: 25 mg, 50 mg, 100 mg
Oral suspension: 25 mg/5 ml

Indications, route, and dosage
Anxiety, tension, hyperkinesia
Adults: 50 to 100 mg P.O. q.i.d.
Children over age 6: 50 to 100 mg P.O. daily in divided doses.
Children under age 6: 50 mg P.O. daily in divided doses.
Preoperative and postoperative adjunctive sedation; to control emesis; adjunct to asthma treatment
Adults: 25 to 100 mg I.M. q 4 to 6 hours.
Children: 1.1 mg/kg I.M. q 4 to 6 hours.

Pharmacodynamics
Anxiolytic and sedative actions: Hydroxyzine produces its sedative and antianxiety effects through suppression of activity at subcortical levels; analgesia occurs at high doses.

Antipruritic action: Drug is a direct competitor of histamine for binding at cellular receptor sites.

Other actions: Hydroxyzine is used as a preoperative and postoperative adjunct for its sedative, antihistaminic, and anticholinergic activity.

Pharmacokinetics
• *Absorption:* Absorbed rapidly and completely after oral administration. Peak serum levels occur within 2 to 4 hours. Sedation and other clinical effects are usually noticed in 15 to 30 minutes.
• *Distribution:* Not well understood.
• *Metabolism:* Drug is metabolized almost completely in the liver.
• *Excretion:* Drug metabolites are excreted primarily in urine; small amounts of drug and metabolites are found in feces. Half-life of drug is 3 hours. Sedative effects can last for 4 to 6 hours, and antihistaminic effects can persist for up to 4 days.

Contraindications and precautions
Contraindicated in patients hypersensitive to drug and during early pregnancy. Use cautiously with adjustments in dosage in elderly or debilitated patients.

Interactions
Hydroxyzine may add to or potentiate the effects of *alcohol, barbiturates, opioids, tranquilizers,* and other *CNS depressants;* the dose of *CNS depressants* should be reduced by 50%.

Concomitant use with other *anticholinergic drugs* causes additive anticholinergic effects.

Hydroxyzine may block the vasopressor action of *epinephrine.* If a vasoconstrictor is needed, use *norepinephrine* or *phenylephrine.*

Effects on diagnostic tests
Drug therapy causes falsely elevated urinary 17-hydroxycorticosteroid levels. It also may cause false-negative skin allergen tests by attenuating or inhibiting the cutaneous response to histamine.

Adverse reactions
CNS: *drowsiness,* involuntary motor activity.
GI: *dry mouth.*
Other: marked discomfort at I.M. injection site, ***hypersensitivity reactions*** (wheezing, dyspnea, chest tightness).

Overdose and treatment
Clinical manifestations of overdose include excessive sedation and hypotension; ***seizures*** may occur.

Treatment is supportive only. For recent oral ingestion, empty gastric contents through emesis or lavage. Correct hypotension with fluids and vasopressors (phenylephrine or metaraminol). Do not give epinephrine, because hydroxyzine may counteract its effect.

☑ Special considerations
• Observe patients for excessive sedation, especially those receiving other CNS depressants.

- Inject deep I.M. only; not for I.V., intra-arterial, or S.C. use. Aspirate injection carefully to prevent inadvertent intravascular administration.

Patient education

- Tell patient to avoid tasks that require mental alertness or physical coordination until CNS effects of drug are known; advise against use of other CNS depressants with hydroxyzine unless prescribed. Patient should avoid alcohol ingestion.
- Instruct patient to seek medical approval before taking OTC cold or allergy preparations that contain antihistamine, which may potentiate the effects of hydroxyzine.
- Advise patient to use sugarless gum or candy to help relieve dry mouth and to drink plenty of water to help with dry mouth or constipation.

Geriatric use

- Elderly patients may experience greater CNS depression and anticholinergic effects. Lower doses are indicated.

Breast-feeding

- It is unknown if drug occurs in breast milk. Safe use has not been established in breast-feeding women.

hyoscyamine

Cystospaz

hyoscyamine sulfate

Anaspaz, Cystospaz-M, Levsin, Levsin Drops, Levsinex Timecaps, Neoquess

Pharmacologic classification: belladonna alkaloid
Therapeutic classification: anticholinergic
Pregnancy risk category C

How supplied

Available by prescription only
hyoscyamine
Tablets: 0.15 mg
hyoscyamine sulfate
Tablets: 0.125 mg
Capsules (extended-release): 0.375 mg
Oral solution: 0.125 mg/ml
Elixir: 0.125 mg/5 ml
Injection: 0.5 mg/ml

Indications, route, and dosage

GI tract disorders caused by spasm; adjunctive therapy for peptic ulcers
Adults: 0.125 to 0.25 mg P.O. or S.L. q.i.d. before meals and h.s.; 0.375 to 0.75 mg P.O. (extended-release form) q 12 hours; or 0.25 to 0.5 mg I.M., I.V., or S.C. q 4 hours b.i.d. to q.i.d. (Substitute oral medication when symptoms are controlled.)
Children age 2 to 12: 0.033 mg at approximately 22 lb (10 kg); at approximately 44 lb (20 kg), 0.0625 mg; at approximately 88 lb (40 kg), 0.0938 mg; at approximately 110 lb (50 kg), 0.125 mg.
Children under age 2: 0.0125 mg at approximately 5 lb (2.3 kg); at approximately 7.5 lb (3.4 kg), 0.0167 mg; at approximately 11 lb (5 kg), 0.02 mg; at approximately 15 lb (6.8 kg), 0.025 mg; at approximately 22 lb (10 kg), 0.033 mg; at approximately 33 lb (15 kg), 0.05 mg.

Pharmacodynamics

Antispasmodic and antiulcer action: Hyoscyamine competitively blocks acetylcholine at cholinergic neuroeffector sites, decreasing GI motility and inhibiting gastric acid secretion.

Pharmacokinetics

- *Absorption:* Drug is well absorbed when taken orally; onset of action usually occurs in 20 to 30 minutes with tablets and 5 to 20 minutes with the elixir. Onset of action with parenteral administration usually occurs in 2 to 3 minutes.
- *Distribution:* Drug is well distributed throughout the body and crosses the blood-brain barrier. About 50% of dose binds to plasma proteins.
- *Metabolism:* Metabolized in the liver. Usual duration of effect is up to 4 hours with standard oral and parenteral administration and up to 12 hours for the extended-release preparation.
- *Excretion:* Drug and metabolites are excreted in the urine.

Contraindications and precautions

Contraindicated in patients with glaucoma, obstructive uropathy, obstructive disease of the GI tract, severe ulcerative colitis, myasthenia gravis, hypersensitivity to anticholinergics, paralytic ileus, intestinal atony, unstable CV status in acute hemorrhage, or toxic megacolon.

Use cautiously in patients with autonomic neuropathy, hyperthyroidism, coronary artery disease, arrhythmias, heart failure, hypertension, hiatal hernia with reflux esophagitis, hepatic or renal disease, and ulcerative colitis. Also use cautiously in hot or humid environments where drug-induced heat stroke can occur.

Interactions

Concomitant use with *amantadine* may increase such adverse anticholinergic effects as confusion and hallucinations. Concomitant use with *haloperidol* or *phenothiazines* may reduce the antipsychotic effectiveness of these drugs, possibly by direct CNS antagonism; *phenothiazines* may also increase hyoscyamine's adverse anticholinergic effects. *Antacids* and *antidiarrheals* may decrease hyoscyamine's absorption. Administer hyoscyamine 1 hour before these agents.

Effects on diagnostic tests

None reported.

Adverse reactions

CNS: headache, insomnia, drowsiness, dizziness, nervousness, weakness; *confusion, excitement* (in elderly patients).
CV: *palpitations,* tachycardia.
EENT: *blurred vision,* mydriasis, increased intraocular pressure, cycloplegia, photophobia.

GI: *dry mouth,* dysphagia, *constipation,* heartburn, loss of taste, nausea, vomiting, *paralytic ileus.*
GU: *urinary hesitancy, urine retention,* impotence.
Skin: urticaria, decreased sweating or possible anhidrosis, other dermal manifestations.
Other: fever, allergic reactions.

Note: Overdose may cause curare-like effects, such as ***respiratory paralysis.***

Overdose and treatment

Clinical signs of overdose include curare-like symptoms, central stimulation followed by depression, and such psychotic symptoms as disorientation, confusion, hallucinations, delusions, anxiety, agitation, and restlessness. Peripheral effects may include dilated, nonreactive pupils; blurred vision; flushed, hot, dry skin; dryness of mucous membranes; dysphagia; decreased or absent bowel sounds; urine retention, hyperthermia; headache; tachycardia; hypertension; and increased respiration.

Treatment is primarily symptomatic and supportive, as needed. Maintain patent airway. If patient is alert, induce emesis (or use gastric lavage) and follow with a saline cathartic and activated charcoal to prevent further drug absorption. In severe cases, physostigmine may be administered to block antimuscarinic effects. Give fluids as needed, to treat shock; diazepam to control psychotic symptoms; and pilocarpine (instilled into the eyes) to relieve mydriasis. If urine retention occurs, catheterization may be necessary.

☑ Special considerations

Besides those relevant to all *anticholinergics,* consider the following recommendations.

- Drug is usually administered P.O. but may be given I.V., I.M., S.C., or S.L. when therapeutic effect is needed or if oral administration is not possible.
- Titrate drug based on patient's response and tolerance.

Patient education

- Advise patient to avoid driving or preforming other hazardous activities if drowsiness, dizziness, or blurred vision occurs.
- Tell patient to drink fluids to avoid constipation.
- Instruct patient to report rash or other skin eruptions.

Geriatric use

- Use drug cautiously to elderly patients; lower doses are indicated.

Breast-feeding

- Drug may be excreted in breast milk, possibly resulting in infant toxicity. Avoid use in breast-feeding patients. Drug may also decrease milk production.

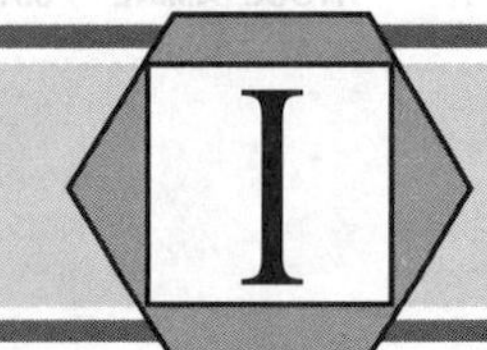

ibuprofen

Advil, Children's Advil, Medipren, Motrin, Motrin IB, Nuprin, PediaProfen, Rufen, Trendar

Pharmacologic classification: NSAID
Therapeutic classification: nonnarcotic analgesic, antipyretic, anti-inflammatory
Pregnancy risk category B (D in third trimester)

How supplied

Available without a prescription
Tablets: 200 mg
Tablets (chewable): 50 mg, 100 mg
Oral suspension: 100 mg/5 ml

Available by prescription only
Tablets: 100 mg, 300 mg, 400 mg, 600 mg, 800 mg
Oral suspension: 100 mg/5 ml
Oral drops: 40 mg/ml

Indications, route, and dosage

Arthritis, gout, and postextraction dental pain
Adults: 300 to 800 mg P.O. t.i.d. or q.i.d. Do not exceed 3,200 mg as total daily dose.
Primary dysmenorrhea
Adults: 400 mg P.O. q 4 to 6 hours.
Mild to moderate pain
Adults: 400 mg P.O. q 4 to 6 hours.
Children: 10 mg/kg P.O. q 6 to 8 hours; maximum dosage, 40 mg/kg.
Juvenile arthritis
Children: 20 to 40 mg/kg/day P.O., divided into three or four doses. For mild disease, 20 mg/kg/day in divided doses.
Fever reduction
Adults: 200 to 400 mg P.O. q 4 to 6 hours p.r.n. Do not exceed 1,200 mg/day or take more than 3 days.
Children age 6 months to 12: 5 mg/kg P.O. q 6 to 8 hours p.r.n. if baseline temperature is 102.5° F (39.2° C) or below; 10 mg/kg P.O. if baseline temperature is over 102.5° F. Recommended daily maximum dose, 40 mg/kg. Alternatively, use the accompanying dosage table.

Pharmacodynamics

Analgesic, antipyretic, and anti-inflammatory actions: Mechanisms of action are unknown; ibuprofen is thought to inhibit prostaglandin synthesis.

Pharmacokinetics

- *Absorption:* 80% of an oral dose is absorbed from the GI tract.
- *Distribution:* Ibuprofen is highly protein-bound.
- *Metabolism:* Drug undergoes biotransformation in the liver.
- *Excretion:* Excreted mainly in urine, with some biliary excretion. Plasma half-life ranges from 2 to 4 hours.

Contraindications and precautions

Contraindicated in patients with hypersensitivity to drug or in those who have the syndrome of nasal polyps, angioedema, and bronchospastic reaction to aspirin or other NSAIDs.

Use cautiously in patients with impaired renal or hepatic function, GI disorders, peptic ulcer disease, cardiac decompensation, hypertension, or known coagulation defects. Because chewable tablets contain aspartame, use cautiously in patients with phenylketonuria.

Interactions

Concomitant use of ibuprofen with *anticoagulants* and *thrombolytic drugs* (*coumarin derivatives, heparin, streptokinase, urokinase*) may potentiate anticoagulant effects. Bleeding problems may occur if ibuprofen is used with other drugs that inhibit platelet aggregation, such as parenteral *aspirin, carbenicillin, cefamandole, cefoperazone, dextran, dipyridamole, mezlocillin, piperacillin, plicamycin, salicylates, sulfinpyrazone, ticarcillin, valproic acid,* or other *anti-inflammatory agents.* Concomitant use with *salicylates, anti-inflammatory agents, alcohol, corticotropin,* or *steroids* may cause increased GI adverse effects, including ulceration and hemorrhage. *Aspirin* may decrease the bioavailability of ibuprofen.

Because of the influence of prostaglandins on glucose metabolism, concomitant use with *insulin* or *oral antidiabetic agents* may potentiate hypoglycemic effects. Ibuprofen may displace highly protein-bound drugs from binding sites. Toxicity may occur with *coumarin derivatives, nifedipine, phenytoin,* or *verapamil.* Increased nephrotoxicity may occur with *gold compounds*, other anti-inflammatory agents, or *acetaminophen.*

Ibuprofen may decrease the renal clearance of *lithium* and *methotrexate. Antacids* may decrease the absorption of ibuprofen. Ibuprofen may decrease effectiveness of *diuretics* and *antihypertensives.* Concomitant use with *diuretics* may increase nephrotoxicity. Concomitant use with *furosemide* and *thiazides* may decrease their effectiveness. Ibuprofen may reduce the blood pressure response to *ACE inhibitors* and may result in an acute reduction in renal function.

Effects on diagnostic tests

Ibuprofen's physiologic effects may prolong bleeding time; decrease blood glucose concentrations

CHILDREN'S DOSAGE OF IBUPROFEN

AGE	WEIGHT (lb)	MG	TEASPOONS
5 mg/kg for fever < 102.5° F (39.2° C)			
6 to 11 months	13 to 17	25	¼
12 to 23 months	18 to 23	50	½
2 to 3 years	24 to 35	75	¾
4 to 5 years	36 to 47	100	1
6 to 8 years	48 to 59	125	1¼
9 to 10 years	60 to 71	150	1½
11 to 12 years	72 to 95	200	2
10 mg/kg for fever > 102.5° F (39.2° C)			
6 to 11 months	13 to 17	50	½
12 to 23 months	18 to 23	100	1
2 to 3 years	24 to 35	150	1½
4 to 5 years	36 to 47	200	2
6 to 8 years	48 to 59	250	2½
9 to 10 years	60 to 71	300	3
11 to 12 years	72 to 95	350	4

(note that each ml of suspension contains 0.3 g sucrose); increase BUN, serum creatinine, and serum potassium levels; decrease serum uric acid, hemoglobin, and hematocrit levels; prolong PT; and increase serum alkaline phosphatase, serum LD, and serum transaminase levels.

Adverse reactions

CNS: *headache, dizziness,* nervousness, aseptic meningitis.
CV: *peripheral edema,* fluid retention, edema.
EENT: *tinnitus.*
GI: *epigastric distress, nausea, occult blood loss, peptic ulceration,* diarrhea, constipation, dyspepsia, flatulence, heartburn, decreased appetite.
GU: *acute renal failure*, azotemia, cystitis, hematuria.
Hematologic: prolonged bleeding time, anemia, ***neutropenia, pancytopenia, thrombocytopenia, aplastic anemia, leukopenia, agranulocytosis.***
Hepatic: elevated enzymes.
Respiratory: ***bronchospasm.***
Skin: pruritus, *rash*, urticaria, ***Stevens-Johnson syndrome***.

Overdose and treatment

Clinical manifestations of overdose include dizziness, drowsiness, paresthesia, vomiting, nausea, abdominal pain, headache, sweating, nystagmus, apnea, and cyanosis.

To treat drug overdose, empty stomach immediately by inducing emesis with ipecac syrup or by gastric lavage. Administer activated charcoal via nasogastric tube. Provide symptomatic and supportive measures (respiratory support and correction of fluid and electrolyte imbalances). Monitor laboratory parameters and vital signs closely. Alkaline diuresis may enhance renal excretion. Dialysis is of minimal value because ibuprofen is strongly protein-bound.

☑ Special considerations

Besides those relevant to all *NSAIDs,* consider the following recommendations.

- Maximum results in arthritis may require 1 to 2 weeks of continuous therapy with ibuprofen. Improvement may be seen, however, within 7 days.
- Administer drug on an empty stomach, 1 hour before or 2 hours after meals for maximum absorption. However, it may be administered with meals to lessen GI upset.
- Monitor cardiopulmonary status closely; monitor vital signs, especially heart rate and blood pressure. Observe for possible fluid retention.
- Establish safety measures, including raised side rails and supervised walking, to prevent possible injury from CNS effects.
- Monitor auditory and ophthalmic functions periodically during ibuprofen therapy.

Patient education

- Instruct patient to seek medical approval before taking OTC medications.
- Advise patient not to self-medicate with ibuprofen for longer than 10 days for analgesic use and not to exceed maximum dosage of six tablets (1.2 g) daily for self-medication. Caution patient not to take drug if fever lasts longer than 3 days unless prescribed.
- Tell patient to report adverse reactions. They are usually dose-related.
- Instruct patient in safety measures to prevent injury. Caution him to avoid hazardous activities that require mental alertness until CNS effects are known.
- Encourage patient to adhere to prescribed drug regimen and stress importance of medical follow-up.

Geriatric use

- Patients over age 60 may be more susceptible to the toxic effects of ibuprofen, especially adverse GI reactions. Use lowest possible effective dose.
- The effect of drug on renal prostaglandins may cause fluid retention and edema, a significant drawback for elderly patients, especially those with heart failure.

Pediatric use

- Safety and efficacy in children under age 6 months have not been established.

Breast-feeding

- Drug does not enter breast milk in significant quantities. However, manufacturer recommends alternative feeding methods during drug therapy.

ibutilide fumarate

Corvert

Pharmacologic classification: ibutilide derivative
Therapeutic classification: supraventricular antiarrhythmic
Pregnancy risk category C

How supplied

Available by prescription only
Injection: 0.1 mg/ml

Indications, route, and dosage

Rapid conversion of atrial fibrillation or atrial flutter of recent onset to sinus rhythm

Adults weighing 132 lb (60 kg) or more: 1 mg I.V. over 10 minutes.

Adults weighing below 132 lb: 0.01 mg/kg I.V. over 10 minutes.

Note: Infusion should be stopped if presenting arrhythmia is terminated or if sustained or nonsustained ventricular tachycardia or marked prolongation of QT or QTc occurs. If arrhythmia does not terminate within 10 minutes after infusion ends, a second 10-minute infusion of equal strength may be administered.

Pharmacodynamics

Antiarrhythmic action: An antiarrhythmic drug with predominantly class III properties, ibutilide prolongs action potential duration in isolated cardiac myocytes and increases both atrial and ventricular refractoriness.

Pharmacokinetics

- *Absorption:* Ibutilide is only given I.V.
- *Distribution:* Highly distributed and about 40% protein-bound.
- *Metabolism:* Not clearly defined.
- *Excretion:* Drug is excreted mainly in urine with the rest in feces; half-life of drug is about 6 hours.

Contraindications and precautions

Contraindicated in patients with hypersensitivity to drug or its components and history of polymorphic ventricular tachycardia, such as torsades de pointes. Use cautiously in patients with hepatic or renal dysfunction.

Interactions

Class Ia antiarrhythmic drugs (*disopyramide, quinidine, procainamide*) and other *class III drugs* (*amiodarone, sotalol)* increase the potential for prolonged refractoriness. Avoid concomitant administration and for at least five half-lives before administration of ibutilide and for 4 hours after ibutilide dosing. Supraventricular arrhythmias may mask the cardiotoxicity associated with excessive digoxin levels. Use cautiously.

Phenothiazines, tricyclic antidepressants, tetracyclic antidepressants, H_1*-receptor antagonist antihistamines*, and *other drugs that prolong QT interval* increase the risk for proarrhythmia. Monitor patient closely.

Effects on diagnostic tests

None reported.

Adverse reactions

CNS: headache.
CV: ventricular extrasystoles, nonsustained ventricular tachycardia, hypotension, bundle branch block, ***sustained ventricular tachycardia***, AV block, hypertension, QT-segment prolongation, ***bradycardia,*** palpitation, tachycardia.
GI: nausea.

Overdose and treatment

Overdosage could exaggerate the expected prolongation of repolarization seen at usual clinical doses. Treatment should be supportive and appropriate for the condition.

☑ Special considerations

- Patients with atrial fibrillation of more than 2 to 3 days' duration must be given adequate anticoagulants, generally for at least 2 weeks.
- Proper equipment and facilities, including cardiac monitoring, intracardiac pacing facilities, cardioverter-defibrillator, and medication for treatment of sustained ventricular tachycardia, should be available during and after drug administration.

• Hypokalemia and hypomagnesemia should be corrected before therapy begins to reduce the potential for proarrhythmia.
• Administer drug undiluted or diluted in 50 ml diluent; may add to 0.9% NaCl injection or D_5W injection before infusion. The contents of one 10-ml vial (0.1 mg/ml) may be also added to a 50-ml infusion bag to form an admixture of about 0.017 mg/ml ibutilide fumarate. Aseptic technique should be strictly followed during preparation of admixture. Drug is compatible with use of polyvinyl chloride plastic bags or polyolefin bags.
• Admixtures of the product, with approved diluents, are chemically and physically stable for 24 hours at room temperature and for 48 hours at refrigerated temperatures.
• Inspect parenteral drug products visually for particulate matter and discoloration before administration.
• Monitor patient's ECG continuously throughout drug administration and for at least 4 hours afterward or until QTc has returned to baseline because drug can induce or worsen ventricular arrhythmias in some patients. Longer monitoring is required if arrhythmic activity is noted.

Patient education
• Tell patient to report adverse reactions immediately.
• Instruct patient to report discomfort at I.V. injection site.

Pediatric use
• Safety and effectiveness in children under age 18 have not been established.

Breast-feeding
• It is not known if drug is excreted in breast milk; therefore, breast-feeding should be discouraged during drug therapy.

idarubicin
Idamycin

Pharmacologic classification: antibiotic antineoplastic
Therapeutic classification: antineoplastic
Pregnancy risk category D

How supplied
Available by prescription only
Injection: 5 mg, 10 mg, 20 mg (lyophilized powder) in single-dose vials with 50-, 100-, or 200-mg lactose

Indications, route, and dosage
Treatment of acute myelocytic leukemia in adults, including French-American-British classifications M1 through M7, in combination with other approved antileukemic agents
Adults: 12 mg/m² daily by slow I.V. injection (over 10 to 15 minutes) for 3 days. Administer in combination with cytarabine 100 mg/m² daily by continuous infusion for 7 days, or give cytarabine as a 25-mg/m² bolus followed by 200 mg/m² daily by continuous I.V. infusion for 5 days. A second course may be administered if needed.
✦ ***Dosage adjustment.*** If patient experiences severe mucositis, delay administration until recovery is complete and reduce dosage by 25%. Also reduce dosage in patients with hepatic or renal impairment. Idarubicin should not be given if bilirubin level is above 5 mg/dl.

Dosage and indications may vary. Check current literature for recommended protocol.

Pharmacodynamics
Antineoplastic action: Idarubicin inhibits nucleic acid synthesis by intercalation and interacts with the enzyme topoisomerase II. It is highly lipophilic, which results in an increased rate of cellular uptake.

Pharmacokinetics
• *Absorption:* Peak cellular concentrations are achieved within minutes of I.V. injection.
• *Distribution:* Drug is highly lipophilic and excessively tissue-bound (97%), with highest concentrations in nucleated blood and bone marrow cells. Its metabolite, idarubicinol, is detected in CSF; clinical significance of this is under evaluation.
• *Metabolism:* Extensive extrahepatic metabolism is indicated. Metabolite has cytotoxic activity.
• *Excretion:* Predominantly by biliary excretion as its metabolite and, to a lesser extent, by renal elimination. Mean terminal half-life is 22 hours (range, 4 to 46 hours) when used as a single agent and 20 hours (range, 7 to 38 hours) when combined with cytarabine. Plasma levels of metabolite are sustained for longer than 8 days.

Contraindications and precautions
No known contraindications. Use cautiously in patients with impaired renal or hepatic function and in those with bone marrow suppression induced by previous drug therapy or radiation therapy.

Interactions
None reported.

Effects on diagnostic tests
None reported.

Adverse reactions
CNS: *headache, changed mental status,* peripheral neuropathy, ***seizures.***
CV: ***heart failure,*** atrial fibrillation, chest pain, ***MI,*** asymptomatic decline in left ventricular ejection fraction, ***myocardial insufficiency, arrhythmias, hemorrhage, myocardial toxicity.***
GI: *nausea, vomiting, cramps, diarrhea, mucositis,* ***severe enterocolitis with perforation*** (rare).
GU: decreased renal function.
Hematologic: ***myelosuppression.***
Hepatic: changes in hepatic function.
Skin: *rash, urticaria, bullous erythrodermatous rash on palms and soles,* hives (at injection site), erythema (at previously irradiated sites), tissue necrosis at injection site (if extravasation occurs).
Other: INFECTION, *alopecia, fever,* hyperuricemia, hypersensitivity reactions.

Overdose and treatment
Severe and prolonged myelosuppression and possibly increased severity of GI toxicity are anticipated. Supportive treatment, including platelet transfusions, antibiotics, and treatment of mucositis, is required. Acute cardiac toxicity with severe arrhythmias and delayed cardiac failure may also occur. Peritoneal dialysis or hemodialysis is not effective.

☑ Special considerations
- Idarubicin should not be mixed with other drugs unless specific compatibility data is available. Heparin causes precipitation. Degradation occurs with prolonged contact with alkaline solutions.
- Frequently monitor CBC and hepatic and renal function.
- Hyperuricemia may result from rapid lysis of leukemic cells; take appropriate preventive measures (including adequate hydration) before starting treatment.
- Control systemic infections before therapy.
- Administer drug over 10 to 15 minutes into a free-flowing I.V. infusion of NaCl solution or D_5W, which is running into a large vein.
- If extravasation or signs of extravasation occur, discontinue infusion immediately and restart in another vein. Treat with intermittent ice packs—30 minutes immediately, then 30 minutes four times daily for 4 days—and evaluate affected extremity.
- Antiemetics may be used to prevent or treat nausea and vomiting.
- Reconstitute drug using 5, 10, or 20 ml NaCl solution for the 5-, 10-, or 20-mg vial, respectively, to give a final concentration of 1 mg/ml. Do not use bacteriostatic NaCl.
- Follow usual chemotherapy mixing precautions. Vial is under negative pressure.
- Reconstituted solutions are stable for 3 days (72 hours) at room temperature (59° to 86° F [15° to 30° C]); 7 days, if refrigerated. Discard unused solutions appropriately.

Patient education
- Instruct patient to recognize signs and symptoms of extravasation and to report them if they occur.
- Tell patient to report signs and symptoms of infection, including persistent fever or sore throat.
- Tell patient to minimize dangerous behavior that can cause bleeding and to report bleeding or abnormal bruising.

Pediatric use
- Safety and efficacy in children have not been established.

Breast-feeding
- It is unknown if idarubicin is excreted in breast milk. The potential for serious adverse reactions in the infant must be considered. Breast-feeding should be discontinued before starting therapy with idarubicin.

idoxuridine (IDU)
Herplex Liquifilm

Pharmacologic classification: halogenated pyrimidine
Therapeutic classification: antiviral
Pregnancy risk category C

How supplied
Available by prescription only
Ophthalmic solution: 0.1%

Indications, route, and dosage
Herpes simplex keratitis, ◊ ocular vaccinia infections, ◊ cutaneous herpes simplex
Adults and children: Instill 1 drop of solution into conjunctival sac q 1 hour during day and q 2 hours at night until improvement; then decrease to 1 drop q 2 hours during day and q 4 hours at night. Response should be seen within 7 days; if not, discontinue and begin alternative therapy. Continue therapy 5 to 7 days after healing appears to be complete. Therapy should not be continued longer than 21 days.

Pharmacodynamics
Antiviral action: Idoxuridine interferes with DNA synthesis, blocking viral reproduction.

Pharmacokinetics
- *Absorption:* Drug is poorly absorbed after instillation into the eye.
- *Distribution:* Unknown.
- *Metabolism:* Metabolized to iodouracil and iodide in the liver.
- *Excretion:* Drug is excreted by the kidney.

Contraindications and precautions
Contraindicated in patients with hypersensitivity to drug.

Interactions
When used concomitantly with *boric acid preparations,* local irritation may occur. Avoid concomitant use.

Effects on diagnostic tests
None reported.

Adverse reactions
EENT: irritation, pain, burning, or inflammation of eye; mild edema of eyelid or cornea; photophobia; small punctate defects in corneal epithelium; corneal ulceration; slowed corneal wound healing (with ointment).
Other: hypersensitivity reactions.

Overdose and treatment
Overdosage will not ordinarily cause acute problems. Should accidental overdosage in eye(s) occur, flush with water or 0.9% NaCl solution. No untoward consequences should be expected from accidental ingestion, even of the entire bottle of solution. Metabolic breakdown and excretion occur rapidly. Have patient drink fluids to dilute.

☑ Special considerations
- Drug is not intended for long-term use because it may damage corneal epithelium or inhibit ulcer healing. Do not use for more than 7 days after healing is complete, or 21 days total.
- Do not mix with other medications; do not use old solution, which may cause ocular burning and has no antiviral activity.
- Clean eye area of excessive exudate before application.

Patient education
- Tell patient to watch for signs of sensitivity, such as itching lids or constant burning, and to stop drug and report them immediately.
- Inform patient to avoid sharing washcloths and towels with family members.
- Advise patient to wash hands before and after applying solution.
- Tell patient to apply finger pressure to inside corner of the eyes for 1 minute after solution instillation, to minimize systemic absorption; patient should not close eyes tightly or blink more than usual.
- Because drug may cause sensitivity to light, advise patient to wear sunglasses in bright light.
- Tell patient to call if improvement does not occur after 14 days.

Breast-feeding
- No data available; however, breast-feeding probably should be avoided during idoxuridine therapy.

ifosfamide
Ifex

Pharmacologic classification: alkylating agent (cell cycle–phase nonspecific)
Therapeutic classification: antineoplastic
Pregnancy risk category D

How supplied
Injection: 1-g, 3-g vials

Indications, route, and dosage
Germ cell testicular cancer, ◇ lung cancer, ◇ Hodgkin's and ◇ malignant lymphoma, ◇ breast cancer, ◇ acute and ◇ chronic lymphocytic leukemia, ◇ ovarian cancer, ◇ gastric cancer, ◇ pancreatic cancer, ◇ sarcomas
Adults: 1.2 g/m²/day I.V. for 5 days. Regimen is usually repeated q 3 weeks.

Drug may be given by slow I.V. push, by intermittent infusion over at least 30 minutes, or by continuous infusion.

Dosage and indications may vary. Check current literature for recommended protocol.

Pharmacodynamics
Antineoplastic action: Ifosfamide requires activation by hepatic microsomal enzymes to exert its cytotoxic activity. The active compound cross-links strands of DNA and also breaks the DNA chain.

Pharmacokinetics
- *Absorption:* Ifosfamide is not administered orally.
- *Distribution:* Ifosfamide crosses the blood-brain barrier along with its metabolites.
- *Metabolism:* Approximately 50% of a dose is metabolized in the liver.
- *Excretion:* Drug and its metabolites are excreted primarily in the urine. The terminal half-life is reported to be about 7 hours at doses of 1.6 to 2.4 g/m²/day and about 15 hours at a single dose of 3.8 to 5 g/m².

Contraindications and precautions
Contraindicated in patients with severe bone marrow suppression or hypersensitivity to drug. Use cautiously in patients with renal or hepatic impairment, compromised bone marrow reserve as indicated by granulocytopenia, bone marrow metastases, prior radiation therapy, or therapy with cytotoxic agents.

Interactions
Concomitant use with *chloral hydrate, phenobarbital,* and *phenytoin* may increase the activity of ifosfamide by induction of hepatic microsomal enzymes, increasing the conversion of ifosfamide to its active form. Be alert for possible combined drug actions, desirable or undesirable, involving ifosfamide even though ifosfamide has been used successfully concurrently with other drugs, including *other cytotoxic drugs.*

Effects on diagnostic tests
Drug therapy may increase serum concentrations of AST, ALT, bilirubin, LD, creatinine, BUN, and alkaline phosphatase.

Adverse reactions
CNS: *somnolence, confusion,* ***coma, seizures,*** ataxia, hallucinations, depressive psychosis, dizziness, disorientation, cranial nerve dysfunction.
GI: *nausea, vomiting.*
GU: *hemorrhagic cystitis, hematuria,* ***nephrotoxicity.***
Hematologic: ***leukopenia, thrombocytopenia, myelosuppression.***
Hepatic: elevated liver enzyme levels, liver dysfunction.
Other: *alopecia, metabolic acidosis,* infection, phlebitis.

Overdose and treatment
Clinical manifestations of overdose include myelosuppression, nausea, vomiting, alopecia, and hemorrhagic cystitis.

Treatment is usually supportive and includes transfusion of blood components, antiemetics, and bladder irrigation.

☑ Special considerations
- Follow all established procedures for the safe handling, administration, and disposal of chemotherapeutic agents.
- To reconstitute 1-g vial, use 20 ml of sterile water; for a 3-g vial, use 60 ml of sterile water for in-

jection to give a concentration of 50 mg/ml. 0.9% NaCl solution may also be used for reconstitution.
- Push fluids (3 L daily) and administer with mesna (Mesnex) to prevent hemorrhagic cystitis. Avoid giving drug at bedtime, because infrequent voiding during the night may increase the possibility of cystitis. Bladder irrigation with 0.9% NaCl solution may decrease the possibility of cystitis.
- Dilutions not prepared with bacteriostatic water for injection (benzyl alcohol or parabenz preserved) should be refrigerated and used within 6 hours.
- Drug can be further diluted with D_5W or 0.9% NaCl solution for I.V. infusion. This solution is stable for 7 days at room temperature and 6 weeks at 41° F (5° C).
- Drug may be given by I.V. push injection in a minimum of 75 ml 0.9% NaCl solution over 30 minutes.
- Infusing each dose over 2 hours or longer will decrease possibility of cystitis.
- Sterile phlebitis may occur at the injection site; apply warm compresses.
- Assess patient for changes in mental status and cerebellar dysfunction. Dose may have to be decreased.
- Monitor CBC and renal and liver function tests.

Patient education
- Encourage patient to void every 2 hours during the day and twice during the night. Catheterization should be required for patient unable to void.
- Tell patient to ensure adequate fluid intake to prevent bladder toxicity and to facilitate excretion of uric acid.
- Warn patient to avoid exposure to people with infections. Tell him to report signs of infection or unusual bleeding immediately.
- Reassure patient that hair should grow back after treatment has ended.
- Tell patient to call immediately if blood appears in the urine.
- Advise both male and female patient to use contraceptive measures during therapy.

Pediatric use
- Safety and effectiveness in children have not been established.

Breast-feeding
- Ifosfamide is excreted in breast milk. Because of the potential for serious adverse reactions, mutagenicity, and carcinogenicity in the infant, breast-feeding is not recommended.

imiglucerase
Cerezyme

Pharmacologic classification: glycosidase
Therapeutic classification: replacement enzyme
Pregnancy risk category C

How supplied
Available by prescription only
Injection: 200 units/vial

Indications, route, and dosage
Long-term endogenous enzyme (glucosylceramidase) replacement therapy in patients with confirmed type I Gaucher's disease
Adults and children: Individualize dosage; initially, 2.5 to 60 U/kg I.V. administered over 1 to 2 hours. Frequency of dosing typically is once q 2 weeks, but may range from three times weekly to once monthly depending on dosage and disease severity. Dosage may be reduced for maintenance therapy at intervals of 3 to 6 months while response parameters are carefully monitored.

Pharmacodynamics
Enzymatic action: Imiglucerase catalyzes the hydrolysis of glucocerebroside to glucose and ceramide (part of the normal degradation pathway for lipids) and thus prevents the sequelae of Gaucher's disease, which are normally due to the accumulation of glucocerebroside.

Pharmacokinetics
- *Absorption:* During 1-hour I.V. infusions of four doses, steady-state enzymatic activity was achieved in 30 minutes.
- *Distribution:* Volume of distribution, based on patient weight, is 0.09 to 0.15 L/kg.
- *Metabolism:* Unknown.
- *Excretion:* Half-life is 3.6 to 10.4 minutes. Patient may develop immunoglobulin g antibodies to imiglucerase, which decrease distribution and clearance and increase elimination half-life.

Contraindications and precautions
No known contraindications. Use cautiously in patients who have exhibited symptoms of hypersensitivity to product or alglucerase and in those who have previously been treated with alglucerase or have developed antibodies to alglucerase.

Interactions
None reported.

Effects on diagnostic tests
None reported.

Adverse reactions
CNS: headache, dizziness.
CV: mild hypotension.
GI: nausea, abdominal discomfort.
GU: decreased urinary frequency.
Skin: pruritus, rash.
Other: hypersensitivity reaction.

Overdose and treatment
No information available.

☑ Special considerations
- Reconstitute each vial with 5.1 ml sterile water for injection USP. Inspect solution before use, and discard if particulate matter or discoloration exists. Dilute solution further with 0.9% NaCl to a final volume of 100 to 200 ml. Because imiglucerase is preservative-free, use immediately. Administer by I.V. infusion over 1 to 2 hours.

• When diluted to 50 ml, drug has been shown to be stable for up to 24 hours when stored at 36° to 46° F (2° to 8° C).
• Monitor response parameters to determine lowest effective dose.

Breast-feeding

• It is unknown if drug occurs in breast milk. Use with caution in breast-feeding women.

imipenem-cilastatin sodium

Primaxin I.M., Primaxin I.V.

Pharmacologic classification: carbapenem (thienamycin class); beta-lactam antibiotic
Therapeutic classification: antibiotic
Pregnancy risk category C

How supplied

Available by prescription only
Powder (for I.M. injection): 500-mg, 750-mg vial
Injection: 250-mg, 500-mg vials, ADD-Vantage, and infusion bottles

Indications, route, and dosage

Mild to moderate lower respiratory tract, skin and skin-structure, or gynecologic infections
Adults weighing at least 154 lb (70 kg): 500 to 750 mg I.M. q 12 hours.
Mild to moderate intra-abdominal infections
Adults weighing at least 154 lb: 750 mg I.M. q 12 hours.
Serious respiratory and urinary tract infections; intra-abdominal, gynecologic, bone, joint, or skin infections; bacterial septicemia; endocarditis
Adults weighing at least 154 lb: 250 mg to 1 g by I.V. infusion q 6 to 8 hours. Maximum daily dosage is 50 mg/kg/day or 4 g/day, whichever is less.
◊ *Children:* 15 to 25 mg/kg q 6 hours.
✦ ***Dosage adjustment.*** In patients with renal failure and creatinine clearance of 6 to 20 ml/minute/1.73 m^2, 125 to 250 mg I.V. q 12 hours for most pathogens. There may be an increased risk of seizures when doses of 500 mg q 12 hours are administered to these patients. When creatinine clearance is 5 ml/minute/1.73 m^2 or less, drug should not be given unless hemodialysis is instituted within 48 hours.

Note: In patients weighing less than 154 lb or those with impaired renal function, dosages vary. Check current literature for recommended protocol.

Pharmacodynamics

Antibacterial action: A bactericidal drug, imipenem inhibits bacterial cell wall synthesis. Its spectrum of antimicrobial activity includes many gram-positive, gram-negative, and anaerobic bacteria, including *Staphylococcus* and *Streptococcus species, Escherichia coli, Klebsiella, Proteus, Enterobacter* species, *Pseudomonas aeruginosa,* and *Bacteroides* species, including *B. fragilis.* Resistant bacteria include methicillin-resistant staphylococci, *Clostridium difficile,* and other *Pseudomonas* species.

Cilastatin inhibits imipenem's enzymatic breakdown in the kidneys, making it effective in treating urinary tract infections.

Pharmacokinetics

• *Absorption:* Following I.M. administration, imipenem blood levels peak within 2 hours; cilastatin levels reach their peak within 1 hour. After I.V. administration, peak levels of both agents appear in about 20 minutes. Imipenem is about 75% bioavailable and cilastatin is about 95% bioavailable after I.M. administration compared with I.V. administration.
• *Distribution:* Imipenem-cilastatin is distributed rapidly and widely. Approximately 20% of imipenem is protein-bound; 40% of cilastatin is protein-bound.
• *Metabolism:* Imipenem is metabolized by kidney dehydropeptidase I, resulting in low urine concentrations. Cilastatin inhibits this enzyme, thereby reducing imipenem's metabolism.
• *Excretion:* About 70% of imipenem-cilastatin dose is excreted unchanged by the kidneys (when imipenem is combined with cilastatin) by tubular secretion and glomerular filtration. Imipenem is cleared by hemodialysis; therefore, a supplemental dose is required after this procedure. Half-life of drug is about 1 hour after I.V. administration. The prolonged absorption that occurs after I.M. administration results in a longer half-life (2 to 3 hours).

Contraindications and precautions

Contraindicated in patients with hypersensitivity to drug. Imipenem and cilastatin sodium reconstituted with lidocaine hydrochloride for I.M. injection is contraindicated in patients with known hypersensitivity to local anesthetics of the amide type and in patients with severe shock or heart block.

Use cautiously in patients with impaired renal function, seizure disorders, or allergy to penicillins or cephalosporins.

Interactions

Chloramphenicol may impede the bactericidal effects of imipenem; give chloramphenicol a few hours after imipenem-cilastatin. *Probenecid* may prevent tubular secretion of cilastatin (but not imipenem) and thereby prolong plasma cilastatin half-life. Generalized seizures have occurred in several patients during combined imipenem-cilastatin and *ganciclovir* therapy.

Effects on diagnostic tests

Serum levels of AST, ALT, alkaline phosphatase, LD, and bilirubin may be elevated, and erythrocyte, platelet, and leukocyte counts reduced during drug therapy.

Adverse reactions

CNS: ***seizures***, dizziness, somnolence.
CV: hypotension.
GI: nausea vomiting, diarrhea, *pseudomembranous colitis.*
Hematologic: ***agranulocytosis,*** thrombocytosis.

Skin: rash, urticaria, pruritus.
Other: ***hypersensitivity reactions (anaphylaxis);*** *thrombophlebitis, pain at injection site,* fever, transient increases in liver enzymes.

Overdose and treatment

If overdosage occurs, discontinue drug, treat symptomatically, and institute supportive measures as required. Although imipenem-cilastatin sodium is hemodialyzable, its use in treating drug overdose is questionable.

☑ Special considerations

- Culture and sensitivity tests should be done before starting therapy.
- When reconstituting powder, shake until solution is clear. Solution may range from colorless to yellow; color variations within this range do not affect drug potency. After reconstitution, solution remains stable for 10 hours at room temperature and for 48 hours when refrigerated.
- Do not administer drug by direct I.V. bolus injection. Infuse 250- or 500-mg dose over 20 to 30 minutes; infuse 1-g dose over 40 to 60 minutes. If nausea occurs, slow infusion.
- Continue use of anticonvulsants in patients with known seizure disorders. Patients who exhibit CNS toxicity should receive phenytoin or benzodiazepines. Reduce dosage or discontinue drug if CNS toxicity continues.
- Drug has broadest antibacterial spectrum of any available antibiotic. It is most valuable for empiric treatment of unidentified infections and for mixed infections that would otherwise require combination of antibiotics, possibly including an aminoglycoside.
- Prolonged use may result in overgrowth of nonsusceptible organisms. In addition, use of imipenem-cilastatin as a sole course of therapy has resulted in resistance during therapy.
- Drug may be physically incompatible with aminoglycosides; avoid mixing together.

Geriatric use

- Administer cautiously to elderly patients because they may also have renal dysfunction.

Pediatric use

- Safety and effectiveness in children under age 12 have not been established; however, drug has been used in children age 3 months to 13 years. Dosage range is 15 to 25 mg/kg every 6 hours.

Breast-feeding

- It is not known if imipenem is distributed into breast milk. Administer cautiously to breast-feeding women.

imipramine hydrochloride

Apo-Imipramine*, Impril*, Novopramine*, Tofranil

imipramine pamoate

Tofranil-PM

Pharmacologic classification: dibenzazepine tricyclic antidepressant
Therapeutic classification: antidepressant
Pregnancy risk category B

How supplied

Available by prescription only
imipramine hydrochloride
Tablets: 10 mg, 25 mg, 50 mg
Injection: 25 mg/2 ml
imipramine pamoate
Capsules: 75 mg, 100 mg, 125 mg, 150 mg

Indications, route, and dosage

Depression
Adults: Initially, 75 to 100 mg P.O. or I.M. daily in divided doses, with 25- to 50-mg increments, up to 200 mg. Alternatively, some patients can start with lower doses (25 mg P.O.) and titrate slowly in 25-mg increments every other day. Maximum dosage, 300 mg daily. Alternatively, entire dosage may be given h.s. (I.M. route rarely used.) Maximum dosage is 200 mg/day for outpatients, 300 mg/day for inpatients, 100 mg/day for elderly patients.
◊ ***Childhood enuresis***
Children age 6 and over: 25 to 75 mg P.O. daily, 1 hour before bedtime. Usual dose 1.5 mg/kg/day in three divided doses. Maximum dosage, 5 mg/kg/day.

Pharmacodynamics

Antidepressant action: Imipramine is thought to exert its antidepressant effects by inhibiting reuptake of norepinephrine and serotonin in CNS nerve terminals (presynaptic neurons), which results in increased concentrations and enhanced activity of these neurotransmitters in the synaptic cleft. Drug also has anticholinergic activity and is used to treat nocturnal enuresis in children over age 6.

Pharmacokinetics

- *Absorption:* Absorbed rapidly from the GI tract and muscle tissue after oral and I.M. administration.
- *Distribution:* Imipramine is distributed widely into the body, including the CNS and breast milk. Drug is 90% protein-bound. Peak effect occurs in ½ to 2 hours; steady state is achieved within 2 to 5 days. Therapeutic plasma levels (parent drug and metabolite) are thought to range from 150 to 300 ng/ml.
- *Metabolism:* Metabolized by the liver to the active metabolite desipramine. A significant first-pass effect may explain variability of serum concentrations in different patients taking the same dosage.
- *Excretion:* Mostly excreted in urine.

Contraindications and precautions

Contraindicated during acute recovery phase of MI, in patients with hypersensitivity to drug, and in those receiving MAO inhibitors.

Use cautiously in patients at risk for suicide; in those with impaired renal or hepatic function, history of urine retention, angle-closure glaucoma, increased intraocular pressure, CV disease, hyperthyroidism, seizure disorders, or allergy to sulfites (injectable form only); and in patients receiving thyroid medications.

Interactions

Concomitant use of imipramine with *sympathomimetics*, including *epinephrine, phenylephrine, phenylpropanolamine*, and *ephedrine* (often found in nasal sprays), may increase blood pressure; use with *warfarin* may prolong PT and cause bleeding. Concomitant use with *pimozide, thyroid medication*, and *antiarrhythmic agents* (*quinidine, disopyramide, procainamide*) may increase incidence of arrhythmias and conduction defects.

Imipramine may decrease hypotensive effects of *centrally acting antihypertensive drugs*, such as *clonidine, guanabenz, guanadrel, guanethidine, methyldopa*, and *reserpine*. Concomitant use with *disulfiram* or *ethchlorvynol* may cause delirium and tachycardia.

Additive effects are likely after concomitant use of imipramine with *CNS depressants*, including *alcohol, analgesics, barbiturates, narcotics, tranquilizers*, and *anesthetics* (oversedation); *atropine* or other *anticholinergic drugs*, including *antihistamines, meperidine, phenothiazines*, and *antiparkinsonian agents* (oversedation, paralytic ileus, visual changes, and severe constipation); or *metrizamide* (increased risk of seizures).

Barbiturates and *heavy smoking* induce imipramine metabolism and decrease therapeutic efficacy; *haloperidol* and *phenothiazines* decrease its metabolism, decreasing therapeutic efficacy. *Beta blockers, cimetidine, methylphenidate, oral contraceptives*, and *propoxyphene* may inhibit imipramine metabolism, increasing plasma levels and toxicity.

Effects on diagnostic tests

Imipramine may prolong conduction time (elongation of QT and PR intervals, flattened T waves on ECG); it also may elevate liver function test results, decrease WBC counts, and decrease or increase serum glucose levels.

Adverse reactions

CNS: *drowsiness, dizziness*, excitation, tremor, confusion, hallucinations, anxiety, ataxia, paresthesia, nervousness, EEG changes, ***seizures***, extrapyramidal reactions.
CV: *orthostatic hypotension, tachycardia, ECG changes*, hypertension, ***MI, stroke, arrhythmias, heart block, precipitation of heart failure.***
EENT: blurred vision, tinnitus, mydriasis.
Endocrine: gynecomastia (in males), galactorrhea and breast enlargement (in females), altered libido, impotence, testicular swelling, increased or decreased blood sugars, inappropriate antidiuretic hormone secretion syndrome.
GI: *dry mouth, constipation*, nausea, vomiting, anorexia, paralytic ileus, abdominal cramps.
GU: *urine retention.*
Skin: rash, urticaria, photosensitivity, pruritus.
Other: *diaphoresis*, ***hypersensitivity reaction.***

After abrupt withdrawal of long-term therapy: nausea, headache, malaise (does not indicate addiction).

Overdose and treatment

Drug overdose is frequently life-threatening, particularly when combined with alcohol. The first 12 hours after acute ingestion are a stimulatory phase characterized by excessive anticholinergic activity (agitation, irritation, confusion, hallucinations, hyperthermia, parkinsonian symptoms, seizure, urine retention, dry mucous membranes, pupillary dilatation, constipation, and ileus). This is followed by CNS depressant effects, including hypothermia, decreased or absent reflexes, sedation, hypotension, cyanosis, and cardiac irregularities, including tachycardia, conduction disturbances, and quinidine-like effects on the ECG.

Severity of overdose is best indicated by widening of the QRS complex, which usually represents a serum level in excess of 1,000 ng/ml; serum concentrations are usually not helpful. Metabolic acidosis may follow hypotension, hypoventilation, and seizures.

Treatment is symptomatic and supportive, including maintaining airway, stable body temperature, and fluid or electrolyte balance. Induce emesis if patient is conscious; follow with gastric lavage and activated charcoal to prevent further absorption. Dialysis is of little use.

Treat seizures with parenteral diazepam or phenytoin and arrhythmias with parenteral phenytoin or lidocaine. Quinidine, procainamide, and atropine are not to be used during an overdose. Treat acidosis with sodium bicarbonate. Do not give barbiturates; these may enhance CNS and respiratory depressant effects.

☑ Special considerations

Besides those relevant to all *tricyclic antidepressants*, consider the following recommendations.
- Drug may be used to treat nocturnal enuresis in children.
- Imipramine is associated with a high incidence of orthostatic hypotension. Check sitting and standing blood pressures after initial dose.
- Drug should not be withdrawn abruptly, but tapered gradually over time.
- Tolerance to drug's sedative effects usually develops over several weeks.
- Drug should be discontinued at least 48 hours before surgical procedures.

Patient education

- Tell patient to take drug exactly as prescribed.
- Explain that full effects of drug may not become apparent for up to 4 to 6 weeks after initiation of therapy.
- Warn patient not to discontinue drug abruptly, not to share drug with others, and not to drink alcoholic beverages while taking drug.
- Advise patient to take drug with food or milk if it causes stomach upset.

• Suggest relieving dry mouth with sugarless chewing gum or hard candy. Encourage good dental prophylaxis because persistent dry mouth may lead to increased incidence of dental caries.
• Encourage patient to report unusual or troublesome effects immediately, including confusion, movement disorders, rapid heartbeat, dizziness, fainting, or difficulty urinating.

Geriatric use
• Recommended dosage is 30 to 40 mg P.O. daily, not to exceed 100 mg daily. Initiate therapy at low doses (10 mg) and titrate slowly. Elderly patients may be at greater risk for adverse cardiac reactions.

Pediatric use
• Drug is not recommended for treating depression in patients under age 12. Do not use pamoate salt for enuresis in children.

Breast-feeding
• Imipramine is excreted in breast milk in low concentrations. The potential benefit to the mother should outweigh possible risks to the infant.

immune globulin (gamma globulin, IG, immune serum globulin, ISG)

immune globulin for I.M. use (IGIM)
Gamastan, Gammar

immune globulin for I.V. use (IGIV)
Gamimune N (5%, 10%), Gammagard S/D, Gammar- P IV, Iveegam, Polygam S/D, Sandoglobulin, Venoglobulin-I, Venoglobulin-S

Pharmacologic classification: immune serum
Therapeutic classification: stimulates antibody production
Pregnancy risk category C

How supplied
Available by prescription only
IGIM
Injection: 2-ml, 10-ml vials
IGIV
I.V.: Gamimune N—5% and 10% solution in 10-ml, 50-ml, 100-ml, and 250-ml single-use vials; Gammagard S/D—2.5-g, 5-g, and 10-g single-use vials for reconstitution; Gammar-P IV—1-g, 2.5-g, and 5-g vials with diluent and 10-g vials with administration set and diluent; Iveegam—1-g, 2.5-g, and 5-g vials with diluent; Polygam S/D—2.5-g, 5-g, and 10-g single-use vials with diluent; Sandoglobulin—1-g, 3-g, 6-g, and 12-g vials or kits with diluent or bulk packs without diluent; Venoglobulin-I—2.5-g and 5-g vials with or without reconstitution kits with sterile water, 10-g vials with reconstitution kit and administration set, and 0.5-g vials with reconstitution kit; Venoglobulin-S—5% and 10% in 50-ml, 100-ml, and 200-ml vials.

Indications, route, and dosage
Agammaglobulinemia, hypogammaglobulinemia, immune deficiency (IGIV)
Adults and children: For Gamimune N only, 100 to 200 mg/kg or 2 to 4 ml/kg I.V. infusion monthly. Infusion rate is 0.01 to 0.02 ml/kg/minute for 30 minutes. Rate can then be increased to maximum of 0.08 ml/kg/minute for remainder of infusion.

For Gammagard S/D only, initially 200 to 400 mg/kg I.V., followed by 100 mg/kg monthly. Initiate infusion at 0.5 ml/kg/hour, gradually increasing to maximum of 4 ml/kg/hour.

For Gammar-P IV only, 200 to 400 mg/kg q 3 to 4 weeks. Infusion rate is 0.01 ml/kg/minute, increasing to 0.02 ml/kg/minute after 15 to 30 minutes, with gradual increase to 0.06 ml/kg/minute.

For Iveegam only, 200 mg/kg I.V. monthly. If response is inadequate, doses may be increased up to 800 mg/kg or the drug may be administered more frequently. Infuse at 1 to 2 ml/minute.

For Polygam S/D only, 100 mg/kg I.V. monthly. An initial dose of 200 to 400 mg/kg may be administered. Initiate infusion at 0.5 ml/kg/hour, gradually increasing to maximum of 4 ml/kg/hour.

For Sandoglobulin only, 200 mg/kg I.V. monthly. Start with 0.5 to 1 ml/minute of a 3% solution; increase up to 2.5 ml/minute gradually after 15 to 30 minutes.

For Venoglobulin-I only, 200 mg/kg I.V. monthly; may be increased to 300 to 400 mg/kg and may be repeated more frequently than once monthly. Infuse at 0.01 to 0.02 ml/kg/minute for 30 minutes, then increase to 0.04 ml/kg/minute or higher if tolerated.

For Venoglobulin-S only, 200 mg/kg I.V. monthly. Increase dose to 300 to 400 mg/kg monthly or administer more frequently if adequate IgI levels are not achieved. Initiate infusion at 0.01 to 0.02 ml/kg/minute for 30 minutes, then increase 5% solutions to 0.04 ml/kg/minute and 10% solutions to 0.05 ml/kg/minute if tolerated.
Hepatitis A exposure (IGIM)
Adults and children: 0.02 to 0.04 ml/kg I.M. as soon as possible after exposure. Up to 0.1 ml/kg may be given after prolonged or intense exposure.
Measles exposure (IGIM)
Adults and children: 0.25 ml/kg within 6 days after exposure.
Postexposure prophylaxis of measles (IGIM)
Adults and children: 0.5 ml/kg I.M. within 6 days after exposure.
Chickenpox exposure (IGIM)
Adults and children: 0.6 to 1.2 ml/kg I.M. as soon as exposed.
Rubella exposure in first trimester of pregnancy (IGIM)
Women: 0.55 ml/kg I.M. as soon as exposed.
Idiopathic thrombocytopenic purpura (IGIV)
Adults and children: 400 mg/kg Sandoglobulin I.V. for 2 to 5 consecutive days; or 400 mg/kg Gamimune N 5% for 5 days or 1,000 mg/kg Gamimune N 10% for 1 to 2 days. Maintenance dose is 400 to 1,000

mg/kg I.V. of Gamimune N 10% as a single infusion to maintain a platelet count greater than 30,000/mm³.

Bone marrow transplantation (IGIV)

Adults over age 20: Gamimune N 10%, 500mg/kg on day 7 and day 2 before transplantation; then weekly through 90 days posttransplant.

Pharmacodynamics

Immune action: Immune globulin provides passive immunity by increasing antibody titer. The mechanism by which IGIV increases platelet counts in idiopathic thrombocytopenic purpura is not fully known.

Pharmacokinetics

- *Absorption:* After slow I.M. absorption, serum concentrations peak within 2 days.
- *Distribution:* Distributes evenly between intravascular and extravascular spaces.
- *Metabolism:* Unknown.
- *Excretion:* Serum half-life is reportedly 21 to 24 days in immunocompetent patients.

Contraindications and precautions

Contraindicated in patients hypersensitive to drug.

Interactions

Concomitant use of immune globulin may interfere with the immune response to live *virus vaccines* (for example, *measles, mumps, rubella*). Do not administer live virus vaccines within 3 months after administration of immune globulin.

Effects on diagnostic tests

None reported.

Adverse reactions

CNS: headache.
GI: nausea, vomiting.
Respiratory: dyspnea, shortness of breath.
Skin: erythema, urticaria.
Other: malaise, fever, ***anaphylaxis,*** chills, chest pain, hip pain, faintness, chest tightness, joint pain, muscle stiffness (at injection site).

Overdose and treatment

Excessively rapid I.V. infusion rate can precipitate an anaphylactoid reaction.

☑ Special considerations

- Obtain a thorough history of allergies and reactions to immunizations.
- Epinephrine solution 1:1,000 should be available to treat allergic reactions.
- Inject I.M. formulation into different sites, preferably into buttocks. Do not inject more than 3 ml per injection site.
- Do not give for hepatitis A exposure if 2 weeks or more have elapsed since exposure or after onset of clinical illness.
- Closely monitor blood pressure in patient receiving IGIV, especially if it is patient's first infusion of immune globulin.
- Immune globulin has not been associated with an increased frequency of AIDS. It is devoid of HIV. Immune globulin recipients do not develop antibodies to HIV.
- Although pregnancy is not a contraindication to use, it is unknown if immune globulin can cause fetal harm.
- Store Sandoglobulin and Gammagard S/D at room temperature not exceeding 77° F (25° C); Gamimune-N and Iveegam, at 36° to 46° F (2° to 8° C) but do not freeze; Gammar-P IV, at room temperature below 86° F (30° C) but do not freeze; Venoglobulin- at room temperature below 86° F.
- Immune globulin has been studied in the treatment of various conditions, including Kawasaki disease, asthma, allergic disorders, autoimmune neutropenia, myasthenia gravis, and platelet transfusion rejection. It also has been used in the prophylaxis of infections in immunocompromised patients.
- Gamimune N can be diluted with D_5W.
- Reconstitute Gammagard S/D with diluent (sterile water for injection) and transfer device provided by manufacturer. Administration set (provided) contains a 15-micron in-line filter that must be used during administration.
- Reconstitute Sandoglobulin with diluent supplied (0.9% NaCl).

Patient education

- Explain that patient's chances of getting AIDS or hepatitis after receiving immune globulin are minute.
- Tell patient what to expect after vaccination: some local pain, swelling, and tenderness at the injection site. Recommend acetaminophen to ease minor discomfort.
- Instruct patient to promptly report headache, skin changes, or difficulty breathing.

Breast-feeding

- It is not known if immune globulin distributes into breast milk. Use with caution in breast-feeding women.

indapamide

Lozol

Pharmacologic classification: thiazide-like diuretic
Therapeutic classification: diuretic, antihypertensive
Pregnancy risk category B

How supplied

Available by prescription only
Tablets: 1.25 mg, 2.5 mg

Indications, route, and dosage

Edema of heart failure

Adults: 2.5 mg P.O. as a single daily dose taken in the morning; increase dosage to 5 mg daily after 1 week if response is poor.

Hypertension

Adults: 1.25 mg P.O. as a single daily dose taken in the morning; increase dosage to 2.5 mg daily after 4 weeks if response is poor. Maximum daily dose, 5 mg.

Pharmacodynamics

Diuretic action: Indapamide increases urinary excretion of sodium and water by inhibiting sodium reabsorption in the cortical diluting tubule of the nephron, thus relieving edema.

Antihypertensive action: Exact mechanism of indapamide's antihypertensive effect is unknown. This effect may result from direct arteriolar vasodilatation, via calcium channel blockade. Indapamide also reduces total body sodium.

Pharmacokinetics

- *Absorption:* After oral administration, drug is absorbed completely from the GI tract; peak serum levels occur at 2 to 2½ hours
- *Distribution:* Distributes widely into body tissues because of its lipophilicity; drug is 71% to 79% plasma protein-bound.
- *Metabolism:* Indapamide undergoes significant hepatic metabolism.
- *Excretion:* About 60% of a dose of drug is excreted in urine within 48 hours; approximately 16% to 23% is excreted in feces.

Contraindications and precautions

Contraindicated in patients with anuria or hypersensitivity to other sulfonamide-derived drugs. Use cautiously in patients with severe impaired renal or hepatic function and progressive hepatic disease.

Interactions

Indapamide potentiates the hypotensive effects of most other *antihypertensive drugs*; this may be used to therapeutic advantage.

Indapamide may potentiate hyperglycemic, hypotensive, and hyperuricemic effects of *diazoxide*, and its hyperglycemic effect may increase *insulin* or *sulfonylurea* requirements in diabetic patients.

Indapamide may reduce renal clearance of *lithium*, elevating serum lithium levels, and may necessitate reduction in lithium dosage by 50%.

Indapamide turns urine slightly more alkaline and may decrease urinary excretion of some amines, such as *amphetamine* and *quinidine*; alkaline urine may also decrease therapeutic efficacy of *methenamine compounds* such as *methenamine mandelate.*

Cholestyramine and *colestipol* may bind indapamide, preventing its absorption; give drugs 1 hour apart.

Effects on diagnostic tests

Indapamide therapy may alter serum electrolyte levels and may increase serum urate, glucose, cholesterol, and triglyceride levels. It also may interfere with tests for parathyroid function and should be discontinued before such tests.

Adverse reactions

CNS: headache, nervousness, dizziness, lightheadedness, weakness, vertigo, restlessness, drowsiness, fatigue, anxiety, depression, numbness of extremities, irritability, agitation.
CV: volume depletion and dehydration, orthostatic hypotension, palpitations, premature ventricular contractions, irregular heartbeat, vasculitis.
GI: anorexia, nausea, epigastric distress, vomiting, abdominal pain, diarrhea, constipation.
GU: nocturia, polyuria, frequent urination, impotence.
Skin: *rash*, pruritus, flushing.
Other: muscle cramps and spasms; asymptomatic hyperuricemia; fluid and electrolyte imbalances, including dilutional hyponatremia and hypochloremia, metabolic alkalosis, hypokalemia; gout; rhinorrhea; weight loss.

Overdose and treatment

Clinical signs of overdose include GI irritation and hypermotility, diuresis, and lethargy, which may progress to coma.

Treatment is mainly supportive; monitor and assist respiratory, CV, and renal function as indicated. Monitor fluid and electrolyte balance. Induce vomiting with ipecac in conscious patient; otherwise, use gastric lavage to avoid aspiration. Do not give cathartics; these promote additional loss of fluids and electrolytes.

☑ Special considerations

Recommendations for use of indapamide and for care and teaching of the patient during therapy are the same as those for all *thiazide* and *thiazide-like diuretics.*

Geriatric use

- Elderly and debilitated patients require close observation and may require reduced dosages. They are more sensitive to excess diuresis because of age-related changes in CV and renal function. Excess diuresis promotes orthostatic hypotension, dehydration, hypovolemia, hyponatremia, hypomagnesemia, and hypokalemia.

Pediatric use

- Safety and effectiveness in children have not been established.

Breast-feeding

- Drug is distributed into breast milk; its safety and effectiveness in breast-feeding women have not been established.

indinavir sulfate

Crixivan

Pharmacologic classification: HIV protease inhibitor
Therapeutic classification: antiviral
Pregnancy risk category C

How supplied

Available by prescription only
Capsules: 200 mg, 400 mg

Indications, route, and dosage

Treatment of patients with HIV infection when antiretroviral therapy is warranted
Adults: 800 mg P.O. q 8 hours.

✦ ***Dosage adjustment.*** Reduce dosage to 600 mg P.O. q 8 hours in patients with mild to moderate hepatic insufficiency due to cirrhosis.

Pharmacodynamics

Antiviral action: Indinavir sulfate is an inhibitor of HIV protease, an enzyme required for the proteolytic cleavage of the viral polyprotein precursors into the individual functional proteins found in infectious HIV. Indinavir binds to the protease active site and inhibits the activity of the enzyme. This inhibition prevents cleavage of the viral polyproteins, resulting in the formation of immature noninfectious viral particles.

Pharmacokinetics

- *Absorption:* Indinavir is rapidly absorbed in the GI tract when it is administered on an empty stomach. A meal high in calories, fat, and protein significantly interferes with drug absorption, whereas lighter meals do not.
- *Distribution:* About 60% of drug is plasma protein-bound.
- *Metabolism:* Indinavir is metabolized to at least seven metabolites. Cytochrome P-450 3A4 (CYP3A4) is the major enzyme responsible for formation of the oxidative metabolites.
- *Excretion:* Less than 20% of drug is excreted unchanged in urine.

Contraindications and precautions

Contraindicated in patients with hypersensitivity to any component of drug. Use cautiously in patients with hepatic insufficiency due to cirrhosis.

Interactions

Indinavir should not be administered concurrently with *astemizole, cisapride, midazolam,* or *triazolam,* because competition for CYP3A4 by indinavir could result in inhibition of the metabolism of these drugs and create the potential for serious or life-threatening events, such as arrhythmias or prolonged sedation.

Indinavir causes an increase in the plasma concentrations of *rifabutin.* Therefore, a dosage reduction of rifabutin is necessary if administered concomitantly with indinavir. Because rifampin is a potent inducer of CYP3A4, which could markedly diminish plasma concentrations of indinavir, coadministration of indinavir and rifampin is not recommended.

Ketoconazole causes an increase in the plasma concentrations of indinavir. A dosage reduction of indinavir should be considered when they are coadministered.

If indinavir and *didanosine* are administered concomitantly, they should be administered at least 1 hour apart on an empty stomach; a normal (acidic) gastric pH may be necessary for optimum absorption of indinavir, whereas acid rapidly degrades didanosine, which is formulated with buffering agents to increase pH.

Effects on diagnostic tests

None reported.

Adverse reactions

CNS: headache, insomnia, dizziness, somnolence, asthenia, fatigue.
GI: abdominal pain, *nausea,* diarrhea, vomiting, acid regurgitation, anorexia, dry mouth.
GU: nephrolithiasis.
Hematologic: decreased hemoglobin, platelet count, or neutrophil count.
Other: *hyperbilirubinemia; flank* pain; malaise; back pain; taste perversion; elevations in ALT, AST, and serum amylase.

Overdose and treatment

No information available.

☑ Special considerations

- Dosage of indinavir is the same whether drug is used alone or in combination with other antiretroviral agents. However, antiretroviral activity of indinavir may be increased when used in combination with approved reverse transcriptase inhibitors.
- Drug must be taken at 8-hour intervals.
- When administering rifabutin concomitantly, the dose of rifabutin should be reduced by half. However, when administering ketoconazole concomitantly, dosage of indinavir should be decreased to 600 mg q 8 hours.
- Drug may cause nephrolithiasis. If signs and symptoms of nephrolithiasis occur, consider stopping drug for 1 to 3 days during the acute phase. To prevent nephrolithiasis, patient should maintain adequate hydration.

Patient education

- Inform patient that indinavir is not a cure for HIV infection. He may continue to develop opportunistic infections and other complications associated with HIV disease. Drug has also not been shown to reduce risk of transmitting HIV to others through sexual contact or blood contamination.
- Caution patient not to adjust dosage or discontinue indinavir therapy without medical approval.
- Advise patient that if a dose of indinavir is missed, he should take the next dose at the regularly scheduled time and should not double the dose.
- Instruct patient to take drug on an empty stomach with water 1 hour before or 2 hours after a meal. Alternatively, he may take it with other liquids (such as skim milk, juice, coffee, or tea) or with a light meal. Inform patient that a meal high in calories, fat, and protein reduces the absorption of indinavir.
- Tell patient to store capsules in the original container and to keep the desiccant in the bottle because the capsules are sensitive to moisture.
- Instruct patient to consume at least 1.5 L of fluid daily.

Pediatric use

- Safety and effectiveness in children have not been established.

Breast-feeding

- Indinavir may be excreted in breast milk. Because of the potential for indinavir to cause adverse effects in nursing infants, breast-feeding is not recommended. In addition, an HIV-positive woman should not breast-feed to prevent transmitting the infection to the infant.

indomethacin, indomethacin sodium trihydrate

Apo-Indomethacin*, Indameth, Indochron E-R, Indocid*, Indocin, Indocin SR, Novomethacin*

Pharmacologic classification: NSAID
Therapeutic classification: nonnarcotic analgesic, antipyretic, anti-inflammatory
Pregnancy risk category NR

How supplied

Available by prescription only
Capsules: 25 mg, 50 mg
Capsules (sustained-release): 75 mg
Suspension: 25 mg/5 ml
Injection: 1-mg vials
Suppositories: 50 mg

Indications, route, and dosage

Moderate to severe arthritis, ankylosing spondylitis
Adults: 25 mg P.O. b.i.d. or t.i.d. with food or antacids; may increase dose by 25 to 50 mg daily q 7 days up to 200 mg daily; or 50 mg P.R. q.i.d. Alternatively, sustained-release capsules may be given: 75 mg to start, in the morning or h.s., followed, if necessary, by 75 mg b.i.d.

Acute gouty arthritis
Adults: 50 mg t.i.d. Reduce dose as soon as possible, then stop it. Do not use sustained-release capsules for this condition.

To close a hemodynamically significant patent ductus arteriosus in premature infants (I.V. form only)
Newborn age under 48 hours: 0.2 mg/kg I.V. followed by 2 doses of 0.1 mg/kg at 12- to 24-hour intervals.
Newborn age 2 to 7 days: 0.2 mg/kg I.V. followed by 2 doses of 0.2 mg/kg at 12- to 24-hour intervals.
Newborn over age 7 days: 0.2 mg/kg I.V. followed by 2 doses of 0.25 mg/kg at 12- to 24-hour intervals.

Acute shoulder pain
Adults: 75 to 150 mg P.O. b.i.d. or t.i.d. with food or antacids; usual treatment is 7 to 14 days.

◊ ***Dysmenorrhea***
Adults: 25 mg P.O. t.i.d. with food or antacids.

◊ ***Bartter's syndrome***
Adults: 150 mg/day P.O. with food or antacids.
Children: 0.5 to 2 mg/kg in divided doses.

Pharmacodynamics

Analgesic, antipyretic, and anti-inflammatory actions: Exact mechanisms of action are unknown; indomethacin is thought to produce its analgesic, antipyretic, and anti-inflammatory effects by inhibiting prostaglandin synthesis and possibly by inhibiting phosphodiesterase.

Closure of patent ductus arteriosus: Exact mechanism of action is unknown, but is believed to be through inhibition of prostaglandin synthesis.

Pharmacokinetics

- *Absorption:* Drug is absorbed rapidly and completely from the GI tract.
- *Distribution:* Drug is highly protein-bound.
- *Metabolism:* Metabolized in the liver.
- *Excretion:* Mainly in urine; some biliary excretion.

Contraindications and precautions

Contraindicated in patients with hypersensitivity to drug or history of aspirin- or NSAID-induced asthma, rhinitis, or urticaria; in pregnancy or while breast-feeding. Also contraindicated in infants with untreated infection, active bleeding, coagulation defects or thrombocytopenia, congenital heart disease in whom patency of the ductus arteriosus is necessary for satisfactory pulmonary or systemic blood flow, necrotizing enterocolitis, or impaired renal function. Suppositories contraindicated in patients with history of proctitis or recent rectal bleeding.

Use cautiously in the elderly and in patients with history of GI disease, impaired renal or hepatic function, epilepsy, parkinsonism, CV disease, infection, mental illness, or depression.

Interactions

Concomitant use of indomethacin with *anticoagulants* and *thrombolytic drugs* (such as *coumarin derivatives, heparin, streptokinase, urokinase*) may potentiate anticoagulant effects. Bleeding problems may occur if indomethacin is used with other drugs that inhibit platelet aggregation, such as *aspirin, parenteral carbenicillin, cefamandole, cefoperazone, dextran, dipyridamole, mezlocillin, piperacillin, plicamycin, salicylates, sulfinpyrazone, ticarcillin, valproic acid,* or *other anti-inflammatory agents.* Concomitant use with *salicylates, anti-inflammatory agents, alcohol, corticotropin,* or *steroids* may cause increased GI adverse effects, including ulceration and hemorrhage. *Aspirin* may decrease the bioavailability of indomethacin.

Because of the influence of prostaglandins on glucose metabolism, concomitant use with *insulin* or *oral antidiabetic agents* may potentiate hypoglycemic effects. Indomethacin may displace highly protein-bound drugs from binding sites. Toxicity may occur with *coumarin derivatives, nifedipine, phenytoin,* or *verapamil.* Increased nephrotoxicity may occur with *gold compounds, other anti-inflammatory agents,* or *acetaminophen.* Indomethacin may decrease the renal clearance of *methotrexate* and *lithium.*

Concurrent use with *antihypertensives* and *diuretics* may decrease their effectiveness. Concurrent use with *triamterene* not recommended due to potential nephrotoxicity. Other *diuretics* may also predispose patients to nephrotoxicity.

Effects on diagnostic tests

Drug therapy may interfere with dexamethasone suppression test results. It may also interfere with urinary 5-hydroxyindoleacetic acid determinations.

Adverse reactions

Oral and rectal forms:
CNS: *headache, dizziness,* depression, drowsiness, confusion, somnolence, fatigue, peripheral

neuropathy, ***seizures,*** psychic disturbances, syncope, *vertigo.*
CV: hypertension, *edema, **heart failure.***
EENT: blurred vision, corneal and retinal damage, hearing loss, tinnitus.
GI: *nausea,* anorexia, *diarrhea, peptic ulceration, **GI bleeding,*** constipation, dyspepsia, ***pancreatitis.***
GU: hematuria, ***acute renal failure,*** proteinuria, interstitial nephritis.
Hematologic: ***hemolytic anemia, aplastic anemia, agranulocytosis, leukopenia, thrombocytopenic purpura,*** iron-deficiency anemia.
Skin: pruritus, urticaria, ***Stevens-Johnson syndrome.***
Other: hypersensitivity (rash, respiratory distress, ***anaphylaxis, angioedema***), hyperkalemia.
I.V. form:
GU: proteinuria, interstitial nephritis.

Overdose and treatment

Clinical manifestations of overdose include dizziness, nausea, vomiting, intense headache, mental confusion, drowsiness, tinnitus, sweating, blurred vision, paresthesias, and seizures.

To treat indomethacin overdose, empty stomach immediately by inducing emesis with ipecac syrup or by gastric lavage. Administer activated charcoal via nasogastric tube. Provide symptomatic and supportive measures (respiratory support and correction of fluid and electrolyte imbalances). Monitor laboratory parameters and vital signs closely. Dialysis may be of little value because indomethacin is strongly protein-bound.

☑ Special considerations

Besides those relevant to all *NSAIDs,* consider the following recommendations.

- Do not mix oral suspension with liquids or antacids before administering.
- Patient should retain suppository in the rectum for at least 1 hour after insertion to ensure maximum absorption.
- Reconstitute 1 mg vial of I.V. dose with 1 to 2 ml of sterile water for injection or 0.9% NaCl injection. Prepare solution immediately before use to prevent deterioration. Do not use solution if it is discolored or contains a precipitate.
- Administer drug by direct I.V. injection over 5 to 10 seconds. Use a large vein to prevent extravasation.
- Monitor I.V. site for complications.
- Monitor cardiopulmonary status for significant changes. Watch for signs and symptoms of fluid overload. Check weight and intake and output daily.
- Monitor renal function studies before start of therapy and frequently during therapy to prevent adverse effects.
- Severe headache may occur. If headache persists, dose should be decreased.
- I.V. administration should be used only for premature neonates with patent ductus arteriosus. Do not administer a second or third I.V. dose if anuria or marked oliguria exists.
- If ductus arteriosus reopens, a second course of one to three doses may be given. If ineffective, surgery may be necessary.
- Monitor carefully for bleeding and for reduced urine output.

Patient education

- Instruct patient in proper administration of dosage form prescribed, such as suppository, sustained-release capsule, or suspension.
- Advise patient to seek medical approval before taking OTC medications.
- Caution patient to avoid hazardous activities that require alertness or concentration. Instruct him in safety measures to prevent injury.
- Tell patient to report signs and symptoms of adverse reactions. Encourage patient to adhere to prescribed drug regimen and recommended follow-up.

Geriatric use

- Patients over age 60 may be more susceptible to the toxic effects of indomethacin.
- The effect of drug on renal prostaglandins may cause fluid retention and edema, a significant drawback for elderly patients and those with heart failure.

Pediatric use

- Safety of long-term drug use in children under age 14 has not been established.
- Use of I.V. indomethacin in premature infants for patent ductus arteriosus is considered an alternative to surgery.

Breast-feeding

- Drug is secreted into breast milk in concentrations similar to those in maternal plasma; avoid use in breast-feeding women.

influenza virus vaccine, 1998-1999 trivalent types A & B (purified surface antigen)

Fluvirin

influenza virus vaccine, 1998-1999 trivalent types A & B (subvirion or purified subvirion)

Fluogen, FluShield, Fluzone

influenza virus vaccine, 1998-1999 trivalent types A & B (whole virion)

Fluzone

Pharmacologic classification: vaccine
Therapeutic classification: viral vaccine
Pregnancy risk category C

How supplied

Available by prescription only
Injection: 0.5 ml prefilled syringe; 5-ml vials

Indications, route, and dosage

Annual influenza prophylaxis in high-risk patients

Adults and children age 9 and over: 0.5 ml I.M.
Children age 3 to 8: 0.5 ml I.M.
Children age 6 to 35 months: 0.25 ml I.M.
Note: Second dose may be given in previously unvaccinated children under age 9 at least 1 month after first dose.

Check package insert for annual changes and additional dosing recommendations.

Pharmacodynamics

Influenza prophylaxis: Vaccine promotes active immunity to influenza by inducing antibody production. Protection is provided only against those strains of virus from which the vaccine is prepared (or closely related strains).

Pharmacokinetics

- *Absorption:* Duration of immunity varies widely but usually lasts about 1 year.
- *Distribution:* No information available.
- *Metabolism:* No information available.
- *Excretion*: No information available.

Contraindications and precautions

Contraindicated in patients with hypersensitivity to chicken eggs or any component of the vaccine such as thimersol. Defer vaccination in patients with acute respiratory or other active infection and delay immunization in those with an active neurologic disorder.

Interactions

Concomitant use of influenza vaccine with *corticosteroids* or *immunosuppressants* may impair the immune response to the vaccine.

Influenza vaccine may decrease serum *phenytoin* and *aminopyrine* levels and increase serum *theophylline* levels.

Rarely, patients receiving *warfarin* concomitantly with influenza vaccine have demonstrated prolonged PT, GI bleeding, transient gross hematuria, and epistaxis.

Effects on diagnostic tests

No information available.

Adverse reactions

Other: ***anaphylaxis,*** fever, malaise, myalgia, erythema, induration, and *soreness at injection site.*

Fever and malaise reactions occur most often in children and in others not exposed to influenza viruses. Severe reactions in adults are rare.

Overdose and treatment

No information available.

☑ Special considerations

- Annual influenza prophylaxis is recommended for elderly persons and for adults and children with chronic CV, pulmonary, or renal disorders; metabolic disease; severe anemia; or compromised immune function. Vaccine also is recommended for medical personnel who have extensive contact with high-risk patients, residents of nursing homes or other chronic care facilities, and teenagers or children (age 6 months through 18 years) who are receiving long-term aspirin therapy and may be at risk of Reye's syndrome after influenza. Also, vaccine should be given to persons who wish to reduce their risk of acquiring an influenza infection.
- Obtain a thorough history of allergies, especially to eggs or chicken feathers, and of reactions to previous immunizations.
- Patients with a known or suspected hypersensitivity to egg protein should have a skin test to assess sensitivity to vaccine. Administer a scratch test with 0.05 to 0.1 ml of a 1:100 dilution in 0.9% NaCl solution for injection. Patients with positive skin test reactions should not receive the influenza virus vaccine.
- Epinephrine solution 1:1,000 should be available to treat allergic reactions.
- Influenza vaccine should not be administered to patients with active influenza infection. Such infection should be treated with amantadine.
- Preferred I.M. injection site is the deltoid muscle in adults and older children and the anterolateral thigh in infants and young children.
- To reduce the frequency of adverse reactions, use only the split-virus or purified surface antigen vaccine in children.
- Pneumococcal vaccine, DTP, or live attenuated measles virus vaccine may be given simultaneously but at a different injection site.
- Store vaccine between 36° and 46° F (2° and 8° C). Do not freeze.

Patient education

- Tell patient that he may experience discomfort at the injection site after immunization; he also may develop fever, malaise, and muscle aches 6 to 12 hours after vaccination that may persist for several days. Recommend acetaminophen to alleviate these effects.
- Encourage patient to report distressing adverse reactions promptly.
- Warn patient that many cases of Guillain-Barré syndrome were reported after vaccination for the swine flu of 1976. This condition usually causes reversible paralysis and muscle weakness, but it can be fatal in some individuals. Influenza vaccines made after 1976 have not been associated with as high an incidence of Guillain-Barré syndrome, but the condition still occurs, albeit rarely. Patients with history of Guillain-Barré syndrome have a greater risk for repeat episodes.
- Tell patient that he will need to be vaccinated annually.

Geriatric use

- Annual vaccination is highly recommended for patients over age 65.

Pediatric use

- Influenza vaccine is contraindicated in children under age 6 months.

Breast-feeding

• Breast-feeding is not a contraindication for receiving vaccine.

insulin (regular)

Humulin-R, Novolin R, Novolin R PenFill, Pork Regular Iletin II, Regular Iletin I, Regular (Concentrated) Iletin II, Regular Insulin, Regular Purified Pork Insulin, Velosulin Human

insulin (lispro)

Humalog

prompt insulin zinc suspension (semilente)

Iletin Semilente*

isophane insulin suspension (NPH)

Humulin N, NPH Iletin*, NPH Iletin I, NPH Insulin*, NPH-N, Novolin N, Novolin N PenFill, Pork NPH Iletin II

insulin zinc suspension (lente)

Humulin L, Lente Iletin I, Lente Iletin II, Lente L, Novolin L

protamine zinc insulin suspension (PZI)

Iletin PZI*

extended zinc insulin suspension (ultralente)

Humulin U Ultralente, Ultralente*

isophane insulin suspension and insulin injection (70% isophane insulin and 30% insulin injection)

Humulin 70/30, Novolin 70/30, Novolin 70/30 PenFill

isophane insulin suspension and insulin injection (50% isophane insulin and 50% insulin injection)

Humulin 50/50

Pharmacologic classification: pancreatic hormone
Therapeutic classification: antidiabetic
Pregnancy risk category NR

How supplied

Available without a prescription
insulin (regular)
Injection (pork): 100 units/ml, 500 units/ml
Injection (beef, pork): 100 units/ml
Injection (human): 100 units/ml
insulin (lispro)
Injection (human): 100 units/ml
Cartridge (human): 1.5 ml
prompt insulin zinc suspension (semilente)
Injection (beef, pork): 100 units/ml
isophane insulin suspension (NPH)
Injection (pork): 100 units/ml
Injection (beef, pork): 100 units/ml
Injection (human): 100 units/ml
insulin zinc suspension (lente)
Injection (pork): 100 units/ml
Injection (beef): 100 units/ml
Injection (beef, pork): 100 units/ml
Injection (human): 100 units/ml
PZI
Injection (beef, pork): 100 units/ml
extended zinc insulin suspension (ultralente)
Injection (pork): 100 units/ml
Injection (beef, pork): 100 units/ml
Injection (human): 100 units/ml
Available by prescription only
regular (concentrated) Iletin II insulin
Injection (pork): 500 units/ml

Indications, route, and dosage

Diabetic ketoacidosis (regular insulin)
Adults: Administer loading dose of 0.15 units/kg I.V. followed by 0.1 units/kg/hour as a continuous infusion. Rate of insulin infusion should be decreased when plasma glucose concentration reaches 300 mg/dl. Infusion of D_5W should be started separately from the insulin infusion when plasma glucose reaches 250 mg/dl. Thirty minutes before discontinuing insulin infusion, a dose of insulin should be administered S.C.; intermediate-acting insulin is recommended.

Alternative dosage schedule is 50 to 100 units I.V. and 50 to 100 units S.C. immediately; subsequent doses should be based on therapeutic response and glucose, acetone, or ketone levels monitored at 1- to 2-hour intervals, or 2.4 to 7.2 units I.V. loading dose followed by 2.4 to 7.2 units/hour.
Children: 0.5 to 1 unit/kg in two divided doses, one given I.V. and the other S.C., followed by 0.5 to 1 unit/kg I.V. q 1 to 2 hours; or 0.1 unit/kg I.V. bolus, then 0.1 unit/kg/hour continuous I.V. infusion until blood sugar drops to 250 mg/dl; then start S.C. insulin.

Ketosis-prone and juvenile-onset diabetes mellitus, diabetes mellitus inadequately controlled by diet and oral antidiabetics
Adults and children: Individualized dosage adjusted based on patient's blood and urine glucose levels.

Hyperkalemia
Adults: 5 to 10 units of regular insulin with 50 ml of D_5W over 5 minutes. Alternatively, 25 units of regular insulin given S.C. and an infusion of 1,000 ml dextrose 10% in water with 90 mEq sodium bicarbonate; infuse 330 ml over 30 minutes and the balance over 3 hours.

Provocative test for growth hormone secretion
Adults: Rapid I.V. injection of regular insulin 0.05 to 0.15 units/kg.

Pharmacodynamics

Antidiabetic action: Insulin is used as a replacement for the physiologic production of endogenous insulin in patients with insulin-dependent diabetes mellitus (IDDM) and diabetes mellitus inadequately controlled by diet and oral hypoglycemic agents. Insulin increases glucose transport across muscle and fat-cell membranes to reduce blood glucose levels. It also promotes conversion of glucose to its storage form, glycogen; triggers amino acid uptake and conversion to protein in muscle cells and inhibits protein degradation; stimulates triglyceride formation and inhibits release of free fatty acids from adipose tissue; and stimulates lipoprotein lipase activity, which converts circulating lipoproteins to fatty acids. Insulin is available in various forms and these differ mainly in onset, peak, and duration of action. Characteristics of the various insulin preparations are compared in the chart on the next page.

Pharmacokinetics

- *Absorption:* Insulin must be given parenterally because it is destroyed in the GI tract. Commercially available preparations are formulated to differ in onset, peak, and duration after subcutaneous administration. They are classified as rapid-acting (½ to 1-hour onset), intermediate-acting (1- to 2-hour onset), and long-acting (4- to 8-hour onset). The accompanying chart summarizes major pharmacokinetic differences.
- *Distribution:* Insulin is distributed widely throughout the body.
- *Metabolism:* Some insulin is bound and inactivated by peripheral tissues, but the majority appears to be degraded in the liver and kidneys.
- *Excretion:* Insulin is filtered by the renal glomeruli and undergoes some tubular reabsorption. Plasma half-life is about 9 minutes after I.V. administration.

Contraindications and precautions

None reported.

Interactions

Alcohol, anabolic steroids, beta blockers, clofibrate, fenfluramine, MAO inhibitors, salicylates, and *tetracycline* can cause a prolonged hypoglycemic effect. Monitor blood glucose carefully.

Corticosteroids, dextrothyroxine sodium, epinephrine, and *thiazide diuretics* can diminish insulin response. Monitor for hyperglycemia.

Effects on diagnostic tests

The physiologic effects of insulin may decrease serum magnesium, potassium, or inorganic phosphate concentrations.

Adverse reactions

Skin: urticaria, pruritus, swelling, redness, stinging, warmth at injection site.

Other: *lipoatrophy, lipohypertrophy,* hypersensitivity reactions ***(anaphylaxis,*** rash), ***hypoglycemia,*** hyperglycemia (rebound, or Somogyi, effect).

Overdose and treatment

Insulin overdose may produce signs and symptoms of hypoglycemia (tachycardia, palpitations, anxiety, hunger, nausea, diaphoresis, tremors, pallor, restlessness, headache, and speech and motor dysfunction). Treatment is directed toward treating hypoglycemia. Treatment is based on patient's symptoms. If patient is responsive, give 10 to 15 g of a fast-acting oral carbohydrate. If patient's signs and symptoms persist after 15 minutes, give an additional 10 g carbohydrate. If patient is unresponsive, an I.V. bolus of dextrose 50% solution should immediately increase blood glucose. Some prefer to use dextrose 25% in water because it is less irritating should extravasation occur. A common infusion rate is based on glucose content: 10 to 20 mg/kg/minute. Parenteral glucagon or epinephrine S.C. may also be given; both drugs raise blood glucose levels in a few minutes by stimulating glycogenolysis. Fluid and electrolyte imbalance may require I.V. fluids and electrolyte (such as potassium) replacement.

☑ Special considerations

- Accuracy of measurement is very important, especially with regular insulin concentrated. Aids, such as magnifying sleeve, dose magnifier, or cornwall syringe, may help improve accuracy.
- With regular insulin concentrated, a secondary hypoglycemic reaction may occur 18 to 24 hours after injection. This may be caused by a repository effect of drug and the high concentration of insulin in the preparation (500 units/ml).
- Dosage is always expressed in USP units.
- Human insulin may be advantageous for patients who are allergic to pork or beef forms, for noninsulin-dependent patients requiring intermittent or short-term therapy (such as pregnancy, surgery, infection, or total parenteral nutrition therapy), for patients with insulin resistance, or for those who develop lipoatrophy.
- Do not interchange single-source beef or pork insulins without considering the need for dosage adjustment.
- Lente, semilente, and ultralente insulins may be mixed in any proportion.
- Regular insulin may be mixed with NPH or lente insulins in any proportion. However, in vitro binding will occur over time until an equilibrium is reached. These mixtures should be administered either immediately after preparation or after stability occurs (15 minutes for NPH regular, 24 hours for lente regular) in order to minimize variability in patient response. Note that switching from separate injections to a prepared mixture also may alter the patient's response. When mixing two insulins, always draw regular insulin into the syringe first.
- Lispro insulin may be mixed with Humulin N or Humulin U and should be given within 15 minutes before a meal to prevent a hypoglycemic reaction. The effects of mixing lispro insulin with insulins of animal source or insulin preparations produced by other manufacturers have not been studied and may require a change in dosage.

COMPARING INSULIN PREPARATIONS

The chart below lists the various forms of insulin and their times of onset, peak, and duration. Individual responses can vary.

PREPARATION	PURIFIED*	ONSET	PEAK	DURATION
Rapid-acting insulins				
insulin injection (regular, crystalline zinc)				
Regular Iletin I	No	½ hr	2 to 4 hr	6 to 8 hr
Regular Insulin	No	½ hr	2½ to 5 hr	8 hr
Pork Regular Iletin II	Yes	½ hr	2 to 4 hr	6 to 8 hr
Velosulin BR Human	Yes	½ hr	1 to 3 hr	8 hr
Regular Purified Pork Insulin	Yes	½ hr	2½ to 5 hr	8 hr
Humulin R	N.A.	½ hr	2 to 4 hr	6 to 8 hr
Novolin R/Novolin R PenFill	N.A.	½ hr	2½ to 5 hr	8 hr
insulin injection (lispro)				
Humalog	Yes	< ½ hr	½ to 1½ hr	< 6 hr
prompt insulin zinc suspension (semilente)				
Iletin Semilente	No	1 to 3 hr	2 to 8 hr	12 to 16 hr
Intermediate-acting insulins				
isophane insulin suspension (NPH)				
NPH Iletin I	No	1 to 2 hr	6 to 12 hr	18 to 24 hr
NPH Insulin	No	1½ hr	4 to 12 hr	24 hr
Pork NPH Iletin II	Yes	1 to 2 hr	6 to 12 hr	18 to 24 hr
Humulin N	N.A.	1 to 2 hr	6 to 12 hr	18 to 24 hr
Novolin N/Novolin N PenFill	N.A.	1½ hr	4 to 12 hr	24 hr
insulin zinc suspension (lente)				
Lente Iletin I	No	1 to 3 hr	6 to 12 hr	18 to 24 hr
Lente Iletin II	Yes	1 to 3 hr	6 to 12 hr	18 to 24 hr
Lente L	Yes	2½ hr	7 to 15 hr	22 hr
Humulin L	N.A.	1 to 3 hr	6 to 12 hr	18 to 24 hr
Novolin L	N.A.	2½ hr	7 to 15 hr	22 hr
isophane (NPH) 70%, regular insulin 30%				
Humulin 70/30	N.A.	½ hr	4 to 8 hr	24 hr
Novolin 70/30/Novolin 70/30 PenFill	N.A.	½ hr	2 to 12 hr	24 hr
isophane (NPH) 50%, regular insulin 50%				
Humulin 50/50	N.A.	½ hr	4 to 8 hr	24 hr
Long-acting insulins				
protamine zinc insulin suspension				
Iletin PZI	No	4 to 8 hr	14 to 24 hr	36 hr or more
extended insulin zinc suspension (ultralente)				
Ultralente	No	4 hr	10 to 30 hr	36 hr
Humulin U Ultralente	Yes	4 to 6 hr	8 to 20 hr	24 to 28 hr

N.A. indicates not applicable.
*Purified insulins contain < 10 ppm proinsulin.

• Store insulin in cool area. Refrigeration desirable but not essential, except with regular insulin concentrated.
• Do not use insulin that has changed color or becomes clumped or granular in appearance.
• Check expiration date on vial before using contents.
• Administration route is S.C. because it allows slower absorption and causes less pain than I.M. injections. Ketosis-prone, juvenile-onset, severely ill, and newly diagnosed diabetics with very high blood sugar levels may require hospitalization and I.V. treatment with regular fast-acting insulin. Ketosis-resistant diabetics may be treated as outpatients with intermediate-acting insulin after they have received instructions on how to alter dosage according to self-performed urine or blood glucose determinations. Some patients, primarily pregnant or brittle diabetics, may use a dextrometer to perform fingerstick blood glucose tests at home.
• Press but do not rub site after injection. Rotate injection sites. Record sites to avoid overuse of one area. However, unstable diabetics may achieve better control if injection site is rotated within same anatomic region.
• To mix insulin suspension, swirl vial gently or rotate between palms or between palm and thigh. Do not shake vigorously; this causes bubbling and air in syringe.
• In pregnant diabetic patients, insulin requirements increase, sometimes drastically, then decline immediately postpartum.
• Some patients may develop insulin resistance and require large insulin doses to control symptoms of diabetes. U-500 insulin is available for such patients as Purified Pork Iletin Regular Insulin, U-500. Although every pharmacy may not normally stock it, it is readily available. Patient should notify pharmacist several days before prescription refill is needed. Give hospital pharmacy sufficient notice before refill of inhouse prescription. Never store U-500 insulin in same area with other insulin preparations because of danger of severe overdose if given accidentally to other patients. U-500 insulin must be administered with a U-100 syringe because no syringes are made for this drug.
• Human insulin may be advantageous in patients who are allergic to pork or beef forms. Humulin is synthesized by a genetically altered strain of Escherichia coli. Novolin brands are derived by enzymatic alteration of pork insulin.

Patient education

• Be sure patient knows that insulin therapy relieves symptoms but does not cure the disease.
• Tell patient about nature of disease, importance of following therapeutic regimen, specific diet, weight reduction, exercise, personal hygiene, avoiding infection, and timing of injection and eating.
• Instruct patient to strictly adhere to manufacturer's instructions regarding assembly, administration, and care of specialized delivery systems, such as insulin pumps.
• Emphasize importance of regular meal times and that meals must not be omitted.
• Teach patient that blood glucose monitoring is an essential guide to correct dosage and to therapeutic success.
• Emphasize importance of recognizing hypoglycemic symptoms because insulin-induced hypoglycemia is hazardous and may cause brain damage if prolonged.
• Advise patient to always wear a medical identification bracelet or pendant, to carry ample insulin supply and syringes on trips, to have carbohydrates (sugar or candy) on hand for emergency, and to note time-zone changes for dose schedule when traveling.
• Instruct patient not to change the order of mixing insulins or change the model or brand of syringe or needle. Be sure he knows when mixing two insulins, always draw regular insulin into the syringe first.
• Inform patient that use of marijuana may increase insulin requirements.
• Inform patient that cigarette smoking decreases absorption of insulin administered S.C. Advise him not to smoke within 30 minutes after insulin injection.

interferon alfa-n3

Alferon N

Pharmacologic classification: biological response modifier
Therapeutic classification: antineoplastic
Pregnancy risk category C

How supplied

Available by prescription only
Injection: 5 million IU/ml in 1-ml vials

Indications, route, and dosage

Treatment of condylomata acuminata
Adults: 0.05 ml (250,000 IU) per wart injected using a 30G needle into the base of each wart twice weekly for up to 8 weeks. For large warts, inject at several points around the periphery of the wart using a total dose of 0.5 ml per wart. Maximum dose for each treatment is 0.5 ml per wart.

Note: Be sure to check literature for current protocol.

Pharmacodynamics

Antineoplastic action: The interferons are naturally occurring small-protein molecules produced and secreted by cells in response to viral infections and biological inducers. They bind to specific membrane receptors on cell surfaces to initiate a series of events that include induction of protein synthesis, which is then followed by various cellular responses (inhibition of virus replication, suppression of cell proliferation, immunomodulation, enhanced phagocytosis, augmentation of lymphocytic cytotoxicity, and enhancement of human leukocyte antigen expression). Exact mechanism of action is undetermined.

Pharmacokinetics

- *Absorption:* After intralesional injection, plasma concentrations are below detectable levels, but systemic effects indicate that some systemic absorption does occur.
- *Distribution:* Unknown.
- *Metabolism:* Unknown.
- *Excretion:* Unknown.

Contraindications and precautions

Contraindicated in patients hypersensitive to interferon alfa and in those with history of anaphylactic reactions to murine (mouse) immunoglobulin, egg protein, or neomycin. Use cautiously in patients with debilitating illnesses such as heart failure, unstable angina, pulmonary disease, coagulation or seizure disorders, myelosuppression, or diabetes mellitus with ketoacidosis.

Interactions

None reported.

Effects on diagnostic tests

Decreases in WBC counts have been reported. The following laboratory values were abnormal in cancer patients: hemoglobin, WBC count, platelet counts, gamma-glutamyl transferase, AST, alkaline phosphatase, and total bilirubin.

Adverse reactions

CNS: dizziness, light-headedness, insomnia, depression.
CV: hypotension.
GI: dyspepsia, heartburn, vomiting, nausea, diarrhea.
Other: *acute hypersensitivity reactions with mild to moderate flulike syndrome (myalgia, fever, chills, fatigue, headache), arthralgia, back pain, malaise, soreness at injection site, chest pains.*

Overdose and treatment

No information available.

☑ Special considerations

- Interferon alfa-n3 has been used for many unlabeled indications: hairy cell leukemia, bladder tumors, carcinoid tumors, chronic myelogenous leukemia, cutaneous T-cell lymphoma, essential thrombocythemia, malignant lymphoma (low grade), cervical carcinoma, chronic lymphocytic leukemia, acute leukemias, osteosarcoma, Kaposi's sarcoma related to acquired immunodeficiency syndrome, malignant gliomas, melanoma, multiple myeloma, nasopharyngeal sarcoma, ovarian carcinoma, renal carcinoma, cutaneous warts, cytomegaloviruses, herpes keratoconjunctivitis, herpes simplex, papillomaviruses, rhinoviruses, vaccinia virus, varicella zoster, viral hepatitis B, and chronic hepatitis C.
- Different brands of interferons may not be therapeutically interchangeable.
- Almost all patients experience flulike symptoms, which diminish with continued therapy.
- Genital warts usually begin to disappear after several weeks of therapy, but treatment should continue for the full 8 weeks. In patients who experience partial resolution during treatment, further resolution occurs after treatment ends. Of those patients who experienced complete resolution, half had complete resolution by the end of treatment; the rest within 3 months post-treatment.
- Do not administer further treatment for 3 months after first course of therapy unless warts enlarge or new warts appear.
- Flulike symptoms are relieved by acetaminophen.
- Interferon alfa-n3 is manufactured from pooled units of human leukocytes induced by incomplete infection with an avian virus. Donors are screened to minimize risk of HIV and hepatitis B. There are no reported incidents of HIV or hepatitis B transmission.
- Store drug in refrigerator; do not freeze. Do not shake.
- Use 30G needle to administer drug.

Patient education

- Tell patient to watch for signs of anaphylaxis (local or generalized hives, tightness of the chest, wheezing, and dizziness or weakness) and to report them if they occur.
- Advise patient of risks and benefits of therapy.

Pediatric use

- Safety and efficacy in children have not been established.

Breast-feeding

- It is unknown if drug is excreted in breast milk; the potential for serious adverse reactions in the infant must be considered.

interferon alfa-2a, recombinant

Roferon-A

interferon alfa-2b, recombinant

Intron A

Pharmacologic classification: biological response modifier
Therapeutic classification: antineoplastic
Pregnancy risk category C

How supplied

Available by prescription only
alfa-2a
Solution for injection: 3 million IU/vial, 9 million IU/vial, 9 million IU/multidose vial, 18 million IU/multidose vial, 36 million IU/multidose vial
Powder for injection with diluent: 18 million IU/multidose vial
alfa-2b
Powder for injection with diluent: 3 million IU/vial; 5 million IU/vial; 10 million IU/vial; 18 million IU/multidose vial; 25 million IU/vial; 50 million IU/vial
Solution for injection: 10 million IU/vial, 18 million IU/multidose vial, 25 million IU/vial

Indications, route, and dosage

Hairy cell leukemia

alfa-2a

Adults: For induction, 3 million IU S.C. or I.M. daily for 16 to 24 weeks. For maintenance, 3 million IU S.C. or I.M. three times weekly.

alfa-2b

Adults: For induction and maintenance, 2 million IU/m^2 I.M. or S.C. three times weekly.

Condylomata acuminata

alfa-2b

Adults: 1 million IU per lesion, intralesionally, three times weekly for 3 weeks.

Kaposi's sarcoma

alfa-2a

Adults: For induction, 36 million IU S.C. or I.M. daily for 10 to 12 weeks; for maintenance, 36 million IU three times weekly.

alfa-2b

Adults: 30 million IU/m^2 S.C. or I.M. three times weekly. Maintain dose unless disease progresses rapidly or intolerance occurs.

Chronic hepatitis C

Adults: 3 million IU (alfa-2b) S.C. or I.M. three times weekly. If response occurs, continue therapy for 6 months. If no response by 16 weeks, discontinue therapy.

Chronic hepatitis B

Adults: 30 to 35 million IU (alfa-2b) S.C. or I.M. weekly either as 5 million IU daily or 10 million IU three times weekly for 16 weeks.

Pharmacodynamics

Antineoplastic action: Interferon alfa is a sterile protein product produced by recombinant DNA techniques applied to genetically engineered *Escherichia coli* bacteria. The interferons are naturally occurring small protein molecules produced and secreted by cells in response to viral infections or synthetic and biological inducers. Their exact mechanism of action is unknown but appears to involve direct antiproliferative action against tumor cells or viral cells to inhibit replication and modulation of host immune response by enhancing the phagocytic activity of macrophages and augmenting specific cytotoxicity of lymphocytes for target cells. To date, three major classes of interferons have been identified: alfa, beta, and gamma.

Pharmacokinetics

- *Absorption:* More than 80% of dose is absorbed after I.M. or S.C. injection.
- *Distribution:* Not applicable.
- *Metabolism:* Drug appears to be metabolized in the liver and kidney.
- *Excretion:* Drug is reabsorbed from glomerular filtrate with minor biliary elimination.

Contraindications and precautions

Contraindicated in patients hypersensitive to drug or to murine (mouse) immunoglobulin. Use cautiously in patients with CV or pulmonary disease, diabetes mellitus, coagulation disorders, or myelosuppression.

Interactions

When used concomitantly, interferons may enhance the CNS effects of *CNS depressants.*

Concurrent use with a *live virus vaccine* may potentiate replication of vaccine virus, increase adverse effects, and decrease patient's antibody response.

Bone marrow depressant effects may be increased when used with *blood dyscrasia–causing medications, bone marrow depressant therapy,* or *radiation therapy.* Dosage reduction may be required. Interferon may substantially increase the half-life of *methylxanthines* (including *aminophylline, theophylline*), perhaps by interfering with the cytochrome P-450 drug metabolizing enzymes.

Effects on diagnostic tests

Interferon therapy may cause mild and transient alterations of blood pressure (hypotension is likely). Interferons may decrease hemoglobin, hematocrit, leukocyte counts, platelets, and neutrophils (dose-related; recovery occurs within several days or weeks after withdrawal of interferon). Interferons may prolong PT and partial thromboplastin time (dose-related); ALT, AST, LD, and alkaline phosphatase levels (dose-related; reversible on withdrawal of interferon); and serum calcium, serum phosphorus, and fasting blood glucose levels.

Adverse reactions

CNS: *dizziness, confusion,* paresthesia, numbness, lethargy, *depression, decreased mental status,* forgetfulness, ***coma,*** nervousness, insomnia, sedation, apathy, anxiety, irritability, fatigue, vertigo, gait disturbances, incoordination.

CV: hypotension, chest pain, ***arrhythmias,*** palpitations, syncope, ***heart failure,*** hypertension, edema, ***MI.***

EENT: *dryness or inflammation of the oropharynx,* rhinorrhea, sinusitis, conjunctivitis, earache, eye irritation.

GI: *anorexia, nausea, diarrhea, vomiting,* abdominal fullness, *abdominal pain,* flatulence, constipation, hypermotility, gastric distress, *weight loss, change in taste.*

GU: transient impotence.

Hematologic: ***leukopenia, mild thrombocytopenia.***

Hepatic: ***hepatitis.***

Respiratory: *cough, dyspnea.*

Skin: *rash, dryness, pruritus, partial alopecia,* urticaria, flushing.

Other: inflammation at injection site (rare), flulike syndrome (fever, fatigue, *myalgia, headache, chills, arthralgia),* diaphoresis, excessive salivation, cyanosis, night sweats, hot flashes.

Overdose and treatment

No information available.

☑ Special considerations

- When preparing antineoplastic agents for injection, take special precautions because of their potential for carcinogenicity and mutagenicity. Use of a biological containment cabinet is recommended. Do not shake vials.

• S.C. administration route should be used in patients whose platelet count is below 50,000/mm³.
• Different brands of interferons may not be therapeutically interchangeable.
• Almost all patients experience flulike symptoms at the beginning of therapy; these effects tend to diminish with continued therapy.
• Make sure patient is well hydrated, especially during initial stages of treatment. Premedicate patient with acetaminophen to minimize flulike symptoms.
• Dosage reduction may be needed if headache persists. Hypotension may result from fluid depletion; may require supportive treatment.
• Administration of drug at bedtime minimizes inconvenience of fatigue.
• Monitor blood pressure, BUN, hematocrit, platelet count, ALT, AST, LD, alkaline phosphatase, serum bilirubin, creatinine, uric acid, total and differential leukocyte count, and ECG.
• Monitor for CNS adverse reactions, such as decreased mental status and dizziness. Periodic neuropsychiatric monitoring is recommended.
• Special precautions required for patients who develop thrombocytopenia: exercise extreme care in performing invasive procedures; inspect injection site and skin frequently for signs of bruising; limit frequency of I.M. injections; test urine, emesis fluid, stool, and secretions for occult blood.
• When using interferon alfa-2b for condylomata acuminata by intralesional injection, use only the 10 million-IU vial reconstituted with 1 ml of diluent. Using other strengths or more diluent would produce a hypertonic solution. For administration, use a 25G to 30G needle and a tuberculin syringe. Up to five lesions may be treated simultaneously.
• The following indications are not included in U.S. labeling, but drug may be used for these applications: chronic myelocytic leukemia; treatment of renal carcinoma or superficial bladder carcinoma; treatment of malignant lymphomas, especially nodular, poorly differentiated types; malignant melanoma; multiple myeloma; mycosis fungoides; papillomas; and laryngeal papillomatosis (interferon alfa-2b).

Patient education
• Review patient instruction sheet if patient is to self-administer, to ensure patient understanding of when and how to take medication. Stress importance of drinking extra fluids to prevent hypotension from fluid loss.
• Instruct patient in proper oral hygiene during treatment, because the bone marrow depressant effects of interferon may result in increased incidence of microbial infection, delayed healing, and gingival bleeding. A decrease in salivary flow may also occur.
• Advise patient not to take a missed dose or to double the next dose, but to call for further instructions.
• If patient is to self-administer drug, teach him to prepare injection, how to use disposable syringe, proper administration technique, and stability of drug.
• Inform patient to store drug in refrigerator; keep from freezing.
• Caution patient against driving or performing tasks requiring alertness until response to medication is known.
• Advise patient to seek medical approval before taking OTC medications for colds, coughs, allergies, and similar disorders; explain that interferons commonly cause flulike symptoms and patient may need to take acetaminophen before each dose.
• Emphasize need to follow instructions about taking and recording temperature, and how and when to take acetaminophen; not to have any immunization; and to avoid contact with persons who have taken oral polio vaccine. Because the body's resistance may be compromised, infection may occur.
• Tell patient drug may cause temporary loss of some hair. Normal hair growth should return when drug is discontinued.
• Inform patient to avoid use of aspirin and chronic alcohol intake because these may increase risk of GI bleeding.

Geriatric use
• Neurotoxicity and cardiotoxicity are more common in elderly patients, especially those with underlying CNS or cardiac impairment.

Pediatric use
• Safety and efficacy in children under age 18 have not been established.

Breast-feeding
• Risk-to-benefit ratio must be considered. Drug is usually not recommended in breast-feeding women because of the potential for serious adverse effects on breast-fed infants.

interferon beta-1a
Avonex

Pharmacologic classification: biological response modifier
Therapeutic classification: antiviral, immunoregulator
Pregnancy risk category C

How supplied
Available by prescription only
Lyophilized powder for injection: 33 mcg (6.6 million IU) of interferon beta-1a

Indications, route, and dosage
To slow progression of physical disability and decrease the frequency of clinical exacerbations in relapsing multiple sclerosis
Adults: 30 mcg I.M. once weekly.

Pharmacodynamics
Antiviral/immunoregulator actions: The mechanisms by which interferon beta-1a exerts its actions in multiple sclerosis are not clearly understood. However, it is known that the biological response-modifying properties of interferon beta-1a are mediated through its interactions with specific cell receptors found on the surface of human cells. The binding to these receptors induces the expression of a num-

ber of interferon-induced gene products that are believed to be the mediators of the biological actions of interferon beta-1a.

Pharmacokinetics

- *Absorption:* No information available.
- *Distribution:* No information available.
- *Metabolism:* No information available.
- *Excretion:* No information available.

Contraindications and precautions

Contraindicated in patients with history of hypersensitivity to natural or recombinant interferon beta, human albumin, or any other component of the formulation. Use cautiously in patients with depression, seizure disorders, or severe cardiac conditions.

Interactions

None reported.

Effects on diagnostic tests

None reported.

Adverse reactions

CNS: *headache, sleep difficulty, dizziness,* syncope, suicidal tendency, seizure, speech disorder, ataxia.
CV: chest pain, vasodilation.
EENT: otitis media, decreased hearing.
GI: *nausea, diarrhea, dyspepsia,* anorexia, abdominal pain.
GU: ovarian cyst, vaginitis.
Hematologic: anemia, elevated eosinophil levels, decreased hematocrit.
Musculoskeletal: *muscle ache,* muscle spasm, arthralgia.
Respiratory: *upper respiratory tract infection,* sinusitis, dyspnea.
Skin: ecchymosis (at injection site), urticaria, alopecia, nevus, herpes zoster, herpes simplex.
Other: *flulike symptoms, pain, fever, asthenia, chills, infection,* injection site reaction, malaise, hypersensitivity reaction, elevated AST levels.

Overdose and treatment

No information available.

☑ Special considerations

- Safety and efficacy of interferon beta-1a in chronic progressive multiple sclerosis have not been evaluated.
- Use of interferon beta-1a may cause depression and suicidal ideation. It is not known whether these symptoms may be related to the underlying neurologic basis of multiple sclerosis, to interferon beta-1a treatment, or to a combination of both. Closely monitor patient for these symptoms and consider cessation of therapy if they occur.
- Monitor patient with cardiac disease, such as angina, heart failure, or arrhythmia, for worsening of clinical condition during initiation of therapy. Although drug does not have any known direct-acting cardiac toxicity, it does cause flulike symptoms, which may be stressful to patients with severe cardiac conditions.
- Exert caution when administering drug to patients with preexisting seizure disorders.
- The following laboratory tests are recommended before initiating therapy and at periodic intervals thereafter: complete and differential WBC counts, platelet counts, and blood chemistries, including liver function tests.
- To reconstitute drug, inject 1.1 ml of the supplied diluent (sterile water for injection) into vial and gently swirl to dissolve drug. Do not shake.
- Use drug as soon as possible or within 6 hours after being reconstituted if stored at 36° to 46° F (2° to 8° C).
- Vials of drug should be stored in the refrigerator. If refrigeration is unavailable, drug can be stored at 77° F (25° C) for up to 30 days. Do not expose drug to high temperatures or freezing.

Patient education

- Teach patient or family member how to administer I.M. injections, including solution preparation, use of aseptic technique, rotation of injection sites, and equipment disposal. Periodically reevaluate patient's or family member's technique.
- Caution patient not to change dosage or administration schedule. If a dose is missed, tell him to take it as soon as he remembers. The regular schedule may then be resumed, but two injections should not be administered within 2 days of each other.
- Instruct patient how to store drug properly.
- Inform patient that flulike symptoms are not uncommon following initiation of therapy. Recommend use of acetaminophen to lessen the impact of these symptoms.
- Advise patient to report depression, suicidal ideation, or other adverse reactions.
- Tell patient to keep syringes and needles away from children. Also instruct patient not to reuse needles or syringes but to discard them in a syringe disposal unit.
- Advise women of childbearing age not to become pregnant while taking interferon beta-1a because of the abortifacient potential of drug. If pregnancy does occur, instruct her to discontinue treatment and call immediately.

Pediatric use

- Safety and effectiveness in children under age 18 have not been established.

Breast-feeding

- It is not known if drug is excreted in breast milk. Because of the potential for serious adverse reactions in breast-fed infants, a decision whether to discontinue breast-feeding or drug must be made.

interferon beta-1b

Betaseron

Pharmacologic classification: biological response modifier
Therapeutic classification: antiviral, immunoregulator
Pregnancy risk category C

How supplied

Available by prescription only
Powder for injection, lyophilized: 9.6 million IU (0.3 mg)

Indications, route, and dosage

Reduction of the frequency of exacerbations in relapsing-remitting multiple sclerosis
Adults: 8 million IU (0.25 mg) S.C. every other day.

Pharmacodynamics

Antiviral/immunoregulator actions: The mechanisms by which interferon beta-1b exerts its actions in multiple sclerosis are not clearly understood. However, it is known that the biological response-modifying properties of interferon beta-1b are mediated through its interactions with specific cell receptors found on the surface of human cells. The binding to these receptors induces the expression of a number of interferon-induced gene products that are believed to be the mediators of the biological actions of interferon beta-1b.

Pharmacokinetics

- *Absorption:* Serum levels are undetectable after the recommended dose; after higher doses, serum levels peak within 1 to 8 hours after S.C. administration.
- *Distribution:* Information not available.
- *Metabolism:* Information not available.
- *Excretion:* Information not available on patients with multiple sclerosis; however, in clinical studies involving healthy patients elimination half-life ranged from 8 minutes to 4 hours.

Contraindications and precautions

Contraindicated in patients hypersensitive to interferon beta or human albumin. Use cautiously in women of childbearing age.

Interactions

None significant.

Effects on diagnostic tests

None reported.

Adverse reactions

CNS: depression, anxiety, emotional lability, depersonalization, ***suicidal tendencies,*** confusion, somnolence, *hypertonia, asthenia, migraine,* ***seizures****, headache, dizziness.*
CV: palpitations, hypertension, tachycardia, peripheral vascular disorder, hemorrhage.
EENT: laryngitis, *sinusitis, conjunctivitis,* abnormal vision.
Endocrine: Cushing's syndrome, diabetes insipidus, diabetes mellitus, hypothyroidism, SIADH secretion.
GI: *diarrhea, constipation, abdominal pain, vomiting.*
GU: *menstrual disorders (bleeding or spotting, early or delayed menses, fewer days of menstrual flow, menorrhagia).*
Hematologic: *decreased WBC and absolute neutrophil counts.*
Respiratory: dyspnea.
Other: *flulike symptoms (fever, chills, malaise, myalgia, diaphoresis); elevated ALT levels; elevated bilirubin levels;* breast pain; *pelvic pain; inflammation, pain, and necrosis at injection site; lymphadenopathy;* generalized edema; *myasthenia; diaphoresis, alopecia.*

Overdose and treatment

No information available.

☑ Special considerations

- Drug is being investigated in the treatment of AIDS, AIDS-related Kaposi's sarcoma, metastatic renal-cell carcinoma, malignant melanoma, cutaneous T-cell lymphoma, and acute hepatitis C as unlabeled uses.
- Safety and efficacy in chronic progressive multiple sclerosis have not been evaluated.
- Drug use may cause depression and suicidal ideation. Other mental disorders have been observed and can include anxiety, emotional lability, depersonalization, and confusion. It is not known whether these symptoms may be related to the underlying neurologic basis of multiple sclerosis, to interferon beta-1b treatment, or to a combination of both. Closely monitor patient with these symptoms and consider stopping therapy.
- Perform the following laboratory tests before initiating therapy and at periodic intervals thereafter: hemoglobin, complete and differential WBC counts, platelet counts, and blood chemistries, including liver function tests.
- Having patient take drug at bedtime may minimize mild flulike symptoms that commonly occur.
- To reconstitute, inject 1.2 ml of supplied diluent (0.45% NaCl injection) into vial and gently swirl to dissolve drug. Do not shake. Reconstituted solution will contain 8 million IU (0.25 mg)/ml. Discard vial containing particulate material or discolored solution.
- Drug should be injected immediately after preparation.
- Refrigerate drug or reconstituted product (up to 3 hours) at 36° to 46° F (2° to 8° C). Do not freeze.

Patient education

- Because photosensitization may occur, caution patient to take protective measures (for example, sunscreens, protective clothing) against exposure to ultraviolet light or sunlight until tolerance is determined.
- Teach patient how to self-administer S.C. injections, including solution preparation, use of aseptic technique, rotation of injection sites, and equipment disposal. Periodically reevaluate patient's technique.
- Instruct patient to rotate injection sites to minimize local reactions.
- Inform patient that flulike symptoms are not uncommon following initiation of therapy. Recommend taking drug at bedtime to help minimize the symptoms.
- Caution patient not to change dosage or schedule of administration without medical consultation.
- Advise patient to report depression or suicidal ideation.

• Inform women of childbearing age about drug's abortifacient potential.

Pediatric use
• Safety and efficacy in children under age 18 have not been established.

Breast-feeding
• It is not known if drug is excreted in breast milk. Because of the potential for serious adverse reactions in breast-fed infants, a decision whether to discontinue breast-feeding or drug, taking into account the importance of drug to the mother, must be made.

interferon gamma-1b
Actimmune

Pharmacologic classification: biological response modifier
Therapeutic classification: antineoplastic
Pregnancy risk category C

How supplied
Available by prescription only
Injection: 100 mcg (3 million units)/0.5 ml in single-dose vials

Indications, route, and dosage
To decrease the frequency and severity of serious infection of chronic granulomatous disease
Adults with body surface area over 0.5 m^2: 50 mcg/m^2 (1.5 million units/m^2) S.C. three times weekly (for example, Monday, Wednesday, and Friday).
Adults with body surface area of 0.5 m^2 or less: 1.5 mcg/kg S.C. three times weekly (for example, Monday, Wednesday, and Friday).

Pharmacodynamics
Antineoplastic action: Interferon gamma-1b is a single-chain polypeptide containing 140 amino acids, produced by fermentation of genetically engineered *Escherichia coli.* It has potent phagocytic activity not seen with other interferons. Exact mechanism of action is unknown, but growing evidence suggests it interacts functionally with other interleukin molecules and all form part of a complex lymphokine network. A broad range of biological activities have been noted, including enhancement of oxidative metabolism of tissue macrophages, antibody-dependent cellular cytotoxicity, natural killer cell activity, and effects on Fc receptor expression on monocytes and major histocompatibility antigen expression. In chronic granulomatous disease, interferon gamma-1b provides enhancement of phagocyte function, including elevation of superoxide levels and improved killing of *Staphylococcus aureus.*

Pharmacokinetics
• *Absorption:* About 90% is absorbed after S.C. injection. Peak plasma concentrations are reached after 7 hours; no accumulation is noted after 12 consecutive daily doses.
• *Distribution:* Unknown.
• *Metabolism:* Unknown.
• *Excretion:* Unknown. Mean elimination half-life after S.C. dosing is 5.9 hours.

Contraindications and precautions
Contraindicated in patients hypersensitive to drug or to genetically engineered products derived from *Escherichia coli.* Use cautiously in patients with CV disease (arrhythmias, heart failure, or ischemia), compromised CNS function, or seizure disorders and in those receiving myelosuppressive agents.

Interactions
Drug can decrease hepatic microsomal cytochrome P-450 concentrations, which could lead to decreased metabolism of drugs that use this metabolic degradation pathway.

Use with caution in patients receiving *myelosuppressive agents.*

Effects on diagnostic tests
None reported.

Adverse reactions
CNS: *fatigue,* decreased mental status, gait disturbance, dizziness.
GI: *nausea, vomiting, diarrhea,* abdominal pain.
Hematologic: ***neutropenia, thrombocytopenia.***
Metabolic: elevated liver enzyme levels (at high doses).
Skin: rash; *erythema, tenderness* (at injection site).
Other: flulike syndrome (headache, fever, chills, myalgia, arthralgia), weight loss, back pain, proteinuria.

Overdose and treatment
No information available.

☑ Special considerations
• Optimum injection sites are the right and left deltoids and anterior thigh.
• Flulike symptoms may be minimized by administering at bedtime and may be treated with acetaminophen.
• If acute hypersensitivity reaction occurs, discontinue drug immediately and institute symptomatic and supportive treatment.
• Transient cutaneous rash has not required discontinuation of therapy.
• If home use is appropriate, instruct patient, family, and caregiver on safe and effective use of drug. Help them review contents of patient information package insert.
• Store drug in refrigerator immediately; do not freeze. Avoid excessive or vigorous agitation. Do not shake. Unopened or unentered vials should not be left at room temperature longer than 12 hours before use. Do not return vials that exceed these limits to refrigerator; they should be discarded.
• Each vial is designed for single use only. Discard unused portions of vials.
• Do not use after the stated expiration date on vial.

• If severe adverse reactions occur, dose should be reduced by 50% or therapy discontinued until reaction subsides.

Patient education
• Thoroughly review the patient information package insert with patient.
• For home use, teach correct procedures for collection and disposal of medical waste.

Pediatric use
• Safety and efficacy have not been established in children under age 1.

Breast-feeding
• It is unknown if drug is excreted in breast milk. Because of the potential for serious adverse reactions in infants, a decision must be made whether to continue breast-feeding.

ipecac syrup

Pharmacologic classification: alkaloid emetic
Therapeutic classification: emetic
Pregnancy risk category C

How supplied
Available with and without a prescription
Syrup: 70 mg powdered ipecac/ml

Indications, route, and dosage
To induce vomiting in poisoning
Adults: 15 to 30 ml P.O., followed by 200 to 300 ml of water.
Children age 1 or older: 15 ml P.O., followed by about 200 ml of water or milk.
Children under age 1: 5 to 10 ml P.O., followed by 100 to 200 ml of water or milk.

May repeat dose once after 20 minutes, if necessary.

Pharmacodynamics
Emetic action: Ipecac syrup directly irritates the GI mucosa and directly stimulates the chemoreceptor trigger zone through the effects of emetine and cephalin, its two alkaloids.

Pharmacokinetics
• *Absorption:* Ipecac syrup is absorbed in significant amounts mainly when it does not produce emesis. Onset of action usually occurs in 20 minutes.
• *Distribution:* Unknown.
• *Metabolism:* Unknown.
• *Excretion:* Emetine is excreted in urine slowly, over a period lasting up to 60 days. Duration of effect is 20 to 25 minutes.

Contraindications and precautions
Contraindicated in semicomatose or unconscious patients or those with severe inebriation, seizures, shock, or loss of gag reflex. Do not give after ingestion of gasoline, kerosene, volatile oils, or caustic substances (lye).

Interactions
Activated charcoal may inactivate ipecac syrup; concomitant use with *antiemetics* or *milk* (or *milk products*) may decrease ipecac syrup's therapeutic effectiveness. Concomitant use with *carbonated beverages* may cause abdominal distention. *Vegetable oil* will delay absorption.

Effects on diagnostic tests
None reported.

Adverse reactions
CNS: depression, *drowsiness.*
CV: ***arrhythmias,*** bradycardia, hypotension; atrial fibrillation, ***fatal myocarditis*** (with excessive doses).
GI: diarrhea.

Overdose and treatment
Clinical effects of overdose include diarrhea, persistent nausea or vomiting (longer than 30 minutes), stomach cramps or pain, arrhythmias, hypotension, myocarditis, difficulty breathing, and unusual fatigue or weakness.

Toxicity from chronic ipecac overdosage usually involves use of the concentrated fluid extract in dosage appropriate for the syrup. Clinical effects of cardiotoxicity include tachycardia, T-wave depression, atrial fibrillation, depressed myocardial contractility, heart failure, and myocarditis. Other toxic effects include bloody stools and vomitus, hypotension, shock, seizures, and coma. Heart failure is the usual cause of death.

Treatment requires discontinuation of drug followed by symptomatic and supportive care, which may include digitalis and pacemaker therapy to treat cardiotoxic effects. However, no antidote exists for the cardiotoxic effects of ipecac, which may be fatal despite intensive treatment.

☑ Special considerations
• Administer ipecac syrup before giving activated charcoal, not after. Follow dose with 1 or 2 glasses of water. If vomiting does not occur after second dose, give activated charcoal to adsorb both ipecac syrup and ingested poison. Follow with gastric lavage.
• Inspect emesis for ingested substances, such as tablets or capsules.
• Ipecac syrup usually empties the stomach completely within 30 minutes (in over 90% of patients); average emptying time is 20 minutes.
• Be careful not to confuse ipecac syrup with ipecac fluid extract, which is rarely used but 14 times more potent. Never store these two drugs together—the wrong drug could cause death.
• In antiemetic toxicity, ipecac syrup is usually effective if less than 1 hour has passed since ingestion of antiemetic.
• Little if any systemic toxicity occurs with doses of 30 ml or less.
• Drug may be abused by patients with eating disorders (such as bulimia or anorexia nervosa).
• Ipecac syrup also may be used in small amounts as an expectorant in cough preparations; however, this use has doubtful therapeutic benefit.

Patient education
- Advise patient to seek medical attention immediately when poisoning is suspected.
- Caution patient to call poison information center before taking ipecac syrup.
- Warn patient to avoid drinking milk or carbonated beverages with ipecac syrup because they may decrease drug's effectiveness; instead, instruct him to take syrup with 1 or 2 glasses of water.
- Advise patient to take activated charcoal only after vomiting has stopped.

Pediatric use
- Advise parents to keep ipecac syrup at home at all times but to keep it out of children's reach.

Breast-feeding
- Safety in breast-feeding infants has not been established; possible risks must be weighed against drug's benefits.

ipratropium bromide
Atrovent

Pharmacologic classification: anticholinergic
Therapeutic classification: bronchodilator
Pregnancy risk category B

How supplied
Available by prescription only
Inhaler: each metered dose supplies 18 mcg
Inhalation solution: 2.5 ml
Nasal spray: 0.03%, 0.06%

Indications, route, and dosage
Bronchospasm in chronic bronchitis and emphysema
Adults: Usually, 2 inhalations (36 mcg) q.i.d.; patient may take additional inhalations p.r.n., but should not exceed 12 inhalations in 24 hours or 500 mcg q 6 to 8 hours via oral nebulizer.
Rhinorrhea associated with allergic and nonallergic perennial rhinitis
0.03% nasal spray
Adults and children age 12 and older: 2 sprays (42 mcg) per nostril b.i.d. or t.i.d.
Rhinorrhea associated with the common cold
0.06% nasal spray
Adults and children age 12 and older: 2 sprays (84 mcg) per nostril t.i.d. or q.i.d.

Pharmacodynamics
Anticholinergic action: Ipratropium appears to inhibit vagally mediated reflexes by antagonizing the action of acetylcholine. Anticholinergics prevent the increases in intracellular concentration of cyclic guanosine monophosphate (cyclic GMP) that result from interaction of acetylcholine with the muscarinic receptor on bronchial smooth muscle.

The bronchodilation following inhalation is primarily a local, site-specific effect, not a systemic one.

Pharmacokinetics
- *Absorption:* Drug is not readily absorbed into the systemic circulation either from the surface of the lung or from the GI tract as confirmed by blood levels and renal excretion studies. Much of an inhaled dose is swallowed as shown by fecal excretion studies.
- *Distribution:* Not applicable.
- *Metabolism:* Hepatic; elimination half-life is about 2 hours.
- *Excretion:* Most of an administered dose is excreted unchanged in feces. Absorbed drug is excreted in urine and bile.

Contraindications and precautions
Contraindicated in patients with hypersensitivity to drug or atropine or its derivatives and in those with a history of hypersensitivity to soya lecithin or related food products, such as soybeans and peanuts. Use cautiously in patients with angle-closure glaucoma, prostatic hyperplasia, and bladder-neck obstruction.

Interactions
Concurrent use of ipratropium with *antimuscarinic agents*, including *ophthalmic preparations*, may produce additive effects. Increased risk of fluorocarbon toxicity may result from too-closely timed administration of ipratropium and other *fluorocarbon propellant–containing oral inhalants*, such as *adrenocorticoids, cromolyn, glucocorticoids,* or *sympathomimetics.* A 5-minute interval between such agents is recommended.

Effects on diagnostic tests
None reported.

Adverse reactions
CNS: dizziness, headache, nervousness.
CV: palpitations.
EENT: cough, blurred vision, rhinitis, sinusitis.
GI: nausea, GI distress, dry mouth.
Respiratory: *upper respiratory tract infection, bronchitis,* cough, dyspnea, pharyngitis, bronchospasm, increased sputum.
Skin: rash.
Other: pain, back pain, chest pain, flulike symptoms.

Overdose and treatment
Acute overdosage by inhalation is unlikely because ipratropium is not well-absorbed systemically after aerosol or oral administration.

☑ Special considerations
- Because of delayed onset of bronchodilation, drug is not recommended to treat acute respiratory distress.

Patient education
- Tell patient to shake drug well before using.
- Initial nasal spray pump requires priming with 7 actuations of the pump. If used regularly as recommended, no further priming is needed. If not used for over 24 hours, the pump will require 2 ac-

tuations. If not used for over 7 days, the pump will require 7 actuations to reprime.

- Instruct patient to store drug away from heat and direct sunlight, and to protect it from freezing.
- Tell patient that temporary blurred vision may result if aerosol is sprayed into eyes.
- Advise patient to allow 1 minute between inhalations.
- Instruct patient to take a missed dose as soon as possible—unless it is almost time for the next scheduled dose, in which case he should skip the missed dose. Warn him to never double-dose.
- Suggest sugarless hard candy, gum, ice, or saliva substitute to relieve dry mouth. Tell patient to report dry mouth if it persists longer than 2 weeks.
- Instruct patient to call if he experiences no benefits within 30 minutes after administration, or if condition worsens.

Pediatric use

- Safety and efficacy in children under age 12 have not been established.

Breast-feeding

- It is not known if drug is excreted in breast milk. Although lipid-insoluble quaternary bases pass into breast milk, ipratropium is unlikely to reach the infant, especially when taken by aerosol. However, use caution when administering to breast-feeding women.

irbesartan

Avapro

Pharmacologic classification: angiotensin II receptor antagonist
Therapeutic classification: antihypertensive
Pregnancy risk category C (D in second and third trimesters)

How supplied

Available by prescription only
Tablets: 75 mg, 150 mg, 300 mg

Indications, route, and dosage

Treatment of hypertension—alone, or in combination with other antihypertensives

Adults: initially 150 mg P.O. once daily, increased to maximum of 300 mg once daily if necessary, without regard to food.

✦ ***Dosage adjustment.*** In volume- and salt-depleted patients, 75 mg P.O. initially.

Pharmacodynamics

Antihypertensive action: Blocks the vasoconstrictor and aldosterone-secreting effects of angiotensin II by selectively blocking the binding of angiotensin II to its receptor sites.

Pharmacokinetics

- *Absorption:* Drug is absorbed rapidly and completely. The average absolute bioavailability is 60% to 80% and is not affected by food. Peak plasma concentrations occur 1½ to 2 hours after ingestion.
- *Distribution:* Irbesartan is 90% bound to plasma proteins. It may cross the blood brain barrier and placenta. Steady state is achieved within 3 days. Drug is widely distributed.
- *Metabolism:* Irbesartan is metabolized by conjugation and oxidation. Cytochrome P-450 2C9 is the major enzyme responsible for formation of the oxidative metabolites. Metabolites do not appear to add significantly to the drug's pharmacologic activity.
- *Excretion:* Excreted in the bile and urine. 20% is excreted in the urine and the rest in the feces. Drug may also be excreted in breast milk. Elimination half-life is 11 to 15 hours.

Contraindications and precautions

Contraindicated in patients who are hypersensitive to drug or its components and in pregnant or breast-feeding patients.

Use cautiously in volume- or salt-depleted patients, in patients whose renal function may depend on the activity of the renin-angiotensin-aldosterone system (for example, patients with severe heart failure), and in those with unilateral or bilateral renal artery stenosis.

Interactions

None reported.

Effects on diagnostic tests

Drug therapy may cause a minor increase in BUN or serum creatinine levels.

Adverse reactions

CNS: fatigue, anxiety, dizziness, headache.
CV: chest pain, edema, tachycardia.
EENT: pharyngitis, rhinitis, sinus abnormality.
GI: diarrhea, dyspepsia, abdominal pain, nausea, vomiting.
GU: urinary tract infection.
Respiratory: upper respiratory infection.
Skin: rash.
Other: musculoskeletal trauma or pain.

Overdose and treatment

No information available. The most likely clinical manifestations of an overdose are expected to be hypotension and tachycardia, and possibly bradycardia. Drug is not removed by hemodialysis. If hypotension occurs, place patient in supine position and, if necessary, give an I.V. infusion of normal saline.

☑ Special considerations

- Pharmacokinetics of drug are not altered in patients with renal impairment or in patients on hemodialysis. Irbesartan is not removed by hemodialysis. Dosage adjustment is not necessary in patients with mild to severe renal impairment unless patient with renal impairment is also volume depleted.
- Dosage adjustment is not necessary in patients with hepatic insufficiency.
- Patients not adequately treated by the maximum 300-mg once-daily dose are unlikely to derive ad-

ditional benefit from a higher dose or twice-daily dosing.
• Monitor blood pressure regularly. A transient hypotensive response is not a contraindication to further treatment. Therapy can usually be continued once blood pressure has stabilized.

Patient education
• Warn female patient that drug is contraindicated during pregnancy because of potential danger to the fetus. Advise her to call immediately if pregnancy occurs or if she plans to become pregnant.
• Tell patient the drug may be taken once daily with or without food.
• Advise patient that if a dose is missed to take it as soon as possible, but not to take double doses.
• Warn patient about symptoms of hypotension and what to do.
• Caution patient not to discontinue drug without medical approval.

Geriatric use
• Dosage adjustment is not necessary.

Pediatric use
• Safety and effectiveness in children under age 18 have not been established.

Breast-feeding
• Because of the potential for serious adverse reactions in breast-fed infants, breast-feeding should be discontinued during drug therapy.

irinotecan hydrochloride
Camptosar

Pharmacologic classification: topoisomerase inhibitor
Therapeutic classification: antineoplastic
Pregnancy risk category D

How supplied
Available by prescription only
Injection: 100-mg vial

Indications, route, and dosage
Treatment of metastatic carcinoma of the colon or rectum in which the disease has recurred or progressed following fluorouracil (5-FU)-based therapy
Adults: Initially, 125 mg/m^2 I.V. infusion over 90 minutes. Recommended treatment regimen is 125 mg/m^2 I.V. administered once weekly for 4 weeks, followed by a 2-week rest period. Thereafter, additional courses of treatment may be repeated q 6 weeks (4 weeks on therapy, followed by 2 weeks off therapy). Subsequent doses may be adjusted to as high as 150 mg/m^2 or to as low as 50 mg/m^2 in 25- to 50-mg/m^2 increments depending on patient's tolerance. Treatment with additional courses may continue indefinitely in patients who attain a response or in those whose disease remains stable provided intolerable toxicity does not occur.

Pharmacodynamics
Antineoplastic action: Irinotecan is a derivative of camptothecin. Camptothecins interact specifically with the enzyme topoisomerase I, which relieves torsional strain in DNA by inducing reversible single-strand breaks. Irinotecan and its active metabolite bind to the topoisomerase I–DNA complex and prevent religation of these single-strand breaks.

Pharmacokinetics
• *Absorption:* Drug is only administered I.V.
• *Distribution:* Irinotecan is about 30% to 68% bound to plasma protein, whereas its active metabolite, SN-38, is about 95% bound.
• *Metabolism:* Drug undergoes metabolic conversion in the liver to its active metabolite SN-38.
• *Excretion:* A small amount of drug and SN-38 are excreted in urine. Terminal half-life of irinotecan is 6 hours in patients who are age 65 and older and 5½ hours in patients under age 65; mean terminal elimination half-life of SN-38 is about 10 hours.

Contraindications and precautions
Contraindicated in patients with hypersensitivity to drug. Use cautiously in elderly patients and in those who have previously received pelvic or abdominal irradiation because of increased risk of severe myelosuppression.

Interactions
Other *antineoplastic agents* may cause additive adverse effects such as myelosuppression and diarrhea.

Effects on diagnostic tests
None reported.

Adverse reactions
CNS: *insomnia, dizziness, asthenia, headache.*
CV: *vasodilation, edema.*
GI: **DIARRHEA,** *nausea, vomiting, anorexia, constipation, flatulence, stomatitis, dyspepsia, abdominal cramping and pain, abdominal enlargement.*
Hematologic: **LEUKOPENIA,** *anemia,* **NEUTROPENIA.**
Metabolic: *weight loss, dehydration, increased alkaline phosphatase, increased AST levels.*
Respiratory: *dyspnea, increased coughing, rhinitis.*
Skin: *alopecia, sweating, rash.*
Other: *fever, pain, back pain, chills, minor infection.*

Overdose and treatment
The adverse effects of overdosage are similar to those reported with the recommended dosage and regimen. There is no known antidote for drug overdosage. Institute maximum supportive care to prevent dehydration because of diarrhea and to treat any infectious complications.

☑ Special considerations
• Premedicate patient with antiemetic agents on day of treatment starting at least 30 minutes before drug administration. In clinical studies, most patients received 10 mg of dexamethasone conjunction with another antiemetic agent, such as a

5-HT3 blocker (such as ondansetron or granisetron). Patients should also receive an antiemetic regimen (prochlorperazine) for subsequent use as needed.
• Irinotecan is packaged in a backing/plastic blister to protect against inadvertent breakage and leakage. Inspect vial for damage and visible signs of leaks before removing the backing/plastic blister. If damaged, incinerate the unopened package. Store vial at room temperature of 59° to 86° F (15° to 30° C) and protect from light. Do not remove vial and backing/plastic blister from carton until time of use.
• Exercise caution in handling and preparing infusion solutions of irinotecan. Gloves should be worn. If drug solution comes into contact with skin, wash skin immediately and thoroughly with soap and water. If drug solution contacts the mucous membranes, flush thoroughly with water.
• Irinotecan must be diluted before infusion with D_5W injection (preferred) or 0.9% NaCl injection to a final concentration range of 0.12 to 1.1 mg/ml.
• Drug solution is stable for up to 24 hours at room temperature of 77° F (25° C) and in ambient fluorescent lighting. Store solutions diluted in D_5W in refrigerator (35° to 46° F [2° to 8° C]) and protect from light; these are stable for 48 hours. However, because of possible microbial contamination during dilution, use admixture within 24 hours if refrigerated or within 6 hours if kept at room temperature. Refrigeration of admixtures using 0.9% NaCl is not recommended due to a low and sporadic incidence of visible particulates.
• Avoid freezing of drug and admixtures because drug may precipitate.
• Do not add other drugs to drug infusion.
• Avoid drug extravasation. If extravasation occurs, flush site with sterile water and apply ice.
• Withhold diuretic therapy during dosing with irinotecan and during periods of active vomiting or diarrhea because of potential risk of dehydration secondary to vomiting or diarrhea induced by irinotecan.
• Irinotecan can induce severe forms of diarrhea. Diarrhea occurring within 24 hours of drug administration may be preceded by complaints of diaphoresis and abdominal cramping and may be ameliorated by giving 0.25 to 1 mg of atropine I.V. unless contraindicated. Diarrhea occurring more than 24 hours after drug administration can be prolonged, may lead to dehydration and electrolyte imbalance, and can be life-threatening. Late diarrhea should be treated promptly with loperamide (4 mg at onset and then 2 mg every 2 hours until patient is diarrhea-free for at least 12 hours; during the night, patient may take 4 mg of loperamide every 4 hours). Premedication with loperamide is not recommended. Monitor patient with severe diarrhea and give fluid and electrolyte replacement if dehydration occurs. Drug therapy should be interrupted if severe diarrhea occurs.
• Therapy should be temporarily discontinued if neutropenic fever occurs or if the absolute neutrophil count drops below 500/mm³. Drug dose should be reduced if there is a clinically significant decrease in the total WBC count (less than 2,000/mm³), neutrophil count (below 1,000/mm³), hemoglobin (under 8 g/dl), or platelet count (under 100,000/mm³). Consult manufacturer for dosage guidelines in these situations.
• Routine administration of a colony-stimulating factor is not necessary but may be helpful in patients experiencing significant neutropenia.
• Careful monitoring of the WBC count with differential, hemoglobin, and platelet count is recommended before each dose of irinotecan.

Patient education
• Advise women of childbearing age to avoid pregnancy because drug may cause fetal harm.
• Inform patient about risk of diarrhea and when and how to treat it if it occurs. Tell patient to have loperamide readily available and to begin treatment for diarrhea that occurs more than 24 hours after drug administration at the first episode of poorly formed or loose stools or the earliest onset of bowel movements more frequent than normally expected for the patient. Instruct patient to notify primary health care provider if diarrhea occurs and to avoid use of drugs with laxative properties.
• Tell patient to call if vomiting occurs, fever or evidence of infection develops, or symptoms of dehydration (fainting, light-headedness, or dizziness) occur following drug administration.
• Warn patient that alopecia may occur.

Geriatric use
• Use caution when administering drug to elderly patients.

Pediatric use
• Safety and effectiveness in children have not been established.

Breast-feeding
• It is not known if drug is excreted in breast milk. Because of the potential for serious adverse reactions in breast-fed infants, it is recommended that breast-feeding be discontinued during irinotecan therapy.

iron dextran
DexFerrum, InFeD

Pharmacologic classification: parenteral iron supplement
Therapeutic classification: hematinic
Pregnancy risk category C

How supplied
Available by prescription only
Injection: 50 mg elemental iron/ml in 2-ml single dose vials

Indications, route, and dosage
Iron-deficiency anemia
Adults and children: Dosage is highly individualized and is based on patient's weight and hemoglobin level. Drug is usually given I.M.; preservative-free solution can be given I.V. Check current literature for recommended protocol.

Pharmacodynamics
Hematinic action: Iron dextran is a complex of ferric hydroxide and dextran in a colloidal solution. After I.M. injection, 10% to 50% remains in the muscle for several months; remainder enters bloodstream, increasing plasma iron concentration for up to 2 weeks. Iron is an essential component of hemoglobin.

Pharmacokinetics
- *Absorption:* I.M. doses are absorbed in two stages: 60% after 3 days, and up to 90% by 3 weeks. Remainder is absorbed over several months or longer.
- *Distribution:* During first 3 days, local inflammation facilitates passage of drug into the lymphatic system; drug is then ingested by macrophages, which enter lymph and blood.
- *Metabolism:* After I.M. or I.V. administration, iron dextran is cleared from plasma by reticuloendothelial cells of the liver, spleen, and bone marrow.
- *Excretion:* In doses of 500 mg or less, half-life is 6 hours. Traces are excreted in breast milk, urine, bile, and feces. Drug cannot be removed by hemodialysis.

Contraindications and precautions
Contraindicated in patients with hypersensitivity to drug, in those with all anemias except iron-deficiency anemia, and in those with acute infectious renal disease. Use cautiously in patients with impaired hepatic function, rheumatoid arthritis, and other inflammatory diseases.

Interactions
None significant.

Effects on diagnostic tests
Large doses (over 250 mg iron) may color the serum brown.

Iron dextran may cause false elevations of serum bilirubin level and false reductions in serum calcium level.

Iron dextran prevents meaningful measurement of serum iron concentration and total iron binding capacity for up to 3 weeks; I.M. injection may cause dense areas of activity on bone scans using technetium 99m diphosphonate, for 1 to 6 days.

Adverse reactions
CNS: headache, transitory paresthesia, arthralgia, myalgia, dizziness, malaise.
CV: *hypotensive reaction, peripheral vascular flushing (with overly rapid I.V. administration).*
GI: nausea, anorexia.
Respiratory: ***bronchospasm,*** dyspnea.
Skin: rash, urticaria, purpura.
Other: *soreness, inflammation, brown skin discoloration (at I.M. injection site); local phlebitis (at I.V. injection site),* sterile abscess, necrosis, atrophy, fibrosis, ***anaphylaxis***, delayed sensitivity reactions, fever, chills.

Overdose and treatment
Injected iron has much greater bioavailability than oral iron, but data on acute overdose is limited.

☑ Special considerations
- Discontinue oral iron before giving iron dextran.
- Use 10-ml multidose vial only for I.M. injections, because it contains phenol as a preservative; use only 2- or 5-ml ampule without preservative for I.V. administration.
- Administer test dose of 0.5 ml iron dextrose I.M. or I.V. Be alert for anaphylaxis on test dose; monitor vital signs for drug reaction. Keep epinephrine (0.5 ml of a 1:1,000 solution) readily available for such an emergency.
- Inject I.M. preparation deeply into upper outer quadrant of buttocks (never an arm or other exposed area) using a 2- to 3-inch (5- to 8-cm), 19G or 20G needle. Use Z-track technique to avoid leakage into S.C. tissue and skin stains, and minimize staining by using a separate needle to withdraw drug from its container.
- I.V. use is controversial, and some health care facilities do not allow it.
- Give drug I.V. if patient has insufficient muscle mass for deep injection, impaired absorption from muscle because of stasis or edema, a risk of uncontrolled I.M. bleeding from trauma (as in hemophilia), or need for massive and prolonged parenteral therapy (as in chronic substantial blood loss). Do not administer more than 50 mg of iron/minute (1 ml/minute) if using drug undiluted.
- After I.V. iron dextran administration, flush vein with 10 ml 0.9% NaCl injection to minimize local irritation. Have patient rest for 15 to 30 minutes, because orthostatic hypotension may occur.
- Monitor hemoglobin, hematocrit, and reticulocyte count during therapy. An increase of about 1 g/dl weekly in hemoglobin is usual.

Patient education
- Warn patient of possibility of skin staining with I.M. injections.

Pediatric use
- Drug is not recommended for use in children under age 4 months.

Breast-feeding
- Traces of unmetabolized iron dextran are excreted in breast milk; impact on neonate is unknown.

isoetharine hydrochloride
Arm-a-Med Isoetharine, Beta-2, Bisorine, Bronkosol

isoetharine mesylate
Bronkometer

Pharmacologic classification: adrenergic
Therapeutic classification: bronchodilator
Pregnancy risk category C

How supplied
Available by prescription only
Nebulizer inhaler: 0.062%, 0.08%, 0.1%, 0.125%, 0.167%, 0.17%, 0.2%, 0.25%, 1% solution
Aerosol inhaler: 340 mcg/metered spray

Indications, route, and dosage

Bronchial asthma and reversible bronchospasm that may occur with bronchitis and emphysema

isoetharine hydrochloride

Adults: Administered by oxygen aerosolization, 0.5 ml (range 0.25 to 0.5 ml) of a 1% solution diluted 1:3. Administered by IPPB solution, 0.5 ml (range 0.25 to 1 ml) of a 1% solution diluted 1:3. Administered by hand-nebulizer, 4 inhalations (range 3 to 7 inhalations) of undiluted 1% solution.

isoetharine mesylate

Adults: Administered by metered aerosol, 1 to 2 inhalations. Occasionally, more may be required.

Pharmacodynamics

Bronchodilating action: Isoetharine relaxes bronchial smooth muscle by direct action on $beta_2$-adrenergic receptors, resulting in relief of bronchospasm, increased vital capacity, and decreased airway resistance. It may also inhibit release of histamine. Isoetharine also relaxes the smooth muscles of the peripheral vasculature.

Pharmacokinetics

- *Absorption:* Absorbed rapidly from the respiratory tract after oral inhalation. Bronchodilation occurs immediately, peaks in 5 to 15 minutes, and persists 1 to 4 hours.
- *Distribution:* Distributed widely throughout the body.
- *Metabolism:* Drug is metabolized in lungs, liver, GI tract, and other tissues.
- *Excretion:* Isoetharine is excreted in urine as unchanged drug and metabolites.

Contraindications and precautions

Contraindicated in patients with hypersensitivity to drug. Use cautiously in patients with hyperthyroidism, hypertension, or coronary artery disease and in those with sensitivity to sympathomimetics.

Interactions

Concomitant use with *epinephrine* or other *sympathomimetics* may produce additive adverse CV effects. *Beta-adrenergic blocking agents* (such as *propranolol*) antagonize isoetharine's bronchodilating, cardiac, and vasodilating effects.

Effects on diagnostic tests

None reported.

Adverse reactions

CNS: *tremor, headache,* dizziness, excitement, anxiety.
CV: *palpitations,* increased heart rate, alterations in blood pressure.
GI: nausea, vomiting.

Overdose and treatment

Clinical manifestations of overdose include exaggeration of common adverse reactions, particularly nausea and vomiting, arrhythmias, hypertension, and extreme tremors.

Treatment includes symptomatic and supportive measures. Monitor vital signs closely. Sedatives may be used to treat restlessness. Cardioselective beta blockers (such as metoprolol) may be used to treat arrhythmias, but with caution (may induce asthmatic attack).

☑ Special considerations

Besides those relevant to all *adrenergics* used as bronchodilators, consider the following recommendations.

- Tolerance may develop after prolonged or excessive use.
- Therapy should be administered upon arising in the morning and before meals to reduce fatigue from activity.
- Paradoxical airway resistance (sudden worsening of dyspnea) may follow repeated excessive use. If this occurs, patient or family should discontinue isoetharine and call for alternative therapy (such as epinephrine).
- Alternating therapy with isoetharine inhalation and epinephrine may be helpful. However, these drugs should not be administered simultaneously because of danger of excessive cardiac stimulation.
- Protect solutions from light, freezing, and heat. Store at controlled room temperature.
- Ask patient about sensitivity to sulfites.

Patient education

- Instruct patient in correct use of inhaler.
- Tell patient to use only as directed, to take no more than two inhalations at one time with 1- to 2-minute intervals between, and to save applicator; refills may be available.
- Instruct patient to wait 1 full minute after initial one to two inhalations (Bronkometer) before inhaling another dose. Action should begin immediately and peak within 5 to 15 minutes.
- Warn patient to keep spray away from eyes.
- Urge patient to use inhalation therapy as prescribed. If symptoms persist or worsen, patient should call for further instructions. Excessive use may decrease desired effect and cause distressing tachycardia, palpitations, headache, nausea, and dizziness.
- Tell patient to store drug away from heat and light (not in bathroom medicine cabinet where heat and humidity can cause drug to deteriorate) and out of children's reach.

Geriatric use

- Elderly patients may be more sensitive to isoetharine's effects; lower dose may be needed.

Pediatric use

- Pediatric dosage recommendations not established by the manufacturer; however, some believe pediatric dosage is the same as the adult dosage.

Breast-feeding

- It is unknown if drug is excreted in breast milk; therefore, use with caution in breast-feeding women.

isoniazid (INH)

Isotamine*, Laniazid, Laniazid C.T., Nydrazid, PMS Isoniazid*, Rimifon*

Pharmacologic classification: isonicotinic acid hydrazine
Therapeutic classification: antitubercular
Pregnancy risk category C

How supplied

Available by prescription only
Tablets: 50 mg, 100 mg, 300 mg
Oral solution: 50 mg/5 ml
Injection: 100 mg/ml

Indications, route, and dosage

Primary treatment against actively growing tubercle bacilli

Adults: 5 mg/kg P.O. or I.M. daily in a single dose, up to 300 mg/day, continued for 9 months to 2 years.
Infants and children: 10 mg/kg P.O. or I.M. daily in a single dose, up to 300 mg/day, continued for 18 months to 2 years. Concomitant administration of at least one other effective antitubercular drug is recommended.

Prophylaxis against tubercle bacilli of those closely exposed or with positive skin test

Adults: 300 mg P.O. daily single dose, continued for 6 months to 1 year.
Infants and children: 10 mg/kg P.O. daily single dose, up to 300 mg/day, continued for 6 months to 1 year.

Pharmacodynamics

Antitubercular action: INH interferes with lipid and DNA synthesis, thus inhibiting bacterial cell wall synthesis. Its action is bacteriostatic or bactericidal, depending on organism susceptibility and drug concentration at infection site. INH is active against *Mycobacterium tuberculosis, M. bovis,* and some strains of *M. kansasii.*

Resistance by *M. tuberculosis* develops rapidly when INH is used to treat tuberculosis, and it is usually combined with another antitubercular agent to prevent or delay resistance. During prophylaxis, however, resistance is not a problem and isoniazid can be used alone.

Pharmacokinetics

• *Absorption:* Rapidly and completely absorbed from the GI tract after oral administration; peak serum concentrations occur 1 to 2 hours after ingestion. INH also is absorbed readily after I.M. injection.
• *Distribution:* INH is distributed widely into body tissues and fluids, including ascitic, synovial, pleural, and cerebrospinal fluids; lungs and other organs; and sputum and saliva. Drug crosses the placenta and enters breast milk in concentrations similar to plasma.
• *Metabolism:* INH is inactivated primarily in the liver by genetically controlled acetylation. Rate of metabolism varies individually; fast acetylators metabolize drug five times as rapidly as others. About 50% of Blacks and Whites are slow acetylators of INH, whereas over 80% of Chinese, Japanese, and Eskimos are fast acetylators.
• *Excretion:* About 75% of a dose is excreted in urine as unchanged drug and metabolites in 24 hours; some drug is excreted in saliva, sputum, feces, and breast milk. Plasma half-life in adults is 1 to 4 hours, depending on metabolic rate. Drug is removed by peritoneal dialysis or hemodialysis.

Contraindications and precautions

Contraindicated in patients with acute hepatic disease or drug-associated hepatic damage. Use cautiously in the elderly and in patients with severe, non-INH-associated hepatic disease, seizure disorders (especially those taking phenytoin), severe renal impairment, or chronic alcoholism.

Interactions

Concomitant daily use of *alcohol* may increase incidence of INH-induced hepatitis and seizures.

Concomitant use with *cycloserine* increases hazard of CNS toxicity, drowsiness, and dizziness from cycloserine.

INH-induced inhibition of metabolism and elevation of serum concentrations increases toxicity of *benzodiazepines* (such as *diazepam*), *carbamazepine* and *phenytoin.*

Concomitant use of INH and *disulfiram* may cause coordination difficulties and psychotic episodes.

Concomitant use with *antacids* decreases oral absorption of INH; use with *corticosteroids* may decrease INH efficacy; use with *rifampin* may accelerate INH metabolism to hepatotoxic metabolites, because of rifampin-induced enzyme production; use with *anticoagulants* may increase anticoagulant activity.

Effects on diagnostic tests

INH alters results of urine glucose tests that use cupric sulfate method (Benedict's reagent, Diastix, or Chemstrip uG).

Elevated liver function study results occur in about 15%; most abnormalities are mild and transient, but some persist throughout treatment.

Adverse reactions

CNS: *peripheral neuropathy* (dose-related and especially in patients who are malnourished, alcoholic, diabetic, or slow acetylators), usually preceded by paresthesia of hands and feet, seizures, toxic encephalopathy, memory impairment, toxic psychosis.
EENT: optic neuritis, atrophy.
GI: nausea, vomiting, epigastric distress.
Hematologic: ***agranulocytosis,*** hemolytic anemia, ***aplastic anemia***, eosinophilia, ***thrombocytopenia***, sideroblastic anemia.
Hepatic: ***hepatitis*** (occasionally severe and sometimes fatal, especially in elderly patients), jaundice, *elevated serum transaminase levels,* bilirubinemia.
Other: rheumatic and lupuslike syndromes, hypersensitivity reactions (fever, rash, lymphadenopathy, vasculitis), hyperglycemia, metabolic acidosis, pyridoxine deficiency, hypocalcemia, hypophosphatemia, gynecomastia, irritation at I.M. injection site.

Overdose and treatment

Early signs of overdose include nausea, vomiting, slurred speech, dizziness, blurred vision, and visual hallucinations, occurring 30 minutes to 3 hours after ingestion; gross overdose causes CNS depression progressing from stupor to coma, with respiratory distress, intractable seizures, and death.

To treat, establish ventilation; control seizures with diazepam. Pyridoxine is administered to equal dose of INH. Initial dose is 1 to 4 g pyridoxine I.V., followed by 1 g every 30 minutes thereafter, until the entire dose is given. Clear drug with gastric lavage after seizure control and correct acidosis with parenteral sodium bicarbonate; force diuresis with I.V. fluids and osmotic diuretics, and, if necessary, enhance clearance of the drug with hemodialysis or peritoneal dialysis.

☑ Special considerations

- At least 12 months of preventive therapy is recommended for persons with past tuberculosis and HIV-infected individuals.
- If compliance is a problem, twice-weekly supervised drug administration may be effective. Recommended twice-weekly dose for adults is 15 mg/kg P.O., not to exceed 900 mg.
- Oral doses should be taken on empty stomach for maximum absorption, or with food if gastric irritation occurs.
- Aluminum-containing antacids or laxatives should be taken 1 hour after oral dose of INH.
- Obtain specimens for culture and sensitivity testing before first dose, but therapy may begin before test results are complete; repeat periodically to detect drug resistance.
- Monitor blood, renal, and hepatic function studies before and periodically during therapy to minimize toxicity; assess visual function periodically.
- Observe patient for adverse effects, especially hepatic dysfunction, CNS toxicity, and optic neuritis. Establish safety measures, in case postural hypotension occurs.
- Drug may hinder stabilization of serum glucose level in patients with diabetes mellitus.
- Improvement usually evident after 2 to 3 weeks of therapy.
- Some recommend pyridoxine 50 mg P.O. daily to prevent peripheral neuropathy from large doses of INH. It may also be useful in patients at risk of developing peripheral neuropathy (malnourished patients, diabetics, and alcohol abusers). Pyridoxine (50 to 200 mg daily) has been used to treat drug-induced neuropathy.
- Because drug is dialyzable, patients undergoing hemodialysis or peritoneal dialysis may need dosage adjustments.
- Hepatotoxicity appears to be age-related and may limit use for prophylaxis. Alcohol consumption and history of alcohol-related liver disease also increases risk of hepatotoxicity.

Patient education

- Explain disease process and rationale for long-term therapy.
- Teach signs and symptoms of hypersensitivity and other adverse reactions, particularly visual disturbances, and emphasize need to report these; urge patient to report any unusual effects.
- Warn patient not to use alcohol; explain hazard of serious CNS toxicity and increased hazard of hepatitis.
- Teach patient how and when to take drug; instruct patient to take INH on an empty stomach, at least 1 hour before or 2 hours after meals. If GI irritation occurs, drug may be taken with food.
- Urge patient to comply with and complete prescribed regimen. Advise patient not to discontinue drug without medical approval; explain importance of follow-up appointments.
- Inform patient that drug therapy is usually continued for 18 months to 2 years for treatment of active tuberculosis; 12 months for prophylaxis; 9 months if INH and rifampin therapy are combined.
- Emphasize importance of uninterrupted therapy to prevent relapse and spread of infection.

Geriatric use

- Use with caution in elderly patients; incidence of hepatic effects is increased after age 35. Drug prophylaxis in patients with a positive purified protein derivative (PPD) test may not be indicated in older patients because of risk of hepatotoxicity.

Pediatric use

- Infants and children tolerate larger doses of drug.

Breast-feeding

- Drug is excreted in breast milk; use with caution in breast-feeding women and monitor infants for possible INH-induced toxicity.

---

isoproterenol
Isuprel

isoproterenol hydrochloride
Isuprel, Isuprel Glossets, Isuprel Mistometer, Norisodrine

isoproterenol sulfate
Medihaler-Iso

Pharmacologic classification: adrenergic
Therapeutic classification: bronchodilator, cardiac stimulant
Pregnancy risk category C

How supplied

Available by prescription only
isoproterenol
Nebulizer inhaler: 0.25%, 0.5%, 1%
isoproterenol hydrochloride
Tablets (S.L.): 10 mg, 15 mg
Aerosol inhaler: 120 mcg/metered spray, 131 mcg/metered spray
Injection: 200 mcg/ml
isoproterenol sulfate
Aerosol inhaler: 80 mcg/metered spray

Indications, route, and dosage

Complete heart block after closure of ventricular septal defect
Adults: I.V. bolus, 0.02 to 0.06 mg (1 to 3 ml of a 1:50,000 dilution).
Children: I.V. bolus, 0.01 to 0.03 mg (0.5 to 1.5 ml of a 1:50,000 dilution).
To prevent heart block
Adults: 10 to 30 mg S.L. four to six times daily.
Maintenance therapy of AV block
Adults: Initially, 10 mg S.L., followed by 5 to 50 mg p.r.n. Alternatively, 5 mg (half of a 10-mg tablet) administered P.R., followed by 5 to 15 mg p.r.n.
Bronchospasm during mild acute asthma attacks
isoproterenol hydrochloride
Adults and children: Via aerosol inhalation, 1 inhalation initially, repeated p.r.n. after 1 to 5 minutes, to maximum 6 inhalations daily. Maintenance dose is 1 to 2 inhalations four to six times daily at 3- to 4-hour intervals. Via hand-bulb nebulizer, 5 to 15 deep inhalations of a 0.5% solution; if needed, may be repeated in 5 to 10 minutes. May be repeated up to five times daily.

Alternatively, 3 to 7 deep inhalations of a 1% solution, repeated once in 5 to 10 minutes if needed. May be repeated up to five times daily.
isoproterenol sulfate
Adults and children: For acute dyspneic episodes, 1 inhalation initially; repeated if needed after 2 to 5 minutes. Maximum 6 inhalations daily. Maintenance dosage is 1 to 2 inhalations up to six times daily.
Bronchospasm in COPD
isoproterenol hydrochloride
Adults and children: Via hand-bulb nebulizer: 5 to 15 deep inhalations of a 0.5% solution, or 3 to 7 deep inhalations of a 1% solution no more frequently than q 3 to 4 hours.
Bronchospasm during mild acute asthma attacks or in COPD
isoproterenol hydrochloride
Adults and children: Oral inhalation of 2 ml of 0.125% solution or 2.5 ml of 0.1% solution up to five times daily.
Acute asthma attacks unresponsive to inhalation therapy or control of bronchospasm during anesthesia
isoproterenol hydrochloride
Adults: 0.01 to 0.02 mg (0.5 to 1 ml of a 1:50,000 dilution) I.V. Repeat if needed.
For bronchodilation
isoproterenol hydrochloride
Adults: 10 to 20 mg S.L., not to exceed 60 mg daily.
Children: 5 to 10 mg S.L., not to exceed 30 mg daily.
Emergency treatment of arrhythmias
isoproterenol hydrochloride
Adults: Initially, 0.02 to 0.06 mg I.V. bolus. Subsequent doses 0.01 to 0.2 mg I.V. Alternatively, 5 mcg/minute titrated to patient's response. Range, 2 to 20 mcg/minute. Alternatively, 0.2 mg I.M. or S.C.; subsequent doses 0.02 to 1 mg I.M. or 0.15 to 0.2 mg S.C. In extreme cases, 0.02 mg (0.1 of 1:5,000) intracardiac injection.
Children: May give half of initial adult dose.
Immediate temporary control of atropine-resistant hemodynamically significant bradycardia
isoproterenol hydrochloride
Adults: 2 to 10 mcg/minute I.V. infusion, titrated to patient's response.
Children: 0.1 mcg/kg/minute, titrated to patient's response. Maximum rate 1 mcg/kg/minute.
Heart block, Stokes-Adams attacks, and shock
isoproterenol hydrochloride
Adults and children: 0.5 to 5 mcg/minute by continuous I.V. infusion titrated to patient's response; or 0.02 to 0.06 mg I.V. boluses with 0.01 to 0.2 mg additional doses; or 0.2 mg I.M. or S.C. with 0.02 to 1 mg I.M. or 0.15 to 0.2 mg additional doses.

Pharmacodynamics

Bronchodilator action: Isoproterenol relaxes bronchial smooth muscle by direct action on $beta_2$-adrenergic receptors, relieving bronchospasm, increasing vital capacity, decreasing residual volume in lungs, and facilitating passage of pulmonary secretions. It also produces relaxation of GI and uterine smooth muscle via stimulation of $beta_2$ receptors. Peripheral vasodilation, cardiac stimulation, and relaxation of bronchial smooth muscle are the main therapeutic effects.

Cardiac stimulant action: Isoproterenol acts on $beta_1$-adrenergic receptors in the heart, producing a positive chronotropic and inotropic effect; it usually increases cardiac output. In patients with AV block, isoproterenol shortens conduction time and the refractory period of the AV node and increases the rate and strength of ventricular contraction.

Pharmacokinetics

• *Absorption:* After injection or oral inhalation, drug is absorbed rapidly; after sublingual or rectal administration, absorption is variable and often unreliable. Onset of action is prompt after oral inhalation and persists up to 1 hour. Effects persist for a few minutes after I.V. injection, up to 2 hours after S.C. or sublingual administration, and up to 4 hours after rectal administration of sublingual tablet.
• *Distribution:* Distributed widely throughout the body.
• *Metabolism:* Isoproterenol is metabolized by conjugation in the GI tract and by enzymatic reduction in liver, lungs, and other tissues.
• *Excretion:* Excreted primarily in urine as unchanged drug and its metabolites.

Contraindications and precautions

Contraindicated in patients with tachycardia caused by digitalis intoxication, in patients with preexisting arrhythmias (other than those that may respond to treatment with isoproterenol), and in those with angina pectoris. Use cautiously in the elderly and in patients with impaired renal function, CV disease, coronary insufficiency, diabetes, hyperthyroidism, or a sensitivity to sympathomimetic amines.

Interactions

Concomitant use of isoproterenol with *epinephrine* and other *sympathomimetics* may cause additive

CV reactions. However, these drugs may be used together if at least 4 hours elapse between administration of the two drugs. Use with *beta-adrenergic blockers* antagonizes isoproterenol's cardiac-stimulating, bronchodilating, and vasodilating effects. Use with *ergot alkaloids* may increase blood pressure.

Arrhythmias may occur more readily when drug is administered to patients receiving a *cardiac glycoside, potassium-depleting drugs,* or *other drugs that affect cardiac rhythm.* Isoproterenol should be used with caution in patients receiving *cyclopropane* or *halogenated hydrocarbon general anesthetics.*

Effects on diagnostic tests

Isoproterenol may reduce the sensitivity of spirometry in the diagnosis of asthma.

Adverse reactions

CNS: *headache, mild tremor,* weakness, dizziness, *nervousness,* insomnia, ***Stokes-Adams seizures.***
CV: palpitations, *tachycardia, anginal pain,* ***arrhythmias, cardiac arrest****, rapid rise and fall in blood pressure.*
GI: *nausea, vomiting, heartburn.*
Respiratory: ***bronchospasm,*** bronchitis, sputum increase, pulmonary edema.
Other: diaphoresis, hyperglycemia; swelling of parotid glands (with prolonged use).

Overdose and treatment

Clinical manifestations of overdose include exaggeration of common adverse reactions, particularly arrhythmias, extreme tremors, nausea, vomiting, and profound hypotension.

Treatment includes symptomatic and supportive measures. Monitor vital signs closely. Sedatives (barbiturates) may be used to treat CNS stimulation. Use cardioselective beta blocker to treat tachycardia and arrhythmias. These agents should be used with caution; they may induce asthmatic attack.

☑ Special considerations

Besides those relevant to all *adrenergics,* consider the following recommendations.

- Drug does not replace administration of blood, plasma, fluids, or electrolytes in patients with blood volume depletion.
- Severe paradoxical airway resistance may follow oral inhalations.
- Hypotension must be corrected before isoproterenol is administered.
- If three to five treatments within 6 to 12 hours provide minimal or no relief, re-evaluate therapy.
- Continuously monitor ECG during I.V. administration.
- Carefully monitor response to therapy by frequent determinations of heart rate, ECG pattern, blood pressure, and central venous pressure, as well as (for patients in shock) urine volume, blood pH, and Pco_2 levels.
- Prescribed I.V. infusion rate should include specific guidelines for regulating flow or terminating infusion in relation to heart rate, premature beats, ECG changes, precordial distress, blood pressure, and urine flow. Because of danger of precipitating arrhythmias, rate of infusion is usually decreased or infusion may be temporarily discontinued if heart rate exceeds 110 beats/minute.
- Constant-infusion pump prevents sudden infusion of excessive amounts of drug.
- Sublingual doses should not be given more frequently than every 3 to 4 hours nor more than three times daily.
- Sublingual tablet may be administered rectally, if indicated.
- Monitor patient for rebound bronchospasm when drug's effects end.
- Isoproterenol has also been used to aid diagnosis of coronary artery disease and of mitral regurgitation.
- Do not inject solutions intended for oral inhalation.

Patient education

- Remind patient to save applicator; refills may be available.
- Urge patient to call if no relief is gained or condition worsens.
- Advise patient to store oral forms away from heat and light (not in bathroom medicine cabinet where heat and moisture will cause deterioration of the drug). Keep drug out of the reach of children.

Inhalation

- Give patient instructions on proper use of inhaler.
- Tell patient that saliva and sputum may appear red or pink after oral inhalation, because isoproterenol turns red on exposure to air.
- Advise patient to rinse mouth with water after drug is absorbed completely and between doses.

Sublingual

- Tell patient to allow sublingual tablet to dissolve under tongue, without sucking, and not to swallow saliva (may cause epigastric pain) until drug has been absorbed completely.
- Warn patient that frequent use of sublingual tablets may damage teeth due to acidity of drug.

Geriatric use

- Elderly patients may be more sensitive to therapeutic and adverse effects of drug.

Pediatric use

- Use with caution in children.

Breast-feeding

- It is unknown if drug is excreted in breast milk; therefore, use cautiously in breast-feeding women.

isosorbide

Ismotic

Pharmacologic classification: osmotic diuretic
Therapeutic classification: antiglaucoma
Pregnancy risk category B

How supplied

Available by prescription only
Oral solution: 45% in 220-ml containers

Indications, route, and dosage
Short-term reduction of intraocular pressure from glaucoma
Adults: Initially, 1.5 g/kg P.O. b.i.d. to q.i.d. as indicated. Usual dosage range, 1 to 3 g/kg.

Pharmacodynamics
Diuretic action: Increases osmolarity of fluid presented to the kidney, decreasing reabsorption of water and resulting in diuresis. In the eye, isosorbide creates an osmotic gradient between plasma and ocular fluids.

Pharmacokinetics
- *Absorption:* Drug is absorbed rapidly after oral administration. Action begins within 10 to 30 minutes and peaks at 60 to 90 minutes.
- *Distribution:* Drug achieves good ocular penetration and is distributed to total body water.
- *Metabolism:* None.
- *Excretion:* Drug is eliminated unchanged by the kidney. Duration of action is 5 to 6 hours, and half-life is 7 to 8 hours.

Contraindications and precautions
Contraindicated in patients with anuria caused by severe renal disease, severe dehydration, acute pulmonary edema, and hemorrhagic glaucoma. Use cautiously in patients with diseases associated with sodium retention such as heart failure.

Interactions
None significant.

Effects on diagnostic tests
None reported.

Adverse reactions
CNS: vertigo, light-headedness, lethargy, headache, confusion, disorientation, irritability, syncope, dizziness.
GI: gastric discomfort, nausea, vomiting.
Other: hypernatremia, hyperosmolality, thirst.

Overdose and treatment
Clinical effects of overdose include hypoglycemia, hyperuricemia, fluid and electrolyte imbalances, weakness, hyporeflexia, and arrhythmias.

Emesis may be indicated after substantial ingestion unless the patient is obtunded or comatose. Monitor the patient's fluid and electrolyte status closely.

☑ Special considerations
- Isosorbide carries less risk of nausea and vomiting than other oral hyperosmotics. Serving over cracked ice seems to improve palatability.
- Monitor patient for 5 to 10 minutes after drug administration.
- Drug may be used to interrupt acute attack of glaucoma before laser or surgical treatment.
- Additional antiemetics (I.M.) may be needed when isosorbide is used to lower intraocular pressure.

Patient education
- Tell patient to sip medication to improve palatability.
- Inform patient that drug may cause him to feel thirsty.

Geriatric use
- Use drug with caution in elderly patients because of increased risk of fluid and electrolyte imbalances.

Pediatric use
- Use drug with caution in children because of increased risk of fluid and electrolyte imbalances.

isosorbide dinitrate
Apo-ISDN*, Coronex*, Dilatrate-SR, Iso-Bid, Isonate, Isordil, Isordil Tembids, Isordil Titradose, Isotrate, Novosorbide*, Sorbitrate, Sorbitrate SA

Pharmacologic classification: nitrate
Therapeutic classification: antianginal, vasodilator
Pregnancy risk category C

How supplied
Available by prescription only
Tablets: 5 mg, 10 mg, 20 mg, 30 mg, 40 mg
Tablets (S.L.): 2.5 mg, 5 mg, 10 mg
Tablets (extended-release): 40 mg
Tablets (chewable): 5 mg, 10 mg
Capsules (extended-release): 40 mg

Indications, route, and dosage
Treatment or prophylaxis of acute anginal attacks; treatment of chronic ischemic heart disease (by preload reduction)
Adults: S.L. form—2.5 to 10 mg under tongue for prompt relief of angina pain, repeated q 2 to 3 hours during acute phase, or q 4 to 6 hours for prophylaxis.

Chewable form—2.5 to 10 mg. p.r.n., for acute attack or q 2 to 3 hours for prophylaxis, but only after initial test dose of 5 mg to determine risk of severe hypotension.

Oral form—10 to 20 mg P.O. t.i.d. or q.i.d. for prophylaxis only (use smallest effective dose).

Extended-release forms—20 to 40 mg P.O. q 8 to 12 hours.

◊ ***Adjunctive treatment of heart failure***
Adults: 5 to 10 mg S.L. q 3 to 4 hours. Alternatively, give 20 to 40 mg P.O. (or chewable tablets) q 4 hours. Usually administered with vasodilators.

◊ ***Diffuse esophageal spasm without gastroesophageal reflux***
Adults: 10 to 30 mg P.O. q 4 hours.

Pharmacodynamics
Antianginal action: Drug reduces myocardial oxygen demand through peripheral vasodilation, resulting in decreased venous filling pressure (preload) and, to a lesser extent, decreased arterial impedance (afterload). These combined effects result in decreased cardiac work and, consequently, reduced myocardial oxygen demands. Drug also re-

distributes coronary blood flow from epicardial to subendocardial regions.

Vasodilating action: Drug dilates peripheral vessels (primarily venous), helping to manage pulmonary edema and heart failure caused by decreased venous return to the heart (preload). Arterial vasodilatory effects also decrease arterial impedance (afterload) and thus left ventricular work, benefiting the failing heart. These combined effects may help some patients with acute MI. (Use of isosorbide dinitrate in patients with heart failure and acute MI is currently unapproved.)

Pharmacokinetics

• *Absorption:* Oral form is well absorbed from the GI tract but undergoes first-pass metabolism, resulting in bioavailability of about 50% (depending on dosage form used). With S.L. and chewable forms, onset of action is 3 minutes; with other oral forms, 30 minutes; with extended-release forms, 1 hour.
• *Distribution:* Limited information is available on drug's plasma protein binding and distribution. Like nitroglycerin, it is distributed widely throughout the body.
• *Metabolism:* Drug is metabolized in the liver to active metabolites.
• *Excretion:* Metabolites are excreted in the urine; elimination half-life is about 5 to 6 hours with oral administration; 2 hours with S.L. administration. About 80% to 100% of absorbed dose is excreted in the urine within 24 hours. Duration of effect is longer than that of S.L. preparations. With S.L. and chewable forms, duration of effect is 30 minutes to 2 hours; with other oral forms, 5 to 6 hours.

Contraindications and precautions

Contraindicated in patients with hypersensitivity or idiosyncrasy to nitrates, severe hypotension, shock, or acute MI with low left ventricular filling pressure. Use cautiously in patients with hypotension or blood volume depletion (such as from diuretic therapy).

Interactions

Concomitant use of isosorbide with *alcohol, antihypertensive drugs, calcium channel blockers, phenothiazines,* or *vasodilators* may cause additive hypotensive effects.

Effects on diagnostic tests

Isosorbide dinitrate may interfere with serum cholesterol determination tests using the Zlatkis-Zak color reaction, causing a falsely decreased value.

Adverse reactions

CNS: *headache* (sometimes with throbbing), dizziness, weakness.
CV: *orthostatic hypotension, tachycardia, palpitations, ankle edema,* fainting.
GI: nausea, vomiting.
Skin: cutaneous vasodilation, *flushing,* rash.
Other: hypersensitivity reactions, sublingual burning.

Overdose and treatment

Clinical effects of overdose result primarily from vasodilation and methemoglobinemia and include hypotension, persistent throbbing headache, palpitations, visual disturbance, flushing of the skin and sweating (with skin later becoming cold and cyanotic), nausea and vomiting, colic and bloody diarrhea, orthostatism, initial hyperpnea, dyspnea, slow respiratory rate, bradycardia, heart block, increased intracranial pressure with confusion, fever, paralysis, and tissue hypoxia, which can lead to cyanosis, metabolic acidosis, coma, clonic seizures, and circulatory collapse. Death may result from circulatory collapse or asphyxia.

Treatment includes gastric lavage followed by administration of activated charcoal to remove remaining gastric contents. Blood gas measurements and methemoglobin levels should be monitored, as indicated. Supportive care includes respiratory support and oxygen administration, passive movement of extremities to aid venous return, recumbent positioning (Trendelenburg position, if necessary), maintenance of adequate body temperature, and administration of I.V. fluids.

An I.V. adrenergic agonist (such as phenylephrine) may be considered if further treatment is required. For methemoglobinemia, methylene blue (1 to 2 mg/kg I.V.) may be given. (Epinephrine and related compounds are contraindicated in isosorbide dinitrate overdose.)

☑ Special considerations

• Drug may cause headache, especially at first. Dose may need to be reduced temporarily, but tolerance usually develops to this effect. In the interim, patient may relieve headache with aspirin or acetaminophen.
• Additional dose may be given before anticipated stress or at bedtime if angina is nocturnal.
• Monitor blood pressure and intensity and duration of patient's response to drug.
• Drug may cause orthostatic hypotension. To minimize this, have patient change to upright position slowly, walk up and down stairs carefully, and lie down at first sign of dizziness.
• Do not discontinue drug abruptly because this may cause coronary vasospasm.
• Store drug in cool place, in tightly closed container away from light.
• Maintenance of continuous 24-hour plasma levels may result in refractory tolerance. Dosing regimens should include dose-free intervals, which vary based on form of drug used.

Patient education

• Instruct patient to take medication regularly, as prescribed, and to keep it easily accessible at all times. Drug is physiologically necessary but not addictive.
• Warn patient that headache may occur initially, but may respond to usual headache remedies or dosage reduction. Assure patient that headache usually subsides gradually with continued treatment.
• If patient is taking oral tablet, tell him to take it on empty stomach, either 30 minutes before or 1 to 2

hours after meals; to swallow oral tablets whole; and to chew chewable tablets thoroughly before swallowing.
- Advise patient to sit when self-administering S.L. tablets. He should lubricate tablet with saliva or place a few milliliters of fluid under tongue with tablet. If patient experiences tingling sensation with drug placed sublingually, he may try to hold tablet in buccal pouch. Dose may be repeated every 10 to 15 minutes for maximum of three doses. If no relief occurs, he should call or go to hospital emergency room.
- Warn patient to make positional changes gradually to avoid excessive dizziness.
- Instruct patient to avoid alcohol while taking drug because severe hypotension and CV collapse may occur.
- Advise patient to report blurred vision, dry mouth, or persistent headache.
- Caution patient not to stop long-term therapy abruptly.

Pediatric use
- Methemoglobinemia may occur in infants receiving large doses of isosorbide dinitrate.

Breast-feeding
- It is not known if drug is excreted in breast milk. Use cautiously in breast-feeding patients.

isosorbide mononitrate
Imdur, ISMO, Monoket

Pharmacologic classification: nitrate
Therapeutic classification: antianginal
Pregnancy risk category C

How supplied
Available by prescription only
Tablets: 10 mg, 20 mg
Tablets (extended-release): 30 mg, 60 mg, 120 mg

Indications, route, and dosage
Prevention of angina pectoris due to coronary artery disease (but not to abort acute anginal attacks)
Adults: 20 mg P.O. b.i.d., with doses 7 hours apart and first dose on awakening. For extended-release tablets, 30 to 60 mg P.O. once daily, on arising; after several days, dosage may be increased to 120 mg once daily; rarely, 240 mg may be required; extended-release tablets should not be crushed or chewed.

Pharmacodynamics
Antianginal action: Drug is the major active metabolite of isosorbide dinitrate. It relaxes vascular smooth muscle and consequently dilates peripheral arteries and veins. Dilation of the veins promotes peripheral pooling of blood and decreases venous return to the heart, thereby reducing left ventricular end-diastolic pressure and pulmonary capillary wedge pressure (preload). Arteriolar relaxation reduces systemic vascular resistance, systolic arterial pressure, and mean arterial pressure (afterload). Dilation of the coronary arteries also occurs.

Pharmacokinetics
- *Absorption:* Drug's absolute bioavailability is almost 100%. Maximum serum concentrations are achieved 30 to 60 minutes after ingestion.
- *Distribution:* Volume of distribution of isosorbide mononitrate is approximately 0.6 L/kg. Less than 4% is bound to plasma proteins.
- *Metabolism:* Drug is not subject to first-pass metabolism in the liver.
- *Excretion:* Less than 1% of isosorbide mononitrate is eliminated in urine. Overall elimination half-life of drug is about 5 hours.

Contraindications and precautions
Contraindicated in patients with hypersensitivity or idiosyncrasy to nitrates, severe hypotension, shock, or acute MI with low left ventricular filling pressure. Use cautiously in patients with hypotension or blood volume depletion (such as from diuretic therapy).

Interactions
Drug's vasodilating effects may be additive with those of other *vasodilators*, especially *alcohol*. Marked symptomatic orthostatic hypotension has been reported when *calcium channel blockers* and *organic nitrates* were used in combination. Dose adjustments of either class of agents may be necessary.

Effects on diagnostic tests
None reported.

Adverse reactions
CNS: *headache* (sometimes with throbbing), dizziness, weakness.
CV: *orthostatic hypotension, tachycardia, palpitations, ankle edema,* fainting.
GI: nausea, vomiting.
Musculoskeletal: arthralgia.
Respiratory: bronchitis, pneumonia, upper respiratory tract infection.
Skin: cutaneous vasodilation, *flushing,* rash.
Other: hypersensitivity reactions, sublingual burning.

Overdose and treatment
Symptoms of overdose may include increased intracranial pressure; persistent, throbbing headache; confusion; moderate fever; vertigo; palpitations; visual disturbances; nausea and vomiting (possibly with colic and even bloody diarrhea); syncope (especially with upright position); air hunger; dyspnea, later followed by reduced ventilatory effort; diaphoresis, with skin either flushed or cold and clammy; heart block and bradycardia; paralysis; coma; seizures; and death.

No specific antagonist to drug's vasodilator effects is known. However, drug is significantly removed from the blood during hemodialysis.

If drug is ingested, induce emesis or perform gastric lavage followed by activated charcoal administration. Because drug is rapidly and completely absorbed, however, gastric lavage may be effective only with recent ingestion. Treat severe hypotension and reflex tachycardia by elevating legs and administering I.V. fluids. Epinephrine is ineffective in reversing severe hypotension associated with overdosage, and epinephrine and related compounds are contraindicated. Administer oxygen and artificial ventilation if necessary. Monitor methemoglobin levels as indicated.

☑ Special considerations

• Drug-free interval sufficient to avoid tolerance to drug is not completely defined. The recommended regimen involves two daily doses given 7 hours apart, with a gap of 17 hours between the second dose of 1 day and the first dose of the next day. Considering the relatively long half-life of drug, this result is consistent with those obtained for other organic nitrates.
• The asymmetric twice-daily regimen successfully avoids significant rebound or withdrawal effects. In studies of other nitrates, the incidence and magnitude of such phenomena appear to be highly dependent on the schedule of nitrate administration.
• Onset of action of oral drug is not sufficiently rapid to be useful in aborting an acute anginal episode.
• Benefits of drug in patients with acute MI or heart failure have not been established. Because drug's effects are difficult to terminate rapidly, its use is not recommended in such patients. If it is used, however, careful clinical or hemodynamic monitoring must be performed to avoid the hazards of hypotension and tachycardia.
• Methemoglobinemia has occurred in patients receiving other organic nitrates and probably could occur as an adverse reaction. Significant methemoglobinemia has occurred in association with moderate overdoses of organic nitrates. Suspect methemoglobinemia in patients who exhibit signs of impaired oxygen delivery despite adequate cardiac output and adequate PaO_2. Classically, methemoglobinemic blood is chocolate brown, without color change on exposure to air. Treatment of choice for methemoglobinemia is methylene blue, 1 to 2 mg/kg I.V.

Patient education

• Tell patient to follow prescribed dosing schedule carefully (two doses taken 7 hours apart) to maintain antianginal effect and to prevent tolerance.
• Warn patient that daily headaches sometimes accompany treatment with nitrates, including isosorbide mononitrate, and are a marker of drug activity. Patient should not alter treatment schedule, because loss of headache may be associated with simultaneous loss of antianginal efficacy. Tell patient to treat headaches with aspirin or acetaminophen.
• Warn patient to avoid alcohol while taking drug because of increased risk of light-headedness.
• Tell patient to rise slowly from recumbent or seated position to avoid light-headedness caused by sudden drop in blood pressure.

Pediatric use

• Safety and effectiveness in children have not been established.

Breast-feeding

• Excretion of drug in breast milk is unknown. Use caution when administering to a breast-feeding patient.

isotretinoin

Accutane

Pharmacologic classification: retinoic acid derivative
Therapeutic classification: antiacne, keratinization stabilizer
Pregnancy risk category X

How supplied

Available by prescription only
Capsules: 10 mg, 20 mg, 40 mg

Indications, route, and dosage

Severe recalcitrant nodular acne
Adults and adolescents: 0.5 to 2 mg/kg P.O. daily given in two divided doses and continued for 15 to 20 weeks.
◊ ***Keratinization disorders resistant to conventional therapy,*** ◊ ***prevention of skin cancer***
Adults: Dosage varies with specific disease and severity of the disorder; dosages up to 2 to 4 mg/kg P.O. daily have been used. Consult current literature for specific recommendations.
◊ ***Squamous cell cancer of the head and neck***
Adults: 50 to 100 mg/m^2.

Pharmacodynamics

Antiacne action: Exact mechanism of action is unknown; isotretinoin decreases the size and activity of sebaceous glands, which decreases secretion and probably explains the rapid clinical improvement. A reduction in *Propionibacterium acnes* in the hair follicles occurs as a secondary result of decreased nutrients.

Keratinizing action: Isotretinoin has anti-inflammatory and keratinizing effects. The mechanism is unknown.

Pharmacokinetics

• *Absorption:* When administered orally, drug is absorbed rapidly from the GI tract. Peak concentrations occur in 3 hours, with peak concentrations of the metabolite 4-oxo-isotretinoin occurring in 6 to 20 hours. Therapeutic range for isotretinoin has not been established.
• *Distribution:* Drug is distributed widely. In animals, it is found in most organs and is known to cross the placenta. In humans, degree of placental transfer and the degree of secretion in breast milk are unknown. Isotretinoin is 99.9% protein-bound, primarily to albumin.
• *Metabolism:* Isotretinoin is metabolized in the liver and possibly in the gut wall. The major metabolite is 4-oxo-isotretinoin, with tretinoin and 4-oxo-tretinoin also found in the blood and urine.
• *Excretion:* Elimination process is not fully known, although renal and biliary pathways are known to be used.

Contraindications and precautions
Contraindicated in women of childbearing age unless patient has had a negative serum pregnancy test within 2 weeks before beginning therapy, will begin drug therapy on day 2 or 3 of next menstrual period, and will comply with stringent contraceptive measures for 1 month before therapy, during therapy, and for at least 1 month after therapy. Severe fetal abnormalities may occur if used during pregnancy. Also contraindicated in patients hypersensitive to parabens, which are used as preservatives.

Interactions
Isotretinoin will have a cumulative drying effect when used with *medicated soaps and cleansers, medicated "cover-ups," topical resorcinol peeling agents* (*benzoyl peroxide*), and *alcohol-containing preparations*. Concurrent use of *vitamin A products* may have an additive toxic effect. *Tetracyclines* may increase the potential for the development of pseudotumor cerebri. *Alcohol* intake may increase plasma triglyceride levels. Coadministration of *carbamazapine* and isotretinoin has resulted in decreased carbamazapine levels in plasma.

Effects on diagnostic tests
Drug's physiologic effects may alter liver function tests, blood counts, and blood glucose, uric acid, cholesterol, and triglyceride levels. Drug may cause elevation of erythrocyte sedimentation rate.

Adverse reactions
CNS: headache, fatigue, *pseudotumor cerebri* (benign intracranial hypertension).
EENT: *conjunctivitis,* corneal deposits, dry eyes, visual disturbances, *epistaxis, dry nose.*
GI: nonspecific GI symptoms, gum bleeding and inflammation, *nausea, vomiting,* anorexia, *dry mouth, abdominal pain.*
Hematologic: anemia, elevated platelet count.
Hepatic: elevated AST, ALT, and alkaline phosphatase levels.
Skin: *cheilosis, rash, dry skin, facial skin desquamation,* peeling of palms and toes, skin infection, photosensitivity, *cheilitis, pruritus, fragility.*
Other: *hypertriglyceridemia, musculoskeletal pain (skeletal hyperostosis), drying of mucous membranes, petechiae, nail brittleness,* thinning of hair, hyperglycemia.

Overdose and treatment
Clinical manifestations of overdose are rare and would be extensions of adverse reactions.

☑ Special considerations
- Therapy usually lasts 15 to 20 weeks, followed by at least 8 weeks off drug before beginning a second course.
- Contact lenses may become uncomfortable during treatment; recommend use of artificial tears.
- Administer drug with or shortly after meals.
- Monitor patient for visual problems.
- Drug has been used in a limited number of patients to treat psoriasis (combined with psoralen and ultraviolet light); it has also been used to treat cutaneous neoplasms.

Patient education
- Recommend taking drug with or shortly after meals to ease GI discomfort; also, chewing gum may relieve dryness of mouth.
- Warn patient that acne may worsen during initial course of therapy and to call if irritation becomes severe.
- Warn patient not to donate blood or become pregnant while taking medication and for 30 days after discontinuing drug.
- Caution against alcohol ingestion, to reduce risk of hypertriglyceridemia.
- Warn patient to be cautious when driving, particularly at night because drug causes decreased night vision.
- Instruct patient not to crush capsules.
- Advise patient not to take vitamin supplements containing vitamin A while taking drug.
- Inform patient to avoid prolonged exposure to sunlight or sun lamps to prevent photosensitivity.

Special instructions for female patients
- Isotretinoin is a potent teratogen and should not be given to female patients who are pregnant or may become pregnant during therapy. Patient selection is important — informed consent must be obtained from patient or her legal guardian before initiating therapy. The patient or responsible adult must fully understand the consequences of fetal exposure to isotretinoin.
- Reliable methods of contraception are essential for sexually active females who are taking isotretinoin.
- Negative blood tests for pregnancy must be obtained before therapy.
- Schedule follow-up visits monthly during therapy. Do not prescribe more than a 6-week supply at a time. Pregnancy tests must be repeated monthly.

Breast-feeding
- It is unknown if drug passes into breast milk; breast-feeding is not recommended during drug therapy.

isradipine
DynaCirc

Pharmacologic classification: calcium channel blocker
Therapeutic classification: antihypertensive
Pregnancy risk category C

How supplied
Available by prescription only
Capsules: 2.5 mg, 5 mg

Indications, route, and dosage
Management of hypertension
Adults: Individualize dosage. Initially, 2.5 mg P.O. b.i.d. alone or with thiazide diuretic. Maximal response may require 2 to 4 weeks; therefore, dosage adjustments of 5 mg daily should be made at 2- to 4-week intervals up to maximum of 20 mg daily. Dosages of 10 mg or more per day have not been shown to be more effective but rather to lead to in-

creased incidence of adverse reactions. Same starting dosage is used in elderly, hepatic-impaired, and renal-impaired patients.

Pharmacodynamics

Antihypertensive action: A dihydropyridine calcium channel blocker, isradipine binds to calcium channels and inhibits calcium flux into cardiac and smooth muscle, which results in dilation of arterioles. This dilation reduces systemic resistance and lowers blood pressure while producing small increases in resting heart rate.

Pharmacokinetics

- *Absorption:* 90% to 95% absorbed after oral administration; peak concentrations are reached in 1½ hours.
- *Distribution:* 95% is bound to plasma protein.
- *Metabolism:* Isradipine is completely metabolized before elimination with extensive first-pass metabolism.
- *Excretion:* 60% to 65% of drug is excreted in urine; 25% to 30%, in feces.

Contraindications and precautions

Contraindicated in patients with hypersensitivity to drug. Use cautiously in patients with heart failure, especially if combined with a beta blocker.

Interactions

Severe hypotension has been reported with concomitant use of a *beta blocker* and a *calcium channel blocker* during *fentanyl anesthesia* but has not been seen with isradipine. Additive negative inotropic effects are possible when used with a beta blocker in patients with some degree of heart failure.

Effects on diagnostic tests

None reported.

Adverse reactions

CNS: dizziness, *headache,* fatigue.
CV: edema, flushing, syncope, angina, tachycardia.
GI: nausea, diarrhea, abdominal discomfort, vomiting.
Respiratory: dyspnea.
Skin: rash.

Overdose and treatment

No well-documented cases of overdose have been reported; however, presumably excessive peripheral vasodilation with marked and prolonged systemic hypotension may occur. Symptomatic and supportive treatment should be provided, including active CV support, monitoring of input and output and cardiac and respiratory function, elevation of lower extremities, and fluid replacement as needed. Vasoconstrictors should be used only when not specifically contraindicated.

☑ Special considerations

- Drug has no significant effect on heart rate and no adverse effects on cardiac contractility, conduction or digitalis clearance, or lipid or renal function.
- Administration with food significantly increases the time to reach peak concentrations by about 1 hour. However, food has no effect on total bioavailability of drug.
- Elevated liver function test results have been reported in some patients.
- Individualize dosage. Allow 2 to 4 weeks between dosage adjustments.

Patient education

- Instruct patient to report irregular heartbeat, shortness of breath, swelling of hands or feet, pronounced dizziness, constipation, nausea, or hypotension.

Geriatric use

- No age-related problems have been reported.

Pediatric use

- Safety and efficacy have not been established in children under age 18.

Breast-feeding

- It is unknown if isradipine is excreted in breast milk. Consider the potential risk of serious adverse reactions in the infant.

itraconazole

Sporanox

Pharmacologic classification: synthetic triazole
Therapeutic classification: antifungal
Pregnancy risk category C

How supplied

Available by prescription only
Capsules: 100 mg

Indications, route, and dosage

Treatment of blastomycosis (pulmonary and extrapulmonary), histoplasmosis (including chronic cavitary pulmonary disease and disseminated nonmeningeal histoplasmosis)
Adults: 200 mg P.O. once daily. If condition does not improve or shows evidence of progressive fungal disease, increase dose in 100-mg increments to maximum of 400 mg daily. Give doses over 200 mg/day in two divided doses.
Aspergillosis (pulmonary and extrapulmonary) in patients who are intolerant of or refractory to amphotericin B therapy
Adults: 200 to 400 mg P.O. daily.
◇ ***Treatment of superficial mycoses (dermatophytoses, pityriasis versicolor, sebopsoriasis, candidiasis [vaginal, oral, or chronic mucocutaneous], onychomycosis),*** ◇ ***systemic mycoses (candidiasis, cryptococcal infections [meningitis, disseminated],*** ◇ ***dimorphic infections [paracoccidioidomycosis, coccidioidomycosis]),*** ◇ ***subcutaneous mycoses (sporotrichosis, chromomycosis),*** ◇ ***cutaneous leishmaniasis,*** ◇ ***fungal keratitis,*** ◇ ***alternariatoxicosis, and*** ◇ ***zygomycosis***
Adults: 50 to 400 mg P.O. daily. Duration of therapy varies from 1 day to greater than 6 months, depending on the condition and mycologic response.

Note: Discontinue drug if patient develops clinical signs and symptoms consistent with liver disease that may be attributable to itraconazole.

Pharmacodynamics

Antifungal action: Itraconazole is a synthetic triazole antifungal agent. In vitro, itraconazole inhibits the cytochrome P-450 dependent synthesis of ergosterol, a vital component of fungal cell membranes.

Pharmacokinetics

- *Absorption:* Oral bioavailability of drug is maximal when taken with food; absolute oral bioavailability is 55%.
- *Distribution:* Plasma protein binding of drug is 99.8%; 99.5% for its metabolite, hydroxyitraconazole.
- *Metabolism:* Drug is extensively metabolized by the liver into a large number of metabolites, including hydroxyitraconazole, the major metabolite.
- *Excretion:* Fecal excretion of parent drug varies between 3% and 18% of the dose. Renal excretion of parent drug is less than 0.03% of dose. About 40% of dose is excreted as inactive metabolites in the urine. Drug is not removed by hemodialysis.

Contraindications and precautions

Contraindicated in patients with hypersensitivity to drug, in patients receiving terfenadine or astemizole, and in breast-feeding patients because drug is excreted in breast milk. Coadministration with cisapride is contraindicated because serious CV events (prolonged QT interval), including death, have occurred in patients taking itraconazole with cisapride.

Use cautiously in patients with hypochlorhydria or HIV infection and in those receiving medications that are highly protein-bound.

Interactions

Itraconazole can increase plasma levels of the *nonsedating antihistamines* (such as *astemizole*), resulting in rare instances of life-threatening arrhythmias and death. Avoid concurrent use. Itraconazole may increase *cyclosporine* plasma levels. Reduce cyclosporine dosage by 50% when using itraconazole doses greater than 100 mg/day, and monitor cyclosporine levels. Itraconazole also may increase *digoxin* levels. Monitor digoxin levels. Hypoglycemia may occur when itraconazole and *sulfonylureas* are used concurrently. Monitor blood glucose. The anticoagulant effect of *warfarin* may be enhanced by itraconazole. Monitor PT. *H_2 antagonists, isoniazid, phenytoin,* and *rifampin* may reduce plasma itraconazole levels. Itraconazole may alter *phenytoin* metabolism. Monitor phenytoin levels. Itraconazole can increase levels of *cisapride*, causing prolongation of the QT interval and, rarely, serious ventricular arrhythmias. Avoid concurrent use.

Effects on diagnostic tests

None reported.

Adverse reactions

CNS: headache, dizziness, somnolence.
CV: hypertension.
GI: *nausea*, vomiting, diarrhea, abdominal pain, anorexia.
GU: albuminuria.
Hepatic: impaired hepatic function.
Skin: rash, pruritus.
Other: edema, fatigue, fever, malaise, decreased libido, hypokalemia, impotence.

Overdose and treatment

In the event of accidental overdosage, employ supportive measures, including gastric lavage with sodium bicarbonate. Itraconazole is not removed by dialysis.

☑ Special considerations

- In life-threatening situations, the recommended loading dose is 200 mg three times daily (600 mg/day) for first 3 days. Continue treatment for minimum of 3 months and until clinical parameters and laboratory tests indicate that the active fungal infection has subsided. An inadequate period of treatment may lead to recurrence of active infection.
- Obtain specimens for fungal cultures and other relevant laboratory studies (wet mount, histopathology, serology) before therapy to isolate and identify causative organisms. Therapy may be instituted before results of cultures and other laboratory studies are known; once results become available, adjust anti-infective therapy accordingly.
- The clinical course of histoplasmosis in HIV-infected patients is more severe and usually requires maintenance therapy to prevent relapse. Because hypochlorhydria has occurred in HIV-infected patients, absorption of itraconazole may be decreased.
- Monitor hepatic enzyme test values in patients with preexisting hepatic function abnormalities.

Patient education

- Instruct patient to take drug with food to enhance absorption.
- Tell patient to report signs and symptoms that may suggest liver dysfunction (jaundice, unusual fatigue, anorexia, nausea, vomiting, dark urine, pale stool) so that appropriate laboratory testing can be performed.

Pediatric use

- Safety and effectiveness in children have not been established.

Breast-feeding

- Because drug is excreted in breast milk, its use is contraindicated in breast-feeding patients.

ivermectin

Stromectol

Pharmacologic classification: broad-spectrum antiparasitic agent
Therapeutic classification: anthelmintic
Pregnancy risk category C

How supplied

Available by prescription only
Tablets (scored): 6 mg

Indications, route, and dosage

Strongyloidiasis of intestinal tract (nondisseminated)

Adults: 200 mcg/kg P.O. as a single dose.

Onchoceriasis

Adults: 150 mcg/kg P.O. as a single dose. The most common dose interval in mass distribution campaigns is 12 months; retreatment of individual patients may be considered at intervals as short as 3 months.

Pharmacodynamics

Anthelmintic action: Drug binds to glutamate-gated chloride ion channels in invertebrate nerve and muscle cells. This increases the permeability of the cell membranes to chloride and hyperpolarization of the nerve or muscle cell occurs, resulting in paralysis and death of the parasite. Ivermectin has a selective toxicity because it has a lower affinity for mammalian ligand-gated chloride channels and not all mammals have glutamate-gated chloride channels.

Drug is active against various life-cycle stages of most, but not all, nematodes. Ivermectin is active against the tissue microfilariae of Onchocerca volvulus but not against the adult form. Its activity against Strongyloides stercoralis is limited to the intestinal stages.

Pharmacokinetics

- *Absorption:* Following oral administration, plasma concentrations are proportional to dose ingested. Peak plasma levels occur approximately 4 hours after dosing.
- *Distribution:* Not reported.
- *Metabolism:* Drug is metabolized in the liver.
- *Excretion:* Apparent plasma half-life of ivermectin following oral administration is approximately at least 16 hours. Drug and its metabolites are excreted in the feces over 12 days; less than 1% of dose is excreted in the urine.

Contraindications and precautions

Contraindicated in patients hypersensitive to any components of product. Patients with hyperreactive onchodermatitis (sowda) may be at increased risk for serious adverse reactions, especially edema and aggravation of onchodermatitis, following treatment with microfilarcidal drugs.

Interactions

None reported.

Effects on diagnostic tests

Drug may cause increased hemoglobin and ALT and AST levels, decreased leukocyte count, and eosinophilia.

Adverse reactions

CNS: dizziness.
CV: peripheral edema, orthostatic hypotension, tachycardia.
EENT: limbitis; punctate opacity.
GI: diarrhea, nausea.
Respiratory: worsened bronchial asthma.
Skin: *pruritis; edema, papular and pustular or frank urticarial rash.*
Other: arthralgia, facial edema, *fever,* headache, *lymph node enlargement,* lymph node tenderness, myalgia, synovitis.

Overdose and treatment

In accidental poisonings or exposures to unknown quantities of veterinary formulations of ivermectin in humans, the most commonly reported effects are rash, edema, headache, dizziness, asthenia, nausea, vomiting, and diarrhea. Seizure, ataxia, dyspnea, abdominal pain, paresthesia, and urticaria have also been reported.

Induction of emesis and gastric lavage promptly, followed by purgatives, may be indicated to prevent absorption of ingested material. Provide supportive therapy, if indicated, including parenteral fluids and electrolytes, respiratory support, and pressor agents if clinically significant hypotension is present.

☑ Special considerations

- Patients with onchocerciasis may experience cutaneous or systemic reactions of varying severity (the Mazzotti reaction) as well as ophthalmologic reactions. These reactions are probably due to allergic and inflammatory responses to the death of the microfilariae.
- In clinical trials for onchocerciasis, worsening of the Mazzotti reactions in first 4 days post-treatment were reported.
- For treatment of onchocerciasis, drug does not kill adult onchocerca parasites; repeated follow-up and retreatment is usually required. Surgical excision of S.C. nodules containing adult parasites may be considered.
- Oral hydration, recumbency, I.V. 0.9% NaCl, or parenteral corticosteroids have been used to treat postural hypotension. Antihistamines and aspirin have also been used for most mild to moderate cases.
- Repeated courses of therapy (2-week intervals) may be required to treat intestinal strongyloidiasis in immunocompromised (including human immunodeficiency virus-infected) patients, and cure may not be achievable. Suppressive therapy (once monthly) may be helpful.
- Obtain follow-up stool examinations to document eradication of infection in patients with strongyloidiasis (three stool examinations over 3 months following treatment).

Patient education

- Tell patient to take drug with a glass of water.

Pediatric use

- Safety and efficacy in patients weighing below 33 lb (15 kg) have not been established.

Breast-feeding

- Drug is excreted in breast milk in low concentrations. Treatment in breast-feeding patients should be undertaken only when risk of delayed treatment to patient outweighs possible risk to newborn.

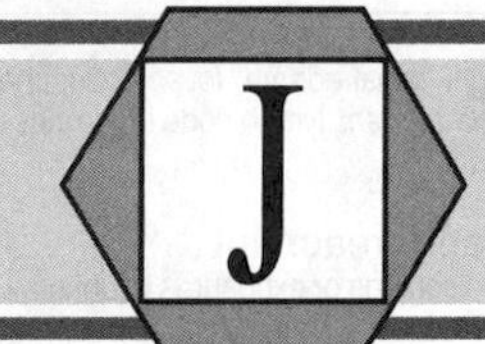

Japanese encephalitis virus vaccine, inactivated

JE-VAX

Pharmacologic classification: vaccine
Therapeutic classification: virus vaccine
Pregnancy risk category C

How supplied

Available by prescription only
Injection: 1-ml, 10-ml vials

Indications, route, and dosage

Active immunization against Japanese encephalitis (JE)

Primary immunization schedule

Adults and children age 3 and older: 1 ml S.C. on days 0, 7, and 30.
Children age 1 to 3: 0.5 ml S.C. on days 0, 7, and 30.

Booster doses

Adults and children age 3 and older: 1 ml S.C. after 2 years.
Children age 1 to 3: 0.5 ml S.C. after 2 years.

Pharmacodynamics

Immunostimulant action: JE vaccine, inactivated, promotes active immunity against JE. Immunity is not permanent or entirely predictable.

Pharmacokinetics

- *Absorption:* No information available.
- *Distribution:* No information available.
- *Metabolism:* No information available.
- *Excretion:* No information available.

Contraindications and precautions

Contraindicated in patients hypersensitive to drug or thimerosal (a preservative) and in those who exhibited severe adverse reactions, such as generalized urticaria or angioedema, to a prior dose of vaccine. Because vaccine is derived from mouse brain, its use is contraindicated in patients hypersensitive to substances of murine or neural origin.

Use cautiously in elderly, breast-feeding, or pregnant patients and in those with history of urticaria after drugs or insect stings.

Interactions

None reported.

Effects on diagnostic tests

None reported.

Adverse reactions

CNS: *headache, dizziness.*
GI: *nausea, vomiting, abdominal pain.*
Respiratory: ***respiratory distress.***
Other: ***anaphylaxis,*** *rash,* generalized urticaria, *local tenderness and swelling at injection site, fever, malaise, chills, myalgia;* ***angioedema*** of the face, oropharynx, extremities, or lips.

Overdose and treatment

No information available.

☑ Special considerations

- Before using vaccine, weigh risks of adverse effects against risks of exposure and illness as well as the availability, acceptability, and efficacy of repellents and other alternative protective measures.
- Vaccine has been associated with a moderate incidence of local and mild systemic adverse effects. Local tenderness and swelling have been reported in up to 20% of those receiving the vaccine; systemic effects, such as fever, headache, malaise, or rash, in up to 10%. Serious reactions, such as generalized urticaria or angioedema, are uncommon (1% or less of those vaccinated).
- Generalized urticaria or angioedema may occur within minutes of vaccination. However, adverse reactions that may be related to vaccine have occurred as late as 17 days after the injection. Most reactions occur within the first 10 days, with the majority occurring within 48 hours. Monitor patient closely for 30 minutes after injection. Warn him about possibility of delayed generalized urticaria or delayed angioedema of the extremities, face, oropharynx or, especially, lips.
- Attempts have been made to characterize the time course of adverse reactions. Reactions to the first dose have occurred a median of 12 hours after injection (88% happened within 3 days). The delay between the second dose and adverse effects was usually longer, with a median of 3 days and some effects not seen for 2 weeks. Some patients exhibited adverse reactions to the second or third dose, even when the first or second dose was well tolerated.
- Encourage patient and parents to report adverse effects after vaccination. Health care providers should report these adverse effects to the U.S. Department of Health and Human Services (DHHS) Vaccine Adverse Event Reporting System (VAERS). Contact VAERS at (800) 822-7967 for information about the system and reporting forms.
- Vaccine should be used to provide protection against JE in persons planning to travel or reside in areas where the virus is endemic. It's not indicated for all persons traveling to or residing in Asia. For most travelers to Asia, the risk for acquiring JE is extremely low. Contact the Centers for Disease

Control and Prevention at (404) 332-4555 for current travel advisories.
• When it is not possible to follow the regular immunization schedule, a two-dose regimen with injections on days 0 and 7 may be used. Antibodies will be induced in about 80% of patients with this schedule. Avoid use of a two-dose regimen unless circumstances are unusual.
• Keep epinephrine 1:1,000 and other resuscitative equipment and drugs available to treat anaphylaxis and other adverse reactions.
• To prepare vaccine for injection, use supplied diluent (sterile water for injection). Add 1.3 ml diluent to the single-dose vial; 11 ml diluent to the 10-dose vial. Shake vial thoroughly to ensure dissolution of vaccine. After reconstitution, vaccine may be stored in the refrigerator at 36° to 46° F (2° to 8° C) for 8 hours.

Patient education
• Because of possibility of delayed reactions, warn patient to remain in areas where medical care is available for 10 days after injection. Caution against international travel during this time.
• Advise patient to seek medical assistance as soon as reaction appears.
• Teach patient personal precautions that may help avoid exposure to mosquito bites, such as using insect repellents and wearing protective clothing. Avoiding outdoor activities, especially during twilight periods and in the evening, will further reduce risk.
• Tell patient to follow the recommended three-dose schedule for best results. When time constraints prohibit use of this schedule, an abbreviated schedule with injections on days 0, 7, and 14 may be used.

Geriatric use
• JE vaccine should be used cautiously in elderly patients.

Pediataric use
• Safety and efficacy of JE vaccine in infants under age 1 have not been established.

Breast-feeding
• It is not known if JE vaccine is excreted in breast milk. Therefore, caution should be exercised when JE vaccine is administered to breast-feeding women.

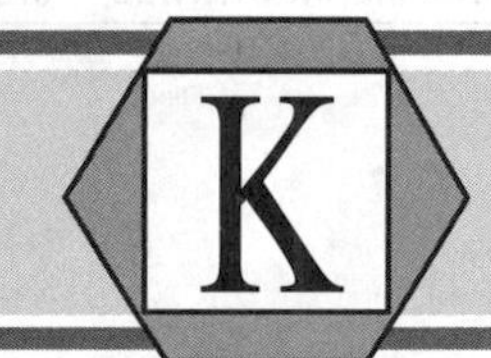

ketamine hydrochloride

Ketalar

Pharmacologic classification: dissociative anesthetic
Therapeutic classification: intravenous anesthetic
Pregnancy risk category NR

How supplied

Available by prescription only
Injection: 10 mg/ml, 50 mg/ml, 100 mg/ml

Indications, route, and dosage

Induction of general anesthesia, especially for short diagnostic or surgical procedures not requiring skeletal muscle relaxation; adjunct to other general anesthetics or low-potency agents, such as nitrous oxide
Adults and children: 1 to 4.5 mg/kg I.V. administered over 60 seconds; or 6.5 to 13 mg/kg I.M. To maintain anesthesia, repeat in increments of half to full initial dose.

Pharmacodynamics

Anesthetic action: Ketamine induces a profound sense of dissociation from the environment by direct action on the cortex and limbic system.

Pharmacokinetics

- *Absorption:* Absorbed rapidly and well after I.M. injection. Drug induces surgical anesthesia in 30 seconds after I.V. administration, which lasts 5 to 10 minutes. After I.M. injection, anesthesia begins in 3 to 4 minutes and lasts 12 to 25 minutes.
- *Distribution:* Drug rapidly enters the CNS.
- *Metabolism:* Metabolized by the liver to an active metabolite with one-third the potency of parent drug.
- *Excretion:* Drug is excreted in the urine.

Contraindications and precautions

Contraindicated in patients with schizophrenia or other acute psychosis because it may exacerbate the condition; in those with CV disease in which a sudden rise in blood pressure would be harmful; and in patients allergic to drug.

Interactions

Ketamine's CV effects may be blocked by concomitant use of *halothane* and, to a lesser extent, by *enflurane*, leading to significant myocardial depression and hypotension. Prolonged recovery time may occur if ketamine is used with *barbiturates* or *narcotics.* Ketamine may increase the neuromuscular effects of *tubocurarine* and other *nondepolarizing muscle relaxants* if used concomitantly. This may result in prolonged respiratory depression. Concomitant use with *thyroid hormones* may cause hypertension and tachycardia.

Effects on diagnostic tests

None reported.

Adverse reactions

CNS: tonic-clonic movements, hallucinations, confusion, excitement, dreamlike states, irrational behavior, psychic abnormalities.
CV: *hypertension; tachycardia;* hypotension, ***bradycardia*** (if used with halothane); ***arrhythmias.***
EENT: diplopia, nystagmus, laryngospasm.
GI: mild anorexia, nausea, vomiting, excessive salivation.
Respiratory: respiratory depression in high doses, apnea (if administered too rapidly).
Skin: transient erythema, measles-like rash.

Note: Discontinue drug if hypersensitivity, laryngospasm, or severe hypotension or hypertension occurs.

Overdose and treatment

Clinical signs include respiratory depression. Support respiration, using mechanical ventilation if necessary.

☑ Special considerations

- Patients require physical support because of rapid induction; monitor vital signs perioperatively. Blood pressure begins to rise shortly after injection, peaks at 10% to 50% above preanesthetic levels, and returns to baseline within 15 minutes. Ketamine's effects on blood pressure make it particularly useful in hypovolemic patients as an induction agent that supports blood pressure.
- Keep verbal, tactile, and visual stimulation to a minimum during induction and recovery. Emergence reactions occur in 12% of patients, including dreams, visual imagery, hallucinations, and delirium and may occur for up to 24 hours postoperatively. They may be reduced by using lower dosage of ketamine with I.V. diazepam and can be treated with short- or ultrashort-acting barbiturates. Incidence is lower in patients under age 15 or over age 65 and when drug is given I.M.
- Dissociative and hallucinatory adverse effects have led to drug abuse.
- Barbiturates are incompatible in the same syringe.
- For direct injection, dilute 100 mg/ml concentration with an equal volume of sterile water for injection, 0.9% NaCl, or D_5W. For continuous infusion, prepare a 1 mg/ml solution by adding 5 ml from the 100 mg/ml vial to 500 ml of D_5W or 0.9% NaCl.

Patient education
- Warn patient to avoid tasks requiring motor coordination and mental alertness for 24 hours after anesthesia.

Geriatric use
- Use drug with caution, especially in patients with suspected stroke, hypertension, or cardiac disease.

Pediatric use
- Drug is safe and especially useful in managing minor surgical or diagnostic procedures or in repeated procedures that require large amounts of analgesia, such as the changing of burn dressings.

ketoconazole
Nizoral

Pharmacologic classification: imidazole derivative
Therapeutic classification: antifungal
Pregnancy risk category C

How supplied
Available by prescription only
Tablets: 200 mg
Cream: 2%
Shampoo: 2%

Indications, route, and dosage
Severe fungal infections caused by susceptible organisms
Adults: Initially, 200 mg P.O. daily as a single dose. Dosage may be increased to 400 mg once daily in patients who do not respond to lower dosage.
Children over age 2: 3.3 to 6.6 mg/kg P.O. daily as a single dose.
Topical treatment of tinea corporis, tinea cruris, tinea versicolor, and tinea pedis
Adults and children: Apply once or b.i.d. for about 2 weeks; for tinea pedis apply for 6 weeks.
Seborrheic dermatitis
Adults and children: Apply b.i.d. for about 4 weeks.
Dandruff
Adults: Apply for 1 minute, rinse, then reapply for 3 minutes. Shampoo twice weekly for 4 weeks with at least 3 days between shampoos.
◊ ***Prostatic carcinoma***
Adults: 400 mg P.O. q 8 hours.

Pharmacodynamics
Antifungal action: Drug is fungicidal and fungistatic, depending on concentrations. It inhibits demethylation of lanosterol, thereby altering membrane permeability and inhibiting purine transport. The in vitro spectrum of activity includes most pathogenic fungi. However, CSF concentrations following oral administration are not predictable. It should not be used to treat fungal meningitis, and specimens should be obtained for susceptibility testing before therapy. Currently available tests may not accurately reflect in vivo activity, so interpret results with caution.

Drug is used orally to treat disseminated or pulmonary coccidiomycosis, paracoccidiomycosis, or histoplamosis; oral candidiasis; and candiduria (but low renal clearance may limit its usefulness).

It is also useful in some dermatophytoses, including tinea capitis, tinea cruris, tinea pedis, tinea manus, and tinea unguium (onychomycosis) caused by *Epidermophyton, Microsporum,* or *Trichophyton.*

Pharmacokinetics
- *Absorption:* Ketoconazole is converted to the hydrochloride salt before absorption. Absorption is erratic; it is decreased by raised gastric pH and may be increased in extent and consistency by food. Peak plasma concentrations occur at 1 to 4 hours.
- *Distribution:* Drug is distributed into bile, saliva, cerumen, synovial fluid, and sebum; CSF penetration is erratic and considered minimal. It is 84% to 99% bound to plasma proteins.
- *Metabolism:* Drug is converted into several inactive metabolites in the liver.
- *Excretion:* Over 50% of a dose is excreted in feces within 4 days; drug and metabolites are secreted in bile. About 13% is excreted unchanged in urine. It is probably excreted in breast milk. Half-life is biphasic, initially 2 hours, with a terminal half-life of 8 hours.

Contraindications and precautions
Contraindicated in patients with hypersensitivity to drug and in those taking astemizole, or cisapride due to potential for serious CV adverse events. Use oral form cautiously in patients with hepatic disease. Because CSF concentrations of ketoconazole are unpredictable following oral administration, do not use drug alone to treat fungal meningitis.

Interactions
Concomitant use of ketoconazole with *drugs that raise gastric pH* (*antacids, antimuscarinic agents, cimetidine, famotidine, ranitidine*) decreases absorption of ketoconazole; *rifampin* may decrease ketoconazole's serum concentration to ineffective levels.

Ketoconazole may enhance the toxicity of other *hepatotoxic drugs* and the anticoagulant effects of *warfarin.*

Ketoconazole may interfere with the metabolism of *cyclosporine* and thus raise serum levels of cyclosporine; concomitant use with *phenytoin* may alter serum levels of both drugs.

Ketoconazole may intensify the effects of *oral sulfonylureas* and may interact with *alcohol* to cause a disulfiram-like reaction.

Concomitant use with *corticosteroids* may result in increased plasma concentrations of the corticosteroid.

Effects on diagnostic tests
Drug has been reported to cause transient elevations of AST, ALT, and alkaline phosphatase levels; it has also been reported to cause transient alterations of serum cholesterol and triglyceride levels.

Adverse reactions

CNS: headache, nervousness, dizziness, somnolence, photophobia, ***suicidal tendencies***, severe depression (with oral administration).
GI: *nausea, vomiting,* abdominal pain, diarrhea (with oral administration).
Hematologic: ***thrombocytopenia,*** hemolytic anemia, leukopenia (with oral administration).
Hepatic: elevated liver enzymes, ***fatal hepatotoxicity*** (with oral administration).
Skin: pruritus; severe irritation, stinging (with topical administration).
Other: gynecomastia with tenderness, fever, chills, impotence (with oral administration).

Overdose and treatment

Overdose may cause dizziness, tinnitus, headache, nausea, vomiting, or diarrhea; patients with adrenal hypofunction or patients on long-term corticosteroid therapy may show signs of adrenal crisis.

Treatment includes induced emesis and sodium bicarbonate lavage, followed by activated charcoal and a cathartic, and supportive measures as needed.

☑ Special considerations

- Identify organism, but do not delay therapy for results of laboratory tests.
- Give drug with citrus juice.
- Monitor for signs of hepatotoxicity: persistent nausea, unusual fatigue, jaundice, dark urine, and pale stools.
- Drug requires acidity for absorption and is ineffective in patients with achlorhydria.

Patient education

- Teach achlorhydric patients how to take ketoconazole: dissolve each tablet in 4 ml of 0.2N hydrochloric acid solution or take with 200 ml of 0.1N hydrochloric acid, and administer through a glass or plastic straw to avoid damaging enamel on patient's teeth. Tell patient to drink a glass of water after each dose.
- Tell patient to avoid driving or performing other hazardous activities if dizziness or drowsiness occur; these often occur early in treatment but abate as treatment continues.
- Caution patient not to alter dose or dosage interval or to discontinue drug without medical approval. Explain that therapy must continue until active fungal infection is completely eradicated, to prevent recurrence.
- Reassure patient that nausea will subside; to minimize reaction, patient may take drug with food or may divide dosage into two doses.
- Advise patient to avoid self-prescribed preparations for GI distress (for example, antacids); some may alter gastric pH levels and interfere with drug action.
- Encourage patient to get specific medical approval before taking other drugs with ketoconazole.

Pediatric use

- Safe use in children under age 2 has not been established. Use in pediatric patients should be considered only when the benefits outweigh the risks.

Breast-feeding

- Drug may be distributed in breast milk. Alternative feeding methods are recommended.

ketoprofen

Actron, Orudis, Orudis KT, Oruvail

Pharmacologic classification: NSAID
Therapeutic classification: nonnarcotic analgesic, antipyretic, anti-inflammatory
Pregnancy risk category B

How supplied

Available by prescription only
Capsules: 25 mg, 50 mg, 75 mg
Capsules (extended-release): 100 mg, 150 mg, 200 mg

Available without a prescription
Tablets: 12.5 mg

Indications, route, and dosage

Rheumatoid arthritis and osteoarthritis
Adults: Usual dose is 75 mg t.i.d. or 50 mg q.i.d. P.O. Maximum dosage is 300 mg/day; or 200 mg (extended-release capsules) P.O. daily.
Mild to moderate pain; dysmenorrhea
Adults: 25 to 50 mg P.O. q 6 to 8 hours p.r.n.
Temporary relief of mild aches and pain, fever (self-medication)
Adults: 12.5 mg q 4 to 6 hours. Do not exceed 75 mg in a 24-hour period.

Pharmacodynamics

Analgesic, antipyretic, and anti-inflammatory actions: Mechanisms of action are unknown; ketoprofen is thought to inhibit prostaglandin synthesis.

Pharmacokinetics

- *Absorption:* Absorbed rapidly and completely from the GI tract.
- *Distribution:* Drug is highly protein-bound. Extent of body tissue fluid distribution not known, but therapeutic levels range from 0.4 to 6 mcg/ml.
- *Metabolism:* Metabolized in the liver.
- *Excretion:* Excreted in urine as parent drug and its metabolites.

Contraindications and precautions

Contraindicated in patients with hypersensitivity to drug or history of aspirin- or NSAID-induced asthma, urticaria, or other allergic-type reactions. Use cautiously in patients with impaired renal or hepatic function, peptic ulcer disease, heart failure, hypertension, or fluid retention.

Interactions

Concomitant use of ketoprofen with *anticoagulants* and *thrombolytic drugs* (such as *coumarin derivatives, heparin, streptokinase, urokinase*) may potentiate anticoagulant effects. Bleeding problems may occur if ketoprofen is used with other *drugs that inhibit platelet aggregation*, such as *aspirin, parenteral carbenicillin, cefamandole, cefoperazone, dextran, dipyridamole, mezlocillin, piperacillin, plicamycin, salicylates, sulfinpyrazone, ticarcillin, valproic acid*, or *other anti-inflammatory agents*. Concomitant use with *salicylates, anti-inflammatory agents, alcohol, corticotropin*, or *steroids* may cause increased GI adverse effects, including ulceration and hemorrhage. *Aspirin* may decrease the bioavailability of ketoprofen.

Because of the influence of prostaglandins on glucose metabolism, concomitant use with *insulin* or *oral antidiabetic agents* may potentiate hypoglycemic effects. Ketoprofen may displace highly protein-bound drugs from binding sites. Toxicity may occur with *coumarin derivatives, nifedipine, phenytoin*, or *verapamil*. Increased nephrotoxicity may occur with *gold compounds, other anti-inflammatory agents*, or *acetaminophen*. Ketoprofen may decrease the renal clearance of *lithium* and *methotrexate*. Ketoprofen may decrease the effectiveness of *antihypertensive agents* and *diuretics*. Concomitant use with diuretics may increase nephrotoxic potential. Concomitant use with diuretics or antihypertensives may decrease their effectiveness.

Effects on diagnostic tests

In vitro interactions with glucose determinations have been reported with glucose oxidase and peroxidase methods.

Drug may interfere with serum iron determination (false increases or decreases depending on method used) and produce false increases in serum bilirubin levels. These interactions were reported with drug concentrations above those seen clinically (60 mg/ml).

Adverse reactions

CNS: *headache, dizziness, CNS excitation* or depression.
EENT: tinnitus, visual disturbances.
GI: *nausea, abdominal pain, diarrhea, constipation, flatulence,* ***peptic ulceration,*** dyspepsia, anorexia, vomiting, stomatitis.
GU: ***nephrotoxicity,*** elevated BUN.
Hematologic: prolonged bleeding time, ***thrombocytopenia, agranulocytosis.***
Hepatic: elevated liver enzymes.
Respiratory: dyspnea, ***bronchospasm, laryngeal edema.***
Skin: rash, photosensitivity, ***exfoliative dermatitis.***
Other: peripheral edema.

Overdose and treatment

Clinical manifestations of overdose include nausea and drowsiness. To treat drug overdose, empty stomach immediately by inducing emesis with ipecac syrup or by gastric lavage. Administer activated charcoal via nasogastric tube. Provide symptomatic and supportive measures (respiratory support and correction of fluid and electrolyte imbalances). Monitor laboratory parameters and vital signs closely. Hemodialysis may be useful in removing ketoprofen and assisting in care of renal failure.

☑ Special considerations

Besides those relevant to all *NSAIDs*, consider the following recommendations.

- Administer tablets on an empty stomach either 30 minutes before or 2 hours after meals to ensure adequate absorption.
- Capsules may be taken with foods or antacids to minimize GI distress.
- Store suppositories in refrigerator.
- Monitor CNS effects of drug. Institute safety measures, such as assisted walking, raised side rails, and gradual position changes, to prevent injury.
- Watch for possible photosensitivity reactions.
- Monitor laboratory test results for abnormalities.

Patient education

- Instruct patient in prescribed drug regimen and proper medication administration.
- Tell patient to seek medical approval before taking OTC medications (especially aspirin and aspirin-containing products).
- Caution patient to avoid activities that require alertness or concentration. Instruct him in safety measures to prevent injury.
- Advise patient of potential photosensitivity reactions. Recommend use of sunscreen.
- Instruct patient to report adverse reactions.
- Advise patient to avoid alcoholic beverages during therapy.

Geriatric use

- Patients over age 60 may be more susceptible to the toxic effects of ketoprofen. Use with caution.
- The effects of drug on renal prostaglandins may cause fluid retention and edema, a significant drawback for elderly patients and those with heart failure. The manufacturer recommends that initial dose be reduced by 33% to 50% in geriatric patients.

Pediatric use

- Safe use in children under age 12 has not been established.

Breast-feeding

- Most NSAIDs are distributed into breast milk; however, distribution of ketoprofen is unknown. Avoid use of ketoprofen in breast-feeding women.

ketorolac tromethamine

Toradol

Pharmacologic classification: NSAID
Therapeutic classification: analgesic
Pregnancy risk category C

How supplied

Available by prescription only
Tablets: 10 mg
Injection: 15 mg/ml (1-ml cartridge and vial), 30 mg/ml (1-ml and 2-ml cartridges and vials)

Indications, route, and dosage

Short-term management of pain

Adults under age 65: Dosage should be based on patient response. Initially, 60 mg I.M. or 30 mg I.V. as a single dose, or multiple doses of 30 mg I.M. or I.V. q 6 hours. Maximum daily dose should not exceed 120 mg.

✦ ***Dosage adjustment.*** In adults age 65 or older, renally impaired patients, and those weighing less than 110 lb (50 kg) body weight, 30 mg I.M. or 15 mg I.V. initially as a single dose, or multiple doses of 15 mg I.M. or I.V. q 6 hours. Maximum daily dose should not exceed 60 mg.

Short-term management of moderately severe, acute pain when switching from parenteral to oral administration

Adults under age 65: 20 mg P.O. as a single dose followed by 10 mg P.O. q 4 to 6 hours, not to exceed 40 mg/day.

✦ ***Dosage adjustment.*** In adults age 65 or older, renally impaired patients, and those weighing less than 110 lb (50 kg) body weight, 10 mg P.O. as a single dose, followed by 10 mg P.O. q 4 to 6 hours, not to exceed 40 mg/day.

Pharmacodynamics

Analgesic action: Ketorolac is an NSAID that acts by inhibiting the synthesis of prostaglandins.

Pharmacokinetics

• *Absorption:* Completely absorbed after I.M. administration. After oral administration, food delays absorption but does not decrease total amount of drug absorbed.

• *Distribution:* Mean peak plasma levels occur about 30 minutes after a 50-mg dose and range from 2.2 to 3 mcg/ml. Over 99% of drug is protein-bound.

• *Metabolism:* Primarily hepatic; a para-hydroxy metabolite and conjugates have been identified; less than 50% of a dose is metabolized. Liver impairment does not substantially alter drug clearance.

• *Excretion:* Primary excretion is in the urine (over 90%); the rest in feces. Terminal plasma half-life is 3.8 to 6.3 hours (average 4.5 hours) in young adults; it is substantially prolonged in patients with renal failure.

Contraindications and precautions

Contraindicated in patients with hypersensitivity to drug, active peptic ulcer disease, recent GI bleeding or perforation, advanced renal impairment, risk for renal impairment due to volume depletion, suspected or confirmed cerebrovascular bleeding, hemorrhagic diathesis, incomplete hemostasis, or high risk of bleeding.

Also contraindicated in patients with history of peptic ulcer disease or GI bleeding, past allergic manifestations to aspirin or other NSAIDs, and during labor and delivery or breast-feeding. In addition, drug is contraindicated as prophylactic analgesic before major surgery or intraoperatively when hemostasis is critical; in patients receiving aspirin, an NSAID, or probenecid; and in those requiring analgesics to be administered epidurally or intrathecally.

Use cautiously in patients with impaired renal or hepatic function.

Interactions

Ketorolac may increase the levels of free (unbound) *salicylates* or *warfarin* in the blood. Clinical significance is unknown. NSAIDs increase *lithium* levels; they decrease *methotrexate* clearance and increase its toxicity. Concomitant use with *diuretics* may decrease efficacy of diuretic and enhance nephrotoxicity.

Effects on diagnostic tests

Like other NSAIDs, ketorolac has been associated with borderline elevations of one or more liver function test results. Meaningful elevations of AST or ALT—three times the upper normal limit—occur in less than 1% of patients. Because drug inhibits platelet aggregation, it can prolong bleeding time.

Adverse reactions

CNS: *drowsiness, sedation,* dizziness, *headache.*

CV: edema, hypertension, palpitations, ***arrhythmias.***

GI: *nausea, dyspepsia, GI pain,* diarrhea, peptic ulceration, vomiting, constipation, flatulence, stomatitis.

GU: ***renal failure.***

Hematologic: decreased platelet adhesion, purpura, ***thrombocytopenia.***

Other: pain (at injection site), pruritus, rash, diaphoresis.

Overdose and treatment

There is no experience with overdose in humans. Animal studies revealed that high doses (above 100 mg/kg) decreased motor activity and caused diarrhea, pallor, crackles, labored breathing, and vomiting.

Withhold drug and provide supportive treatment.

☑ Special considerations

• Drug is intended for short-term management of pain. The rate and severity of adverse reactions should be less than that observed in patients taking NSAIDs on a chronic basis.

• I.M. injections in patients with coagulopathies or those receiving anticoagulants may cause bleeding and hematoma at the site of injection.

• The combined duration of ketorolac I.M., I.V., or P.O. should not exceed 5 days. Oral use is only for continuation of I.V. or I.M. therapy.

• Hypovolemia should be corrected before initiating therapy with ketorolac.

Patient education

• Warn patient that GI ulceration, bleeding, and perforation can occur at any time, with or without warning, in anyone taking NSAIDs on a chronic basis. Teach patient how to recognize the signs and symptoms of GI bleeding.

• Instruct patient to avoid aspirin, aspirin-containing products, and alcoholic beverages during therapy.

Geriatric use

- Use lower initial doses (30 mg I.M.) in patients over age 65 or weighing less than 110 lb. In clinical trials, elderly subjects have exhibited a longer terminal half-life of drug (average 7 hours in elderly patients compared with 4.5 hours in healthy young adults).

Pediatric use

- Drug is not recommended for use in children because safety and efficacy have not been established.

Breast-feeding

- Because drug is distributed in breast milk, its use is contraindicated in breast-feeding patients.

ketorolac tromethamine (ophthalmic)

Acular

Pharmacologic classification: NSAID
Therapeutic classification: ophthalmic anti-inflammatory
Pregnancy risk category C

How supplied

Available by prescription only
Ophthalmic solution: 0.5%

Indications, route, and dosage

Relief of ocular itching caused by seasonal allergic conjunctivitis
Adults: Instill 1 drop (0.25 mg) in conjunctival sac q.i.d. Efficacy has not been established beyond 1 week of continued use.

Pharmacodynamics

Anti-inflammatory action: Ketorolac tromethamine's anti-inflammatory action is thought to be a result, in part, of its ability to inhibit prostaglandin biosynthesis. Drug reduces prostaglandin E_2 levels in aqueous humor with ocular administration. It has also demonstrated analgesic and antipyretic activity because of the same mechanism of action.

Pharmacokinetics

- *Absorption:* Information not available.
- *Distribution:* Information not available.
- *Metabolism:* Information not available.
- *Excretion:* Information not available.

Contraindications and precautions

Contraindicated in patients hypersensitive to any component of the formulation and in those wearing soft contact lenses. Use cautiously in patients with hypersensitivity to other NSAIDs or aspirin and in those with bleeding disorders.

Interactions

None reported.

Effects on diagnostic tests

None reported.

Adverse reactions

EENT: *transient stinging and burning on instillation,* superficial keratitis, superficial ocular infections, ocular irritation.
Other: hypersensitivity reactions.

Overdose and treatment

Overdosage will not ordinarily cause acute problems. If accidentally ingested, have the patient drink fluids to dilute.

☑ Special considerations

- Know that ophthalmic solution has been safely administered in conjunction with other ophthalmic medications, such as antibiotics, beta blockers, carbonic anhydrase inhibitors, cycloplegics, and mydriatics.
- Store drug at controlled room temperature and protect from light.

Patient education

- Teach patient how to administer eye drops and stress importance of not touching dropper to eye or surrounding area.
- Advise patient not to use more drops than prescribed or to use drug for other eye problems unless prescribed.
- Instruct patient to discard drug when outdated or no longer needed.

Pediatric use

- Safety and efficacy in children have not been established.

Breast-feeding

- Use cautiously in breast-feeding women.

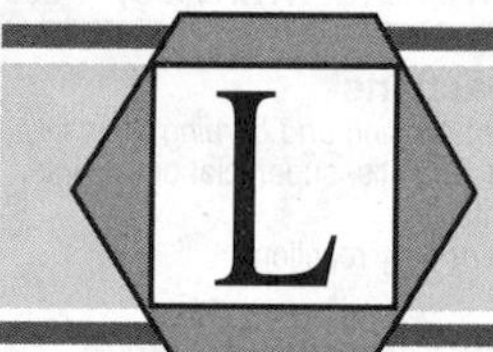

labetalol hydrochloride

Normodyne, Trandate

Pharmacologic classification: alpha- and beta-adrenergic blocker
Therapeutic classification: antihypertensive
Pregnancy risk category C

How supplied

Available by prescription only
Tablets: 100 mg, 200 mg, 300 mg
Injection: 5 mg/ml in 20-ml, 40-ml, and 60-ml vials and 4-ml and 8-ml disposable syringes

Indications, route, and dosage

Hypertension

Adults: 100 mg P.O. b.i.d. with or without a diuretic. Dosage may be increased by 100 mg b.i.d. q 2 or 4 days until optimum response is reached. Usual maintenance dosage is 200 to 400 mg b.i.d.; maximum daily dose is 2,400 mg.

Severe hypertension and hypertensive emergencies; ◊ pheochromocytoma; ◊ clonidine withdrawal hypertension

Adults: Initially, 20-mg I.V. bolus slowly over 2 minutes; may repeat injections of 40 to 80 mg q 10 minutes to maximum dose of 300 mg.

Alternatively, may be given continuous I.V. infusion, at an initial rate of 2 mg/minute until satisfactory response is obtained. Usual cumulative dose is 50 to 200 mg.

◊ Intraoperative hypertension

Adults: Initially, 10 to 30 mg I.V. bolus slowly; may repeat injections of 5 to 10 mg I.V. p.r.n.

Pharmacodynamics

Antihypertensive action: Labetalol inhibits catecholamine access to both beta- and postsynaptic alpha-adrenergic receptor sites. Drug may also have a vasodilating effect.

Pharmacokinetics

- *Absorption:* Oral absorption is high (90% to 100%); however, drug undergoes extensive first-pass metabolism in the liver and only about 25% of an oral dose reaches systemic circulation unchanged. Antihypertensive effect occurs in 20 minutes to 2 hours, peaking in 1 to 4 hours. After direct I.V. administration, antihypertensive effect occurs in 2 to 5 minutes; maximal effect occurs in 5 to 15 minutes.
- *Distribution:* Drug is distributed widely throughout the body; it is approximately 50% protein-bound.
- *Metabolism:* Orally administered drug is metabolized extensively in the liver and possibly in GI mucosa.
- *Excretion:* Approximately 5% of a dose is excreted unchanged in urine; rest is excreted as metabolites in urine and feces (biliary elimination). Antihypertensive effect of an oral dose persists for about 8 to 24 hours; after I.V. administration, it lasts about 2 to 4 hours. Plasma half-life is about 5½ hours after I.V. administration or 6 to 8 hours after oral administration.

Contraindications and precautions

Contraindicated in patients with bronchial asthma, overt cardiac failure, greater than first-degree heart block, cardiogenic shock, severe bradycardia, other conditions associated with severe and prolonged hypotension, and hypersensitivity to drug.

Use cautiously in patients with heart failure, hepatic failure, chronic bronchitis, emphysema, preexisting peripheral vascular disease, and pheochromocytoma.

Interactions

Labetalol may potentiate antihypertensive effects of *diuretics* and *other antihypertensive agents*; concomitant use of I.V. labetalol and *halothane* may result in synergistic antihypertensive effect.

Oral *cimetidine* may increase bioavailability of oral labetalol; therefore, if used concomitantly, labetalol dosage should be adjusted. *Glutethimide* may decrease bioavailability of oral labetalol, requiring adjustment in labetalol dosage.

Labetalol may antagonize bronchodilation produced by *beta-adrenergic agonists*.

Concomitant use with *tricyclic antidepressants* may increase incidence of labetalol-induced tremor.

Labetalol blunts the reflex tachycardia produced by *nitroglycerin* without preventing its hypotensive effect. If used with nitroglycerin in patients with angina, additional antihypertensive effects may occur.

Effects on diagnostic tests

Drug therapy may cause a false-positive increase of urine free and total catecholamine levels when measured by a nonspecific trihydroxindole fluorometric method.

Adverse reactions

CNS: vivid dreams, fatigue, headache, paresthesia, syncope, transient scalp tingling.
CV: *orthostatic hypotension, dizziness,* ***ventricular arrhythmias.***
EENT: nasal stuffiness.
GI: nausea, vomiting, diarrhea.
GU: sexual dysfunction, urine retention.
Respiratory: dyspnea, ***bronchospasm.***

Skin: rash.
Other: muscle spasm, toxic myopathy.

Overdose and treatment
Clinical signs of overdose include severe hypotension, bradycardia, heart failure, and bronchospasm.

After acute ingestion, empty stomach by induced emesis or gastric lavage, and give activated charcoal to reduce absorption. Subsequent treatment is usually symptomatic and supportive.

☑ Special considerations
Besides those relevant to all *beta-adrenergic blockers,* consider the following recommendations.
- Unlike other beta blockers, labetalol does not decrease resting heart rate or cardiac output.
- Dosage may need to be reduced in patients with hepatic insufficiency.
- Dizziness is the most troublesome adverse effect; it tends to occur in early stages of treatment and in patients taking diuretics or receiving higher doses.
- Transient scalp tingling occurs occasionally at beginning of drug therapy. This usually subsides quickly.
- Investigational uses include managing chronic stable angina pectoris, excessive sympathetic activity associated with tetanus, and uncontrolled hypertension before and during anesthesia. Labetalol also may be used (with halothane anesthesia) to produce controlled hypotension.
- Do not mix labetalol with 5% sodium bicarbonate injection because of incompatibility.
- When titrating hospitalized patients from parenteral to oral labetalol, begin with 200 mg, then give 200 to 400 mg P.O. after 6 to 12 hours. Oral dosage may then be increased in usual increments at 1-day intervals, if necessary, to achieve the desired blood pressure control. Daily dose may be given twice or three times daily.

Patient education
- Advise patient that transient scalp tingling may occur during initiation of therapy.

Geriatric use
- Elderly patients may require lower maintenance dosages of labetalol because of increased bioavailability or delayed metabolism; they also may experience enhanced adverse effects. Use drug with caution in elderly patients.

Pediatric use
- Safety and efficacy in children have not been established; use drug only if potential benefit outweighs risk.

Breast-feeding
- Small amounts of labetalol are distributed into breast milk; use drug with caution in breast-feeding women.

lactulose
Cephulac, Cholac, Chronulac, Constilac, Constulose, Duphalac, Enulose

Pharmacologic classification: disaccharide
Therapeutic classification: laxative
Pregnancy risk category B

How supplied
Available by prescription only
Syrup: 10 g/15 ml
Rectal solution: 3.33 g/5 ml

Indications, route, and dosage
Constipation
Adults: 15 to 30 ml P.O. daily (may increase to 60 ml if needed).
To prevent and treat portal-systemic encephalopathy, including hepatic precoma and coma in patients with severe hepatic disease
Adults: Initially, 20 to 30 g (30 to 45 ml) P.O. t.i.d. or q.i.d., until two or three soft stools are produced daily. Usual dosage is 60 to 100 g daily in divided doses; can also be given by retention enema. Mix 300 ml of lactulose with 700 ml of water or 0.9% NaCl solution and retain for 60 minutes. May repeat q 4 to 6 hours.
Infants: Initially, 2.5 to 10 ml daily in divided doses. Adjust doses q 1 to 2 days to produce two to three loose stools daily.
Older children and adolescents: Initially, 40 to 90 ml daily in divided doses. Adjust doses q 1 to 2 days to produce two to three loose stools daily.
◇ ***After barium meal examination***
Adults: 5 to 10 ml P.O. b.i.d. for 1 to 4 weeks.
◇ ***To restore bowel movements after hemorrhoidectomy***
Adults: 15 ml P.O. twice during day before surgery and for 5 days postoperatively.

Pharmacodynamics
Laxative action: Because lactulose is indigestible, it passes through the GI tract to the colon unchanged; there, it is digested by normally occurring bacteria. The weak acids produced in this manner increase the stool's fluid content and cause distention, thus promoting peristalsis and bowel evacuation.

Lactulose also is used to reduce serum ammonia levels in patients with hepatic disease. Lactulose breakdown acidifies the colon; this, in turn, converts ammonia (NH_3) to ammonium (NH_4^+), which is not absorbed and is excreted in the stool. Furthermore, this "ion trapping" effect causes ammonia to diffuse from the blood into the colon, where it is excreted as well.

Pharmacokinetics
- *Absorption:* Drug is absorbed minimally.
- *Distribution:* Distributed locally, primarily in the colon.
- *Metabolism:* Drug is metabolized by colonic bacteria (absorbed portion is not metabolized).

• *Excretion:* Mostly excreted in feces; absorbed portion is excreted in urine.

Contraindications and precautions
Contraindicated in patients on a low-galactose diet. Use cautiously in patients with diabetes mellitus.

Interactions
When used concomitantly, *neomycin* and other *antibiotics* may theoretically decrease lactulose effectiveness by eliminating bacteria needed to digest it into the active form. *Nonabsorbable antacids* may decrease lactulose effectiveness by preventing a decrease in the pH of the colon.

Effects on diagnostic tests
None reported.

Adverse reactions
GI: *abdominal cramps, belching, diarrhea, gaseous distention, flatulence,* nausea, vomiting, diarrhea (with excessive dosage).

Overdose and treatment
No cases of overdose have been reported. Clinical effects include diarrhea and abdominal cramps.

☑ Special considerations
• After administration of drug via nasogastric tube, the tube should be flushed with water to clear it and ensure drug's passage to stomach.
• Dilute drug with water or fruit juice to minimize its sweet taste.
• For administration by retention enema, patient should retain drug for 30 to 60 minutes. If retained less than 30 minutes, dose should be repeated immediately. Begin oral therapy before discontinuing retention enemas.
• Monitor frequency and consistency of stools.
• Do not administer drug with other laxatives because the loose stools produced may be falsely interpreted as an indication that an adequate dosage of lactulose has been achieved.

Patient education
• Advise patient to take drug with juice to improve taste.

Geriatric use
• Monitor patient's serum electrolyte levels; elderly patients are more sensitive to possible hypernatremia.

lamivudine
Epivir

Pharmacologic classification: synthetic nucleoside analogue
Therapeutic classification: antiviral
Pregnancy risk category C

How supplied
Available by prescription only
Tablets: 150 mg
Oral solution: 10 mg/ml

Indications, route, and dosage
Treatment of patients with HIV infection concomitantly with zidovudine
Adults weighing 110 lb (50 kg) or more and children age 12 and older: 150 mg P.O. b.i.d.
Adults weighing under 110 lb: 2 mg/kg P.O. b.i.d.
Children age 3 months to 12 years: 4 mg/kg P.O. b.i.d. Maximum dosage is 150 mg b.i.d.
✦ ***Dosage adjustment.*** In patients with renal failure, refer to chart.

Creatinine clearance (ml/min)	Recommended dosage
≥ 50	150 mg b.i.d.
30 to 49	150 mg once daily
15 to 29	150 mg first dose; then 100 mg once daily
5 to 14	150 mg first dose; then 50 mg once daily
< 5	50 mg first; then 25 mg once daily

Pharmacodynamics
Antiviral action: Lamivudine inhibits HIV reverse transcription via viral DNA chain termination. RNA- and DNA-dependent DNA polymerase activities are also inhibited.

Pharmacokinetics
• *Absorption:* Drug is rapidly absorbed after oral administration in HIV-infected patients.
• *Distribution:* Lamivudine is believed to distribute into extravascular spaces. Volume of distribution is independent of dose and does not correlate with body weight. Less than 36% is bound to plasma proteins.
• *Metabolism:* Metabolism of lamivudine is a minor route of elimination. The only known metabolite is the trans-sulfoxide metabolite.
• *Excretion:* Primarily eliminated unchanged in urine. Mean elimination half-life ranges from 5 to 7 hours.

Contraindications and precautions
Contraindicated in patients with hypersensitivity to drug. Drug should be used with extreme caution, and only if there is no satisfactory alternative therapy, in pediatric patients with history of pancreatitis or other significant risk factors for developing pancreatitis. Treatment with lamivudine should be stopped immediately if clinical signs, symptoms, or laboratory abnormalities suggesting pancreatitis occur.

Use cautiously in patients with impaired renal function; dosage reduction in these patients is necessary.

Interactions
Trimethoprim/sulfamethoxazole may cause increased blood levels of lamivudine because of a decreased clearance of lamivudine. The clinical significance of this interaction is not known. Monitor patient closely.

Effects on diagnostic tests
None reported.

Adverse reactions
Note: Adverse reactions are related to the combination therapy of lamivudine and zidovudine.
CNS: *headache, fatigue, neuropathy, dizziness, insomnia and other sleep disorders,* depressive disorders.
EENT: *nasal symptoms.*
GI: *nausea, diarrhea, vomiting, anorexia,* abdominal pain, abdominal cramps, dyspepsia, pancreatitis (in children age 3 months to 12 years).
Hematologic: ***neutropenia,*** anemia, ***thrombocytopenia.***
Respiratory: *cough.*
Skin: rash.
Other: *malaise, fever, chills, musculoskeletal pain,* myalgia, arthralgia, elevated liver enzymes and bilirubin levels.

Overdose and treatment
No information available.

☑ Special considerations
- Drug must be administered concomitantly with zidovudine. It is not intended for use as monotherapy.
- Monitor patient's CBC, platelet count, and liver function studies throughout therapy because abnormalities may occur.
- An Antiretroviral Pregnancy Registry has been established to monitor maternal-fetal outcomes of pregnant women exposed to lamivudine. Pregnant patients can be registered by calling 1-800-722-9292, extension 38465.

Patient education
- Inform patient that long-term effects of drug are unknown.
- Tell patient that tablets and oral solution are for oral ingestion only.
- Stress importance of taking drug exactly as prescribed.
- Instruct parents of children receiving drug about the signs and symptoms of pancreatitis and tell them to report such occurrences immediately.

Pediatric use
- There are no data on the use of lamivudine in combination with zidovudine in children under age 12.

Breast-feeding
- To avoid transmitting HIV to the infant, HIV-positive women should not breast-feed.

lamivudine/zidovudine
Combivir

Pharmacologic classification: reverse transcriptase inhibitor
Therapeutic classification: antiretroviral
Pregnancy risk category C

How supplied
Available by prescription only
Tablets: each tablet contains 150 mg lamivudine and 300 mg zidovudine

Indications, route, and dosage
Treatment of HIV infection
Adults and children over age 12 and weighing 50 kg (110 lb or more): one tablet P.O. b.i.d.

Pharmacodynamics
Antiretroviral action: Lamivudine and zidovudine are phosphorylated intracellularly to active metabolites that inhibit reverse transcriptase via DNA chain termination. Both drugs are also weak inhibitors of mammalian DNA polymerase. Together, they have synergistic antiretroviral activity. Combination therapy with lamivudine and zidovudine is targeted at suppressing or delaying the emergence of phenotypic and genotypic resistant strains that can occur with retroviral monotherapy, because dual resistance requires multiple mutations.

Pharmacokinetics
- *Absorption:* Both lamivudine and zidovudine are rapidly absorbed following oral administration with respective oral bioavailability of 86% and 64%.
- *Distribution:* Both drugs are extensively distributed and exhibit low protein binding.
- *Metabolism:* Only about 5% of lamivudine is metabolized whereas zidovudine is primarily (74%) metabolized in the liver.
- *Excretion:* Lamivudine is primarily eliminated unchanged in the urine. Zidovudine and its major metabolite are primarily eliminated in the urine. Elimination half-lives of lamivudine and zidovudine are 5 to 7 hours and ½ to 3 hours, respectively. Because renal excretion is a principle route of elimination, dosage adjustments are necessary in patients with compromised renal function making this fixed ratio combination unsuitable. Hemodialysis and peritoneal dialysis have negligible effect on the removal of zidovudine but removal of its metabolite, GZDV, is enhanced. The effect of dialysis on lamivudine is unknown.

Contraindications and precautions
Contraindicated in patients with known hypersensitivity to drug's components and in those with low body weight (under 110 lb), creatinine clearance below 50 ml/minute, or those experiencing dose-limiting adverse effects.

Use combination with caution in patients with bone marrow suppression or renal insufficiency. Lactic acidosis and severe hepatomegaly with steatosis have been reported in patients receiving lamivudine and zidovudine alone and in combination. Stop treatment if signs of lactic acidosis or hepatotoxicity develop. Hepatotoxic events may be more severe in patients with decompensated liver function due to hepatitis B. Myopathy and myositis associated with prolonged use of zidovudine may occur.

Interactions
Increased bioavailability of lamivudine can occur with coadministration of *nelfinavir* or *trimetho-*

prim/sulfamethoxazole and of zidovudine with coadministration of *atovaquone, fluconazole, methadone, probenecid,* and *valproic acid.* Decreased bioavailability of zidovudine may occur with concurrent administration of *nelfinavir* and *ritonavir.* However, dosage modifications of lamivudine and zidovudine are not needed with co-administration of any of these drugs. *Ganciclovir, interferon-alpha,* and other *bone marrow suppressive* or *cytotoxic agents* may increase zidovudine's hematologic toxicity. Most drug interaction studies have not been completed. Use cautiously as with other reverse transcriptase inhibitors.

Effects on diagnostic tests

None reported.

Adverse reactions

CNS: *headache,* malaise, *fatigue, insomnia, dizziness, neuropathy,* depression.
GI: *nausea, diarrhea, vomiting, anorexia,* abdominal pain, abdominal cramps, dyspepsia, ***pancreatitis.***
EENT: *nasal signs and symptoms, cough.*
Hematologic: ***neutropenia,*** anemia.
Musculoskeletal: *musculoskeletal pain,* myalgia, arthralgia, myopathy, myositis.
Skin: rash.
Other: *fever, chills.*

Overdose and treatment

A case report of overdosage (6 g) wtih lamivudine showed normal hematologic tests and no clinical signs or symptoms. Overdoses of zidovudine, with exposure up to 50 g, reported only nausea and vomiting and all patients recovering. There is no known antidote for lamivudine/zidovudine overdosage.

☑ Special considerations

- Do not use combination drug therapy in patients requiring dosage adjustments such as those with renal dysfunction or pediatric patients.
- Monitor for bone marrow toxicity with frequent blood counts, particularly in patients with advanced HIV infection.
- Monitor patients for signs of lactic acidosis and hepatotoxicity.
- Monitor patient's fine motor skills and peripheral sensation for evidence of peripheral neuropathies.
- Combination may be administered with or without food.

Patient education

- Advise patient that combination drug therapy is not a cure for HIV infections, and that he may continue to experience illness including opportunistic infections.
- Warn patient that transmission of HIV virus can still occur with drug therapy.
- Teach patient signs and symptoms of neutropenia and anemia and instruct him to report such occurrences.
- Advise patient to consult primary health care provider before taking other medications.
- Warn patient to report abdominal pain immediately.
- Stress importance of taking combination drug therapy exactly as prescribed to reduce the development of resistance.

Geriatric use

- Safety and effectiveness in patients over age 65 have not been established.

Pediatric use

- Do not use in patients under age 12 because this fixed-dose combination treatment cannot be adjusted for this patient group.

Breast-feeding

- Although zidovudine has been reported in breast milk at concentrations similar to serum, no data are available for the presence of lamivudine and zidovudine.

lamotrigine

Lamictal

Pharmacologic classification: phenyltriazine
Therapeutic classification: anticonvulsant
Pregnancy risk category C

How supplied

Available by prescription only
Tablets: 25 mg, 100 mg, 150 mg, 200 mg

Indications, route, and dosage

Adjunct therapy in treatment of partial seizures caused by epilepsy
Adults: 50 mg P.O. daily for 2 weeks, followed by 100 mg daily in two divided doses for 2 weeks. Thereafter, usual maintenance dose is 300 to 500 mg P.O. daily given in two divided doses. For patients also taking valproic acid, give 25 mg P.O. every other day for 2 weeks, followed by 25 mg P.O. daily for 2 weeks. Thereafter, maximum dosage is 150 mg P.O. daily in two divided doses.

Pharmacodynamics

Anticonvulsant action: Unknown. It is believed to relate to an inhibition of the release of glutamate and aspartate in the brain. This may occur by acting on voltage-sensitive sodium channels.

Pharmacokinetics

- *Absorption:* Drug is rapidly and completely absorbed from the GI tract with negligible first-pass metabolism. Absolute bioavailability is 98%.
- *Distribution:* About 55% is bound to plasma proteins.
- *Metabolism:* Drug is metabolized predominantly by glucuronic acid conjugation; the major metabolite is an inactive 2-N-glucuronide conjugate.
- *Excretion:* Excreted primarily in urine with only a small portion being excreted in feces.

Contraindications and precautions

Contraindicated in patients with hypersensitivity to drug. Use cautiously in patients with impaired renal, hepatic, or cardiac function.

Interactions
Carbamazepine, phenobarbital, phenytoin, and *primidone* decrease lamotrigine's steady state concentrations. Monitor patient closely.

Folate inhibitors (such as *co-trimoxazole, methotrexate*) may be affected by lamotrigine because it inhibits dihydrofolate reductase, an enzyme involved in the synthesis of folic acid. Monitor patient closely because drug may have an additive effect. *Valproic acid* decreases lamotrigine's clearance, which increases drug's steady-state concentrations. Monitor patient closely for toxicity.

Effects on diagnostic tests
None reported.

Adverse reactions
CNS: *dizziness, headache, ataxia, somnolence,* incoordination, insomnia, tremor, depression, anxiety, seizures, irritability, speech disorder, decreased memory, concentration disturbance, sleep disorder, emotional lability, vertigo, mind racing, ***suicidal attempts.***
CV: palpitations.
EENT: *diplopia, blurred vision,* vision abnormality, nystagmus.
GI: *nausea, vomiting,* diarrhea, dyspepsia, abdominal pain, constipation, tooth disorder, anorexia, dry mouth.
Respiratory: rhinitis, pharyngitis, cough, dyspnea.
Skin: ***Stevens-Johnson syndrome****, rash,* pruritus, hot flashes, alopecia, acne.
Other: dysarthria, muscle spasm, flulike syndrome, fever, infection, neck pain, malaise, chills, dysmenorrhea, vaginitis, amenorrhea, photosensitivity.

Overdose and treatment
Limited information available. One patient became comatose and remained in a coma for 8 to 12 hours; a second patient experienced dizziness, headache, and somnolence. Both patients recovered without sequelae. Following a suspected overdosage, treatment should be supportive. Emesis should be induced or gastric lavage performed, if necessary. It is not known if hemodialysis is effective.

☑ Special considerations
- Do not discontinue drug abruptly because of risk of increasing seizure frequency. Instead, taper drug over at least 2 weeks.
- Stop drug immediately if drug-induced rash occurs.
- If lamotrigine is added to a multidrug regimen that includes valproate, reduce dose of lamotrigine. Use a lower maintenance dosage in patients with severe renal impairment.
- Evaluate patient for reduction in the frequency and duration of seizures. Periodic evaluation of adjunct anticonvulsant's serum levels should be done.

Patient education
- Inform patient that rash may occur, especially during first 6 weeks of therapy and in pediatric patients. Combination therapy of valproic acid and lamotrigine is likely to precipitate a serious rash. Although it may resolve with continued therapy, tell patient to report it immediately in case drug needs to be discontinued.
- Warn patient not to perform hazardous activities until CNS effects are known.
- Advise patient to take protective measures against photosensitivity reactions until tolerance is known.

Geriatric use
- Safety and effectiveness in patients over age 65 have not been established.

Pediatric use
- Safety and effectiveness in children under age 16 have not been established.

Breast-feeding
- Drug use in breast-feeding women is not recommended.

lansoprazole
Prevacid

Pharmacologic classification: acid (proton pump inhibitor
Therapeutic classification: antiulcer
Pregnancy risk category B

How supplied
Available by prescription only
Capsules (delayed-release): 15 mg, 30 mg

Indications, route, and dosage
Short-term treatment of active duodenal ulcer
Adults: 15 mg P.O. daily before meals for 4 weeks.
Short-term treatment of erosive esophagitis
Adults: 30 mg P.O. daily before meals for up to 8 weeks. If healing does not occur, an additional 8 weeks of therapy may be needed.
Long-term treatment of pathologic hypersecretory conditions, including Zollinger-Ellison syndrome
Adults: Initially 60 mg P.O. once daily. Increase dosage p.r.n. Daily dosages exceeding 120 mg should be administered in divided doses.

Pharmacodynamics
Antiulcer action: Lansoprazole inhibits activity of the acid (proton) pump and binds to hydrogen-potassium ATPase, located at the secretory surface of the gastric parietal cells, to block the formation of gastric acid.

Pharmacokinetics
- *Absorption:* Rapidly absorbed with absolute bioavailability of over 80%.
- *Distribution:* Lansoprazole is 97% bound to plasma proteins.
- *Metabolism:* Drug is extensively metabolized in the liver.
- *Excretion:* About two-thirds of dose is excreted in feces one third in urine.

Contraindications and precautions
Contraindicated in patients with hypersensitivity to drug.

Interactions
Lansoprazole may interfere with the absorption of *ampicillin esters, iron salts,* and *ketoconazole.* Monitor patient closely. *Sucralfate* delays lansoprazole absorption. Give lansoprazole at least 30 minutes prior to sucralfate.

Theophylline may cause mild increase in theophylline excretion. Use together cautiously. Dosage adjustment of theophylline may be necessary when lansoprazole is started or stopped.

Effects on diagnostic tests
None reported.

Adverse reactions
CNS: headache, agitation, amnesia, anxiety, apathy, confusion, depression, dizziness or syncope, hallucinations, hemiplegia, aggravated hostility, decreased libido, nervousness, paresthesia, thinking abnormality.
CV: chest pain, edema, angina, ***CVA,*** hypertension or hypotension, ***MI, shock,*** palpitations, vasodilation, ***cardiospasm.***
EENT: amblyopia, deafness, epistaxis, eye pain, visual field deficits, otitis media, taste perversion, tinnitus.
GI: *diarrhea, nausea, abdominal pain,* halitosis, melena, anorexia, cholelithiasis, constipation, dry mouth, thirst, dyspepsia, dysphagia, eructation, esophageal stenosis, esophageal ulcer, esophagitis, fecal discoloration, flatulence, gastric nodules, fundic gland polyps, gastroenteritis, GI hemorrhage, hematemesis, increased appetite, increased salivation, rectal hemorrhage, stomatitis, tenesmus, ulcerative colitis.
GU: hematuria, impotence, kidney calculus, albuminuria, abnormal menses, breast tenderness, breast enlargement or gynecomastia.
Hematologic: anemia, hemolysis.
Hepatic: abnormal liver function tests.
Metabolic: diabetes mellitus, goiter, hyperglycemia, hypoglycemia, gout, weight gain or loss.
Musculoskeletal: arthritis, arthralgia, musculoskeletal pain, myalgia.
Respiratory: asthma, bronchitis, increased cough, dyspnea, hemoptysis, hiccups, pneumonia, upper respiratory tract inflammation.
Skin: acne, alopecia, pruritus, rash, urticaria.
Other: asthenia, candidiasis, fever, flulike syndrome, infection, malaise.

Overdose and treatment
No adverse effects have been reported with drug overdosage. Drug is not removed from the circulation by hemodialysis. If required, treatment should be supportive.

☑ Special considerations
- Dosage adjustment is not necessary in the elderly or in patients with renal insufficiency; however, it may be required for patients with severe liver disease.
- Drug should not be used as maintenance therapy for patients with duodenal ulcer disease or erosive esophagitis.

Patient education
- Instruct patient to take drug before meals.
- Caution patient not to open, chew, or crush capsules; capsules should be swallowed whole.

Geriatric use
- Although initial dosing regimen need not be altered for elderly patients, subsequent doses over 30 mg/day should not be administered unless additional gastric acid suppression is necessary.

Pediatric use
- Safety and effectiveness in children have not been established.

Breast-feeding
- Because it is not known if lansoprazole is excreted in breast milk, a decision to discontinue breast-feeding or drug should be made.

latanoprost
Xalatan

Pharmacologic classification: prostaglandin analogue
Therapeutic classification: antiglaucoma; ocular antihypertensive
Pregnancy risk category C

How supplied
Available by prescription only
Ophthalmic solution: 0.005%

Indications, route, and dosage
Treatment of increased intraocular pressure (IOP) in patients with ocular hypertension or open-angle glaucoma who are intolerant of other IOP-lowering medications or insufficiently responsive to another IOP-lowering medication
Adults: Instill 1 drop in the conjunctival sac of the affected eye(s) once daily in the evening.

Pharmacodynamics
Antiglaucoma/ocular antihypertensive actions: Although exact mechanism of latanoprost's ability to lower IOP is unknown, it is believed to occur by increasing the outflow of aqueous humor.

Pharmacokinetics
- *Absorption:* Drug is absorbed through the cornea. Peak concentration in the aqueous humor occurs about 2 hours after topical administration.
- *Distribution:* Latanoprost's distribution volume is about 0.16 L/kg. The acid of latanoprost could be measured in aqueous humor during first 4 hours and in plasma only during first hour after local administration.
- *Metabolism:* Drug is hydrolyzed by esterases in the cornea to the biologically active acid. The ac-

tive acid of drug reaching the systemic circulation is primarily metabolized by the liver.
• *Excretion:* Metabolites are mainly eliminated in urine.

Contraindications and precautions
Contraindicated in patients with hypersensitivity to drug, benzalkonium chloride, or other ingredients in the product. Use cautiously when administering to patients with impaired renal or hepatic function.

Interactions
Precipitation occurs when eyedrops containing *thimerosal* are mixed with latanoprost. If such drugs are used concomitantly, they should be administered at least 5 minutes apart.

Effects on diagnostic tests
None reported.

Adverse reactions
EENT: blurred vision; burning; stinging; itching; conjunctival hyperemia; foreign body sensation; increased pigmentation of iris; punctate epithelial keratopathy; dry eye; excessive tearing; photophobia; conjunctivitis; diplopia; eye pain or discharge; retinal artery embolus (rare); retinal detachment (rare); vitreous hemorrhage from diabetic retinopathy (rare); lid crusting, edema, erythema, discomfort, or pain.
Other: upper respiratory tract infection, cold, flu; muscle, joint, back, or chest pain; angina pectoris; rash; allergic skin reaction.

Overdose and treatment
Apart from ocular irritation and conjunctival or episcleral hyperemia, the ocular effects of latanoprost administered at high doses are not known. Treatment should be symptomatic if overdosage occurs.

☑ Special considerations
• Latanoprost may gradually change eye color, increasing the amount of brown pigment in the iris. The change in iris color occurs slowly and may not be noticeable for several months to years. The increased pigmentation may be permanent.

Patient education
• Inform patient about potential of change in iris color. Patients who are receiving treatment in only one eye should be told about the potential for increased brown pigmentation in the treated eye and thus, heterochromia between the eyes.
• Teach patient to instill drops. Advise him to wash hands before and after instilling solution, and warn him not to touch dropper or tip to eye or surrounding tissue.
• Advise patient to apply light finger pressure on lacrimal sac for 1 minute after instillation to minimize systemic absorption of drug.
• Instruct patient to report ocular reactions, especially conjunctivitis and lid reactions.
• Tell patient using contact lenses to remove them before administration of the solution and not to reinsert the contact lenses until 15 minutes have elapsed after administration.
• Advise patient that if more than one topical ophthalmic drug is being used, the drugs should be administered at least 5 minutes apart.
• Stress importance of compliance with recommended therapy.

Pediatric use
• Safety and effectiveness in children have not been established.

Breast-feeding
• It is not known if drug is excreted into breast milk. Exercise caution when administering drug to breast-feeding women.

letrozole
Femara

Pharmacologic classification: aromatase inhibitor
Therapeutic classification: hormone
Pregnancy risk category D

How supplied
Available by prescription only
Tablets: 2.5 mg

Indications, route, & dosage
Treatment of metastatic breast cancer in postmenopausal women with disease progression following antiestrogen therapy
Adults and elderly: 2.5 mg P.O. as a single daily dose, without regard to meals.

Pharmacodynamics
Hormone action: Inhibits conversion of androgens to estrogens by competitive inhibition of the aromatase enzyme system. Decreased estrogens are likely to lead to decreased tumor mass or delayed progression of tumor growth in some women.

Pharmacokinetics
• *Absorption:* Rapidly and completely absorbed. Food does not affect bioavailability. Steady-state plasma levels are reached in 2 to 6 weeks after daily dosing.
• *Distribution:* Drug has a large volume of distribution (1.9 L/kg). It is weakly protein bound
• *Metabolism:* Slowly metabolized to an inactive form. In human liver microsomes, letrozole strongly inhibited cytochrome P450 isozyme 2A6 and moderately inhibited isozyme 2C19.
• *Excretion:* The inactive glucuronide metabolite is eliminated in the urine.

Contraindications and precautions
Contraindicated in patients with known hypersensitivity to drug or its components. Avoid use in pregnant patients because drug may cause fetal harm. Use cautiously in patients with severe liver impairment.

Interactions
None reported.

Effects on diagnostic tests
Drug may cause alterations in liver function tests.

Adverse reactions
CNS: headache, somnolence, dizziness, fatigue, asthenia.
CV: hypertension, ***thromboembolism,*** chest pain.
GI: *nausea,* vomiting, constipation, diarrhea, abdominal pain, anorexia, dyspepsia.
Musculoskeletal: *bone pain, extremities and back pain,* arthralgias.
Respiratory: dyspnea, coughing.
Skin: hot flashes, rash, pruritus.
Other: edema, weight gain, hypercholesterolemia, viral infections.

Overdose and treatment
There have been no reports of overdose during clinical trials with letrozole.

If overdose occurs, consider inducing emesis if patient is alert; provide supportive care and monitor vital signs frequently.

☑ Special considerations
- No dosage adjustment is needed in patients with mild to moderate liver dysfunction or in renally impaired patients with creatinine clearance of 10 ml/minute or more.
- Patients treated with letrozole do not need glucocorticoid or mineralocorticoid replacement therapy. Letrozole significantly lowers serum estrone, estradiol, and estrone sulfate, but has not been shown to significantly affect adrenal corticosteroid synthesis, aldosterone synthesis, or synthesis of thyroid hormones.

Patient education
- Instruct patient to take drug exactly as prescribed.
- Tell patient that drug can be taken with or without food.
- Advise patient that drug treatment is chronic, and stress importance of follow-up appointments.
- Tell patient to inform primary health care provider if pregnancy is suspected or is being planned.

Breast-feeding
- It is unknown if letrozole is excreted in breast excretion. Use caution when administering letrozole to a nursing mother.

leucovorin calcium (citrovorum factor or folinic acid)
Wellcovorin

Pharmacologic classification: formyl derivative (active reduced form of folic acid)
Therapeutic classification: vitamin, antidote
Pregnancy risk category C

How supplied
Available by prescription only
Tablets: 5 mg, 15 mg, 25 mg
Injection: 1-ml ampule (3 mg/ml with 0.9% benzyl alcohol, 5 mg/ml with methyl and propyl parabens); 50-mg, 100-mg, and 350-mg vials for reconstitution (contain no preservatives)

Indications, route, and dosage
Overdose of folic acid antagonist
Adults and children: P.O., I.M., or I.V. dose equivalent to weight of antagonist given as soon as possible after the overdose.
Leucovorin rescue after large methotrexate dose in treatment of cancer
Adults and children: Administer 24 hours after last dose of methotrexate according to protocol. Give 15 mg I.M., I.V., or P.O. q 6 hours until methotrexate serum level is less than 5×10^{-8} M.
Toxic effects of methotrexate used to treat severe psoriasis
Adults and children: 4 to 8 mg I.M. 2 hours after methotrexate dose.
Hematologic toxicity from pyrimethamine or trimethoprim therapy
Adults and children: 5 to 15 mg P.O. or I.M. daily.
Advanced colorectal cancer
Adults: 200 mg/m^2 by slow I.V. injection over 3 minutes followed by 5-fluorouracil (5-FU) or 20 mg/m^2 by slow I.V. injection over 3 minutes followed by 5-FU. Repeat treatment for 5 days. May repeat course at 4-week intervals for two courses and then at 4- to 5-week intervals provided the patient has recovered from toxic effects of previous treatment.
Megaloblastic anemia from congenital enzyme deficiency
Adults and children: 3 to 6 mg I.M. daily, then 1 mg P.O. daily for life.
Folate-deficient megaloblastic anemias
Adults and children: Up to 1 mg of leucovorin P.O. or I.M. daily. Duration of treatment depends on hematologic response.

Pharmacodynamics
Reversal of folic acid antagonism: Leucovorin is a derivative of tetrahydrofolic acid, the reduced form of folic acid. Leucovorin performs as a cofactor in 1-carbon transfer reactions in the biosynthesis of purines and pyrimidines of nucleic acids. Impairment of thymidylate synthesis in patients with folic acid deficiency may account for defective DNA synthesis, megaloblast formation, and megaloblastic and macrocytic anemias. Leucovorin is a potent antidote for the hematopoietic and reticuloendothelial toxic effects of folic acid antagonists (trimethoprim, pyrimethamine, and methotrexate). "Leucovorin rescue" is used to prevent or decrease toxicity of massive methotrexate doses. Folinic acid "rescues" normal cells without reversing the oncolytic effect of methotrexate.

Pharmacokinetics
- *Absorption:* After oral administration, leucovorin is absorbed rapidly; peak serum folate concentrations occur less than 2 hours following a 15-mg dose. The increase in plasma and serum folate activity after oral administration is mainly from 5-methyltetrahydrofolate (the major transport and storage form of folate in the body).

• *Distribution:* Tetrahydrofolic acid and its derivatives are distributed throughout the body; the liver contains approximately half of the total body folate stores.
• *Metabolism:* Leucovorin is metabolized in the liver.
• *Excretion:* Drug is excreted by the kidneys as 10-formyl tetrahydrofolate and 5,10-methenyl tetrahydrofolate. Duration of action is 3 to 6 hours.

Contraindications and precautions

Contraindicated in patients with pernicious anemia and other megaloblastic anemias secondary to the lack of vitamin B_{12}.

Interactions

Concomitant use of leucovorin with *phenytoin* will decrease serum phenytoin concentrations and increase frequency of seizures. Although this interaction has occurred solely in patients receiving folic acid, it should be considered when leucovorin is administered. The mechanism by which this occurs appears to be an increased metabolic clearance of phenytoin or a redistribution of phenytoin in the CSF and brain. Phenytoin and *primidone* may decrease serum folate levels, producing symptoms of folate deficiency. After chemotherapy with *folic acid antagonists*, parenteral administration is preferable to oral dosing because vomiting may cause loss of the leucovorin. To treat an overdose of folic acid antagonists, leucovorin should be administered within 1 hour if possible; it is usually ineffective after a 4-hour delay. Leucovorin has no effect on other methotrexate toxicities. When given concomitantly, leucovorin will increase toxicity of *fluorouracil*; lower doses of fluorouracil should be used.

Effects on diagnostic tests

Leucovorin may mask the diagnosis of pernicious anemia.

Adverse reactions

Skin: hypersensitivity reactions (urticaria, ***anaphylactoid reactions***).

Overdose and treatment

Leucovorin is relatively nontoxic; no specific recommendations for overdose are reported. However, an excessive amount of leucovorin may nullify the chemotherapeutic effect of folic acid antagonists such as methotrexate.

☑ Special considerations

• Drug administration continues until plasma methotrexate levels are below 5×10^{-8} M.
• To prepare drug for parenteral use, add 5 ml of bacteriostatic water for injection to vial containing 50 mg of base drug.
• Maximum rate of leucovorin infusion should not exceed 160 mg/minute because of calcium concentration of solution.
• Do not use as sole treatment of pernicious anemia or vitamin B_{12} deficiency.
• To treat overdose of folic acid antagonists, use the drug within 1 hour; it is not effective after a 4-hour delay.
• Monitor patient for signs of drug allergy, such as rash, wheezing, pruritus, and urticaria.
• Monitor serum creatinine levels daily to detect possible renal function impairment.
• When giving more than 25 mg, drug should be administered parenterally.
• Store at room temperature in a light-resistant container, not in high-moisture areas.

Patient education

• Emphasize importance of taking leucovorin only under medical supervision.

Pediatric use

• Drug may increase frequency of seizures in susceptible children.
• Do not use diluents containing benzyl alcohol when reconstituting drug for neonates.

Breast-feeding

• It is unknown if leucovorin is distributed into breast milk; use with caution in breast-feeding women.

leuprolide acetate

Lupron, Lupron Depot, Lupron Depot-Ped, Lupron Depot-3 Month

Pharmacologic classification: gonadotropin-releasing hormone
Therapeutic classification: antineoplastic; luteinizing hormone-releasing hormone (LHRH) analogue
Pregnancy risk category X

How supplied

Available by prescription only
Injection: 5 mg/ml in 2.8-ml multiple-dose vials
Suspension for depot injection: 3.75 mg, 7.5 mg, 11.25 mg, 15 mg, 22.5 mg

Indications, route, and dosage

Dosage and indications may vary. Check current literature for recommended protocol.

Management of advanced prostate cancer
Adults: 7.5 mg I.M. (depot injection) once monthly or 1 mg S.C. daily; or 22.5 mg I.M. q 3 months.

Treatment of endometriosis
Adults: 3.75 mg I.M. (depot injection) once monthly for a maximum of 6 months.

◊ ***Central precocious puberty***
Children: starting dose 50 mcg/kg/day, given as a single S.C. injection. May titrate upward by 10 mcg/kg/day until total downregulation is achieved. This becomes the maintenance dose.

Pharmacodynamics

Antineoplastic action: Leuprolide is a synthetic analogue of LHRH. It inhibits gonadotropin secretion and androgen or estrogen synthesis. Because of this effect leuprolide may inhibit the growth of hormone-dependent tumors.

Hormonal action: Because leuprolide lowers levels of sex hormones, it causes a decrease in the size of endometrial implants, resulting in decreased dysmenorrhea and pelvic pain in women with endometriosis.

Pharmacokinetics

• *Absorption:* Leuprolide is a polypeptide molecule that is destroyed in the GI tract. After S.C. administration, drug is rapidly, and essentially completely, absorbed.
• *Distribution:* Distribution in humans has not been determined; however, it is suggested that high concentrations distribute into kidney, liver, pineal, and pituitary tissue. Approximately 7% to 15% of a dose is bound to plasma proteins.
• *Metabolism:* Unclear, but drug may be metabolized in the anterior pituitary and hypothalamus, similar to endogenous gonadotropin-releasing hormone.
• *Excretion:* Plasma elimination half-life has been reported to be 3 hours.

Contraindications and precautions

Contraindicated in patients hypersensitive to drug or other gonadotropin-releasing hormone analogues, during pregnancy or lactation, and in women with undiagnosed vaginal bleeding. Use cautiously in patients with hypersensitivity to benzyl alcohol.

Interactions

None reported.

Effects on diagnostic tests

Serum acid phosphatase and testosterone levels initially increase then decrease with continued therapy.

Adverse reactions

CNS: *dizziness, depression, headache, pain,* insomnia.
CV: ***arrhythmias,*** angina, ***MI,*** *peripheral edema, ECG changes,* hypertension, murmur.
GI: *nausea, vomiting,* anorexia, constipation.
GU: *impotence, vaginitis,* urinary frequency, hematuria, urinary tract infection, gynecomastia.
Hepatic: elevated liver enzyme levels.
Respiratory: dyspnea, sinus congestion, pulmonary fibrosis.
Other: transient bone pain during first week of treatment, *hot flashes,* skin reactions at injection site, *androgen-like effects,* joint disorder, myalgia, neuromuscular disorder, *weight gain or loss,* anemia, dermatitis, *asthenia.*

Overdose and treatment

No information available.

☑ Special considerations

• Use a 22G needle for monthly injection and a 23G needle for 3-month injection.
• When treating endometriosis, administer for a maximum of 6 months. Safety and efficacy of retreatment is unknown.
• Discard solution if particulate matter is visible or if the solution is discolored.
• Erythema or induration may develop at injection site.
• When used to treat prostate cancer, leuprolide may produce worsening of signs and symptoms of disease during first 1 to 2 weeks of therapy. Temporary paresthesia and weakness may occur during first week of therapy.
• Measure serum testosterone and acid phosphatase levels before and during therapy.
• No unusual adverse effects were observed in patients who had received 20 mg daily for 2 years.
• Refrigerate drug until used. Do not freeze. Reconstituted suspension is stable for 24 hours.

Patient education

• Reassure patient that bone pain is transient and will disappear after about 1 week.
• Inform patient that a temporary reaction of burning, itching, and swelling at injection site may occur. Tell him to report persistent reactions.
• Advise patient to continue taking drug even if he experiences a sense of well-being.
• Instruct female patient of childbearing age to use an effective nonhormonal method of contraception during therapy.

levamisole hydrochloride

Ergamisol

Pharmacologic classification: immunomodulator
Therapeutic classification: antineoplastic
Pregnancy risk category C

How supplied

Available by prescription only
Tablets: 50 mg

Indications, route, and dosage

Adjuvant treatment in combination with fluorouracil after surgical resection in patients with Dukes' stage C colon cancer
Adults: Initially, 50 mg P.O. q 8 hours for 3 days starting 7 to 30 days after surgery. Repeat q 14 days for 1 year. Administer with fluorouracil 450 mg/m^2 daily by rapid I.V. push for 5 days concomitant with a 3-day course of levamisole, starting 21 to 34 days after surgery.

If levamisole therapy begins 7 to 20 days after surgery, start fluorouracil with the second course of levamisole at 21 to 24 days. If levamisole is initiated 21 to 30 days after surgery, start fluorouracil simultaneously with the first course of therapy.

Maintenance dose is 50 mg P.O. q 8 hours for 3 days q 2 weeks. Give with fluorouracil 450 mg/m^2 daily by rapid I.V. push weekly beginning 28 days after initiation of the 5-day course.

Note: If an acute neurologic syndrome occurs, immediate discontinuation of therapy should be considered.

Pharmacodynamics

Antineoplastic action: Levamisole is an immunomodulator, and its mechanism of action in combination with fluorouracil is unknown. Its effects on the immune system are complete, but it appears to restore depressed immune function rather than stimulate response to above-normal levels. It can also stimulate antibody formation; enhance T-cell responses by stimulating T-cell activation and proliferation; potentiate monocyte and macrophage formation, including phagocytosis and chemotaxis; increase neutrophil mobility adherence and chemotaxis; and inhibit alkaline phosphatase. Levamisole also has cholinergic activity.

Pharmacokinetics

- *Absorption:* Drug is rapidly absorbed from the GI tract with peak plasma levels obtained within 1½ to 2 hours.
- *Distribution:* Unknown.
- *Metabolism:* Extensively metabolized by the liver.
- *Excretion:* 70% of metabolites are excreted in urine over 3 days; 5%, in feces; less than 5% of unchanged drug is excreted in urine; less than 2%, in feces.

Contraindications and precautions

Contraindicated in patients hypersensitive to drug.

Interactions

Disulfiram-like reaction occurs if used concurrently with *alcohol.* Concomitant administration with *phenytoin* has increased phenytoin levels. Monitor plasma phenytoin levels and decrease dosage as needed. Concomitant administration with *warfarin* may result in excessive prolongation of PT.

Adverse reactions

CNS: *dizziness, headache, paresthesia, somnolence, depression, nervousness, insomnia, anxiety, fatigue, fever.*
CV: chest pain, edema.
EENT: blurred vision, conjunctivitis, *stomatitis, dysgeusia, altered sense of smell.*
GI: *nausea, diarrhea, vomiting, anorexia, abdominal pain, constipation, flatulence, dyspepsia.*
Hematologic: ***agranulocytosis, leukopenia, thrombocytopenia,*** anemia.
Skin: dermatitis, ***exfoliative dermatitis,*** *pruritus, urticaria.*
Other: hyperbilirubinemia, rigors, *alopecia, infection, arthralgia, myalgia.*

Overdose and treatment

Fatalities have been reported after ingestion of 15 mg/kg by a 3-year-old child and of 32 mg/kg by an adult. No further clinical information is available. Gastric lavage is recommended along with symptomatic and supportive measures.

☑ Special considerations

- Drug should not be used in higher than recommended dosage or administered more frequently than indicated.
- Before drug therapy begins, patient should be ambulatory, maintain normal oral nutrition, have well-healed wounds, fully recovered from any postsurgical complications, and not be hospitalized.
- If WBC count is 2,500 to 3,500/mm³, defer fluorouracil dose until it is over 3,500/mm³. If WBC count is below 2,500/mm³, defer fluorouracil until WBC count is above 3,500/mm³ and then reduce dose by 20%. If WBC count remains below 2,500/mm³ for more than 10 days even after deferring fluorouracil, discontinue drug. Defer both if platelet counts are below 100,000/mm³.
- If stomatitis or diarrhea develops during initial fluorouracil administration schedule, discontinue course before full five doses are administered. If stomatitis or diarrhea occurs during weekly maintenance therapy, defer next dose of fluorouracil until it subsides. If adverse reactions are moderate to severe, reduce fluorouracil by 20% when treatment is resumed.
- Flulike syndrome frequently accompanies the onset of agranulocytosis but may also occur in the absence of agranulocytosis. Instruct patient to report flulike symptoms immediately.
- Obtain CBC with differential, platelet counts, electrolytes, and liver function tests before initiation of therapy. CBC with differential and platelet counts should be performed weekly before each fluorouracil treatment; electrolyte and liver function tests, every 3 months for 1 year. Modify doses as needed.

Patient education

- Advise patient to use a soft toothbrush and electric razor to avoid trauma and excessive bleeding.
- Tell patient to report unusual bruising or bleeding, persistent fever or flulike symptoms, sore throat, or weakness.
- Advise patient to avoid exposure to persons with infection.

Pediatric use

- Safety and efficacy in children have not been established.

Breast-feeding

- It is unknown if drug occurs in breast milk. The potential for serious adverse reactions in infants must be considered.

levobunolol hydrochloride

AKBeta, Betagan

Pharmacologic classification: beta-adrenergic blocker
Therapeutic classification: antiglaucoma
Pregnancy risk category C

How supplied

Available by prescription only
Ophthalmic solution: 0.25%, 0.5%

Indications, route, and dosage

Chronic open-angle glaucoma and ocular hypertension

Adults: Instill 1 to 2 drops (0.5% solution) daily or 1 to 2 drops (0.25% solution) b.i.d. in eye(s).

Pharmacodynamics

Antiglaucoma action: Levobunolol is a nonselective beta-adrenergic blocking agent that reduces intraocular pressure. Exact mechanisms are unknown, but the drug appears to reduce formation of aqueous humor.

Pharmacokinetics

- *Absorption:* Onset of activity usually occurs within 60 minutes; peak effect, 2 to 6 hours.
- *Distribution:* Unknown.
- *Metabolism:* Unknown.
- *Excretion:* Duration of effect is 24 hours.

Contraindications and precautions

Contraindicated in patients with hypersensitivity to drug, bronchial asthma, history of bronchial asthma or severe COPD, sinus bradycardia, second- or third-degree AV block, cardiac failure, and cardiogenic shock. Use cautiously in patients with chronic bronchitis, emphysema, diabetes mellitus, hyperthyroidism, and myasthenia gravis.

Interactions

Levobunolol may increase the systemic effect of *oral beta blockers*, enhance the hypotensive and bradycardiac effects of *reserpine* and *catecholamine-depleting agents,* and increase reductions in intraocular pressure induced by *epinephrine, pilocarpine,* or *carbonic anhydrase inhibitors.*

Effects on diagnostic tests

Although oral beta blockers have been reported to decrease serum glucose levels from blockage of normal glycogen release after hypoglycemia, such instances have not been reported with the use of ophthalmic beta blockers.

Adverse reactions

CNS: headache, depression, insomnia.
CV: slight reduction in resting heart rate.
EENT: *transient eye stinging and burning,* tearing, erythema, itching, keratitis, corneal punctate staining, photophobia; decreased corneal sensitivity (with long-term use).
GI: nausea.
Skin: urticaria.
Other: evidence of beta blockade and systemic absorption (*hypotension,* ***bradycardia,*** *syncope,* ***asthmatic attacks in patients with history of asthma, heart failure).***

Overdose and treatment

Overdose is extremely rare with ophthalmic use. However, usual manifestations include bradycardia, hypotension, bronchospasm, heart block, and cardiac failure.

After accidental ingestion, emesis is most effective if initiated within 30 minutes, providing patient is not obtunded, comatose, or having seizures. Follow with activated charcoal. Treat bradycardia, conduction defects, and hypotension with I.V. fluids, glucagon, atropine, or isoproterenol. Treat bronchoconstriction with I.V. aminophylline, and seizures with I.V. diazepam.

☑ Special considerations

- Cardiac output is reduced in both healthy patients and those with heart disease. Drug may decrease heart rate and blood pressure and produces beta blockade in bronchi and bronchioles. No effect on pupil size or accommodation has been noted.
- In some patients, a few weeks' treatment may be required to stabilize pressure-lowering response; determine intraocular pressure after 4 weeks of treatment.
- Levobunolol is faster-acting than timolol.

Patient education

- Warn patient not to touch dropper to eye or surrounding tissue.
- Show patient how to instill drug. Teach him to press lacrimal sac lightly for 1 minute after drug administration, to decrease chance of systemic absorption.
- Remind patient not to blink more than usual or to close eyes tightly during treatment.
- Although transient stinging and discomfort are common, tell patient to call if reaction is severe.

Geriatric use

- Drug should be used with caution in elderly patients with cardiac or pulmonary disease, who may experience exacerbation of symptoms, depending on extent of systemic absorption.

levocabastine hydrochloride

Livostin

Pharmacologic classification: cyclohexylpiperidine derivative
Therapeutic classification: antihistamine (H_1-receptor antagonist), antiallergic ophthalmic
Pregnancy risk category C

How supplied

Available by prescription only
Ophthalmic suspension: 0.05%

Indications, route, and dosage

Allergic conjunctivitis
Adults and children age 12 and older: Instill 1 drop in affected eye(s) q.i.d. Treatment may be continued for up to 2 weeks.

Pharmacodynamics

Antihistamine action: Levocabastine competes with histamine for H_1-receptor sites and suppresses histamine-induced allergic symptoms.

Pharmacokinetics

- *Absorption:* After instillation in the eye, levocabastine is systemically absorbed. However, amount of systemically absorbed drug after therapeutic ocular doses is low.
- *Distribution:* Unknown.
- *Metabolism:* Drug is metabolized minimally in the liver to an acylgluconide metabolite.
- *Excretion:* From 65% to 70% of absorbed drug is excreted unchanged in the urine, with an additional 10% appearing as the acylgluconide metabolite. Up to 20% of an absorbed dose is excreted in the feces.

Contraindications and precautions
Contraindicated in patients hypersensitive to drug or its components and in those wearing soft contact lenses.

Interactions
None reported.

Effects on diagnostic tests
None reported.

Adverse reactions
CNS: headache, fatigue, somnolence.
EENT: *transient eye discomfort upon instillation (burning, stinging), eye discharge,* dryness, pain, or redness; lacrimation; eyelid edema; visual disturbances; pharyngitis.
GI: dry mouth, nausea.
Respiratory: cough, dyspnea.
Skin: rash.

Overdose and treatment
No information available.

☑ Special considerations
- Drug is for ophthalmic use only, not for injection.
- Shake well before use.
- Keep tightly closed when not in use and store at room temperature.
- Do not use if suspension is discolored.

Patient education
- Instruct patient how to instill eye drops and stress importance of not touching dropper to eye or surrounding area.
- Tell patient to shake suspension well before use.
- Instruct patient to keep bottle tightly closed when not in use and store at room temperature.
- Advise patient that drug should not be used if the suspension is discolored.

Pediatric use
- Safety and efficacy in children under age 12 have not been established.

Breast-feeding
- Use cautiously in breast-feeding women. An analysis of breast milk from a patient revealed a daily dose of levocabastine present to be about 0.5 mcg.

levocarnitine
Carnitor, L-Carnitine, VitaCarn

Pharmacologic classification: amino acid derivative
Therapeutic classification: nutritional supplement
Pregnancy risk category B

How supplied
Available by prescription only
Carnitor
Tablets: 330 mg
Oral solution: 100 mg/ml in 118-ml multiple-dose bottle
Injection: 1 g/5 ml

Available without a prescription
L-Carnitine
Tablets: 250 mg, 500 mg
VitaCarn
Oral solution: 100 mg/ml in 118-ml multiple-dose bottle

Indications, route, and dosage
Primary systemic carnitine deficiency
Adults: 990 mg P.O. b.i.d. or t.i.d., using 330-mg tablets. For oral solution, initially, 1 g/day (10 ml/day); increase slowly to 3 g/day (30 ml/day) as needed and tolerated.
Children: Initially, 50 mg/kg/day P.O. in divided doses, then increased p.r.n. Maximum dosage, 3 g/day.
Acute and chronic treatment in patients with an inborn error of metabolism that results in secondary carnitine deficiency
Adults: 50 mg/kg I.V. bolus over 2 to 3 minutes or by infusion daily. An I.V. loading dose is commonly given to patients with severe metabolic crisis, followed by an equivalent dose over the next 24 hours. The 50 mg/kg/day dose should be divided so that doses are administered q 3 or 4 hours and never less than q 6 hours either by infusion or by I.V. injection. Subsequent daily doses should be in the range of 50 mg/kg or as therapy requires. The highest dose administered has been 300 mg/kg.
Dietary supplement for renal patients
Adults: 500 to 1,500 mg P.O. daily or as directed by primary health care provider, registered dietitian, or nutritionist.

Pharmacodynamics
Nutrient action: Levocarnitine is a naturally occurring substance required in human energy metabolism. It facilitates transport of long-chain fatty acids into cellular mitochondria. The fatty acids are then used to produce energy.

Pharmacokinetics
- *Absorption:* Following oral administration, time to peak concentration is about 3.3 hours.
- *Distribution:* Drug is not bound to plasma proteins or albumin.
- *Metabolism:* Major metabolites are trimethylamine N-oxide, primarily found in urine (8% to 49% of the administered dose), and gamma butyrobetaine, primarily found in feces (0.44% to 45% of administered dose).
- *Excretion:* Drug is eliminated primarily in urine; less so in feces.

Contraindications and precautions
No known contraindications.

Interactions
None significant.

Effects on diagnostic tests
None reported.

Adverse reactions
GI: *nausea, vomiting, cramps, diarrhea.*
Other: *body odor.*

Overdose and treatment
There have been no reports of drug overdosage. Large doses may cause diarrhea. Overdosage should be treated with supportive care.

☑ Special considerations
- Obtain a plasma carnitine level before beginning therapy, and then at weekly and monthly intervals. Monitoring should include blood chemistries, vital signs, plasma carnitine levels (plasma free-carnitine level should be between 35 and 60 micromoles/L), and overall clinical status.
- Inspect parenteral drug products visually for particulate matter and discoloration before administration when solution and container permit.
- Store ampules in carton at room temperature to protect from light. Discard unused portions of opened ampules because they lack preservatives.
- Monitor patient for tolerance during first week of administration and after dosage increase.
- Because of dietary restrictions and other factors, renal dialysis patients have a limited intake of this essential nutrient. Thus, a dietary supplement of this nutrient may become necessary.

Patient education
- Instruct patient to drink oral solution slowly because GI reactions may result from too-rapid consumption.
- Tell patient that oral solution may be consumed alone or put in drinks or other liquids to mask taste.
- Instruct patient to space doses evenly throughout the day (every 3 to 4 hours) during or after meals to maximize tolerance.

Breast-feeding
- It is not known if drug is excreted in breast milk. Because many drugs are excreted in breast milk, a decision should be made whether to discontinue breast-feeding or drug, taking into account the importance of drug to the mother.

levodopa
Dopar, Larodopa

Pharmacologic classification: dopamine precursor
Therapeutic classification: antiparkinsonian
Pregnancy risk category C

How supplied
Available by prescription only
Tablets: 100 mg, 250 mg, 500 mg
Capsules: 100 mg, 250 mg, 500 mg

Indications, route, and dosage
Parkinsonism
Levodopa is indicated in treating idiopathic, postencephalitic, arteriosclerotic parkinsonism and symptomatic parkinsonism that may follow injury to the nervous system by carbon monoxide intoxication and manganese intoxication.

Adults: Initially, 0.5 to 1 g P.O. daily, given b.i.d., t.i.d., or q.i.d. with food; increase by no more than 0.75 g daily q 3 to 7 days, as tolerated. The usual optimal dose is 3 to 6 g daily divided into three doses. Do not exceed 8 g daily, except for exceptional patients. A significant therapeutic response may not be obtained for 6 months. Larger dose requires close supervision.

Pharmacodynamics
Antiparkinsonian action: Precise mechanism has not been established. A small percentage of each dose crossing the blood-brain barrier is decarboxylated. The dopamine then stimulates dopaminergic receptors in the basal ganglia to enhance the balance between cholinergic and dopaminergic activity, resulting in improved modulation of voluntary nerve impulses transmitted to the motor cortex.

Pharmacokinetics
- *Absorption:* Drug is absorbed rapidly from the small intestine by an active amino acid transport system, with 30% to 50% reaching general circulation.
- *Distribution:* Distributed widely to most body tissues, but not to the CNS, which receives less than 1% of dose because of extensive metabolism in the periphery.
- *Metabolism:* 95% of levodopa is converted to dopamine by l-aromatic amino acid decarboxylase enzyme in the lumen of the stomach and intestines and on the first pass through the liver.
- *Excretion:* Excreted primarily in urine; 80% of dose is excreted within 24 hours as dopamine metabolites. Half-life is 1 to 3 hours.

Contraindications and precautions
Contraindicated in concurrent therapy with MAO inhibitors within 14 days, and in hypersensitivity to drug, acute angle-closure glaucoma, melanoma, or undiagnosed skin lesions.

Use cautiously in patients with severe renal, CV, hepatic, and pulmonary disorders; peptic ulcer; psychiatric illness; MI with residual arrhythmias; bronchial asthma; emphysema; and endocrine disorders.

Interactions
Concomitant use with *amantadine, benztropine, procyclidine*, or *trihexyphenidyl* may increase the efficacy of levodopa. *Bromocriptine* may produce additive effects, allowing reduced levodopa dosage. *Anesthetics* or *hydrocarbon inhalation* may cause arrhythmias because of increased endogenous dopamine concentration. (Levodopa should be discontinued 6 to 8 hours before administration of anesthetics such as halothane.)

Antacids containing calcium, magnesium, or sodium bicarbonate may increase absorption of levodopa.

Concurrent use of *anticonvulsants* (such as *hydantoins, phenytoin*), *benzodiazepines, haloperidol, papaverine, phenothiazines, rauwolfia alka-*

loids, or *thioxanthenes* may decrease therapeutic effects of levodopa.

Antihypertensives used concurrently with levodopa may produce increased hypotensive effect.

Methyldopa may alter the antiparkinsonian effects of levodopa and may produce additive toxic CNS effects.

Combined use with *MAO inhibitors* may cause a hypertensive crisis. MAO inhibitors should be discontinued for 2 to 4 weeks before starting levodopa.

Pyridoxine in a small dose (10 mg) reverses the antiparkinsonian effects of levodopa.

Sympathomimetics may increase the risk of arrhythmias (dosage reduction of the sympathomimetic is recommended; the administration of *carbidopa* with levodopa reduces the tendency of sympathomimetics to cause dopamine-induced arrhythmias).

Anticholinergics used with levodopa may produce a mild synergy and increased efficacy (gradual reduction in anticholinergic dosage is necessary).

Tricyclic antidepressants may increase sympathetic activity, with sinus tachycardia and hypertension.

Effects on diagnostic tests

Coombs' test occasionally becomes positive during extended therapy. Colorimetric test for uric acid has shown false elevations. False-positive results have been noted on tests for urine glucose using the copper-reduction method; false-negative results have occurred with the glucose oxidase method. Levodopa also may interfere with tests for urine ketones, urine norepinephrine and urine protein determinations.

Adverse reactions

CNS: *aggressive behavior; choreiform, dystonic, and dyskinetic movements; involuntary grimacing, head movements, myoclonic body jerks,* ***seizures,*** ataxia, tremor, muscle twitching; bradykinetic episodes; psychiatric disturbances; mood changes, nervousness, anxiety, disturbing dreams, euphoria, malaise, fatigue; severe depression, ***suicidal tendencies,*** dementia, delirium, hallucinations (may require reduction or withdrawal of drug).

CV: *orthostatic hypotension,* cardiac irregularities, phlebitis.

EENT: blepharospasm, blurred vision, diplopia, mydriasis or miosis, activation of latent Horner's syndrome, oculogyric crises, excessive salivation.

GI: dry mouth, bitter taste, *nausea, vomiting, anorexia,* weight loss (at start of therapy), constipation, flatulence, diarrhea, abdominal pain.

GU: urinary frequency, urine retention, incontinence, darkened urine, priapism.

Hematologic: ***hemolytic anemia, leukopenia, agranulocytosis.***

Hepatic: elevated liver enzymes, ***hepatotoxicity.***

Other: dark perspiration, hyperventilation, hiccups.

Overdose and treatment

Clinical manifestations of overdose include spasm or closing of eyelids, irregular heartbeat, or palpitations. Treatment includes immediate gastric lavage, maintenance of an adequate airway, and judicious administration of I.V. fluids and may include antiarrhythmic drugs if necessary. Pyridoxine 10 to 25 mg P.O. has been reported to reverse toxic and therapeutic effects of levodopa. (Its usefulness has not been established in acute overdose.)

☑ Special considerations

- Drug should be given between meals and with low-protein snack to maximize drug absorption and minimize GI upset. Foods high in protein appear to interfere with transport of drug.
- Maximum effectiveness of drug may not occur for several weeks or months after therapy begins.
- Monitor patient also receiving antihypertensive medication for possible drug interactions. Discontinue MAO inhibitors at least 2 weeks before levodopa therapy begins.
- Adjust dosage based on patient's response and tolerance. Observe and monitor vital signs, especially while adjusting dose.
- Monitor patient for muscle twitching and blepharospasm (twitching of eyelids), which may be an early sign of drug overdose.
- Test patients on long-term therapy regularly for diabetes and acromegaly; check blood tests and liver and kidney function studies periodically for adverse effects. Leukopenia may require cessation of therapy.
- Because of risk of precipitating a symptom complex resembling neuroleptic malignant syndrome, observe patient closely if levodopa dosage is reduced abruptly or discontinued.
- If restarting therapy after a long period of interruption, adjust drug dosage gradually to previous level.
- Patients undergoing surgery should continue levodopa as long as oral intake is permitted, usually 6 to 24 hours before surgery. Drug should be resumed as soon as patient is able to take oral medication.
- Protect drug from heat, light, and moisture. If preparation darkens, it has lost potency and should be discarded.
- Monitor serum laboratory tests periodically. Coombs' test occasionally becomes positive during extended use. Expect uric acid elevation with colorimetric method but not with uricase method.
- Alkaline phosphatase, AST, ALT, LD, bilirubin, BUN, and protein-bound iodine levels show transient elevations in patients receiving levodopa; WBC, hemoglobin, and hematocrit levels show occasional reduction.
- Although controversial, a medically supervised period of drug discontinuance (drug holiday) may reestablish the effectiveness of a lower dose regimen.
- Combination of levodopa-carbidopa usually reduces amount of levodopa needed, thus reducing incidence of adverse reactions.
- Levodopa has also been used to relieve pain of herpes zoster.
- Tablets and capsules may be crushed and mixed with applesauce or baby-food fruits for patients who have difficulty swallowing pills.

Patient education

- Warn patient and family not to increase drug dose without specific instruction. (They may be tempted to do this as disease symptoms of parkinsonism progress.)
- Explain that therapeutic response may not occur for up to 6 months.
- Advise patient and family that multivitamin preparations, fortified cereals, and certain OTC products may contain pyridoxine (vitamin B_6), which can reverse the effects of levodopa.
- Warn patient of possible dizziness and orthostatic hypotension, especially at start of therapy. Tell patient to change position slowly and dangle legs before getting out of bed. Instruct patient in use of elastic stockings to control this adverse reaction if appropriate.
- Inform patient of signs and symptoms of adverse reactions and therapeutic effects and need to report changes.
- Tell patient to take a missed dose as soon as possible; skip dose if next scheduled dose is within 2 hours, but do not double up doses.
- Advise patient not to take drug with food, but that eating something about 15 minutes after administration may help reduce GI upset.
- Warn patient of possible darkening of urine, sweat, and other body fluids.

Geriatric use

- Smaller doses may be required because of reduced tolerance to drug's effects.
- Elderly patients, especially those with osteoporosis, should resume normal activity gradually, because increased mobility may increase risk of fractures.
- Elderly patients are more likely to develop psychic adverse effects, such as anxiety, confusion, or nervousness; those with preexisting heart disease are more susceptible to levodopa's cardiac effects.

Pediatric use

- Safe use of levodopa in children under age 12 has not been established.

Breast-feeding

- Drug may inhibit lactation and should not be used by breast-feeding patients.

levodopa-carbidopa

Sinemet, Sinemet CR

Pharmacologic classification: decarboxylase inhibitor dopamine precursor combination
Therapeutic classification: antiparkinsonian
Pregnancy risk category C

How supplied

Available by prescription only
Tablets: 10 mg carbidopa with 100 mg levodopa (Sinemet 10-100), 25 mg carbidopa with 100 mg levodopa (Sinemet 25-100), 25 mg carbidopa with 250 mg levodopa (Sinemet 25-250)
Tablets (sustained-release): 50 mg carbidopa with 200 mg levodopa (Sinemet CR 50-200), 25 mg carbidopa with 100 mg levodopa (Sinemet CR 25-100)

Indications, route, and dosage

Parkinsonism

Adults: Most patients respond to a 25 mg/100 mg combination (1 tablet t.i.d.). Dose may be increased q 1 or 2 days; or 1 tablet of 10 mg/100 mg t.i.d. or q.i.d. up to 2 tablets q.i.d.; or 1 sustained-release tablet b.i.d. at intervals at least 6 hours apart. Intervals may be adjusted based on patient response. Usual dose is 2 to 8 tablets daily in divided doses of 4 to 8 hours while awake.

Maintenance therapy must be carefully adjusted based on patient tolerance and desired therapeutic response.

Usual maintenance dose is 3 to 6 tablets of 25 mg carbidopa/250 mg levodopa daily in divided doses. Do not exceed 8 tablets of 25 mg carbidopa/250 mg levodopa daily. Optimum daily dosage must be determined by careful titration for each patient.

Daily dose of carbidopa should be 70 mg or above to suppress the peripheral metabolism of levodopa but should not exceed 200 mg.

Pharmacodynamics

Decarboxylase inhibiting action: Carbidopa inhibits the peripheral decarboxylation of levodopa, thus slowing its conversion to dopamine in extracerebral tissues. This results in an increased availability of levodopa for transport to the brain, where it undergoes decarboxylation to dopamine.

Pharmacokinetics

- *Absorption:* 40% to 70% of dose is absorbed after oral administration. Plasma levodopa concentrations are increased when carbidopa and levodopa are administered concomitantly because carbidopa inhibits the peripheral metabolism of levodopa.
- *Distribution:* Carbidopa is distributed widely in body tissues except the CNS. Levodopa is also distributed into breast milk.
- *Metabolism:* Carbidopa is not metabolized extensively. It inhibits metabolism of levodopa in the GI tract, thus increasing its absorption from the GI tract and its concentration in plasma.
- *Excretion:* 30% of dose is excreted unchanged in urine within 24 hours. When given with carbidopa, the amount of levodopa excreted unchanged in urine is increased by about 6%. Half-life is 1 to 2 hours.

Contraindications and precautions

Contraindicated in patients with hypersensitivity to drug, acute angle-closure glaucoma, melanoma, or undiagnosed skin lesions, and within 14 days of MAO inhibitor therapy.

Use cautiously in patients with severe CV, endocrine, pulmonary, renal, or hepatic disorders; peptic ulcer; psychiatric illness; MI with residual arrhythmias; bronchial asthma; emphysema; and well-controlled chronic open-angle glaucoma.

Photoguide to tablets and capsules

This photoguide provides full-color photographs of some of the most commonly prescribed tablets and capsules in the United States. Shown in actual size, the drugs are organized alphabetically by trade or generic name for quick reference.

Accupril

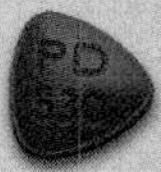

10 mg

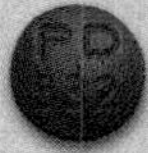

20 mg

Adalat

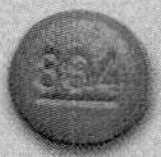

30 mg (extended-release)

Allegra

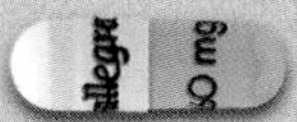

60 mg

Altace

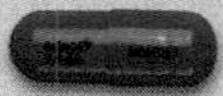

2.5 mg

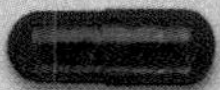

5 mg

Ambien

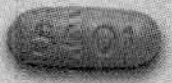

5 mg

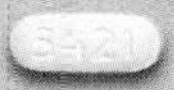

10 mg

amitriptyline hydrochloride

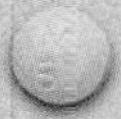

25 mg

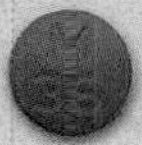

50 mg

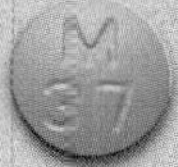

75 mg

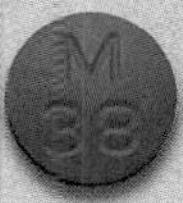

100 mg

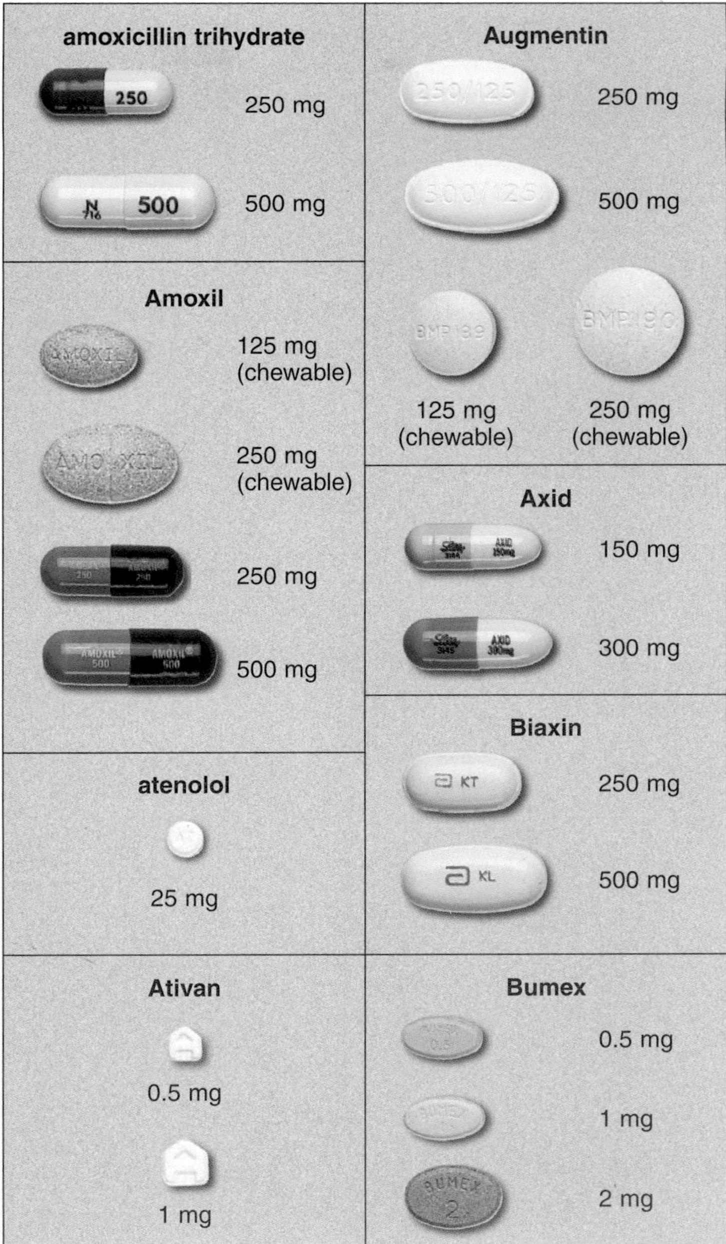
amoxicillin trihydrate
250 mg
500 mg
Amoxil
125 mg (chewable)
250 mg (chewable)
250 mg
500 mg
atenolol
25 mg
Ativan
0.5 mg
1 mg
Augmentin
250 mg
500 mg
125 mg (chewable)
250 mg (chewable)
Axid
150 mg
300 mg
Biaxin
250 mg
500 mg
Bumex
0.5 mg
1 mg
2 mg

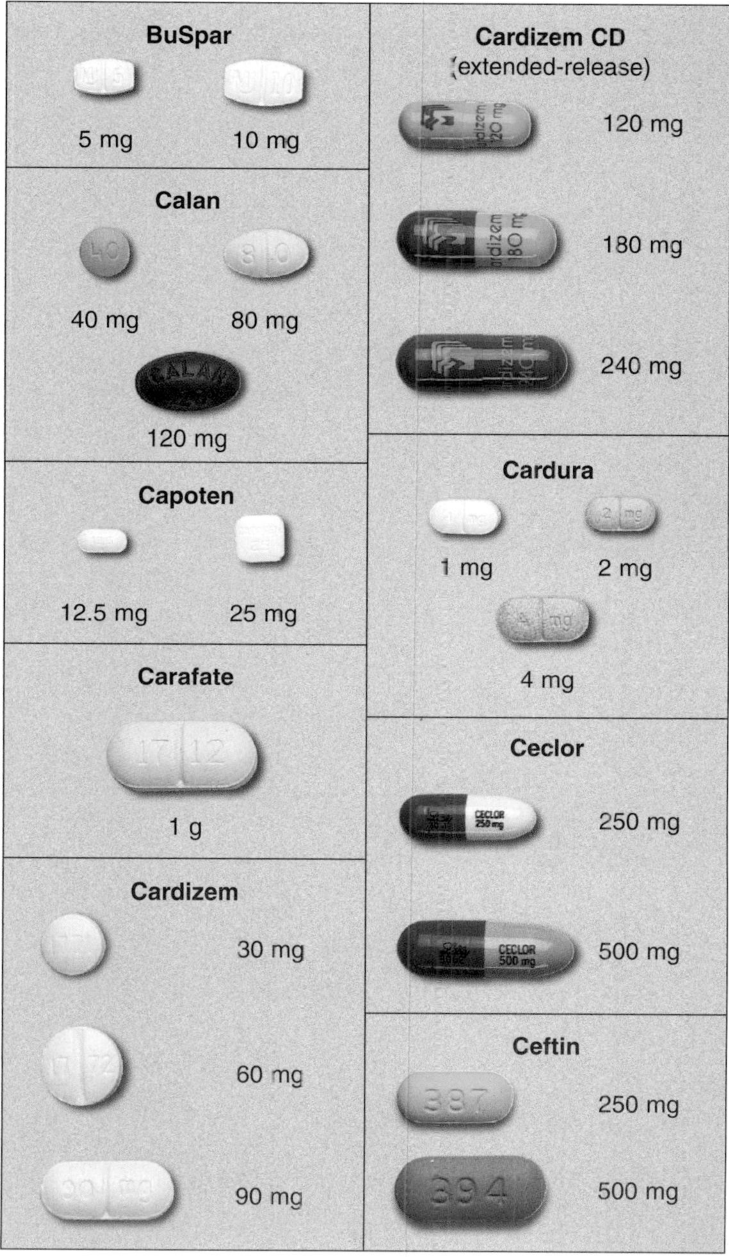
BuSpar
5 mg
10 mg
Calan
40 mg
80 mg
120 mg
Capoten
12.5 mg
25 mg
Carafate
1 g
Cardizem
30 mg
60 mg
90 mg
Cardizem CD
(extended-release)
120 mg
180 mg
240 mg
Cardura
1 mg
2 mg
4 mg
Ceclor
250 mg
500 mg
Ceftin
250 mg
500 mg

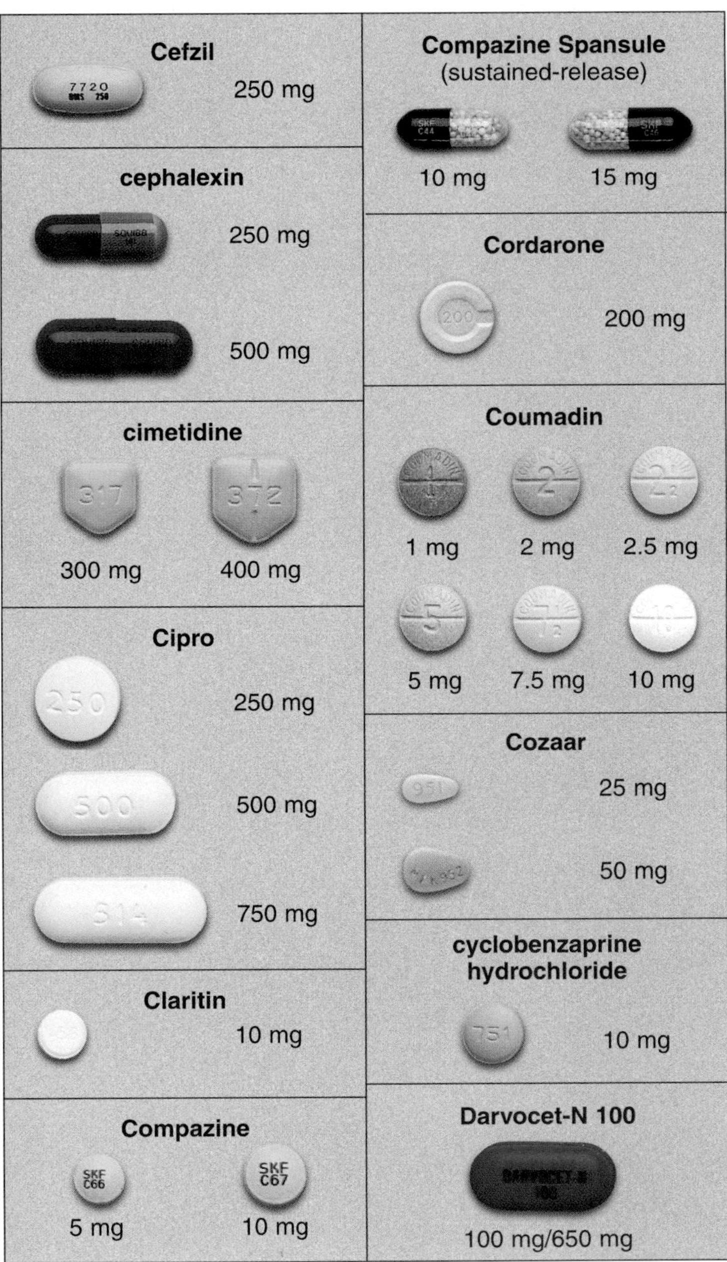
Cefzil
7720
BMS 750
250 mg
cephalexin
SQUIBB
250 mg
500 mg
cimetidine
317
372
300 mg
400 mg
Cipro
250
250 mg
500
500 mg
514
750 mg
Claritin
10 mg
Compazine
SKF
C66
SKF
C67
5 mg
10 mg
Compazine Spansule
(sustained-release)
SKF
C44
SKF
C46
10 mg
15 mg
Cordarone
200
200 mg
Coumadin
1 mg
2 mg
2.5 mg
5 mg
7.5 mg
10 mg
Cozaar
951
25 mg
50 mg
cyclobenzaprine
hydrochloride
751
10 mg
Darvocet-N 100
DARVOCET-N
100
100 mg/650 mg

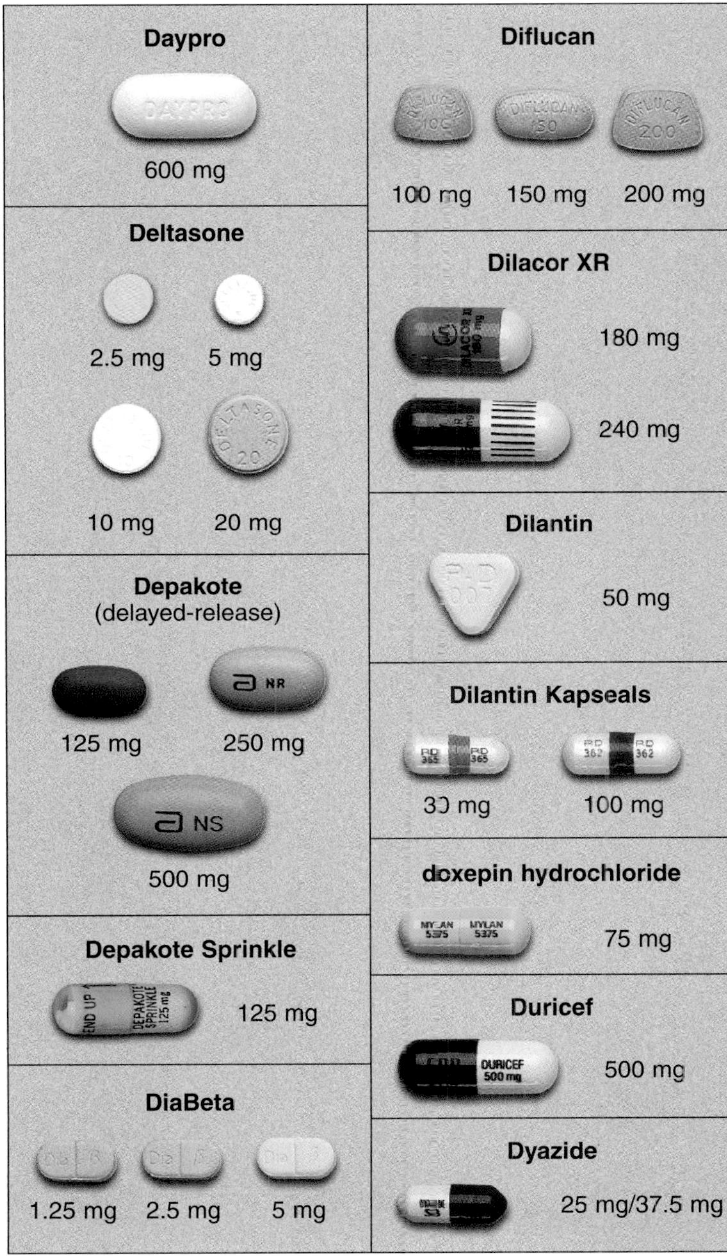
Daypro
600 mg
Deltasone
2.5 mg
5 mg
10 mg
20 mg
Depakote
(delayed-release)
125 mg
250 mg
500 mg
Depakote Sprinkle
125 mg
DiaBeta
1.25 mg
2.5 mg
5 mg
Diflucan
100 mg
150 mg
200 mg
Dilacor XR
180 mg
240 mg
Dilantin
50 mg
Dilantin Kapseals
30 mg
100 mg
doxepin hydrochloride
75 mg
Duricef
500 mg
Dyazide
25 mg/37.5 mg

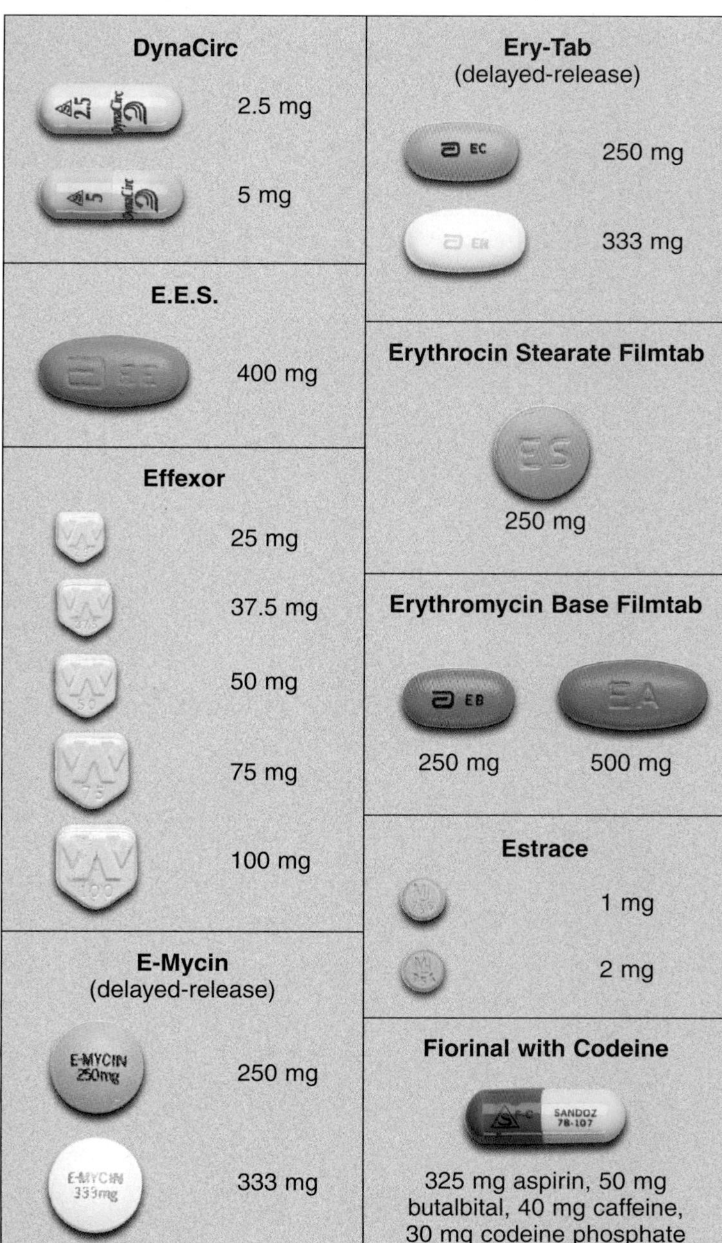
DynaCirc
2.5 mg
5 mg
E.E.S.
400 mg
Effexor
25 mg
37.5 mg
50 mg
75 mg
100 mg
E-Mycin
(delayed-release)
250 mg
333 mg
Ery-Tab
(delayed-release)
250 mg
333 mg
Erythrocin Stearate Filmtab
250 mg
Erythromycin Base Filmtab
250 mg
500 mg
Estrace
1 mg
2 mg
Fiorinal with Codeine
325 mg aspirin, 50 mg butalbital, 40 mg caffeine, 30 mg codeine phosphate

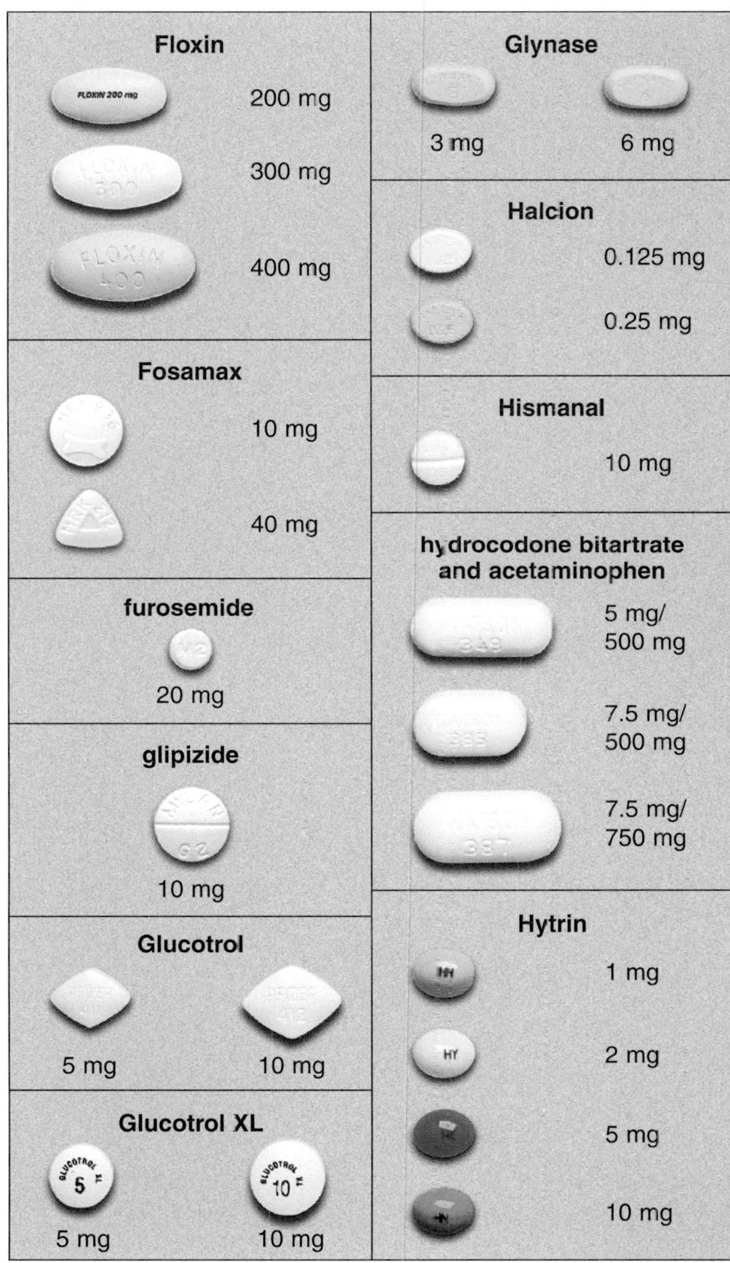
Floxin
200 mg
300 mg
400 mg
Fosamax
10 mg
40 mg
furosemide
20 mg
glipizide
10 mg
Glucotrol
5 mg
10 mg
Glucotrol XL
5 mg
10 mg
Glynase
3 mg
6 mg
Halcion
0.125 mg
0.25 mg
Hismanal
10 mg
hydrocodone bitartrate and acetaminophen
5 mg/ 500 mg
7.5 mg/ 500 mg
7.5 mg/ 750 mg
Hytrin
1 mg
2 mg
5 mg
10 mg

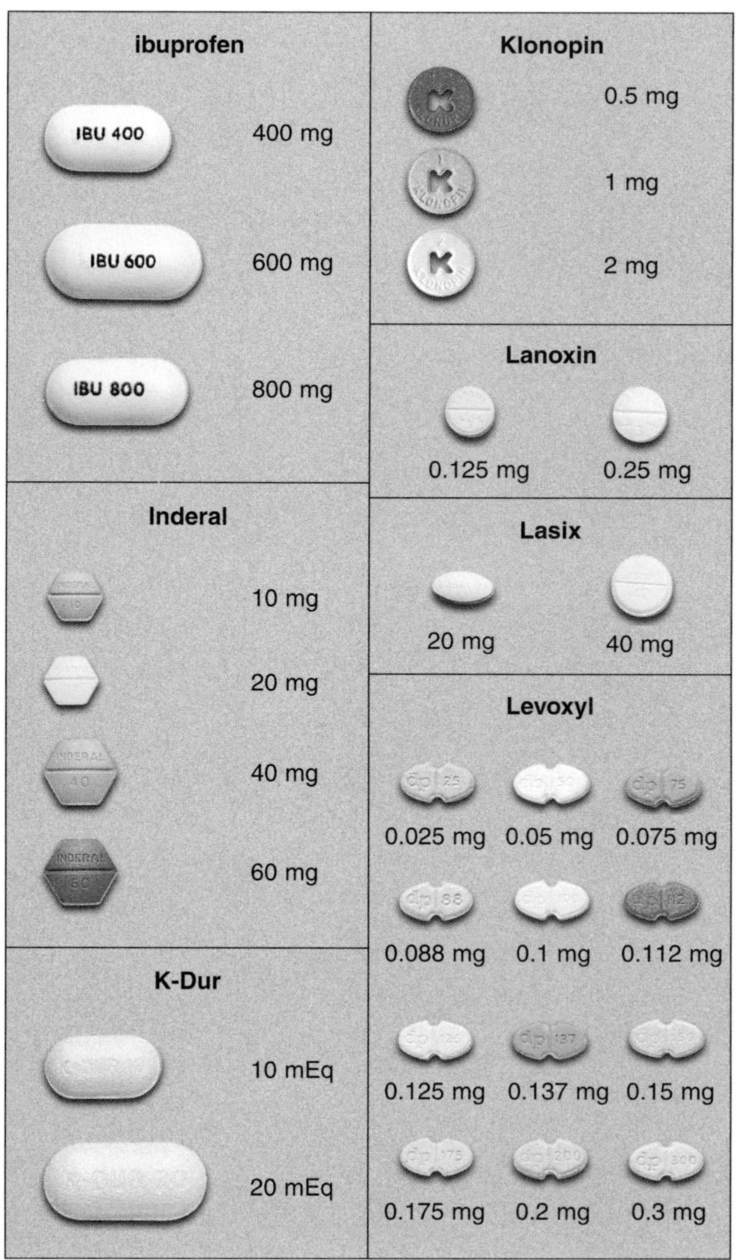
ibuprofen
IBU 400
400 mg
IBU 600
600 mg
IBU 800
800 mg
Klonopin
0.5 mg
1 mg
2 mg
Lanoxin
0.125 mg
0.25 mg
Lasix
20 mg
40 mg
Inderal
10 mg
20 mg
INDERAL 40
40 mg
INDERAL 60
60 mg
Levoxyl
0.025 mg
0.05 mg
0.075 mg
0.088 mg
0.1 mg
0.112 mg
0.125 mg
0.137 mg
0.15 mg
0.175 mg
0.2 mg
0.3 mg
K-Dur
10 mEq
20 mEq

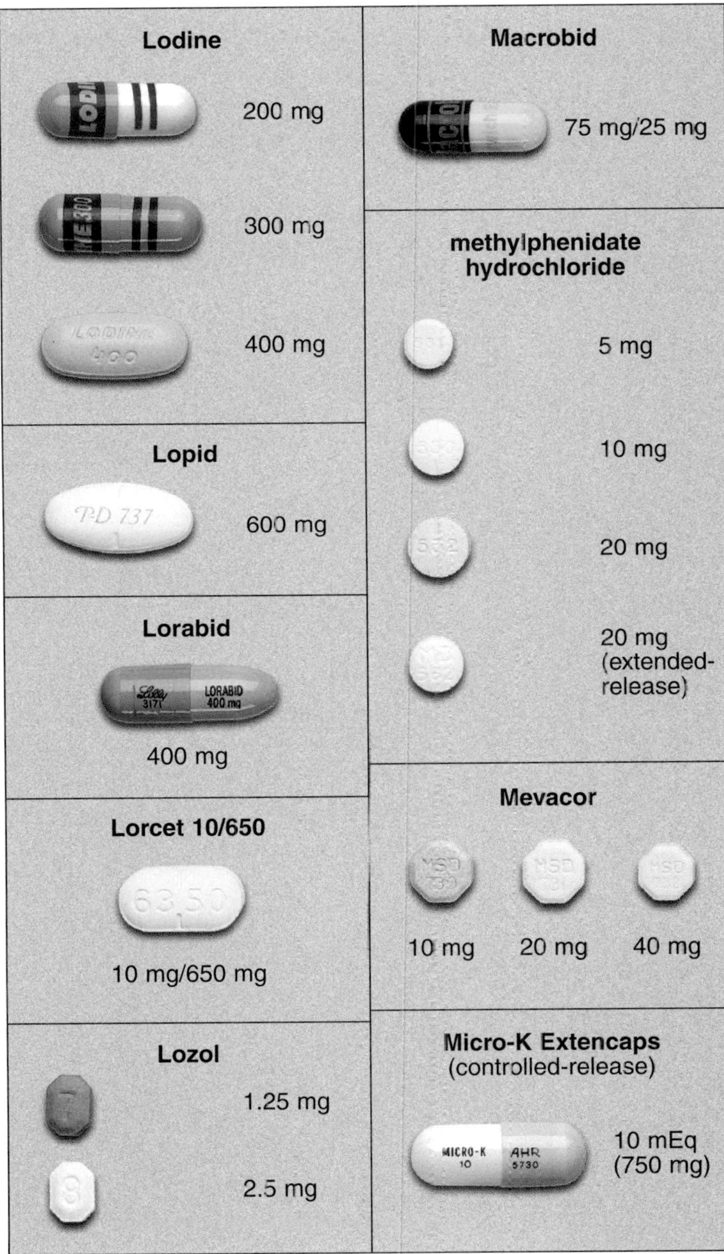
Lodine
200 mg
300 mg
400 mg
Lopid
P-D 737
600 mg
Lorabid
LORABID
400 mg
400 mg
Lorcet 10/650
10 mg/650 mg
Lozol
1.25 mg
2.5 mg
Macrobid
75 mg/25 mg
methylphenidate hydrochloride
5 mg
10 mg
20 mg
20 mg (extended-release)
Mevacor
10 mg
20 mg
40 mg
Micro-K Extencaps (controlled-release)
MICRO-K 10
AHR 5730
10 mEq (750 mg)

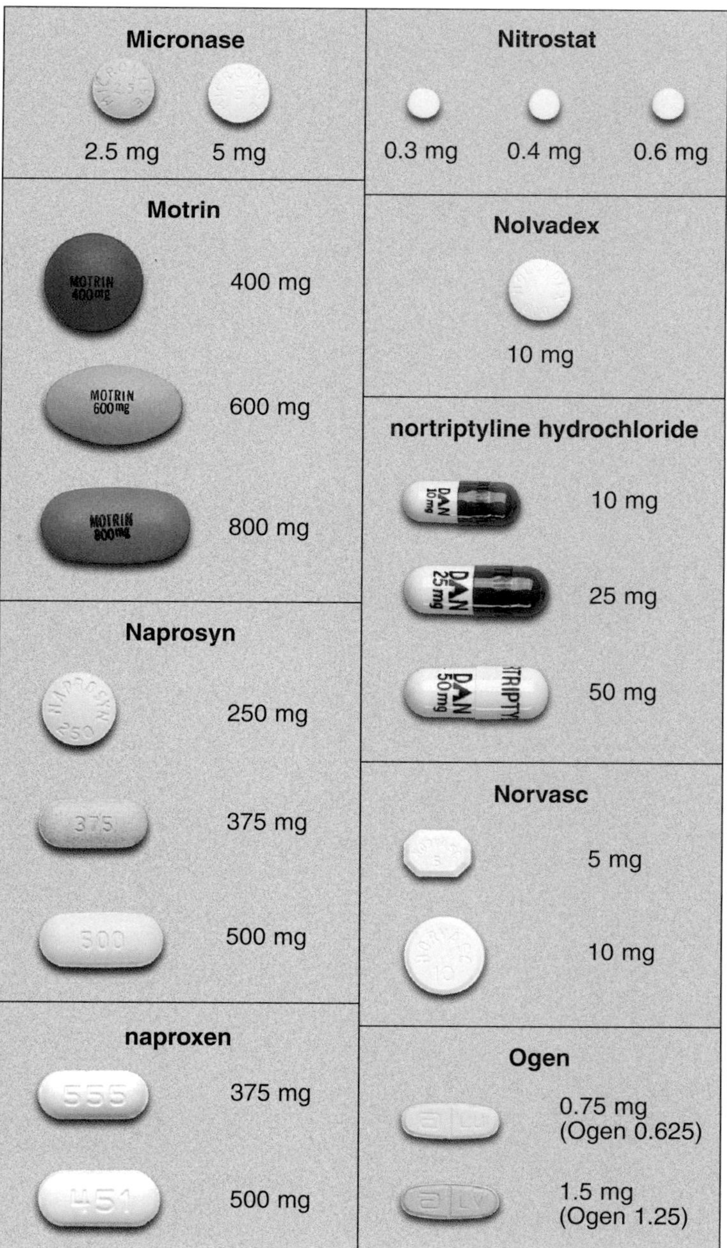
Micronase
2.5 mg
5 mg
Nitrostat
0.3 mg
0.4 mg
0.6 mg
Motrin
MOTRIN 400 mg
400 mg
MOTRIN 600 mg
600 mg
MOTRIN 800 mg
800 mg
Nolvadex
10 mg
nortriptyline hydrochloride
DAN 10 mg
10 mg
DAN 25 mg
25 mg
DAN 50 mg
50 mg
Naprosyn
NAPROSYN 250
250 mg
375
375 mg
500
500 mg
Norvasc
5 mg
10 mg
naproxen
555
375 mg
451
500 mg
Ogen
0.75 mg
(Ogen 0.625)
1.5 mg
(Ogen 1.25)

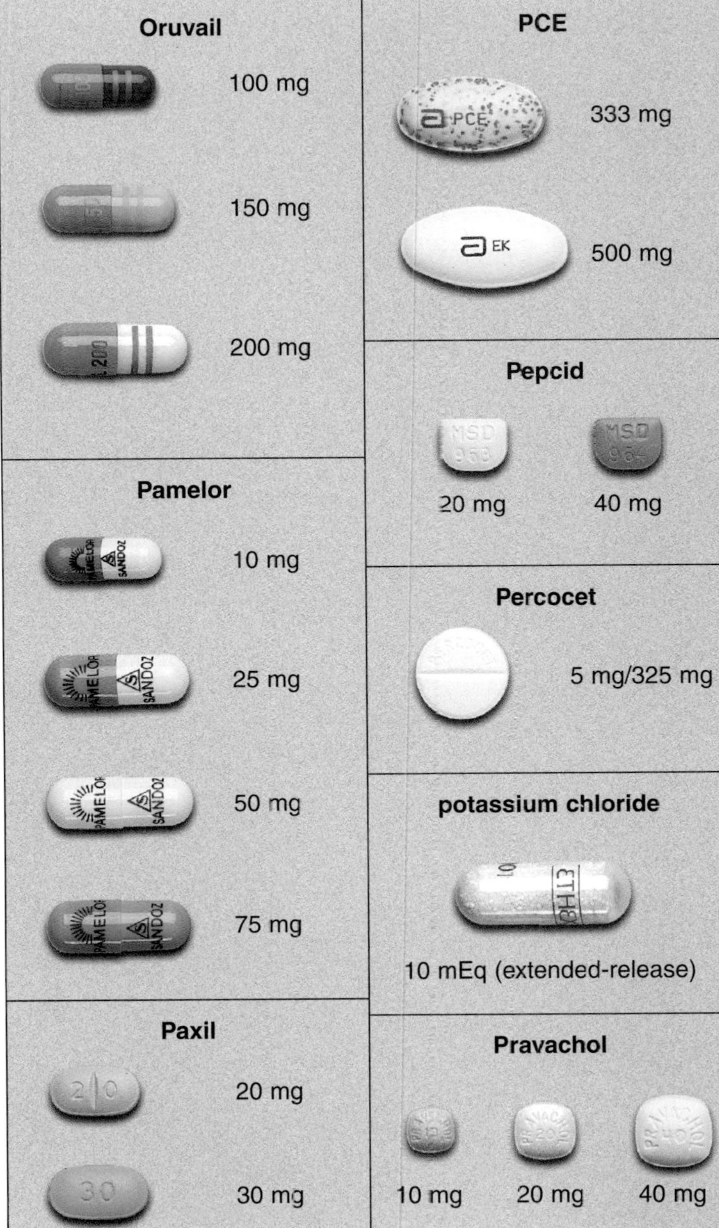
Oruvail
100 mg
150 mg
200 mg
Pamelor
10 mg
25 mg
50 mg
75 mg
Paxil
20 mg
30 mg
PCE
333 mg
500 mg
Pepcid
20 mg
40 mg
Percocet
5 mg/325 mg
potassium chloride
10 mEq (extended-release)
Pravachol
10 mg
20 mg
40 mg

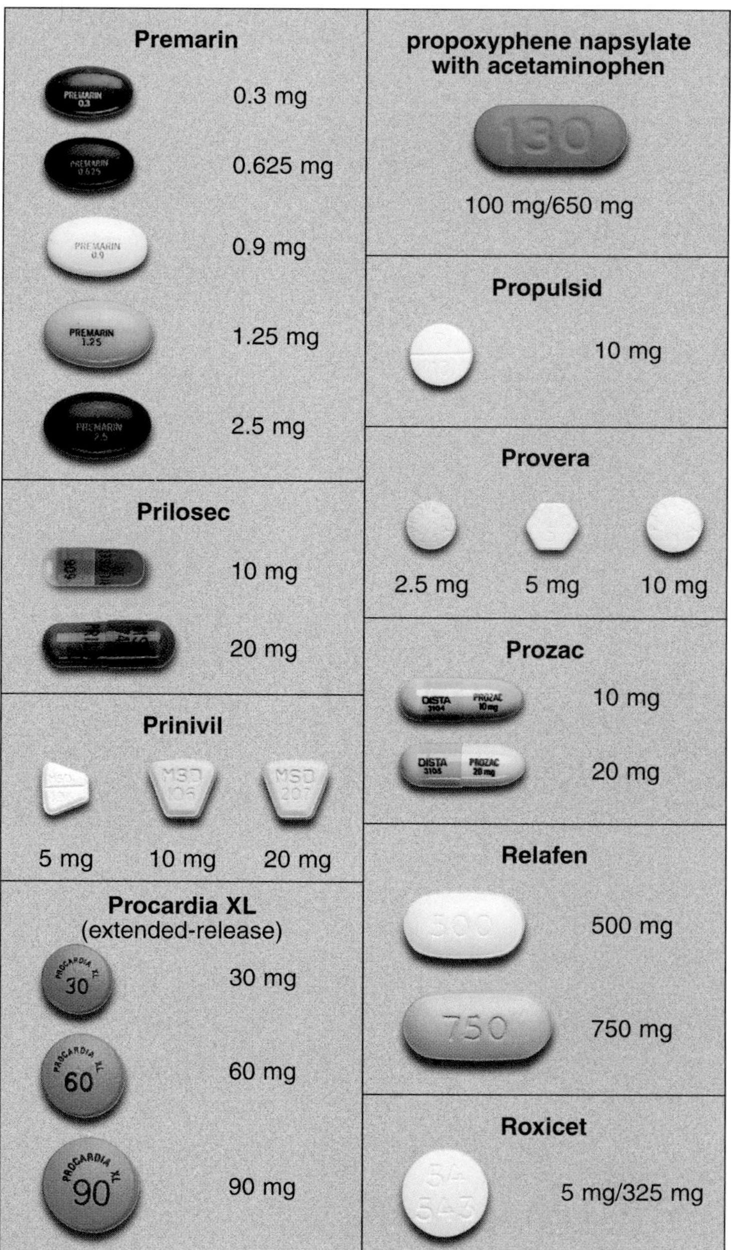
Premarin
0.3 mg
0.625 mg
0.9 mg
1.25 mg
2.5 mg
Prilosec
10 mg
20 mg
Prinivil
5 mg
10 mg
20 mg
Procardia XL
(extended-release)
30 mg
60 mg
90 mg
propoxyphene napsylate with acetaminophen
100 mg/650 mg
Propulsid
10 mg
Provera
2.5 mg
5 mg
10 mg
Prozac
10 mg
20 mg
Relafen
500 mg
750 mg
Roxicet
5 mg/325 mg

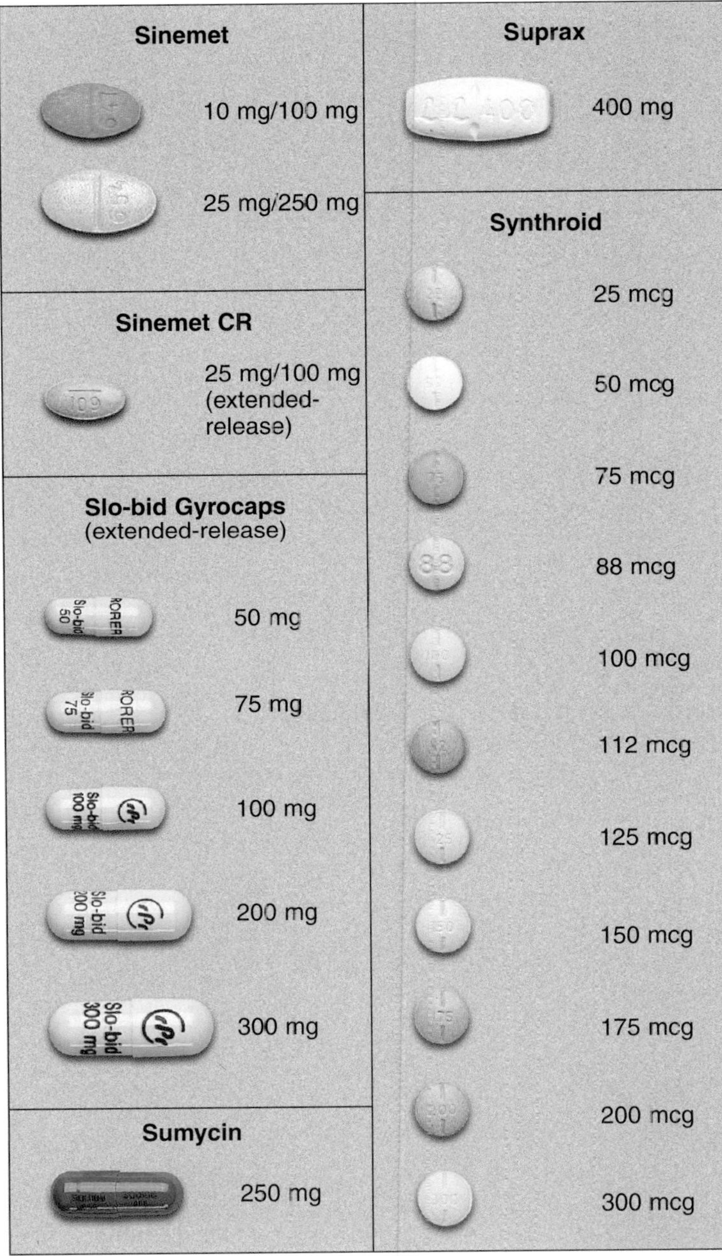
Sinemet
10 mg/100 mg
25 mg/250 mg
Sinemet CR
25 mg/100 mg (extended-release)
Slo-bid Gyrocaps
(extended-release)
50 mg
75 mg
100 mg
200 mg
300 mg
Sumycin
250 mg
Suprax
400 mg
Synthroid
25 mcg
50 mcg
75 mcg
88 mcg
100 mcg
112 mcg
125 mcg
150 mcg
175 mcg
200 mcg
300 mcg

Tagamet

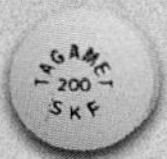

200 mg

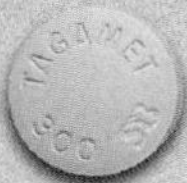

300 mg

Tenormin

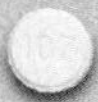

25 mg

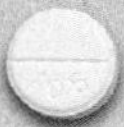

50 mg

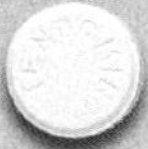

100 mg

Theo-Dur
(extended-release)

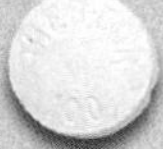

100 mg

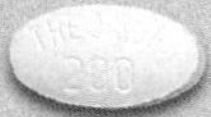

200 mg

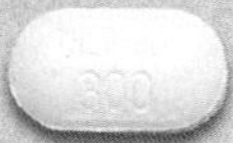

300 mg

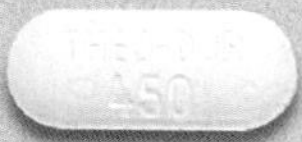

450 mg

Ticlid

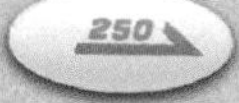

250 mg

Toprol XL

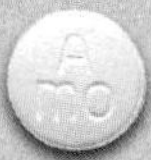

50 mg

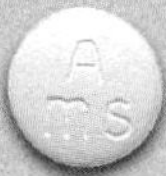

100 mg

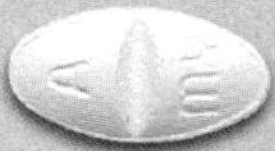

200 mg

Toradol

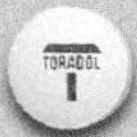

10 mg

Trental

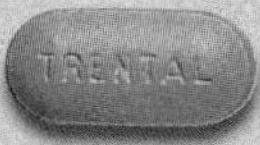

400 mg

Trimox

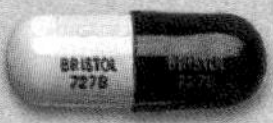

250 mg

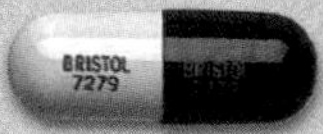

500 mg

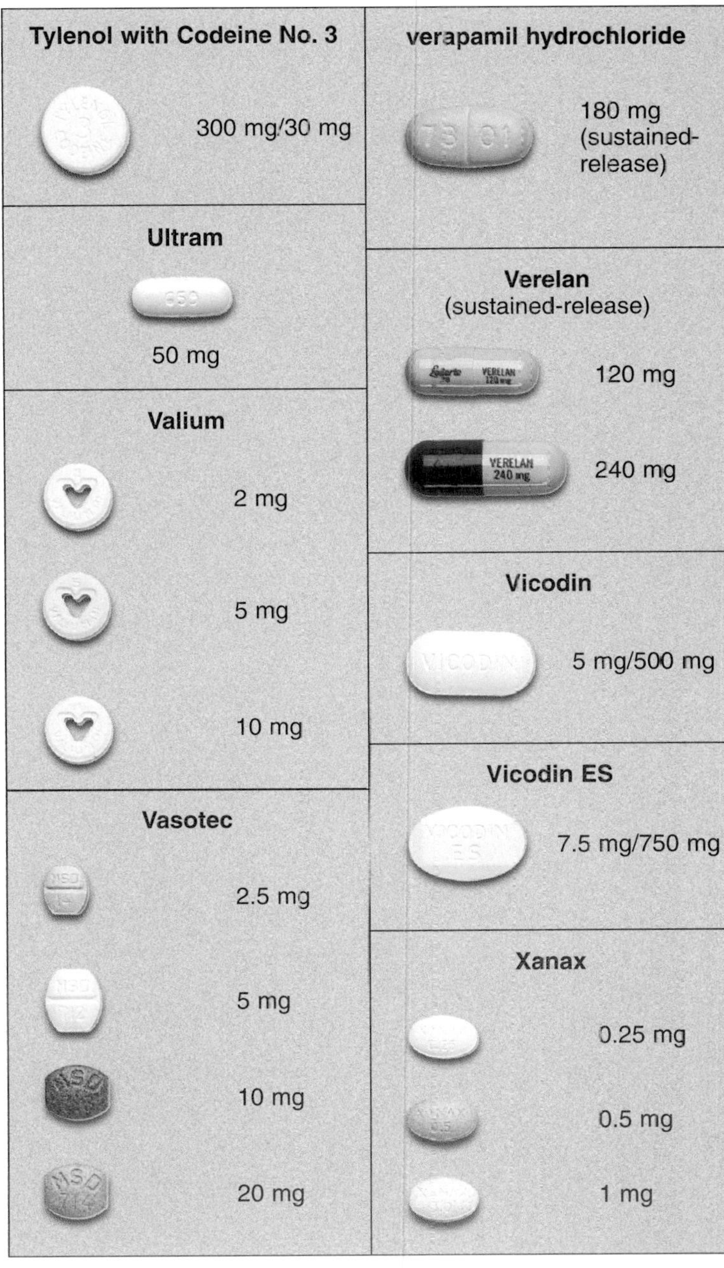
Tylenol with Codeine No. 3
300 mg/30 mg
Ultram
50 mg
Valium
2 mg
5 mg
10 mg
Vasotec
2.5 mg
5 mg
10 mg
20 mg
verapamil hydrochloride
180 mg (sustained-release)
Verelan
(sustained-release)
120 mg
240 mg
Vicodin
5 mg/500 mg
Vicodin ES
7.5 mg/750 mg
Xanax
0.25 mg
0.5 mg
1 mg

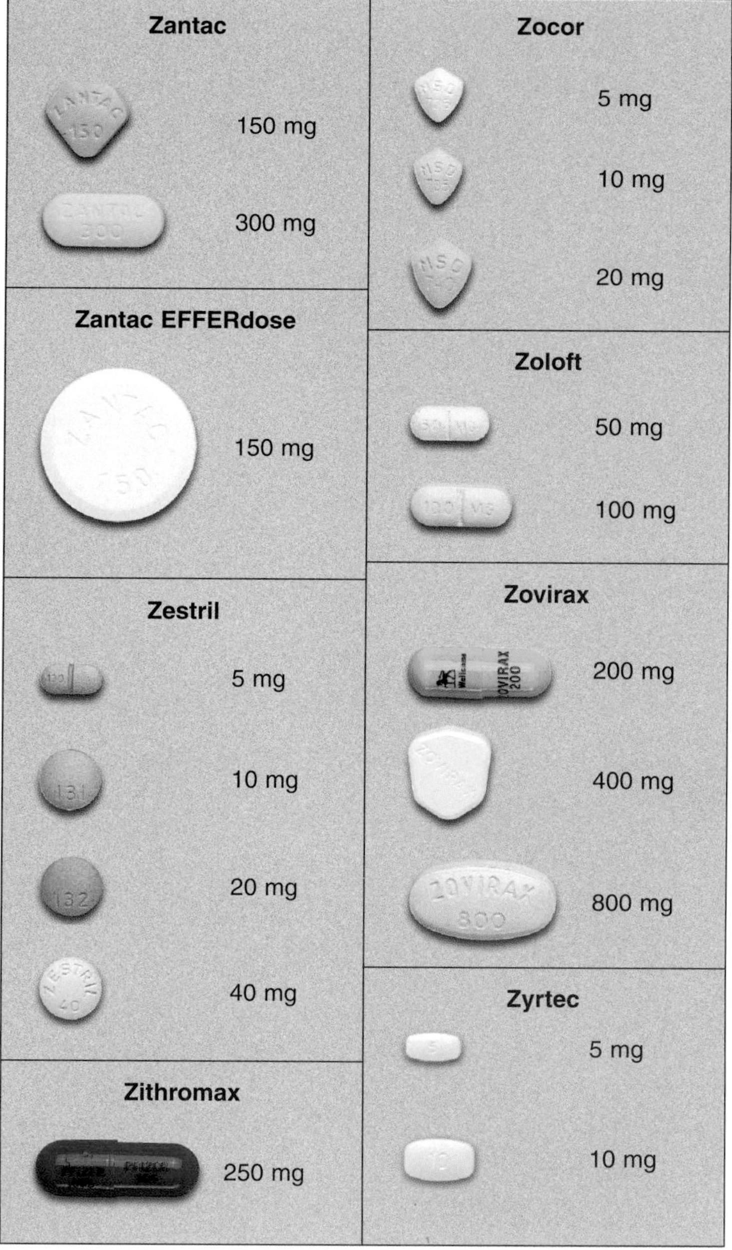
Zantac
150 mg
300 mg
Zantac EFFERdose
150 mg
Zestril
5 mg
10 mg
20 mg
40 mg
Zithromax
250 mg
Zocor
5 mg
10 mg
20 mg
Zoloft
50 mg
100 mg
Zovirax
200 mg
400 mg
800 mg
Zyrtec
5 mg
10 mg

Interactions

Concomitant use with *amantadine, benztropine, procyclidine*, or *trihexyphenidyl* may increase the efficacy of levodopa. *Bromocriptine* may produce additive effects, allowing reduced levodopa dosage.

Anesthetics or hydrocarbon inhalation may cause arrhythmias because of increased endogenous dopamine concentration. (Levodopa-carbidopa should be discontinued 6 to 8 hours before administration of anesthetics such as halothane.)

Antacids containing calcium, magnesium, or sodium bicarbonate may increase absorption of levodopa.

Concurrent use of *anticonvulsants (hydantoin), benzodiazepines, droperidol, haloperidol, loxapine, metyrosine, papaverine, phenothiazines, rauwolfia alkaloids*, and *thioxanthenes* may decrease therapeutic effects of levodopa.

Concomitant use with *antihypertensives* may increase the hypotensive effect.

Methyldopa may alter the antiparkinsonian effects of levodopa and may produce additive toxic CNS effects. *Molindone* may inhibit antiparkinsonian effects of levodopa by blocking dopamine receptors in the brain.

Concurrent use of *MAO inhibitors* may cause a hypertensive crisis. Discontinue MAO inhibitors for 2 to 4 weeks before starting levodopa-carbidopa.

Sympathomimetics may increase risk of arrhythmias (reduced dosage of the sympathomimetic is recommended; however, administration of carbidopa with levodopa reduces the tendency of sympathomimetics to cause dopamine-induced arrhythmias).

Effects on diagnostic tests

Antiglobulin determinations (Coombs' test) are occasionally positive after long-term use. Thyroid function determinations may inhibit thyroid-stimulating hormone response to protirelin.

Levodopa-carbidopa therapy may elevate serum gonadotropin levels. Serum and urine uric acid determinations may show false elevations.

Urine glucose determinations using copper reduction method may show false-positive results; with the glucose oxidase method, false-negative results. Urine ketone determination using dip-stick method, urine norepinephrine determinations, and urine protein determinations using Lowery test may show false-positive results.

Systemic effects of drug may elevate levels of BUN, ALT, AST, alkaline phosphatase, serum bilirubin, LD, and serum protein-bound iodine.

Adverse reactions

CNS: *choreiform, dystonic, dyskinetic movements; involuntary grimacing, head movements, myoclonic body jerks, ataxia,* tremor, muscle twitching; bradykinetic episodes; psychiatric disturbances, anxiety, disturbing dreams, euphoria, malaise, fatigue; severe depression, ***suicidal tendencies,*** dementia, delirium, hallucinations (may necessitate reduction or withdrawal of drug), confusion, insomnia, agitation.

CV: *orthostatic hypotension,* ***cardiac irregularities,*** phlebitis.

EENT: blepharospasm, blurred vision, diplopia, mydriasis or miosis, oculogyric crises, excessive salivation.

GI: *dry mouth,* bitter taste, *nausea, vomiting, anorexia,* weight loss may occur at start of therapy; constipation; flatulence; diarrhea; abdominal pain.

GU: urinary frequency, urine retention, urinary incontinence, darkened urine, priapism.

Hematologic: ***hemolytic anemia, thrombocytopenia, leukopenia, agranulocytosis.***

Hepatic: ***hepatotoxicity.***

Other: dark perspiration, hyperventilation, hiccups.

Overdose and treatment

There have been no reports of overdosage with carbidopa. Clinical manifestations of levodopa overdose are irregular heartbeat and palpitations, severe continuous nausea and vomiting, spasm or closing of eyelids.

Treatment of overdose includes immediate gastric lavage and antiarrhythmic medication if necessary. Pyridoxine is not effective in reversing the actions of carbidopa and levodopa combinations.

☑ Special considerations

- Carefully monitor patient also receiving antihypertensive or hypoglycemic agents. Discontinue MAO inhibitors at least 2 weeks before therapy begins.
- Adjust dosage based on patient's response and tolerance to drug. Therapeutic and adverse reactions occur more rapidly with levodopa-carbidopa combination than with levodopa alone. Observe and monitor vital signs, especially while dosage is being adjusted.
- Muscle twitching and blepharospasm (twitching of eyelids) may be an early sign of overdose.
- Test patients on long-term therapy regularly for diabetes and acromegaly; periodically repeat blood test and liver and kidney function studies.
- If patient is being treated with levodopa, discontinue at least 8 hours before starting levodopa-carbidopa.
- The combination drug usually reduces the amount of levodopa needed by 75%, thereby reducing the incidence of adverse reactions.
- Pyridoxine (vitamin B_6) does not reverse beneficial effects of levodopa-carbidopa. Multivitamins can be taken without fear of losing control of symptoms.
- If therapy is interrupted temporarily, usual daily dosage may be given as soon as patient resumes oral medications.
- Maximum effectiveness of drug may not occur for several weeks or months after therapy begins.
- Sustained-release tablets may be split, never crushed or chewed.

Patient education

- Instruct patient to report adverse reactions and therapeutic effects.
- Warn patient of possible dizziness or orthostatic hypotension, especially at start of therapy. Tell patient to change position slowly and dangle legs before getting out of bed. Elastic stockings may be helpful in some patients.

• Tell patient to take food shortly after taking drug to relieve gastric irritation.
• Inform patient that drug may cause urine or sweat to darken.
• Tell patient to take a missed dose as soon as possible, to skip a missed dose if next scheduled dose is within 2 hours, and never to double-dose.

Geriatric use
• In elderly patients, smaller doses may be required because of reduced tolerance to the effects of levodopa-carbidopa. Elderly patients, especially those with osteoporosis, should resume normal activity gradually because increased mobility may increase the risk of fractures.
• Elderly patients are especially vulnerable to CNS adverse effects, such as anxiety, confusion, or nervousness; those with preexisting heart disease are more susceptible to cardiac effects.

Pediatric use
• Safe use of drug in children under age 18 has not been established.

Breast-feeding
• Because levodopa may inhibit lactation, do not use drug in breast-feeding women.

levofloxacin
Levaquin

Pharmacologic classification: fluoroquinolone
Therapeutic classification: broad-spectrum antibiotic
Pregnancy risk category C

How supplied
Tablets: 250, 500 mg
Single-use vials: 500 mg
Infusion (premixed): 250 mg in 50 ml D_5W, 500 mg in 100 ml D_5W

Indications, route, and dosage
***Acute maxillary sinusitis caused by susceptible strains of* Streptococcus pneumoniae, Moraxella catarrhalis, *or* Haemophilus influenzae**
Adults: 500 mg P.O. or I.V. daily for 10 to 14 days.
***Acute bacterial exacerbation of chronic bronchitis caused by* Staphylococcus aureus, S. pneumoniae, M. catarrhalis, H. influenzae, *or* H. parainfluenzae**
Adults: 500 mg P.O. or I.V. daily for 7 days.
Community-acquired pneumonia caused by* S. aureus, S. pneumoniae, M. catarrhalis, H. influenzae, H. parainfluenzae, Klebsiella pneumoniae, Chlamydia pneumoniae, Legionella pneumophila, *or Mycoplasma pneumoniae
Adults: 500 mg P.O. or I.V. daily for 7 to 14 days.
***Uncomplicated skin and skin structure infections (mild to moderate) caused by* S. aureus or Streptococcus pyogenes**
Adults: 500 mg P.O. or I.V. daily for 7 to 10 days.
✦ ***Dosage adjustment.*** If creatinine clearance is 20 to 49 ml/minute, subsequent dosages are half the initial dose. If creatinine clearance is 10 to 19 ml/minute, subsequent dosages are half the initial dose and the interval is prolonged to q 48 hours.
***Complicated urinary tract infections (mild to moderate) caused by* Enterococcus faecalis, Enterobacter cloacae, Escherichia coli, K. pneumoniae, Proteus mirabilis, *or* Pseudomonas aeruginosa**
Adults: 250 mg P.O. or I.V. daily for 10 days.
***Acute pyelonephritis (mild to moderate) caused by* E. coli**
Adults: 250 mg P.O. or I.V. daily for 10 days.
✦ ***Dosage adjustment.*** If creatinine clearance is 10 to 19 ml/minute, dosage interval is increased to q 48 hours.

Pharmacodynamics
Antibactericidal action: Drug inhibits bacterial DNA gyrase, an enzyme required for DNA replication, transcription, repair, and recombination in susceptible bacteria.

Pharmacokinetics
• *Absorption:* The plasma concentration after I.V. administration is comparable to that observed for equivalent oral doses (on a mg/mg basis). Therefore, oral and I.V. routes can be considered interchangeable. Plasma levels peak within 1 to 2 hours after oral dosing. Steady state is reached within 48 hours on a 500 mg/day regimen.
• *Distribution:* Mean volume of distribution ranges from 89 to 112 L after single and multiple 500-mg doses, indicating widespread distribution into body tissues. Drug also penetrates well into lung tissues; lung tissue levels were generally two- to five-fold higher than plasma concentrations.
• *Metabolism:* Drug undergoes limited metabolism in humans. The only identified metabolites are the desmethyl and N-oxide metabolites, which have little relevant pharmacologic activity.
• *Excretion:* Primarily excreted unchanged in the urine. Mean terminal half-life is approximately 6 to 8 hours.

Contraindications and precautions
Contraindicated in patients with hypersensitivity to drug, its components, or quinolone antimicrobials. Safety and efficacy of levofloxacin in children, adolescents (under age 18), and pregnant and breast-feeding women have not been established.

Use cautiously in patients with history of seizure disorders or other CNS diseases, such as cerebral arteriosclerosis, because quinolones can cause CNS stimulation and increased intracranial pressure, which may lead to seizures (lowered seizure threshold), toxic psychoses, tremors, restlessness, anxiety, light-headedness, confusion, hallucinations, paranoia, depression, nightmares, insomnia and, rarely, suicidal thoughts or acts. These can occur after the first dose.

Interactions
Antacids containing aluminum or magnesium, iron salts, products containing zinc, and *sucralfate* may

interfere with GI absorption of levofloxacin. Administer at least 2 hours apart. *Antidiabetic agents* may alter blood glucose levels. Monitor glucose levels closely. *NSAIDs* may increase CNS stimulation. Monitor for seizure activity.

Warfarin and derivatives may cause increased effect of oral anticoagulant with some fluoroquinolones. Monitor PT and INR. *Theophylline* coadministration may result in decreased clearance of theophylline. Monitor theophylline levels.

Effects on diagnostic tests
Levofloxacin may cause abnormal EEG and a decreased glucose level and lymphocyte count.

Adverse reactions
CNS: headache, insomnia, dizziness, encephalopathy, paresthesia, ***seizures.***
CV: chest pain, palpitations, vasodilation.
GI: nausea, diarrhea, constipation, vomiting, abdominal pain, dyspepsia, flatulence, ***pseudomembranous colitis.***
GU: vaginitis.
Hematologic: eosinophilia, hemolytic anemia.
Musculoskeletal: back pain, tendon rupture.
Respiratory: allergic pneumonitis.
Skin: rash, photosensitivity, pruritus, erythema multiforme, ***Stevens-Johnson syndrome.***
Other: pain, ***hypersensitivity reactions,*** injection site reaction, ***anaphylaxis, multisystem organ failure.***

Overdose and treatment
No information available. If acute overdosage occurs, empty the stomach, maintain hydration, and observe. Drug is not effectively removed by hemodialysis or peritoneal dialysis.

☑ Special considerations
- If patient experiences symptoms of excessive CNS stimulation (restlessness, tremor, confusion, hallucinations), discontinue medication. Institute seizure precautions.
- Ruptures of tendons and tendonitis have occurred with quinolone therapy. Discontinue drug if pain, inflammation, or rupture of a tendon occurs. These ruptures can occur after therapy has been stopped.
- Because a rapid or bolus administration may result in hypotension, I.V. levofloxacin should only be administered by slow infusion over 60 minutes.
- Avoid excessive exposure to sunlight.

Patient education
- Tell patient to take drug as prescribed, even if symptoms disappear.
- Advise patient to take drug with plenty of fluids and to avoid antacids, sucralfate, and products containing iron or zinc for at least 2 hours before and after each dose.
- Warn patient to avoid hazardous tasks until adverse CNS effects of drug are known.
- Advise patient to use sunblock and wear protective clothing when exposed to excessive sunlight.
- Tell patient to stop drug and call if rash or other signs of hypersensitivity develop.
- Tell patient to report pain or inflammation.
- Tell diabetic patient to monitor blood glucose levels and report if a hypoglycemic reaction occurs.

Geriatric use
- Dosage adjustment based on age alone is not necessary.

Pediatric use
- Safety and effectiveness in children below age 18 have not been established.

Breast-feeding
- Drug has not been measured in breast milk. Based on data from ofloxacin, it can be presumed that levofloxacin will be excreted in breast milk. Because of potential for serious adverse reactions in breast-fed infants, a decision should be made whether to discontinue breast-feeding or drug.

levomethadyl acetate hydrochloride
Orlaam

Pharmacologic classification: synthetic diphenylheptane derivative
Therapeutic classification: opiate agonist
Controlled substance schedule II
Pregnancy risk category C

How supplied
Available by prescription only
Oral solution: 10 mg/ml

Indications, route, and dosage
Management of opiate dependence
Adults: Dosage is highly individualized. Initially, 20 to 40 mg P.O. Each subsequent dose, administered at 48- to 72-hour intervals, may be adjusted in increments of 5 to 10 mg until steady state is reached, usually within 1 to 2 weeks. Most patients are stable on 60 to 90 mg P.O. three times weekly. Maximum dosage is 140 mg three times weekly.

Pharmacodynamics
Opiate agonist action: Levomethadyl is a synthetic opiate agonist structurally similar to methadone. It suppresses symptoms of withdrawal in opiate-dependent individuals by cross-substituting for opiate agonists of the morphine type. Long-term administration may produce sufficient tolerance to block the euphoric effects of opiate agonists.

Pharmacokinetics
- *Absorption:* Onset of action occurs in 2 to 4 hours and has a duration of 48 to 72 hours, which permits administration three times weekly.
- *Distribution:* About 80% of drug is bound to plasma proteins, primarily an alpha-globulin. Evidence suggests that persistence of plasma levels may be related in part to binding to tissue proteins.
- *Metabolism:* Drug undergoes first-pass metabolism to its demethylated metabolite nor-LAAM, which is sequentially N-demethylated to dinor-LAAM. These metabolites also are opioid agonists and are more potent than parent drug.

• *Excretion:* Drug is excreted in urine, primarily as metabolites.

Contraindications and precautions
Contraindicated in patients hypersensitive to drug. Use cautiously in patients with cardiac conduction disorders or with hepatic or renal failure.

Interactions
Carbamazepine, phenobarbital, phenytoin, and *rifampin* increase hepatic enzyme activity, which may increase levomethadyl's peak activity or shorten its duration of action. Monitor patient closely for withdrawal symptoms.

Cimetidine, erythromycin, and *ketoconazole* inhibit hepatic enzyme activity, which may decrease levomethadyl's peak activity or prolong its duration of action. Patients should be monitored closely.

Narcotic antagonists (such as *naloxone*) and *agonist-antagonists* (such as *pentazocine*) may precipitate abstinence syndrome. Don't use together. In addition, such agonists as *meperidine* and *propoxyphene* should not be used in patients taking levomethadyl; to be effective, these agonists would have to be given in such high doses that the risk of toxic effects would be unacceptable.

Effects on diagnostic tests
None reported.

Adverse reactions
CNS: drowsiness, sedation, anxiety, abnormal dreams, insomnia, nervousness.
CV: bradycardia, edema, prolonged QT interval.
EENT: blurred vision, rhinitis.
GI: *abdominal pain, diarrhea, constipation, dry mouth, nausea, vomiting.*
GU: *impotence, difficulty with ejaculation.*
Respiratory: *cough.*
Skin: *rash, diaphoresis.*
Other: yawning, arthralgia, asthenia, back pain, chills, flulike syndrome, malaise, abstinence syndrome with sudden withdrawal.

Overdose and treatment
In the event of an overdose, naloxone should be used to reverse the effects of levomethadyl. This antagonist must be used carefully because of the potential for severe withdrawal effects. Because drug's duration is much longer than that of naloxone, repeated dosing with or continuous I.V. infusion of naloxone is likely to be required.

☑ Special considerations
• Drug should only be used by licensed and approved clinics. There are no recognized clinical uses for drug outside of addiction treatment programs. Drug may be dispensed only by treatment programs approved by the FDA, DEA, and designated state authority. By law, take-home doses of drug are forbidden.
• Do not administer drug on a daily basis because of risk of fatal overdose.
• When used to replace methadone, recommended initial dose is 1.2 to 1.3 times the daily methadone dose, three times weekly. Initial dose should not exceed 120 mg. Adjust dosage based on clinical response. The crossover to methadone should be done in a single dose rather than decreasing doses of methadone and increasing doses of levomethadyl.
• Always dilute drug before administration and mix with diluent before dispensing.
• Most patients can tolerate the 72-hour interval between weekly regimens. If withdrawal is a problem during this interval, increase the preceding dose or switch to an every-other-day schedule. Never give drug on 2 consecutive days; instead, give small supplemental doses of methadone. Consider risk of drug diversion before giving patient take-home methadone.
• If patient is of childbearing age, monthly pregnancy tests are recommended. Switch patient to methadone if pregnancy occurs.

Patient education
• Inform patient that drug is intended for use as part of a comprehensive treatment plan that also includes appropriate medical evaluation, treatment planning, and counseling. Tell patient the therapeutic goal is to reduce illicit opioid use early in treatment and that drug is comparable to treatment with methadone in attaining this goal.
• Warn patient that drug can cause CNS effects and impair mental and physical abilities required for such potentially hazardous tasks as driving a car or operating machinery.
• Stress importance of avoiding other CNS depressants, including alcohol, because interactions may result in serious, even fatal, complications.
• Explain importance of compliance with dosage regimen. Tell patient that daily administration would risk excessive accumulation and overdosage.
• Inform patient that tolerance and physical dependence will develop with repeated administration.
• Tell patient that because of drug's slow onset of action, full effects of drug will not occur for at least several days.

Pediatric use
• Use in children under age 18 is not recommended.

Breast-feeding
• Use of drug in breast-feeding women is not recommended.

levonorgestrel implants
Norplant System

Pharmacologic classification: progestin
Therapeutic classification: contraceptive
Pregnancy risk category X

How supplied
Available by prescription only
Implants: 36 mg in each of 6 silastic capsules; kits also include trocar, scalpel, forceps, syringe, two needles, package of skin closures, three packages of gauze sponges, stretch bandages, and surgical drape

Indications, route, and dosage

Long-term (up to 5 years), reversible prevention of pregnancy

Adults: Six silastic capsules containing 36 mg each for a total of 216 mg are surgically implanted in the superficial plane beneath the skin of a woman's upper arm.

Pharmacodynamics

Contraceptive action: Levonorgestrel is a synthetic, biologically active progestin, exhibiting no significant estrogenic activity. A continuous low dose of levonorgestrel is diffused through the wall of each capsule. Pregnancy is prevented by at least two mechanisms: inhibition of ovulation and thickening of the cervical mucus.

Pharmacokinetics

- *Absorption:* Maximum or near maximum concentrations are reached within 24 hours of implantation. Drug is 100% bioavailable. Plasma concentrations average 0.3 ng/ml over 5 years but are highly variable as a function of individual metabolism and body weight.
- *Distribution:* Drug is bound by the circulating protein sex hormone-binding globulin (SHBG).
- *Metabolism:* Metabolized by the liver.
- *Excretion:* Metabolites are excreted in the urine.

Contraindications and precautions

Contraindicated in patients with active thrombophlebitis or thromboembolic disorders, undiagnosed abnormal genital bleeding, acute liver disease, malignant or benign liver tumors, known or suspected breast cancer and in known or suspected pregnancy, history of idiopathic intracranial hypertension, and hypersensitivity to levonorgestrel or components of the Norplant System.

Use cautiously in diabetic and prediabetic patients and in those with history of depression or hyperlipidemia.

Interactions

Use in women taking *carbamazepine* or *phenytoin* results in reduced efficacy of levonorgestrel, which increases risk of pregnancy.

Effects on diagnostic tests

Decreased SHBG and thyroxine concentrations and increased T_3 uptake have been reported.

Adverse reactions

CNS: headache, nervousness, dizziness, depression, tingling, numbness.
GI: nausea, *abdominal discomfort*, appetite change.
GU: *amenorrhea, many days of bleeding or prolonged bleeding, spotting, irregular onset of bleeding, frequent onset of bleeding, scanty bleeding, cervicitis, vaginitis, leukorrhea.*
Skin: dermatitis, acne, hirsutism, hypertrichosis, alopecia; infection, transient pain, itching (at implant site).
Other: adnexal enlargement, mastalgia, weight gain, *musculoskeletal pain, removal difficulty, breast discharge.*

Overdose and treatment

Overdose can occur if more than six silastic capsules are in situ, resulting in fluid retention with its associated effects and uterine bleeding irregularities. All previously implanted capsules should be removed before insertion of a new set.

☑ Special considerations

- The total implanted dose is 216 mg. Implantation of all six capsules should be performed during the first 7 days of menstrual cycle. Insertion is subdermal in the midportion of the inside of the upper arm, 8 to 10 cm above the elbow crease.
- Each capsule is 2.4 mm in diameter and 34 mm in length.
- Determine if patient has allergies to the antiseptic or anesthetic to be used or contraindications to progestin-only contraception.
- During insertion, pay special attention to asepsis and correct placement of capsules; use careful technique, to minimize tissue trauma.
- Provide copy of patient information booklet; carefully review potential adverse reactions, risk and benefit of use of system, and other forms of contraception.

Patient education

- Tell patient that altered bleeding patterns tend to become more regular after 9 to 12 months.
- Warn patient to report heavy bleeding.
- Advise patient to avoid bumping or wetting the insertion site for at least 3 days after insertion.
- Explain that some tenderness in the implant area may occur for 1 to 2 days.
- Tell patient that insertion usually takes 10 to 15 minutes and causes little or no discomfort because of the local anesthetic.
- Advise patient that, when laboratory studies are ordered, she should inform all health care providers that levonorgestrel implants are being used.
- Tell patient who takes phenytoin or carbamazepine that she may need to use additional contraceptive measures.
- Advise patient to thoroughly review patient information booklet.

levothyroxine sodium (T_4 or L-thyroxine sodium)

Eltroxin, Levo-T, Levothroid, Levoxine, Levoxyl, Synthroid

Pharmacologic classification: thyroid hormone
Therapeutic classification: thyroid hormone replacement
Pregnancy risk category A

How supplied

Available by prescription only
Tablets: 25 mcg, 50 mcg, 75 mcg, 88 mcg, 100 mcg, 112 mcg, 125 mcg, 137 mcg, 150 mcg, 175 mcg, 200 mcg, 300 mcg
Injection: 200 mcg/vial, 500 mcg/vial

Indications, route, and dosage

Cretinism

Children under age 1: Initially, 25 to 50 mcg P.O. daily, increased to 50 mcg (in 4 to 6 weeks).

Myxedema coma

Adults: 300 to 500 mcg I.V. If no response occurs in 24 hours, give an additional 100 to 300 mcg I.V. in 48 hours. A maintenance dose of 50 to 200 mcg may be given until condition stabilizes and drug can be given orally.

Thyroid hormone replacement for atrophy of gland, surgical removal, excessive radiation or antithyroid drugs, or congenital defect

Adults: For mild hypothyroidism—initially, 50 mcg P.O. daily, increased by 25 to 50 mcg P.O. daily q 2 to 4 weeks until desired response is achieved; may be administered I.V. or I.M. when P.O. ingestion is precluded for long periods.

For severe hypothyroidism—12.5 to 25 mcg daily, increased by 25 to 50 mcg daily q 2 to 4 weeks until desired response is achieved.

✦ ***Dosage adjustment.*** For geriatric patients and those with CV disease, start at 12.5 to 25 mcg daily and increase in 12.5- to 25-mcg increments q 2 to 8 weeks.

Children: Therapy may be initiated at the full therapeutic dose. Incremental doses are not usually needed.

Children over age 12: Over 150 mcg or 2 to 3 mcg/kg/day.

Children age 6 to 12: 100 to 150 mcg or 4 to 5 mcg/kg/day.

Children age 1 to 5: 75 to 100 mcg or 5 to 6 mcg/kg/day.

Children age 6 to 12 months: 50 to 75 mcg or 6 to 8 mcg/kg/day.

Children up to 6 months: 25 to 50 mcg or 8 to 10 mcg/kg/day.

Pharmacodynamics

Thyroid hormone replacement: Drug affects protein and carbohydrate metabolism, promotes gluconeogenesis, increases the use and mobilization of glycogen stores, stimulates protein synthesis, and regulates cell growth and differentiation. Major effect of drug is to increase the metabolic rate of tissue.

Pharmacokinetics

• *Absorption:* Absorption is varied from 50% to 80% from the GI tract. Full effects do not occur for 1 to 3 weeks after oral therapy begins. After I.M. administration, absorption is variable and poor. After an I.V. dose in patients with myxedema coma, increased responsiveness may occur within 6 to 8 hours, but maximum therapeutic effect may not occur for up to 24 hours.

• *Distribution:* Not fully described; however, drug is distributed into most body tissues and fluids. The highest levels are found in the liver and kidneys; 99% is protein-bound.

• *Metabolism:* Drug is metabolized in peripheral tissues, primarily in the liver, kidneys, and intestines. About 85% of levothyroxine metabolized is deiodinated.

• *Excretion:* Fecal excretion eliminates 20% to 40% of levothyroxine. Half-life is 6 to 7 days.

Contraindications and precautions

Contraindicated in patients with hypersensitivity to drug, acute MI uncomplicated by hypothyroidism, untreated thyrotoxicosis, or uncorrected adrenal insufficiency. Use cautiously in the elderly and in patients with renal impairment, angina pectoris, hypertension, ischemia, or other CV disorders.

Interactions

Concomitant use of levothyroxine with *corticotropin* causes changes in thyroid status. Decreased *theophylline* clearance can be expected in hypothyroid patients; clearance returns to normal when euthyroid state is achieved. Changes in levothyroxine dosages may require dosage changes in corticotropin as well. Concomitant use with an *anticoagulant* may alter anticoagulant effect; an increase in levothyroxine dosage may necessitate a decrease in anticoagulant dosage. Concomitant use of levothyroxine with *tricyclic antidepressants* or *sympathomimetics* may increase the effects of any or all of these drugs and may lead to coronary insufficiency or arrhythmias.

Concomitant use of levothyroxine with *oral antidiabetic agents* or *insulin* may affect the dosage requirements of these agents. *Beta blockers* may decrease the conversion of levothyroxine to liothyronine. *Cholestyramine* may delay absorption of levothyroxine. *Estrogens,* which increase serum thyroxine-binding globulin levels, increase levothyroxine requirements. *Hepatic enzyme inducers* (such as *phenytoin*) may increase hepatic degradation of levothyroxine and raise dosage requirements of levothyroxine. Concomitant use with *somatrem* may accelerate epiphyseal maturation.

Effects on diagnostic tests

Levothyroxine therapy alters radioactive iodine (^{131}I) thyroid uptake, protein-bound iodine levels, and liothyronine uptake.

Adverse reactions

CNS: *nervousness, insomnia, tremor,* headache.
CV: *tachycardia,* palpitations, ***arrhythmias,*** *angina pectoris,* ***cardiac arrest.***
GI: diarrhea, vomiting.
Other: weight loss, diaphoresis, heat intolerance, fever, menstrual irregularities, allergic skin reactions.

Overdose and treatment

Clinical manifestations of overdose include signs and symptoms of hyperthyroidism, including weight loss, increased appetite, palpitations, nervousness, diarrhea, abdominal cramps, sweating, tachycardia, increased blood pressure, widened pulse pressure, angina, arrhythmias, tremor, headache, insomnia, heat intolerance, fever, and menstrual irregularities.

Treatment of overdose requires reduction of GI absorption and efforts to counteract central and peripheral effects, primarily sympathetic activity. Use gastric lavage or induce emesis (followed by activated charcoal up to 4 hours after ingestion). If the patient is comatose or is having seizures, inflate cuff on endotracheal tube to prevent aspiration. Treatment may include oxygen and artificial ventilation as needed to support respiration. It also should include appropriate measures to treat heart failure and to control fever, hypoglycemia, and fluid loss. Propranolol (or another beta blocker) may be used to combat many of the effects of increased sympathetic activity. Levothyroxine should be gradually withdrawn over 2 to 6 days, then resumed at a lower dose.

☑ Special considerations

Besides those relevant to all *thyroid hormones*, consider the following recommendations.

- Administer as a single dose before breakfast.
- Carefully observe patient for adverse effects during initial titration phase.
- Monitor for aggravation of concurrent diseases, such as Addison's disease or diabetes mellitus.
- Patient with history of lactose intolerance may be sensitive to Levothroid, which contains lactose.
- Synthroid 100- and 300-mcg tablets contain tartrazine, a dye that causes allergic reactions in susceptible individuals.
- When switching from levothyroxine to liothyronine, levothyroxine dosage should stop when liothyronine treatment begins. After residual effects of levothyroxine have disappeared, liothyronine dosage can be increased in small increments. When switching from liothyronine to levothyroxine, levothyroxine therapy should begin several days before withdrawing liothyronine to avoid relapse.
- Patient taking levothyroxine who requires ^{131}I uptake studies must discontinue drug 4 weeks before test.
- Protect drug from moisture and light. Prepare I.V. dose immediately before injection. Do not mix with other I.V. solutions.
- Levothyroxine has predictable effects because of standard hormonal content; therefore, it is the usual drug of choice for thyroid hormone replacement.

Patient education

- Instruct patient to take drug at same time each day; encourage morning dosing to avoid insomnia.
- Tell patient to report headache, diarrhea, nervousness, excessive sweating, heat intolerance, chest pain, increased pulse rate, or palpitations.
- Encourage patient to use the same product consistently because all brands do not have equal bioavailability.
- Advise patient not to store drug in warm, humid areas, such as the bathroom, to prevent deterioration of product.
- Replacement therapy is to be taken essentially for life, except in cases of transient hypothyroidism.

Geriatric use

- Elderly patients are more sensitive to effects of drug. In patients over age 60, initial dosage should be 25% lower than usual recommended dosage.

Pediatric use

- Partial hair loss may occur during the first few months of therapy. Reassure child and parents that this is temporary.

Breast-feeding

- Minimal amounts of drug are excreted in breast milk. Use with caution in breast-feeding women.

lidocaine (lignocaine)

Xylocaine

lidocaine hydrochloride

Anestacon, Dilocaine, L-caine, Lidoject, LidoPen Auto-Injector, Nervocaine, Xylocaine, Xylocaine 10% Oral, Xylocaine Viscous

Pharmacologic classification: amide derivative
Therapeutic classification: ventricular antiarrhythmic, local anesthetic
Pregnancy risk category B

How supplied

Available without a prescription
Ointment: 2.5%
Liquid: 2.5%
Cream: 0.5%
Spray: 0.5%

Available by prescription only
Injection: 5 mg/ml, 10 mg/ml, 15 mg/ml, 20 mg/ml, 40 mg/ml, 100 mg/ml, 200 mg/ml
Premixed solutions: 2 mg/ml, 4 mg/ml, 8 mg/ml in D_5W
Ointment: 5%
Topical solution: 2%, 4%
Jelly: 2%
Spray: 10%

Indications, route, and dosage

Ventricular arrhythmias from MI, cardiac manipulation, or cardiac glycosides

Adults: 50 to 100 mg (1 to 1.5 mg/kg) I.V. bolus at 25 to 50 mg/minute. Repeat bolus q 3 to 5 minutes until arrhythmias subside or adverse effects develop. Do not exceed 300-mg total bolus during a 1-hour period. Simultaneously, begin constant infusion of 1 to 4 mg/minute. If single bolus has been given, repeat smaller bolus (usually ½ initial bolus) 5 to 10 minutes after start of infusion to maintain therapeutic serum level. After 24 hours of continuous infusion, decrease rate by ½.

✦ ***Dosage adjustment.*** Give half the bolus amount to elderly or lightweight patients and to those with heart failure or hepatic disease. Use slower infusion rate in elderly patients, those with heart failure or hepatic disease, or patients weighing under 110 lb (50 kg).

For I.M. administration: 300 mg (4.3 mg/kg) in deltoid muscle has been used in early stages of acute MI.

Children: 0.5 to 1 mg/kg by I.V. bolus, followed by infusion of 20 to 50 mcg/kg/minute.

◊ ***Status epilepticus***
Adults: 1 mg/kg I.V. bolus; then, if seizure continues, administer 0.5 mg/kg 2 minutes after first dose; infusion at 30 mcg/kg/minute may be used.
Local anesthesia of skin or mucous membranes, pain from dental extractions, stomatitis
Adults and children: Apply 2% to 5% solution or ointment or 15 ml of Xylocaine Viscous q 3 to 4 hours to oral or nasal mucosa.
Local anesthesia in procedures involving the male or female urethra
Adults: Instill about 15 ml (male) or 3 to 5 ml (female) into urethra.
Pain, burning, or itching caused by burns, sunburn, or skin irritation
Adults and children: Apply liberally.

Pharmacodynamics
Ventricular antiarrhythmic action: One of the oldest antiarrhythmics, lidocaine remains among the most widely used drugs for treating acute ventricular arrhythmias. According to the Advanced Cardiac Life Support guidelines (American Heart Association, 1994), lidocaine is drug of choice to treat ventricular tachycardia and fibrillation. As a class IB antiarrhythmic, it suppresses automaticity and shortens the effective refractory period and action potential duration of His-Purkinje fibers and suppresses spontaneous ventricular depolarization during diastole. Therapeutic concentrations do not significantly affect conductive atrial tissue and AV conduction. Unlike quinidine and procainamide, lidocaine does not significantly alter hemodynamics when given in usual doses. Drug seems to act preferentially on diseased or ischemic myocardial tissue; exerting its effects on the conduction system, it inhibits reentry mechanisms and halts ventricular arrhythmias.

Local anesthetic action: As a local anesthetic, lidocaine acts to block initiation and conduction of nerve impulses by decreasing the permeability of the nerve cell membrane to sodium ions.

Pharmacokinetics
- *Absorption:* Drug is absorbed after oral administration; however, a significant first-pass effect occurs in the liver and only about 35% of drug reaches the systemic circulation. Oral doses high enough to achieve therapeutic blood levels result in an unacceptable toxicity, probably from high concentrations of lidocaine.
- *Distribution:* Distributed widely throughout the body; it has a high affinity for adipose tissue. After I.V. bolus administration, an early, rapid decline in plasma levels occurs; this is associated mainly with distribution into highly perfused tissues, such as the kidneys, lungs, liver, and heart, followed by a slower elimination phase in which metabolism and redistribution into skeletal muscle and adipose tissue occur. The first (early) distribution phase occurs rapidly, calling for initiation of a constant infusion after an initial bolus dose. Distribution volume declines in patients with liver or hepatic disease, resulting in toxic concentrations with usual doses. About 60% to 80% of circulating drug is bound to plasma proteins. Usual therapeutic drug level is 1.5 to 5 mcg/ml. Although toxicity may occur within this range, levels greater than 5 mcg/ml are considered toxic and warrant dosage reduction.
- *Metabolism:* Lidocaine is metabolized in the liver to two active metabolites. Less than 10% of a parenteral dose escapes metabolism and reaches the kidneys unchanged. Metabolism is affected by hepatic blood flow, which may decrease after MI and with heart failure. Liver disease also may limit metabolism.
- *Excretion:* Drug's half-life undergoes a biphasic process, with an initial phase of 7 to 30 minutes followed by a terminal half-life of 1.5 to 2 hours. Elimination half-life may be prolonged in patients with heart failure or liver disease. Continuous infusions longer than 24 hours also may cause an apparent half-life increase.

Contraindications and precautions
Contraindicated in patients with hypersensitivity to amide-type local anesthetics, Stokes-Adams syndrome, Wolff-Parkinson-White syndrome, and severe degrees of SA, AV, or intraventricular block in absence of artificial pacemaker. Also contraindicated in patients with inflammation or infection in puncture region, septicemia, severe hypertension, spinal deformities, and neurologic disorders.

Use cautiously in the elderly; in patients with renal or hepatic disease, complete or second-degree heart block, sinus bradycardia, or heart failure; and in those weighing less than 110 lb.

Interactions
Concomitant use of lidocaine with cimetidine or *beta blockers* may cause lidocaine toxicity from reduced hepatic clearance. Concomitant use of high-dose lidocaine with *succinylcholine* may increase succinylcholine's neuromuscular effects. Concomitant use with other *antiarrhythmic agents*, including *phenytoin, procainamide, propranolol*, and *quinidine*, may cause additive or antagonist effects as well as additive toxicity.

Effects on diagnostic tests
Because I.M. lidocaine therapy may increase CK levels, isoenzyme tests should be performed for differential diagnosis of acute MI.

Adverse reactions
CNS: anxiety, nervousness, lethargy, somnolence, paresthesia, muscle twitching; *confusion, tremor, stupor, restlessness, light-headedness,* hallucinations, ***seizures*** (with systemic form); apprehension, seizures followed by drowsiness, unconsciousness, ***respiratory arrest***, confusion, tremors, stupor, restlessness, slurred speech, euphoria, depression, light-headedness, ***seizures*** (with topical use).
CV: bradycardia, **CARDIAC ARREST;** *hypotension,* ***new or worsened arrhythmias*** (with systemic form); hypotension, myocardial depression, ***arrhythmias*** (with topical use).
EENT: *tinnitus, blurred or double vision* (with systemic form); tinnitus, blurred or double vision (with topical use).
GI: nausea, vomiting (with topical use).

Skin: dermatologic reactions, sensitization, rash (with topical use).
Other: ***anaphylaxis***; soreness at injection site, sensation of cold (with systemic form); edema, ***status asthmaticus***, diaphoresis (with topical use).

Overdose and treatment

Clinical effects of overdose include signs and symptoms of CNS toxicity, such as seizures or respiratory depression, and CV toxicity (as indicated by hypotension).

Treatment includes general supportive measures and drug discontinuation. A patent airway should be maintained and other respiratory support measures carried out immediately. Diazepam or thiopental may be given to treat any seizures. To treat significant hypotension, vasopressors (including dopamine and norepinephrine) may be administered.

☑ Special considerations

- Monitor patient receiving I.V. lidocaine infusion and on cardiac monitor at all times. Use infusion pump or microdrip system and timer to monitor infusion precisely. Never exceed infusion rate of 4 mg/minute, if possible. A faster rate greatly increases risk of toxicity.
- Do not administer lidocaine with epinephrine (for local anesthesia) to treat arrhythmias. Use solutions with epinephrine cautiously in CV disorders and in body areas with limited blood supply (ears, nose, fingers, toes).
- Monitor vital signs and serum electrolyte, BUN, and creatinine levels.
- Monitor ECG constantly if administering drug I.V., especially in patients with liver disease, heart failure, hypoxia, respiratory depression, hypovolemia, or shock, because these conditions may affect drug metabolism, excretion, or distribution volume, predisposing patient to drug toxicity.
- Monitor for signs of excessive depression of cardiac conductivity (such as sinus node dysfunction, PR-interval prolongation, QRS-interval widening, and appearance or exacerbation of arrhythmias). If they occur, reduce dosage or discontinue drug.
- In many severely ill patients, seizures may be the first sign of toxicity. However, severe reactions are usually preceded by somnolence, confusion, and paresthesias. Regard all signs and symptoms of toxicity as serious, and promptly reduce dosage or discontinue therapy. Continued infusion could lead to seizures and coma. Give oxygen via nasal cannula, if not contraindicated. Keep oxygen and CPR equipment handy.
- Doses of up to 400 mg I.M. have been advocated in prehospital phase of acute MI.
- Patient receiving lidocaine I.M. will show a sevenfold increase in serum CK level. Such CK originates in skeletal muscle, not the heart. Test isoenzyme levels to confirm MI, if using I.M. route.
- Do not use solutions containing preservatives for spinal, epidural, or caudal block.
- With epidural use, inject a 2- to 5-ml test dose at least 5 minutes before giving total dose, to check for intravascular or subarachnoid injection. Motor paralysis and extensive sensory anesthesia indicate subarachnoid injection.
- Therapeutic serum levels range from 2 to 5 mcg/ml.
- Discard partially used vials containing no preservatives.
- Drug has been used investigationally to treat refractory status epilepticus.

Geriatric use

- Use drug with caution in elderly patients, those weighing below 110 lb, and those with heart failure or renal or hepatic disease. Such patients will need dosage reduction.
- Because of prevalence of concurrent disease states and declining organ system function in elderly patients, conservative lidocaine doses should be used.

Pediatric use

- Safety and effectiveness in children have not been established. Use of an I.M. autoinjector device is not recommended.

lindane (gamma benzene hexachloride)

G-well, Kwell, Scabene

Pharmacologic classification: chlorinated hydrocarbon insecticide
Therapeutic classification: scabicide, pediculicide
Pregnancy risk category B

How supplied

Available by prescription only
Cream: 1%
Lotion: 1%
Shampoo: 1%

Indications, route, and dosage

Note: In no case should more than 2 oz be used by one person in one application.
Scabies
Adults and children: After bathing with soap and water, apply a thin layer of cream or lotion and gently massage it on all skin surfaces, moving from the neck to the toes. After 8 to 12 hours, remove drug by bathing and scrubbing well. Treatment may be repeated after 1 week if needed.
Pediculosis
Adults and children: Apply shampoo to dry, affected area and wait 4 minutes. Then add a small amount of water and lather for 4 to 5 minutes; rinse thoroughly. Comb hair to remove nits. Treatment may be repeated after 1 week if needed.

Pharmacodynamics

Scabicide and pediculicide action: Lindane is toxic to the parasitic arthropod *Sarcoptes scabiei* and its eggs, and to *Pediculus capitis, Pediculus corporis*, and *Phthirus pubis*. Drug is absorbed through the organism's exoskeleton and causes its death.

Pharmacokinetics
• *Absorption:* 10% of topical dose may be absorbed in 24 hours.
• *Distribution:* Lindane is stored in body fat.
• *Metabolism:* Metabolism occurs in the liver.
• *Excretion:* Lindane is excreted in urine and feces.

Contraindications and precautions
Contraindicated in patients hypersensitive to drug, when skin is raw or inflamed, or in patients with seizure disorders. Also contraindicated in premature infants. Use cautiously in infants and young patients, who are at highest risk for CNS toxicity.

Interactions
None reported.

Effects on diagnostic tests
None reported.

Adverse reactions
CNS: *dizziness, **seizures.***
Skin: *irritation* (with repeated use).

Overdose and treatment
Accidental ingestion may cause extreme CNS toxicity; reported symptoms include CNS stimulation, dizziness, and seizures. To treat lindane ingestion, empty stomach by appropriate measures (emesis or lavage); follow with saline catharsis (do not use oil laxative). Treat seizures with pentobarbital, phenobarbital, or diazepam, as needed.

☑ Special considerations
• Make sure patient's body is clean (scrubbed well) and dry before application.
• Avoid applying drug to acutely inflamed skin or raw, weeping surfaces.
• Place hospitalized patient in isolation with linen-handling precautions.

Patient education
• Explain correct use of drug.
• Warn patient that itching may continue for several weeks, even if treatment is effective, especially in scabies infestation.
• If drug accidentally contacts eyes, tell patient to flush with water and call for further instructions. He should avoid inhaling vapor.
• Explain that reapplication usually is not necessary unless live mites are found; advise reapplication if drug is accidentally washed off, but caution against overuse.
• Tell patient he may use drug to clean combs and brushes, and to wash them thoroughly afterward; advise patient that all clothing and bed linen that may have been contaminated by him within the past 2 days should be machine washed in hot water and dried in hot dryer or dry-cleaned to avoid reinfestation or transmission of organism.
• Discourage repeated use of drug, which may irritate skin and cause systemic toxicity.
• Caution patient to avoid concomitant use of other oils or ointments.
• Advise patient that family and close contacts, including sexual contacts, should be treated concurrently.
• Warn patient not to use if open wounds, cuts, or sores are present on scalp or groin, unless directed by primary health care provider.

Pediatric use
• Use with caution, especially in infants and small children, who are much more susceptible to CNS toxicity. Discourage thumb-sucking in children using lindane, to prevent ingestion of drug. The Centers for Disease Control and Prevention recommends other scabicide therapies for children under age 10.

Breast-feeding
• Because drug is secreted in breast milk in low concentrations, an alternative method of feeding may be used for 4 days if there is any concern.

liothyronine sodium (T_3)
Cytomel, Triostat

Pharmacologic classification: thyroid hormone
Therapeutic classification: thyroid hormone replacement
Pregnancy risk category A

How supplied
Available by prescription only
Tablets: 5 mcg, 25 mcg, 50 mcg
Injection: 10 mcg/ml

Indications, route, and dosage
Cretinism
Children: 5 mcg P.O. daily, increased by 5 mcg q 3 to 4 days until desired response occurs.
Myxedema
Adults: Initially, 5 mcg daily, increased by 5 to 10 mcg q 1 to 2 weeks. Maintenance dosage is 50 to 100 mcg daily.
Myxedema coma, precoma
Adults: Initially, 25 to 50 mcg I.V.; reassess after 4 to 12 hours, then switch to P.O. as soon as possible. Patients with known or suspected cardiac disease should receive 10 to 20 mcg I.V.
Nontoxic goiter
Adults: Initially, 5 mcg P.O. daily; may be increased by 5 to 10 mcg daily at intervals of 1 to 2 weeks until dosage of 25 mcg daily is reached. Thereafter, dosage may be increased by 12.5 to 25 mcg daily at intervals of 1 to 2 weeks until desired response is noted. Usual maintenance dosage is 75 mcg daily.
Adults over age 65: Initially, 5 mcg P.O. daily, increased by 5-mcg increments q 1 to 2 weeks until dosage of 25 mcg is reached. Thereafter, dosage may be increased by 12.5 to 25 mcg daily q 1 to 2 weeks.
Children: Initially, 5 mcg P.O. daily, increased by 5-mcg increments at weekly intervals until desired response is achieved.

Thyroid hormone replacement
Adults: Initially, 25 mcg P.O. daily, increased by 12.5 to 25 mcg q 1 to 2 weeks until satisfactory response is achieved. Usual maintenance dosage is 25 to 75 mcg daily.
Liothyronine suppression test to differentiate hyperthyroidism from euthyroidism
Adults: 75 to 100 mcg daily for 7 days.

Pharmacodynamics
Thyroid hormone replacement: Liothyronine is usually a second-line drug in the treatment of hypothyroidism, myxedema, and cretinism. This component of thyroid hormone affects protein and carbohydrate metabolism, promotes gluconeogenesis, increases the utilization and mobilization of glycogen stores, stimulates protein synthesis, and regulates cell growth and differentiation. The major effect of liothyronine is to increase the metabolic rate of tissue. It may be most useful in syndromes of thyroid hormone resistance.

Pharmacokinetics
- *Absorption:* Liothyronine is 95% absorbed from the GI tract. Peak effect occurs within 24 to 72 hours.
- *Distribution:* Drug is highly protein-bound. Its distribution has not been fully described.
- *Metabolism:* Not fully understood.
- *Excretion:* Half-life is 1 to 2 days.

Contraindications and precautions
Contraindicated in patients with hypersensitivity to drug, acute MI uncomplicated by hypothyroidism, untreated thyrotoxicosis, or uncorrected adrenal insufficiency. Use cautiously in the elderly and in patients with angina pectoris, hypertension, ischemia, other CV disorders, renal insufficiency, diabetes, or myxedema.

Interactions
Concomitant use of liothyronine with *adrenocorticoids* or *corticotropin* alters thyroid status. Changes in liothyronine dosages may require dosage changes in the adrenocorticoid or corticotropin as well.

Concomitant use of liothyronine with *anticoagulants* may impair the latter's effects; an increase in liothyronine dosage may require a lower dosage of the anticoagulant. Concomitant use of liothyronine with *tricyclic antidepressants* or *sympathomimetics* may increase the effects of any or all of these medications, causing coronary insufficiency or arrhythmias. Concomitant use of liothyronine with *oral antidiabetic agents* or *insulin* may affect dosage requirements of these agents. *Estrogens*, which increase serum thyroxine-binding globulin levels, increase liothyronine requirements.

Effects on diagnostic tests
Liothyronine therapy alters radioactive iodine (^{131}I) uptake, protein-bound iodine levels, and liothyronine uptake.

Adverse reactions
CNS: *nervousness, insomnia, tremor,* headache.
CV: *tachycardia,* ***arrhythmias***, angina pectoris, ***cardiac decompensation and collapse.***
GI: diarrhea, vomiting.
Other: weight loss, heat intolerance, diaphoresis, accelerated bone maturation in infants and children, menstrual irregularities, skin reactions.

Overdose and treatment
Clinical manifestations of overdose include signs and symptoms of hyperthyroidism, including weight loss, increased appetite, palpitations, diarrhea, nervousness, abdominal cramps, sweating, headache, tachycardia, increased blood pressure, widened pulse pressure, angina, arrhythmias, tremor, insomnia, heat intolerance, fever, and menstrual irregularities.

Treatment of overdose reduces GI absorption and counteracts central and peripheral effects, primarily sympathetic activity. Use gastric lavage or induce emesis (followed by activated charcoal up to 4 hours after ingestion). If patient is comatose or having seizures, inflate the cuff on an endotracheal tube to prevent aspiration. Treatment may include oxygen and ventilation to maintain respiration. It also should include appropriate measures to treat heart failure and to control fever, hypoglycemia and fluid loss. Propranolol (or another beta blocker) may be used to counteract many of the effects of increased sympathetic activity. Liothyronine should be withdrawn gradually over 2 to 6 days, then resumed at a lower dose.

☑ Special considerations
Besides those relevant to all *thyroid hormones*, consider the following recommendations.
- Liothyronine may be preferred when rapid effect is desired or when GI absorption or peripheral conversion of levothyroxine to liothyronine is impaired.
- Oral absorption may be reduced in patients with heart failure.
- When switching from levothyroxine to liothyronine, discontinue levothyroxine and start liothyronine at low dosage, increasing in small increments after residual effects of levothyroxine have disappeared. When switching from liothyronine to levothyroxine, start levothyroxine several days before withdrawing liothyronine to avoid relapse.
- Discontinue drug 7 to 10 days before patient undergoes radioactive iodine uptake studies.

Patient education
- Tell patient to report headache, diarrhea, nervousness, excessive sweating, heat intolerance, chest pain, increased pulse rate, or palpitations.
- Advise patient not to store drug in warm, humid areas, such as the bathroom, to prevent deterioration of drug.
- Encourage patient to take drug at the same time each day, preferably in the morning, to avoid insomnia.

Geriatric use
- Elderly patients are more sensitive to drug's effects. In patients over age 60, initial dosage should be 25% lower than usual recommended dosage.

Pediatric use
• Partial hair loss may occur during first few months of therapy. Reassure child and parents that this is temporary.
• Infants and children may experience an accelerated rate of bone maturation.

Breast-feeding
• Minimal amounts of drug are excreted in breast milk. Use with caution in breast-feeding women.

liotrix
Euthroid, Thyrolar

Pharmacologic classification: thyroid hormone
Therapeutic classification: thyroid hormone replacement
Pregnancy risk category A

How supplied
Available by prescription only
Tablets: Euthroid-1/2—levothyroxine sodium 30 mcg and liothyronine sodium 7.5 mcg
Euthroid-1—levothyroxine sodium 60 mcg and liothyronine sodium 15 mcg
Euthroid-2—levothyroxine sodium 120 mcg and liothyronine sodium 30 mcg
Euthroid-3—levothyroxine sodium 180 mcg and liothyronine sodium 45 mcg
Thyrolar-1/4—levothyroxine sodium 12.5 mcg and liothyronine sodium 3.1 mcg
Thyrolar-1/2—levothyroxine sodium 25 mcg and liothyronine sodium 6.25 mcg
Thyrolar-1—levothyroxine sodium 50 mcg and liothyronine sodium 12.5 mcg
Thyrolar-2—levothyroxine sodium 100 mcg and liothyronine sodium 25 mcg
Thyrolar-3—levothyroxine sodium 150 mcg and liothyronine sodium 37.5 mcg

Indications, route, and dosage
Hypothyroidism
Dosages must be individualized to approximate deficit in patient's thyroid secretion.
Adults: Initially, 15 to 30 mg thyroid equivalent P.O. daily, increased by 15 to 30 mg thyroid equivalent q 1 to 2 weeks until desired response is achieved.
Children over age 12: 2 to 3 mcg/kg/day.
Children age 6 to 12: 4 to 5 mcg/kg/day.
Children age 1 to 5: 5 to 6 mcg/kg/day.
Children age 6 to 12 months: 6 to 8 mcg/kg/day.
Children under age 6 months: 8 to 10 mcg/kg/day.

Pharmacodynamics
Thyroid stimulant and replacement: Liotrix affects protein and carbohydrate metabolism, promotes gluconeogenesis, increases the use and mobilization of glycogen stores, stimulates protein synthesis, and regulates cell growth and differentiation. The major effect of liotrix is to increase the metabolic rate of tissue. It is used to treat hypothyroidism (myxedema, cretinism, and thyroid hormone deficiency).

Liotrix is a synthetic preparation combining levothyroxine sodium and liothyronine sodium. Such combination products were developed because circulating T_3 was assumed to result from direct release from the thyroid gland. About 80% of T_3 is now known to be derived from deiodination of T_4 in peripheral tissues, and patients receiving only T_4 have normal serum T_3 and T_4 levels. Therefore, there is no clinical advantage to combining thyroid agents; actually, it could result in excessive T_3 concentration.

Pharmacokinetics
• *Absorption:* About 50% to 95% is absorbed from the GI tract.
• *Distribution:* Distribution is not fully understood.
• *Metabolism:* Liotrix is metabolized partially in peripheral tissues (liver, kidneys, and intestines).
• *Excretion:* Drug is excreted partially in feces.

Contraindications and precautions
Contraindicated in patients with hypersensitivity to drug, acute MI uncomplicated by hypothyroidism, untreated thyrotoxicosis, or uncorrected adrenal insufficiency.

Use cautiously in the elderly and in patients with impaired renal function, ischemia, angina pectoris, hypertension, other CV disorders, myxedema, and diabetes mellitus or insipidus.

Interactions
Concomitant use of liotrix with *corticotropin* or an *adrenocorticoid* alters thyroid status; changes in liotrix dosage may require adrenocorticoid or corticotropin dosage changes as well. Concomitant use with an *anticoagulant* may alter anticoagulant effect; an increase in liotrix dosage may require a lower anticoagulant dose. Concomitant use of liotrix with *sympathomimetics* or *tricyclic antidepressants* may increase the effects of any or all of these drugs and may lead to coronary insufficiency or arrhythmias. Concomitant use with *insulin* or *oral antidiabetic agents* may affect dosage requirements of these agents. *Beta blockers* may decrease the conversion of T_4 to T_3. Cholestyramine may delay absorption of T_4. *Estrogens*, which increase serum thyroxine-binding globulin levels, increase liotrix dosage requirements. *Hepatic enzyme inducers* (such as *phenytoin*) may increase hepatic degradation of T_4, resulting in increased requirements of T_4. Concomitant use with *somatrem* may accelerate epiphyseal maturation.

Effects on diagnostic tests
Liotrix therapy alters radioactive iodine (^{131}I) thyroid uptake, protein-bound iodine levels, and T_3 uptake.

Adverse reactions
CNS: *nervousness, insomnia, tremor,* headache.
CV: *tachycardia,* ***arrhythmias,*** angina pectoris, ***cardiac decompensation and collapse.***
GI: diarrhea, vomiting.
Other: weight loss, heat intolerance, diaphoresis, accelerated rate of bone maturation in infants and

children, menstrual irregularities, allergic skin reactions.

Overdose and treatment

Clinical manifestations of overdose include signs and symptoms of hyperthyroidism, including weight loss, increased appetite, palpitations, nervousness, diarrhea, abdominal cramps, sweating, tachycardia, increased pulse rate and blood pressure, angina, arrhythmias, tremor, headache, insomnia, heat intolerance, fever, and menstrual irregularities.

Treatment requires reduction of GI absorption and efforts to counteract central and peripheral effects, primarily sympathetic activity. Use gastric lavage or induce emesis, then follow with activated charcoal, if less than 4 hours since ingestion. If patient is comatose or having seizures, inflate the cuff on an endotracheal tube to prevent aspiration. Treatment may include oxygen and artificial ventilation as needed to maintain respiration. It should also include appropriate measures to treat heart failure and to control fever, hypoglycemia, and fluid loss. Propranolol (or atenolol, metoprolol, acebutolol, nadolol, or timolol) may be used to combat many of the effects of increased sympathetic activity. Thyroid therapy should be withdrawn gradually over 2 to 6 days, then resumed at a lower dosage.

☑ Special considerations

Besides those relevant to all *thyroid hormones*, consider the following recommendations.

- Note that T_4 is drug of choice for hypothyroidism. Hepatic conversion of T_4 to T_3 is usually adequate. Excessive exogenous supplementation of T_3 is usually associated with toxicity.
- The two commercially prepared liotrix brands contain different amounts of each ingredient; do not change from one brand to the other without considering the differences in potency.
- Monitor patient's pulse rate and blood pressure.
- Protect drug from heat and moisture.

Patient education

- Tell patient to report headache, diarrhea, nervousness, excessive sweating, heat intolerance, chest pain, increased pulse rate, or palpitations.
- Advise patient not to store liotrix in warm and humid areas, such as the bathroom.
- Encourage patient to take a single daily dose in the morning to avoid insomnia.

Geriatric use

- Elderly patients are more sensitive to drug's effects and may require a lower dosage.

Pediatric use

- Partial hair loss may occur during first few months of therapy. Reassure child and parents that this is temporary.
- Infants and children may experience accelerated rate of bone maturation.

Breast-feeding

- Minimal amounts of drug are excreted in breast milk. Use with caution in breast-feeding women.

lisinopril

Prinivil, Zestril

Pharmacologic classification: ACE inhibitor
Therapeutic classification: antihypertensive
Pregnancy risk category C (D second and third trimesters)

How supplied

Available by prescription only
Tablets: 2.5 mg, 5 mg, 10 mg, 20 mg, 40 mg

Indications, route, and dosage

Mild to severe hypertension
Adults: Initially, 10 mg P.O. daily. Most patients are well-controlled on 20 to 40 mg daily as a single dose. Doses up to 80 mg have been used.
Heart failure
Adults: Initially, 5 mg P.O. daily. Most patients are well-controlled on 5 to 20 mg daily as a single dose.
Acute MI
Adults: Initially, 5 mg P.O.; then give 5 mg after 24 hours, 10 mg after 48 hours, and 10 mg daily for 6 weeks.

In patients with acute MI with low systolic blood pressure (below 120 mm Hg), give 2.5 mg P.O. when treatment is started or during the first 3 days after an infarct. If hypotension occurs, a daily maintenance dose of 5 mg may be given with temporary reductions to 2.5 mg if needed.

✦ ***Dosage adjustment.*** In adults with renal failure, initially, 5 mg/day P.O. if creatinine clearance is between 10 and 30 ml/minute, and 2.5 mg/day P.O. if it is less than 10 ml/minute. Dosage may be titrated upward until blood pressure is controlled or to maximum of 40 mg daily. Dosage for patients with heart failure who have a creatinine clearance of below 30 ml/minute is 2.5 mg/day P.O.

Pharmacodynamics

Antihypertensive action: Lisinopril inhibits ACE, preventing the conversion of angiotensin I to angiotensin II, a potent vasoconstrictor. Reduced formation of angiotensin II decreases peripheral arterial resistance and aldosterone secretion, thereby reducing sodium and water retention and blood pressure.

Pharmacokinetics

- *Absorption:* Variable absorption occurs after oral administration; an average of about 25% of an oral dose has been absorbed by test subjects. Peak serum levels occur in about 7 hours. Onset of antihypertensive activity occurs in about 1 hour and peaks in about 6 hours.
- *Distribution:* Drug is distributed widely in tissues. Plasma protein binding appears insignificant. Minimal amounts enter the brain. Preclinical studies indicate that it crosses the placenta.
- *Metabolism:* Lisinopril is not metabolized.
- *Excretion:* Excreted unchanged in the urine.

Contraindications and precautions

Contraindicated in patients with hypersensitivity to ACE inhibitors or history of angioedema related to previous treatment with ACE inhibitor. Use cautiously in patients at risk for hyperkalemia or in those with impaired renal function.

Interactions

Concurrent use with *diuretics* may cause excessive hypotension. *Indomethacin* may attenuate the hypotensive effect of lisinopril. Concomitant use with *potassium-sparing diuretics, potassium supplements*, or *potassium-containing salt substitutes* may lead to hyperkalemia. Concurrent use with *lithium* may increase plasma lithium levels.

Effects on diagnostic tests

Drug's physiologic effects may lead to elevations of serum potassium, serum creatinine, BUN, and serum bilirubin levels; minor reductions of hemoglobin and hematocrit; and changes in liver enzymes.

Adverse reactions

CNS: *dizziness, headache, fatigue, paresthesia.*
CV: hypotension, *orthostatic hypotension,* chest pain.
EENT: *nasal congestion.*
GI: *diarrhea,* nausea, dyspepsia.
GU: impotence.
Hematologic: ***neutropenia, agranulocytopenia.***
Respiratory: *dry, persistent, tickling, nonproductive cough;* dyspnea.
Skin: rash.
Other: ***angioedema, anaphylaxis,*** hyperkalemia.

Overdose and treatment

The most likely manifestation of overdose would be hypotension. Recommended treatment is I.V. infusion of 0.9% NaCl solution.

☑ Special considerations

Besides those relevant to all *ACE inhibitors,* consider the following recommendations.

- Drug absorption is unaffected by food.
- Lisinopril attenuates potassium loss of thiazide diuretics. If patient is taking a diuretic, discontinue diuretic 2 to 3 days before lisinopril therapy, or reduce lisinopril dosage to 5 mg once daily.
- If drug does not adequately control blood pressure, diuretics may be added.
- Review WBC and differential counts before treatment, every 2 weeks for 3 months, and periodically thereafter.
- Lower dosage is necessary in patients with impaired renal function.
- Beneficial effects of lisinopril may require several weeks of therapy.

Patient education

- Tell patient to report light-headedness, especially in first few days of treatment, so dose can be adjusted; signs of infection such as sore throat or fever, because drug may decrease WBC count; facial swelling or difficulty breathing, because drug may cause angioedema; and loss of taste, which may necessitate discontinuation of drug.
- Advise patient to avoid sudden postural changes to minimize orthostatic hypotension.
- Warn patient to seek medical approval before taking OTC cold preparations.
- Instruct patient to avoid potassium-containing salt substitutes.

Geriatric use

- Elderly patients may require lower doses due to impaired drug clearance. They may also be more sensitive to drug's hypotensive effects.

Pediatric use

- Safety and efficacy in children have not been established; use only if potential benefits outweigh risks.

Breast-feeding

- Drug may be distributed into breast milk, but effect on breast-feeding infant is unknown; use with caution in breast-feeding women.

lithium carbonate

Carbolith*, Duralith*, Eskalith, Eskalith CR, Lithane, Lithizine*, Lithobid, Lithonate, Lithotabs

lithium citrate

Cibalith-S

Pharmacologic classification: alkali metal
Therapeutic classification: antimanic, antipsychotic
Pregnancy risk category D

How supplied

Available by prescription only
lithium carbonate
Capsules: 150 mg, 300 mg, 600 mg
Tablets: 300 mg
Tablets (sustained-release): 300 mg, 450 mg
lithium citrate
Syrup (sugarless): 300 mg/5 ml (with 0.3% alcohol)

Indications, route, and dosage

Prevention or control of mania; prevention of depression in patients with bipolar illness
Adults: Acute and maintenance dosage, 900 mg (sustained-release tablet) P.O. in morning and h.s., or 600 mg (tablet or capsule) in the morning, noon, and h.s.
◊ ***Major depression,*** ◊ ***schizoaffective disorder,*** ◊ ***schizophrenic disorder,*** ◊ ***alcohol dependence***
Adults: 300 mg lithium carbonate P.O. t.i.d. or q.i.d.
◊ ***Apparent mixed bipolar disorder in children***
Children: Initially, 15 to 60 mg/kg or 0.5 to 1.5 g/m² lithium carbonate P.O. daily in three divided doses. Do not exceed usual adult dosage. Adjust dosage based on patient response and serum lithium levels; usual dosage range is 150 to 300 mg daily in divided doses.

◇ ***Chemotherapy-induced neutropenia in children and patients with AIDS receiving zidovudine***
Adults and children: 300 to 1,000 mg P.O. daily.

Pharmacodynamics

Antimanic action: Lithium is thought to exert its antipsychotic and antimanic effects by competing with other cations for exchange at the sodium-potassium ion pump, thus altering cation exchange at the tissue level. It also inhibits adenyl cyclase, reducing intracellular levels of cyclic adenosine monophosphate (cAMP) and to a lesser extent, cyclic guanosine monophosphate (cGMP).

Pharmacokinetics

- *Absorption:* Rate and extent of absorption vary with dosage form; absorption is complete within 6 hours of oral administration from conventional tablets and capsules.
- *Distribution:* Distributed widely into the body, including breast milk; concentrations in thyroid gland, bone, and brain tissue exceed serum levels. Peak effects occur at 30 minutes to 3 hours; liquid peaks at 15 minutes to 1 hour. Steady-state serum level achieved in 12 hours: therapeutic effect begins in 5 to 10 days and is maximal within 3 weeks. Therapeutic and toxic serum levels and therapeutic effects show good correlation. Therapeutic range is 0.6 to 1.2 mEq/L; adverse reactions increase as level reaches 1.5 to 2 mEq/L—such concentrations may be necessary in acute mania. Toxicity usually occurs at levels above 2 mEq/L.
- *Metabolism:* Lithium is not metabolized.
- *Excretion:* Excreted 95% unchanged in urine; about 50% to 80% of a given dose is excreted within 24 hours. Level of renal function determines elimination rate.

Contraindications and precautions

Contraindicated if therapy cannot be closely monitored and during pregnancy. Use cautiously in the elderly; in patients with thyroid disease, seizure disorders, renal or CV disease, severe dehydration or debilitation, or sodium depletion; and in those receiving neuroleptics, neuromuscular blockers, and diuretics.

Interactions

Concomitant use of lithium with *thiazide diuretics* may decrease renal excretion and enhance lithium toxicity; diuretic dosage may need to be reduced by 30%. *Indomethacin, phenylbutazone, piroxicam,* and *other NSAIDs* also decrease renal excretion of lithium and may require a 30% reduction in lithium dosage.

Carbamazepine, mazindol, methyldopa, phenytoin, and *tetracyclines,* may increase lithium toxicity. *Fluoxetine* increases lithium serum levels. *Antacids* and *other drugs containing aminophylline, caffeine, calcium, sodium,* or *theophylline* may increase lithium excretion by renal competition for elimination, thus decreasing lithium's therapeutic effect.

Lithium may interfere with pressor effects of *sympathomimetic agents*, especially *norepinephrine*; may potentiate the effects of *neuromuscular blocking agents* (such as *atracurium, pancuronium, succinylcholine*); and may decrease the effects of *chlorpromazine*.

Concomitant use with *haloperidol* may result in severe encephalopathy characterized by confusion, tremors, extrapyramidal effects, and weakness. Use this combination with caution.

Dietary sodium may alter the renal elimination of lithium. Increased sodium intake may increase elimination of drug; decreased intake may decrease elimination.

Acute neurotoxicity with delirium has occurred in patients receiving lithium and *electroconvulsive therapy (ECT)*. Lithium dosage should be reduced or withdrawn before ECT.

Effects on diagnostic tests

Drug therapy causes false-positive test results on thyroid function tests. Drug also elevates neutrophil count.

Adverse reactions

CNS: tremors, drowsiness, headache, confusion, restlessness, dizziness, psychomotor retardation, lethargy, ***coma,*** blackouts, ***epileptiform seizures***, EEG changes, worsened organic mental syndrome, impaired speech, ataxia, muscle weakness, incoordination.
CV: *reversible ECG changes,* ***arrhythmias,*** hypotension, bradycardia, ***peripheral vascular collapse*** (rare).
EENT: tinnitus, blurred vision.
GI: dry mouth, metallic taste, nausea, vomiting, anorexia, diarrhea, *thirst,* abdominal pain, flatulence, indigestion.
GU: *polyuria,* glycosuria, renal toxicity with long-term use, decreased creatinine clearance, albuminuria.
Hematologic: *leukocytosis with WBC count of 14,000 to 18,000/mm³* (reversible).
Skin: pruritus, rash, diminished or absent sensation, drying and thinning of hair, psoriasis, acne, alopecia.
Other: transient hyperglycemia, goiter, hypothyroidism (lowered T_3, T_4, and protein-bound iodine, but elevated ^{131}I uptake), hyponatremia, ankle and wrist edema.

Overdose and treatment

Vomiting and diarrhea occur within 1 hour of acute ingestion (induce vomiting in noncomatose patients if it is not spontaneous). Death has occurred in patients who have ingested 10 to 60 g of lithium; patients have ingested 6 g with minimal toxic effects. Serum lithium levels above 3.4 mEq/L are potentially fatal.

Overdose with chronic lithium ingestion may follow altered pharmacokinetics, drug interactions, or volume or sodium depletion; sedation, confusion, hand tremors, joint pain, ataxia, muscle stiffness, increased deep tendon reflexes, visual changes, and nystagmus may occur. Symptoms may progress to coma, movement abnormalities, tremors, seizures, and CV collapse.

Treatment is symptomatic and supportive; closely monitor vital signs. If emesis is not feasible, treat with gastric lavage. Monitor fluid and electrolyte balance; correct sodium depletion with 0.9% NaCl solution. Institute hemodialysis if serum level is above 3 mEq/L, and in severely symptomatic patients unresponsive to fluid and electrolyte correction, or if urine output decreases significantly. Serum rebound of tissue lithium stores (from high volume distribution) commonly occurs after dialysis and may necessitate prolonged or repeated hemodialysis. Peritoneal dialysis may help but is less effective.

☑ Special considerations

- Shake syrup formulation before administration.
- Discontinue drug before ECT therapy.
- Administer drug with food or milk to reduce GI upset.
- Monitor baseline ECG, thyroid and renal studies, and electrolyte levels. Monitor lithium blood levels 8 to 12 hours after first dose, usually before morning dose, two or three times weekly the first month, then weekly to monthly on maintenance therapy.
- Determination of serum drug levels is crucial to safe use of drug. Do not use drug in patients who cannot have regular serum drug level checks. Be sure patient or responsible family member can comply with instructions.
- When lithium blood levels are below 1.5 mEq/L, adverse reactions usually remain mild.
- Monitor fluid intake and output, especially when surgery is scheduled.
- Expect lag of 1 to 3 weeks before drug's beneficial effects are noticed. Other psychotropic medications (for example, chlorpromazine) may be necessary during interim period.
- Monitor for signs of edema or sudden weight gain.
- Adjust fluid and salt ingestion to compensate if excessive loss occurs through protracted sweating or diarrhea. Patient should have fluid intake of 2,500 to 3,000 ml daily and a balanced diet with adequate salt intake.
- Arrange for outpatient follow-up of thyroid and renal functions every 6 to 12 months. Thyroid should be palpated to check for enlargement.
- Check urine for specific gravity level below 1.015, which may indicate diabetes insipidus.
- Drug may alter glucose tolerance in diabetic patients. Monitor blood glucose levels closely.
- Lithium is used investigationally to increase WBC count in patients undergoing cancer chemotherapy. It has also been used investigationally to treat cluster headaches, aggression, organic brain syndrome, and tardive dyskinesia. Drug has been used to treat SIADH.
- Monitor serum levels and signs of impending toxicity.
- Lithane tablets contain tartrazine, a dye that may precipitate an allergic reaction in certain individuals, particularly asthmatics sensitive to aspirin.
- Monitor drug dosing carefully when patient's initial manic symptoms begin to subside because the ability to tolerate high serum lithium levels decreases as symptoms resolve.
- EEG changes include diffuse slowing, widening of frequency spectrum, potentiation, and disorganization of background rhythm.

Patient education

- Explain that lithium has a narrow therapeutic margin of safety. A serum drug level that is even slightly high can be dangerous.
- Warn patient and family to watch for signs of toxicity (diarrhea, vomiting, dehydration, drowsiness, muscle weakness, tremor, fever, and ataxia) and to expect transient nausea, polyuria, thirst, and discomfort during first few days. If toxic symptoms occur, tell patient to withhold one dose and call promptly.
- Warn ambulatory patient to avoid activities that require alertness and good psychomotor coordination until CNS response to drug is determined.
- Advise patient to maintain adequate water intake and adequate—but not excessive—salt in diet.
- Explain importance of regular follow-up visits to measure lithium serum levels.
- Tell patient to avoid large amounts of caffeine, which will interfere with drug's effectiveness.
- Advise patient to seek medical approval before initiating weight-loss program.
- Tell patient not to switch brands of lithium or take other prescription or OTC drugs without medical approval. Different brands may not provide equivalent effect.
- Tell patient to take drug with food or milk.
- Warn patient against stopping drug abruptly.
- Tell patient to explain to close friend or family members the signs of lithium overdose, in case emergency aid is needed.
- Instruct patient to carry identification and instruction card with toxicity and emergency information.

Geriatric use

- Elderly patients are more susceptible to chronic overdose and toxic effects, especially dyskinesias. These patients usually respond to a lower dosage.

Pediatric use

- Drug is not recommended for use in children under age 12.

Breast-feeding

- Lithium level in breast milk is 33% to 50% that of maternal serum level. Breast-feeding should be avoided during treatment with lithium.

lodoxamide tromethamine
Alomide

Pharmacologic classification: cromolyn-like mast cell stabilizer
Therapeutic classification: antiallergic ophthalmic
Pregnancy risk category B

How supplied
Available by prescription only
Ophthalmic solution: 0.1%

Indications, route, and dosage

Treatment of vernal keratoconjunctivitis, vernal conjunctivitis, vernal keratitis

Adults and children age 2 and older: 1 to 2 drops in affected eye(s) t.i.d. for up to 3 months.

Pharmacodynamics

Ocular antiallergy action: Lodoxamide's precise mechanism of action is unknown. However, it is thought that the drug may prevent calcium influx into mast cells upon antigen stimulation. Lodoxamide has no intrinsic vasoconstrictor, antihistaminic, cyclooxygenase inhibition or other anti-inflammatory activity.

Pharmacokinetics

- *Absorption:* Unknown.
- *Distribution:* Unknown.
- *Metabolism:* Unknown.
- *Excretion:* Urinary excretion; the elimination half-life is 8½ hours.

Contraindications and precautions

Contraindicated in patients hypersensitive to drug or its components.

Interactions

None reported.

Effects on diagnostic tests

None reported.

Adverse reactions

CNS: headache, dizziness, somnolence.
EENT: *transient eye discomfort on instillation (burning, stinging);* blepharitis; blurred vision; chemosis; corneal erosion, ulcer, or abrasion; crystalline deposits; epitheliopathy; sensation of foreign body, stickiness, or warmth; hyperemia; keratitis; keratopathy; ocular edema, discharge, swelling, fatigue, itching, or allergy; pruritus; scales on eyelids or eyelashes; tearing; dry nose.
GI: nausea, stomach discomfort.
Skin: rash, heat sensation.

Overdose and treatment

No information available.

☑ Special considerations

- Drug is for ophthalmic use only, not for injection.
- Continuous drug treatment may be required for as long as 3 months.

Patient education

- Instruct patient how to instill eye drops and stress importance of not touching dropper to eye or surrounding area.
- Inform patient that transient burning or stinging may occur on instillation. Advise patient to call if these symptoms persist.
- Instruct patient not to wear contact lenses during drug treatment.

Pediatric use

- Safety and efficacy in children under age 2 have not been established.

Breast-feeding

- It is unknown if drug is excreted in breast milk. Use caution when administering drug to breast-feeding women.

lomefloxacin hydrochloride

Maxaquin

Pharmacologic classification: fluoroquinolone
Therapeutic classification: broad-spectrum antibiotic
Pregnancy risk category C

How supplied

Available by prescription only
Tablets: 400 mg

Indications, route, and dosage

***Acute bacterial exacerbations of chronic bronchitis caused by* Haemophilus influenzae *or* Moraxella (Branhamella) catarrhalis**

Adults: 400 mg P.O. daily for 10 days.

***Uncomplicated urinary tract infections (cystitis) caused by* Escherichia coli, Klebsiella pneumoniae, Proteus mirabilis, *or* Staphylococcus saprophyticus**

Adults: 400 mg P.O. daily for 10 days.

***Complicated urinary tract infections caused by* E. coli, K. pneumoniae, P. mirabilis, *or* Pseudomonas aeruginosa*; possibly effective against infections caused by* Citrobacter diversus *or* Enterobacter cloacae**

Adults: 400 mg P.O. daily for 14 days.

Prophylaxis of infections after transurethral surgical procedures

Adults: 400 mg P.O. 2 to 6 hours before surgery as a single dose.

✦ ***Dosage adjustment.*** In adults with renal failure and creatinine clearance of 10 to 40 ml/minute/1.73 m^2, give loading dose of 400 mg P.O. on first day, followed by 200 mg P.O. daily for duration of therapy. Periodic determination of blood drug levels is recommended. Hemodialysis removes negligible amounts of drug.

Pharmacodynamics

Antibiotic action: Lomefloxacin inhibits bacterial DNA gyrase, an enzyme necessary for bacterial replication. Drug is bactericidal.

Pharmacokinetics

- *Absorption:* Rapidly absorbed from the GI tract; absolute bioavailability is 95% to 98%. Food impairs absorption by reducing total amount absorbed and slowing absorption rate.
- *Distribution:* Only 10% of drug is bound to plasma proteins.
- *Metabolism:* Drug is metabolized in the liver.
- *Excretion:* Mostly excreted unchanged in urine; about 10% is excreted as metabolites. Solubility in urine is pH dependent. About 10% of a dose appears unchanged in the feces. Half-life is 8 hours. Steady state is reached after 2 days of once-daily therapy.

Contraindications and precautions
Contraindicated in patients with hypersensitivity to drug or other fluoroquinolones. Use cautiously in patients with known or suspected CNS disorders, such as seizures or cerebral arteriosclerosis.

Interactions
Antacids and *sucralfate* bind with lomefloxacin in the GI tract and impair its absorption. Administer no less than 4 hours before or 2 hours after a dose. *Probenecid* decreases excretion of lomefloxacin.

When administered with *cimetidine*, other quinolones show substantially increased plasma half-lives. Other quinolones also increase the effects or serum levels of *cyclosporine* and *warfarin*. Lomefloxacin has not been tested for these effects, however. Monitor for toxicity.

Effects on diagnostic tests
None reported.

Adverse reactions
CNS: *dizziness, headache,* abnormal dreams, fatigue, malaise, asthenia, agitation, anorexia, anxiety, confusion, depersonalization, depression, increased appetite, insomnia, nervousness, somnolence, seizures, coma, hyperkinesia, tremor, vertigo, paresthesia, arthralgia, myalgia.
CV: flushing, hypotension, hypertension, edema, syncope, ***arrhythmia,*** tachycardia, ***bradycardia***, extrasystoles, cyanosis, angina pectoris, ***MI***, ***cardiac failure***, ***pulmonary embolism***, cerebrovascular disorder, cardiomyopathy, phlebitis.
EENT: epistaxis, abnormal vision, conjunctivitis, eye pain, earache, tinnitus, tongue discoloration, taste perversion.
GI: *diarrhea, nausea,* dry mouth, pseudomembranous colitis, abdominal pain, dyspepsia, vomiting, flatulence, constipation, inflammation, dysphagia, bleeding.
GU: dysuria, hematuria, anuria, leukorrhea, epididymitis, orchitis, vaginitis, vaginal moniliasis, intermenstrual bleeding, perineal pain.
Hematologic: thrombocythemia, ***thrombocytopenia***, lymphadenopathy, increased fibrinolysis.
Respiratory: dyspnea, ***bronchospasm,*** respiratory disorder or infection, increased sputum, stridor.
Skin: pruritus, skin disorder, skin exfoliation, eczema, rash, urticaria, *photosensitivity.*
Other: ***anaphylaxis***, increased diaphoresis, leg cramps, thirst, chest or back pain, chills, allergic reaction, facial edema, flulike symptoms, decreased heat tolerance, hypoglycemia, elevated liver enzymes, gout.

Overdose and treatment
Treatment of overdose includes emptying the stomach by induced vomiting or gastric lavage, observing patient closely, and providing supportive care. Drug is not significantly removed by hemodialysis or peritoneal dialysis.

☑ Special considerations
- Drug should not be used for empiric treatment of acute exacerbations of chronic bronchitis when suspected pathogen is *Streptococcus pneumoniae* because this organism demonstrates resistance to drug. Because blood drug levels do not readily exceed the minimum inhibitory concentration against *Pseudomonas aeruginosa,* drug should not be used to treat bacteremia caused by this organism, but it has been used successfully to treat complicated urinary tract Pseudomonas infections.

Patient education
- Remind patient to take all of drug prescribed, even after he feels better.
- Advise patient to take drug on an empty stomach.
- Tell patient to avoid hazardous tasks that require alertness, such as driving, until adverse CNS effects of drug are known.
- Instruct patient to avoid sunlight or artificial ultraviolet light, and to call immediately if signs of photosensitivity occur.
- Caution patient to avoid mineral supplements or vitamins with iron or minerals within the 2-hour period before or after taking drug.
- Tell patient that sucralfate or antacids containing magnesium or aluminum should not be taken within 4 hours before or 2 hours after taking drug.
- Instruct patient to drink fluids liberally.

Pediatric use
- Because studies have shown that quinolones can cause arthropathy in immature animals, these drugs should be avoided in children.

Breast-feeding
- It is unknown if drug is excreted in breast milk. Because of risk of serious adverse effects on the infant, a decision should be made whether to discontinue the drug or breast-feeding.

lomustine (CCNU)
CeeNU, CeeNU Dose Pack

Pharmacologic classification: alkylating agent, nitrosourea (cell cycle–phase nonspecific)
Therapeutic classification: antineoplastic
Pregnancy risk category D

How supplied
Available by prescription only
Capsules: 10 mg, 40 mg, 100 mg
Dose pack: 2 capsules lomustine 10 mg, 2 capsules lomustine 40 mg, 2 capsules lomustine 100 mg

Indications, route, and dosage
Dosage and indications may vary. Check current literature for recommended protocol.
Brain, colon, lung, and renal cell cancer; Hodgkin's disease; lymphomas; melanomas; multiple myeloma
Adults and children: 100 to 130 mg/m² P.O. as single dose q 6 weeks.

✦ ***Dosage adjustment.*** Reduce dose according to bone marrow depression using the following guidelines:

Nadir after prior dose		% of prior dose to be given
WBCs/mm³	***Platelets/ mm³***	
> 4,000	100,000	100%
3,000 to 3,999	75,000 to 99,999	100%
2,000 to 2,999	25,000 to 74,999	70%
< 2,000	< 25,000	50%

Repeat doses should not be given until WBC count is more than 4,000/mm³ and platelet count is more than 100,000/mm³.

Pharmacodynamics

Antineoplastic action: Lomustine exerts its cytotoxic activity through alkylation, resulting in the inhibition of DNA and RNA synthesis. As with other nitrosourea compounds, lomustine is known to modify cellular proteins and alkylate proteins, resulting in an inhibition of protein synthesis. Cross-resistance exists between lomustine and carmustine.

Pharmacokinetics

- *Absorption:* Drug is rapidly and well absorbed across the GI tract after oral administration.
- *Distribution:* Distributed widely into body tissues. Because of its high lipid solubility, drug and its metabolites cross the blood-brain barrier to a significant extent.
- *Metabolism:* Metabolized rapidly and extensively in the liver. Some of the metabolites have cytotoxic activity.
- *Excretion:* Metabolites of lomustine are excreted primarily in urine, with smaller amounts excreted in feces and through the lungs. Plasma elimination of drug is biphasic, with an initial phase half-life of 6 hours and a terminal phase of 1 to 2 days. Extended half-life of the terminal phase is thought to be caused by enterohepatic circulation and protein-binding.

Contraindications and precautions

Contraindicated in patients with hypersensitivity to drug. Use cautiously in patients with decreased platelet, WBC, or RBC counts and in those receiving other myelosuppressants.

Interactions

None reported.

Effects on diagnostic tests

Lomustine therapy may cause transient increases in liver function tests.

Adverse reactions

CNS: disorientation, lethargy, ataxia.
GI: *nausea, vomiting,* stomatitis.
GU: ***nephrotoxicity,*** progressive azotemia, ***renal failure.***
Hematologic: *anemia,* ***leukopenia,*** delayed up to 6 weeks, lasting 1 to 2 weeks; thrombocytopenia, delayed up to 4 weeks, lasting 1 to 2 weeks; ***bone marrow suppression,*** delayed up to 6 weeks.
Other: ***hepatotoxicity, secondary malignant disease,*** pulmonary fibrosis, alopecia.

Overdose and treatment

Clinical manifestations of overdose include myelosuppression, nausea, and vomiting. Treatment is usually supportive and includes antiemetics and transfusion of blood components.

☑ Special considerations

- Give drug 2 to 4 hours after meals. Drug is more completely absorbed if taken when the stomach is empty. To avoid nausea, give antiemetic before administering.
- Anorexia may persist for 2 to 3 days after a given dose.
- Dose modification may be required in patients with decreased platelet, WBC, or RBC count.
- Monitor CBC weekly. Drug is usually not administered more often than every 6 weeks; bone marrow toxicity is cumulative and delayed.
- Frequently assess renal and hepatic status.
- Avoid all I.M. injections when platelet count is below 100,000/mm³.
- Use anticoagulants cautiously. Watch closely for signs of bleeding.
- Because drug crosses the blood-brain barrier, it may be used to treat primary brain tumors.

Patient education

- Emphasize importance of continuing medication despite nausea and vomiting.
- Emphasize importance of taking the exact dose.
- Tell patient to call immediately if vomiting occurs shortly after a dose is taken.
- Advise patient to avoid exposure to people with infections.
- Caution patient to avoid alcoholic beverages for a short period after taking drug.
- Warn patient to avoid aspirin-containing products.
- Tell patient to promptly report a sore throat, fever, or unusual bruising or bleeding.
- Advise patient to use effective contraceptive measures during drug therapy.

Breast-feeding

- Metabolites of lomustine have been found in breast milk. Breast-feeding should be discontinued because of increased risk of serious adverse reactions, mutagenicity, and carcinogenicity in the infant.

loperamide hydrochloride

Imodium, Imodium A-D, Kaopectate II, Maalox Anti-Diarrheal, Pepto Diarrhea Control

Pharmacologic classification: piperadine derivative
Therapeutic classification: antidiarrheal
Pregnancy risk category B

How supplied

Available by prescription only
Capsules: 2 mg

Available without a prescription
Tablets: 2 mg
Solution: 1 mg/5 ml

Indications, route, and dosage

Acute, nonspecific diarrhea

Adults and children over age 12: Initially, 4 mg P.O., then 2 mg after each unformed stool. Maximum dosage, 16 mg daily.
Children age 9 to 11: 2 mg t.i.d. on first day.
Children age 6 to 8: 2 mg b.i.d. on first day.
Children age 2 to 5: 1 mg t.i.d. on first day.

Maintenance dose is one-third to one-half the initial dose.

Chronic diarrhea

Adults: Initially, 4 mg P.O., then 2 mg after each unformed stool until diarrhea subsides. Adjust dose to individual response.

Directions for patient self-medication

Adults: 4 teaspoons or 2 tablets after the first loose bowel movement, followed by 2 teaspoons or 1 tablet after each subsequent loose bowel movement. Do not exceed 8 teaspoons daily.
Children age 9 to 11 (60 to 95 lb [27 to 43 kg]): 2 teaspoons or 1 tablet after first loose bowel movement, followed by 1 teaspoon or 1/2 tablet after each subsequent loose bowel movement. Do not exceed 6 teaspoons daily.
Children age 6 to 8 (48 to 59 lb [22 to 27 kg]): 2 teaspoons or 1 tablet after first loose bowel movement, followed by 1 teaspoon or 1/2 tablet after each subsequent loose bowel movement. Do not exceed 4 teaspoons daily
Children age 2 to 5 (24 to 47 lb [11 to 21 kg]): 1 teaspoon after first loose bowel movement, followed by 1 teaspoon after each subsequent loose bowel movement. Do not exceed 3 teaspoons daily.

Pharmacodynamics

Antidiarrheal action: Loperamide reduces intestinal motility by acting directly on intestinal mucosal nerve endings; tolerance to antiperistaltic effect does not develop. Drug also may inhibit fluid and electrolyte secretion by an unknown mechanism. Although it is chemically related to opiates, it has not shown any physical dependence characteristics in humans, and it possesses no analgesic activity.

Pharmacokinetics

- *Absorption:* Drug is absorbed poorly from the GI tract.
- *Distribution:* Not well characterized.
- *Metabolism:* Absorbed loperamide is metabolized in the liver.
- *Excretion:* Drug is excreted primarily in feces; less than 2% is excreted in urine.

Contraindications and precautions

Contraindicated in children under age 2 and in patients with hypersensitivity or when constipation must be avoided. Also, OTC use is contraindicated in patients with a fever exceeding 101° F (38.3° C) or if blood is present in the stool. Use cautiously in patients with hepatic impairment.

Interactions

Concomitant use with an opioid analgesic may cause severe constipation.

Effects on diagnostic tests

None reported.

Adverse reactions

CNS: drowsiness, fatigue, dizziness.
GI: dry mouth; abdominal pain, distention, or discomfort; *constipation;* nausea; vomiting.
Skin: rash, hypersensitivity reactions.

Overdose and treatment

Clinical effects of overdose include constipation, GI irritation, and CNS depression.

Treatment is with activated charcoal if ingestion was recent. If patient is vomiting, activated charcoal may be given in a slurry when patient can retain fluids. Alternatively, gastric lavage may be performed, followed by administration of activated charcoal slurry. Monitor for CNS depression; treat respiratory depression with naloxone.

☑ Special considerations

- After administration via nasogastric tube, tube should be flushed to clear it and ensure drug's passage to stomach.

Patient education

- Warn patient to take drug only as directed and not to exceed recommended dose.
- Caution patient to avoid driving and other tasks requiring alertness because drug may cause drowsiness and dizziness.
- Instruct patient to call if no improvement occurs in 48 hours or if fever develops.

Pediatric use

- Drug is approved for use in children age 2 and older; however, children may be more susceptible to untoward CNS effects.

Breast-feeding

- It is unknown if drug is excreted in breast milk. Use with caution.

loracarbef
Lorabid

Pharmacologic classification: synthetic beta-lactam antibiotic of carbacephem class
Therapeutic classification: antibiotic
Pregnancy risk category B

How supplied
Available by prescription only
Pulvules: 200 mg
Powder for oral suspension: 100 mg/5 ml, 200 mg/5 ml

Indications, route, and dosage
Secondary bacterial infections of acute bronchitis
Adults: 200 to 400 mg P.O. q 12 hours for 7 days.
Acute bacterial exacerbations of chronic bronchitis
Adults: 400 mg P.O. q 12 hours for 7 days.
Pneumonia
Adults: 400 mg P.O. q 12 hours for 14 days.
Pharyngitis or tonsillitis
Adults: 200 mg P.O. q 12 hours for 10 days.
Children age 6 months to 12 years: 15 mg/kg P.O. daily in divided doses q 12 hours for 10 days.
Sinusitis
Adults: 400 mg P.O. q 12 hours for 10 days.
Acute otitis media
Children: 30 mg/kg (oral suspension) P.O. daily in divided doses q 12 hours for 10 days.
Uncomplicated skin and skin-structure infections
Adults: 200 mg P.O. q 12 hours for 7 days.
Impetigo
Children: 15 mg/kg P.O. daily in divided doses q 12 hours for 7 days.
Uncomplicated cystitis
Adults: 200 mg P.O. daily for 7 days.
Uncomplicated pyelonephritis
Adults: 400 mg P.O. q 12 hours for 14 days.
✦ ***Dosage adjustment.*** Adults and children with renal failure and creatinine clearance of 50 ml/minute or more do not require dose and interval changes. In patients with creatinine clearance of 10 to 49 ml/minute, half usual dose at same interval or normal recommended dose at twice the usual dosage interval; in those with creatinine clearance below 10 ml/minute, usual dose q 3 to 5 days. Hemodialysis patients should be given another dose after dialysis.

Pharmacodynamics
Antibiotic action: Loracarbef exerts its bactericidal action by binding to essential target proteins of the bacterial cell wall, leading to inhibition of cell-wall synthesis. Loracarbef is active against gram-positive aerobes, such as *Staphylococcus aureus, S. saprophyticus, Streptococcus pneumoniae,* and *S. pyogenes,* and gram-negative aerobes, such as *Escherichia coli, Haemophilus influenzae,* and *Moraxella (Branhamella) catarrhalis.*

Pharmacokinetics
- *Absorption:* After oral administration, drug is approximately 90% absorbed from the GI tract. When pulvules are taken with food, peak plasma concentrations are 50% to 60% of those achieved on an empty stomach. (Effect of food on rate and extent of absorption of suspension form has not been studied to date.) Absorption of suspension form is greater than that of pulvule. Average peak plasma concentrations of pulvule form occur in approximately 1.2 hours; those of suspension form occur in approximately 0.8 hours.
- *Distribution:* Approximately 25% of circulating drug is bound to plasma proteins.
- *Metabolism:* Drug does not appear to be metabolized.
- *Excretion:* Drug is eliminated primarily in urine. Elimination half-life in patients with normal renal function averages 1 hour.

Contraindications and precautions
Contraindicated in patients with hypersensitivity to drug or other cephalosporins and in patients with diarrhea caused by pseudomembranous colitis. Use cautiously in pregnant and breast-feeding patients.

Interactions
Probenecid decreases the excretion of loracarbef, causing increased plasma levels. Monitor for toxicity.

Effects on diagnostic tests
Drug can cause prolonged PT, positive direct Coombs' test, elevated LD, pancytopenia, and neutropenia.

Adverse reactions
CNS: headache, somnolence, nervousness, insomnia, dizziness.
CV: vasodilation.
GI: diarrhea, nausea, vomiting, abdominal pain, anorexia, ***pseudomembranous colitis.***
GU: vaginal candidiasis, transient increases in BUN and creatinine levels.
Hematologic: ***transient thrombocytopenia, leukopenia,*** eosinophilia.
Skin: rash, urticaria, pruritus, ***erythema multiforme.***
Other: hypersensitivity reactions, including ***anaphylaxis*** transient elevations in AST, ALT, and alkaline phosphatase levels.

Overdose and treatment
Toxic symptoms after overdose of beta-lactams, such as loracarbef, may include nausea, vomiting, epigastric distress, and diarrhea. Forced diuresis, peritoneal dialysis, hemodialysis, or hemoperfusion have not been established as beneficial for an overdose of loracarbef. Hemodialysis is effective in hastening the elimination of loracarbef from plasma in patients with chronic renal failure.

☑ Special considerations
- The increased rate of absorption should be considered if oral suspension is to be substituted for

pulvule. Pulvules should not be substituted for oral suspension when treating otitis media.
• Pseudomembranous colitis has been reported with nearly all antibacterial agents and may range from mild to life-threatening. Therefore, diagnosis must be considered in patients who present with diarrhea subsequent to drug administration.
• Obtain specimen for culture and sensitivity tests before giving first dose. Therapy may begin pending test results.
• Drug may cause overgrowth of nonsusceptible bacteria or fungi. Monitor for signs and symptoms of superinfection.
• To reconstitute powder for oral suspension, add 30 ml of water in two portions to the 50-ml bottle or 60 ml of water in two portions to the 100-ml bottle; shake after each addition.
• After reconstitution, oral suspension is stable for 14 days at room temperature (59° to 86° F [15° to 30° C]).

Patient education
• Instruct patient to take drug at least 1 hour before or at least 2 hours after eating.
• Tell patient to take drug exactly as prescribed, even after he feels better.
• Inform patient that oral suspension can be stored at room temperature for 14 days. Instruct patient to discard unused portion after 14 days.

Pediatric use
• Safety and effectiveness in infants under age 6 months have not been established.

Breast-feeding
• It is not known if drug occurs in breast milk. Use caution when administering drug to breast-feeding women.

loratadine
Claritin

Pharmacologic classification: tricyclic antihistamine
Therapeutic classification: antihistaminic
Pregnancy risk category B

How supplied
Available by prescription only
Tablets: 10 mg
Tablets (rapidly distintegrating): 10 mg
Syrup: 1 mg/ml

Indications, route, and dosage
Symptomatic treatment of seasonal allergic rhinitis and indicated for treatment of idiopathic chronic urticaria
Adults and children age 6 and older: 10 mg P.O. daily.
✦ **Dosage adjustment.** In patients with liver failure or glomerular filtration rate below 30 ml/ minute, adjust dose to 10 mg every other day.

Pharmacodynamics
Antihistaminic action: Loratadine is a long-acting tricyclic antihistamine with selective peripheral H_1-receptor antagonistic activity.

Pharmacokinetics
• *Absorption:* Drug is readily absorbed, with onset of action beginning within 1 to 3 hours, reaching maximum at 8 to 12 hours, and lasting in excess of 24 hours. Because peak plasma concentration may be delayed by 1 hour with a meal, drug should be administered on an empty stomach.
• *Distribution:* About 97% bound to plasma protein. Drug does not readily cross the blood-brain barrier.
• *Metabolism:* Extensively metabolized to an active metabolite (descarboethoxyloratadine). The specific enzyme systems responsible for metabolism have not been identified.
• *Excretion:* Approximately 80% of total dose administered can be found equally distributed between urine and feces. Mean elimination half-life is 8.4 hours for loratadine. Drug is not eliminated by hemodialysis; it is unknown if drug is eliminated by peritoneal dialysis.

Contraindications and precautions
Contraindicated in patients with hypersensitivity to drug. Use cautiously in patients with hepatic impairment and in breast-feeding women.

Interactions
Drugs known to inhibit hepatic metabolism should be coadministered with caution until definitive interaction studies can be completed.

Effects on diagnostic tests
None reported.

Adverse reactions
CNS: headache, somnolence, fatigue.
GI: dry mouth.

Overdose and treatment
Somnolence, tachycardia, and headache have been reported with overdoses greater than 10 mg (40 to 180 mg). If overdosage occurs, institute symptomatic and supportive measures promptly and maintain for as long as necessary.

Treatment consists of emesis (ipecac syrup), except in patients with impaired consciousness, followed by administration of activated charcoal to adsorb any remaining drug. If vomiting is unsuccessful or contraindicated, gastric lavage should be performed with 0.9% NaCl. Saline cathartics also may be of value for rapid dilution of bowel contents.

☑ Special considerations
• No information exists to indicate that drug abuse or dependency occurs.

Patient education
• Instruct patient to take drug on an empty stomach at least 2 hours after a meal and to avoid eating for at least 1 hour after taking drug.

• Tell patient to take drug only once daily. Tell him to call if symptoms persist or worsen.
• Warn patient to stop taking drug 4 days before allergy skin tests to preserve accuracy of tests.

Pediatric use
• Safety and effectiveness in children under age 6 have not been established.

Breast-feeding
• Loratadine passes easily into breast milk. Antihistamine therapy is contraindicated in breast-feeding women.

lorazepam
Apo-Lorazepam*, Ativan, Novo-Lorazem*

Pharmacologic classification: benzodiazepine
Therapeutic classification: antianxiety, sedative-hypnotic
Controlled substance schedule IV
Pregnancy risk category D

How supplied
Available by prescription only
Tablets: 0.5 mg, 1 mg, 2 mg
Tablets (S.L.):* 1 mg, 2 mg
Injection: 2 mg/ml, 4 mg/ml

Indications, route, and dosage
Anxiety, tension, agitation, irritability, especially in anxiety neuroses or organic (especially GI or CV) disorders
Adults: 2 to 6 mg P.O. daily in divided doses; maximum dosage, 10 mg/day.
Insomnia
Adults: 2 to 4 mg P.O. h.s.
Preoperatively
Adults: 0.05 mg/kg I.M. 2 hours before surgery (maximum, 4 mg). Alternatively, 0.044 mg/kg (maximum total dose, 2 mg) I.V. 15 to 20 minutes before surgery; in adults below age 50 dosage may be increased to 0.05 mg/kg (maximum, 4 mg) when increased lack of recall of preoperative events is desired.

Pharmacodynamics
Anxiolytic and sedative actions: Lorazepam depresses the CNS at the limbic and subcortical levels of the brain. It produces an antianxiety effect by influencing the effect of the neurotransmitter gamma-aminobutyric acid (GABA) on its receptor in the ascending reticular activating system, which increases inhibition and blocks both cortical and limbic arousal after stimulation of the reticular formation.

Pharmacokinetics
• *Absorption:* When administered orally, drug is well absorbed through the GI tract. Peak levels occur in 2 hours.
• *Distribution:* Distributed widely throughout the body. Drug is about 85% protein-bound.
• *Metabolism:* Drug is metabolized in the live inactive metabolites.
• *Excretion:* The metabolites of lorazepam are excreted in urine as glucuronide conjugates.

Contraindications and precautions
Contraindicated in patients with acute angle-closure glaucoma or hypersensitivity to drug, other benzodiazepines, or its vehicle (used in parenteral dosage form).

Use cautiously in patients with pulmonary, renal, or hepatic impairment and in elderly, acutely ill, or debilitated patients. Do not use in pregnant patients, especially during the first trimester of pregnancy.

Interactions
Lorazepam potentiates the CNS depressant effects of *alcohol, antidepressants, antihistamines, barbiturates, general anesthetics, MAO inhibitors, narcotics,* and *phenothiazines.*

Concomitant use with *cimetidine* and possibly *disulfiram* causes diminished hepatic metabolism of lorazepam, which increases its plasma concentration.

Heavy smoking accelerates lorazepam's metabolism, thus lowering clinical effectiveness.

Combined use of parenteral lorazepam and *scopolamine* may be associated with an increased incidence of hallucinations, irrational behavior, and increased sedation.

Effects on diagnostic tests
Drug therapy may elevate liver function test results.

Adverse reactions
CNS: *drowsiness,* amnesia, insomnia, agitation, *sedation,* dizziness, weakness, unsteadiness, disorientation, depression, headache.
EENT: visual disturbances.
GI: abdominal discomfort, nausea, change in appetite.
Other: ***acute withdrawal syndrome*** (after sudden discontinuation in physically dependent persons).

Overdose and treatment
Clinical manifestations of overdose include somnolence, confusion, coma, hypoactive reflexes, dyspnea, labored breathing, hypotension, bradycardia, slurred speech, and unsteady gait or impaired coordination.

Treatment requires support of blood pressure and respiration until drug effects subside; monitor vital signs. Mechanical ventilatory assistance via endotracheal tube may be required to maintain a patent airway and support adequate oxygenation. Flumazenil, a specific benzodiazepine antagonist, may be useful. Use I.V. fluids and vasopressors such as dopamine and phenylephrine to treat hypotension, if necessary. If patient is conscious, induce emesis. Use gastric lavage if ingestion was recent, but only if an endotracheal tube is present to prevent aspiration. After emesis or lavage, administer activated charcoal with a cathartic as a single dose. Dialysis is of limited value.

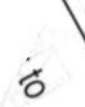

derations
...ant to all *benzodiazepines,* con-
...ving recommendations.
...pam is one of the preferred benzodi-
...pines for patients with hepatic disease.

- Use lowest possible effective dose to avoid oversedation.
- Parenteral lorazepam appears to possess potent amnestic effects.
- Administer oral drug in divided doses, with the largest dose given before bedtime.
- Arteriospasm may result from intra-arterial injection of lorazepam. Do not administer by this route.
- For I.V. administration, dilute lorazepam with an equal volume of a compatible diluent, such as D_5W, sterile water for injection, or 0.9% NaCl solution.
- Drug may be injected directly into a vein or into the tubing of a compatible I.V. infusion, such as 0.9% NaCl solution or D_5W solution. The rate of lorazepam I.V. injection should not exceed 2 mg/minute. Emergency resuscitative equipment should be available when administering I.V.
- Administer diluted lorazepam solutions immediately.
- Do not use drug solutions if they are discolored or contain a precipitate.
- Administer I.M. dose of lorazepam undiluted, deep into a large muscle mass.
- Periodically assess hepatic function studies to prevent cumulative effects and to ensure adequate drug metabolism.

Patient education

- Caution patient not to make changes in drug regimen without specific instructions.
- As appropriate, teach safety measures to protect from injury, such as gradual position changes and supervised walking.
- Advise patient of possible retrograde amnesia after I.V. or I.M. use.
- Tell patient to avoid large amounts of caffeine-containing products, which may interfere with drug's effectiveness.
- Advise patient of potential for physical and psychological dependence with chronic use.
- Tell patient to discontinue drug slowly (over 8 to 12 weeks) after long-term therapy.

Geriatric use

- Elderly patients are more sensitive to lorazepam's CNS depressant effects. They may require supervision with ambulation and activities of daily living during initiation of therapy or after an increase in dose.
- Lower doses usually are effective in elderly patients because of decreased elimination.
- Parenteral administration of drug is more likely to cause apnea, hypotension, bradycardia, and cardiac arrest in elderly patients.

Pediatric use

- Safe use of oral lorazepam in children under age 12 has not been established.
- Safe use of sublingual or parenteral lorazepam in children under age 18 has not been established.
- Closely observe neonate for withdrawal symptoms if mother took lorazepam for a prolonged period during pregnancy.

Breast-feeding

- Drug may be excreted in breast milk. Do not administer to breast-feeding women.

losartan potassium
Cozaar

Pharmacologic classification: angiotensin II receptor antagonist
Therapeutic classification: antihypertensive
Pregnancy risk category C (D second and third trimesters)

How supplied
Available by prescription only
Tablets: 25 mg, 50 mg

Indications, route, and dosage
Hypertension
Adults: Initially, 25 to 50 mg P.O. daily. Maintenance dosage is 25 to 100 mg P.O. once daily or b.i.d.

Pharmacodynamics
Antihypertensive action: Losartan is an angiotensin II receptor antagonist that blocks the vasoconstrictor and aldosterone-secreting effects of angiotensin II by selectively blocking the binding of angiotensin II to its receptor sites found in many tissues, including vascular smooth muscle.

Pharmacokinetics
- *Absorption:* Drug is well absorbed and undergoes substantial first-pass metabolism; systemic bioavailability is about 33%.
- *Distribution:* Both losartan and its active metabolite are highly bound to plasma proteins, primarily albumin.
- *Metabolism:* Cytochrome P-450 2C9 and 3A4 are involved in the biotransformation of drug to its metabolites.
- *Excretion:* Drug and its metabolites are primarily excreted in feces with a small amount excreted in urine.

Contraindications and precautions
Contraindicated in patients with hypersensitivity to drug. Use cautiously in patients with impaired renal or hepatic function.

Interactions
Concomitant administration of *cimetidine* increases bioavailability without affecting pharmacokinetics of active metabolite. Concomitant administration with *phenobarbital* decreases bioavailability of losartan and active metabolite.

Effects on diagnostic tests
None reported.

Adverse reactions
CNS: dizziness, insomnia.
GI: diarrhea, dyspepsia.
Musculoskeletal: muscle cramps, myalgia, back or leg pain.
Respiratory: nasal congestion, cough, upper respiratory infection, sinus disorder, sinusitis.

Overdose and treatment
The most likely manifestation is hypotension and tachycardia; bradycardia could occur from parasympathetic stimulation. If symptomatic hypotension occurs, supportive treatment should be initiated. Neither losartan nor its active metabolite can be removed by hemodialysis.

☑ Special considerations
- Drugs such as losartan that act directly on the renin-angiotensin system can cause fetal and neonatal morbidity and death when administered to pregnant women; these problems have not been detected when exposure has been limited to the first trimester. If pregnancy is suspected, drug should probably be discontinued.
- Use lowest dosage (25 mg) initially in patients with impaired hepatic function and in those who are intravascularly volume-depleted (receiving diuretic therapy).
- Drug can be used alone or in combination with other antihypertensive agents.
- If antihypertensive effect measured at trough (using once-daily dosing) is inadequate, a twice-daily regimen at the same total daily dose or an increased dose may give a more satisfactory response.
- Monitor patient taking diuretics concurrently in treatment of hypertension for symptomatic hypotension.
- Regularly assess patient's renal function (serum creatinine and BUN levels).
- Patients with severe heart failure whose renal function depends on the angiotensin-aldosterone system have experienced acute renal failure during therapy with ACE inhibitors. Manufacturer of losartan states that drug would be expected to do the same. Closely monitor patient, especially during first few weeks of therapy.

Patient education
- Instruct patient not to discontinue drug abruptly.
- Tell patient to avoid sodium substitutes; these products may contain potassium, which can cause hyperkalemia in patients taking losartan.
- Inform female patient of childbearing age about the consequences of second- and third-trimester exposure to losartan and instruct her to call immediately if pregnancy is suspected.

Pediatric use
- Safety and effectiveness in children have not been established.

Breast-feeding
- It is not known if drug is excreted in breast milk. Because of the potential for adverse effects on the breast-fed infant, a decision should be made whether to discontinue the drug or breast-feeding, taking into account the importance of drug to the mother.

lovastatin
Mevacor

Pharmacologic classification: lactone; HMG-CoA reductase inhibitor
Therapeutic classification: cholesterol-lowering agent
Pregnancy risk category X

How supplied
Available by prescription only
Tablets: 10 mg, 20 mg, 40 mg

Indications, route, and dosage
Reduction of low-density lipoprotein and total cholesterol levels in patients with primary hypercholesterolemia (types IIa and IIb), atherosclerosis
Adults: Initially, 20 mg once daily with evening meal. For patients with severely elevated cholesterol levels (for example, over 300 mg/dl), initial dose should be 40 mg. Recommended range is 20 to 80 mg in single or divided doses.

Pharmacodynamics
Antilipemic action: Lovastatin, an inactive lactone, is hydrolyzed to the beta-hydroxy acid, which specifically inhibits 3-hydroxy-3-methylglutaryl-coenzyme A reductase (HMG-CoA reductase). This enzyme is an early (and rate-limiting) step in the synthetic pathway of cholesterol. At therapeutic doses, the enzyme is not blocked, and biologically necessary amounts of cholesterol can still be synthesized.

Pharmacokinetics
- *Absorption:* Animal studies indicate that about 30% of an oral dose is absorbed. Administration of drug with food improves plasma concentrations of total inhibitors by about 30%. Onset of action is about 3 days, with maximal therapeutic effects seen in 4 to 6 weeks.
- *Distribution:* Less than 5% of an oral dose reaches the systemic circulation because of extensive first-pass hepatic extraction; the liver is the drug's principal site of action. Both the parent compound and its principal metabolite are highly bound (more than 95%) to plasma proteins. Animal studies indicate that lovastatin can cross the placenta and the blood-brain barrier.
- *Metabolism:* Drug is converted to the active B hydroxy acid form in the liver. Other metabolites include the 6' hydroxy derivative and two unidentified compounds.
- *Excretion:* About 80% of lovastatin is excreted primarily in feces, about 10% in urine.

Contraindications and precautions
Contraindicated in patients with hypersensitivity to drug, in those with active liver disease or conditions associated with unexplained persistent elevations of serum transaminase levels, in pregnant

and breast-feeding patients, and in women of childbearing age unless there is no risk of pregnancy.

Use cautiously in patients who consume excessive amounts of alcohol or have history of liver disease.

Interactions

Concomitant administration with *cholestyramine* or *colestipol* may enhance lipid-reducing effects but may decrease bioavailability of lovastatin. Concomitant administration of *cyclosporine, erythromycin, gemfibrozil,* or *niacin* may increase risk of severe myopathy or rhabdomyolysis. Lovastatin may increase the anticoagulant effects of *warfarin. Isradipine* may increase clearance of lovastatin and its metabolites. *Itraconazole* co-administration with lovastatin increases HMG-CoA reductase inhibitor levels. Therapy with lovastatin should be temporarily interrupted if *systemic azole antifungal treatment* is required.

Effects on diagnostic tests

Lovastatin may elevate serum CK or serum transaminase levels.

Adverse reactions

CNS: headache, dizziness, peripheral neuropathy, insomnia.
EENT: blurred vision.
GI: constipation, diarrhea, dyspepsia, flatulence, abdominal pain or cramps, heartburn, nausea, vomiting.
Skin: rash, pruritus, alopecia.
Other: muscle cramps, myalgia, myositis, ***rhabdomyolysis,*** elevated serum transaminase levels, abnormal liver test results, chest pain, photosensitivity.

Overdose and treatment

No information available.

☑ Special considerations

- Initiate drug therapy only after diet and other nonpharmacologic therapies have proven ineffective. Patient should be on a standard cholesterol-lowering diet and continue on this diet during therapy.
- Administer drug with evening meal; absorption is enhanced and cholesterol biosynthesis is greater in the evening.
- Therapeutic response occurs in about 2 weeks, with maximum effects in 4 to 6 weeks.
- Monitor for signs of myositis; have patient report muscle aches and pains.
- Perform liver function tests frequently during initiation of therapy and periodically thereafter.
- Store tablets at room temperature in a light-resistant container.
- Do not exceed 20 mg/day if patient is receiving immunosuppressive drugs.

Patient education

- Stress importance of lowering cholesterol.
- Advise patient to restrict alcohol intake.
- Instruct patient to take drug with evening meal.
- Tell patient to report adverse reactions, particularly muscle aches and pains, and to take precautions with exposure to sun and other ultraviolet light until tolerance is determined.

Pediatric use

- Safety and efficacy in children have not been established.

Breast-feeding

- An alternative feeding method is recommended during therapy with lovastatin.

loxapine hydrochloride

Loxitane C, Loxitane IM

loxapine succinate

Loxapac*, Loxitane

Pharmacologic classification: dibenzoxazepine
Therapeutic classification: antipsychotic
Pregnancy risk category NR

How supplied

Available by prescription only
Capsules: 5 mg, 10 mg, 25 mg, 50 mg
Oral concentrate: 25 mg/ml
Injection: 50 mg/ml

Indications, route, and dosage

Psychotic disorders

Adults: 10 mg P.O. b.i.d. to q.i.d., rapidly increasing to 60 to 100 mg P.O. daily for most patients (dose varies from patient to patient) or 12.5 to 50 mg I.M. q 4 to 6 hours. Maximum daily dosage, 250 mg. Do not administer drug I.V.

Pharmacodynamics

Antipsychotic action: Loxapine is the only tricyclic antipsychotic; it is structurally similar to amoxapine. Loxapine is thought to exert its antipsychotic effects by postsynaptic blockade of CNS dopamine receptors, thus inhibiting dopamine-mediated effects. Loxapine has many other central and peripheral effects; its most prominent adverse reactions are extrapyramidal.

Pharmacokinetics

- *Absorption:* Drug is absorbed rapidly and completely from the GI tract. Sedation occurs in 30 minutes.
- *Distribution:* Distributed widely into the body, including breast milk. Peak effect occurs at 1½ to 3 hours; steady-state serum level is achieved within 3 to 4 days. Drug is 91% to 99% protein-bound.
- *Metabolism:* Drug is metabolized extensively by the liver, forming a few active metabolites; duration of action is 12 hours.
- *Excretion:* Mostly excreted as metabolites in urine; some is excreted in feces via the biliary tract. About 50% of drug is excreted in urine and feces within 24 hours.

Contraindications and precautions

Contraindicated in patients with hypersensitivity to dibenzoxazepines and in patients experiencing coma, severe CNS depression, or drug-induced depressed states. Use cautiously in patients with seizure or CV disorders, glaucoma, or history of urine retention.

Interactions

Concomitant use of loxapine with *sympathomimetics*, including *epinephrine, phenylephrine, phenylpropanolamine*, and *ephedrine* (often found in nasal sprays), and with *appetite suppressants* may decrease their stimulatory and pressor effects. Loxapine may cause epinephrine reversal, an inhibition of epinephrine's vasopressor effect.

Loxapine may inhibit blood pressure response to *centrally acting antihypertensive drugs*, such as *clonidine, guanabenz, guanadrel, guanethidine, methyldopa*, and *reserpine*. Loxapine may antagonize therapeutic effect of *bromocriptine* on prolactin secretion; it may also decrease the vasoconstricting effects of high-dose *dopamine*, and may decrease effectiveness and increase toxicity of *levodopa* (by dopamine blockade).

Additive effects are likely after concomitant use of loxapine and *CNS depressants*, including *alcohol, analgesics, barbiturates, narcotics, tranquilizers, anesthetics* (general, spinal, and epidural), and *parenteral magnesium sulfate* (oversedation, respiratory depression, and hypotension); *antiarrhythmic agents, disopyramide, quinidine*, and *procainamide* (increased incidence of arrhythmias and conduction defects); *atropine* and *other anticholinergic drugs*, including *antidepressants, antihistamines, MAO inhibitors, meperidine, phenothiazines*, and *antiparkinson agents* (oversedation, paralytic ileus, visual changes, and severe constipation); and *nitrates* (hypotension).

Beta-blocking agents may inhibit loxapine metabolism, increasing plasma levels and toxicity.

Concomitant use with *lithium* may result in severe neurologic toxicity with an encephalitis-like syndrome and in decreased therapeutic response to loxapine. *Aluminum- and magnesium-containing antacids* and *antidiarrheals* decrease loxapine absorption and, thus, its therapeutic effects.

Effects on diagnostic tests

Drug causes false-positive test results for urinary porphyrins, urobilinogen, amylase, and 5-hydroxyindoleacetic acid (5-HIAA) because of darkening of urine by metabolites; it also causes false-positive urine pregnancy test results using human chorionic gonadotropin.

Loxapine elevates test results for liver enzymes and protein-bound iodine, and causes quinidine-like effects on the ECG.

Adverse reactions

CNS: *extrapyramidal reactions, sedation, drowsiness,* ***seizures***, numbness, confusion, syncope, *tardive dyskinesia*, pseudoparkinsonism, EEG changes, dizziness.
CV: *orthostatic hypotension,* ***tachycardia***, ECG changes, hypertension.
EENT: *blurred vision*, nasal congestion.
GI: *dry mouth, constipation*, nausea, vomiting, paralytic ileus.
GU: *urine retention*, menstrual irregularities, gynecomastia.
Hematologic: leukopenia, ***agranulocytosis, thrombocytopenia.***
Skin: *mild photosensitivity*, allergic reactions, rash, pruritus.
Other: weight gain, ***neuroleptic malignant syndrome,*** jaundice.

Overdose and treatment

CNS depression is characterized by deep, unarousable sleep and possible coma, hypotension or hypertension, extrapyramidal symptoms, abnormal involuntary muscle movements, agitation, seizures, arrhythmias, ECG changes, hypothermia or hyperthermia, and autonomic nervous system dysfunction.

Treatment is symptomatic and supportive, including maintaining vital signs, airway, stable body temperature, and fluid and electrolyte balance.

Do not induce vomiting: drug inhibits cough reflex, and aspiration may occur. Use gastric lavage, then activated charcoal and saline cathartics; hemodialysis may be helpful. Regulate body temperature as needed. Treat hypotension with I.V. fluids: do not give epinephrine. Treat seizures with parenteral diazepam or barbiturates; arrhythmias with parenteral phenytoin (1 mg/kg with rate titrated to blood pressure); and extrapyramidal reactions with benztropine at 1 to 2 mg or parenteral diphenhydramine at 10 to 50 mg.

☑ Special considerations

- Assess patient periodically for abnormal body movement.
- Tardive dyskinesia may occur, usually after prolonged use. It may not appear until months or years after treatment and may disappear spontaneously or persist for life.
- Avoid combining drug with alcohol or other depressants.
- Obtain baseline blood pressure measurements before starting therapy and monitor regularly.
- Dilute liquid concentrate with orange or grapefruit juice just before giving.
- Periodic ophthalmic tests are recommended.
- Dose of 10 mg is therapeutic equivalent of 100 mg chlorpromazine.
- Photosensitivity warnings may apply with loxapine.

Patient education

- Warn against activities that require alertness and good psychomotor coordination until CNS response to drug is determined. Drowsiness and dizziness usually subside after first few weeks.
- Recommend sugarless gum or candy, mouthwash, ice chips, or artificial saliva to help alleviate dry mouth.
- Advise patient to get up slowly to avoid orthostatic hypotension.

Geriatric use

- Elderly patients are highly sensitive to antimuscarinic, hypotensive, and sedative effects of drug and have a higher risk of developing extrapyramidal adverse reactions, such as parkinsonism and tardive dyskinesia. These patients develop higher plasma concentrations and therefore require lower initial dosage and more gradual titration.

Pediatric use

• Drug is not recommended for children under age 16.

lymphocyte immune globulin (antithymocyte globulin [equine], ATG)

Atgam

Pharmacologic classification: immunoglobulin
Therapeutic classification: immunosuppressive
Pregnancy risk category C

How supplied

Available by prescription only
Injection: 50 mg of equine IgG per ml, in 5-ml ampules

Indications, route, and dosage

Prevention of acute renal allograft rejection
Adults and children: 15 mg/kg/day I.V. for 14 days, then same dosage every other day for next 14 days (to a total of 21 doses in 28 days). The first dose of ATG should be administered within 24 hours before or after transplantation.

Treatment of acute renal allograft rejection
Adults and children: 10 to 15 mg/kg/day for 14 days; if necessary, same dosage may be given every other day for another 14 days (to a total of 21 doses in 28 days). Therapy with ATG should begin at the first sign of acute rejection.

Aplastic anemia
Adults and children: 10 to 20 mg/kg I.V. daily for 8 to 14 days, followed by alternate day therapy for an additional 14 days (total of 21 doses in 28 days).

◊ ***Skin allotransplantation***
Adults: 10 mg/kg 24 hours before allograft; then 10 to 15 mg/kg every other day. Maintenance dosage is variable and can range from 5 to 40 mg/ kg/day, based on clinical response and clinical indicators of immunosuppressive activity. Therapy usually continues until allografts cover less than 20% of total body surface area; often, this requires 40 to 60 days of treatment.

Bone marrow allotransplantation; ◊ ***graft-versus-host disease after bone marrow transplantation***
Adults: 7 to 10 mg/kg I.V. every other day for six doses.

◊ ***Agranulocytosis***
Adults: 100 g over a 30-month period.

Pharmacodynamics

Immunosuppressive action: The exact mechanism has not been fully defined but may involve elimination of antigen-reactive T cells (T lymphocytes) in peripheral blood or alteration of T-cell function. The effects of antilymphocyte preparations, including ATG, on T cells are variable and complex. Whether the effects of ATG are mediated through a specific subset of T cells has not been determined.

Pharmacokinetics

• *Absorption:* Peak plasma levels of equine IgG after I.V. administration of ATG vary, depending on patient's ability to catabolize foreign IgG.
• *Distribution:* Distribution of ATG into body fluids and tissues has not been fully described. Because antilymphocyte serum reportedly is poorly distributed into lymphoid tissues (for example, spleen, lymph nodes), it is likely that ATG is also poorly distributed into these tissues.

No information is available on transplacental distribution of ATG. However, such distribution is likely because other immunoglobulins cross the placenta. Virtually all transplacental passage of immunoglobulins occurs during the last 4 weeks of pregnancy.

• *Metabolism:* Not known.
• *Excretion:* Plasma half-life of equine IgG reportedly averages about 6 days (range 1.5 to 13 days). Approximately 1% of a dose of ATG is excreted in urine, principally as unchanged equine IgG. In one report, mean urinary concentration of equine IgG was approximately 4 mcg/ml after approximately 21 doses of ATG over 28 days.

Contraindications and precautions

Contraindicated in patients hypersensitive to drug. An intradermal skin test is recommended at least 1 hour before first dose. Marked local swelling or erythema larger than 10 mm indicates an increased potential for severe systemic reaction, such as anaphylaxis. Severe reactions to skin test, such as hypotension, tachycardia, dyspnea, generalized rash, or anaphylaxis, usually preclude further administration of drug.

Use cautiously in patients receiving other immunosuppressive medications, such as corticosteroids or azathioprine.

Interactions

Concomitant use of ATG with other *immunosuppressive therapy (azathioprine, corticosteroids, graft irradiation),* may intensify immunosuppression, an effect that can be used to therapeutic advantage; however, such therapy may increase vulnerability to infection and possibly the risk of lymphoma or lymphoproliferative disorders.

Effects on diagnostic tests

None reported.

Adverse reactions

CNS: malaise, ***seizures***, *headache.*
CV*:* ***hypotension,*** chest pain, thrombophlebitis, tachycardia, edema, iliac vein obstruction, renal artery stenosis.
EENT: ***laryngospasm.***
GI: *nausea, vomiting, diarrhea,* hiccups, epigastric pain, abdominal distention, stomatitis.
Hematologic: LEUKOPENIA, THROMBOCYTOPENIA, ***hemolysis, aplastic anemia.***

Hepatic: elevated liver enzyme level.
Respiratory: *dyspnea, **pulmonary edema.***
Skin: *rash, pruritus, urticaria.*
Other: *febrile reactions,* serum sickness, ***anaphylaxis***, *infections,* night sweats, lymphadenopathy, hyperglycemia, *chills, myalgia, arthralgia.*

Overdose and treatment

No information available.

☑ Special considerations

- Dilute drug concentrate for injection before I.V. infusion. Dilute required dose of ATG in 0.9% NaCl or 0.45% NaCl injection (usually 250 to 1,000 ml); final concentration preferably should not exceed 1 mg of equine IgG per ml. Infuse over at least 4 hours.
- Infusion in dextrose or highly acidic solutions is not recommended.
- Invert I.V. infusion solution container into which ATG concentrate is added to prevent contact of undiluted ATG with air inside the container. Refrigerate diluted solutions of ATG at 36° to 46° F (2° to 8° C) if administration is delayed. Reconstituted solutions should not be used after 12 hours (including actual infusion time), even if stored at 36° to 46° F.
- Because of risk of severe systemic reaction (anaphylaxis), manufacturer recommends an intradermal skin test before administration of initial dose of ATG. The skin test procedure consists of intradermal injection of 0.1 ml of a 1:1,000 dilution of ATG concentrate for injection in 0.9% NaCl injection (5 mcg of equine IgG). A control test using 0.9% NaCl injection should be administered in the other arm to facilitate interpretation of the results. If a wheal or area of erythema exceeding 10 mm in diameter (with or without pseudopod formation) and itching or marked local swelling develops, infusion of ATG requires extreme caution; severe and potentially fatal systemic reactions can occur in patients with a positive skin test. A systemic reaction to the skin test such as generalized rash, tachycardia, dyspnea, hypotension, or anaphylaxis rules out further administration of ATG. The predictive value of the ATG skin test has not been clearly established, and an allergic reaction may occur despite a negative skin test.
- Anaphylaxis may occur at any time during drug therapy and may be indicated by hypotension, respiratory distress, or pain in the chest, flank, or back.
- The manufacturer has not yet determined the total number of ATG doses (10 to 20 mg/kg per dose) that can be administered safely to a patient. Some renal allograft recipients have received up to 50 doses in 4 months; others, up to four 28-day courses of 21 doses each without an increased incidence of adverse effects.
- Drug has been used to treat aplastic anemia, and as an adjunct in bone marrow and skin allotransplantation.
- Observe patient receiving drug for signs of leukopenia, thrombocytopenia, and concurrent infection.
- To minimize risks of leukopenia and infection, some clinicians recommend that azathioprine and corticosteroid dosages be reduced by 50% when ATG is used concomitantly with these drugs for the prevention or treatment of renal allograft rejection.
- Monitor patients for signs of infection during ATG therapy.
- Some clinicians elect to administer prophylactic platelet transfusion in patients receiving drug for aplastic anemia because of high risk of thrombocytopenia.

Patient education

- Warn patient that a febrile reaction is likely.

Pediatric use

- Safety and efficacy in children have not been established. Drug has had limited use in children age 3 months to 19 years.

Breast-feeding

- Although it is unknown if drug occurs in breast milk, other immunoglobulins are distributed into breast milk. Breast-feeding women should consider an alternative feeding method.

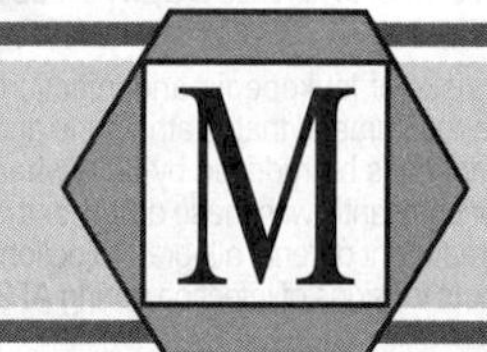

mafenide
Sulfamylon

Pharmacologic classification: synthetic anti-infective
Therapeutic classification: topical antibacterial
Pregnancy risk category C

How supplied
Available by prescription only
Cream: 8.5%

Indications, route, and dosage
Adjunctive treatment of second- and third-degree burns
Adults and children: Apply a thickness of 1/16″ with a sterile gloved hand daily or b.i.d. to cleaned, debrided wounds. Reapply p.r.n. to keep burned area covered.

Pharmacodynamics
Antibacterial action: Mechanism of action is undetermined; however, it appears that drug interferes with bacterial cellular metabolism. Mafenide has a wide spectrum of activity and is bacteriostatic against many gram-negative and gram-positive organisms, including *Pseudomonas aeruginosa,* and several strains of anaerobes.

Pharmacokinetics
- *Absorption:* Drug diffuses through devascularized areas and is absorbed quickly.
- *Distribution:* Drug is distributed rapidly after topical application.
- *Metabolism:* Drug is metabolized rapidly to a weak carbonic anhydrase inhibitor metabolite.
- *Excretion:* Excreted in the urine.

Contraindications and precautions
No known contraindications. Use cautiously in burn patients with renal failure or pulmonary dysfunction and in those with sensitivity to drug or sulfonamides.

Interactions
None reported.

Effects on diagnostic tests
None reported.

Adverse reactions
Hematologic: eosinophilia, bone marrow depression, DIC.
Respiratory: tachypnea, decreased $Paco_2$.
Skin: pain, *burning sensation,* rash, pruritus, swelling, urticaria, blisters, erythema.
Other: *metabolic acidosis,* facial edema.

Overdose and treatment
Accidental ingestion may cause diarrhea. To treat local overapplication, discontinue drug and clean skin thoroughly.

☑ Special considerations
- Apply to clean, debrided wound with sterile gloved hand, covering wound to approximately 1/16″; reapply to areas if removed. Keep burned areas covered with cream at all times. Dressings usually are not required; if necessary, apply only a thin layer of dressing.
- Patient should be bathed daily to aid debridement; prior layer of cream should be removed before reapplication; whirlpool baths are extremely effective.
- Continue treatment until site is healed or ready for grafting.
- Monitor patient for overgrowth of nonsusceptible organisms; severe prolonged pain may indicate allergy.
- Monitor acid-base balance closely, especially in patients with pulmonary or renal dysfunction; if metabolic acidosis develops, discontinue drug for 24 to 48 hours.

Patient education
- Instruct patient in proper care of burn sites; stress importance of calling promptly if condition worsens or adverse reactions occur.

Breast-feeding
- It is not known if drug is excreted in breast milk. Because of potential for adverse effects, a decision should be made whether to discontinue breast-feeding or drug.

magaldrate (aluminum magnesium hydroxide)
Iosopan, Lowsium, Magaldrate, Riopan

Pharmacologic classification: aluminum-magnesium salt
Therapeutic classification: antacid
Pregnancy risk category C

How supplied
Available without a prescription
Tablets: 480 mg
Tablets (chewable): 480 mg
Suspension: 540 mg/5 ml

Indications, route, and dosage
Indigestion or hyperacidity associated with peptic ulcer, gastritis, peptic esophagitis, hiatal hernia
Adults: 5 to 10 ml (suspension) between meals and h.s. with water.

For oral form, 480 to 960 mg (tablets) P.O. with water between meals and h.s.; or 1 to 2 chewable tablets (chewed before swallowing) between meals and h.s.

Pharmacodynamics
Antacid action: Magaldrate neutralizes gastric acid, reducing the direct acid irritant effect. This increases gastric pH, which inactivates pepsin. Magaldrate also enhances mucosal barrier integrity and improves gastroesophageal sphincter tone.

Pharmacokinetics
- *Absorption:* Aluminum may be absorbed systemically. Magnesium also may be absorbed, posing a risk to patients with renal failure. Absorption is unrelated to mechanism of action.
- *Distribution:* Primarily local.
- *Metabolism:* None.
- *Excretion:* Excreted in feces; some aluminum and magnesium may be excreted in breast milk. Duration of action is prolonged.

Contraindications and precautions
Contraindicated in patients with severe renal disease. Use cautiously in patients with mild renal impairment.

Interactions
When used concomitantly, magaldrate may increase *levodopa* absorption, increasing risk of toxicity.

Drug may inhibit absorption of *phenothiazines* (especially *chlorpromazine*) and may decrease absorption of *anticoagulants, antimuscarinics, coumadin chenodiol, chlordiazepoxide, diazepam, digoxin, isoniazid, phosphates, quinolones, tetracycline,* and *vitamin A* thus lessening their effectiveness.

Magaldrate also may cause premature release of *enterically coated drugs.* Separate use of magaldrate and all oral drugs by 1 to 2 hours.

Effects on diagnostic tests
Drug may antagonize pentagastrin's effect during gastric acid secretion tests; drug may decrease serum potassium levels, and increase serum gastrin and urine pH levels.

Adverse reactions
GI: mild constipation, diarrhea.

Overdose and treatment
No information available.

☑ Special considerations
- Shake suspension well; give with small amounts of water or fruit juice.
- After administration through nasogastric tube, flush tube with water to clear it and ensure drug's passage to stomach.
- Give drug at least 1 hour apart from enterically coated medications.
- Suspension contains saccharin and sorbitol; chewable tablets contain sorbitol.
- Monitor renal function and serum phosphate, potassium, and magnesium levels in patients with renal disease.
- Most formulations contain less than 0.5 mg of sodium per tablet (or 5 ml of liquid).

Patient education
- Caution patient to take drug only as directed and 1 or 2 hours apart from other oral medications.
- Remind patient to shake suspension well or to chew tablets thoroughly.
- Warn patient not to take more than 18 teaspoonfuls or 20 tablets in a 24-hour period.

Pediatric use
- Use of drug as an antacid in children under age 6 requires a well-established diagnosis because children typically give vague descriptions of symptoms.

Breast-feeding
- Some aluminum and magnesium may be excreted in breast milk. However, no problems have been associated with use in breast-feeding women.

magnesium hydroxide (milk of magnesia)
Milk of Magnesia, Phillips' Milk of Magnesia, Concentrated Philips' Milk of Magnesia

Pharmacologic classification: magnesium salt
Therapeutic classification: antacid, antiulcer agent, laxative
Pregnancy risk category NR

How supplied
Available without a prescription
Tablets: 300 mg, 600 mg
Tablets (chewable): 311 mg
Liquid: 400 mg/5 ml, 800 mg/5 ml
Suspension (concentrated): 10 ml (equivalent to 30 ml of milk of magnesia)
Suspension: 77.5 mg/g

Indications, route, and dosage
Constipation, bowel evacuation before surgery
Adults and children over age 6: 10 to 20 ml concentrated milk of magnesia P.O.; 15 to 60 ml milk of magnesia P.O.
Laxative
Adults: 30 to 60 ml P.O., usually h.s.
Children age 6 to 12: 15 to 30 ml P.O.
Children age 2 to 6: 5 to 15 ml P.O.
Antacid
Adults: 5 to 15 ml (liquid) P.O. p.r.n., up to q.i.d.; 2.5 to 7.5 ml (liquid concentrate) P.O. p.r.n., up to q.i.d.; 2 to 4 tablets P.O. p.r.n., up to q.i.d.
Children: 2.5 to 5 ml P.O. p.r.n.

Pharmacodynamics

Antiulcer action: Magnesium hydroxide neutralizes gastric acid, decreasing the direct acid irritant effect. This increases pH, which, in turn, leads to pepsin inactivation. Magnesium hydroxide also enhances mucosal barrier integrity and improves gastric and esophageal sphincter tone.

Antacid action: Drug reacts rapidly with hydrochloric acid in the stomach to form magnesium chloride and water.

Laxative action: Magnesium hydroxide produces its laxative effect by increasing the osmotic gradient in the gut and drawing in water, causing distention that stimulates peristalsis and bowel evacuation.

Pharmacokinetics

- *Absorption:* About 15% to 30% of magnesium may be absorbed systemically (posing a potential risk to patients with renal failure).
- *Distribution:* None.
- *Metabolism:* None.
- *Excretion:* Unabsorbed drug is excreted in feces; absorbed drug is excreted rapidly in urine.

Contraindications and precautions

Contraindicated in patients with abdominal pain, nausea, vomiting, or other symptoms of appendicitis or acute surgical abdomen and in those with myocardial damage, heart block, fecal impaction, rectal fissures, intestinal obstruction or perforation, renal disease, and patients about to deliver.

Use cautiously in patients with rectal bleeding.

Interactions

When used concomitantly, magnesium hydroxide may decrease absorption of *quinolones* and *tetracyclines* and may cause premature release of *enterically coated drugs.*

Concomitant use of magnesium hydroxide with *aluminum hydroxide* may decrease the absorption rate and extent of *chlordiazepoxide, chlorpromazine, dicumarol, digoxin, iron salts,* and *isoniazid.* Absorption of *buffered or enteric-coated aspirin* is increased by simultaneous administration.

Effects on diagnostic tests

None reported.

Adverse reactions

GI: *abdominal cramping, nausea, diarrhea,* laxative dependence (with long-term or excessive use).
Other: fluid and electrolyte disturbances (with daily use).

Overdose and treatment

No information available.

☑ Special considerations

- Give drug at least 1 hour apart from enterically coated medications; shake suspension well.
- After administration of the drug through nasogastric tube, tube should be flushed with water to clear it.
- Monitor for signs and symptoms of hypermagnesemia, especially if patient has impaired renal function.

Patient education

- Caution patient to avoid overuse to prevent laxative dependence.
- Instruct patient to shake suspension well or to chew tablets well.

Pediatric use

- Use of drug as an antacid in children under age 6 needs a well-established diagnosis because children tend to give vague descriptions of symptoms.

Breast-feeding

- Some magnesium may be excreted in breast milk, but no problems have been reported with use by breast-feeding women.

magnesium salicylate

Doan's Extra Strength Caplets, Doan's Regular Caplets, Magan, Mobidin

Pharmacologic classification: salicylate
Therapeutic classification: nonnarcotic analgesic, antipyretic, anti-inflammatory
Pregnancy risk category C

How supplied

Available by prescription only
Tablets: 545 mg, 600 mg

Available without a prescription
Tablets: 325 mg, 500 mg

Indications, route, and dosage

Arthritis
Adults: 545 mg to 1.2 g t.i.d. or q.i.d.
Analgesia and antipyresis
Adults and children over age 11: 300 to 600 mg P.O. q 4 hours p.r.n.
Analgesia (self-medicated)
Adults and children over age 11: 500 mg to 1 g P.O. initially, then 500 mg q 4 hours p.r.n., not to exceed 3.5 g in 24 hours. Absorption of buffered or enteric-coated aspirin is increased by simultaneous administration. Use with caution in children; may receive the following doses q 4 hours p.r.n., not to exceed five doses in 24 hours.
Children age 11: 450 mg P.O.
Children age 9 to 10: 375 mg P.O.
Children age 6 to 8: 300 mg P.O.
Children age 4 to 5: 225 mg P.O.
Children age 2 to 3: 150 mg P.O.
Children below age 2: must be individualized.

Pharmacodynamics

Analgesic action: Drug produces analgesia by an ill-defined effect on the hypothalamus (central action) and by blocking generation of pain impulses (peripheral action). The peripheral action may involve inhibition of prostaglandin synthesis.

Anti-inflammatory action: Drug is thought to exert its anti-inflammatory effect by inhibiting prostaglandin synthesis; it may also inhibit the synthesis or action of other mediators of inflammation.

Antipyretic action: Drug relieves fever by acting on the hypothalamic heat-regulating center to produce peripheral vasodilation. This increases peripheral blood supply and promotes sweating, which leads to loss of heat and to cooling by evaporation.

Pharmacokinetics

- *Absorption:* Magnesium salicylate is absorbed rapidly and completely from the GI tract.
- *Distribution:* Drug is highly protein-bound.
- *Metabolism:* Drug is hydrolyzed in the liver.
- *Excretion:* Metabolites are excreted in urine.

Contraindications and precautions

Contraindicated in patients with hypersensitivity to drug, salicylates, or NSAIDs or those with severe chronic renal insufficiency because of risk of magnesium toxicity. Also contraindicated in patients with bleeding disorders. Use cautiously in patients with hypoprothrombinemia or vitamin K deficiency.

Interactions

Anticoagulants and *thrombolytic drugs* may to some degree potentiate the platelet-inhibiting effects of magnesium salicylate. Monitor therapy closely for both drugs. Concomitant use of magnesium salicylate with *drugs that are highly protein-bound* (such as *phenytoin, sulfonylureas, warfarin*) may cause displacement of either drug, and adverse effects. Monitor therapy closely for both drugs. Concomitant use with other *GI-irritant drugs (antibiotics, steroids, other NSAIDs)* may potentiate the adverse GI effects of magnesium salicylate. Use together with caution.

Ammonium chloride and *other urine acidifiers* increase magnesium salicylate blood levels; monitor for magnesium salicylate toxicity. *Antacids in high doses*, and other *urine alkalizers*, decrease magnesium salicylate blood levels; monitor for decreased salicylate effect. *Corticosteroids* enhance magnesium salicylate elimination.

Food and *antacids* delay and decrease absorption of magnesium salicylate.

Effects on diagnostic tests

High doses of drug may cause false-positive urine glucose test results using copper sulfate method; it may cause false-negative urine glucose test results using glucose enzymatic method. False increases or decreases have been seen in urine vanillylmandelic acid tests; false increases in serum uric acid have been seen. Magnesium salicylate may interfere with the Gerhardt test for urine aceto-acetic acid. Drug may increase serum levels of AST, ALT, alkaline phosphatase, and bilirubin.

Adverse reactions

EENT: *tinnitus, hearing loss.*
GI: *nausea, vomiting, GI distress.*
Hepatic: abnormal liver function studies, hepatitis.
Skin: *rash*, bruising.
Other: hypersensitivity reactions (***anaphylaxis***, asthma), ***Reye's syndrome.***

Overdose and treatment

Clinical manifestations of overdose include metabolic acidosis with respiratory alkalosis, hyperpnea, and tachypnea from increased carbon dioxide production and direct stimulation of the respiratory center.

To treat overdose of magnesium salicylate, empty stomach immediately by inducing emesis with ipecac syrup if patient is conscious, or by gastric lavage. Administer activated charcoal via nasogastric tube. Provide symptomatic and supportive measures, such as respiratory support and correction of fluid and electrolyte imbalances. Monitor laboratory parameters and vital signs closely. Alkaline diuresis may enhance renal excretion.

☑ Special considerations

Besides those relevant to all *salicylates*, consider the following recommendations.

- Drug has been associated with a lower incidence of GI disturbances.
- Drug has a less profound effect on inhibiting platelet aggregation than other salicylates.
- Obtain hemoglobin and PT tests periodically.
- Monitor serum magnesium levels to prevent magnesium toxicity, especially in patients with renal insufficiency.

Patient education

- Instruct patient to follow prescribed regimen and to report problems.
- Advise patient not to take drug longer than 10 days without medical supervision.
- Caution patient to keep drug out of children's reach.

Geriatric use

- Patients over age 60 may be more susceptible to the toxic effects of this drug. Use with caution.
- The effects of salicylates on renal prostaglandins may cause fluid retention and edema, a significant drawback for elderly patients and those with heart failure.

Pediatric use

- Safety of long-term magnesium salicylate use in children has not been established.
- Because of epidemiologic association with Reye's syndrome, the Centers for Disease Control and Prevention recommends that children with chickenpox or flulike symptoms should not be given salicylates.
- Febrile, dehydrated children can develop toxicity rapidly.

Breast-feeding

- Salicylates are distributed in breast milk; avoid use in breast-feeding women.

magnesium sulfate

Pharmacologic classification: mineral/electrolyte
Therapeutic classification: anticonvulsant
Pregnancy risk category A

How supplied

Injectable solutions: 10%, 12.5%, 20%, 50% in

2-ml, 5-ml, 8 ml, 10-ml, 20-ml, 30-ml, and 50-ml ampules, vials, and prefilled syringes

Indications, route, and dosage

Hypomagnesemic seizures

Adults: 1 to 2 g (as 10% solution) I.V. over 15 minutes, then 1 g I.M. q 4 to 6 hours, based on patient's response and magnesium blood levels.

Seizures secondary to hypomagnesemia in acute nephritis

Children: 0.2 ml/kg of 50% solution I.M. q 4 to 6 hours, p.r.n., or 100 mg/kg of 10% solution I.V. given slowly. Titrate dosage according to magnesium blood levels and seizure response.

Life-threatening arrhythmias

Adults: For patient with sustained ventricular tachycardia or torsades de pointes, give 2 to 6 g I.V. over several minutes followed by 3 to 20 mg/minute I.V. infusion for 5 to 48 hours depending on patient response and serum magnesium concentrations. For patients with paroxysmal atrial tachycardia, give 3 to 4 g I.V. over 30 seconds.

Prevention or control of seizures in preeclampsia or eclampsia

Adults: Initially, 4 g I.V. in 250 ml D_5W and 4 to 5 g deep I.M. each buttock; then 4 g deep I.M. into alternate buttock q 4 hours, p.r.n. Alternatively, 4 g I.V. as a loading dose followed by 1 to 2 g hourly as an I.V. infusion. Maximum daily dose, 40 g.

Barium poisoning, ◊ asthma

Adults: 1 to 2 g I.V.

Mild hypomagnesemia

Adults: 1 g I.M. q 4 to 6 hours; or 5 g in 1 L of D_5W or dextrose 5% in 0.9% NaCl solution I.V. over 3 hours.

Pharmacodynamics

Anticonvulsant action: Magnesium sulfate has CNS and respiratory depressant effects. It acts peripherally, causing vasodilation; moderate doses cause flushing and sweating, whereas high doses cause hypotension. It prevents or controls seizures by blocking neuromuscular transmission.

Drug is sometimes used in pregnant women to prevent or control preeclamptic or eclamptic seizures; it also is used to treat hypomagnesemic seizures in adults, and in children with acute nephritis.

Pharmacokinetics

- *Absorption:* I.V. magnesium sulfate acts immediately; effects last about 30 minutes. After I.M. injection, it acts within 60 minutes and lasts for 3 to 4 hours. Effective anticonvulsant serum levels are 2.5 to 7.5 mEq/L.
- *Distribution:* Magnesium sulfate is distributed widely throughout the body.
- *Metabolism:* None.
- *Excretion:* Excreted unchanged in urine; some is excreted in breast milk.

Contraindications and precautions

Parenteral administration of drug contraindicated in patients with heart block or myocardial damage. Use cautiously in patients with impaired renal function and in women in labor. Do not give in toxemia of pregnancy during the two hours preceding delivery.

Interactions

Concomitant use with *alcohol, antidepressants, antipsychotics, anxiolytics, barbiturates, general anesthetics, hypnotics,* or *narcotics* may increase CNS depressant effects; reduced dosages may be required. Concomitant use of magnesium sulfate with succinylcholine or tubocurarine potentiates and prolongs neuromuscular blocking action of these drugs; use with caution.

Extreme caution should be used when magnesium sulfate is used concomitantly with *cardiac glycosides*; changes in cardiac conduction in digitalized patients may lead to heart block if I.V. calcium is administered.

Effects on diagnostic tests

None reported.

Adverse reactions

CNS: drowsiness, *depressed reflexes,* flaccid paralysis, hypothermia.
CV: *hypotension, flushing,* ***circulatory collapse***, depressed cardiac function.
Other: diaphoresis, ***respiratory paralysis***, hypocalcemia.

Overdose and treatment

Clinical manifestations of overdose with magnesium sulfate include a sharp drop in blood pressure and respiratory paralysis, ECG changes (increased PR, QRS, and QT intervals), heart block, and asystole.

Treatment requires artificial ventilation and I.V. calcium salt to reverse respiratory depression and heart block. Usual dosage is 5 to 10 mEq of calcium (10 to 20 ml of a 10% calcium gluconate solution).

☑ Special considerations

- I.V. bolus must be injected slowly (to avoid respiratory or cardiac arrest).
- If available, administer by constant infusion pump; maximum infusion rate is 150 mg/minute. Rapid drip causes feeling of heat.
- Discontinue drug as soon as needed effect is achieved.
- Concentration of magnesium sulfate for I.V. administration should not exceed 20% at a rate no greater than 150 mg/minute (1.5 ml of a 10% concentration or equivalent). For I.M. administration in adults, concentrations of 25% or 50% are generally used; in infants and children, concentrations should not exceed 20%.
- When giving repeated doses, test knee jerk reflex before each dose; if absent, discontinue magnesium. Use of drug beyond this point risks respiratory center failure.
- Respiratory rate must be 16 breaths per minute or more before each dose. Keep I.V. calcium salts on hand.
- To calculate grams of magnesium in a percentage of solution: X% = X g/100 ml (for example, 25% = 25 g/100 ml = 250 mg/ml).

• Monitor serum magnesium load and clinical status to avoid overdose.
• After use in toxemic women within 24 hours before delivery, watch newborn for signs of magnesium toxicity, including neuromuscular and respiratory depression.

Pediatric use
• Drug is not indicated for pediatric use.

Breast-feeding
• Drug is excreted in breast milk; in patients with normal renal function, all magnesium sulfate is excreted within 24 hours of discontinuing drug. Alternative feeding method is recommended during therapy.

mannitol
Osmitrol, Resectisol

Pharmacologic classification: osmotic diuretic
Therapeutic classification: diuretic, prevention and management of acute renal failure or oliguria, reduction of intracranial or intraocular pressure, treatment of drug intoxication
Pregnancy risk category C

How supplied
Available by prescription only
Injection: 5%, 10%, 15%, 20%, 25%
Urogenital solution: 5 g/100 ml distilled water

Indications, route, and dosage
Test dose for marked oliguria or suspected inadequate renal function
Adults and children over age 12: 200 mg/kg or 12.5 g as a 15% or 20% solution I.V. over 3 to 5 minutes. Response is adequate if 30 to 50 ml urine/hour is excreted over 2 to 3 hours.
◊ *Children under age 12:* 0.2 g/kg or 6 g/m² I.V. over 3 to 5 minutes.
Treatment of oliguria
Adults and children over age 12: 50 to 100 g as a 15% to 20% solution I.V. over 90 minutes to several hours.
Children under age 12: 2 g/kg or 60 g/m² I.V.
Prevention of oliguria or acute renal failure
Adults and children over age 12: 50 to 100 g followed by a 5% to 10% solution I.V. Exact concentration is determined by fluid requirements.
Treatment of edema and ascites
Adults and children over age 12: 100 g as a 10% to 20% solution I.V. over 2 to 6 hours.
◊ *Children under age 12:* 2 g/kg or 60 g/m² I.V. as a 15% to 20% solution over 2 to 6 hours.
To reduce intraocular pressure or intracranial pressure
Adults and children over age 12: 1.5 to 2 g/kg as a 15% to 25% solution I.V. over 30 to 60 minutes administered 60 to 90 minutes before surgery.
◊ *Children under age 12:* 2 g/kg or 60 g/m² I.V. as a 15% to 20% solution over 30 to 60 minutes.
To promote diuresis in drug intoxication
Adults and children over age 12: 25 g loading dose followed by an infusion maintaining 100 to 500 ml urine output/hour and positive fluid balance. For patients with barbiturate poisoning, give 0.5 g/kg followed by a 5% to 10% solution.
◊ *Children under age 12:* 5% to 10% solution to maintain a 100 to 500 ml urine output/hour and positive fluid balance.
Urologic irrigation
Adults: 2.5% solution.

Pharmacodynamics
Diuretic action: Mannitol increases the osmotic pressure of glomerular filtrate, inhibiting tubular reabsorption of water and electrolytes, thus promoting diuresis. This action also promotes urinary elimination of certain drugs. This effect is useful for prevention and management of acute renal failure or oliguria. This action is also useful for reduction of intracranial or intraocular pressure because mannitol elevates plasma osmolality, enhancing flow of water into extracellular fluid.

Pharmacokinetics
• *Absorption:* Drug is not absorbed from the GI tract. I.V. mannitol lowers intracranial pressure in 15 minutes and intraocular pressure in 30 to 60 minutes; it produces diuresis in 1 to 3 hours.
• *Distribution:* Mannitol remains in the extracellular compartment. It does not cross the blood-brain barrier.
• *Metabolism:* Metabolized minimally to glycogen in the liver.
• *Excretion:* Drug is filtered by the glomeruli; half-life in adults with normal renal function is about 100 minutes.

Contraindications and precautions
Contraindicated in patients with hypersensitivity to drug and in those with anuria, severe pulmonary congestion, frank pulmonary edema, severe heart failure, severe dehydration, metabolic edema, progressive renal disease or dysfunction, or active intracranial bleeding except during craniotomy. Use cautiously in pregnant patients.

Interactions
Mannitol may enhance renal excretion of *lithium* and lower serum lithium levels. Concurrent use with *cardiac glycosides* may enhance the possibility of digitalis toxicity. Mannitol may increase the effects of other *diuretics*, including *carbonic anhydrase inhibitors*.

Effects on diagnostic tests
Drug therapy alters electrolyte balance. It also may interfere with tests for inorganic phosphorus concentration or blood ethylene glycol.

Adverse reactions
CNS: ***seizures,*** dizziness, headache.
CV: edema, thrombophlebitis, hypotension, hypertension, ***heart failure,*** tachycardia, angina-like chest pain.
EENT: blurred vision, rhinitis, dry mouth.

GI: thirst, nausea, vomiting, *diarrhea*.
GU: urine retention.
Other: fluid and electrolyte imbalance, dehydration, local pain, fever, chills, urticaria.

Overdose and treatment
Clinical manifestations of overdose include polyuria, cellular dehydration, hypotension, and CV collapse.

Discontinue infusion and institute supportive measures. Hemodialysis removes mannitol and decreases serum osmolality.

☑ Special considerations
Besides those relevant to all *osmotic diuretics*, consider the following recommendations.
- Use with extreme caution in patients with compromised renal function; monitor vital signs (including CVP) hourly and input and output, weight, renal function, fluid balance, and serum and urinary sodium and potassium levels daily.
- For maximum pressure reduction during surgery, give drug 1 to 1½ hours preoperatively.
- Drug should be administered I.V. via an in-line filter, with great care to avoid extravasation.
- Do not administer with whole blood; agglutination will occur.
- Mannitol solutions commonly crystallize at low temperatures; place crystallized solutions in a hot water bath, shake vigorously to dissolve crystals, and cool to body temperature before use. Do not use solutions with undissolved crystals.

Patient education
- Tell patient he may feel thirsty or experience mouth dryness, and emphasize importance of drinking only the amount of fluids provided.
- With initial doses, warn patient to change position slowly, especially when rising from lying or sitting position, to prevent dizziness from orthostatic hypotension.
- Instruct patient to immediately report pain in the chest, back, or legs; shortness of breath; or apnea.

Geriatric use
- Elderly or debilitated patients will require close observation and may require lower dosages. Excessive diuresis promotes rapid dehydration, leading to hypovolemia, hypokalemia, and hyponatremia.

Pediatric use
- Dosage for children under age 12 has not been established.

Breast-feeding
- Safety of drug in breast-feeding women has not been established.

measles, mumps, and rubella virus vaccine, live
M-M-R II

Pharmacologic classification: vaccine
Therapeutic classification: viral vaccine
Pregnancy risk category C

How supplied
Available by prescription only
Injection: Single-dose vial containing not less than 1,000 $TCID_{50}$ (tissue culture infective doses) of attenuated measles virus derived from Enders' attenuated Edmonston strain (grown in chick embryo culture); 20,000 $TCID_{50}$ of the Jeryl Lynn (B level) mumps strain (grown in chick embryo culture); and 1,000 $TCID_{50}$ of the Wistar RA 27/3 strain of rubella virus (propagated in human diploid cell culture)

Indications, route, and dosage
Measles, mumps, and rubella immunization
Adults (born after 1957) and children: 0.5 ml S.C. in outer aspect of the upper arm. Two doses are recommended for children. Give first dose, 0.5 ml S.C., when child is age 15 months or older and give the second dose when child enters school or first grade (age 4 to 6). Some local health officials may elect to give the second dose at an older age.

Pharmacodynamics
Measles, mumps, and rubella prophylaxis: This vaccine promotes active immunity to measles (rubeola), mumps, and German measles (rubella) by inducing production of antibodies.

Pharmacokinetics
- *Absorption:* Antibodies are usually evident 2 to 3 weeks after injection. Duration of vaccine-induced immunity is expected to be lifelong.
- *Distribution:* No information available.
- *Metabolism:* No information available.
- *Excretion:* No information available.

Contraindications and precautions
Contraindicated in immunosuppressed patients; in those with cancer, blood dyscrasias, gamma globulin disorders, fever, active untreated tuberculosis, or anaphylactic or anaphylactoid reactions to neomycin or eggs; in those receiving corticosteroid or radiation therapy; and in pregnant patients.

Interactions
Concomitant use of measles, mumps, and rubella virus vaccine with *immune serum globulin* or *transfusions of blood or blood products* may interfere with the immune response to the vaccine. Whenever possible, vaccination should be deferred for 3 months in these situations.

Administration of *immunosuppressive agents* may interfere with the response to vaccine.

Effects on diagnostic tests
Measles, mumps, and rubella vaccine may temporarily decrease the response to tuberculin skin testing. If a tuberculin skin test is necessary, administer it either before or simultaneously with this vaccine.

Adverse reactions
GI: diarrhea.
Skin: urticaria, rash.
Other: fever, regional lymphadenopathy, ***anaphylaxis***, vasculitis, erythema at injection site, otitis

media, conjunctivitis, syncope, malaise, sore throat, cough, headache, vomiting.

Overdose and treatment
No information available.

☑ Special considerations
- Obtain a thorough history of allergies, especially to antibiotics, eggs, chicken, or chicken feathers, and of reactions to immunizations.
- Perform a skin test to assess vaccine sensitivity (against a control of 0.9% NaCl solution in the opposing extremity) in patients with history of anaphylactoid reactions to egg ingestion. Administer a prick (intracutaneous) or scratch test with a 1:10 dilution. Read results after 5 to 30 minutes. A positive reaction is a wheal with or without pseudopodia and surrounding erythema.
- Epinephrine solution 1:1,000 should be available to treat allergic reactions.
- Most adults born before 1957 are believed to have been infected with naturally occurring disease, and vaccination is not necessary; however, vaccination should be offered if they are considered susceptible.
- Do not administer I.V. Use a 25G, ⅝″ needle and inject S.C., preferably into the outer aspect of the upper arm. Use a sterile syringe free of preservatives, antiseptics, and detergents for each injection, because these substances may inactivate the live virus vaccine.
- Solution may be used if red, pink, or yellow, but it must be clear.
- Use only the diluent supplied. Discard reconstituted solution after 8 hours.
- Vaccine should not be given less than 1 month before or after immunization with other live virus vaccines—except for monovalent or trivalent live oral poliovirus vaccine, which may be administered simultaneously at separate sites using separate syringes.
- Vaccine may not offer any protection when given within a few days after exposure to natural measles, mumps, or rubella.
- Give passive immunization with immune serum globulin, if necessary, when immediate protection against measles is required in patients who cannot receive the measles vaccine component. Do not administer any live virus vaccine component simultaneously with immune serum globulin.
- Revaccination is unnecessary if the child received two doses of vaccine at least 1 month apart, beginning after the first birthday.
- Store vaccine at 36° to 46° F (2° to 8° C) and protect from light.

Patient education
- Tell patient what to expect after vaccination: tingling sensations in the extremities or joint aches and pains that may resemble arthritis, beginning several days to several weeks after vaccination. These symptoms usually resolve within 1 week. Other effects include pain and inflammation at the injection site and a low-grade fever, rash, or difficulty breathing. Recommend acetaminophen to alleviate adverse reactions, such as fever.
- Tell patient to report distressing adverse reactions.
- Advise women of childbearing age not to become pregnant for 3 months after receiving vaccine.

Pediatric use
- Children under age 15 months may not respond to one, two or all three of vaccine components, because retained maternal antibodies may interfere with immune response. However, vaccination at age 12 months is recommended if child lives in a high-risk area, because the benefits outweigh the risk of a slightly lower efficacy of vaccine.

Breast-feeding
- No data are available regarding distribution of measles or mumps virus components in breast milk. Some reports have demonstrated transfer of rubella virus or virus antigen into breast milk in approximately 68% of patients.
- Few adverse effects have been associated with breast-feeding after immunization with rubella-containing vaccines. The risk-benefit ratio suggests that breast-feeding women may be immunized with the rubella component if necessary.

measles and rubella virus vaccine, live, attenuated
M-R-Vax II

Pharmacologic classification: vaccine
Therapeutic classification: viral vaccine
Pregnancy risk category C

How supplied
Available by prescription only
Injection: Single-dose vial containing not less than 1,000 $TCID_{50}$ (tissue culture infective doses) each of attenuated measles virus derived from Enders' attenuated Edmonston strain (grown in chick embryo culture) and the Wistar RA 27/3 strain of rubella virus (propagated in human diploid cell culture)

Note: 10-dose and 50-dose vials are available to government agencies and institutions only.

Indications, route, and dosage
Measles and rubella immunization
Adults and children age 15 months and over: 0.5 ml in outer aspect of the upper arm. For adequate protection against measles, a two-dose schedule is recommended (at least 1 month between doses).

Pharmacodynamics
Measles and rubella prophylaxis: Vaccine promotes active immunity to measles (rubeola) and German measles (rubella) virus by inducing production of antibodies.

Pharmacokinetics
- *Absorption:* Antibodies are usually detectable 2 to 3 weeks after injection. Duration of vaccine-induced immunity is expected to be lifelong.
- *Distribution:* No information available.
- *Metabolism:* No information available.
- *Excretion:* No information available.

Contraindications and precautions

Contraindicated in immunosuppressed patients; in those with cancer, blood dyscrasias, gamma globulin disorders, fever, active untreated tuberculosis, or anaphylactic or anaphylactoid reactions to eggs or neomycin; in those receiving corticosteroid or radiation therapy; and in pregnant patients.

Interactions

Concomitant use of measles and rubella vaccine with *immune serum globulin* or *transfusions of blood or blood products* may interfere with immune response to vaccine. Defer vaccination for 3 months in these situations whenever possible.

The administration of *immunosuppressive agents* may interfere with response to vaccine.

Effects on diagnostic tests

Measles and rubella vaccine may temporarily decrease response to tuberculin skin testing. If a tuberculin skin test is necessary, administer it either before or simultaneously with measles and rubella vaccine.

Adverse reactions

Other: rash, fever, lymphadenopathy, erythema, burning, or stinging (at injection site); vasculitis, syncope, malaise, cough, sore throat, headache, vomiting, diarrhea, ***anaphylaxis.***

Overdose and treatment

No information available.

☑ Special considerations

- Obtain a thorough history of allergies (especially to antibiotics, eggs, chicken, or chicken feathers) and of reactions to immunizations.
- Perform skin testing to assess vaccine sensitivity (against a control of 0.9% NaCl solution in the opposing extremity) in patients with history of anaphylactoid reactions to eggs. Administer a prick (intracutaneous) or scratch test with a 1:10 dilution. Read results after 5 to 30 minutes. A positive reaction is a wheal with or without pseudopodia and surrounding erythema.
- Epinephrine solution 1:1,000 should be available to treat allergic reactions.
- Do not administer I.V. Use a 25G, ⅝" needle and inject S.C., preferably into the outer aspect of the upper arm.
- Use a sterile syringe free of preservatives, antiseptics, and detergents for each injection because these substances may inactivate the live virus vaccine.
- Use only diluent supplied. Discard reconstituted solution after 8 hours.
- Store vaccine at 36° to 46° F (2° to 8° C), and protect from light. Solution may be used if red, pink, or yellow, but it must be clear.
- Vaccine should not be given less than 1 month before or after immunization with other live virus vaccines, except for mumps virus vaccine and monovalent or trivalent live oral poliovirus vaccine, which may be administered simultaneously.
- Vaccine may not offer protection when given within a few days' exposure to natural measles or rubella.
- According to Centers for Disease Control and Prevention recommendations, measles, mumps and rubella (MMR) is the preferred vaccine.
- Give passive immunization with immune serum globulin when immediate protection against measles is required in patients who cannot receive the measles vaccine component. Do not administer either vaccine component simultaneously with immune serum globulin.
- Revaccination is not necessary if primary vaccine is given at or after age 15 months.

Patient education

- Tell patient what to expect: tingling sensations in the extremities or joint aches and pains that may resemble arthritis, beginning several days to several weeks after vaccination. These symptoms usually resolve within 1 week. Other effects include pain and inflammation at the injection site and a low-grade fever, rash, or difficulty breathing. Recommend acetaminophen for relief of fever.
- Encourage patient to report distressing adverse reactions.
- Advise women of childbearing age not to become pregnant for 3 months after receiving the vaccine.

Pediatric use

- Children under age 15 months may not respond to one or both of the vaccine components because retained maternal antibodies may interfere with the immune response.

Breast-feeding

- No data are available regarding distribution of measles and rubella virus components in breast milk. Some reports have demonstrated transfer of rubella virus or virus antigen into breast milk in approximately 68% of patients.
- Few adverse effects have been associated with breast-feeding after immunization with rubella-containing vaccines. The risk-benefit ratio suggests that breast-feeding women may be immunized with the rubella component if necessary.

measles virus vaccine, live, attenuated

Attenuvax

Pharmacologic classification: vaccine
Therapeutic classification: viral vaccine
Pregnancy risk category C

How supplied

Available by prescription only
Injection: Single-dose vial containing not less than 1,000 $TCID_{50}$ (tissue culture infective doses) per 0.5 ml of attenuated measles virus derived from Enders' attenuated Edmonston strain grown in chick embryo culture (10- and 50-dose vials available to government agencies and institutions only)

Indications, route, and dosage

Immunization

Adults and children age 15 months and over: 0.5 ml (1,000 units) S.C. in outer aspect of the upper arm. Administer two doses at least 1 month apart. For children, usual schedule is the first dose at age 15 months and a second dose at the entry of school (age 4 to 6 years).

Pharmacodynamics

Measles prophylaxis: Measles virus vaccine promotes active immunity to measles virus by inducing production of antibodies.

Pharmacokinetics

- *Absorption:* Antibodies are usually evident 2 to 3 weeks after injection. Duration of vaccine-induced immunity is at least 13 to 16 years and probably lifelong in most immunized persons.
- *Distribution:* No information available.
- *Metabolism:* No information available.
- *Excretion:* No information available.

Contraindications and precautions

Contraindicated in immunosuppressed patients; in those with cancer, blood dyscrasias, gamma globulin disorders, fever, active untreated tuberculosis, or anaphylactic or anaphylactoid reactions to neomycin or eggs; in those receiving corticosteroid or radiation therapy; and in pregnant patients.

Interactions

Concomitant use of measles vaccine with *immune serum globulin* or *transfusions of blood or blood products* may interfere with immune response to vaccine. Defer vaccination for 3 months in these situations.

Administration of *immunosuppressive agents* (such as *interferon*) may interfere with response to vaccine. Concurrent administration of *meningococcal vaccine* can result in a reduced seroconversion rate to meningococci.

Effects on diagnostic tests

Measles vaccine temporarily may decrease the response to tuberculin skin testing. Should a tuberculin skin test be necessary, administer it either before or simultaneously with the measles vaccine.

Adverse reactions

CNS: febrile seizures (in susceptible children).
GI: anorexia.
Hematologic: leukopenia.
Skin: rash, erythema, swelling, tenderness (at injection site).
Other: fever, lymphadenopathy, ***anaphylaxis.***

Overdose and treatment

No information available.

☑ Special considerations

- Obtain a thorough history of allergies, especially to antibiotics, eggs, chicken, or chicken feathers, and of reactions to immunizations.
- Patients with a history of anaphylactoid reactions to eggs should first have a skin test to assess vaccine sensitivity (against a control of 0.9% NaCl solution in the other arm). Administer a prick (intracutaneous) or scratch test with a 1:10 dilution. Read results after 5 to 30 minutes. A positive reaction is a wheal with or without pseudopodia and surrounding erythema.
- Epinephrine solution 1:1,000 should be available to treat allergic reactions.
- Do not administer I.V. Use a 25G, ⅝" needle and inject S.C., preferably into the outer aspect of the upper arm. Use a sterile syringe free of preservatives, antiseptics, and detergents for each injection, because these substances may inactivate the live virus vaccine.
- Use diluent supplied. Discard reconstituted solution after 8 hours.
- Measles vaccine should not be given less than 1 month before or after immunization with other live virus vaccines—except for mumps virus vaccine, rubella virus vaccine, or monovalent or trivalent live oral poliovirus vaccine, which may be administered simultaneously.
- Vaccine may offer some protection when given within a few days after exposure to natural measles and substantial protection when given a few days before exposure.
- According to Centers for Disease Control and Prevention recommendations, measles, mumps, and rubella (MMR) is the preferred vaccine.
- Give passive immunization with immune serum globulin if immediate protection against measles is required in patients who cannot receive the measles vaccine.
- Revaccination is unnecessary if primary vaccine is given at age 15 months or older.
- Store vaccine at 35° to 46° F (2° to 8° C), and protect from light. Solution may be used if red, pink, or yellow, but it must be clear.

Patient education

- Tell patient what to expect after vaccination: pain and inflammation at the injection site, fever, rash, general malaise, or difficulty breathing. Recommend acetaminophen for relief of fever.
- Encourage patient to report distressing adverse reactions.
- Advise women of childbearing age not to become pregnant for 3 months after receiving the vaccine.

Pediatric use

- Children under age 15 months may not respond to the vaccine, because retained maternal antibodies may interfere with the immune response.

Breast-feeding

- It is unknown if vaccine is distributed into breast milk. Use with caution in breast-feeding women.

mebendazole

Vermox

Pharmacologic classification: benzimidazole
Therapeutic classification: anthelmintic
Pregnancy risk category C

How supplied

Available by prescription only
Tablets (chewable): 100 mg

Indications, route, and dosage

Pinworm infestations
Adults and children over age 2: 100 mg P.O. as a single dose. If infection persists 3 weeks later, repeat treatment.
Other roundworm, whipworm, and hookworm infestations
Adults and children over age 2: 100 mg P.O. b.i.d. for 3 days. If infection persists 3 weeks later, repeat treatment.
◊ ***Trichinosis (second-line agent)***
Adults: 200 to 400 mg P.O. t.i.d. for 3 days, then 400 to 500 mg t.i.d. for 10 days.
◊ ***Capillariasis***
Adults: 200 mg b.i.d. for 20 days.
◊ ***Toxocariasis***
Adults: 100 to 200 mg b.i.d. for 5 days.
◊ ***Dracunculiasis***
Adults: 400 to 800 mg daily for 6 days.
◊ ***Mansonella perstans infestations***
Adults: 100 mg b.i.d. for 30 days.
◊ ***Angiostrongylus cantonensis infestations***
Adults and children: 100 mg b.i.d. for 5 days.

Pharmacodynamics

Anthelmintic action: Mebendazole inhibits uptake of glucose and other low-molecular weight nutrients in susceptible helminths, depleting the glycogen stores they need for survival and reproduction. It has a broad spectrum and may be useful in mixed infections. It is considered a drug of choice in the treatment of ascariasis, capillariasis, enterobiasis, trichuriasis, and uncinariasis; it has been used investigationally to treat echinococciasis, onchocerciasis, and trichinosis.

Pharmacokinetics

- *Absorption:* About 5% to 10% of an administered dose of mebendazole is absorbed; peak plasma concentrations occur at 2 to 4 hours. Absorption varies widely among patients.
- *Distribution:* Drug is highly bound to plasma proteins; it crosses the placenta.
- *Metabolism:* Mebendazole is metabolized to inactive 2-amino-5(6)-benzimidazolyl phenylketone.
- *Excretion:* Most of a mebendazole dose is excreted in feces; 2% to 10% is excreted in urine in 48 hours as either unchanged drug or the 2-amine metabolite. Half-life is 3 to 9 hours. It is unknown if drug is excreted in breast milk.

Contraindications and precautions

Contraindicated in patients with hypersensitivity to drug.

Interactions

Concomitant use with *anticonvulsants*, including *carbamazepine* and *phenytoin*, may enhance the metabolism of mebendazole and decrease its efficacy. *Cimetidine* inhibits mebendazole metabolism and may result in increased plasma concentrations of drug.

Effects on diagnostic tests

None reported.

Adverse reactions

GI: occasional, transient abdominal pain and diarrhea in massive infection and expulsion of worms.
Other: fever.

Overdose and treatment

Signs and symptoms of overdose may include GI disturbances and altered mental status. No specific recommendations exist; treatment is supportive. After recent ingestion (within 4 hours), empty stomach by induced emesis or gastric lavage. Follow with activated charcoal to decrease absorption.

☑ Special considerations

- Tablets may be chewed, swallowed whole, or crushed and mixed with food.
- Laxatives, enemas, or dietary restrictions are unnecessary.
- Collect stool specimens in a clean, dry container and transfer to a properly labeled container to send to laboratory; ova may be destroyed by toilet bowl water, urine, and some drugs.
- High-dose treatment of hydatid disease and trichinosis is investigational. Frequently monitor WBC counts to detect drug toxicity, especially during initial therapy.

Patient education

- Teach patient and family members personal hygiene measures to prevent reinfection: washing perianal area and changing undergarments and bedclothes daily; washing hands and cleaning fingernails before meals and after defecation; and sanitary disposal of feces.
- Advise patient to bathe often, by showering, if possible.
- Advise patient to keep hands away from mouth, to keep fingernails short, and to wear shoes to avoid hookworm; explain that ova are easily transmitted directly and indirectly by hands, food, or contaminated articles. Washing clothes in household washing machine will destroy ova.
- Instruct patient to handle bedding carefully, because shaking will send ova into the air, and to disinfect toilet facilities and vacuum or damp-mop floors daily to reduce number of ova.
- Encourage patient's family and contacts to be checked for infestation and treated, if necessary.

Pediatric use
• Drug should be given to children under age 2 only when potential benefits justify risks.

Breast-feeding
• Safety in breast-feeding women has not been established.

mechlorethamine hydrochloride (nitrogen mustard)
Mustargen
Pharmacologic classification: alkylating agent (cell cycle–phase nonspecific)
Therapeutic classification: antineoplastic
Pregnancy risk category D

How supplied
Available by prescription only
Injection: 10-mg vials

Indications, route, and dosage
Dosage and indications may vary. Check current literature for recommended protocols.
Hodgkin's disease, bronchogenic carcinoma, chronic lymphocytic leukemia, chronic myelocytic leukemia, lymphosarcoma, polycythemia vera
Adults: 0.4 mg/kg I.V. per course of therapy as a single dose or 0.1 to 0.2 mg/kg on 2 to 4 successive days q 3 to 6 weeks. Give through running I.V. infusion. Dose reduced in prior radiation or chemotherapy to 0.2 to 0.4 mg/kg. Dose based on ideal or actual body weight, whichever is less.
Intracavitary doses for neoplastic effusions
Adults: 0.2 to 0.4 mg/kg.

Pharmacodynamics
Antineoplastic action: Mechlorethamine exerts its cytotoxic activity through the basic processes of alkylation. Drug causes cross-linking of DNA strands, single-strand breakage of DNA, abnormal base pairing, and interruption of other intracellular processes, resulting in cell death.

Pharmacokinetics
• *Absorption:* Well absorbed after oral administration; however, because the drug is very irritating to tissue, it must be administered I.V. After intracavitary administration, mechlorethamine is absorbed incompletely, probably from deactivation by body fluids in the cavity.
• *Distribution:* Drug does not cross the blood-brain barrier.
• *Metabolism:* Drug undergoes rapid chemical transformation and reacts quickly with various cellular components before being deactivated.
• *Excretion:* Metabolites are excreted in urine. Less than 0.01% of an I.V. dose is excreted unchanged in urine.

Contraindications and precautions
Contraindicated in patients with hypersensitivity to drug and with known infectious diseases.

Use cautiously in patients with severe anemia or depressed neutrophil or platelet count and in those who have recently undergone chemotherapy or radiation therapy.

Interactions
None reported.

Effects on diagnostic tests
Drug therapy may increase blood and urine uric acid levels. Renal, hepatic, and bone marrow function abnormalities have been reported.

Adverse reactions
CNS: weakness, vertigo.
EENT: tinnitus; deafness (with high doses).
GI: *nausea, vomiting, anorexia* (beginning within minutes, lasting 8 to 24 hours).
Hematologic: ***thrombocytopenia***, lymphocytopenia, ***agranulocytosis***, nadir of myelosuppression occurring by days 4 to 10 and lasting 10 to 21 days; mild anemia begins in 2 to 3 weeks.
Skin: rash, sloughing, severe irritation (if drug extravasates or touches skin).
Other: *alopecia,* precipitation of herpes zoster, ***anaphylaxis***, hyperuricemia, *thrombophlebitis,* amyloidosis, jaundice, menstrual irregularities, impaired spermatogenesis.

Overdose and treatment
Clinical manifestations of overdose include severe leukopenia, anemia, thrombocytopenia, and a hemorrhagic diathesis with subsequent delayed bleeding. Death may follow.

Treatment is usually supportive and includes transfusion of blood components and antibiotic treatment of complicating infections.

☑ Special considerations
• To reconstitute powder, use 10 ml of sterile water for injection or 0.9% NaCl solution to give a concentration of 1 mg/ml.
• When reconstituted, drug is a clear colorless solution. Do not use if solution is discolored or if droplets of water are visible within vial before reconstitution.
• Solution is very unstable. Prepare immediately before infusion and use within 15 minutes. Discard unused solution.
• Drug may be administered I.V. push over a few minutes into the tubing of a freely flowing I.V. infusion.
• Dilution of drug into a large volume of I.V. solution is not recommended, because it may react with the diluent and is not stable for a prolonged period.
• Treatment of extravasation includes local injections of a 1/6 M sodium thiosulfate solution. Prepare solution by mixing 4 ml of sodium thiosulfate 10% with 6 ml of sterile water for injection. Also, apply ice packs for 6 to 12 hours to minimize local reactions.
• During intracavitary administration, patient should be turned from side to side every 15 minutes for 1 hour to distribute drug.

• Avoid contact with skin or mucous membranes. Wear gloves when preparing solution and during administration to prevent accidental skin contact. If contact occurs, wash with copious amounts of water.
• Monitor uric acid levels, CBC, and liver function tests.
• To prevent hyperuricemia with resulting uric acid nephropathy, allopurinol may be given; keep patient well hydrated.
• Anticoagulants should be used cautiously. Watch closely for signs of bleeding.
• Avoid all I.M. injections when platelet count is low.
• Drug has been used topically to treat mycosis fungoides.

Patient education

• Tell patient to avoid exposure to people with infections.
• Adequate fluid intake is very important to facilitate excretion of uric acid.
• Reassure patient that hair should grow back after treatment has ended.
• Tell patient to promptly report signs or symptoms of bleeding or infection.
• Advise patient to use contraception while using drug.

Breast-feeding

• It is not known if drug distributes into breast milk. However, because of the potential for serious adverse reactions, mutagenicity, and carcinogenicity in the infant, breast-feeding is not recommended.

meclizine hydrochloride

Antivert, Antivert/25, Antrizine, Bonine, Dizmiss, Meclizine, Meni-D, Ru-Vert-M

Pharmacologic classification: piperazine-derivative antihistamine
Therapeutic classification: antiemetic, antivertigo
Pregnancy risk category B

How supplied

Available with or without a prescription
Tablets: 12.5 mg, 25 mg, 50 mg
Tablets (chewable): 25 mg
Capsules: 25 mg, 30 mg

Indications, route, and dosage

Dizziness
Adults and children age 12 or older: 25 to 100 mg P.O. daily in divided doses. Dosage varies with patient response.
Motion sickness
Adults and children age 12 or older: 25 to 50 mg P.O. 1 hour before travel; may repeat dose daily for duration of journey.

Pharmacodynamics

Antiemetic action: Meclizine probably inhibits nausea and vomiting by centrally decreasing sensitivity of labyrinth apparatus that relays stimuli to the chemoreceptor trigger zone and stimulates the vomiting center in the brain.

Antivertigo action: Drug decreases labyrinth excitability and conduction in vestibular-cerebellar pathways.

Pharmacokinetics

• *Absorption:* Onset of action is about 60 minutes.
• *Distribution:* Well distributed throughout the body and crosses the placenta.
• *Metabolism:* Meclizine probably is metabolized in the liver.
• *Excretion:* Half-life is about 6 hours; action persists for 8 to 24 hours. Drug is excreted unchanged in feces; metabolites are found in urine.

Contraindications and precautions

Contraindicated in patients hypersensitive to drug. Use cautiously in patients with asthma, glaucoma, or prostatic hyperplasia.

Interactions

Additive sedative and CNS depressant effects may occur when meclizine is used concomitantly with other *CNS depressants*, such as *alcohol, barbiturates, sleeping agents, tranquilizers,* and *antianxiety agents*; drug should not be given to patients taking *ototoxic medications*, such as *aminoglycosides, cisplatin, loop diuretics, salicylates,* and *vancomycin*, because meclizine may mask signs of ototoxicity.

Effects on diagnostic tests

Meclizine should be discontinued 4 days before diagnostic skin tests, to avoid preventing, reducing, or masking test response.

Adverse reactions

CNS: *drowsiness,* restlessness, excitation, nervousness, auditory and visual hallucinations.
CV: hypotension, palpitations, tachycardia.
EENT: blurred vision, diplopia, tinnitus, dry nose and throat.
GI: dry mouth, constipation, anorexia, nausea, vomiting, diarrhea.
GU: urine retention, urinary frequency.
Skin: urticaria, rash.

Overdose and treatment

Clinical manifestations of moderate overdose may include hyperexcitability alternating with drowsiness. Seizures, hallucinations, and respiratory paralysis may occur in profound overdose. Anticholinergic symptoms, such as dry mouth, flushed skin, fixed and dilated pupils, and GI symptoms, are common, especially in children.

Treat overdose by administering gastric lavage to empty stomach contents; emesis with ipecac syrup may be ineffective. Treat hypotension with vasopressors, and control seizures with diazepam or phenytoin. Do not give stimulants.

☑ Special considerations

Besides those relevant to all *antihistamines,* consider the following recommendations.

• Tablets may be placed in mouth and allowed to dissolve without water, or they may be chewed or swallowed whole.
• Abrupt withdrawal of drug after long-term use may cause paradoxical reactions or sudden reversal of improved state.

Patient education
• Instruct patient to avoid activities that require mental alertness and physical coordination, such as driving and operating dangerous machinery.

Geriatric use
• Elderly patients are usually more sensitive to adverse effects of antihistamines and are especially likely to experience a greater degree of dizziness, sedation, hyperexcitability, dry mouth, and urine retention than younger patients.

Pediatric use
• Safety and efficacy for use in children have not been established. Do not use in children under age 12; infants and children under age 6 may experience paradoxical hyperexcitability.

Breast-feeding
• Safety in breast-feeding has not been established.

medium-chain triglycerides
MCT Oil

Pharmacologic classification: modular supplement
Therapeutic classification: enteral nutrition therapy
Pregnancy risk category C

How supplied
Available without a prescription
Oil: 960 ml (115 calories/15 ml)

Indications, route, and dosage
Inadequate digestion or absorption of food fats
Adults: 15 ml P.O. t.i.d. or q.i.d. Maximum, 100 ml/day.

Pharmacodynamics
Metabolic action: Medium-chain triglycerides are indicated as a supplementary fat source when conventional fats are not tolerated. Medium-chain triglycerides are more rapidly hydrolyzed than conventional food fat, require less bile for digestion, are carried by the portal circulation, and are not dependent on chylomicron formation or lymphatic transport. Medium-chain triglycerides are a useful energy source in malabsorption patients but do not provide essential fatty acids.

Pharmacokinetics
• *Absorption:* Medium-chain triglycerides are absorbed by the portal circulation; they are not dependent on chylomicron formation or lymphatic transport for absorption. Compared with dietary fat, they require less bile acid for digestion.
• *Distribution:* Triglycerides are transported by lipoproteins to storage sites in adipose tissue.
• *Metabolism:* Triglycerides are broken down by lipase to free fatty acids and glycerol. The free fatty acids are used to produce energy through the fatty acid cycle.
• *Excretion:* Excess fat is excreted in feces; ketone bodies may appear in urine.

Contraindications and precautions
No known contraindications. Use cautiously in patients with hepatic cirrhosis and complications, such as portacaval shunts or tendency to encephalopathy.

Interactions
No reported.

Effects on diagnostic tests
None reported.

Adverse reactions
CNS: reversible ***coma*** in susceptible patients (such as those with advanced hepatic cirrhosis).
GI: nausea, vomiting, diarrhea, abdominal distention, cramps.

Overdose and treatment
No information available.

☑ Special considerations
• Medium-chain triglycerides provide 7.7 calories/ml.
• To minimize GI adverse effects, give smaller doses more frequently with meals, or mixed with salad dressing or chilled fruit juice.
• Use metal, glass, or ceramic containers and utensils.
• Medium-chain triglycerides do not provide essential fatty acids.

Patient education
• Provide counseling with dietitian so patient can learn how to incorporate this substance into his diet.

medroxyprogesterone acetate
Amen, Curretab, Cycrin, Depo-Provera, Provera

Pharmacologic classification: progestin
Therapeutic classification: progestin, antineoplastic
Pregnancy risk category X

How supplied
Available by prescription only
Tablets: 2.5 mg, 5 mg, 10 mg
Injection: 150 mg/ml, 400 mg/ml

Indications, route, and dosage
Abnormal uterine bleeding from hormonal imbalance
Adults: 5 to 10 mg P.O. daily for 5 to 10 days beginning on day 16 or 21 of menstrual cycle. If pa-

tient has received estrogen, then 10 mg P.O. daily for 10 days beginning on day 16 of cycle.
Secondary amenorrhea
Adults: 5 to 10 mg P.O. daily for 5 to 10 days.
Endometrial or renal carcinoma
Adults: 400 to 1,000 mg I.M. weekly.
◊ ***Paraphilia in males***
Adults: Initially, 200 mg I.M. b.i.d. or t.i.d. or 500 mg I.M. weekly. Adjust dosage based on response.
Contraception in females
Adults: 150 mg I.M. q 3 months; give first injection on first 5 days of menstrual cycle.

Pharmacodynamics
Progestational action: Parenteral medroxyprogesterone suppresses ovulation, causes thickening of cervical mucus, and induces sloughing of the endometrium.

Antineoplastic action: Drug may inhibit growth progression of progestin-sensitive endometrial or renal cancer tissue by an unknown mechanism.

Pharmacokinetics
- *Absorption:* Slow absorption after I.M. administration.
- *Distribution:* Not well characterized.
- *Metabolism:* Primarily hepatic; not well characterized.
- *Excretion:* Primarily renal; not well characterized.

Contraindications and precautions
Contraindicated in patients with hypersensitivity to drug, active thromboembolic disorders, or past history of thromboembolic disorders or of cerebral vascular disease or apoplexy, breast cancer, undiagnosed abnormal vaginal bleeding, missed abortion, or hepatic dysfunction and during pregnancy. Tablets are also contraindicated in patients with liver dysfunction or known or suspected malignant disease of the genital organs.

Use cautiously in patients with diabetes mellitus, seizures, migraines, cardiac or renal disease, asthma, or mental depression.

Interactions
In patients receiving *bromocriptine*, progestins may cause amenorrhea or galactorrhea, thus interfering with the action of bromocriptine. Concurrent use of these drugs is not recommended. *Aminoglutethimide* may increase the hepatic metabolism of medroxyprogesterone, possibly decreasing its therapeutic effect.

Effects on diagnostic tests
Pregnanediol excretion may decrease; serum alkaline phosphatase and amino acid levels may increase. Glucose tolerance has been shown to decrease in a small percentage of patients.

Adverse reactions
CNS: depression.
CV: thrombophlebitis, ***pulmonary embolism***, edema, ***thromboembolism, CVA.***
EENT: exophthalmos, diplopia.
GU: breakthrough bleeding, dysmenorrhea, amenorrhea, cervical erosion, abnormal secretions.
Hepatic: cholestatic jaundice.
Skin: rash, pain, induration, sterile abscesses, acne, pruritus, melasma, alopecia, hirsutism.
Other: breast tenderness, enlargement, or secretion; changes in weight.

Overdose and treatment
No information available.

☑ Special considerations
Besides those relevant to all *progestins,* consider the following recommendations.
- Parenteral form is for I.M. administration only. Inject deep into large muscle mass, preferably the gluteal muscle. Monitor for development of sterile abscesses. Suspension must be shaken vigorously immediately before each use to ensure complete suspension of drug.
- Drug has been used to treat obstructive sleep apnea and to manage paraphilia.
- When used as a long-acting contraceptive in females, rule out pregnancy before initiating therapy.

Breast-feeding
- Detectable amounts of drug have been identified in breast milk. In nursing mothers treated with medroxyprogesterone, the milk composition, quality and amount are not adversely affected. Infants exposed to drug via breast milk have been studied for developmental and behavioral effects through puberty; no adverse effects have been noted.

medrysone
HMS Liquifilm Ophthalmic

Pharmacologic classification: corticosteroid
Therapeutic classification: ophthalmic anti-inflammatory
Pregnancy risk category C

How supplied
Available by prescription only
Ophthalmic suspension: 1%

Indications, route, and dosage
Allergic conjunctivitis, vernal conjunctivitis, episcleritis, ophthalmic epinephrine sensitivity reaction
Adults and children: Instill 1 drop in conjunctival sac b.i.d. to q.i.d. May use hourly during first 1 to 2 days if needed.

Pharmacodynamics
Anti-inflammatory action: Medrysone, a synthetic corticosteroid, stimulates the synthesis of enzymes needed to decrease the inflammatory response. Conjunctival administration of medrysone effectively reduces local inflammation. Because medrysone has not been proven to be effective in iritis and uveitis, it is not recommended for treatment of these conditions.

Pharmacokinetics
• *Absorption:* After ophthalmic administration, medrysone is absorbed through the aqueous humor. Because of the low doses used, very little drug is absorbed systemically.
• *Distribution:* Drug is distributed through the local tissue layers. Any drug that is absorbed into circulation is distributed rapidly into muscle, liver, skin, intestines, and kidneys.
• *Metabolism:* Medrysone is primarily metabolized locally. The small amount that is absorbed into systemic circulation is metabolized primarily in the liver to inactive compounds.
• *Excretion:* Inactive metabolites are excreted by the kidneys, primarily as glucuronides and sulfates, but also as unconjugated products. Small amounts of the metabolites are also excreted in feces.

Contraindications and precautions
Contraindicated in patients with vaccinia, varicella, acute superficial herpes simplex (dendritic keratitis), viral diseases of conjunctiva and cornea, ocular tuberculosis, fungal or viral eye diseases, iritis, uveitis, or any acute, purulent, untreated eye infection. Use cautiously in patients with corneal abrasions.

Interactions
None reported.

Effects on diagnostic tests
None reported.

Adverse reactions
EENT: thinning of cornea, interference with corneal wound healing, increased susceptibility to viral or fungal corneal infection, corneal ulceration; discharge, discomfort, ocular pain, foreign body sensation, glaucoma exacerbation, cataracts, visual acuity and visual field defects, optic nerve damage (with excessive or long-term use).
Other: systemic effects, adrenal suppression (with excessive or long-term use).

Overdose and treatment
No information available.

☑ Special considerations
• Advise patient to apply light finger pressure on lacrimal sac for 1 minute after instillation.

mefloquine hydrochloride
Lariam

Pharmacologic classification: quinine derivative
Therapeutic classification: antimalarial
Pregnancy risk category C

How supplied
Available by prescription only
Tablets: 250 mg

Indications, route, and dosage
Treatment of malaria
Adults: 5 tablets (1,250 mg) P.O. as a single dose. Patients with Plasmodium vivax infections should receive subsequent therapy with primaquine (an 8-aminoquinolone) to avoid relapse.
Prophylaxis for malaria
Adults: 250 mg P.O. once weekly for 4 weeks, then 250 mg every other week. Initiate prophylaxis 1 week before entering endemic area, and continue for 4 weeks after return. For prolonged visits to endemic areas, prophylaxis should continue for three doses after return.
Children: Initiate prophylaxis 1 week before entering endemic area, and continue for 4 weeks after return. Give ¼ tablet to children weighing between 33 and 42 lb (15 and 19 kg); ½ tablet for those weighing 44 to 66 lb (20 to 30 kg); ¾ tablet for those weighing 68 to 99 lb (31 to 45 kg); and 1 tablet for those weighing more than 99 lb (45 kg). Take dose at same time each day.

Pharmacodynamics
Antimalarial action: Mefloquine acts as a blood schizonticide. Its exact mechanism of action has not been identified. Drug is effective against all human types of malaria, including chloroquine-resistant malaria, and *Plasmodium falciparum* and *P. vivax* infections.

Pharmacokinetics
• *Absorption:* Well absorbed after oral administration.
• *Distribution:* Mefloquine concentrates in the RBCs and is approximately 98% protein-bound.
• *Metabolism:* Drug is metabolized by the liver.
• *Excretion:* Drug is primarily excreted via the liver. Small amounts can be found in the urine and breast milk. Half-life in normal adults is approximately 21 days.

Contraindications and precautions
Contraindicated in patients with hypersensitivity to drug or related compounds. Use cautiously in patients with cardiac disease or seizure disorders. Mefloquine should be used in pregnancy only if potential benefit justifies the potential risk to the fetus.

Interactions
Mefloquine may have CV effects when taken with *beta blockers (propranolol).* To prevent cardiac problems resulting from concomitant use with *quinine* or *quinidine,* mefloquine dose should follow the last quinine dose by at least 12 hours. Seizures may occur with concomitant use of mefloquine and *chloroquine;* loss of seizure control may occur with concomitant use of *valproic acid.* Do not use with *halofantrine* because of danger of a potentially fatal prolongation of the QTc interval.

Effects on diagnostic tests
Drug may cause decreased hematocrit and elevations in transaminases, leukopenia, and thrombocytopenia.

Adverse reactions
CNS: dizziness, syncope, headache, psychotic manifestations, hallucinations, confusion, anxiety, fatigue, vertigo, depression, ***seizures.***
CV: extrasystoles.
EENT: tinnitus, visual disturbances.
GI: loss of appetite, vomiting, *nausea,* loose stools, diarrhea, abdominal discomfort or pain.
Skin: rash.
Other: fever, chills, myalgia.

Overdose and treatment
Treatment usually includes induced vomiting and management of symptoms. Major problems are related to cardiotoxic effects. Treat vomiting or diarrhea with standard fluid therapy.

☑ Special considerations
- Monitor liver function tests with prolonged therapy.
- Ophthalmologic examinations are recommended during prolonged therapy because ocular lesions have been noted in laboratory animals.

Patient education
- Advise patient to use caution when performing potentially hazardous tasks because drug may cause dizziness and altered sense of balance.
- To facilitate compliance, advise patient taking mefloquine for prophylaxis to take drug on same day of week.
- Instruct patient taking drug for prophylaxis to discontinue drug if signs or symptoms of unexplained anxiety, depression, confusion, or restlessness occur. These symptoms may indicate impending toxicity.
- Tell patient not to take drug on an empty stomach and always to take it with a full (at least 8 oz) glass of water.

Pediatric use
- Safety and efficacy in children have not been demonstrated.

megestrol acetate
Megace

Pharmacologic classification: progestin
Therapeutic classification: antineoplastic
Pregnancy risk category X

How supplied
Available by prescription only
Tablets: 20 mg, 40 mg
Suspension: 200 mg/5 ml

Indications, route, and dosage
Dosage and indications may vary. Check current literature for recommended protocol.
Palliative treatment of breast carcinoma
Adults: 40 mg (tablets) P.O. q.i.d.
Palliative treatment of endometrial carcinoma
Adults: 10 to 80 mg (tablets) P.O. q.i.d.
Anorexia, cachexia, or weight loss in patients with AIDS
Adults: 800 mg (suspension) P.O. daily in divided doses; 100 to 400 mg for AIDS-related cachexia.

Pharmacodynamics
Antineoplastic action: Megestrol inhibits growth and causes regression of progestin-sensitive breast and endometrial cancer tissue by an unknown mechanism.

Treatment of anorexia, cachexia, or weight loss: Mechanism for weight gain is unknown. It may stimulate appetite by interfering with the production of mediators such as cachectin.

Pharmacokinetics
- *Absorption:* Well absorbed across the GI tract after oral administration.
- *Distribution:* Megestrol appears to be stored in fatty tissue and is highly bound to plasma proteins.
- *Metabolism:* Drug is completely metabolized in the liver.
- *Excretion:* Metabolites are eliminated primarily through the kidneys.

Contraindications and precautions
Contraindicated in patients hypersensitive to drug and during pregnancy (especially first 4 months). Use cautiously in patients with history of thrombophlebitis.

Interactions
Concomitant use with *bromocriptine* may cause amenorrhea or galactorrhea, thus interfering with the action of bromocriptine. Concurrent use of these drugs is not recommended.

Effects on diagnostic tests
Pregnanediol excretion may decrease; serum alkaline phosphatase and amino acid concentrations may increase. Glucose tolerance has been shown to decrease in a small percentage of patients receiving megestrol.

Adverse reactions
CV: thrombophlebitis, hypertension, edema, chest pain.
GI: nausea, vomiting, diarrhea, flatulence.
GU: breakthrough menstrual bleeding, impotence, decreased libido.
Hepatic: hepatomegaly.
Respiratory: ***pulmonary embolism***, dyspnea, pneumonia, cough, pharyngitis.
Skin: rash, pruritus, candidiasis.
Other: weight gain, increased appetite, carpal tunnel syndrome, alopecia, hyperglycemia.

Overdose and treatment
No information available.

☑ Special considerations
Recommendations for administration of megestrol and for care and teaching of the patient during therapy are the same as those for all *progestins.*

melphalan (phenylalanine mustard)

Alkeran

Pharmacologic classification: alkylating agent (cell cycle–phase nonspecific)
Therapeutic classification: antineoplastic
Pregnancy risk category D

How supplied

Available by prescription only
Tablets (scored): 2 mg
Powder for injection: 50 mg

Indications, route, and dosage

Dosage and indications may vary. Check current literature for recommended protocol.

Multiple myeloma
Adults: 6 mg P.O. daily for 2 to 3 weeks; then stop therapy for 4 weeks. When WBC and platelet count begin to rise, start maintenance dose of 2 mg P.O. daily. Alternatively, give 0.15 mg/kg/day P.O. for 7 days administered at 2- to 6-week intervals or 0.25 mg/kg/day P.O. for 4 days at 4- to 6-week intervals; monitor patient's blood counts.

For I.V. administration, give 16 mg/m^2 over 15 to 20 minutes once at 2-week intervals for four doses. Monitor patient's blood counts and reduce dose as necessary.

Epithelial ovarian cancer
Adults: 200 mcg/kg/day P.O. for 5 days, repeated q 4 to 6 weeks if blood counts return to normal.

Pharmacodynamics

Antineoplastic action: Melphalan exerts its cytotoxic activity by forming cross-links of strands of DNA and RNA and inhibiting protein synthesis.

Pharmacokinetics

- *Absorption:* Absorption from GI tract is incomplete and variable. One study found that absorption ranged from 25% to 89% after an oral dose of 0.6 mg/kg.
- *Distribution:* Drug distributes rapidly and widely into total body water. Drug is initially 50% to 60% bound to plasma proteins and eventually increases to 80% to 90% over time.
- *Metabolism:* Extensively deactivated by the process of hydrolysis.
- *Excretion:* Elimination of drug has been described as biphasic, with an initial half-life of 8 minutes and a terminal half-life of 2 hours. Melphalan and its metabolites are excreted primarily in urine, with 10% of an oral dose excreted as unchanged drug.

Contraindications and precautions

Contraindicated in patients with hypersensitivity to drug and in those whose disease is known to be resistant to drug. Patients hypersensitive to chlorambucil may have cross-sensitivity to melphalan.

Use cautiously in patients with impaired renal function, severe leukopenia, thrombocytopenia, anemia, or chronic lymphocytic leukemia.

Interactions

Melphalan may increase cyclosporine-induced nephrotoxicity. Monitor renal function closely in patients receiving melphalan and *cyclosporine* concomitantly or melphalan and *cisplatin* concomitantly. *Interferon alpha* may cause a decrease in melphalan serum concentrations.

Food decreases bioavailability of drug. *Fever* may enhance elimination of melphalan. *Cimetidine* inhibits GI absorption.

Effects on diagnostic tests

Melphalan therapy may increase blood and urine levels of uric acid.

Adverse reactions

CV: hypotension, tachycardia, edema.
GI: nausea, vomiting, diarrhea, oral ulceration.
Hematologic: ***thrombocytopenia, leukopenia, bone marrow suppression,*** hemolytic anemia.
Respiratory: ***pneumonitis, pulmonary fibrosis,*** dyspnea, bronchospasm.
Skin: pruritus, alopecia, urticaria.
Other: ***anaphylaxis,*** hypersensitivity, ***hepatotoxicity.***

Overdose and treatment

Clinical manifestations of overdose include myelosuppression, hypocalcemia, severe nausea, vomiting, ulceration of the mouth, decreased consciousness, seizures, muscular paralysis, and cholinomimetic effects.

Treatment is usually supportive and includes transfusion of blood components.

☑ Special considerations

- Oral dose may be taken all at one time.
- Administer drug on an empty stomach because absorption is decreased by food.
- Frequent hematologic monitoring, including CBC, is necessary for accurate dosage adjustments and prevention of toxicity.
- Discontinue therapy temporarily or reduce dosage if WBC count falls below 3,000/mm^3 or platelet count falls below 100,000/mm^3.
- Avoid I.M. injections when platelet count is below 100,000/mm^3.
- Dosage reduction should be considered in patients with renal failure receiving I.V. melphalan. Increased bone marrow suppression was observed in patients with BUN concentrations of 30 mg/dl or more.
- Anticoagulants, aspirin, and aspirin-containing products should be used cautiously.

Patient education

- Instruct patient to continue taking drug despite nausea and vomiting.
- Tell patient to call immediately if vomiting occurs shortly after taking a dose.
- Explain that adequate fluid intake is important to facilitate excretion of uric acid.
- Instruct patient to avoid exposure to people with infections.
- Reassure patient that hair should grow back after treatment has ended.

- Tell patient to promptly report signs and symptoms of infection or bleeding.
- Advise women of childbearing age to avoid becoming pregnant while receiving drug therapy.

Breast-feeding
- It is not known if drug distributes into breast milk. However, because of the potential for serious adverse reactions, mutagenicity, and carcinogenicity in the infant, breast-feeding is not recommended.

meningococcal polysaccharide vaccine
Menomune-A/C/Y/W-135

Pharmacologic classification: vaccine
Therapeutic classification: bacterial vaccine
Pregnancy risk category C

How supplied
Available by prescription only
Injection: a killed bacterial vaccine in single-dose, 10-dose, and 50-dose vials with vial of diluent

Indications, route, and dosage
Meningococcal meningitis prophylaxis
Adults and children over age 2: 0.5 ml S.C.

Pharmacodynamics
Meningitis prophylaxis: Vaccine promotes active immunity to meningitis caused by *Neisseria meningitidis.*

Pharmacokinetics
- *Absorption:* No information available.
- *Distribution:* No information available.
- *Metabolism:* No information available.
- *Excretion:* No information available.

Contraindications and precautions
Contraindicated in immunosuppressed and pregnant patients and those hypersensitive to thimerosal. Defer vaccination in patients with acute illness.

Interactions
None reported.

Effects on diagnostic tests
None reported.

Adverse reactions
CNS: headache.
Other: *pain, tenderness, erythema, induration* (at injection site); ***anaphylaxis***, malaise, chills, fever, muscle cramps.

Overdose and treatment
No information available.

☑ Special considerations
- Obtain a thorough history of allergies and reactions to immunizations.
- Do not give meningitis vaccine intradermally, I.M., or I.V.
- Epinephrine solution 1:1,000 should be available to treat allergic reactions.
- Reconstitute vaccine with diluent provided. Shake until dissolved. Discard reconstituted solution after 5 days.
- Store vaccine between 36° and 46° F (2° and 8° C).
- Protective antibody levels may be achieved within 10 to 14 days after vaccination.

Patient education
- Tell patient that pain and inflammation may occur at injection site. Recommend acetaminophen to alleviate adverse reactions, such as fever.
- Encourage patient to report distressing adverse reactions.
- Advise patient on use of contraceptive information if necessary.
- Explain that vaccine will provide immunity only to meningitis caused by one type of bacteria.

Pediatric use
- Vaccine is not recommended for children under age 2.

Breast-feeding
- It is unknown if vaccine is distributed into breast milk. Use with caution in breast-feeding women.

menotropins
Humegon, Pergonal

Pharmacologic classification: gonadotropin
Therapeutic classification: ovulation stimulant, spermatogenesis stimulant
Pregnancy risk category X

How supplied
Available by prescription only
Injection: 75 IU of luteinizing hormone (LH) and 75 IU of follicle-stimulating hormone (FSH) activity per ampule; 150 IU of LH and 150 IU of FSH activity per ampule

Indications, route, and dosage
Production of follicular maturation
Adults: 75 IU each of FSH and LH I.M. daily for 7 to 12 days, followed by 5,000 to 10,000 USP units human chorionic gonadotropin (HCG) I.M. 1 day after last dose of menotropins; repeat for two more menstrual cycles. Then, if ovulation or follicular development does not occur, increase to 150 IU each of FSH and LH I.M. daily for 7 to 12 days, followed by 5,000 to 10,000 USP units HCG I.M. 1 day after last dose of menotropins; repeat for two menstrual cycles.
Stimulation of spermatogenesis
Adults: After 4 to 6 months of treatment with HCG, 1 ampule (75 IU FSH/LH) I.M. three times weekly (given concomitantly with 2,000 USP units HCG twice weekly) for at least 4 months. If no improvement occurs after 4 months, treatment may continue with 75 IU FSH/LH three times weekly or 150 IU FSH/LH three times weekly.

Pharmacodynamics

Ovulation stimulant action: Menotropins causes growth and maturation of the ovarian follicle in women who do not have primary ovarian failure by mimicking the action of endogenous LH and FSH. Additional treatment with HCG is usually required to achieve ovulation.

Spermatogenesis stimulant action: Menotropins causes spermatogenesis when coadministered with HCG in men with primary or secondary pituitary hypofunction.

Pharmacokinetics

- *Absorption:* Drug must be administered parenterally for effectiveness.
- *Distribution:* Unknown.
- *Metabolism:* Not fully known.
- *Excretion:* Excreted in the urine.

Contraindications and precautions

Contraindicated in patients hypersensitive to drug; in women with primary ovarian failure, uncontrolled thyroid or adrenal dysfunction, pituitary tumor, abnormal uterine bleeding, uterine fibromas, or ovarian cysts or enlargement; in pregnant patients; and in men with normal pituitary function, primary testicular failure, or infertility disorders other than hypogonadotropic hypogonadism.

Interactions

None reported.

Effects on diagnostic tests

None reported.

Adverse reactions

CNS: headache, malaise, dizziness.
CV: *stroke,* tachycardia.
GI: nausea, vomiting, diarrhea, abdominal cramps, bloating.
GU: *ovarian enlargement with pain and abdominal distention, multiple births, ovarian hyperstimulation syndrome* (sudden severe abdominal pain, distention, nausea, vomiting, weight gain, and dyspnea followed by hypovolemia, hemoconcentration, electrolyte imbalance, pleural effusion, ascites, and hemoperitoneum), ovarian cysts, ectopic pregnancy.
Respiratory: *atelectasis, acute respiratory distress syndrome, pulmonary embolism, pulmonary infarction, arterial occlusion,* dyspnea, tachypnea.
Other: fever, gynecomastia, ***hypersensitivity and anaphylactic reactions***, chills, musculoskeletal aches, joint pains, rash.

Overdose and treatment

The most common dose-related adverse effect appears to be ovarian hyperstimulation syndrome. Drug should be discontinued. Symptomatic and supportive care include bed rest, fluid and electrolyte replacement, and analgesics.

☑ Special considerations

- Drug is administered by I.M. route only.
- Reconstitute drug with 1 to 2 ml of sterile NaCl injection. Use immediately.
- Pregnancies that follow ovulation induced with menotropins show a relatively high frequency of multiple births.

Patient education

- Teach patient signs and tests that indicate time of ovulation, such as increase in basal body temperature and increase in the appearance and volume of cervical mucus.
- Warn patient to immediately report symptoms of ovarian hyperstimulation syndrome, such as abdominal distention and pain, dyspnea, and vaginal bleeding.
- Tell patient multiple births are possible. Ectopic pregnancy and congenital malformations have been reported in pregnancies following treatment.
- In infertility, encourage daily intercourse from day before HCG is given until ovulation occurs.
- Advise patient that she should be examined at least every other day for signs of excessive ovarian stimulation during therapy and for 2 weeks after treatment is discontinued.

Breast-feeding

- Drug is not indicated for use in breast-feeding women.

meperidine hydrochloride (pethidine hydrochloride)

Demerol

Pharmacologic classification: opioid
Therapeutic classification: analgesic, adjunct to anesthesia
Controlled substance schedule II
Pregnancy risk category C

How supplied

Available by prescription only
Tablets: 50 mg, 100 mg
Liquid: 50 mg/5 ml
Injection: 10 mg/ml, 25 mg/ml, 50 mg/ml, 75 mg/ml, 100 mg/ml

Indications, route, and dosage

Moderate to severe pain
Adults: 50 to 150 mg P.O., I.M., I.V., or S.C. q 3 to 4 hours.
Children: 0.5 to 0.8 mg/lb P.O., I.M., I.V., or S.C. q 3 to 4 hours or 175 mg/m² daily in six divided doses. Maximum single dose for children should not exceed 100 mg.
Preoperatively
Adults: 50 to 100 mg I.M., I.V., or S.C. 30 to 90 minutes before surgery.
Children: 0.5 to 1 mg/lb I.M., I.V., or S.C. 30 to 90 minutes before surgery. Do not exceed adult dose.
Support of anesthesia
Adults: Repeated slow I.V. injections of fractional doses (10 mg/ml) or continuous I.V. infusion of 1 mg/ml. Dose should be titrated to meet patient's needs.
Obstetric analgesia
Adults: 50 to 100 mg I.M. or S.C. when pain becomes regular; may repeat at 1- to 3-hour intervals.

Pharmacodynamics

Analgesic action: Meperidine is a narcotic agonist with actions and potency similar to those of morphine, with principle actions at the opiate receptors. It is recommended for the relief of moderate to severe pain.

Pharmacokinetics

- *Absorption:* Meperidine given orally is only half as effective as it is parenterally. Onset of analgesia occurs within 10 to 45 minutes. Duration of action is 2 to 4 hours.
- *Distribution:* Drug is distributed widely throughout the body and is 60% to 80% bound to plasma proteins.
- *Metabolism:* Metabolized primarily by hydrolysis in the liver to an acute metabolite, normeperidine.
- *Excretion:* About 30% of dose is excreted in the urine as the N-demethylated derivative; about 5% is excreted unchanged. Excretion is enhanced by acidifying the urine. Half-life of parent compound is 3 to 5 hours and the half-life of metabolite is 8 to 21 hours.

Contraindications and precautions

Contraindicated in patients with hypersensitivity to drug and in those who have received MAO inhibitors within the past 14 days.

Use cautiously in elderly or debilitated patients and in those with increased intracranial pressure, head injury, asthma, other respiratory conditions, supraventricular tachycardia, seizures, acute abdominal conditions, renal or hepatic disease, hypothyroidism, Addison's disease, urethral stricture, and prostatic hyperplasia.

Interactions

Concomitant use with other *CNS depressants* (*alcohol, narcotic analgesics, general anesthetics, antihistamines, barbiturates, benzodiazepines, muscle relaxants, phenothiazines, sedative-hypnotics,* and *tricyclic antidepressants*) potentiates drug's respiratory and CNS depression, sedation, and hypotensive effects. Concomitant use with *cimetidine* may also increase respiratory and CNS depression, causing confusion, disorientation, apnea, or seizures; such use requires reduced dosage of meperidine.

Drug accumulation and enhanced effects may result from concomitant use with other *drugs that are extensively metabolized in the liver* (*rifampin, phenytoin,* and *digitoxin*); combined use with *anticholinergics* may cause paralytic ileus.

Patients who become physically dependent on drug may experience acute withdrawal syndrome if given a narcotic antagonist.

Severe CV depression may result from concomitant use with *general anesthetics*; meperidine can potentiate the adverse effects of *isoniazid.*

Concomitant use with *MAO inhibitors* may precipitate unpredictable and occasionally fatal reactions, even in patients who may receive MAO inhibitors within 14 days of receiving meperidine. Some reactions have been characterized by coma, respiratory depression, cyanosis, and hypotension; in others, hyperexcitability, seizures, tachycardia, hyperpyrexia, and hypertension have occurred.

Effects on diagnostic tests

Drug increases plasma amylase or lipase levels through increased biliary tract pressure; levels may be unreliable for 24 hours after meperidine administration.

Adverse reactions

CNS: *sedation, somnolence, clouded sensorium, euphoria, dizziness,* paradoxical excitement, tremor, ***seizures*** (with large doses), headache, hallucinations, syncope, *light-headedness.*
CV: *hypotension,* bradycardia, tachycardia, ***cardiac arrest, shock.***
GI: *constipation,* ileus, dry mouth, *nausea, vomiting,* biliary tract spasms.
GU: *urine retention.*
Respiratory: ***respiratory depression, respiratory arrest.***
Skin: pruritus, urticaria, *diaphoresis.*
Other: physical dependence, muscle twitching; phlebitis (after I.V. delivery); pain (at injection site); local tissue irritation, induration (after S.C. injection).

Overdose and treatment

The most common signs and symptoms of meperidine overdose are CNS depression, respiratory depression, skeletal muscle flaccidity, cold and clammy skin, mydriasis, bradycardia, and hypotension. Other acute toxic effects include hypothermia, shock, apnea, cardiopulmonary arrest, circulatory collapse, pulmonary edema, and seizures.

To treat acute overdose, first establish adequate respiratory exchange via a patent airway and ventilation as needed; administer a narcotic antagonist (naloxone) to reverse respiratory depression. (Because the duration of action of meperidine is longer than that of naloxone, repeated dosing is necessary.) Naloxone should not be given unless the patient has clinically significant respiratory or CV depression. Monitor vital signs closely.

If patient presents within 2 hours of ingestion of an oral overdose, empty the stomach immediately by inducing emesis (ipecac syrup) or using gastric lavage. Use caution to avoid risk of aspiration. Administer activated charcoal via nasogastric tube for further removal of meperidine, and acidify urine to help remove drug.

Provide symptomatic and supportive treatment (continued respiratory support, correction of fluid or electrolyte imbalance). Monitor laboratory parameters, vital signs, and neurologic status closely.

☑ Special considerations

Besides those relevant to all *opioids,* consider the following recommendations.

- Drug may be administered to some patients who are allergic to morphine.
- Drug and its active metabolite normeperidine accumulate. Monitor for neurotoxic effects, especially in burn patients and those with poor renal function, sickle cell anemia, or cancer.

• Because drug toxicity commonly appears after several days of treatment, this drug is not recommended for treatment of chronic pain.
• Drug may be given slow I.V., preferably as a diluted solution. S.C. injection is very painful. During I.V. administration, tachycardia may occur, possibly as a result of drug's atropine-like effects.
• Oral dose is less than half as effective as parenteral dose. Give I.M. if possible. When changing from parenteral to oral route, dosage should be increased.
• Syrup has local anesthetic effect. Give with water.
• Alternating meperidine with a peripherally active nonnarcotic analgesic (aspirin, acetaminophen, NSAIDs) may improve pain control while allowing lower narcotic dosages.
• Injectable meperidine is compatible with sodium chloride and D_5W solutions and their combinations, and with lactated Ringer's and sodium lactate solution.
• Question patient carefully regarding possible use of MAO inhibitors within the past 14 days.

Geriatric use

• Lower doses are usually indicated for elderly patients, because they may be more sensitive to the therapeutic and adverse effects of drug.

Pediatric use

• Drug should not be administered to infants under age 6 months.

Breast-feeding

• Drug is excreted in breast milk; use with caution in breast-feeding women.

mephenytoin

Mesantoin

Pharmacologic classification: hydantoin derivative
Therapeutic classification: anticonvulsant
Pregnancy risk category NR

How supplied

Available by prescription only
Tablets: 100 mg

Indications, route, and dosage

Generalized tonic-clonic or complex-partial seizures

Adults: 50 to 100 mg P.O. daily; may increase by 50 to 100 mg at weekly intervals, up to 200 mg P.O. q 8 hours. Dosages up to 800 mg/day may be required.
Children: Initial dosage is 50 to 100 mg P.O. daily. May increase slowly by 50 to 100 mg at weekly intervals up to 200 mg P.O. t.i.d., divided q 8 hours. Dosage must be adjusted individually. Usual maintenance dosage is 100 to 400 mg/day (or 3 to 15 mg/kg/day or 100 to 450 mg/m^2/day) administered in three equally divided doses.

Pharmacodynamics

Anticonvulsant action: Like other hydantoin derivatives, mephenytoin stabilizes the neuronal membranes and limits seizure activity either by increasing efflux or by decreasing influx of sodium ions across cell membranes in the motor cortex during generation of nerve impulses. Like phenytoin, mephenytoin appears to have antiarrhythmic effects.

Mephenytoin is used for prophylaxis of tonic-clonic (grand mal), psychomotor, focal, and jacksonian-type partial seizures in patients refractory to less toxic agents. It is usually combined with phenytoin, phenobarbital, or primidone; phenytoin is preferred because it causes less sedation than barbiturates. Mephenytoin also is used with succinimides to control combined absence and tonic-clonic disorders; combined use with oxazolidinediones is not recommended because of the increased hazard of blood dyscrasias.

Pharmacokinetics

• *Absorption:* Mephenytoin is absorbed from the GI tract. Onset of action occurs in 30 minutes and persists for 24 to 48 hours.
• *Distribution:* Drug is distributed widely throughout the body; good seizure control without toxicity occurs when serum concentrations of drug and major metabolite reach 25 to 40 mcg/ml.
• *Metabolism:* Mephenytoin is metabolized by the liver.
• *Excretion:* Drug and its metabolites are excreted in urine.

Contraindications and precautions

Contraindicated in patients with hydantoin hypersensitivity.

Interactions

Mephenytoin's therapeutic effects and toxicity may be increased by concomitant use with *oral anticoagulants, antihistamines, chloramphenicol, cimetidine, diazepam, diazoxide, disulfiram, isoniazid, phenylbutazone, salicylates, sulfamethizole,* or *valproate.* Mephenytoin's therapeutic effects may be decreased by concomitant use of *alcohol* or *folic acid.* Mephenytoin may decrease the effects of *oral contraceptives.*

Effects on diagnostic tests

Mephenytoin may elevate liver function test results.

Adverse reactions

CNS: ataxia, *drowsiness,* fatigue, irritability, choreiform movements, depression, tremor, insomnia, dizziness (usually transient).
EENT: conjunctivitis, diplopia, nystagmus, gingival hyperplasia (with prolonged use).
GI: nausea and vomiting (with prolonged use).
Hematologic: ***neutropenia, agranulocytosis, thrombocytopenia,*** eosinophilia, leukocytosis.
Skin: rash, ***exfoliative dermatitis, Stevens-Johnson syndrome, fatal dermatitides leukopenia.***
Other: edema, lymphadenopathy, polyarthropathy, ***pulmonary fibrosis.***

Overdose and treatment

Signs of acute mephenytoin toxicity may include restlessness, dizziness, drowsiness, nausea, vomiting, nystagmus, ataxia, dysarthria, tremor, and slurred speech; hypotension, respiratory depression, and coma may follow. Death may result from respiratory and circulatory depression.

Treat overdose with gastric lavage or emesis and follow with supportive treatment. Carefully monitor vital signs and fluid and electrolyte balance. Forced diuresis is of little or no value. Hemodialysis or peritoneal dialysis may be helpful.

☑ Special considerations

Besides those relevant to all *hydantoin derivatives,* consider the following recommendations.

- Decreased alertness and coordination are most pronounced at start of treatment. Patient may need help with walking and other activities for first few days.
- Drug should not be discontinued abruptly. Transition from mephenytoin to other anticonvulsant drug should progress over 6 weeks.
- CBC and platelet counts should be performed before therapy, after 2 weeks of initial therapy, and after 2 weeks on maintenance dose; they should be repeated every month for 1 year and, subsequently, at 3-month intervals.
- Safe use of mephenytoin during pregnancy has not been established. Drug should be used during pregnancy only when clearly needed.

Patient education

- Tell patient never to discontinue drug or change dosage except as prescribed and to avoid alcohol, which decreases effectiveness of drug and increases sedative effects.
- Explain that follow-up laboratory tests are essential for safe use.
- Instruct patient to report unusual changes immediately (cutaneous reaction, sore throat, glandular swelling, fever, mucous membrane swelling).

Pediatric use

- Children usually require from 100 to 400 mg/day.

Breast-feeding

- Safe use in breast-feeding has not been established. Alternative feeding method is recommended during therapy with mephenytoin.

meprobamate

Apo-Meprobamate*, Equanil, Meprospan, Miltown, Neuramate

Pharmacologic classification: carbamate
Therapeutic classification: antianxiety
Controlled substance schedule IV
Pregnancy risk category D

How supplied

Available by prescription only
Tablets: 200 mg, 400 mg, 600 mg
Capsules (sustained-release): 200 mg, 400 mg

Indications, route, and dosage

Anxiety and tension

Adults: 1.2 to 1.6 g P.O. daily in three or four equally divided doses. Maximum dosage, 2.4 g daily (sustained-release capsules, 400 to 800 mg b.i.d.).
Children age 6 to 12: 100 to 200 mg P.O. b.i.d. or t.i.d. Not recommended for children under age 6 (sustained-release capsules, 200 mg b.i.d.).

Pharmacodynamics

Anxiolytic action: While the cellular mechanism is unknown, drug causes nonselective CNS depression similar to that seen with use of barbiturates. Meprobamate acts at multiple sites in the CNS, including the thalamus, hypothalamus, limbic system, and spinal cord, but not the medulla or reticular activating system.

Pharmacokinetics

- *Absorption:* After oral administration, drug is well absorbed; peak serum levels occur in 1 to 3 hours. Sedation usually occurs within 1 hour.
- *Distribution:* Meprobamate is distributed throughout the body; 20% is protein-bound. Drug occurs in breast milk at two to four times the serum concentration; meprobamate crosses the placenta.
- *Metabolism:* Metabolized rapidly in the liver to inactive glucuronide conjugates. Half-life of drug is 6 to 17 hours.
- *Excretion:* Metabolites of drug and 10% to 20% of a single dose as unchanged drug are excreted in urine.

Contraindications and precautions

Contraindicated in patients hypersensitive to meprobamate or related compounds (such as carisoprodol, mebutamate, tybamate, and carbromal) and in those with porphyria. Avoid use of drug during first trimester of pregnancy.

Use cautiously in elderly or debilitated patients and in those with impaired renal or hepatic function, seizure disorders, or suicidal tendencies.

Interactions

Meprobamate may add to or potentiate the effects of *alcohol, antihistamines, barbiturates, narcotics, tranquilizers,* or *other CNS depressants.*

Effects on diagnostic tests

Drug therapy may falsely elevate urinary 17-ketosteroids, 17-ketogenic steroids (as determined by the Zimmerman reaction), and 17-hydroxycorticosteroid levels (as determined by the Glenn-Nelson technique).

Adverse reactions

CNS: *drowsiness,* ataxia, dizziness, slurred speech, headache, vertigo, ***seizures.***
CV: palpitations, tachycardia, hypotension, ***arrhythmias,*** syncope.
GI: nausea, vomiting, diarrhea.
Hematologic: *aplastic anemia, thrombocytopenia, agranulocytosis.*
Skin: pruritus, urticaria, erythematous maculopapular rash, ***hypersensitivity reactions.***

After abrupt withdrawal of long-term therapy, severe generalized tonic-clonic seizures may occur.

Overdose and treatment

Clinical manifestations of overdose include drowsiness, lethargy, ataxia, coma, hypotension, shock, and respiratory depression.

Treatment of overdose is supportive and symptomatic, including maintaining adequate ventilation and a patent airway, with mechanical ventilation if needed.

Treat hypotension with fluids and vasopressors as needed. Empty gastric contents by emesis or lavage if ingestion was recent, followed by activated charcoal and a cathartic. Treat seizures with parenteral diazepam. Peritoneal dialysis and hemodialysis may effectively remove drug. Serum levels above 100 mcg/ml may be fatal.

☑ Special considerations

- Assess level of consciousness and vital signs frequently.
- Impose safety precautions, such as raised bed rails, especially for elderly patients, when initiating treatment, or increasing the dose. Patient may need assistance when walking.
- Periodic evaluation of CBC is recommended during long-term therapy.
- Drug abuse and addiction may occur.
- Withdraw drug gradually; otherwise, withdrawal symptoms may occur if patient has been taking drug for a long time.

Patient education

- Tell patient to avoid alcohol and other CNS depressants, such as antihistamines, narcotics, and tranquilizers, while taking drug, unless prescribed.
- Advise patient not to increase dose or frequency and not to abruptly discontinue or decrease dose unless prescribed.
- Tell patient to avoid tasks that require mental alertness or physical coordination until drug's CNS effects are known.
- Recommend sugarless candy or gum or ice chips to relieve dry mouth.
- Advise patient to report sore throat, fever, or unusual bleeding or bruising.
- Inform patient of potential for physical or psychological dependence with chronic use.

Geriatric use

- Elderly patients may have more pronounced CNS effects. Use lowest dose possible.

Pediatric use

- Safety has not been established in children under age 6.

Breast-feeding

- Drug is found in breast milk at two to four times the serum concentration. Do not use in breast-feeding women.

mercaptopurine (6-MP)

Purinethol

Pharmacologic classification: antimetabolite (cell cycle–phase specific, S phase)
Therapeutic classification: antineoplastic
Pregnancy risk category D

How supplied

Available by prescription only
Tablets (scored): 50 mg

Indications, route, and dosage

Dosage and indications may vary. Check current literature for recommended protocols.

Acute lymphoblastic leukemia (in children), acute myeloblastic leukemia, chronic myelocytic leukemia

Adults: 2.5 mg/kg P.O. daily as a single dose, up to 5 mg/kg daily. Maintenance dosage 1.5 to 2.5 mg/kg daily.

Children age 5 and over: 2.5 mg/kg P.O. daily. Maintenance dosage, 1.5 to 2.5 mg/kg daily.

◇ ***Treatment of regional enteritis (Crohn's disease) and ulcerative colitis***

Adults: Usual dosage is 1.5 mg/kg/day, gradually increased to 2.5 mg/kg/day if tolerated.

Pharmacodynamics

Antineoplastic action: Mercaptopurine is converted intracellularly to its active form, which exerts its cytotoxic antimetabolic effects by competing for an enzyme required for purine synthesis. This results in inhibition of DNA and RNA synthesis. Cross-resistance exists between mercaptopurine and thioguanine.

Pharmacokinetics

- *Absorption:* Absorption after an oral dose is incomplete and variable; approximately 50% of a dose is absorbed. Peak serum levels occur 2 hours after a dose.
- *Distribution:* Distributes widely into total body water. Drug crosses the blood-brain barrier, but the CSF concentration is too low for treatment of meningeal leukemias.
- *Metabolism:* Drug is extensively metabolized in the liver. It appears to undergo extensive first-pass metabolism, contributing to its low bioavailability.
- *Excretion:* Drug and its metabolites are excreted in urine.

Contraindications and precautions

Contraindicated in patients whose disease has shown resistance to drug. Use cautiously after chemotherapy or radiation therapy in patients with depressed neutrophil or platelet counts and in those with impaired renal or hepatic function.

Interactions

The concomitant use of *allopurinol* at doses of 300 to 600 mg/day, increases the toxic effects of mercaptopurine, especially myelosuppression. This interaction is due to the inhibition of mercaptopurine metabolism by allopurinol. Reduce dosage of mercaptopurine to 25% to 30% when administering concomitantly with allopurinol.

Concomitant use with mercaptopurine decreases the anticoagulant activity of *warfarin*. The mechanism of this interaction is unknown. Enhanced marrow suppression has occurred when mercaptopurine has been used with *trimethoprim-sulfamethoxazole*.

Drug should be used cautiously with *other hepatotoxic drugs* because of the increased potential for hepatotoxicity.

Effects on diagnostic tests

Drug may also cause falsely elevated serum glucose and uric acid values when sequential multiple analyzer is used.

Adverse reactions

GI: *nausea, vomiting, anorexia, painful oral ulcers, diarrhea, **pancreatitis**, GI ulceration.*
Hematologic: ***leukopenia, thrombocytopenia***, anemia (all may persist several days after drug is stopped).
Hepatic: *jaundice, **hepatotoxicity**.*
Skin: rash, hyperpigmentation.
Other: hyperuricemia.

Overdose and treatment

Clinical manifestations of overdose include myelosuppression, nausea, vomiting, and hepatic necrosis.

Treatment is usually supportive and includes transfusion of blood components and antiemetics. Hemodialysis is thought to be of marginal use because of the rapid intracellular incorporation of mercaptopurine into active metabolites with long persistence.

☑ Special considerations

- Monitor weekly blood counts; watch for precipitous fall.
- Store tablets at room temperature and protect from light.
- Dose modifications may be required following chemotherapy or radiation therapy, in depressed neutrophil or platelet count, and in impaired hepatic or renal function.
- Monitor intake and output. Push fluids (3 L/day).
- Drug is sometimes called 6-mercaptopurine or 6-MP.
- Monitor hepatic function and hematologic values weekly during therapy.
- Monitor serum uric acid levels. If allopurinol is necessary, use very cautiously.
- Observe for signs of bleeding and infection.
- Hepatic dysfunction is reversible when drug is stopped. Watch for jaundice, clay-colored stools, and frothy dark urine. Drug should be stopped if hepatic tenderness occurs.
- Avoid all I.M. injections when platelet count is below 100,000/mm^3.

Patient education

- Warn patient that improvement may take 2 to 4 weeks or longer.
- Tell patient to continue medication despite nausea and vomiting.
- Instruct patient to call immediately if vomiting occurs shortly after taking a dose.
- Warn patient to avoid alcoholic beverages while taking drug.
- Urge patient to ensure adequate fluid intake, to increase urine output and facilitate the excretion of uric acid.
- Advise patient to avoid exposure to people with infections. Tell patient to call immediately if signs of unusual bleeding or infection occur.
- Advise women of childbearing age not to become pregnant while receiving drug.

Pediatric use

- Adverse GI reactions are less common in children than in adults.

Breast-feeding

- It is not known if drug distributes into breast milk. However, because of the potential for serious adverse reactions, mutagenicity, and carcinogenicity in the infant, breast-feeding is not recommended.

meropenem

Merrem I.V.

Pharmacologic classification: carbapenem derivative
Therapeutic classification: antibiotic
Pregnancy risk category B

How supplied

Available by prescription only
Powder for injection: 500 mg/15 ml, 500 mg/20 ml, 500 mg/100 ml, 1 g/15 ml, 1 g/30 ml, 1 g/100 ml

Indications, route, and dosage

***Complicated appendicitis and peritonitis caused by viridans group streptococci,* Escherichia coli, Klebsiella pneumoniae, Pseudomonas aeruginosa, Bacteroides fragilis, B. thetaiotaomicron, *and* Peptostreptococcus species*; bacterial meningitis caused by* Streptococcus pneumoniae, Haemophilus influenzae, *and* Neisseria meningitidis**

Adults: Administer 1 g I.V. q 8 hours over 15 to 30 minutes as I.V. infusion or over about 3 to 5 minutes as I.V. bolus injection (5 to 20 ml).

Children age 3 months and older: Give 20 mg/kg (intra-abdominal infection) or 40 mg/kg (bacterial meningitis) q 8 hours over 15 to 30 minutes as I.V. infusion or over about 3 to 5 minutes as I.V. bolus injection (5 to 20 ml).

Note: For children weighing over 110 lb (50 kg) give 1 g q 8 hours for treating intra-abdominal infections and 2 g q 8 hours for treating meningitis.

✦ ***Dosage adjustment.*** In adults with renal failure, give 1 g q 12 hours if creatinine clearance is 26 to 50 ml/minute, 500 mg q 12 hours if it is 10 to 25 ml/minute, and 500 mg q 24 hours if it is below 10 ml/minute. There is no experience in children with renal impairment.

Pharmacodynamics

Antibiotic action: Meropenem inhibits cell wall synthesis in bacteria. It readily penetrates the cell wall of most gram-positive and gram-negative bacteria to reach penicillin-binding protein targets.

Pharmacokinetics

- *Absorption:* Meropenem is only given I.V.
- *Distribution:* Drug is distributed into most body fluids and tissues, including CSF. It is only about 2% bound to plasma protein.
- *Metabolism:* Drug is thought to undergo minimal metabolism. One inactive metabolite has been identified.
- *Excretion:* Excreted unchanged primarily in urine. Drug's elimination half-life in adults with normal renal function and children age 2 and older is about 1, and 1½ hours in children age 3 months to 2 years.

Contraindications and precautions

Contraindicated in patients with hypersensitivity to any component of drug or other drugs in the same class and in those who have demonstrated anaphylactic reactions to beta-lactams. Use cautiously in patients with history of seizure disorders or impaired renal function.

Interactions

Probenecid competes with meropenem for active tubular secretion and thus inhibits the renal excretion of meropenem. This significantly increases the elimination half-life of meropenem and the extent of systemic exposure. Therefore, the coadministration of probenecid with meropenem is not recommended.

Effects on diagnostic tests

None reported.

Adverse reactions

CNS: headache, syncope, insomnia, agitation, delirium, confusion, dizziness, ***seizure***, nervousness, paresthesia, hallucinations, somnolence, anxiety, depression.
CV: ***heart failure, cardiac arrest, MI, pulmonary embolism***, tachycardia, hypertension, ***bradycardia***, hypotension.
GI: diarrhea, nausea, vomiting, constipation, abdominal pain or enlargement, oral moniliasis, anorexia.
GU: dysuria, ***kidney failure***, increased creatinine clearance or BUN levels, presence of RBCs in urine.
Hematologic: anemia, increased or decreased platelet count, increased eosinophil count, prolonged or shortened PT or partial thromboplastin time, positive direct or indirect Coombs' test, decreased hemoglobin or hematocrit, decreased WBC count.
Hepatic: ***hepatic failure***, cholestatic jaundice, jaundice, flatulence, ileus; increased levels of ALT, AST, alkaline phosphatase, LD, and bilirubin.
Respiratory: ***apnea, hypoxia,*** respiratory disorder, dyspnea.
Skin: rash, pruritus, urticaria, sweating.
Other: ***hypersensitivity and anaphylactic reactions;*** inflammation, pain, edema, phlebitis, or thrombophlebitis at injection site; bleeding events, pain, chest pain, ***sepsis***, ***shock***, fever, back pain, peripheral edema.

Overdose and treatment

Clinical manifestations and treatment of overdosage are unknown. If overdose occurs, discontinue drug and give general supportive treatment until renal elimination occurs. Meropenem and its metabolite are readily dialyzable and effectively removed by hemodialysis.

☑ Special considerations

- Do not use to treat methicillin-resistant staphylococci.
- Obtain specimen for culture and sensitivity tests before giving first dose. Therapy may begin pending test results.
- For I.V. bolus administration, add 10 ml of sterile water for injection to 500 mg/20 ml vial size or 20 ml to 1 g/30 ml vial size. Shake to dissolve and let stand until clear.
- For I.V. infusion, infusion vials (500 mg/100 ml and 1 g/100 ml) may be directly reconstituted with a compatible infusion fluid. Alternatively, an injection vial may be reconstituted, then the resulting solution added to an I.V. container and further diluted with an appropriate infusion fluid. ADD-Vantage vials should not be used.
- For ADD-Vantage vials, reconstitute only with half 0.45% NaCl injection, 0.9% NaCl injection, or 5% dextrose injection in 50-, 100-, or 250-ml Abbott ADD-Vantage flexible diluent containers. Follow manufacturer guidelines closely when using ADD-Vantage vials.
- Do not mix with or physically add meropenem to solutions containing other drugs.
- Use freshly prepared solutions of meropenem immediately whenever possible. Stability of drug varies with type of drug used (injection vial, infusion vial, or ADD-Vantage container). Consult manufacturer's literature for details.
- Serious and occasionally fatal hypersensitivity (anaphylactic) reactions have been reported in patients receiving therapy with beta-lactams. Before therapy is initiated, ascertain if previous hypersensitivity reactions to penicillins, cephalosporins, other beta-lactams, and other allergens have occurred.
- Discontinue drug immediately if an allergic reaction occurs. Serious anaphylactic reactions require immediate, emergency treatment with epinephrine, oxygen, I.V. steroids, and airway management. Other therapy may also be required as indicated by the patient's condition.
- Seizures and other CNS adverse reactions associated with meropenem therapy commonly occur in patients with CNS disorders, bacterial meningitis, and compromised renal function.
- If seizures occur during meropenem therapy, decrease dosage or discontinue meropenem.
- Drug may cause overgrowth of nonsusceptible bacteria or fungi. Monitor patient for signs and symptoms of superinfection.
- Periodic assessment of organ system functions, including renal, hepatic, and hematopoietic, is recommended during prolonged therapy.

Geriatric use
• Use cautiously in elderly patients because of decreased renal function. Dosage adjustment is recommended in patients with advanced age whose creatinine clearance levels are below 50 ml/minute.

Pediatric use
• Safety and effectiveness have not been established for pediatric patients under age 3 months.

Breast-feeding
• It is not known if drug is excreted in breast milk; use cautiously in breast-feeding women.

mesalamine
Asacol, Pentasa, Rowasa

Pharmacologic classification: salicylate
Therapeutic classification: anti-inflammatory
Pregnancy risk category B

How supplied
Available by prescription only
Capsules (controlled-release): 250 mg
Tablets (delayed-release): 400 mg
Suppositories: 500 mg
Rectal suspension: 4 g/60 ml, in units of 7 disposable bottles

Indications, route, and dosage
Active mild to moderate distal ulcerative colitis, proctosigmoiditis, proctitis
Adults: 800 mg (delayed-release tablets) P.O. t.i.d. for 6 weeks or 1 g (controlled-release capsules) q.i.d. for up to 8 weeks.

Alternatively, use 1 rectal suppository b.i.d. for 3 to 6 weeks. For maximum benefit, the suppository should be retained for 1 to 3 hours or longer. Usual dosage of mesalamine suspension enema in 60-ml units is one rectal instillation (4 g) once daily, preferably h.s., retained for approximately 8 hours.

◊ Lower doses of suspension enemas of 4 g q 2 to 3 nights or 1 g daily have been effective.

Pharmacodynamics
Anti-inflammatory action: Mechanism of action of mesalamine (and sulfasalazine) is unknown, but appears to be topical rather than systemic. Mucosal production of arachidonic acid (AA) metabolites, both through cyclooxygenase pathways (for example, prostaglandins [PGs]) and through lipoxygenase pathways (for example, leukotrienes [LTs] and hydroxyeicosatetraenoic acids [HETEs]) is increased in patients with chronic inflammatory bowel disease; possibly, mesalamine may diminish inflammation by blocking cyclooxygenase and inhibiting PG production in the colon.

Sulfasalazine is split by bacterial action in the colon into sulfapyridine (SP) and mesalamine (5-ASA). The mesalamine component is considered therapeutically active in ulcerative colitis. The usual oral dose of sulfasalazine for active ulcerative colitis in adults is 3 to 4 g per day in divided doses; 4 g of sulfasalazine provide 1.6 g of free mesalamine to the colon.

Pharmacokinetics
• *Absorption:* Drug administered rectally as a suppository or suspension enema is poorly absorbed from the colon. Extent of absorption depends on retention time, with considerable individual variation. Oral tablets are coated with an acrylic resin that delays the release of drug until tablet is beyond the terminal ileum. About 72% of a dose reaches the colon; 28% of a dose is absorbed. Absorption is not affected by food. Capsules are formulated to release therapeutic concentrations throughout the GI tract. About 20% to 30% is absorbed.
• *Distribution:* Maximum plasma levels of oral mesalamine and N-acetyl 5-aminosalicylic acid are about twice as high as those seen with sulfasalazine therapy. At steady state, approximately 10% to 30% of daily 4-g rectal dose can be recovered in cumulative 24-hour urine collections.
• *Metabolism:* Drug undergoes acetylation, but site is unknown. Most absorbed drug is excreted in urine as the N-acetyl-5-ASA metabolite. Elimination half-life of drug is ½ to 1½ hours; half-life of acetylated metabolite is 5 to 10 hours. Steady-state plasma levels show no accumulation of either free or metabolized drug during repeated daily administrations.
• *Excretion:* After rectal administration, drug is mostly excreted in the feces as parent drug and metabolite. After oral administration, drug is mostly excreted in the urine as metabolite.

Contraindications and precautions
Contraindicated in patients hypersensitive to drug, its components (sulfite in rectal preparation), or salicylates. Use cautiously in patients with impaired renal function.

Interactions
None reported.

Effects on diagnostic tests
None reported.

Adverse reactions
CNS: headache, dizziness, fatigue, malaise, asthenia, chills, anxiety, depression, hyperesthesia, paresthesia, tremor.
GI: abdominal pain, cramps, discomfort, flatulence, diarrhea, rectal pain, bloating, nausea, *pancolitis*, vomiting, constipation, eructation.
Respiratory: wheezing.
Skin: itching, rash, urticaria, hair loss.
Other: ***anaphylaxis*** (rare), fever, arthralgia, chest pain, myalgia, back pain, hypertonia, dysuria, hematuria, urinary urgency.

Overdose and treatment
No information available.

☑ Special considerations
• While drug's effects may be evident in 3 to 21 days, usual course of therapy is 3 to 6 weeks de-

pending on symptoms and sigmoidoscopic findings. Clinical studies have not determined if suspension enema will modify relapse rates after the 6-week, short-term treatment.

Patient education

- Tell patient to swallow the tablets whole and not to crush or chew them.
- For maximum effectiveness, tell patient to retain suppository as long as possible (at least 1 to 3 hours).
- Instruct patient in correct use of rectal suspension:

– Shake the bottle well to make sure the suspension is homogeneous.

– Remove the protective sheath from the applicator tip. Holding the bottle at the neck will not cause medication to be discharged.

– To administer, lie on the left side (to facilitate migration into the sigmoid colon) with the lower leg extended and the upper right leg flexed forward for balance; or may use the knee-chest position.

– Gently insert the applicator tip in the rectum, pointing toward the umbilicus.

– Steadily squeeze the bottle to discharge the preparation into the colon.

- Patient instructions are included with every 7 units.

Pediatric use

- Safety and efficacy for use in children have not been established.

Breast-feeding

- It is not known if drug or its metabolites are excreted in breast milk. Avoid breast-feeding during therapy because many drugs are excreted in breast milk.

mesna

Mesnex

Pharmacologic classification: thiol derivative
Therapeutic classification: uroprotectant
Pregnancy risk category B

How supplied

Available by prescription only
Injection: 100 mg/ml in 2- and 10-ml ampules

Indications, route, and dosage

Prevention of ifosfamide-induced hemorrhagic cystitis

Adults: Calculate daily dose as 60% of the ifosfamide dose. Administer in three equally divided bolus doses: Give first dose at time of ifosfamide injection. Subsequent doses are given at 4 and 8 hours following ifosfamide.

Protocols that use 1.2 g/m² ifosfamide would employ 240 mg/m² mesna at 0, 4, and 8 hours after ifosfamide.

◊ ***Prophylaxis in bone marrow recipients receiving cyclophosphamides***

Adults: 60% to 160% of the cyclophosphamide daily dose given in three to five divided doses or by continuous infusion.

Pharmacodynamics

Uroprotectant action: Mesna disulfide is reduced to mesna in the kidney and reacts with the urotoxic metabolites of ifosfamide to detoxify the drug and protect the urinary system.

Pharmacokinetics

- *Absorption:* Mesna is administered I.V.
- *Distribution:* Remains in the vascular compartment. Mesna doesn't distribute through tissues.
- *Metabolism:* Rapidly metabolized to mesna disulfide, its only metabolite.
- *Excretion:* In the kidneys, 33% of the dose is eliminated in the urine in 24 hours; half-life of mesna and mesna disulfide are 0.36 and 1.17 hours, respectively.

Contraindications and precautions

Contraindicated in patients hypersensitive to mesna or thiol-containing compounds.

Interactions

None reported.

Effects on diagnostic tests

Mesna may produce a false-positive test for urinary ketones. A red-violet color will return to violet with the addition of acetic acid.

Adverse reactions

CNS: headache, fatigue.
GI: soft stools, nausea, vomiting, diarrhea, dysgeusia.
Other: limb pain, hypotension, allergy.

Note: Because mesna is used concomitantly with ifosfamide and other chemotherapeutic agents, it is difficult to determine adverse reactions attributable solely to mesna.

Overdose and treatment

No information available. There is no known antidote.

☑ Special considerations

- Mesnex multidose vials may be stored and used for up to 8 days.
- Discard unused mesna from open ampules. It will form an inactive oxidation product (dimesna) upon exposure to oxygen.
- Dilute appropriate dose in 5% dextrose injection, 0.9% NaCl solution injection, or lactated Ringer's injection to a concentration of 20 mg/ml. Once diluted, solution is stable for 24 hours at room temperature.
- Mesna is physically incompatible with cisplatin. Do not add mesna to cisplatin infusions.

Patient education

- Instruct patient to report hematuria or allergy immediately.

Pediatric use

- Safety in children has not been established.

Breast-feeding

- It is not known if mesna is excreted in breast milk.

mesoridazine besylate

Serentil

Pharmacologic classification: phenothiazine (piperidine derivative)
Therapeutic classification: antipsychotic
Pregnancy risk category NR

How supplied

Available by prescription only
Tablets: 10 mg, 25 mg, 50 mg, 100 mg
Oral concentrate: 25 mg/ml (0.6% alcohol)
Injection: 25 mg/ml

Indications, route, and dosage

Psychoneurotic manifestations (anxiety)
Adults and children over age 12: 10 mg P.O. t.i.d. up to maximum of 150 mg/day.

Schizophrenia
Adults and children over age 12: Initially, 50 mg P.O. t.i.d. to maximum of 400 mg/day; or 25 mg I.M. repeated in 30 to 60 minutes, p.r.n., not to exceed 200 mg I.M. daily.

Alcoholism
Adults and children over age 12: 25 mg P.O. b.i.d., up to maximum of 200 mg/day.

Behavioral problems associated with chronic brain syndrome
Adults and children over age 12: 25 mg P.O. t.i.d., up to maximum of 300 mg/day. I.M. dosage form is irritating.

Pharmacodynamics

Antipsychotic action: Mesoridazine, a metabolite of thioridazine, is thought to exert its antipsychotic effects by postsynaptic blockade of CNS dopamine receptors, thereby inhibiting dopamine-mediated effects.

Drug has many other central and peripheral effects; it produces both alpha and ganglionic blockade and counteracts histamine- and serotonin-mediated activity. Its most prominent adverse reactions are antimuscarinic and sedative; it causes fewer extrapyramidal effects than other antipsychotics.

Pharmacokinetics

- *Absorption:* Drug appears to be well absorbed from the GI tract following oral administration. I.M. dosage form is absorbed rapidly.
- *Distribution:* Distributed widely into the body, including breast milk. Peak effects occur at 2 to 4 hours; steady-state serum level is achieved within 4 to 7 days. Drug is 91% to 99% protein-bound.
- *Metabolism:* Drug is metabolized extensively by the liver; no active metabolites are formed. Duration of action is 4 to 6 hours.
- *Excretion:* Mostly excreted as metabolites in urine; some is excreted in feces via the biliary tract.

Contraindications and precautions

Contraindicated in patients with hypersensitivity to drug or in those experiencing severe CNS depression or comatose states.

Interactions

Concomitant use of mesoridazine with *sympathomimetics*, including *epinephrine, phenylephrine, phenylpropanolamine*, and *ephedrine* (often found in nasal sprays), or *appetite suppressants* may decrease their stimulatory and pressor effects. *Phenothiazines* can cause epinephrine reversal and produce hypotension when epinephrine is used as a pressor agent.

Mesoridazine may inhibit blood pressure response to *centrally acting antihypertensive drugs*, such as *clonidine, guanabenz, guanadrel, guanethidine, methyldopa*, and *reserpine*. Additive effects are likely after concomitant use of mesoridazine with *CNS depressants*, including *alcohol, analgesics, barbiturates, narcotics, tranquilizers*, and *general, spinal, or epidural anesthetics*, or *parenteral magnesium sulfate* (oversedation, respiratory depression, and hypotension); *antiarrhythmic agents, disopyramide, procainamide*, or *quinidine* (increased incidence of cardiac arrhythmias and conduction defects); *atropine* and *other anticholinergic drugs*, including *antidepressants, antihistamines, MAO inhibitors, meperidine, phenothiazines*, and *antiparkinson agents* (oversedation, paralytic ileus, visual changes, and severe constipation); *nitrates* (hypotension); and *metrizamide* (increased risk of seizures).

Beta-blocking agents may inhibit mesoridazine metabolism, increasing plasma levels and toxicity. Concomitant use with *propylthiouracil* increases risk of agranulocytosis; concomitant use with *lithium* may result in severe neurologic toxicity with an encephalitis-like syndrome, and a decreased therapeutic response to mesoridazine.

Pharmacokinetic alterations and subsequent decreased therapeutic response to mesoridazine may follow concomitant use with *phenobarbital* (enhanced renal excretion); *aluminum- and magnesium-containing antacids and antidiarrheals* (decreased absorption); *caffeine*; or *heavy smoking* (increased metabolism).

Mesoridazine may antagonize therapeutic effect of *bromocriptine* on prolactin secretion; it also may decrease the vasoconstricting effects of *high-dose dopamine*, and may decrease effectiveness and increase toxicity of *levodopa* (by dopamine blockade). Mesoridazine may inhibit metabolism and increase toxicity of *phenytoin*.

Effects on diagnostic tests

Mesoridazine causes false-positive test results for urinary porphyrins, urobilinogen, amylase, and 5-hydroxyindoleacetic acid, because of darkening of urine by metabolites; it also causes false-positive urine pregnancy test results using human chorionic gonadotropin.

Drug elevates tests for liver function and protein-bound iodine and causes quinidine-like effects on the ECG.

Adverse reactions

CNS: extrapyramidal reactions, *tardive dyskinesia, sedation, drowsiness, tremor, rigidity, weakness, EEG changes, dizziness.*
CV: *hypotension, tachycardia, ECG changes.*

EENT: *ocular changes, blurred vision, retinitis pigmentosa, nasal congestion.*
GI: *dry mouth, constipation, nausea, vomiting.*
GU: *urine retention, menstrual irregularities, gynecomastia, inhibited ejaculation.*
Hematologic: leukopenia, ***agranulocytosis, aplastic anemia***, eosinophilia, ***thrombocytopenia.***
Hepatic: jaundice, abnormal liver function test results.
Skin: *mild photosensitivity, allergic reactions, pain at I.M. injection site, sterile abscess, rash.*
Other: weight gain, ***neuroleptic malignant syndrome.***

After abrupt withdrawal of long-term therapy: gastritis, nausea, vomiting, dizziness, tremor, feeling of warmth or cold, diaphoresis, tachycardia, headache, insomnia.

Overdose and treatment

CNS depression is characterized by deep, unarousable sleep and possible coma, hypotension or hypertension, extrapyramidal symptoms, abnormal involuntary muscle movements, agitation, seizures, arrhythmias, ECG changes, hypothermia or hyperthermia, and autonomic nervous system dysfunction.

Treatment is symptomatic and supportive, including maintaining vital signs, airway, stable body temperature, and fluid and electrolyte balance.

Do not induce vomiting: drug inhibits cough reflex, and aspiration may occur. Use gastric lavage, then activated charcoal and sodium chloride cathartics; dialysis does not help. Regulate body temperature as needed. Treat hypotension with I.V. fluids: do not give epinephrine. Treat seizures with parenteral diazepam or barbiturates; arrhythmias, with parenteral phenytoin (1 mg/kg with rate titrated to blood pressure); extrapyramidal reactions, with benztropine at 1 to 2 mg or parenteral diphenhydramine at 10 to 50 mg.

☑ Special considerations

Recommendations for administration of mesoridazine, for care and teaching of the patient during therapy, and for use in elderly and breast-feeding patients are the same as those for all *phenothiazines.*

Pediatric use

- Drug not recommended in children under age 12.

metaproterenol sulfate

Alupent, Metaprel

Pharmacologic classification: adrenergic
Therapeutic classification: bronchodilator
Pregnancy risk category C

How supplied

Available by prescription only
Tablets: 10 mg, 20 mg
Syrup: 10 mg/5 ml
Aerosol inhaler: 0.65 mg/metered spray
Nebulizer inhaler: 0.4%, 0.6%, 5% solution

Indications, route, and dosage

Bronchial asthma and reversible bronchospasm
Oral
Adults and children over age 9 or weighing over 60 lb (27 kg): 20 mg P.O. t.i.d. or q.i.d.
Children age 6 to 9 or weighing below 60 lb: 10 mg P.O. t.i.d. or q.i.d.
Inhalation
Adults and children age 12 and older: Administered by metered aerosol, 2 or 3 inhalations, with at least 2 minutes between inhalations; no more than 12 inhalations in 24 hours. Administered by hand-bulb nebulizer, 10 inhalations of an undiluted 5% solution or alternatively, administered by IPPB, 0.3 ml (range, 0.2 to 0.3 ml of a 5% solution diluted in approximately 2.5 ml of a 0.9% NaCl solution or 2.5 ml of a commercially available 0.4% or 0.6% solution for nebulization).

Pharmacodynamics

Bronchodilator action: Metaproterenol relaxes bronchial smooth muscle and peripheral vasculature by stimulating $beta_2$-adrenergic receptors, thus decreasing airway resistance via bronchodilation. It has lesser effect on $beta_1$ receptors and has little or no effect on alpha-adrenergic receptors. In high doses, it may cause CNS and cardiac stimulation, resulting in tachycardia, hypertension, or tremors.

Pharmacokinetics

- *Absorption:* Well-absorbed from the GI tract. Onset of action occurs within 1 minute after oral inhalation, 5 to 30 minutes after nebulization, and 15 to 30 minutes after oral administration, with peak effects seen in about 1 hour. Duration of action after oral inhalation is 1 to 4 hours after single dose; 1 to 2½ hours after multiple doses; after nebulization, 2 to 6 hours after single dose, 4 to 6 hours after repeated doses; after oral administration, 1 to 4 hours.
- *Distribution:* Drug is widely distributed throughout the body.
- *Metabolism:* Extensively metabolized on first pass through the liver.
- *Excretion:* Drug is excreted in urine, mainly as glucuronic acid conjugates.

Contraindications and precautions

Contraindicated in patients with hypersensitivity to drug or its ingredients, in use during anesthesia with cyclopropane or halogenated hydrocarbon general anesthetics, and in those with tachycardia and arrhythmias associated with tachycardia, peripheral or mesenteric vascular thrombosis, profound hypoxia, or hypercapnia.

Use cautiously in patients with hypertension, hyperthyroidism, heart disease, diabetes, or cirrhosis and in those receiving cardiac glycosides.

Interactions

Concomitant use with *other sympathomimetics* may produce additive effects and toxicity. Use of metaproterenol with *general anesthetics* (especially *chloroform, cyclopropane, halothane,* and *trichlorethylene*), *cardiac glycosides, levodopa, theophylline derivatives, other sympathomimetics,* or *thyroid hormones* may increase the potential for cardiac effects, including severe ventricular tachycardia, cardiac arrhythmias, and coronary insufficiency.

Beta-adrenergic blockers, especially *propranolol*, antagonize metaproterenol's bronchodilating effects.

Increased CNS stimulation may result from concomitant use with *xanthines, other sympathomimetics,* and *other CNS stimulating drugs.*

Concomitant use of *MAO inhibitors* or *tricyclic antidepressants* may potentiate the CV actions.

Effects on diagnostic tests

Drug may reduce sensitivity of spirometry in diagnosis of asthma.

Adverse reactions

CNS: *nervousness, weakness, drowsiness, tremor, vertigo, headache.*
CV: *tachycardia, hypertension, palpitations;* ***cardiac arrest*** (with excessive use).
GI: *vomiting, nausea, heartburn, dry mouth.*
Respiratory: paradoxical bronchiolar constriction with excessive use, cough, dry and irritated throat.
Skin: rash, hypersensitivity reactions.

Overdose and treatment

Clinical manifestations of overdose include exaggeration of common adverse reactions, particularly nausea and vomiting, cardiac arrhythmias, angina, hypertension, and seizures.

Treatment includes supportive and symptomatic measures. Monitor vital signs closely. Support CV status. Use cardioselective $beta_1$-adrenergic blockers (acebutolol, atenolol, metoprolol) to treat symptoms with extreme caution; they may induce severe bronchospasm or asthmatic attack.

☑ Special considerations

Besides those relevant to all *adrenergics,* consider the following recommendations.

- Adverse reactions are dose-related and characteristic of sympathomimetics and may persist a long time because of the long duration of action of metaproterenol.
- Excessive or prolonged use may lead to decreased effectiveness.
- Avoid simultaneous administration of adrenocorticoid inhalation aerosol. Allow at least 5 minutes to lapse between using the two aerosols.
- Monitor patient for signs and symptoms of toxic effects (nausea and vomiting, tremors, and cardiac arrhythmias).
- Aerosol treatments may be used with oral tablet dosing.

Patient education

- Instruct patient to use only as directed and to take no more than two inhalations at one time with 1- to 2-minute intervals between. Remind patient to save applicator; refills may be available.
- Tell patient to take missed dose if remembered within 1 hour. If beyond 1 hour, patient should skip dose and resume regular schedule. The patient should not double dose.
- Tell patient to store drug away from heat and light, and safely out of children's reach.
- Inform patient to call immediately if no relief occurs or condition worsens.
- Warn patient to avoid simultaneous use of adrenocorticoid aerosol and to allow at least 5 minutes to lapse between using the two aerosols.
- Tell patient that he may experience bad taste in mouth after using oral inhaler.
- Instruct patient to shake container, exhale through nose as completely as possible, then administer aerosol while inhaling deeply through mouth, and hold breath for 10 seconds before exhaling slowly. Patient should wait 1 to 2 minutes before repeating inhalations.
- Tell patient that drug may have shorter duration of action after prolonged use. Advise patient to report failure to respond to usual dose.
- Warn patient not to increase dose or frequency unless prescribed; serious adverse reactions are possible.

Geriatric use

- Elderly patients may be more sensitive to the therapeutic and adverse effects of drug.

Pediatric use

- Oral inhalation in children under 12 is not recommended as safety and efficacy have not been established. Safety and efficacy of oral preparations in children under age 6 have not been established.

metaraminol bitartrate

Aramine

Pharmacologic classification: adrenergic
Therapeutic classification: vasopressor
Pregnancy risk category C

How supplied

Available by prescription only
Injection: 10 mg/ml

Indications, route, and dosage

Prevention of hypotension
Adults: 2 to 10 mg I.M. or S.C.
Children: 0.1 mg/kg or 3 mg/m² S.C. or I.M.
Hypotension in severe shock
Adults: 0.5 to 5 mg direct I.V. followed by I.V. infusion. If necessary, mix 15 to 100 mg (up to 500 mg has been used) in 500 ml 0.9% NaCl solution or D_5W; titrate infusion based on blood pressure response.
Children: 0.01 mg/kg or 0.3 mg/m² direct I.V. followed by I.V. infusion, if necessary, of 0.4 mg/kg or 12 mg/m² diluted and titrated to maintain desired blood pressure.
◊ ***Priapism***
Adults: 1 to 2 mg injected into corpus cavernosum of the penis.

Pharmacodynamics

Vasopressor action: Drug acts predominantly by direct stimulation of alpha-adrenergic receptors, which constrict both capacitance and resistance blood vessels, resulting in increased total peripheral resistance; increased systolic and diastolic blood pressure; decreased blood flow to vital organs, skin, and skeletal muscle; and constriction of renal blood vessels, which reduces renal blood flow. It also has a direct stimulating effect on $beta_1$ receptors of the heart, producing a positive inotropic response, and an indirect effect, releasing norepinephrine from its storage sites, which, with repeated use, may result in tachyphylaxis. Metaraminol also acts as a weak or false neurotransmitter by replacing norepinephrine in sympathetic nerve endings. Its main effects are vasoconstriction and cardiac stimulation. It does not usually cause CNS stimulation but may cause contraction of pregnant uterus and uterine blood vessels because of its alpha-adrenergic effects.

Pharmacokinetics

- *Absorption:* Onset of action after I.M. injection occurs within 10 minutes; after I.V. injection, within 1 to 2 minutes; after S.C. injection, 5 to 20 minutes. Pressor effects may persist 20 to 90 minutes, depending on route of administration and patient variability.
- *Distribution:* Not completely known.
- *Metabolism:* In vitro tests suggest that metaraminol is not metabolized. Effects appear to be terminated by uptake of drug into tissues and by urinary excretion.
- *Excretion:* Drug is excreted in urine; may be accelerated by acidifying urine.

Contraindications and precautions

Contraindicated in patients with hypersensitivity to drug and in those receiving anesthesia with cyclopropane and halogenated hydrocarbon anesthetics.

Use cautiously in patients with cardiac or thyroid disease, hypertension, peripheral vascular disease, cirrhosis, history of malaria, or sulfite sensitivity; in those receiving cardiac glycosides; and during pregnancy.

Interactions

Concomitant use may prolong and intensify cardiac stimulant and vasopressor effects of *MAO inhibitors.* Do not administer metaraminol until 14 days after MAO inhibitors have been discontinued.

Increased cardiac effects may result when metaraminol is used with *general anesthetics, cardiac glycosides, levodopa, maprotiline, other sympathomimetics*, or *thyroid hormones.*

When metaraminol is used with the *alpha-adrenergic blocking agents*, pressor effects may be decreased (but not completely blocked). When metaraminol is used with *doxapram, ergot alkaloids, mazindol, methylphenidate,* or *trimethaphan,* pressor effects may be increased.

Concomitant use of *beta blockers* with metaraminol may result in mutual inhibition of therapeutic effects with increased potential for hypertension, and excessive bradycardia with possible heart block.

Metaraminol may also decrease the hypotensive effects of *guanadrel, guanethidine, rauwolfia alkaloids,* and *diuretics* used as antihypertensives. Concomitant use with *atropine* blocks the reflex bradycardia caused by metaraminol and enhances its pressor response.

Effects on diagnostic tests

None reported.

Adverse reactions

CNS: apprehension, dizziness, headache, tremor.
CV: hypertension; hypotension; palpitations; ***arrhythmias***, including sinus or ***ventricular tachycardia***; ***cardiac arrest.***
GI: nausea.
Skin: flushing, diaphoresis.
Other: abscess, necrosis, sloughing upon extravasation.

Overdose and treatment

Clinical manifestations of overdose include severe hypertension, arrhythmias, seizures, cerebral hemorrhage, acute pulmonary edema, and cardiac arrest.

Treatment requires discontinuation of drug followed by supportive and symptomatic measures. Monitor vital signs closely. Use atropine for reflex bradycardia and propranolol for arrhythmias. Use a sympatholytic agent to relieve hypertension.

☑ Special considerations

Besides those relevant to all *adrenergics,* consider the following recommendations.

- Monitor blood pressure and heart rate and rhythm during and after metaraminol administration until patient is stable.
- Correct blood volume depletion before administration. Metaraminol is not a substitute for blood, plasma, fluids, or electrolyte replacement.
- Drug must be diluted before I.V. use. Preferred solutions for dilution are 0.9% NaCl solution or dextrose 5% injection. Select injection site carefully. I.V. route is preferred, using large veins. Avoid extravasation. Monitor infusion rate; use of infusion-controlling device preferred. Withdraw drug gradually; recurrent hypotension may follow abrupt withdrawal.
- When administering I.M. or S.C, allow at least 10 minutes to elapse before administering additional doses because maximum effect is not immediately apparent.
- To treat extravasation, infiltrate site promptly with 10 to 15 ml 0.9% NaCl solution containing 5 to 10 mg phentolamine, using fine needle.
- Cumulative effect possible after prolonged use. Excessive vasopressor response may persist after drug is withdrawn.
- Keep emergency drugs on hand to reverse effect of metaraminol: atropine for reflex bradycardia, phentolamine for extravasation, and propranolol for arrhythmias.
- Monitor diabetic patients closely. Insulin adjustments may be needed.
- Closely monitor fluid and electrolyte status.
- Do not mix in bag or syringe with other medications.

Patient education
- Ask patient about allergy to sulfites before administering drug.
- Inform patient that he will need frequent assessment of vital signs.
- Tell patient to report adverse reactions.

Geriatric use
- Elderly patients may be more sensitive to drug's effects.

Pediatric use
- Because safety has not been fully established, use cautiously.

Breast-feeding
- It is not known if drug is distributed in breast milk; use cautiously in breast-feeding patients.

metformin hydrochloride
Glucophage

Pharmacologic classification: biguanide
Therapeutic classification: antidiabetic
Pregnancy risk category B

How supplied
Available by prescription only
Tablets: 500 mg, 850 mg

Indications, route, and dosage
Adjunct to diet and exercise to lower blood glucose in patients with non-insulin-dependent diabetes mellitus
Adults: Initially, give 500 mg P.O. b.i.d. with morning and evening meals or 850 mg P.O. once daily with morning meal. When 500-mg dosage used, increase dosage by 500 mg weekly to maximum dosage of 2,500 mg daily p.r.n. When 850-mg dosage used, increase dosage 850 mg every other week to maximum daily dosage of 2,550 mg p.r.n.

Pharmacodynamics
Antidiabetic action: Drug decreases hepatic glucose production and intestinal absorption of glucose and improves insulin sensitivity (increases peripheral glucose uptake and utilization).

Pharmacokinetics
- *Absorption:* Absorbed from GI tract with absolute bioavailability being about 50% to 60%. Food decreases the extent and slightly delays absorption.
- *Distribution:* Drug is negligibly bound to plasma proteins. It partitions into erythrocytes, most likely as a function of time.
- *Metabolism:* Metformin is not metabolized.
- *Excretion:* 90% is excreted in urine. Elimination half-life in plasma is about 6.2 to 17.6 hours in blood.

Contraindications and precautions
Contraindicated in patients with hypersensitivity to drug, renal disease, or metabolic acidosis. Drug should be temporarily withheld in patients undergoing radiologic studies involving parenteral administration of iodinated contrast materials because use of such products may result in acute renal dysfunction. Discontinue drug if patient develops a hypoxic state. Avoid use in patients with hepatic disease.

Use cautiously in elderly, debilitated, or malnourished patients and in those with adrenal or pituitary insufficiency because of increased susceptibility to developing hypoglycemia.

Interactions
Calcium channel blockers, corticosteroids, estrogens, isoniazid, nicotinic acid, oral contraceptives, phenothiazines, phenytoin, sympathomimetics, thiazides or other diuretics, and *thyroid agents* may produce hyperglycemia. Monitor patient's glycemic control. Metformin dosage may need to be increased.

Cationic drugs such as *amiloride, cimetidine, digoxin, morphine, procainamide, quinidine, quinine, ranitidine, triamterene, trimethoprim,* and *vancomycin* have the potential to compete for common renal tubular transport systems, which may increase metformin plasma levels. Monitor patient's blood glucose level. *Nifedipine* increases metformin plasma levels. Monitor patient closely. Metformin dosage may need to be decreased.

Effects on diagnostic tests
None reported.

Adverse reactions
GI: diarrhea, nausea, vomiting, abdominal bloating, flatulence, anorexia.
Hematologic: ***megaloblastic anemia.***
Skin: rash, dermatitis.
Other: ***lactic acidosis***, unpleasant or metallic taste.

Overdose and treatment
Hypoglycemia has not been observed with ingestion of up to 85 g of metformin, although lactic acidosis has occurred. Hemodialysis may be useful for removing accumulated drug from patients in whom metformin overdosage is suspected.

☑ Special considerations
- Assess patient's renal function before beginning therapy and then annually thereafter. If renal impairment is detected, give another antidiabetic agent.
- Administer drug with meals; once-daily dosage should be administered with breakfast, twice-daily dosage should be administered with breakfast and dinner.
- When transferring patients from standard oral hypoglycemic agents other than chlorpropamide to metformin, no transition period is necessary. When transferring patients from chlorpropamide, exercise care during the first 2 weeks because of prolonged retention of chlorpropamide in the body, increasing risk of hypoglycemia during this time.
- Monitor patient's blood glucose level regularly to evaluate effectiveness.
- If patient does not respond to 4 weeks of maximum dose of metformin, add an oral sulfonylurea while continuing metformin at the maximum dose.

If patient still does not respond after several months of concomitant therapy at maximum doses, discontinue both agents and initiate insulin therapy.

- Monitor patient closely during times of increased stress, such as infection, fever, surgery, or trauma. Insulin therapy may be required in these situations.
- Incidence of drug-induced lactic acidosis is very low. Reported cases have occurred primarily in diabetic patients with significant renal insufficiency, multiple concomitant medical or surgical problems, and multiple concomitant medications. Risk of lactic acidosis increases with advanced age and degree of renal impairment.
- Discontinue drug immediately if patient develops conditions associated with hypoxemia or dehydration because of risk of lactic acidosis associated with these conditions.
- Suspend therapy temporarily for surgical procedures (except minor procedures not associated with restricted intake of food and fluids) or radiologic procedures involving parenteral administration of iodinated contrast, and do not restart until patient's oral intake has resumed and renal function is normal.
- Monitor patient's hematologic status for megaloblastic anemia. Patients with inadequate vitamin B_{12} or calcium intake or absorption appear to be predisposed to developing subnormal vitamin B_{12} levels. These patients should have serum vitamin B_{12} levels checked routinely at 2- to 3-year intervals.

Patient education

- Instruct patient to discontinue drug immediately and report unexplained hyperventilation, myalgia, malaise, unusual somnolence, or other nonspecific symptoms of early lactic acidosis.
- Warn patient not to consume excessive amounts of alcohol while taking metformin.
- Instruct patient about nature of diabetes, importance of following therapeutic regimen; adhering to specific diet, weight reduction, exercise and personal hygiene programs; and avoiding infection. Explain how and when to perform self-monitoring of blood glucose level, and teach recognition of hypoglycemia and hyperglycemia.
- Tell patient not to change drug dosage without medical approval. Encourage him to report abnormal blood glucose levels.
- Advise patient not to take other medications, including OTC drugs, without calling first.
- Instruct patient to carry medical identification regarding diabetic status.

Geriatric use

- Because aging is associated with decreased renal function, administer cautiously to elderly patients.

Pediatric use

- Safety and effectiveness in pediatric patients have not been established. Studies in maturity-onset diabetes of the young have not been conducted.

Breast-feeding

- It is not known if metformin is excreted in breast milk. Because of the potential for serious adverse effects in nursing infants, drug should not be administered to breast-feeding women.

methadone hydrochloride

Dolophine, Methadose, Physeptone*

Pharmacologic classification: opioid
Therapeutic classification: analgesic, narcotic detoxification adjunct
Controlled substance schedule II
Pregnancy risk category C

How supplied

Available by prescription only
Tablets: 5 mg, 10 mg, 40 mg for oral solution (for narcotic abstinence syndrome)
Oral solution: 5 mg/5 ml, 10 mg/5 ml, 10 mg/ml (concentrate)
Injection: 10 mg/ml

Indications, route, and dosage

Severe pain

Adults: 2.5 to 10 mg P.O., I.M., or S.C. q 3 to 4 hours, p.r.n. or around-the-clock.

Narcotic abstinence syndrome

Adults: 15 to 20 mg P.O. daily (highly individualized).

Maintenance dosage is 20 to 120 mg P.O. daily. Adjust dose p.r.n. Daily doses above 120 mg require special state and federal approval. If patient feels nauseated, give ¼ of total P.O. dose in two injections, S.C. or I.M.

Pharmacodynamics

Analgesic action: Methadone is an opiate agonist that has analgesic activity via an affinity for the opiate receptors similar to that of morphine. It is recommended for severe, chronic pain and is also used in detoxification and maintenance of patients with opiate abstinence syndrome.

Pharmacokinetics

- *Absorption:* Methadone is well absorbed from the GI tract. Oral administration delays onset and prolongs duration of action as compared to parenteral administration. Onset of action occurs within ½ to 1 hour; peak effect is seen at ½ to 1 hour.
- *Distribution:* Drug is highly bound to tissue protein, which may explain its cumulative effects and slow elimination.
- *Metabolism:* Methadone is metabolized primarily in the liver by N-demethylation.
- *Excretion:* Duration of action is 4 to 6 hours. Half-life is prolonged (7 to 11 hours) in patients with hepatic dysfunction. Urinary excretion, the major route, is dose-dependent. Methadone metabolites are also excreted in the feces via the bile.

Contraindications and precautions

Contraindicated in patients with hypersensitivity to drug. Use cautiously in elderly or debilitated patients and in those with severe renal or hepatic impairment, acute abdominal conditions, hypothyroidism, Addison's disease, prostatic hyperplasia, urethral stricture, head injury, increased intracranial pressure, asthma, or other respiratory disorders.

Interactions
Concomitant use with *other CNS depressants* (*alcohol, narcotic analgesics, general anesthetics, antidepressants, antihistamines, barbiturates, benzodiazepines, muscle relaxants, phenothiazines,* and *sedative-hypnotics*) potentiates drug's respiratory and CNS depression, sedation, and hypotensive effects. Concomitant use with *cimetidine* may also increase respiratory and CNS depression, causing confusion, disorientation, apnea, or seizures. Such use usually requires reduced dosage of methadone.

Drug accumulation and enhanced effects may result from concomitant use with *other drugs that are extensively metabolized in the liver* (*digitoxin, phenytoin,* and *rifampin*); combined use with *anticholinergics* may cause paralytic ileus.

Patients who become physically dependent on drug may experience acute withdrawal syndrome if given a *narcotic antagonist.* Use with caution, and monitor closely.

Concurrent use with *rifampin* may reduce blood concentration of methadone.

Effects on diagnostic tests
Methadone increases plasma amylase levels.

Adverse reactions
CNS: *sedation, somnolence, clouded sensorium, euphoria, dizziness, choreic movements,* ***seizures*** (with large doses), headache, insomnia, agitation, *light-headedness,* syncope.
CV: *hypotension, bradycardia,* ***shock, cardiac arrest,*** palpitations.
EENT: visual disturbances.
GI: *nausea, vomiting, constipation, ileus, dry mouth, anorexia, biliary tract spasm.*
GU: *urine retention, decreased libido.*
Respiratory: ***respiratory depression, respiratory arrest.***
Skin: *diaphoresis,* pruritus, urticaria, edema.
Other: physical dependence; pain at injection site; tissue irritation, induration (after S.C. injection).

Overdose and treatment
The most common signs and symptoms of drug overdose are CNS depression, respiratory depression, and miosis (pinpoint pupils). Others include hypotension, bradycardia, hypothermia, shock, apnea, cardiopulmonary arrest, circulatory collapse, pulmonary edema, and seizures. Toxicity may result from accumulation of drug over several weeks.

To treat acute overdose, first establish adequate respiratory exchange via a patent airway and ventilation as needed; administer a narcotic antagonist (naloxone) to reverse respiratory depression. (Because the duration of action of methadone is longer than that of naloxone, repeated naloxone dosing is necessary.) The antagonist naloxone should not be given unless the patient has clinically significant respiratory or CV depression. Monitor vital signs closely.

If patient presents within 2 hours of ingestion of an oral overdose, empty the stomach immediately by inducing emesis (ipecac syrup) or using gastric lavage. Use caution to avoid risk of aspiration. Administer activated charcoal via nasogastric tube for further removal of drug in an oral overdose.

Provide symptomatic and supportive treatment (continued respiratory support, correction of fluid or electrolyte imbalance). Monitor laboratory parameters, vital signs, and neurologic status closely.

☑ Special considerations
Besides those relevant to all *opioids,* consider the following recommendations.

- Verify that patient is in a methadone maintenance program for management of narcotic addiction and, if so, at what dosage, and continue that program appropriately.
- Dispersable tablets may be dissolved in 4 oz (120 ml) of water or fruit juice; oral concentrate must be diluted to at least 3 oz (90 ml) with water before administration.
- Oral liquid form (not tablets) is legally required and is the only form available in drug maintenance programs.
- Regimented scheduling (around-the-clock) is beneficial in severe, chronic pain. When used for severe, chronic pain, tolerance may develop with long-term use, requiring a higher dose to achieve the same degree of analgesia.
- Patient treated for narcotic abstinence syndrome will usually require an additional analgesic if pain control is necessary.
- If used with general anesthetics, tranquilizers, sedatives, hypnotics, alcohol, tricyclic antidepressants, or MAO inhibitors, respiratory depression, hypotension, profound sedation, or coma may occur. Use together with extreme caution. Monitor patient's response.
- Physical and psychological tolerance or dependence may occur. Be aware of potential for abuse.

Patient education
- If appropriate, tell patient that constipation is often severe during maintenance with methadone. Instruct him to take a stool softener or other laxative.
- Caution patient to avoid activities that require full alertness, such as driving and operating machinery, because of potential for drowsiness.

Geriatric use
- Lower doses are usually indicated for elderly patients, because they may be more sensitive to the therapeutic and adverse effects of drug.

Pediatric use
- Drug is not recommended for use in children. Safe use as maintenance drug in adolescent addicts not established.

Breast-feeding
- Methadone is excreted in breast milk; it may cause physical dependence in breast-feeding infants of women on methadone maintenance therapy.

methamphetamine hydrochloride

Desoxyn

Pharmacologic classification: amphetamine

Therapeutic classification: CNS stimulant, short-term adjunctive anorexigenic agent, sympathomimetic amine

Controlled substance schedule II

Pregnancy risk category C

How supplied

Available by prescription only

Tablets: 5 mg

Tablets (long-acting): 5 mg, 10 mg, 15 mg

Indications, route, and dosage

Attention deficit hyperactivity disorder

Children age 6 and older: Initially, 5 mg P.O. once daily or b.i.d., with 5-mg increments weekly, p.r.n. Usual effective dosage is 20 to 25 mg daily.

Short-term adjunct in exogenous obesity

Adults: 10 to 15 mg/day P.O. in morning. Do not use for more than a few weeks.

Pharmacodynamics

CNS stimulant action: Amphetamines are sympathomimetic amines with CNS stimulant activity; in hyperactive children, they have a paradoxical calming effect.

Anorexigenic action: Anorexigenic effects are thought to occur in the hypothalamus, where decreased smell and taste acuity decreases appetite; they may involve other systemic and metabolic effects. They may be tried for short-term control of refractory obesity, with caloric restriction and behavior modification.

The cerebral cortex and reticular activating system appear to be the primary sites of activity; amphetamines release nerve terminal stores of norepinephrine, promoting nerve impulse transmission. At high dosages, effects are mediated by dopamine.

Amphetamines are used to treat narcolepsy and as adjuncts to psychosocial measures in attention deficit disorder in children. The precise mechanisms of action in these conditions are unknown.

Pharmacokinetics

- *Absorption:* Drug is rapidly absorbed from the GI tract after oral administration; effects last 6 to 12 hours.
- *Distribution:* Widely distributed throughout the body. Crosses the placenta and enters breast milk.
- *Metabolism:* Metabolized in the liver to at least seven metabolites.
- *Excretion:* Excreted in urine.

Contraindications and precautions

Contraindicated in patients with moderate to severe hypertension, hyperthyroidism, symptomatic CV disease, advanced arteriosclerosis, glaucoma, hypersensitivity or idiosyncrasy to sympathomimetic amines, or history of drug abuse; within 14 days of MAO inhibitor therapy; and in agitated patients.

Use cautiously in elderly, debilitated, asthenic, or psychopathic patients and in those with history of suicidal or homicidal tendencies.

Interactions

Concomitant use with *MAO inhibitors* (or drugs with MAO-inhibiting activity, such as *furazolidone*), or within 14 days of such therapy, may cause hypertensive crisis; use with *antihypertensives* may antagonize their effects.

Concomitant use with *acetazolamide, antacids,* or *sodium bicarbonate* enhances reabsorption of methamphetamine and prolongs duration of action, whereas use with *ascorbic acid* enhances methamphetamine excretion and shortens duration of action. Use with *phenothiazines* or *haloperidol* decreases methamphetamine effects; *barbiturates* antagonize methamphetamine by CNS depression, whereas *caffeine* or *other CNS stimulants* produce additive effects.

Patients using methamphetamine have an increased risk of arrhythmias during *general anesthesia.* Drug may alter *insulin* requirements.

Effects on diagnostic tests

Drug may elevate plasma corticosteroid levels and may interfere with urinary steroid determinations.

Adverse reactions

CNS: *nervousness, insomnia, irritability,* talkativeness, dizziness, headache, hyperexcitability, tremor, euphoria.
CV: hypertension, *tachycardia, palpitations,* ***arrhythmias.***
EENT: blurred vision, mydriasis.
GI: dry mouth, metallic taste, diarrhea, constipation, anorexia.
GU: impotence.
Skin: urticaria.
Other: altered libido.

Overdose and treatment

Symptoms of overdose include increasing restlessness, tremor, hyperreflexia, tachypnea, confusion, aggressiveness, hallucinations, and panic; fatigue and depression usually follow the excitement stage. Other symptoms may include arrhythmias, shock, alterations in blood pressure, nausea, vomiting, diarrhea, and abdominal cramps; death is usually preceded by seizures and coma.

Treat overdose symptomatically and supportively: if ingestion is recent (within 4 hours), use gastric lavage or emesis and sedate with barbiturate; monitor vital signs and fluid and electrolyte balance. I.V. phentolamine is suggested for treatment of severe acute hypertension. Chlorpromazine is useful in decreasing CNS stimulation and sympathomimetic effects. Urinary acidification may enhance excretion. Sodium chloride catharsis (magnesium citrate) may hasten GI evacuation of unabsorbed long-acting forms. Hemodialysis or peritoneal dialysis may be effective in severe cases.

☑ Special considerations

- Drug is not recommended for first-line treatment of obesity.
- Do not crush long-acting dosage forms.
- When treating behavioral disorders in children, consider a periodic discontinuation of the drug to evaluate effectiveness and the need for continued therapy.
- Rapid withdrawal of drug after prolonged use may lead to depression, somnolence, and increased appetite.

Patient education

- Warn patient that potential for abuse is high. Discourage use to combat fatigue.
- Advise patient to avoid caffeine-containing drinks and alcohol, to take drug 1 hour before next meal, and to take last daily dose at least 6 hours before bedtime to prevent insomnia.
- Warn patient not to increase dosage unless prescribed.
- Inform patient that methamphetamine may impair ability to engage in potentially hazardous activities, such as operating machinery or driving a motor vehicle.

Geriatric use

- Elderly or debilitated patients may be especially sensitive to methamphetamine's effects. Drug should be used with caution.

Pediatric use

- Drug is not recommended for weight reduction in children under age 12.

Breast-feeding

- Because amphetamines are excreted in breast milk, an alternative method of feeding should be used.

methazolamide

Neptazane

Pharmacologic classification: carbonic anhydrase inhibitor
Therapeutic classification: adjunctive treatment for open-angle glaucoma, perioperatively for acute angle-closure glaucoma
Pregnancy risk category C

How supplied

Available by prescription only
Tablets: 25 mg, 50 mg

Indications, route, and dosage

Glaucoma (open-angle or preoperatively in obstructive or angle-closure)
Adults: 50 to 100 mg P.O. b.i.d. or t.i.d.

Pharmacodynamics

Anti-glaucoma action: In open-angle glaucoma and perioperatively for acute angle-closure glaucoma, methazolamide decreases the formation of aqueous humor, lowering intraocular pressure. Drug has a weak diuretic effect.

Pharmacokinetics

- *Absorption:* Methazolamide is absorbed more slowly than acetazolamide.
- *Distribution:* Drug distributes into plasma, erythrocytes, extracellular fluid, bile, aqueous humor, and CSF.
- *Metabolism:* Partially metabolized by the liver.
- *Excretion:* About 20% to 30% of dose is excreted in urine.

Contraindications and precautions

Contraindicated for long-term use in acute angle-closure glaucoma and in patients with depressed serum sodium or potassium levels, renal or hepatic disease or dysfunction, adrenal gland dysfunction, or hyperchloremic acidosis. Use cautiously in patients with emphysema and pulmonary obstruction.

Interactions

Methazolamide alkalizes urine, thus decreasing excretion of *amphetamines, flecainide, procainamide,* and *quinidine.* Methazolamide increases excretion of *lithium, phenobarbital,* and *salicylates,* lowering plasma levels of these drugs and necessitating dosage adjustments. Drug may augment the effects of *thiazide diuretics.* Use with *steroids* may potentiate hypokalemia.

Effects on diagnostic tests

Because methazolamide alkalizes urine, it may cause false-positive proteinuria when Albustix or Albutest tests are performed. Methazolamide also may decrease iodine uptake by the thyroid.

Adverse reactions

CNS: drowsiness, paresthesia, fatigue, malaise, confusion.
EENT: transient myopia, hearing dysfunction, tinnitus.
GI: nausea, vomiting, anorexia, taste alteration, diarrhea.
GU: crystalluria, renal calculi.
Skin: urticaria.
Other: metabolic acidosis, electrolyte imbalance, ***anaphylaxis.***

Overdose and treatment

Specific recommendations are unavailable. Treatment is supportive and symptomatic. Carbonic anhydrase inhibitors increase bicarbonate excretion and may cause hypokalemia and hyperchloremic acidosis. Induce emesis or perform gastric lavage. Do not induce catharsis because this may exacerbate electrolyte disturbances. Monitor fluid and electrolyte levels.

☑ Special considerations

- Advise patient to comply with prescribed dosage to lessen risk of metabolic acidosis. Effects may decrease in acidosis.
- Monitor patients with glaucoma for eye pain to ensure drug efficacy.

Geriatric use

• Elderly and debilitated patients require close observation because they are more susceptible to drug-induced diuresis. Excessive diuresis promotes rapid dehydration, hypovolemia, hypokalemia, and hyponatremia and may cause circulatory collapse. Reduced dosages may be indicated.

Breast-feeding

• Safety of drug in breast-feeding women has not been established.

methicillin sodium

Staphcillin

Pharmacologic classification: penicillinase-resistant penicillin
Therapeutic classification: antibiotic
Pregnancy risk category B

How supplied

Available by prescription only
Injection: 1 g, 4 g, 6 g
Pharmacy bulk package: 10 g
I.V. infusions piggyback: 1 g, 4 g

Indications, route, and dosage

Systemic infections caused by susceptible organisms
Adults: 4 to 12 g I.M. or I.V. daily, divided into doses given q 4 to 6 hours.
Children: 100 to 300 mg/kg I.M. or I.V. daily, divided into doses given q 4 to 6 hours.
Infants over 7 days and weighing over 4 lb 7 oz (2,013 g): 100 mg/kg daily, divided into doses given q 6 hours; for meningitis, give 200 mg/kg daily.
Infants over 7 days and weighing below 4 lb 7 oz: 75 mg/kg daily, divided into doses given q 8 hours; for meningitis, give 150 mg/kg daily.
Infants under 7 days and weighing over 4 lb 7 oz: 75 mg/kg daily, divided into doses given q 8 hours; for meningitis, give 150 mg/kg daily.
Infants under 7 days and weighing below 4 lb 7 oz: 50 mg/kg daily, divided into doses given q 12 hours; for meningitis, give 100 mg/kg daily.
✦ ***Dosage adjustment.*** In adults with renal failure with creatinine clearance of 10 ml/minute or less, give 1 g I.M. or I.V. q 8 to 12 hours.

Pharmacodynamics

Antibiotic action: Methicillin is bactericidal; it adheres to bacterial penicillin-binding proteins, thus inhibiting bacterial cell wall synthesis. Methicillin resists the effects of penicillinase enzymes that inactivate penicillin and is thus active against many strains of penicillinase-producing bacteria. This activity is most important against penicillinase-producing staphylococci; some strains may remain resistant. Methicillin is also active against certain gram-positive aerobic and anaerobic bacilli but has no significant effect on gram-negative bacilli.

Pharmacokinetics

• *Absorption:* Methicillin is inactivated by gastric secretions and must be given parenterally. Peak plasma concentrations occur 30 to 60 minutes after I.M. injection.
• *Distribution:* Distributed widely. CSF penetration is poor but enhanced by meningeal inflammation. Methicillin crosses the placenta; it is 30% to 50% protein-bound.
• *Metabolism:* Methicillin is metabolized only partially.
• *Excretion:* Drug and metabolites are excreted in urine by renal tubular secretion and glomerular filtration. They are also excreted in breast milk and in bile. Elimination half-life in adults is about ½ hour, prolonged to 2½ hours in severe renal impairment; it is prolonged to 4 to 6 hours in anuric patients.

Contraindications and precautions

Contraindicated in infants and in patients with hypersensitivity to drug or other penicillins. Use cautiously in patients with other drug allergies, especially to cephalosporins.

Interactions

Concomitant use of methicillin with *aminoglycosides* produces synergistic bactericidal effects against *Staphylococcus aureus*. However, drugs are physically and chemically incompatible and are inactivated when mixed or given together.

Probenecid blocks renal tubular secretion of methicillin, raising its serum concentrations.

Effects on diagnostic tests

Methicillin falsely shows increases in serum uric acid concentration levels (copper-chelate method); it interferes with measurement of 17-hydroxycorticosteroids (Porter-Silber test). Positive Coombs' tests have been reported. Methicillin may cause transient reductions in RBC, WBC, and platelet counts. Abnormal urinalysis result may indicate drug-induced interstitial nephritis. Methicillin may falsely decrease serum aminoglycoside concentrations.

Adverse reactions

CNS: neuropathy, ***seizures***, lethargy, hallucinations, anxiety, confusion, agitation, depression, dizziness, fatigue.
GI: glossitis, stomatitis, nausea, vomiting, enterocolitis, pseudomembranous colitis.
GU: interstitial nephritis, nephropathy, hematuria, ***hemorrhagic cystitis.***
Hematologic: ***agranulocytosis***, *eosinophilia*, hemolytic anemia, transient ***neutropenia***, anemia, ***leukopenia, thrombocytopenia.***
Other: ***Stevens-Johnson syndrome***, *hypersensitivity reactions* (chills, fever, edema, rash, urticaria, ***anaphylaxis***), overgrowth of nonsusceptible organisms, vein irritation, thrombophlebitis.

Overdose and treatment

Clinical signs of overdose include neuromuscular irritability or seizures. Drug can be removed by gastric lavage, but is not appreciably removed by hemodialysis or peritoneal dialysis.

☑ Special considerations

Besides those relevant to all *penicillins*, consider the following recommendations.

- Schedule for administration around the clock to maintain adequate plasma levels.
- Frequently monitor results of urinalysis for signs of adverse renal effects.
- Monitor neurologic status. High blood concentrations may cause seizures.
- Periodically check renal, hepatic, and hematopoietic function during prolonged therapy.

Patient education

- Encourage patient to report all adverse reactions.

Pediatric use

- Elimination of drug is reduced in neonates; safety in neonates has not been established.

Breast-feeding

- Methicillin is excreted in breast milk; use with caution in breast-feeding women.

methimazole

Tapazole

Pharmacologic classification: thyroid hormone antagonist
Therapeutic classification: antihyperthyroid
Pregnancy risk category D

How supplied

Available by prescription only
Tablets: 5 mg, 10 mg

Indications, route, and dosage

Hyperthyroidism, preparation for thyroidectomy, thyrotoxic crisis

Adults: 15 mg P.O. daily if mild; 30 to 40 mg P.O. daily if moderately severe; 60 mg P.O. daily if severe; all are given in three equally divided doses q 8 hours. Continue until patient is euthyroid, then start maintenance dosage of 5 to 15 mg daily.
Children: 0.4 mg/kg/day divided q 8 hours. Continue until patient is euthyroid, then start maintenance dosage of 0.2 mg/kg/day divided q 8 hours.

Pharmacodynamics

Antithyroid action: In treating hyperthyroidism, methimazole inhibits synthesis of thyroid hormone by interfering with the incorporation of iodide into tyrosyl. Methimazole also inhibits the formation of iodothyronine. As preparation for thyroidectomy, methimazole inhibits synthesis of the thyroid hormone and causes a euthyroid state, reducing surgical problems during thyroidectomy; as a result, the mortality for a single-stage thyroidectomy is low. Iodide reduces the vascularity of the gland, making it less friable. For treating thyrotoxic crisis (thyrotoxicosis), propylthiouracil (PTU) theoretically is preferred over methimazole because it inhibits peripheral deiodination of thyroxine to triiodothyronine.

Pharmacokinetics

- *Absorption:* Absorbed rapidly from the GI tract (80% to 95% bioavailable). Peak plasma levels are reached within 1 hour.
- *Distribution:* Drug readily crosses the placenta and is distributed into breast milk. It is concentrated in the thyroid. Drug is not protein-bound.
- *Metabolism:* Methimazole undergoes hepatic metabolism.
- *Excretion:* About 80% of drug and its metabolites are excreted renally; 7% is excreted unchanged. Half-life is between 5 and 13 hours.

Contraindications and precautions

Contraindicated in patients with hypersensitivity to drug and in breast-feeding patients. Use cautiously in pregnant patients.

Interactions

Concomitant use of methimazole with *PTU* and *adrenocorticoids* or *corticotropin* may require a dosage adjustment of the steroid when thyroid status changes. Concomitant use with *other bone marrow depressant agents* causes an increased risk of agranulocytosis. Concomitant use with *other hepatotoxic agents* increases the risk of hepatotoxicity. Concurrent use with *iodinated glycerol, lithium,* or *potassium iodide* may potentiate hypothyroid and goitrogenic effects.

Antivitamin K action of methimazole potentiates the action of *anticoagulants.*

Effects on diagnostic tests

Methimazole therapy alters selenomethionine (^{75}Se) uptake by the pancreas and ^{123}I or ^{131}I uptake by the thyroid. Hepatotoxicity may be evident by elevations of PT and of serum ALT, serum AST, bilirubin, alkaline phosphatase, and LD levels.

Adverse reactions

CNS: headache, drowsiness, vertigo, paresthesia, neuritis, neuropathies, CNS stimulation, depression.
EENT: loss of taste.
GI: diarrhea, nausea, vomiting (may be dose-related), salivary gland enlargement, epigastric distress.
GU: nephritis.
Hematologic: ***agranulocytosis, leukopenia, thrombocytopenia, aplastic anemia.***
Hepatic: jaundice, hepatic dysfunction, hepatitis.
Skin: rash, urticaria, discoloration, pruritus, erythema nodosum, exfoliative dermatitis, lupuslike syndrome.
Other: arthralgia, myalgia, fever, lymphadenopathy, hypothyroidism (mental depression; cold intolerance; hard, nonpitting edema; hypoprothrombinemia and bleeding).

Overdose and treatment

Clinical manifestations of overdose include nausea, vomiting, epigastric distress, fever, headache, arthralgia, pruritus, edema, and pancytopenia. Treatment is supportive; gastric lavage should be performed or emesis should be induced if possible. If bone marrow depression develops, fresh whole blood, corticosteroids, and anti-infectives may be required.

☑ Special considerations

- Best response occurs if dosage is administered around-the-clock and given at the same time each day with respect to meals.
- Dosages of over 40 mg/day increase the risk of agranulocytosis.
- A beta blocker, most often propranolol, is usually given to manage the peripheral signs of hyperthyroidism, primarily tachycardia.
- Euthyroid state may take several months to develop.

Patient education

- Tell patient to take drug at regular intervals around-the-clock and to take it at the same time each day in relation to meals.
- If GI upset occurs, tell patient to take drug with meals.
- Tell patient to call promptly if fever, sore throat, malaise, unusual bleeding, yellowing of eyes, nausea, or vomiting occurs.
- Advise patient not to store drug in bathroom; heat and humidity cause it to deteriorate.
- Tell patient to inform other doctors and dentists of drug use.
- Teach patient how to recognize the signs of hyperthyroidism and hypothyroidism and what to do if they occur.

Breast-feeding

- Patient should discontinue breast-feeding before beginning therapy because drug occurs in breast milk. However, if breast-feeding is necessary, PTU is the preferred antithyroid agent.

methocarbamol

Robaxin

Pharmacologic classification: carbamate derivative of guaifenesin
Therapeutic classification: skeletal muscle relaxant
Pregnancy risk category C

How supplied

Available by prescription only
Tablets: 500 mg, 750 mg
Injection: 100 mg/ml

Indications, route, and dosage

Adjunct in acute, painful musculoskeletal conditions

Adults: 1.5 g P.O. q.i.d. for 2 to 3 days. Maintenance dosage, 4 to 4.5 g P.O. daily in three to six divided doses. Alternatively, 1 g I.M. or I.V. Maximum dosage, 3 g daily I.M. or I.V. for 3 consecutive days.

Supportive therapy in tetanus management

Adults: 1 to 2 g I.V. push (300 mg/minute) and an additional 1 to 2 g may be added to I.V. solution. Total initial I.V. dosage, 3 g. Repeat I.V. infusion of 1 to 2 g q 6 hours until nasogastric tube can be inserted.

Children: 15 mg/kg or 500 mg/m^2 I.V. Don't inject faster than 180 mg/m^2/minute. May be repeated q 6 hours if necessary to total dosage of 1.8 g/m^2 daily for 3 consecutive days.

Pharmacodynamics

Skeletal muscle relaxant action: Drug does not relax skeletal muscle directly. Its effects appear to be related to its sedative action; however, the exact mechanism of action is unknown.

Pharmacokinetics

- *Absorption:* Rapidly and completely absorbed from the GI tract. Onset of action after single oral dose is within 30 minutes. Onset of action after single I.V. dose is achieved immediately.
- *Distribution:* Methocarbamol is widely distributed throughout the body.
- *Metabolism:* Extensively metabolized in liver via dealkylation and hydroxylation. Half-life of drug is between 0.9 and 1.8 hours.
- *Excretion:* Drug is rapidly and almost completely excreted in urine, mainly as its glucuronide and sulfate metabolites (40% to 50%), as unchanged drug (10% to 15%), and the rest as unidentified metabolites.

Contraindications and precautions

Contraindicated in patients with hypersensitivity to drug, impaired renal function (injectable form), or seizure disorder (injectable form). Safe use of methocarbamol in regard to fetal development has not been established. Therefore, drug should not be used in women who are or may become pregnant, especially during early pregnancy unless the benefits outweigh the possible hazards.

Interactions

Concomitant use of methocarbamol with *other CNS depressant drugs*, including *alcohol, anxiolytics, narcotics, psychotics*, and *tricyclic antidepressants*, may cause additive CNS depression. When used with *other depressants*, exercise care to avoid overdose. Patients with myasthenia gravis who receive *anticholinesterase agents* may experience severe weakness if given methocarbamol.

Effects on diagnostic tests

Methocarbamol therapy alters results of laboratory tests for urine 5-hydroxyindoleacetic acid (5-HIAA) using quantitative method of Udenfriend (false-positive) and for urine vanillylmandelic acid (false-positive when Gitlow screening test used; no problem when quantitative method of Sunderman used).

Adverse reactions

CNS: drowsiness, dizziness, light-headedness, headache, syncope, mild muscular incoordination (with I.M. or I.V. use), ***seizures*** (with I.V. use only), vertigo.
CV: hypotension, bradycardia (with I.M. or I.V. use).
EENT: blurred vision, conjunctivitis, nystagmus, diplopia.
GI: nausea, GI upset, metallic taste.

GU: hematuria (with I.V. use only), discoloration of urine.
Skin: urticaria, pruritus, rash.
Respiratory: thrombophlebitis.
Other: extravasation (with I.V. use only), fever, flushing, ***anaphylactic reactions*** (with I.M. or I.V. use).

Overdose and treatment

Clinical manifestations of overdose include extreme drowsiness, nausea and vomiting, and arrhythmias.

Treatment includes symptomatic and supportive measures. If ingestion is recent, empty stomach by emesis or gastric lavage (may reduce absorption). Maintain adequate airway; monitor urine output and vital signs; and administer I.V. fluids if needed.

☑ Special considerations

- Do not administer S.C. Give I.V. undiluted at a rate not exceeding 300 mg per minute. May also be given by I.V. infusion after diluting in D_5W or 0.9% NaCl solution.
- Patient should be supine during and for at least 10 to 15 minutes after I.V. injection.
- To give via nasogastric tube, crush tablets and suspend in water or 0.9% NaCl solution.
- When used in tetanus, follow manufacturer's instructions.
- Patient's urine may turn black, blue, brown, or green if left standing.
- Patient needs assistance in walking after parenteral administration.
- Extravasation of I.V. solution may cause thrombophlebitis and sloughing from hypertonic solution.
- Oral administration should replace parenteral use as soon as feasible.
- Adverse reactions after oral administration are usually mild and transient and subside with dosage reduction.
- For I.M. administration, do not give more than 500 mg in each gluteal region.

Patient education

- Tell patient urine may turn black, blue, green, or brown.
- Warn patient drug may cause drowsiness. Patient should avoid hazardous activities that require alertness until degree of CNS depression can be determined.
- Advise patient to make position changes slowly, particularly from recumbent to upright position, and to dangle legs before standing.
- Advise patient to avoid alcoholic beverages and use OTC cold or cough preparations carefully because some contain alcohol.
- Tell patient to store drug away from heat and light (not in bathroom medicine cabinet) and safely out of reach of children.
- Tell patient to take missed dose if remembered within 1 hour. Beyond 1 hour, patient should skip that dose and resume regular schedule. Do not double dose.
- Inform athletes that skeletal muscle relaxants are banned in competition and tested for by the U.S. Olympic Committee and the National Collegiate Athletic Association.

Geriatric use

- Lower doses are indicated, because elderly patients are more sensitive to drug's effects.

Pediatric use

- For children under age 12, use only as recommended for tetanus.

Breast-feeding

- Drug is excreted in breast milk in small amounts. Patient should not breast-feed during treatment with methocarbamol.

methohexital sodium

Brevital Sodium, Brietal Sodium*

Pharmacologic classification: barbiturate
Therapeutic classification: I.V. anesthetic
Controlled substance schedule IV
Pregnancy risk category B

How supplied

Available by prescription only
Injection: 500 mg, 2.5 g, 5 g powder for injection

Indications, route, and dosage

Induction of anesthesia; anesthesia for short procedures (such as electroconvulsive therapy [ECT])
Dosage is highly individualized.
Adults and children: For induction of anesthesia, a 1% solution is administered at a rate of about 1 ml/5 seconds, possibly with inhalant anesthetics or skeletal muscle relaxants, or both. Induction dose may vary from 50 to 120 mg or more but averages about 70 mg; it usually provides anesthesia for 5 to 7 minutes. Maintenance of anesthesia may be achieved via intermittent injections of about 20 to 40 mg (2 to 4 ml of 1% solution), as needed, usually q 4 to 7 minutes; or by continuous I.V infusion of a 0.2% solution (average rate of about 3 ml of a 0.2% solution per minute [1 drop/second]).

Pharmacodynamics

Anesthetic action: Methohexital produces anesthesia by direct depression of the polysynaptic midbrain reticular activating system; drug decreases presynaptic (via decreased neurotransmitter release) and postsynaptic excitation. These effects may be subsequent to increased gamma-aminobutyric acid (GABA), enhancement of GABA's effects, or a direct effect on GABA receptor sites.

Pharmacokinetics

- *Absorption:* Drug is only given I.V.; it is an ultra-short-acting barbiturate; peak concentrations in the brain occur between 30 seconds and 2 minutes after administration.
- *Distribution:* Drug distributes throughout the body; highest initial concentrations occur in vascular areas of the brain, primarily gray matter.
- *Metabolism:* Metabolized extensively in the liver.
- *Excretion:* Excretion of metabolites occurs via the kidneys through glomerular filtration. Duration of action depends on tissue redistribution.

Contraindications and precautions

Contraindicated in patients with acute intermittent or variegate porphyria or known hypersensitivity to drug and whenever general anesthesia is contraindicated.

Use cautiously in patients with circulatory, cardiac, renal, hepatic, endocrine, or pulmonary dysfunction; severe anemia; marked obesity or status asthmaticus (use extremely cautiously) because drug worsens these conditions. Also, use cautiously in patients with a full stomach because it blocks airway reflexes and may predispose the patient to aspiration.

Interactions

Methohexital may potentiate or add to CNS depressant effects of *alcohol, antihistamines, benzodiazepines, hypnotics, narcotics, phenothiazines,* and *sedatives.*

Concomitant use with *ketamine* for anesthesia may cause profound respiratory depression, because ketamine potentiates methohexital.

Effects on diagnostic tests

Methohexital causes dose-dependent alteration of EEG patterns.

Adverse reactions

CNS: skeletal muscle hyperactivity, anxiety, restlessness, headache, emergence delirium.
CV: transient hypotension, tachycardia, ***circulatory depression, peripheral vascular collapse.***
GI: abdominal pain, nausea, vomiting, excessive salivation.
Respiratory: *respiratory arrest, respiratory depression, apnea, laryngospasm, bronchospasm,* hiccups.
Skin: pain, swelling; ulceration, necrosis (on extravasation).
Other: thrombophlebitis, pain (at injection site); injury to adjacent nerves; ***hypersensitivity reaction.***

Note: Discontinue drug if peripheral vascular collapse, respiratory arrest, or hypersensitivity reaction occurs.

Overdose and treatment

Clinical signs of overdose include respiratory depression, respiratory arrest, hypotension, and shock. Treat supportively, using, as needed, mechanical ventilation and I.V. fluids or vasopressors (dopamine, phenylephrine) for hypotension. Monitor vital signs closely.

☑ Special considerations

- Avoid extravasation or intra-arterial injection because of possible tissue necrosis and gangrene.
- Drug is physically incompatible with lactated Ringer's solution; with acidic solutions, such as atropine, metocurine, and succinylcholine; and with silicone. Avoid contact with rubber stoppers or parts of syringes that have been treated with silicone. The preferred diluent is sterile water, but D_5W or 0.9% NaCl may be used. Do not use bacteriostatic diluents.
- Maintenance of patent airway and adequate ventilation must be ensured during induction and maintenance of anesthesia.

Geriatric use

- Lower doses may be indicated.

Pediatric use

- Safety and efficacy in children have not been established.

Breast-feeding

- Use cautiously in breast-feeding patients.

methotrexate, methotrexate sodium

Folex, Mexate, Mexate-AQ, Rheumatrex

Pharmacologic classification: antimetabolite (cell cycle–phase specific, S phase)
Therapeutic classification: antineoplastic
Pregnancy risk category X

How supplied

Available by prescription only
Tablets (scored): 2.5 mg
Injection: 20-mg, 25-mg, 50-mg, 100-mg, 250-mg, 1-g vials, lyophilized powder, preservative-free; 25-mg/ml vials, preservative-free solution; 2.5-mg/ml, 25-mg/ml vials, lyophilized powder, preserved

Indications, route, and dosage

Dosage and indications may vary. Check current literature for recommended protocols.

Trophoblastic tumors (choriocarcinoma, hydatidiform mole)
Adults: 15 to 30 mg P.O. or I.M. daily for 5 days. Repeat after 1 or more weeks, according to response or toxicity.

Acute lymphoblastic leukemia
Adults and children: 3.3 mg/m² P.O. daily for 4 to 6 weeks or until remission occurs; then 20 to 30 mg/m² P.O. or I.M. twice weekly or 2.5 mg/kg I.V. q 14 days. (Used in combination with prednisone.)

Meningeal leukemia
Adults and children: 12 mg/m² intrathecally to a maximum dose of 15 mg q 2 to 5 days until CSF is normal. Use only vials of powder with no preservatives; dilute using 0.9% NaCl solution injection without preservatives. Use only new vials of drug and diluent. Use immediately after reconstitution.

Burkitt's lymphoma (stage I or II)
Adults: 10 to 25 mg P.O. daily for 4 to 8 days with 7- to 10-day rest intervals.

Lymphosarcoma (stage III; malignant lymphoma)
Adults: 0.625 to 2.5 mg/kg daily P.O., I.M., or I.V.

Mycosis fungoides (advanced)
Adults: 2.5 to 10 mg P.O. daily or 50 mg I.M. weekly; or 25 mg I.M. twice weekly.

Psoriasis (severe)
Adults: 10 to 25 mg P.O., I.M., or I.V. as single weekly dose.

Rheumatoid arthritis (severe, refractory)
Adults: 7.5 to 15 mg weekly P.O. in single or divided doses.
Adjunct treatment in osteosarcoma
Adults: Give 12 to 15 g/m² as a 4-hour I.V. infusion.

Pharmacodynamics
Antineoplastic action: Methotrexate exerts its cytotoxic activity by tightly binding with dihydrofolic acid reductase, an enzyme crucial to purine metabolism, resulting in an inhibition of DNA, RNA, and protein synthesis.

Pharmacokinetics
- *Absorption:* Absorption across the GI tract appears to be dose related. Lower doses are essentially completely absorbed, while absorption of larger doses is incomplete and variable. Intramuscular doses are absorbed completely. Peak serum levels are achieved 30 minutes to 2 hours after an intramuscular dose and 1 to 4 hours after an oral dose.
- *Distribution:* Methotrexate is distributed widely throughout the body, with the highest concentrations found in the kidneys, gallbladder, spleen, liver, and skin. Drug crosses the blood-brain barrier but does not achieve therapeutic levels in the CSF. Approximately 50% of the drug is bound to plasma protein.
- *Metabolism:* Drug is metabolized only slightly in the liver.
- *Excretion:* Excreted primarily into urine as unchanged drug. Elimination has been described as biphasic, with a first phase half-life of 45 minutes and a terminal phase half-life of 4 hours.

Contraindications and precautions
Contraindicated in patients hypersensitive to drug and during pregnancy or breast-feeding. Also contraindicated in patients with psoriasis or rheumatoid arthritis who also have alcoholism, alcoholic liver, chronic liver disease, immunodeficiency syndromes, or preexisting blood dyscrasias.

Use cautiously in very young or elderly or debilitated patients and in those with impaired renal or hepatic function, bone marrow suppression, aplasia, leukopenia, thrombocytopenia, anemia, folate deficiency, infection, peptic ulcer, or ulcerative colitis.

Interactions
Concomitant use with *probenecid* increases the therapeutic and toxic effects of methotrexate by inhibiting the renal tubular secretion of methotrexate; *salicylates* also increase the therapeutic and toxic effects of methotrexate by the same mechanism. Combined use of these agents requires a lower dosage of methotrexate.

NSAIDs, salicylates, sulfonamides, and *sulfonylureas* may increase the therapeutic and toxic effects of methotrexate by displacing methotrexate from plasma proteins, increasing the concentrations of free methotrexate. Concurrent use of these agents with methotrexate should be avoided if possible.

Immunizations may not be effective when given during methotrexate therapy. Because of the risk of disseminated infections, live virus vaccines are generally not recommended during therapy.

Phenytoin serum levels may be decreased by chemotherapeutic regimens that employ methotrexate, resulting in an increased risk of seizures.

Folic acid may decrease the effectiveness of methotrexate. Pyrimethamine should not be given concurrently because of similar pharmacologic action.

Oral antibiotics, such as *chloramphenicol, tetracycline,* and *nonabsorbable broad-spectrum antibiotics,* may decrease absorption of the drug.

Effects on diagnostic tests
Drug therapy may increase blood and urine concentrations of uric acid. Methotrexate may alter results of the laboratory assay for folate by inhibiting the organism used in the assay, thus interfering with the detection of folic acid deficiency.

Adverse reactions
CNS: ***arachnoiditis*** (within hours of intrathecal use), subacute ***neurotoxicity*** (may begin a few weeks later), ***necrotizing demyelinating leukoencephalopathy*** (may occur a few years later), malaise, fatigue, dizziness, headache, drowsiness, ***seizures.***
EENT: pharyngitis, gingivitis, blurred vision.
GI: stomatitis, diarrhea, abdominal distress, anorexia, GI ulceration and bleeding, enteritis, *nausea, vomiting.*
GU: nephropathy, *tubular necrosis,* ***renal failure,*** hematuria, menstrual dysfunction, defective spermatogenesis, cystitis.
Hematologic: WBC and platelet count nadirs occurring on day 7; anemia, ***leukopenia, thrombocytopenia*** (all dose-related).
Hepatic: acute toxicity (elevated transaminase level), *chronic toxicity (cirrhosis,* ***hepatic fibrosis****).*
Respiratory: ***pulmonary fibrosis, pulmonary interstitial infiltrates,*** pneumonitis; dry, nonproductive cough.
Skin: *urticaria, pruritus, hyperpigmentation, erythematous rash, ecchymoses, psoriatic lesions (aggravated by exposure to sun), rash, photosensitivity.*
Other: alopecia, osteoporosis (in children, with long-term use), fever, chills, reduced resistance to infection, septicemia, hyperuricemia, arthralgia, myalgia, diabetes, ***sudden death.***

Overdose and treatment
Clinical manifestations of overdose include myelosuppression, anemia, nausea, vomiting, dermatitis, alopecia, and melena.

The antidote for the hematopoietic toxicity of methotrexate is calcium leucovorin, started within 1 hour after the administration of methotrexate. The dosage of leucovorin should be high enough to produce plasma concentrations higher than those of methotrexate.

☑ Special considerations
- Methotrexate may be given undiluted by I.V. push injection.

• Drug can be diluted to a higher volume with 0.9% NaCl solution for I.V. infusion.
• Use reconstituted solutions of preservative-free drug within 24 hours after mixing.
• For intrathecal administration, use preservative-free formulations only. Dilute with unpreserved 0.9% NaCl.
• Dose modification may be required in impaired hepatic or renal function, bone marrow depression, aplasia, leukopenia, thrombocytopenia, or anemia. Use cautiously in infection, peptic ulcer, ulcerative colitis, and in very young, old, or debilitated patients.
• GI adverse reactions may require drug discontinuation.
• Rash, redness, or ulcerations in mouth or pulmonary adverse reactions may signal serious complications.
• Monitor uric acid levels.
• Monitor intake and output daily. Force fluids (2 to 3 L daily).
• Alkalinize urine by giving sodium bicarbonate tablets to prevent precipitation of drug, especially with high doses. Maintain urine pH at more than 6.5. Reduce dose if BUN level is 20 to 30 mg/dl or serum creatinine level is 1.2 to 2 mg/dl. Stop drug if BUN level is more than 30 mg/dl or serum creatinine level is more than 2 mg/dl.
• Watch for increases in AST, ALT, and alkaline phosphatase levels, which may signal hepatic dysfunction. Methotrexate should not be used when the potential for "third spacing" exists.
• Watch for bleeding (especially GI) and infection.
• Monitor temperature daily, and watch for cough, dyspnea, and cyanosis.
• Avoid all I.M. injections in patients with thrombocytopenia.
• Leucovorin rescue is necessary with high-dose protocols (doses greater than 100 mg).

Patient education

• Emphasize importance of continuing drug despite nausea and vomiting. Advise patient to call immediately if vomiting occurs shortly after taking a dose.
• Encourage patient to maintain adequate fluid intake to increase urine output, to prevent nephrotoxicity, and to facilitate excretion of uric acid.
• Warn patient to avoid alcoholic beverages during therapy.
• Caution patient to avoid conception during and immediately after therapy because of possible abortion or congenital anomalies.
• Tell patient to avoid prolonged exposure to sunlight and to use a highly protective sunscreen when exposed to sunlight.
• Teach patient good mouth care to prevent superinfection of oral cavity.
• Advise patient that hair should grow back after treatment has ended.
• Recommend salicylate-free analgesics for pain relief or fever reduction.
• Tell patient to avoid exposure to people with infections and to report signs of infection immediately.
• Advise patient to report unusual bruising or bleeding promptly.

Breast-feeding

• Drug occurs in breast milk. Therefore, because of potential for serious adverse reactions, mutagenicity, and carcinogenicity in the infant, breast-feeding should be discontinued.

methoxsalen

8-MOP, Oxsoralen, Oxsoralen-Ultra

Pharmacologic classification: psoralen derivative
Therapeutic classifications: pigmenting, antipsoriatic
Pregnancy risk category C

How supplied

Available by prescription only
Capsules: 10 mg
Lotion: 1%

Indications, route, and dosage

Induce repigmentation in vitiligo
Adults and children over age 12: 20 mg P.O. (maximum 0.6 mg/kg) 2 to 4 hours before measured periods of exposure to sunlight or ultraviolet (UV) light on alternate days. Alternatively, for small, well-defined lesions, apply lotion 1 to 2 hours before exposure to UV light, no more than once weekly. Wear gloves while applying lotion.

Psoriasis
Adults: Give dose P.O. 1½ to 2 hours before exposure to high-intensity ultraviolet A light, two or three times weekly, at least 48 hours apart. Dosage is based upon patient's weight.

Weight (kg)	Dose (mg)
< 30	10
30 to 50	20
51 to 65	30
66 to 80	40
81 to 90	50
91 to 115	60
> 115	70

◊ ***Cutaneous T-cell lymphoma***
Adults: 0.6 mg/kg P.O. if serum methoxsalen level is less than 50 ng/ml. Give initial dose and an additional 10 mg after 24 hours.

Pharmacodynamics

Pigmenting action: Exact mechanism of action of methoxsalen is not known; it is dependent on the presence of functioning melanocytes and UV light. Methoxsalen may stimulate the enzymes that catalyze melanin precursors. Also, the inflammatory response generated may stimulate melanin production.

Antipsoriatic action: Methoxsalen probably exerts its antipsoriatic effects by inhibiting DNA synthesis and decreasing cell proliferation. Cell-regulating, leukocyte, and vascular effects may also be involved in this action.

Oral dosage form produces greater erythemic and melanogenic effects, while the topical preparation causes a more intense photosensitizing response.

Pharmacokinetics

- *Absorption:* Following oral administration, drug is absorbed well but variably, with peak serum concentrations in 1½ to 3 hours. Food increases both absorption and peak concentration. Extent of topical absorption has not been determined. Skin sensitivity to UV light occurs in about 1 to 2 hours, reaches a maximum effect in 1 to 4 hours, and persists for 3 to 8 hours. Topical administration yields a UV sensitivity in 1 to 2 hours, which may persist for several days.
- *Distribution:* Methoxsalen is distributed throughout the body, with epidermal cells preferentially taking up drug; 75% to 91% is bound to serum proteins, most commonly albumin. Distribution across the placenta or in breast milk is unknown.
- *Metabolism:* Methoxsalen is activated by long-wavelength UV light and is metabolized in the liver.
- *Excretion:* Excreted almost entirely as metabolites in the urine, with 80% to 90% eliminated within the first 8 hours.

Contraindications and precautions

Contraindicated in patients sensitive to psoralen compounds and in patients with diseases associated with photosensitivity (such as porphyria, acute lupus erythematosus, xeroderma, or hydromorphic and polymorphic light eruptions). Also contraindicated in patients with melanoma, invasive squamous cell carcinoma, and aphakia.

Oxsoralen capsules contain tartrazine; therefore, use cautiously in patients with tartrazine or aspirin sensitivity.

Use cautiously in patients with familial history of sunlight allergy, GI diseases, or chronic infection.

Interactions

Methoxsalen reacts with *other photosensitizing drugs* and *foods,* including *coal tar products, griseofulvin, nalidixic acid, phenothiazines, sulfonamides, tetracyclines, thiazides,* and *trioxsalen,* to yield an additive photosensitizing effect. Avoid foods such as *carrots, celery, figs, limes, mustard, parsley,* and *parsnips* because they contain *furocoumarin,* which may cause an additive effect. No serious reactions have been reported with these foods, but caution should be exercised.

Effects on diagnostic tests

Abnormal liver function test results have been reported, but the exact relationship is unknown.

Adverse reactions

CNS: dizziness, headache, depression, nervousness, trouble sleeping.
GI: *nausea,* abdominal discomfort, diarrhea.
Skin: burns, blistering, peeling, swelling of extremities, itching, erythema, photosensitivity.
Other: cataracts, ***toxic hepatitis,*** leg cramps.

Note: Discontinue drug if signs of overexposure to sunlight occur.

Overdose and treatment

Clinical manifestations of overdose include serious burning and blistering of skin, which may occur from overdose of drug or overexposure to UV light. Treat acute oral overdose with gastric lavage, which, however, is effective only in the first 2 to 3 hours. Place patient in a darkened room for 8 to 24 hours or until cutaneous reactions subside. Treat burns as necessary.

☑ Special considerations

- Never dispense lotion to patient. It should be applied only by medically trained staff under controlled conditions.
- Wear gloves when applying lotion to patient.
- Temporary withdrawal of therapy is the recommended procedure in case of burning or blistering of the skin.
- Oxsoralen-Ultra should not be used interchangeably with regular Oxsoralen because it exhibits significantly greater bioavailability.
- Treatment regimen of psoralens and ultraviolet radiation in the range of 320 to 400 nm wavelength (UVA) is known as PUVA. Preleukemia and acute myeloid leukemia have been associated with PUVA therapy.
- CBC with differential, antinuclear antibody, liver function, BUN, and creatinine tests should be performed at baseline and repeated every 6 months.
- Patient should wear UVA protective glasses for several hours after treatment.
- Periodic ophthalmologic exams are recommended during therapy.

Patient education

- Teach patient how and when to use product; tell patient to wear gloves to avoid photosensitization and possible burns. Stress adherence to correct dosage schedule. If a dose is missed, patient should not increase the next dose. If more than one dose is missed, a proportionately lower dose should be given when therapy is resumed.
- Advise patient to take drug with food and milk to reduce GI irritation and, possibly, increase absorption.
- Tell patient to use proper protective precautions, including sunglasses and sunscreens. However, sunscreens may be only partially effective. Tell patient to protect skin for 8 hours after oral administration.
- Explain that drug may take several months to work. Tell patient not to increase the dose or UV light exposure during this time.

Pediatric use

- Use in children under age 12 is not recommended.

Breast-feeding
• It is unknown if drug is distributed in breast milk; therefore, the drug should be used cautiously in breast-feeding women.

methylcellulose
Citrucel, Methylcellulose Tablets

Pharmacologic classification: adsorbent
Therapeutic classification: bulk-forming laxative
Pregnancy risk category C

How supplied
Available without a prescription
Powder: 105 mg/g, 364 mg/g
Tablets: 500 mg

Indications, route, and dosage
Chronic constipation
Adults: Maximum dose is 6 g daily, divided into 0.45 to 3 g/dose.
Children age 6 to 12: Maximum dose is 3 g daily, divided into 0.45 to 1.5 g/dose.

Pharmacodynamics
Laxative action: Methylcellulose adsorbs intestinal fluid and serves as a source of indigestible fiber, stimulating peristaltic activity.

Pharmacokinetics
• *Absorption:* Methylcellulose is not absorbed. Action begins in 12 to 24 hours, but full effect may not occur for 2 to 3 days.
• *Distribution:* Distributed locally, in the intestine.
• *Metabolism:* None.
• *Excretion:* Excreted in feces.

Contraindications and precautions
Contraindicated in patients with abdominal pain, nausea, vomiting, or other symptoms of appendicitis or acute surgical abdomen and in those with intestinal obstruction or ulceration, disabling adhesions, or difficulty swallowing.

Interactions
When used concomitantly, methylcellulose may absorb *oral medications*; separate administration by at least 1 hour.

Effects on diagnostic tests
None reported.

Adverse reactions
GI: *nausea, vomiting, diarrhea* (with excessive use); *esophageal, gastric, small intestinal, or colonic strictures* (when drug is chewed or taken in dry form); *abdominal cramps, especially in severe constipation; laxative dependence (with long-term or excessive use).*

Overdose and treatment
No information available.

☑ Special considerations
• Administer drug with water or juice (at least 8 oz).
• Drug may absorb oral medications; schedule at least 1 hour apart from all other drugs.
• Bulk laxatives most closely mimic natural bowel function and do not promote laxative dependence.
• Drug is especially useful in patients with postpartum constipation, chronic laxative abuse, irritable bowel syndrome, diverticular disease, or colostomies; in debilitated patients; and to empty colon before barium enema examinations.

Patient education
• Instruct patient to take other oral medications 1 hour before or after methylcellulose.
• Explain that drug's full effect may not occur for 2 to 3 days.

Breast-feeding
• Because drug is not absorbed, use probably poses no risk to breast-feeding infants.

methyldopa
Aldomet, Apo-Methyldopa*, Dopamet*, Novomedopa*

Pharmacologic classification: centrally acting antiadrenergic
Therapeutic classification: antihypertensive
Pregnancy risk category B

How supplied
Available by prescription only
Tablets: 125 mg, 250 mg, 500 mg
Oral suspension: 250 mg/5 ml
Injection (as methyldopate hydrochloride): 250 mg/5 ml in 5-ml vials

Indications, route, and dosage
Moderate to severe hypertension
Adults: Initially, 250 mg P.O. b.i.d. or t.i.d. in first 48 hours, then increased or decreased p.r.n. q 2 days. Alternatively, 250 to 500 mg I.V. q 6 hours (maximum dose, 1 g q 6 hours). Adjust dosage if other antihypertensive drugs are added to or deleted from therapy.

Maintenance dose is 500 mg to 2 g P.O. daily in two to four divided doses. Maximum recommended daily dosage is 3 g. I.V. infusion dosage is 250 to 500 mg given over 30 to 60 minutes q 6 hours. Maximum I.V. dosage, 1 g q 6 hours.
Children: Initially, 10 mg/kg P.O. daily or 300 mg/m^2 P.O. daily in two to four divided doses; or 20 to 40 mg/kg I.V. daily or 0.6 to 1.2 g/m^2 I.V. daily in four divided doses. Increase dosage at least q 2 days until desired response occurs. Maximum daily dosage is 65 mg/kg, 2 g/m^2, or 3 g, whichever is least.

Pharmacodynamics
Antihypertensive action: Exact mechanism of antihypertensive effect is unknown; it is thought to be caused by methyldopa's metabolite, alpha-methylnorepinephrine, which stimulates central inhibito-

ry alpha-adrenergic receptors, decreasing total peripheral resistance; drug may act as a false neurotransmitter. Drug may also reduce plasma renin activity.

Pharmacokinetics

• *Absorption:* Methyldopa is absorbed partially from the GI tract. Absorption varies, but usually about 50% of an oral dose is absorbed. After oral administration, maximal decline in blood pressure occurs in 3 to 6 hours; however, full effect is not evident for 2 to 3 days. No correlation exists between plasma concentration and antihypertensive effect. After I.V. administration, blood pressure usually begins to fall in 4 to 6 hours.
• *Distribution:* Distributed throughout the body and is bound weakly to plasma proteins.
• *Metabolism:* Methyldopa is metabolized extensively in the liver and intestinal cells.
• *Excretion:* Drug and its metabolites are excreted in urine; unabsorbed drug is excreted unchanged in feces. Elimination half-life is approximately 2 hours. Antihypertensive activity usually persists up to 24 hours after oral administration and 10 to 16 hours after I.V. administration.

Contraindications and precautions

Contraindicated in patients with hypersensitivity to drug or active hepatic disease (such as acute hepatitis) and active cirrhosis. Also contraindicated if previous methyldopa therapy has been associated with liver disorders. Use cautiously in patients with impaired hepatic function, in those receiving MAO inhibitors, and in breast-feeding women.

Interactions

Methyldopa may potentiate the antihypertensive effects of *other antihypertensive agents* and the pressor effects of *sympathomimetic amines* such as *phenylpropanolamine.*

Concomitant use with *phenothiazines* or *tricyclic antidepressants* may cause a reduction in antihypertensive effects; use with *haloperidol* may produce dementia and sedation; use with *phenoxybenzamine* may cause reversible urinary incontinence.

Methyldopa may impair *tolbutamide* metabolism, enhancing tolbutamide's hypoglycemic effect. Patients undergoing surgery may require reduced dosages of *anesthetics.*

Diuretics may increase hypotensive effect of methyldopa. Concomitant use of *lithium* may increase risk of lithium toxicity.

Oral iron therapy may decrease hypotensive effects and increase serum levels of levodopa.

Effects on diagnostic tests

Methyldopa alters urine uric acid, serum creatinine, and AST levels; it may also cause falsely high levels of urine catecholamines, interfering with the diagnosis of pheochromocytoma. A positive direct antiglobulin (Coombs') test may also occur.

Adverse reactions

CNS: *sedation, headache, weakness, dizziness,* decreased mental acuity, paresthesia, parkinsonism, involuntary choreoathetoid movements, psychic disturbances, depression, nightmares.
CV: ***bradycardia,*** *orthostatic hypotension, aggravated angina,* ***myocarditis***, edema.
EENT: *nasal congestion.*
GI: nausea, vomiting, diarrhea, ***pancreatitis,*** *dry mouth,* constipation.
Hematologic: ***hemolytic anemia, thrombocytopenia, leukopenia,*** bone marrow depression.
Hepatic: ***hepatic necrosis***, abnormal liver function tests, ***hepatitis.***
Skin: rash.
Other: gynecomastia, galactorrhea, drug-induced fever, amenorrhea, impotence, decreased libido.

Overdose and treatment

Clinical signs of overdose include sedation, hypotension, impaired atrioventricular conduction, and coma.

After recent (within 4 hours) ingestion, empty stomach by induced emesis or gastric lavage. Give activated charcoal to reduce absorption; then treat symptomatically and supportively. In severe cases, hemodialysis may be considered.

☑ Special considerations

• Patients with impaired renal function may require smaller maintenance dosages of drug.
• Methyldopate hydrochloride is administered I.V.; I.M. or S.C. administration is not recommended because of unpredictable absorption.
• Patients receiving methyldopa may become hypertensive after dialysis because drug is dialyzable.
• At the initiation of, and periodically throughout therapy, monitor hemoglobin, hematocrit, and RBC count for hemolytic anemia; also monitor liver function tests.
• Take blood pressure in supine, sitting, and standing positions during dosage adjustment; take blood pressure at least every 30 minutes during I.V. infusion until patient is stable.
• Sedation and drowsiness usually disappear with continued therapy; bedtime dosage will minimize this effect. Orthostatic hypotension may indicate a need for dosage reduction. Some patients tolerate receiving the entire daily dose in the evening or h.s.
• Monitor intake and output and daily weights to detect sodium and water retention; voided urine exposed to air may darken because of the breakdown of methyldopa or its metabolites.
• Tolerance may develop after 2 to 3 weeks.
• Signs of hepatotoxicity may occur 2 to 4 weeks after therapy begins.
• Monitor for signs and symptoms of drug-induced depression.

Patient education

• Teach patient signs and symptoms of adverse effects, such as "jerky" movements, and about the need to report them; he should also report excessive weight gain (5 lb [2.25 kg] weekly), signs of infection, or fever.
• Teach patient to minimize adverse effects by taking drug at bedtime until tolerance develops to sedation, drowsiness, and other CNS effects; by avoid-

ing sudden position changes to minimize orthostatic hypotension; and by using ice chips, hard candy, or gum to relieve dry mouth.
- Warn patient to avoid hazardous activities that require mental alertness until sedative effects subside.
- Instruct patient to call for instructions before taking OTC cold preparations.

Geriatric use
- Dosage reductions may be necessary in elderly patients because they are more sensitive to sedation and hypotension.

Pediatric use
- Safety and efficacy in children have not been established; use only if potential benefits outweigh risks.

Breast-feeding
- Drug is distributed into breast milk; the American Academy of Pediatrics considers methyldopa to be compatible with breast-feeding.

methylergonovine maleate
Methergine

Pharmacologic classification: ergot alkaloid
Therapeutic classification: oxytocic
Pregnancy risk category C

How supplied
Available by prescription only
Tablets: 0.2 mg
Injection: 0.2 mg/ml ampule

Indications, route, and dosage
Prevention and treatment of postpartum hemorrhage due to uterine atony or subinvolution
Adults: 0.2 mg I.M. or I.V. q 2 to 4 hours for maximum five doses. Following initial I.M. or I.V. dose, may give 0.2 to 0.4 mg P.O. q 6 to 12 hours for maximum of 7 days. Decrease dose if severe cramping occurs.
◊ ***Diagnosis of coronary artery spasm***
Adults: 0.1 to 0.4 mg I.V.

Pharmacodynamics
Oxytocic action: Drug stimulates contractions of uterine and vascular smooth muscle. The intense uterine contractions are followed by periods of relaxation. Drug produces vasoconstriction primarily of capacitance blood vessels, causing increased central venous pressure and elevated blood pressure. Drug increases the amplitude and frequency of uterine contractions and tone, which therefore impedes uterine blood flow.

Pharmacokinetics
- *Absorption:* Absorption is rapid, with 60% of an oral dose appearing in the bloodstream. Peak plasma concentrations occur in approximately 3 hours. Onset of action is immediate for I.V., 2 to 5 minutes for I.M., and 5 to 15 minutes for oral doses.
- *Distribution:* Appears to be rapidly distributed into tissues.
- *Metabolism:* Extensive first-pass metabolism precedes hepatic metabolism.
- *Excretion:* Excreted primarily in the feces, with a small amount in urine.

Contraindications and precautions
Contraindicated in patients with hypertension, toxemia, or sensitivity to ergot preparations and in pregnant patients. Use cautiously in patients with renal or hepatic disease, sepsis, or obliterative vascular disease and during the first stage of labor.

Interactions
Drug enhances the vasoconstrictor potential of other *ergot alkaloids* and *sympathomimetic amines.* Combined use of *local anesthetics* with *vasoconstrictors* (*lidocaine* with *epinephrine*) or *smoking* (*nicotine*) will enhance vasoconstriction.

Effects on diagnostic tests
Drug therapy may decrease serum prolactin concentrations.

Adverse reactions
CNS: dizziness, headache, ***seizures***, ***CVA*** (with I.V. use), hallucinations.
CV: hypertension, transient chest pain, palpitations, hypotension.
EENT: tinnitus, nasal congestion, foul taste.
GI: *nausea, vomiting, diarrhea.*
GU: hematuria.
Respiratory: dyspnea.
Other: diaphoresis, thrombophlebitis, leg cramps.

Overdose and treatment
Clinical manifestations of overdose include seizures and gangrene, with nausea, vomiting, diarrhea, dizziness, fluctuations in blood pressure, weak pulse, chest pain, tingling, and numbness and coldness in extremities.

Treatment of oral overdose requires that the patient drink tap water, milk, or vegetable oil to delay absorption, then follow with gastric lavage or emesis, then activated charcoal and cathartics. Treat seizures with anticonvulsants and hypercoagulability with heparin; use vasodilators to improve blood flow as required. Gangrene may require surgical amputation.

☑ Special considerations
- Contractions begin 5 to 15 minutes after P.O. administration, 2 to 5 minutes after I.M. injection, and immediately following I.V. injection; continue 3 hours or more after P.O. or I.M. administration, 45 minutes after I.V.
- Monitor blood pressure, pulse rate, and uterine response; watch for sudden change in vital signs or frequent periods of uterine relaxation, and character and amount of vaginal bleeding.
- Do not administer I.V. routinely because of the possibility of inducing sudden hypertensive and CV accidents.
- Store tablets in tightly closed, light-resistant containers. Discard if discolored.

- Store I.V. solutions below 77° F (25° C). Administer only if solution is clear and colorless.
- If I.V. administration is considered essential as a life-saving measure, give slowly over no less than 60 seconds.

Patient education
- Advise patient to avoid smoking while taking drug.
- Advise patient of adverse reactions.

Breast-feeding
- Ergot alkaloids inhibit lactation. Drug is excreted in breast milk, and ergotism has been reported in breast-fed infants.

methylphenidate hydrochloride
Ritalin, Ritalin-SR

Pharmacologic classification: piperidine CNS stimulant
Therapeutic classification: CNS stimulant (analeptic)
Controlled substance schedule II
Pregnancy risk category NR

How supplied
Available by prescription only
Tablets: 5 mg, 10 mg, 20 mg
Tablets (sustained-release): 20 mg

Indications, route, and dosage
Attention deficit hyperactivity disorder (ADHD)
Children age 6 and older: Initially, 5 to 10 mg P.O. daily before breakfast and lunch, increased in 5- to 10-mg increments weekly p.r.n. until an optimum daily dosage of 2 mg/kg is reached, not to exceed 60 mg/day. Usual effective daily dosage, 20 to 30 mg.
Narcolepsy
Adults: 10 mg P.O. b.i.d. or t.i.d. 30 to 45 minutes before meals. Dosage varies with patient needs; average dosage is 40 to 60 mg/day.

When using sustained-release tablets, calculate regular dose in q 8-hour intervals and administer as such.

Pharmacodynamics
Analeptic action: The cerebral cortex and reticular activating system appear to be the primary sites of activity; methylphenidate releases nerve terminal stores of norepinephrine, promoting nerve impulse transmission. At high doses, effects are mediated by dopamine.

Drug is used to treat narcolepsy and as an adjunctive to psychosocial measures in ADHD. Like amphetamines, it has a paradoxical calming effect in hyperactive children.

Pharmacokinetics
- *Absorption:* Absorbed rapidly and completely after oral administration; peak plasma concentrations occur at 1 to 2 hours. Duration of action is usually 4 to 6 hours (with considerable individual variation); sustained-release tablets may act for up to 8 hours.
- *Distribution:* Unknown.
- *Metabolism:* Methylphenidate is metabolized by the liver.
- *Excretion:* Drug is excreted in urine.

Contraindications and precautions
Contraindicated in patients with hypersensitivity to drug, glaucoma, motor tics, family history of or diagnosis of Tourette syndrome, or history of marked anxiety, tension, or agitation. Use cautiously in patients with history of seizures, drug abuse, hypertension, or EEG abnormalities.

Interactions
Concomitant use with *caffeine* may decrease efficacy of methylphenidate in ADHD; use with *MAO inhibitors* (or drugs with MAO-inhibiting activity) or within 14 days of such therapy may cause severe hypertension.

Methylphenidate may inhibit metabolism and increase the serum levels of *anticonvulsants* (*phenobarbital, phenytoin, primidone*), *coumarin anticoagulants*, *phenylbutazone*, and *tricyclic antidepressants*; it also may decrease the hypotensive effects of *bretylium* and *guanethidine*.

Caffeine may enhance methylphenidate's CNS stimulant effects. Avoid concomitant use.

Effects on diagnostic tests
None reported.

Adverse reactions
CNS: *nervousness, insomnia, Tourette syndrome,* dizziness, headache, akathisia, dyskinesia, ***seizures***, drowsiness.
CV: *palpitations, angina, tachycardia, changes in blood pressure and pulse rate,* ***arrhythmias.***
GI: nausea, abdominal pain, anorexia, weight loss.
Hematologic: ***thrombocytopenia***, ***thrombocytopenic purpura, leukopenia,*** anemia.
Skin: rash, urticaria, ***exfoliative dermatitis, erythema multiforme.***

Overdose and treatment
Symptoms of overdose may include euphoria, confusion, delirium, coma, toxic psychosis, agitation, headache, vomiting, dry mouth, mydriasis, self-injury, fever, diaphoresis, tremors, hyperreflexia, muscle twitching, seizures, flushing, hypertension, tachycardia, palpitations, and arrhythmias.

Treat overdose symptomatically and supportively: use gastric lavage or emesis in patients with intact gag reflex. Maintain airway and circulation. Closely monitor vital signs and fluid and electrolyte balance. Maintain patient in cool room, monitor temperature, minimize external stimulation, and protect him against self-injury. External cooling blankets may be needed.

☑ Special considerations
- Methylphenidate is the drug of choice for ADHD. Therapy is usually discontinued after puberty.
- Monitor initiation of therapy closely; drug may precipitate Tourette syndrome.
- If paradoxical aggravation of symptoms occurs during therapy, reduce dosage or discontinue drug.

• Check vital signs regularly for increased blood pressure or other signs of excessive stimulation; avoid late-day or evening dosing, especially of long-acting dosage forms, to minimize insomnia.
• Drug may decrease seizure threshold in seizure disorders.
• Monitor CBC, differential, and platelet counts when patient is taking drug long-term.
• Intermittent drug-free periods when stress is least evident (weekends, school holidays) may help prevent development of tolerance and permit decreased dosage when drug is resumed. Sustained-release form allows convenience of single, at-home dosing for school children.
• Drug has abuse potential; discourage use to combat fatigue. Some abusers dissolve tablets and inject drug.
• After high-dose and long-term use, abrupt withdrawal may unmask severe depression. Lower dosage gradually to prevent acute rebound depression.
• Drug impairs ability to perform tasks requiring mental alertness.
• Be sure patient obtains adequate rest; fatigue may result as drug wears off.
• Monitor height and weight; drug has been associated with growth suppression.
• Discourage methylphenidate use for analeptic effect; CNS stimulation superimposed on CNS depression may cause neuronal instability and seizures.
• Do not administer drug to women of childbearing age unless potential benefits outweigh the possible risks.

Patient education
• Explain rationale for therapy and the risks and benefits that may be anticipated.
• Tell patient to avoid drinks containing caffeine to prevent added CNS stimulation and not to alter dosage unless prescribed.
• Advise narcoleptic patient to take first dose on awakening; advise ADHD patient to take last dose several hours before bedtime to avoid insomnia.
• Tell patient not to chew or crush sustained-release dosage forms.
• Warn patient not to use drug to mask fatigue, to be sure to obtain adequate rest, and to call if excessive CNS stimulation occurs.
• Advise patient to avoid hazardous activities that require mental alertness until degree of sedative effect is determined.

Pediatric use
• Drug is not recommended for ADHD in children under age 6. It has been associated with growth suppression; all patients should be monitored.

methylprednisolone
Medrol

methylprednisolone acetate
depMedalone-40, depMedalone-80, Depoject-40, Depoject-80, Depo-Medrol, Depo-Predate-40, Depo-Predate-80, Duralone-40, Duralone-80, Medralone, Rep-Pred-40, Rep-Pred-80

methylprednisolone sodium succinate
A-methaPred, Solu-Medrol

Pharmacologic classification: glucocorticoid
Therapeutic classification: anti-inflammatory, immunosuppressant
Pregnancy risk category C

How supplied
Available by prescription only
methylprednisolone
Tablets: 2 mg, 4 mg, 8 mg, 16 mg, 24 mg, 32 mg
methylprednisolone acetate
Injection: 20 mg/ml, 40 mg/ml, 80 mg/ml suspension
methylprednisolone sodium succinate
Injection: 40 mg, 125 mg, 500 mg, 1,000 mg, 2,000 mg/vial

Indications, route, and dosage
Multiple sclerosis
methylprednisolone (systemic)
Adults: 200 mg P.O. daily for 1 week, followed by 80 mg every other day for 1 month.
Inflammation
methylprednisolone
Adults: 2 to 60 mg P.O. daily in four divided doses, depending on disease being treated.
Children: Administer 0.117 to 1.66 mg/kg daily or 3.3 to 50 mg/m² P.O. daily in three or four divided doses.
methylprednisolone acetate
Adults: 10 to 80 mg I.M. daily; or 4 to 80 mg into joints and soft tissue p.r.n. q 1 to 5 weeks; or 20 to 60 mg intralesionally.
methylprednisolone sodium succinate
Adults: 10 to 250 mg I.M. or I.V. q 4 hours.
Children: 0.03 to 0.2 mg/kg or 1 to 6.25 mg/m² I.M. or I.V. daily in divided doses.
Shock
methylprednisolone sodium succinate
Adults: 100 to 250 mg I.V. at 2- to 6-hour intervals.
◊ ***Severe lupus nephritis***
Adults: 1 g I.V. over 1 hour for 3 days.
◊ ***Treatment or minimization of motor and sensory defects caused by acute spinal cord injury***
Adults: Initially, 30 mg/kg I.V. over 15 minutes followed in 45 minutes by I.V. infusion of 5.4 mg/kg/hour for 23 hours.

* Canada only ◊ Unlabeled clinical use

Pharmacodynamics

Anti-inflammatory action: Methylprednisolone stimulates the synthesis of enzymes needed to decrease the inflammatory response. It suppresses the immune system by reducing activity and volume of the lymphatic system, thus producing lymphocytopenia (primarily of T lymphocytes), decreasing immunoglobulin and complement concentrations, decreasing passage of immune complexes through basement membranes, and possibly by depressing reactivity of tissue to antigen-antibody interactions.

Drug is an intermediate-acting glucocorticoid. It has essentially no mineralocorticoid activity but is a potent glucocorticoid, with five times the potency of an equal weight of hydrocortisone. It is used primarily as an anti-inflammatory agent and immunosuppressant.

Methylprednisolone may be administered orally. Methylprednisolone sodium succinate may be administered by I.M. or I.V. injection or by I.V. infusion, usually at 4- to 6-hour intervals. Methylprednisolone acetate suspension may be administered by intra-articular, intrasynovial, intrabursal, intralesional, or soft tissue injection. It has a slow onset but a long duration of action. Injectable forms are usually used only when the oral dosage forms cannot be used.

Pharmacokinetics

- *Absorption:* Absorbed readily after oral administration. After oral and I.V. administration, peak effects occur in about 1 to 2 hours. The acetate suspension for injection has a variable absorption over 24 to 48 hours, depending on whether it is injected into an intra-articular space or a muscle, and on the blood supply to that muscle.
- *Distribution:* Drug is distributed rapidly to muscle, liver, skin, intestines, and kidneys. Adrenocorticoids are distributed into breast milk and through the placenta.
- *Metabolism:* Methylprednisolone is metabolized in the liver to inactive glucuronide and sulfate metabolites.
- *Excretion:* Inactive metabolites and small amounts of unmetabolized drug are excreted by the kidneys. Insignificant quantities of drug are excreted in feces. Biological half-life of methylprednisolone is 18 to 36 hours.

Contraindications and precautions

Contraindicated in patients allergic to any component of the formulation, in those with systemic fungal infections, and in premature infants (acetate and succinate).

Use cautiously in patients with renal disease, GI ulceration, hypertension, osteoporosis, diabetes mellitus, hypothyroidism, cirrhosis, diverticulitis, nonspecific ulcerative colitis, recent intestinal anastomoses, thromboembolic disorders, seizures, myasthenia gravis, heart failure, tuberculosis, emotional instability, ocular herpes simplex, and psychotic tendencies.

Interactions

When used concomitantly, adrenocorticoids may decrease the effects of *oral anticoagulants* by unknown mechanisms.

Glucocorticoids increase the metabolism of *isoniazid* and *salicylates*; cause hyperglycemia, requiring dosage adjustment of *insulin* or *oral antidiabetic agents* in diabetic patients; and may enhance hypokalemia associated with *amphotericin B* or *diuretic* therapy. The hypokalemia may increase the risk of toxicity in patients concurrently receiving *cardiac glycosides*.

Barbiturates, phenytoin, and *rifampin* may cause decreased corticosteroid effects because of increased hepatic metabolism. *Antacids, cholestyramine,* and *colestipol* decrease the corticosteroid effect by adsorbing the corticosteroid, decreasing the amount absorbed.

Concomitant use with *estrogens* may reduce the metabolism of corticosteroids by increasing the concentration of transcortin. The half-life of the corticosteroid is then prolonged because of increased protein binding. Concomitant administration of *ulcerogenic drugs* such as *NSAIDs* may increase the risk of GI ulceration.

Methylprednisolone may interact with *anticholinesterase*, causing profound weakness. Drug may decrease effectiveness of *vaccines*. Levels of *cyclosporine* may increase.

Effects on diagnostic tests

Drug suppresses reactions to skin tests; causes false-negative results in the nitroblue tetrazolium test for systemic bacterial infections; decreases ^{131}I uptake and protein-bound iodine concentrations in thyroid function tests; may increase glucose and cholesterol levels; may decrease serum potassium, calcium, thyroxine, and triiodothyronine levels; and may increase urine glucose and calcium levels.

Adverse reactions

Most adverse reactions to corticosteroids are dose-dependent or duration-dependent.

CNS: *euphoria, insomnia,* psychotic behavior, pseudotumor cerebri, vertigo, headache, paresthesia, ***seizures.***

CV: ***heart failure***, hypertension, edema, ***arrhythmias,*** thrombophlebitis, ***thromboembolism***, ***fatal arrest or circulatory collapse*** (following rapid administration of large I.V. doses).

EENT: cataracts, glaucoma.

GI: *peptic ulceration,* GI irritation, increased appetite, pancreatitis, nausea, vomiting.

Skin: delayed wound healing, acne, various skin eruptions.

Other: muscle weakness, osteoporosis, hirsutism, susceptibility to infections, hypokalemia, hyperglycemia, carbohydrate intolerance, growth suppression in children, menstrual irregularities, cushingoid state (moonface, buffalo hump, central obesity), ***acute adrenal insufficiency that may occur with increased stress (infection, surgery, or trauma) or abrupt withdrawal after long-term therapy.***

After abrupt withdrawal: rebound inflammation, fatigue, weakness, arthralgia, fever, dizziness, lethargy, depression, fainting, orthostatic hypotension, dyspnea, anorexia, hypoglycemia. ***After prolonged use, sudden withdrawal may be fatal.***

Overdose and treatment

Acute ingestion, even in massive doses, is rarely a clinical problem. Toxic signs and symptoms rarely occur if drug is used for less than 3 weeks, even at large doses. However, chronic use causes adverse physiologic effects, including suppression of the hypothalamus-pituitary-adrenal axis, cushingoid appearance, muscle weakness, and osteoporosis.

☑ Special considerations

Recommendations for use of methylprednisolone and for care and teaching of patients during therapy are the same as those for all *systemic adrenocorticoids.*

Pediatric use

• Chronic use of adrenocorticoids in children and adolescents may delay growth and maturation.

---

methyltestosterone

Android-10, Android-25, Oreton Methyl, Testred, Virilon

Pharmacologic classification: androgen
Therapeutic classification: androgen replacement
Controlled substance schedule III
Pregnancy risk category X

How supplied

Available by prescription only
Tablets: 10 mg, 25 mg
Tablets (buccal): 10 mg
Capsules: 10 mg

Indications, route, and dosage

Breast cancer in women
Adults: 50 to 200 mg P.O. daily, or 25 to 100 mg buccal daily.
Male hypogonadism
Adults and adolescents: 10 to 50 mg P.O. daily, or 5 to 25 mg buccal daily.

Pharmacodynamics

Androgenic action: Drug mimics action of endogenous androgen testosterone by stimulating receptors in androgen-responsive organs and tissues. It exerts inhibitory, antiestrogenic effects on hormone-responsive breast tumors and metastases.

Pharmacokinetics

• *Absorption:* No information available.
• *Distribution:* No information available.
• *Metabolism:* Drug is metabolized by the liver.
• *Excretion:* Excreted as metabolites in urine.

Contraindications and precautions

Contraindicated in pregnant and breast-feeding patients and in males with breast cancer or prostate cancer. Use cautiously in the elderly; in patients with cardiac, renal, or hepatic disease; in healthy males with delayed puberty; and in those with a tartrazine allergy or sensitivity to mercury compounds.

Interactions

In patients with diabetes, decreased blood glucose levels may require adjustment of *insulin* or *oral antidiabetic* drug dosage.

Methyltestosterone may potentiate the effects of *warfarin-type anticoagulants*, resulting in increased PT. Use with *adrenocorticosteroids* or *corticotropin* increases potential for fluid and electrolyte accumulation. Coadministration of *imipramine* with methyltestosterone resulted in a dramatic paranoid response in four of five patients.

Effects on diagnostic tests

Drug may cause abnormal results of fasting plasma glucose, glucose tolerance, and metyrapone tests. Sulfobromophthalein (BSP) retention may be increased. Thyroid function test results (protein-bound iodine, radioactive iodine uptake, thyroid-binding capacity) and 17-ketosteroid levels may decrease. Liver function test results, PT (especially in patients on anticoagulant therapy), and serum creatinine may be elevated. Because of drug's anabolic activity, serum sodium, potassium, calcium, phosphate, and cholesterol levels may all rise.

Adverse reactions

CNS: headache, anxiety, depression, paresthesia, sleep apnea syndrome.
CV: edema.
EENT: irritation of oral mucosa (with buccal administration).
GI: nausea.
GU: hypoestrogenic effects in women (flushing; diaphoresis; vaginitis, including itching, dryness, and burning; vaginal bleeding; nervousness; emotional lability; menstrual irregularities), excessive hormonal effects in men (prepubertal premature epiphyseal closure, *acne, priapism,* growth of body and facial hair, phallic enlargement; postpubertal testicular atrophy, oligospermia, decreased ejaculatory volume, impotence, gynecomastia, epididymitis).
Hepatic: reversible jaundice, cholestatic hepatitis, abnormal liver enzyme levels.
Other: hypercalcemia, polycythemia, hypersensitivity skin manifestations, suppression of clotting factors, muscle cramps or spasms, androgenic effects in women (acne, edema, *weight gain, hirsutism, hoarseness, clitoral enlargement,* decreased breast size, deepening voice, changes in libido, male-pattern baldness, oily skin or hair).

Overdose and treatment

No information available.

☑ Special considerations

Besides those relevant to all *androgens,* consider the following recommendations.

• Carefully observe female patient for signs of excessive virilization. If possible, discontinue therapy at first sign of virilization because some adverse

effects (deepening of the voice, clitoral enlargement) are irreversible.
- Observe for signs and symptoms of hypoglycemia in patients with diabetes, and for signs and symptoms of bleeding such as ecchymoses or petechiae in patients receiving oral anticoagulants.
- Do not administer drug for more than 6 months. After 6 months, stop for 3 to 4 weeks, then restart treatment.

Patient education
- Tell patient to place buccal tablets in upper or lower buccal pouch between cheek and gum and to allow 30 to 60 minutes to dissolve. Advise him to change tablet absorption site with each buccal dose to minimize risk of buccal irritation; tablets should never be chewed or swallowed.
- Advise patient not to eat, drink, chew, or smoke while buccal tablet is in place, and to rinse mouth with water after use of buccal tablets.
- Instruct patient to report inflamed or painful oral membranes or discomfort. Emphasize good oral hygiene.
- Advise patient to report signs and symptoms of virilization (in females), too frequent or persistent erections (in males), or GI distress immediately.

Geriatric use
- Observe elderly male patients for the development of prostatic hypertrophy. Development of prostatic hypertrophy or prostatic carcinoma mandates discontinuing drug.

Pediatric use
- Use with extreme caution in children to avoid precocious puberty and premature closure of the epiphyses. X-ray examinations every 6 months are recommended to assess skeletal maturation.

Breast-feeding
- Drug is contraindicated in breast-feeding women.

methysergide maleate
Sansert

Pharmacologic classification: ergot alkaloid
Therapeutic classification: vasoconstrictor
Pregnancy risk category X

How supplied
Available by prescription only
Tablets: 2 mg

Indications, route, and dosage
Prevention of vascular headaches, including migraine and cluster headaches
Adults: 4 to 8 mg P.O. daily in divided doses with meals.
◇ ***To control diarrhea in patients with carcinoid disease***
Adults: 2 mg P.O. t.i.d. Adjust dosage as needed and tolerated. Usual dosage range is 4 to 16 mg P.O. t.i.d.

Pharmacodynamics
Vasoconstrictor action: Drug competitively blocks serotonin peripherally and may act as a serotonin agonist in the CNS (brain stem). Its antiserotonin effects result in inhibition of peripheral vasoconstrictor and pressor effects of serotonin, inflammation induced by serotonin, and a reduction in the increased rate of platelet aggregation caused by serotonin.

The mechanism involved in prophylaxis of vascular headaches by methysergide is unknown; however, its effectiveness may result from humoral factors affecting the pain threshold and from its central serotonin-agonist effect.

Pharmacokinetics
- *Absorption:* Rapidly absorbed from the GI tract.
- *Distribution:* Methysergide is widely distributed in body tissues.
- *Metabolism:* Drug is metabolized in the liver to methylergonovine and glucuronide metabolites.
- *Excretion:* 56% of a dose is excreted in urine as unchanged drug and its metabolites. Plasma elimination half-life is 10 hours.

Contraindications and precautions
Contraindicated in patients with severe hypertension or arteriosclerosis, peripheral vascular insufficiency, renal or hepatic disease, coronary artery disease, phlebitis or cellulitis of lower limbs, collagen diseases, fibrotic processes, or valvular heart disease; in debilitated patients; and during pregnancy.

Use cautiously in patients with peptic ulcer or suspected coronary artery disease and in those with aspirin or tartrazine allergies.

Interactions
Drug may reverse the analgesic activity of *narcotic analgesics.* Concurrent therapy with *beta blockers* may result in peripheral ischemia manifested by cold extremities with possible peripheral gangrene.

Effects on diagnostic tests
None reported.

Adverse reactions
CNS: insomnia, drowsiness, *euphoria, vertigo, ataxia,* light-headedness, hyperesthesia, weakness, hallucinations or feelings of dissociation, rapid speech, lethargy.
CV: *fibrotic thickening of cardiac valves and aorta, inferior vena cava, and common iliac branches (retroperitoneal fibrosis);* vasoconstriction, causing chest pain, abdominal pain, vascular insufficiency of lower limbs; cold, numb, painful extremities with or without paresthesia and diminished or absent pulses; orthostatic hypotension; tachycardia; peripheral edema; murmurs; bruits.
GI: nausea, vomiting, diarrhea, constipation, heartburn.
Hematologic: neutropenia, eosinophilia.
Respiratory: ***pulmonary fibrosis*** (causing dyspnea, tightness and pain in chest, pleural friction rubs, and effusion).

Skin: hair loss, flushing, rash.
Other: arthralgia, myalgia.

Overdose and treatment

Clinical manifestations of overdose include hyperactivity, euphoria, dizziness, peripheral vasospasm with diminished or absent pulses, and coldness, mottling, and cyanosis of extremities.

Treatment requires supportive measures with prolonged and careful monitoring. If patient is conscious and ingestion recent, induce emesis; if unconscious, insert cuffed endotracheal tube and perform gastric lavage followed by sodium chloride (magnesium sulfate) cathartic. Administer I.V. fluids if needed. Monitor vital signs.

Apply warmth (not direct heat) to ischemic extremities if vasospasm occurs. Administer vasodilators (nitroprusside, tolazoline, or prazosin) if needed.

Contact local or regional poison control center for more information.

☑ Special considerations

Besides those relevant to all *ergot alkaloids,* consider the following recommendations.
- GI effects may be reduced by gradual introduction of medication and by giving with food or milk.
- Do not use drug to treat acute episodes of migraine, vascular headache, or muscle contraction headache.
- Dosage should be reduced gradually for 2 to 3 weeks before discontinuing drug.
- If drug is given for cluster headaches, it is usually administered only during the cluster.
- Drug has also been used to control diarrhea in patients with carcinoid disease.
- Protective effect develops in 1 to 2 days and persists for 1 to 2 days after drug is discontinued.

Patient education

- Inform patient not to take drug for longer than 6 months at any one time and to wait 3 to 4 weeks before restarting.
- Tell patient to report immediately signs of numbness or tingling in hands or feet; red or violet blisters on hands and feet; flank or chest pain; shortness of breath; leg cramps when walking; or any other signs or symptoms of impaired circulation.
- Warn patient to avoid alcoholic beverages, because alcohol may worsen headaches; to avoid smoking, because it may increase adverse effects of drug; and to avoid prolonged exposure to very cold temperatures, because cold may increase adverse effects of drug.
- Tell patient to report illness or infection, which may increase sensitivity to drug effects.
- Explain that after discontinuing drug, his body may need time to adjust depending on the amount used and the duration of time involved.
- Tell patient to take drug with food.
- Inform patient that drug may cause drowsiness and to use caution when driving or performing other tasks requiring alertness.
- Caution patient regarding caloric intake to avoid excessive weight gain.
- Drug may contain tartrazine, which can cause an allergic reaction.

Geriatric use

- Use with caution.

Pediatric use

- Drug is not recommended for use in children because of risk of fibrosis.

Breast-feeding

- Drug may occur in breast milk. Breast-feeding should be avoided during treatment with methysergide.

metipranolol hydrochloride

OptiPranolol

Pharmacologic classification: beta-adrenergic blocker
Therapeutic classification: antiglaucoma
Pregnancy risk category C

How supplied

Available by prescription only
Ophthalmic solution: 0.3% in 5- or 10-ml dropper bottles with 0.004% benzalkonium chloride and ethylenediaminetetraacetic acid

Indications, route, and dosage

Treatment of ocular conditions in which lowering of intraocular pressure (IOP) would be beneficial (ocular hypertension, chronic open-angle glaucoma)
Adults: Instill 1 drop into affected eye(s) b.i.d. Larger dosage or more frequent administration is not known to be of benefit. If IOP is not satisfactory, concomitant therapy to lower IOP may be instituted.

Pharmacodynamics

Antiglaucoma action: Exact mechanism of ocular antihypertensive action is not known but appears to be a reduction of aqueous humor production. A slight increase in outflow facility has been demonstrated with metipranolol. Like other noncardioselective beta blockers, metipranolol does not have significant local anesthetic (membrane-stabilizing) actions or intrinsic sympathomimetic activity. It does reduce elevated and normal IOP with or without glaucoma with little or no effect on pupil size or accommodation. In patients with IOP above 24 mm Hg, pressure is reduced an average of 20% to 26%.

Pharmacokinetics

- *Absorption:* Drug is intended to act locally, but some systemic absorption may occur. Onset of action occurs in less than 30 minutes.
- *Distribution:* Local.
- *Metabolism:* Unknown.
- *Excretion:* Unknown; maximium effect occurs in about 2 hours; duration of effect is 12 to 24 hours.

Contraindications and precautions

Contraindicated in patients hypersensitive to drug or its components and in those with bronchial asthma, history of bronchial asthma or severe COPD, sinus bradycardia, second- or third-degree AV block, cardiac failure, and cardiogenic shock.

Use cautiously in patients with nonallergic bronchospasm, chronic bronchitis, emphysema, diabetes mellitus, hyperthyroidism, or cerebrovascular insufficiency.

Interactions

Use with caution in patients taking *systemic beta blockers* because of potential for additive effects. The following agents may interact with systemic beta blockers, and thus may interact with ophthalmic beta blockers: *antithyroid agents, calcium channel blockers, catecholamine-depleting drugs, cimetidine, clonidine, oral contraceptives, digoxin, haloperidol, hydralazine, insulin, lidocaine, morphine, nondepolarizing neuromuscular blocking agents, NSAIDs, phenobarbital, phenothiazines, prazosin, rifampin, salicylates, sympathomimetics, theophylline*, and *thyroid hormones*.

Smoking may also interfere with drug's effect.

Effects on diagnostic tests

None reported.

Adverse reactions

CNS: headache, anxiety, dizziness, depression, somnolence, nervousness, asthenia, brow ache.
CV: hypertension, ***MI,*** atrial fibrillation, angina, palpitations, bradycardia.
EENT: transient local eye discomfort, tearing, conjunctivitis, eyelid dermatitis, blurred vision, blepharitis, abnormal vision, photophobia, eye edema, rhinitis, epistaxis.
GI: nausea.
Respiratory: dyspnea, bronchitis, cough.
Skin: rash.
Other: hypersensitivity reactions, myalgia.

Overdose and treatment

If ocular overdose occurs, flush eye(s) with copious amounts of water or 0.9% NaCl solution.

Systemic overdose, after accidental ingestion, may cause bradycardia, hypotension, bronchospasm, or acute cardiac failure. Discontinue therapy, institute supportive and symptomatic measures, and decrease further absorption, for example, by gastric lavage.

☑ Special considerations

- Concomitant pilocarpine and other miotics, dipivefrin, or systemic carbonic anhydrase inhibitors may be administered if IOP is not adequately controlled.
- Proper administration is essential for optimal therapeutic response; instruct patient in correct techniques.
- The normal eye can retain only about 10 microliters (mcl) of fluid; the average dropper delivers 25 to 50 mcl/drop. Thus, the value of more than 1 drop is questionable. If multiple-drop therapy is indicated, the best interval between drops is 5 minutes.

Patient education

- Tell patient to wash hands thoroughly before administration and then to follow these directions:
  - Tilt head back or lie down and gaze upward.
  - Gently grasp lower eyelid below eyelashes and pull eyelid away from eye to form a "pouch."
  - Place dropper directly over eye, avoiding contact of dropper with eye or any surface.
  - Look up just before applying drop; look down for several seconds after applying drop. Slowly release eyelid.
  - Close eyes gently for 1 to 2 minutes. Closing eyes tightly after instillation may expel medication from "pouch." Apply gentle pressure to inside corner of eye at bridge of nose to retard drainage of solution from intended area.
- Tell patient to avoid rubbing the eye and to minimize blinking.
- Tell patient not to rinse dropper after use.
- Advise patient to check expiration date on bottle before use and not to use eyedrops that have changed color.
- Tell patient who must use more than one medication to wait at least 5 minutes between instillations.

Pediatric use

- Safety and efficacy have not been established.

Breast-feeding

- It is unknown if drug is excreted in breast milk. Use with caution in breast-feeding women because systemic beta blockers are excreted in breast milk.

metoclopramide hydrochloride

Apo-Metoclop*, Clopra, Emex*, Maxeran*, Maxolon, Octamide PFS, Reclomide, Reglan

Pharmacologic classification: para-aminobenzoic acid (PABA) derivative
Therapeutic classification: antiemetic, GI stimulant
Pregnancy risk category B

How supplied

Available by prescription only
Tablets: 5 mg, 10 mg
Syrup: 5 mg/5 ml
Injection: 5 mg/ml
Solution: 10 mg/ml

Indications, route, and dosage

Prevention or reduction of nausea and vomiting induced by highly emetogenic chemotherapy
Adults: 1 to 2 mg/kg I.V. q 2 hours for two doses, beginning 30 minutes before emetogenic chemotherapy drug administration, then q 3 hours for three doses.
Facilitation of small-bowel intubation and to aid in radiologic examinations
Adults: 10 mg I.V. as a single dose over 1 to 2 minutes.

Children age 6 to 14: 2.5 to 5 mg I.V.
Children under age 6: 0.1 mg/kg I.V.
Delayed gastric emptying secondary to diabetic gastroparesis
Adults: 10 mg P.O. 30 minutes before meals and h.s. for 2 to 8 weeks, depending on response; or 10 mg I.V. over 2 minutes.
Gastroesophageal reflux
Adults: 10 to 15 mg P.O. q.i.d., p.r.n., taken 30 minutes before meals and h.s.
Postoperative nausea and vomiting
Adults: 10 to 20 mg I.M. near end of surgical procedure, repeated q 4 to 6 hours p.r.n.
◇ ***Vomiting***
Adults: 10 mg P.O. taken 30 minutes before meals.

Pharmacodynamics

Antiemetic action: Metoclopramide inhibits dopamine receptors in the brain's chemoreceptor trigger zone to inhibit or reduce nausea and vomiting.

GI stimulant action: Drug relieves esophageal reflux by increasing lower esophageal sphincter tone and reduces gastric stasis by stimulating motility of the upper GI tract, thus reducing gastric emptying time.

Pharmacokinetics

- *Absorption:* After oral administration, drug is absorbed rapidly and thoroughly from the GI tract; action begins in ½ to 1 hour. After I.M. administration, about 74% to 96% of drug is bioavailable; action begins in 10 to 15 minutes. After I.V. administration, onset of action occurs in 1 to 3 minutes.
- *Distribution:* Distributed to most body tissues and fluids, including the brain. Drug crosses the placenta and is distributed in breast milk.
- *Metabolism:* Drug is not metabolized extensively; a small amount is metabolized in the liver.
- *Excretion:* Drug is mostly excreted in urine and feces. Hemodialysis and renal dialysis remove minimal amounts. Duration of effect is 1 to 2 hours.

Contraindications and precautions

Contraindicated in patients in whom stimulation of GI motility might be dangerous (for example, those with hemorrhage, obstruction, or perforation) and in those with hypersensitivity to drug, pheochromocytoma, or seizure disorders. Use cautiously in patients with history of depression, Parkinson's disease, and hypertension.

Interactions

Metoclopramide may increase or decrease absorption of other drugs, depending on changes in transit time through the intestinal tract; it may increase absorption of *acetaminophen, aspirin, diazepam, ethanol, levodopa, lithium,* and *tetracycline* and may decrease absorption of *digoxin.* A faster gastric emptying time may allow for an increase in *cyclosporine* absorption, possibly increasing its immunosuppressive and toxic effects.

Anticholinergics and *opiates* may antagonize metoclopramide's effect on GI motility. Concomitant use with *antihypertensives* and *CNS depressants* (such as *alcohol, sedatives,* and *tricyclic antidepressants*) may lead to increased CNS depression.

Concomitant use with *butyrophenone antipsychotics* and *phenothiazine* may potentiate extrapyramidal reactions.

Metoclopramide releases catecholamines in patients with essential hypertension. Use with caution, if at all, in patients receiving *MAO inhibitors.*

Effects on diagnostic tests

Metoclopramide may increase serum aldosterone and prolactin levels.

Adverse reactions

CNS: *restlessness, anxiety, drowsiness, fatigue, lassitude, depression, akathisia, insomnia, confusion,* ***suicide ideation, seizures,*** hallucinations, headache, dizziness, extrapyramidal symptoms, tardive dyskinesia, dystonic reactions.
CV: transient hypertension, hypotension, supraventricular tachycardia, bradycardia.
GI: nausea, bowel disturbances, diarrhea.
Hematologic: ***neutropenia, agranulocytosis.***
Respiratory: ***bronchospasm.***
Skin: rash, urticaria.
Other: fever, prolactin secretion, loss of libido, urinary frequency, incontinence, porphyria.

Overdose and treatment

Clinical effects of overdose (which is rare) include drowsiness, dystonia, seizures, and extrapyramidal effects.

Treatment includes administration of antimuscarinics, antiparkinsonian agents, or antihistamines with antimuscarinic activity (for example, 50 mg diphenhydramine, given I.M.).

☑ Special considerations

- Do not use drug for more than 12 weeks.
- For I.V. push administration, use undiluted and inject over a 1- to 2-minute period. For I.V. infusion, dilute with 50 ml of D_5W, dextrose 5% in 0.45% NaCl, NaCl injection, Ringer's injection, or lactated Ringer's injection, and infuse over at least 15 minutes
- Administer by I.V. infusion 30 minutes before chemotherapy.
- Drug may be used to facilitate nasoduodenal tube placement.
- Diphenhydramine may be used to counteract extrapyramidal effects of high-dose metoclopramide.
- Drug is not recommended for long-term use.
- Drug has been used investigationally to treat anorexia nervosa, dizziness, migraine, intractable hiccups, and to promote postpartum lactation; oral dose form is being used investigationally to treat nausea and vomiting.

Patient education

- Warn patient to avoid driving for 2 hours after each dose because drug may cause drowsiness. Until extent of CNS effect is known, advise patient not to consume alcohol.
- Tell patient to report twitching or involuntary movement.

• Instruct patient to take medication 30 minutes before each meal.

Geriatric use

• Use drug with caution, especially if patient has impaired renal function; dosage may need to be decreased. Elderly patients are more likely to experience extrapyramidal symptoms and tardive dyskinesia.

Pediatric use

• Children have an increased incidence of adverse CNS effects.

Breast-feeding

• Because drug is distributed in breast milk, use caution when administering it to breast-feeding women.

metolazone

Mykrox, Zaroxolyn

Pharmacologic classification: quinazoline derivative (thiazide-like) diuretic
Therapeutic classification: diuretic, antihypertensive
Pregnancy risk category B

How supplied

Available by prescription only
Tablets: 2.5 mg, 5 mg, 10 mg
Tablets (rapid-acting): 0.5 mg (Mykrox)

Indications, route, and dosage

Tablets
Edema (heart failure)
Adults: 5 to 10 mg P.O. daily.
Edema (renal disease)
Adults: 5 to 20 mg P.O. daily.
Hypertension
Adults: 2.5 to 5 mg P.O. daily; maintenance dosage based on patient's blood pressure.
Rapid-acting tablets
Hypertension
Adults: 0.5 mg once daily; may be increased to maximum of 1 mg daily.

Pharmacodynamics

Diuretic action: Metolazone increases urinary excretion of sodium and water by inhibiting sodium reabsorption in the cortical diluting tubule of the nephron, thus relieving edema. Metolazone may be more effective in edema associated with impaired renal function than thiazide or thiazide-like diuretics.

Antihypertensive action: Exact mechanism of metolazone's antihypertensive effect is unknown; it may result from direct arteriolar vasodilatation. Metolazone also reduces total body sodium levels and total peripheral resistance.

Pharmacokinetics

• *Absorption:* About 65% of a given dose of metolazone is absorbed after oral administration to healthy subjects; in cardiac patients, absorption falls to 40%. However, rate and extent of absorption vary among preparations.
• *Distribution:* Metolazone is 50% to 70% erythrocyte-bound and about 33% protein-bound.
• *Metabolism:* Insignificant.
• *Excretion:* About 70% to 95% of metolazone is excreted unchanged in urine. Half-life is about 14 hours in healthy subjects; it may be prolonged in patients with decreased creatinine clearance.

Contraindications and precautions

Contraindicated in patients with anuria, hepatic coma or precoma, or hypersensitivity to thiazides or other sulfonamide-derived drugs. Use cautiously in patients with impaired renal or hepatic function.

Interactions

Metolazone potentiates the hypotensive effects of most other *antihypertensive drugs*; this may be used to therapeutic advantage. Concurrent administration with *furosemide* may cause excessive volume and electrolyte depletion.

Metolazone may potentiate hyperglycemic, hypotensive, and hyperuricemic effects of *diazoxide*, and its hyperglycemic effect may increase *insulin* or *sulfonylurea* requirements in diabetic patients.

Drug may reduce renal clearance of *lithium*, elevating serum lithium levels, and may necessitate a 50% reduction in lithium dosage.

Metolazone turns urine slightly more alkaline and may decrease urinary excretion of some *amines*, such as *amphetamine* and *quinidine*; alkaline urine may also decrease therapeutic efficacy of *methenamine compounds* such as *methenamine mandelate*.

Cholestyramine and *colestipol* may bind metolazone, preventing its absorption; give drugs 1 hour apart.

Metolazone may cause electrolyte disturbances and increase risk of *digoxin* toxicity.

Effects on diagnostic tests

Drug therapy may alter serum electrolyte levels and may increase serum urate, glucose, cholesterol, and triglyceride levels. It also may interfere with tests for parathyroid function and should be discontinued before such tests.

Adverse reactions

CNS: *dizziness, headache, fatigue, vertigo, paresthesia, weakness, restlessness, drowsiness, anxiety, depression, nervousness, blurred vision.*
CV: volume depletion and dehydration, orthostatic hypotension, palpitations, vasculitis.
GI: anorexia, nausea, *pancreatitis,* epigastric distress, vomiting, abdominal pain, diarrhea, constipation, dry mouth.
GU: nocturia, polyuria, frequent urination, impotence.
Hematologic: ***aplastic anemia, agranulocytosis***, leukopenia.
Hepatic: jaundice, hepatitis.
Skin: dermatitis, photosensitivity, rash, purpura, pruritus, urticaria.

Other: hyperglycemia and glucose tolerance impairment; fluid and electrolyte imbalances, including hypokalemia, dilutional hyponatremia and hypochloremia, metabolic alkalosis, hypercalcemia; muscle cramps.

Overdose and treatment

Clinical signs of overdose include orthostatic hypotension, dizziness, electrolyte abnormalities, GI irritation and hypermotility, diuresis, and lethargy, which may progress to coma.

Treatment is mainly supportive; monitor and assist respiratory, CV, and renal function as indicated. Monitor fluid and electrolyte balance. Induce vomiting with ipecac in conscious patient; otherwise, use gastric lavage to avoid aspiration. Do not give cathartics; these promote additional loss of fluids and electrolytes.

☑ Special considerations

Besides those relevant to all *thiazide* and *thiazide-like diuretics,* consider the following recommendations.

- Drug is effective in patients with decreased renal function.
- Metolazone is used as an adjunct in furosemide-resistant edema.
- Drug has been used concomitantly with furosemide to induce diuresis in patients who did not respond to either diuretic alone.
- Rapid-acting form (Mykrox) is not interchangeable with other forms of metolazone. Dosage and uses vary.

Geriatric use

- Elderly and debilitated patients require close observation and may require reduced dosages. They are more sensitive to excess diuresis because of age-related changes in CV and renal function. Excess diuresis promotes orthostatic hypotension, dehydration, hypovolemia, hyponatremia, hypomagnesemia, and hypokalemia.

Pediatric use

- Safety and effectiveness have not been established.

Breast-feeding

- Drug may be distributed in breast milk; its safety and effectiveness in breast-feeding women have not been established.

metoprolol tartrate

Lopressor, Toprol XL

Pharmacologic classification: beta-adrenergic blocker
Therapeutic classification: antihypertensive, adjunctive treatment of acute MI
Pregnancy risk category C

How supplied

Available by prescription only
Tablets: 50 mg, 100 mg
Tablets (extended-release): 50 mg, 100 mg, 200 mg
Injection: 1 mg/ml in 5-ml ampules or prefilled syringes

Indications, route, and dosage

Mild to severe hypertension

Adults: Initially, 100 mg P.O. daily in single or divided doses; usual maintenance dosage is 100 to 450 mg daily. Alternatively, 50 to 100 mg P.O. extended-release tablets daily (maximum dose, 400 mg daily).

Early intervention in acute MI

Adults: Three 5-mg I.V. boluses q 2 minutes. Then, beginning 15 minutes after last dose, 50 mg P.O. q 6 hours for 48 hours. Maintenance dose, 100 mg P.O. b.i.d. or 25 to 50 mg P.O. q 6 hours. (Late treatment 100 mg P.O. b.i.d.)

Angina

Adults: 100 mg in two divided doses. Maintenance dose, 100 to 400 mg daily. Alternatively, 100 mg P.O. extended-release tablets daily (maximum dose, 400 mg daily).

Pharmacodynamics

Antihypertensive action: Metoprolol is classified as a cardioselective $beta_1$ antagonist; exact mechanism of metoprolol's antihypertensive effect is unknown. Drug may reduce blood pressure by blocking adrenergic receptors, thus decreasing cardiac output; by decreasing sympathetic outflow from the CNS; or by suppressing renin release.

Action after acute MI: The exact mechanism by which metoprolol decreases mortality after MI is unknown. In patients with MI, metoprolol reduces heart rate, systolic blood pressure, and cardiac output. Drug also appears to decrease the occurrence of ventricular fibrillation in these patients.

Pharmacokinetics

- *Absorption:* Orally administered metoprolol is absorbed rapidly and almost completely from GI tract; food enhances absorption. Peak plasma concentrations occur in 90 minutes. After I.V. administration, maximum beta blockade occurs in 20 minutes. Maximum therapeutic effect occurs after 1 week of treatment.
- *Distribution:* Distributed widely throughout the body; about 12% is protein-bound.
- *Metabolism:* Drug is metabolized in the liver.
- *Excretion:* About 95% of a given dose of metoprolol is excreted in urine within 72 hours.

Contraindications and precautions

Contraindicated in patients with hypersensitivity to drug or other beta blockers. Also contraindicated in patients with sinus bradycardia, heart block greater than first-degree, cardiogenic shock, or overt cardiac failure when used to treat hypertension or angina.

When used to treat MI, metoprolol also is contraindicated in patients with heart rate less than 45 beats/minute, second- or third-degree heart block, PR interval of 0.24 second or longer with first-degree heart block, systolic blood pressure less than 100 mm Hg, or moderate to severe heart failure.

Use cautiously in patients with impaired hepatic or respiratory function, diabetes, or heart failure.

Interactions
Metoprolol may potentiate antihypertensive effects of *diuretics* or other *antihypertensive agents.* Metoprolol may antagonize the beta-adrenergic effects of *sympathomimetic agents.*

Metoprolol may enhance bradycardia of *cardiac glycosides.*

Verapamil may decrease the bioavailability of metoprolol when administered with antiarrhythmic medications.

Effects on diagnostic tests
Metoprolol may elevate serum transaminase, alkaline phosphatase, LD, and uric acid levels.

Adverse reactions
CNS: *fatigue, dizziness,* depression.
CV: ***bradycardia,*** *hypotension,* ***heart failure.***
GI: nausea, diarrhea.
Respiratory: dyspnea, ***bronchospasm.***
Skin: rash.

Overdose and treatment
Clinical signs of overdose include severe hypotension, bradycardia, heart failure, and bronchospasm.

After acute ingestion, empty stomach by induced emesis or gastric lavage, and give activated charcoal to reduce absorption. Subsequent treatment is usually symptomatic and supportive.

☑ Special considerations
Besides those relevant to all *beta-adrenergic blockers,* consider the following recommendations.
- Metoprolol may be administered daily as a single dose or in divided doses. If a dose is missed, patient should take only the next scheduled dose.
- Administer drug with meals to enhance absorption.
- Reduce dosage in patients with impaired hepatic function.
- Avoid late-evening doses to minimize insomnia.
- Observe patient for signs of mental depression.

Geriatric use
- Elderly patients may require lower maintenance dosages of metoprolol because of delayed metabolism; they may also experience enhanced adverse effects. Use with caution.

Pediatric use
- Safety and efficacy in children have not been established. No dosage recommendation exists for children.

Breast-feeding
- Metoprolol is distributed into breast milk. An alternative feeding method is recommended during therapy.

metronidazole (systemic)
Apo-Metronidazole*, Flagyl, Metric-21, Novonidazol*, Protostat

metronidazole hydrochloride
Flagyl I.V., Flagyl I.V. RTU, Metro I.V

Pharmacologic classification: nitroimidazole
Therapeutic classification: antibacterial, antiprotozoal, amebicide
Pregnancy risk category B

How supplied
Available by prescription only
Tablets: 250 mg, 500 mg
Tablets (film-coated): 250 mg, 500 mg
Capsules: 375 mg
Powder for injection: 500-mg single-dose vials
Injection: 500 mg/100 ml ready to use

Indications, route, and dosage
Amebic hepatic abscess
Adults: 500 to 750 mg P.O. t.i.d. for 5 to 10 days.
Children: 35 to 50 mg/kg P.O. daily (in three doses) for 10 days.
Intestinal amebiasis
Adults: 750 mg P.O. t.i.d. for 5 to 10 days. Centers for Disease Control and Prevention recommends addition of iodoquinol 650 mg P.O. t.i.d. for 20 days.
◊ *Children:* 35 to 50 mg/kg daily (in three doses) for 5 to 10 days. Follow this therapy with oral iodoquinol.
Trichomoniasis
Adults (both men and women concurrently): 375 mg-capsule P.O. b.i.d. for 7 days, or 500-mg tablet P.O. b.i.d. for 7 days or a single dose of 2 g P.O. or divided into two doses given on same day.
◊ *Children:* 15 mg/kg daily (in three doses) for 7 to 10 days.
Refractory trichomoniasis
Adults (women): 500 mg P.O. b.i.d. for 7 days.
Bacterial infections caused by anaerobic microorganisms
Adults: Loading dose is 15 mg/kg I.V. infused over 1 hour (approximately 1 g for a 154-lb [70-kg] adult). Maintenance dose is 7.5 mg/kg I.V. or P.O. q 6 hours (approximately 500 mg for a 70-kg adult). First maintenance dose should be administered 6 hours after the loading dose. Maximum dosage should not exceed 4 g daily.
Children: 7.5 mg/kg I.V. q 6 hours.
◊ ***Giardiasis***
Adults: 250 mg P.O. t.i.d. for 5 days, or 2 g once daily for 3 days.
Children: 5 mg/kg P.O. t.i.d. for 5 days.
Prevention of postoperative infection in contaminated or potentially contaminated colorectal surgery
Adults: 15 mg/kg infused over 30 to 60 minutes and completed approximately 1 hour before surgery. Then 7.5 mg/kg infused over 30 to 60 minutes at 6 and 12 hours after initial dose.

◊ ***Bacterial vaginosis***
Adults: 500 mg P.O. b.i.d. for 7 days; or 2 g P.O. as a single dose.
◊ ***Pelvic inflammatory disease***
Adults: 500 mg P.O. b.i.d. for 14 days (given with 400 mg b.i.d. of ofloxacin).
◊ ***Clostridium difficile***
Adults: 750 mg to 2 g P.O. daily, in three to four divided doses for 7 to 14 days.
◊ ***Helicobacter pylori associated with peptic ulcer disease***
Adults: 250 to 500 mg P.O. t.i.d. (in combination with other medications).
Children: 15 to 20 mg/kg P.O. daily, divided in two doses for 4 weeks (in combination with other medications).

Pharmacodynamics
Bactericidal, amebicidal, and trichomonicidal action: The nitro group of metronidazole is reduced inside the infecting organism; this reduction product disrupts DNA and inhibits nucleic acid synthesis. Drug is active in intestinal and extraintestinal sites. It is active against most anaerobic bacteria and protozoa, including *Bacteroides fragilis, B. melaninogenicus, Fusobacterium, Veillonella, Clostridium, Peptococcus, Peptostreptococcus, Entamoeba histolytica, Trichomonas vaginalis, Giardia lamblia,* and *Balantidium coli.*

Pharmacokinetics
- *Absorption:* About 80% of an oral dose is absorbed, with peak serum concentrations occurring at about 1 hour; food delays the rate but not the extent of absorption.
- *Distribution:* Drug is distributed into most body tissues and fluids, including CSF, bone, bile, saliva, pleural and peritoneal fluids, vaginal secretions, seminal fluids, middle ear fluid, and hepatic and cerebral abscesses. CSF levels approach serum levels in patients with inflamed meninges; they reach about 50% of serum levels in patients with uninflamed meninges. Less than 20% of metronidazole is bound to plasma proteins. It readily crosses the placenta.
- *Metabolism:* Metabolized to an active 2-hydroxymethyl metabolite and also to other metabolites.
- *Excretion:* About 60% to 80% of dose is excreted as parent compound or its metabolites. About 20% of a metronidazole dose is excreted unchanged in urine; about 6% to 15% is excreted in feces. Drug's half-life is 6 to 8 hours in adults with normal renal function; its half-life may be prolonged in patients with impaired hepatic function.

Contraindications and precautions
Contraindicated in patients with hypersensitivity to drug or other nitroimidazole derivatives. Use cautiously in patients with history of blood dyscrasia or alcoholism, hepatic disease, retinal or visual field changes, or CNS disorders and in those receiving hepatotoxic drugs.

Interactions
Concomitant use of metronidazole with *oral anticoagulants* prolongs PT. Concomitant use with *alcohol* inhibits alcohol dehydrogenase activity, causing a disulfiram-like reaction (nausea, vomiting, headache, abdominal cramps, and flushing) in some patients; it is not recommended. Concomitant use with *disulfiram* may precipitate psychosis and confusion and should be avoided.

Concomitant use with *barbiturates* and *phenytoin* may diminish the antimicrobial effectiveness of metronidazole by increasing its metabolism and may require higher doses of metronidazole.

Concomitant use with *cimetidine* may decrease the clearance of metronidazole, thereby increasing its potential for causing adverse effects.

Metronidazole may interact with *astemizole* resulting in serious CV effects. Use with *lithium* may increase lithium levels.

Effects on diagnostic tests
Drug may interfere with the chemical analyses of aminotransferases and triglyceride, leading to falsely decreased values. Rarely, it has been reported to flatten the T waves on ECGs.

Metronidazole may interfere with AST, ALT, LD, and glucose levels.

Adverse reactions
CNS: vertigo, headache, ataxia, dizziness, syncope, incoordination, confusion, irritability, depression, weakness, insomnia, ***seizures***, peripheral neuropathy.
CV: ECG change (flattened T wave), edema (with I.V. RTU preparation).
GI: abdominal cramping, stomatitis, epigastric distress, nausea, vomiting, anorexia, diarrhea, constipation, proctitis, dry mouth.
GU: darkened urine, polyuria, dysuria, cystitis, decreased libido, dyspareunia, dryness of vagina and vulva, vaginal candidiasis.
Hematologic: ***transient leukopenia, neutropenia.***
Skin: flushing, rash.
Other: overgrowth of nonsusceptible organisms, especially *Candida* (glossitis, furry tongue); metallic taste; fever; thrombophlebitis (after I.V. infusion); fleeting joint pain, sometimes resembling serum sickness.

Overdose and treatment
Clinical signs of overdose include nausea, vomiting, ataxia, seizures, and peripheral neuropathy.

There is no known antidote for metronidazole; treatment is supportive. If patient does not vomit spontaneously, induced emesis or gastric lavage is indicated for an oral overdose; activated charcoal and a cathartic may be used. Diazepam or phenytoin may be used to control seizures.

☑ Special considerations
- Trichomoniasis should be confirmed by wet smear and amebiasis by culture before giving drug.
- If indicated during pregnancy for trichomoniasis, the 7-day regimen is preferred over the single-dose regimen. Treatment with metronidazole should be avoided during the first trimester.
- I.V. form should be administered by slow infusion only; if used with a primary I.V. fluid system, dis-

continue the primary fluid during the infusion; do not give by I.V. push.

- Monitor patient on I.V. metronidazole for candidiasis.
- When treating amebiasis, monitor number and character of stools; send fecal specimens to laboratory promptly; infestation is detectable only in warm specimens. Repeat fecal examinations at 3-month intervals to ensure elimination of amebae.
- When preparing powder for injection, follow manufacturer's instructions carefully; use solution prepared from powder within 24 hours. I.V. solutions must be prepared in three steps: reconstitution with 4.4 ml of 0.9% NaCl solution injection (with or without bacteriostatic water); dilution with lactated Ringer's injection, D_5W, or 0.9% NaCl solution; and neutralization with sodium bicarbonate, 5 mEq per 500 mg metronidazole.

Patient education

- Inform patient that drug may cause metallic taste and discolored (red-brown) urine.
- Tell patient to take tablets with meals to minimize GI distress and that tablets may be crushed to facilitate swallowing.
- Counsel patient on need for medical follow-up after discharge.
- Advise patient to report adverse effects.
- Tell patient to avoid alcohol and alcohol-containing medications during therapy and for at least 48 hours after the last dose to prevent disulfiram-like reaction.

Amebiasis patients:

- Explain to patient that follow-up examinations of stool specimens are necessary for 3 months after treatment is discontinued, to ensure elimination of amebae.
- To help prevent reinfection, instruct patient and family members in proper hygiene, including disposal of feces and hand washing after defecation and before handling, preparing, or eating food, and about the risks of eating raw food and the control of contamination by flies.
- Encourage other household members and suspected contacts to be tested and, if necessary, treated.

Trichomoniasis patients:

- Teach correct personal hygiene, including perineal care.
- Explain that asymptomatic sexual partners of patients being treated for trichomoniasis should be treated simultaneously to prevent reinfection; patient should refrain from intercourse during therapy or have partner use condom.

Pediatric use

- Neonates may eliminate drug more slowly than older infants and children.

Breast-feeding

- Patient should discontinue breast-feeding while taking drug.

metronidazole (topical)

MetroGel, MetroGel-Vaginal, MetroCream, Noritate

Pharmacologic classification: nitroimidazole

Therapeutic classification: antiprotozoal, antibacterial

Pregnancy risk category B

How supplied

Available by prescription only
Topical gel: 0.75%
Topical cream: 0.75%, 1%
Vaginal gel: 0.75%

Indications, route, and dosage

Topical treatment of acne rosacea, ◊ pressure ulcer, inflammatory papules or pustules

Adults: Apply a thin film b.i.d. to affected area during the morning and evening (once daily for Noritate). Significant results should be seen within 3 weeks and continue for first 9 weeks of therapy.

Topical treatment of bacterial vaginosis

Adults: One applicator b.i.d., vaginally, for 5 days.

Pharmacodynamics

Anti-inflammatory action: Although its exact mechanism of action is unknown, topical metronidazole probably exerts an anti-inflammatory effect through its antibacterial and antiprotozoal actions.

Pharmacokinetics

- *Absorption:* Under normal conditions, serum levels of metronidazole after topical administration are negligible; 20% to 25% is absorbed vaginally with peak serum concentrations in 6 to 12 hours.
- *Distribution:* Drug is less than 20% bound to plasma proteins.
- *Metabolism:* Unknown.
- *Excretion:* Unknown after topical or intravaginal application.

Contraindications and precautions

Contraindicated in patients hypersensitive to drug or its ingredients (such as parabens) and other nitroimidazole derivatives. Use cautiously in patients with history of blood dyscrasia. Use vaginal form cautiously in patients with history of CNS disease because risk of seizures or peripheral neuropathy exists.

Interactions

Concomitant use with *oral anticoagulants* may potentiate the anticoagulant effect. Monitor patient for potential adverse effects.

Effects on diagnostic tests

None reported.

Adverse reactions

CNS: dizziness, light-headedness, headache (with vaginal form).
EENT: lacrimation (if topical gel is applied around the eyes).

GI: cramps, pain, nausea, diarrhea, constipation, metallic or bad taste in mouth (with vaginal form).
GU: *cervicitis, vaginitis,* urinary frequency (with vaginal form).
Skin: rash, *transient redness, dryness, mild burning, stinging* (with vaginal form).
Other: overgrowth of nonsusceptible organisms, decreased appetite (with vaginal form).

Overdose and treatment
None reported. Overdose after topical application is unlikely.

☑ Special considerations
- Topical metronidazole therapy has not been associated with the adverse reactions observed with parenteral or oral metronidazole therapy (including disulfiram-like reaction following alcohol ingestion). However, some of the drug can be absorbed following topical use. Limited clinical experience has not shown any of these adverse effects.

Patient education
- Advise patient to cleanse area thoroughly before applying the drug. Patient may use cosmetics after applying the drug.
- Instruct patient to avoid use of drug on eyelids and to apply it cautiously if drug must be used around the eyes.
- If local reactions occur, advise patient to apply drug less frequently or to discontinue use and call for specific instructions.

Pediatric use
- Safety has not been established.

Breast-feeding
- Drug is excreted in breast milk. A decision should be made whether to discontinue drug or breast-feeding, after assessing the importance of drug to mother.

mexiletine hydrochloride
Mexitil

Pharmacologic classification: lidocaine analogue, sodium channel antagonist
Therapeutic classification: ventricular antiarrhythmic
Pregnancy risk category C

How supplied
Available by prescription only
Capsules: 150 mg, 200 mg, 250 mg

Indications, route, and dosage
Life-threatening documented ventricular arrhythmias, including ventricular tachycardia
Adults: 200 mg P.O. q 8 hours. May increase or decrease dose in increments of 50 to 100 mg q 8 hours if satisfactory control is not obtained. Alternatively, give a loading dose of 400 mg with maintenance dose of 200 mg P.O. q 8 hours. Some patients may respond well to 450 mg q 12 hours. Maximum daily dose should not exceed 1,200 mg.

◊ ***Diabetic neuropathy***
Adults: 150 mg daily for 3 days; then, 300 mg daily for 3 days followed by 10 mg/kg daily.

Pharmacodynamics
Antiarrhythmic action: Mexiletine is structurally similar to lidocaine and exerts similar electrophysiologic and hemodynamic effects. A class IB antiarrhythmic, it suppresses automaticity and shortens the effective refractory period and action potential duration of His-Purkinje fibers and suppresses spontaneous ventricular depolarization during diastole. At therapeutic serum levels, the drug does not affect conductive atrial tissue or AV conduction.

Unlike quinidine and procainamide, mexiletine does not significantly alter hemodynamics when given in usual doses. Its effects on the conduction system inhibit reentry mechanisms and halt ventricular arrhythmias. Drug does not have a significant negative inotropic effect.

Pharmacokinetics
- *Absorption:* About 90% of drug is absorbed from the GI tract; peak serum levels occur in 2 to 3 hours. Absorption rate decreases with conditions that speed gastric emptying.
- *Distribution:* Widely distributed throughout the body. About 50% to 60% of circulating drug is bound to plasma proteins. Usual therapeutic drug level is 0.5 to 2 mcg/ml. Although toxicity may occur within this range, levels above 2 mcg/ml are considered toxic and are associated with an increased frequency of adverse CNS effects, warranting dosage reduction.
- *Metabolism:* Metabolized in the liver to relatively inactive metabolites. Less than 10% of a parenteral dose escapes metabolism and reaches the kidneys unchanged. Metabolism is affected by hepatic blood flow, which may be reduced in patients who are recovering from MI and in those with heart failure. Liver disease also limits metabolism.
- *Excretion:* In healthy patients, drug's half-life is 10 to 12 hours. Elimination half-life may be prolonged in patients with heart failure or liver disease. Urinary excretion increases with urine acidification and slows with urine alkalinization.

Contraindications and precautions
Contraindicated in patients with cardiogenic shock or preexisting second- or third-degree AV block in the absence of an artificial pacemaker. Use cautiously in patients with hypotension, heart failure, first-degree heart block, ventricular pacemaker, preexisting sinus node dysfunction, or seizure disorders.

Interactions
Concomitant use of mexiletine with *drugs that alter gastric emptying time* (such as *antacids containing aluminum-magnesium hydroxide, atropine* and *narcotics*) may delay mexiletine absorption; concomitant use with *metoclopramide* may increase absorption.

Concomitant use with *drugs that alter hepatic enzyme function* (such as *phenobarbital, phenytoin, rifampin*) may induce hepatic metabolism of mexiletine and thus reduce serum drug levels. Concomitant use with *cimetidine* may decrease mexiletine metabolism, resulting in increased serum levels. Concomitant use with *drugs that acidify the urine* (such as *ammonium chloride*) enhances mexiletine excretion; concomitant use with *drugs that alkalinize urine* (such as *high-dose antacids, carbonic anhydrase inhibitors, sodium bicarbonate*) decreases mexiletine excretion.

When used with *theophylline*, mexiletine may increase serum theophylline levels.

Effects on diagnostic tests
Liver function test results may be transiently altered during mexiletine therapy.

Adverse reactions
CNS: *tremor, dizziness, blurred vision, diplopia, confusion*, light-headedness, incoordination, changes in sleep habits, paresthesia, weakness, fatigue, speech difficulties, tinnitus, depression, *nervousness, headache.*
CV: ***new or worsened arrhythmias,*** palpitations, chest pain, nonspecific edema, angina.
GI: *nausea, vomiting, upper GI distress, heartburn, diarrhea, constipation, dry mouth, changes in appetite, abdominal pain.*
Skin: rash.

Overdose and treatment
Clinical effects of overdose are primarily extensions of adverse CNS effects. Seizures are the most serious effect.

Treatment usually involves symptomatic and supportive measures. In acute overdose, emesis induction or gastric lavage should be performed. Urine acidification may accelerate drug elimination. If patient has bradycardia and hypotension, atropine may be given.

☑ Special considerations
- Dosage should be administered with meals, if possible.
- Because of proarrhythmic effects, drug is generally not recommended for non life-threatening arrhythmias.
- Avoid administering drug within 1 hour of antacids containing aluminum-magnesium hydroxide.
- When changing from lidocaine to mexiletine, stop infusion when first mexiletine dose is given. Keep infusion line open, however, until arrhythmia appears to be satisfactorily controlled.
- Patients who are not controlled by dosing every 8 hours may respond to dosing every 6 hours.
- Many patients who respond well to mexiletine (300 mg or less every 8 hours) can be maintained on an every 12-hour schedule. The same total daily dose is divided into twice-daily doses, which improves patient compliance.
- Monitor blood pressure and heart rate and rhythm for significant change.
- Tremor (usually a fine hand tremor) is commonly evident in patients taking higher doses of mexiletine.

Patient education
- Tell patient to take drug with food to reduce risk of nausea.
- Instruct patient to report if the following occur: unusual bleeding or bruising, signs of infection (such as fever, sore throat, stomatitis, or chills), or fatigue.

Geriatric use
- Most elderly patients require reduced dosages, because of reduced hepatic blood flow and therefore, decreased metabolism. Elderly patients also may be more susceptible to CNS adverse effects.

Breast-feeding
- Drug is excreted in breast milk. Alternative feeding method should be used during therapy.

mezlocillin sodium
Mezlin

Pharmacologic classification: extended-spectrum penicillin, acyclaminopenicillin
Therapeutic classification: antibiotic
Pregnancy risk category B

How supplied
Available by prescription only
Injection: 1 g, 2 g, 3 g, 4 g
Infusion: 2 g, 3 g, 4 g
Pharmacy bulk package: 20 g

Indications, route, and dosage
Infections caused by susceptible organisms
Adults: 200 to 300 mg/kg I.V. or I.M. daily given in four to six divided doses. Usual dose is 3 g q 4 hours or 4 g q 6 hours. For serious infections, up to 24 g daily may be administered.
Children under age 12: 200 to 300 mg/kg/day I.M. or I.V. in divided doses q 4 to 6 hours.
✦ ***Dosage adjustment.*** In adult patients with renal failure with creatinine clearance of 10 to 30 ml/minute, give 3 g q 6 to 8 hours for life-threatening or serious infection. For urinary tract infection (UTI), give 1.5 g q 6 to 8 hours. If creatinine clearance is below 10 ml/minute, give 2 g q 6 to 8 hours for life-threatening or serious infection. For UTI, give 1.5 g q 8 hours.

Patients on hemodialysis should be given 3 to 4 g after each dialysis session, then q 12 hours. Patients on peritoneal dialysis may receive 3 g q 12 hours.

Pharmacodynamics
Antibiotic action: Mezlocillin is bactericidal; it adheres to bacterial penicillin-binding proteins, thereby inhibiting bacterial cell wall synthesis.

Extended-spectrum penicillins are more resistant to inactivation by certain beta-lactamases, especially those produced by gram-negative organisms, but are still liable to inactivation by certain others.

Drug's spectrum of activity includes many gram-negative aerobic and anaerobic bacilli, many gram-positive and gram-negative aerobic cocci, and some gram-positive aerobic and anaerobic bacilli, but a large number of these organisms are resistant to mezlocillin. Mezlocillin may be effective against some strains of carbenicillin-resistant and ticarcillin-resistant gram-negative bacilli. Mezlocillin should not be used as sole therapy because of the rapid development of resistance. Some clinicians feel that there is no evidence that it has any advantages over ticarcillin or carbenicillin, at least with respect to cure rates. Drug is less active against *Pseudomonas aeruginosa* than other members of this class, such as piperacillin.

Pharmacokinetics

• *Absorption:* After an I.M. dose, peak plasma concentrations occur at ¾ to 1½ hours.
• *Distribution:* Drug is distributed widely. It penetrates minimally into CSF with uninflamed meninges, crosses the placenta, and is 16% to 42% protein-bound.
• *Metabolism:* Partially metabolized; about 15% of a dose is metabolized to inactive metabolites.
• *Excretion:* Excreted primarily (39% to 72%) in urine by glomerular filtration and renal tubular secretion; up to 30% of a dose is excreted in bile, and some is excreted in breast milk. Elimination half-life in adults is ¾ to 1½ hours; in extensive renal impairment, half-life is extended to 2 to 14 hours. Mezlocillin is removed by hemodialysis but not by peritoneal dialysis.

Contraindications and precautions

Contraindicated in patients with hypersensitivity to drug or other penicillins. Use cautiously in patients with bleeding tendencies, uremia, hypokalemia, or allergy to cephalosporins.

Interactions

Concomitant use with *aminoglycoside antibiotics* results in a synergistic bactericidal effect against *Pseudomonas aeruginosa, Escherichia coli, Klebsiella, Citrobacter, Enterobacter, Serratia,* and *Proteus mirabilis.* However, the drugs are physically and chemically incompatible and are inactivated when mixed or given together.

Concomitant use of mezlocillin (and other extended-spectrum penicillins) with *clavulanic acid* also produces a synergistic bactericidal effect against certain beta-lactamase–producing bacteria.

Probenecid blocks tubular secretion of penicillins, raising their serum concentrations.

Large doses of penicillins may interfere with renal tubular secretion of *methotrexate,* thus delaying elimination and elevating serum concentrations of methotrexate.

Mezlocillin may prolong neuromuscular blockade in *vecuronium bromide.*

Effects on diagnostic tests

Drug alters tests for urinary or serum proteins; it interferes with turbidimetric methods that use sulfosalicylic acid, trichloroacetic acid, acetic acid, or nitric acid.

Mezlocillin does not interfere with tests using bromo-phenol blue (Albustix, Albutest, MultiStix).

Positive Coombs' tests have been reported in patients taking carbenicillin disodium.

Mezlocillin may prolong PTs; it may also cause transient elevations in liver function studies and transient reductions in RBC, WBC, and platelet counts.

Adverse reactions

CNS: neuromuscular irritability, ***seizures.***
GI: nausea, diarrhea, vomiting, abnormal taste sensation, pseudomembranous colitis.
GU: interstitial nephritis.
Hematologic: ***bleeding*** (with high doses), ***neutropenia, thrombocytopenia,*** eosinophilia, ***leukopenia, hemolytic anemia.***
Other: hypersensitivity reactions (***anaphylaxis,*** edema, fever, chills, rash, pruritus, urticaria), overgrowth of nonsusceptible organisms, *hypokalemia, pain at injection site, vein irritation, phlebitis.*

Overdose and treatment

Clinical signs of overdose include neuromuscular sensitivity or seizures; a 4- to 6-hour hemodialysis will remove 20% to 30% of mezlocillin.

☑ Special considerations

Beside those relevant to all *penicillins,* consider the following recommendations.
• Mezlocillin may be more suitable than carbenicillin or ticarcillin for patients on salt-free diets; mezlocillin contains only 1.85 mEq of sodium per gram.
• Monitor serum potassium level and liver function studies.
• Monitor patient with high serum concentrations for seizures.
• Drug is almost always used with another antibiotic, such as an aminoglycoside, in life-threatening infections.
• Inject I.M. dose slowly over 12 to 15 seconds to minimize pain. Do not exceed 2 g per site.
• If precipitate forms during refrigerated storage, warm to 98.6° F (37° C) in warm water bath and shake well. Solution should be clear.
• Because drug is partially dialyzable, dosage may need adjustment in patients undergoing hemodialysis.

Geriatric use

• Half-life may be prolonged in elderly patients because of impaired renal function.

Breast-feeding

• Drug occurs in breast milk; safe use in breast-feeding women has not been established. Alternative feeding method is recommended during therapy.

miconazole

Monistat I.V.

miconazole nitrate

Femizol-M, Micatin, Monistat 3, Monistat 7, Monistat-Derm

Pharmacologic classification: imidazole derivative
Therapeutic classification: antifungal
Pregnancy risk category B (C for I.V. form)

How supplied

Available by prescription only
Injection: 10 mg/ml
Vaginal suppositories: 200 mg
Vaginal cream: 2%
Cream: 2%

Available without a prescription
Cream: 2%
Powder: 2%
Spray: 2%
Vaginal cream: 2%
Vaginal suppositories: 100 mg, 200 mg

Indications, route, and dosage

Systemic fungal infections caused by susceptible organisms

Adults: 200 to 3,600 mg daily. I.V. dosages may vary with diagnosis and with infective agent. May divide daily dosage over three infusions, 200 to 1,200 mg per infusion. Dilute in at least 200 ml of 0.9% NaCl solution. Repeated courses may be needed because of relapse or reinfection.

Children over age 1: 20 to 40 mg/kg daily. Maximum dose per infusion, 15 mg/kg.

Children under age 1: 15 to 30 mg/kg daily given in three or four divided doses.

Bladder instillation: 200 mg diluted and instilled into the bladder b.i.d. to q.i.d. or by continuous irrigation.

Fungal meningitis

Adults: 20 mg intrathecally q 1 to 2 days if S.C. ventricular reservoir is used, or q 3 to 7 days if a reservoir is not used, as an adjunct to I.V. administration.

Cutaneous or mucocutaneous fungal infections caused by susceptible organisms

Topical use

Adults: Cover affected areas b.i.d. for 2 to 4 weeks.

Vaginal use

Adults: Insert 200-mg suppository h.s. for 3 days, or 100-mg suppository or 1 applicatorful of vaginal cream h.s. for 7 days.

Pulmonary coccidioidomycosis

Adults: Give nebulized form, 20 mg q.i.d. for 17 days.

Pharmacodynamics

Antifungal action: Miconazole is both fungistatic and fungicidal, depending on drug concentration, in *Coccidioides immitis, Candida albicans, Cryptococcus neoformans, Histoplasma capsulatum, Candida tropicalis, Candida parapsilosis, Paracoccidioides brasiliensis, Sporothrix schenckii, Aspergillus flavus, A. ustus, Microsporum canis, Curvularia, Pseudallescheria boydii,* dermatophytes, and some gram-positive bacteria. Miconazole causes thickening of the fungal cell wall, altering membrane permeability; it also may kill the cell by interference with peroxisomal enzymes, causing accumulation of peroxide within the cell wall. It attacks virtually all pathogenic fungi.

Drug is considered an alternative to amphotericin B to treat coccidiomycosis, but ketoconazole is preferred. Its clinical effectiveness in blastomycosis and histoplasmosis is highly variable. Its broad spectrum of activity makes it useful in treating superficial cutaneous infections and vaginal candidal infections.

Pharmacokinetics

- *Absorption:* About 50% of an oral miconazole dose is absorbed; however, no oral dosage form is currently available. A small amount of drug is systemically absorbed after vaginal administration.
- *Distribution:* Drug penetrates well into inflamed joints, vitreous humor, and the peritoneal cavity. Distribution into sputum and saliva is poor, and CSF penetration is unpredictable. Over 90% is bound to plasma proteins.
- *Metabolism:* Miconazole is metabolized in the liver, predominantly to inactive metabolites.
- *Excretion:* Miconazole elimination is triphasic; terminal half-life is about 24 hours. Between 10% and 14% of an oral dose is excreted in urine; 50%, in feces. Up to 1% of a vaginal dose is excreted in urine; 14% to 22% of an I.V. dose is excreted in urine. It is unknown whether it is excreted in breast milk.

Contraindications and precautions

Topical form contraindicated in patients with hypersensitivity to drug. Use cautiously in patients with hepatic insufficiency and during initial I.V. administration because of risk of anaphylaxis.

Interactions

Miconazole enhances the anticoagulant effect of *warfarin.* It may antagonize the effects of *amphotericin B.* Drug may increase phenytoin levels.

Effects on diagnostic tests

Miconazole may cause a transient decrease in hematocrit levels and an increase or decrease in platelet counts; it frequently causes erythrocyte aggregation. Miconazole also may cause hyponatremia, hyperlipidemia, and hypertriglyceridemia; abnormalities in lipoprotein and immunoelectrophoretic patterns are from the polyoxyl 35 castor oil vehicle.

Adverse reactions

CNS: dizziness, drowsiness (with injected form); headache (with topical administration).
GI: *nausea, vomiting, diarrhea (with injected form).*
GU: vulvovaginal burning, pruritus, or irritation with vaginal cream; pelvic cramps (with topical administration).
Hematologic: transient decrease in hematocrit, ***thrombocytopenia*** (with injected form).
Skin: *pruritic rash* (with injected form); irritation, burning, maceration, allergic contact dermatitis (with topical administration).
Other: ***anaphylactoid reactions***, fever, chills, transient decrease in serum sodium, ***phlebitis at injection site*** (with injected form).

Overdose and treatment

Symptoms of overdose include GI complaints and altered mental status. Treatment after recent oral ingestion (within 4 hours) includes emesis or lavage followed by activated charcoal and an osmotic cathartic; subsequent care is supportive.

☑ Special considerations

- Identify causative organism by culture and sensitivity studies before I.V. or topical therapy is started.
- Initial I.V. therapy requires direct medical supervision; cardiorespiratory arrest has been reported with first dose.
- Check for possible hypersensitivity to drug before I.V. infusion; be prepared for anaphylaxis.
- Infuse over 30 to 60 minutes; rapid injection of undiluted miconazole may cause arrhythmias.
- Premedication with an antiemetic may lessen nausea and vomiting.
- Monitor CBC and electrolyte, triglyceride, and cholesterol levels before and frequently throughout therapy to detect adverse effects.
- Pruritic rash may persist for weeks after drug is discontinued; it may be controlled with oral or I.V. diphenhydramine.
- Clean affected area before applying cream. After application, massage area gently until cream disappears.
- Continue topical therapy for at least 1 month; improvement should begin in 1 to 2 weeks. If no improvement occurs by 4 weeks, reevaluate diagnosis.
- Insert vaginal applicator high into vagina.
- Patients with fungal meningitis require I.V. and intrathecal therapy.

Patient education

- Teach patient the symptoms of fungal infection, and explain treatment rationale.
- Encourage patient to adhere to prescribed regimen and follow-up visits and to report adverse effects.
- Teach patient correct procedure for intravaginal or topical applications.
- To prevent vaginal reinfection, teach correct perineal hygiene and recommend that patient abstain from sexual intercourse during therapy.

Pediatric use

- Safe use in children under age 1 has not been established.

Breast-feeding

- Safety has not been established.

midazolam hydrochloride

Versed

Pharmacologic classification: benzodiazepine
Therapeutic classification: preoperative sedative, agent for conscious sedation, adjunct for induction of general anesthesia, amnesic agent
Controlled substance schedule IV
Pregnancy risk category D

How supplied

Available by prescription only
Injection: 1 mg/ml in 2-ml, 5-ml, and 10-ml vials; 5 mg/ml in 1-ml, 2-ml, 5-ml, and 10-ml vials; 5 mg/ml in 2-ml disposable syringe

Indications, route, and dosage

Preoperative sedation (to induce sleepiness or drowsiness and relieve apprehension)
Adults under age 60: 0.07 to 0.08 mg/kg I.M. approximately 1 hour before surgery. May be administered with atropine or scopolamine and reduced doses of narcotics.
♦ ***Dosage adjustment.*** Reduce dosage in patients over age 60, those with COPD, those considered to be high-risk surgical patients and in those who have received concomitant narcotics or other depressants.

Conscious sedation
Adults under age 60: Initially, 1 to 2.5 mg I.V. administered over at least 2 minutes; repeat in 2 minutes, if needed, in small increments of initial dose over at least 2 minutes to achieve desired effect. Total dose up to 5 mg may be used. Additional doses to maintain desired level of sedation may be given by slow titration in increments of 25% of dose used to reach the sedation endpoint.
Adults age 60 and over: 1.5 mg or less over at least 2 minutes. If additional titration is needed, give at a rate not exceeding 1 mg over 2 minutes. Total doses exceeding 3.5 mg are not usually necessary.

Induction of general anesthesia
Unpremedicated adults under age 55: 0.3 to 0.35 mg/kg I.V. over 20 to 30 seconds if patient has not received preanesthesia medication, or 0.2 to 0.25 mg/kg I.V. over 20 to 30 seconds if patient has received preanesthesia medication. Additional increments of 25% of the initial dose may be needed to complete induction.
Unpremedicated adults age 55 and over: Initially, 0.3 mg/kg. For debilitated patients, initial dose is 0.2 to 0.25 mg/kg. For premedicated patients, 0.15 mg/kg may be sufficient.

Continuous infusion for sedation of intubated and mechanically ventilated patients as a component of anesthesia or during treatment in the critical care setting
Adults: If a loading dose is necessary to rapidly initiate sedation, give 0.01 to 0.05 mg/kg slowly or infused over several minutes, with dose repeated at 10- to 15-minute intervals until adequate sedation is achieved. For maintenance of sedation, usual infusion rate is 0.02 to 0.10 mg/kg/hour (1 to 7 mg/hour). Infusion rate should be titrated to the desired amount of sedation. Drug can be titrated up or down by 25% to 50% of the initial infusion rate to achieve optimal sedation without oversedation.
Children: After a loading dose of 0.05 to 0.2 mg/kg over 2 to 3 minutes in intubated patients only, an infusion may be initiated at 0.06 to 0.12 mg/kg/ hour (1 to 2 mcg/kg/minute). Dose may be titrated up or down by 25% of the initial or subsequent infusion rate to obtain optimal sedation.
Neonates: Use only on intubated neonates. No loading dose is used in neonates. Neonates less

than 32 weeks receive infusion rates of 0.03 mg/kg/hour (0.5 mcg/kg/minute). In neonates older than 32 weeks, infusion rates are 0.06 mg/kg/hour (1 mcg/kg/minute). Infusion may be run more rapidly in the first few hours to obtain a therapeutic blood level. Rate of infusion should be frequently and carefully reassessed to administer the lowest possible amount of drug.

Pharmacodynamics

Sedative and anesthetic action: Although exact mechanism is unknown, midazolam, like other benzodiazepines, is thought to facilitate the action of gamma-aminobutyric acid (GABA) to provide a short-acting CNS depressant action.

Amnesic action: Mechanism of action by which midazolam causes amnesia is not known.

Pharmacokinetics

- *Absorption:* Absorption after I.M. administration appears to be 80% to 100%; peak serum concentrations occur in 45 minutes and are about one-half of those after I.V. administration. Sedation begins within 15 minutes after an I.M. dose and within 2 to 5 minutes after I.V. injection. After I.V. administration, induction of anesthesia occurs in 1½ to 2½ minutes.
- *Distribution:* Drug has a large volume of distribution and is approximately 97% protein-bound. Drug crosses the placenta and enters fetal circulation.
- *Metabolism:* Midazolam is metabolized in the liver.
- *Excretion:* Metabolites of midazolam are excreted in urine. Half-life of drug is 1.2 to 12.3 hours. Duration of sedation is usually 1 to 4 hours.

Contraindications and precautions

Contraindicated in patients with hypersensitivity to drug or acute angle-closure glaucoma and in those experiencing shock, coma, or acute alcohol intoxication. Use cautiously in patients with uncompensated acute illnesses and in elderly or debilitated patients.

Interactions

Midazolam may add to or potentiate the effects of *alcohol, antidepressants, antihistamines, barbiturates, narcotics, tranquilizers,* and other *CNS and respiratory depressants. Erythromycin* may decrease plasma clearance of midazolam.

Droperidol, fentanyl, and *narcotics*, used as preoperative medications, potentiate the hypnotic effect of midazolam. Midazolam may decrease the needed dose of *inhaled anesthetics* by depressing respiratory drive. *Isoniazid* may decrease the metabolism of midazolam.

Effects on diagnostic tests

None reported.

Adverse reactions

CNS: headache, oversedation, drowsiness, amnesia.
CV: variations in blood pressure (hypotension) and pulse rate, ***cardiac arrest.***
GI: *nausea,* vomiting, *hiccups.*
Respiratory: *decreased respiratory rate,* ***apnea, respiratory arrest.***
Other: *pain, tenderness (at injection site).*

Overdose and treatment

Clinical manifestations of overdose include confusion, stupor, coma, respiratory depression, and hypotension.

Treatment is supportive. Maintain patent airway, and ensure adequate ventilation with mechanical support if necessary. Monitor vital signs. Use I.V. fluids or ephedrine to treat hypotension. Flumazenil, a specific benzodiazepine-receptor antagonist, is indicated for complete or partial reversal of the sedative effects.

☑ Special considerations

Besides those relevant to all *benzodiazepines,* consider the following recommendations.

- Individualize dosage; use smallest effective dose possible. Use with extreme caution and reduced dosage in elderly and debilitated patients.
- Medical personnel who administer midazolam should be familiar with airway management. Close monitoring of cardiopulmonary function is required. Continuously monitor patients who have received midazolam to detect potentially life-threatening respiratory depression.
- Solutions of D_5W, 0.9% NaCl solution, and lactated Ringer's solution are compatible with midazolam.
- Before I.V. administration, ensure the immediate availability of oxygen and resuscitative equipment. Apnea and death have been reported with rapid I.V. administration. Avoid intra-arterial injection because the hazards of this route are unknown. Avoid extravasation. Administer I.V. dose slowly to prevent respiratory depression.
- Know that there is a potential for adverse effects, (hypotension, metabolic acidosis, kernicterus) related to neonate metabolism of benzyl alcohol. Take into account the amount of benzyl alcohol when giving high doses of drugs (including midazolam) containing the preservative.
- Administer I.M. dose deep into a large muscle mass to prevent tissue injury.
- Do not use solution that is discolored or contains a precipitate.
- Hypotension occurs more frequently in patients premedicated with narcotics. Monitor vital signs closely.
- Laryngospasm and bronchospasm may occur rarely; countermeasures should be available.
- Midazolam can be mixed in the same syringe with morphine, meperidine, atropine, and scopolamine.

Patient education

- Advise patient to postpone tasks that require mental alertness or physical coordination until the drug's effects have worn off.
- As necessary, instruct patient in safety measures, such as supervised walking and gradual position changes, to prevent injury.
- Advise patient to call for instructions before taking OTC drugs.

Geriatric use
• Elderly or debilitated patients, especially those with COPD, are at significantly increased risk for respiratory depression and hypotension. Lower doses are indicated. Use with caution.

Pediatric use
• Safety and efficacy have not been established in children.

Breast-feeding
• It is unknown if drug passes into breast milk; it should be used with caution in breast-feeding women.

milrinone lactate
Primacor

Pharmacologic classification: bipyridine phosphodiesterase inhibitor
Therapeutic classification: inotropic vasodilator
Pregnancy risk category C

How supplied
Available by prescription only
Solution: 1 mg/ml in 10-ml and 20-ml vials
Cartridge: 5 ml

Indications, route, and dosage
Short-term I.V. therapy for heart failure
Adults: Initial loading dose of 50 mcg/kg I.V. over 10 minutes, followed by continuous infusion/maintenance dose of 0.375 to 0.75 mcg/kg/minute. Adjust infusion dose based on hemodynamic and clinical response.
✦ ***Dosage adjustment.*** Refer to chart for dosing instructions for patients with renal impairment.

Creatinine clearance (ml/min/1.73 m²)	Infusion rate (mcg/kg/min)
5	0.20
10	0.23
20	0.28
30	0.33
40	0.38
50	0.43

Note: If hypotension occurs, administration of milrinone should be reduced or temporarily discontinued until patient's condition stabilizes.

Pharmacodynamics
Inotropic/vasodilator action: Milrinone is a selective inhibitor of peak III cAMP phosphodiesterase isozyme in cardiac and vascular muscle. This inhibitory action is consistent with cAMP-mediated increases in intracellular ionized calcium and contractile force in cardiac muscle, as well as with cAMP-dependent contractile protein phosphorylation and relaxation in vascular muscle. In addition to increasing myocardial contractility, milrinone improves diastolic function, shown by improvements in left ventricular diastolic relaxation.

Pharmacokinetics
• *Absorption:* Not applicable.
• *Distribution:* Drug is approximately 70% bound to human plasma protein.
• *Metabolism:* About 12% of dose is metabolized to a glucuronide metabolite.
• *Excretion:* After I.V. administration, about 90% of drug is excreted unchanged in the urine within 8 hours.

Contraindications and precautions
Contraindicated in patients with hypersensitivity to drug, severe aortic or pulmonic valvular disease in place of surgical correction, or during the acute phase of an MI. Use cautiously in patients with atrial fibrillation or flutter.

Interactions
None reported.

Effects on diagnostic tests
None reported.

Adverse reactions
CNS: headache.
CV: ***ventricular arrhythmias,*** *ventricular ectopic activity, nonsustained ventricular tachycardia,* **SUSTAINED VENTRICULAR TACHYCARDIA, VENTRICULAR FIBRILLATION,** hypotension, angina.

Overdose and treatment
Hypotension may occur with milrinone overdosage because of its vasodilator effect. No specific antidote is known, but general measures for circulatory support should be taken.

☑ Special considerations
• Drug therapy is not recommended for patients in acute phase of post-MI; clinical studies in this population are lacking.
• Monitor renal function and fluid and electrolyte changes during milrinone therapy. Correct hypokalemia with potassium supplements before or during use of milrinone.
• Duration of therapy depends on patient responsiveness. Patients have been maintained on infusions of milrinone for up to 5 days.
• When furosemide is injected into an I.V. line containing milrinone, an immediate chemical interaction occurs, as evidenced by the formation of a precipitate. Therefore, furosemide should not be administered in an I.V. line that contains milrinone.

Pediatric use
• Safety and efficacy in children have not been established.

Breast-feeding
• Excretion of drug into breast milk is not known. Use caution when administering drug to breast-feeding women.

mineral oil

Agoral, Fleet Enema Mineral Oil, Kondremul*, Kondremul Plain, Lansoyl*, Milkinol, Neo-Cultol, Nujol*, Petrogalar Plain, Zymenol

Pharmacologic classification: lubricant oil
Therapeutic classification: laxative
Pregnancy risk category C

How supplied

Available without a prescription
Jelly: 180 ml
Emulsion: 2.5 ml/5 ml, 1.4 g /5 ml
Suspension: 1.4 ml/5 ml, 2.75 ml/5 ml, 4.75 ml/5 ml
Rectal oil enema: 120 ml

Indications, route, and dosage

Constipation, preparation for bowel studies or surgery
Adults and children age 12 and older: 15 to 45 ml P.O. as a single dose or in divided doses, or 120-ml enema.
Children age 6 to 11: 5 to 15 ml P.O. daily as a single dose or in divided doses, or 30- to 60-ml enema.
Children over age 2 to 6: 30- to 60-ml enema.

Pharmacodynamics

Laxative action: Mineral oil acts mainly in the colon, lubricating the intestine and retarding colonic fluid absorption.

Pharmacokinetics

- *Absorption:* Mineral oil normally is absorbed minimally; with emulsified drug form, significant absorption occurs. Action begins in 6 to 8 hours.
- *Distribution:* Mineral oil is distributed locally, primarily in the colon.
- *Metabolism:* None.
- *Excretion:* Mineral oil is excreted in feces.

Contraindications and precautions

Contraindicated in patients with abdominal pain, nausea, vomiting, or other symptoms of appendicitis or acute surgical abdomen and in those with fecal impaction or intestinal obstruction or perforation. Contraindicated in patients with colostomy, ileostomy, ulcerative colitis and diverticulitis. Use cautiously in elderly or debilitated patients and in the young.

Interactions

Stool softeners such as *docusate* increase mineral oil absorption to potentially toxic levels; avoid concomitant use, which may cause lipoid pneumonia. Mineral oil may impair absorption of *fat-soluble vitamins* (*A, D, E,* and *K*), *anticoagulants, oral contraceptives, cardiac glycosides,* and *sulfonamides,* thus lessening their therapeutic effects.

Effects on diagnostic tests

None reported.

Adverse reactions

GI: *nausea; vomiting; diarrhea* (with excessive use); abdominal cramps, especially in severe constipation; decreased absorption of nutrients and fat-soluble vitamins, resulting in deficiency; slowed healing after hemorrhoidectomy.
Other: laxative dependence (with long-term or excessive use), anal pruritus, anal irritation, hemorrhoids, perianal discomfort, ***lipid pneumonia.***

Overdose and treatment

No information available.

☑ Special considerations

- Avoid administering drug to patients lying flat because if drug is aspirated into the lungs, pneumonitis may result.
- Do not give drug with food because this may delay gastric emptying, resulting in delayed drug action and increased aspiration risk. Separate by at least 2 hours.
- To improve taste, give emulsion and suspension with fruit juice or carbonated beverages.
- Prescribe cleansing enema 30 minutes to 1 hour after retention enema.
- Reduce or divide dose or use emulsified drug form to avoid leakage through anal sphincter.
- Mineral oil may impair absorption of fat-soluble vitamins (A, D, E, and K).

Patient education

- Instruct patient not to take mineral oil with stool softeners.
- Warn patient that mineral oil may leak through anal sphincter, especially with repeated use or with enema form. Undergarment protection may be desired.

Geriatric use

- Because of increased aspiration risk, use caution when administering drug to elderly patients.

Pediatric use

- Mineral oil is not recommended for children under age 6 because of risk of aspiration. Enema form is contraindicated in children under age 2.

minocycline hydrochloride

Dynacin, Minocin

Pharmacologic classification: tetracycline
Therapeutic classification: antibiotic
Pregnancy risk category NR

How supplied

Available by prescription only
Capsules: 50 mg, 100 mg
Tablets: 50 mg, 100 mg
Suspension: 50 mg/5 ml
Injection: 100 mg/vial

Indications, route, and dosage

Infections caused by sensitive organisms
Adults: Initially, 200 mg P.O., I.V.; then 100 mg q 12 hours or 50 mg P.O. q 6 hours.

Children over age 8: Initially, 4 mg/kg P.O., I.V.; then 4 mg/kg P.O. daily, divided q 12 hours. Give I.V. in 500 to 1,000 ml solution without calcium, over 6 hours.

Gonorrhea in patients sensitive to penicillin
Adults: Initially, 200 mg; then 100 mg q 12 hours for 4 days.

Syphilis in patients sensitive to penicillin
Adults: Initially, 200 mg; then 100 mg q 12 hours for 10 to 15 days.

Meningococcal carrier state
Adults: 100 mg P.O. q 12 hours for 5 days.

Uncomplicated urethral, endocervical, or rectal infection
Adults: 100 mg P.O. q 12 hours for at least 7 days.

Uncomplicated gonoccocal urethritis in men
Adults: 100 mg P.O. q 12 hours for 5 days.

Mycobacterium marinum
Adults: 100 mg P.O. q 12 hours for 6 to 8 weeks.

Cholera
Adults: Initially, 200 mg P.O.; then 100 mg P.O. q 12 hours for 72 hours.

Acne
Adults: 50 mg P.O. daily, b.i.d. or t.i.d.

◊ ***Nocardiosis***
Adults: Usual dose for 12 to 18 months.

◊ ***Sclerosis agent for pleural effusions***
Adults: 300 mg mixed in 40 to 50 ml 0.9% NaCl solution, instilled through a thoracostomy tube.

Pharmacodynamics

Antibacterial action: Minocycline is bacteriostatic; it binds reversibly to ribosomal units, thus inhibiting bacterial protein synthesis.

Minocycline is active against many gram-negative and gram-positive organisms, *Mycoplasma, Rickettsia, Chlamydia,* and spirochetes; it may be more active against staphylococci than other tetracyclines.

The potential vestibular toxicity and cost of minocycline limit its usefulness. It may be more active than other tetracyclines against Nocardia asteroides; it is also effective against *Mycobacterium marinum* infections. It has been used for meningococcal meningitis prophylaxis because of its activity against Neisseria meningitidis.

Pharmacokinetics

- *Absorption:* About is 90% to 100% absorbed after oral administration; peak serum levels occur at 2 to 3 hours.
- *Distribution:* Widely distributed into body tissues and fluids, including synovial, pleural, prostatic, and seminal fluids, bronchial secretions, saliva, and aqueous humor; CSF penetration is poor. Drug crosses the placenta; it is 55% to 88% protein-bound.
- *Metabolism:* Minocycline is metabolized partially.
- *Excretion:* Excreted primarily unchanged in urine by glomerular filtration. Plasma half-life is 11 to 22 hours in adults with normal renal function. Some drug is excreted in breast milk.

Contraindications and precautions

Contraindicated in patients with hypersensitivity to drug or other tetracyclines. Use cautiously in patients with impaired renal or hepatic function, in children under age 8, and during the last half of pregnancy.

Interactions

Concomitant use of minocycline with *antacids containing aluminum, calcium, or magnesium* or with *laxatives containing magnesium* decreases oral absorption of minocycline (because of chelation); concomitant use with *oral iron products* or *sodium bicarbonate* also decreases absorption. *Foods* and *milk* and other *dairy products* may also decrease absorption of minocycline, but less so than with other tetracyclines.

Tetracyclines may antagonize bactericidal effects of *penicillin,* inhibiting cell growth through bacteriostatic action; administer penicillin 2 to 3 hours before minocycline.

Concomitant use of minocycline necessitates lowered dosage of *oral anticoagulants* due to enhanced effects, and lowered dose of *digoxin* due to increased bioavailability.

Oral contraceptives may be less effective when administered with minocycline.

Effects on diagnostic tests

Drug causes false-negative results in urine glucose tests using glucose oxidase reagent (Clinistix or glucose enzymatic test strip).

Minocycline causes false elevations in fluorometric test results for urinary catecholamines.

Adverse reactions

CNS: headache, ***intracranial hypertension (pseudotumor cerebri),*** light-headedness, dizziness, vertigo.
CV: pericarditis.
EENT: dysphagia, glossitis.
GI: *anorexia, epigastric distress, oral candidiasis, nausea, vomiting, diarrhea,* enterocolitis, inflammatory lesions in anogenital region.
Hematologic: ***neutropenia,*** eosinophilia, ***thrombocytopenia***, hemolytic anemia.
Skin: *maculopapular and erythematous rashes, photosensitivity, increased pigmentation, urticaria.*
Other: hypersensitivity reactions ***(anaphylaxis);*** elevated liver enzymes; increased BUN level; permanent discoloration of teeth, enamel defects, and bone growth retardation if used in children under age 8; superinfection; *thrombophlebitis.*

Overdose and treatment

Clinical signs of overdose are usually limited to GI tract; give antacids or empty stomach by gastric lavage if ingestion occurred within the preceding 4 hours.

☑ Special considerations

Besides those relevant to all *tetracyclines,* consider the following recommendations.

- Reconstitute 100 mg powder with 5 ml sterile water for injection, with further dilution of 500 to 1,000 ml for I.V. infusion.

• Reconstituted solution is stable for 24 hours at room temperature. However, final diluted solution should be used immediately.

Pediatric use
• Drug is not recommended for use in children under age 9.

Breast-feeding
• Avoid use in breast-feeding women.

minoxidil (systemic)
Loniten

Pharmacologic classification: peripheral vasodilator
Therapeutic classification: antihypertensive
Pregnancy risk category C

How supplied
Available by prescription only
Tablets: 2.5 mg, 10 mg

Indications, route, and dosage
Severe hypertension
Adults and children older than age 12: Initially, 5 mg P.O. as a single daily dose. Effective dosage range is usually 10 to 40 mg daily. Maximum dosage is 100 mg/day.
Children under age 12: 0.2 mg/kg (maximum 5 mg) as a single daily dose. Effective dosage range is usually 0.25 to 1 mg/kg daily in one or two doses. Maximum dosage is 50 mg/day.

Pharmacodynamics
Antihypertensive action: Drug produces its antihypertensive effect by a direct vasodilating effect on vascular smooth muscle; the effect on resistance vessels (arterioles and arteries) is greater than that on capacitance vessels (venules and veins).

Pharmacokinetics
• *Absorption:* Minoxidil is absorbed rapidly from the GI tract; antihypertensive effect occurs in 30 minutes, peaking at 2 to 3 hours.
• *Distribution:* Drug is distributed widely into body tissues; it is not bound to plasma proteins.
• *Metabolism:* Approximately 90% of a given dose is metabolized.
• *Excretion:* Drug and metabolites are excreted primarily in urine. Antihypertensive action persists for approximately 3 days.

Contraindications and precautions
Contraindicated in patients with pheochromocytoma or hypersensitivity to drug. Use cautiously in patients with impaired renal function or after acute MI.

Interactions
Concomitant use with *diuretics* or *guanethidine* may cause profound orthostatic hypotension.

Effects on diagnostic tests
Minoxidil may elevate serum alkaline phosphatase, serum creatinine, and BUN levels, as well as antinuclear antibody titers; drug may transiently decrease hemoglobin and hematocrit levels. Minoxidil may also alter direction and magnitude of T waves on ECG.

Adverse reactions
CV: *edema, tachycardia, pericardial effusion and tamponade,* ***heart failure***, ECG changes, rebound hypertension.
GI: nausea, vomiting.
Skin: rash, ***Stevens-Johnson syndrome.***
Other: *hypertrichosis (elongation, thickening, and enhanced pigmentation of fine body hair), breast tenderness, weight gain.*

Overdose and treatment
Clinical signs of overdose include hypotension, tachycardia, headache, and skin flushing.

After acute ingestion, empty stomach by induced emesis or gastric lavage, and give activated charcoal to reduce absorption. Further treatment is usually symptomatic and supportive. Administer 0.9% NaCl solution I.V. to maintain blood pressure. Sympathomimetic drugs, such as epinephrine and norepinephrine, should be avoided because of their excessive cardiac stimulating action.

☑ Special considerations
• Drug therapy is usually given concomitantly with other antihypertensive drugs, such as diuretics, beta blockers, or sympathetic nervous system suppressants.
• Monitor blood pressure and pulse after administration, and report significant changes; assess intake, output, and body weight for sodium and water retention.
• Monitor for heart failure, pericardial effusion, and cardiac tamponade; have phenylephrine, dopamine, and vasopressin on hand to treat hypotension.
• Patients with renal failure or on dialysis may require smaller maintenance doses of minoxidil. Because minoxidil is removed by dialysis, it is recommended that on the day of dialysis, the drug be administered immediately after dialysis if dialysis is at 9 a.m.; if dialysis is after 3 p.m., the daily dose is given at 7 a.m. (8 hours before dialysis).

Patient education
• Explain that drug is usually taken with other antihypertensive medications; emphasize importance of taking drug as prescribed.
• Caution patient to report the following cardiac symptoms promptly: increased heart rate (over 20 beats/minute over normal), rapid weight gain, shortness of breath, chest pain, severe indigestion, dizziness, light-headedness, or fainting.
• Tell patient to call for instructions before taking OTC cold preparations.
• Advise patient that hypertrichosis will disappear 1 to 6 months after stopping drug.

Geriatric use
• Elderly patients may be sensitive to drug's antihypertensive effects. Dosage adjustment may be necessary because of altered drug clearance.

Pediatric use
• Because of limited experience in children, use with caution. Cautious drug titration is necessary.

Breast-feeding
• Drug occurs in breast milk. An alternative feeding method is recommended during therapy.

minoxidil (topical)
Rogaine

Pharmacologic classification: direct-acting vasodilator
Therapeutic classification: hair-growth stimulant
Pregnancy risk category C

How supplied
Available without a prescription
Topical solution: 2%, 5%

Indications, route, and dosage
Male pattern baldness (alopecia androgenetica), diffuse hair loss or thinning in women, ◊ adjunct to hair transplantation
Adults: Apply 1 ml to affected area b.i.d. for 4 months or longer.

Pharmacodynamics
Hair-growth stimulation: Exact mechanism by which drug promotes hair growth is unknown. It may alter androgen metabolism in the scalp, or it may exert a local vasodilatation and enhance the microcirculation around the hair follicle. It may also directly stimulate the hair follicle.

Pharmacokinetics
• *Absorption:* Poorly absorbed through intact skin. Approximately 0.3% to 4.5% of a topically applied dose reaches the systemic circulation.
• *Distribution:* Serum levels are generally negligible.
• *Metabolism:* Not fully described.
• *Excretion:* Eliminated primarily by the kidneys. About 95% of a topically applied dose is eliminated after 4 days.

Contraindications and precautions
Contraindicated in patients hypersensitive to drug or any component of the solution or during pregnancy. Use cautiously in patients with renal, cardiac, or hepatic disease and in those over age 50.

Interactions
None reported. Theoretically, absorbed minoxidil may potentiate orthostatic hypotension in patients taking *guanethidine* and *diuretics.*

Effect on diagnostic tests
None reported.

Adverse reactions
CNS: headache, dizziness, faintness, light-headedness.
CV: edema, chest pain, hypertension, hypotension, palpitations, increased or decreased pulse rate.
EENT: sinusitis.
GI: diarrhea, nausea, vomiting.
GU: urinary tract infection, renal calculi, urethritis.
Respiratory: bronchitis, upper respiratory infection.
Skin: irritant dermatitis, allergic contact dermatitis, eczema, hypertrichosis, local erythema, pruritus, dry skin or scalp, flaking, alopecia, exacerbation of hair loss.
Other: back pain, tendinitis, edema, weight gain.

Overdose and treatment
No information available. However, if topical use produces systemic adverse effects, wash application site thoroughly with soap and water and treat symptoms, as appropriate. Treatment is symptomatic. Clinical signs of oral overdose include hypotension, tachycardia, headache, and skin flushing.

After acute ingestion, empty stomach by induced emesis or gastric lavage and give activated charcoal to reduce absorption. Further treatment is usually symptomatic and supportive.

☑ Special considerations
• Do not use with other topical agents such as corticosteroids, retinoids, and petrolatum or agents that enhance percutaneous absorption. Rogaine is for topical use only; each ml contains 20 mg or 50 mg minoxidil and accidental ingestion could cause adverse systemic effects.
• Monitor patient 1 month after starting topical drug therapy and at least every 6 months afterward. Discontinue topical minoxidil if systemic effects occur.
• The alcohol base will burn and irritate the eye and other sensitive surfaces (eye, abraded skin, and mucous membranes). If topical minoxidil contacts sensitive areas, flush with copious cool water.
• Before starting treatment, check that patient has a normal, healthy scalp. Local abrasion or dermatitis may increase absorption and the risk of adverse effects.
• Before treatment with topical minoxidil, patient should have a history and physical and should be advised of potential risks; a risk-benefit decision should be made. Patients with cardiac disease should realize that adverse effects may be especially serious. Alert patient to possibility of tachycardia and fluid retention, and monitor for increased heart rate, weight gain, or other systemic effects.

Patient education
• Tell patient to avoid inhaling the spray.
• Teach patient to apply topical minoxidil as follows: Hair and scalp should be dry before application. One ml should be applied to the total affected areas twice daily. Total daily dose should not exceed 2 ml. If the fingertips are used to apply the drug, wash the hands afterwards.
• Encourage patient to carefully review patient information leaflet, which is included with each package and in the full product information.

• Inform patient that 4 months of use may be required before results become apparent.

Pediatric use
• Safety and effectiveness have not been established for patients under age 18.

Breast-feeding
• Topical minoxidil should not be administered to breast-feeding women.

mirtazapine
Remeron

Pharmacologic classification: piperazinoazepine
Therapeutic classification: tetracyclic antidepressant
Pregnancy risk category C

How supplied
Available by prescription only
Tablets: 15 mg, 30 mg

Indications, route, and dosage
Depression
Adults: Initially, 15 mg P.O. h.s. Maintenance dosage ranges from 15 mg to 45 mg daily. Dosage adjustments should be made at intervals no less than 1 to 2 weeks apart.

Pharmacodynamics
Antidepressant action: Unknown.

Pharmacokinetics
• *Absorption:* Mirtazapine is rapidly and completely absorbed from the GI tract. Absolute bioavailability of drug is about 50%.
• *Distribution:* About 85% bound to plasma protein.
• *Metabolism:* Extensively metabolized in the liver.
• *Excretion:* Drug is predominantly eliminated in urine (75%) with 15% being excreted in feces. Half-life is between 20 and 40 hours.

Contraindications and precautions
Contraindicated in patients with hypersensitivity to drug. Coadministration with MAO inhibitors is contraindicated.

Use cautiously in patients with CV or cerebrovascular disease, seizure disorders, suicidal ideation, impaired hepatic and renal function, or history of mania or hypomania. Also, use cautiously in patients with conditions that predispose them to hypotension, such as dehydration, hypovolemia, or treatment with antihypertensive medication.

Interactions
Alcohol, diazepam, and other *CNS depressants* may cause additive CNS effects when administered with mirtazapine. Avoid concomitant use. Mirtazapine should not be used in combination with *MAO inhibitor* or within 14 days of initiating or discontinuing therapy with MAO inhibitor because of potential serious, and sometimes fatal, reactions.

Effects on diagnostic tests
Nonfasting cholesterol increases greater than or equal to the upper limits of normal were observed in 15% of patients treated with mirtazapine.

Adverse reactions
CNS: *somnolence,* dizziness, asthenia, abnormal dreams, abnormal thinking, tremor, confusion.
GI: nausea, *increased appetite, dry mouth, constipation.*
GU: urinary frequency.
Hematologic: ***agranulocytosis*** (rare).
Respiratory: dyspnea.
Other: *weight gain,* back pain, flu syndrome, edema, peripheral edema, myalgia.

Overdose and treatment
Overdosage may result in disorientation, drowsiness, impaired memory, and tachycardia. If overdosage occurs, treatment should be that for any antidepressant overdosage. If patient is unconscious, establish an airway and provide adequate oxygenation. Gastric lavage, induced emesis, or both should be considered. Activated charcoal should also be considered. Monitor cardiac and vital signs and provide general symptomatic and supportive measures.

☑ Special considerations
• Although incidence of agranulocytosis is rare, discontinue drug and monitor patient closely if he develops a sore throat, fever, stomatitis, or other signs of infection together with a low WBC count.
• Monitor patient closely because it is not known if mirtazapine causes physical or psychological dependence.

Patient education
• Caution patient not to perform hazardous activities if somnolence occurs with drug use.
• Instruct patient not to use alcohol or other CNS depressants while taking drug because of additive effect.
• Tell patient to report signs and symptoms of infection such as fever, chills, sore throat, mucous membrane ulceration, or other possible signs of infection including any flulike complaints.
• Stress importance of compliance with mirtazapine therapy.
• Instruct patient not to take any concomitant medication without medical approval.
• Tell women of childbearing age to report suspected pregnancy immediately.

Geriatric use
• Administer mirtazapine cautiously to elderly patients because pharmacokinetic studies reveal a decreased clearance in the elderly.

Pediatric use
• Safety and effectiveness in children have not been established.

Breast-feeding
• It is not known if drug occurs in breast milk; use cautiously in breast-feeding women.

misoprostol
Cytotec

Pharmacologic classification: prostaglandin E_1 analogue
Therapeutic classification: antiulcer, gastric mucosal protectant
Pregnancy risk category X

How supplied
Available by prescription only
Tablets: 100 mcg, 200 mcg

Indications, route, and dosage
Prevention of gastric ulcer induced by NSAIDs
Adults: 200 mcg P.O. q.i.d with meals and h.s. Reduce dosage to 100 mcg P.O. q.i.d. in patients who cannot tolerate this dosage.
◇ ***Duodenal or gastric ulcer***
Adults: 100 to 200 mcg P.O. q.i.d. with meals and h.s.
◇ ***Prevention of acute graft rejection in renal transplantation***
Adults: 200 mcg P.O. q.i.d. for 2 weeks.

Pharmacodynamics
Antiulcer action: Misoprostol enhances the production of gastric mucus and bicarbonate, and decreases basal, nocturnal, and stimulated gastric acid secretion.

Pharmacokinetics
• *Absorption:* Rapid after oral administration.
• *Distribution:* Drug is less than 90% bound to plasma proteins. Peak levels are reached in about 12 minutes.
• *Metabolism:* Rapidly de-esterified to misoprostol acid, the biologically active metabolite. The de-esterified metabolite undergoes further oxidation in several body tissues.
• *Excretion:* About 15% of an oral dose appears in the feces; the balance is excreted in the urine. Terminal half-life is 20 to 40 minutes.

Contraindications and precautions
Contraindicated in pregnant or breast-feeding patients and in those with a known allergy to prostaglandins.

Interactions
Misoprostol levels are diminished by concomitant administration with *food* or *antacid*, and misoprostol diminishes the availability of *aspirin*. None of these effects is believed to be significant.

Effects on diagnostic tests
Misoprostol produces a modest decrease in basal pepsin secretion.

Adverse reactions
CNS: headache.
GI: *diarrhea, abdominal pain, nausea, flatulence, dyspepsia, vomiting, constipation.*
Other: hypermenorrhea, dysmenorrhea, spotting, cramps, menstrual disorders.

Overdose and treatment
There has been little clinical experience with overdose. Cumulative daily doses of 1,600 mcg have been administered, with only minor GI discomfort noted. Treatment should be supportive.

☑ Special considerations
• Misoprostol should not be prescribed for a female patient of childbearing age unless she:
– needs NSAID therapy, and is at high risk of developing gastric ulcers.
– is capable of complying with effective contraception.
– has received both oral and written warnings regarding the hazards of misoprostol therapy, the risk of possible contraception failure, and the hazards this drug would pose to other women of childbearing age who might take this drug by mistake.
– has had a negative serum pregnancy test within 2 weeks before beginning therapy, and she will begin therapy on the second or third day of her next normal menstrual period.
• Diarrhea is usually dose-related and develops within the first 2 weeks of therapy. It can be minimized by administering the drug after meals and at bedtime, and by avoiding magnesium-containing antacids.
• Drug has been used for treatment and prophylaxis of reflux esophagitis, alcohol-induced gastritis, hemorrhagic gastritis, and fat malabsorption in cystic fibrosis.

Patient education
• Explain importance of not giving drug to anyone else. Make sure patient understands that a miscarriage could result if drug is taken by a pregnant woman.

Pediatric use
• Safety has not been established in children under age 18.

Breast-feeding
• Breast-feeding is not recommended because of potential for drug-induced diarrhea in infant.

mitomycin (mitomycin-C; MTC)
Mutamycin

Pharmacologic classification: antineoplastic antibiotic (cell cycle–phase nonspecific)
Therapeutic classification: antineoplastic
Pregnancy risk category NR

How supplied
Available by prescription only
Injection: 5-mg, 20-mg, 40-mg vials

Indications, route, and dosage

Dosage and indications may vary. Check current literature for recommended protocol. Not indicated as a single-agent primary therapy.

Stomach and pancreatic adenocarcinoma (in conjunction with other chemotherapeutic agents); ◊ breast, ◊ colon, ◊ rectum, ◊ head, ◊ neck, ◊ lung, ◊ cervix, and ◊ bladder cancer

Adults: 20 mg/m² as a single dose. Repeat cycle q 6 to 8 weeks, adjusting dose, if needed, according to the following guidelines.

✦ ***Dosage adjustment.***

Nadir after prior dose		% of prior dose to be given
WBC/mm³	*Platelets/ mm³*	
> 4,000	>100,000	100%
3,000 to 3,999	75,000 to 99,999	100%
2,000 to 2,999	25,000 to 74,999	70%
< 2,000	< 25,000	50%

Stop drug if WBC count is below 4,000/mm³ or platelet count is below 100,000/mm³. No repeat dose should be given until blood counts have recovered above these levels.

Pharmacodynamics

Antineoplastic action: Mitomycin exerts its cytotoxic activity by a mechanism similar to that of the alkylating agents. The drug is converted to an active compound which forms cross-links between strands of DNA, inhibiting DNA synthesis. Mitomycin also inhibits RNA and protein synthesis to a lesser extent.

Pharmacokinetics

- *Absorption:* Because of its vesicant nature, drug must be administered I.V.
- *Distribution:* Drug distributes widely into body tissues; animal studies show that the highest concentrations are found in the kidneys followed by the muscle, eyes, lungs, intestines, and stomach. It does not cross the blood-brain barrier.
- *Metabolism:* Mitomycin is metabolized by hepatic microsomal enzymes and is also deactivated in the kidneys, spleen, brain, and heart.
- *Excretion:* Drug and its metabolites are excreted in urine. A small portion is eliminated in bile and feces.

Contraindications and precautions

Contraindicated in patients with hypersensitivity to drug, thrombocytopenia, coagulation disorders, or an increase in bleeding tendency due to other causes. Contraindicated as primary therapy as a single agent to replace surgery or radiotherapy.

Interactions

Acute shortness of breath and severe bronchospasm have occurred following use of *vinca alkaloids* in patients who had previously or simultaneously received mitomycin.

Effects on diagnostic tests

Mitomycin therapy, through drug-induced renal toxicity, may increase serum creatinine and BUN concentrations.

Adverse reactions

CNS: headache, neurologic abnormalities, confusion, drowsiness, fatigue.
GI: *nausea, vomiting, anorexia, diarrhea.*
Hematologic: ***thrombocytopenia***, ***leukopenia*** (may be delayed up to 8 weeks and may be cumulative with successive doses); ***microangiopathic hemolytic anemia, characterized by thrombocytopenia***, ***renal failure,*** and hypertension.
Respiratory: ***interstitial pneumonitis,*** pulmonary edema, dyspnea, nonproductive cough, adult respiratory distress syndrome.
Other: desquamation, induration, pruritus, pain at injection site; ***septicemia;*** cellulitis, ulceration, sloughing with extravasation; *reversible alopecia;* fever; blurred vision, pain.

Overdose and treatment

Clinical manifestations of overdose include myelosuppression, nausea, vomiting, and alopecia.

Treatment is usually supportive and includes transfusion of blood components, antiemetics, and antibiotics for infections that may develop.

☑ Special considerations

- To reconstitute 5-mg vial, use 10 ml of sterile water for injection; to reconstitute 20-mg vial, use 40 ml of sterile water for injection; to reconstitute a 40-mg vial, use 80 ml sterile water water for injection, to give a concentration of 0.5 mg/ml. Allow to stand at room temperature until complete dissolution occurs.
- Drug may be administered by I.V. push injection slowly over 5 to 10 minutes into the tubing of a freely flowing I.V. infusion.
- Drug can be further diluted to 100 to 150 ml with 0.9% NaCl solution or D_5W for I.V. infusion (over 30 to 60 minutes or longer).
- Reconstituted solution remains stable for 1 week at room temperature and for 2 weeks if refrigerated.
- Mitomycin has been used intra-arterially to treat certain tumors, for example, into hepatic artery for colon cancer. It has also been given as a continuous daily infusion.
- An unlabeled use of drug is to treat small bladder papillomas. It is instilled directly into the bladder in a concentration of 20 mg/20 ml sterile water.
- Ulcers caused by extravasation develop late and dorsal to the extravasation site. Apply cold compresses for at least 12 hours.
- Continue CBC and blood studies at least 7 weeks after therapy is stopped. Monitor for signs of bleeding.

Patient education
- Tell patient to avoid exposure to people with infections.
- Warn patient not to receive immunizations during therapy and for several weeks afterward. Members of the same household should not receive immunizations during the same period.
- Reassure patient that hair should grow back after treatment has been discontinued.
- Tell patient to call promptly if he develops a sore throat or fever or notices unusual bruising or bleeding.

Breast-feeding
- It is not known if drug distributes into breast milk. However, because of the potential for serious adverse reactions, mutagenicity, and carcinogenicity in the infant, breast-feeding is not recommended.

mitotane
Lysodren

Pharmacologic classification: chlorophenothane (DDT) analogue
Therapeutic classification: antineoplastic, antiadrenal
Pregnancy risk category C

How supplied
Available by prescription only
Tablets (scored): 500 mg

Indications, route, and dosage
Dosage and indications may vary. Check current literature for recommended protocol.

Inoperable adrenocortical cancer
Adults: Initially, 2 to 6 g P.O. daily in divided doses t.i.d. or q.i.d. Increase to 9 to 10 g daily as tolerated. If severe adverse reactions appear, reduce dosage until maximum tolerated dosage is achieved (varies from 2 to 19 g daily but is usually 8 to 10 g daily).

◊ ***Cushing's syndrome***
Adults: 1 to 12 g P.O. daily in divided doses; usual initial dose is 3 to 6 g daily in 3 to 4 divided doses, maintenance dosage ranges from 500 mg twice weekly to 2 g daily.

Pharmacodynamics
Antineoplastic action: Exact mechanism of mitotane's activity is unclear. Possibly, a metabolite binds to mitochondrial proteins in the adrenal cortex, resulting in cell death.

Adrenocortical action: Mitotane also inhibits the production of corticosteroids and alters extra-adrenal metabolism of endogenous and exogenous steroids.

Pharmacokinetics
- *Absorption:* After oral administration, 35% to 40% of a dose is absorbed across the GI tract.
- *Distribution:* Widely distributed in body tissue; fatty tissue is the primary storage site. Slow release of mitotane from fatty tissue into the plasma occurs after the drug is discontinued. A metabolite of mitotane has been detected in the CSF.
- *Metabolism:* Metabolized in the liver and other tissue.
- *Excretion:* Drug and its metabolites are excreted in urine and bile. Plasma elimination half-life is reported to be 18 to 159 days.

Contraindications and precautions
Contraindicated in patients hypersensitive to drug. Do not use drug in patients in shock or who have suffered trauma.

Use cautiously in patients with hepatic disease. All tumor tissues should be surgically removed before drug administration to avoid infarction and hemorrhage in the tumor because of rapid cytotoxic effect of drug.

Interactions
When used concomitantly, mitotane may decrease the effect of *barbiturates, coumarin anticoagulants,* and *phenytoin* through the induction of hepatic microsomal enzymes, increasing the metabolism of these agents to inactive compounds. Concomitant use with *CNS depressants* can cause an additive CNS depression. *Spironolactone* may block the actions of mitotane.

Effects on diagnostic tests
Mitotane therapy may decrease concentrations of urinary 17-hydroxycorticosteroid, plasma cortisol, protein-bound iodine, and serum uric acid.

Adverse reactions
CNS: *depression, somnolence, lethargy, vertigo; brain damage and dysfunction in long-term, high-dose therapy.*
CV: hypertension.
EENT: visual disturbances.
GI: *severe nausea, vomiting, diarrhea, anorexia.*
GU: hemorrhagic cystitis.
Skin: dermatitis, *maculopapular rash.*
Other: increased serum cholesterol level, adrenal insufficiency.

Overdose and treatment
Clinical manifestations of overdose include vomiting, weakness, numbness of extremities, diarrhea, apprehension, and excitement.

Treatment is usually supportive and includes activated charcoal, sodium chloride cathartic, induction of emesis with ipecac, intestinal lavage with mannitol 20%, and appropriate symptomatic therapy.

☑ Special considerations
- Drug can be administered with or without food in the stomach. Avoid administering drug with a fatty meal because it distributes mostly to body fat.
- Give an antiemetic before administering mitotane, to reduce nausea.
- Dosage may be reduced if GI or skin reactions are severe.
- Dose modification may be required in hepatic disease.

- Obese patients may need higher dosage and may have longer-lasting adverse reactions, because drug distributes mostly to body fat.
- Evaluate efficacy by reduction in pain, weakness, anorexia, and tumor mass.
- Monitor for symptoms of hepatotoxicity.
- Drug should not be used in a patient with shock or trauma. Use of corticosteroids may avoid acute adrenocorticoid insufficiency.
- Glucocorticoid therapy is usually required. During periods of physiologic stress (such as infection or surgery), glucocorticoid dosage should be increased.
- Monitor behavioral and neurologic signs daily throughout therapy.
- Adequate trial is at least 3 months, but therapy can continue if clinical benefits are observed.

Patient education

- Stress importance of continuing drug despite nausea and vomiting.
- Warn patient to avoid alcoholic beverages after taking a dose of medication because excessive drowsiness may occur.
- Tell patient drug may cause drowsiness. Patient should use caution when performing activities that require mental alertness.
- Instruct patient to call immediately if vomiting occurs shortly after taking a dose.
- Tell patient to report injury, infection, or other illness that may require supplemental steroid use.

Breast-feeding

- It is not known if drug distributes into breast milk. However, because of the potential for serious adverse reactions in the infant, breast-feeding is not recommended.

mitoxantrone hydrochloride

Novantrone

Pharmacologic classification: antibiotic antineoplastic
Therapeutic classification: antineoplastic
Pregnancy risk category D

How supplied

Available by prescription only
Injection: 2 mg mitoxantrone base/ml in 10-ml, 12.5-ml, 15-ml vials

Indications, route, and dosage

Initial treatment in combination with other approved drugs for acute nonlymphocytic leukemia

Adults: For induction (in combination chemotherapy), 12 mg/m² daily by I.V. infusion on days 1 to 3, and 100 mg/m² of cytosine arabinoside by continuous I.V. infusion (over 24 hours) on days 1 to 7 for 7 days.

Most complete remissions follow initial course of induction therapy. A second course may be given if antileukemic response is incomplete: give mitoxantrone for 2 days and cytosine for 5 days using the same daily dosage levels. Second course of therapy should be withheld until toxicity clears if severe or life-threatening nonhematologic toxicity occurs.

Combined initial therapy for pain related to advanced hormone-refractory prostate cancer

Adults: 12 to 14 mg/m² I.V. infusion over 15 to 30 minutes q 21 days.

Pharmacodynamics

Antineoplastic action: Mitoxantrone's mechanism of action is not completely established. It is a DNA-reactive agent that has cytocidal effects on proliferating and nonproliferating cells, suggestive of lack of cell-phase specificity.

Pharmacokinetics

- *Absorption:*. Drug is only administered by I.V. infusion.
- *Distribution:* Drug is 78% plasma protein-bound.
- *Metabolism:* Metabolized by the liver.
- *Excretion:* Excretion is via renal and hepatobiliary systems; 6% to 11% of dose is excreted in urine within 5 days: 65% is unchanged drug; 35% is two inactive metabolites. Within 5 days, 25% of dose is excreted in feces.

Contraindications and precautions

Contraindicated in patients hypersensitive to mitoxantrone. Use cautiously in patients with prior exposure to anthracyclines or other cardiotoxic drugs.

Interactions

None reported.

Effects on diagnostic tests

None reported.

Adverse reactions

CNS: ***seizures,*** headache.
EENT: conjunctivitis.
CV: ***heart failure, arrhythmias,*** tachycardia.
GI: *bleeding, abdominal pain, diarrhea, nausea, mucositis, vomiting,* stomatitis.
GU: ***renal failure.***
Hematologic: ***myelosuppression.***
Hepatic: jaundice.
Respiratory: *dyspnea, cough.*
Skin: *petechiae, ecchymoses.*
Other: *alopecia,* hyperuricemia, *sepsis, fungal infections, fever.*

Overdose and treatment

Accidental overdoses have occurred and have caused severe leukopenia with infection. Monitor hematologic parameters and treat symptomatically. Antimicrobial therapy may be necessary.

☑ Special considerations

- Close and frequent monitoring of hematologic and chemical laboratory parameters, including serial CBC and liver function tests, with frequent patient observation is recommended.
- Safety of administration by routes other than I.V. has not been established. Do not use drug intrathecally.

• Hyperuricemia may result from rapid lysis of tumor cells. Monitor serum uric acid levels. Institute hypouricemic therapy before antileukemic therapy.
• Transient elevations of AST and ALT have occurred 4 to 24 days after mitoxantrone therapy.
• To prepare, dilute solutions to at least 50 ml with either 0.9% NaCl solution or D_5W. Inject slowly into tubing of a freely running I.V. solution of 0.9% NaCl solution or D_5W over not less than 3 minutes. Discard unused infusion solutions appropriately. Do not mix for infusion with heparin; a precipitate may form. Specific compatibility data are not available.
• If extravasation occurs, discontinue I.V. and restart in another vein. Mitoxantrone is a nonvesicant and the possibility of severe local reactions is minimal.
• Urine may appear blue-green for 24 hours after administration.
• Bluish discoloration of sclera may occur. Teach patient that this is sign of myelosuppression.

Patient education
• Tell patient urine may appear blue-green for 24 hours after administration and sclera may appear bluish.
• Advise patient to call promptly if signs and symptoms of myelosuppression develop (fever, sore throat, easy bruising, or excessive bleeding).
• Advise patient to use contraception; tell patient to call if pregnancy is suspected.
• Tell patient to drink fluids to minimize uric acid nephropathy.

Pediatric use
• Safety and efficacy have not been established.

Breast-feeding
• It is unknown if drug is excreted in breast milk. Because of potential for serious adverse reactions in infants, breast-feeding should be discontinued before therapy.

mivacurium chloride
Mivacron

Pharmacologic classification: nondepolarizing neuromuscular blocker
Therapeutic classification: skeletal muscle relaxant
Pregnancy risk category C

How supplied
Available by prescription only
Injection: 2 mg/ml in 5-ml and 10-ml vials
Infusion: 0.5 mg/ml, in 50 ml D_5W

Indications, route, and dosage
Adjunct to general anesthesia, to facilitate endotracheal intubation, and to provide skeletal muscle relaxation during surgery or mechanical ventilation
Dosage is highly individualized. Note that all times of onset and duration of neuromuscular blockade are averages and considerable individual variation is normal.

Adults: Usually, 0.15 mg/kg I.V. push over 5 to 15 seconds provides adequate muscle relaxation within 2½ minutes for endotracheal intubation. Clinically sufficient neuromuscular blockade usually lasts approximately 15 to 20 minutes. Supplemental doses of 0.1 mg/kg I.V. q 15 minutes usually maintain muscle relaxation. Alternatively, maintain neuromuscular blockade with a continuous infusion of 4 mcg/kg/minute started simultaneously with initial dose, or 9 to 10 mcg/kg/minute started after evidence of spontaneous recovery of initial dose. When used with isoflurane or enflurane anesthesia, dosage is usually reduced about 35% to 40%.
✦ ***Dosage adjustment.*** Infusion rate needs to be reduced by 50% in end-stage renal and liver patients.
Children age 2 to 12: 0.20 mg/kg I.V. push administered over 5 to 15 seconds.

Neuromuscular blockade is usually evident in less than 2 minutes. Although supplemental doses of 0.1 mg/kg I.V. q 15 minutes usually maintain muscle relaxation in adults, maintenance doses are usually required more frequently in children. Alternatively, maintain neuromuscular blockade with a continuous infusion titrated to effect. Most children respond to 5 to 31 mcg/kg/minute (average, 14 mcg/kg/minute).

Pharmacodynamics
Neuromuscular blocking action: Mivacurium competes with acetylcholine for receptor sites at the motor end-plate. Because this action may be antagonized by cholinesterase inhibitors, mivacurium is considered a competitive antagonist. Drug is a mixture of three stereoisomers, each possessing neuromuscular blocking activity: the cis-trans isomer (36% of the total) and the trans-trans isomer (57% of the total) are about 10 times as potent as the cis-cis isomer (only 6% of the total). The isomers do not interconvert in vivo.

Pharmacokinetics
• *Absorption:* Absorption is rapid; may produce neuromuscular blockade in approximately 3.3 minutes with sufficient neuromuscular blockade lasting 15 to 20 minutes.
• *Distribution:* Mivacurium's volume of distribution is small, indicating that it does not extensively distribute to tissues.
• *Metabolism:* Rapidly hydrolyzed by plasma pseudocholinesterase to inactive components.
• *Excretion:* Drug metabolites are excreted in bile and urine. Of the highly active isomers, the cis-trans and trans-trans isomers each have an elimination half-life of under 2.3 minutes. The less active cis-cis isomer, which is only a small portion of the total drug, has an elimination half-life of 55 minutes.

Contraindications and precautions
Contraindicated in patients with hypersensitivity to drug. Use cautiously in patients with significant CV disease, metastatic cancer, severe electrolyte disturbances, or neuromuscular disease; in those who may be adversely affected by the release of histamine; and in those in whom neuromuscular block-

ade reversibility is difficult, such as patients with myasthenia gravis or myasthenic syndrome. Use with extreme caution in patients with reduced plasma cholinesterase activity; may cause prolonged neuromuscular blockade.

Interactions

Administration to patients receiving *aminoglycosides* (*gentamicin, kanamycin, neomycin, streptomycin*), *bacitracin, colistimethate, colistin, magnesium salts, polymyxin B,* or *tetracyclines* may result in increased muscle weakness. *Carbamazepine* and *phenytoin* may prolong the time to maximal block or shorten the duration of blockade with neuromuscular blockers.

Quinidine or *inhalational anesthetics* (especially *enflurane, isoflurane*) may enhance the activity (or prolong action) of nondepolarizing neuromuscular blockers.

Mivacurium is physically incompatible with *alkaline solutions* (such as *barbiturate solutions*) and may form a precipitate. Do not administer through the same I.V. line with any of these drugs.

Plasma cholinesterase activity may be diminished by chronic use of *oral contraceptives, glucocorticosteroids*, or *MAO inhibitors*.

Effects on diagnostic tests

None reported.

Adverse reactions

CNS: dizziness.
CV: *flushing, tachycardia, bradycardia,* ***arrhythmias,*** *hypotension.*
Respiratory: ***bronchospasm,*** wheezing, ***respiratory insufficiency or apnea.***
Skin: rash, urticaria, erythema.
Other: prolonged muscle weakness, phlebitis, muscle spasms.

Overdose and treatment

Overdosage may result in prolonged neuromuscular blockade. Maintain a patent airway and control respirations until patient recovers neuromuscular function. Antagonists should not be administered until there is some evidence of spontaneous recovery. In clinical trials, administration of 0.03 to 0.064 mg/kg neostigmine methylsulfate or 0.5 mg/kg edrophonium chloride to patients with spontaneous recovery of muscle function resulted in increased muscle strength of about 10% recovery to about 95% recovery within 10 minutes.

☑ Special considerations

- When mivacurium is administered I.V. push to adults receiving anesthetic combinations of nitrous oxide and opiates, neuromuscular blockade usually lasts 15 to 20 minutes; most patients recover 95% of muscle strength in 25 to 30 minutes.
- Duration of drug effect is increased about 150% in patients with end-stage renal disease and 300% in patients with hepatic dysfunction.
- Dosage should be adjusted to ideal body weight in obese patients (patients 30% or more above their ideal weight) because of reported prolonged neuromuscular blockade.
- A nerve stimulator and train-of-four monitoring are recommended to document antagonism of neuromuscular blockade and recovery of muscle strength. Before attempting pharmacologic reversal with neostigmine methylsulfate or edrophonium chloride, some evidence of spontaneous recovery should be evident.
- Experimental evidence suggests that acid-base and electrolyte balance may influence actions of and response to nondepolarizing neuromuscular blockers. Alkalosis may counteract paralysis; acidosis may enhance it.
- Note that mivacurium, like other neuromuscular blockers, does not have an effect on consciousness or pain threshold. To avoid patient distress, this drug should not be administered until the patient's consciousness is obtunded by the general anesthetic.
- Drug is compatible with D_5W, 0.9% NaCl solution injection, dextrose 5% in 0.9% NaCl solution injection, lactated Ringer's injection, and dextrose 5% in lactated Ringer's injection. Diluted solutions are stable for 24 hours at room temperature.
- When diluted as directed, mivacurium is compatible with alfentanil, fentanyl, sufentanil, droperidol, and midazolam.
- Drug is available as premixed infusion in D_5W. After removing the protective outer wrap, check container for minor leaks by squeezing the bag before administering. Do not add other drugs to the container, and do not use the container in series connections.

Pediatric use

- Like other neuromuscular blockers, dosage requirements for children are higher on a mg/kg basis as compared with adults. Onset and recovery of neuromuscular blockade occur more rapidly in children.

Breast-feeding

- It is unknown if drug is excreted in breast milk. Use with caution in breast-feeding women.

moexipril hydrochloride

Univasc

Pharmacologic classification: ACE inhibitor
Therapeutic classification: antihypertensive
Pregnancy risk category C (D second and third trimesters)

How supplied

Available by prescription only
Tablets: 7.5 mg, 15 mg

Indications, route, and dosage

Hypertension

Adults: Initially, 7.5 mg P.O. once daily before meals for patients not receiving diuretics. If control is not adequate, dose can be increased or divided dosing may be attempted. Recommended dosage range is 7.5 to 30 mg daily, administered in one or two divided doses 1 hour before meals. For patients receiving diuretics, give 3.75 mg P.O. once daily before meals. Make subsequent dosage adjustments according to blood pressure response.

Pharmacodynamics

Antihypertensive action: Exact mechanism is unknown. Moexipril's action is thought to result primarily from suppression of the renin-angiotensin-aldosterone system. Moexipril's metabolite, moexiprilat, inhibits ACE and thereby inhibits the production of angiotensin II (a potent vasoconstrictor and stimulator of aldosterone secretion). Other mechanisms may also be involved.

Pharmacokinetics

- *Absorption:* Drug is incompletely absorbed from the GI tract with a bioavailability of about 13%. Food significantly decreases drug's bioavailability.
- *Distribution:* About 50% protein-bound.
- *Metabolism:* Metabolized extensively to the active metabolite, moexiprilat.
- *Excretion:* Drug is excreted primarily in feces with a small amount being excreted in urine. Half-life of drug is over 2 to 9 hours.

Contraindications and precautions

Contraindicated in patients with hypersensitivity to drug, history of angioedema related to previous treatment with an ACE inhibitor, and during pregnancy. Use cautiously in patients with impaired renal function, heart failure, or renal artery stenosis and in breast-feeding women.

Interactions

Because *diuretics* increase risk of excessive hypotension, they should be discontinued or dose of moexipril lowered. Moexipril increases serum *lithium* levels and lithium toxicity. Avoid concomitant use. *Potassium-sparing diuretics, potassium supplements,* and *sodium substitutes containing potassium* increase risk of hyperkalemia. Monitor serum potassium closely.

Effects on diagnostic tests

Moexipril may cause minor elevations in creatinine and BUN. Elevations of liver enzymes and uric acid may also occur.

Adverse reactions

CNS: *dizziness,* headache, fatigue.
CV: peripheral edema, hypotension, orthostatic hypotension, chest pain, flushing.
EENT: pharyngitis, rhinitis, sinusitis.
GI: diarrhea, dyspepsia, nausea.
GU: urinary frequency.
Hematologic: ***neutropenia.***
Respiratory: *dry, persistent, tickling, nonproductive cough.*
Skin: rash.
Other: myalgia, ***anaphylactoid reactions, angioedema,*** hyperkalemia, flu syndrome, upper respiratory tract infection, pain.

Overdose and treatment

Although no information is available on overdosage of moexipril, it is believed that it would be similiar to other ACE inhibitors with hypotension being the principal adverse reaction. Because the hypotensive effect of moexipril is achieved through vasodilation and effective hypovolemia, it is reasonable to treat moexipril overdose by infusion of 0.9% NaCl solution. In addition, renal function and serum potassium should be monitored.

☑ Special considerations

- Monitor patient for hypotension. Excessive hypotension can occur when drug is given with diuretics. If possible, discontinue diuretic therapy 2 to 3 days before starting moexipril to decrease potential for excessive hypotensive response. If drug does not adequately control blood pressure, reinstitute diuretic therapy with care.
- Measure blood pressure at trough (just before a dose) to verify adequate blood pressure control. Be aware that drug is less effective in reducing trough blood pressures in blacks than in nonblacks.
- Assess renal function before treatment and periodically throughout therapy. Monitor serum potassium levels.
- Other ACE inhibitors have been associated with agranulocytosis and neutropenia. Monitor CBC with differential counts before therapy, especially in patients who have collagen vascular disease with impaired renal function.
- Because angioedema associated with involvement of the tongue, glottis, or larynx may cause a fatal airway obstruction, have appropriate therapy, such as S.C. epinephrine 1:1,000 (0.3 to 0.5 ml), and equipment to ensure a patent airway is available.
- In patients undergoing major surgery or anesthesia with agents that produce hypotension, moexipril may block the compensatory renin release. Hypotension can be treated with volume expansion.

Patient education

- Instruct patient to take drug on an empty stomach; meals, particularly those that are high in fat, can impair absorption.
- Tell patient to avoid sodium substitutes; these products may contain potassium, which can cause hyperkalemia in patients taking this drug.
- Inform patient that light-headedness can occur, especially during the first few days of therapy. Tell him to rise slowly to minimize this effect and to report symptoms. If fainting occurs, tell patient to stop drug and call immediately.
- Instruct patient to use caution in hot weather and during exercise. Inadequate fluid intake, vomiting, diarrhea, and excessive perspiration can lead to light-headedness and syncope.
- Advise patient to report signs of infection, such as fever and sore throat. Also tell patient to report the following signs or symptoms: easy bruising or bleeding; swelling of tongue, lips, face, eyes, mucous membranes, or extremities; difficulty swallowing or breathing; and hoarseness.
- Tell female patient to report suspected pregnancy immediately. Drug will need to be discontinued.

Pediatric use

- Safety and effectiveness in children have not been established.

Breast-feeding

- It is not known if moexipril is excreted in breast milk; use with caution in breast-feeding women.

molindone hydrochloride

Moban

Pharmacologic classification: dihydroindolone
Therapeutic classification: antipsychotic
Pregnancy risk category NR

How supplied

Available by prescription only
Tablets: 5 mg, 10 mg, 25 mg, 50 mg, 100 mg
Oral solution: 20 mg/ml

Indications, route, and dosage

Psychotic disorders

Adults: 50 to 75 mg P.O. daily, increased 100 mg daily in 3 to 4 days to a maximum of 225 mg daily. Maintenance dose for mild disease is 5 to 15 mg t.i.d. or q.i.d., moderate disease is 10 to 25 mg t.i.d. or q.i.d., and severe disease is 225 mg daily.

Pharmacodynamics

Antipsychotic action: Molindone is unrelated to all other antipsychotic drugs; it is thought to exert its antipsychotic effects by postsynaptic blockade of CNS dopamine receptors, thereby inhibiting dopamine-mediated effects.

Molindone has many other central and peripheral effects; it also produces alpha and ganglionic blockade. Its most prominent adverse reactions are extrapyramidal.

Pharmacokinetics

- *Absorption:* Data are limited, but absorption appears rapid; peak effects occur within 1½ hours.
- *Distribution:* Molindone is distributed widely into the body.
- *Metabolism:* Molindone is metabolized extensively; drug effects persist for 24 to 36 hours.
- *Excretion:* Most of drug is excreted as metabolites in urine; some is excreted in feces via the biliary tract. Overall, 90% of a given dose is excreted within 24 hours.

Contraindications and precautions

Contraindicated in patients with hypersensitivity to drug and in those experiencing coma or severe CNS depression. Use cautiously in patients at risk for seizures or when high physical activity is harmful to patient.

Interactions

Concomitant use with *sympathomimetics*, including *epinephrine, phenylephrine, phenylpropanolamine*, and *ephedrine* (often found in nasal sprays), or *appetite suppressants* may decrease their stimulatory and pressor effects. Because of its alpha-blocking potential, molindone may cause *epinephrine* reversal, a hypotensive response to epinephrine.

Molindone may inhibit blood pressure response to *centrally acting antihypertensive drugs*, such as *clonidine, guanabenz, guanadrel, guanethidine, methyldopa*, and *reserpine*. Additive effects are likely after concomitant use of molindone with *CNS depressants*, including *alcohol, analgesics, barbiturates, narcotics, tranquilizers*, and *general, spinal, or epidural anesthetics*, or *parenteral magnesium sulfate* (oversedation, respiratory depression, and hypotension); *antiarrhythmic agents, disopyramide, quinidine*, or *procainamide* (increased incidence of cardiac arrhythmias and conduction defects); *atropine* or other *anticholinergic drugs*, including *antidepressants, antihistamines, MAO inhibitors, meperidine, phenothiazines*, and *antiparkinson agents* (oversedation, paralytic ileus, visual changes, and severe constipation); *nitrates* (hypotension); and *metrizamide* (increased risk of seizures).

Beta-blocking agents may inhibit molindone metabolism, increasing plasma levels and toxicity.

Concomitant use with *propylthiouracil* increases risk of agranulocytosis and decreases therapeutic response to molindone.

Decreased therapeutic response to molindone may follow concomitant use with *calcium-containing drugs*, such as *phenytoin* and *tetracyclines, aluminum- and magnesium-containing antacids*, or *antidiarrheals* (decreased absorption); or *caffeine* (increased metabolism).

Molindone may antagonize therapeutic effect of *bromocriptine* on prolactin secretion; it may also decrease the vasoconstricting effects of *high-dose dopamine* and may decrease effectiveness and increase toxicity of *levodopa* (by dopamine blockade). *Calcium sulfate* in molindone tablets may inhibit the absorption of phenytoin or tetracyclines.

Effects on diagnostic tests

Drug causes false-positive results in urine pregnancy tests using human chorionic gonadotropin and additive potential for causing seizures with metrizamide myelography.

Molindone elevates levels of liver enzymes (AST and ALT), free fatty acids, and BUN; drug may alter WBC counts and may increase or decrease serum glucose levels.

Adverse reactions

CNS: *extrapyramidal reactions, tardive dyskinesia, sedation, drowsiness, depression, euphoria, pseudoparkinsonism, EEG changes, dizziness.*
CV: *orthostatic hypotension, tachycardia, ECG changes.*
EENT: *blurred vision.*
GI: *dry mouth, constipation, nausea.*
GU: *urine retention, menstrual irregularities, gynecomastia, inhibited ejaculation.*
Hematologic: ***leukopenia,*** leukocytosis.
Hepatic: jaundice, abnormal liver function test results.
Skin: *mild photosensitivity, allergic reactions.*
Other: ***neuroleptic malignant syndrome*** (rare).

Overdose and treatment

CNS depression is characterized by deep, unarousable sleep and possible coma, hypotension or hypertension, extrapyramidal symptoms, abnormal involuntary muscle movements, agitation, seizures, arrhythmias, ECG changes, hypothermia or hyperthermia, and autonomic nervous system dysfunction.

Treatment is symptomatic and supportive, including maintaining vital signs, airway, stable body temperature, and fluid/electrolyte balance.

Do not induce vomiting: drug inhibits cough reflex, and aspiration may occur. Use gastric lavage, then activated charcoal and sodium chloride cathartics; dialysis does not help. Regulate body temperature as needed. Treat hypotension with I.V. fluids: do not give epinephrine. Treat seizures with parenteral diazepam or barbiturates; arrhythmias, with parenteral phenytoin (1 mg/kg with rate titrated to blood pressure); extrapyramidal reactions, with benztropine at 1 to 2 mg or parenteral diphenhydramine at 10 to 50 mg.

☑ Special considerations

- Drug may cause GI distress and should be administered with food or fluids.
- Dilute concentrate in 2 to 4 oz of liquid, preferably soup, water, juice, carbonated drinks, milk, or puddings.
- Drug may cause pink to brown discoloration of urine.
- Protect liquid form from light.

Patient education

- Explain risks of dystonic reaction and tardive dyskinesia, and advise him to report abnormal body movements.
- Warn patient to avoid spilling liquid preparation on the skin; rash and irritation may result.
- Advise patient to avoid temperature extremes (hot or cold baths, sunlamps, or tanning beds) because drug may cause thermoregulatory changes.
- Suggest sugarless gum or candy, ice chips, or artificial saliva to relieve dry mouth.
- Warn patient not to take drug with antacids or antidiarrheals; not to drink alcoholic beverages or take other drugs that cause sedation; not to stop taking drug or take any other drug except as instructed; and to take drug exactly as prescribed, without doubling after missing a dose.
- Warn patient about sedative effect. Tell him to report difficult urination, sore throat, dizziness, or fainting.
- Advise patient to get up slowly from a recumbent or seated position to minimize effects of light-headedness.
- Tell patient that drug may contain sodium metabisulfite, which can cause an allergic reaction to those with a sulfite allergy.

Geriatric use

- Lower doses are recommended; 30% to 50% of usual dose may be effective. Elderly patients are at greater risk for tardive dyskinesia and other extrapyramidal effects.

Pediatric use

- Drug is not recommended for children under age 12.

montelukast sodium

Singulair

Pharmacologic classification: leukotriene receptor antagonist
Therapeutic classification: antiasthmatic
Pregnancy risk category B

How supplied

Available by prescription only
Tablets: 10 mg
Tablets (chewable): 5 mg

Indications, route, and dosage

For prophylaxis and chronic treatment of asthma
Adults and adolescents: 10 mg P.O. once daily in evening.
Children age 6 to 14: 5 mg (chewable tablet) P.O. once daily in the evening.

Pharmacodynamics

Antiasthmatic action: Montelukast causes inhibition of airway cysteinyl leukotriene receptors. Drug binds with high affinity and selectivity to the $CysLT_1$ receptor, and inhibits the physiologic action of the cysteinyl leukotriene LTD_4. This receptor inhibition reduces early- and late-phase bronchoconstriction due to antigen challenge.

Pharmacokinetics

- *Absorption*: Rapidly absorbed after oral administration with mean peak plasma concentrations achieved in 3 to 4 hours, and mean oral bioavailability of 64%. Food does not affect absorption of drug. For chewable tablet, peak levels are reached in 2 to 2½ hours and mean oral bioavailability is 73%.
- *Distribution*: Drug is minimally distributed to the tissues with a steady-state volume of distribution of 8 to 11 L. Over 99% bound to plasma proteins.
- *Metabolism:* Extensively metabolized, but plasma concentrations of metabolites at therapeutic doses are undetectable. In vitro studies with human liver microsomes demonstrate metabolism involvement by cytochromes P-450 3A4 and 2C9.
- *Excretion:* Approximately 86% of an oral dose is metabolized and excreted in the feces, indicating drug and its metabolites are excreted almost exclusively in the bile. Half life is 2.7 to 5.5 hours.

Contraindications and precautions

Contraindicated in patients with hypersensitivity to drug or its components. Also contraindicated in patients with acute asthmatic attacks or status asthmaticus. Although airway function is improved in patients with known aspirin hypersensitivity, these patients should avoid aspirin and NSAIDs.

Interactions
Use caution when montelukast is used with *drugs known to inhibit 3A4 and 2C9 enzymes.* Clinical monitoring may be needed when drug is given with *phenobarbital* or *rifampin,* which induce hepatic metabolism.

Effects on diagnostic tests
Drug therapy may increase ALT and AST levels.

Adverse reactions
CNS: *headache,* dizziness, fatigue, asthenia.
EENT: nasal congestion, dental pain.
GI: dyspepsia, infectious gastroenteritis, abdominal pain.
Respiratory: cough, influenza.
Skin: rash.
Other: fever, trauma.

Overdose and treatment
No specific information is available on treatment of drug overdose. Provide supportive measures for overdose such as removal of unabsorbed material from the GI tract and clinical monitoring.

☑ Special considerations
- Although dose of inhaled corticosteroids may be reduced gradually, montelukast should not be abruptly substituted for inhaled or oral corticosteroids.
- Drug should not be used as monotherapy for management of exercise-induced bronchospasm.
- No added benefit is achieved with doses above 10 mg daily.

Patient education
- Advise patient to take drug daily, even if asymptomatic, and to contact primary health care provider if asthma is not well controlled.
- Warn patient that drug is not beneficial in acute asthma attacks, or in exercise-induced bronchospasm and advise him to keep appropriate rescue medications available.
- Advise patient with known aspirin sensitivity not to take aspirin and NSAIDs.
- Warn patient with phenylketonuria that chewable tablet contains phenylalanine, a component of aspartame.
- Advise patients to seek medical attention if short-acting bronchodilators are needed more often than usual or prescribed.

Geriatric use
- No difference in safety and effectiveness of drug has been reported between elderly and younger patient populations.

Pediatric use
- Safety and efficacy in children under age 6 has not been established.

Breast-feeding
- It is not known if drug is excreted in breast milk. Use drug with caution in breast-feeding patients.

moricizine hydrochloride
Ethmozine

Pharmacologic classification: sodium channel blocker
Therapeutic classification: antiarrhythmic
Pregnancy risk category: B

How supplied
Available by prescription only
Tablets: 200 mg, 250 mg, 300 mg

Indications, route, and dosage
Treatment of documented, life-threatening ventricular arrhythmias when benefit of treatment outweighs risks
Adults: Dosage must be individualized. Usual range is 600 to 900 mg daily given q 8 hours in equally divided doses. Dosage may be adjusted within this range in increments of 150 mg daily at 3-day intervals until desired effect is obtained. Hospitalization is recommended for initiation of therapy because patient will be at high risk.

Pharmacodynamics
Antiarrhythmic action: Although moricizine is chemically related to the neuroleptic phenothiazines, it has no demonstrated dopaminergic activities. It does have potent local anesthetic activity and myocardial membrane stabilizing effects. A class I antiarrhythmic agent, it reduces the fast inward current carried by sodium ions. In patients with ventricular tachycardia, moricizine prolongs AV conduction but has no significant effect on ventricular repolarization. Intra-atrial conduction or atrial effective refractory periods are not consistently affected and moricizine has minimal effect on sinus cycle length and sinus node recovery time. This may be significant in patients with sinus node dysfunction.

In patients with impaired left ventricular function, moricizine has minimal effects on measurements of cardiac performance: cardiac index, stroke volume, pulmonary capillary wedge pressure, systemic or pulmonary vascular resistance, and ejection fraction either at rest or during exercise. A small but consistent increase in resting blood pressure and heart rate are seen. Moricizine has no effect on exercise tolerance in patients with ventricular arrhythmias, heart failure, or angina pectoris.

Moricizine has antiarrhythmic activity similar to that of disopyramide, propranolol, and quinidine. Arrhythmia "rebound" is not noted after discontinuation of therapy.

Pharmacokinetics
- *Absorption:* Peak plasma concentrations are usually reached within ½ to 2 hours. Administration within ½ hour of mealtime delays absorption and lowers peak plasma levels but has no effect on extent of absorption.
- *Distribution:* Moricizine is 95% plasma protein-bound.
- *Metabolism:* Drug undergoes significant first-pass metabolism resulting in an absolute bioavailability of approximately 38%. At least 26 metabolites have

been identified with no single one representing at least 1% of the administered dose. It has been shown to induce its own metabolism.
• *Excretion:* 56% is excreted in feces; 39%, in urine; some is also recycled through enterohepatic circulation.

Contraindications and precautions
Contraindicated in patients with cardiogenic shock and in those with hypersensitivity to drug, preexisting second- or third-degree AV block or right bundle branch block when associated with left hemiblock (bifascicular block) unless an artificial pacemaker is present. Discontinue breast-feeding or drug because drug is detected in breast milk.

Use cautiously in patients with impaired renal or hepatic function, sick sinus syndrome, coronary artery disease, or left ventricular function.

Interactions
Concomitant use with *cimetidine* decreases moricizine clearance by 49%; no significant changes in efficacy or tolerance were observed. Patients should receive decreased doses of cimetadine (not more than 600 mg/day). Use with *propranolol* may produce a small additive increase in the PR interval. *Theophylline* clearance increases and plasma half-life decreases with concomitant therapy; monitor when moricizine is added or discontinued. Concomitant *digoxin* therapy prolongs the PR interval.

Effects on diagnostic tests
Drug may elevate liver function test results.

Adverse reactions
CNS: *dizziness, headache, fatigue,* hyperesthesia, anxiety, asthenia, nervousness, paresthesia, sleep disorders.
CV: ***proarrhythmic events (ventricular tachycardia, premature ventricular contractions, supraventricular arrhythmias),*** ECG abnormalities (including *conduction defects, sinus pause, junctional rhythm,* or ***AV block***), ***heart failure***, palpitations, chest pain, ***cardiac death***, hypotension, hypertension, vasodilation, cerebrovascular events.
EENT: blurred vision.
GI: *nausea, vomiting, abdominal pain, dyspepsia, diarrhea, dry mouth.*
GU: urine retention, urinary frequency, dysuria.
Respiratory: dyspnea.
Skin: rash.
Other: drug-induced fever, diaphoresis, musculoskeletal pain, thrombophlebitis.

Overdose and treatment
Symptoms of overdose include emesis, lethargy, coma, syncope, hypotension, conduction disturbances, exacerbation of heart failure, MI, sinus arrest, arrhythmias, and respiratory failure. No specific antidote has been identified.

Treatment should be supportive and include careful monitoring of cardiac, respiratory, and CNS changes. Gastric evacuation with care to avoid aspiration may be used as well.

☑ Special considerations
• When transferring from another antiarrhythmic to moricizine, previous therapy should be withdrawn one to two half-lives before initiating moricizine.
• Initial dosage for patients with renal or hepatic impairment is 600 mg daily or lower. Monitor patient (with ECG) before making dosage adjustments.
• Correct electrolyte imbalances before starting therapy; hypokalemia, hyperkalemia, or hypomagnesemia may alter drug's effects.

Pediatric use
• Safety and efficacy have not been established.

Breast-feeding
• Drug is excreted in breast milk. Because of the potential for adverse reactions in the breast-fed infant, a decision whether or not to continue therapy must be made.

morphine hydrochloride*
Morphitec*, M.O.S.*

morphine sulfate
Astramorph PF, Duramorph, Epimorph*, Infumorph, MS Contin, MSIR, MS/L, MS/S, OMS Concentrate, Oramorph SR, RMS Uniserts, Roxanol, Statex*

Pharmacologic classification: opioid
Therapeutic classification: narcotic analgesic
Controlled substance schedule II
Pregnancy risk category C

How supplied
Available by prescription only
morphine hydrochloride*
Tablets: 10 mg, 20 mg, 40 mg, 60 mg
Syrup: 1 mg/ml, 5 mg/ml, 10 mg/ml, 20 mg/ml, 50 mg/ml
Suppositories: 20 mg, 30 mg
morphine sulfate
Tablets: 15 mg, 30 mg
Tablets (extended-release): 15 mg, 30 mg, 60 mg, 100 mg, 200 mg
Tablets (soluble): 10 mg, 15 mg, 30 mg
Oral solution: 4 mg/ml, 10 mg/5 ml, 20 mg/5 ml, 20 mg/ml, 100 mg/5 ml
Injection (with preservative): 1 mg/ml, 2 mg/ml, 3 mg/ml, 4 mg/ml, 5 mg/ml, 8 mg/ml, 10 mg/ml, 15 mg/ml, 25 mg/ml, 50 mg/ml
Injection (without preservative): 500 mcg/ml, 1 mg/ml, 10 mg/ml, 25 mg/ml
Suppositories: 5 mg, 10 mg, 20 mg, 30 mg

Indications, route, and dosage
Severe pain
Adults: 10 mg q 4 hours S.C. or I.M., or 10 to 30 mg P.O., or 10 to 20 mg P.R. q 4 hours, p.r.n. or around the clock. May be injected slow I.V. (over 4 to 5 minutes) 2.5 to 15 mg diluted in 4 to 5 ml water for injection. May also administer controlled-release tablets 30 mg q 8 to 12 hours. As an epidural injection, 5 mg via an epidural catheter q 24 hours.

Children: 0.1 to 0.2 mg/kg S.C. q 4 hours. Maximum dose is 15 mg. In some situations, morphine may be administered by continuous I.V. infusion or by intraspinal and intrathecal injection.

Preoperative sedation and adjunct to anesthesia
Adults: 8 to 10 mg I.M., S.C., or I.V.

Control of pain associated with acute MI
Adults: 8 to 15 mg I.M., S.C., or I.V. Additional, smaller doses may be given in 3- to 4-hour intervals p.r.n.

Adjunctive treatment of acute pulmonary edema
Adults: 10 to 15 mg I.V. at a rate not exceeding 2 mg/minute.

Pharmacodynamics

Analgesic action: Morphine is the principal opium alkaloid, the standard for opiate agonist analgesic activity. Mechanism of action is thought to be via the opiate receptors, altering patient's perception of pain. Morphine is particularly useful in severe, acute pain or severe, chronic pain. Morphine also has a central depressant effect on respiration and on the cough reflex center.

Pharmacokinetics

- *Absorption:* Variable absorption from the GI tract. Onset of analgesia occurs within 15 to 60 minutes. Peak analgesia occurs ½ to 1 hour after dosing.
- *Distribution:* Morphine is distributed widely through the body.
- *Metabolism:* Drug is metabolized primarily in the liver.
- *Excretion:* Duration of action is 3 to 7 hours. Morphine is excreted in the urine and bile.

Contraindications and precautions

Contraindicated in patients with hypersensitivity to drug or conditions that would preclude administration of opioids by I.V. route (acute bronchial asthma or upper airway obstruction).

Use cautiously in elderly or debilitated patients and in those with head injury, increased intracranial pressure, seizures, pulmonary disease, prostatic hyperplasia, hepatic or renal disease, acute abdominal conditions, hypothyroidism, Addison's disease, or urethral strictures.

Interactions

Concomitant use with other *CNS depressants* (*alcohol, narcotic analgesics, general anesthetics, antihistamines, barbiturates, benzodiazepines, MAO inhibitors, muscle relaxants, phenothiazines, sedative-hypnotics, tricyclic antidepressants*) potentiates drug's respiratory and CNS depression, sedation, and hypotensive effects. Concomitant use with *cimetidine* also may increase respiratory and CNS depression, causing confusion, disorientation, apnea, or seizures. Reduced dosage of morphine is usually necessary.

Drug accumulation and enhanced effects may result from concomitant use with other *drugs that are extensively metabolized in the liver* (*digitoxin, phenytoin, rifampin*); combined use with anticholinergics may cause paralytic ileus.

Patients who become physically dependent on this drug may experience acute withdrawal syndrome if given a *narcotic antagonist.*

Severe CV depression may result from concomitant use with *general anesthetics.*

Effects on diagnostic tests

Morphine increases plasma amylase levels.

Adverse reactions

CNS: *sedation, somnolence, clouded sensorium, euphoria,* ***seizures*** (with large doses), *dizziness, nightmares (with long-acting oral forms),* light-headedness, hallucinations, nervousness, depression, syncope.
CV: *hypotension, bradycardia,* ***shock, cardiac arrest,*** tachycardia, hypertension.
GI: *nausea, vomiting, constipation, ileus, dry mouth, biliary tract spasms, anorexia.*
GU: *urine retention, decreased libido.*
Hematologic: ***thrombocytopenia.***
Respiratory: ***respiratory depression***, apnea, ***respiratory arrest.***
Skin: pruritus, skin flushing (with epidural administration); *diaphoresis; edema.*
Other: *physical dependence.*

Overdose and treatment

Rapid I.V. administration may result in overdose because of the delay in maximum CNS effect (30 minutes). The most common signs and symptoms of morphine overdose is respiratory depression with or without CNS depression, and miosis (pinpoint pupils). Other acute toxic effects include hypotension, bradycardia, hypothermia, shock, apnea, cardiopulmonary arrest, circulatory collapse, pulmonary edema, and seizures.

To treat acute overdose, first establish adequate respiratory exchange via a patent airway and ventilation as needed; administer a narcotic antagonist (naloxone) to reverse respiratory depression. (Because duration of action of morphine is longer than that of naloxone, repeated naloxone dosing is necessary.) Naloxone should not be given in the absence of clinically significant respiratory or CV depression. Monitor vital signs closely.

If patient presents within 2 hours of ingestion of an oral overdose, empty the stomach immediately by inducing emesis (ipecac syrup) or using gastric lavage. Use caution to avoid risk of aspiration. Administer activated charcoal via nasogastric tube for further removal of drug in an oral overdose.

Provide symptomatic and supportive treatment (continued respiratory support, correction of fluid or electrolyte imbalance). Monitor laboratory parameters, vital signs, and neurologic status closely.

☑ Special considerations

Besides those relevant to all *opioids,* consider the following recommendations.

- Morphine is drug of choice in relieving pain of MI; may cause transient decrease in blood pressure.
- Regimented scheduling (around-the-clock) is beneficial in severe, chronic pain.
- Oral solutions of various concentrations are available, as well as a new intensified oral solution.

• Note the disparity between oral and parenteral doses.
• For S.L. administration, measure out oral solution with tuberculin syringe, and administer dose a few drops at a time to allow maximal sublingual absorption and to minimize swallowing.
• Refrigeration of rectal suppositories is not necessary. Note that in some patients, rectal and oral absorption may not be equivalent.
• Preservative-free preparations are now available for epidural and intrathecal administration. The use of the epidural route is increasing.
• Epidural morphine has proven to be an excellent analgesic for patients with postoperative pain. After epidural administration, monitor closely for respiratory depression up to 24 hours after the injection. Check respiratory rate and depth according to protocol (for example, every 15 minutes for 2 hours, then hourly for 18 hours). Some clinicians advocate a dilute naloxone infusion (5 to 10 mcg/kg/hour) during the first 12 hours to minimize respiratory depression without altering pain relief.
• Morphine may worsen or mask gallbladder pain.

Patient education
• Tell patient that oral liquid form of morphine may be mixed with a glass of fruit juice immediately before it is taken, if desired, to improve the taste.
• Tell patient taking long-acting morphine tablets to swallow them whole. Tablets should not be broken, crushed, or chewed before swallowing.

Geriatric use
• Lower doses are usually indicated for elderly patients, who may be more sensitive to the therapeutic and adverse effects of drug.

Breast-feeding
• Morphine is excreted in breast milk. A woman should wait 2 to 3 hours after last dose before breast-feeding to avoid sedation in the infant.

mumps skin test antigen
MSTA

Pharmacologic classification: viral antigen
Therapeutic classification: skin test antigen
Pregnancy risk category C

How supplied
Available by prescription only
Injection: 40 complement-fixing units/ml suspension; 10 tests/1-ml vial

Indications, route, and dosage
Assessment of cell-mediated immunity
Adults and children: 0.1 ml intradermally into the inner surface of the forearm.

Pharmacodynamics
Antigenic action: Mumps skin test is not indicated for the immunization, diagnosis, or treatment of mumps virus infection.

The status of cell-mediated immunity can be determined from use of mumps with other antigens. In vitro tests (such as lymphocyte stimulation and assays for T and B cells) are necessary to diagnose a specific disorder.

Pharmacokinetics
• *Absorption:* After intradermal injection of mumps skin test antigen, the test site should be examined in 48 to 72 hours.
• *Distribution:* Injection must be given intradermally; S.C. injection invalidates the test.
• *Metabolism:* Not applicable.
• *Excretion:* Not applicable.

Contraindications and precautions
Contraindicated in persons sensitive to avian protein (chicken, eggs, or feathers) and in those hypersensitive to thimerosal. Use cautiously in elderly patients and in patients who are immunosuppressed.

Interactions
Long-term use of *cimetidine* may augment or enhance delayed-sensitivity responses, which may be suppressed in patients receiving *immunosuppressants* or *viral vaccines.*

Effects on diagnostic tests
None reported.

Adverse reactions
CNS: headache, drowsiness.
GI: nausea, anorexia.
Other: tenderness, pruritus, and rash occur at injection site. Occasionally, a severe delayed-hypersensitivity reaction will produce vesiculation, local tissue necrosis, abscess, and scar formation, ***anaphylaxis***, Arthus reaction, urticaria, ***angioedema***, shortness of breath, excessive perspiration.

Overdose and treatment
Administer epinephrine 1:1,000 if anaphylaxis occurs.

☑ Special considerations
• Obtain history of allergies and reactions to skin tests. In patients hypersensitive to feathers, eggs, or chicken, a severe reaction may follow administration of mumps skin test antigen.
• After injection of mumps skin test antigen, observe patient for 15 minutes for possible immediate-type systemic allergic reaction. Keep epinephrine 1:1,000 available.
• Accurate dosage (0.1 ml) and administration are essential with the use of mumps skin test antigen.
• Examine injection site within 48 to 72 hours, interpreting as follows:
Positive reaction: Induration of 5 mm or more, with or without erythema, indicates sensitivity.
Negative reaction: Induration less than 5 mm means the individual has not been sensitized to mumps or is anergic.
• Reactivity to this test may be depressed or suppressed for as long as 6 weeks in individuals who have received concurrent virus vaccines, in those

who are receiving a corticosteroid or other immunosuppressive agents, in those who have had viral infections, and in malnourished patients.
- Mumps skin test antigen is not used to assess exposure to mumps. It is used in assessing T-cell function for immunocompetence since most normal individuals will exhibit a positive reaction.
- Cold packs or topical steroids may give relief from the symptoms of pain, pruritus, and discomfort if a local reaction occurs.
- Store vial in refrigerator.

Patient education
- Tell patient to report unusual adverse effects.
- Explain that induration will disappear in a few days.

Geriatric use
- Elderly patients who do not react to test are considered anergic.

Breast-feeding
- Benefit of the mumps skin test to breast-feeding patient should be weighed against possible risk to the infant.

mumps virus vaccine, live
Mumpsvax

Pharmacologic classification: vaccine
Therapeutic classification: viral vaccine
Pregnancy risk category C

How supplied
Available by prescription only
Injection: single-dose vial containing not less than 20,000 $TCID_{50}$ (tissue culture infective doses) of attenuated mumps virus derived from Jeryl Lynn mumps strain (grown in chick embryo culture), and vial of diluent

Indications, route, and dosage
Immunization
Adults and children over age 1: 1 vial (0.5 ml) S.C. in outer aspect of the upper arm.

Pharmacodynamics
Mumps prophylaxis: Vaccine promotes active immunity to mumps.

Pharmacokinetics
- *Absorption:* Antibodies usually are evident 2 to 3 weeks after injection. Duration of vaccine-induced immunity is at least 20 years and probably lifelong.
- *Distribution:* No information available.
- *Metabolism:* No information available.
- *Excretion:* No information available.

Contraindications and precautions
Contraindicated in immunosuppressed patients; in those with cancer, blood dyscrasias, gamma globulin disorders, fever, untreated active tuberculosis, or anaphylactic or anaphylactoid reactions to neomycin or eggs; in those receiving corticosteroid or radiation therapy; and in pregnant patients.

Interactions
Concomitant use of mumps vaccine with *immune serum globulin* or *transfusions of blood or blood products* may interfere with immune response to vaccine. If possible, vaccination should be deferred for 3 months in these situations.

Coadministration of *immunosuppressive agents* may interfere with response to vaccine.

Effects on diagnostic tests
Vaccine temporarily may decrease the response to tuberculin skin testing. If a tuberculin skin test is necessary, administer it either before or simultaneously with mumps vaccine.

Adverse reactions
CNS: ***febrile seizures*** (rare).
Other: *slight fever, rash, malaise, mild allergic reactions, mild lymphadenopathy, diarrhea, injection-site reaction.*

Overdose and treatment
No information available.

☑ Special considerations
- Mumps vaccine should not be used in delayed hypersensitivity (anergy) skin testing.
- Obtain a thorough history of allergies, especially to antibiotics, eggs, chicken, or chicken feathers, and of reactions to immunizations.
- Perform skin testing to assess vaccine sensitivity (against a control of 0.9% NaCl solution in the opposite arm) in patients with history of anaphylactoid reactions to egg ingestion. Administer an intradermal or scratch test with a 1:10 dilution. Read results after 5 to 30 minutes. A positive reaction is a wheal with or without pseudopodia and surrounding erythema. If sensitivity test is positive, consider desensitization.
- Epinephrine solution 1:1,000 should be available to treat allergic reactions.
- Do not administer vaccine I.V. Use a 25G, ⅝" needle and inject S.C., preferably into the outer aspect of the upper arm.
- Use only diluent supplied. Discard reconstituted solution after 8 hours.
- Store in refrigerator and protect from light. Solution may be used if red, pink, or yellow, but it must be clear.
- Do not give vaccine less than 1 month before or after immunization with other live virus vaccines—except for live, attenuated measles virus vaccine, live rubella virus vaccine, or monovalent or trivalent live oral poliovirus vaccine, which may be administered simultaneously.
- Vaccine does not offer protection when given after exposure to natural mumps.
- Revaccination is not required if primary vaccine was given at age 1 or older.

Patient education
- Tell patient that he may experience pain and inflammation at the injection site and a low-grade fever, rash, or general malaise.
- Encourage patient to report distressing adverse reactions.

• Recommend acetaminophen to alleviate adverse reactions, such as fever.
• Tell female patient of childbearing age to avoid pregnancy for 3 months after vaccination. Provide contraceptive information if necessary.

Pediatric use
• Vaccine is not recommended for children under age 1 because retained maternal mumps antibodies may interfere with immune response.

Breast-feeding
• It is unknown if vaccine occurs in breast milk. No problems have been reported. Use vaccine cautiously in breast-feeding women.

mupirocin (pseudomonic acid A)
Bactroban, Bactroban Nasal

Pharmacologic classification: antibiotic
Therapeutic classification: topical antibacterial
Pregnancy risk category B

How supplied
Available by prescription only
Ointment: 2% (1-g single-use tubes, 15 g, 30 g)

Indications, route, and dosage
***Topical treatment of impetigo due to* Staphylococcus aureus, beta-hemolytic Streptococcus, *and* Streptococcus pyogenes**
Adults and children: Apply a small amount to affected area, t.i.d. The area treated may be covered with a gauze dressing if desired.
***Eradication of nasal colonization of methicillin-resistant* Staphylococcus aureus**
Adults: Apply one-half of a single-use tube to each nostril b.i.d. for 5 days.

Pharmacodynamics
Antibacterial action: Mupirocin is structurally unrelated to other agents and is produced by fermentation of the organism *Pseudomonas fluorescens.* Mupirocin inhibits bacterial protein synthesis by reversibly and specifically binding to bacterial isoleucyl transfer-RNA synthetase. Mupirocin shows no cross-resistance with chloramphenicol, erythromycin, gentamicin, lincomycin, methicillin, neomycin, novobiocin, penicillin, streptomycin, or tetracycline.

Pharmacokinetics
• *Absorption:* Normal subjects showed no absorption after 24-hour application under occlusive dressings.
• *Distribution:* Mupirocin is highly protein-bound (about 95%). A substantial decrease in activity can be expected in the presence of serum (as in exudative wounds).
• *Metabolism:* Drug is slightly metabolized locally in the skin to monic acid.
• *Excretion:* Eliminated locally by desquamation of the skin.

Contraindications and precautions
Contraindicated in patients hypersensitive to drug. Use cautiously in patients with burns or impaired renal function.

Interactions
None reported.

Effects on diagnostic tests
None reported.

Adverse reactions
CNS: headache (with nasal use).
EENT: rhinitis, upper respiratory congestion, pharyngitis, taste perversion, burning, cough (with nasal use).
Skin: burning, pruritus, stinging, rash, pain, erythema (with topical administration).

Overdose and treatment
No information available.

☑ Special considerations
• Reevaluate patients not showing a clinical response within 3 to 5 days.
• If sensitivity or chemical irritation occurs, discontinue treatment and institute appropriate alternative therapy.
• When used on burns or to treat extensive open wounds, absorption of polyethylene glycol vehicle is possible and may result in serious renal toxicity.
• Monitor for superinfection. Use of antibiotics (prolonged or repeated) may result in bacterial or fungal overgrowth of nonsusceptible organisms. Such overgrowth may lead to a secondary infection.

Patient education
• Advise patient to wash and dry affected areas thoroughly. Then apply thin film, rubbing in gently.
• For nasal application, use single-use tube for one application only, then discard tube. Apply one-half of the ointment from the tube into one nostril and the remaining into the other nostril, in the morning and evening.
• Avoid contact around eyes and mucous membranes.

Breast-feeding
• It is not known if drug is present in breast milk. Use with caution.

muromonab-CD3
Orthoclone OKT3

Pharmacologic classification: monoclonal antibody
Therapeutic classification: immunosuppressive
Pregnancy risk category C

How supplied
Injection: 5 mg/5 ml in 5-ml ampules

Indications, route, and dosage

Treatment of acute allograft rejection in renal, cardiac, and hepatic transplant patients

Adults: 5 mg/day, for 10 to 14 days. Begin treatment once acute renal rejection is diagnosed.

Note: A "first-dose" reaction is common within ½ to 6 hours after the first dose, consisting of significant fever, chills, dyspnea, and malaise. Pulmonary edema may occur if patient is not pretreated with a corticosteroid.

Pharmacodynamics

Immunosuppressive action: Muromonab-CD3 reverses graft rejection, probably by interfering with T cell function that promotes acute renal rejection. It interacts with, and prevents the function of, the T cell antigen receptor complex in the cellular membrane, which influences antigen recognition and is essential for signal transduction. Muromonab-CD3 reacts with most peripheral T cells in blood and in body tissues, and blocks all known T cell functions.

Pharmacokinetics

- *Absorption:* Immediate after I.V. administration.
- *Distribution:* Unknown.
- *Metabolism:* Unknown.
- *Excretion:* Unknown.

Contraindications and precautions

Contraindicated in pregnant and breast-feeding patients. Also contraindicated in patients with hypersensitivity to drug or to other products of murine (mouse) origin and in those with antimurine antibody titers of 1:1,000 or more; fluid overload, as evidenced by chest radiograph or a weight gain greater than 3% within week before treatment; or history of seizures or predisposition to seizures.

Interactions

Muromonab-CD3 may potentiate immunosuppressive effects of other *immunosuppressant drugs* (*azathioprine, cyclosporine*).

Effects on diagnostic tests

None reported.

Adverse reactions

CNS: *tremor, headache,* ***seizures, encephalopathy, cerebral edema, coma.***

CV: *chest pain, tachycardia, hypertension,* ***cardiac arrest.***

GI: *nausea, vomiting, diarrhea.*

Respiratory: ***severe pulmonary edema, respiratory arrest***, dyspnea, wheezing.

Other: *fever, chills, tremors,* ***infection, anaphylaxis***, increased serum creatinine, ***cytokine release syndrome*** (from flulike symptoms to shock), ***aseptic meningitis, risk of neoplasia.***

Overdose and treatment

No information available.

☑ Special considerations

- Preparation of solution: Draw solution into a syringe through a low protein-binding 0.2 or 0.22 micrometer (mcm) filter. Discard filter and attach needle for I.V. bolus injection.
- Because drug is a protein solution, it may develop a few fine translucent particles, which do not affect its potency.
- Administer as an I.V. bolus in less than 1 minute. Do not give by I.V. infusion or combined with other drug solutions.
- The manufacturer recommends that if patient's temperature exceeds 100° F (37.8° C), lower it with antipyretics before drug administration.
- Chest radiograph taken within 24 hours before treatment must be clear of fluid; monitor WBCs and differentials at intervals during treatment. Monitor drug's effect on circulating T cells using flow cytometry or by expressing the CD3 antigen by in vitro assay.
- Immunosuppressive therapy increases susceptibility to infection and to lymphoproliferative disorders. Lymphomas may follow immunosuppressive therapy; their occurrence seems related to the intensity and duration of immunosuppression rather than the use of specific agents since most patients receive a combination of treatments.
- Reduce concomitant immunosuppressive therapy to daily dose of prednisone 0.5 mg/kg and azathioprine 25 mg. Reduce or discontinue cyclosporine. Maintenance immunosuppression can resume 3 days before stopping muromonab-CD3.
- Refrigerate drug at 36° to 46° F (2° to 8° C). Do not freeze or shake.

Patient education

- Inform patients of expected first-dose effects (fever, chills, dyspnea, chest pain, nausea, vomiting).

Pediatric use

- Safety and efficacy in children have not been established. Patients as young as age 2 have had no unexpected adverse effects.

Breast-feeding

- Safety in breast-feeding women has not been established.

mycophenolate mofetil

CellCept

Pharmacologic classification: mycophenolic acid derivative
Therapeutic classification: immunosuppressive
Pregnancy risk category C

How supplied

Available by prescription only
Capsules: 250 mg

Indications, route, and dosage

Prophylaxis of organ rejection in patients receiving allogeneic renal transplants

Adults: 1 g P.O. b.i.d. started within 72 hours following transplantation. Use in combination with corticosteroids and cyclosporine.

Pharmacodynamics

Immunosuppressive action: Mycophenolate inhibits proliferative responses of T- and B-lymphocytes, suppresses antibody formation by B-lymphocytes, and may inhibit recruitment of leukocytes into sites of inflammation and graft rejection.

Pharmacokinetics

- *Absorption:* Absorbed from the GI tract. Absolute bioavailability of drug is 94%.
- *Distribution:* About 97% of drug is bound to plasma protein.
- *Metabolism:* Drug undergoes complete presystemic metabolism to mycophenolic acid.
- *Excretion:* Primarily excreted in urine with a small amount excreted in feces. Half-life is about 17.9 hours.

Contraindications and precautions

Contraindicated in patients with hypersensitivity to drug, mycophenolic acid, or any component of drug product. Drug should not be used during pregnancy unless the benefits outweigh the risks. Use cautiously in patients with GI disorders.

Interactions

Acyclovir and *ganciclovir* increase risk of toxicity for both drugs. Monitor patient closely. *Antacids with magnesium and aluminum hydroxides* decrease the absorption of mycophenolate mofetil. Separate dosages. *Cholestyramine* may interfere with enterohepatic recirculation, causing a decrease in mycophenolate bioavailability. Do not administer concurrently. Mycophenolate may affect efficacy of *oral contraceptives.* Advise patient to use alternative contraceptive measure.

Effects on diagnostic tests

None reported.

Adverse reactions

CNS: *tremor,* insomnia, dizziness, *headache.*
CV: *chest pain, hypertension, edema.*
GI: *diarrhea, constipation, nausea, dyspepsia, vomiting, oral moniliasis, abdominal pain.*
GU: *urinary tract infection, hematuria,* kidney tubular necrosis.
Hematologic: *anemia,* LEUKOPENIA, THROMBOCYTOPENIA, hypochromic anemia, leukocytosis.
Metabolic: *hypercholesteremia, hypophosphatemia, hypokalemia,* hyperkalemia, hyperglycemia.
Respiratory: *dyspnea, cough,* pharyngitis, bronchitis, pneumonia.
Skin: *acne,* rash.
Other: *pain, fever, sepsis, asthenia, back pain, possible immunosuppression-induced infection or lymphoma.*

Overdose and treatment

Although there is no reported experience of overdosage in humans, doses of 4 to 5 g/day compared with 3 g/day caused an increase in nausea, vomiting, or diarrhea and occasional hematologic abnormalities in some patients. Treatment includes use of bile acid sequestrants to increase the excretion of drug.

☑ Special considerations

- Avoid doses exceeding 1 g b.i.d. in patients with severe chronic renal impairment (glomerular filtration rate below 25 ml/minute) outside the immediate post-transplant period.
- Because of potential teratogenic effects, do not open or crush capsules. Also avoid inhalation or direct contact with skin or mucous membranes of the powder contained in the capsules. If such contact occurs, wash thoroughly with soap and water, rinse eyes with plain water.
- Monitor patient's CBC regularly. If neutropenia develops, interrupt therapy, reduce dose, perform appropriate diagnostic tests, or give additional treatment.
- Immunosuppression-induced infection or lymphoma may occur.

Patient education

- Warn patient not to open or crush capsules but to swallow capsules whole on an empty stomach.
- Instruct patient of need for repeated appropriate laboratory tests during drug therapy.
- Give patient complete dosage instructions and inform him of increased risk of lymphoproliferative diseases and other malignancies.
- Explain that drug is used with other drug therapies. Stress importance of not interrupting or stopping these drugs without medical approval.
- Inform female patient that a pregnancy test should be done within 1 week before beginning therapy and that effective contraception must be used before, during, and for 6 weeks after therapy is completed, even when there is history of infertility (unless due to hysterectomy). Also, two forms of contraception must be used simultaneously unless abstinence is chosen. If pregnancy occurs despite these measures, she must contact primary health care provider immediately.

Pediatric use

- Safety and effectiveness have not been established.

Breast-feeding

- Because it is unknown if drug is excreted in breast milk, its use in breast-feeding women is not recommended.

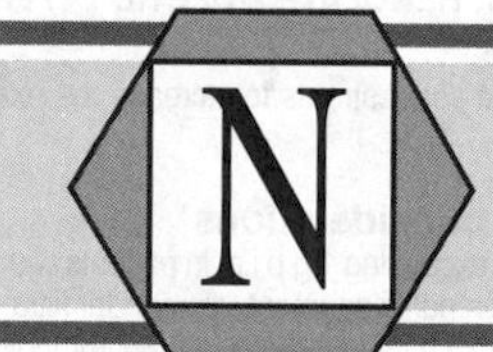

nabumetone
Relafen

Pharmacologic classification: NSAID
Therapeutic classification: antiarthritic
Pregnancy risk category C

How supplied
Available by prescription only
Tablets: 500 mg, 750 mg

Indications, route, and dosage
Acute and chronic treatment of rheumatoid arthritis or osteoarthritis
Adults: Initially, 1,000 mg P.O. daily as a single dose or in divided doses b.i.d. Adjust dosage based on patient response. Maximum recommended daily dose, 2,000 mg.

Pharmacodynamics
Anti-inflammatory action: Nabumetone probably acts by inhibiting the synthesis of prostaglandins. Drug also has analgesic and antipyretic action.

Pharmacokinetics
- *Absorption:* Drug is well absorbed from the GI tract. After absorption, about 35% is rapidly transformed to 6-methoxy-2-naphthylacetic acid (6MNA), the principal active metabolite; the balance is transformed to unidentified metabolites. Administration with food increases the absorption rate and peak levels of 6MNA but does not change total drug absorbed.
- *Distribution:* 6MNA is more than 99% bound to plasma proteins.
- *Metabolism:* 6MNA is metabolized to inactive metabolites in the liver.
- *Excretion:* Metabolites are excreted primarily in the urine. About 9% appears in the feces. Elimination half-life is about 24 hours. Half-life is increased in patients with renal failure.

Contraindications and precautions
Contraindicated in patients with hypersensitivity reactions, history of aspirin- or NSAID-induced asthma, urticaria, or other allergic-type reactions and during third trimester of pregnancy.

Use cautiously in patients with impaired renal or hepatic function, heart failure, hypertension, conditions that predispose to fluid retention, and history of peptic ulcer disease.

Interactions
Concomitant use with *drugs that are highly bound to plasma proteins* (such as *warfarin*) increase the risk of adverse reactions because nabumetone may displace drug. Use together with caution.

Effects on diagnostic tests
None reported.

Adverse reactions
CNS: *dizziness, headache,* fatigue, insomnia, nervousness, somnolence.
CV: vasculitis, edema.
EENT: *tinnitus.*
GI: *diarrhea, dyspepsia, abdominal pain, constipation, flatulence, nausea,* dry mouth, gastritis, stomatitis, anorexia, vomiting, ***bleeding,*** ulceration.
Respiratory: dyspnea, pneumonitis.
Skin: *pruritus, rash,* increased diaphoresis.

Overdose and treatment
After an accidental overdose, empty the stomach by induced emesis or lavage. Activated charcoal may limit the amount of drug absorbed.

☑ Special considerations
Besides those relevant to all *NSAIDs,* consider the following recommendations.
- Because NSAIDs impair the synthesis of renal prostaglandins, they can decrease renal blood flow and lead to reversible renal function impairment, especially in patients with preexisting renal failure, liver dysfunction, and heart failure; in elderly patients; and in those taking diuretics. Monitor these patients closely during therapy.
- During long-term therapy, periodically monitor renal and liver function, CBC, and hematocrit. Monitor carefully for signs and symptoms of GI bleeding.

Patient education
- Tell patient to take drug with food, milk, or antacids to enhance drug absorption.
- Stress importance of follow-up examinations to detect adverse GI effects.
- Teach patient signs and symptoms of GI bleeding, and tell him to report them immediately.
- Advise patient to limit alcohol intake because of risk of additive GI toxicity.

Geriatric use
- No differences in safety or efficacy have been noted in elderly patients.

Pediatric use
- Safety and efficacy have not been established.

Breast-feeding

• The active metabolite of nabumetone, 6MNA, has been found in the milk of laboratory rats. Because of risk of serious toxicity to the infant, use in breast-feeding women is not recommended.

nadolol

Corgard

Pharmacologic classification: beta-adrenergic blocker
Therapeutic classification: antihypertensive, antianginal
Pregnancy risk category C

How supplied

Available by prescription only
Tablets: 20 mg, 40 mg, 80 mg, 120 mg, 160 mg

Indications, route, and dosage

Hypertension
Adults: Initially, 20 to 40 mg P.O. once daily. Dosage may be increased in 40- to 80-mg increments daily at 2- to 14-day intervals until optimum response occurs. Usual maintenance dosage is 40 or 80 mg once daily. Doses of up to 240 or 320 mg daily may be necessary.

Long-term prophylactic management of chronic stable angina pectoris
Adults: Initially, 40 mg P.O. once daily. Dosage may be increased in 40- to 80-mg increments daily at 3- to 7-day intervals until optimum response occurs. Usual maintenance dosage is 40 or 80 mg once daily. Doses of up to 160 or 240 mg daily may be needed.

◇ ***Arrhythmias***
Adults: 60 to 160 mg daily.

◇ ***Prophylaxis of vascular headache***
Adults: 20 to 40 mg once daily; may gradually increase 120 mg daily if necessary.

✦ **Dosage adjustment.** In renally impaired patients, refer to following dosing chart.

Creatinine clearance (ml/min/1.73 m²)	Dosing interval
> 50	q 24 hr
31 to 50	q 24 to 36 hr
10 to 30	q 24 to 48 hr
< 10	q 40 to 60 hr

Pharmacodynamics

Antihypertensive action: Mechanism of antihypertensive effect is unknown. Drug may reduce blood pressure by blocking adrenergic receptors, thus decreasing cardiac output; by decreasing sympathetic outflow from the CNS; or by suppressing renin release.

Antianginal action: Nadolol decreases myocardial oxygen consumption, thus relieving angina, by blocking catecholamine-induced increases in heart rate, myocardial contraction, and blood pressure.

Pharmacokinetics

• *Absorption:* From 30% to 40% of a dose of nadolol is absorbed from the GI tract; peak plasma concentrations occur in 2 to 4 hours. Absorption is not affected by food.
• *Distribution:* Nadolol is distributed throughout the body; drug is about 30% protein-bound.
• *Metabolism:* None.
• *Excretion:* Most of a given dose is excreted unchanged in urine; the remainder is excreted in feces. Plasma half-life is about 20 hours. Antihypertensive and antianginal effects persist for about 24 hours.

Contraindications and precautions

Contraindicated in patients with bronchial asthma, sinus bradycardia and greater than first-degree heart block, and cardiogenic shock. Use cautiously in patients with hyperthyroidism, heart failure, diabetes, chronic bronchitis, emphysema, and impaired renal or hepatic function and in those receiving general anesthesia before undergoing surgery.

Interactions

Concomitant use with *other antiarrhythmic agents* may have additive or antagonistic cardiac effects and additive toxic effects.

Nadolol may potentiate antihypertensive effects of *diuretics* and *other antihypertensive agents* and, at high doses, the neuromuscular blocking effect of *tubocurarine* and related agents.

Nadolol may antagonize beta-adrenergic stimulating effects of *sympathomimetic agents* such as *isoproterenol*; concomitant use with *epinephrine* may cause a decrease in pulse rate with first- and second-degree heart block and hypertension.

Antimuscarinic agents such as *atropine* may antagonize nadolol-induced bradycardia.

Cocaine use may inhibit the therapeutic effects of nadolol.

Effects on diagnostic tests

None reported.

Adverse reactions

CNS: fatigue, dizziness.
CV: *bradycardia, hypotension,* ***heart failure,*** peripheral vascular disease, rhythm and conduction disturbances.
GI: nausea, vomiting, diarrhea, abdominal pain, constipation, anorexia.
Respiratory: *increased airway resistance.*
Skin: rash.
Other: fever.

Overdose and treatment

Clinical signs of overdose include severe hypotension, bradycardia, heart failure, and bronchospasm.

After acute ingestion, empty stomach by induced emesis or gastric lavage, and give activated charcoal to reduce absorption. Magnesium sulfate may be given orally as a cathartic. Subsequent treatment is usually symptomatic and supportive.

☑ Special considerations
Besides those relevant to all *beta-adrenergic blockers,* consider the following recommendations.
- Dosage adjustments may be necessary in patients with renal impairment.
- Nadolol has been used as an antiarrhythmic agent and as a prophylactic agent for migraine headaches.
- If long-term therapy is used, gradually decrease dose over 1 to 2 weeks before discontinuing drug. Abrupt withdrawal can exacerbate angina and cause an MI.

Patient education
- Tell patient not to discontinue nadolol abruptly. Drug should be tapered.

Geriatric use
- Elderly patients may require lower maintenance dosages of nadolol because of increased bioavailability or delayed metabolism; they also may experience enhanced adverse effects.

Pediatric use
- Safety and efficacy in children have not been established; use only if potential benefit outweighs risk.

Breast-feeding
- Drug occurs in breast milk; an alternative feeding method is recommended during therapy.

nafarelin acetate
Synarel

Pharmacologic classification: synthetic decapeptide
Therapeutic classification: gonadotropin-releasing hormone (GnRH) analogue
Pregnancy risk category X

How supplied
Available by prescription only
Nasal solution: 2 mg/ml (200 mcg/metered spray)

Indications, route, and dosage
Management of endometriosis, pain relief, reduction of endometriotic lesions
Adults: Usual daily dose is 400 mcg administered as one 200-mcg spray into one nostril in morning and one 200-mcg spray into the other nostril at night. If menstruation persists after 2 months, may increase dose to 800 mcg daily as one spray in each nostril in morning and one spray in each nostril at night. Treatment should begin on days 2 to 4 of menstrual cycle.

Recommended duration of therapy is 6 months. Retreatment is not recommended; safety data for retreatment not available. Clinical experience is limited to women age 18 and older.

Central precocious puberty
Children: Two sprays (400 mcg) into each nostril in the morning and at night, or three sprays (600 mcg) into alternating nostrils t.i.d. for a total of nine sprays daily to achieve 1,600 to 1,800 mcg daily.

Pharmacodynamics
Hormonal action: Nafarelin stimulates release of luteinizing hormone and follicle-stimulating hormone, which temporarily increases ovarian steroid production. Repeated dosing abolishes the stimulatory effect on the pituitary gland; after about 4 weeks, decreased secretion of gonadal steroids results in quiescence of the tissues and functions that depend on gonadal steroids.

Pharmacokinetics
- *Absorption:* After intranasal administration, nafarelin is rapidly absorbed through the nasal mucosa into systemic circulation. Maximum serum concentrations are achieved in 10 to 40 minutes. Average serum half-life is about 3 hours.
- *Distribution:* 80% is bound to plasma proteins.
- *Metabolism:* Degraded by peptidase.
- *Excretion:* Unknown.

Contraindications and precautions
Contraindicated in patients hypersensitive to GnRH analogues or any components of the formulation (benzalkonium chloride, sorbitol, purified water, glacial acetic acid, hydrochloric acid, or sodium hydroxide), in those with undiagnosed vaginal bleeding, in breast-feeding patients, and during pregnancy.

Interactions
None reported.

Effects on diagnostic tests
Tests of pituitary gonadotropin and gonadal functions may be misleading during treatment and for as long as 4 to 8 weeks after treatment.

Adverse reactions
CNS: *headache, emotional lability, insomnia,* depression.
CV: edema.
EENT: *nasal irritation.*
Skin: *acne,* seborrhea, hirsutism.
Other: *hot flashes, increased or decreased libido, myalgia, reduced breast size,* weight gain or loss, decreased bone density, *vaginal dryness.*

Overdose and treatment
No information available.

☑ Special considerations
- Pregnancy must be excluded before treatment.
- No evidence of favorable or adverse effects on pregnancy rates.
- Loss of bone density may not be reversible after treatment; chronic use of alcohol and tobacco, strong family history of osteoporosis, and chronic use of corticosteroid or anticonvulsant drugs represent major risk factor for loss of bone density.

Patient education
- Instruct patient to carefully read information packet included in drug package.
- Tell patient that regular menstruation should stop with continued use of drug.

• Instruct patient to call if menstruation continues after 2 months of treatment.
• Inform patient that breakthrough bleeding may occur, especially if successive doses are missed.
• Tell patient to discontinue use if she suspects that she has become pregnant and to call promptly. Inform patient of potential risk to fetus and instruct her to use nonhormonal contraception during therapy.
• Explain adverse effects of hypoestrogenism.
• Instruct patient to report intercurrent rhinitis. If rhinitis requires a topical nasal decongestant, it must be used at least 2 hours after nafarelin dose.
• Tell patient to avoid sneezing during or immediately following dosing because it may impair drug absorption.

Breast-feeding

• It is not known if drug is excreted in breast milk; however, use in breast-feeding women is not recommended.

nafcillin sodium

Nafcil, Nallpen, Unipen

Pharmacologic classification: penicillinase-resistant penicillin
Therapeutic classification: antibiotic
Pregnancy risk category B

How supplied

Available by prescription only
Capsules: 250 mg
Tablets: 500 mg
Injection: 500 mg, 1 g, 2 g
Pharmacy bulk package: 10 g
I.V. infusion piggyback: 1 g, 2 g

Indications, route, and dosage

***Systemic infections caused by susceptible organisms (methicillin-sensitive* Staphylococcus aureus)**
Adults: 2 to 4 g P.O. daily, divided into doses given q 6 hours; 2 to 12 g I.M. or I.V. daily, divided into doses given q 4 to 6 hours.
Children: 25 to 50 mg/kg P.O. daily, divided into doses given q 6 hours.
Neonates: 25 mg/kg I.V. b.i.d.

Pharmacodynamics

Antibiotic action: Nafcillin is bactericidal; it adheres to bacterial penicillin-binding proteins, thus inhibiting bacterial cell wall synthesis.

Nafcillin resists the effects of penicillinases—enzymes that inactivate penicillin—and is thus active against many strains of penicillinase-producing bacteria; this activity is most important against penicillinase-producing staphylococci; some strains may remain resistant. Nafcillin is also active against a few gram-positive aerobic and anaerobic bacilli but has no significant effect on gram-negative bacilli.

Pharmacokinetics

• *Absorption:* Absorbed erratically and poorly from the GI tract; peak serum levels occur at ½ to 2 hours after an oral dose and 30 to 60 minutes after an I.M. dose. Food decreases absorption.
• *Distribution:* Nafcillin is distributed widely; CSF penetration is poor but enhanced by meningeal inflammation. Drug crosses the placenta and is 70% to 90% protein-bound.
• *Metabolism:* Drug is metabolized primarily in the liver; it undergoes enterohepatic circulation. Dosage adjustment is not necessary for patients in renal failure.
• *Excretion:* Nafcillin and metabolites are excreted primarily in bile; about 25% to 30% is excreted in urine unchanged. It may also be excreted in breast milk. Elimination half-life in adults is ½ to 1 ½ hours.

Contraindications and precautions

Contraindicated in patients with hypersensitivity to drug or other penicillins. Use cautiously in patients with GI distress or sensitivity to cephalosporins.

Interactions

Concomitant use of nafcillin with *aminoglycosides* produces synergistic bactericidal effects against *S. aureus.* However, the drugs are physically and chemically incompatible and are inactivated when mixed or given together.

Probenecid blocks renal tubular secretion of penicillins; however, this interaction has only a small effect on the excretion of nafcillin.

Concurrent use of *hepatotoxic medications* may increase the risk of hepatotoxicity.

Effects on diagnostic tests

Nafcillin alters tests for urinary and serum proteins; turbidimetric urine and serum proteins are often falsely positive or elevated in tests using sulfosalicylic acid or trichloroacetic acid.

Nafcillin may cause transient reductions in RBC, WBC, and platelet counts. Abnormal urinalysis results may indicate drug-induced interstitial nephritis.

Adverse reactions

GI: *nausea,* vomiting, diarrhea, ***pseudomonas colitis.***
Hematologic: transient leukopenia, ***neutropenia, granulocytopenia, thrombocytopenia*** with high doses.
Other: hypersensitivity reactions (chills, fever, rash, pruritus, urticaria, ***anaphylaxis***), vein irritation, thrombophlebitis.

Overdose and treatment

Clinical signs of overdose include neuromuscular irritability or seizures. No specific recommendations. Treatment is supportive. After recent ingestion (4 hours or less), empty stomach by induced emesis or gastric lavage; follow with activated charcoal to reduce absorption. Nafcillin is not appreciably removed by hemodialysis.

☑ Special considerations

Besides those relevant to all *penicillins,* consider the following recommendations.

• Drug should be given with water only; acid in fruit juice or carbonated beverage may inactivate drug.
• Give dose on empty stomach; food decreases absorption.
• Renal, hepatic, and hematologic systems should be evaluated periodically during prolonged nafcillin therapy.

Patient education
• Tell patient to report severe diarrhea or allergic reactions promptly.

Geriatric use
• Half-life may be prolonged in elderly patients because of impaired hepatic and renal function.

Pediatric use
• Nafcillin that has been reconstituted with bacteriostatic water for injection with benzyl alcohol should not be used in neonates because of toxicity.

Breast-feeding
• Nafcillin is excreted into breast milk; drug should be used with caution in breast-feeding women.

nalbuphine hydrochloride
Nubain

Pharmacologic classification: narcotic agonist-antagonist; opioid partial agonist
Therapeutic classification: analgesic; adjunct to anesthesia
Pregnancy risk category NR

How supplied
Available by prescription only
Injection: 10 mg/ml, 20 mg/ml

Indications, route, and dosage
Moderate to severe pain
Adults: 10 to 20 mg S.C., I.M., or I.V. q 3 to 6 hours, p.r.n. or around the clock. Maximum dosage, 160 mg/day.
Supplement to anesthesia
Adults: 0.3 mg/kg to 3 mg/kg I.V. over 10 to 15 minutes; maintenance dose, 0.25 to 0.5 mg/kg I.V.

Pharmacodynamics
Analgesic action: Believed to result from drug's action at opiate receptor sites in the CNS, relieving moderate to severe pain. The narcotic antagonist effect may result from competitive inhibition at opiate receptors. Like other opioids, nalbuphine causes respiratory depression, sedation, and miosis. In patients with coronary artery disease or MI, it appears to produce no substantial changes in heart rate, pulmonary artery or wedge pressure, left ventricular end-diastolic pressure, pulmonary vascular resistance, or cardiac index.

Pharmacokinetics
• *Absorption:* When administered orally, drug is about one fifth as effective as an analgesic as it is when given I.M., apparently because of "first-pass" metabolism in the GI tract and liver. Onset of action is within 15 minutes, with peak effect seen at ½ to 1 hour.
• *Distribution:* Nalbuphine is not appreciably bound to plasma proteins.
• *Metabolism:* Drug is metabolized in the liver; duration of action is 3 to 6 hours.
• *Excretion:* Excreted in urine and to some degree in bile.

Contraindications and precautions
Contraindicated in patients with hypersensitivity to drug. Use cautiously in patients with history of drug abuse, emotional instability, head injury, increased intracranial pressure, impaired ventilation, MI accompanied by nausea and vomiting, upcoming biliary surgery, and hepatic or renal disease.

Interactions
If administered within a few hours of *barbiturate anesthetics* such as *thiopental,* nalbuphine may produce additive CNS and respiratory depressant effects and, possibly, apnea.

According to some reports, *cimetidine* may increase narcotic nalbuphine toxicity, causing disorientation, respiratory depression, apnea, and seizures. Because data are limited, this combination is not contraindicated; however, be prepared to administer a narcotic antagonist if toxicity occurs.

Reduced doses of nalbuphine are usually necessary when drug is used concomitantly with *other CNS depressants (alcohol, antihistamines, barbiturates, benzodiazepines, muscle relaxants, narcotic analgesics, phenothiazines, sedative-hypnotics, tricyclic antidepressants),* which may potentiate the drug's respiratory and CNS depression, sedation, and hypotensive effects; use with *general anesthetics* may also cause severe CV depression.

Drug accumulation and enhanced effects may result if drug is given concomitantly with other drugs that are extensively metabolized in the liver *(digitoxin, phenytoin, rifampin).*

Patients who become physically dependent on drug may experience acute withdrawal syndrome if given high doses of a narcotic antagonist. Use with caution, and monitor closely.

Effects on diagnostic tests
None reported.

Adverse reactions
CNS: *headache, sedation, dizziness, vertigo,* nervousness, depression, restlessness, crying, euphoria, hostility, unusual dreams, confusion, hallucinations, speech difficulty, delusions.
CV: hypertension, hypotension, tachycardia, bradycardia.
EENT: blurred vision, *dry mouth.*
GI: cramps, dyspepsia, bitter taste, *nausea, vomiting,* constipation, biliary tract spasms.
GU: urinary urgency.
Respiratory: ***respiratory depression,*** dyspnea, asthma, ***pulmonary edema.***
Skin: pruritus, burning, urticaria, *clamminess.*

Overdose and treatment
The most common signs and symptoms of nalbuphine overdose are CNS depression, respiratory depression, and miosis (pinpoint pupils). Other acute toxic effects include hypotension, bradycardia, hypothermia, shock, apnea, cardiopulmonary arrest, circulatory collapse, pulmonary edema, and seizures.

To treat acute overdose, first establish adequate respiratory exchange via a patent airway and ventilation as needed; administer a narcotic antagonist (naloxone) to reverse respiratory depression. Because the duration of action of nalbuphine is longer than that of naloxone, repeated naloxone dosing is necessary. Naloxone should not be given in the absence of clinically significant respiratory or CV depression. Monitor vital signs closely.

Provide symptomatic and supportive treatment (continued respiratory support, correction of fluid or electrolyte imbalance). Monitor laboratory parameters, vital signs, and neurologic status closely.

☑ Special considerations
Besides those relevant to all *opioid (narcotic) agonist-antagonists,* consider the following recommendations.

- Nalbuphine may obscure the signs and symptoms of an acute abdominal condition or worsen gallbladder pain.
- Drug may cause orthostatic hypotension in ambulatory patients.
- When drug is used during labor and delivery, neonate must be observed for signs of respiratory depression.
- Before administration, visually inspect all parenteral products for particulate matter and discoloration.
- Parenteral administration of drug provides better analgesia than oral administration. I.V. doses should be given by slow I.V. injection, preferably in diluted solution. Rapid I.V. injection increases the incidence of adverse effects.
- Drug causes respiratory depression, which at 10 mg is equal to the respiratory depression produced by 10 mg of morphine.
- Drug also acts as a narcotic antagonist; it may precipitate abstinence syndrome in narcotic-dependent patients.

Patient education
- Instruct patient to avoid driving or operating machinery because drug may cause dizziness and fatigue.

Geriatric use
- Lower doses are usually indicated for elderly patients, who may be more sensitive to the therapeutic and adverse effects of the drug.

Pediatric use
- Safety in children under age 18 is not established.

Breast-feeding
- It is not known if drug is excreted in breast milk; it should be used with caution in breast-feeding women.

nalidixic acid
NegGram

Pharmacologic classification: quinolone antibiotic
Therapeutic classification: urinary tract anti-infective
Pregnancy risk category B

How supplied
Available by prescription only
Tablets: 250 mg, 500 mg, 1 g
Suspension: 250 mg/5 ml

Indications, route, and dosage
Acute and chronic urinary tract infections caused by susceptible gram-negative organisms
Adults: 1 g P.O. q.i.d. for 7 to 14 days; 2 g P.O. daily for long-term use. Up to 6 g daily has been used for severe urinary tract infection.
Children over age 3 months: 55 mg/kg P.O. daily divided q. .d. for 7 to 14 days; 33 mg/kg P.O. daily divided q. .d. for long-term use.

Pharmacodynamics
Antimicrobial action: Drug is bactericidal and inhibits microbial synthesis of DNA. Spectrum of action includes most gram-negative organisms except *Pseudomonas.* (Approximately 2% to 14% of patients develop nalidixic acid–resistant organisms during therapy.)

Pharmacokinetics
- *Absorption:* Nalidixic acid is well absorbed from the GI tract; peak concentrations occur in 1 to 2 hours.
- *Distribution:* Nalidixic acid concentrates in renal tissue and seminal fluid; it does not penetrate prostatic tissue and only minimal amounts appear in CSF and the placenta. Drug is highly protein-bound.
- *Metabolism:* Drug acid is metabolized to the more active hydroxynalidixic acid and inactive conjugates in the liver.
- *Excretion:* 13% of metabolites and 2% to 3% of unchanged drug are excreted via the kidneys. In patients with normal renal function, plasma half-life of nalidixic acid is 1 to 2½ hours. In anuric patients, half-life is prolonged up to 21 hours.

Contraindications and precautions
Contraindicated in patients with hypersensitivity to drug, in those with seizure disorders, and in infants under age 3 months.

Use cautiously in patients with impaired renal or hepatic function, pulmonary disease, or severe cerebral arteriosclerosis and in prepubertal children.

Interactions
When used concomitantly with *dicumarol* or *warfarin,* nalidixic acid may displace clinically significant amounts of these anticoagulants from serum albumin binding sites, possibly causing excessive anticoagulation. When taken with other *photosensitizing drugs,* additive effects may occur.

Use with *antacids* may decrease absorption of nalidixic acid.

Effects on diagnostic tests
False-positive reactions may occur in urine glucose tests using cupric sulfate reagents (such as Benedict's test, Fehling's test, and Clinitest), from reaction between glucuronic acid (liberated by urinary metabolites of nalidixic acid) and cupric sulfate. Urine 17-ketosteroid and urine 17-ketogenic steroid levels may be falsely elevated because nalidixic acid interacts with *m*-dinitrobenzene, used to measure these urine metabolites. Urinary vanillylmandelic acid levels may also be falsely elevated.

Circulating erythrocyte, platelet, and leukocyte counts may decrease transiently during nalidixic acid therapy.

Adverse reactions
CNS: drowsiness, weakness, headache, dizziness, vertigo, ***seizures,*** malaise, confusion, hallucinations, psychosis.
EENT: sensitivity to light, change in color perception, diplopia, blurred vision.
GI: *abdominal pain, nausea, vomiting,* diarrhea.
Hematologic: eosinophilia, ***leukopenia, thrombocytopenia,*** hemolytic anemia.
Skin: pruritus, photosensitivity, urticaria, rash.
Other: angioedema, ***increased intracranial pressure and bulging fontanelles in infants and children,*** arthralgia, joint stiffness, anaphylactoid reaction.

Overdose and treatment
Clinical effects of overdose include toxic psychosis, seizures, increased intracranial pressure, metabolic acidosis, lethargy, nausea, and vomiting. However, because nalidixic acid is rapidly excreted, such reactions usually resolve in 2 to 3 hours.

Gastric lavage may be performed after recent ingestion. However, if drug absorption has occurred, supportive measures, including increased fluid administration, should be initiated. Anticonvulsants may be used to treat drug-induced seizures; however, this measure is rarely required.

☑ Special considerations
- Obtain culture and sensitivity tests before starting therapy, and repeat as needed.
- Obtain CBC and renal and liver function studies periodically during long-term therapy.
- Drug is ineffective against *Pseudomonas* infection or infection found outside urinary tract.
- Resistant bacteria may emerge after first 48 hours of therapy (especially if inadequate doses are prescribed).
- Although CNS toxicity is rare, brief seizures, increased intracranial pressure, and toxic psychosis may occur in infants, children, and elderly patients.
- Drug can be used during the second and third trimesters of pregnancy; however, safety has not been established for use in the first trimester.

Patient education
- Instruct patient to report visual disturbances; these usually disappear with dosage reduction.
- Warn patient that exposure to sunlight may cause photosensitivity. Inform him that photosensitivity reactions usually resolve within 2 to 8 weeks after drug therapy ends. Also warn that bullae may continue to follow subsequent exposure to sunlight or mild skin trauma for up to 3 months after drug therapy ends.
- Advise patient that he may take drug with food or milk to avoid GI upset.
- Warn patient to observe caution while driving because drug may produce drowsiness or blurred vision.

Pediatric use
- Do not administer drug to infants under age 3 months because safety has not been established; do not administer to prepubertal children because drug can produce erosions to cartilage in weight-bearing joints.

Breast-feeding
- Drug is excreted in breast milk in low concentrations. In one case, hemolytic anemia occurred in infant of uremic mother taking 1 g q.i.d. Lower drug excretion and elevated serum level resulted in higher excretion in milk.

naloxone hydrochloride
Narcan

Pharmacologic classification: narcotic (opioid) antagonist
Therapeutic classification: narcotic antagonist
Pregnancy risk category B

How supplied
Available by prescription only
Injection: 0.4 mg/ml, 1 mg/ml with preservatives and 0.02 mg/ml, 0.4 mg/ml and 1 mg/ml paraben-free

Indications, route, and dosage
Known or suspected narcotic-induced respiratory depression, including that caused by natural and synthetic narcotics, methadone, nalbuphine, pentazocine, and propoxyphene
Adults: 0.4 to 2 mg I.V., S.C., or I.M., repeated q 2 to 3 minutes, p.r.n. If no response is observed after 10 mg have been administered, diagnosis of narcotic-induced toxicity should be questioned.
Children: 0.01 mg/kg I.V.; give a subsequent dose of 0.1 mg/kg if needed. Dosage for continuous infusion is 0.024 to 0.16 mg/kg/hour. If I.V. route not available, dose may be given I.M. or S.C. in divided doses.
Postoperative narcotic depression
Adults: 0.1 to 0.2 mg I.V. q 2 to 3 minutes, p.r.n. until desired response is obtained.
Children: 0.005 to 0.01 mg/kg dose I.M., I.V., or S.C., repeated q 2 to 3 minutes p.r.n. until desired degree of reversal.
Neonates (asphyxia neonatorum): 0.01 mg/kg I.V. into umbilical vein repeated q 2 to 3 minutes for three doses. Concentration for use in neonates and children is 0.02 mg/ml.

Naloxone challenge for diagnosing opiate dependence
Adults: 0.16 mg I.M. naloxone; if no signs of withdrawal after 20 to 30 minutes, give second dose of 0.24 mg I.V.

Pharmacodynamics
Narcotic (opioid) antagonism: Naloxone is essentially a pure antagonist. In patients who have received an opioid agonist or other analgesic with narcotic-like effects, naloxone antagonizes most of the opioid effects, especially respiratory depression, sedation, and hypotension. Because the duration of action of naloxone in most cases is shorter than that of the opioid, opiate effects may return as those of naloxone dissipate. Naloxone does not produce tolerance or physical or psychological dependence. The precise mechanism of action is unknown, but is thought to involve competitive antagonism of more than one opiate receptor in the CNS.

Pharmacokinetics
- *Absorption:* Naloxone is rapidly inactivated after oral administration; therefore, it is given parenterally. Its onset of action is 1 to 2 minutes after I.V. administration and 2 to 5 minutes after I.M. or S.C. administration. The duration of action is longer after I.M. use and higher doses, when compared with I.V. use and lower doses.
- *Distribution:* Drug is rapidly distributed into body tissues and fluids.
- *Metabolism:* Naloxone is rapidly metabolized in the liver, primarily by conjugation.
- *Excretion:* Duration of action is approximately 45 minutes, depending on route and dose. Drug is excreted in urine. Plasma half-life has been reported to be from 60 to 90 minutes in adults and 3 hours in neonates.

Contraindications and precautions
Contraindicated in patients with hypersensitivity to drug. Use cautiously in patients with cardiac irritability and opiate addiction.

Interactions
When given to a *narcotic* addict, naloxone may produce an acute abstinence syndrome. Use with caution, and monitor closely.

Patients receiving *cardiotoxic drugs* may have serious CV effects with concomitant use of naloxone.

Effects on diagnostic tests
None reported.

Adverse reactions
CV: tachycardia, hypertension (with higher-than-recommended doses); hypotension, ***ventricular fibrillation, cardiac arrest.***
GI: nausea, vomiting (with higher-than-recommended doses).
Other: tremors and withdrawal symptoms in narcotic-dependent patients with higher-than-recommended doses, diaphoresis, ***seizures,*** pulmonary edema.

Overdose and treatment
No serious adverse reactions to naloxone overdose are known except those of acute abstinence syndrome in narcotic-dependent persons.

☑ Special considerations
- Before administration, visually inspect all parenteral products for particulate matter and discoloration.
- Take a careful drug history to rule out possible narcotic addiction, to avoid inducing withdrawal symptoms (apply cautions also to the baby of an addicted woman).
- Because naloxone's duration of activity is shorter than that of most narcotics, vigilance and repeated doses are usually necessary in the management of an acute narcotic overdose in a nonaddicted patient.
- Avoid depending on drug too much; that is, do not neglect attention to the airway, breathing, and circulation. Maintain adequate respiratory and CV status at all times. Respiratory "overshoot" may occur; monitor patient for respiratory rate higher than before respiratory depression. Respiratory rate increases in 1 to 2 minutes, and effect lasts 1 to 4 hours.
- Naloxone is not effective in treating respiratory depression caused by nonopioid drugs.
- Naloxone can be diluted in dextrose 5% or 0.9% NaCl solution. Use within 24 hours after mixing.
- Naloxone is the safest drug to use when cause of respiratory depression is uncertain.
- Naloxone may be administered by continuous I.V. infusion, which is necessary in many cases to control the adverse effects of epidurally administered morphine. Usual dose is 2 mg in 500 ml of D_5W or 0.9% NaCl solution.

Geriatric use
- Lower doses are usually indicated for elderly patients, because they may be more sensitive to the therapeutic and adverse effects of drug.

Breast-feeding
- It is not known if naloxone is excreted in breast milk.

naltrexone hydrochloride
ReVia

Pharmacologic classification: narcotic (opioid) antagonist
Therapeutic classification: narcotic detoxification adjunct
Pregnancy risk category C

How supplied
Available by prescription only
Tablets: 50 mg

Indications, route, and dosage
Adjunct for maintenance of opioid-free state in detoxified individuals
Adults: Do not attempt treatment until naloxone challenge is negative (0.2 mg I.V., if no signs of

withdrawal after 30 seconds, give additional 0.6 mg I.V.; alternatively, administer 0.8 mg S.C. and observe for 20 minutes for signs of withdrawal). Do not attempt treatment until patient has remained opioid-free for 7 to 10 days, verified by analyzing urine for opioids. Initially, 25 mg P.O. If no withdrawal signs occur within 1 hour, administer an additional 25 mg. Once patient has been started on 50 mg q 24 hours, flexible maintenance schedule may be used. From 50 to 150 mg may be given daily, depending on the schedule prescribed, but the average daily dose is 50 mg.

Alcoholism

Adults: 50 mg P.O. daily.

Pharmacodynamics

Opioid antagonism: Naltrexone is essentially a pure opiate (narcotic) antagonist. Like naloxone, it has little or no agonist activity. Its precise mechanism of action is unknown, but it is thought to involve competitive antagonism of more than one opiate receptor in the CNS. When administered to patients who have not recently received opiates, it exhibits little or no pharmacologic effect. At oral doses of 30 to 50 mg daily, it produces minimal analgesia, only slight drowsiness, and no respiratory depression. However, pharmacologic effects, including psychotomimetic effects, increased systolic or diastolic blood pressure, respiratory depression, and decreased oral temperature, which are suggestive of opiate agonist activity, have reportedly occurred in a few patients. In patients who have received single or repeated large doses of opiates, naltrexone attenuates or produces a complete but reversible block of the pharmacologic effects of the narcotic. Naltrexone does not produce physical or psychological dependence, and tolerance to its antagonist activity reportedly does not develop.

Pharmacokinetics

- *Absorption:* Naltrexone is well absorbed after oral administration, reaching peak plasma levels after 1 hour, although it does undergo extensive first-pass hepatic metabolism (only 5% to 20% of an oral dose reaches the systemic circulation unchanged). Peak effect occurs within 1 hour.
- *Distribution:* Drug is approximately 21% to 28% protein-bound. Extent and duration of drug's antagonist activity appear directly related to plasma and tissue concentrations of drug. It is widely distributed throughout the body, but considerable interindividual variation exists.
- *Metabolism:* Oral naltrexone undergoes extensive first-pass hepatic metabolism. Its major metabolite is believed to be a pure antagonist also, and may contribute to its efficacy. Drug and hepatic metabolites may undergo enterohepatic recirculation.
- *Excretion:* Naltrexone is excreted primarily by the kidneys. Elimination half-life is about 4 hours; that of its major active metabolite is about 13 hours.

Contraindications and precautions

Contraindicated in patients receiving opioid analgesics, in opioid-dependent patients, in patients in acute opioid withdrawal, in those with positive urine screen for opioids, or in those with acute hepatitis or liver failure. Also contraindicated in patients with hypersensitivity to drug.

Use cautiously in patients with mild hepatic disease or history of hepatic impairment.

Interactions

When naltrexone is taken with *opioid-containing medications (cough* and *cold preparations, antidiarrheals, opioid analgesics),* opioid activity will be attenuated. Because naltrexone can precipitate potentially severe opiate withdrawal, it should not be used in patients receiving *opiates* or in nondetoxified patients physically dependent on opiates.

Because naltrexone is metabolized in the liver, *other drugs that alter hepatic metabolism* may increase or decrease serum naltrexone levels.

Effects on diagnostic tests

Because of its hepatotoxicity, naltrexone may alter the results of liver function tests. Lymphocytosis also may occur.

Adverse reactions

CNS: *insomnia, anxiety, nervousness, headache,* depression, dizziness, fatigue, somnolence, ***suicide ideation.***

GI: *nausea, vomiting,* anorexia, *abdominal pain,* constipation, increased thirst.

GU: delayed ejaculation, decreased potency.

Hepatic: hepatotoxicity.

Skin: rash.

Other: *muscle and joint pain,* chills.

Overdose and treatment

Naltrexone overdose has not been documented. In one study, subjects who received 800 mg/day (16 tablets) for up to 1 week showed no evidence of toxicity.

In case of overdose, provide symptomatic and supportive treatment in a closely supervised environment. Contact the local or regional poison control center for further information.

☑ Special considerations

- Administer a naloxone (Narcan) challenge test to the patient before naltrexone use. Naloxone (0.8 mg S.C. or I.V., incremental doses) is administered and the patient closely monitored for signs and symptoms of opiate withdrawal. If acute abstinence signs and symptoms are present, do not administer naltrexone.
- Before administering, take a careful drug history to rule out possible narcotic use. Do not attempt treatment until the patient has been opiate-free for 7 to 10 days. Verify self-reporting of abstinence from narcotics by urinalysis. No withdrawal signs or symptoms should be reported by patient or be evident.
- Perform liver function tests before naltrexone use to establish a baseline and to evaluate possible drug-induced hepatotoxicity. In an emergency situation requiring analgesia that can only be achieved with opiates, patient who has been receiving naltrexone may need a higher dose than usual of nar-

cotic, and the resulting respiratory depression may be deeper and more prolonged.
• Drug can cause hepatocellular injury if given at higher than recommended doses. Naltrexone can precipitate or exacerbate signs and symptoms of abstinence in anyone not completely opioid-free.

Patient education
• Inform patient that opioid medications, such as cough and cold preparations, antidiarrheal products, and narcotic analgesics may not be effective; recommend nonnarcotic alternative if available.
• Warn patient not to self-administer narcotics while taking naltrexone because serious injury, coma, or death may result.
• Explain that drug has no tolerance or dependence liability.
• Tell patient to report withdrawal signs and symptoms (tremors, vomiting, bone or muscle pains, sweating, abdominal cramps).
• Tell patient to carry an identification card that alerts medical personnel that naltrexone is taken, and to inform new primary health care provider that he is receiving drug.

Geriatric use
• Use in elderly patients is not documented, but they would probably require reduced dosage.

Pediatric use
• Safe use of naltrexone in patients under age 18 has not been established.

Breast-feeding
• It is unknown if drug is excreted in breast milk. It should be used with caution in breast-feeding women, especially because of its known hepatotoxicity.

nandrolone decanoate
Androlone-D 200, Deca-Durabolin, Hybolin Decanoate-50, Hybolin Decanoate-100, Neo-Durabolic

nandrolone phenpropionate
Durabolin, Hybolin Improved, Nandrobolic

Pharmacologic classification: anabolic steroid
Therapeutic classification: erythropoietic (nandrolone decanoate), anabolic (nandrolone decanoate), antineoplastic (nandrolone phenpropionate)
Controlled substance schedule III
Pregnancy risk category X

How supplied
Available by prescription only
decanoate
Injection: 50 mg/ml, 100 mg/ml, 200 mg/ml (in oil)
phenpropionate
Injection: 25 mg/ml, 50 mg/ml (in oil)

Indications, route, and dosage
Anemia associated with renal insufficiency
decanoate
Adults: 100 to 200 mg I.M. weekly in males; 50 to 100 mg/week in females.
Children age 2 to 13: 25 to 50 mg I.M. q 3 to 4 weeks.
Metastatic breast cancer
phenpropionate
Adults: 50 to 100 mg I.M. weekly.

Pharmacodynamics
Androgenic action: Nandrolone exerts inhibitory effects on hormone-responsive breast tumors and metastases.

Erythropoietic action: Nandrolone stimulates the kidneys' production of erythropoietin, leading to increases in red blood cell mass and volume.

Anabolic action: Nandrolone may reverse corticosteroid-induced catabolism and promote tissue development in severely debilitated patients.

Pharmacokinetics
• *Absorption:* Peak concentrations occur 1 to 6 days after I.M. administration.
• *Distribution:* Drug is slowly released from I.M. depot following injection, and is hydrolyzed to free nandrolone by plasma esterase.
• *Metabolism:* Nandrolone is metabolized in the liver.
• *Excretion:* Both unchanged drug and its metabolites are excreted in the urine. Elimination half-life of nandrolone is 6 to 8 days.

Contraindications and precautions
Contraindicated in patients with hypersensitivity to anabolic steroids, in males with breast cancer or prostate cancer, in patients with nephrosis, in those experiencing the nephrotic phase of nephritis, in women with breast cancer and hypercalcemia, during pregnancy, or in breast-feeding patients.

Use cautiously in patients with renal, cardiac, or hepatic disease; diabetes; epilepsy; migraine; or other conditions that may be aggravated by fluid retention

Interactions
In patients with diabetes, decreased blood glucose levels may require adjustment *of insulin* or *oral antidiabetic drug* dosage.

Nandrolone decanoate may potentiate the effects of *warfarin-type anticoagulants,* causing increases in PT. Use with *adrenocorticosteroids* or *adrenocorticotropic hormone* increases the potential for fluid and electrolyte retention.

Effects on diagnostic tests
Nandrolone may cause abnormal results of fasting plasma glucose, glucose tolerance, and metyrapone tests. Thyroid function test results (protein-bound iodine, radioactive iodine uptake, thyroid-binding capacity) and 17-ketosteroid levels may decrease. Liver function test results, PT (especially in patients receiving anticoagulant therapy), and serum creatinine levels may be elevated. Because of drug's

anabolic activity, serum sodium, potassium, calcium, phosphate, and cholesterol levels may all rise.

Adverse reactions

CNS: excitation, insomnia, habituation, depression.
CV: edema.
GI: nausea, vomiting, diarrhea.
GU: bladder irritability, *hypoestrogenic effects in women (flushing; diaphoresis; vaginitis, including itching, dryness, and burning; vaginal bleeding; nervousness; emotional lability; menstrual irregularities), excessive hormonal effects in men (prepubertal—premature epiphyseal closure,* acne, priapism, *growth of body and facial hair,* phallic enlargement; postpubertal—testicular atrophy, oligospermia, decreased ejaculatory volume, impotence, gynecomastia, epididymitis).
Hematologic: elevated serum lipid levels, suppression of clotting factors.
Hepatic: reversible jaundice, peliosis hepatitis, elevated liver enzyme levels, ***liver cell tumors.***
Skin: pain and induration at injection site.
Other: androgenic effects in women (acne, edema, *weight gain, hirsutism,* hoarseness, clitoral enlargement, *decreased breast size,* changes in libido, male-pattern baldness, *oily skin or hair*).

Overdose and treatment

No information available.

☑ Special considerations

- Nandrolone injections should be administered deeply into the gluteal muscle.
- An adequate iron intake is necessary for maximum response when patient is receiving nandrolone decanoate injections.

Patient education

- Instruct diabetic patient to monitor glucose closely as glucose tolerance may be altered.
- Tell female patient to report menstrual irregularities, acne, deepening of voice, male-pattern baldness, or hirsutism.
- Tell patient to notify primary health care provider if persistent GI upset, nausea, vomiting, changes in skin color, or ankle swelling occur.

Geriatric use

- Observe elderly male patients for the development of prostatic hypertrophy and prostatic carcinoma.

Pediatric use

- The adverse consequences of giving androgens to young children is not fully understood, but the possibility of serious disturbances (premature epiphyseal closure, masculinization of females, or precocious development in males) exists; weigh the possible benefits before instituting therapy in young children.

Breast-feeding

- It is not known if anabolic steroids are excreted in breast milk. Because of the potential for serious adverse reactions in breast-fed infants, a decision to discontinue breast-feeding or drug needs to be reached.

naphazoline hydrochloride

AK-Con, Albalon Liquifilm, Allerest, Clear Eyes, Comfort Eye Drops, Degest 2, I-Naphline, Muro's Opcon, Naphcon, Naphcon-A, Naphcon Forte, Privine, VasoClear, Vasocon

Pharmacologic classification: sympathomimetic
Therapeutic classification: decongestant, vasoconstrictor
Pregnancy risk category C

How supplied

Available by prescription only
Ophthalmic solution: 0.1%

Available without a prescription
Ophthalmic solution: 0.012%, 0.02%, 0.025% (generic), 0.03%
Nasal drops or sprays: 0.05% (solution)

Indications, route, and dosage

Ocular congestion, irritation, itching
Adults: Instill 1 to 3 drops (0.1% solution) or 1 to 2 drops (0.012% to 0.03% solution) in eye daily to q.i.d.
Nasal congestion
Adults and children over age 12: 1 or 2 drops or sprays (0.05% solution) p.r.n. Do not use drops more than q 3 hours or spray more often than q 4 to 6 hours.
Children age 6 to 12: 1 to 2 drops or sprays (0.025% solution) p.r.n.

Pharmacodynamics

Decongestant action: Naphazoline produces vasoconstriction by local and alpha-adrenergic action on blood vessels of the conjunctiva or nasal mucosa; therefore, it reduces blood flow and nasal congestion.

Pharmacokinetics

- *Absorption:* Following intranasal application, local vasoconstriction occurs within 5 to 10 minutes and persists for 5 to 6 hours with a gradual decline over the next 6 hours.
- *Distribution:* Unknown.
- *Metabolism:* Unknown.
- *Excretion:* Unknown.

Contraindications and precautions

Contraindicated in patients with hypersensitivity to drug's ingredients and in those with acute angle-closure glaucoma. Use of 0.1% solution is contraindicated in children. Use cautiously in patients with hyperthyroidism, cardiac disease, hypertension, or diabetes mellitus.

Interactions

Concomitant use with *MAO inhibitors* may result in an increased adrenergic response and hypertensive crisis.

Effects on diagnostic tests
None reported.

Adverse reactions
CNS: headache, dizziness, nervousness, weakness (with ophthalmic form).
CV: hypertension, cardiac irregularities.
EENT: transient eye stinging, pupillary dilation, eye irritation, photophobia, blurred vision, increased intraocular pressure, keratitis, lacrimation (with ophthalmic form); rebound nasal congestion (with excessive or long-term use), sneezing, stinging, dryness of mucosa (with nasal administration).
GI: nausea (with ophthalmic form).
Other: diaphoresis (with ophthalmic form); systemic effects in children after excessive or long-term use, marked sedation (with nasal administration).

Overdose and treatment
Clinical manifestations of overdose include CNS depression, sweating, decreased body temperature, bradycardia, shocklike hypotension, decreased respirations, CV collapse, and coma.

Activated charcoal or gastric lavage may be used initially to treat accidental ingestion (administer early before sedation occurs). Monitor vital signs and ECG, as ordered. Treat seizures with I.V. diazepam.

☑ Special considerations
- Naphazoline is the most widely used ocular decongestant.
- Monitor for blurred vision, pain, or lid edema.
- Do not shake container.

Patient education
- Teach patient how to instill ophthalmic or nasal medication; tell him not to share drug with others.
- Advise patient to report blurred vision, eye pain, or lid swelling that occurs when using ophthalmic product.
- Inform patient using ophthalmic solution that photophobia may follow pupil dilation; tell patient to report this effect promptly.
- Warn patient not to exceed recommended dosage; rebound nasal congestion and conjunctivitis also may occur with frequent or prolonged use.
- Tell patient to call if nasal congestion persists after 5 days of using nasal solution.

Geriatric use
- Use drug with caution in elderly patients with severe cardiac disease or poorly controlled hypertension and in diabetics prone to diabetic ketoacidosis.

Pediatric use
- Use in infants and children may result in CNS depression, leading to coma and marked reduction in body temperature. Although available without a prescription, parents should not use nasal solution containing 0.025% naphazoline hydrochloride in children under age 6, and 0.05% naphazoline hydrochloride in children under age 12.

naproxen
Naprosyn

naproxen sodium
Aleve, Anaprox

Pharmacologic classification: NSAID
Therapeutic classification: nonnarcotic analgesic, antipyretic, anti-inflammatory
Pregnancy risk category B

How supplied
Available by prescription only
naproxen
Tablets: 250 mg, 375 mg, 500 mg
Tablets (delayed-release): 375 mg, 500 mg
Oral suspension: 125 mg/5 ml
naproxen sodium
Tablets (film-coated): 275 mg, 550 mg

Note: 220 mg, 275 mg, 550 mg of naproxen sodium = 200 mg, 250 mg, or 500 mg of naproxen, respectively.

Available without a prescription
naproxen sodium
Tablets, capsules: 220 mg

Indications, route, and dosage
Mild to moderately severe musculoskeletal or soft tissue irritation
naproxen
Adults: 250 to 500 mg P.O. b.i.d. Alternatively, 250 mg in the morning and 500 mg in the evening.
naproxen sodium
Adults: 275 to 550 mg P.O. b.i.d. Alternatively, 275 mg in the morning and 550 mg in the evening.
Mild to moderate pain; primary dysmenorrhea
naproxen
Adults: 500 mg P.O. to start, followed by 250 mg P.O. q 6 to 8 hours p.r.n. Maximum daily dose should not exceed 1.25 g naproxen.
naproxen sodium
Adults: 550 mg P.O. to start, followed by 275 mg P.O. q 6 to 8 hours p.r.n. Maximum daily dose is 1.375 g naproxen sodium.
Self-medication: 220 mg q 8 to 12 hours. Maximum daily dose is 440 mg for adults age 65 and older, or three tablets for adults below age 65. Do not self-medicate for more than 10 days.
Acute gout
naproxen
Adults: 750 mg initially, then 250 mg q 8 hours until episode subsides.
naproxen sodium
Adults: 825 mg initially, then 275 mg q 8 hours until attack has subsided.
Juvenile rheumatoid arthritis
naproxen
Children: 10 mg/kg/day in two divided doses.

Pharmacodynamics
Analgesic, antipyretic, and anti-inflammatory actions: Mechanisms of action are unknown; naproxen is thought to inhibit prostaglandin synthesis.

Pharmacokinetics

• *Absorption:* Absorbed rapidly and completely from the GI tract. Effect peaks at 2 to 4 hours.
• *Distribution:* Drug is highly protein-bound. It crosses the placenta and is distributed into the milk.
• *Metabolism:* Naproxen is metabolized in the liver.
• *Excretion:* Drug is excreted in urine. Half-life is 10 to 20 hours.

Contraindications and precautions

Contraindicated in patients with hypersensitivity to drug or asthma, rhinitis, or nasal polyps. Use cautiously in the elderly and in patients with history of peptic ulcer disease or renal, CV, GI, or hepatic disease.

Interactions

Concomitant use of naproxen with *anticoagulants* and *thrombolytic drugs (coumadin derivatives, heparin, streptokinase, urokinase)* may potentiate anticoagulant effects. Bleeding problems may occur if used with other drugs that inhibit platelet aggregation, such as *aspirin, parenteral carbenicillin, cefamandole, cefoperazone, dextran, dipyridamole, mezlocillin, piperacillin, plicamycin, sulfinpyrazone, ticarcillin, valproic acid, salicylates, or other anti-inflammatory agents.* Concomitant use with *alcohol, anti-inflammatory agents, corticotropin, salicylates,* or steroids may increase GI adverse reactions, including ulceration and hemorrhage. *Aspirin* may decrease the bioavailability of naproxen.

Because of the influence of prostaglandins on glucose metabolism, concomitant use with *insulin* or *oral antidiabetic agents* may potentiate hypoglycemic effects. Naproxen may displace highly protein-bound drugs from binding sites. Toxicity may occur with *coumadin derivatives, nifedipine, phenytoin,* or *verapamil.* Increased nephrotoxicity may occur with *acetaminophen, gold compounds*, or *other anti-inflammatory agents.* Naproxen may decrease the renal clearance of *lithium* and *methotrexate.* Naproxen may decrease the clinical effectiveness of *antihypertensive agents* and *diuretics.* Concomitant use may increase risk of nephrotoxicity.

Effects on diagnostic tests

Naproxen and its metabolites may interfere with urinary 5-hydroxyindoleacetic acid and 17-hydroxycorticosteroid determinations. The physiologic effects of naproxen may lead to an increase in bleeding time (may persist for 4 days after withdrawal of drug); serum creatinine and potassium, BUN, and serum transaminase levels may also increase.

Adverse reactions

CNS: *headache, drowsiness, dizziness,* vertigo.
CV: *edema,* palpitations.
EENT: visual disturbances, *tinnitus,* auditory disturbances.
GI: *epigastric distress, occult blood loss, nausea,* ***peptic ulceration***, constipation, dyspepsia, heartburn, diarrhea, stomatitis, thirst.
GU: nephrotoxicity.
Hematologic: ***thrombocytopenia,*** eosinophilia, ***agranulocytosis***, neutropenia.
Hepatic: elevated liver enzyme levels.
Respiratory: dyspnea.
Skin: *pruritus, rash,* urticaria, ecchymosis, diaphoresis, purpura.

Overdose and treatment

Clinical manifestations of overdose include drowsiness, heartburn, indigestion, nausea, and vomiting.

To treat overdose of naproxen, empty stomach immediately by inducing emesis with ipecac syrup or by gastric lavage. Administer activated charcoal via nasogastric tube. Provide symptomatic and supportive measures (respiratory support and correction of fluid and electrolyte imbalances). Monitor laboratory parameters and vital signs closely. Hemodialysis is ineffective in naproxen removal.

☑ Special considerations

Besides those relevant to all *NSAIDs,* consider the following recommendations.
• Use lowest possible effective dose; 250 mg of naproxen is equivalent to 275 mg of naproxen sodium.
• Relief usually begins within 2 weeks after beginning therapy with naproxen.
• Institute safety measures to prevent injury resulting from possible CNS effects.
• Monitor fluid balance. Monitor for signs and symptoms of fluid retention, especially significant weight gain.

Patient education

• Caution patient to avoid concomitant use of OTC drugs.
• Teach patient signs and symptoms of possible adverse reactions and tell him to report them promptly.
• Instruct patient to check his weight every 2 to 3 days and to report any gain of 3 lb (1.4 kg) or more within 1 week.
• Instruct patient in safety measures; advise him to avoid activities that require alertness until CNS effects are known.
• Warn patient against combining naproxen (Naprosyn) with naproxen sodium (Anaprox) because both agents circulate in the blood as naproxen anion.

Geriatric use

• Patients over age 60 are more sensitive to the adverse effects (especially GI toxicity) of drug.
• Naproxen's effect on renal prostaglandins may cause fluid retention and edema. This may be significant in elderly patients, especially those with heart failure.

Pediatric use

• Safe use of naproxen in children under age 2 has not been established. Safe use of naproxen sodium in children has not been established. No age-related problems reported.

Breast-feeding

- Because they are distributed into breast milk, naproxen and naproxen sodium should be avoided during breast-feeding.

naratriptan hydrochloride

Amerge

Pharmacologic classification: a selective 5-hydroxytryptamine$_1$ (5-HT$_1$) receptor subtype agonist
Therapeutic classification: antimigraine
Pregnancy risk category C

How supplied

Available by prescription only
Tablets: 1 mg, 2.5 mg

Indications, route, and dosage

Treatment of acute migraine headache attacks with or without aura

Adults: 1 or 2.5 mg P.O. as a single dose. Dose should be individualized, depending on the possible benefit of the 2.5-mg dose and the greater risk of adverse events. If headache returns or if only partial response occurs, may repeat dose after 4 hours, for maximum dose of 5 mg within 24 hours.

✦ ***Dosage adjustment.*** In patients with mild to moderate renal or hepatic impairment, consider a lower initial dose; do not exceed maximum dose of 2.5 mg over a 24-hour period. Do not use in patients with severe renal or hepatic impairment.

Pharmacodynamics

Antimigraine action: Naratriptan binds with high affinity to 5-HT$_{1D}$ and 5-HT$_{1B}$ receptors. One theory suggests that activation of 5-HT$_{1D/1B}$ receptors located on intracranial blood vessels leads to vasoconstriction, which is associated with the migraine relief. Another hypothesis suggests that activation of 5-HT$_{1D/1B}$ receptors on sensory nerve endings in the trigeminal system results in the inhibition of pro-inflammatory neuropeptide release.

Pharmacokinetics

- *Absorption:* Well absorbed with approximately 70% oral bioavailability. Peak plasma concentrations occur in 2 to 4 hours.
- *Distribution:* Steady-state volume of distribution is 170 L. Plasma protein binding is 28% to 31%.
- *Metabolism:* In vitro, naratriptan is metabolized by many P-450 cytochrome isoenzymes to inactive metabolites.
- *Excretion:* Naratriptan is predominantly eliminated in the urine, with 50% of dose recovered unchanged and 30% as metabolites. Mean elimination half-life is 6 hours.

Contraindications and precautions

Contraindicated in patients with hypersensitivity to drug or its components and in those with history, symptoms, or signs of ischemic cardiac, cerebrovascular (such as stroke or transient ischemic attack), or peripheral vascular syndromes (such as ischemic bowel disease). Also contraindicated in patients with significant underlying CV diseases, including angina pectoris, MI, and silent myocardial ischemia.

Contraindicated in patients with severe renal (creatinine clearance below 15 ml/minute) or hepatic (Child-Pugh grade C) impairment and in those with hemiplegic or basilar migraine.

Drug or other 5-HT$_1$ agonists are also contraindicated in patients with potential risk factors for coronary artery disease, such as hypertension, hypercholesterolemia, obesity, diabetes, strong family history of coronary artery disease, females with surgical or physiologic menopause, males over age 40, or smoking.

Interactions

Ergot-containing or *ergot-type drugs* or *other 5-HT$_1$ agonists* have been reported to cause prolonged vasospastic reactions because their actions may be additive; use of these drugs within 24 hours of naratriptan is contraindicated.

Rarely, *selective serotonin reuptake inhibitors (SSRIs)* (such as *fluoxetine, fluvoxamine, paroxetine, sertraline)* have been reported to cause weakness, hyperreflexia, and incoordination when coadministered with 5-HT$_1$ agonists. If concomitant therapy with naratriptan and a SSRI is needed, monitor patient.

Concomitant use of *oral contraceptives* with naratriptan resulted in slightly higher concentrations of naratriptan.

Smoking increases the clearance of naratriptan by 30%.

Effects on diagnostic tests

None reported.

Adverse reactions

CNS: paresthesias, dizziness, drowsiness, malaise, fatigue, vertigo.
CV: palpitations, increased blood pressure, tachyarrhythmias, ***abnormal ECG changes (PR, QT wave prolongation, ST/T wave abnormalities, premature ventricular contractions, atrial flutter and/or fibrillation),*** syncope.
EENT: ear, nose and throat infections, photophobia.
GI: nausea, hyposalivation, vomiting.
Other: warm or cold temperature sensations; pressure, tightness, heaviness sensations.

Overdose and treatment

A significant increase in blood pressure has been observed with an overdose, occurring between 30 minutes and 6 hours after ingestion of drug. Blood pressure returned to normal within 8 hours without pharmacologic intervention in some patients, whereas in others antihypertensive drug treatment was necessary.

No specific antidote exists. Perform ECG monitoring for evidence of ischemia. Monitor patient for at least 24 hours after an overdose or while symptoms persist. The effect of hemodialysis or peritoneal dialysis is unknown.

☑ Special considerations

- Use drug only when a clear diagnosis of migraine has been established. It is not intended for prophylactic therapy of migraines or for use in the management of hemiplegic or basilar migraine.
- Administer first dose in a medically equipped facility for patients at risk for coronary artery disease but determined to have a satisfactory CV evaluation. Consider ECG monitoring.
- Perform periodic cardiac re-evaluation in patients who have or develop risk factors for coronary artery disease.
- Safety and effectiveness have not been established for cluster headaches.

Patient education

- Tell patient that drug is intended to relieve, and not prevent, migraine headaches.
- Instruct patient not to use drug if pregnancy is suspected or during pregnancy itself.
- Teach patient to alert primary health care provider of risk factors for coronary artery disease.
- Instruct patient to take dose soon after headache starts. If there is no response to the first tablet, tell patient to seek medical approval before taking second tablet.
- Tell patient that if more relief is needed after the first tablet, such as when a partial response occurs or if the headache returns, he may take a second tablet but not sooner than 4 hours after the first tablet. Inform him not to exceed two tablets within 24 hours.

Geriatric use

- Do not use drug in elderly patients.

Pediatric use

- Safety and effectiveness in children under age 18 have not been established.

Breast-feeding

- Use with caution in breast-feeding patients.

natamycin

Natacyn

Pharmacologic classification: polyene macrolide antibiotic
Therapeutic classification: antifungal
Pregnancy risk category C

How supplied

Available by prescription only
Ophthalmic suspension: 5%

Indications, route, and dosage

Conjunctivitis and keratitis caused by susceptible fungi
Adults: Initially, 1 drop instilled in conjunctival sac q 1 to 2 hours. After 3 to 4 days, reduce dosage to 1 drop six to eight times daily.
Blepharitis caused by susceptible fungi
Adults: 1 drop instilled in conjunctival sac q 4 to 6 hours.

Pharmacodynamics

Antifungal action: Natamycin increases fungal cell membrane permeability, causing leakage of essential cellular contents.

Pharmacokinetics

- *Absorption:* Systemic absorption is unlikely after topical administration; drug is not absorbed from the GI tract.
- *Distribution:* Topical administration produces effective concentrations within the corneal stroma but not in intraocular fluid.
- *Metabolism:* Unknown.
- *Excretion:* Unknown.

Contraindications and precautions

Contraindicated in patients hypersensitive to drug. Because of risk of accelerating the spread of infection, concurrent application of drug and a topical corticosteroid is contraindicated in patients with fungal infections of the eye.

Interactions

None reported.

Effects on diagnostic tests

None reported.

Adverse reactions

EENT: ocular edema, hyperemia, conjunctival chemosis.

Overdose and treatment

The toxicity of ingested natamycin is unknown; if accidentally ingested, use general measures such as emesis, cathartic, or lavage to remove drug from the GI tract. Treat dermal exposure by washing the area with soap and water. Observe the patient closely for possible signs and symptoms.

☑ Special considerations

- Natamycin is the only antifungal available in an ophthalmic preparation; it is the treatment of choice for fungal keratitis.
- Continue therapy for 14 to 21 days or until active disease subsides; then, reduce dosage gradually at 4- to 7-day intervals to assure that organism has been eliminated; if infection does not improve within 7 to 10 days, reevaluate diagnosis.
- Remove excessive exudate before application.

Patient education

- Show patient how to apply drug and to apply light finger pressure on lacrimal sac for 1 minute after drops are instilled. Stress importance of compliance with recommended therapy.
- Advise patient not to share eye medications with family members.
- Instruct patient to shake suspension well before using and to store it in refrigerator or at room temperature.
- Warn patient that drug may cause blurred vision and photosensitivity.

nedocromil sodium

Tilade

Pharmacologic classification: pyranoquinoline
Therapeutic classification: anti-inflammatory respiratory inhalant
Pregnancy risk category B

How supplied

Available by prescription only
Inhalation aerosol: 1.75 mg per actuation in 16.2-g canister (U.S.); 2 mg per actuation in 16.2-g canister (Canada)

Indications, route, and dosage

Maintenance therapy in mild to moderate bronchial asthma

Adults and children age 12 and over: 2 inhalations q.i.d., preferably at regular intervals; may gradually decrease dosing interval to b.i.d.

Pharmacodynamics

Anti-inflammatory/antiallergic action: Inhibits activation and release of inflammatory mediators from various cell types in the lumen and mucosa of the bronchial tree. These mediators, which include the leukotrienes, histamine, and prostaglandins, are preformed or derived from arachidonic acid metabolism. A range of human cells associated with asthma may be involved. As a result, nedocromil exhibits specific anti-inflammatory properties when administered topically to the bronchial mucosa. It has demonstrated a significant inhibitory effect on allergen-induced early and late asthmatic reactions and on bronchial hyperresponsiveness. Nedocromil also may affect sensory nerves in the lung. The result is inhibition of bradykinin-induced bronchoconstriction.

Pharmacokinetics

- *Absorption:* 2% to 3% of amount swallowed after nedocromil inhalation is absorbed. From 6% to 9% of nedocromil deposited in the lungs is completely absorbed. Onset of action occurs within 30 minutes, peaks in 5 to 90 minutes, and lasts 6 to 12 hours.
- *Distribution:* Drug is distributed to plasma only. Approximately 89% is reversibly bound to plasma proteins when plasma concentrations range between 0.5 and 50 mcg/ml.
- *Metabolism:* Nedocromil is not metabolized.
- *Excretion:* Drug is rapidly excreted unchanged in the bile and urine. Half-life is approximately 1.5 to 3.3 hours.

Contraindications and precautions

Contraindicated in patients hypersensitive to the formulation or in patients experiencing an acute asthmatic attack or acute bronchospasm.

Interactions

None reported.

Effects on diagnostic tests

None reported.

Adverse reactions

CNS: headache, dysphagia, fatigue.
GI: nausea, vomiting, dyspepsia, abdominal pain, dry mouth.
Respiratory: upper respiratory tract infection, rhinitis, cough, pharyngitis, increased sputum, bronchitis, dyspnea, ***bronchospasm.***
Other: *unpleasant taste,* chest pain.

Overdose and treatment

Because nedocromil does not pass the blood-brain barrier, symptoms of overdosage probably require nothing more than observation of patient and discontinuation of drug when appropriate.

☑ Special considerations

- Dosage may be reduced to two inhalations three times daily and then twice daily after several weeks, when patient's asthma is under control.
- In maintenance therapy, drug must be used regularly, even during symptom-free periods, to achieve benefit.
- A decrease in severity of clinical symptoms or the need for concomitant therapy is a sign of improvement that usually occurs in the first 2 weeks of therapy if patient responds to therapy.
- When nedocromil is added to an existing regimen of bronchodilators or inhaled or oral corticosteroids, a reduction in dosage of the steroid or bronchodilator may be achieved in some patients. However, reduction should be gradual and under close medical supervision to avoid an exacerbation of asthma.
- Do not exceed 16 mg within 24 hours.
- In some patients, bronchospasm may be prevented by a single dose of nedocromil before activities that precipitate asthma, such as exercise or exposure to cold air, pollutants, or allergens.

Patient education

- Warn patient that drug has no direct bronchodilating action and cannot replace bronchodilators during an acute asthmatic attack.
- Tell patient that drug is an adjunct to the regular bronchodilator regimen and may reduce the need for corticosteroids or bronchodilators.
- Emphasize that drug should be taken regularly for best results. Most patients report benefits after 1 week of use; some require longer treatment before improvement occurs.
- Teach patient how to use the inhaler. Instruct him to shake canister immediately before use and to invert it just before actuation.
- Advise patient to clean inhaler at least twice weekly and to remove canister before rinsing inhaler in hot running water. Allow inhaler to air dry overnight.

Pediatric use

- Safety and efficacy have not been established for children under age 12.

Breast-feeding

- It is unknown if drug occurs in breast milk. Use cautiously when administering drug to breast-feeding women.

nefazodone hydrochloride

Serzone

Pharmacologic classification: phenylpiperazine
Therapeutic classification: antidepressant
Pregnancy risk category C

How supplied

Available by prescription only
Tablets: 100 mg, 150 mg, 200 mg, 250 mg

Indications, route, and dosage

Depression

Adults: Initially, 200 mg/day P.O. divided into two doses. Dosage increased in 100- to 200-mg/day increments at intervals of no less than 1 week p.r.n. Usual dosage range, 300 to 600 mg/day.

Pharmacodynamics

Antidepressive action: Nefazodone's action is not precisely defined. It inhibits neuronal uptake of serotonin and norepinephrine. It also occupies central 5-HT2 (serotonin) and $alpha_1$-adrenergic receptors.

Pharmacokinetics

- *Absorption:* Nefazodone is rapidly and completely absorbed but, because of extensive metabolism, its absolute bioavailability is only about 20%.
- *Distribution:* Over 99% is bound to plasma proteins.
- *Metabolism:* Drug is extensively metabolized by n-dealkylation and aliphatic and aromatic hydroxylation.
- *Excretion:* Nefazodone and its metabolites are excreted in urine. Half-life of drug is 2 to 4 hours.

Contraindications and precautions

Contraindicated in patients with hypersensitivity to drug or other phenylpiperazine antidepressants. Do not use within 14 days of MAO inhibitor therapy and in coadministration with astemizole or cisapride.

Use cautiously in patients with CV or cerebrovascular disease that could be exacerbated by hypotension (such as history of MI, angina, or CVA) and conditions that would predispose patients to hypotension (such as dehydration, hypovolemia, and antihypertensive drug treatment). Also use cautiously in patients with history of mania.

Interactions

Nefazodone, when coadministered with *alprazolam* and *triazolam*, potentiates the effects of these drugs. Do not administer concurrently. However, if necessary, dosage of alprazolam and triazolam may need to be reduced greatly.

Use with *astemizole* or *cisapride* may cause decreased metabolism of these drugs, leading to increased levels and cardiotoxicity. Avoid concomitant use.

Use with *CNS active drugs* may alter CNS activity. Use together cautiously. Nefazodone may increase *digoxin* level. Use together cautiously and monitor digoxin levels.

Use with *MAO inhibitors* may cause severe excitation, hyperpyrexia, seizures, delirium, or coma. Avoid concomitant use.

Nefazodone administered with *other highly plasma protein-bound drugs* may increase incidence and severity of adverse reactions. Monitor patient closely.

Effects on diagnostic tests

None reported.

Adverse reactions

CNS: *headache, somnolence, dizziness, asthenia,* insomnia, *light-headedness, confusion,* memory impairment, paresthesia, abnormal dreams, decreased concentration, ataxia, incoordination, taste perversion, psychomotor retardation, tremor, hypertonia.
CV: orthostatic hypotension, vasodilation, hypotension, peripheral edema.
EENT: *blurred vision, abnormal vision,* pharyngitis, tinnitus, visual field defect.
GI: *dry mouth, nausea, constipation,* dyspepsia, diarrhea, increased appetite, vomiting.
GU: urinary frequency, urinary tract infection, urine retention, vaginitis.
Respiratory: cough.
Skin: pruritus, rash.
Other: infection, flu syndrome, chills, fever, neck rigidity, breast pain, thirst, arthralgia.

Overdose and treatment

Common symptoms associated with overdosage of nefazodone include nausea, vomiting, and somnolence. Other drug-associated adverse reactions may occur. Provide symptomatic and supportive treatment in the case of hypotension or excessive sedation. Use gastric lavage if needed.

☑ Special considerations

- Allow at least 1 week after stopping drug before giving patient an MAO inhibitor. Also, allow at least 14 days before patient is started on nefazodone after MAO inhibitor therapy has been discontinued.
- Record mood changes. Monitor patient for suicidal tendencies, and allow a minimum supply of drug.

Patient education

- Warn patient not to engage in hazardous activities until CNS effects are known.
- Instruct male patient that if prolonged or inappropriate erections occur, he should stop drug immediately and seek medical attention.
- Instruct female patient to report if pregnancy is suspected or is being planned during therapy.
- Instruct patient not to drink alcoholic beverages during therapy.
- Tell patient to report rash, hives, or a related allergic reaction.
- Inform patient that several weeks of therapy may be required to obtain the full antidepressant effect. Once improvement is seen, advise patient not to discontinue drug until directed.

Geriatric use
• Because of increased systemic exposure to nefazodone, initiate treatment at half the usual dose, but titrate upward over the same dosage range as in younger patients. Observe usual precautions in elderly patients who have concomitant medical illnesses or are receiving concomitant drugs.

Pediatric use
• Safety and effectiveness in children under age 18 have not been established.

Breast-feeding
• It is not known if nefazodone is excreted in breast milk; use caution when administering drug to breast-feeding women.

nelfinavir mesylate
Viracept

Pharmacologic classification: HIV protease inhibitor
Therapeutic classification: antiviral
Pregnancy risk category B

How supplied
Available by prescription only
Tablets: 250 mg
Powder: 50 mg/g of powder

Indications, route, and dosage
Treatment of HIV infection when antiretroviral therapy is warranted
Adults: 750 mg P.O. t.i.d with meal or light snack.
Children age 2 to 13: 20 to 30 mg/kg/dose P.O. t.i.d with meal or light snack; do not to exceed 750 mg t.i.d. Recommended pediatric dose given t.i.d. is shown in the following chart.

Body weight (kg)	No. of level 1-g scoops	No. of level tea-spoons	No. of tablets
7 to < 8.5	4	1	-
8.5 to < 10.5	5	1.25	-
10.5 to < 12	6	1.5	-
12 to < 14	7	1.75	-
14 to < 16	8	2	-
16 to < 18	9	2.25	-
18 to < 23	10	2.5	2
≥ 23	15	3.75	3

Pharmacodynamics
Antiviral action: Nelfinavir is an HIV protease inhibitor. Inhibition of the protease enzyme prevents cleavage of the viral polyprotein, resulting in the production of an immature, noninfectious virus.

Pharmacokinetics
• *Absorption:* Absolute bioavailability not determined. Food increases absorption of drug. Peak levels were reached 2 to 4 hours after administration of drug with food.
• *Distribution:* Apparent volume of distribution is 2 to 7 L/kg. Over 98% of drug is bound to plasma protein.
• *Metabolism:* Nelfinavir is metabolized in the liver by multiple cytochrome P-450 isoforms, including CYP3A.
• *Excretion:* Terminal half-life of drug is 3.5 to 5 hours. Drug is primarily excreted in the feces.

Contraindications and precautions
Contraindicated in patients with hypersensitivity to any component of drug.

Use cautiously in patients with hepatic dysfunction or hemophilia types A and B.

Interactions
Do not administer nelfinavir concurrently with *amiodarone, astemizole, cisapride, ergot derivatives, midazolam, quinidine,* or *triazolam* because nelfinavir is expected to produce large increases in plasma levels of these drugs, which may increase risk for serious or life-threatening adverse events.

Nelfinavir dramatically increases *rifabutin* plasma levels. Therefore, reduce dose of rifabutin to one half the usual dose. *Rifampin* decreases nelfinavir plasma levels do not use together.

Carbamazepine, phenobarbital, and *phenytoin* may reduce the effectiveness of nelfinavir by decreasing nelfinavir plasma concentrations.

AntiHIV protease inhibitors (indinavir, ritonavir) may increase nelfinavir plasma levels. Nelfinavir may decrease plasma levels of *oral contraceptives* (*ethinyl estradiol, norethindrone*); advise patient to use alternate or additional contraceptive measures during nelfinavir therapy.

Coadministration of nelfinavir with drugs primarily metabolized by CYP3A (such as *dihydropyridine, calcium channel blockers*) may result in increased concentrations of the other drug and decreased plasma concentration of nelfinavir; use together cautiously.

Antiretroviral activity may be increased when used in combination with approved *reverse transcriptase inhibitors.*

Effects on diagnostic tests
None reported.

Adverse reactions
CNS: anxiety, depression, dizziness, emotional lability, hyperkinesia, insomnia, migraine headache, paresthesia, ***seizures***, sleep disorders, somnolence, ***suicide ideation***.
EENT: iritis, eye disorders, pharyngitis, rhinitis, sinusitis.
GI: abdominal pain nausea, *diarrhea*, flatulence, anorexia dyspepsia, epigastric pain, GI bleeding, pancreatitis, mouth ulceration, vomiting.
GU: sexual dysfunction, kidney calculus, urine abnormality.

Hematologic: anemia, ***leukopenia, thrombocytopenia.***
Hepatic: ***hepatitis.***
Metabolic: dehydration, diabetes mellitus, hyperlipidemia, hyperuricemia, hypoglycemia.
Respiratory: dyspnea.
Skin: rash, dermatitis, folliculitis, fungal dermatitis, pruritus, sweating, urticaria.
Other: fever, malaise, back pain, arthralgia, arthritis, cramps, myalgia, myasthenia, myopathy.

Overdose and treatment
Information is limited. Unabsorbed drug may be removed by emesis or gastric lavage; activated charcoal may also be used. Dialysis is not beneficial.

☑ Special considerations
- Decision to use drug is based on surrogate marker changes in patients who received drug in combination with nucleoside analogues or alone for up to 24 weeks. There are no results from controlled trials evaluating the effect on survival or incidence of opportunistic fungal infections.
- Drug dosage is same whether used alone or in combination with other antiretroviral agents.
- Administer oral powder in children unable to take tablets; may mix oral powder with water, milk, formula, soy formula, soy milk, or dietary supplements. Tell patient to drink entire contents.
- Do not reconstitute with water in its original container.
- Use reconstituted powder within 6 hours.
- Acidic foods or juice are not recommended due to bitter taste.
- Monitor CBC with differential (especially neutrophils) and chemistries; low incidences of laboratory abnormalities were reported in clinical studies. Increases in alkaline phosphatase, amylase, CK, LD, AST, ALT, and gamma glutamyltransferase may occur; monitor closely.

Patient education
- Advise patient to take drug with food.
- Inform patient that drug is not a cure for HIV infection.
- Tell patient that long-term effects of drug are currently unknown and that there is evidence that drug reduces risk of HIV transmission to others.
- Advise patient to take drug daily as prescribed and not to alter dose or discontinue drug without medical approval.
- If patient misses a dose, tell him to take the dose as soon as possible and return to his normal schedule. If a dose is skipped, advise patient not to double dose.
- Tell patient that diarrhea is the most common adverse effect and that it can be controlled with loperamide if necessary.
- Instruct patient taking oral contraceptives to use alternate or additional contraceptive measures.
- Advise patient to report use of other prescribed or OTC drugs.

Pediatric use
- Safety, efficacy, and pharmacokinetics have not been established in children under age 2.

Breast-feeding
- It is not known if drug is excreted in breast milk. Although safety has not been established, advise HIV-infected women not to breast-feed, in order to avoid HIV transmission to the infant.

neomycin sulfate
Mycifradin, Myciguent, Neo-Tabs

Pharmacologic classification: aminoglycoside
Therapeutic classification: antibiotic
Pregnancy risk category C

How supplied
Available by prescription only
Tablets: 500 mg
Oral solution: 125 mg/5 ml
Otic: 5 mg/ml (with polymixin B sulfate 10,000 units/ml and hydrocortisone 1%)

Available without a prescription
Cream: 0.5%
Ointment: 0.5%

Indications, route, and dosage
***Infectious diarrhea caused by enteropathogenic* Escherichia coli**
Adults: 50 mg/kg P.O. daily in four divided doses for 2 to 3 days.
Children: 50 to 100 mg/kg P.O. daily divided q 4 to 6 hours for 2 to 3 days.
Suppression of intestinal bacteria preoperatively
Adults: 1 g P.O. q 1 hour for four doses, then 1 g q 4 hours for rest of 24 hours. A NaCl cathartic should precede therapy.
Children: 40 to 100 mg/kg P.O. daily divided q 4 to 6 hours. First dose should be preceded by NaCl cathartic.
Adjunctive treatment in hepatic coma
Adults: 1 to 3 g P.O. q.i.d. for 5 to 6 days; 200 ml of 1% or 100 ml of 2% solution as enema retained for 20 to 60 minutes q 6 hours.
Children: 50 to 100 mg/kg P.O. daily in divided doses for 5 to 6 days.
External ear canal infection
Adults and children: 2 to 5 drops into ear canal t.i.d. or q.i.d.
Topical bacterial infections, burns, wounds, skin grafts, following surgical procedure, lesions, pruritus, trophic ulcerations, and edema
Adults and children: Rub in small amount gently b.i.d., t.i.d., or as directed.
✦ ***Dosage adjustment.*** Use reduced dosage in adults and children with renal failure. Specific recommendations are not available.

Pharmacodynamics
Antibiotic action: Neomycin is bactericidal; it binds directly to the 30S ribosomal subunit, thus inhibiting bacterial protein synthesis. Its spectrum of action includes many aerobic gram-negative organisms and some aerobic gram-positive organisms. Drug is far less active against many gram-negative

organisms than are tobramycin, gentamicin, amikacin, and netilmicin. Given orally or as retention enema, neomycin inhibits ammonia-forming bacteria in the GI tract, reducing ammonia and improving neurologic status of patients with hepatic encephalopathy. It is rarely given systemically because of its high potential for ototoxicity and nephrotoxicity. The FDA recently revoked licensing of the parenteral preparation for this reason.

Pharmacokinetics

- *Absorption:* Absorbed poorly (about 3%) after oral administration, although oral administration is enhanced in patients with impaired GI motility or mucosal intestinal ulcerations. After oral administration, peak serum levels occur at 1 to 4 hours. Neomycin is not absorbed through intact skin; it may be absorbed from wounds, burns, or skin ulcers.
- *Distribution:* Neomycin crosses the placenta. Oral administration restricts distribution to the GI tract.
- *Metabolism:* Not metabolized.
- *Excretion:* Drug is excreted primarily in urine by glomerular filtration. Elimination half-life in adults is 2 to 3 hours; in severe renal damage, half-life may extend to 24 hours. After oral administration, neomycin is excreted primarily unchanged in feces.

Contraindications and precautions

Contraindicated in patients hypersensitive to drug. Oral form contraindicated in patients sensitive to other aminoglycosides and in those with intestinal obstruction.

Use oral form cautiously in the elderly and in patients with impaired renal function, neuromuscular disorders, or ulcerative bowel lesions. Do not administer drug parenterally. Use topical form cautiously in patients with extensive dermatologic conditions.

Interactions

Concomitant use with the following drugs may increase the hazard of nephrotoxicity, ototoxicity, and neurotoxicity: *amphotericin B, cephalosporins, cisplatin, methoxyflurane, polymyxin B, vancomycin,* and *other aminoglycosides*; hazard of ototoxicity is also increased during use with *bumetanide, ethacrynic acid, furosemide, mannitol,* or *urea. Dimenhydrinate, other antiemetics,* and *antivertigo drugs* may mask neomycin-induced ototoxicity.

Concomitant use with *penicillins* results in a synergistic bactericidal effect against *Pseudomonas aeruginosa, Escherichia coli, Klebsiella, Citrobacter, Enterobacter, Serratia,* and *Proteus mirabilis.* However, the drugs are physically and chemically incompatible and are inactivated when mixed or given together.

Neomycin may potentiate neuromuscular blockade from *general anesthetics* or *neuromuscular blocking agents* such as *succinylcholine* and *tubocurarine.*

Oral neomycin inhibits vitamin K producing bacteria in GI tract and may potentiate action of *oral anticoagulants*; dosage adjustment of anticoagulants may be necessary.

Effects on diagnostic tests

Neomycin-induced nephrotoxicity may elevate levels of BUN, nonprotein nitrogen, or serum creatinine; it may increase urinary excretion of casts, if systemic absorption occurs.

Adverse reactions

EENT: *ototoxicity* (with oral administration).
GI: nausea, vomiting diarrhea, malabsorption syndrome, *Clostridium difficile*–associated colitis (with oral administration).
GU: *nephrotoxicity* (with oral administration).
Skin: *rash, contact dermatitis,* urticaria (with topical administration).
Other: ***neuromuscular blockade*** (with topical administration).

Overdose and treatment

Clinical signs of overdose include ototoxicity, nephrotoxicity, and neuromuscular toxicity. Remove drug by hemodialysis or peritoneal dialysis; treatment with calcium salts or anticholinesterases reverses neuromuscular blockade. After recent ingestion (4 hours or less), empty the stomach by induced emesis or gastric lavage; follow with activated charcoal to reduce absorption.

☑ Special considerations

Besides those relevant to all *aminoglycosides,* consider the following recommendations.

Preoperative bowel contamination

- Provide low-residue diet and cathartic immediately before administration of oral neomycin; follow-up enemas may be necessary to completely empty bowel.

Topical therapy

- Do not apply to more than 20% of body surface.
- Do not apply to any body surface of patient with decreased renal function without considering risk/benefit ratio.
- Monitor patient for hypersensitivity or contact dermatitis.

Otic therapy

- Reculture persistent drainage.
- Drug best used in combination with other antibiotics.
- Avoid touching ear with dropper.

neostigmine bromide

neostigmine methylsulfate

Prostigmin

Pharmacologic classification: cholinesterase inhibitor
Therapeutic classification: muscle stimulant
Pregnancy risk category C

How supplied

Available by prescription only
Tablets: 15 mg
Injection: 0.25 mg/ml, 0.5 mg/ml, 1 mg/ml

Indications, route, and dosage

Antidote for nondepolarizing neuromuscular blocking agents

Adults: 0.5 to 2 mg slow I.V. Repeat p.r.n.; maximum total dose, 5 mg. Give 0.6 to 1.2 mg atropine sulfate I.V. before antidote dose if patient is bradycardic.

Neonates and infants: 0.01 mg/kg to 0.04 mg/kg I.V. with 0.02 mg/kg of atropine sulfate.

Postoperative abdominal distention and bladder atony

Adults: 0.25 to 0.5 mg I.M. or S.C. q 4 to 6 hours for 2 to 3 days.

Diagnosis of myasthenia gravis

Adults: 0.022 mg/kg I.M. If cholinergic reaction occurs, discontinue test and give atropine sulfate 0.4 to 0.6 mg I.V.

Children: 0.025 to 0.04 mg/kg I.M. preceded by 0.011 mg/kg S.C. of atropine sulfate.

Symptomatic control of myasthenia gravis

Adults: 0.5 mg S.C. or I.M. Oral dose can range from 15 to 375 mg/day (average 150 mg in 24 hours). Subsequent dosages must be individualized, based on response and tolerance of adverse effects. Therapy may be required day and night.

Children: 7.5 to 15 mg P.O. t.i.d. or q.i.d.

Pharmacodynamics

Muscle stimulant action: Neostigmine blocks acetylcholine's hydrolysis by cholinesterase, resulting in acetylcholine accumulation at cholinergic synapses. That leads to increased cholinergic receptor stimulation at the myoneural junction.

Pharmacokinetics

- *Absorption:* Drug is poorly absorbed (1% to 2%) from GI tract after oral administration. Action usually begins 2 to 4 hours after oral administration and 10 to 30 minutes after injection.
- *Distribution:* About 15% to 25% of dose binds to plasma proteins.
- *Metabolism:* Drug is hydrolyzed by cholinesterases and metabolized by microsomal liver enzymes. Duration of effect varies considerably, depending on patient's physical and emotional status and on disease severity.
- *Excretion:* About 80% of dose is excreted in urine as unchanged drug and metabolites in the first 24 hours after administration.

Contraindications and precautions

Contraindicated in patients with hypersensitivity to cholinergics or to bromide and in those with peritonitis or mechanical obstruction of the intestine or urinary tract.

Use cautiously in patients with bronchial asthma, bradycardia, seizure disorders, recent coronary occlusion, vagotonia, hyperthyroidism, arrhythmias, and peptic ulcer.

Interactions

Concomitant use with *procainamide* or *quinidine* may reverse neostigmine's cholinergic effect on muscle. *Corticosteroids* may also decrease cholinergic effects; when corticosteroids are stopped, however, neostigmine's cholinergic effects may increase, possibly affecting muscle strength.

Concomitant use with *succinylcholine* may result in prolonged respiratory depression from plasma esterase inhibition, causing delayed succinylcholine hydrolysis; use with *other cholinergic drugs* may cause additive toxicity.

Magnesium has a direct depressant effect on skeletal muscle and may antagonize neostigmine's beneficial effects.

Atropine antagonizes the muscarinic effects of neostigmine.

Effects on diagnostic tests

None reported.

Adverse reactions

CNS: dizziness, headache, muscle weakness, loss of consciousness, drowsiness.
CV: bradycardia, hypotension, tachycardia, AV block, syncope, ***cardiac arrest.***
EENT: blurred vision, lacrimation, miosis.
GI: *nausea, vomiting, diarrhea, abdominal cramps,* excessive salivation, flatulence, increased peristalsis.
GU: urinary frequency.
Respiratory: ***bronchospasm,*** dyspnea, respiratory depression, ***respiratory arrest,*** increased secretions.
Skin: rash, urticaria, diaphoresis, flushing.
Other: *muscle cramps,* muscle fasciculations, arthralgia, hypersensitivity reactions ***(anaphylaxis).***

Overdose and treatment

Clinical signs of overdose include headache, nausea, vomiting, diarrhea, blurred vision, miosis, excessive tearing, bronchospasm, increased bronchial secretions, hypotension, incoordination, excessive sweating, muscle weakness, cramps, fasciculations, paralysis, bradycardia or tachycardia, excessive salivation, and restlessness or agitation.

Support respiration; bronchial suctioning may be performed. Discontinue drug immediately. Atropine may be given to block neostigmine's muscarinic effects but will not counter drug's paralytic effects on skeletal muscle. Avoid atropine overdose, because it may lead to bronchial plug formation.

☑ Special considerations

- Monitor patient's vital signs, particularly the pulse.
- If muscle weakness is severe, determine if this stems from drug toxicity or from exacerbation of myasthenia gravis. A test dose of edrophonium I.V. will aggravate drug-induced weakness but will temporarily relieve weakness resulting from the disease.
- Hospitalized patients may be able to manage a bedside supply of tablets to take themselves.
- Give drug with food or milk to reduce the chance for GI adverse effects.
- When administering drug to patient with myasthenia gravis, schedule largest dose before anticipated periods of fatigue. For example, if patient has dysphagia, schedule this dose 30 minutes before each meal.

• Stop all other cholinergic drugs during neostigmine therapy because of risk of additive toxicity.
• When administering neostigmine to prevent abdominal distention and GI distress, insertion of a rectal tube may be indicated to help passage of gas.
• Administering atropine concomitantly with neostigmine can relieve or eliminate adverse reactions; these symptoms may indicate neostigmine overdose and will be masked by atropine.
• Patients may develop resistance to drug.

Patient education
• Instruct patient to observe and record changes in muscle strength.

Geriatric use
• Elderly patients may be more sensitive to neostigmine's effects. Use with caution.

Pediatric use
• Safety and effectiveness in children have not been fully established.

Breast-feeding
• Neostigmine may be excreted in breast milk, possibly resulting in infant toxicity. Evaluate patient's clinical status to see if breast-feeding or drug should be discontinued.

nevirapine
Viramune

Pharmacologic classification: nonnucleoside reverse transcriptase inhibitor
Therapeutic classification: antiviral
Pregnancy risk category C

How supplied
Available by prescription only
Tablets: 200 mg

Indications, route, and dosage
Adjunct treatment of patients with HIV-1 infection who have experienced clinical or immunologic deterioration
Adults: 200 mg P.O. daily for first 14 days, followed by 200 mg P.O. b.i.d. in combination with nucleoside analogue antiretroviral agents.

Pharmacodynamics
Antiviral action: Nevirapine binds directly to reverse transcriptase and blocks the RNA-dependent and DNA-dependent DNA polymerase activities by causing a disruption of the enzyme's catalytic site.

Pharmacokinetics
• *Absorption:* Nevirapine is readily absorbed.
• *Distribution:* Widely distributed, crosses the placenta, and excreted in breast milk. It is about 60% bound to plasma proteins.
• *Metabolism:* Nevirapine is extensively metabolized in the liver.
• *Excretion:* Metabolites are primarily excreted in urine; a small amount is excreted in feces.

Contraindications and precautions
Contraindicated in patients with hypersensitivity to drug. Use cautiously in patients with impaired renal or hepatic function because the pharmacokinetics of nevirapine have not been evaluated in these patient groups.

Interactions
Nevirapine may lower the plasma concentrations of *drugs that are extensively metabolized by P-450 CYP3A.* Dosage adjustment of these drugs may be required. Nevirapine may decrease plasma concentrations of *protease inhibitors* or *oral contraceptives* and should not be administered concomitantly.

Effects on diagnostic tests
None reported.

Adverse reactions
CNS: headache, peripheral neuropathy, paresthesia.
GI: nausea, diarrhea, abdominal pain, ulcerative stomatitis.
Hematologic: *decreased neutrophil count,* increased ALT, AST, gamma-glutamyl transpeptidase (GGT), and total bilirubin levels.
Hepatic: hepatitis, abnormal liver function test results.
Skin: *rash.*
Other: fever, myalgia.

Overdose and treatment
No information available.

☑ Special considerations
• Perform clinical chemistry tests, including liver function tests, before initiating therapy and regularly throughout therapy.
• Resistant virus emerges rapidly when drug is administered as monotherapy. Therefore, always administer in combination with at least one other antiretroviral agent.
• Discontinue drug if patient develops a severe rash or a rash accompanied by fever, blistering, oral lesions, conjunctivitis, swelling, muscle or joint aches, or general malaise. If rash occurs during the initial 14 days, do not increase dosage until it has resolved. Most rashes occur within the first 6 weeks of therapy.
• Temporarily stop drug in patients experiencing moderate or severe liver function test abnormalities (excluding GGT) until they have returned to baseline. May restart drug at half the previous dose level. If moderate or severe liver function test abnormalities recur, discontinue drug therapy.
• If therapy is interrupted for over 7 days, restart therapy as if receiving drug for first time.
• If disease progresses during therapy, consider altering antiretroviral therapy.

Patient education
• Inform patient that drug is not a cure for HIV, and the illnesses associated with advanced HIV-1 infection may still occur. Also tell patient that drug does not reduce risk of transmission of HIV-1 to

others through sexual contact or blood contamination.
- Instruct patient to report rash immediately. Therapy may need to be stopped temporarily.
- Stress importance of taking drug exactly as prescribed. If a dose is missed, tell patient to take the next dose as soon as possible. However, if a dose is skipped, he should not double the next dose.
- Tell patient not to use other medications without medical approval.
- Advise women of childbearing age to avoid oral contraceptives and other hormonal methods of birth control as a method of contraception during therapy.

Pediatric use
- Safety and effectiveness in children have not been established.

Breast-feeding
- Drug is excreted in breast milk. HIV-infected women should not breast-feed.

niacin (vitamin B_3, nicotinic acid)
Niac, Nico-400, Nicobid, Nicolar, Nicotinex, Slo-Niacin

Pharmacologic classification: B-complex vitamin
Therapeutic classification: vitamin B_3, antilipemic, peripheral vasodilator
Pregnancy risk category A (C if greater than RDA)

How supplied
Available by prescription only
Capsules: 500 mg
Injection: 30-ml vials, 100 mg/ml

Available without a prescription
Tablets: 25 mg, 50 mg, 100 mg, 125 mg, 250 mg, 400 mg, 500 mg
Tablets (timed-release): 250 mg, 500 mg, 750 mg
Capsules (timed-release): 125 mg, 250 mg, 300 mg, 400 mg, 500 mg, 750 mg
Elixir: 50 mg/5 ml

Indications, route, and dosage
Pellagra
Adults: 300 to 500 mg in divided doses P.O., S.C., I.M., or I.V. infusion daily, depending on severity of niacin deficiency. Maximum recommended daily dosage is 500 mg; should be divided into 10 doses, 50 mg each.
Children: Up to 300 mg P.O. daily, depending on severity of niacin deficiency.

To prevent recurrence after symptoms subside, advise adequate nutrition and adequate supplements to meet RDA.
Peripheral vascular disease and circulatory disorders
Adults: 100 to 150 mg P.O. three to five times daily.
Adjunctive treatment of hyperlipidemias, especially those associated with hypercholesterolemia
Adults: 1.5 to 3 g daily in three divided doses with or after meals, increased at intervals to 6 g daily to maximum of 9 g daily.
Dietary supplement
Adults: 10 to 20 mg P.O. daily.

Pharmacodynamics
Vitamin replacement: As a vitamin, niacin functions as a coenzyme essential to tissue respiration, lipid metabolism, and glycogenolysis. Niacin deficiency causes pellagra, which manifests as dermatitis, diarrhea, and dementia; administration of niacin cures pellagra. Niacin lowers cholesterol and triglyceride levels by an unknown mechanism.

Vasodilating action: Niacin acts directly on peripheral vessels, dilating cutaneous vessels and increasing blood flow, predominantly in the face, neck, and chest.

Antilipemic effect: Mechanism of action is unknown. Nicotinic acid inhibits lipolysis in adipose tissues, decreases hepatic esterification of triglyceride, and increases lipoprotein lipase activity. It reduces serum cholesterol and triglyceride levels.

Pharmacokinetics
- *Absorption:* Absorbed rapidly from the GI tract. Peak plasma levels occur in 45 minutes. Cholesterol and triglyceride levels decrease after several days.
- *Distribution:* Niacin coenzymes are distributed widely in body tissues; niacin is distributed in breast milk.
- *Metabolism:* Metabolized by the liver to active metabolites.
- *Excretion:* Niacin is excreted in urine.

Contraindications and precautions
Contraindicated in patients with hepatic dysfunction, active peptic ulcer, severe hypotension, arterial hemorrhage, or hypersensitivity to drug. Use cautiously in patients with history of liver disease, peptic ulcer, allergy, gout, gallbladder disease, diabetes mellitus, or coronary artery disease.

Interactions
Concomitant use with *sympathetic blocking agents* may cause added vasodilation and hypotension. Concomitant use with *aspirin* may decrease the metabolic clearance of nicotinic acid.

Effects on diagnostic tests
Niacin therapy alters fluorometric test results for urine catecholamines and results for urine glucose tests using cupric sulfate (Benedict's reagent).

Adverse reactions
Most reactions are dose-dependent.
CV: *excessive peripheral vasodilation,* hypotension, atrial fibrillation, ***arrhythmias.***
GI: *nausea, vomiting, diarrhea,* possible activation of peptic ulceration, epigastric or substernal pain.
Hepatic: ***hepatic dysfunction.***
Skin: ***flushing,*** pruritus, dryness, tingling.

Other: hyperglycemia, hyperuricemia, toxic amblyopia.

Overdose and treatment
Niacin is a water-soluble vitamin; these seldom cause toxicity in patients with normal renal function.

☑ Special considerations
- RDA of niacin in adult males is 19 mg; in adult females, 15 mg; and in children, 5 to 20 mg.
- For I.V. infusion, use concentration of 10 mg/ml or dilute in 500 ml 0.9% NaCl solution; give slowly, no faster than 2 mg/minute.
- I.V. administration of niacin may cause fibrinolysis, metallic taste in mouth, and anaphylactic shock.
- Megadoses of niacin are not usually recommended.
- Monitor hepatic function and blood glucose levels during initial therapy.
- Aspirin may reduce flushing response.

Patient education
- Explain disease process and rationale for therapy; stress that use of niacin to treat hyperlipidemia or to dilate peripheral vessels is not simply "taking a vitamin," but serious medicine. Emphasize importance of complying with therapy.
- Instruct patient not to substitute sustained-release (timed) tablets for intermediate-release tablets in equivalent doses. Severe hepatic toxicity, including necrosis, has occurred.
- Explain that cutaneous flushing and warmth commonly occur in the first 2 hours; they will cease on continued therapy.
- Advise patient not to make sudden postural changes to minimize effects of postural hypotension.
- Instruct patient to avoid hot liquids when initially taking drug to reduce flushing response.
- Advise patient to take drug with meals to minimize GI irritation.

Breast-feeding
- There have been no reports of problems in breast-feeding patients taking normal daily doses as dietary requirement.

niacinamide (nicotinamide)

Pharmacologic classification: B-complex vitamin
Therapeutic classification: vitamin B_3
Pregnancy risk category C

How supplied
Available without a prescription
Tablets: 50 mg, 100 mg, 125 mg, 250 mg, 500 mg

Indications, route, and dosage
Pellagra
Adults: 150 to 500 mg P.O. depending on severity of niacin deficiency. Maximum recommended daily dose is 500 mg; should be divided into 50-mg doses.
Children: Up to 300 mg P.O. daily, depending on severity of niacin deficiency.

To prevent recurrence after symptoms subside, advise adequate nutrition and supplements to meet RDA.

Pharmacodynamics
Vitamin replacement. Niacinamide is used by the body as a source of niacin; it is essential for tissue respiration, lipid metabolism, and glycogenolysis, but lacks the vasodilating and antilipemic effects of niacin.

Pharmacokinetics
- *Absorption:* Readily absorbed from the GI tract.
- *Distribution:* Drug is distributed widely in body tissues.
- *Metabolism:* Metabolized in the liver.
- *Excretion:* Excreted in the urine.

Contraindications and precautions
Contraindicated in patients with hepatic dysfunction, active peptic ulcer, severe hypotension, arterial hemorrhage, or hypersensitivity to drug. Use cautiously in patients with gallbladder disease, diabetes mellitus, or coronary artery disease and in those with history of liver disease, peptic ulcer, allergy, or gout.

Interactions
None reported.

Effects on diagnostic tests
Niacinamide alters liver function and serum bilirubin test results.

Adverse reactions
Most reactions are dose-dependent.
CV: *excessive peripheral vasodilation,* hypotension, atrial fibrillation, ***arrhythmias.***
GI: *nausea, vomiting, diarrhea,* possible activation of peptic ulceration, epigastric or substernal pain.
Hepatic: ***hepatic dysfunction.***
Skin: ***flushing,*** pruritus, dryness, tingling.
Other: hyperglycemia, hyperuricemia, toxic amblyopia.

Overdose and treatment
Niacinamide is a water-soluble vitamin; these seldom cause toxicity in patients with normal renal function.

☑ Special considerations
- Megadoses of niacinamide are not usually recommended.
- Monitor hepatic function and blood glucose levels during initial therapy.
- Niacinamide has no vasodilating or antilipemic effects.

Patient education
- Advise patient to take drug with meals to minimize GI irritation.

Breast-feeding

• There have been no reports of problems in breast-feeding patients taking normal daily doses as dietary requirement.

nicardipine hydrochloride

Cardene, Cardene SR

Pharmacologic classification: calcium channel blocker
Therapeutic classification: antianginal, antihypertensive
Pregnancy risk category C

How supplied

Available by prescription only
Capsules: 20 mg, 30 mg
Capsules (extended-release): 30 mg, 45 mg, 60 mg
Injection: 2.5 mg/ml in 10-ml ampules

Indications, route, and dosage

Hypertension; management of chronic stable angina

Adults: Initially, 20 mg P.O. t.i.d. Titrate dosage based on patient response. Usual dosage range, 20 to 40 mg t.i.d. Extended-release capsules (for hypertension only) can be initiated at 30 mg b.i.d. Usual dose, 30 to 60 mg b.i.d.

Short-term management of hypertension when oral therapy is not feasible or possible

Adults: Initially 5 mg/hour I.V. infusion; titrate infusion upward by 2.5 mg/hour q 15 minutes up to a maximum of 15 mg/hour, p.r.n.

Pharmacodynamics

Antihypertensive and antianginal action: Nicardipine inhibits the transmembrane flux of calcium ions into cardiac and smooth muscle cells. Drug appears to act specifically on vascular muscle, and may cause a smaller decrease in cardiac output than other calcium channel blockers because of its vasodilatory effect.

Pharmacokinetics

• *Absorption:* Completely absorbed after oral administration. Plasma levels are detectable within 20 minutes, and peak in about 1 hour. Absorption may be decreased if drug is taken with food. Therapeutic serum levels are 28 to 50 ng/ml.
• *Distribution:* Extensively (more than 95%) bound to plasma proteins.
• *Metabolism:* A substantial first-pass effect reduces absolute bioavailability to about 35%. Drug is extensively metabolized in the liver, and the process is saturable. Increasing dosage yields nonlinear increases in plasma levels.
• *Excretion:* Elimination half-life is about 8.6 hours after steady state levels are reached.

Contraindications and precautions

Contraindicated in patients with hypersensitivity to drug and in those with advanced aortic stenosis. Use cautiously in patients with impaired renal or hepatic function, cardiac conduction disturbances, hypotension, or heart failure.

Interactions

Concomitant administration of *cimetidine* results in higher plasma levels of nicardipine. Serum levels of *digoxin* should be carefully monitored because some *calcium channel blockers* may increase plasma levels of *cardiac glycosides.*

Concomitant administration of *cyclosporine* results in increased plasma levels of cyclosporine. Careful monitoring is recommended.

Severe hypotension has been reported in patients taking *calcium channel blockers* who undergo *fentanyl* anesthesia.

Effects on diagnostic tests

None reported.

Adverse reactions

CNS: *dizziness, light-headedness, headache, paresthesia, asthenia.*
CV: *peripheral edema, palpitations,* angina, tachycardia.
GI: nausea, abdominal discomfort, dry mouth.
Skin: rash, *flushing.*

Overdose and treatment

Overdosage may produce hypotension, bradycardia, drowsiness, confusion, and slurred speech. Treatment is supportive, with vasopressors administered as needed. I.V. calcium gluconate may be useful to counteract the effects of drug.

☑ Special considerations

Besides those relevant to all *calcium channel blockers,* consider the following recommendations.
• Allow at least 3 days between oral dosage changes to ensure achievement of steady state plasma levels.
• When treating patients with chronic stable angina, S.L. nitroglycerin, prophylactic nitrate therapy, and beta blockers may be continued.
• When treating hypertension, measure blood pressure during times of plasma level trough (approximately 8 hours after dose, or immediately before subsequent doses). Because of prominent effects that may occur during plasma level peaks, measure blood pressure 1 to 2 hours after dose.
• In patients with hepatic dysfunction, therapy should begin at 20 mg P.O. twice-daily; carefully titrate subsequent dosage based on patient response.
• Dilute solution in ampule before I.V. infusion.
• Monitor blood pressure during I.V. administration because nicardipine I.V. decreases peripheral resistance.

Pediatric use

• Safe use in children under age 18 has not been established.

Breast-feeding

• Substantial levels of drug have been found in the milk of animals given nicardipine. Breast-feeding is not recommended.

nicotine

Habitrol, Nicoderm, Nicotrol, Nicotrol NS, ProStep

Pharmacologic classification: nicotinic cholinergic agonist
Therapeutic classification: smoking cessation aid
Pregnancy risk category D

How supplied

Available with or without a prescription
Transdermal system: designed to release nicotine at a fixed rate
Habitrol: 21 mg/day, 14 mg/day, 7 mg/day
Nicoderm: 21 mg/day, 14 mg/day, 7 mg/day
Nicotrol: 15 mg/day, 10 mg/day, 5 mg/day
ProStep: 22 mg/day, 11 mg/day
Nasal spray: metered spray pump
Nicotrol NS: 10 ml/ml

Indications, route, and dosage

Relief of nicotine withdrawal symptoms in patients attempting smoking cessation
Adults: One transdermal system applied to a nonhairy part of the upper trunk or upper outer arm. Dosage varies slightly with product selected.
Habitrol, Nicoderm
Initially, apply one 21-mg/day system daily for 6 weeks. After 24 hours, the system should be removed and a new system applied to a different site. Then, taper dosage to 14 mg/day for 2 to 4 weeks. Finally, taper dosage to 7 mg/day if necessary. Nicotine substitution and gradual withdrawal should take 8 to 12 weeks.
✦ ***Dosage adjustment.*** Patients who weigh under 100 lb (45 kg), have CV disease, or who smoke less than half a pack of cigarettes daily should start therapy with the 14-mg/day system.
Nicotrol
Initially, apply one 15-mg/day system daily for 12 weeks. The system should be applied upon waking and removed h.s. Then, taper dosage to 10 mg/day for 2 weeks. Finally, taper dosage to 5 mg/day for 2 weeks if necessary. Alternatively, dosage may be reduced in patients who have successfully abstained from smoking q 2 to 4 weeks until 5-mg/day dosage has been used for 2 weeks. Nicotine substitution and gradual withdrawal should take 14 to 20 weeks.
Nicotrol NS
Adults: Initially, 1 or 2 doses/hour (1 dose = 2 sprays—one in each nostril). Encourage patient to use at least the recommended minimum of 8 doses/day. Maximum recommended dose is 40 mg or 80 sprays/day. Duration of treatment should not exceed 3 months.
ProStep
Initially, apply one 22-mg/day system daily for 4 to 8 weeks. After 24 hours, system should be removed and a new system applied to a different site. In patients weighing under 100 lb (45 kg), start therapy with the 11-mg/day system; those who have successfully stopped smoking during this period may discontinue drug. If therapy was initiated with the 22-mg/day system, treatment may continue for an additional 2 to 4 weeks at lower dosage (11 mg/day). Nicotine substitution and gradual withdrawal should take 6 to 12 weeks.

Pharmacodynamics

Nicotinic cholinergic action: Nicotine transdermal system and nasal spray provide nicotine, the chief stimulant alkaloid found in tobacco products, which stimulates nicotinic acetylcholine receptors in the CNS, neuromuscular junction, autonomic ganglia, and adrenal medulla.

Pharmacokinetics

- *Absorption:* Drug is rapidly absorbed.
- *Distribution:* Plasma protein-binding of drug is below 5%.
- *Metabolism:* Drug is metabolized by the liver, kidney, and lung. Over 20 metabolites have been identified. Primary metabolites are cotinine (15%) and trans-3-hydroxycotinine (45%).
- *Excretion:* Drug is excreted primarily in the urine as metabolites; about 10% is excreted unchanged. With high urine flow rates or acidified urine, up to 30% can be excreted unchanged.

Contraindications and precautions

Contraindicated in patients with hypersensitivity to nicotine or any components. Also contraindicated in nonsmokers and in patients with recent MI, life-threatening arrhythmias, and severe or worsening angina pectoris.

Use cautiously in patients with hyperthyroidism, pheochromocytoma, insulin-dependent diabetes, or peptic ulcer disease.

Interactions

Cessation of smoking may decrease induction of hepatic enzymes responsible for metabolizing certain drugs, such as *acetaminophen, caffeine, imipramine, oxazepam, pentazocine, propranolol,* and *theophylline*; dosage reduction of such drugs may be necessary. Cessation of smoking may increase the amount of subcutaneous *insulin* absorbed and may require reduction of insulin dosage.

Cessation of smoking may decrease levels of circulating catecholamines and may require lower doses of *adrenergic antagonists* (such as *labetalol, prazosin*) or higher doses of *adrenergic agonists* (such as *isoproterenol, phenylephrine*).

Effects on diagnostic tests

None reported.

Adverse reactions

CNS: somnolence, dizziness, *headache, insomnia,* paresthesia, abnormal dreams, nervousness.
EENT: pharyngitis, sinusitis.
GI: abdominal pain, constipation, dyspepsia, nausea, diarrhea, vomiting, dry mouth.
GU: dysmenorrhea.
Respiratory: increased cough.
Skin: *local or systemic erythema, pruritus, burning at application site,* cutaneous hypersensitivity, rash.

Other: back pain, myalgia, diaphoresis, hypertension.

Overdose and treatment

Overdosage could produce symptoms associated with acute nicotine poisoning, including nausea, vomiting, diarrhea, weakness, respiratory failure, hypotension, and seizures. Treat symptomatically. Barbiturates or benzodiazepines may be used to treat seizures, and atropine may attenuate excessive salivation or diarrhea. Administer fluids to treat hypotension; increase urine flow to enhance elimination of drug.

☑ Special considerations

- Discourage use of transdermal system for more than 3 months. Chronic nicotine consumption by any route can be dangerous and habit-forming.
- Patients who cannot stop cigarette smoking during the initial 4 weeks of therapy will probably not benefit from continued use of drug. Patients who were unsuccessful may benefit from counseling to identify factors that led to the unsuccessful attempt. Encourage patient to minimize or eliminate the factors that contributed to treatment failure and to try again, possibly after some interval, before the next attempt.
- Healthcare workers' exposure to the nicotine within the transdermal systems should be minimal; however, avoid unnecessary contact with the system. After contact, wash hands with water alone because soap can enhance absorption.
- Nicotrol NS is not recommended in patients with chronic nasal disorders or severe reactive airway disease.

Patient education

- Tell patient to discontinue use of patch and to call immediately if a generalized rash or persistent or severe local skin reactions (pruritus, edema, or erythema) occur.
- Make sure patient understands that nicotine can evaporate from the transdermal system once it is removed from its protective packaging. The patch should not be altered in any way (folded or cut) before it is applied. It should be applied promptly after removal of the system's protective packaging. Tell patient not to store patch at temperatures above 86° F (30° C).
- Teach patient how to dispose of transdermal system. After removal, fold the patch in half, bringing the adhesive sides together. If the system comes in a protective pouch, dispose of the used patch in the pouch that contained the new system. Careful disposal is necessary to prevent accidental poisoning of children or pets.
- Be sure that patient reads and understands the patient information that is dispensed with drug when the prescription is filled.
- Inform patient to refrain from smoking while using the system; he may experience adverse effects from the increased nicotine levels.
- Explain that patient is likely to experience nasal irritation, which may become less bothersome with continued use of Nicotrol NS.

Pediatric use

- Safety and efficacy in children have not been established. Note that the amount of nicotine contained in a patch could prove fatal to a child if ingested; even used patches contain a substantial amount of residual nicotine. Patients should take care to ensure that both used and unused transdermal systems and metered spray bottles are kept out of the reach of children.

Breast-feeding

- Nicotine passes freely into breast milk and is readily absorbed after oral administration. Weigh the infant's risk of exposure to nicotine against his risk of exposure from continued smoking by the mother.

nicotine polacrilex (nicotine resin complex)

Nicorette

Pharmacologic classification: nicotinic agonist
Therapeutic classification: smoking cessation aid
Pregnancy risk category X

How supplied

Available with and without a prescription
Chewing gum: 2 mg, 4 mg nicotine resin complex per square

Indications, route, and dosage

Aid in managing nicotine dependence
Serves as a temporary aid to smoker seeking to give up smoking while participating in a behavior modification program under medical supervision. Generally, smoker with the "physical" type of nicotine dependence is most likely to benefit from use of nicotine chewing gum.
Adults: Chew one piece of gum slowly and intermittently for 30 minutes whenever the urge to smoke occurs. Most patients require approximately 10 pieces of gum daily during first month. Patients using the 2-mg strength should not exceed 30 pieces of gum daily; those using the 4-mg strength should not exceed 20 pieces of gum daily.

Pharmacodynamics

Nicotine replacement action: Nicotine is an agonist at the nicotinic receptors in the peripheral nervous system and CNS and produces both behavioral stimulation and depression. It acts on the adrenal medulla to aid in overcoming physical dependence on nicotine during withdrawal from habitual smoking.

Nicotine's CV effects are usually dose-dependent. Nonsmokers have experienced CNS-mediated symptoms of hiccuping, nausea, and vomiting, even with a small dose. A smoker chewing a 2-mg piece of gum every hour usually does not experience CV adverse effects.

Pharmacokinetics

• *Absorption:* Nicotine is bound to ion-exchange resin and is released only during chewing. The blood level depends upon the vigor with which the gum is chewed.
• *Distribution:* Nicotine's distribution into tissues has not been fully characterized. It crosses the placenta and occurs in breast milk.
• *Metabolism:* Metabolized mainly by the liver and less so by the kidneys and lungs. Main metabolites are cotinine and nicotine-19-N-oxide.
• *Excretion:* Both nicotine and its metabolites are excreted in urine, with approximately 10% to 20% excreted unchanged. Excretion of nicotine is increased in acid urine and by high urine output.

Contraindications and precautions

Contraindicated in nonsmokers; in patients with recent MI, life-threatening arrhythmias, severe or worsening angina pectoris, or active temporomandibular joint disease; and during pregnancy.

Use cautiously in patients with hyperthyroidism, pheochromocytoma, insulin-dependent diabetes, peptic ulcer disease, history of esophagitis, oral or pharyngeal inflammation, or dental conditions that might be exacerbated by chewing gum.

Interactions

Smoking may increase the metabolism of the following drugs: *caffeine, imipramine, pentazocine,* and *theophylline.* Smoking cessation either with or without nicotine substitutes may reverse this effect. Smoking cessation may reduce the first-pass metabolism of *propoxyphene.*

Nicorette gum and smoking can increase the circulating levels of *cortisol* and *catecholamines.* Therapy with *adrenergic agonists* or *adrenergic blockers* may require adjustments.

Effects on diagnostic tests

None reported.

Adverse reactions

CNS: dizziness, light-headedness, irritability, insomnia, headache, paresthesia.
CV: atrial fibrillation.
EENT: throat soreness, jaw muscle ache (from chewing).
GI: nausea, vomiting, indigestion, eructation, anorexia, excessive salivation.
Other: hiccups, sweating.

Overdose and treatment

The risk of overdose is minimized by early nausea and vomiting that result from excessive nicotine intake. Poisoning manifests as nausea, vomiting, salivation, abdominal pain, diarrhea, cold sweats, headache, dizziness, disturbed hearing and vision, mental confusion, and weakness.

Treatment includes emesis—give ipecac syrup if it has not occurred. A NaCl cathartic will speed the gum's passage through the GI tract. Give gastric lavage followed by activated charcoal in unconscious patients. Provide supportive treatment of respiratory paralysis and CV collapse as needed.

☑ Special considerations

• Patients most likely to benefit from Nicorette gum are smokers with a high physical dependence. Typically, they smoke over 15 cigarettes daily; prefer brands of cigarettes with high nicotine levels; usually inhale the smoke; smoke the first cigarette within 30 minutes of arising; and find the first morning cigarette the hardest to give up.
• Instruct patient to chew gum slowly and intermittently for about 30 minutes to promote slow and even buccal absorption of nicotine. Fast chewing allows faster absorption and produces more adverse reactions.
• At the initial visit, instruct patient to chew one piece of gum whenever the urge to smoke occurs instead of having a cigarette. Most patients will require approximately 10 pieces of gum daily during first month of treatment.
• Tell patient who has successfully abstained to gradually withdraw gum use after 3 months; he should not use gum for longer than 6 months.
• Inform patient that gum is sugar-free and usually does not stick to dentures.

Breast-feeding

• Nicotine passes freely into breast milk and is readily absorbed after oral administration. Weigh the infant's risk of exposure to nicotine from a transdermal patch against his risk of exposure from continued smoking by the mother.

nifedipine

Adalat, Adalat CC, Procardia, Procardia XL

Pharmacologic classification: calcium channel blocker
Therapeutic classification: antianginal
Pregnancy risk category C

How supplied

Available by prescription only
Capsules: 10 mg, 20 mg
Tablets (extended-release): 30 mg, 60 mg, 90 mg

Indications, route, and dosage

Management of Prinzmetal's or variant angina or chronic stable angina pectoris
Adults: Starting dose is 10 mg P.O. t.i.d. Usual effective dosage range is 10 to 20 mg t.i.d. Some patients may require up to 30 mg q.i.d. Maximum daily dose for capsules is 180 mg; for extended-release tablets, 120 mg.

Hypertension
Adults: Initially, 30 to 60 mg P.O. once daily (extended-release tablets). Adjust dosage at 7- to 14-day intervals based on patient tolerance and response. Maximum daily dosage is 120 mg.

◊ ***Quick reduction of blood pressure***
Adults: 10 to 20 mg q 20 to 30 minutes; capsule should be bitten and then swallowed.

Pharmacodynamics

Antianginal action: Nifedipine dilates systemic arteries, resulting in decreased total peripheral resistance and modestly decreased systemic blood pressure with a slightly increased heart rate, decreased afterload, and increased cardiac index. Reduced afterload and the subsequent decrease in myocardial oxygen consumption probably account for nifedipine's value in treating chronic stable angina. In Prinzmetal's angina, nifedipine inhibits coronary artery spasm, increasing myocardial oxygen delivery.

Pharmacokinetics

- *Absorption:* Approximately 90% of a dose is absorbed rapidly from the GI tract after oral administration; however, only about 65% to 70% of drug reaches the systemic circulation because of a significant first-pass effect in the liver. Peak serum levels occur in about 30 minutes to 2 hours. Hypotensive effects may occur 5 minutes after S.L. administration. Therapeutic serum levels are 25 to 100 ng/ml.
- *Distribution:* About 92% to 98% of circulating nifedipine is bound to plasma proteins.
- *Metabolism:* Drug is metabolized in the liver.
- *Excretion:* Excreted in the urine and feces as inactive metabolites. Elimination half-life is 2 to 5 hours. Duration of effect ranges from 4 to 12 hours.

Contraindications and precautions

Contraindicated in patients with hypersensitivity to drug. Use cautiously in the elderly and in patients with heart failure or hypotension. Use extended-release form cautiously in patients with GI narrowing. Use with caution in patients with unstable angina who are not currently taking a beta blocker because a higher incidence of MI has been reported.

Interactions

Concomitant use of nifedipine with *beta blockers* may exacerbate angina, heart failure, and hypotension. Concomitant use with *fentanyl* may cause excessive hypotension. Concomitant use with *digoxin* may cause increased serum digoxin levels. Use with *hypotensive agents* may precipitate excessive hypotension.

Cimetidine may decrease metabolism of nifedipine and therefore increase drug levels of nifedipine. Use together cautiously. Drug may increase *phenytoin* levels.

Effects on diagnostic tests

Mild to moderate increase in serum concentrations of alkaline phosphate, LD, AST, and ALT have been noted.

Adverse reactions

CNS: *dizziness, light-headedness, flushing, headache, weakness,* syncope, nervousness.
CV: *peripheral edema,* hypotension, palpitations, ***heart failure, MI, pulmonary edema.***
EENT: nasal congestion.
GI: *nausea,* diarrhea, constipation, abdominal discomfort.
Respiratory: dyspnea, cough.
Skin: rash, pruritus.
Other: muscle cramps, hypokalemia.

Overdose and treatment

Clinical effects of overdose are extensions of drug's pharmacologic effects, primarily peripheral vasodilation and hypotension.

Treatment includes such basic support measures as hemodynamic and respiratory monitoring. If patient requires blood pressure support by a vasoconstrictor, norepinephrine may be administered. Extremities should be elevated and any fluid deficit corrected.

☑ Special considerations

- Initial doses or dosage increase may exacerbate angina briefly. Reassure patient that this symptom is temporary.
- Nifedipine is not available in S.L. form. No advantage has been found in S.L. or intrabuccal use. It is recommended that capsule be bitten, then swallowed.
- Monitor blood pressure regularly, especially if patient is also taking beta blockers or antihypertensives.
- Although rebound effect has not been observed when drug is stopped, reduce dosage slowly.

Patient education

- Instruct patient to swallow capsules whole without breaking, crushing, or chewing them unless instructed otherwise.
- Tell patient that he may experience annoying hypotensive effects during titration of dose and urge compliance with therapy.

Geriatric use

- Use drug with caution in elderly patients because they may be more sensitive to drug's effects and duration of effect may be prolonged.

nilutamide

Nilandron

Pharmacologic classification: nonsteroidal antiandrogen
Therapeutic classification: antineoplastic
Pregnancy risk category C

How supplied

Available by prescription only
Tablets: 50 mg

Indications, route, and dosage

Adjunct therapy with surgical castration for treatment of metastatic prostate cancer (stage D_2)
Adults: Six tablets (50 mg each) P.O. once daily for total of 300 mg/day for 30 days; then three tablets once daily for total of 150 mg/day. For optimal benefit, initiate therapy on day of or day after surgical castration.

Pharmacodynamics

Antineoplastic action: Nonsteroidal antiandrogen interacts with the androgen receptor and prevents normal androgenic response. Prostate cancer is known to be androgen sensitive and responds to androgen ablation.

Pharmacokinetics

- *Absorption:* Rapidly and completely absorbed after oral administration.
- *Distribution:* Moderate binding to plasma proteins and low binding to erythrocytes.
- *Metabolism:* Extensively metabolized to at least five metabolites with less than 2% of drug excreted unchanged in the urine.
- *Excretion:* Excreted in the urine. Half-life ranges from 38 to 59 hours.

Contraindications and precautions

Contraindicated in patients with hypersensitivity to drug and severe hepatic or respiratory disease.

Interactions

Vitamin K antagonists, phenytoin, and *theophylline* may possibly delay elimination and toxicity of drug. Doses should be modified. Drug may inhibit liver cytochrome P450 isoenzymes and reduce the metabolism of compounds requiring these systems.

Effects on diagnostic tests

None reported.

Adverse reactions

CNS: dizziness.
CV: hypertension.
EENT: abnormal vision, *impaired adaptation to darkness.*
GI: nausea, constipation.
GU: urinary tract infection.
Hepatic: elevated liver enzymes.
Respiratory: dyspnea, ***interstitial pneumonitis.***
Other: *hot flashes.*

Overdose and treatment

No clinical signs or symptoms or changes in parameters such as transaminases or chest X-ray were reported in an attempted suicide in which 13 g of nilutamide (43 times maximum dosage) was ingested. Doses of 600 and 900 mg/day were associated with GI disorders, malaise, headache, and dizziness. General supportive care with frequent monitoring of vital signs is indicated. Dialysis is not useful.

☑ Special considerations

- Obtain baseline liver enzymes and periodically, at 3-month intervals. Discontinue drug if transaminase levels exceed three times upper limit of normal.
- Obtain a baseline chest radiograph before initiating therapy. Monitor patient, especially if he is Asian, for signs of interstitial pneumonitis.

Patient education

- Tell patient that drug should be started on day of or day after surgical castration.
- Explain purpose of drug, how it is given, and importance of not stopping treatment without medical approval.
- Tell patient to report dyspnea or aggravation of preexisting dyspnea immediately.
- Inform patient of possibility of developing hepatitis and to report symptoms of nausea, vomiting, abdominal pain, or jaundice. Tell patient to avoid alcohol because of possibility of intolerance (facial flushes, hypotension, malaise).
- Warn patient that visual disturbances, such as delayed ability to adapt to darkness, may affect driving at night or through tunnels; recommend use of tinted glasses to alleviate this effect.

Pediatric use

- Safety and effectiveness have not been determined.

Breast-feeding

- It is unknown if drug appears in breast milk.

nimodipine

Nimotop

Pharmacologic classification: calcium channel blocker
Therapeutic classification: cerebral vasodilator
Pregnancy risk category C

How supplied

Available by prescription only
Capsules. 30 mg

Indications, route, and dosage

Improvement of neurologic deficits after subarachnoid hemorrhage from ruptured congenital aneurysms

Adults: 60 mg P.O. q 4 hours for 21 days. Therapy should begin within 96 hours of subarachnoid hemorrhage.

✦ ***Dosage adjustment.*** In adults with hepatic impairment, 30 mg P.O. q 4 hours.

◊ ***Migraine headache***

Adults: 120 mg P.O. daily, 1 hour before or within 2 hours after meals.

Pharmacodynamics

Neuronal-sparing action: Nimodipine inhibits calcium ion influx across cardiac and smooth muscle cells, thus decreasing myocardial contractility and oxygen demand, and dilates coronary arteries and arterioles. Although the action is not completely known, it is believed that dilation of the small cerebral resistance vessels with increased collateral circulation is possible.

Pharmacokinetics

- *Absorption:* Well absorbed after oral administration. However, because of extensive first-pass metabolism, bioavailability is only about 3% to 30%.
- *Distribution:* Greater than 95% protein-bound.
- *Metabolism:* Extensively metabolized in the liver. Drug and metabolites undergo enterohepatic recycling.
- *Excretion:* Less than 1% as parent drug. Elimination half-life is 1 to 9 hours.

Contraindications and precautions

No known contraindications. Use cautiously in patients with hepatic failure.

Interactions
Concomitant use with *antihypertensives* may enhance the hypotensive effect; use with *calcium channel blocking agents* may enhance these drugs' CV effects. Drug may increase *phenytoin* levels.

Effects on diagnostic tests
None reported.

Adverse reactions
CNS: headache, psychic disturbances.
CV: decreased blood pressure, flushing, edema, tachycardia.
GI: nausea, diarrhea, abdominal discomfort.
Respiratory: dyspnea.
Skin: dermatitis, rash.
Other: muscle cramps.

Overdose and treatment
Nausea, weakness, drowsiness, confusion, bradycardia, and decreased cardiac output can be expected. Treatment should be supportive. Administer pressor amines to counter hypotension; cardiac pacing, atropine, or sympathomimetics to treat bradycardia. Calcium gluconate I.V. has been used to treat calcium channel blocker overdose.

☑ Special considerations
Besides those relevant to all *calcium channel blockers,* consider the following recommendations.
- Unlike other calcium channel blockers, drug is not used for angina pectoris or hypertension.
- Use lower doses in patients with hepatic failure. Initiate therapy at 30 mg P.O. every 4 hours, and closely monitor blood pressure and heart rate.
- Monitor blood pressure and heart rate in all patients, especially during initiation of therapy.
- If patient cannot swallow capsules, puncture the ends of liquid-filled capsule with an 18G needle and draw the contents into a syringe. Instill dose into patient's nasogastric tube and rinse tube with 30 ml of 0.9% NaCl.

Patient education
- Advise patient to rise from supine position slowly to avoid dizziness and hypotension, especially at beginning of therapy.

Pediatric use
- Safety and efficacy have not been established.

Breast-feeding
- Substantial amounts of drug occur in milk of lactating animals. Avoid breast-feeding during therapy.

nisoldipine
Sular

Pharmacologic classification: calcium channel blocker
Therapeutic classification: antihypertensive
Pregnancy risk category C

How supplied
Available by prescription only
Tablets (extended-release): 10 mg, 20 mg, 30 mg, 40 mg

Indications, route, and dosage
Hypertension
Adults: Initially, 20 mg P.O. once daily, then increased by 10 mg/week or at longer intervals, p.r.n. Usual maintenance dosage, 20 to 40 mg once daily. Do not exceed 60 mg daily.
✦ ***Dosage adjustment.*** In patients over age 65 or those with hepatic dysfunction, give starting dose of 10 mg P.O. once daily. Monitor blood pressure closely during any dosage adjustment.

Pharmacodynamics
Antihypertensive action: Nisoldipine prevents the entry of calcium ions into vascular smooth muscle cells, thereby causing dilation of the arterioles, which in turn decreases peripheral vascular resistance.

Pharmacokinetics
- *Absorption:* Drug is relatively well absorbed from the GI tract. High-fat foods significantly affect release of drug from the coat-core formulation.
- *Distribution:* About 99% is bound to plasma protein.
- *Metabolism:* Extensively metabolized with five major metabolites identified.
- *Excretion:* Drug is excreted in urine; half-life ranges from 7 to 12 hours.

Contraindications and precautions
Contraindicated in patients with hypersensitivity to dihydropyridine calcium channel blockers. Use cautiously in patients receiving beta blockers or in those who have compromised ventricular or hepatic function and heart failure.

Interactions
Cimetidine increases bioavailability (rate or extent of absorption) of nisoldipine as well as increasing peak concentration.

Quinidine decreases bioavailability but not peak concentration of nisoldipine.

Effects on diagnostic tests
None reported.

Adverse reactions
CNS: *headache,* dizziness.
CV: vasodilation, palpitations, chest pain.
EENT: pharyngitis, sinusitis.
GI: nausea.
Skin: rash.
Other: *peripheral edema.*

Overdose and treatment
Although there is no experience with drug overdosage, that with similar drugs leads to pronounced hypotension. Treatment should focus on CV support, including monitoring of CV and respiratory function, elevation of extremities, and judicious use of calcium infusion, pressor agents, and fluids.

☑ Special considerations

- Monitor patient carefully. Some patients, especially those with severe obstructive coronary artery disease, have developed increased frequency, duration, or severity of angina or even acute MI after initiation of calcium channel blocker therapy or at time of dosage increase.
- Monitor blood pressure regularly, especially during initial administration and titration of drug.

Patient education

- Tell patient to take drug exactly as prescribed, even if he feels well.
- Instruct patient to swallow tablet whole and not to chew, divide, or crush tablets.
- Tell patient not to take drug with a high-fat meal or with grapefruit products.
- Advise patient to rise slowly from supine position to avoid dizziness and hypotension, especially at beginning of therapy.

Geriatric use

- Elderly patients may have two- to threefold higher plasma concentrations than younger patients, which requires cautious dosing.

Pediatric use

- Safety and effectiveness in children have not been established.

Breast-feeding

- It is not known if drug is excreted in breast milk. Use of drug in breast-feeding women is not recommended.

nitrofurantoin macrocrystals

Macrobid, Macrodantin

nitrofurantoin

Furadantin

Pharmacologic classification: nitrofuran
Therapeutic classification: urinary tract anti-infective
Pregnancy risk category B

How supplied

Available by prescription only
macrocrystals
Capsules: 25 mg, 50 mg, 100 mg
Capsules (dual-release): 100 mg
microcrystals
Suspension: 25 mg/5 ml

Indications, route, and dosage

Initial or recurrent urinary tract infections caused by susceptible organisms

Adults and children over age 12: 50 to 100 mg P.O. q.i.d. or 100 mg dual-release capsules q 12 hours.
Children age 1 month to 12 years: 5 to 7 mg/kg/24 hours P.O. daily, divided q.i.d.

Long-term suppression therapy

Adults: 50 to 100 mg P.O. daily h.s. as a single dose.
Children: As low as 1 mg/kg/day in a single dose or two divided doses.

Pharmacodynamics

Antibacterial action: Nitrofurantoin has bacteriostatic action in low concentrations and possible bactericidal action in high concentrations. Although its exact mechanism of action is unknown, it may inhibit bacterial enzyme systems interfering with bacterial carbohydrate metabolism. Drug is most active at an acidic pH.

Drug's spectrum of activity includes many common gram-positive and gram-negative urinary pathogens, including *Escherichia coli, Staphylococcus aureus,* enterococci, and certain strains of *Klebsiella* and *Enterobacter.* Organisms that usually resist nitrofurantoin include *Pseudomonas, Acinetobacter, Serratia, Providencia,* and *Proteus.*

Pharmacokinetics

- *Absorption:* When administered orally, drug is well absorbed (mainly by the small intestine) from GI tract. Presence of food aids drug's dissolution and speeds absorption. The macrocrystal form exhibits slower dissolution and absorption; it causes less GI distress.
- *Distribution:* Drug crosses into bile and placenta. 60% binds to plasma proteins. Plasma half-life is approximately 20 minutes. Peak urine concentrations occur in about 30 minutes when drug is given as microcrystals, somewhat later when given as macrocrystals.
- *Metabolism:* Metabolized partially in the liver.
- *Excretion:* About 30% to 50% of dose is eliminated by glomerular filtration and tubular secretion into urine as unchanged drug within 24 hours. Some drug may be excreted in breast milk.

Contraindications and precautions

Contraindicated in pregnant patients at term (38 to 42 weeks' gestation), during labor and delivery, or when the onset of labor is imminent. Contraindicated in children age 1 month and less and in patients with moderate to severe renal impairment, anuria, oliguria, or creatinine clearance under 60 ml/minute.

Use cautiously in patients with impaired renal function, anemia, diabetes mellitus, electrolyte abnormalities, vitamin B deficiency, debilitating disease, or G6PD deficiency.

Interactions

When used concomitantly, *probenecid* and *sulfinpyrazone* reduce renal excretion of nitrofurantoin, leading to increased serum and decreased urine nitrofurantoin concentrations. Increased serum concentration may lead to increased toxicity; decreased urine concentration may reduce drug's antibacterial effectiveness.

Concomitant use with *magnesium trisilicate antacids* may decrease nitrofurantoin absorption.

Anticholinergic drugs and foods enhance nitrofurantoin's bioavailability by slowing GI motility, thereby increasing the drug's dissolution and absorption.

Concomitant use with *quinolone derivatives (cinoxacin, ciprofloxacin, nalidixic acid, norfloxacin)* may antagonize the anti-infective effects.

Effects on diagnostic tests

Nitrofurantoin may cause false-positive results in urine glucose tests using cupric sulfate reagents (such as Benedict's test, Fehling's test, or Clinitest) because it reacts with these reagents.

Serum glucose may be decreased; bilirubin and alkaline phosphatase may be elevated.

Adverse reactions

CNS: ***peripheral neuropathy,*** headache, dizziness, drowsiness, *ascending polyneuropathy* (with high doses or renal impairment).

GI: *anorexia, nausea, vomiting,* abdominal pain, *diarrhea.*

Hematologic: ***hemolysis in patients with G6PD deficiency*** (reversed after stopping drug), ***agranulocytosis, thrombocytopenia.***

Hepatic: ***hepatitis, hepatic necrosis.***

Respiratory: ***pulmonary sensitivity reactions*** (cough, chest pain, fever, chills, dyspnea, pulmonary infiltration with consolidation or pleural effusion), ***asthmatic attacks in patients with history of asthma.***

Skin: maculopapular, erythematous, or eczematous eruption; pruritus; urticaria; ***exfoliative dermatitis;*** Stevens-Johnson syndrome.

Other: hypersensitivity reactions ***(anaphylaxis),*** transient alopecia, drug fever, overgrowth of nonsusceptible organisms in the urinary tract.

Overdose and treatment

Acute overdosage may result in nausea and vomiting. Treat symptomatically. No specific antidote is known. Increase fluid intake to promote urinary excretion of drug. Nitrofurantoin is dialyzable.

☑ Special considerations

- Obtain culture and sensitivity tests before starting therapy, and repeat as needed.
- Oral suspension may be mixed with water, milk, fruit juice, and formulas.
- Monitor CBC regularly.
- Monitor fluid intake and output and pulmonary status.
- Drug may turn urine brown or rust-yellow.
- Continue treatment for at least 3 days after sterile urine specimens have been obtained.
- Long-term therapy may cause overgrowth of nonsusceptible organisms, especially *Pseudomonas.*

Patient education

- Instruct patient to take drug with food or milk to minimize GI distress.
- Caution patient that drug may cause false-positive results in urine glucose tests using cupric sulfate reduction method (Clinitest) but not in glucose oxidase test (glucose enzymatic test strip, Diastix, or Chemstrip uG).
- Emphasize that bedtime dose is important because drug will remain in bladder longer.
- Warn patient that drug may turn urine brown or rust-yellow.

Pediatric use

- Contraindicated in infants under age 1 month because their immature enzyme systems increase risk of hemolytic anemia.

Breast-feeding

- Safety has not been established. Although drug is excreted in low concentrations in breast milk, no adverse reactions have been reported, except in infants with G6PD deficiency, who may develop hemolytic anemia.

nitrofurazone

Furacin

Pharmacologic classification: synthetic antibacterial nitrofuran derivative
Therapeutic classification: topical antibacterial
Pregnancy risk category C

How supplied

Available by prescription only
Topical solution: 0.2%
Ointment: 0.2% soluble dressing
Cream: 0.2%

Indications, route, and dosage

Adjunct for major burns (especially when resistance to other anti-infectives occurs); prevention of skin graft infection before or after surgery

Adults and children: Apply directly to lesion or to dressings used to cover affected area daily or as indicated, depending on severity of burn. Apply once daily or every few days, depending on dressing technique.

Pharmacodynamics

Antibacterial action: Exact mechanism of action is unknown. However, it appears that drug inhibits bacterial enzymes involved in carbohydrate metabolism. Nitrofurazone has a broad spectrum of activity.

Pharmacokinetics

- *Absorption:* Limited with topical use.
- *Distribution:* None.
- *Metabolism:* None.
- *Excretion:* None.

Contraindications and precautions

Contraindicated in patients hypersensitive to drug. Use cautiously in patients with known or suspected renal impairment.

Interactions

None reported.

Effects on diagnostic tests

None reported.

Adverse reactions

Skin: *erythema, pruritus,* burning, edema, severe reactions (vesiculation, denudation, ulceration), *allergic contact dermatitis.*

Overdose and treatment

Discontinue use and cleanse area with mild soap and water.

☑ Special considerations

- Avoid contact with eyes and mucous membranes.
- Monitor patient for overgrowth of nonsusceptible organisms, including fungi.
- Use diluted solutions within 24 hours after preparation; discard diluted solution that becomes cloudy.

Patient education

- Teach patient proper application of drug and to apply directly on lesion or place on gauze.
- Tell patient to avoid exposure of drug to direct sunlight, excessive heat, strong fluorescent lighting, and alkaline materials.

Breast-feeding

- Safety has not been established. Potential benefits to mother must be weighed against risks to infant.

nitroglycerin (glyceryl trinitrate)

Oral, extended-release
Niong, Nitro-Bid, Nitroglyn, Nitrong, Nitrong SR*

S.L.
Nitrostat

Translingual
Nitrolingual

I.V.
Nitro-Bid IV, Tridil

Topical
Nitro-Bid, Nitrol

Transdermal
Deponit, Minitran, Nitro-Derm, Nitrodisc, Nitro-Dur, NTS, Transderm-Nitro

Transmucosal
Nitrogard

Pharmacologic classification: nitrate
Therapeutic classification: antianginal, vasodilator
Pregnancy risk category C

How supplied

Available by prescription only
Tablets (sustained-release): 2.6 mg, 6.5 mg, 9 mg
Tablets (S.L.): 0.15 mg, 0.3 mg, 0.4 mg, 0.6 mg
Tablets (buccal, controlled-release): 1 mg, 2 mg, 3 mg
Capsules (sustained-release): 2.5 mg, 6.5 mg, 9 mg, 13 mg
Aerosol (lingual): 0.4 mg/metered spray
I.V.: 0.5 mg/ml, 0.8 mg/ml, 5 mg/ml
I.V. premixed solutions in dextrose: 100 mcg/ml, 200 mcg/ml, 400 mcg/ml
Topical: 2% ointment
Transdermal: 0.1-mg, 0.2-mg, 0.3-mg, 0.4-mg, 0.6 mg/hour systems

Indications, route, and dosage

Prophylaxis against chronic anginal attacks
Adults: One sustained-release capsule q 8 to 12 hours; or 2% ointment. Start with ½" ointment, increasing with ½" increments until headache occurs, then decreasing to previous dose. Range of dosage with ointment is 2" to 5". Usual dose is 1" to 2". Alternatively, transdermal disc or pad may be applied to hairless site once daily. However, to prevent tolerance, topical forms should not be worn overnight.
Relief of acute angina pectoris, prophylaxis to prevent or minimize anginal attacks when taken immediately before stressful events
Adults: One S.L. tablet dissolved under the tongue or in the buccal pouch immediately on indication of angina attack. May repeat q 5 minutes for 15 to 30 minutes. Or, using Nitrolingual spray, spray one or two doses into mouth, preferably onto or under the tongue. May repeat q 3 to 5 minutes to a maximum of three doses within a 15-minute period. Or, transmucosally, 1 to 3 mg q 3 to 5 hours during waking hours.
Hypertension, heart failure, angina
Nitroglycerin is indicated to control hypertension associated with surgery, to treat heart failure associated with MI, to relieve angina pectoris in acute situations, and to produce controlled hypotension during surgery (by I.V. infusion).
Adults: Initial infusion rate is 5 mcg/minute. May be increased by 5 mcg/minute q 3 to 5 minutes until a response is noted. If a 20-mcg/minute rate doesn't produce desired response, dosage may be increased by as much as 20 mcg/minute q 3 to 5 minutes.
◊ ***Hypertensive crisis***
Adults: Infuse at 5 to 100 mcg/minute.

Pharmacodynamics

Antianginal action: Nitroglycerin relaxes vascular smooth muscle of both the venous and arterial beds, resulting in a net decrease in myocardial oxygen consumption. It also dilates coronary vessels, leading to redistribution of blood flow to ischemic tissue. Drug's systemic and coronary vascular effects (which may vary slightly with the various nitroglycerin forms) probably account for its value in treating angina.

Vasodilating action: Nitroglycerin dilates peripheral vessels, making it useful (in I.V. form) in producing controlled hypotension during surgical procedures and in controlling blood pressure in perioperative hypertension. Because peripheral vasodilation decreases venous return to the heart (preload), nitroglycerin also helps to treat pulmonary edema and heart failure. Arterial vasodilation decreases arterial impedance (afterload), thereby decreasing left ventricular work and aiding the failing heart. These combined effects may prove valuable in treating some patients with acute MI.

Pharmacokinetics

• *Absorption:* Drug is well absorbed from the GI tract. However, because it undergoes first-pass metabolism in the liver, it is incompletely absorbed into the systemic circulation. Onset of action for oral preparations is slow (except for sublingual tablets). After sublingual administration, absorption from the oral mucosa is relatively complete. Nitroglycerin also is well absorbed after topical administration as an ointment or transdermal system. Onset of action for various preparations is as follows: I.V.,1 to 2 minutes; S.L., 1 to 3 minutes; translingual spray, 2 minutes; transmucosal tablet, 3 minutes; ointment, 20 to 60 minutes; oral (sustained-release), 40 minutes; transdermal, 40 to 60 minutes.
• *Distribution:* Nitroglycerin is distributed widely throughout the body. About 60% of circulating drug is bound to plasma proteins.
• *Metabolism:* Metabolized in the liver and serum to 1,3 glyceryl dinitrate; 1,2 glyceryl dinitrate; and glyceryl mononitrate. Dinitrate metabolites have a slight vasodilatory effect.
• *Excretion:* Metabolites are excreted in the urine; elimination half-life is about 1 to 4 minutes. Duration of effect for various preparations is as follows: I.V., 3 to 5 minutes; S.L., up to 30 minutes; translingual spray, 30 to 60 minutes; transmucosal tablet, 5 hours; ointment, 3 to 6 hours; oral (sustained-release), 4 to 8 hours; transdermal, 18 to 24 hours.

Contraindications and precautions

Contraindicated in patients with hypersensitivity to nitrates and in those with early MI (S.L. form), severe anemia, increased intracranial pressure, angle-closure glaucoma, postural hypotension, and allergy to adhesives (transdermal form). I.V. form is contraindicated in patients with hypersensitivity to I.V. form, cardiac tamponade, restrictive cardiomyopathy, or constrictive pericarditis. Extended-release preparations should not be used in patients with organic or functional GI hypermotility or malabsorption syndrome.

Use cautiously in patients with hypotension or volume depletion.

Interactions

Concomitant use of nitroglycerin with *alcohol, antihypertensive drugs,* or *phenothiazines* may cause additive hypotensive effects. Concomitant use with *ergot alkaloids* may precipitate angina. Oral nitroglycerin may increase the bioavailability of ergot alkaloids.

Effects on diagnostic tests

Nitroglycerin may interfere with serum cholesterol determination tests using the Zlatkis-Zak color reaction, resulting in falsely decreased values.

Adverse reactions

CNS: *headache, sometimes with throbbing; dizziness;* weakness.
CV: *orthostatic hypotension, tachycardia, flushing, palpitations,* fainting.
GI: nausea, vomiting.
Skin: cutaneous vasodilation, contact dermatitis (patch), rash.
Other: hypersensitivity reactions, S.L. burning.

Overdose and treatment

Clinical effects of overdose result primarily from vasodilation and methemoglobinemia and include hypotension, persistent throbbing headache, palpitations, visual disturbances, flushing of the skin, sweating (with skin later becoming cold and cyanotic), nausea and vomiting, colic, bloody diarrhea, orthostasis, initial hyperpnea, dyspnea, slow respiratory rate, bradycardia, heart block, increased intracranial pressure with confusion, fever, paralysis, tissue hypoxia (from methemoglobinemia) leading to cyanosis, and metabolic acidosis, coma, clonic seizures, and circulatory collapse. Death may result from circulatory collapse or asphyxia.

Treatment includes gastric lavage followed by administration of activated charcoal to remove remaining gastric contents. Blood gas measurements and methemoglobin levels should be monitored, as indicated. Supportive care includes respiratory support and oxygen administration, passive movement of the extremities to aid venous return, and recumbent positioning.

☑ Special considerations

• Use only S.L. and translingual forms to relieve acute angina attack.
• To apply ointment, spread in uniform thin layer to hairless part of skin except distal parts of arms or legs, because absorption will not be maximal at these sites. Do not rub in. Cover with plastic film to aid absorption and to protect clothing. If using Tape-Surrounded Appli-Ruler (TSAR) system, keep TSAR on skin to protect patient's clothing and ensure that ointment remains in place. If serious adverse effects develop in patients using ointment or transdermal system, remove product at once or wipe ointment from skin. Be sure to avoid contact with ointment.
• Administration as I.V. infusion requires special nonabsorbent tubing supplied by manufacturer, because regular plastic tubing may absorb up to 80% of drug. Infusion should be prepared in glass bottle or container.
• If drug causes headache (especially likely with initial doses), aspirin or acetaminophen may be indicated. Dosage may need to be reduced temporarily.
• S.L. dose may be administered before anticipated stress or at bedtime if angina is nocturnal.
• Drug may cause orthostatic hypotension. To minimize this, patient should change to upright position slowly, go up and down stairs carefully, and lie down at the first sign of dizziness.
• When administering drug to patients during initial days after acute MI, monitor hemodynamic and clinical status carefully.
• Monitor blood pressure and intensity and duration of patient's response to drug.
• Be sure to remove transdermal patch before defibrillation. Because of patch's aluminum backing, electric current may cause patch to explode.

• When terminating transdermal nitroglycerin treatment for angina, gradually reduce dosage and frequency of application over 4 to 6 weeks.
• To prevent withdrawal symptoms, reduce dosage gradually after long-term use of oral or topical preparations.
• Store drug in cool, dark place in tightly closed container. To ensure freshness, replace supply of S.L. tablets every 3 months. Remove cotton from container because it absorbs drug.

Patient education

• Instruct patient to take medication regularly, as prescribed and to keep S.L. form accessible at all times. Drug is physiologically necessary but not addictive.
• Teach patient to take oral tablet on empty stomach, either 30 minutes before or 1 to 2 hours after meals, to swallow oral tablets whole, and to chew chewable tablets thoroughly before swallowing.
• Instruct patient to take S.L. tablet at first sign of angina attack. Tell him to wet tablet with saliva, place it under the tongue until completely absorbed, and sit down and rest. If no relief occurs after three tablets, he should call or go to hospital emergency room. If he complains of tingling sensation with drug placed sublingually, he may try holding tablet in buccal pouch.
• Advise patient to store S.L. tablets in original container or other container specifically approved for this use away from heat and light. Keep cap to bottle tightly closed.
• Instruct patient to place transmucosal tablet under upper lip or in buccal pouch, to let it dissolve slowly over a 3- to 5-hour period, and not to chew or swallow tablet. Advise him that dissolution rate may increase if he touches tablet with tongue or drinks hot liquids.
• If patient is receiving nitroglycerin lingual aerosol (Nitrolingual), instruct him how to use this device correctly. Remind him not to inhale spray but to release it onto or under the tongue. Also tell him not to swallow immediately after administering the spray but to wait about 10 seconds before swallowing.
• Caution patient to use care when wearing transdermal patch near microwave oven because leaking radiation may heat patch's metallic backing and cause burns.
• Warn patient that headache may follow initial doses but that this symptom may respond to usual headache remedies or dosage reduction (however, dose should be reduced only with medical approval). Assure patient that headache usually subsides gradually with continued treatment.
• Instruct patient to avoid alcohol while taking drug because severe hypotension and CV collapse may occur.
• Warn patient that drug may cause dizziness or flushing and to move to an upright position slowly.
• Tell patient to report blurred vision, dry mouth, or persistent headache.

Pediatric use

• Methemoglobinemia may occur in infants receiving large doses of nitroglycerin.

nitroprusside sodium

Nipride*, Nitropress

Pharmacologic classification: vasodilator
Therapeutic classification: antihypertensive
Pregnancy risk category C

How supplied

Available by prescription only
Injection: 50 mg/2-ml, 50 mg/5-ml vials

Indications, route, and dosage

Hypertensive emergencies
Adults and children: I.V. infusion titrated to blood pressure, with a range of 0.3 to 10 mcg/kg/minute. Maximum infusion rate is 10 mcg/kg/minute for 10 minutes.
Acute heart failure
Adults and children: I.V. infusion titrated to cardiac output and systemic blood pressure. Same dosage range as for hypertensive emergencies.

Pharmacodynamics

Antihypertensive action: Nitroprusside acts directly on vascular smooth muscle, causing peripheral vasodilation.

Pharmacokinetics

• *Absorption:* Drug is administered by I.V. route. I.V. infusion of nitroprusside reduces blood pressure almost immediately.
• *Distribution:* Unknown.
• *Metabolism:* Nitroprusside is metabolized rapidly in erythrocytes and tissues to a cyanide radical and then converted to thiocyanate in the liver.
• *Excretion:* Excreted primarily as metabolites in the urine. Blood pressure returns to pretreatment level 1 to 10 minutes after completion of infusion.

Contraindications and precautions

Contraindicated in patients with hypersensitivity to drug, compensatory hypertension (such as in arteriovenous shunt or coarctation of the aorta), inadequate cerebral circulation, congenital optic atrophy, or tobacco-induced amblyopia.

Use cautiously in patients with renal or hepatic disease, increased intracranial pressure, hypothyroidism, hyponatremia, or low vitamin B_{12} concentrations.

Interactions

Nitroprusside may potentiate antihypertensive effects of *other antihypertensive medications;* its antihypertensive effects may be potentiated by *general anesthetics*, particularly *enflurane* and *halothane*. *Pressor agents* such as *epinephrine* may cause an increase in blood pressure during nitroprusside therapy.

Effects on diagnostic tests

An increase in serum creatinine concentration may occur during therapy.

Adverse reactions

CNS: *headache, dizziness,* loss of consciousness, apprehension, ***increased intracranial pressure,*** *restlessness.*
CV: bradycardia, hypotension, tachycardia, palpitations, ECG changes.
GI: *nausea, abdominal pain,* ileus.
Skin: pink color, flushing, rash, *diaphoresis.*
Other: acidosis, ***thiocyanate toxicity, methemoglobinemia, cyanide toxicity,*** venous streaking, irritation at infusion site, hypothyroidism, *muscle twitching.*

Overdose and treatment

Clinical manifestations of overdose include the adverse reactions listed above and increased tolerance to the drug's antihypertensive effects.

Treat overdose by giving nitrites to induce methemoglobin formation. Discontinue drug and administer amyl nitrite inhalations for 15 to 30 seconds each minute until a 3% sodium nitrite solution can be prepared. Administer amyl nitrite cautiously to minimize risk of additional hypotension secondary to vasodilation. Then administer the sodium nitrite solution by I.V. infusion at a rate not exceeding 2.5 to 5 ml/minute up to a total dose of 10 to 15 ml. Follow with I.V. sodium thiosulfate infusion (12.5 g in 50 ml of D_5W solution) over 10 minutes. If necessary, repeat infusions of sodium nitrite and sodium thiosulfate at half the initial doses. Further treatment involves symptomatic and supportive care.

☑ Special considerations

- Check blood pressure at least every 5 minutes at start of infusion and every 15 minutes thereafter during infusion.
- Prepare solution using D_5W solution; do not use bacteriostatic water for injection or sterile NaCl solution for reconstitution; because of light sensitivity, foil-wrap I.V. solution (but not tubing). Fresh solutions have faint brownish tint; discard after 24 hours.
- Infuse drug with infusion pump.
- Drug is best run piggyback through a peripheral line with no other medications; do not adjust rate of main I.V. line while drug is running because even small boluses can cause severe hypotension.
- Nitroprusside can cause cyanide toxicity; therefore, check serum thiocyanate levels every 72 hours; levels above 100 mcg/ml are associated with cyanide toxicity, which can produce profound hypotension, metabolic acidosis, dyspnea, ataxia, and vomiting. If such symptoms occur, discontinue infusion and re-evaluate therapy.
- Drug also may be used to produce controlled hypotension during anesthesia, to reduce bleeding from surgical procedure.
- Hypertensive patients are more sensitive to nitroprusside than normotensive patients. Also, patients taking other antihypertensive drugs are extremely sensitive to nitroprusside. Nitroprusside has been used in patients with acute MI, refractory heart failure, and severe mitral regurgitation. It has also been used orally as an antihypertensive.

Patient education

- Ask patient to report CNS symptoms (such as headache or dizziness) promptly.

Geriatric use

- Elderly patients may be more sensitive to drug's antihypertensive effects.

Breast-feeding

- It is not known if drug is distributed into breast milk; administer with caution to breast-feeding women.

nizatidine

Axid, Axid AR

Pharmacologic classification: H_2-receptor antagonist
Therapeutic classification: antiulcer
Pregnancy risk category B

How supplied

Available by prescription only
Capsules: 150 mg, 300 mg
Available without a prescription
Capsules: 75 mg

Indications, route, and dosage

Treatment of active duodenal ulcer
Adults: 300 mg P.O. once daily h.s. Alternatively, may give 150 mg P.O. b.i.d.
Maintenance therapy for duodenal ulcer patients
Adults: 150 mg P.O. once daily h.s.
Gastroesophageal reflux disease
Adults: 150 mg P.O. b.i.d.
Heartburn (self-medication)
Adults: One 75-mg capsule P.O. ½ hour before meals; use up to b.i.d.
✦ ***Dosage adjustment.*** In adults with renal failure, refer to following dosing chart.

Creatinine clearance (ml/min)	Active duodenal ulcer	Maintenance
20 to 50	150 mg/day	150 mg q other day
< 20	150 mg q other day	150 mg q 3 days

Pharmacodynamics

Antiulcer action: Nizatidine is a competitive, reversible inhibitor of H_2 receptors, particularly those in the gastric parietal cells.

Pharmacokinetics

- *Absorption:* Nizatidine is well absorbed (more than 90%) after oral administration. Absorption may be slightly enhanced by food, and slightly impaired by antacids.
- *Distribution:* Approximately 35% of nizatidine is bound to plasma protein. Peak plasma concentra-

tions occur ½ to 3 hours after the dose is administered.
• *Metabolism:* Nizatidine probably undergoes hepatic metabolism. About 40% of excreted drug is metabolized; the remainder is excreted unchanged.
• *Excretion:* More than 90% of an oral dose of nizatidine is excreted in the urine within 12 hours. Renal clearance is about 500 ml/minute, which indicates excretion by active tubular secretion. Less than 6% of an administered dose is eliminated in the feces.

Elimination half-life is 1 to 2 hours. Moderate to severe renal impairment significantly prolongs half-life and decreases clearance of nizatidine. In anephric persons, half-life is 3½ to 11 hours; plasma clearance is 7 to 14 L/hour.

Contraindications and precautions
Contraindicated in patients hypersensitive to H_2-receptor antagonists. Use cautiously in patients with impaired renal function.

Interactions
Because nizatidine does not inhibit the cytochrome P-450–linked drug metabolizing enzyme system, drug interactions mediated by inhibition of hepatic metabolism are not expected. Concomitant use of high doses of *aspirin* (3,900 mg/day) with nizatidine (150 mg twice-daily) increases serum salicylate levels.

Effects on diagnostic tests
False-positive tests for urobilinogen may occur during nizatidine therapy.

Adverse reactions
CNS: somnolence.
CV: ***arrhythmias.***
Hematologic: eosinophilia.
Skin: *diaphoresis,* rash, urticaria.
Other: hyperuricemia, fever, hepatocellular injury, elevated liver function tests.

Overdose and treatment
Expected clinical effects of overdose are cholinergic, including lacrimation, salivation, emesis, miosis, and diarrhea. Treatment may include use of activated charcoal, emesis, or lavage, with clinical monitoring and supportive therapy.

☑ Special considerations
• Because drug is excreted primarily by the kidneys, reduce dosage in patients with moderate to severe renal insufficiency.
• Nizatidine is partially metabolized in the liver. In patients with normal renal function and uncomplicated hepatic dysfunction, the disposition of nizatidine is similar to that in patients with normal hepatic function.
• For patients on maintenance therapy, consider that effects of continuous drug therapy for over 1 year are not known.

Patient education
• Advise patient not to smoke as this may increase gastric acid secretion and worsen the disease.

Geriatric use
• Safety and efficacy appear similar to those in younger patients. However, consider that elderly patients have reduced renal function.

Pediatric use
• Safety and efficacy in children have not been established.

Breast-feeding
• Use with caution in women who are breast-feeding. Consider that nizatidine is secreted and concentrated in the milk of lactating rats.

norepinephrine bitartrate (formerly levarterenol bitartrate)
Levophed

Pharmacologic classification: adrenergic (direct-acting)
Therapeutic classification: vasopressor
Pregnancy risk category C

How supplied
Available by prescription only
Injection: 1 mg/ml parenteral

Indications, route, and dosage
To maintain blood pressure in acute hypotensive states
Adults: Initially, 8 to 12 mcg/minute I.V. infusion, then titrated to maintain desired blood pressure; maintenance dosage, 2 to 4 mcg/minute.
Children: Initially, 2 mcg/minute or 2 mcg/m²/minute I.V. infusion, then titrated to maintain desired blood pressure. For advanced cardiac life support, initial infusion rate is 0.1 mcg/kg/minute.
◊ ***GI bleeding***
Adults: 8 mg in 250 ml 0.9% NaCl solution given intraperitoneally, or 8 mg in 100 ml 0.9% NaCl solution given via a nasogastric tube q hour for 6 to 8 hours then q 2 hours for 4 to 6 hours.

Pharmacodynamics
Vasopressor action: Norepinephrine acts predominantly by direct stimulation of alpha-adrenergic receptors, constricting both capacitance and resistance blood vessels. That results in increased total peripheral resistance; increased systolic and diastolic blood pressure; decreased blood flow to vital organs, skin, and skeletal muscle; and constriction of renal blood vessels, which reduces renal blood flow. It also has a direct stimulating effect on $beta_1$ receptors of the heart, producing a positive inotropic response. Its main therapeutic effects are vasoconstriction and cardiac stimulation.

Pharmacokinetics
• *Absorption:* Pressor effect occurs rapidly after infusion, is of short duration, and stops within 1 to 2 minutes after infusion is stopped.
• *Distribution:* Drug localizes in sympathetic nerve tissues. It crosses the placenta but not the blood-brain barrier.

• *Metabolism:* Norepinephrine is metabolized in the liver and other tissues to inactive compounds.
• *Excretion:* Excreted in urine primarily as sulfate and glucuronide conjugates. Small amounts are excreted unchanged in urine.

Contraindications and precautions
Contraindicated in patients with mesenteric or peripheral vascular thrombosis, profound hypoxia, hypercapnia, or hypotension resulting from blood volume deficit and during cyclopropane and halothane anesthesia.

Use cautiously in patients with sulfite allergies or in those receiving MAO inhibitors or triptyline- or imipramine-type antidepressants.

Interactions
When used concomitantly with *general anesthetics*, norepinephrine may cause increased arrhythmias; when used with *tricyclic antidepressants, some antihistamines, parenteral ergot alkaloids, guanethidine, MAO inhibitors,* and *methyldopa*, norepinephrine may cause severe, prolonged hypertension.

Use with *beta blockers* may result in an increased potential for hypertension. (Propranolol may be used to treat arrhythmias occurring during norepinephrine administration.) Use with *furosemide* or *other diuretics* may decrease arterial responsiveness.

Concomitant use with *atropine* blocks the reflex bradycardia caused by norepinephrine and enhances its pressor effects.

Effects on diagnostic tests
None reported.

Adverse reactions
CNS: anxiety, weakness, dizziness, tremor, restlessness, insomnia.
CV: bradycardia, ***severe hypertension, arrhythmias.***
Respiratory: respiratory difficulties, ***asthmatic episodes.***
Other: ***anaphylaxis,*** irritation with extravasation.

Overdose and treatment
Clinical manifestations of overdose include severe hypertension, photophobia, retrosternal or pharyngeal pain, intense sweating, vomiting, cerebral hemorrhage, seizures, and arrhythmias. Monitor vital signs closely.

Treatment includes supportive and symptomatic measures. Use atropine for reflex bradycardia, phentolamine for extravasation, and propranolol for arrhythmias.

☑ Special considerations
Besides those relevant to all *adrenergics*, consider the following recommendations.
• Correct blood volume depletion before administration. Norepinephrine is not a substitute for blood, plasma, fluid, or electrolyte replacement.
• Select injection site carefully. Administration by I.V. infusion requires an infusion pump or other device to control flow rate. If possible, infuse into antecubital vein of the arm or the femoral vein. Change injection sites for prolonged therapy. Must be diluted before use with 5% dextrose or with NaCl. (Dilution with NaCl alone not recommended.) Monitor infusion rate. Withdraw drug gradually; recurrent hypotension may follow abrupt withdrawal.
• Prepare infusion solution by adding 4 mg norepinephrine to 1 L of 5% dextrose. The resultant solution contains 4 mcg/ml.
• To treat extravasation, infiltrate site promptly with 10 to 15 ml NaCl solution containing 5 to 10 mg phentolamine, using a fine needle.
• Some clinicians add phentolamine (5 to 10 mg) to each liter of infusion solution as a preventive against sloughing, should extravasation occur.
• Monitor intake and output. Norepinephrine reduces renal blood flow, which may cause decreased urine output initially.
• Monitor patient constantly during administration of norepinephrine. Obtain baseline blood pressure and pulse before therapy, and repeat every 2 minutes until stabilization; repeat every 5 minutes during drug administration.
• In addition to vital signs, monitor patient's mental state, skin temperature of extremities, and skin color (especially earlobes, lips, and nail beds).
• In patients with previously normal blood pressure, adjust flow rate to maintain blood pressure at low normal (usually 80 to 100 mm Hg systolic); in hypertensive patients, maintain systolic no higher than 40 mm Hg below preexisting pressure level.
• Protect solution from light. Discard solution that is discolored or contains a precipitate.

Patient education
• Inform patient of need for frequent monitoring of vital signs.
• Tell patient to report adverse reactions.

Geriatric use
• Elderly patients are more sensitive to drug's effects. Decreased cardiac output may be harmful to elderly patients with poor cerebral or coronary circulation.

Pediatric use
• Use with caution in children.

norethindrone
Micronor, Nor-Q.D.

norethindrone acetate
Aygestin, Norlutate*

Pharmacologic classification: progestin
Therapeutic classification: contraceptive
Pregnancy risk category X

How supplied
Available by prescription only
norethindrone
Tablets: 0.35 mg
norethindrone acetate
Tablets: 5 mg

Indications, route, and dosage

Amenorrhea, abnormal uterine bleeding, endometriosis

norethindrone acetate

Adults: 2.5 to 10 mg P.O. daily on days 5 to 10 of second half of menstrual cycle or on days 5 through 25 of menstrual cycle.

Endometriosis

norethindrone acetate

Adults: 5 mg P.O. daily for 14 days, then increase by 2.5 mg/day q 2 weeks up to 15 mg/day. Daily therapy may be continued consecutively for 6 to 9 months; if breakthrough bleeding occurs, therapy should be temporarily discontinued.

Contraception

Adults: 0.35 mg norethindrone P.O. daily, beginning day 1 of menstrual cycle and continuing uninterrupted thereafter.

Pharmacodynamics

Contraceptive action: Norethindrone suppresses ovulation, causes thickening of cervical mucus, and induces sloughing of the endometrium.

Pharmacokinetics

- *Absorption:* Well absorbed after oral administration.
- *Distribution:* Distributed widely. It is about 80% protein-bound and distributes into bile and breast milk.
- *Metabolism:* Primarily hepatic metabolism; drug undergoes extensive first-pass metabolism.
- *Excretion:* Drug is excreted primarily in feces. Elimination half-life is 5 to 14 hours.

Contraindications and precautions

Contraindicated in patients with thromboembolic disorders, cerebral apoplexy, or history of these conditions; hypersensitivity to drug; breast cancer, undiagnosed abnormal vaginal bleeding; severe hepatic disease, or missed abortion and during pregnancy.

Use cautiously in patients with diabetes mellitus, seizures, migraine, cardiac or renal disease, asthma, or mental depression.

Interactions

Concomitant use with *bromocriptine* may cause amenorrhea or galactorrhea, thus interfering with the action of bromocriptine. Concurrent use of these drugs is not recommended.

Effects on diagnostic tests

Pregnanediol excretion may decrease; serum alkaline phosphatase and amino acid levels may increase. Glucose tolerance has been shown to decrease in a small percentage of patients receiving this drug.

Adverse reactions

CNS: depression.
CV: thrombophlebitis, ***pulmonary embolism,*** edema, ***thromboembolism, CVA.***
EENT: exophthalmos, diplopia.
GU: breakthrough bleeding, dysmenorrhea, amenorrhea, cervical erosion, abnormal secretions.
Hepatic: cholestatic jaundice.
Skin: melasma, rash, acne, pruritus.
Other: breast tenderness, enlargement, or secretion; changes in weight.

Overdose and treatment

No information available.

☑ Special considerations

Recommendations for administration of norethindrone, and for care and teaching of the patient during therapy, are the same as those for all *progestins.*

norfloxacin (systemic)

Noroxin

Pharmacologic classification: fluoroquinolone
Therapeutic classification: broad-spectrum antibiotic
Pregnancy risk category C

How supplied

Available by prescription only
Tablets: 400 mg

Indications, route, and dosage

Complicated and uncomplicated urinary tract infections caused by various gram-negative and gram-positive bacteria

Adults: For complicated infection, 400 mg P.O. b.i.d. for 10 to 21 days; for uncomplicated infection, 400 mg P.O. b.i.d. for 3 to 10 days. Do not exceed 800 mg/day. Patients with creatinine clearance below 30 ml/minute should receive 400 mg/day for appropriate duration of therapy.

Uncomplicated gonorrhea

Adults: 800 mg P.O. as a single dose.

Prostatitis

Adults: 400 mg P.O. q 12 hours for 28 days.

◊ ***Gastroenteritis***

Adults: 400 mg P.O. b.i.d. for 5 days.

◊ ***Treatment of traveler's diarrhea***

Adults: 400 mg P.O. b.i.d. for up to 3 days.

Pharmacodynamics

Antibacterial action: Norfloxacin is generally bactericidal. It inhibits DNA gyrase, blocking DNA synthesis. Drug's spectrum of activity includes most aerobic gram-positive and gram-negative urinary pathogens, including *Pseudomonas aeruginosa.*

Pharmacokinetics

- *Absorption:* About 30% to 40% of dose is absorbed from the GI tract (as dose increases, percentage of absorbed drug decreases). Food may reduce absorption.
- *Distribution:* Drug is distributed into renal tissue, liver, gallbladder, prostatic fluid, testicles, seminal fluid, bile, and sputum. From 10% to 15% binds to plasma proteins.
- *Metabolism:* Unknown.
- *Excretion:* Most systemically absorbed drug is excreted by the kidneys, with about 30% appearing in feces. In patients with normal renal function,

plasma half-life is 3 to 4 hours; up to 8 hours in severe renal impairment.

Contraindications and precautions

Contraindicated in patients with hypersensitivity to fluoroquinolones. Use cautiously in patients with renal impairment or conditions predisposing them to seizure disorders, such as cerebral arteriosclerosis.

Interactions

When used concomitantly, *probenecid* may increase serum norfloxacin levels. Concomitant use with *nitrofurantoin* antagonizes norfloxacin's antibacterial activity. Concomitant use with *antacids* is not recommended by manufacturer. Food interferes with norfloxacin's absorption.

Concomitant use with *xanthine derivatives (aminophylline, theophylline)* may increase theophylline concentration and the risk of xanthine-related toxicities.

Norfloxacin may prolong PT in patients also on *warfarin* therapy. *Multivitamins* containing *divalent* or *trivalent* cations may interfere with absorption of norfloxacin.

Effects on diagnostic tests

Hematocrit may decrease and eosinophilia and neutropenia may occur during therapy with norfloxacin.

Adverse reactions

CNS: fatigue, somnolence, headache, dizziness, ***seizures,*** depression, insomnia.
GI: nausea, constipation, flatulence, heartburn, dry mouth, abdominal pain, diarrhea, vomiting, anorexia.
GU: increased serum creatinine and BUN levels, crystalluria.
Hematologic: eosinophilia.
Musculoskeletal: back pain, tendinitis.
Skin: photosensitivity.
Other: hypersensitivity reactions (rash, ***anaphylactoid reaction***), transient elevations of AST, ALT, and alkaline phosphatase; fever; hyperhidrosis.

Overdose and treatment

No information available.

☑ Special considerations

- Obtain culture and sensitivity tests before starting therapy, and repeat as needed throughout therapy.
- Make sure patient is well hydrated before and during therapy to avoid crystalluria.
- Arrange for baseline and follow-up BUN, creatinine clearance, CBC, and liver function tests.
- Evaluate patient for signs and symptoms of resistant infection or reinfection.

Patient education

- Instruct patient to continue taking drug as directed, even if he feels better.
- Advise patient to take drug 1 hour before or 2 hours after meals and antacids.
- Warn patient that drug may cause dizziness that impairs his ability to perform tasks that require alertness and coordination.
- Instruct patient to avoid excessive exposure to sunlight.

Pediatric use

- Contraindicated in children because animal studies suggest a potential risk of arthropathy.

Breast-feeding

- Safety has not been established; alternative feeding method is recommended during treatment with norfloxacin.

norfloxacin (ophthalmic)

Chibroxin

Pharmacologic classification: fluoroquinolone
Therapeutic classification: broad-spectrum antibiotic
Pregnancy risk category C

How supplied

Available by prescription only
Ophthalmic solution: 0.3% in 5-ml containers

Indications, route, and dosage

Conjunctivitis caused by susceptible strains of bacteria

Adults and children age 1 and over: 1 or 2 drops in the affected eye q.i.d. for up to 7 days. If condition warrants, 2 drops may be applied q 2 hours during the waking hours of first day of treatment.

Pharmacodynamics

Antibiotic action: Ophthalmic norfloxacin inhibits bacterial DNA gyrase, an enzyme necessary for bacterial replication. Drug is bacteriostatic or bactericidal, depending on concentration.

Pharmacokinetics

- *Absorption:* Systemic absorption of ophthalmic norfloxacin is limited.
- *Distribution:* No information available.
- *Metabolism:* No information available.
- *Excretion:* No information available.

Contraindications and precautions

Contraindicated in patients with a history of hypersensitivity to norfloxacin or other fluoroquinolone antibiotics. Do not inject drug into eye.

Interactions

Drug interactions with the ophthalmic form have not been studied. Systemically administered drug interferes with metabolism of *caffeine, cyclosporine,* and *theophylline*; it may also enhance the effects of *oral anticoagulants.* Use cautiously in patients receiving these drugs.

Effects on diagnostic tests

None reported.

Adverse reactions

EENT: local burning or discomfort, itching, chemosis, photophobia, conjunctival hyperemia, white crystalline precipitates, lid margin crusting, bad or bitter taste in mouth, hypersensitivity reactions.
GI: nausea.

Overdose and treatment

A topical overdose of the drug may be flushed from the eye with warm tap water.

☑ Special considerations

- Drug is indicated for treatment of conjunctivitis when caused by susceptible bacteria. Known susceptible strains include *Acinetobacter calcoaceticus, Aeromonas hydrophila, Haemophilus influenzae, Proteus mirabilis, Serratia marcescens, Staphylococcus aureus, S. epidermidis, S. warneri,* and *Streptococcus pneumoniae.*

Patient education

- Teach patient how to instill drug correctly. Remind him not to touch the tip of the bottle with his hands and to avoid contact of the tip with the eye or surrounding tissue.
- Instruct patient not to share washcloths or towels with other family members to avoid spreading infection. Tell him not to share norfloxacin with others.
- Advise patient to wash hands before and after instilling solution.
- Tell patient to store drug at room temperature and to protect it from light.
- Advise patient not to wear contact lenses during therapy.

Pediatric use

- Systemically administered quinolones have caused arthropathy in young animals; however, ophthalmic norfloxacin has not produced this adverse effect.

Breast-feeding

- It is unknown if drug is excreted in breast milk. Use with caution in breast-feeding women.

norgestrel

Ovrette

Pharmacologic classification: progestin
Therapeutic classification: contraceptive
Pregnancy risk category X

How supplied

Available by prescription only
Tablets: 0.075 mg

Indications, route, and dosage

Contraception
Adults: 1 tablet P.O. daily, beginning on first day of menstruation.

Pharmacodynamics

Contraceptive action: Norgestrel suppresses ovulation and causes thickening of cervical mucus.

Pharmacokinetics

- *Absorption:* Well absorbed after oral administration.
- *Distribution:* No information available.
- *Metabolism:* No information available.
- *Excretion:* No information available.

Contraindications and precautions

Contraindicated in patients with thromboembolic disorders, cerebral apoplexy, or history of these conditions; hypersensitivity to drug; breast cancer; undiagnosed abnormal vaginal bleeding; severe hepatic disease; and missed abortion and during pregnancy.

Use cautiously in patients with renal or cardiac disease, diabetes mellitus, migraine, seizures, asthma, or mental depression.

Interactions

Concomitant use with *bromocriptine* may cause amenorrhea or galactorrhea, thus interfering with the action of bromocriptine. Concurrent use of these drugs is not recommended.

Effects on diagnostic tests

Pregnanediol excretion may decrease; serum alkaline phosphatase and amino acid levels may increase. Glucose tolerance has been shown to decrease in a small percentage of patients receiving drug.

Adverse reactions

CNS: cerebral thrombosis or hemorrhage, migraine, depression.
CV: thrombophlebitis, ***pulmonary embolism,*** edema, ***thromboembolism, CVA.***
EENT: exophthalmos, diplopia.
GU: *breakthrough bleeding, change in menstrual flow,* dysmenorrhea, spotting, amenorrhea, cervical erosion.
Hepatic: cholestatic jaundice.
Skin: melasma, rash, acne, pruritus.
Other: breast tenderness, enlargement, or secretion; changes in weight.

Overdose and treatment

No information available.

☑ Special considerations

Besides those relevant to all *progestins,* consider the following recommendations.

- Failure rate of the progestin-only contraceptive is about three times higher than that of the combination contraceptives.
- Ovrette tablets contain tartrazine. Use cautiously in patients with tartrazine or aspirin sensitivity.

Patient education

- Tell patient to take drug at the same time every day, even during menstruation. Norgestrel is also known as the "minipill."
- Advise patient of increased risk of serious CV adverse reactions associated with heavy smoking, especially while taking oral contraceptives.
- Tell patient that risk of pregnancy increases with each tablet missed. If one tablet is missed, she

should take it as soon as she remembers and then take the next tablet at the regular time. If two tablets are missed, she should take one as soon as she remembers and then take the next regular dose at the usual time; she should use a nonhormonal method of contraception in addition to norgestrel until 14 tablets have been taken. If three or more tablets are missed, she should discontinue drug and use a nonhormonal method of contraception until after her period. Instruct patient to do a pregnancy test if her menstrual period does not occur within 45 days.
• Advise patient to report excessive bleeding or bleeding between menstrual cycles immediately.
• Instruct patient to use a second method of birth control for the first cycle on norgestrel, or for 3 weeks after starting the hormonal contraceptive, to ensure full protection.
• Advise patient who wishes to become pregnant to wait at least 3 months after discontinuing norgestrel, to prevent birth defects.

Breast-feeding

• If possible, advise breast-feeding patient not to use oral contraceptives until infant is completely weaned because drug may interfere with lactation by decreasing the quantity and quality of breast milk. Recommend other means of contraception.

nortriptyline hydrochloride

Aventyl, Pamelor

Pharmacologic classification: tricyclic antidepressant
Therapeutic classification: antidepressant
Pregnancy risk category NR

How supplied

Available by prescription only
Capsules: 10 mg, 25 mg, 50 mg, 75 mg
Solution: 10 mg/5 ml (4% alcohol)

Indications, route, and dosage

Depression,* ◊ *panic disorder
Adults: 25 mg P.O. t.i.d. or q.i.d., gradually increasing to a maximum of 150 mg/day. Alternatively, entire dosage may be given h.s.
Elderly or adolescents: 30 to 50 mg P.O. daily or in divided doses.

Pharmacodynamics

Antidepressant action: Drug is thought to exert its antidepressant effects by inhibiting reuptake of norepinephrine and serotonin in CNS nerve terminals (presynaptic neurons), which results in increased concentrations and enhanced activity of these neurotransmitters in the synaptic cleft. Nortriptyline inhibits reuptake of serotonin more actively than norepinephrine; it is less likely than other tricyclic antidepressants to cause orthostatic hypotension.

Pharmacokinetics

• *Absorption:* Absorbed rapidly from the GI tract after oral administration.
• *Distribution:* Drug is distributed widely into the body, including the CNS and breast milk. It is 95% protein-bound. Peak plasma levels occur within 8 hours after a given dose; steady-state serum levels are achieved within 2 to 4 weeks. Therapeutic serum level ranges from 50 to 150 ng/ml.
• *Metabolism:* Metabolized by the liver; a significant first-pass effect may account for variability of serum concentrations in different patients taking the same dosage.
• *Excretion:* Mostly excreted in urine; some in feces, via the biliary tract.

Contraindications and precautions

Contraindicated during acute recovery phase of MI and in patients with hypersensitivity to drug or MAO therapy within past 14 days. Use cautiously in patients with history of urine retention or seizures, glaucoma, suicidal tendencies, CV disease, or hyperthyroidism and in those receiving thyroid medication.

Interactions

Concomitant use of nortriptyline with *sympathomimetics,* including *epinephrine, phenylephrine, phenylpropanolamine,* and *ephedrine* (often found in nasal sprays), may increase blood pressure; use with *warfarin* may increase PT and cause bleeding. Concomitant use with *pimozide, thyroid medication,* or *antiarrhythmic agents (disopyramide, procainamide, quinidine)* may increase incidence of arrhythmias and conduction defects.

Nortriptyline may decrease hypotensive effects of *centrally acting antihypertensive drugs,* such as *clonidine, guanabenz, guanadrel, guanethidine, methyldopa,* and *reserpine.*

Concomitant use with *disulfiram* or *ethchlorvynol* may cause delirium and tachycardia.

Additive effects are likely after concomitant use of nortriptyline with *CNS depressants,* including *alcohol, analgesics, barbiturates, narcotics, tranquilizers,* and *anesthetics* (oversedation); *atropine* and *other anticholinergic drugs,* including *antihistamines, meperidine, phenothiazines,* and *antiparkinson agents* (oversedation, paralytic ileus, visual changes, and severe constipation); and *metrizamide* (increased risk of seizures).

Barbiturates and heavy smoking induce nortriptyline metabolism and decrease therapeutic efficacy; *phenothiazines* and *haloperidol* decrease its metabolism, decreasing therapeutic efficacy; *beta blockers, cimetidine, methylphenidate, oral contraceptives,* and *propoxyphene* may inhibit nortriptyline metabolism, increasing plasma levels and toxicity.

Effects on diagnostic tests

Nortriptyline may prolong conduction time (elongation of QT and PR intervals, flattened T waves on ECG); it also may elevate liver function test results, decrease WBC count, and decrease or increase serum glucose levels.

Adverse reactions

CNS: *drowsiness, dizziness,* ***seizures,*** tremor, weakness, confusion, headache, nervousness,

EEG changes, extrapyramidal reactions, insomnia, nightmares, hallucinations, paresthesia, ataxia, agitation.
CV: *tachycardia,* hypertension, hypotension, ***MI,*** heart block, ***stroke.***
EENT: *blurred vision,* tinnitus, mydriasis.
GI: dry mouth, *constipation,* nausea, vomiting, anorexia, paralytic ileus.
GU: *urine retention.*
Hematologic: bone marrow depression, ***agranulocytosis,*** eosinophilia, ***thrombocytopenia.***
Skin: rash, urticaria, photosensitivity.
Other: *diaphoresis,* hypersensitivity reaction.

After abrupt withdrawal of long-term therapy: nausea, headache, malaise (does not indicate addiction).

Overdose and treatment

The first 12 hours after acute ingestion are a stimulatory phase characterized by excessive anticholinergic activity (agitation, irritation, confusion, hallucinations, hyperthermia, parkinsonian symptoms, seizures, urine retention, dry mucous membranes, pupillary dilation, constipation, and ileus). This is followed by CNS depressant effects, including hypothermia, decreased or absent reflexes, sedation, hypotension, cyanosis, and cardiac irregularities, including tachycardia, conduction disturbances, and quinidine-like effects on the ECG.

Severity of overdose is best indicated by prolonging QRS complex beyond 100 ms, which usually indicates a serum level above 1,000 ng/ml. Metabolic acidosis may follow hypotension, hypoventilation, and seizures.

Treatment is symptomatic and supportive, including maintaining a patent airway, stable body temperature, and fluid and electrolyte balance. Induce emesis with ipecac syrup if patient is conscious; follow with gastric lavage and activated charcoal to prevent further absorption. Dialysis is usually ineffective. Consider use of cardiac glycosides or physostigmine if serious CV abnormalities or cardiac failure occurs. Treat seizures with parenteral diazepam or phenytoin; arrhythmias with parenteral phenytoin or lidocaine; and acidosis with sodium bicarbonate. *Do not give barbiturates;* these may enhance CNS and respiratory depressant effects.

☑ Special considerations

Besides those relevant to all *tricyclic antidepressants,* consider the following recommendations.

- Drug may be administered at bedtime to reduce daytime sedation. Tolerance to sedative effects usually develops over the initial weeks of therapy.
- Withdraw drug gradually over a few weeks; however, it should be discontinued at least 48 hours before surgical procedures.
- Drug is available in liquid form.
- In patients with bipolar disorders, drug may cause symptoms of the manic phase to emerge.

Patient education

- Explain that full effects of drug therapy may not occur for up to 4 weeks after start of therapy.
- Warn patient about sedative effects.
- Recommend taking full daily dose at bedtime to prevent daytime sedation.
- Instruct patient to avoid drinking alcoholic beverages, doubling doses after missing one, and discontinuing drug abruptly, unless instructed.
- Warn patient about possible dizziness. Tell patient to lie down for about 30 minutes after each dose at start of therapy and to avoid sudden postural changes, to avoid dizziness. Postural hypotension is usually less severe than with amitriptyline.
- Urge patient to report unusual reactions promptly: confusion, movement disorders, fainting, rapid heartbeat, or difficulty urinating.
- Tell patient to store drug away from children.
- Suggest relieving dry mouth with sugarless chewing gum or candy.
- Advise patient to avoid activities that require physical and mental alertness, such as driving a car or operating machinery.

Geriatric use

- Lower dosages may be indicated. Elderly patients are at greater risk for adverse cardiac effects.

Pediatric use

- Drug is not recommended for children. Lower dosages may be indicated for adolescents.

Breast-feeding

- Nortriptyline is excreted in breast milk in low concentrations; potential benefit to mother should outweigh potential harm to infant.

nystatin

Mycostatin, Nilstat, Nystex

Pharmacologic classification: polyene macrolide
Therapeutic classification: antifungal
Pregnancy risk category B

How supplied

Available by prescription only
Tablets: 500,000 units
Suspension: 100,000 units/ml
Vaginal suppositories: 100,000 units
Cream: 100,000 units/g
Ointment: 100,000 units/g
Powder: 100,000 units/g
Lozenges: 200,000 units

Indications, route, and dosage

GI infections
Adults: 500,000 to 1 million units as oral tablets, t.i.d.
Oral, vaginal, and intestinal infections caused by susceptible organisms
Adults: 500,000 to 1 million units of oral suspension t.i.d. for oral candidiasis. Alternatively, give 200,000 to 400,000 units (lozenges) four to five times daily; allow to dissolve in mouth.
Children and infants over age 3 months: 250,000 to 500,000 units of oral suspension q.i.d.

Newborn and premature infants: 100,000 units of oral suspension q.i.d.
Cutaneous or mucocutaneous candidal infections
Topical use: Apply to affected areas b.i.d. or t.i.d. until healing is complete.
Vaginal use: 100,000 units, as vaginal tablets, inserted high into vagina daily or b.i.d. for 14 days.

Pharmacodynamics
Antifungal action: Nystatin is both fungistatic and fungicidal. It binds to sterols in the fungal cell membrane, altering its permeability and allowing leakage of intracellular components. It acts against various yeasts and fungi, including *Candida albicans.*

Pharmacokinetics
- *Absorption:* Nystatin is not absorbed from the GI tract, nor through the intact skin or mucous membranes.
- *Distribution:* No detectable amount of drug is available for tissue distribution.
- *Metabolism:* No detectable amount of drug is systemically available for metabolism.
- *Excretion:* Oral nystatin is excreted almost entirely unchanged in feces.

Contraindications and precautions
Contraindicated in patients with hypersensitivity to drug.

Interactions
None reported.

Effects on diagnostic tests
None reported.

Adverse reactions
GI: transient nausea, diarrhea (usually with large oral dosage), vomiting (with oral administration or vaginal tablets).
Skin: occasional contact dermatitis from preservatives in some forms (with topical administration or vaginal tablets).

Overdose and treatment
Nystatin overdose may result in nausea, vomiting, and diarrhea. Treatment is unnecessary because toxicity is negligible.

☑ Special considerations
- Vaginal tablets may be used by pregnant women up to 6 weeks before term.
- Avoid hand contact with drug; hypersensitivity is rare but can occur.
- For treatment of oral candidiasis, patient should have clean mouth, and should hold suspension in mouth for several minutes before swallowing; for infant thrush, medication should be swabbed on oral mucosa.
- May give immunosuppressed patient vaginal tablets (100,000 units) orally to provide prolonged drug contact with oral mucosa; alternatively, use clotrimazole troche.
- For candidiasis of the feet, patient should dust powder on shoes and stockings as well as feet for maximal contact and effectiveness.
- Avoid occlusive dressings or ointment on moist covered body areas that favor yeast growth.
- To prevent maceration, use cream on intertriginous areas, and powder on moist lesions.
- Clean affected skin gently before topical application; cool, moist compresses applied for 15 minutes between applications help soothe dry skin.
- Cleansing douches may be used by nonpregnant women for esthetic reasons; they should use preparations that do not contain antibacterials, which may alter flora and promote reinfection.
- Protect drug from light, air, and heat.
- Drug is ineffective in systemic fungal infection.

Patient education
- Teach patient signs and symptoms of candidal infection. Inform patient about predisposing agents: use of antibiotics, oral contraceptives, and corticosteroids; diabetes; infected sexual partners; and tight-fitting pantyhose and undergarments.
- Teach good oral hygiene. Explain that overuse of mouthwash and poorly fitting dentures, especially in elderly patients, may alter flora and promote infection.
- Tell patient to continue using vaginal cream through menstruation; emphasize importance of washing applicator thoroughly after each use.
- Advise patient to change stockings and undergarments daily; teach good skin care.
- Teach patient how to administer each dosage form prescribed.
- Tell patient to continue drug for at least 48 hours after symptoms clear, to prevent reinfection.

Breast-feeding
- Safety has not been established.

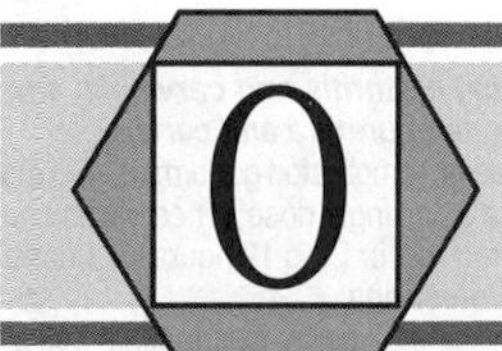

octreotide acetate
Sandostatin

Pharmacologic classification: synthetic octapeptide
Therapeutic classification: somatotropic hormone
Pregnancy risk category B

How supplied
Available by prescription only
Injection: 0.05 mg/ml, 0.1 mg/ml, 0.2 mg/ml, 0.5 mg/ml, 1 mg/ml

Indications, route, and dosage
Symptomatic treatment of flushing and diarrhea associated with carcinoid tumors
Adults: Initially, 100 to 600 mcg daily S.C. in two to four divided doses for first 2 weeks of therapy (usual daily dosage, 300 mcg). Subsequent dosage based on individual response.
Symptomatic treatment of watery diarrhea associated with Vasoactive Intestinal Peptide-secreting tumors (VIPomas)
Adults: Initially, 200 to 300 mcg daily S.C. in two to four divided doses for first 2 weeks of therapy. Subsequent dosage based on individual response, but usually will not exceed 450 mcg daily.
Acromegaly
Adults: Initially, 50 mcg t.i.d. S.C. Subsequent dosage based on individual response. Usual dosage is 100 mcg S.C. t.i.d. but some patients may require up to 500 mcg t.i.d. for maximum effectiveness.
◊ ***Decrease output of rectal or pancreatic fistulas***
Adults: 50 to 200 mcg S.C. q 8 hours.
◊ ***Variceal bleeding***
Adults: 25 to 50 mcg/hour via a continuous I.V. infusion.
◊ ***Diarrheal states***
Adults: 100 to 500 mcg S.C. t.i.d.
◊ ***Irritable bowel syndrome***
Adults: 100 mcg S.C. as a single dose to 125 mcg S.C. b.i.d.
◊ ***Dumping syndrome***
Adults: 50 to 150 mcg S.C. daily.

Pharmacodynamics
Antidiarrheal action: Octreotide mimics the action of naturally occurring somatostatin and decreases the secretion of gastroenterohepatic peptides that may contribute to the adverse signs and symptoms seen in patients with metastatic carcinoid tumors and VIPomas. It is not known if drug affects the tumor directly.

Pharmacokinetics
• *Absorption:* Octreotide is absorbed rapidly and completely after injection. Peak plasma levels occur in less than ½ hour.
• *Distribution:* Drug is distributed to the plasma, where it binds to serum lipoprotein and albumin.
• *Metabolism:* Eliminated from the plasma at a slower rate than the naturally occurring hormone. Apparent half-life is about 1½ hours, with a duration of effect of up to 12 hours.
• *Excretion:* About 35% of drug appears unchanged in the urine.

Contraindications and precautions
Contraindicated in patients hypersensitive to drug or its components.

Interactions
Octreotide may decrease plasma levels of *cyclosporine.* Concomitant use with *insulin, oral antidiabetic agents (sulfonylureas)*, or *oral diazoxide* may require dosage adjustments. Use with octreotide may require dosage adjustment of other drugs used to control symptoms of the disease (such as *beta blockers, calcium channel blockers,* and *electrolyte-controlling agents*).

Effects on diagnostic tests
Octreotide suppresses secretion of growth hormone and of the gastroenterohepatic peptides gastrin, VIP, insulin, glucagon, secretin, motilin, and pancreatic polypeptide.

Adverse reactions
CNS: dizziness, light-headedness, fatigue, headache.
CV: sinus bradycardia, conduction abnormalities, ***arrhythmias.***
EENT: blurred vision.
GI: *nausea, diarrhea, abdominal pain* or *discomfort, loose stools,* vomiting, fat malabsorption, gallstones or biliary sludge, flatulence, constipation.
GU: pollakiuria, urinary tract infection.
Skin: flushing, edema, wheals, erythema or pain at injection site, alopecia.
Other: hyperglycemia, hypoglycemia, hypothyroidism, pain or burning at the S.C. injection site, cold symptoms, backache, joint pain, flulike symptoms.

Overdose and treatment
Doses of 1,000 mcg have been administered as an I.V. bolus in volunteers without adverse effects. Drug may produce metabolic changes in certain patients.

☑ Special considerations

- Fluid and electrolyte balance may be altered after initiation of octreotide therapy.
- Half-life may be altered in patients with end-stage renal failure who are undergoing dialysis. Dosage adjustment may be necessary.
- Obtain baseline and periodic tests of thyroid function because drug's long-term effects on hypothalamic-pituitary function are not known.
- Monitor laboratory values during therapy, such as urinary 5-hydroxyindoleacetic acid, plasma serotonin, plasma substance P for carcinoid tumors, and plasma VIP for VIPomas.
- Mild, transient hypoglycemia or hyperglycemia may occur during therapy. Observe patient for signs of glucose imbalance and monitor closely.
- Drug may alter fat absorption and aggravate fat malabsorption. Perform periodic assessment of 72-hour fecal fat and serum carotene.
- Drug may decrease vitamin B levels during chronic treatment. Monitor patient's vitamin B levels.

Patient education

- Because drug may cause gallstones, tell patient to report abdominal discomfort promptly.

Pediatric use

- Doses of 1 to 10 mcg/kg appear to be well-tolerated in children.

Breast-feeding

- Safety has not been established. It is not known if drug is excreted in breast milk.

ofloxacin

Floxin, Ocuflox

Pharmacologic classification: fluoroquinolone
Therapeutic classification: antibiotic
Pregnancy risk category C

How supplied

Available by prescription only
Tablets: 200 mg, 300 mg, 400 mg
Injection: 200 mg in 50 ml D_5W; 400 mg in water for injection in 10- and 20-ml single-use vials; 400 mg in 100 ml D_5W.
Ophthalmic solution: 0.3%

Indications, route, and dosage

Conjunctivitis caused by known organism
Adults and children over age 1: Instill 1 to 2 drops in conjunctival sac q 2 to 4 hours, while awake, for first 2 days and then q.i.d. for up to 5 additional days.

Acute bacterial exacerbations of chronic bronchitis and pneumonia caused by susceptible organisms, mild to moderate skin and skin-structure infections, and community-acquired pneumonia
Adults: 400 mg P.O. or I.V. q 12 hours for 10 days.

Sexually transmitted diseases, such as acute uncomplicated urethral and cervical gonorrhea, nongonococcal urethritis and cervicitis, and mixed infections of urethra and cervix
Adults: For acute uncomplicated gonorrhea, 400 mg P.O. or I.V. once as a single dose; for cervicitis and urethritis, 300 mg P.O. or I.V. q 12 hours for 7 days.

Urinary tract infections
Adults: For cystitis caused by *Escherichia coli* or *Klebsiella pneumoniae,* 200 mg P.O. or I.V. q 12 hours for 3 days; for cystitis caused by other organisms, 200 mg P.O. or I.V. q 12 hours for 7 days.

Complicated urinary tract infections
Adults: 200 mg P.O. or I.V. q 12 hours for 10 days.

Prostatitis
Adults: 300 mg P.O. or I.V. q 12 hours for 6 weeks.

◊ ***Adjunct in Brucella infections***
Adults: 400 mg P.O. daily.

◊ ***Peritonitis in patients receiving continuous ambulatory peritoneal dialysis***
Adults: 400 mg P.O. loading dose, then 300 mg P.O. daily for 7 to 10 days.

◊ ***Typhoid fever***
Adults: 200 to 400 mg P.O. q 12 hours for 7 to 14 days.

◊ ***Antituberculosis agent***
Adults: 300 mg P.O. daily.

◊ ***Treatment of postoperative sternotomy or soft-tissue wounds caused by* Mycobacterium fortuitum**
Adults: 300 to 600 mg P.O. daily for 3 to 6 months.

◊ ***Leprosy***
Adults: 400 mg P.O. daily for 8 weeks.

◊ ***Acute Q fever pneumonia***
Adults: 600 mg P.O. daily for up to 16 days.

◊ ***Mediterranean spotted fever***
Adults: 200 mg P.O. q 12 hours for 7 days.

✦ ***Dosage adjustment.*** In patients with renal failure and creatinine clearance of 50 ml/minute or less, adjust dosage. Give initial dose as recommended; additional doses as follows: If creatinine clearance is 10 to 50 ml/minute, no dosage adjustment at 24-hour intervals; if below 10 ml/ minute, 50% of recommended dose q 24 hours.

Maximum daily dosage in patients with hepatic function disorders is 400 mg.

Pharmacodynamics

Antibacterial action: Ofloxacin interferes with DNA gyrase, which is needed for synthesis of bacterial DNA.

Pharmacokinetics

- *Absorption:* Drug is well absorbed after oral administration, with maximum serum concentrations achieved within 1 to 2 hours. Because the oral bioavailability is about 98%, oral and I.V. dosage is the same.
- *Distribution:* Widely distributed to body tissues and fluids.
- *Metabolism:* Less than 10% of a single dose is metabolized.
- *Excretion:* 70% to 80% is excreted unchanged in urine; less than 5%, in feces.

Contraindications and precautions

Contraindicated in patients with hypersensitivity to drug or other fluoroquinolones. Use oral and I.V.

forms cautiously in patients with seizure disorders, CNS diseases (such as cerebral arteriosclerosis), hepatic disorders, or renal failure and during pregnancy.

Interactions

Concomitant therapy with *theophylline* may prolong theophylline half-life, increase serum theophylline levels, and risk theophylline-related adverse effects. Monitor closely and adjust theophylline dosage as needed. Concomitant administration with *antacids* interferes with GI absorption of ofloxacin, resulting in decreased serum levels; separate administration by 2 to 4 hours.

Patients receiving *warfarin* may have prolonged PT. Ofloxacin taken with *antidiabetic agents* may affect blood glucose levels, causing hypoglycemia or hyperglycemia.

Effects on diagnostic tests

Drug may increase blood glucose levels.

Adverse reactions

CNS: dizziness; headache, fatigue, lethargy, malaise, drowsiness, sleep disorders, nervousness, insomnia, visual disturbances, ***seizures*** (with oral or I.V. form).
CV: chest pain (with oral or I.V. form).
EENT: *transient ocular burning or discomfort,* stinging, redness, itching, photophobia, lacrimation, eye dryness (with ophthalmic form).
GI: *nausea,* ***pseudomembranous colitis,*** anorexia, abdominal pain or discomfort, diarrhea, vomiting, constipation, dry mouth, flatulence, dysgeusia (with oral or I.V. form).
GU: vaginitis, vaginal discharge, genital pruritus (with oral or I.V. form).
Musculoskeletal: trunk pain (with oral or I.V. form).
Skin: rash, pruritus, photosensitivity (with oral or I.V. form).
Other: hypersensitivity reactions ***(anaphylactoid reaction),*** elevated liver enzymes, fever, phlebitis (with oral or I.V. form).

Overdose and treatment

In case of overdose, empty the stomach and maintain hydration. Observe patient and treat symptomatically.

☑ Special considerations

- Perform periodic assessment of organ system functions during prolonged therapy.
- Give I.V. ofloxacin by slow infusion only; do not give I.M., S.C., intrathecally, or by intraperitoneal injection. Administer over at least 60 minutes and avoid rapid or bolus injection. Compatible with most common I.V. solutions, including D_5W injection, 0.9% NaCl injection, dextrose 5% in 0.9% NaCl injection, dextrose 5% in 0.45% NaCl injection, 5% dextrose in lactated Ringer's solution, and 5% sodium bicarbonate injection.
- Drug is not recommended for syphilis.

Patient education

- Advise patient to drink fluids liberally.
- Advise patient to separate doses of antacids, vitamins, and ofloxacin by 2 hours.
- Advise patient to take on an empty stomach ½ hour before or 2 hours after meals.
- Tell patient dizziness and light-headedness may occur. Advise caution when driving or operating hazardous machinery until effects of drug are known.
- Warn patient that hypersensitivity reactions may follow first dose; he should discontinue drug at first sign of rash or other allergic reaction and notify primary health care provider immediately.
- Advise patient to avoid prolonged exposure to direct sunlight and to use a sunscreen when outdoors.

Pediatric use

- Safety and efficacy in children under age 18 have not been established. Similar drugs have caused arthropathy in juvenile animals.

Breast-feeding

- Safety has not been established. Ofloxacin is excreted in breast milk in levels similar to those found in plasma.

---

olanzapine

Zyprexa

Pharmacologic classification: thienobenzodiazepine derivative
Therapeutic classification: antipsychotic
Pregnancy risk category C

How supplied

Available by prescription only
Tablets: 5 mg, 7.5 mg, 10 mg

Indications, route, and dosage

Management of manifestations of psychotic disorders

Adults: Initially, 5 to 10 mg P.O. once daily. Adjust dosage in 5-mg daily increments at intervals of not less than 1 week. Most patients respond to 10 mg/day; do not exceed 20 mg/day.

Pharmacodynamics

Unknown. Acts as an antagonist at dopamine (D_{1-4}) and serotonin ($5-HT_{2A/2C}$) receptors; may also exhibit antagonist-binding at adrenergic, cholinergic, and histaminergic receptors.

Pharmacokinetics

- *Absorption:* Peak levels occur approximately 6 hours after an oral dose. Food does not affect rate or extent of absorption. Approximately 40% of dose is eliminated by first-pass metabolism.
- *Distribution:* Extensively distributed throughout the body, with a volume of distribution of approximately 1,000 L. Drug is 93% protein bound, primarily to albumin and $alpha_1$-acid glycoprotein.
- *Metabolism:* Direct glucuronidation and cytochrome P-450–mediated oxidation
- *Excretion:* Approximately 57% of drug appears in the urine and 30% in feces as metabolites. Only

7% of dose is recovered in the urine unchanged. Elimination half-life ranges from 21 to 54 hours.

Contraindications and precautions

Contraindicated in patients with known hypersensitivity to drug. Use cautiously in patients with heart disease, cerebrovascular disease, conditions that predispose to hypotension (gradual titration of therapy minimizes the risk), history of seizures or conditions that might lower the seizure threshold, and hepatic impairment. Also use cautiously in elderly patients, in those with history of paralytic ileus, significant prostatic hypertrophy, or narrow-angle glaucoma, or those at risk for aspiration pneumonia.

Interactions

Alcohol, antihypertensives, and *diazepam* may potentiate hypotensive effects. Monitor blood pressure closely.

Coadministration with *carbamazepine, omeprazole,* and *rifampin* may cause increased clearance of olanzapine; monitor patient.

Concurrent use with *levodopa* and *dopamine agonists* may cause antagonized effects of these agents. Monitor patient. *Fluvoxamine* may inhibit olanzapine elimination.

Effects on diagnostic tests

Olanzapine may cause asymptomatic increases in ALT, AST, gamma glutamyltransferase, serum prolactin, eosinophil count, and CK.

Adverse reactions

CNS: *somnolence, agitation, insomnia, headache, nervousness, hostility, parkinsonism, dizziness,* anxiety, personality disorder, *akathesia,* hypertonia, tremor, amnesia, articulation impairment, euphoria, stuttering, dystonic/dyskinetic events, tardive dyskinesia.
CV: orthostatic hypotension, tachycardia, chest pain, hypotension, edema.
EENT: amblyopia, blepharitis, corneal lesion.
GI: constipation, dry mouth, abdominal pain, increased appetite, increased salivation, nausea, vomiting, thirst.
GU: premenstrual syndrome, hematuria, metrorrhagia, urinary incontinence, urinary tract infection.
Musculoskeletal: joint pain, extremity pain, back pain, neck rigidity, twitching.
Respiratory: *rhinitis,* increased cough, pharyngitis, dyspnea.
Skin: vesiculobullous rash.
Other: weight gain or loss, fever, intentional injury, flu syndrome, suicide attempt.

Overdose and treatment

Symptoms of overdose may include drowsiness and slurred speech. There is no specific antidote to olanzapine, and treatment should be symptomatic. Monitor patient for hypotension, circulatory collapse, obtundation, seizures, or dystonic reactions. Gastric lavage with activated charcoal and sorbitol may be effective. Drug is not removed by dialysis. Avoid epinephrine, dopamine, or other sympathomimetics with beta-agonist activity.

☑ Special considerations

- Monitor patient for signs of neuroleptic malignant syndrome (hyperpyrexia, muscle rigidity, altered mental status, autonomic instability), a rare but frequently fatal adverse reaction that can occur with the administration of antipsychotic drugs. Drug should be stopped immediately and patient monitored and treated.
- Initiate therapy with 5 mg in patients who are debilitated, predisposed to hypotension, or have an alteration in metabolism due to smoking status, gender, or age or who are pharmacologically sensitive to drug.
- Efficacy for long-term use (over 6 weeks) has not been established.
- Obtain baseline and periodic liver function tests.

Patient education

- Warn patient to avoid hazardous tasks until adverse CNS effects of drug are known.
- Caution patient against exposure to extreme heat; drug may impair body's ability to reduce core temperature.
- Instruct patient to avoid alcohol.
- Tell patient to rise slowly to avoid orthostatic hypotension.
- Advise patient to use ice chips or sugarless candy or gum to relieve dry mouth.
- Inform patient not to take prescription or OTC drugs without medical approval because of potential drug interactions.

Geriatric use

- Drug may be initiated at lower dose because clearance may be decreased. Half-life is 1.5 times greater in this population.

Pediatric use

- Safety and efficacy in children under age 18 have not been established.

Breast-feeding

- Animal studies have shown that drug is excreted in breast milk. Advise breast-feeding patient to seek alternative feeding method during therapy.

olsalazine sodium

Dipentum

Pharmacologic classification: salicylate
Therapeutic classification: anti-inflammatory
Pregnancy risk category C

How supplied

Available by prescription only
Capsules: 250 mg

Indications, route, and dosage

Maintenance of remission of ulcerative colitis in patients intolerant of sulfasalazine
Adults: 1 g P.O. daily in two divided doses.

Pharmacodynamics
Anti-inflammatory action: Mechanism of action is unknown but appears to be topical rather than systemic. Drug is converted to mesalamine (5-aminosalicylic acid; 5-ASA) in the colon. Presumably, mesalamine diminishes inflammation by blocking cyclooxygenase and inhibiting prostaglandin production in the colon.

Pharmacokinetics
- *Absorption:* After oral administration, approximately 2.4% of a single dose is absorbed; maximum concentrations appear in about 2 hours.
- *Distribution:* Once metabolized to 5-ASA, it is absorbed slowly from the colon, resulting in very high local concentrations.
- *Metabolism:* 0.1% is metabolized in the liver; remainder will reach the colon, where it is rapidly converted to 5-ASA by colonic bacteria.
- *Excretion:* Less than 1% is recovered in urine.

Contraindications and precautions
Contraindicated in patients hypersensitive to salicylates. Use cautiously in patients with existing renal disease.

Interactions
Olsalazine increases PT in patients receiving *warfarin* therapy.

Effects on diagnostic tests
None reported.

Adverse reactions
CNS: headache, depression, vertigo, dizziness, fatigue.
GI: *diarrhea,* nausea, *abdominal pain,* dyspepsia, bloating, anorexia, stomatitis.
Skin: rash, itching.
Other: arthralgia.

Overdose and treatment
Decreased motor activity and diarrhea can occur. Treat overdosage symptomatically and supportively.

☑ Special considerations
- Diarrhea was noted in 17% of patients, but it is difficult to distinguish from underlying condition.
- Monitor CBC with differential and liver function tests periodically.

Patient education
- Advise patient to take drug with food and in evenly divided doses.
- Inform patient to call if diarrhea develops.

Pediatric use
- Safety and efficacy have not been established.

Breast-feeding
- It is unknown if drug is excreted in breast milk. Use with caution.

omeprazole
Prilosec

Pharmacologic classification: substituted benzimidazole
Therapeutic classification: gastric acid suppressant
Pregnancy risk category C

How supplied
Available by prescription only
Capsules (delayed-release): 10 mg, 20 mg

Indications, route, and dosage
Active duodenal ulcer
Adults: 20 mg P.O. daily for 4 to 8 weeks.
Helicobacter pylori *eradication for the reduction of the risk of duodenal ulcer recurrence*
– Triple therapy (omeprazole/clarithromycin/amoxicillin)
Adults: 20 mg P.O. b.i.d. plus 500 mg clarithromycin P.O. b.i.d. plus 1000 mg amoxicillin P.O. b.i.d. for 10 days. In patients with an ulcer present at the time of initiation of therapy, an additional 18 days of omeprazole 20 mg once daily is recommended alone for ulcer healing and symptom relief.

Note: Refer to entries on clarithromycin and amoxicillin.

– Dual therapy (omeprazole/clarithromycin)
Adults: 40 mg each morning plus 500 mg clarithromycin t.i.d. for 14 days followed by 14 days of omeprazole 20 mg daily.

Note: Refer to entry on clarithromycin.

Severe erosive esophagitis; symptomatic, poorly responsive gastroesophageal reflux disease (GERD)
Adults: 20 mg P.O. daily for 4 to 8 weeks. Patients with GERD should have failed initial therapy with a H_2 antagonist. Dosages up to 40 mg daily may be necessary.
Pathological hypersecretory conditions (such as Zollinger-Ellison syndrome)
Adults: Initial dosage is 60 mg P.O. daily; titrate dosage based on patient response. Administer daily dosages exceeding 80 mg in divided doses. Doses up to 120 mg t.i.d. have been administered. Continue therapy as long as clinically indicated.
Gastric ulcer
Adults: 40 mg P.O. daily for 4 to 8 weeks.

Pharmacodynamics
Antisecretory action: Omeprazole inhibits the activity of the acid (proton) pump, H+/K+ adenosine triphosphatase (ATPase), located at the secretory surface of the gastric parietal cell. This blocks the formation of gastric acid.

Pharmacokinetics
- *Absorption:* Omeprazole is acid-labile, and the formulation contains enteric-coated granules that permit absorption after drug leaves the stomach. Absorption is rapid, with peak levels occurring in less than 3½ hours. Bioavailability is about 40% because of instability in gastric acid as well as a substantial first-pass effect. Bioavailability increas-

es slightly with repeated dosing, possibly because of drug's effect on gastric acidity.
• *Distribution:* Protein binding is about 95%.
• *Metabolism:* Metabolism is primarily hepatic.
• *Excretion:* Primarily renal. Plasma half-life is ½ to 1 hour, but drug effects may persist for days.

Contraindications and precautions
Contraindicated in patients hypersensitive to drug or its components.

Interactions
Elimination of drugs metabolized by hepatic oxidation, including *diazepam, phenytoin*, and *warfarin*, may be impaired by omeprazole. Patients taking these drugs or others that are metabolized by the hepatic microsomal enzyme system (including *propranolol, theophylline*) should be monitored closely.

Drugs that depend on low gastric pH for absorption (including *ampicillin esters, iron derivatives, ketoconazole*) may exhibit poor bioavailability in patients taking omeprazole.

Effects on diagnostic tests
Serum gastrin levels rise in most patients during first 2 weeks of therapy.

Adverse reactions
CNS: headache, dizziness, asthenia.
GI: diarrhea, abdominal pain, nausea, vomiting, constipation, flatulence.
Respiratory: cough, upper respiratory infection.
Skin: rash.
Other: back pain.

Overdose and treatment
There are rare reports of overdose; symptoms include confusion, drowsiness, blurred vision, tachycardia, nausea, vomiting, diaphoresis, dry mouth, and headache. Dosages up to 360 mg daily have been well-tolerated. Dialysis is believed to be of little value because of the extent of binding to plasma proteins. Treatment should be symptomatic and supportive.

☑ Special considerations
• Drug increases its own bioavailability with repeated administration. It is labile in gastric acid; less of it is lost to hydrolysis because drug raises gastric pH.
• Dosage adjustments are not required for patients with impaired renal function; however, they are needed in those with hepatic impairment.
• Capsule should not be crushed.

Patient education
• Explain importance of taking drug exactly as prescribed.
• Tell patient to take before meals and not to crush capsules.

Pediatric use
• Safe use in children has not been established.

Breast-feeding
• It is not known if drug is excreted in breast milk. Avoid breast-feeding during therapy.

ondansetron hydrochloride
Zofran

Pharmacologic classification: serotonin ($5\text{-}HT_3$) receptor antagonist
Therapeutic classification: antiemetic
Pregnancy risk category B

How supplied
Available by prescription only
Tablets: 4 mg, 8 mg
Injection: 2 mg/ml in 20-ml multidose vials, 2-ml single-dose vials
Injection, premixed: 32 mg/50 ml in 5% dextrose single-dose vial

Indications, route, and dosage
Prevention of nausea and vomiting associated with initial and repeat courses of emetogenic cancer chemotherapy, including high-dose cisplatin
Adults and children age 4 and older: Three I.V. doses of 0.15 mg/kg with first dose infused over 15 minutes beginning 30 minutes before start of chemotherapy with subsequent doses of 0.15 mg/kg administered 4 and 8 hours after first dose. May also administer as a single dose of 32 mg 30 minutes before start of chemotherapy.
Adults and children over age 12: 8 mg P.O. b.i.d. starting 30 minutes before start of chemotherapy, with subsequent dose 8 hours after first dose, then 8 mg q 12 hours for 1 to 2 days after completion of chemotherapy.
Children age 4 to 12: 4 mg P.O. t.i.d. dosed the same times as for adults.
Prevention of radiation-induced nausea and vomiting
Adults: 8 mg P.O. t.i.d.
Prevention of postoperative nausea and vomiting
Adults: 16 mg P.O. 1 hour before anesthesia or 4 mg I.V. immediately before anesthesia or shortly postoperatively.

Pharmacodynamics
Antiemetic action: Mechanism of action is not fully defined; however, ondansetron is *not* a dopamine-receptor antagonist. Because serotonin receptors of the $5\text{-}HT_3$ type are present both peripherally on vagal nerve terminals and centrally in the chemoreceptor trigger zone, it is not certain if ondansetron's antiemetic action is mediated centrally, peripherally, or in both sites.

Pharmacokinetics
• *Absorption:* Absorption is variable with oral administration with the time to peak concentration reached within 2 hours and bioavailability of 50% to 60%.
• *Distribution:* 70% to 76% is plasma protein-bound.

• *Metabolism:* Extensively metabolized by hydroxylation on the indole ring, followed by glucuronide or sulfate conjugation.
• *Excretion:* 5% of dose is recovered in urine as parent compound.

Contraindications and precautions
Contraindicated in patients hypersensitive to drug. Use cautiously in patients with hepatic failure.

Interactions
Ondansetron is metabolized by cytochrome P-450; thus, *inducers or inhibitors of cytochrome P-450 enzyme* may change clearance and half-life of ondansetron; however, no dosage adjustment is required. *Carmustine, cisplatin,* and *etoposide* do not affect ondansetron's pharmacokinetics.

Effects on diagnostic tests
Drug may increase serum levels of ALT and AST.

Adverse reactions
CNS: *headache, malaise, fatigue, dizziness, sedation.*
GI: *diarrhea, constipation,* abdominal pain, xerostomia.
Hepatic: transient elevations in AST and ALT levels.
Skin: rash.
Other: *musculoskeletal pain,* chills, urine retention, chest pain, injection-site reaction, fever, hypoxia, gynecologic disorders.

Overdose and treatment
Doses more than 10 times the recommended dose have been given without incident. There is no recommended antidote. If overdose is suspected, manage with supportive therapy.

☑ Special considerations
• Ondansetron is stable at room temperature for 48 hours after dilution with 0.9% NaCl, D_5W, 5% dextrose and 0.9% NaCl, 5% dextrose and 0.45% NaCl, or 3% NaCl.

Geriatric use
• No age-related problems have been reported.

Pediatric use
• Little information is available for use in children age 3 and under.

Breast-feeding
• It is unknown if drug is excreted in breast milk; caution is recommended.

opium tincture (laudanum)

opium tincture, camphorated (paregoric)

Pharmacologic classification: opiate
Therapeutic classification: antidiarrheal
Controlled substance schedule II or III (depending on amount of opium contained in product)
Pregnancy risk category B (D for high doses or long term)

How supplied
Available by prescription only
opium tincture
Alcoholic solution: equivalent to morphine 10 mg/ml
opium tincture, camphorated
Alcoholic solution: Each 5 ml contains morphine, 2 mg; anise oil, 0.2 ml; benzoic acid, 20 mg; camphor, 20 mg; glycerin, 0.2 ml; and ethanol to make 5 ml

Indications, route, and dosage
Acute, nonspecific diarrhea
Do not confuse doses of opium tincture and camphorated opium tincture.
Adults: 0.6 ml opium tincture (range, 0.3 to 1 ml) P.O. q.i.d. (maximum dosage, 6 ml daily), or 5 to 10 ml camphorated opium tincture daily, b.i.d., t.i.d., or q.i.d. until diarrhea subsides.
Children: 0.25 to 0.5 ml/kg camphorated opium tincture daily, b.i.d., t.i.d., or q.i.d. until diarrhea subsides.

Opium tincture has been used to treat withdrawal symptoms in infants whose mothers are narcotic addicts.

Pharmacodynamics
Antidiarrheal action: Opium, derived from the opium poppy, contains several ingredients. The most active ingredient, morphine, increases GI smooth-muscle tone, inhibits motility and propulsion, and diminishes secretions. By inhibiting peristalsis, the drug delays passage of intestinal contents, increasing water resorption and relieving diarrhea.

Pharmacokinetics
• *Absorption:* Morphine is absorbed variably from the gut.
• *Distribution:* Although opium alkaloids are distributed widely in the body, the low doses used to treat diarrhea act primarily in the GI tract. Camphor crosses the placenta.
• *Metabolism:* Opium is metabolized rapidly in the liver.
• *Excretion:* Opium is excreted in urine; opium alkaloids (especially morphine) enter breast milk. Drug effect persists 4 to 5 hours.

Contraindications and precautions
Contraindicated in patients with acute diarrhea caused by poisoning until toxic material is removed from GI tract or in those with diarrhea caused by organisms that penetrate intestinal mucosa. Use

cautiously in patients with asthma, prostatic hyperplasia, hepatic disease, and history of opium dependence.

Interactions
When used concomitantly with other *CNS depressants*, opium tincture and camphorated opium tincture result in an additive effect. Concomitant use with *metoclopramide* may antagonize the effects of metoclopramide.

Effects on diagnostic tests
Opium tincture and camphorated opium tincture may prevent delivery of technetium-99m disofenin to the small intestine during hepatobiliary imaging tests; delay test until 24 hours after last dose. Drugs also may increase serum amylase and lipase levels by inducing contractions of the sphincter of Oddi and increasing biliary tract pressure.

Adverse reactions
CNS: dizziness, light-headedness.
GI: nausea, vomiting, physical dependence (after long-term use).

Overdose and treatment
Clinical effects of overdose include drowsiness, hypotension, seizures, and apnea. Empty stomach by induced emesis or gastric lavage; maintain patent airway. Use naloxone to treat respiratory depression. Monitor patient for signs and symptoms of CNS or respiratory depression.

☑ Special considerations
- Mix drug with sufficient water to ensure passage to stomach.
- Opium tincture is 25 times more potent than camphorated opium tincture (paregoric); take care not to confuse these drugs.
- Monitor vital signs.
- Monitor bowel function.
- Risk of physical dependence on drug increases with long-term use.
- Do not refrigerate drug.

Patient education
- Warn patient that physical dependence may result from long-term use.
- Warn patient to use caution when driving a car or performing other tasks requiring alertness because drug may cause drowsiness, dizziness, and blurred vision.
- Because drug is indicated only for short-term use, instruct patient to report diarrhea that persists longer than 48 hours.
- Advise patient to take drug with food if it causes nausea, vomiting, or constipation.
- Instruct patient to call immediately if he has difficulty breathing or shortness of breath.
- Instruct patient to drink adequate fluids while diarrhea persists.

Breast-feeding
- Because opium alkaloids (especially morphine) are excreted in breast milk, drug's possible risks must be weighed against benefits.

oprelvekin
Neumega

Pharmacologic classification: recombinant human interleukin eleven (rhIL-11)
Therapeutic classification: human thrombopoietic growth factor
Pregnancy risk category C

How supplied
Available by prescription only
Injection: 5 mg single-dose vial with diluent

Indications, route and dosage
Prevention of severe thrombocytopenia and reduction of need for platelet transfusions following myelosuppressive chemotherapy in patients with nonmyeloid malignancies who are at high risk for severe thrombocytopenia
Adults: 50 mcg/kg S.C. once daily. Begin dosing 6 to 24 hours after completion of chemotherapy and discontinue at least 2 days before starting the next planned cycle of chemotherapy. Continue dosing until the postnadir platelet count is 50,000 cells/mcl or more.

Pharmacodynamics
Thrombopoietic growth factor action: Oprelvekin is a thrombopoetic growth factor that directly stimulates the proliferation of hematopoietic stem cells and megakaryocyte progenitor cells. The primary activity of oprelvekin is stimulation of megakaryocytopoiesis and thrombopoiesis. Platelets produced in response to oprelvekin posess a normal life-span and are functionally normal. Bone-forming and bone-resorbing cells are potential targets for oprelvekin. In human studies, platelet counts began to increase relative to baseline between 5 and 9 days after the start of oprelvekin therapy. After treatment ceased, platelet counts continued to increase for up to 7 days; platelet counts returned to baseline within 14 days.

Pharmacokinetics
- *Absorption:* Administered S.C., the absolute bioavailability of oprelvekin is over 80%.
- *Distribution:* Peak plasma concentrations of oprelvekin occur 3 to 5 hours after an S.C. dose.
- *Metabolism:* Mostly metabolized before excretion; routes of metabolism are unknown.
- *Excretion:* Excreted primarily by the kidneys; terminal half-life is about 6.9 hours.

Contraindications and precautions
Contraindicated in patients with history of hypersensitivity to drug or its components.

Use cautiously in patients with heart failure, in those at risk for the development of clinical heart failure, and in patients with history of heart failure that is currently well controlled. Also use cautiously in patients with history of papilledema, atrial arrhythmias, or CNS tumors. Use with caution in patients receving cardiac medications or with previous treatment with doxorubicin and in the elderly.

Interactions
None reported.

Effects on diagnostic tests
Drug may cause a decrease in hemoglobin, serum albumin, other proteins (transferrin and gamma globulins), and calcium levels. These effects are due to plasma expansion. A twofold increase in plasma fibrinogen has been observed. Von Willebrand factor concentrations also increased.

Adverse reactions
CNS: *asthenia, headache, insomnia, dizziness,* paresthesia.
CV: *tachycardia, vasodilation, palpitations,* ATRIAL FLUTTER OR FIBRILLATION, *syncope.*
EENT: blurred vision, *conjunctival injection, pharyngitis, rhinitis,* eye hemorrhage.
GI: *oral moniliasis, nausea, vomiting, diarrhea, mucositis.*
Hematologic: NEUTROPENIC FEVER.
Respiratory: *dyspnea, cough,* PLEURAL EFFUSIONS.
Skin: *rash,* skin discoloration, exfoliative dermatitis, transient rash at injection site.
Other: dehydration, *edema, fever.*

Overdose and treatment
No information available. Large doses of drug may be associated with an increased incidence of cardiac events. If overdose occurs, discontinue drug and observe patient for cardiac signs of toxicity.

☑ Special considerations
- Administer S.C. in the abdomen, thigh, hip, or upper arm.
- Store drug and diluent in the refrigerator until ready to use.
- Reconsititute single-dose vial with 1 ml of supplied diluent. Avoid excessive or vigorous agitation. Discard unused drug.
- Use reconstituted drug within 3 hours.
- Closely monitor fluid and electrolyte status (especially potassium levels) in patients receiving chronic diuretic therapy. Severe hypokalemia resulting in death has occurred in patients concomitantly receiving diuretics or ifosfamide and oprelvekin; use with caution.
- Obtain a CBC before chemotherapy and at regular intervals during drug therapy.
- Some patients may develop antibodies to drug.

Patient education
- Provide patient with the information leaflet that is available from the manufacturer. A copy can also be obtained from the drug package insert.
- If patient is to self-administer, instruct him how to prepare and administer drug.
- Advise patient to administer each dose at about same time each day.
- Tell patient to keep drug refrigerated before reconsititution and not to reconstitute until ready to use. Also inform patient that reconstituted drug is stable at room temperature or in the refrigerator for up to 3 hours.
- Tell patient not to reuse vial that has been reconstituted and entered by a syringe, and to discard remaining solution after dose is administered.
- Instruct patient to call primary health care provider immediately if swelling, chest pain, irregular heart beat, blurred vision, difficulty breathing, or fatigue occurs.

Pediatric use
- Efficacy trials in pediatric patients have not been conducted.

Breast-feeding
- It is not known if drug occurs in breast milk. Depending on the importance of drug to mother, a decision should be made whether to discontinue breast-feeding or drug.

orphenadrine citrate
Banflex, Flexoject, Flexon, Myolin, Myotrol, Norflex

orphenadrine hydrochloride
Disipal*

Pharmacologic classification: diphenhydramine analogue
Therapeutic classification: skeletal muscle relaxant
Pregnancy risk category C

How supplied
Available by prescription only
Tablets: 50 mg, 100 mg
Tablets (extended-release): 100 mg
Injection: 30 mg/ml parenteral

Indications, route, and dosage
Adjunct in painful, acute musculoskeletal conditions
Adults: 100 mg P.O. b.i.d., or 60 mg I.V. or I.M. q 12 hours.
◊ ***Leg cramps***
Adults: 100 mg P.O. h.s.

Pharmacodynamics
Skeletal muscle relaxant action: Orphenadrine does not relax skeletal muscle directly. Atropine-like central action on cerebral motor centers or on the medulla may be the mechanism by which it reduces skeletal muscle spasm. Its reported analgesic effect may add to its skeletal muscle relaxant properties.

Pharmacokinetics
- *Absorption:* Rapidly absorbed from the GI tract; onset of action occurs within 1 hour, peaks within 2 hours, and persists for 4 to 6 hours.
- *Distribution:* Widely distributed throughout the body.
- *Metabolism:* Unknown, but drug is almost completely metabolized to at least eight metabolites.
- *Excretion:* Excreted in urine, mainly as its metabolites. Small amounts are excreted unchanged. Its half-life is about 14 hours.

* Canada only ◊ Unlabeled clinical use

Contraindications and precautions
Contraindicated in patients with hypersensitivity to drug; glaucoma; prostatic hyperplasia; pyloric, duodenal, or bladder neck obstruction; myasthenia gravis; and peptic ulceration.

Use cautiously in elderly or debilitated patients or in those with tachycardia, cardiac disease, arrhythmias, or sulfite allergy.

Interactions
Concomitant use with *propoxyphene* or *CNS depressants (alcohol, antipsychotics, anxiolytics, tricyclic antidepressants)* may produce additive CNS effects; concurrent use requires reduction of both agents. Use with other *anticholinergic agents* may increase anticholinergic effects; with *MAO inhibitors*, may increase CNS adverse effects.

Effects on diagnostic tests
None reported.

Adverse reactions
CNS: weakness, *drowsiness,* light-headedness, confusion, agitation, tremor, headache, dizziness, hallucinations.
CV: palpitations, tachycardia, syncope.
EENT: dilated pupils, blurred vision, difficulty swallowing, increased intraocular pressure.
GI: constipation, *dry mouth,* nausea, vomiting, epigastric distress.
GU: urinary hesitancy, urine retention.
Hematologic: ***aplastic anemia.***
Skin: urticaria, pruritus.
Other: ***anaphylaxis.***

Overdose and treatment
Clinical manifestations of overdose include dry mouth, blurred vision, urine retention, tachycardia, confusion, paralytic ileus, deep coma, seizures, shock, respiratory arrest, cardiac arrhythmias, and death.

Treatment includes symptomatic and supportive measures. If ingestion is recent, induce emesis or gastric lavage followed by activated charcoal. Monitor vital signs and fluid and electrolyte balance.

☑ Special considerations
- Perform periodic blood, urine, and liver function tests during prolonged therapy.
- Monitor vital signs, especially intake and output, noting urine retention.
- When giving drug I.V., inject slowly over 5 minutes. Keep patient supine during and 5 to 10 minutes after injection. Paradoxical initial bradycardia may occur when giving I.V.; usually disappears in 2 minutes.
- Some commercially available orphenadrine citrate injection formulations may contain sodium bisulfite, a sulfite that can cause allergic-type reactions, including anaphylaxis.

Patient education
- Recommend ice chips, sugarless gum, hard candy, or saliva substitutes to relieve dry mouth.
- Tell patient to avoid hazardous activities that require alertness or physical coordination until CNS depressant effects can be determined.
- Warn patient to avoid alcoholic beverages and to use cough and cold preparations cautiously, because some contain alcohol.
- Tell patient to store drug away from heat and light (not in bathroom medicine cabinet) and safely out of reach of children.
- Instruct patient to take missed dose if remembered within 1 hour. If beyond 1 hour, patient should skip that dose and return to regular schedule. Do not double dose.

Geriatric use
- Elderly patients may be more sensitive to drug's effects.

Pediatric use
- Safety and efficacy in children under age 12 have not been established.

oxacillin sodium
Bactocill, Prostaphlin

Pharmacologic classification: penicillinase-resistant penicillin
Therapeutic classification: antibiotic
Pregnancy risk category B

How supplied
Available by prescription only
Capsules: 250 mg, 500 mg
Oral solution: 250 mg/5 ml (after reconstitution)
Injection: 250 mg, 500 mg, 1 g, 2 g, 4 g
Pharmacy bulk package: 10 g
I.V. infusion: 1 g, 2 g, 4 g

Indications, route, and dosage
***Systemic infections caused by* Staphylococcus aureus**
Adults and children weighing over 88 lb (40 kg): 2 to 6 g P.O. daily, divided into doses given q 4 to 6 hours; 1 to 12 g I.M. or I.V. daily, divided into doses given q 4 to 6 hours. Doses vary based on severity of infection.
Children over age 1 month weighing below 88 lb: 50 to 100 mg/kg P.O. daily, divided into doses given q 4 to 6 hours; 50 to 200 mg/kg I.M. or I.V. daily, divided into doses given q 4 to 6 hours. Doses vary based on severity of infection.
✦ ***Dosage adjustment.*** In adults with creatinine clearance below 10 ml/minute, 1 g I.M. or I.V. q 4 to 6 hours.

Pharmacodynamics
Antibiotic action: Oxacillin is bactericidal; it adheres to bacterial penicillin-binding proteins, thus inhibiting bacterial cell wall synthesis. Oxacillin resists the effects of penicillinases—enzymes that inactivate penicillin—and is thus active against many strains of penicillinase-producing bacteria; this activity is most important against penicillinase-producing staphylococci; some strains may remain resistant. Oxacillin is also active against a few gram-

positive aerobic and anaerobic bacilli but has no significant effect on gram-negative bacilli.

Pharmacokinetics

- *Absorption:* Drug is absorbed rapidly but incompletely from the GI tract; it is stable in an acid environment. Peak serum concentrations occur within ½ to 2 hours after an oral dose and 30 minutes after an I.M. dose. Food decreases absorption.
- *Distribution:* Oxacillin is distributed widely. CSF penetration is poor but enhanced by meningeal inflammation. Oxacillin crosses the placenta; it is 89% to 94% protein-bound.
- *Metabolism:* Drug is metabolized partially.
- *Excretion:* Drug and metabolites are excreted primarily in urine by renal tubular secretion and glomerular filtration; it is also excreted in breast milk and in small amounts in bile. Elimination half-life in adults is ½ to 1 hour, extended to 2 hours in severe renal impairment. Dosage adjustments are not required in patients with creatinine clearance below 10 ml/minute.

Contraindications and precautions

Contraindicated in patients with hypersensitivity to drug or other penicillins. Use cautiously in patients with other drug allergies (especially to cephalosporins), in neonates, and in infants.

Interactions

Concomitant use of oxacillin with *aminoglycosides* produces synergistic bactericidal effects against *S. aureus.* However, the drugs are physically and chemically incompatible and are inactivated when mixed or given together. In vivo inactivation has been reported when aminoglycosides and penicillins are used concomitantly.

Probenecid blocks renal tubular secretion of penicillins, raising their serum levels.

Effects on diagnostic tests

Oxacillin alters tests for urinary and serum proteins; turbidimetric urine and serum proteins are often falsely positive or elevated in tests using sulfosalicylic acid or trichloroacetic acid.

Drug may cause transient reductions in RBC, WBC, and platelet counts. Elevations in liver function tests may indicate drug-induced hepatitis or cholestasis. Abnormal urinalysis results may indicate drug-induced interstitial nephritis.

Oxacillin may falsely decrease serum aminoglycoside concentrations.

Adverse reactions

CNS: neuropathy, neuromuscular irritability, ***seizures,*** lethargy, hallucinations, anxiety, confusion, agitation, depression, dizziness, fatigue.
GI: oral lesions, nausea, vomiting, diarrhea, enterocolitis, pseudomembranous colitis.
GU: interstitial nephritis, nephropathy.
Hematologic: ***thrombocytopenia,*** eosinophilia, ***hemolytic anemia, neutropenia,*** anemia, ***agranulocytosis.***
Other: hypersensitivity reactions (fever, chills, rash, urticaria, ***anaphylaxis,*** overgrowth of nonsusceptible organisms, elevated liver enzymes, *thrombophlebitis*).

Overdose and treatment

Clinical signs of overdose include neuromuscular sensitivity or seizures. No specific recommendations. Treatment is supportive. After recent ingestion (within 4 hours), empty the stomach by induced emesis or gastric lavage; follow with activated charcoal to reduce absorption. Oxacillin is not appreciably removed by peritoneal dialysis or hemodialysis.

☑ Special considerations

Besides those relevant to all *penicillins,* consider the following recommendations.

- Give oral drug with water only; acid in fruit juice or carbonated beverage may inactivate drug.
- Give oral dose on empty stomach; food decreases absorption.
- Except in osteomyelitis, do not give I.M. or I.V. unless patient cannot take oral dose.
- Assess renal and hepatic function; watch for elevated AST and ALT and report significant changes.

Patient education

- Explain need to take oral preparations without food and to follow with water only because of acid content of fruit juice and carbonated beverages.
- Tell patient to report allergic reactions or severe diarrhea promptly.
- Emphasize importance of completing the full course of therapy.

Geriatric use

- Half-life may be prolonged in elderly patients because of impaired renal function.

Pediatric use

- Elimination of oxacillin is reduced in neonates. Transient hematuria, azotemia, and albuminuria have occurred in some neonates receiving oxacillin; monitor renal function closely.

Breast-feeding

- Oxacillin is excreted into breast milk; drug should be used with caution in breast-feeding women.

oxaprozin

Daypro

Pharmacologic classification: NSAID
Therapeutic classification: nonnarcotic analgesic, antipyretic, anti-inflammatory
Pregnancy risk category C

How supplied

Available by prescription only
Caplets: 600 mg

Indications, route, and dosage

Management of acute or chronic osteoarthritis or rheumatoid arthritis
Adults: Initially, 1,200 mg P.O. daily. Individualize to smallest effective dosage to minimize adverse re-

actions. Smaller patients or those with mild symptoms may require only 600 mg daily. Maximum daily dosage is 1,800 mg or 26 mg/kg, whichever is lower, in divided doses.

Pharmacodynamics

Analgesic, antipyretic, and *anti-inflammatory actions:* Oxaprozin's exact mechanism of action is not clearly defined. It inhibits several steps along the arachidonic acid pathway of prostaglandin synthesis. One of the modes of action is presumed to be a result of the inhibition of cyclooxygenase activity and prostaglandin synthesis at the site of inflammation.

Pharmacokinetics

- *Absorption:* Drug demonstrates high oral bioavailability (95%) with peak plasma concentrations occurring between 3 and 5 hours after dosing. Food may reduce the rate of absorption, but extent of absorption is unchanged.
- *Distribution:* Approximately 99.9% is bound to albumin in plasma.
- *Metabolism:* Drug is primarily metabolized in the liver by microsomal oxidation (65%) and glucuronic acid conjugation (35%).
- *Excretion:* Glucuronide metabolites are excreted in urine (65%) and feces (35%).

Contraindications and precautions

Contraindicated in patients with hypersensitivity to drug or with the syndrome of nasal polyps, angioedema, and bronchospastic reaction to aspirin or other NSAIDs. Use cautiously in patients with renal or hepatic dysfunction, history of peptic ulcer, hypertension, CV disease, or conditions predisposing to fluid retention.

Interactions

Concomitant administration of oxaprozin and *aspirin* is not recommended because oxaprozin displaces salicylates from plasma protein binding, increasing the risk of salicylate toxicity.

Oral anticoagulants may increase the risk of bleeding when administered concomitantly with oxaprozin. Concomitant use with *beta blockers,* such as *metoprolol,* may cause a transient increase in blood pressure after 14 days of therapy. Therefore, routine blood pressure monitoring should be considered when starting oxaprozin therapy.

Effects on diagnostic tests

Oxaprozin can affect platelet aggregation and prolong bleeding time. It also may decrease hemoglobin levels, causing anemia, and elevate liver function studies.

Adverse reactions

CNS: depression, sedation, somnolence, confusion, sleep disturbances.
EENT: tinnitus, blurred vision.
GI: *nausea, dyspepsia, diarrhea, constipation,* abdominal pain or distress, anorexia, flatulence, vomiting, ***hemorrhage,*** stomatitis, ulcer.
GU: dysuria, urinary frequency.
Hepatic: elevated liver function test results (with chronic use), ***severe hepatic dysfunction*** (rare).
Skin: *rash,* photosensitivity.

Overdose and treatment

No information specific to oxaprozin overdose is available. Common symptoms of acute overdose with other NSAIDs (lethargy, drowsiness, nausea, vomiting, and epigastric pain) are generally reversible with supportive care. GI bleeding and coma have occurred after NSAID overdose. Hypertension, acute renal failure, and respiratory depression are rare. Gut decontamination may be indicated in symptomatic patients seen within 4 hours of ingestion or after a large overdose (5 to 10 times the usual dose). This is accomplished via emesis or activated charcoal with an osmotic cathartic.

☑ Special considerations

- Serious GI toxicity, including peptic ulceration and bleeding, can occur in patients taking NSAIDs despite the absence of GI symptoms. Patients at risk for developing peptic ulceration and bleeding are those with history of serious GI events, alcoholism, smoking, or other factors associated with peptic ulcer disease.
- Elevations of liver function tests can occur after chronic use. These abnormal findings may persist, worsen, or resolve with continued therapy. Rarely, patients may progress to severe hepatic dysfunction. Periodically monitor liver function tests in patients receiving long-term therapy, and closely monitor patients with abnormal test results.
- Anemia may occur in patients receiving oxaprozin. Obtain hemoglobin level or hematocrit in patients with prolonged therapy at intervals appropriate for their clinical situation.
- Dosages above 1,200 mg/day should be used for patients who weigh more than 110 lb (50 kg), who have normal renal and hepatic function, who are at low risk of peptic ulceration, and whose severity of disease justifies maximal therapy.
- Most patients tolerate once-daily dosing. Divided doses may be tried in patients unable to tolerate single doses.

Patient education

- Warn patient to call immediately if signs and symptoms of GI bleeding or visual or auditory adverse reactions occur.
- Tell patient to take drug with milk or meals if adverse GI reactions occur.
- Because photosensitivity reactions may occur, advise patient to use a sunblock, wear protective clothing, and avoid prolonged exposure to sunlight.

Geriatric use

- Elderly patients may need a reduced dose because of low body weight or disorders associated with aging.
- Elderly patients are less likely than younger patients to tolerate adverse reactions associated with oxaprozin.

Pediatric use
• Safety and effectiveness in children have not been established.

Breast-feeding
• Studies of oxaprozin excretion in human milk have not been conducted. Therefore, use caution when administering drug to a breast-feeding woman.

oxazepam
Apo-Oxazepam*, Novoxapam*, Ox-pam*, Serax, Zapex*

Pharmacologic classification: benzodiazepine
Therapeutic classification: antianxiety agent, sedative-hypnotic
Controlled substance schedule IV
Pregnancy risk category D

How supplied
Available by prescription only
Tablets: 15 mg
Capsules: 10 mg, 15 mg, 30 mg

Indications, route, and dosage
Alcohol withdrawal, severe anxiety
Adults: 15 to 30 mg P.O. t.i.d. or q.i.d.
Tension, mild to moderate anxiety
Adults: 10 to 15 mg P.O. t.i.d. or q.i.d.
➜ ***Dosage adjustment.*** In older adults, give 10 mg P.O. t.i.d.; then increase to 15 mg t.i.d. or q.i.d. p.r.n.

Pharmacodynamics
Anxiolytic and sedative-hypnotic action: Oxazepam depresses the CNS at the limbic and subcortical levels of the brain. It produces an antianxiety effect by enhancing the effect of the neurotransmitter gamma-aminobutyric acid on its receptor in the ascending reticular activating system, which increases inhibition and blocks both cortical and limbic arousal.

Pharmacokinetics
• *Absorption:* When administered orally, oxazepam is well absorbed through the GI tract. Peak levels occur in 3 hours after dosing. Onset of action occurs at 1 to 2 hours.
• *Distribution:* Distributed widely throughout the body. Drug is 85% to 95% protein-bound.
• *Metabolism:* Metabolized in the liver to inactive metabolites.
• *Excretion:* Metabolites of oxazepam are excreted in urine as glucuronide conjugates. Half-life of drug is 5.7 to 10.9 hours.

Contraindications and precautions
Contraindicated in patients with psychosis or hypersensitivity to drug. Use cautiously in elderly or debilitated patients; in those with history of drug abuse; and in those in whom a decrease in blood pressure is associated with cardiac problems.

Interactions
Oxazepam potentiates the CNS depressant effects of *alcohol, general anesthetics, antidepressants, antihistamines, barbiturates, MAO inhibitors, narcotics,* and *phenothiazines.*

Concomitant use with *cimetidine* and possibly *disulfiram* causes diminished hepatic metabolism of oxazepam, which increases its plasma concentration.

Heavy smoking accelerates oxazepam metabolism, thus lowering clinical effectiveness. *Antacids* may decrease the rate of oxazepam absorption. Oxazepam may inhibit the therapeutic effects of *levodopa.*

Effects on diagnostic tests
Oxazepam therapy may increase liver function test results. Changes in EEG patterns, usually low-voltage, fast activity, may occur during and after oxazepam therapy.

Adverse reactions
CNS: *drowsiness, lethargy,* dizziness, vertigo, headache, syncope, tremor, slurred speech.
CV: edema.
GI: nausea.
Hematologic: ***leukopenia*** (rare).
Hepatic: ***hepatic dysfunction.***
Skin: rash.
Other: altered libido.

Overdose and treatment
Clinical manifestations of overdose include somnolence, confusion, coma, hypoactive reflexes, dyspnea, labored breathing, hypotension, bradycardia, slurred speech, and unsteady gait or impaired coordination.

Support blood pressure and respiration until the drug effects have subsided; monitor vital signs. Mechanical ventilatory assistance via endotracheal tube may be required to maintain a patent airway and support adequate oxygenation. Flumazenil, a specific benzodiazepine antagonist, may be useful. As needed, use I.V. fluids and vasopressors, such as dopamine and phenylephrine, to treat hypotension. If the patient is conscious, induce emesis. Use gastric lavage if ingestion was recent, but only if an endotracheal tube is present to prevent aspiration. After emesis or lavage, administer activated charcoal with a cathartic as a single dose. Dialysis is of limited value.

☑ Special considerations
Besides those relevant to all *benzodiazepines,* consider the following recommendations.
• Monitor hepatic and renal function studies to ensure normal function.
• Oxazepam tablets contain tartrazine dye; check patient's history for allergy to this substance.
• Store drug in a cool, dry place away from light.
• Inform patient to reduce dosage gradually (over 8 to 12 weeks) after long-term use.

Patient education
• Advise patient not to change part of drug regimen without medical approval.
• Instruct patient in safety measures, such as gradual position changes and supervised ambulation, to prevent injury.

• Because sleepiness may not occur for up to 2 hours after taking oxazepam, tell patient to wait before taking an additional dose.
• Advise patient of potential for physical and psychological dependence with chronic use of oxazepam.
• Tell patient not to discontinue drug suddenly if he's been taking it for prolonged periods.

Geriatric use
• Elderly patients are more susceptible to the CNS depressant effects of oxazepam. Some may require supervision with ambulation and activities of daily living during initiation of therapy or after an increase in dose.
• Lower doses are usually effective in elderly patients because of decreased elimination.

Pediatric use
• Safe use in children under age 12 has not been established. Closely observe neonate for withdrawal symptoms if mother took oxazepam for a prolonged period during pregnancy.

Breast-feeding
• The breast-fed infant of a mother who uses oxazepam may become sedated, have feeding difficulties, or lose weight; avoid use in breast-feeding women.

oxiconazole nitrate
Oxistat

Pharmacologic classification: ergosterol synthesis inhibitor
Therapeutic classification: antifungal
Pregnancy risk category B

How supplied
Available by prescription only
Lotion: 1%
Topical cream: 1%

Indications, route, and dosage
Topical treatment of dermal infections caused by* Trichophyton rubrum *and* T. mentagrophytes *(tinea pedis, tinea cruris, and tinea corporis)
Adults and children: Apply to affected area once to twice daily (in the evening) for 2 weeks (1 month for tinea pedis).

Pharmacodynamics
Antifungal action: Oxiconazole inhibits ergosterol synthesis in susceptible fungal organisms, thereby weakening cytoplasmic membrane integrity.

Pharmacokinetics
• *Absorption:* Systemic absorption is low. Less than 0.3% is recovered in the urine up to 5 days after application.
• *Distribution:* Most of drug concentrates in the epidermis, with smaller amounts in the upper and deeper corneum.
• *Metabolism:* Unknown.
• *Excretion:* Urine recovery of drug has been demonstrated. It is unknown if drug is excreted in the feces.

Contraindications and precautions
Contraindicated in patients hypersensitive to drug.

Interactions
None reported.

Effects on diagnostic tests
None reported.

Adverse reactions
Skin: pruritus, burning, stinging, contact dermatitis, irritation, scaling, tingling, pain, eczema, folliculitis.

Overdose and treatment
Oral or parenteral administration to animals resulted in CNS stimulation and tissue irritation. Specific treatment recommendations are unavailable.

☑ Special considerations
• If patient shows no response after treatment for 2 weeks to 1 month, review the diagnosis.

Patient education
• Make sure patient understands that drug is for external use only.
• Instruct patient not to use drug near the eyes or vagina.
• Tell patient to complete prescribed therapy and to call if condition does not improve.

Breast-feeding
• Animal studies have shown that drug is excreted in breast milk. Use caution when prescribing drug to breast-feeding women.

oxtriphylline
Apo-Oxtriphylline*, Choledyl, Choledyl SA

Pharmacologic classification: xanthine derivative
Therapeutic classification: bronchodilator
Pregnancy risk category C

How supplied
Available by prescription only
Tablets (delayed release): 100 mg, 200 mg
Tablets (sustained release): 400 mg, 600 mg
Syrup: 50 mg/5 ml*
Elixir: 100 mg/5 ml*

Indications, route, and dosage
To relieve acute bronchial asthma and reversible bronchospasm associated with chronic bronchitis and emphysema
Adults (nonsmokers): 4.7 mg/kg P.O. q 8 hours
Adults (smokers) and children age 9 to 16: 4.7 mg/kg q 6 hours
Children age 1 to 9: 6.2 mg/kg P.O. q 6 hours.

For all patients, if total daily maintenance dosage is established at approximately 800 to 1,200 mg, one sustained-action tablet q 12 hours may be substituted.

Pharmacodynamics

Bronchodilating action: Oxtriphylline exerts its bronchodilating action after it is converted to theophylline. (Oxtriphylline is 64% anhydrous theophylline.) Theophylline antagonizes adenosine receptors in the bronchi, and may inhibit phosphodiesterase and increase levels of cyclic adenosine monophosphate, thus relaxing smooth muscle of the respiratory tract.

Pharmacokinetics

- *Absorption:* Drug is well absorbed; rate of absorption and onset of action depend on dosage form.
- *Distribution:* Distributed rapidly throughout body fluids and tissues.
- *Metabolism:* Oxtriphylline, the choline salt of theophylline, is converted to theophylline, then metabolized to inactive compounds.
- *Excretion:* Drug is excreted in the urine as theophylline (10%) and theophyllic metabolites.

Contraindications and precautions

Contraindicated in patients with hypersensitivity to xanthines (caffeine, theobromine) and in those with preexisting arrhythmias, especially tachyarrhythmias.

Use cautiously in the young, in elderly patients, and in those with impaired renal or hepatic function, peptic ulcer, COPD, cardiac failure, cor pulmonale, glaucoma, severe hypoxemia, hypertension, compromised cardiac or circulatory function, angina, acute MI, sulfite sensitivity, hyperthyroidism, or diabetes mellitus.

Interactions

When used concomitantly, oxtriphylline increases the excretion of *lithium. Allopurinol* (high dose), *cimetidine, macrolides (erythromycin, troleandomycin), propranolol,* and *quinolones* may increase serum concentration of oxtriphylline by decreasing hepatic clearance.

Aminoglutethimide, barbiturates, marijuana, and *nicotine* decrease effects of oxtriphylline by enhancing its metabolism. *Beta blockers* exert antagonistic pharmacologic effect.

Effects on diagnostic tests

Oxtriphylline may falsely elevate serum uric acid levels measured by colorimetric methods. Theophylline levels may be falsely elevated in patients using furosemide, phenylbutazone, probenecid, some cephalosporins, sulfa medications, theobromine, caffeine, tea, chocolate, cola beverages, and acetaminophen, depending on assay method used.

Adverse reactions

CNS: *restlessness, dizziness,* headache, *insomnia,* irritability, ***seizures,*** muscle twitching.
CV: *palpitations, sinus tachycardia,* extrasystoles, flushing, marked hypotension, ***arrhythmias.***
GI: *nausea, vomiting,* epigastric pain, diarrhea.
Respiratory: tachypnea, ***respiratory arrest.***
Skin: rash, flushing.

Overdose and treatment

Clinical manifestations of overdose include nausea, vomiting, insomnia, irritability, tachycardia, extrasystoles, tachypnea, or tonic-clonic seizures. The onset of toxicity may be sudden and severe, with arrhythmias and seizures as the first signs. Induce emesis except in convulsing patients; follow with activated charcoal and cathartics. Treat arrhythmias with lidocaine and seizures with I.V. benzodiazepine; support CV and respiratory systems.

☑ Special considerations

- Do not crush sustained-release tablets.
- Monitor vital signs and intake and output. Observe for CNS stimulation and CV adverse reactions.
- Store drug at 59° to 86° F (15° to 30° C) away from heat and light.

Patient education

- Instruct patient about drug and dosage schedule; if a dose is missed, he should take it as soon as possible. However, he should never double-dose.
- Advise patient of adverse effects and possible signs of toxicity, and to report signs of excessive CNS stimulation (nervousness, tremors, akathisia).
- Warn patient to avoid consuming large quantities of xanthine-containing foods and beverages.

Geriatric use

- Decrease dose and monitor closely.

Pediatric use

- Use with caution in neonates.

Breast-feeding

- Drug is excreted in breast milk and may cause irritability, insomnia, or fretfulness in the breast-fed infant.

oxybutynin chloride

Ditropan

Pharmacologic classification: synthetic tertiary amine
Therapeutic classification: antispasmodic
Pregnancy risk category B

How supplied

Available by prescription only
Tablets: 5 mg
Syrup 5 mg/5 ml

Indications, route, and dosage

For the relief of symptoms of bladder instability associated with voiding in patients with uninhibited and reflex neurogenic bladder
Adults: 5 mg P.O. b.i.d. to t.i.d. to maximum of 5 mg q.i.d.
Children over age 5: 5 mg P.O. b.i.d. to maximum of 5 mg t.i.d.

Pharmacodynamics

Antispasmodic action: Oxybutynin reduces the urge to void, increases bladder capacity, and reduces the frequency of contractions to the detrusor muscle. Drug exerts a direct spasmolytic action and an antimuscarinic action on smooth muscle.

Pharmacokinetics

- *Absorption:* Drug is absorbed rapidly, with peak levels occurring in 3 to 6 hours. Action begins in 30 to 60 minutes and persists for 6 to 10 hours.
- *Distribution:* No information available.
- *Metabolism:* Drug is metabolized by the liver.
- *Excretion:* Drug is excreted principally in urine.

Contraindications and precautions

Contraindicated in patients with hypersensitivity to drug, myasthenia gravis, GI obstruction, glaucoma, adynamic ileus, megacolon, severe colitis, ulcerative colitis when megacolon is present, or obstructive uropathy; in elderly or debilitated patients with intestinal atony; and in hemorrhaging patients with unstable CV status.

Use cautiously in the elderly and in patients with impaired renal or hepatic function, autonomic neuropathy, or reflux esophagitis.

Interactions

Concomitant use with *digoxin* may increase digoxin levels. Worsening of schizophrenia, decreased serum concentrations of *haloperidol,* and development of tardive dyskinesia may occur when oxybutynin is given with haloperidol. Increased incidence of anticholinergic adverse effects with *phenothiazine* may occur. There is a possibility of an additive sedative effect with other *CNS depressants.*

Effects on diagnostic tests

None reported.

Adverse reactions

CNS: dizziness, insomnia, restlessness, hallucinations, asthenia.
CV: *palpitations, tachycardia,* vasodilation.
EENT: mydriasis, cycloplegia, decreased lacrimation, amblyopia.
GI: nausea, vomiting, *constipation, dry mouth,* decreased GI motility.
GU: *urinary hesitancy, urine retention.*
Skin: rash.
Other: decreased diaphoresis, fever, suppressed lactation.

Overdose and treatment

Clinical manifestations of overdose include restlessness, excitement, psychotic behavior, flushing, hypotension, circulatory failure, and fever. In severe cases, paralysis, respiratory failure, and coma may occur. Treatment requires gastric lavage. Activated charcoal may be administered as well as a cathartic. Physostigmine may be considered to reverse symptoms of anticholinergic intoxication. Treat hyperpyrexia symptomatically with ice bags or other cold applications and alcohol sponges. Maintain artificial respiration if paralysis of respiratory muscles occurs.

A slow I.V. infusion of 2% thiopental sodium or a 2% solution of chloral hydrate (100 to 200 ml) rectally may be needed to control extreme excitement.

☑ Special considerations

- Discontinue drug periodically to determine if patient still requires medication.

Patient education

- Instruct patient regarding medication and dosage schedule; tell him to take a missed dose as soon as possible and not to double up on doses.
- Warn patient about possibility of decreased mental alertness or visual changes.
- Remind patient to use drug cautiously when in warm climates to minimize risk of heatstroke that may occur because of decreased sweating.

Geriatric use

- Elderly patients may be more sensitive to the antimuscarinic effects. Drug is contraindicated in elderly and debilitated patients with intestinal atony.

Pediatric use

- Dosage guidelines have not been established for children under age 5.

Breast-feeding

- It is not known if drug is excreted in breast milk. Exercise caution when administering to a breast-feeding woman.

oxycodone hydrochloride

OxyContin, Roxicodone, Supeudol*

Pharmacologic classification: opioid
Therapeutic classification: analgesic
Controlled substance schedule II
Pregnancy risk category C

How supplied

Available by prescription only
Tablets: 5 mg
Tablets (sustained-release): 10 mg, 20 mg, 40 mg
Oral solution: 5 mg/ml
Suppositories: 10 mg, 20 mg

Indications, route, and dosage

Moderate to severe pain
Adults: 5 mg P.O. q 6 hours; alternatively, 10 to 40 mg P.R. p.r.n., t.i.d. or q.i.d.
Chronic pain
Adults: Initially, 10 mg sustained-release tablet q 12 hours; may increase dose q 1 to 2 days. Dosing frequency should not be increased.

Pharmacodynamics

Analgesic action: Oxycodone acts on opiate receptors providing analgesia for moderate to moderately severe pain. Episodes of acute pain, rather than chronic pain, appear to be more responsive to treatment with oxycodone.

Pharmacokinetics
• *Absorption:* After oral administration, onset of analgesic effect occurs within 15 to 30 minutes and peak effect is reached within 1 hour.
• *Distribution:* Rapid.
• *Metabolism:* Drug is metabolized in the liver.
• *Excretion:* Oxycodone is excreted principally by the kidneys. Duration of analgesia is 6 hours and for sustained-release tablets is 12 hours.

Contraindications and precautions
Contraindicated in patients with hypersensitivity to drug. Use cautiously in elderly or debilitated patients and in those with head injury, increased intracranial pressure, seizures, asthma, COPD, prostatic hyperplasia, severe hepatic or renal disease, acute abdominal conditions, urethral stricture, hypothyroidism, Addison's disease, or arrhythmias.

Interactions
Concomitant with other *CNS depressants (alcohol, general anesthetics, antihistamines, barbiturates, benzodiazepines, muscle relaxants, narcotic analgesics, phenothiazines, sedative-hypnotics, tricyclic antidepressants),* potentiates drug's respiratory and CNS depression, sedation, and hypotensive effects. Concomitant use with *cimetidine* may also increase respiratory and CNS depression, causing confusion, disorientation, apnea, or seizures.

Drug accumulation and enhanced effects may result from concomitant use with other drugs that are extensively metabolized in the liver *(digitoxin, phenytoin, rifampin);* combined use with *anticholinergics* may cause paralytic ileus.

Patients who become physically dependent on this drug may experience acute withdrawal syndrome if given high doses of an *opioid agonist-antagonist* or a *single dose of an antagonist.*

Severe CV depression may result from concomitant use with *general anesthetics.*

Oxycodone products containing *aspirin* may increase anticoagulant's effect. Monitor clotting times, and use together cautiously.

Effects on diagnostic tests
Oxycodone increases plasma amylase and lipase and liver enzyme levels.

Adverse reactions
CNS: *sedation, somnolence, clouded sensorium, euphoria, dizziness, light-headedness,* ***seizures.***
CV: *hypotension,* bradycardia.
GI: *nausea, vomiting, constipation,* ileus.
GU: *urine retention.*
Respiratory: ***respiratory depression.***
Skin: *diaphoresis,* pruritus, rash.
Other: physical dependence.

Overdose and treatment
The most common signs and symptoms of a severe overdose are CNS depression, respiratory depression, and miosis (pinpoint pupils). Other acute toxic effects include hypotension, bradycardia, hypothermia, shock, apnea, cardiopulmonary arrest, circulatory collapse, pulmonary edema, and convulsions.

To treat acute overdose, first establish adequate respiratory exchange via a patent airway and ventilation as needed; administer a narcotic antagonist (naloxone) to reverse respiratory depression. (Because the duration of action of oxycodone is longer than that of naloxone, repeated naloxone dosing is necessary.) Naloxone should not be given unless patient has clinically significant respiratory or CV depression. Monitor vital signs closely.

If patient presents within 2 hours of ingestion of an oral overdose, empty the stomach immediately by inducing emesis (ipecac syrup) or using gastric lavage. Use caution to avoid any risk of aspiration. Administer activated charcoal via nasogastric tube for further removal of the drug in an oral overdose.

Provide symptomatic and supportive treatment (continued respiratory support, correction of fluid or electrolyte imbalance). Monitor laboratory parameters, vital signs, and neurologic status closely.

Dialysis may be helpful if combination products with aspirin or acetaminophen are involved.

☑ Special considerations
Besides those relevant to all *opioids,* consider the following recommendations.
• Single-agent oxycodone solution or tablets is ideal for patients who cannot take aspirin or acetaminophen.
• Oxycodone has high abuse potential.
• Drug may obscure signs and symptoms of an acute abdominal condition or worsen gallbladder pain.
• Consider prescribing a stool softener for patients on long-term therapy.

Patient education
• For full analgesic effect, teach patient to take drug before he has intense pain.
• Warn patient about possibility of decreased alertness or visual changes.

Geriatric use
• Lower doses are usually indicated for elderly patients, who may be more sensitive to the therapeutic and adverse effects of the drug.

Pediatric use
• Dosage may be individualized for children; however, safety and effectiveness in children have not been established.

Breast-feeding
• It is unknown if drug is excreted in breast milk; use with caution in breast-feeding women.

oxymetazoline hydrochloride

Afrin, Allerest 12-Hour Nasal Spray, Dristan Long Lasting, Duramist Plus, Duration, 4-Way Long Lasting Spray, Neo-Synephrine 12 Hour Nasal Spray, Nostrilla Long Acting Nasal Decongestant, NTZ Long Acting Decongestant Nasal Spray, OcuClear, Sinarest 12 Hour Nasal Spray, Visine L.R.

Pharmacologic classification: sympathomimetic
Therapeutic classification: decongestant, vasoconstrictor
Pregnancy risk category C

How supplied

Available without a prescription
Nasal solution: 0.025% (drops) for children
Nasal drops or spray: 0.05%
Ophthalmic solution: 0.025%

Indications, route, and dosage

Nasal congestion
Adults and children over age 6: Apply 2 to 3 drops or sprays of 0.05% solution in each nostril b.i.d.; should not be used for more than 3 to 5 days.
Children age 2 to 6: Apply 2 to 3 drops of 0.025% solution to nasal mucosa b.i.d. Use no more than 3 to 5 days. Dosage for younger children has not been established.
Relief of minor eye redness
Adults and children over age 6: Apply 1 to 2 drops in the conjunctival sac b.i.d. to q.i.d. (space at least 6 hours apart).

Pharmacodynamics

Decongestant action: Produces local vasoconstriction of arterioles through alpha receptors to reduce blood flow and nasal congestion.

Pharmacokinetics

- *Absorption:* Following intranasal application, local vasoconstriction occurs within 5 to 10 minutes and persists for 5 to 6 hours with a gradual decline over the next 6 hours.
- *Distribution:* Unknown.
- *Metabolism:* Unknown.
- *Excretion:* Unknown.

Contraindications and precautions

Contraindicated in patients with hypersensitivity to drug. Ophthalmic form contraindicated in patients with angle-closure glaucoma.

Use cautiously in patients with hyperthyroidism, cardiac disease, or hypertension and in those receiving MAO inhibitors. Use nasal solution cautiously in patients with diabetes mellitus. Ophthalmic form should be used cautiously in those with eye disease, infection, or injury.

Interactions

Oxymetazoline hydrochloride may potentiate the pressor effects of *tricyclic antidepressants* from significant systemic absorption of the decongestant. In ophthalmic form, *local anesthetics* can increase absorption and *beta blockers* can increase systemic adverse effects.

Effects on diagnostic tests

None reported.

Adverse reactions

CNS: headache, insomnia; drowsiness, dizziness, possible sedation (with nasal form); light-headedness, nervousness (with ophthalmic form).
CV: palpations; ***CV collapse,*** hypertension (with nasal form); tachycardia, irregular heartbeat (with ophthalmic form).
EENT: rebound nasal congestion or irritation with excessive or long-term use, dryness of nose and throat, increased nasal discharge, stinging, sneezing (with nasal form); *transient stinging upon instillation,* blurred vision, reactive hyperemia, keratitis, lacrimation, increased intraocular pressure (with ophthalmic form).
Other: systemic effects in children (with excessive or long-term use, with nasal form); trembling (with ophthalmic form).

Overdose and treatment

Clinical manifestations of overdose include somnolence, sedation, sweating, CNS depression with hypertension, bradycardia, decreased cardiac output, rebound hypertension, CV collapse, depressed respirations, coma.

If ingested, emesis is not recommended, unless given early, because of rapid onset of sedation. Activated charcoal or gastric lavage may be used initially. Monitor vital signs and ECG. Treat seizures with I.V. diazepam.

☑ Special considerations

- Monitor carefully for adverse reactions in patients with CV disease, diabetes mellitus, or prostatic hypertrophy because systemic absorption can occur.

Patient education

- Emphasize that only one person should use dropper bottle or nasal spray.
- Advise patient not to exceed recommended dosage and to use drug only when needed.
- Tell patient to discontinue drug and call if symptoms persist after 3 days of self-medication.
- Tell patient nasal mucosa may sting, burn, or become dry.
- Warn patient that excessive use may cause bradycardia, hypotension, dizziness, and weakness.
- Show patient how to apply: have him bend head forward and sniff spray briskly or apply light pressure on lacrimal sac after instillation of eyedrop.

Geriatric use

- Use drug with caution in elderly patients with cardiac disease, poorly controlled hypertension, or diabetes mellitus.

Pediatric use

- Children may exhibit increased adverse effects from systemic absorption; 0.05% nasal solution is contraindicated in children under age 6; 0.025% nasal solution should be used in children under age 2 only under medical direction and supervision.

oxymorphone hydrochloride

Numorphan

Pharmacologic classification: opioid
Therapeutic classification: analgesic
Controlled substance schedule II
Pregnancy risk category C

How supplied

Available by prescription only
Injection: 1 mg/ml, 1.5 mg/ml
Suppository: 5 mg

Indications, route, and dosage

Moderate to severe pain

Adults: 1 to 1.5 mg I.M. or S.C. q 4 to 6 hours, p.r.n., or around the clock; 0.5 mg I.V. q 4 to 6 hours, p.r.n. or around the clock; or 1 suppository administered P.R. q 4 to 6 hours, p.r.n., or around the clock.

Note: Parenteral administration of drug is also indicated for preoperative medication, for support of anesthesia, for obstetric analgesia, and for relief of anxiety in dyspnea associated with acute left-sided heart failure and pulmonary edema.

Pharmacodynamics

Analgesic action: Oxymorphone effectively relieves moderate to severe pain via agonist activity at the opiate receptors. It has little or no antitussive effect.

Pharmacokinetics

- *Absorption:* Oxymorphone is well absorbed after P.R., S.C., I.M., or I.V. administration. Onset of action occurs within 5 to 10 minutes. Peak analgesic effect is seen at ½ to 1 hour.
- *Distribution:* Drug is widely distributed.
- *Metabolism:* Primarily metabolized in the liver.
- *Excretion:* Duration of action is 3 to 6 hours. Drug is excreted primarily in the urine as oxymorphone hydrochloride.

Contraindications and precautions

Contraindicated in patients with hypersensitivity to drug. Use cautiously in elderly or debilitated patients and in those with head injury, increased intracranial pressure, seizures, asthma, COPD, acute abdomen conditions, prostatic hyperplasia, severe renal or kidney disease, urethral stricture, respiratory depression, Addison's disease, arrhythmias, or hypothyroidism.

Interactions

Concomitant use with other *CNS depressants (alcohol, general anesthetics, antihistamines, barbiturates, benzodiazepines, muscle relaxants, opiates, phenothiazines, sedative-hypnotics, tricyclic antidepressants)* potentiates drug's respiratory and CNS depression, sedation, and hypotensive effects.

Concomitant use with *cimetidine* may also increase respiratory and CNS depression, causing confusion, disorientation, apnea, or seizures. Reduced dosage of oxymorphone is usually necessary.

Drug accumulation and enhanced effects may result from concomitant use with other drugs that are extensively metabolized in the liver *(digitoxin, phenytoin, rifampin);* combined use with *anticholinergics* may cause paralytic ileus.

Patients who become physically dependent on drug may experience acute withdrawal syndrome if given a *narcotic antagonist.*

Severe CV depression may result from concomitant use with *general anesthetics.*

Effects on diagnostic tests

Oxymorphone increases plasma amylase levels.

Adverse reactions

CNS: *sedation, somnolence, clouded sensorium, euphoria,* dizziness, ***seizures*** (with large doses), light-headedness, headache.
CV: *hypotension,* bradycardia.
GI: *nausea, vomiting, constipation,* ileus.
GU: *urine retention.*
Respiratory: ***respiratory depression.***
Skin: pruritus.
Other: physical dependence.

Overdose and treatment

The most common signs and symptoms of oxymorphone overdose are CNS depression (extreme somnolence progressing to stupor and coma), respiratory depression, and miosis (pinpoint pupils). Other acute toxic effects include hypotension, bradycardia, hypothermia, shock, apnea, cardiopulmonary arrest, circulatory collapse, pulmonary edema, and seizures.

To treat acute overdose, first establish adequate respiratory exchange via a patent airway and ventilation as needed; administer a narcotic antagonist (naloxone) to reverse respiratory depression. (Because drug's duration of action is longer than that of naloxone, repeated naloxone dosing is necessary.) Naloxone should not be given unless the patient has clinically significant respiratory or CV depression. Monitor vital signs closely.

Provide symptomatic and supportive treatment (continued respiratory support, correction of fluid or electrolyte imbalance). Monitor laboratory parameters, vital signs, and neurologic status closely.

☑ Special considerations

Besides those relevant to all *opioids,* consider the following recommendations.

- Refrigerate oxymorphone suppositories.
- Drug is well absorbed P.R. and is an alternative to opioids with more limited dosage forms.
- Drug may worsen gallbladder pain.

Geriatric use

- Lower doses are usually indicated for elderly patients, who may be more sensitive to the therapeutic and adverse effects of the drug.

Pediatric use
• Do not use in children under age 12.

Breast-feeding
• It is not known if drug is excreted in breast milk; use with caution in breast-feeding women.

oxytocin
Pitocin, Syntocinon

Pharmacologic classification: exogenous hormone
Therapeutic classification: oxytocic, lactation stimulant
Pregnancy risk category C

How supplied
Available by prescription only
Injection: 10-units/ml ampules, vials, and Tubex
Nasal solution: 40 units/ml

Indications, route, and dosage
Induction of labor
Adults: Initially, no more than 1 to 2 milliunits/minute I.V. infusion. Rate of infusion may be increased slowly. Decrease rate when labor is firmly established.
Augmentation of labor
Adults: Initially, 2 milliunits/minute I.V. infusion. Rate of infusion may be increased slowly to maximum of 20 milliunits/minute.
Reduction of postpartum bleeding after expulsion of placenta
Adults: 10 to 40 milliunits/minute I.V. infusion (or 10 units I.M.) after delivery of the placenta.
To induce abortion
Adults: 10 units mixed in 500 ml D_5W or 0.9% NaCl solution I.V. at 10 to 20 milliunits (20 to 40 drops)/minute.
To promote initial milk ejection
Adults: One spray or one drop nasal solution into one or both nostrils 2 or 3 minutes before breast-feeding or pumping breasts.
◇ ***Oxytocin challenge test to assess fetal distress in high-risk pregnancies greater than 31 weeks' gestation***
Adults: Prepare solution by adding 5 to 10 units oxytocin to 1 L of 5% dextrose injection (yielding a solution of 5 to 10 milliunits per ml). Infuse 0.5 milliunits/minute, gradually increasing at 15-minute intervals to maximum infusion of 20 milliunits/minute. Discontinue infusion when three moderate uterine contractions occur in a 10-minute interval.

Pharmacodynamics
Oxytocic action: Oxytocin increases the sodium permeability of uterine myofibrils, indirectly stimulating the contraction of uterine smooth muscle. The threshold for response is lowered in the presence of high estrogen concentrations. Uterine response increases with the length of the pregnancy and increases further during active labor. Response mimics labor contractions.

Lactation stimulation: By contracting the myoepithelial cells surrounding the alveoli of the breasts, oxytocin forces milk from the alveoli into the larger ducts and facilitates milk ejection.

Pharmacokinetics
• *Absorption:* Onset is immediate following I.V. injection and occurs within 3 to 5 minutes of an I.M. injection. Absorption through nasal mucosa is rapid but may be erratic; it acts within a few minutes. Oxytocin is destroyed in the GI tract.
• *Distribution:* Drug is distributed throughout the extracellular fluid; small amounts may enter the fetal circulation.
• *Metabolism:* Oxytocin is metabolized rapidly in the kidneys and liver. In early pregnancy, a circulating enzyme, oxytocinase, can inactivate the drug.
• *Excretion:* Only small amounts are excreted in the urine as oxytocin. Half-life is 3 to 5 minutes and duration of action is 1 hour following I.V. infusion; 2 to 3 hours I.M.; and 20 minutes intranasal.

Contraindications and precautions
Systemic form contraindicated when cephalopelvic disproportion is present or when delivery requires conversion, as in transverse lie; in fetal distress when delivery isn't imminent, prematurity, and other obstetric emergencies; and in patients with severe toxemia, hypertonic uterine patterns, hypersensitivity to drug, total placenta previa, and vasoprevia. Nasal form contraindicated in patients with hypersensitivity to drug and during pregnancy.

Use systemic form cautiously during first and second stages of labor and in patients with history of cervical or uterine surgery (including cesarean section), grand multiparity, uterine sepsis, traumatic delivery, overdistended uterus, and invasive cervical cancer.

Interactions
Cyclopropane anesthesia may modify oxytocin's CV effects. It may also delay the induction of *thiopental anesthesia.*

Concomitant use of *sympathomimetics* may increase pressor effects, possibly resulting in postpartum hypertension.

Effects on diagnostic tests
None reported.

Adverse reactions
Maternal:
CNS: ***subarachnoid hemorrhage*** (from hypertension), ***seizures or coma*** (from water intoxication) (with systemic administration).
CV: *hypertension,* increased heart rate, systemic venous return, and cardiac output, ***arrhythmias*** (with systemic administration).
EENT: nasal irritation, rhinorrhea, lacrimation (with nasal form).
GI: nausea, vomiting (with systemic administration).
Hematologic: ***afibrinogenemia*** (with systemic administration; may be related to postpartum bleeding).
Other: hypersensitivity reactions ***(anaphylaxis),*** tetanic uterine contractions, ***abruptio placentae, impaired uterine blood flow, water retention,***

pelvic hematoma, ***increased uterine motility, uterine rupture, postpartum hemorrhage*** (with systemic administration); uterine bleeding, uterine contractions (with nasal form).
Fetal:
CV: bradycardia, ***premature ventricular contractions, arrhythmias*** (with systemic administration).
Respiratory: ***anoxia, asphyxia*** (with systemic administration).
Other: ***infant brain damage, death, jaundice, low Apgar scores,*** retinal hemorrhage (with systemic administration).

Overdose and treatment

Clinical manifestations of overdose include hyperstimulation of the uterus, causing tetanic contractions and possible uterine rupture, cervical laceration, abruptio placentae, impaired uterine blood flow, amniotic fluid embolism, and fetal trauma. Drug has a very short half-life; therefore, therapy should be halted and supportive care initiated.

☑ Special considerations

- Administer by I.V. infusion, not I.V. bolus injection.
- Never give oxytocin by more than one route simultaneously.
- Monitor and record uterine contractions, heart rate, blood pressure, intrauterine pressure, fetal heart rate, and character of blood loss every 15 minutes.
- When administering oxytocin challenge test, monitor fetal heart rate and uterine contractions immediately before and during infusion. If fetal heart rate does not change during test, repeat in 1 week. If late deceleration in fetal heart rate is noted, consider terminating pregnancy.
- Drug may produce an antidiuretic effect; monitor fluid intake and output.
- During long infusions, watch for signs of water intoxication.
- Have magnesium sulfate (20% solution) available for relaxation of the myometrium.
- Drug is not recommended for routine I.M. use. However, 10 units may be administered I.M. after delivery of the placenta to control postpartum uterine bleeding.
- Solution containing 10 milliunits/ml may be prepared by adding 10 units of oxytocin to 1 L of 0.9% NaCl solution or D_5W. Solution containing 20 milliunits/ml may be prepared by adding 10 units of oxytocin to 500 ml of 0.9% NaCl solution or D_5W.

Patient education

- Explain possible adverse effects of drug.
- For patient using nasal route, instruct patient to clear nasal passages before using drug. With head in vertical position, tell him to hold squeeze bottle upright and eject solution into nostril. If preferred, the solution can be instilled in drop form by inverting the squeeze bottle and exerting gentle pressure.

Breast-feeding

- Minimal amounts of drug enter breast milk. Risks must be evaluated.

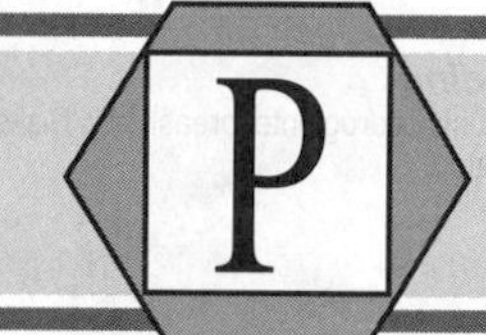

paclitaxel

Taxol

Pharmacologic classification: novel antimicrotubule
Therapeutic classification: antineoplastic
Pregnancy risk category D

How supplied

Available by prescription only
Injection: 30 mg/5 ml

Indications, route, and dosage

Metastatic ovarian cancer after failure of first-line or subsequent chemotherapy
Adults: 135 or 175 mg/m^2 I.V. over 3 hours q 3 weeks. Subsequent courses should not be repeated until neutrophil count is at least 1,500 cells/mm^3 and platelet count is at least 100,000 cells/mm^3.
Breast carcinoma after failure of combination chemotherapy for metastatic disease or relapse within 6 months of adjuvant chemotherapy (prior therapy should have included an anthracycline unless clinically contraindicated)
Adults: 175 mg/m^2 I.V. over 3 hours q 3 weeks.

Pharmacodynamics

Antineoplastic action: Paclitaxel prevents depolymerization of cellular microtubules, thus inhibiting the normal reorganization of the microtubule network necessary for mitosis and other vital cellular functions.

Pharmacokinetics

- *Absorption:* Unknown.
- *Distribution:* Approximately 89% to 98% of paclitaxel is bound to serum proteins.
- *Metabolism:* May be metabolized in the liver.
- *Excretion:* Excretion in humans is not fully understood.

Contraindications and precautions

Contraindicated in patients with hypersensitivity to drug or polyoxyethylated castor oil, a vehicle used in drug solution, and in those with baseline neutrophil counts below 1,500/mm^3. Use cautiously in patients who have received radiation therapy.

Interactions

Myelosuppression may be greater when *cisplatin* is administered before rather than after paclitaxel. *Ketoconazole* may inhibit paclitaxel metabolism. Use these two drugs together cautiously.

Effects on diagnostic tests

Paclitaxel alters hematologic studies because of its suppressive effect on bone marrow.

Adverse reactions

CNS: *peripheral neuropathy.*
CV: *bradycardia, hypotension, abnormal ECG.*
GI: *nausea, vomiting, diarrhea, mucositis.*
Hematologic: NEUTROPENIA, LEUKOPENIA, THROMBOCYTOPENIA, anemia, *bleeding.*
Hepatic: *elevated liver enzyme levels.*
Other: *hypersensitivity reactions* ***(anaphylaxis),*** *alopecia, myalgia, arthralgia, phlebitis, cellulitis at injection site, infections.*

Overdose and treatment

Primary complications of overdosage would probably include bone marrow suppression, peripheral neurotoxicity, and mucositis. No specific antidote for paclitaxel overdosage is known.

☑ Special considerations

- Severe hypersensitivity reactions characterized by dyspnea, hypotension, angioedema, and generalized urticaria have occurred in 2% of patients receiving paclitaxel. To reduce the incidence or severity of these reactions, pretreat patients with corticosteroids (such as dexamethasone), antihistamines (such as diphenhydramine), and H_2-receptor antagonists (such as cimetidine or ranitidine).
- Do not rechallenge patients who experience severe hypersensitivity reactions to paclitaxel.
- In patients who experience severe neutropenia (neutrophil count below 500 cells/mm^3 for 1 week or longer) or severe peripheral neuropathy during drug therapy, reduce dosage by 20% for subsequent courses. Incidence and severity of neurotoxicity and hematologic toxicity increase with dose, especially above 190 mg/m^2.
- Bone marrow toxicity is the most frequent and dose-limiting toxicity. Frequent blood count monitoring is necessary during therapy. Packed RBC or platelet transfusions may be necessary in severe cases. Institute bleeding precautions as appropriate.
- If patient develops significant conduction abnormalities during drug administration, administer appropriate therapy and monitor cardiac function continuously during subsequent drug therapy.
- Use caution during preparation and administration of paclitaxel. Use of gloves is recommended. If solution contacts skin, wash skin immediately and thoroughly with soap and water. If drug contacts mucous membranes, flush membranes thoroughly with water. Mark all waste materials with CHEMOTHERAPY HAZARD labels.
- Concentrate must be diluted before infusion. Compatible solutions include 0.9% NaCl injection, D_5W,

dextrose 5% in 0.9% NaCl injection, and 5% dextrose in lactated Ringer's injection. Dilute to a final concentration of 0.3 to 1.2 mg/ml. Diluted solutions are stable for 27 hours at room temperature.

- Prepare and store infusion solutions in glass containers. Undiluted concentrate should not contact polyvinyl chloride I.V. bags or tubing. Store diluted solution in glass or polypropylene bottles, or use polypropylene or polyolefin bags. Administer through polyethylene-lined administration sets, and use an in-line filter with a microporous membrane not exceeding 0.22 microns.
- Continuously monitor patient for 30 minutes after initiating the infusion. Continue close monitoring throughout infusion.

Patient education

- Advise female patient of childbearing age to avoid becoming pregnant during therapy with paclitaxel because of potential harm to the fetus.
- Warn patient that alopecia occurs in almost all patients.
- Teach patient to recognize and immediately report signs and symptoms of peripheral neuropathy, such as tingling, burning, or numbness in the extremities. Although mild symptoms are common, severe symptoms occur infrequently. Dosage reduction may be necessary.

Pediatric use

- Safety and effectiveness in children have not been established.

Breast-feeding

- Because of potential for serious adverse reactions in breast-fed infants, breast-feeding should be discontinued during paclitaxel therapy.

pamidronate disodium

Aredia

Pharmacologic classification: bisphosphonate; pyrophosphate analogue
Therapeutic classification: antihypercalcemic
Pregnancy risk category C

How supplied

Available by prescription only
Injection: 30 mg/vial, 60 mg/vial, 90 mg/vial

Indications, route, and dosage

Moderate to severe hypercalcemia associated with malignancy (with or without metastases)
Adults: Dosage depends on severity of hypercalcemia. Serum calcium levels should be corrected for serum albumin. Corrected serum calcium (CCa) is calculated using the following formula:

$$\frac{\text{CCa}}{(\text{mg/dl})} = \frac{\text{serum Ca}}{(\text{mg/dl})} + \frac{0.8\ (4 - \text{serum albumin})}{(\text{g/dl})}$$

✦ ***Dosage adjustment.*** Patients with moderate hypercalcemia (CCa levels of 12 to 13.5 mg/dl) may receive 60 to 90 mg by I.V. infusion over 24 hours. Patients with severe hypercalcemia (CCa levels over 13.5 mg/dl) may receive 90 mg as the initial dose.

Paget's disease
Adults: 30 mg I.V. daily over 4 hours for 3 consecutive days for total dose of 90 mg.

Osteolytic bone lesions of multiple myeloma
Adults: 90 mg I.V. daily over 4 hours once monthly.

Pharmacodynamics

Antihypercalcemic action: Pamidronate inhibits the resorption of bone. Drug adsorbs to hydroxyapatite crystals in bone and may directly block the dissolution of calcium phosphate. Drug apparently does not inhibit bone formation or mineralization.

Pharmacokinetics

- *Absorption:* Rapid onset of action; duration of action up to 3 months in bone.
- *Distribution:* After I.V. administration in animals, about 50% to 60% of a dose is rapidly absorbed by bone; drug is also taken up by the kidneys, liver, spleen, teeth, and tracheal cartilage.
- *Metabolism:* None.
- *Excretion:* Drug is excreted by the kidneys; an average of 51% of a dose is excreted in urine within 72 hours of administration.

Contraindications and precautions

Contraindicated in patients hypersensitive to drug or other bisphosphonates, such as etidronate. Use with extreme caution in patients with impaired renal function.

Interactions

Pamidronate may form a precipitate when mixed with solutions that contain *calcium.*

Effects on diagnostic tests

Pamidronate therapy may alter serum electrolyte levels, including serum calcium, potassium, magnesium, and phosphate.

Adverse reactions

CNS: seizures, fatigue, headache, somnolence.
CV: atrial fibrillation, syncope, tachycardia, *hypertension.*
GI: *abdominal pain, anorexia, constipation, nausea, vomiting,* GI hemorrhage.
Hematologic: *leukopenia,* ***thrombocytopenia,*** *anemia.*
Musculoskeletal: *bone pain.*
Other: *hypophosphatemia, hypokalemia, hypomagnesemia, hypocalcemia, fever, infusion-site reaction, generalized pain.*

Overdose and treatment

Symptomatic hypocalcemia could result from overdosage; treat with I.V. calcium. In one reported case, a 209-lb (95-kg) woman who received 285 mg daily for 3 days experienced hyperpyrexia (103° F [39.4° C]), hypotension, and transient taste perversion. Fever and hypotension were rapidly corrected with steroids.

☑ Special considerations

- Because drug can cause electrolyte disturbances, careful monitoring of serum electrolytes (especially calcium, phosphate, and magnesium) is essential. Short-term administration of calcium may be necessary in patients with severe hypocalcemia. Also monitor creatinine, CBC, differential, hematocrit, and hemoglobin levels.
- Carefully monitor patients with preexisting anemia, leukopenia, or thrombocytopenia during first 2 weeks after therapy.
- Monitor patient's temperature. In trials, 27% of patients experienced a slightly elevated temperature for 24 to 48 hours after therapy.
- Reconstitute vial with 10 ml sterile water for injection. Once drug is completely dissolved, add to 1,000 ml 0.45% or 0.9% NaCl injection or D_5W. Do not mix with infusion solutions that contain calcium, such as Ringer's injection or lactated Ringer's injection. Administer in a single I.V. solution, in a separate line from all other drugs. Visually inspect for precipitate before administering.
- Injection solution is stable for 24 hours when refrigerated. Give only by I.V. infusion. Animal studies have shown evidence of nephropathy when drug is given as a bolus.
- Consider retreatment if hypercalcemia recurs; allow a minimum of 7 days to elapse before retreatment to allow for full response to the initial dose.

Pediatric use

- Safety and efficacy in children have not been established.

Breast-feeding

- It is unknown if drug is excreted in breast milk. Use with caution in breast-feeding women.

pancreatin

Dizymes, Donnazyme, Entozyme, Hi-Vegi-Lip, 4X Pancreatin, 8X Pancreatin, Pancrezyme 4X

Pharmacologic classification: pancreatic enzyme
Therapeutic classification: digestant
Pregnancy risk category C

How supplied

Available without a prescription
Dizymes
Tablets (enteric-coated): 250 mg pancreatin; 6,750 units lipase; 41,250 units protease; 43,750 units amylase
Hi-Vegi-Lip
Tablets (enteric-coated): 2,400 mg pancreatin; 4,800 units lipase; 60,000 units protease; 60,000 units amylase
4X Pancreatin, Pancrezyme 4X
Tablets (enteric-coated): 2,400 mg pancreatin; 12,000 units lipase; 60,000 units protease; 60,000 units amylase
8X Pancreatin
Tablets (enteric-coated): 7,200 mg pancreatin; 22,500 units lipase; 180,000 units protease; 180,000 units amylase

Available by prescription only
Donnazyme
Tablets: 500 mg pancreatin; 1,000 units lipase; 12,500 units protease; 12,500 units amylase
Entozyme
Tablets: 300 mg pancreatin; 600 units lipase; 7,500 units protease; 7,500 units amylase

Indications, route, and dosage

Exocrine pancreatic secretion insufficiency, digestive aid in cystic fibrosis, steatorrhea, and other disorders of fat metabolism secondary to insufficient pancreatic enzymes
Adults and children: 1 to 2 tablets P.O. with meals.

Pharmacodynamics

Digestive action: The proteolytic, amylolytic, and lipolytic enzymes enhance the digestion of proteins, starches, and fats. This agent is sensitive to acids and is more active in neutral or slightly alkaline environments.

Pharmacokinetics

- *Absorption:* Drug is not absorbed; it acts locally in the GI tract.
- *Distribution:* None.
- *Metabolism:* None.
- *Excretion:* Drug is excreted in feces.

Contraindications and precautions

Contraindicated in patients with hypersensitivity to drug or pork protein or enzymes, acute pancreatitis, and acute exacerbations of chronic pancreatitis. Use cautiously in pregnant or breast-feeding patients.

Interactions

Pancreatin activity may be reduced *by calcium-* or *magnesium-containing antacids*; however, *antacids* or *H_2 blockers* (such as *cimetidine*) may reduce the inactivation of the enzymes by gastric acid. Drug decreases absorption of *iron-containing products.*

Effects on diagnostic tests

Pancreatin, particularly in large doses, increases serum uric acid concentrations.

Adverse reactions

GI: nausea, diarrhea (with high doses).
Other: allergic reactions, perianal irritation, rash.

Overdose and treatment

Clinical manifestations of overdose include hyperuricosuria, hyperuricemia, diarrhea, abdominal cramps, and transient intestinal upset.

☑ Special considerations

- For maximal effect, administer dose just before or during a meal.
- Tablets may not be crushed or chewed; follow with a glass of water to ensure complete swallowing.

• Diet should balance fat, protein, and starch intake properly to avoid indigestion. Dosage varies according to degree of maldigestion and malabsorption, amount of fat in diet, and enzyme activity of individual preparations.
• Adequate replacement decreases number of bowel movements and improves stool consistency.
• Use only after confirmed diagnosis of exocrine pancreatic insufficiency. Not effective in GI disorders unrelated to pancreatic enzyme deficiency.
• Enteric coating may reduce availability of enzyme in upper portion of jejunum.

Patient education

• Explain use of drug, and advise storage away from heat and light.
• Be sure patient or family understands special dietary instructions for the particular disease. Tell him not to change brands without medical approval.

pancrelipase

Cotazym, Cotazym-S, Creon 10, Creon 20, Ilozyme, Ku-Zyme HP, Pancrease, Pancrease MT4, Pancrease MT10, Pancrease MT16, Pancrease MT20, Pancrelipase, Protilase, Ultrase MT12, Ultrase MT20, Ultrase MT24, Viokase, Zymase

Pharmacologic classification: pancreatic enzyme
Therapeutic classification: digestant
Pregnancy risk category C

How supplied

Available by prescription only
Cotazym
Capsules: 8,000 units lipase; 30,000 units protease; 30,000 units amylase
Cotazym-S
Capsules: 5,000 units lipase; 20,000 units protease; 20,000 units amylase
Creon 10
Capsules (delayed-release): 10,000 units lipase; 37,500 units protease; 33,200 units amylase
Creon 20
Capsules (delayed-release): 20,000 units lipase; 75,000 units protease; 66,400 units amylase
Ilozyme
Tablets: 11,000 units lipase; 30,000 units protease; 30,000 units amylase
Ku-Zyme HP
Capsules: 8,000 units lipase; 30,000 units protease; 30,000 units amylase
Pancrease
Capsules: 4,000 units lipase; 25,000 units protease; 20,000 units amylase
Pancrease MT4
Capsules (enteric-coated microtablets): 4,000 units lipase; 12,000 units protease; 12,000 units amylase
Pancrease MT10
Capsules (enteric-coated microtablets): 10,000 units lipase; 30,000 units protease; 30,000 units amylase
Pancrease MT16
Capsules (enteric-coated microtablets): 16,000 units lipase; 48,000 units protease; 48,000 units amylase
Pancrease MT20
Capsules (enteric-coated microtablets): 20,000 units lipase; 44,000 units protease; 56,000 units amylase
Pancrelipase and Protilase
Capsules: 4,000 units lipase; 25,000 units protease; 20,000 units amylase
Ultrase MT12
Capsules: 12,000 units lipase; 39,000 units protease; 39,000 units amylase
Ultrase MT20
Capsules: 20,000 units lipase; 65,000 units protease; 65,000 units amylase
Ultrase MT24
Capsules: 24,000 units lipase; 78,000 units protease; 78,000 units amylase
Viokase
Powder: 16,800 units lipase; 70,000 units protease; 70,000 units amylase
Zymase
Capsules: 12,000 units lipase; 24,000 units protease; 24,000 units amylase

Indications, route, and dosage

Exocrine pancreatic secretion insufficiency, cystic fibrosis in adults and children, steatorrhea, and other disorders of fat metabolism secondary to insufficient pancreatic enzymes
Adults: 4,000 to 48,000 units lipase with meals and snacks. Dose must be titrated to patient's response.
Children age 7 to 12: 4,000 to 12,000 units lipase with meals and snacks. Dose must be titrated to patient's response.
Children age 1 to 6: 4,000 to 8,000 units lipase with meals and 4,000 units with snacks. Dose must be titrated to patient's response.
Children age 6 to 12 months: 2,000 units lipase with meals and snacks. Dose must be titrated to patient's response.
Patients with pancreatectomy or obstructive pancreatic duct
Adults: 8,000 to 16,000 units lipase at 2-hour intervals; may increase dose to 64,000 to 88,000 units in severe cases.

Pharmacodynamics

Digestive action: The proteolytic, amylolytic, and lipolytic enzymes enhance the digestion of proteins, starches, and fats. This agent is sensitive to acids and is more active in neutral or slightly alkaline environments.

Pharmacokinetics

• *Absorption:* Drug is not absorbed and acts locally in the GI tract.
• *Distribution:* None.
• *Metabolism:* None.
• *Excretion:* Drug is excreted in feces.

Contraindications and precautions

Contraindicated in patients with severe hypersensitivity to pork, acute pancreatitis, or acute exacerbations of chronic pancreatic diseases. Use cautiously in pregnant or breast-feeding women.

Interactions
When used concomitantly, pancrelipase activity may be reduced *by calcium-* or *magnesium-containing antacids*; however, *antacids* or *H_2 blockers* (such as *cimetidine*) may reduce inactivation of the enzymes by gastric acid. Pancrelipase decreases absorption of *iron-containing products.*

Effects on diagnostic tests
Pancrelipase therapy increases serum uric acid concentrations, particularly with large doses.

Adverse reactions
GI: *nausea,* cramping, diarrhea (high doses).
Other: allergic reaction.

Overdose and treatment
Clinical manifestations of overdose include hyperuricosuria, hyperuricemia, diarrhea, and transient GI upset.

☑ Special considerations
- For maximal effect, administer dose just before or during a meal. Patient should drink a glass of water or juice to ensure complete swallowing.
- Preparations may not be crushed or chewed.
- Use only after confirmed diagnosis of exocrine pancreatic insufficiency. Not effective in GI disorders unrelated to enzyme deficiency.
- For young children, mix powders (including content of capsules) with applesauce and give at mealtime. Avoid inhalation of powder. Older children may swallow capsules with food.
- Dosage varies with degree of maldigestion and malabsorption, amount of fat in diet, and enzyme activity of individual preparations.
- Adequate replacement decreases number of bowel movements and improves stool consistency.
- Enteric coating on some products may reduce availability of enzyme in upper portion of jejunum.

Patient education
- Teach patient or family proper use of drug, and advise storage away from heat and light.
- Be sure patient or family understands special dietary instructions for the particular disease.
- Tell patient not to change brands without medical approval.

Pediatric use
- Capsules may be opened to facilitate swallowing. They may be sprinkled on food, but a pH of 5.5 or greater is necessary to ensure stability. Dosage for children under age 6 months has not been established.

pancuronium bromide
Pavulon

Pharmacologic classification: nondepolarizing neuromuscular blocker
Therapeutic classification: skeletal muscle relaxant
Pregnancy risk category C

How supplied
Available by prescription only
Injection: 1 mg/ml, 2 mg/ml parenteral

Indications, route, and dosage
Adjunct to anesthesia to induce skeletal muscle relaxation, facilitate intubation and ventilation, and to weaken muscle contractions in induced seizures
Dose depends on anesthetic used, individual needs, and response. Doses are representative and must be adjusted.
Adults and children over age 1 month: Initially, 0.04 to 0.1 mg/kg I.V.; then 0.01 mg/kg q 25 to 60 minutes if needed.

Pharmacodynamics
Skeletal muscle relaxant action: Pancuronium prevents acetylcholine (ACh) from binding to the receptors on the motor end-plate, thus blocking depolarization. It may increase heart rate through direct blocking effect on the ACh receptors of the heart; increase is dose-related. Pancuronium causes little or no histamine release and no ganglionic blockade.

Pharmacokinetics
- *Absorption:* After I.V. administration, onset of action occurs within 30 to 45 seconds, with peak effects seen in 3 to 4½ minutes. Onset and duration are dose-related. After 0.06 mg/kg dose, effects begin to subside in 35 to 45 minutes. Repeated doses may increase the magnitude and duration of action.
- *Distribution:* Pancuronium is 87% bound to plasma proteins.
- *Metabolism:* Unknown metabolism; small amounts may be metabolized by the liver.
- *Excretion:* Mainly excreted unchanged in urine; some through biliary excretion.

Contraindications and precautions
Contraindicated in patients with hypersensitivity to bromides or preexisting tachycardia and in those for whom even a minor increase in heart rate is undesirable.

Use cautiously in elderly or debilitated patients and in those with impaired renal, pulmonary, or hepatic function; respiratory depression; myasthenia gravis; myasthenic syndrome of lung or bronchogenic cancer; dehydration; thyroid disorders; collagen diseases; porphyria; electrolyte disturbances; hyperthermia; or toxemic states. Also use large doses cautiously in patients undergoing cesarean section.

Interactions
Concomitant use of pancuronium with *succinylcholine* may enhance and prolong neuromuscular blocking effects of pancuronium. The effects of pancuronium may also be potentiated by *aminoglycoside antibiotics, general anesthetics, beta-blocking agents, clindamycin, furosemide, lincomycin, lithium, parenteral magnesium salts, depolarizing neuromuscular blocking agents, other nondepolarizing neuromuscular blocking agents, polymyx-*

in antibiotics, quinidine or *quinine, thiazide diuretics,* and *potassium-depleting agents.* Concomitant use with *opioid analgesics* may increase respiratory depression.

Effects on diagnostic tests
None reported.

Adverse reactions
CV: tachycardia, increased blood pressure.
Respiratory: ***prolonged, dose-related respiratory insufficiency or apnea.***
Skin: transient rashes.
Other: excessive salivation, residual muscle weakness, allergic or idiosyncratic hypersensitivity reactions.

Overdose and treatment
Clinical manifestations of overdose include prolonged respiratory depression, apnea, and CV collapse.

Use a peripheral nerve stimulator to monitor response and to evaluate neuromuscular blockade. Maintain an adequate airway and manual or mechanical ventilation until patient can maintain adequate ventilation unassisted. Neostigmine, edrophonium, or pyridostigmine may be used to reverse effects.

☑ Special considerations
- Monitor baseline electrolyte levels, intake and output, and vital signs, especially heart rate and respiration.
- Administration requires direct medical supervision, with emergency respiratory support available.
- If using succinylcholine, allow its effects to subside before administering pancuronium.
- Store drug in refrigerator and not in plastic container or syringes. Plastic syringes may be used to administer dose.
- Do not mix in same syringe or give through same needle with barbiturates or other alkaline solutions.
- Use fresh solution only.
- Reduce dosage when ether or other inhalation anesthetics that enhance neuromuscular blockade are used.
- Large doses may increase frequency and severity of tachycardia.
- Drug does not relieve pain or affect consciousness; be sure to assess need for analgesic or sedative.

Geriatric use
- The usual adult dose must be individualized depending on response.

Pediatric use
- Dosage for neonates under age 1 month must be carefully individualized. For infants over age 1 month and children, see adult dosage.

Breast-feeding
- It is unknown if pancuronium is excreted in breast milk. Use with caution in breast-feeding women.

papaverine hydrochloride
Cerespan, Genabid, Pavabid, Pavabid Plateau Caps, Pavacels, Pavacot, Pavagen, Pavarine, Pavased, Pavatine, Pavatym, Paverolan

Pharmacologic classification: benzylisoquinoline derivative, opiate alkaloid
Therapeutic classification: peripheral vasodilator
Pregnancy risk category C

How supplied
Available by prescription only
Tablets: 30 mg, 60 mg, 100 mg, 150 mg, 200 mg, 300 mg
Tablets (sustained-release): 200 mg
Capsules (sustained-release): 150 mg
Injection: 30 mg/ml in 2- and 10-ml ampules

Indications, route, and dosage
Relief of cerebral and peripheral ischemia associated with arterial spasm and myocardial ischemia; treatment of coronary occlusion and certain cerebral angiospastic states
Adults: 75 to 300 mg P.O. three to five times daily or 150 to 300 mg sustained-release preparations q 8 to 12 hours; 30 to 120 mg I.M. or I.V. q 3 hours, as indicated. In treatment of extrasystoles, give two doses 10 minutes apart.
Children: 6 mg/kg I.M.or I.V. q.i.d.
◊ ***Impotence***
Adults: 2.5 to 60 mg injected intracavernously.

Pharmacodynamics
Vasodilating action: Papaverine relaxes smooth muscle directly by inhibiting phosphodiesterase, thus increasing concentration of cyclic adenosine monophosphate. There is considerable controversy regarding the clinical effectiveness of papaverine. Some clinicians find little objective evidence of any clinical value.

Pharmacokinetics
- *Absorption:* 54% of orally administered papaverine is bioavailable. Peak plasma levels occur 1 to 2 hours after an oral dose; half-life varies from ½ to 24 hours, but levels can be maintained by giving drug at 6-hour intervals. Sustained-release forms are sometimes absorbed poorly and erratically.
- *Distribution:* Papaverine tends to localize in adipose tissue and in the liver; the remainder is distributed throughout the body. About 90% of drug is protein-bound.
- *Metabolism:* Drug is metabolized by the liver.
- *Excretion:* Excreted in urine as metabolites.

Contraindications and precautions
I.V. use is contraindicated in patients with Parkinson's disease or complete AV block. Use cautiously in patients with glaucoma.

Interactions
Papaverine may decrease the antiparkinsonian effects of *levodopa* and exacerbate such symptoms

as rigidity and tremors. Heavy *tobacco* smoking may interfere with the therapeutic effect of papaverine because nicotine constricts the blood vessels. Papaverine's effects may be potentiated by *CNS depressants* and may have a synergic response with *morphine.*

Effects on diagnostic tests
Drug therapy alters serum concentrations of eosinophils, ALT, alkaline phosphatase, and bilirubin. Elevated serum bilirubin levels signal hepatic hypersensitivity to papaverine.

Adverse reactions
CNS: *headache,* vertigo, drowsiness, sedation, malaise.
CV: *increased heart rate, increased blood pressure* (with parenteral use), depressed AV and intraventricular conduction, ***arrhythmias.***
GI: constipation, *nausea,* anorexia, abdominal pain, diarrhea.
Hepatic: ***hepatitis*** (jaundice, eosinophilia, abnormal liver function tests), ***cirrhosis.***
Respiratory: increased depth and rate of respiration.
Skin: *diaphoresis, flushing,* rash.

Overdose and treatment
Clinical signs of overdose include drowsiness, weakness, nystagmus, diplopia, incoordination, and lassitude, progressing to coma with cyanosis and respiratory depression.

To slow drug absorption, give activated charcoal, tap water, or milk; then evacuate stomach contents by gastric lavage or emesis, and follow with catharsis. If coma and respiratory depression occur, take appropriate measures; maintain blood pressure. Hemodialysis may be helpful.

☑ Special considerations
- Papaverine is an opiate; however, it has strikingly different pharmacologic properties than other drugs in this group.
- Drug may be given orally, I.M. or, when immediate effect is needed, by slow I.V. injection. Inject I.V. slowly over 1 to 2 minutes; arrhythmias and fatal apnea may follow rapid injection.
- Papaverine injection is incompatible with lactated Ringer's injection; a precipitate will form.

Patient education
- Advise patient to avoid sudden postural changes to minimize possible orthostatic hypotension.
- Instruct patient to report nausea, abdominal distress, anorexia, constipation, diarrhea, jaundice, rash, sweating, tiredness, or headache.

Geriatric use
- Elderly patients are at greater risk of papaverine-induced hypothermia.

Pediatric use
- Children's doses are administered parenterally.

Breast-feeding
- Safety in breast-feeding women has not been established.

para-aminosalicylate sodium (PAS)
PAS Sodium

Pharmacologic classification: aminobenzoic acid analogue
Therapeutic classification: antitubercular
Pregnancy risk category C

How supplied
Available by prescription only
Tablets: 500 mg, 1 g
Powder: 4.18-g packets

Indications, route, and dosage
Adjunctive treatment of tuberculosis
Adults: 14 to 16 g P.O. daily, divided in two to three doses.
Children: 275 to 420 mg/kg P.O. daily, divided in three or four doses.

Pharmacodynamics
Antibiotic action: PAS is bacteriostatic; it interferes with folic acid synthesis by enzyme inhibition. PAS is active only against *Mycobacterium tuberculosis.*

PAS is considered adjunctive therapy in tuberculosis and is given with another antitubercular agent to prevent or delay development of drug resistance by *M. tuberculosis.*

Pharmacokinetics
- *Absorption:* PAS is absorbed readily from the GI tract.
- *Distribution:* Widely distributed in the body, especially in pleural and caseous tissue.
- *Metabolism:* PAS is metabolized in the liver.
- *Excretion:* 80% of drug is excreted via the kidneys as metabolites and free acid. Half-life of drug is 1 hour.

Contraindications and precautions
Contraindicated in patients with known hypersensitivity to aminosalicylic acid or its salts. Use cautiously in patients with hepatic or renal disease, history of gastric ulcer, and heart failure or G6PD deficiency in whom excess sodium could be harmful.

Interactions
Aminosalicylic acid and its salts may decrease oral absorption of *rifampin* and *vitamin B_{12};* PAS may increase effects of *oral anticoagulants.*

Probenecid increases aminosalicylic acid serum concentrations by blocking renal tubular secretion. *Diphenhydramine* decreases oral absorption of PAS.

Ascorbic acid and *ammonium chloride* may acidify urine in PAS-treated patients, causing crystalluria. PAS may decrease absorption of *digoxin.*

Effects on diagnostic tests
PAS alters urine glucose testing by cupric sulfate method (Benedict's reagent or Clinitest) and may

cause false-positive elevations of urine urobilinogen (Ehrlich's reagent method), urinary protein, and vanillylmandelic acid.

Adverse reactions

CNS: ***encephalopathy.***
CV: vasculitis.
GI: *nausea, vomiting, diarrhea, abdominal pain,* peptic ulcer, gastric ulcer, malabsorption (folic acid, vitamin B_{12}, iron, lipids).
GU: albuminuria, *hematuria, crystalluria.*
Hematologic: leukopenia, ***agranulocytosis,*** eosinophilia, ***thrombocytopenia, hemolytic anemia.***
Hepatic: jaundice, ***hepatitis.***
Metabolic: acidosis, hypokalemia, goiter.
Skin: rash, pruritus.
Other: infectious mononucleosis-like syndrome, fever, lymphadenopathy.

Note: Drug should be discontinued if patient shows signs of hypersensitivity reaction, bone marrow toxicity, or hepatic failure.

Overdose and treatment

Signs of overdose include nausea, vomiting, hypokalemia, and acidosis. No specific recommendations for treatment are available. Treatment is supportive. After recent ingestion (within 4 hours), empty the stomach by induced emesis or gastric lavage. Follow with activated charcoal to decrease absorption.

It is not known if drug is removed by hemodialysis or peritoneal dialysis.

☑ Special considerations

- Drug may be taken with or after meals or with antacids to avoid gastric irritation.
- Obtain specimens for culture and sensitivity testing before giving first dose. Therapy may begin before test results are completed; repeat tests periodically to detect drug resistance.
- Observe patients for adverse reactions and monitor serum electrolyte levels and hematologic, renal, and liver function studies to minimize toxicity.
- Avoid PAS in patients on sodium-restricted diets; a 15-g dose contains 1.6 g sodium.
- Observe patient for edema.
- Store drug in tight, light-resistant container in a dry place. Drug deteriorates rapidly with exposure to heat, air, or moisture. Discard if drug turns brown or purple.

Patient education

- Explain disease process and rationale for long-term therapy.
- Teach signs and symptoms of hypersensitivity and other adverse reactions, and emphasize need to report unusual effects.
- Tell patient to call promptly if loss of appetite, fatigue, malaise, jaundice, dark urine, rash, or itching occurs.
- Teach patient how and when to take drug and to discard drug if it turns brown or purple.
- To prevent bitter aftertaste, tell patient to rinse mouth with clear water or to chew sugarless gum after taking drug.
- Urge patient to comply with prescribed regimen and not to discontinue drug without medical approval; explain importance of follow-up appointments.

Breast-feeding

- Drug may be excreted in breast milk; use with caution in breast-feeding women.

paromomycin sulfate

Humatin

Pharmacologic classification: aminoglycoside
Therapeutic classification: antibacterial, amebicide
Pregnancy risk category C

How supplied

Available by prescription only
Capsules: 250 mg

Indications, route, and dosage

Intestinal amebiasis (acute and chronic)
Adults and children: 25 to 35 mg/kg P.O. daily in three doses for 5 to 10 days after meals.
Tapeworm (fish, beef, pork, and dog) infections in patients who cannot take praziquantel or niclosamide
Adults: 1 g P.O. q 15 minutes for four doses.
Children: 11 mg/kg P.O. q 15 minutes for four doses.
Adjunctive management of hepatic coma
Adults: 4 g P.O. daily in two to four divided doses for 5 to 6 days. Higher daily doses (up to 8 g) have been used, but usually cause serious adverse effects.
◇ **Dientamoeba fragilis *infections,*** ◇ ***giardiasis***
Adults and children: 25 to 30 mg/kg P.O. daily in three divided doses for 7 days.
◇ ***Cryptosporidiosis in patients with AIDS***
Adults: 1.5 to 2.25 g P.O. daily in three to six divided doses for 10 to 14 days.
◇ **Hymenolepis nana *infection***
Adults: 45 mg/kg P.O. daily for 5 to 7 days.
◇ ***Treatment of cestodiasis caused by* Diphyllobothrium latum, Taenia saginata, T. solium, *and* Dipylidium caninum**
Adults: 1 g P.O. q 15 minutes for four doses.
Children: 11 mg/kg P.O. q 15 minutes for four doses.

Pharmacodynamics

Amebicidal action: Paromomycin acts on contact in the intestinal lumen by an unknown mechanism. It is effective against the trophozoite and encysted forms of *Entamoeba histolytica* and against *Diphyllobothrium latum* (fish tapeworm), *Dipylidium caninum* (dog and cat tapeworm), *Hymenolepis nana* (dwarf tapeworm), *Taenia saginata* (beef tapeworm), and *T. solium* (pork tapeworm).

Adjunct in hepatic coma: Paromomycin inhibits nitrogen-forming bacteria in the GI tract by inhibiting protein synthesis at the 30S subunit of the ribosome.

Pharmacokinetics

- *Absorption:* Very small amounts of an oral dose of paromomycin are absorbed by the intact GI tract; however, larger amounts may be absorbed in patients with ulcerative intestinal disorders or renal insufficiency.
- *Distribution:* Distribution has not been characterized adequately.
- *Metabolism:* No metabolites detected.
- *Excretion:* Almost 100% of drug is excreted unchanged in the feces; systemically absorbed drug is excreted in urine and may accumulate in patients with renal dysfunction. It is unknown if paromomycin is excreted in breast milk.

Contraindications and precautions

Contraindicated in patients with hypersensitivity to drug and in those with impaired renal function or intestinal obstruction. Use cautiously in patients with ulcerative lesions of the bowel.

Interactions

Concomitant use of aminoglycosides with *anticoagulants* may result in warfarin-induced hypoprothrombinemia. Aminoglycosides can decrease absorption of *digoxin* and *methotrexate* and can decrease serum retinol and plasma levels. Aminoglycosides can enhance *neuromuscular blockers* and increase risk of respiratory paralysis and renal dysfunction when administered concurrently with *polypeptide antibiotics.*

Effects on diagnostic tests

None reported.

Adverse reactions

CNS: headache, vertigo.
EENT: ototoxicity (potential).
GI: anorexia, nausea, vomiting, epigastric pain and burning, abdominal cramps, diarrhea, increased motility, steatorrhea, pruritus ani, malabsorption syndrome.
GU: hematuria, ***nephrotoxicity*** (potential).
Hematologic: eosinophilia.
Skin: rash, exanthema.
Other: overgrowth of nonsusceptible organisms.

Overdose and treatment

Paromomycin overdose may affect CV and respiratory function. Treatment is largely supportive. After recent ingestion (within 4 hours), empty stomach by induced emesis or gastric lavage. Follow with activated charcoal to decrease absorption. Osmotic cathartics also may help.

☑ Special considerations

- Administer paromomycin after meals to prevent GI upset.
- Watch for signs of bacterial or fungal superinfection.
- Monitor patients with GI ulceration or renal dysfunction; increased drug absorption and decreased drug clearance may result.
- Criterion of cure is absence of fecal amebae in specimen examined weekly for 6 weeks after discontinuation of treatment and thereafter monthly for 2 years.
- Drug is not effective in the treatment of extraintestinal amebiasis.
- Many clinicians prefer praziquantel or niclosamide for the treatment of tapeworm infection. Paromomycin may cause disintegration of worm segments and, possibly, release of viable eggs.

Patient education

- Counsel patient on need for medical follow-up after discharge.
- Advise patient to report adverse effects.
- Teach patient how disease is transmitted.
- To help prevent reinfection, instruct patient in proper hygiene, including disposal of feces and hand washing after defecation and before eating, and about the risks of eating raw food and the control of contamination by flies. Advise patient not to prepare, process, or serve food until treatment is completed.
- Advise patient to use liquid soap or reserved bar of soap to prevent cross-contamination.
- Tell patient to encourage other household members and suspected contacts to be tested and, if necessary, treated.
- Tell patient that isolation is unnecessary.

Geriatric use

- Drug should be used with caution because of the possibility of decreased renal function and baseline hearing impairment in this age-group.

Breast-feeding

- Safety has not been established.

paroxetine hydrochloride

Paxil

Pharmacologic classification: selective serotonin reuptake inhibitor
Therapeutic classification: antidepressant
Pregnancy risk category B

How supplied

Available by prescription only
Tablets: 10 mg, 20 mg, 30 mg, 40 mg

Indications, route, and dosage

Depression
Adults: Initially, 20 mg P.O. daily, preferably in the morning. Increase dosage by 10 mg/day at 1-week intervals, to maximum of 50 mg daily, if necessary.
✦ ***Dosage adjustment.*** For elderly or debilitated patients or patients with severe hepatic or renal disease, 10 mg P.O. daily, preferably in the morning. Increase dosage by 10 mg/day at 1-week intervals, p.r.n., to maximum of 40 mg daily.
Obsessive-compulsive disorder (OCD)
Adults: Initially, 20 mg P.O. daily, preferably in the morning. Increase dosage by 10 mg/day at 1-week intervals to target dose of 40 mg/day. Maximum dose, 60 mg/day.
Panic disorder
Adults: Initially, 10 mg P.O. daily, preferably in the morning. Increase dosage by 10 mg/day at 1-week

intervals, to target dose of 40 mg/day. Maximum dose, 60 mg/day.

Pharmacodynamics

Antidepressant action: Action is presumed to be linked to potentiation of serotonergic activity in the CNS, resulting from inhibition of neuronal reuptake of serotonin.

Pharmacokinetics

• *Absorption:* Paroxetine is completely absorbed after oral dosing.
• *Distribution:* Drug distributes throughout the body, including the CNS, with only 1% remaining in the plasma. Approximately 93% to 95% of paroxetine is bound to plasma protein.
• *Metabolism:* Approximately 36% of drug is metabolized in the liver. The principal metabolites are polar and conjugated products of oxidation and methylation, which are readily cleared.
• *Excretion:* Approximately 64% is excreted in urine (2% as parent compound and 62% as metabolite).

Contraindications and precautions

Contraindicated in patients taking MAO inhibitors. Use cautiously in patients with history of seizures or mania; in those with severe, concurrent systemic illness; or in those at risk for volume depletion.

Interactions

Cimetidine decreases hepatic metabolism of paroxetine, leading to risk of toxicity; dosage adjustments may be necessary. Paroxetine may decrease *digoxin* levels; monitor the patient closely.

Concurrent use of an *MAO inhibitor* and paroxetine may increase the risk of serious, sometimes fatal, adverse reactions and should be avoided. *Phenobarbital* induces paroxetine metabolism, thereby reducing plasma levels of drug. Paroxetine may alter the pharmacokinetics of *phenytoin,* requiring dosage adjustment.

Paroxetine may increase *procyclidine* levels; monitor the patient for excessive anticholinergic effects. Concomitant use of paroxetine and *tryptophan* may increase the incidence of adverse reactions, such as diaphoresis, headache, nausea, and dizziness; avoid concomitant use. Paroxetine may increase risk of bleeding when used concomitantly with *warfarin;* monitor INR.

Effects on diagnostic tests

None reported.

Adverse reactions

CNS: *somnolence, dizziness, insomnia, tremor, nervousness,* anxiety, paresthesia, confusion, *headache,* agitation.
CV: palpitations, vasodilation, postural hypotension.
EENT: lump or tightness in throat, dysgeusia.
GI: *dry mouth, nausea, constipation, diarrhea,* flatulence, vomiting, dyspepsia, increased or decreased appetite, abdominal pain.
GU: ejaculatory disturbances, male genital disorders (including anorgasmia, erectile difficulties, delayed ejaculation or orgasm, impotence, and sexual dysfunction), urinary frequency, other urinary disorders, female genital disorders (including anorgasmia, difficulty with orgasm).
Skin: rash, pruritus.
Other: *asthenia, diaphoresis,* myopathy, myalgia, myasthenia, decreased libido, yawning.

Overdose and treatment

Signs and symptoms associated with drug overdose may include nausea, vomiting, drowsiness, sinus tachycardia, and dilated pupil. Treatment should consist of general measures used in management of overdosage with any antidepressant. Gastric evacuation by emesis, lavage, or both should be performed. In most cases, 20 to 30 g of activated charcoal may then be administered every 4 to 6 hours during the first 24 to 48 hours after ingestion. Supportive care, frequent monitoring of vital signs, and careful observation are indicated. ECG and cardiac function monitoring are warranted with evidence of any abnormality.

Special caution must be taken with a patient who currently receives or recently received paroxetine if the patient ingests an excessive quantity of a tricyclic antidepressant. In such cases, accumulation of the parent tricyclic and its active metabolite may increase the possibility of clinically significant sequelae and extend the time needed for close medical observation.

☑ Special considerations

• At least 14 days should elapse between discontinuation of an MAO inhibitor and initiation of drug therapy. Similarly, at least 14 days should elapse between discontinuation of paroxetine and initiation of an MAO inhibitor.
• Hyponatremia may occur with paroxetine use, especially in elderly patients, those taking diuretics, and those who are otherwise volume depleted. Monitor serum sodium levels.
• If signs of psychosis occur or increase, reduce dosage. Monitor patients for suicidal tendencies and allow them only a minimum supply of drug.

Patient education

• Caution patient not to operate hazardous machinery, including automobiles, until reasonably certain that paroxetine therapy does not affect ability to engage in such activity.
• Tell patient that he may notice improvement in 1 to 4 weeks but that he must continue with the prescribed regimen to obtain continued benefits.
• Instruct patient to call before taking other medications, including OTC preparations, while receiving paroxetine therapy.
• Tell patient to abstain from alcohol while taking paroxetine.

Geriatric use

• Use cautiously and in lower dosages in elderly patients.

Pediatric use

• Safety and effectiveness in children have not been established.

Breast-feeding
• Paroxetine is excreted in breast milk. Caution should be exercised when drug is administered to a breast-feeding woman.

pegaspargase (PEG-L-asparaginase)
Oncaspar

Pharmacologic classification: modified version of the enzyme L-asparaginase
Therapeutic classification: antineoplastic
Pregnancy risk category C

How supplied
Available by prescription only
Injection: 750 IU/ml in single-use vial

Indications, route, and dosage
Acute lymphoblastic leukemia (ALL) in patients who require L-asparaginase but have developed hypersensitivity to the native forms of L-asparaginase
Adults and children with body surface area of at least 0.6 m^2: 2,500 IU/m^2 I.M. or I.V. q 14 days.
Children with body surface area less than 0.6 m^2: 82.5 IU/kg I.M. or I.V. q 14 days.

Note: Moderate to life-threatening hypersensitivity reactions necessitate discontinuation of L-asparaginase treatment.

Pharmacodynamics
Antineoplastic action: Pegaspargase is a modified version of the enzyme L-asparaginase, which exerts its cytotoxic activity by inactivating the amino acid asparagine. Because leukemic cells cannot synthesize their own asparagine, protein synthesis and eventually synthesis of DNA and RNA are inhibited.

Pharmacokinetics
• *Absorption:* No information available.
• *Distribution:* No information available.
• *Metabolism:* No information available.
• *Excretion:* No information available.

Contraindications and precautions
Contraindicated in patients with pancreatitis or a history of pancreatitis; in those who have had significant hemorrhagic events associated with prior L-asparaginase therapy; and in those with previous serious allergic reactions, such as generalized urticaria, bronchospasm, laryngeal edema, hypotension, or other unacceptable adverse reactions to pegaspargase.

Use cautiously in patients with hepatic dysfunction and during pregnancy.

Interactions
Depletion of serum protein by pegaspargase may increase the toxicity of other *protein-bound drugs.* Additionally, during its inhibition of protein synthesis and cell replication, pegaspargase may interfere with the action of drugs, such as *methotrexate,* that require cell replication for their lethal effects. Pegaspargase may interfere with the enzymatic detoxification of other drugs, particularly in the liver.

Concurrent administration of pagaspargase with such drugs as *aspirin, dipyridamole, heparin, NSAIDs,* or *warfarin* may cause imbalances in coagulation factors, predisposing the patient to bleeding or thrombosis.

Effects on diagnostic tests
None reported.

Adverse reactions
CNS: seizures, headache, paresthesia, ***status epilepticus,*** somnolence, coma, mental status changes, dizziness, emotional lability, mood changes, parkinsonism, confusion, disorientation, fatigue.
CV: hypotension, tachycardia, chest pain, subacute bacterial endocarditis, hypertension.
EENT: epistaxis.
Endocrine: hyperglycemia, hypoglycemia.
GI: nausea, vomiting, abdominal pain, anorexia, diarrhea, constipation, indigestion, flatulence, GI pain, mucositis, ***pancreatitis (sometimes fulminant and fatal),*** increased serum amylase and lipase levels, severe colitis.
GU: increased BUN level, increased creatinine level, increased urinary frequency, hematuria, severe hemorrhagic cystitis, renal dysfunction, renal failure.
Hematologic: ***thrombosis;*** prolonged PT, prolonged partial thromboplastin time, decreased antithrombin III; ***DIC;*** decreased fibrinogen; hemolytic anemia; ***leukopenia; pancytopenia; agranulocytosis; thrombocytopenia;*** increased thromboplastin; easy bruising; ecchymoses; ***hemorrhage*** (may be fatal).
Hepatic: jaundice, abnormal liver function test results, bilirubinemia, increased ALT and AST, ascites, hypoalbuminemia, fatty changes in liver, ***liver failure.***
Metabolic: hyperuricemia, hyponatremia, uric acid nephropathy, hypoproteinemia, proteinuria, weight loss, metabolic acidosis, increased blood ammonia level, hyperglycemia, hypoglycemia.
Musculoskeletal: arthralgia, myalgia, musculoskeletal pain, joint stiffness, cramps.
Respiratory: cough, ***severe bronchospasm,*** upper respiratory tract infection.
Skin: itching, alopecia, fever blister, purpura, hand whiteness, fungal changes, nail whiteness and ridging, erythema simplex, petechial rash, injection pain or reaction, localized edema.
Other: hypersensitivity reactions, including ***anaphylaxis,*** rash, erythema, edema, pain, fever, chills, urticaria, dyspnea, or bronchospasm; pain in extremities; peripheral edema; malaise; night sweats; mouth tenderness; infection; ***sepsis, septic shock.***

Overdose and treatment
Only three cases of overdosage (10,000 IU/m^2 as an I.V. infusion) have been reported. One patient experienced a slight increase in liver enzymes, one developed a rash, and one experienced no adverse effects. No other information is available.

☑ Special considerations

• I.M. is the preferred administration route because it has a lower incidence of hepatotoxicity, coagulopathy, and GI and renal disorders than the I.V. route.
• Drug should not be administered if it has ever been frozen. Although there may not be an apparent change in drug's appearance, its activity is destroyed after freezing.
• Avoid excessive agitation; do *not* shake. Keep refrigerated at 36° to 46° F (2° to 8° C). Do not use if cloudy, if precipitate is present, or if stored at room temperature for more than 48 hours. Do not freeze. Discard unused portions. Use only one dose per vial; do not re-enter the vial. Do not save unused drug for later administration.
• When administering I.M., limit volume at a single injection site to 2 ml. If the volume to be administered is greater than 2 ml, use multiple injection sites.
• When administered I.V., give over 1 to 2 hours in 100 ml of NaCl or 5% dextrose injection through an infusion that is already running.
• Pegaspargase should be the sole induction agent only when a combined regimen using other chemotherapeutic agents is inappropriate because of toxicity or other specific patient-related factors or in patients refractory to other therapy.
• Hypersensitivity reactions to pegaspargase, including life-threatening anaphylaxis, may occur during therapy, especially in patients with known hypersensitivity to other forms of L-asparaginase. As a precaution, observe patient for 1 hour and have resuscitation equipment and other agents necessary to treat anaphylaxis available.
• A decrease in circulating lymphoblasts is common after initiating therapy. This may be accompanied by a marked rise in serum uric acid. As a guide to the effects of therapy, monitor patient's peripheral blood count and bone marrow. Obtain frequent serum amylase determinations to detect early evidence of pancreatitis. Monitor blood glucose during therapy because hyperglycemia may occur. When using pegaspargase with hepatotoxic chemotherapy, monitor patient for liver dysfunction. Pegaspargase may affect some plasma proteins; therefore, monitoring of fibrinogen, PT, and partial thromboplastin time may be indicated.
• Pegaspargase may be a contact irritant, and the solution must be handled and administered with care. Gloves are recommended. Inhalation of vapors and contact with skin or mucous membranes, especially those of the eyes, must be avoided. In case of contact, wash with copious amounts of water for at least 15 minutes.

Patient education

• Tell patient to report hypersensitivity reactions immediately.
• Instruct patient not to take other drugs, including OTC preparations, without obtaining medical approval; pegaspargase increases the risk of bleeding when given concomitantly with certain drugs, such as aspirin, and may increase the toxicity of other medications.
• Instruct patient to report signs and symptoms of infection (fever, chills, malaise); drug may have immunosuppressive activity.

Breast-feeding

• Because of potential for serious adverse reactions in breast-fed infants, a decision must be made whether to discontinue breast-feeding or drug, taking into account the importance of drug to mother.

pemoline

Cylert

Pharmacologic classification: oxazolidinedione derivative, CNS stimulant
Therapeutic classification: analeptic
Controlled substance schedule IV
Pregnancy risk category B

How supplied

Available by prescription only
Tablets: 18.75 mg, 37.5 mg, 75 mg
Tablets (chewable and containing povidine): 37.5 mg

Indications, route, and dosage

Attention deficit hyperactivity disorder (ADHD)
Children age 6 and older: Initially, 37.5 mg P.O. given in the morning. Daily dosage can be raised by 18.75 mg weekly. Effective dosage range, 56.25 to 75 mg daily; maximum, 112.5 mg daily.

Note: Because of its association with life-threatening hepatic failure, pemoline should not be considered as first-line therapy for ADHD.

◊ ***Narcolepsy***
Adults: 50 to 200 mg daily, in divided doses after breakfast and lunch.

Pharmacodynamics

Analeptic action: Pemoline differs structurally from methylphenidate and amphetamines; however, like those drugs, pemoline has a paradoxical calming effect in children with ADHD.

Pemoline's mechanism of action is unknown; it may be mediated through dopaminergic mechanisms. Investigationally, its CNS stimulant effect has been studied in narcolepsy in adults, in fatigue, in depressed and schizophrenic states, and in elderly patients.

Pharmacokinetics

• *Absorption:* Well absorbed after oral administration. Peak therapeutic effects occur within 4 hours and persist for about 8 hours.
• *Distribution:* Distribution is unknown. Drug is 50% protein-bound.
• *Metabolism:* Pemoline is metabolized by the liver to active and inactive metabolites.
• *Excretion:* Drug and its metabolites are excreted in urine; 75% of an oral dose is excreted within 24 hours.

Contraindications and precautions

Contraindicated in patients with hepatic dysfunction and hypersensitivity or idiosyncrasy to drug. Use cautiously in patients with impaired renal function. Should not be used as first-line therapy in ADHD.

Interactions
Concomitant use with *caffeine* may decrease efficacy of pemoline in ADHD; concomitant use with *anticonvulsants* may decrease the seizure threshold.

Effects on diagnostic tests
Drug may cause abnormalities in liver function test results.

Adverse reactions
CNS: *insomnia,* dyskinetic movements, irritability, fatigue, mild depression, dizziness, headache, drowsiness, hallucinations, ***seizures,*** *Tourette's syndrome,* abnormal oculomotor function.
GI: anorexia, abdominal pain, nausea.
Hematologic: ***aplastic anemia.***
Hepatic: elevated liver enzymes, ***hepatic failure.***
Skin: rash.

Overdose and treatment
Symptoms of overdose may include irregular respiration, hyperreflexia, restlessness, tachycardia, hallucinations, excitement, and agitation.

Treat overdose symptomatically and supportively: use gastric lavage if symptoms are not severe (hyperexcitability or coma). Monitor vital signs and fluid and electrolyte balance. Maintain patient in a cool room, monitor temperature, and minimize external stimulation; protect patient from self-injury. Chlorpromazine or haloperidol usually can reverse CNS stimulation. Hemodialysis may help.

☑ Special considerations
- Monitor initiation of therapy closely; drug may precipitate Gilles de la Tourette's syndrome.
- Check vital signs regularly for increased blood pressure or other signs of excessive stimulation.
- Give drug in a single morning dose for maximum daytime benefit and to minimize insomnia.
- Monitor blood and urine glucose levels in diabetic patients; drug may alter insulin requirements.
- Monitor CBC, differential, and platelet counts while patient is on long-term therapy.
- Determine baseline and periodically assess liver function tests. If abnormalities occur, discontinue therapy.
- Explain that therapeutic effects may not appear for 3 to 4 weeks and that intermittent drug-free periods when stress is least evident (weekends, school holidays) may help assess patient's condition, prevent development of tolerance, and permit decreased dosage when drug is resumed.
- Monitor height and weight; drug has been associated with growth suppression.
- Abrupt withdrawal after high-dose long-term use may unmask severe depression. Lower dosage gradually to prevent acute rebound depression.
- Drug impairs ability to perform tasks requiring mental alertness.
- Be sure patient obtains adequate rest; fatigue may result as drug wears off.
- Discourage pemoline use for analeptic effect, as drug has abuse potential; CNS stimulation superimposed on CNS depression may cause neuronal instability and seizures.
- Carefully follow manufacturer's directions for reconstitution, storage, and administration of all preparations. Pemoline has been used to treat narcolepsy in adults (50 to 200 mg divided twice-daily) as well as depression and schizophrenia, but these uses are controversial.

Patient education
- Explain rationale for therapy and the anticipated risks and benefits; teach signs and symptoms of adverse reactions and need to report these.
- Tell patient to avoid drinks containing caffeine, to prevent added CNS stimulation, and not to alter dosage without medical approval.
- Warn patient not to use drug to mask fatigue, to be sure to obtain adequate rest, and to report excessive CNS stimulation.
- Advise diabetic patient to monitor blood glucose levels because drug may alter insulin needs.
- Advise patient to avoid tasks that require mental alertness until degree of sedative effect is determined.

Pediatric use
- Drug is not recommended for ADHD in children under age 6.

penbutolol sulfate
Levatol

Pharmacologic classification: beta-adrenergic blocker
Therapeutic classification: antihypertensive
Pregnancy risk category C

How supplied
Available by prescription only
Tablets: 20 mg

Indications, route, and dosage
Treatment of mild to moderate hypertension
Adults: 20 mg P.O. once daily. Usually given with other antihypertensive agents, such as thiazide diuretics. Dosages as high as 40 to 80 mg daily and as low as 10 mg daily have been effective.

Pharmacodynamics
Antihypertensive action: Penbutolol blocks both beta$_1$- and beta$_2$-adrenergic receptors. Its antihypertensive effects may be related to its peripheral antiadrenergic effects that lead to decreased cardiac output, a central effect that leads to decreased sympathetic tone, or decreased renin secretion by the kidneys.

Pharmacokinetics
- *Absorption:* Penbutolol is almost completely absorbed after oral administration. Peak plasma levels occur 2 to 3 hours after administration.

• *Distribution:* 80% to 98% of drug is bound to plasma proteins.
• *Metabolism:* Drug is metabolized by the liver. Several metabolites have been identified; some retain partial pharmacologic activity.
• *Excretion:* Average elimination half-life of the parent drug is 5 hours; some metabolites persist for 20 hours or more. Most metabolites are excreted in the urine.

Contraindications and precautions

Contraindicated in patients with hypersensitivity to drug or other beta blockers and in those with sinus bradycardia, cardiogenic shock, overt cardiac failure, greater than first-degree heart block, bronchial asthma, bronchospastic disease, or chronic bronchitis.

Use cautiously in patients with heart failure controlled by drug therapy, diabetes, or history of bronchospastic disease.

Interactions

Oral calcium antagonists may enhance the hypotensive effects of beta-adrenergic blocking agents as well as predispose the patient to bradycardia and arrhythmias. *Clonidine* may cause paradoxical hypertension when combined with beta-adrenergic blocking agents. Also, beta blockers may enhance rebound hypertension when clonidine is withdrawn.

Beta-adrenergic blocking agents may alter the hypoglycemic response to *insulin* or *oral antidiabetic agents.* Monitor patient closely.

Beta blockers may enhance the "first dose" orthostatic hypotension seen with *doxazosin, prazocin,* and *terazocin.* Avoid the concomitant use of *reserpine* or *other catecholamine-depleting drugs.*

Penbutolol has been shown to increase the volume of distribution of *lidocaine* in normal patients, implying that it may increase the loading dose requirements in some patients.

Effects on diagnostic tests

Drug may interfere with glucose or insulin tolerance tests.

Adverse reactions

CNS: *dizziness,* headache, fatigue, insomnia, asthenia.
CV: chest pain, *bradycardia,* ***heart failure.***
GI: nausea, diarrhea, dyspepsia.
GU: impotence.
Respiratory: cough, dyspnea.
Skin: excessive diaphoresis.

Note: The potential for adverse effects associated with other beta blockers should be considered.

Overdose and treatment

Clinical signs of overdose may include bradycardia, bronchospasm, heart failure, and severe hypotension.

After emptying the stomach by lavage (for acute oral ingestion), administer symptomatic and supportive care. Bradycardia may be treated with atropine or cautious use of isoproterenol. Cardiac glycosides, glucagon hydrochloride, dobutamine, and diuretics may be useful in treating heart failure, and vasopressors (such as epinephrine or alpha-adrenergic agonists) may be used to counter severe hypotension. In refractory cases of hypotension, administration of glucagon hydrochloride may be useful. Treat bronchospasm with aminophylline or isoproterenol.

☑ Special considerations

Besides those relevant to all *beta-adrenergic blockers,* consider the following recommendations.
• Like other beta blockers, penbutolol may cause patients to exhibit hypersensitivity to catecholamines upon withdrawal.
• To discontinue drug, slowly taper dosage over a period of 1 to 2 weeks, especially in patients with ischemic heart disease. If symptoms of angina develop, immediately reinstitute therapy, at least temporarily, and take steps to control the patient's unstable angina.

Patient education

• Advise patient not to discontinue drug abruptly, because sudden withdrawal of other beta blockers has precipitated angina and MI.
• Tell patient to report adverse effects immediately, particularly slow heart rate, chest congestion, cough, wheezing, or shortness of breath from mild exertion.
• Teach patient about disease and therapy. Explain why it is important to continue taking drug, even when feeling well.
• Advise patient to report unpleasant adverse effects promptly.
• Inform patient to call before taking OTC medications.

Geriatric use

• Pharmacokinetic studies indicate no difference in plasma half-life in healthy elderly patients compared with patients on renal dialysis.

Pediatric use

• Safety and effectiveness in children have not been established.

Breast-feeding

• It is not known if penbutolol is excreted in breast milk. Use with caution in breast-feeding women.

penicillamine

Cuprimine, Depen

Pharmacologic classification: chelating agent
Therapeutic classification: heavy metal antagonist, antirheumatic
Pregnancy risk category NR

How supplied

Available by prescription only
Capsules: 125 mg, 250 mg
Tablets: 250 mg

Indications, route, and dosage

Wilson's disease

Adults: 250 mg P.O. q.i.d. 0.5 to 1 hour before meals and at least 2 hours after evening meal. Adjust dosage to achieve urinary copper excretion of 0.5 to 1 mg daily. Dosage over 2 g is seldom necessary.

Children: 20 mg/kg P.O. daily divided q.i.d. 0.5 to 1 hour before meals and at least 2 hours after evening meal. Adjust dosage to achieve a minimum urinary copper excretion of 0.5 to 1 mg daily.

Cystinuria

Adults: 250 mg P.O. daily in four divided doses, then gradually increasing dosage. Usual dosage, 2 g daily (range, 1 to 4 g daily). Adjust dosage to achieve urinary cystine excretion of less than 100 mg daily when renal calculi are present, or 100 to 200 mg daily when no calculi are present.

Children: 30 mg/kg daily P.O. divided q.i.d. 0.5 to 1 hour before meals and at least 2 hours after evening meal. Adjust dosage to achieve urinary cystine excretion of less than 100 mg daily when renal calculi are present, or 100 to 200 mg daily when no calculi are present.

Rheumatoid arthritis, ◇ Felty's syndrome

Adults: Initially, 125 to 250 mg P.O. daily, with increases of 125 to 250 mg daily at 1- to 3-month intervals if necessary. Maximum dosage is 1.5 g daily.

◇ Adjunctive treatment of heavy metal poisoning

Adults: 500 to 1,500 mg P.O. daily for 1 to 2 months.

Children: 30 to 40 mg/kg or 600 to 750 mg/m² P.O. daily for 1 to 6 months.

◇ Primary biliary cirrhosis

Adults: Initially, 250 mg P.O. daily, with increases of 250 mg q 2 weeks. Maximum dosage, 1 g daily in divided doses.

Pharmacodynamics

Antirheumatic action: Mechanism of action in rheumatoid arthritis is unknown; penicillamine depresses circulating IgM rheumatoid factor (but not total circulating immunoglobulin levels) and depresses T-cell but not B-cell activity. It also depolymerizes some macroglobulins (for example, rheumatoid factor).

Chelating agent: Penicillamine forms stable, soluble complexes with copper, iron, mercury, lead, and other heavy metals that are excreted in urine; it is particularly useful in chelating copper in patients with Wilson's disease. Penicillamine also combines with cystine to form a complex more soluble than cystine alone, thereby reducing free cystine below the level of urinary stone formation.

Pharmacokinetics

- *Absorption:* Drug is well absorbed after oral administration; peak serum levels occur at 1 hour.
- *Distribution:* Limited data available.
- *Metabolism:* Metabolized by liver to inactive compounds.
- *Excretion:* Only small amounts of penicillamine are excreted unchanged; after 24 hours, about 50% of drug is excreted in urine and about 50% in feces.

Contraindications and precautions

Contraindicated in patients with known hypersensitivity to drug, history of penicillamine-related aplastic anemia or agranulocytosis, or significant renal or hepatic insufficiency; in pregnant women; and in patients receiving gold salts, immunosuppressants, antimalarials, or phenylbutazone because of the increased risk of serious hematologic effects.

Use cautiously in patients allergic to penicillin (cross reaction is rare); in those who receive a second course of therapy and who may have become sensitized and are more likely to have allergic reactions; and in patients who develop proteinuria not associated with Goodpasture's syndrome.

Interactions

Iron salts and *antacids* decrease absorption of penicillamine. *Gold therapy, antimalarial* or *cytotoxic* agents should not be given concurrently. Both are associated with serious hematologic and renal effects. *Digoxin* levels may be decreased when given concurrently.

Effects on diagnostic tests

Drug therapy may cause positive test results for antinuclear antibody with or without clinical systemic lupus erythematosus-like syndrome.

Adverse reactions

EENT: oral ulcerations, glossitis, cheilosis, tinnitus, optic neuritis.

GI: anorexia, nausea, vomiting, dyspepsia, diarrhea, dysgeusia, *hypogeusia.*

Hematologic: eosinophilia, leukopenia, ***thrombocytopenia, aplastic anemia, agranulocytosis,*** thrombotic thrombocytopenia, purpura, hemolytic anemia or iron deficiency anemia, lupus-like syndrome.

Hepatic: cholestatic jaundice, ***pancreatitis,*** hepatic dysfunction.

Skin: *pruritus; erythematous rash;* intensely pruritic rash with scaly, macular lesions on trunk; pemphigoid reactions; urticaria; ***exfoliative dermatitis;*** increased skin friability; purpuric or vesicular ecchymoses; wrinkling.

Other: *proteinuria,* arthralgia, lymphadenopathy, pneumonitis, alteration in sense of taste (salty and sweet), metallic taste, Goodpasture's syndrome, alopecia, drug fever, thyroiditis, myasthenia gravis (with prolonged use).

Note: Discontinue drug if patient has signs of hypersensitivity or drug fever, usually in conjunction with other allergic manifestations (if Wilson's disease, may rechallenge); or if the following occur: rash developing 6 months or more after start of therapy; pemphigoid reaction; hematuria or proteinuria with hemoptysis or pulmonary infiltrates; gross or persistent microscopic hematuria or proteinuria greater than 2 g/day in patients with rheumatoid arthritis; platelet count below 100,000/mm³ or leukocyte count below 3,500/mm³, or if either shows three consecutive decreases (even within normal range).

Overdose and treatment

There are no reports of significant drug overdose. Induce emesis unless unconscious or gag reflex is absent; otherwise empty stomach by gastric lavage and then administer activated charcoal and sorbitol. Thereafter, treat supportively. Treat seizures with diazepam (or pyridoxine if previously successful). Hemodialysis will remove penicillamine.

☑ Special considerations

- Perform urinalyses, CBC including differential blood count every 2 weeks for 4 to 6 months, then monthly; kidney and liver functions studies also should be performed, usually every 6 months. Report fever or allergic reactions (rash, joint pain, easy bruising) immediately. Check routinely for proteinuria, and handle patient carefully to avoid skin damage.
- About one third of patients receiving drug experience an allergic reaction. Monitor patient for signs and symptoms of allergic reaction.
- Patients with Wilson's disease or cystinuria may require daily pyridoxine (vitamin B_6) supplementation.
- Prescribe drug to be taken 1 hour before or 2 hours after meals or other medications to facilitate absorption.
- For initial treatment of Wilson's disease, 10 to 40 mg of sulfurated potash should be administered with each meal during penicillamine therapy for 6 months to 1 year, then discontinued.
- Drug also has been used to treat lead poisoning and primary biliary cirrhosis.

Patient education

- Provide health education for patients with Wilson's disease, rheumatoid arthritis, or cystinuria; explain disease process and rationale for therapy and explain that clinical results may not be evident for 3 months.
- Encourage patient compliance with therapy and follow-up visits.
- Stress importance of immediate reporting of fever, chills, sore throat, bruising, bleeding, or allergic reaction.
- Tell patient to take drug on an empty stomach 30 minutes to 1 hour before meals or 2 hours after ingesting food, antacids, mineral supplements, vitamins, or other medications. Tell patient to drink large amounts of water, especially at night.
- Advise patient receiving drug for rheumatoid arthritis that an exacerbation of disease may occur during therapy. This usually can be controlled by the concomitant administration of NSAIDs.
- Advise patient taking penicillamine for Wilson's disease to maintain a low-copper (less than 2 mg daily) diet by excluding foods with high copper content, such as chocolate, nuts, liver, and broccoli. Also, sulfurated potash may be administered with meals to minimize copper absorption.

Geriatric use

- Lower doses may be indicated. Monitor renal and hepatic function closely.

Pediatric use

- Check for possible iron deficiency resulting from chronic use. Safety and efficacy of penicillamine in juvenile rheumatoid arthritis have not yet been established in children.

Breast-feeding

- Safety has not been established in breast-feeding; alternative feeding method is recommended during therapy.

penicillin G benzathine

Bicillin L-A, Megacillin Suspension*, Permapen

penicillin G potassium

Pfizerpen

penicillin G procaine

Ayercillin*, Bicillin C-R, Crysticillin A.S., Pfizerpen-AS, Wycillin

penicillin G sodium

Pharmacologic classification: natural penicillin
Therapeutic classification: antibiotic
Pregnancy risk category B

How supplied

Available by prescription only
penicillin G benzathine
Suspension: 250,000 units/5 ml*; 500,000 units/ml*
Injection: 300,000 units/ml; 600,000 units/ml; 1.2 million units/2 ml; 2.4 million units/4 ml
penicillin G potassium
Powder for injection: 1 million units, 5 million units, 10 million units, 20 million units
Injection (premixed, frozen): 1 million units/50 ml, 2 million units/50 ml, 3 million units/50 ml
penicillin G procaine
Injection: 300,000 units/ml; 500,000 units/ml; 600,000 units/ml
penicillin G sodium
Powder for injection: 1 million units*, 5 million units, 10 million units*

Indications, route, and dosage

Congenital syphilis
penicillin G benzathine
Children under age 2: 50,000 units/kg I.M. as a single dose.
Group A streptococcal upper respiratory infections, ◇ diphtheria, ◇ yaws, pinta, and bejel
penicillin G benzathine
Adults: 1.2 million units I.M. in a single injection.
Children who weigh 59 lb (27 kg) or more: 900,000 units I.M. in a single injection.
Children under 59 lb: 300,000 to 600,000 units I.M. in a single injection.
Prophylaxis of poststreptococcal rheumatic fever
penicillin G benzathine
Adults and children: 1.2 million units I.M. once monthly or 600,000 units twice monthly.
Syphilis of less than 1 year's duration
penicillin G benzathine
Adults: 2.4 million units I.M. in a single dose.

* Canada only ◇ Unlabeled clinical use

Syphilis of more than 1 year's duration
penicillin G benzathine
Adults: 2.4 million units I.M. weekly for 3 successive weeks.
Moderate to severe systemic infections
penicillin G potassium, sodium
Adults: 12 to 24 million units I.M. or I.V. daily, given in divided doses q 4 hours.
Children: 25,000 to 300,000 units/kg I.M. or I.V. daily, given in divided doses q 4 hours.
Moderate to severe systemic infections, pneumococcal pneumonia
penicillin G procaine
Adults: 600,000 to 1.2 million units I.M. daily as a single dose or q 6 to 12 hours.
Children: 300,000 units I.M. daily as a single dose.
Uncomplicated gonorrhea
penicillin G procaine
Adults and children over age 12: 1 g probenecid, then 30 minutes later, 4.8 million units of penicillin G procaine I.M., divided into two injection sites.
✦ ***Dosage adjustment.*** In patients with renal failure, refer to following dosing chart.

Creatinine clearance (ml/min)	Dosage (after full loading dose)
10 to 50	50% of usual dose q 4 to 5 hr; or, give usual dose q 8 to 12 hr
< 10	50% of usual dose q 8 to 12 hr; or, give usual dose q 12 to 18 hr

Pharmacodynamics
Antibiotic action: Penicillin G is bactericidal; it adheres to penicillin-binding proteins, thus inhibiting bacterial cell wall synthesis. Penicillin G's spectrum of activity includes most nonpenicillinase-producing strains of gram-positive and gram-negative aerobic cocci; spirochetes; and some gram-positive aerobic and anaerobic bacilli.

Pharmacokinetics
Penicillin G is available as four salts, each having the same bactericidal action, but designed to offer greater oral stability (potassium salt) or to prolong duration of action by slowing absorption after I.M. injection (benzathine and procaine salts).
• *Absorption:* Oral—penicillins are hydrolyzed by gastric acids; only 15% to 30% of an oral dose of penicillin G potassium is absorbed; the remainder is hydrolyzed by gastric secretions. Peak serum concentrations of penicillin G potassium occur at 30 minutes. Food in stomach reduces rate and extent of absorption. Penicillin V is absorbed better after oral administration than penicillin G potassium.

I.M.—sodium and potassium salts of penicillin G are absorbed rapidly after I.M. injection; peak serum concentrations occur within 15 to 30 minutes. Absorption of other salts is slower. Peak serum concentrations of penicillin G procaine occur at 1 to 4 hours, with drug detectable in serum for 1 to 2 days; peak serum concentrations of penicillin G benzathine occur at 13 to 24 hours, with serum concentrations detectable for 1 to 4 weeks.
• *Distribution:* Penicillin G is distributed widely into synovial, pleural, pericardial, and ascitic fluids and bile, and into liver, skin, lungs, kidneys, muscle, intestines, tonsils, maxillary sinuses, saliva, and erythrocytes. CSF penetration is poor but is enhanced in patients with inflamed meninges. Pencillin G crosses the placenta; it is 45% to 68% protein-bound.
• *Metabolism:* Between 16% and 30% of an I.M. dose of penicillin G is metabolized to inactive compounds.
• *Excretion:* Penicillin G is excreted primarily in urine by tubular secretion; 20% to 60% of dose is recovered in 6 hours. Some drug is excreted in breast milk. Elimination half-life in adults is about ½ to 1 hour. Severe renal impairment prolongs half-life; penicillin G is removed by hemodialysis and is only minimally removed by peritoneal dialysis.

Contraindications and precautions
Contraindicated in patients with hypersensitivity to drug or other penicillins. Use cautiously in patients with drug allergies (especially to cephalosporins or imipenem). Penicillin G potassium is contraindicated in patients with renal failure.

Interactions
Concomitant use with *aminoglycosides* produces synergistic therapeutic effects, chiefly against enterococci; this combination is most effective in enterococcal bacterial endocarditis. However, drugs are physically and chemically incompatible and are inactivated when mixed or given together. In vivo inactivation has been reported when aminoglycosides and penicillins are used concomitantly.

Probenecid blocks tubular secretion of penicillin, raising its serum concentrations. Concomitant use of penicillin G with *clavulanate* appears to enhance effect of penicillin G against certain beta-lactamase-producing bacteria.

Large doses of penicillin may interfere with renal tubular secretion of *methotrexate*, thus delaying elimination and elevating serum concentrations of methotrexate.

Concomitant use of penicillin G with some *NSAIDs* prolongs penicillin half-life by competition for urinary excretion or displacement of penicillin from protein-binding sites; similarly, concomitant use with *sulfinpyrazone*, which inhibits tubular secretion of penicillin G, also prolongs its half-life.

Concomitant use of parenteral penicillin G potassium with *potassium-sparing diuretics* may cause hyperkalemia. Penicillins may decrease effectiveness of *oral contraceptives*.

Effects on diagnostic tests
Penicillin G alters test results for urine and serum protein levels; it interferes with turbidimetric methods using sulfosalicylic acid, trichloracetic acid, acetic acid, and nitric acid. Penicillin G does not interfere with tests using bromophenol blue (Albustix, Albutest, Multistix).

Penicillin G alters urine glucose testing using cupric sulfate (Benedict's reagent); use Diastix,

Chemstrip uG, or glucose enzymatic test strip instead. Penicillin G may cause falsely elevated results of urine specific gravity tests in patients with low urine output and dehydration, and falsely elevated Norymberski and Zimmermann test results for 17-ketogenic steroids; it causes false-positive CSF protein test results (Folin-Ciocalteau method) and may cause positive Coombs' test results.

Penicillin G may falsely decrease serum aminoglycoside concentrations. Adding beta-lactamase to the sample inactivates the penicillin, rendering the assay more accurate. Alternatively, the sample can be spun down and frozen immediately after collection.

Adverse reactions

CNS: neuropathy, ***seizures*** (with high doses), lethargy, hallucinations, anxiety, confusion, agitation, depression, dizziness, fatigue.
GI: nausea, vomiting, enterocolitis, pseudomembranous colitis.
GU: interstitial nephritis, nephropathy.
Hematologic: eosinophilia, hemolytic anemia, ***thrombocytopenia,*** leukopenia, anemia, ***agranulocytosis.***
Other: hypersensitivity reactions (maculopapular and ***exfoliative dermatitis,*** chills, fever, edema, ***anaphylaxis***), pain and sterile abscess at injection site; overgrowth of nonsusceptible organisms (with penicillin G potassium and procaine); possible severe potassium poisoning with high doses (hyperreflexia, ***seizures, coma***), thrombophlebitis (with penicillin G potassium only).

Overdose and treatment

Clinical signs of overdose include neuromuscular irritability or seizures. No specific recommendations available. Treatment is supportive. After recent ingestion (within 4 hours), empty stomach by induced emesis or gastric lavage. Follow with activated charcoal to decrease absorption. Penicillin G can be removed by hemodialysis.

☑ Special considerations

Besides those relevant to all *penicillins,* consider the following recommendations.

- Give oral drug on empty stomach for maximum drug absorption because food may interfere with absorption; follow drug only with water because acid in citrus juices and carbonated beverages impairs absorption.
- Monitor closely for possible hypernatremia with sodium salt or hyperkalemia with potassium salt.
- Patients with poor renal function are predisposed to high blood concentrations, which may cause seizures. Monitor renal function.
- Have emergency equipment on hand to manage possible anaphylaxis.
- Because penicillins are dialyzable, patients undergoing hemodialysis may need dosage adjustments.
- Administer by deep I.M. injection in upper outer quadrant of buttock. In infants and small children, use the midlateral aspect of thigh.
- Drug can be administered as a continuous infusion for meningitis.

Geriatric use

- Half-life is prolonged in elderly patients because of impaired renal function.

Breast-feeding

- Drug is excreted in breast milk; use in breast-feeding women may sensitize infant to penicillin.

penicillin V

penicillin V potassium

Betapen-VK, Ledercillin VK, Nadopen-V*, Pen Vee K, PVF K*, Robicillin VK, V-Cillin K, Veetids

Pharmacologic classification: natural penicillin
Therapeutic classification: antibiotic
Pregnancy risk category B

How supplied

Available by prescription only
penicillin V
Tablets: 125 mg, 250 mg, 500 mg
Solution: 125 mg/5 ml, 250 mg/5 ml (after reconstitution)
penicillin V potassium
Tablets: 125 mg, 250 mg, 500 mg
Tablets (film-coated): 250 mg, 500 mg
Solution: 125 mg/5 ml, 250 mg/5 ml (after reconstitution)

Indications, route, and dosage

Mild to moderate susceptible infections
Adults and children age 12 and over: 125 to 500 mg (200,000 to 800,000 units) P.O. q 6 hours.
Children age 1 month to 12 years: 15 to 50 mg/kg (25,000 to 90,000 units/kg) P.O. daily, divided into doses given q 6 to 8 hours.
Endocarditis prophylaxis for dental surgery
Adults: 2 g P.O. 30 to 60 minutes before procedure, then 1 g 6 hours later.
Children under 66 lb (30 kg): Half the adult dose.
Necrotizing ulcerative gingivitis
Adults: 250 to 500 mg P.O. q 6 to 8 hours.
◇ ***Lyme disease***
Adults: 250 to 500 mg P.O. q.i.d. for 10 to 20 days.
◇ ***Prophylaxis for pneumococcal infection***
Adults: 250 mg P.O. b.i.d.
Children over age 5: 125 mg P.O. b.i.d.

Pharmacodynamics

Antibiotic action: Penicillin V is bactericidal; it adheres to penicillin-binding proteins, thus inhibiting bacterial cell wall synthesis. Penicillin V's spectrum of activity includes most nonpenicillinase-producing strains of gram-positive and gram-negative aerobic cocci; spirochetes; and some gram-positive aerobic and anaerobic bacilli.

Pharmacokinetics

- *Absorption:* Penicillin V has greater acid stability and is absorbed more completely than penicillin G after oral administration. About 60% to 75% of an oral dose of penicillin V is absorbed. Peak serum

concentrations occur at 60 minutes in fasting subjects; food has no significant effect.
• *Distribution:* Drug is distributed widely into synovial, pleural, pericardial, and ascitic fluids and bile, and into liver, skin, lungs, kidneys, muscle, intestines, tonsils, maxillary sinuses, saliva, and erythrocytes. CSF penetration is poor but is enhanced in patients with inflamed meninges. Penicillin V crosses the placenta; it is 75% to 89% protein-bound.
• *Metabolism:* Between 35% and 70% of a dose is metabolized to inactive compounds.
• *Excretion:* Excreted primarily in urine by tubular secretion; 26% to 65% of dose is recovered in 6 hours. Some drug is excreted in breast milk. Elimination half-life in adults is ½ hour. Severe renal impairment prolongs half-life.

Contraindications and precautions
Contraindicated in patients with hypersensitivity to drug or other penicillins. Use cautiously in patients with drug allergies (especially to cephalosporins or imipenem).

Interactions
Penicillin V may decrease efficacy of *estrogen-containing oral contraceptives*; breakthrough bleeding may occur.

Concomitant use with *aminoglycosides* produces synergistic therapeutic effects, chiefly against enterococci; however, drugs are physically and chemically incompatible and are inactivated when given together. In vivo inactivation has been reported when aminoglycosides and pencillins are used concomitantly.

Probenecid blocks tubular secretion of penicillin, resulting in higher serum concentrations of drug. Concomitant use of penicillin V with *sulfinpyrazone*, which inhibits tubular secretion of penicillin V, prolongs its half-life. Concomitant use with *some anticoagulants* and *heparin* can increase risk of bleeding.

Effects on diagnostic tests
Penicillin V alters test results for urine and serum protein levels; it interferes with turbidimetric methods using sulfosalicylic acid, trichloracetic acid, acetic acid, and nitric acid. Penicillin V does not interfere with tests using bromophenol blue (Albustix, Albutest, MultiStix). Penicillin V may falsely decrease serum aminoglycoside concentrations.

Adverse reactions
CNS: neuropathy.
GI: *epigastric distress,* vomiting, diarrhea, *nausea,* black "hairy" tongue.
GU: nephropathy.
Hematologic: eosinophilia, hemolytic anemia, leukopenia, ***thrombocytopenia.***
Other: hypersensitivity reactions (rash, urticaria, fever, laryngeal edema, ***anaphylaxis***), overgrowth of nonsusceptible organisms.

Overdose and treatment
Clinical signs of overdose include neuromuscular sensitivity or seizures. No specific recommendations are available. Treatment is supportive. After recent ingestion (within 4 hours), empty stomach by induced emesis or gastric lavage; follow with activated charcoal to reduce absorption.

☑ Special considerations
Besides those relevant to all *penicillins,* consider the following recommendations.
• Give oral dose 1 hour before or 2 hours after meals for maximum absorption.
• After reconstitution, oral solution is stable for 14 days if refrigerated.

Geriatric use
• Half-life may be prolonged in elderly patients because of impaired renal function.

Breast-feeding
• Penicillin V is excreted in breast milk; use in breast-feeding women may sensitize the infant to penicillins.

pentamidine isethionate
NebuPent, Pentam 300

Pharmacologic classification: diamidine derivative
Therapeutic classification: antiprotozoal
Pregnancy risk category C

How supplied
Available by prescription only
Injection: 300-mg vials
Solution for inhalation: 300 mg

Indications, route, and dosage
***Pneumonia caused by* Pneumocystis carinii**
Adults and children: 4 mg/kg I.V. or I.M. once a day for 14 to 21 days. As alternate dose in children, 150 mg/m^2 daily for 5 days, then 100 mg/m^2 for duration of therapy.
Prophylaxis against* Pneumocystis carinii *pneumonia (PCP) in persons at high risk for the disease
Adults: 300 mg by inhalation once q 4 weeks. Aerosol form of drug should be administered by the Respirgard II jet nebulizer.
◊ ***Prophylaxis against* Trypanosoma gambiense**
Adults: 4 mg/kg I.V. or I.M. usually q 3 to 6 months.
◊ ***Leishmaniasis***
Adults: 2 to 4 mg/kg I.V. or I.M. daily or every other day up to 15 doses.

Pharmacodynamics
Antiprotozoal action: Mechanism is unknown. However, pentamidine may work by inhibiting synthesis of RNA, DNA, proteins, or phospholipids. It may also interfere with several metabolic processes, particularly certain energy-yielding reactions and reactions involving folic acid. Drug's spectrum of activity includes *P. carinii* and *Trypanosoma* organisms.

Pharmacokinetics
• *Absorption:* Daily I.M. doses (4 mg/kg) produce surprisingly few plasma level fluctuations. Plasma

levels usually increase slightly 1 hour after I.M. injection. Little information exists regarding pharmacokinetics with I.V. administration. Absorption is limited after aerosol administration.
• *Distribution:* Pentamidine appears to be extensively tissue-bound. CNS penetration is poor. Extent of plasma protein-binding is unknown.
• *Metabolism:* Unknown.
• *Excretion:* Mostly excreted unchanged in the urine. Drug's extensive tissue-binding may account for its appearance in urine 6 to 8 weeks after therapy ends.

Contraindications and precautions
Contraindicated in patients with a history of an anaphylactic reaction to drug. Use cautiously in patients with hepatic or renal dysfunction, hypertension, hypotension, hypoglycemia, hypocalcemia, leukopenia, thrombocytopenia, or anemia.

Interactions
When used concomitantly, pentamidine may have additive nephrotoxic effects with *aminoglycosides, amphotericin B, capreomycin, cisplatin, colistin, methoxyflurane, polymyxin B,* and *vancomycin.*

Effects on diagnostic tests
BUN, serum creatinine, AST, and ALT levels may increase during pentamidine therapy.

Other abnormal findings may include hyperkalemia and hypocalcemia. Hypoglycemia may occur initially (possibly from stimulation of endogenous insulin release); later, hyperglycemia may result from direct pancreatic cell damage.

Adverse reactions
CNS: confusion, hallucinations, *fatigue, dizziness,* headache.
CV: *hypotension, ventricular tachycardia,* chest pain.
GI: nausea, metallic taste, decreased appetite, pharyngitis, vomiting, diarrhea, abdominal pain, anorexia, bad taste in mouth.
GU: *elevated serum creatinine,* ***acute renal failure.***
Hematologic: leukopenia, ***thrombocytopenia,*** anemia.
Hepatic: elevated liver function tests.
Respiratory: *cough, bronchospasm, shortness of breath,* pneumothorax.
Skin: *rash,* ***Stevens-Johnson syndrome.***
Other: ***hypoglycemia,*** hypocalcemia, *sterile abscess, pain or induration at injection site, congestion, night sweats, chills,* edema, myalgia.

Overdose and treatment
No information available.

☑ Special considerations
• Make sure patient is adequately hydrated before administering drug; dehydration may lead to hypotension and renal toxicity.
• I.V. infusion avoids risk of local reactions and proves as safe as I.M. injection when given slowly, over at least 60 minutes. To prepare drug for I.V. infusion, add 3 to 5 ml of sterile water for injection or D_5W to 300-mg vial to yield 100 mg/ml or 60 mg/ml, respectively. Withdraw desired dose and dilute further into 50 to 250 ml of D_5W; infuse over at least 60 minutes. Diluted solution remains stable for 48 hours.
• To prepare drug for I.M. injection, add 3 ml of sterile water for injection to 300-mg vial to yield 100 mg/ml. Withdraw desired dose and inject deep I.M.
• To minimize risk to hypotension, patient should be supine during I.V. administration. Because sudden, severe hypotension may develop after I.M. injection or during I.V. infusion, closely monitor blood pressure during infusion and several times thereafter until patient is stable.
• Keep emergency drugs and equipment (including emergency airway, vasopressors, and I.V. fluids) on hand.
• Monitor daily blood glucose, BUN, and serum creatinine levels.
• Monitor periodic electrolyte levels, CBC, platelet count, and liver function tests.
• Observe patient for signs and symptoms of hypoglycemia.
• When inhalation solution is used for prophylaxis against PCP, high-risk individuals include persons infected with HIV with a history of PCP; patients who have never had an episode of PCP but whose CD4+ T cells are below 20% of total lymphocytes, or whose CD4+ T-cell count is below 200/mm².
• To administer by inhalation, dilute dose in 6 ml of sterile water and deliver at 6 L/minute from a 50-p.s.i. compressed air source until reservoir is dry. Alternate delivery systems (other than the Respirgard II) are under investigation but are currently not recommended.
• Patients who develop wheezing or cough during pentamidine aerosol therapy may benefit by pretreatment (at least 5 minutes before pentamidine administration) with a bronchodilator.

pentazocine hydrochloride
Talwin*, Talwin-Nx (with naloxone hydrochloride)

pentazocine lactate
Talwin

Pharmacologic classification: narcotic agonist–antagonist, opioid partial agonist
Therapeutic classification: analgesic, adjunct to anesthesia
Controlled substance schedule IV
Pregnancy risk category NR (C for Talwin-Nx)

How supplied
Available by prescription only
Tablets: 50 mg
Injection: 30 mg/ml

Indications, route, and dosage
Moderate to severe pain
Adults: 50 to 100 mg P.O. q 3 to 4 hours, p.r.n. or around the clock. Maximum oral dosage, 600 mg daily. Or 30 mg I.M., I.V., or S.C. q 3 to 4 hours,

p.r.n. or around the clock. Maximum parenteral dosage, 360 mg daily. Doses above 30 mg I.V. or 60 mg I.M. or S.C. not recommended.

For patients in labor, give 30 mg I.M. or 20 mg I.V. in 2- to 3-hour intervals.

Pharmacodynamics

Analgesic action: Exact mechanism of action is unknown. It is believed to be a competitive antagonist at some receptors, and an agonist at others, resulting in relief of moderate pain.

Pentazocine can produce respiratory depression, sedation, miosis, and antitussive effects. It also may cause psychotomimetic and dysphoric effects. In patients with coronary artery disease, it elevates mean aortic pressure, left ventricular end-diastolic pressure, and mean pulmonary artery pressure. In patients with acute MI, I.V. pentazocine increases systemic and pulmonary arterial pressures and systemic vascular resistance.

Pharmacokinetics

• *Absorption:* Drug is well absorbed after oral or parenteral administration. However, orally administered drug undergoes first-pass metabolism in the liver and less than 20% of a dose reaches the systemic circulation unchanged. Bioavailability is increased in patients with hepatic dysfunction; patients with cirrhosis absorb 60% to 70% of drug. Onset of analgesia is 15 to 30 minutes, with peak effect at 15 to 60 minutes.
• *Distribution:* Drug appears to be widely distributed in the body.
• *Metabolism:* Metabolized in the liver, mainly by oxidation and secondarily by glucuronidation. Metabolism may be prolonged in patients with impaired hepatic function.
• *Excretion:* Duration of effect is 3 hours. There is considerable interpatient variability in its urinary excretion. Small amounts of drug are excreted in the feces after oral or parenteral administration.

Contraindications and precautions

Contraindicated in patients with hypersensitivity to drug or its components and in children under age 12. Use cautiously in patients with impaired renal or hepatic function, acute MI, head injury, increased intracranial pressure, or respiratory depression.

Interactions

If administered within a few hours of *barbiturates*, such as *thiopental*, pentazocine may produce additive CNS and respiratory depressant effects and, possibly, apnea.

Cimetidine may increase pentazocine toxicity, causing disorientation, respiratory depression, apnea, and seizures. Because data are limited, this combination is not contraindicated; however, be prepared to administer naloxone if toxicity occurs.

Reduced doses of pentazocine usually are necessary when drug is used concomitantly with *other CNS depressants (alcohol, narcotic analgesics, antihistamines, barbiturates, benzodiazepines, muscle relaxants, phenothiazines, sedative-hypnotics, tricyclic antidepressants),* because such use potentiates drug's respiratory and CNS depression, sedation, and hypotensive effects; use with general anesthetics also may cause severe CV depression.

Drug accumulation and enhanced effects may result from concomitant use with other drugs that are extensively metabolized in the liver *(digitoxin, phenytoin, rifampin).*

Patients who become physically dependent on drug may experience acute withdrawal syndrome if given high doses of a *narcotic agonist-antagonist* or a single dose of an antagonist. Use with caution, and monitor closely.

Effects on diagnostic tests

None reported.

Adverse reactions

CNS: *sedation,* visual disturbances, hallucinations, drowsiness, *dizziness, light-headedness,* confusion, *euphoria,* headache, syncope, psychotomimetic effects.
CV: circulatory depression, ***shock,*** hypertension.
EENT: dry mouth.
GI: *nausea, vomiting,* constipation.
GU: urine retention.
Respiratory: ***respiratory depression,*** dyspnea, apnea.
Skin: induration, nodules, sloughing, and sclerosis of injection site; diaphoresis; pruritus.
Other: hypersensitivity reactions ***(anaphylaxis)***, physical and psychological dependence, depression of WBCs.

Overdose and treatment

The signs of pentazocine hydrochloride overdose have not been defined because of a lack of clinical experience with overdosage. If overdose should occur, all supportive measures (oxygen, I.V. fluids, vasopressors) should be used as necessary. Mechanical ventilation should be considered. Parenteral naloxone is an effective antagonist for respiratory depression because of pentazocine.

☑ Special considerations

Besides those relevant to all *opioid (narcotic) agonist-antagonists,* consider the following recommendations.
• Tablets are not well absorbed.
• Do not mix in same syringe with soluble barbiturates.
• Pentazocine may obscure the signs and symptoms of an acute abdominal condition or worsen gallbladder pain.
• Drug may cause orthostatic hypotension in ambulatory patients. Have patient sit down to relieve symptoms.
• Drug possesses narcotic antagonist properties. May precipitate abstinence syndrome in narcotic-dependent patients.
• Talwin-Nx, the available oral pentazocine, contains the narcotic antagonist naloxone, which prevents illicit I.V. use.

Patient education

• Tell patient to report rash, confusion, disorientation, or other serious adverse effects.

• Warn patient that Talwin-Nx is for oral use only. Severe reactions may result if tablets are crushed, dissolved, and injected.
• Tell patient to avoid use of alcohol and other CNS depressants.

Geriatric use
• Lower doses are usually indicated for elderly patients, who may be more sensitive to the therapeutic and adverse effects of drug.

Pediatric use
• Use of drug is not recommended in children under age 12.

Breast-feeding
• It is unknown if drug occurs in breast milk; use with caution in breast-feeding women.

pentobarbital sodium
Nembutal

Pharmacologic classification: barbiturate
Therapeutic classification: anticonvulsant, sedative-hypnotic
Controlled substance schedule II (suppositories schedule III)
Pregnancy risk category D

How supplied
Available by prescription only
Elixir: 18.2 mg/5 ml
Capsules: 50 mg, 100 mg
Injection: 50 mg/ml, 1-ml and 2-ml disposable syringes; 2-ml, 20-ml, and 50-ml vials
Suppositories: 30 mg, 60 mg, 120 mg, 200 mg

Indications, route, and dosage
Sedation
Adults: 20 to 40 mg P.O. b.i.d., t.i.d., or q.i.d.
Children: 2 to 6 mg/kg P.O. daily in divided doses, to maximum of 100 mg/dose.
Insomnia
Adults: 100 mg P.O. h.s. or 150 to 200 mg deep I.M.; 120 to 200 mg P.R.
Children: 2 to 6 mg/kg I.M., up to maximum of 100 mg/dose. Or 30 mg P.R. (age 2 months to 1 year), 30 to 60 mg P.R. (age 1 to 4), 60 mg P.R. (age 5 to 12), 60 to 120 mg P.R. (age 12 to 14).
Preanesthetic medication
Adults: 150 to 200 mg I.M. or P.O. in two divided doses.
Anticonvulsant
Adults: Initially, 100 mg I.V.; after 1 minute additional doses may be given. Maximum dosage, 500 mg.
Children: 50 mg initially; after 1 minute additional small doses may be given until desired effect is obtained.

Pharmacodynamics
Sedative-hypnotic action: Exact cellular site and mechanism(s) of action are unknown. Pentobarbital acts throughout the CNS as a nonselective depressant with a fast onset of action and short duration of action. Particularly sensitive to this drug is the reticular activating system, which controls CNS arousal. Pentobarbital decreases both presynaptic and postsynaptic membrane excitability by facilitating the action of gamma-aminobutyric acid (GABA).

Anticonvulsant action: Pentobarbital suppresses the spread of seizure activity produced by epileptogenic foci in the cortex, thalamus, and limbic systems by enhancing the effect of GABA. Both presynaptic and postsynaptic excitability are decreased, and the seizure threshold is raised.

Pharmacokinetics
• *Absorption:* Absorbed rapidly after oral or rectal administration; onset of action, 10 to 15 minutes. Peak serum concentrations occur between 30 and 60 minutes after oral administration. After I.M. injection, the onset of action occurs within 10 to 25 minutes. After I.V. administration, the onset of action occurs immediately. Serum concentrations needed for sedation and hypnosis are 1 to 5 mcg/ml and 5 to 15 mcg/ml, respectively. After oral or rectal administration, duration of hypnosis is 1 to 4 hours.
• *Distribution:* Distributed widely throughout the body. Approximately 35% to 45% is protein-bound. Drug accumulates in fat with long-term use.
• *Metabolism:* Metabolized in the liver by penultimate oxidation.
• *Excretion:* 99% of pentobarbital is eliminated as glucuronide conjugates and other metabolites in the urine. Terminal half-life ranges from 35 to 50 hours. Duration of action is 3 to 4 hours.

Contraindications and precautions
Contraindicated in patients with hypersensitivity to barbiturates or porphyria or with severe respiratory disease when dyspnea or obstruction is evident. Use cautiously in elderly or debilitated patients and in those with acute or chronic pain, mental depression, suicidal tendencies, history of drug abuse, or impaired hepatic function.

Interactions
Pentobarbital may potentiate or add to CNS and respiratory depressant effects of other *sedative-hypnotics, alcohol, antidepressants, antihistamines, narcotics,* and *tranquilizers.*

Pentobarbital enhances the enzymatic degradation of *warfarin* and *other oral anticoagulants*; patients may require increased doses of the anticoagulants. Drug also enhances hepatic metabolism of some drugs, including *digitoxin* (not digoxin), *corticosteroids, oral contraceptives* and *other estrogens, theophylline* and *other xanthines,* and *doxycycline.* Pentobarbital impairs the effectiveness of *griseofulvin* by decreasing absorption from the GI tract.

Disulfiram, MAO inhibitors, and *valproic acid* decrease the metabolism of pentobarbital and can increase its toxicity. *Rifampin* may decrease pentobarbital levels by increasing hepatic metabolism.

Effects on diagnostic tests
Pentobarbital may cause a false-positive phentolamine test. Drug's physiologic effects may impair

the absorption of cyanocobalamin ^{57}Co; it may decrease serum bilirubin concentrations in neonates, epileptic patients, and patients with congenital nonhemolytic unconjugated hyperbilirubinemia. EEG patterns show a change in low-voltage, fast activity; changes persist for a time after discontinuation of therapy.

Adverse reactions

CNS: *drowsiness, lethargy, hangover,* paradoxical excitement in elderly patients, somnolence, syncope, hallucinations.
CV: bradycardia, hypotension.
GI: nausea, vomiting.
Hematologic: exacerbation of porphyria.
Respiratory: ***respiratory depression.***
Skin: rash, urticaria, **STEVENS-JOHNSON SYNDROME.**
Other: ***angioedema,*** physical and psychological dependence.

Overdose and treatment

Clinical manifestations of overdose include unsteady gait, slurred speech, sustained nystagmus, somnolence, confusion, respiratory depression, pulmonary edema, areflexia, and coma. Typical shock syndrome with tachycardia and hypotension may occur. Jaundice, hypothermia followed by fever, and oliguria also may occur. Serum concentrations greater than 10 mcg/ml may produce profound coma; concentrations greater than 30 mcg/ml may be fatal.

To treat, maintain and support ventilation and pulmonary function as necessary; support cardiac function and circulation with vasopressors and I.V. fluids, as needed. If patient is conscious and gag reflex is intact, induce emesis (if ingestion was recent) by administering ipecac syrup. If emesis is contraindicated, perform gastric lavage while a cuffed endotracheal tube is in place to prevent aspiration. Follow with administration of activated charcoal or sodium chloride cathartic. Measure intake and output, vital signs, and laboratory parameters. Maintain body temperature.

Alkalinization of urine may be helpful in removing drug from the body. Hemodialysis may be useful in severe overdose.

☑ Special considerations

Besides those relevant to all *barbiturates,* consider the following recommendations.

- Reserve I.V. injection for emergency treatment. Be prepared for emergency resuscitative measures.
- Avoid I.V. administration at a rate exceeding 50 mg/minute to prevent hypotension and respiratory depression.
- High-dose therapy for elevated intracranial pressure may require mechanically assisted ventilation.
- Administer I.M. dose deep into large muscle mass. Do not administer more than 5 ml into any one site.
- Discard solution that is discolored or contains precipitate.
- Administration of full loading doses over short periods of time to treat status epilepticus will require ventilatory support in adults.
- To assure accuracy of dosage, do not divide suppositories.
- Drug has no analgesic effect and may cause restlessness or delirium in patients with pain.
- Nembutal tablets contain tartrazine dye, which may cause allergic reactions in susceptible persons.
- To prevent rebound of rapid-eye-movement sleep after prolonged therapy, discontinue gradually over 5 to 6 days.

Patient education

- Advise pregnant patient of potential hazard to fetus or neonate when taking pentobarbital late in pregnancy. Withdrawal symptoms can occur.
- Tell patient not to take drug continuously for longer than 2 weeks.
- Emphasize the dangers of combining drug with alcohol. An excessive depressant effect is possible even if drug is taken the evening before ingestion of alcohol.

Geriatric use

- Elderly patients usually require lower doses because of increased susceptibility to CNS depressant effects of pentobarbital. Confusion, disorientation, and excitability may occur in elderly patients. Use with caution.

Pediatric use

- Barbiturates may cause paradoxical excitement in children. Use with caution.

Breast-feeding

- Pentobarbital passes into breast milk. Do not administer to breast-feeding women.

pentostatin (2′-deoxycoformycin; DCF)

Nipent

Pharmacologic classification: antimetabolite (adenosine deaminase inhibitor)
Therapeutic classification: antineoplastic
Pregnancy risk category D

How supplied

Available by prescription only
Powder for injection: 10 mg/vial

Indications, route, and dosage

Alpha-interferon-refractory hairy cell leukemia
Adults: 4 mg/m² I.V. every other week.

Pharmacodynamics

Antileukemic action: Pentostatin inhibits the enzyme adenosine deaminase (ADA), causing an increase in intracellular levels of deoxyadenosine triphosphate. This increase leads to cell damage and death. Because ADA is most active in cells of the lymphoid system (especially malignant T cells), drug is useful in treating leukemias.

Pharmacokinetics

- *Absorption:* Time to achieve response, 2.9 to 24.1 months; duration of pharmacologic action is more than 1 week after a single dose.

• *Distribution:* Plasma protein-binding is low (about 4%); distribution half-life is about 11 minutes.
• *Metabolism:* Unknown.
• *Excretion:* Over 90% of drug is excreted in urine. Clearance depends on renal function; mean terminal half-life is about 6 hours in patients with normal renal function; increases to 18 hours or more in patients with renal impairment (creatinine clearance below 50 ml/minute).

Contraindications and precautions
Contraindicated in patients hypersensitive to drug.

Interactions
Concomitant use with *fludarabine* increases the risk of severe or fatal pulmonary toxicity. Don't use together. Concomitant use with *vidarabine* increases the incidence or severity of adverse effects associated with either drug.

Effects on diagnostic tests
None reported.

Adverse reactions
CNS: *headache, neurologic symptoms,* anxiety, confusion, depression, dizziness, insomnia, nervousness, paresthesia, somnolence, abnormal thinking, *fatigue.*
CV: **ARRHYTHMIAS,** abnormal ECG, thrombophlebitis, peripheral edema, **HEMORRHAGE.**
EENT: abnormal vision, conjunctivitis, ear pain, eye pain, epistaxis, pharyngitis, rhinitis, sinusitis.
GI: *nausea, vomiting, anorexia, diarrhea,* constipation, flatulence, stomatitis.
GU: hematuria, dysuria, increased BUN and creatinine levels.
Hematologic: ***myelosuppression,*** **LEUKOPENIA,** *anemia,* **THROMBOCYTOPENIA,** lymphadenopathy.
Hepatic: *elevated liver enzyme levels.*
Respiratory: *cough, bronchitis,* dyspnea, lung edema, pneumonia.
Skin: ecchymosis, petechiae, rash, eczema, dry skin, herpes simplex or zoster, maculopapular rash, vesiculobullous rash, pruritus, seborrhea, discoloration, diaphoresis.
Other: *fever,* **INFECTION,** *pain, hypersensitivity reactions, chills,* sepsis, ***death, neoplasm,*** chest pain, abdominal pain, back pain, flulike syndrome, asthenia, malaise, myalgia, arthralgia, weight loss.

Overdose and treatment
High dosage of pentostatin (20 to 50 mg/m² in divided doses over 5 days) has been associated with deaths from severe CNS, hepatic, pulmonary, and renal toxicity. No specific antidote is known. If overdosage occurs, treat symptoms and provide supportive care.

☑ Special considerations
• Use drug only in patients who have hairy cell leukemia refractory to alpha interferon (when disease progresses after a minimum of 3 months of treatment with alpha interferon or does not respond after 6 months of therapy).
• Optimal duration of therapy is unknown. Current recommendations call for two additional courses of therapy after a complete response. If patient hasn't had a partial response after 6 months of therapy, discontinue drug. If patient has had only a partial response, continue drug for another 6 months; if patient has had a complete response, continue for two courses of therapy.
• Store powder for injection in the refrigerator (36° to 46° F [2° to 8° C]). Reconstituted and diluted solutions should be used within 8 hours because drug contains no preservative.
• Follow appropriate guidelines for proper handling, administration, and disposal of chemotherapeutic agents. Treat all spills and waste products with 5% sodium hypochlorite solution. Wear protective clothing and polyethylene gloves. To prepare and administer: Add 5 ml sterile water for injection to the vial containing pentostatin powder for injection. Mix thoroughly to make a solution of 5 mg/ml. Administer drug by I.V. bolus injection, or dilute further in 25 or 50 ml of D_5W or 0.9% NaCl injection and infuse over 20 to 30 minutes.
• Be sure patient is adequately hydrated before therapy. Administer 500 to 1,000 ml of D_5W in 0.45% NaCl injection. Give 500 ml of D_5W after drug is given.
• Before therapy, assess renal function with a serum creatinine or creatinine clearance assay; repeat determinations periodically. Perform baseline and periodic determinations of CBC. Bone marrow aspirates and biopsies may be required at 2- to 3-month intervals to assess response to treatment.

Patient education
• Warn patient to avoid contact with infected persons.
• Tell patient to call immediately if signs of infection or unusual bleeding occur.

Pediatric use
• Safe use in children or adolescents has not been established.

Breast-feeding
• It is unknown if drug is excreted in breast milk. Because of the risk of serious toxicity to the breast-feeding infant, either the drug or breast-feeding should be discontinued.

pentoxifylline
Trental

Pharmacologic classification: xanthine derivative
Therapeutic classification: hemorrheologic
Pregnancy risk category C

How supplied
Available by prescription only
Tablets (extended-release): 400 mg

Indications, route, and dosage
Intermittent claudication from chronic occlusive vascular disease
Adults: 400 mg P.O. t.i.d. with meals.

Pharmacodynamics

Hemorrheologic action: Pentoxifylline improves capillary blood flow by increasing erythrocyte flexibility and reducing blood viscosity.

Pharmacokinetics

• *Absorption:* Drug is absorbed almost completely from the GI tract but undergoes first-pass hepatic metabolism. Absorption is slowed by food. Peak concentrations occur in 2 to 4 hours, but clinical effect requires 2 to 4 weeks of continuous therapy.
• *Distribution:* Unknown; drug is bound to erythrocyte membrane.
• *Metabolism:* Metabolized extensively by erythrocytes and the liver.
• *Excretion:* Metabolites are excreted principally in urine; less than 4% of drug is excreted in feces. Half-life of unchanged drug is about ½ to ¾ hour; half-life of metabolites is about 1 to 1½ hours.

Contraindications and precautions

Contraindicated in patients who are intolerant to methylxanthines, such as caffeine, theophylline, and theobromine, and in patients with recent cerebral or retinal hemorrhage. Use cautiously in elderly patients.

Interactions

Concomitant use of pentoxifylline and *antihypertensives* may increase hypotensive response; some patients taking pentoxifylline have had small decreases in blood pressure.

Although a causal relationship has not been proved, bleeding and prolonged PT have been reported in patients treated with pentoxifylline; patients taking *oral anticoagulants* (such as *warfarin*) or *drugs that inhibit platelet aggregation* with pentoxifylline may have bleeding abnormalities.

Effects on diagnostic tests

None reported.

Adverse reactions

CNS: headache, dizziness.
CV: angina, chest pain.
GI: dyspepsia, nausea, vomiting, flatus, bloating.

Overdose and treatment

Clinical signs of overdose include flushing, hypotension, seizures, somnolence, loss of consciousness, fever, and agitation. There is no known antidote. Empty stomach by gastric lavage and use activated charcoal; treat symptoms and support respiration and blood pressure.

☑ Special considerations

• Monitor blood pressure regularly, especially in patients taking antihypertensive agents; also monitor INR, especially in patients taking anticoagulants such as warfarin.
• If GI and CNS adverse effects occur, decrease dosage to twice daily. If adverse effects persist, drug should be discontinued.
• Drug is useful in patients who are not good candidates for surgery.
• Do not crush or break timed-release tablets; make sure patient swallows them whole.

Patient education

• Explain need for continuing therapy for at least 8 weeks; warn patient not to discontinue drug during this period without medical approval.
• Advise taking drug with meals to minimize GI distress.
• Tell patient to report GI or CNS adverse reactions; they may require dosage reduction.

Geriatric use

• Elderly patients may have increased bioavailability and decreased excretion of drug and, thus, are at higher risk for toxicity; adverse reactions may be more common in the elderly.

Pediatric use

• Safety and efficacy have not been established for patients under age 18.

Breast-feeding

• Pentoxifylline enters breast milk. Alternative feeding method is recommended during therapy.

pergolide mesylate

Permax

Pharmacologic classification: dopaminergic agonist
Therapeutic classification: antiparkinsonian
Pregnancy risk category B

How supplied

Available by prescription only
Tablets: 0.05 mg, 0.25 mg, 1 mg

Indications, route, and dosage

Adjunct to levodopa-carbidopa in the management of Parkinson's disease

Adults: Initially, 0.05 mg P.O. daily for first 2 days. Gradually increase dosage by 0.1 to 0.15 mg q third day over next 12 days of therapy. Subsequent dosage can be increased by 0.25 mg q third day until optimum response occurs. Mean therapeutic daily dose is 3 mg.

Drug is usually administered in divided doses t.i.d. Gradual reductions in levodopa-carbidopa dosage may be made during dosage titration.

Pharmacodynamics

Antiparkinsonian action: Pergolide stimulates dopamine receptors at both D_1 and D_2 sites. It acts by directly stimulating postsynaptic receptors in the nigrostriatal system.

Pharmacokinetics

• *Absorption:* Well absorbed after oral administration.
• *Distribution:* Pergolide is approximately 90% bound to plasma proteins.

• *Metabolism:* Metabolized to at least 10 different compounds, some of which retain some pharmacologic activity.
• *Excretion:* Primarily by the kidneys.

Contraindications and precautions
Contraindicated in patients hypersensitive to drug or to ergot alkaloids. Use cautiously in patients prone to arrhythmias.

Interactions
Concomitant use of drugs that are *dopamine antagonists,* including *butyrophenones, metoclopramide, phenothiazines,* and *thioxanthines* may antagonize the effects of pergolide.

Pergolide is extensively protein-bound; therefore, exercise caution if pergolide is coadministered with other *drugs known to affect protein binding.*

Effects on diagnostic tests
None reported.

Adverse reactions
CNS: headache, asthenia, *dyskinesia, dizziness, hallucinations, dystonia, confusion, somnolence,* insomnia, anxiety, depression, tremor, abnormal dreams, personality disorder, psychosis, abnormal gait, akathisia, extrapyramidal syndrome, incoordination, akinesia, hypertonia, neuralgia, speech disorder, twitching, paresthesia.
CV: *orthostatic hypotension,* vasodilation, palpitations, hypotension, syncope, hypertension, ***arrhythmias, MI.***
EENT: *rhinitis,* epistaxis, abnormal vision, diplopia, eye disorder.
GI: dry mouth, taste perversion, abdominal pain, *nausea, constipation,* diarrhea, dyspepsia, anorexia, vomiting.
GU: urinary frequency, urinary tract infection, hematuria.
Skin: rash, diaphoresis.
Other: flulike syndrome; chest, neck, and back pain; chills; infection; facial, peripheral, or generalized edema; weight gain; arthralgia; bursitis; myalgia; dyspnea; anemia.

Note: The preceding adverse reactions, although not always attributable to drug, occurred in more than 1% of the study population.

Overdose and treatment
One patient who intentionally ingested 60 mg presented with hypotension and vomiting. Other cases of overdose revealed symptoms of hallucinations, involuntary movements, palpitations, and arrhythmias.

Provide supportive treatment. Monitor cardiac function and protect the patient's airway. Antiarrhythmics and sympathomimetics may be necessary to support CV function. Adverse CNS effects may be treated with dopaminergic antagonists (such as phenothiazines). If indicated, gastric lavage or induced emesis may be used to empty the stomach of its contents. Orally administered activated charcoal may be useful in attenuating absorption.

☑ Special considerations
• In early clinical trials, 27% of patients who attempted pergolide therapy did not finish the trial because of adverse effects (primarily hallucinations and confusion).

Patient education
• Inform patient of potential for adverse effects. Warn patient to avoid activities that could expose him to injury secondary to orthostatic hypotension and syncope.
• Caution patient to rise slowly to avoid orthostatic hypotension, particularly at the beginning of therapy.

Pediatric use
• Safety has not been established.

Breast-feeding
• Safety has not been established.

permethrin
Elimite Nix

Pharmacologic classification: synthetic pyrethroid
Therapeutic classification: scabicide, pediculocide
Pregnancy risk category B

How supplied
Available by prescription only
Elimite
Cream: 5%
Available without a prescription
Nix
Liquid: 60 ml (1%)

Indications, route, and dosage
Pediculosis
Adults and children: Apply sufficient volume to saturate the hair and scalp. Allow to remain on the hair for 10 minutes before rinsing.
Scabies
Adults and children: Thoroughly massage into skin from head to soles of feet. Treat infants on the hairline, neck, scalp, temple, and forehead. Remove cream by washing after 8 to 14 hours. One application is curative.

Pharmacodynamics
Scabicide action: Permethrin acts on the parasites' nerve cell membranes to disrupt the sodium channel current and thereby paralyze them.

Pharmacokinetics
• *Absorption:* Not entirely investigated but probably less than 2% of the amount applied.
• *Distribution:* Systemic distribution is unknown.
• *Metabolism:* Rapidly metabolized by ester hydrolysis to inactive metabolites.
• *Excretion:* Metabolites are excreted in the urine. Residual persistence on the hair is detectable for up to 10 days.

Contraindications and precautions
Contraindicated in patients hypersensitive to pyrethrins or chrysanthemums.

Interactions
None reported.

Effects on diagnostic tests
None reported.

Adverse reactions
Skin: pruritus, *burning, stinging,* edema, tingling, numbness or scalp discomfort, mild erythema, scalp rash.

Overdose and treatment
With accidental ingestion, perform gastric lavage and use general supportive measures.

☑ Special considerations
- A single treatment is usually all that is necessary. Combing of nits is not required for effectiveness, but drug package supplies a fine-tooth comb for cosmetic use as desired.
- A second application may be necessary if lice are observed 7 days after the initial application.
- Permethrin has been shown to be at least as effective as lindane (Kwell) in treating head lice.

Patient education
- Tell patient or caregiver to wash hair with shampoo, rinse it thoroughly, and then towel dry.
- Tell patient or caregiver to apply sufficient volume to saturate the hair and scalp.
- Instruct patient to report itching, redness, or swelling of the scalp.
- Advise patient that drug is for external use only and to avoid contact with mucous membranes.

Pediatric use
- Safety and efficacy for use in children under age 2 have not been established.

Breast-feeding
- It is not known whether permethrin is excreted in breast milk. Consider discontinuing breast-feeding temporarily or not using the medication.

perphenazine
Apo-Perphenazine*, Trilafon

Pharmacologic classification: phenothiazine (piperazine derivative)
Therapeutic classification: antipsychotic; antiemetic
Pregnancy risk category NR

How supplied
Available by prescription only
Tablets: 2 mg, 4 mg, 8 mg, 16 mg
Oral concentrate: 16 mg/5 ml
Injection: 5 mg/ml

Indications, route, and dosage
Psychosis
Adults: Initially, 8 to 16 mg P.O. b.i.d., t.i.d., or q.i.d., increasing to 64 mg daily. Alternatively, administer 5 to 10 mg I.M.; change to P.O. as soon as possible.
Children over age 12: 6 to 12 mg P.O. daily in divided doses.
Mental disturbances, acute alcoholism, nausea, vomiting, hiccups
Adults and children over age 12: 5 to 10 mg I.M., p.r.n. Maximum dosage is 15 mg daily in ambulatory patients; 30 mg daily in hospitalized patients; or 8 to 16 mg P.O. daily in divided doses.

Perphenazine may be given slowly by I.V. drip at a rate of 1 mg/2 minutes with continuous blood pressure monitoring (rarely used). A maximum of 5 mg I.V. diluted to 0.5 mg/ml with 0.9% NaCl solution may be given for severe hiccups or vomiting. Extended-release preparation may be given 8 to 16 mg P.O. b.i.d. for outpatients; 8 to 32 mg P.O. b.i.d. for inpatients.

Pharmacodynamics
Antipsychotic action: Perphenazine is thought to exert its antipsychotic effects by postsynaptic blockade of CNS dopamine receptors, thus inhibiting dopamine-mediated effects; antiemetic effects are attributed to dopamine receptor blockade in the medullary chemoreceptor trigger zone. Perphenazine has many other central and peripheral effects: it produces both alpha and ganglionic blockade and counteracts histamine- and serotonin-mediated activity. Its most serious adverse reactions are extrapyramidal.

Pharmacokinetics
- *Absorption:* Rate and extent of absorption vary with administration route: oral tablet absorption is erratic and variable, with onset of action ranging from ½ to 1 hour; oral concentrate absorption is much more predictable. I.M. drug is absorbed rapidly.
- *Distribution:* Distributed widely into the body, including breast milk. Drug is 91% to 99% protein-bound. After oral tablet administration, peak effect occurs at 2 to 4 hours; steady-state serum levels are achieved within 4 to 7 days.
- *Metabolism:* Drug is metabolized extensively by the liver, but no active metabolites are formed.
- *Excretion:* Mostly excreted in urine via the kidneys; some in feces via the biliary tract.

Contraindications and precautions
Contraindicated in patients with hypersensitivity to drug; in patients experiencing coma; in those with CNS depression, blood dyscrasia, bone marrow depression, liver damage, or subcortical damage; and in those receiving large doses of CNS depressants.

Use cautiously in elderly or debilitated patients; in those with alcohol withdrawal, psychic depression, suicidal tendencies, adverse reaction to other phenothiazines, impaired renal function, respiratory disorders; and in patients receiving other CNS depressants or anticholinergics.

Interactions

Concomitant use of perphenazine with *sympathomimetics*, including *epinephrine, phenylephrine, phenylpropanolamine*, and *ephedrine* (commonly found in nasal sprays), and with *appetite suppressants* may decrease their stimulatory and pressor effects.

Phenothiazines can cause epinephrine reversal and a hypotensive response when *epinephrine* is used for its pressor effects.

Perphenazine may inhibit blood pressure response to *centrally acting antihypertensive drugs*, such as *clonidine, guanabenz, guanadrel, guanethidine, methyldopa*, and *reserpine*. Additive effects are likely after concomitant use of perphenazine with *CNS depressants*, including *alcohol, analgesics, barbiturates, narcotics, tranquilizers*, and *general, spinal*, or *epidural anesthetics*, or *parenteral magnesium sulfate* (oversedation, respiratory depression, and hypotension); *antiarrhythmic agents, disopyramide, quinidine*, and *procainamide* (increased incidence of arrhythmias and conduction defects); *atropine* or *other anticholinergic drugs*, including *antidepressants, antihistamines, MAO inhibitors, meperidine, phenothiazines*, and *antiparkinson agents* (oversedation, paralytic ileus, visual changes, and severe constipation); *nitrates* (hypotension); and *metrizamide* (increased risk of seizures).

Beta-blocking agents may inhibit perphenazine metabolism, increasing plasma levels and toxicity. Concomitant use with *propylthiouracil* increases risk of agranulocytosis; concomitant use with *lithium* may result in severe neurologic toxicity with an encephalitis-like syndrome, and a decreased therapeutic response to perphenazine.

Pharmacokinetic alterations and subsequent decreased therapeutic response to perphenazine may follow concomitant use with *phenobarbital* (enhanced renal excretion), *aluminum and magnesium-containing antacids* and *antidiarrheals* (decreased absorption), *caffeine*, or *heavy smoking* (increased metabolism).

Perphenazine may antagonize therapeutic effect of *bromocriptine* on prolactin secretion; it may also decrease vasoconstricting effects of *high-dose dopamine* and may decrease effectiveness and increase toxicity of *levodopa* (by dopamine blockade). Perphenazine may inhibit metabolism and increase toxicity of *phenytoin*.

Effects on diagnostic tests

Perphenazine causes false-positive test results for urinary porphyrins, urobilinogen, amylase, and 5-hydroxyindoleacetic acid because of darkening of urine by metabolites; it also causes false-positive urine pregnancy test results using human chorionic gonadotropin.

Perphenazine elevates test results for liver enzymes and protein-bound iodine and causes quinidine-like effects on the ECG.

Adverse reactions

CNS: *extrapyramidal reactions, tardive dyskinesia*, sedation, pseudoparkinsonism, EEG changes, dizziness, adverse behavioral effects, ***seizures,*** drowsiness.
CV: *orthostatic hypotension*, tachycardia, ECG changes, ***cardiac arrest.***
EENT: ocular changes, *blurred vision*, nasal congestion.
GI: *dry mouth, constipation*, nausea, vomiting, diarrhea, ileus.
GU: *urine retention*, dark urine, menstrual irregularities, gynecomastia, inhibited ejaculation.
Hematologic: leukopenia, galactorrhea, hyperglycemia, hypoglycemia, ***agranulocytosis,*** eosinophilia, ***hemolytic anemia, thrombocytopenia.***
Hepatic: jaundice, abnormal liver function test results.
Skin: *mild photosensitivity*, allergic reactions, pain at I.M. injection site, sterile abscess.
Other: weight gain, SIADH, ***neuroleptic malignant syndrome.***

After abrupt withdrawal of long-term therapy: gastritis, nausea, vomiting, dizziness, tremor, feeling of warmth or cold, diaphoresis, tachycardia, headache, insomnia.

Overdose and treatment

CNS depression is characterized by deep, unarousable sleep and possible coma, hypotension or hypertension, extrapyramidal symptoms, dystonia, abnormal involuntary muscle movements, agitation, seizures, arrhythmias, ECG changes, hypothermia or hyperthermia, and autonomic nervous system dysfunction.

Treatment is symptomatic and supportive, including maintaining vital signs, airway, stable body temperature, and fluid and electrolyte balance.

Do not induce vomiting: Drug inhibits cough reflex, and aspiration may occur. Use gastric lavage, then activated charcoal and sodium chloride cathartics; dialysis is usually ineffective. Regulate body temperature as needed. Treat hypotension with I.V. fluids: *Do not give epinephrine.* Treat seizures with parenteral diazepam or barbiturates; arrhythmias with parenteral phenytoin (1 mg/kg with rate titrated to blood pressure); and extrapyramidal reactions with benztropine at 1 to 2 mg or parenteral diphenhydramine at 10 to 50 mg.

☑ Special considerations

Besides those relevant to all *phenothiazines*, consider the following recommendations.

- Oral formulations may cause stomach upset; administer with food or fluid.
- Dilute the concentrate in 2 to 4 oz (60 to 120 ml) of liquid (water, carbonated drinks, fruit juice, tomato juice, milk, or puddings). Dilute every 5 ml of concentrate with 60 ml of suitable fluid.
- Liquid formulation may cause rash upon contact with skin.
- I.M. injection may cause skin necrosis; avoid extravasation.
- Administer I.M. injection deep into upper outer quadrant of buttocks. Massaging the injection site may prevent formation of abscesses.
- Do not administer drug for injection if it is excessively discolored or contains precipitate.

• Monitor blood pressure before and after parenteral administration.
• Shake oral concentrate before administration.

Patient education

• Explain the risks of dystonic reactions and tardive dyskinesia, and tell patient to report abnormal body movements.
• Instruct patient to avoid sun exposure and to wear sunscreen when going outdoors, to prevent photosensitivity reactions; and to avoid using sun lamps and tanning beds, which may cause burning of the skin or skin discoloration.
• Tell patient to avoid spilling the liquid; contact with skin may cause rash and irritation.
• Warn patient not to take extremely hot or cold baths and to avoid exposure to temperature extremes, sun lamps, or tanning beds; drug may cause thermoregulatory changes.
• Advise patient to take drug exactly as prescribed and not to double dose for missed doses.
• Inform patient that interactions with many other drugs are possible. Advise patient to seek medical approval before taking self-prescribed medication.
• Instruct patient not to stop taking drug suddenly; any adverse reactions may be alleviated by a dosage reduction. Patient should promptly report difficulty urinating, sore throat, dizziness, or fainting.
• Tell patient to avoid hazardous activities that require alertness until drug's effect is established. Reassure patient that sedative effects of drug should become tolerable in several weeks.
• Tell patient not to drink alcohol or take other medications that may cause excessive sedation.
• Explain which fluids are appropriate for diluting the concentrate (not apple juice or caffeine-containing drinks); explain dropper technique of measuring dose.
• Recommend sugarless hard candy or chewing gum, ice chips, or artificial saliva to relieve dry mouth.
• Tell patient not to crush or chew sustained-release form.

Geriatric use

• Use lower doses in elderly patients. Dose must be titrated to effects; 30% to 50% of the usual dose may be effective. Elderly patients are at greater risk for adverse effects, especially tardive dyskinesia and other extrapyramidal effects.

Pediatric use

• Drug is not recommended for children under age 12.

Breast-feeding

• Drug is widely distributed, including in breast milk; use with caution. Potential benefits to the mother should outweigh the potential harm to the infant.

phenazopyridine hydrochloride

Azo-Standard, Baridium, Eridium, Geridium, Phenazo*, Phenazodine, Pyridiate, Pyridium, Urodine, Urogesic

Pharmacologic classification: azo dye
Therapeutic classification: urinary analgesic
Pregnancy risk category B

How supplied

Available by prescription only
Tablets: 100 mg, 200 mg

Available without a prescription
Tablets: 95 mg

Indications, route, and dosage

Pain with urinary tract irritation or infection
Adults: 100 to 200 mg P.O. t.i.d.
Children age 6 to 12: 4 mg/kg t.i.d. for no more than 2 days.
Give drug after meals.

Pharmacodynamics

Analgesic action: Drug has a local anesthetic effect on urinary tract mucosa via an unknown mechanism.

Pharmacokinetics

• *Absorption:* Not described.
• *Distribution:* Traces of drug are thought to enter CSF and cross the placenta.
• *Metabolism:* Drug is metabolized in the liver.
• *Excretion:* Phenazopyridine is excreted by the kidneys; 65% is excreted unchanged in urine. Average time of total excretion of drug is 20.4 hours.

Contraindications and precautions

Contraindicated in patients with hypersenstivity to drug, glomerulonephritis, severe hepatitis, uremia, pyelonephritis during pregnancy, or renal insufficiency.

Interactions

None significant.

Effects on diagnostic tests

Drug may alter results of Diastix, Chemstrip uG, glucose enzymatic test strip, Acetest, and Ketostix. Clinitest should be used to obtain accurate urine glucose test results. Drug may also interfere with Ehrlich's test for urine urobilinogen; phenolsulfonphthalein excretion tests of kidney function; sulfobromophthalein excretion tests of liver function; and urine tests for protein, steroids, or bilirubin.

Adverse reactions

CNS: headache.
GI: nausea, GI disturbances.
Hematologic: hemolytic anemia.
Skin: rash, pruritus.
Other: ***anaphylactoid reactions,*** methemoglobinemia.

Overdose and treatment
Clinical manifestations of overdose include methemoglobinemia (most obvious as cyanosis), along with renal and hepatic impairment and failure.

To treat overdose of phenazopyridine, empty stomach immediately by inducing emesis with ipecac syrup or by gastric lavage. Administer methylene blue, 1 to 2 mg/kg I.V., or 100 to 200 mg ascorbic acid P.O. to reverse methemoglobinemia. Provide symptomatic and supportive measures (respiratory support and correction of fluid and electrolyte imbalances). Monitor laboratory parameters and vital signs closely. Contact local or regional poison information center for specific instructions.

☑ Special considerations
- Drug colors urine red or orange; it may stain fabrics.
- Use only as an analgesic.
- May be used with an antibiotic to treat urinary tract infections.
- Discontinue drug in 2 days with concurrent antibiotic use.

Patient education
- Instruct patient in measures to prevent urinary tract infection.
- Advise patient of possible adverse reactions; caution that drug colors urine red or orange and may stain clothing.
- Tell patient that stains on clothing may be removed with a 0.25% solution of sodium dithionate or hydrosulfite.
- Advise patient to take a missed dose as soon as possible and not to double doses.
- Instruct patient to report symptoms that worsen or do not resolve.

Geriatric use
- Use with caution in elderly patients because of possible decreased renal function.
- Administer with food or fluids to reduce GI upset.
- Evaluate response to medication therapy; assess urinary function, such as output, complaints of burning, pain, and frequency.
- Monitor vital signs, especially temperature.
- Encourage patient to force fluids (if not contraindicated). Monitor intake and output.

Breast-feeding
- Safe use in breast-feeding women has not been established

phenelzine sulfate
Nardil

Pharmacologic classification: MAO inhibitor
Therapeutic classification: antidepressant
Pregnancy risk category C

How supplied
Available by prescription only
Tablets: 15 mg

Indications, route, and dosage
Severe depression, ◊ ***panic disorder***
Adults: 15 mg P.O. t.i.d. Increase rapidly to 60 mg/day maximum daily dose, 90 mg. Onset of maximum therapeutic effect is 2 to 6 weeks. Some clinicians reduce dosage after response occurs; maintenance dosage may be as low as 15 mg daily or every other day.

Pharmacodynamics
Antidepressant action: Depression is thought to result from low CNS concentrations of neurotransmitters, including norepinephrine and serotonin. Phenelzine inhibits MAO, an enzyme that normally inactivates amine-containing substances, thus increasing the concentration and activity of these agents.

Pharmacokinetics
- *Absorption:* Drug is absorbed rapidly and completely from the GI tract.
- *Distribution:* Not yet determined.
- *Metabolism:* Hepatic.
- *Excretion:* Drug is excreted primarily in urine within 24 hours; some drug is excreted in feces via the biliary tract. Half-life is relatively short, but enzyme inhibition is prolonged and unrelated to half-life.

Contraindications and precautions
Contraindicated in patients with hypersensitivity to drug, heart failure, pheochromocytoma, hypertension, liver disease, and CV disease. Also contraindicated during therapy with other MAO inhibitors (isocarboxazid, tranylcypromine) or within 10 days of such therapy or within 10 days of elective surgery requiring general anesthesia, cocaine use, or local anesthesia containing sympathomimetic vasoconstrictors.Contraindicated within 2 weeks of SSRI antidepressant use. Contraindicated by some manufacturers in patients over age 60 because of possibility of existing cerebrosclerosis with damaged vessels.

Use cautiously in patients at risk for diabetes, suicide, or seizures disorders and in those receiving thiazide diuretics or spinal anesthesics.

Interactions
Phenelzine enhances pressor effects of *amphetamines, ephedrine, phenylephrine, phenylpropanolamine,* and related drugs and may result in serious CV toxicity; most *OTC cold, hay fever,* and *weight-reduction products* contain these drugs.

Concomitant use of phenelzine with *disulfiram* may cause tachycardia, flushing, or palpitations. Concomitant use with *general* or *spinal anesthetics,* which are normally metabolized by MAO, may cause severe hypotension and excessive CNS depression.

Phenelzine decreases effectiveness of *local anesthetics (procaine, lidocaine),* resulting in poor nerve block, and should be discontinued for at least 1 week before use of these agents. Concomittant use with *serotonergic drugs (fluoxetine, fluvoxamine, paroxetine, sertraline)* can result in serious adverse effects; at least a 2-week waiting period between drug use is recommended.

Use cautiously and in reduced dosage with *alcohol, barbiturates* and *other sedatives, dextromethorphan, narcotics,* and *tricyclic antidepressants.*

Concomitant use of phenelzine with foods high in *tryptophan, tyramine,* or *caffeine* may precipitate hypertensive crisis. Avoid concomitant use.

Effects on diagnostic tests
Phenelzine therapy elevates liver function test results and urinary catecholamine levels and may elevate WBC count.

Adverse reactions
CNS: *dizziness,* vertigo, headache, hyperreflexia, tremor, muscle twitching, *insomnia,* drowsiness, weakness, fatigue.
CV: postural hypotension, edema.
GI: dry mouth, *anorexia,* nausea, constipation.
Other: diaphoresis, weight gain, sexual disturbances.

Overdose and treatment
Signs of overdose include exacerbations of adverse reactions or exaggerated responses to normal pharmacologic activity; such symptoms become apparent slowly (within 24 to 48 hours) and may persist for up to 2 weeks. Agitation, flushing, tachycardia, hypotension, hypertension, palpitations, increased motor activity, twitching, increased deep tendon reflexes, seizures, hyperpyrexia, cardiorespiratory arrest, and coma may occur. Doses of 375 mg to 1.5 g have been ingested with fatal and nonfatal results.

Treat symptomatically and supportively: Give 5 to 10 mg phentolamine I.V. push for hypertensive crisis; treat seizures, agitation, or tremors with I.V. diazepam; tachycardia, with beta blockers; and fever, with cooling blankets. Monitor vital signs and fluid and electrolyte balance. Use of sympathomimetics (such as norepinephrine or phenylephrine) is contraindicated in hypotension caused by MAO inhibitors.

☑ Special considerations
Besides those relevant to all *MAO inhibitors,* consider the following recommendations.
- Consider the inherent risk of suicide until significant improvement of depressive state occurs. High-risk patients should have close supervision during initial drug therapy. To reduce risk of suicidal overdose, prescribe the smallest quantity of tablets consistent with good management.
- At start of therapy, patient should lie down for about 1 hour after taking phenelzine; to prevent dizziness from orthostatic blood pressure changes, patient should avoid sudden changes to standing position.
- Unlike that with other MAO inhibitors, combination therapy with phenelzine and tricyclic antidepressants is generally well tolerated.

Patient education
- Warn patient not to take alcohol, other CNS depressants, or self-prescribed medications (such as cold, hay fever, or diet preparations) without medical approval.
- Explain that many foods and beverages (such as wine, beer, cheeses, preserved fruits, meats, and vegetables) may interact with drug. A list of foods to avoid can usually be obtained from the dietary department or pharmacy at most hospitals.
- Tell patient to avoid hazardous activities that require alertness until drug's full effect on the CNS is known. Suggest taking drug at bedtime to minimize daytime sedation.
- Instruct patient to take drug exactly as prescribed and not to double dose if a dose is missed.
- Tell patient not to discontinue drug abruptly and to report any problems; dosage reduction can relieve most adverse reactions.

Geriatric use
- Drug is not recommended for patients over age 60.

Pediatric use
- Drug is not recommended for children under age 16.

phenobarbital
Barbita, Solfoton

phenobarbital sodium
Luminal

Pharmacologic classification: barbiturate
Therapeutic classification: anticonvulsant, sedative-hypnotic
Controlled substance schedule IV
Pregnancy risk category D

How supplied
Available by prescription only
Tablets: 8 mg, 15 mg, 16 mg, 30 mg, 32 mg, 60 mg, 65 mg, 100 mg
Capsules: 15 mg, 16 mg
Oral solution: 15 mg/5 ml; 20 mg/5 ml
Elixir: 20 mg/5 ml
Injection: 30 mg/ml, 60 mg/ml, 65 mg/ml, 130 mg/ml
Powder for injection: 120 mg/ampule

Indications, route, and dosage
All forms of epilepsy except absence seizures, febrile seizures in children
Adults: 60 to 100 mg P.O. daily, divided t.i.d. or given as single dose h.s. Alternatively, give 200 to 300 mg I.M. or I.V. and repeat q 6 hours p.r.n.
Children: 1 to 6 mg/kg P.O. daily, usually divided q 12 hours. It can, however, be administered once daily. Alternatively, give 4 to 6 mg/kg I.V. or I.M. daily and monitor patient's blood levels.
Status epilepticus
Adults and children: 10 to 20 mg/kg I.V. over 10 to 15 minutes. Repeat if necessary.
Sedation
Adults: 30 to 120 mg P.O., I.M., or I.V. daily in two or three divided doses.
Children: 8 to 32 mg P.O. daily.
Insomnia
Adults: 100 to 200 mg P.O. or 100 to 320 mg I.M.

Preoperative sedation
Adults: 100 to 200 mg I.M. 60 to 90 minutes before surgery.
Children: 1 to 3 mg/kg I.V. or I.M. 60 to 90 minutes before surgery.

Pharmacodynamics

Anticonvulsant action: Phenobarbital suppresses the spread of seizure activity produced by epileptogenic foci in the cortex, thalamus, and limbic systems by enhancing the effect of gamma-aminobutyric acid (GABA). Both presynaptic and postsynaptic excitability are decreased; also, phenobarbital raises the seizure threshold.

Sedative-hypnotic action: Phenobarbital acts throughout the CNS as a nonselective depressant with a slow onset of action and a long duration of action. Particularly sensitive to this drug is the reticular activating system, which controls CNS arousal. Phenobarbital decreases both presynaptic and postsynaptic membrane excitability by facilitating the action of GABA. The exact cellular site and mechanism(s) of action are unknown.

Pharmacokinetics

- *Absorption:* Drug is well absorbed after oral and rectal administration, with 70% to 90% reaching the bloodstream. Absorption after I.M. administration is 100%. After oral administration, peak serum levels are reached in 1 to 2 hours, and peak levels in the CNS are achieved at 1 to 3 hours. Onset of action occurs 1 hour or longer after oral dosing; onset after I.V. administration is about 5 minutes. A serum concentration of 10 mcg/ml is needed to produce sedation; 40 mcg/ml usually produces sleep. Concentrations of 20 to 40 mcg/ml are considered therapeutic for anticonvulsant therapy.
- *Distribution:* Distributed widely throughout the body. Phenobarbital is approximately 25% to 30% protein-bound.
- *Metabolism:* Metabolized by the hepatic microsomal enzyme system.
- *Excretion:* 25% to 50% of a phenobarbital dose is eliminated unchanged in urine; remainder is excreted as metabolites of glucuronic acid. Drug's half-life is 5 to 7 days.

Contraindications and precautions

Contraindicated in patients with barbiturate hypersensitivity, history of manifest or latent porphyria, hepatic dysfunction, respiratory disease with dyspnea or obstruction, and nephritis.

Use cautiously in elderly or debilitated patients and in those with acute or chronic pain, depression, suicidal tendencies, history of drug abuse, blood pressure alterations, CV disease, shock, or uremia.

Interactions

Phenobarbital may add to or potentiate CNS and respiratory depressant effects of other *sedative-hypnotics, alcohol, antidepressants, antihistamines, narcotics, phenothiazines,* and *tranquilizers.*

Phenobarbital enhances the enzymatic degradation of *warfarin* and *other oral anticoagulants;* patients may require increased doses of the anticoagulant. Drug also enhances hepatic metabolism of some drugs, including *digitoxin* (not digoxin), *corticosteroids, oral contraceptives* and *other estrogens, theophylline* and *other xanthines,* and *doxycycline.*

Phenobarbital impairs the effectiveness of *griseofulvin* by decreasing absorption from the GI tract. *Disulfiram, MAO inhibitors,* and *valproic acid* decrease the metabolism of phenobarbital and can increase its toxicity. *Rifampin* may decrease phenobarbital levels by increasing hepatic metabolism.

Effects on diagnostic tests

Phenobarbital may cause a false-positive phentolamine test. The physiologic effects of drug may impair the absorption of cyanocobalamin ^{57}Co; it may decrease serum bilirubin concentrations in neonates, epileptics, and in patients with congenital nonhemolytic unconjugated hyperbilirubinemia. Barbiturates may increase sulfobromophthalein retention. EEG patterns show a change in low-voltage, fast activity; changes persist for a time after discontinuation of therapy.

Adverse reactions

CNS: *drowsiness, lethargy, hangover,* paradoxical excitement in elderly patients, somnolence.
CV: bradycardia, hypotension.
GI: nausea, vomiting.
Hematologic: exacerbation of porphyria.
Respiratory: ***respiratory depression, apnea.***
Skin: rash, ***erythema multiforme, Stevens-Johnson syndrome,*** urticaria; pain, swelling, thrombophlebitis, necrosis, nerve injury at injection site.
Other: ***angioedema,*** physical and psychological dependence.

Overdose and treatment

Clinical manifestations of overdose include unsteady gait, slurred speech, sustained nystagmus, somnolence, confusion, respiratory depression, pulmonary edema, areflexia, and coma. Typical shock syndrome with tachycardia and hypotension along with jaundice, oliguria, and chills followed by fever may occur.

Treatment is aimed at the maintenance and support of ventilation and pulmonary function as necessary; support of cardiac function and circulation with vasopressors and I.V. fluids as needed. If patient is conscious and gag reflex is intact, induce emesis (if ingestion was recent) by administering ipecac syrup. If emesis is contraindicated, perform gastric lavage while a cuffed endotracheal tube is in place to prevent aspiration. Follow with administration of activated charcoal or sodium chloride cathartic. Measure intake and output, vital signs, and laboratory parameters. Maintain body temperature.

Alkalinization of urine may be helpful in removing drug from the body; hemodialysis may be useful in severe overdose. Oral activated charcoal may enhance phenobarbital elimination regardless of its route of administration.

☑ Special considerations

Besides those relevant to all *barbiturates,* consider the following recommendations.

- Oral solution may be mixed with water or juice to improve taste.
- Do not crush or break extended-release form; this will impair drug action.
- Reconstitute powder for injection with 2.5 to 5 ml sterile water for injection. Roll vial in hands; do not shake.
- Use a larger vein for I.V. administration to prevent extravasation.
- Avoid I.V. administration at a rate exceeding 60 mg/minute to prevent hypotension and respiratory depression. It may take up to 30 minutes after I.V. administration to achieve maximum effect.
- Administer parenteral dose within 30 minutes of reconstitution because phenobarbital hydrolyzes in solution and on exposure to air.
- Keep emergency resuscitation equipment on hand when administering phenobarbital I.V.
- Administer I.M. dose deep into a large muscle mass to prevent tissue injury.
- Only parenteral solutions prepared from powder may be given S.C.; however, this route is not recommended.
- Do not use injectable solution if it contains a precipitate.
- Administration of full loading doses over short periods of time to treat status epilepticus will require ventilatory support in adults.
- Full therapeutic effects are not seen for 2 to 3 weeks, except when loading dose is used.

Patient education

- Advise patient of potential for physical and psychological dependence with prolonged use.
- Warn patient to avoid alcohol and other CNS depressants while taking drug. An excessive depressant effect is possible even if drug is taken the evening before ingestion of alcohol.
- Caution patient not to stop taking drug suddenly because this could cause a withdrawal reaction.
- Advise patient to avoid driving and other hazardous activities that require alertness until the adverse CNS effects of drug are known.

Geriatric use

- Elderly patients are more sensitive to drug's effects and usually require lower doses. Confusion, disorientation, and excitability may occur in elderly patients.

Pediatric use

- Paradoxical hyperexcitability may occur in children. Use with caution. Use of phenobarbital extended-release capsules is not recommended in children under age 12.

Breast-feeding

- Phenobarbital passes into breast milk; avoid administering to breast-feeding women.

phentermine hydrochloride

Adipex-P, Dapex, Fastin, Ionamin, Obe-Nix, Obermine, Parmine, Phentrol

Pharmacologic classification: amphetamine congener
Therapeutic classification: short-term adjunctive anorexigenic, indirect-acting sympathomimetic amine
Controlled substance schedule IV
Pregnancy risk category X

How supplied

Available by prescription only
Capsules and tablets: 8 mg, 15 mg, 18.75 mg, 30 mg, 37.5 mg
Capsules (resin complex, sustained-release): 15 mg, 30 mg, 37.5 mg

Indications, route, and dosage

Short-term adjunct in exogenous obesity
Adults: 8 mg P.O. t.i.d. ½ hour before meals; or 15 to 37.5 mg daily before breakfast; or 15 to 30 mg daily before breakfast (resin complex).

Pharmacodynamics

Anorexigenic action: Phentermine is an indirect-acting sympathomimetic amine; it causes fewer and less severe adverse reactions from CNS stimulation than do amphetamines, and its potential for addiction is lower. Anorexigenic effects are thought to follow direct stimulation of the hypothalamus; they may involve other CNS and metabolic effects.

Pharmacokinetics

- *Absorption:* Absorbed readily after oral administration; therapeutic effects persist for 4 to 6 hours.
- *Distribution:* Drug is distributed widely throughout the body.
- *Metabolism:* Unknown.
- *Excretion:* Excreted in urine.

Contraindications and precautions

Contraindicated in patients with hyperthyroidism, moderate to severe hypertension, advanced arteriosclerosis, symptomatic CV disease, glaucoma, or hypersensitivity or idiosyncrasy to sympathomimetic amines; within 14 days of MAO inhibitor therapy; and in agitated patients. Use cautiously in patients with mild hypertension.

Interactions

Concomitant use with *MAO inhibitors* (or *drugs with MAO-inhibiting effects*) or within 14 days of such therapy may cause hypertensive crisis. Phentermine may decrease hypotensive effects of *guanethidine* and *other antihypertensive agents;* it also may alter *insulin* requirements in diabetic patients. Concomitant use with excessive amounts of *caffeine* may cause additive CNS stimulation.

Concomitant use with *general anesthetics* may result in arrhythmias. *Acetazolamide, antacids,* and *sodium bicarbonate* increase renal reabsorption of phentermine and prolong its duration of action.

Haloperidol and *phenothiazines* decrease phentermine effects.

Effects on diagnostic tests

None reported.

Adverse reactions

CNS: overstimulation, headache, euphoria, dysphoria, dizziness, *insomnia.*
CV: *palpitations, tachycardia,* increased blood pressure.
GI: dry mouth, dysgeusia, constipation, diarrhea, other GI disturbances.
GU: impotence.
Skin: urticaria.
Other: altered libido.

Overdose and treatment

Signs and symptoms of acute overdose include restlessness, tremor, hyperreflexia, fever, tachypnea, dizziness, confusion, aggressive behavior, hallucinations, blood pressure changes, arrhythmias, nausea, vomiting, diarrhea, and cramps. Fatigue and depression usually follow CNS stimulation; seizures, coma, and death may follow.

Treat overdose symptomatically and supportively: sedation may be necessary. Chlorpromazine may antagonize CNS stimulation. Acidification of urine may hasten excretion. Monitor vital signs and fluid and electrolyte balance.

☑ Special considerations

- Intermittent courses of treatment (6 weeks on, followed by 4 weeks off) are equally effective as continuous use.
- Greatest weight loss occurs in the first weeks of therapy and diminishes in succeeding weeks. When such tolerance to drug effect develops, drug should be discontinued instead of increasing the dosage.
- Do not crush sustained-release dosage forms.
- Give morning dose 2 hours after breakfast.

Patient education

- Advise patient to take morning dose 2 hours after breakfast, not to crush or chew sustained-release products, and to avoid caffeine-containing drinks.
- Tell patient to take last daily dose at least 6 hours before bedtime to prevent insomnia.
- Warn patient not to take drug more frequently than prescribed.
- Advise patient that drug may produce dizziness, fatigue, or drowsiness.
- Tell patient to call if palpitations occur.
- Tell diabetic patients to closely monitor blood glucose. Results may require adjustment in eating habits, body weight, and activity and change in dosage of antidiabetic drug.

Pediatric use

- Phentermine is not recommended for children under age 12.

phentolamine mesylate

Regitine

Pharmacologic classification: alpha-adrenergic blocker
Therapeutic classification: antihypertensive for pheochromocytoma; cutaneous vasodilator
Pregnancy risk category C

How supplied

Available by prescription only
Injection: 5 mg/ml in 1-ml vials

Indications, route, and dosage

Aid for diagnosis of pheochromocytoma
Adults: 5 mg I.V. or I.M.
Children: 1 mg I.V., 3 mg I.M., or 0.1 mg/kg or 3 mg/m^2 I.V.
Control or prevention of paroxysmal hypertension immediately before or during pheochromocytomectomy
Adults: 5 mg I.M. or I.V. 1 to 2 hours preoperatively, repeated as necessary; 5 mg I.V. during surgery if indicated.
Children: 1 mg, 0.1 mg/kg, or 3 mg/m^2 I.M. or I.V. 1 to 2 hours preoperatively, repeated as necessary; 1 mg, 0.1 mg/kg, or 3 mg/m^2 I.V. during surgery if indicated
Prevention or treatment of dermal necrosis and sloughing of extravasation after I.V. administration of norepinephrine or ◇ dopamine
Adults and children: Inject 5 to 10 mg in 10 ml of 0.9% NaCl solution into the affected area, or add 10 mg to each liter of I.V. fluids containing norepinephrine
◇ ***Adjunctive treatment of left-sided heart failure secondary to acute MI***
Adults: 170 to 400 mcg/minute by I.V. infusion.
◇ ***Treatment adjunct for males with impotence (neurogenic or vascular)***
Adults: 0.5 to 1 mg by intracavernosal injection. Usually administered with 30 mg papaverine injection.
◇ ***Hypertensive crisis from sympathomimetic amines***
Adults: 5 to 15 mg I.V.

Pharmacodynamics

Antihypertensive action: Phentolamine competitively antagonizes endogenous and exogenous amines at presynaptic and postsynaptic alpha-adrenergic receptors, decreasing both preload and afterload.

Cutaneous vasodilation: Phentolamine blocks epinephrine- and norepinephrine-induced vasoconstriction.

Pharmacokinetics

- *Absorption:* Antihypertensive effect is immediate after I.V. administration.
- *Distribution:* Unknown.
- *Metabolism:* Unknown.
- *Excretion:* About 10% of a given dose is excreted unchanged in urine; excretion of remainder is

unknown. Drug has a short duration of action; plasma half-life is 19 minutes after I.V. administration.

Contraindications and precautions
Contraindicated in patients with angina, coronary artery disease, MI or history of MI, or hypersensitivity to drug. Use cautiously in patients with peptic ulcer or gastritis.

Interactions
Phentolamine antagonizes vasoconstrictor and hypertensive effects of *ephedrine* and *epinephrine.*

Effects on diagnostic tests
None reported.

Adverse reactions
CNS: *dizziness, weakness, flushing,* ***cerebrovascular occlusion,*** cerebrovascular spasm.
CV: *hypotension,* ***shock, arrhythmias,*** tachycardia, ***MI.***
EENT: *nasal congestion.*
GI: *diarrhea, nausea, vomiting.*

Overdose and treatment
Signs and symptoms of overdose include hypotension, dizziness, fainting, tachycardia, vomiting, lethargy, and shock.

Treat supportively and symptomatically. Use norepinephrine if necessary to increase the blood pressure. *Do not* use epinephrine; it stimulates both alpha and beta receptors and will cause vasodilation and a further drop in blood pressure.

☑ Special considerations
Besides those relevant to all *alpha-adrenergic blockers,* consider the following recommendations.
- Usual doses of phentolamine have little effect on the blood pressure of normal individuals or patients with essential hypertension.
- Before test for pheochromocytoma, have patient rest in supine position until blood pressure is stabilized. When phentolamine is administered I.V., inject dose rapidly after effects of the venipuncture on the blood pressure have passed. A marked decrease in blood pressure will be seen immediately, with the maximum effect seen within 2 minutes. Record blood pressure immediately after the injection, at 30-second intervals for the first 3 minutes, and at 1-minute intervals for the next 7 minutes. When drug is administered I.M., maximum effect occurs within 20 minutes. Record blood pressure every 5 minutes for 30 to 45 minutes after injection.
- A positive test response occurs when patient's blood pressure decreases at least 35 mm Hg systolic and 25 mm Hg diastolic; a negative test response occurs when the patient's blood pressure remains unchanged, is elevated, or decreases less than 35 mm Hg systolic and 25 mm Hg diastolic.
- When possible, sedatives, analgesics, and all other medication should be withdrawn at least 24 hours (preferably 48 to 72 hours) before the phentolamine test; antihypertensive drugs should be withdrawn and test should not be performed until blood pressure returns to pretreatment levels; rauwolfia drugs should be withdrawn at least 4 weeks before test.
- Drug has been used to treat hypertension resulting from clonidine withdrawal and to treat the reaction to sympathetic amines or other drugs or foods in patients taking MAO inhibitors.
- Drug has also been used in patients with MI associated with left-sided heart failure in an attempt to reduce infarct size and decrease left ventricular ejection impedance. It also has been used to treat supraventricular premature contractions.

Patient education
- Teach patient about phentolamine test, if indicated.
- Tell patient to report adverse effects at once.
- Tell patient not to take sedatives or narcotics for at least 24 hours before phentolamine test.

Geriatric use
- Administer cautiously.

Pediatric use
- Administer cautiously.

Breast-feeding
- It is not known if drug occurs in breast milk; because of possible adverse reactions in the infant, discontinue either breast-feeding or drug depending on the importance of drug to patient.

phenylephrine hydrochloride
Nasal products
Allerest, Neo-Synephrine, Sinex

Parenteral
Neo-Synephrine

Ophthalmic
Ak-Dilate, Ak-Nefrin, Isopto Frin, Mydfrin, Neo-Synephrine, Prefrin Liquifilm

Pharmacologic classification: adrenergic
Therapeutic classification: vasoconstrictor
Pregnancy risk category C

How supplied
Available by prescription only
Injection: 10 mg/ml
Ophthalmic solution: 0.12%, 2.5%, 10%

Available without a prescription
Nasal solution: 0.125%, 0.16%, 0.25%, 0.5%, 1%
Nasal spray: 0.25%, 0.5%, 1%

Indications, route, and dosage
Hypotensive emergencies during spinal anesthesia
Adults: Initially, 0.1 to 0.2 mg I.V.; subsequent doses should also be low (0.1 mg).
Children: 0.5 to 1 mg/25 lb (11 kg) of body weight.

Prevention of hypotension during spinal or inhalation anesthesia
Adults: 2 to 3 mg S.C. or I.M. 3 to 4 minutes before anesthesia.
Mild to moderate hypotension
Adults: 1 to 10 mg S.C. or I.M. (initial dose should not exceed 5 mg). Additional doses may be given in 1 to 2 hours if needed. Or, 0.1 to 0.5 mg slow I.V. injection (initial dose should not exceed 0.5 mg). Additional doses may be given q 10 to 15 minutes.
Children: 0.1 mg/kg or 3 mg/m² I.M. or S.C.
Paroxysmal supraventricular tachycardia
Adults: Initially, 0.5 mg rapid I.V.; subsequent doses may be increased in increments of 0.1 to 0.2 mg. Maximum dose should not exceed 1 mg.
Prolongation of spinal anesthesia
Adults: 2 to 5 mg added to anesthetic solution.
Adjunct in the treatment of severe hypotension or shock
Adults: 0.1 to 0.18 mcg/minute I.V. infusion. After blood pressure stabilizes, maintain at 0.04 to 0.06 mcg/minute, adjusted to patient response.
Vasoconstrictor for regional anesthesia
Adults: 1 mg phenylephrine added to 20 ml local anesthetic.
Mydriasis (without cycloplegia)
Adults: Instill 1 or 2 drops 2.5% or 10% solution in eye before procedure. May be repeated in 10 to 60 minutes if needed.
Posterior synechia (adhesion of iris)
Adults: Instill 1 drop of 10% solution in eye 3 or more times daily with atropine sulfate.
Diagnosis of Horner's or Raeder's syndrome
Adults: Instill a 1% or 10% solution in both eyes.
Initial treatment of postoperative malignant glaucoma
Adults: Instill 1 drop of a 10% solution with 1 drop of a 1% to 4% atropine sulfate solution 3 or more times daily.
Nasal, ◊ sinus, or eustachian tube congestion
Adults and children over age 12: Apply 2 to 3 drops or 1 to 2 sprays of 0.25% to 1% solution instilled in each nostril; or a small quantity of 0.5% nasal jelly applied into each nostril. Apply jelly or spray to nasal mucosa.
Children age 6 to 12: Apply 2 to 3 drops or 1 to 2 sprays in each nostril.
Children under age 6: Apply 2 to 3 drops or sprays of 0.125% or 0.16% solution in each nostril.

Drops, spray, or jelly can be given q 4 hours, p.r.n.
Conjunctival congestion
Adults: 1 to 2 drops of 0.08% to 0.25% solution applied to conjunctiva q 3 to 4 hours p.r.n.

Pharmacodynamics
Vasopressor action: Phenylephrine acts predominantly by direct stimulation of alpha-adrenergic receptors, which constrict resistance and capacitance blood vessels, resulting in increased total peripheral resistance; increased systolic and diastolic blood pressure; decreased blood flow to vital organs, skin, and skeletal muscle; and constriction of renal blood vessels, reducing renal blood flow. Its main therapeutic effect is vasoconstriction.

It may also act indirectly by releasing norepinephrine from its storage sites. Phenylephrine does not stimulate beta receptors except in large doses (activates $beta_1$ receptors). Tachyphylaxis (tolerance) may follow repeated injections.

Other alpha-adrenergic effects include action on the dilator muscle of the pupil (producing contraction) and local decongestant action in the arterioles of the conjunctiva (producing constriction).

Phenylephrine acts directly on alpha-adrenergic receptors in the arterioles of conjunctiva nasal mucosa, producing constriction. Its vasoconstricting action on skin, mucous membranes, and viscera slows the vascular absorption rate of local anesthetics, which prolongs their action, localizes anesthesia, and decreases the risk of toxicity.

Phenylephrine may cause contraction of pregnant uterus and constriction of uterine blood vessels.

Pharmacokinetics
- *Absorption:* Pressor effects occur almost immediately after I.V. injection and persist 15 to 20 minutes; after I.M. injection, onset is within 10 to 15 minutes, persisting ½ to 2 hours; after S.C. injection, onset is within 10 to 15 minutes, with effects persisting 50 to 60 minutes. Nasal or conjunctival decongestant effects persist ½ to 4 hours. Peak effects for mydriasis are 15 to 60 minutes for the 2.5% solution; 10 to 90 minutes for the 10% solution. Mydriasis recovery time is 3 hours for the 2.5% solution; 3 to 7 hours for the 10% solution.
- *Distribution:* Unknown.
- *Metabolism:* Phenylephrine is metabolized in the liver and intestine by MAO.
- *Excretion:* Unknown.

Contraindications and precautions
All forms are contraindicated in patients with hypersensitivity to drug. Injected form is also contraindicated in those with severe hypertension or ventricular tachycardia. Ophthalmic form is also contraindicated in patients with angle-closure glaucoma and in those who wear soft contact lenses.

Use all forms cautiously in the elderly and in patients with hyperthyroidism or cardiac disease. Use nasal and ophthalmic forms cautiously in patients with type I diabetes mellitus, hypertension, or advanced arteriosclerotic changes and in children who have low body weight. Use injectable form cautiously in patients with severe atherosclerosis, bradycardia, partial heart block, myocardial disease, or allergy to sulfites.

Interactions
Phenylephrine may increase risk of arrhythmias, including tachycardia, when used concomitantly with *epinephrine* or *other sympathomimetics, cardiac glycosides, guanadrel* or *guanethidine, levodopa, MAO inhibitors, tricyclic antidepressants,* or *general anesthetics (cyclopropane, halothane).*

Pressor effects are potentiated when phenylephrine is used with *doxapram, ergot alkaloids, MAO inhibitors, mazindol, methyldopa,* and *oxytocics.*

Decreased pressor response (hypotension) may result when phenylephrine is used with *alpha-adren-*

ergic blockers, antihypertensives, diuretics used as antihypertensives, guanadrel or *guanethidine, rauwolfia alkaloids*, or *nitrates*.

Use of phenylephrine with *thyroid hormones* may increase effects of either drug; with *nitrates*, it may reduce antianginal effects.

The mydriatic response to phenylephrine is decreased in concomitant use of *levodopa* and increased in concomitant use with *cycloplegic antimuscarinic drugs* such as *atropine*.

Effects on diagnostic tests

Phenylephrine may lower intraocular pressure in normal eyes or in open-angle glaucoma. Drug also may cause false-normal tonometry readings.

Adverse reactions

CNS: *headache*; excitability (with injected form); brow ache (with ophthalmic form); tremor, dizziness, nervousness (with nasal form).

CV: bradycardia, ***arrhythmias,*** hypertension (with injected form); *hypertension* (with 10% solution), tachycardia, palpitations, ***PVCs, MI*** (with ophthalmic form); *palpitations, tachycardia,* ***PVCs,*** hypertension, pallor (with nasal form).

EENT: transient eye burning or stinging on instillation, blurred vision, increased intraocular pressure, keratitis, lacrimation, reactive hyperemia of eye, allergic conjunctivitis, rebound miosis (with ophthalmic form); transient burning or stinging, dryness of nasal mucosa, rebound nasal congestion with continued use (with nasal form).

GI: nausea (with nasal form).

Skin: pallor, dermatitis (with ophthalmic form).

Other: tachyphylaxis (may occur with continued use), ***anaphylaxis, asthmatic episodes,*** decreased organ perfusion (with prolonged use), tissue sloughing with extravasation (with injected form); trembling, diaphoresis (with ophthalmic form).

Overdose and treatment

Clinical manifestations of overdose include exaggeration of common adverse reactions, palpitations, paresthesia, vomiting, arrhythmias, and hypertension.

To treat, discontinue drug and provide symptomatic and supportive measures. Monitor vital signs closely. Use atropine sulfate to block reflex bradycardia; phentolamine to treat excessive hypertension; and propranolol to treat arrhythmias, or levodopa to reduce an excessive mydriatic effect of an ophthalmic preparation as necessary.

☑ Special considerations

Besides those relevant to all *adrenergics*, consider the following recommendations.

- Give I.V. through large veins, and monitor flow rate. To treat extravasation ischemia, infiltrate site promptly and liberally with 10 to 15 ml of NaCl solution containing 5 to 10 mg of phentolamine through fine needle. Topical nitroglycerin has also been used.
- During I.V. administration, pulse, blood pressure, and central venous pressure should be monitored every 2 to 5 minutes. Control flow rate and dosage to prevent excessive increases. I.V. overdoses can induce ventricular arrhythmias.
- Hypovolemic states should be corrected before administration of drug; phenylephrine should not be used in place of fluid, blood, plasma, and electrolyte replacement.
- Phenylephrine is chemically incompatible with butacaine, sulfate, alkalies, ferric salts, and oxidizing agents and metals.

Ophthalmic

- Apply digital pressure to lacrimal sac during and for 1 to 2 minutes after instillation to prevent systemic absorption.
- Prolonged exposure to air or strong light may cause oxidation and discoloration. Do not use if solution is brown or contains precipitate.
- To prevent contamination, do not touch applicator tip to any surface. Instruct patient in proper technique.

Nasal

- Prolonged or chronic use may result in rebound congestion and chronic swelling of nasal mucosa.
- To reduce risk of rebound congestion, use weakest effective dose.
- After use, rinse tip of spray bottle or dropper with hot water and dry with clean tissue. Wipe tip of nasal jelly container with clean, damp tissues.

Patient education

- Tell patient to store away from heat, light, and humidity (not in bathroom medicine cabinet) and out of children's reach.
- Warn patient to use only as directed. If using OTC product, patient should follow directions on label and not use more often or in larger doses than prescribed or recommended.
- Caution patient not to exceed recommended dosage regardless of formulation; patient should not double, decrease, or omit doses nor change dosage intervals unless so instructed.
- Tell patient to call if drug provides no relief in 2 days after using phenylephrine ophthalmic solution or 3 days after using the nasal solution.
- Explain that systemic absorption from nasal and conjunctival membranes can occur. Patient should report systemic reactions, such as dizziness and chest pain, and discontinue drug.

Ophthalmic

- Instruct patient not to use if solution is brown or contains a precipitate.
- Tell patient to wash hands before applying and to use finger to apply pressure to lacrimal sac during and for 1 to 2 minutes after instillation to decrease systemic absorption.
- Warn patient to avoid touching tip to any surface to prevent contamination.
- Inform patient that after applying drops, pupils will become unusually large. Patient should use sunglasses to protect eyes from sunlight and other bright lights, and call if effects persist 12 hours or more.

Nasal

- After use, tell patient to rinse tip of spray bottle or dropper with hot water and dry with clean tissue or wipe tip of nasal jelly container with clean, damp tissues.

• Instruct patient to blow nose gently (with both nostrils open) to clear nasal passages well, before using medication.
• Teach patient correct instillation
–drops: Tilt head back while sitting or standing up, or lie on bed and hang head over side. Stay in position a few minutes to permit medication to spread through nose.
–spray: With head upright, squeeze bottle quickly and firmly to produce 1 or 2 sprays into each nostril; wait 3 to 5 minutes, blow nose and repeat dose.
–jelly: Place in each nostril and sniff it well back into nose.
• Tell patient that increased fluid intake helps keep secretions liquid.
• Warn patient to avoid using nonprescription medications with phenylephrine to prevent possible hazardous interactions.

Geriatric use

• Effects may be exaggerated in elderly patients. In patients over age 50, phenylephrine (ophthalmic solution) appears to alter the reponse of the dilator muscle of the pupil so that rebound miosis may occur the day after drug is administered.

Pediatric use

• Infants and children may be more susceptible than adults to drug effects. Because of the risk of precipitating severe hypertension, only ophthalmic solutions containing 0.5% or less should be used in infants under age 1. The 10% ophthalmic solution is contraindicated in infants. Most manufacturers recommend that the 0.5% nasal solution not be used in children under age 12 except under medical supervision, and the 0.25% nasal solution should not be used in children under age 6 except under medical supervision.

Breast-feeding

• It is not known if drug occurs in breast milk; use with caution in breast-feeding women.

phenytoin, phenytoin sodium, phenytoin sodium (extended)

Dilantin, Dilantin Kapseals

phenytoin sodium (prompt)

Pharmacologic classification: hydantoin derivative
Therapeutic classification: anticonvulsant
Pregnancy risk category D

How supplied

Available by prescription only
phenytoin
Tablets (chewable): 50 mg
Oral suspension: 30 mg/5 ml*, 125 mg/5 ml
phenytoin sodium
Injection: 50 mg/ml
phenytoin sodium (extended)
Capsules: 30 mg, 100 mg
phenytoin sodium (prompt)
Capsules: 30 mg, 100 mg

Indications, route, and dosage

Generalized tonic-clonic seizures, status epilepticus, nonepileptic seizures (post-head trauma, Reye's syndrome)
Adults: Loading dosage is 10 to 15 mg/kg I.V. slowly, not to exceed 50 mg/minute; oral loading dosage consists of 1 g divided into three doses (400 mg, 300 mg, 300 mg) given at 2-hour intervals. Maintenance dosage once controlled is 300 mg P.O. daily (extended only); initially use a dose divided t.i.d. (extended or prompt).
Children: Loading dosage is 15 to 20 mg/kg I.V. at 50 mg/minute, or P.O. divided q 8 to 12 hours; then start maintenance dosage of 4 to 8 mg/kg P.O. or I.V. daily, divided q 12 hours.
Neuritic pain (migraine, trigeminal neuralgia, and Bell's palsy)
Adults: 200 to 600 mg P.O. daily in divided doses.
Skeletal muscle relaxant
Adults: 200 to 600 mg P.O. daily p.r.n.
◇ ***Ventricular arrhythmias unresponsive to lidocaine or procainamide, and arrhythmias induced by cardiac glycosides***
Adults: 50 to 100 mg q 10 to 15 minutes p.r.n., not to exceed 15 mg/kg. Infusion rate should never exceed 50 mg/minute (slow I.V. push).
Alternate method: 100 mg I.V. q 15 minutes until adverse effects develop, arrhythmias are controlled, or 1 g has been given. Also may administer entire loading dose of 1 g I.V. slowly at 25 mg/minute. Can be diluted in 0.9% NaCl solution. I.M. dosage is not recommended because of pain and erratic absorption.
Prophylactic control of seizures during neurosurgery
Adults: 100 to 200 mg I.V. at intervals of approximately 4 hours during perioperative and postoperative periods.

Pharmacodynamics

Anticonvulsant action: Like other hydantoin derivatives, phenytoin stabilizes neuronal membranes and limits seizure activity by either increasing efflux or decreasing influx of sodium ions across cell membranes in the motor cortex during generation of nerve impulses. Phenytoin exerts its antiarrhythmic effects by normalizing sodium influx to Purkinje's fibers in patients with cardiac glycoside–induced arrhythmias. It is indicated for generalized tonic-clonic (grand mal) and partial seizures.

Other actions: Phenytoin inhibits excessive collagenase activity in patients with epidermolysis bullosa.

Pharmacokinetics

• *Absorption:* Phenytoin is absorbed slowly from the small intestine; absorption is formulation-dependent and bioavailability may differ among products. Extended-release capsules give peak serum concentrations at 4 to 12 hours; prompt-release products peak at 1½ to 3 hours. I.M. doses are absorbed erratically; about 50% to 75% of I.M. dose is absorbed in 24 hours.

*Canada only ◇ Unlabeled clinical use

• *Distribution:* Drug is distributed widely throughout the body; therapeutic plasma levels are 10 to 20 mcg/ml, although in some patients, they occur at 5 to 10 mcg/ml. Lateral nystagmus may occur at levels above 20 mcg/ml; ataxia usually occurs at levels above 30 mcg/ml; significantly decreased mental capacity occurs at 40 mcg/ml. Phenytoin is about 90% protein-bound, less so in uremic patients.
• *Metabolism:* Metabolized by the liver to inactive metabolites.
• *Excretion:* Drug is excreted in urine and exhibits dose-dependent (zero-order) elimination kinetics; above a certain dosage level, small increases in dosage disproportionately increase serum levels.

Contraindications and precautions

Contraindicated in patients with hydantoin hypersensitivity, sinus bradycardia, SA block, second- or third-degree AV block, or Adams-Stokes syndrome.

Use cautiously in elderly or debilitated patients; in those with hepatic dysfunction, hypotension, myocardial insufficiency, diabetes, or respiratory depression; and in those receiving hydantoin derivatives.

Interactions

Phenytoin interacts with many drugs. Diminished therapeutic effects and toxic reactions commonly are the result of recent changes in drug therapy. Phenytoin's therapeutic effects may be increased by concomitant use with *allopurinol, chloramphenicol, chlorpheniramine, cimetidine, diazepam, disulfiram, ethanol (acute), ibuprofen, imipramine, isoniazid, miconazole, phenacemide, phenylbutazone, salicylates, succinimides, trimethoprim,* or *valproic acid.*

Phenytoin's therapeutic effects may be decreased by *antacids, antineoplastics, barbiturates, calcium, calcium gluconate, carbamazepine, charcoal, diazoxide, ethanol (chronic), folic acid, loxapine, nitrofurantoin, pyridoxine,* or *theophylline.* Other drugs that lower seizure threshold (such as *antipsychotic agents*) may attenuate phenytoin's therapeutic effects.

Phenytoin may decrease the effects of the following drugs by stimulating hepatic metabolism: *corticosteroids, cyclosporine, dicumarol, digitoxin, disopyramide, dopamine, doxycycline, estrogens, furosemide, haloperidol, levodopa, meperidine, methadone, metyrapone, oral contraceptives, quinidine,* or *sulfonylureas.*

Effects on diagnostic tests

Phenytoin may raise blood glucose levels by inhibiting pancreatic insulin release; it may decrease serum levels of protein-bound iodine and may interfere with the 1-mg dexamethasone suppression test.

Adverse reactions

CNS: *ataxia, slurred speech,* dizziness, insomnia, nervousness, twitching, headache, *mental confusion, decreased coordination.*
CV: periarteritis nodosa.
EENT: *nystagmus, diplopia,* blurred vision, *gingival hyperplasia* (especially in children).
GI: *nausea, vomiting,* constipation.
Hematologic: ***thrombocytopenia, leukopenia, agranulocytosis, pancytopenia,*** macrocythemia, megaloblastic anemia.
Hepatic: ***toxic hepatitis.***
Skin: scarlatiniform or morbilliform rash; bullous, ***exfoliative,*** or purpuric dermatitis; ***Stevens-Johnson syndrome;*** lupus erythematosus; *hirsutism;* ***toxic epidermal necrolysis;*** photosensitivity; pain, necrosis, and inflammation at injection site; discoloration of skin ("purple glove syndrome") if given by I.V. push in back of hand.
Other: lymphadenopathy, hyperglycemia, osteomalacia, hypertrichosis.

Overdose and treatment

Early signs and symptoms of overdose may include drowsiness, nausea, vomiting, nystagmus, ataxia, dysarthria, tremor, and slurred speech; hypotension, arrhythmias, respiratory depression, and coma may follow. Death is caused by respiratory and circulatory depression. Estimated lethal dose in adults is 2 to 5 g.

Treat overdose with gastric lavage or emesis and follow with supportive treatment. Carefully monitor vital signs and fluid and electrolyte balance. Forced diuresis is of little or no value. Hemodialysis or peritoneal dialysis may be helpful.

☑ Special considerations

Besides those relevant to all *hydantoin derivatives,* consider the following recommendations.
• Monitoring of serum levels is essential because of dose-dependent excretion.
• Only extended-release capsules are approved for once-daily dosing; all other forms are given in divided doses every 8 to 12 hours.
• Oral or nasogastric feeding may interfere with absorption of oral suspension; separate doses as much as possible from feedings but no less than 1 hour. During continuous tube feeding, tube should be flushed before and after dose.
• If suspension is used, shake well.
• I.M. administration should be avoided; it is painful and drug absorption is erratic.
• Mix I.V. doses in 0.9% NaCl solution and use within 1 hour; mixtures with D_5W will precipitate. Do not refrigerate solution; do not mix with other drugs.
• When giving I.V., continuous monitoring of ECG, blood pressure, and respiratory status is essential.
• Abrupt withdrawal may precipitate status epilepticus.
• If using I.V. bolus, use slow (50 mg/minute) I.V. push or constant infusion; too-rapid I.V. injection may cause hypotension and circulatory collapse. Do not use I.V. push in veins on back of hand; larger veins are needed to prevent discoloration associated with purple glove syndrome.
• Phenytoin commonly is abbreviated as DPH (diphenylhydantoin), an older drug name.

Patient education

• Tell patient to use same brand of phenytoin consistently. Changing brands may change therapeutic effect.

- Instruct patient to take drug with food or milk to minimize GI distress.
- Warn patient not to discontinue drug, except with medical supervision; to avoid hazardous activities that require alertness until CNS effect is determined; and to avoid alcoholic beverages, which can decrease effectiveness of drug and increase adverse reactions.
- Encourage patient to wear a medical identification bracelet or necklace.
- Stress good oral hygiene to minimize overgrowth and sensitivity of gums.

Geriatric use
- Elderly patients metabolize and excrete phenytoin slowly; therefore, they may require lower doses.

Pediatric use
- Special pediatric-strength suspension is available (30 mg/5 ml) is available in Canada only. Take extreme care to use correct strength. Do not confuse with adult strength (125 mg/5 ml).

Breast-feeding
- Drug is excreted in breast milk; an alternative feeding method is recommended during therapy.

physostigmine salicylate
Antilirium

physostigmine sulfate
Eserine, Isopto Eserine

Pharmacologic classification: cholinesterase inhibitor
Therapeutic classification: antimuscarinic antidote, antiglaucoma
Pregnancy risk category C

How supplied
Available by prescription only
Injection: 1 mg/ml
Ophthalmic ointment: 0.25%
Ophthalmic solution: 0.25%, 0.5%

Indications, route, and dosage
Tricyclic antidepressant and anticholinergic poisoning
Adults: 0.5 to 2 mg I.M. or I.V. given slowly (not to exceed 1 mg/minute I.V.). Dosage individualized and repeated p.r.n. q 10 minutes.
Children: Reserve for life-threatening situations only. Initial pediatric I.V. or I.M. dose of physostigmine salicylate is 0.02 mg/kg. Dosage may be repeated at 5- to 10-minute intervals to maximum of 2 mg if no adverse cholinergic signs are present.
Postanesthesia care
Adults: 0.5 to 1 mg I.M. or I.V. given slowly (not to exceed 1 mg/minute I.V.). Dosage individualized and repeated p.r.n. q 10 to 30 minutes.
Open-angle glaucoma
Adults: Instill 2 drops into eye(s) up to q.i.d., or apply ointment to lower fornix up to t.i.d.

Pharmacodynamics
Antimuscarinic action: Physostigmine competitively blocks acetylcholine hydrolysis by cholinesterase, resulting in acetylcholine accumulation at cholinergic synapses; that antagonizes the muscarinic effects of overdose with antidepressants and anticholinergics. With ophthalmic use, miosis and ciliary muscle contraction increase aqueous humor outflow and decrease intraocular pressure.

Pharmacokinetics
- *Absorption:* Well absorbed from the GI tract, mucous membranes, and subcutanoues tissues when given I.M. or I.V., with effects peaking within 5 minutes. After ophthalmic use, drug may be absorbed orally after passage through the nasolacrimal duct.
- *Distribution:* Drug is distributed widely and crosses the blood-brain barrier.
- *Metabolism:* Cholinesterase hydrolyzes physostigmine relatively quickly. Duration of effect is 1 to 2 hours after I.V. administration, 12 to 48 hours after ophthalmic use.
- *Excretion:* Only a small amount of drug is excreted in urine. Exact mode of excretion is unknown.

Contraindications and precautions
Injected form contraindicated in patients with mechanical obstruction of the intestine or urogenital tract, asthma, gangrene, diabetes, CV disease, or vagotonia and in those receiving choline esters or depolarizing neuromuscular blockers.

Ophthalmic form is contraindicated in patients with intolerance to physostigmine, active uveitis, or corneal injury. Use injectable form cautiously during pregnancy.

Interactions
Concomitant use with *succinylcholine* may prolong respiratory depression by inhibiting hydrolysis of succinylcholine by plasma esterases. Concomitant use with *systemic cholinergic agents* may cause additive toxicity.

Effects on diagnostic tests
None reported.

Adverse reactions
CNS: weakness; headache (with ophthalmic form); ***seizures,*** *restlessness, excitability* (with injected form).
CV: slow or irregular heartbeat (with ophthalmic form); bradycardia, hypotension (with injected form).
EENT: blurred vision, eye pain, burning, redness, stinging, eye irritation, twitching of eyelids, watering of eyes (with ophthalmic form); miosis (with injected form).
GI: nausea, vomiting, diarrhea; epigastric pain, *excessive salivation* (with injected form).
GU: loss of bladder control (with ophthalmic form); urinary urgency (with injected form).
Respiratory: ***bronchospasm,*** bronchial constriction, dyspnea (with injected form).
Other: diaphoresis, shortness of breath.

Overdose and treatment
Clinical effects of overdose include headache, nausea, vomiting, diarrhea, blurred vision, miosis, myopia, excessive tearing, bronchospasm, increased bronchial secretions, hypotension, incoordination, excessive sweating, muscle weakness, bradycardia, excessive salivation, restlessness or agitation, and confusion.

Support respiration; bronchial suctioning may be performed. Drug should be discontinued immediately. Atropine may be given to block physostigmine's muscarinic effects. Avoid atropine overdose because it may cause bronchial plug formation.

☑ Special considerations
- Observe solution for discoloration. Do not use if darkened.
- Atropine sulfate injection should always be available as an antagonist and antidote for most of the effects of physostigmine.
- The commercially available formulation of physostigmine salicylate injection contains sodium bisulfite, a sulfite that can cause allergic-type reactions including anaphylaxis and life-threatening or less severe asthmatic episodes in certain susceptible individuals.

Ophthalmic
- Have patient lie down or tilt his head back to facilitate administration of eyedrops.
- Wait at least 5 minutes before administering any other eyedrops.
- Gently pinch patient's nasal bridge for 1 to 2 minutes after administering each dose of eyedrops to minimize systemic absorption.
- After applying ointment, have patient close eyelids and roll eyes.

Patient education
Ophthalmic
- Teach patient how to administer ophthalmic ointment or solution.
- Instruct patient not to close his eyes tightly or blink unnecessarily after instilling the ophthalmic solution.
- Warn patient that he may experience blurred vision and difficulty seeing after initial doses.
- Instruct patient to report abdominal cramps, diarrhea, or excessive salivation.
- Remind patient to wait 5 minutes (if using eyedrops) or 10 minutes (if using ointment) before using another eye preparation.

Geriatric use
- Use caution when administering to elderly patients because they may be more sensitive to drug's effects.

Breast-feeding
- Safety and efficacy have not been established.

pilocarpine hydrochloride
Salagen

Pharmacologic classification: cholinergic agonist
Therapeutic classification: anti-xerostomia
Pregnancy risk category C

How supplied
Available by prescription only
Tablets: 5 mg

Indications, route, and dosage
Treatment of symptoms of xerostomia from salivary gland hypofunction caused by radiotherapy for cancer of the head and neck
Adults: 5 mg P.O. t.i.d. Dosage may be increased to 10 mg P.O. t.i.d., p.r.n.

Pharmacodynamics
Antixerostomia action: Oral pilocarpine increases secretion of the salivary glands, which eliminates dryness.

Pharmacokinetics
- *Absorption:* Pilocarpine is absorbed in the GI tract. A high-fat meal may decrease rate of absorption.
- *Distribution:* Unknown.
- *Metabolism:* Inactivation of pilocarpine is believed to occur at neuronal synapses and probably in plasma.
- *Excretion:* Drug and its minimally active or inactive degradation products are excreted in urine.

Contraindications and precautions
Contraindicated in patients with uncontrolled asthma or known hypersensitivity to pilocarpine and when miosis is undesirable, such as in acute iritis and narrow-angle glaucoma.

Use cautiously in patients with CV disease, controlled asthma, chronic bronchitis, COPD, cholelithiasis, biliary tract disease, nephrolithiasis, and cognitive or psychiatric disturbances.

Interactions
Beta-adrenergic antagonists may increase risk of conduction disturbances. Use together cautiously. *Drugs with parasympathomimetic effects* may result in additive pharmacologic effects. Monitor patient closely.

Drugs with anticholinergic effects may antagonize the anticholinergic effects of oral pilocarpine. Use together cautiously.

Effects on diagnostic tests
None reported.

Adverse reactions
CNS: *dizziness, headache,* tremor.
CV: hypertension, tachycardia.
GI: *nausea,* dyspepsia, diarrhea, abdominal pain, vomiting, dysphagia.
GU: *urinary frequency.*

EENT: *rhinitis,* lacrimation, amblyopia, pharyngitis, voice alteration, conjunctivitis, epistaxis, sinusitis, abnormal vision.
Skin: *flushing,* rash, pruritis.
Other: *sweating, chills, asthenia,* edema, taste perversion, myalgia.

Overdose and treatment

Taking 100 mg of oral pilocarpine is potentially fatal. Treatment is with atropine titration (0.5 mg to 1 mg S.C. or I.V.) and supportive measures to maintain respiration and circulation. Epinephrine (0.3 mg to 1 mg S.C. or I.M.) may also be useful during severe CV depression or bronchoconstriction. It is not known if pilocarpine is dialyzable.

☑ Special considerations

- Patient should undergo careful examination of the fundus before therapy is initiated because retina detachment has been reported with pilocarpine use in patients with preexisting retinal disease.
- Monitor patient for signs and symptoms of pilocarpine toxicity characterized by an exaggeration of its parasympathomimetic effects; these include headache, visual disturbance, lacrimation, sweating, respiratory distress, GI spasm, nausea, vomiting, diarrhea, AV block, tachycardia, bradycardia, hypotension, hypertension, shock, mental confusion, cardiac arrhythmia, and tremors.

Patient education

- Warn patient that drug may cause visual disturbances, especially at night, that could impair his ability to drive safely.
- Tell patient to drink plenty of fluids to prevent dehydration if drug causes excessive sweating. If adequate fluid intake cannot be maintained, tell patient to notify primary health care provider.

Pediatric use

- Safety and effectiveness in children have not been established.

Breast-feeding

- It is unknown if drug occurs in breast milk. Because of the potential for serious adverse reactions in nursing infants, a decision should be made whether to discontinue breast-feeding or drug, taking into account the importance of drug to mother.

pilocarpine hydrochloride (ophthalmic)

Adsorbocarpine, Akarpine, Isopto Carpine, Minims Pilocarpine*, Miocarpine*, Ocusert Pilo, Pilocar, Pilopine HS

pilocarpine nitrate

P.V. Carpine Liquifilm

Pharmacologic classification: cholinergic agonist
Therapeutic classification: miotic
Pregnancy risk category C

How supplied

Available by prescription only
pilocarpine hydrochloride
Solution: 0.25%, 0.5%, 1%, 2%, 3%, 4%, 5%, 6%, 8%, 10%
Gel: 4%
Releasing-system insert: 20 mcg/hour, 40 mcg/hour
pilocarpine nitrate
Solution: 1%, 2%, 4%

Indications, route, and dosage

Chronic open-angle glaucoma; before, or instead of, emergency surgery in acute narrow-angle glaucoma

Adults and children: 1 or 2 drops of 1% to 4% solution in lower conjunctival sac q 4 to 12 hours (dosage based on periodic tonometric readings) or ½" ribbon of 4% gel (Pilopine HS) h.s.

Alternatively, apply one Ocusert Pilo System (20 or 40 mcg/hour) q 7 days.

Emergency treatment of acute narrow-angle glaucoma

Adults and children: 1 drop of 2% solution q 5 minutes for three to six doses, followed by 1 drop q 1 to 3 hours until pressure is controlled.

To counteract mydriatic effects of sympathomimetic agents

Adults: 1 drop of 1% solution in affected eye.

Pharmacodynamics

Miotic action: Pilocarpine stimulates cholinergic receptors on the sphincter muscles of the iris, resulting in miosis. It also produces ciliary muscle contraction, resulting in accommodation with deepening of the anterior chamber, and vasodilation of conjunctival vessels of the outflow tract.

Pharmacokinetics

- *Absorption:* Pilocarpine drops act within 10 to 30 minutes, with peak effect at 2 to 4 hours. With the Ocusert Pilo System, 0.3 to 7 mg of pilocarpine are released during the initial 6-hour period; during the remainder of the 1-week insertion period, the release rate is within ± 20% of the rated value. Effect is seen in 1½ to 2 hours and is maintained for the 1-week life of the insertion.
- *Distribution:* Unknown.
- *Metabolism:* Unknown.
- *Excretion:* Duration of effect of pilocarpine drops is 4 to 6 hours.

Contraindications and precautions

Contraindicated in hypersensitivity to drug or when cholinergic effects such as constriction are undesirable (for example, acute iritis, some forms of secondary glaucoma, pupillary block glaucoma, acute inflammatory disease of the anterior chamber).

Use cautiously in patients with acute cardiac failure, bronchial asthma, peptic ulcer, hyperthyroidism, GI spasm, urinary obstruction, and Parkinson's disease.

Interactions

When used concomitantly, pilocarpine can enhance reductions in intraocular pressure caused by *epinephrine derivatives* and *timolol.*

Demecarium, echothiophate, and *isoflurophate* decrease the pharmacologic effects of pilocarpine.

Effects on diagnostic tests
None reported.

Adverse reactions
CV: hypertension, tachycardia.
EENT: periorbital or supraorbital headache, *myopia,* ciliary spasm, *blurred vision,* conjunctival irritation, transient stinging and burning, keratitis, lens opacity, retinal detachment, lacrimation, changes in visual field, *brow pain.*
GI: nausea, vomiting, diarrhea, salivation.
Respiratory: ***bronchoconstriction, pulmonary edema.***
Other: hypersensitivity reactions, diaphoresis.

Overdose and treatment
Clinical manifestations of overdose include flushing, vomiting, bradycardia, bronchospasm, increased bronchial secretion, sweating, tearing, involuntary urination, hypotension, and tremors. Vomiting is usually spontaneous with accidental ingestion; if not, induce emesis and follow with activated charcoal or a cathartic. Treat dermal exposure by washing the areas twice with water. Use epinephrine to treat the CV responses. Atropine sulfate is the antidote of choice. Flush the eye with water or sodium chloride to treat a local overdose. Doses up to 20 mg are generally considered nontoxic.

☑ Special considerations
- Drug may be used alone or with mannitol, urea, glycerol, or acetazolamide. It also may be used to counteract effects of mydriatic and cycloplegic agents after surgery or ophthalmoscopic examination and may be used alternately with atropine to break adhesions.

Patient education
- Warn patient that vision will be temporarily blurred, that miotic pupil may make surroundings appear dim and reduce peripheral field of vision, and that transient brow ache and myopia are common at first; assure patient that adverse effects subside 10 to 14 days after therapy begins.
- Instruct patient to check for the presence of the pilocarpine ocular system at bedtime and upon arising.
- Tell patient that if systems in both eyes are lost, they should be replaced as soon as possible. If one system is lost, it may either be replaced with a fresh system or the system remaining in the other eye may be removed and both replaced with fresh systems so that both systems will subsequently be replaced on the same schedule.
- Instruct patient that if the Ocusert System falls out of the eye during sleep, he should wash hands, then rinse Ocusert in cool tap water and reposition it in the eye. Do not use the insert if it's deformed.
- Inform patient that systems should be replaced every 7 days.
- Provide patient with a copy of the manufacturer's instructions for the pilocarpine ocular system.
- Tell patient to use caution in night driving and other activities in poor illumination because miotic pupil diminishes side vision and illumination.
- Stress importance of complying with prescribed medical regimen.
- Reassure patient that adverse effects will subside.
- Teach patient the correct way to instill drops and to apply light finger pressure on lacrimal sac for 1 minute after administration to minimize systemic absorption.
- Instruct patient to apply gel at bedtime because it will cause blurred vision.

pimozide
Orap

Pharmacologic classification: diphenylbutylpiperidine
Therapeutic classification: antipsychotic
Pregnancy risk category C

How supplied
Available by prescription only
Tablets: 2 mg

Indications, route, and dosage
Suppression of severe motor and phonic tics in patients with Tourette syndrome
Adults and children over age 12: Initially, 1 to 2 mg/day in divided doses. Then, increase dosage p.r.n. every other day.
Maintenance dose: From 7 to 16 mg/day. Maximum dosage, 20 mg/day.
Children under age 12: 0.05 mg/kg h.s.; increase at 3-day intervals to maximum of 0.2 mg/kg. Maximum dosage, 10 mg/day.

Pharmacodynamics
Antipsychotic action: Mechanism of action in Tourette syndrome is unknown: it is thought to exert its effects by postsynaptic and/or presynaptic blockade of CNS dopamine receptors, thus inhibiting dopamine-mediated effects. Pimozide also has anticholinergic, antiemetic, and anxiolytic effects and produces alpha blockade.

Pharmacokinetics
- *Absorption:* Absorbed slowly and incompletely from the GI tract; bioavailability is about 50%. Peak plasma levels may occur from 4 to 12 hours (usually in 6 to 8 hours).
- *Distribution:* Drug is distributed widely into the body.
- *Metabolism:* Metabolized by the liver; a significant first-pass effect exists.
- *Excretion:* About 40% of a given dose is excreted in urine as parent drug and metabolites in 3 to 4 days; about 15% is excreted in feces via the biliary tract within 3 to 6 days.

Contraindications and precautions
Contraindicated in patients with hypersensitivity to drug, in treatment of simple tics or tics other than those associated with Tourette syndrome, concur-

rent drug therapy known to cause motor and phonic tics, congenital long QT syndrome or history of arrhythmias, patients with severe toxic CNS depression, and patients experiencing coma.

Use cautiously in patients with impaired renal or hepatic function, glaucoma, prostatic hyperplasia, seizure disorders, or EEG abnormalities.

Interactions

Concomitant use of pimozide with *disopyramide, procainamide, quinidine,* and *other antiarrhythmics, phenothiazines, other antipsychotics,* and *antidepressants* may further depress cardiac conduction and prolong QT interval, resulting in serious arrhythmias. Concomitant use with *anticonvulsants (carbamazepine, phenobarbital, phenytoin)* may induce seizures, even in patients previously stabilized on anticonvulsants; an anticonvulsant dosage increase may be required.

Concomitant use with *amphetamines, methylphenidate,* or *pemoline* may induce Tourette-like tic and may exacerbate existing tics.

Concomitant use with *CNS depressants,* including *alcohol, analgesics, anxiolytics, barbiturates, narcotics, parenteral magnesium sulfate, tranquilizers,* and *general, spinal,* or *epidural anesthetics* may cause over-sedation and respiratory depression due to additive CNS depressant effects.

Effects on diagnostic tests

Pimozide causes quinidine-like ECG effects (including prolongation of QT interval and flattened T waves).

Adverse reactions

CNS: *parkinsonian-like symptoms,* drowsiness, headache, insomnia, other extrapyramidal signs and symptoms (dystonia, akathisia, hyperreflexia, opisthotonos, oculogyric crisis), *tardive dyskinesia, sedation, adverse behavioral effects.*
CV: *ECG changes (prolonged QT interval),* hypotension, hypertension, tachycardia.
EENT: visual disturbances.
GI: *dry mouth, constipation.*
GU: impotence, urinary frequency.
Skin: rash, diaphoresis.
Other: ***neuroleptic malignant syndrome,*** muscle rigidity.

Overdose and treatment

Clinical signs of overdose include severe extrapyramidal reactions, hypotension, respiratory depression, coma, and ECG abnormalities, including prolongation of QT interval, inversion or flattening of T waves, and new appearance of U waves.

Treat with gastric lavage to remove unabsorbed drug. Maintain blood pressure with I.V. fluids, plasma expanders, or norepinephrine. *Do not use epinephrine.*

Do not induce vomiting because of the potential for aspiration.

Treat extrapyramidal symptoms with parenteral diphenhydramine. Monitor for adverse effects for at least 4 days because of prolonged half-life (55 hours) of drug.

☑ Special considerations

- Elderly patients may be at greater risk for adverse CV effects.
- Obtain baseline ECG before therapy begins and then periodically to monitor CV effects.
- Maintain patient's serum potassium level within normal range; decreased potassium concentrations increase risk of arrhythmias. Monitor potassium level in patients with diarrhea and those who are taking diuretics.
- Assess patient periodically for abnormal body movement.
- Extrapyramidal reactions develop in about 10% to 15% of patients at normal doses. They are especially likely to occur during early days of therapy.
- If excessive restlessness and agitation occur, therapy with a beta blocker, such as propranolol or metoprolol, may be helpful.

Patient education

- Inform patient of risks, signs, and symptoms of dystonic reactions and tardive dyskinesia.
- Advise patient to take pimozide exactly as prescribed, not to double dose for missed doses, not to share drug with others, and not to stop taking it suddenly.
- Explain that drug's therapeutic effect may not be apparent for several weeks.
- Urge patient to report unusual effects promptly.
- Tell patient not to take pimozide with alcohol, sleeping medications, or other drugs that may cause drowsiness without medical approval.
- Recommend use of sugarless hard candy or chewing gum, ice chips, or artificial saliva to relieve dry mouth.
- To prevent dizziness at start of therapy, tell patient to lie down for 30 minutes after taking each dose and should avoid sudden changes in posture, especially when rising to upright position.
- To minimize daytime sedation, suggest taking entire daily dose at bedtime.
- Warn patient to avoid hazardous activities that require alertness until drug's effects are known.

Geriatric use

- Elderly patients are more likely to develop cardiac toxicity and tardive dyskinesia even at normal doses.

Pediatric use

- Use and efficacy in children under age 12 are limited. Dosage should be kept at the lowest possible level. Use of drug in children for any disorder other than Tourette syndrome is not recommended.

---

pindolol

Visken

Pharmacologic classification: beta-adrenergic blocker
Therapeutic classification: antihypertensive
Pregnancy risk category B

How supplied
Available by prescription only
Tablets: 5 mg, 10 mg

Indications, route, and dosage
Hypertension
Adults: Initially, 5 mg P.O. b.i.d. increased by 10 mg/day q 3 to 4 weeks up to maximum of 60 mg/day. Usual dosage is 10 to 30 mg daily, given in two or three divided doses. In some patients, once-daily dosing may be possible.
◇ ***Angina***
Adults: 15 to 40 mg daily P.O. in three or four divided doses.

Pharmacodynamics
Antihypertensive action: Exact mechanism of antihypertensive action is unknown. Pindolol does not consistently affect cardiac output or renin release, and its other mechanisms such as decreased peripheral resistance probably contribute to its hypotensive effect. Because pindolol has some intrinsic sympathomimetic activity—that is, beta-agonist sympathomimetic activity—it may be useful in patients who develop bradycardia with other beta-blocking agents. It is a nonselective beta-blocking agent, inhibiting both $beta_1$ and $beta_2$ receptors.

Pharmacokinetics
- *Absorption:* After oral administration, pindolol is absorbed rapidly from the GI tract; peak plasma concentrations occur in 1 to 2 hours. Pindolol's effect on the heart rate usually occurs in 3 hours. Food does not reduce bioavailability but may increase the rate of GI absorption.
- *Distribution:* Distributed widely throughout the body and is 40% to 60% protein-bound.
- *Metabolism:* About 60% to 65% of a given dose of pindolol is metabolized by the liver.
- *Excretion:* In adults with normal renal function, 35% to 50% of a given dose is excreted unchanged in urine; half-life is about 3 to 4 hours. Drug's antihypertensive effect usually persists for 24 hours.

Contraindications and precautions
Contraindicated in patients with hypersensitivity to drug, bronchial asthma, severe bradycardia, heart block greater than first degree, cardiogenic shock, or overt cardiac failure.

Use cautiously in patients with heart failure, nonallergic bronchospastic disease, diabetes, hyperthyroidism, and impaired renal or hepatic function.

Interactions
Pindolol may potentiate the antihypertensive effects of *other antihypertensive agents.*

Effects on diagnostic tests
Pindolol may elevate serum transaminase, alkaline phosphatase, lactic dehydrogenase, and uric acid levels.

Adverse reactions
CNS: *insomnia, fatigue, dizziness, nervousness,* vivid dreams, weakness, paresthesia.
CV: *edema,* bradycardia, ***heart failure,*** chest pain.
GI: *nausea,* abdominal discomfort.
Respiratory: *increased airway resistance,* dyspnea.
Skin: rash, pruritus.
Other: *muscle pain, joint pain.*

Overdose and treatment
Clinical signs of overdose include severe hypotension, bradycardia, heart failure, and bronchospasm.

After acute ingestion, empty stomach by induced emesis or gastric lavage, and give activated charcoal to reduce absorption. Subsequent treatment is usually symptomatic and supportive.

☑ Special considerations
Besides those relevant to all *beta-adrenergic blockers,* consider the following recommendation.
- Maximum therapeutic response may not be seen for 2 weeks or more.

Geriatric use
- Elderly patients may require lower maintenance doses of pindolol because of increased bioavailability or delayed metabolism; they also may experience enhanced adverse effects. Half-life of drug may be increased in elderly patients.

Pediatric use
- Safety and efficacy of pindolol in children have not been established; use only if potential benefit outweighs risk.

Breast-feeding
- Pindolol passes into breast milk; an alternative feeding method is recommended during therapy.

pipecuronium bromide
Arduan

Pharmacologic classification: nondepolarizing neuromuscular blocker
Therapeutic classification: skeletal muscle relaxant
Pregnancy risk category C

How supplied
Available by prescription only
Injection: 10 mg/vial

Indications, route, and dosage
To provide skeletal muscle relaxation during surgery as an adjunct to general anesthesia
Adults and children: Dosage is highly individualized. The following doses may serve as a guide, assuming that patient is not obese and has normal renal function. Initially, doses of 70 to 85 mcg/kg I.V. are used to provide conditions considered ideal for endotracheal intubation and will maintain paralysis for 1 to 2 hours. If succinylcholine is used for endotracheal intubation, initial doses of pipecuronium 50 mcg/kg will provide good relaxation for 45 minutes or more. Maintenance doses of 10 to 15 mcg/kg provide relaxation for about 50 minutes.

♦ ***Dosage adjustment.*** In patients with renal failure, refer to the following dosing chart.

Creatinine clearance (ml/min)	Dose (mcg/kg)
100	85
80	70
60	55
40	50

Pharmacodynamics

Muscle relaxant action: Like other nondepolarizing muscle relaxants, pipecuronium competes with acetylcholine for receptor sites at the motor end plate. Because this action may be antagonized by cholinesterase inhibitors, it is considered a competitive antagonist.

Pharmacokinetics

- *Absorption:* No information is available regarding use of drug by any route other than I.V. Maximum onset of action occurs within 5 minutes.
- *Distribution:* Volume of distribution (V_D) is about 0.25 L/kg and increases in patients with renal failure. Other conditions associated with increased V_D (including edema, old age, and CV disease) may delay onset.
- *Metabolism:* Only about 20% to 40% of an administered dose is metabolized, probably in the liver. One metabolite (3-desacetyl pipecuronium) has about 50% of the neuromuscular blocking activity of the parent drug.
- *Excretion:* Primarily renal. In preliminary studies, the half-life of drug has been estimated at 1.7 hours; it may increase to 4 hours or more in patients with severe renal disease.

Contraindications and precautions

Contraindicated in patients with hypersensitivity to drug. Use cautiously in patients with renal failure.

Interactions

Concomitant parenteral or intraperitoneal administration of certain *antibiotics in high doses* has been associated with muscle weakness; this weakness may worsen in the presence of a nondepolarizing neuromuscular blocking agent. These antibiotics include *aminoglycosides (gentamicin, kanamycin, neomycin,* and *streptomycin), bacitracin, colistimethate sodium, colistin, polymyxin B, tetracyclines.*

Some *volatile inhalational anesthetics* may intensify or prolong the action of nondepolarizing neuromuscular blocking agents.

Concomitant use with *quinidine* may prolong the action of nondepolarizing neuromuscular blocking agents. Use with *magnesium salts* such as those used for treatment of toxemia of pregnancy may enhance and prolong neuromuscular blockade.

Experimental evidence suggests that *acid-base balance* may influence the actions of pipecuronium. *Alkalosis* may counteract the paralysis and *acidosis* may enhance it. *Electrolyte disturbances* may also influence response.

Pipecuronium may be administered after succinylcholine when the latter is used to facilitate intubation. There is no evidence to support the safe use of pipecuronium before succinylcholine to decrease adverse effects of the latter drug. Concomitant use with *other nondepolarizing neuromuscular blocking agents* is not recommended.

Effects on diagnostic tests

None reported.

Adverse reactions

CV: hypotension, bradycardia, hypertension, myocardial ischemia, ***CVA,*** thrombosis, atrial fibrillation, ***ventricular extrasystole.***
GU: anuria.
Respiratory: dyspnea, respiratory depression, ***respiratory insufficiency or apnea.***
Skin: rash, urticaria.
Other: prolonged muscle weakness, increased creatinine levels.

Overdose and treatment

No cases have been reported. Provide supportive treatment, and ventilate patient as necessary. Closely monitor vital signs.

Antagonists such as neostigmine should not be used until there is some evidence of spontaneous recovery of neuromuscular function. A nerve stimulator is recommended to document antagonism of neuromuscular blockade.

☑ Special considerations

- Because of its prolonged duration of action, drug is recommended only for procedures that take 90 minutes or longer.
- Adjust dosage to ideal body weight in obese patients.
- Store powder at room temperature or in the refrigerator (36° to 86° F [2° to 30° C]).
- Reconstitute with 10 ml solution before use to yield a solution of 1 mg/ml. Large volumes of diluent or addition of drug to a hanging I.V. solution is not recommended.
- When reconstituted with sterile water for injection or other compatible I.V. solutions, such as 0.9% NaCl injection, D_5W, lactated Ringer's injection, and dextrose 5% in NaCl, drug is stable for 24 hours if refrigerated.
- If reconstituted with solution other than bacteriostatic water for injection, discard unused portions of drug.
- When reconstituted with bacteriostatic water for injection, drug is stable for 5 days at room temperature or in the refrigerator. Note that bacteriostatic water contains benzyl alcohol and is not intended for use in neonates.
- Clinical trials have shown that edrophonium 0.5 mg/kg was not as effective as neostigmine 0.04 mg/kg in reversing the effects of pipecuronium. Higher doses of edrophonium and pyridostigmine have not been studied.

Pediatric use

- Drug is not recommended for use in patients under age 3 months. Limited evidence suggests that children (age 1 to 14) under balanced anesthesia or halothane anesthesia may be less sensitive than adults.

Breast-feeding
• There is no information regarding the distribution of drug in breast milk. Use with caution in breast-feeding women.

piperacillin sodium
Pipracil

Pharmacologic classification: extended-spectrum penicillin, acylaminopenicillin
Therapeutic classification: antibiotic
Pregnancy risk category B

How supplied
Available by prescription only
Injection: 2 g, 3 g, 4 g
Infusion: 2 g, 3 g, 4 g
Pharmacy bulk package: 40 g

Indications, route, and dosage
Infections caused by susceptible organisms
Adults and children over age 12: Serious infection: 12 to 18 g/day I.V. in divided doses q 4 to 6 hours; uncomplicated urinary tract infection (UTI) and community-acquired pneumonia: 6 to 8 g/day I.V. in divided doses q 6 to 12 hours; complicated UTI: 8 to 16 g/day I.V. in divided doses q 6 to 8 hours; and uncomplicated gonorrhea: 2 g I.M. as a single dose. Maximum daily dose, 24 g.
Prophylaxis of surgical infections
Adults: Intra-abdominal surgery: 2 g I.V. before surgery, 2 g during surgery, and 2 g q 6 hours after surgery for no more than 24 hours; vaginal hysterectomy: 2 g I.V. before surgery, 2 g 6 hours after first dose then 2 g 12 hours after second dose; cesarean section: 2 g I.V. after cord is clamped then 2 g q 4 hours for two doses; abdominal hysterectomy: 2 g I.V. before surgery, 2 g in postanesthesia care unit, and 2 g after 6 hours.
✦ ***Dosage adjustment.*** In adult patients with renal failure, refer to the following dosing chart.

Creatinine clearance (ml/min)	Urinary tract infection		Serious systemic infection
	Uncomplicated	Complicated	
> 40	*	*	*
20 to 40	*	3 g q 8 hr	4 g q 8 hr
< 20	3 g q 12 hr	3 g q 12 hr	4 g q 12 hr

*No dosage adjustment necessary

Pharmacodynamics
Antibiotic action: Piperacillin is bactericidal; it adheres to bacterial penicillin-binding proteins, thus inhibiting bacterial cell wall synthesis.

Extended-spectrum penicillins are more resistant to inactivation by certain beta-lactamases, especially those produced by gram-negative organisms, but are still liable to inactivation by certain others. Because of the potential for rapid development of bacterial resistance, it should not be used as a sole agent in the treatment of an infection.

Piperacillin's spectrum of activity includes many gram-negative aerobic and anaerobic bacilli, many gram-positive and gram-negative aerobic cocci, and some gram-positive aerobic and anaerobic bacilli. Piperacillin may be effective against some strains of carbenicillin-resistant and ticarcillin-resistant gram-negative bacilli. Piperacillin is more active against *Pseudomonas aeruginosa* than are other extended-spectrum penicillins.

Pharmacokinetics
• *Absorption:* Peak plasma concentrations occur 30 to 50 minutes after an I.M. dose.
• *Distribution:* Distributed widely after parenteral administration. It penetrates minimally into uninflamed meninges and slightly into bone and sputum. Piperacillin is 16% to 22% protein-bound; it crosses the placenta.
• *Metabolism:* Not significantly metabolized.
• *Excretion:* Drug is excreted primarily (42% to 90%) in urine by renal tubular secretion and glomerular filtration; it is also excreted in bile and in breast milk. Elimination half-life in adults is about ½ to 1½ hours; in extensive renal impairment, half-life is extended to about 2 to 6 hours; in combined hepatorenal dysfunction, half-life may extend from 11 to 32 hours. Drug is removed by hemodialysis but not by peritoneal dialysis.

Contraindications and precautions
Contraindicated in patients with hypersensitivity to drug or other penicillins. Use cautiously in patients with other drug allergies (especially to cephalosporins), bleeding tendencies, uremia, or hypokalemia.

Interactions
Concomitant use of piperacillin with *aminoglycoside antibiotics* results in synergistic bactericidal effects against *Pseudomonas aeruginosa, Escherichia coli, Klebsiella, Citrobacter, Enterobacter, Serratia,* and *Proteus mirabilis.* However, drugs are physically and chemically incompatible and are inactivated when mixed or given together. In vivo inactivation has been reported when aminoglycosides and extended-spectrum penicillins are used concomitantly.

Concomitant use of piperacillin (and other extended-spectrum penicillins) with *clavulanic acid, sulbactam,* or *tazobactam* also produces a synergistic bactericidal effect against certain beta-lactamase–producing bacteria.

Probenecid blocks tubular secretion of piperacillin, raising serum concentrations of drug. Large doses of penicillins may interfere with renal tubular secretion of *methotrexate,* thus delaying elimination and elevating serum concentrations of methotrexate. Penicillins may decrease the efficacy of *oral contraceptives.*

Effects on diagnostic tests
Piperacillin may falsely decrease serum aminoglycoside concentrations. Piperacillin may cause hypokalemia and hypernatremia and may prolong PT; it may also cause transient elevations in liver function studies and transient reductions in RBC, WBC, and platelet counts.

Piperacillin may cause positive Coombs' tests.

Adverse reactions
CNS: ***seizures,*** headache, dizziness, fatigue.
GI: nausea, diarrhea, vomiting, pseudomembranous colitis.
GU: interstitial nephritis.
Hematologic: *bleeding* (with high doses), neutropenia, eosinophilia, leukopenia, ***thrombocytopenia.***
Other: *hypokalemia,* hypersensitivity reactions (edema, fever, chills, rash, pruritus, urticaria, ***anaphylaxis***), overgrowth of nonsusceptible organisms, pain at injection site, vein irritation, phlebitis, prolonged muscle relaxation.

Overdose and treatment
Clinical signs of overdose include neuromuscular hypersensitivity or seizures resulting from CNS irritation by high drug concentrations. A 4- to 6-hour hemodialysis will remove 10% to 50% of piperacillin.

☑ Special considerations
Besides those relevant to all *penicillins,* consider the following recommendations.
- Piperacillin is almost always used with another antibiotic such as an aminoglycoside in life-threatening situations.
- Drug may be more suitable than carbenicillin or ticarcillin for patients on salt-free diets; piperacillin contains only 1.85 mEq of sodium per g.
- Drug may be administered by direct I.V. injection, given slowly over at least 5 minutes; chest discomfort occurs if injection is given too rapidly.
- Patients with cystic fibrosis are most susceptible to fever or rash from piperacillin.
- Monitor serum electrolytes, especially potassium.
- Monitor neurologic status. High serum levels of this drug may cause seizures.
- Use reduced dosage in patients with creatinine clearance below 40 ml/minute.
- Monitor CBC, differential, and platelets. Drug may cause thrombocytopenia. Observe patient carefully for signs of occult bleeding.
- Because drug is dialyzable, patients undergoing hemodialysis may need dosage adjustments.

Geriatric use
- Half-life may be prolonged in elderly patients because of impaired renal function.

Pediatric use
- Safe use of piperacillin in children under age 12 has not been established.

Breast-feeding
- Drug occurs in breast milk; use with caution in breast-feeding women.

piperacillin sodium and tazobactam sodium
Zosyn

Pharmacologic classification: extended-spectrum penicillin/beta-lactamase inhibitor
Therapeutic classification: antibiotic
Pregnancy risk category B

How supplied
Available by prescription only
Powder for injection (equivalent to piperacillin/tazobactam in a ratio of 8 to 1): 2.25 g, 3.375 g, 4.5 g

Indications, route, and dosage
***Treatment of moderate to severe infections caused by piperacillin-resistant, piperacillin/tazobactam-susceptible, beta-lactamase-producing strains of microorganisms in the following conditions: appendicitis (complicated by rupture or abscess) and peritonitis caused by* Escherichia coli, Bacteroides fragilis, B. ovatus, B. thetaiotaomicron, B. vulgatus; *skin and skin structure infections caused by* Staphylococcus aureus; *postpartum endometritis or pelvic inflammatory disease caused by* E. coli; *moderately severe community-acquired pneumonia caused by* Haemophilus influenzae**
Adults: 3.375 g (3.0 g piperacillin/0.375 g tazobactam) q 6 hours as a 30-minute I.V. infusion.
✦ ***Dosage adjustment.*** In patients with renal dysfunction, refer to the following dosing chart.

Creatinine clearance (ml/min)	Recommended dosage
> 40	12 g/1.5 g/day in divided doses of 3.375 g q 6 hr
20 to 40	8 g/1 g/day in divided doses of 2.25 g q 6 hr
< 20	6 g/0.75 g/day in divided doses of 2.25 g q 8 hr

Note: Discontinue therapy if hypersensitivity reactions or bleeding manifestations occur.

Pharmacodynamics
Antibiotic action: Piperacillin is an extended-spectrum penicillin that inhibits cell wall synthesis during microorganism multiplication; tazobactam increases piperacillin effectiveness by inactivating beta-lactamases, which destroy penicillins.

Pharmacokinetics
- *Absorption:* Unknown.
- *Distribution:* Both piperacillin and tazobactam are approximately 30% bound to plasma proteins.
- *Metabolism:* Piperacillin is metabolized to a minor microbiologically active desethyl metabolite. Tazobactam is metabolized to a single metabolite that lacks pharmacologic and antibacterial activities.

• *Excretion:* Both piperacillin and tazobactam are eliminated via the kidneys by glomerular filtration and tubular secretion. Piperacillin is excreted rapidly as unchanged drug (68% of dose) and tazobactam is excreted as unchanged drug (80%) in the urine. Piperacillin, tazobactam, and desethyl piperacillin also are secreted into the bile.

Contraindications and precautions

Contraindicated in patients with hypersensitivity to drug or other penicillins. Use cautiously in patients with drug allergies (especially to cephalosporins), bleeding tendencies, uremia, or hypokalemia.

Interactions

Mixing piperacillin/tazobactam with an *aminoglycoside* can result in substantial inactivation of the aminoglycoside. Do not mix in the same I.V. container. *Probenecid* administered concomitantly with piperacillin/tazobactam increases blood levels of piperacillin/tazobactam.

Coagulation parameters should be tested more frequently and monitored regularly during simultaneous administration of high doses *of heparin, oral anticoagulants*, or *other drugs that may affect the blood coagulation system* or the *thrombocyte function* when used concurrently with piperacillin/tazobactam.

When used concomitantly with *vecuronium*, piperacillin has been implicated in prolonging the neuromuscular blockade of vecuronium. Piperacillin/tazobactam could produce the same phenomenon if given with vecuronium. Monitor patient closely.

Effects on diagnostic tests

As with other penicillins, piperacillin/tazobactam may result in a false-positive reaction for urine glucose using a copper-reduction method such as Clinitest. Glucose tests based on enzymatic glucose oxidase reactions (such as Diastix or glucose enzymatic test strip) are recommended.

Adverse reactions

CNS: *headache, insomnia,* agitation, dizziness, anxiety.
CV: hypertension, tachycardia, chest pain, edema.
EENT: rhinitis.
GI: *diarrhea, nausea, constipation,* vomiting, dyspepsia, stool changes, abdominal pain.
GU: interstitial nephritis.
Hematologic: leukopenia, anemia, eosinophilia, ***thrombocytopenia.***
Respiratory: dyspnea.
Skin: rash (including maculopapular, bullous, urticarial, and eczematoid), pruritus.
Other: fever; pain; moniliasis; inflammation, phlebitis at I.V. site; ***anaphylaxis.***

Overdose and treatment

No information available.

☑ Special considerations

• Obtain specimen for culture and sensitivity tests before giving first dose. Therapy may begin pending results.
• Pseudomembranous colitis has been reported with nearly all antibacterial agents, including piperacillin/tazobactam, and may range in severity from mild to life-threatening. Therefore, consider this diagnosis in patients presenting with diarrhea after piperacillin/tazobactam administration.
• Bacterial and fungal superinfection may occur and warrants appropriate measures.
• Use piperacillin/tazobactam in combination with an aminoglycoside to treat infections caused by *Pseudomonas aeruginosa.*
• Piperacillin/tazobactam contains 2.35 mEq (54 mg) of sodium per g of piperacillin in the combination product. This should be considered when treating patients requiring restricted sodium intake.
• Perform periodic electrolyte determinations in patients with low potassium reserves; hypokalemia can occur when patient with potentially low potassium reserves receives cytotoxic therapy or diuretics.
• As with other semisynthetic penicillins, piperacillin has been associated with increased incidence of fever and rash in patients with cystic fibrosis.
• Reconstitute piperacillin/tazobactam with 5 ml of diluent per 1 g of piperacillin. Appropriate diluents include sterile or bacteriostatic water for injection, 0.9% NaCl injection, bacteriostatic 0.9% NaCl injection, D_5W, dextrose 5% in 0.9% NaCl injection, or dextran 6% in 0.9% NaCl injection. Do not use lactated Ringer's injection. Shake until dissolved. Further dilution can be made to a final desired volume.
• Infuse over at least 30 minutes. Discontinue primary infusion during administration if possible. Do not mix with other drugs.
• Use single-dose vials immediately after reconstitution. Discard unused drug after 24 hours if held at room temperature; 48 hours if refrigerated. Once diluted, drug is stable in I.V. bags for 24 hours at room temperature or 1 week if refrigerated.
• Change I.V. site every 48 hours.

Pediatric use

• Safety and effectiveness in children under age 12 have not been established.

Breast-feeding

• Piperacillin is excreted in low concentrations in breast milk (tazobactam concentrations have not been studied). Use with caution when administering piperacillin/tazobactam to a breast-feeding woman.

pirbuterol acetate

Maxair

Pharmacologic classification: beta-adrenergic agonist
Therapeutic classification: bronchodilator
Pregnancy risk category C

How supplied

Available by prescription only
Inhaler: 0.2 mg per inhalation

Indications, route, and dosage
Prevention and reversal of bronchospasm; asthma
Adults and children age 12 and over: 1 or 2 inhalations (0.2 to 0.4 mg) repeated q 4 to 6 hours. Not to exceed 12 inhalations daily.

Pharmacodynamics
Bronchodilating action: Pirbuterol stimulates $beta_2$-adrenergic receptors and increases the activity of intracellular adenylate cyclase, an enzyme that catalyzes the conversion of adenosine triphosphate to cyclic adenosine monophosphate (cAMP). Elevated cellular cAMP is associated with bronchodilation and inhibition of the cellular release of mediators of immediate hypersensitivity.

Pharmacokinetics
- *Absorption:* Negligible serum levels are achieved after inhalation of the usual dose.
- *Distribution:* Pirbuterol acts locally.
- *Metabolism:* Hepatic.
- *Excretion:* About 50% of an inhaled dose is recovered in the urine as the parent drug and metabolites.

Contraindications and precautions
Contraindicated in patients with hypersensitivity to pirbuterol. Use cautiously in patients with CV disorders, hyperthyroidism, diabetes, or seizure disorders and in those who are sensitive to sympathomimetic amines.

Interactions
Propranolol and *other beta-adrenergic blocking agents* may decrease the bronchodilating effects of *beta agonists.* Administer cautiously to patients receiving *MAO inhibitors* or *tricyclic antidepressants,* because these agents may enhance the vascular effects of beta-adrenergic agonists.

Effects on diagnostic tests
None reported.

Adverse reactions
CNS: tremor, nervousness, dizziness, insomnia, headache, vertigo.
CV: tachycardia, palpitations, chest tightness.
EENT: dry or irritated throat, dry mouth, cough.
GI: nausea, vomiting, diarrhea.

Overdose and treatment
Anginal pain, hypertension, and tachycardia may result from overdose. Treatment is generally supportive. Sedatives or barbiturates may be necessary to counter any adverse CNS effects; cautious use of beta blockers may be useful to counter cardiac effects.

☑ Special considerations
Besides those relevant to all *adrenergics,* consider the following recommendation.
- Do not administer to patients who are receiving other beta-adrenergic bronchodilators.

Patient education
- Warn patient not to exceed recommended maximum dose of 12 inhalations daily. He should seek medical attention if a previously effective dosage does not control symptoms because this may signify a worsening of disease.
- Tell patient to call promptly if he experiences increased bronchospasm after using drug.
- Teach patient how to use metered dose inhaler correctly. Have him shake container, exhale through the nose; administer aerosol while inhaling deeply on mouthpiece of inhaler; hold breath for a few seconds, then exhale slowly. Tell him to allow at least 2 minutes between inhalations, and to wait at least 5 minutes before using his steroid inhalant (if he's taking concomitant inhalational corticosteroids).

Pediatric use
- Use in children under age 12 is not recommended.

Breast-feeding
- It is not known if pirbuterol is excreted in breast milk. Use with caution in breast-feeding women.

piroxicam
Apo-Piroxicam*, Feldene, Novo-Pirocam*

Pharmacologic classification: NSAID
Therapeutic classification: nonnarcotic analgesic, antipyretic, anti-inflammatory
Pregnancy risk category B (D in third trimester or near delivery)

How supplied
Available by prescription only
Capsules: 10 mg, 20 mg

Indications, route, and dosage
Osteoarthritis and rheumatoid arthritis
Adults: 20 mg P.O. once daily. If desired, the dose may be divided.
◊ ***Juvenile rheumatoid arthritis***
Children weighing 33 to 67 lb (15 to 30 kg): 5 mg P.O.
Children weighing 68 to 100 lb (31 to 45 kg): 10 mg P.O.
Children weighing 101 to 121 lb (46 to 55 kg): 15 mg P.O.

Pharmacodynamics
Analgesic, antipyretic, and anti-inflammatory actions: Exact mechanisms of action are unknown, but piroxicam is thought to inhibit prostaglandin synthesis.

Pharmacokinetics
- *Absorption:* Drug is absorbed rapidly from the GI tract. Peak effect is seen 3 to 5 hours after dosing. Food delays absorption.
- *Distribution:* Piroxicam is highly protein-bound.
- *Metabolism:* Metabolized in the liver.
- *Excretion:* Drug is excreted in urine. Its long half-life (about 50 hours) allows for once-daily dosing.

Contraindications and precautions
Contraindicated in patients with hypersensitivity to drug or with bronchospasm or angioedema precipitated by aspirin or NSAIDs and during pregnancy or while breast-feeding.

Use cautiously in the elderly and in patients with GI disorders, history of renal, peptic ulcer, or cardiac disease, hypertension, or conditions predisposing to fluid retention.

Interactions
Concomitant use of piroxicam with *anticoagulants* and *thrombolytic drugs (coumarin derivatives, heparin, other highly protein-bound drugs)* may potentiate anticoagulant effects. Bleeding problems may occur if used with other *drugs that inhibit platelet aggregation*, such as *aspirin, cefamandole, cefoperazone, dextran, dipyridamole, mezlocillin, piperacillin, plicamycin, salicylates, sulfinpyrazone, ticarcillin, valproic acid,* or *other anti-inflammatory agents.* Concomitant use with *alcohol, anti-inflammatory agents, corticotropin, salicylates,* or *steroids* may cause increased GI adverse effects, including ulceration and hemorrhage. *Aspirin* may decrease the bioavailability of piroxicam. Because of the influence of prostaglandins on glucose metabolism, concomitant use with *insulin* or *oral antidiabetic agents* may potentiate hypoglycemic effects.

Piroxicam may displace highly protein-bound drugs from binding sites. Toxicity may occur with *coumarin derivatives, nifedipine, phenytoin,* or *verapamil.* Increased nephrotoxicity may occur with *acetaminophen, gold compounds,* or *other anti-inflammatory agents.* Piroxicam may decrease the renal clearance of *lithium* and *methotrexate.* Piroxicam may decrease the effectiveness of *antihypertensive agents* and *diuretics.* Concomitant use with *diuretics* may increase risk of nephrotoxicity.

Effects on diagnostic tests
The physiologic effects of drug may prolong bleeding time (may persist for 2 weeks after discontinuing drug); increase BUN, creatinine, and potassium levels or PT; decrease hematocrit and serum glucose (in diabetic patients), hemoglobin, or uric acid levels; and increase liver function test (alkaline phosphatase, LD, or transaminase levels).

Adverse reactions
CNS: headache, drowsiness, dizziness, somnolence, vertigo.
CV: peripheral edema.
EENT: auditory disturbances.
GI: *epigastric distress, nausea, occult blood loss,* ***peptic ulceration, severe GI bleeding,*** diarrhea, constipation, abdominal pain, dyspepsia, flatulence, anorexia, stomatitis.
GU: *nephrotoxicity,* elevated BUN level.
Hematologic: prolonged bleeding time, anemia, leukopenia, ***aplastic anemia, agranulocytosis,*** eosinophilia, ***thrombocytopenia.***
Hepatic: elevated liver enzymes.
Skin: pruritus, rash, urticaria, *photosensitivity.*

Overdose and treatment
To treat piroxicam overdose, empty stomach immediately by inducing emesis with ipecac syrup or by gastric lavage. Administer activated charcoal via nasogastric tube. Provide symptomatic and supportive measures (respiratory support and correction of fluid and electrolyte imbalances). Monitor laboratory parameters and vital signs closely.

☑ Special considerations
Besides those relevant to all *NSAIDs,* consider the following recommendations.
- Drug is usually administered as a single dose.
- Adverse skin reactions are more common with piroxicam than with other NSAIDs; photosensitivity reactions are the most common.
- Effectiveness of piroxicam usually is not seen for at least 2 weeks after therapy begins. Evaluate response to drug as evidenced by reduced symptoms.
- Drug has not been proven safe to the human fetus.

Patient education
- Advise patient to seek medical approval before taking OTC medications.
- Caution patient to avoid hazardous activities requiring alertness until CNS effects are known. Instruct patient in safety measures to prevent injury.
- Instruct patient in signs and symptoms of adverse effects. Tell patient to report them immediately.
- Encourage patient to comply with recommended medical follow-up.
- Tell patient to avoid aspirin and alcoholic beverages during therapy.

Geriatric use
- Patients over age 60 are more sensitive to the adverse effects of piroxicam. Use with caution.
- Through its effect on renal prostaglandins, piroxicam may cause fluid retention and edema. This may be significant in elderly patients and those with heart failure.

Pediatric use
- Safe use of long-term piroxicam in children has not been established.

Breast-feeding
- Piroxicam may inhibit lactation. Because piroxicam is distributed into breast milk at 1% of maternal serum concentration, use an alternative feeding method during drug therapy. Avoid use in breast-feeding women.

plague vaccine

Pharmacologic classification: vaccine
Therapeutic classification: bacterial vaccine
Pregnancy risk category C

How supplied
Available by prescription only
Injection: 1.8 to 2.2 x 10^9 per million killed plague bacilli *(Yersinia pestis)* per ml in 20-ml vials

Indications, route, and dosage

Primary immunization and booster

Adults and children over age 10: 1 ml I.M. followed by 0.2 ml in 4 weeks, then 0.2 ml 6 months after first dose. Booster dosage is 0.1 to 0.2 ml q 6 months for three doses and thereafter q 1 to 2 years while in endemic area.

Although its efficacy has not been determined, an accelerated adult immunization schedule can be used: three doses of 0.5 ml each, administered at least 1 week apart.

◇ *Children age 5 to 10:* Three-fifths the adult primary or booster dosage.

◇ *Children age 1 to 4:* Two-fifths the adult primary or booster dosage.

◇ *Children under age 1:* One-fifth the adult primary or booster dosage.

Pharmacodynamics

Plague prophylaxis: Vaccine is used to promote active immunity to plague.

Pharmacokinetics

- *Absorption:* Duration of vaccine-induced immunity is about 6 to 12 months. Booster doses are required to maintain immunity.
- *Distribution:* No information available.
- *Metabolism:* No information available.
- *Excretion:* No information available.

Contraindications and precautions

Contraindicated in immunosuppressed or pregnant patients and in those hypersensitive to beef, soy, casein, phenol, or formaldehyde. Patients who have had severe local or systemic reactions to plague vaccine should not be revaccinated. Also contraindicated in patients with severe thrombocytopenia or any coagulation disorder that would contraindicate I.M. injections.

Use cautiously in patients receiving anticoagulants.

Interactions

Concomitant use with *corticosteroids* or *other immunosuppressants* may impair the immune response to plague vaccine, and vaccination may fail to elicit an arbitrary response in these patients. Antibody determinations may be necessary.

Effects on diagnostic tests

None reported.

Adverse reactions

CNS: headache, malaise.
GI: nausea, vomiting.
Musculoskeletal: arthralgia, myalgia.
Other: ***anaphylaxis,*** leukocytosis, *lymphadenopathy, slight fever,* swelling, *induration, erythema at injection site.*

Overdose and treatment

No information available.

☑ Special considerations

- Obtain a thorough history of allergies and reactions to immunizations.
- Epinephrine solution 1:1,000 should be available to treat allergic reactions.
- Before withdrawing the dose, shake the vial until the suspension is uniform.
- Vaccine is a turbid, whitish liquid with a faint odor.
- Deltoid muscle is the preferred I.M. injection site.
- Never administer plague vaccine I.V.
- Store at 36° to 46° F (2° to 8° C). Do not freeze. Vaccine is stable at room temperature for 15 days.
- Administer to pregnant women only when a high risk of infection exists. There are no data regarding safety and efficacy during pregnancy.

Patient education

- Explain that patient will receive three doses of plague vaccine to develop immunity to plague. Thereafter, he will need a booster every 6 months initially, then every 1 to 2 years.
- Tell patient that he may experience pain and inflammation at the injection site and may develop fever, general malaise, headache, swollen lymph nodes, or difficulty breathing. Encourage him to report distressing adverse reactions.

Breast-feeding

- Adverse effects are unknown. Vaccine should be used with caution in breast-feeding women.

plasma protein fraction

Plasmanate, Plasma-Plex, Plasmatein, Protenate

Pharmacologic classification: blood derivative
Therapeutic classification: plasma volume expander
Pregnancy risk category C

How supplied

Available by prescription only
Injection: 5% solution in 50-ml, 250-ml, 500-ml vials

Indications, route, and dosage

Shock

Adults: Varies with patient's condition and response, but usually 250 to 500 ml (12.5 to 25 g protein) I.V., not to exceed 10 ml/minute.

Children: 22 to 33 ml/kg I.V. infused at rate of 5 to 10 ml/minute.

Small children and infants: 15 ml/lb (2.2 kg) I.V. infused at rate of 5 to 10 ml/minute (Plasma-Plex).

Hypoproteinemia

Adults: 1,000 to 1,500 ml I.V. daily. Maximum infusion rate is 8 ml/minute (500 ml infused in 30 to 45 minutes).

Pharmacodynamics

Plasma-expanding action: Plasma protein fraction (PPF) supplies colloid to the blood and expands plasma volume. It causes fluid to shift from interstitial spaces into the circulation and slightly increases plasma protein concentration. It is comprised mostly of albumin, but may contain up to 17% alpha and beta globulins and not more than 1% gamma globulin.

Pharmacokinetics
The pharmacokinetics of PPF are similar to its chief constituent, albumin (approximately 83% to 90%).

• *Absorption:* Albumin is not adequately absorbed from the GI tract.

• *Distribution:* Albumin accounts for approximately 50% of plasma proteins. It is distributed into the intravascular space and extravascular sites, including skin, muscle, and lungs. In patients with reduced circulating blood volumes, hemodilution secondary to albumin administration persists for many hours; in patients with normal blood volume, excess fluid and protein are lost from the intravascular space within a few hours.

• *Metabolism:* Although albumin is synthesized in the liver, the liver is not involved in clearance of albumin from the plasma in healthy individuals.

• *Excretion:* Little is known about albumin excretion in healthy individuals. Administration of albumin decreases hepatic albumin synthesis and increases albumin clearance if plasma oncotic pressure is high. In certain pathologic states, the liver, kidneys, or intestines may provide elimination mechanisms.

Contraindications and precautions
Contraindicated in patients with severe anemia or heart failure and in those undergoing cardiac bypass. Use cautiously in patients with impaired renal or hepatic function, low cardiac reserve, or restricted salt intake.

Interactions
None significant.

Effects on diagnostic tests
PPF slightly increases plasma protein levels.

Adverse reactions
CNS: headache.
CV: hypotension (after rapid infusion or intra-arterial administration), ***vascular overload*** (after rapid infusion), tachycardia.
GI: nausea, vomiting, hypersalivation.
Respiratory: dyspnea, ***pulmonary edema.***
Skin: rash.
Other: flushing, chills, fever, back pain.

Overdose and treatment
Rapid infusion can cause circulatory overload and pulmonary edema. Watch patient for signs of hypervolemia; monitor blood pressure and central venous pressure. Treatment is symptomatic.

☑ Special considerations
• Do not use solution that is cloudy, contains sediment, or has been frozen. Store at room temperature; freezing may break bottle and allow bacterial contamination.

• Use opened solution promptly, discarding unused portion after 4 hours; solution contains no preservatives and becomes unstable.

• One "unit" is usually considered to be 250 ml of the 5% concentration.

• Avoid rapid I.V. infusion. Rate is individualized according to patient's age, condition, and diagnosis. Maximum dosage is 250 g/48 hours; do not give faster than 10 ml/minute. Decrease infusion rate to 5 to 8 ml/minute as plasma volume approaches normal.

• PPF is also used in treatment of burns; dosage depends on the extent and severity of burn.

• No cross-matching is required. PPF should not be administered with the same administration set of solutions containing protein hydrosylates, amino acid solutions, or alcohol.

• Monitor blood pressure frequently; slow or stop infusion if hypotension suddenly occurs. Vital signs should return to normal gradually.

• Observe patient for signs of vascular overload (heart failure, pulmonary edema, widening pulse pressure indicating increased cardiac output) and signs of hemorrhage or shock (after surgery or trauma); be alert for bleeding sites not evident at lower blood pressure.

• Monitor intake and output (watch especially for decreased output), hemoglobin, hematocrit, and serum protein and electrolyte levels to help determine ongoing dosage.

• If patient is dehydrated, give additional fluids either P.O. or I.V.

• Each liter contains 130 to 160 mEq of sodium before dilution with any additional I.V. fluids; a 250-ml container of the 5% concentration contains approximately 33 to 40 mEq sodium.

plicamycin
Mithracin

Pharmacologic classification: antibiotic antineoplastic (cell cycle–phase nonspecific)
Therapeutic classification: antineoplastic, hypocalcemic
Pregnancy risk category X

How supplied
Available by prescription only
Injection: 2,500-mcg vials

Indications, route, and dosage
Dosage and indications may vary. Check current literature for recommended protocol.

Hypercalcemia
Adults: 25 mcg/kg I.V. daily over 4 to 6 hours for 3 to 4 days. Repeat at intervals of 1 week p.r.n.

Testicular cancer
Adults: 25 to 30 mcg/kg I.V. daily over 4 to 6 hours for up to 10 days (based on ideal body weight or actual weight, whichever is less).

◊ ***Paget's disease***
Adults: 15 mcg/kg I.V. daily over 4 to 6 hours for up to 10 days.

Pharmacodynamics
Antineoplastic action: Plicamycin exerts its cytotoxic activity by intercalating between DNA base pairs and also binding to the outside of the DNA molecule. The result is inhibition of DNA-dependent RNA synthesis.

Hypocalcemic action: The exact mechanism by which plicamycin lowers serum calcium levels is unknown. Plicamycin may block the hypercalcemic effect of vitamin D or may inhibit the effect of parathyroid hormone upon osteoclasts, preventing osteolysis. Both mechanisms reduce serum calcium concentrations.

Pharmacokinetics

- *Absorption:* Drug is not administered orally.
- *Distribution:* Plicamycin distributes mainly into the Kupffer's cells of the liver, into renal tubular cells, and along formed bone surfaces. Drug also crosses the blood-brain barrier and achieves appreciable concentrations in the CSF.
- *Metabolism:* Unclear.
- *Excretion:* Drug is eliminated primarily through the kidneys.

Contraindications and precautions

Contraindicated in patients with thrombocytopenia, bone marrow suppression, or coagulation and bleeding disorders and in women who are or who may become pregnant. Use cautiously in patients with impaired renal or hepatic function.

Interactions

None reported.

Effects on diagnostic tests

Because of drug-induced toxicity, plicamycin therapy may increase serum concentrations of alkaline phosphatase, AST, ALT, LD, and bilirubin; it may also increase serum creatinine and BUN levels through nephrotoxicity.

Adverse reactions

CNS: drowsiness, weakness, lethargy, headache, malaise.
GI: *nausea, vomiting,* anorexia, diarrhea, stomatitis.
GU: increased BUN and serum creatinine levels.
Hematologic: ***leukopenia, thrombocytopenia; bleeding syndrome*** (from epistaxis to generalized hemorrhage).
Hepatic: ***elevated liver enzymes levels,*** hepatotoxicity.
Skin: facial flushing, rash.
Other: ***decreased serum calcium,*** potassium, and phosphorus levels; ***death;*** fever; cellulitis with extravasation; phlebitis.

Overdose and treatment

Clinical manifestations of overdose include myelosuppression, electrolyte imbalance, and coagulation disorders. Treatment is usually supportive and includes transfusion of blood components and appropriate symptomatic therapy. Patient's renal and hepatic status should be closely monitored.

☑ Special considerations

- To reconstitute drug, use 4.9 ml of sterile water to give a concentration of 500 mcg/ml. Reconstitute drug immediately before administration, and discard unused solution.
- Drug may be further diluted with 0.9% NaCl solution or D_5W to a volume of 1,000 ml and administered as an I.V. infusion over 4 to 6 hours.
- Although drug may be administered by I.V. push injection, it is discouraged because of the higher incidence and greater severity of GI toxicity. Nausea and vomiting are greatly diminished as infusion rate is decreased.
- Infusions of plicamycin in 1,000 ml D_5W are stable for up to 24 hours.
- If I.V. infiltrates, infusion should be stopped immediately and ice packs applied before restarting an I.V. in other arm.
- Give antiemetics before administering drug, to reduce nausea.
- Monitor LD, AST, ALT, alkaline phosphatase, BUN, creatinine, potassium, calcium, and phosphorus levels.
- Monitor platelet count and PT before and during therapy.
- Check serum calcium levels. Monitor patient for tetany, carpopedal spasm, Chvostek's sign, and muscle cramps because a precipitous drop in calcium levels is possible.
- Observe for signs of bleeding. Facial flushing may be an early indicator.
- Therapeutic effect in hypercalcemia may not be seen for 24 to 48 hours; may last 3 to 15 days.
- Avoid drug contact with skin or mucous membranes.
- Store lyophilized powder in refrigerator.

Patient education

- Tell patient to use salicylate-free medication for pain relief or fever reduction.
- Instruct patient to avoid exposure to people with infections and to call immediately if signs of infection or unusual bleeding occur.
- Inform patient that he and household members should not receive immunizations during therapy and for several weeks after therapy.
- Advise patient to use contraceptive measures during therapy.

Breast-feeding

- It is not known if drug occurs in breast milk. However, because of potential for serious adverse reactions, mutagenicity, and carcinogenicity in the infant, breast-feeding is not recommended.

pneumococcal vaccine, polyvalent

Pneumovax 23, Pnu-Imune 23

Pharmacologic classification: vaccine
Therapeutic classification: bacterial vaccine
Pregnancy risk category C

How supplied

Available by prescription only
Injection: 25 mcg each of 23 polysaccharide isolates of *Streptococcus pneumoniae* per 0.5-ml dose, in 1-ml and 5-ml vials and disposable syringes.

Indications, route, and dosage

Pneumococcal immunization
Adults and children over age 2: 0.5 ml I.M. or S.C. as a one-time dose.

Pharmacodynamics
Pneumonia prophylaxis: Pneumococcal vaccine promotes active immunity against the 23 most prevalent pneumococcal types.

Pharmacokinetics
• *Absorption:* Protective antibodies are produced within 3 weeks after injection. Duration of vaccine-induced immunity is at least 5 years in adults.
• *Distribution:* No information available.
• *Metabolism:* No information available.
• *Excretion:* No information available.

Contraindications and precautions
Contraindicated in patients hypersensitive to drug or its components (phenol). Also contraindicated in patients with Hodgkin's disease who have received extensive chemotherapy or nodal irradiation.

Interactions
Concomitant use of pneumococcal vaccine with *corticosteroids* or other *immunosuppressants* may impair the immune response to vaccine; therefore, vaccination should be avoided.

Effects on diagnostic tests
None reported.

Adverse reactions
GI: nausea, vomiting.
Other: adenitis, ***anaphylaxis,*** arthralgia, headache, myalgia, rash, serum sickness, *slight fever, soreness at injection site,* severe local reaction associated with revaccination within 3 years.

Overdose and treatment
No information available.

☑ Special considerations
• Obtain a thorough history of allergies and reactions to immunizations.
• Persons with asplenia who received the 14-valent vaccine should be revaccinated with the 23-valent vaccine.
• Epinephrine solution 1:1,000 should be available to treat allergic reactions.
• Use the deltoid or midlateral thigh. Do not inject I.V. Avoid intradermal administration because this may cause severe local reactions.
• Polyvalent pneumococcal vaccine also may be administered to children to prevent pneumococcal otitis media.
• Candidates for pneumococcal vaccine include persons age 65 and older; adults and children age 2 or older with chronic illness, asplenia, or splenic dysfunction; and those with sickle-cell anemia and human immunodeficiency virus infection.
• Vaccine also is recommended for patients awaiting organ transplants, those receiving radiation therapy or cancer chemotherapy, persons in nursing homes and orphanages, and bedridden patients.
• If different sites and separate syringes are used, pneumococcal vaccine may be administered simultaneously with influenza, DTP, poliovirus, or *Haemophilus* b polysaccharide vaccines.
• Store vaccine at 36° to 46° F (2° to 8° C). Reconstitution or dilution is unnecessary.

Patient education
• Tell patient to expect redness, soreness, swelling, and pain at the injection site after vaccination. Patient may also develop fever, joint or muscle aches and pains, rash, itching, general weakness, or difficulty breathing.
• Encourage patient to report distressing adverse reactions promptly.
• Advise patient to use acetaminophen to relieve adverse reactions promptly.

Pediatric use
• Children under age 2 do not respond satisfactorily to pneumococcal vaccine. Vaccine's safety and efficacy in this group have not been established.

Breast-feeding
• It is unknown if vaccine occurs in milk. Use with caution in breast-feeding women.

poliovirus vaccine, live, oral, trivalent (Sabin vaccine, TOPV)
Orimune

Pharmacologic classification: vaccine
Therapeutic classification: viral vaccine
Pregnancy risk category C

How supplied
Available by prescription only
Oral vaccine: mixture of three viruses (types 1, 2, and 3), grown in monkey kidney tissue culture, in 0.5-ml single-dose Dispettes

Indications, route, and dosage
Poliovirus immunization (primary series)
Adolescents and older children: Two 0.5-ml doses administered 8 weeks apart. Give third 0.5-ml dose 6 to 12 months after second dose.
Infants: 0.5 ml at age 2 months, 4 months, and 18 months. Optional dose may be given at 6 months when substantial risk of exposure exists.
Supplementary: All children entering elementary school (age 4 to 6) who have completed the primary series should receive a single follow-up dose of TOPV. Booster vaccination beyond elementary school is not routinely recommended.
Adults age 18 and over: TOPV should not be given to persons age 18 and over who have not received at least one prior dose of TOPV. Enhanced potency inactivated polio vaccine (eIPV) should be used if polio vaccination is indicated.

If less than 4 weeks are available before protection is needed, a single dose of TOPV is recommended, followed by IPV later if the person remains at increased risk.

Persons traveling to countries with endemic or epidemic polio who previously completed a primary series should receive a single follow-up dose of TOPV. Do not administer vaccine to neonates under age 6 weeks.

Pharmacodynamics
Polio prophylaxis: TOPV promotes immunity to poliomyelitis by inducing humoral and secretory antibodies and antibodies in the lymphatic tissue of the GI tract.

Pharmacokinetics
- *Absorption:* Antibody response to vaccine occurs within 7 to 10 days after ingestion and peaks around 21 days. Duration of immunity is thought to be lifelong.
- *Distribution:* No information available.
- *Metabolism:* No information available.
- *Excretion:* No information available.

Contraindications and precautions
Oral vaccine is contraindicated in immunosuppressed patients, in those with cancer or immunoglobulin abnormalities, and in those receiving radiation, antimetabolite, alkylating agent, or corticosteroid therapy. These patients should receive IPV. Injectable vaccine is contraindicated in patients hypersensitive to neomycin, streptomycin, or polymyxin B.

Use cautiously in siblings of children with known immunodeficiency syndrome.

Interactions
Concomitant use of TOPV with *corticosteroids* or other *immunosuppressants* may impair the immune response to the vaccine. Vaccination with TOPV should be deferred until the immunosuppressant is discontinued or, alternatively, inactivated poliovirus vaccine may be used. *Immune serum globulin* and *transfusions of blood or blood products* may also interfere with the immune response to poliovirus vaccine. Defer vaccination for 3 months in these situations.

Effects on diagnostic tests
TOPV may temporarily decrease the response to tuberculin skin testing. If a tuberculin test is necessary, administer either before, simultaneously with, or at least 8 weeks after TOPV.

Adverse reactions
Other: crying, decreased appetite, *fever,* hypersensitivity reactions, ***poliomyelitis,*** sleepiness, erythema, induration, *pain* (at injection site).

Overdose and treatment
No information available.

☑ Special considerations
- Obtain a thorough history of allergies, especially to antibiotics, and of reactions to immunizations.
- Vaccine is not effective in modifying or preventing existing or incubating poliomyelitis.
- Check parents' immunization history when they bring in a child for the vaccine; this is an excellent time for parents to receive booster immunizations.
- Adults and immunocompromised persons who have not been vaccinated should receive IPV (Salk) in three doses, given 1 month apart, before other household contacts are immunized with TOPV.
- Vaccine is not for parenteral use. Dose may be administered directly or mixed with distilled water, chlorine-free tap water, simple syrup USP, or milk. It also may be placed on bread, cake, or a sugar cube.
- Keep vaccine frozen until used. It may be refrigerated up to 30 days once thawed, if unopened. Opened vials may be refrigerated up to 7 days.
- Color change from pink to yellow has no effect on the efficacy of the vaccine as long as the vaccine remains clear. Yellow color results from storage at low temperatures.

Patient education
- Inform patient that risk of vaccine-associated paralysis is extremely small for vaccines, susceptible family members, and other close contacts (about 1 case per 2.6 million patients receiving the vaccines).
- Encourage patient to report distressing adverse reactions promptly.

Pediatric use
- Poliovirus vaccine should not be administered to neonates under age 6 weeks.

Breast-feeding
- Breast-feeding does not interfere with successful immunization; hence, no interruption in the feeding schedule is necessary.

polyethylene glycol-electrolyte solution
Colovage, CoLyte, GoLYTELY, NuLYTELY, OCL

Pharmacologic classification: polyethylene glycol 3350 nonabsorbable solution
Therapeutic classification: laxative and bowel evacuant
Pregnancy risk category C

How supplied
Available by prescription only
Powder for oral solution: polyethylene glycol (PEG) 3350 (6 g), anhydrous sodium sulfate (568 mg), sodium chloride (146 mg), potassium chloride (74.5 mg/100 ml) (Colovage); PEG 3350 (120 g), sodium sulfate (3.36 g), sodium chloride (2.92 g), potassium chloride (1.49 g/2 L) (CoLyte); PEG 3350 (236 g), sodium sulfate (22.74 g), sodium bicarbonate (6.74 g), sodium chloride (5.86 g), potassium chloride (2.97 g/4.8 L) (GoLYTELY); PEG 3350 (420 g), sodium bicarbonate (5.72 g), sodium chloride (11.2 g), potassium chloride (1.48 g/4 L) (NuLYTELY); PEG 3350 (6 g), sodium sulfate decahydrate (1.29 g), sodium chloride (146 mg), potassium chloride (75 mg), polysorbate-80 (30 mg/100 ml) (OCL)

Indications, route, and dosage
Bowel preparation before GI examination
Adults: 240 ml P.O. q 10 minutes until 4 L are consumed or the rectal effluent is clear. Typically, ad-

minister 4 hours before examination, allowing 3 hours for drinking and 1 hour for bowel evacuation.
Children age 3 weeks to 18 years: 25 to 40 ml/kg for 4 to 10 hours.
◇ ***Management of acute iron overdose***
Children under age 3: 0.5 L/hour.

Note: If a patient experiences severe bloating, distention, or abdominal pain, slow or temporarily discontinue administration until symptoms abate.

Pharmacodynamics
Laxative and bowel evacuant action: PEG-ES acts as an osmotic agent. With sodium sulfate as the major sodium source, active sodium absorption is markedly reduced. Diarrhea results, which rapidly cleans the bowel, usually within 4 hours.

Pharmacokinetics
- *Absorption:* PEG-ES is a nonabsorbable solution. Onset of action occurs within 30 to 60 minutes.
- *Distribution:* Not applicable because drug is not absorbed.
- *Metabolism:* Not applicable because drug is not absorbed.
- *Excretion:* PEG-ES is excreted via the GI tract.

Contraindications and precautions
Contraindicated in patients with GI obstruction or perforation, gastric retention, toxic colitis, ileus, or megacolon.

Interactions
Oral medication given within 1 hour before start of therapy may be flushed from the GI tract and not absorbed.

Effects on diagnostic tests
Patient preparation for barium enema may be less satisfactory with this solution because it may interfere with the barium coating of the colonic mucosa using the double-contrast technique.

Adverse reactions
GI: ***nausea, bloating, cramps, vomiting, abdominal fullness.***
Skin: urticaria, dermatitis.
Other: anal irritation, rhinorrhea, ***anaphylaxis.***

Overdose and treatment
No information available.

☑ Special considerations
- Drug may be given via a nasogastric tube (at 20 to 30 ml/minute, or 1.2 to 1.8 L/hour) to patients unwilling or unable to drink the preparation. The first bowel movement should occur within 1 hour.
- Tap water may be used to reconstitute the solution. Shake container vigorously several times to ensure that the powder is completely dissolved. After reconstitution to 4 L with water, the solution contains PEG 3350 17.6 mmol/L, sodium 125 mmol/L, sulfate 40 mmol/L (Colyte 80 mmol/L), chloride 35 mmol/L, bicarbonate 20 mmol/L, and potassium 10 mmol/L (1 mmol/L = 1 mEq/L).
- Store reconstituted solution in refrigerator (chilling before administration improves palatability); use within 48 hours.
- Do not add flavorings or additional ingredients to solution before use.
- No major shifts in fluid or electrolyte balance have been reported.

Patient education
- Instruct patient to fast approximately 3 to 4 hours before ingesting the solution.
- Tell patient never to take solid foods less than 2 hours before solution is administered. Also inform him that no foods except clear liquids are permitted after administration of solution until the examination is completed.

polymyxin B sulfate
Aerosporin

Pharmacologic classification: polymyxin antibiotic
Therapeutic classification: antibiotic
Pregnancy risk category B

How supplied
Available by prescription only
Powder for injection: 500,000-unit vials
Ophthalmic sterile powder for solution: 500,000-unit vials to be reconstituted to 20 to 50 ml

Indications, route, and dosage
Acute urinary tract infections, septicemia, or bacteremia caused by sensitive organisms when other antibiotics are ineffective or contraindicated
Adults and children: 15,000 to 25,000 units/kg daily I.V. infusion, divided q 12 hours; or 25,000 to 30,000 units/kg daily, I.M. divided q 4 to 8 hours. I.M. injection not to be used as first choice because of severe pain at injection site.
Meningitis caused by sensitive* Pseudomonas aeruginosa *or* Haemophilus influenzae *when other antibiotics are ineffective or contraindicated
Adults and children over age 2: 50,000 units intrathecally once daily for 3 to 4 days, then 50,000 units every other day for at least 2 weeks after CSF tests are negative and CSF glucose level is normal.
Children under age 2: 20,000 units intrathecally once daily for 3 to 4 days, then 25,000 units every other day for at least 2 weeks after CSF tests are negative and CSF glucose level is normal.
***Eye infections caused by sensitive* P. aeruginosa**
Adults and children: 1 to 3 drops of a solution containing 10,000 to 25,000 units/ml hourly until favorable response occurs. Do not exceed 25,000 units/kg or 2,000,000 units/day.
✦ ***Dosage adjustment.*** In patients with renal failure, refer to the dosage chart on the next page.

Creatinine clearance (ml/min)	Dosage in adults
> 20	75 to 100% of usual dose in two divided doses q 12 hr
5 to 20	50% of usual dose in two divided doses q 12 hr
< 5	15% of usual dose in two divided doses q 12 hr

Pharmacodynamics

Antibacterial action: Polymyxin B sulfate alters permeability of bacterial cytoplasmic membrane. It is bactericidal against many gram-negative organisms and is indicated for sensitive strains of *P. aeruginosa, Enterobacter aerogenes, Klebsiella pneumoniae,* or *Escherichia coli. Proteus, Neisseria,* and gram-positive organisms resist drug.

Pharmacokinetics

- *Absorption:* Not significantly absorbed from GI tract. With I.M. administration, peak serum levels occur in 2 hours.
- *Distribution:* With systemic administration, drug is distributed widely except in CSF, aqueous humor, and placental and synovial fluids. Minimally bound to plasma proteins.
- *Metabolism:* Unknown.
- *Excretion:* About 60% of dose is excreted renally. In patients with normal renal function, plasma half-life is 4 to 6 hours. In patients with creatinine clearance below 10 ml/minute, half-life is 2 to 3 days. There is no appreciable clearance by either hemodialysis or peritoneal dialysis.

Contraindications and precautions

Contraindicated in patients with hypersensitivity to drug. Use injectable form cautiously in patients with impaired renal function or myasthenia gravis.

Interactions

When used concomitantly, polymyxin B sulfate may prolong, intensify, or reinstate neuromuscular blockade and paralysis induced by *neuromuscular blocking agents* and *some anesthetic agents* (for example, *gallamine, succinylcholine,* and *tubocurarine*).

Concomitant use with *other nephrotoxic drugs* (such as *aminoglycosides, amphotericin B, capreomycin, cisplatin, methoxyflurane,* and *vancomycin*) may increase risk of polymyxin-induced nephrotoxicity.

Effects on diagnostic tests

BUN and serum creatinine levels may increase during polymyxin B therapy. CSF protein and leukocyte levels may increase during intrathecal polymyxin B therapy.

Adverse reactions

CNS: ***neurotoxicity,*** irritability, drowsiness, facial flushing, weakness, ataxia, ***respiratory paralysis,*** headache and meningeal irritation with intrathecal administration, peripheral and perioral paresthesias (with injected form).
EENT: blurred vision (with injected form); eye irritation, conjunctivitis (with ophthalmic form).
GU: *nephrotoxicity* (albuminuria, cylindruria, hematuria, proteinuria, decreased urine output, increased BUN level) (with injected form).
Skin: urticaria (with injected form).
Other: drug fever, pain or thrombophlebitis at injection site (with injected form); overgrowth of nonsusceptible organisms, hypersensitivity reactions (local burning, itching) (with ophthalmic form).

Overdose and treatment

Clinical effects of overdose with polymyxin B may include respiratory paralysis that may resist treatment with neostigmine and edrophonium.

Treatment includes supportive measures until muscle function returns. Calcium chloride may be given. Drug is not dialyzable.

☑ Special considerations

- Obtain culture and sensitivity tests before starting therapy.
- Obtain baseline renal function indices (BUN and serum creatinine levels and urine output), and monitor them during therapy.
- To prepare I.V. infusion, dilute each 500,000-unit vial in 300 to 500 ml D_5W; infuse over 60 to 90 minutes. Prepared solution remains stable for 72 hours when refrigerated.
- To prepare I.M. injection, reconstitute according to package instructions and give deep I.M. Procaine 1% may be used as a diluent (unless patient is allergic to procaine).
- To prepare intrathecal injection, add 10 ml of preservative-free sterile NaCl solution to vial to yield 50,000 units/ml. Withdraw desired dose.
- Ensure adequate fluid intake to maintain urine output at 1,500 ml/day.
- Monitor patient for fever, CNS toxicity, rash, or evidence of renal toxicity.
- Monitor for signs and symptoms of local superinfection.
- If patient is receiving drug concomitantly with neuromuscular blocking agents and certain anesthetic agents (such as gallamine, tubocurarine, succinylcholine, and decamethonium), monitor closely and keep mechanical ventilator available.
- Drug should be administered I.V. only in a facility where patient can be monitored appropriately.
- Patients with renal impairment require reduced dose.
- Patients with meningitis require intrathecal administration to ensure adequate CSF drug levels.

Patient education

- Encourage patient to report severe or unusual adverse effects immediately.

polysaccharide-iron complex

Hytinic, Niferex, Niferex-150, Nu-Iron, Nu-Iron 150

Pharmacologic classification: oral iron supplement
Therapeutic classification: hematinic
Pregnancy risk category NR

How supplied

Available without a prescription
Tablets (film-coated): 50 mg
Capsules: 150 mg
Solution: 100 mg/5 ml

Indications, route, and dosage

Treatment of uncomplicated iron-deficiency anemia

Adults and children age 12 and older: 150 to 300 mg P.O. daily as capsules or tablets or 1 to 2 teaspoonfuls of elixir P.O. daily.

Children age 6 to 12: 150 mg to 300 mg P.O. daily as tablets or 1 teaspoonful of elixir P.O. daily.

Children age 2 to 6: Give ½ teaspoonful of elixir P.O. daily.

Pharmacodynamics

Hematinic action: Polysaccharide-iron complex provides elemental iron, an essential component in the formation of hemoglobin.

Pharmacokinetics

- *Absorption:* Although iron is absorbed from entire length of GI tract, the duodenum and proximal jejunum are the primary absorption sites. Up to 10% of iron is absorbed by healthy individuals; patients with iron-deficiency anemia may absorb up to 60%. Enteric coating and some extended-release formulas have decreased absorption because they are designed to release iron past points in GI tract of highest absorption. Food may decrease absorption by 33% to 50%.
- *Distribution:* Iron is transported through GI mucosal cells directly into the blood where it is immediately bound to a carrier protein, transferrin, and transported to the bone marrow for incorporation into hemoglobin. Iron is highly protein-bound.
- *Metabolism:* Iron is liberated by the destruction of hemoglobin, but is conserved and reused by the body.
- *Excretion:* Healthy individuals lose only small amounts of iron each day. Men and postmenopausal women lose about 1 mg/day and premenopausal women about 1.5 mg/day. Loss usually occurs in nails, hair, feces, and urine; trace amounts are lost in bile and sweat.

Contraindications and precautions

Contraindicated in patients with hypersensitivity to any component of drug and in those with hemochromatosis and hemosiderosis.

Interactions

Antacids, cholestyramine resin, cimetidine, tetracycline, and *vitamin E* decrease iron absorption; separate doses by 2 to 4 hours. *Chloramphenicol* causes a delayed response to iron therapy. Monitor patient carefully. Iron decreases absorption of *fluoroquinolones, levodopa, methyldopa,* and *penicillamine* possibly resulting in decreased serum levels or efficacy. *Vitamin C* may increase iron absorption.

Effects on diagnostic tests

Polysaccaride iron complex may blacken feces and may interfere with test for occult blood in stool; guaiac and orthotoluidine tests may yield false-positive results. Benzidine test is usually not affected. Iron overload may decrease uptake of technetium-99m and, thus, interfere with skeletal imaging.

Adverse reactions

Although nausea, constipation, black stools, and epigastric pain are common adverse reactions associated with iron therapy, few, if any, occur with polysaccharide-iron complex. Iron-containing liquids may cause temporary staining of teeth.

Overdose and treatment

The lethal dose of iron is between 200 and 250 mg/kg; fatalities have occurred with lower doses. Symptoms may follow ingestion of 20 to 60 mg/kg. Clinical signs of acute overdose may occur as follows.

Between ½ and 8 hours after ingestion, patient may experience lethargy, nausea and vomiting, green then tarry stools, weak and rapid pulse, hypotension, dehydration, acidosis, and coma. If death does not immediately ensue, symptoms may clear for about 24 hours.

At 12 to 48 hours, symptoms may return, accompanied by diffuse vascular congestion, pulmonary edema, shock, seizures, anuria, and hyperthermia. Death may follow.

Treatment requires immediate support of airway, respiration, and circulation. Induce emesis with ipecac in conscious patients with intact gag reflex; for unconscious patients, empty stomach by gastric lavage. Follow emesis with lavage, using 1% sodium bicarbonate solution, to convert iron to less irritating, poorly absorbed form. (Phosphate solutions have been used, but carry risk of other adverse effects.) Perform radiographic evaluation of abdomen to determine continued presence of excess iron; if serum iron levels exceed 350 mg/dl, deferoxamine may be used for systemic chelation.

Survivors are likely to sustain organ damage, including pyloric or antral stenosis, hepatic cirrhosis, CNS damage, and intestinal obstruction.

☑ Special considerations

- Administer iron with juice (preferably orange juice) or water, but not with milk or antacids.
- Polysaccaride-iron complex is nontoxic and there are relatively few, if any, of the GI adverse effects associated with other iron preparations.
- Be aware that oral iron may turn stools black. This unabsorbed iron is harmless; however, it could mask melena.
- Monitor hemoglobin level and hematocrit and reticulocyte counts during therapy.

Patient education

- Inform parents that as few as three or four tablets can cause serious iron poisoning in children.
- If patient misses a dose, tell him to take it as soon as he remembers but not to take a double dose.
- Advise patient to avoid certain foods that may impair oral iron absorption, including yogurt, cheese, eggs, milk, whole-grain breads and cereals, tea, and coffee.
- Teach patient dietary measures to follow for preventing constipation.

Geriatric use

- Because iron-induced constipation is common in elderly patients, stress proper diet to minimize this adverse effect. Elderly patients may need higher doses of iron because reduced gastric secretions and achlorhydria may lower capacity for iron absorption.

Pediatric use

- Overdose of iron may be fatal; treat patient immediately.

Breast-feeding

- Iron supplements are often recommended for breast-feeding women; no adverse effects have been documented.

porfimer sodium

Photofrin

Pharmacologic classification: photosensitizing
Therapeutic classification: antineoplastic
Pregnancy risk category C

How supplied

Available by prescription only
Injection: 75 mg/vial

Indications, route, and dosage

Palliative treatment of patients with completely obstructing esophageal cancer or partially obstructing esophageal cancer who, in the primary health care provider's opinion, cannot be satisfactorily treated with laser therapy
Adults: 2 mg/kg I.V. over 3 to 5 minutes (first stage), followed by illumination with laser light 40 to 50 hours later (second stage). Total of three courses (each course consisting of both stages) may be given but must be separated by minimum of 30 days.

Pharmacodynamics

Antineoplastic action: Porfimer is a photosensitizing agent that causes cellular damage because of propagation of radical reactions. Tumor death also occurs through ischemic necrosis secondary to vascular occlusion that appears to be partly mediated by thromboxane A_2 release. Cytotoxic and antitumor actions of porfimer are dependent on light and oxygen.

Pharmacokinetics

- *Absorption:* Porfimer is given only I.V.
- *Distribution:* Drug is about 90% bound to plasma protein. Volume of distribution is about 0.49 L/kg; elimination half-life is about 250 hours.
- *Metabolism:* Unknown.
- *Excretion:* Unknown.

Contraindications and precautions

Contraindicated in patients with porphyria, existing tracheoesophageal or bronchoesophageal fistula, tumors eroding into a major blood vessel, or hypersensitivity to porphyrins.

Interactions

Other photosensitizing agents such as *griseofulvin, phenothiazines, sulfonamides, sulfonylurea antidiabetic agents, tetracyclines,* and *thiazide diuretics* may increase photosensitivity reaction. Use together cautiously.

Effects on diagnostic tests

None reported.

Adverse reactions

CNS: anxiety, confusion, *insomnia.*
CV: hypotension, hypertension, ***heart failure,*** atrial fibrillation, tachycardia.
GI: *constipation, abdominal pain, nausea, vomiting,* diarrhea, dyspepsia, dysphagia, eructation, esophageal edema, esophageal tumor bleeding, esophageal stricture, esophagitis, hematemesis, melena, anorexia.
GU: urinary tract infection.
Hematologic: *anemia.*
Respiratory: coughing, *dyspnea, pharyngitis, pleural effusion, pneumonia,* respiratory insufficiency, tracheoesophageal fistula.
Skin: *photosensitivity reaction* (mostly mild erythema on face and hands).
Other: *back or chest pain,* asthenia, substernal or general pain, edema, fever, surgical complication, dehydration, weight loss, moniliasis.

Overdose and treatment

There is no information available regarding drug overdose. Effects of overdose on the duration of photosensitivity are unknown. Do not give laser treatment if overdose of porfimer is administered. In an overdose, patient should protect eyes and skin from direct sunlight or bright indoor lights for 30 days, after which patient should test for residual photosensitivity. Porfimer is not dialyzable.

☑ Special considerations

- Before each course of treatment, patient should be evaluated for tracheoesophageal or bronchoesophageal fistula.
- Reconstitute each vial of porfimer with 31.8 ml of either 5% dextrose injection or 0.9% NaCl injection, resulting in a final concentration of 2.5 mg/ml. Shake well until dissolved. Do not mix porfimer with other drugs in the same solution. Protect reconstituted product from bright light and use immediately.
- Reconstituted drug is an opaque solution. Inspect carefully for particulate matter and discoloration before administration.

• Take precautions to prevent extravasation at injection site. If extravasation occurs, protect area from light.
• Avoid having drug come into contact with eyes and skin during preparation and administration. If accidental exposure occurs, overexposed person must be protected from bright light.
• Patient must receive 630-nm wavelength laser light therapy 40 to 50 hours after porfimer injection for drug to be effective. A second laser light treatment may be given as early as 96 hours or as late as 120 hours after the initial injection with porfimer. No further injection of porfimer should be given for such retreatment with laser light. Before a second laser light treatment, the residual tumor should be debrided; however, vigorous debridement may cause tumor bleeding. Monitor patient closely.
• Inflammatory responses within the area of treatment may cause substernal chest pain. Pain may be of sufficient intensity to warrant a short-term prescription of opiate analgesics.
• Monitor CBC regularly because anemia may occur due to tumor bleeding as a result of drug and laser therapy.

Patient education
• Instruct patient to avoid direct sunlight and bright indoor light for 30 days following each injection. However, tell patient to expose skin to ambient indoor light.
• Tell patient that before exposing any area of skin to direct sunlight or bright indoor light after 30 days, he should expose a small area of skin (not face) to sunlight for 10 minutes. If no photosensitivity reaction (erythema, edema, blistering) occurs within 24 hours, patient can gradually resume normal outdoor activities. However, he should still continue to exercise caution and gradually allow increased exposure. If some photosensitivity reaction occurs with the limited skin test, patient should continue to exert precautions for another 2 weeks before retesting.
• Inform patient that if he is travelling to geographical area with greater sunshine, he should retest his level of photosensitivity.
• Warn patient that ultraviolet sunscreens are not useful in protecting against photosensitivity reactions because photoactivation is caused by visible light.
• Instruct patient that for the next 30 days, he should wear dark sunglasses when going outside. Sunglasses should have an average white light transmittance of less than 4.
• Instruct female patient of childbearing age to practice an effective method of contraception during therapy. If pregnancy is suspected, tell patient to report it immediately.

Pediatric use
• Safety and effectiveness in children have not been established.

Breast-feeding
• It is not known if drug occurs in breast milk. Because of the potential for serious adverse reactions in breast-fed infants, women receiving porfimer must not breast-feed.

potassium iodide (KI, SSKI)
Iosat, Pima, Thyro-Block

Pharmacologic classification: electrolyte
Therapeutic classification: antihyperthyroid, expectorant
Pregnancy risk category D

How supplied
Available by prescription only
Tablets: 130 mg
Tablets (enteric-coated): 300 mg
Syrup: 325 mg/5 ml
Saturated solution (SSKI): 1 g/ml
Strong iodine solution (Lugol's solution): iodine 50 mg/ml and potassium iodide 100 mg/ml

Indications, route, and dosage
Expectorant
Adults: 300 to 600 mg t.i.d. or q.i.d.
Children: 60 to 250 mg q.i.d.
Preoperative thyroidectomy
Adults and children: 50 to 250 mg (or 1 to 5 drops) SSKI t.i.d.; or 0.1 to 0.3 ml (or 3 to 5 drops) Lugol's solution t.i.d.; give drug for 10 to 14 days before surgery.
Nuclear radiation protection
Adults and children: 0.13 ml P.O. of SSKI (130 mg) immediately before or after initial exposure will block 90% of radioactive iodine. Same dosage given 3 to 4 hours after exposure will provide 50% block. Drug should be administered for up to 10 days under medical supervision.
Infants under age 1: Half the adult dosage.
◊ ***To replenish iodine***
Adults: 5 to 10 mg/day.
Children: 1 mg/day.
Management of thyrotoxic crisis
Adults: 500 mg P.O. q 4 hours (approximately 10 drops of a potassium iodide solution containing 1 g/ml). Alternatively, 1 ml of strong iodine solution P.O. t.i.d.
◊ ***Graves' disease in neonates***
Neonates: 1 drop P.O. of strong iodine solution q 8 hours.
◊ ***Cutaneous sporotrichosis***
Adults: 65 to 325 mg P.O. t.i.d.

Pharmacodynamics
Expectorant action: Exact mechanism of potassium iodide's expectorant effect is unknown; it is believed that potassium iodide reduces viscosity of mucus by increasing respiratory tract secretions.

Antihyperthyroid agent action: Potassium iodide acts directly on the thyroid gland to inhibit synthesis and release of thyroid hormone.

Pharmacokinetics
• *Absorption:* Absorption is similar to iodinated amino acids.
• *Distribution:* Potassium iodide is distributed extracellularly.
• *Metabolism:* No reports available.
• *Excretion:* Drug is excreted by the kidneys.

Contraindications and precautions
Contraindicated in patients with tuberculosis, acute bronchitis, iodide hypersensitivity, or hyperkalemia. Some formulations contain sulfites, which may precipitate allergic reactions in hypersensitive individuals.

Use cautiously in patients with hypocomplementemic vasculitis, goiter, or autoimmune thyroid disease.

Interactions
Lithium potentiates both hypothyroid and goitrogenic effects of potassium iodide. Concomitant use with *potassium-sparing diuretics* or *potassium-containing drugs* may cause hyperkalemia and subsequent arrhythmias or cardiac arrest.

Effects on diagnostic tests
Potassium iodide may alter the results of thyroid function tests.

Adverse reactions
EENT: inflammation of salivary glands, periorbital edema.
GI: GI bleeding (rare), nausea, vomiting, stomach pain, diarrhea, burning mouth and throat, sore teeth and gums, *metallic taste.*
Skin: acneiform rash.
Other: fever; hypersensitivity reactions.

Overdose and treatment
Acute overdose is rare; angioedema, laryngeal edema, and cutaneous hemorrhages may occur. Treat hyperkalemia immediately; salt and fluid intake help eliminate iodide.

Iodism (chronic iodine poisoning) may follow prolonged use; symptoms include metallic taste, sore mouth, swollen eyelids, sneezing, skin eruptions, nausea, vomiting, epigastric pain, and diarrhea. Discontinue drug and treat supportively.

☑ Special considerations
- Monitor serum potassium levels before and during therapy; patients taking any diuretic, especially potassium-sparing diuretics, are at risk for hyperkalemia.
- Dilute with 6 oz (180 ml) of water, fruit juice, or broth to reduce GI distress and disguise strong, salty metallic taste; advise patient to use a straw to avoid tooth discoloration.
- Store in light-resistant container because exposure to light liberates traces of free iodine; if crystals develop in solution, dissolve them by placing container in warm water and carefully agitating it.
- Drug may cause flare-up of adolescent acne or other rash.
- Sudden withdrawal may precipitate thyroid storm.
- Maintain fluid intake when using drug as an expectorant; adequate hydration encourages optimal expectorant action.

Patient education
- Enteric-coated tablets are seldom used because of reports of small-bowel lesions with possible obstruction, perforation, and hemorrhage; when prescribed, give tablet with small amount of water, and tell patient to swallow tablet whole (do not crush or chew) and follow with 8 oz (240 ml) of water or juice.
- Advise patient to drink all of solution prepared and to use a straw to avoid discoloring teeth.
- Review signs of iodism with patient, and instruct patient to report such symptoms, especially abdominal pain, distention, nausea, vomiting, or GI bleeding.
- Caution patient not to use OTC drugs without medical approval; many preparations contain iodides and could potentiate drug. For the same reason, patient should discuss ingestion of iodized salt and shellfish.

Geriatric use
- Serum potassium determinations may be needed in elderly patients with renal dysfunction.

Pediatric use
- Strong iodine solution is used for treating Graves' disease in neonates (1 drop every 8 hours).

Breast-feeding
- Potassium iodide should not be used during breast-feeding; drug occurs in breast milk and may cause rash and thyroid suppression in the infant.

potassium salts, oral

potassium acetate

potassium bicarbonate
K+ Care ET, K-Electrolyte, K-Ide, Klor-Con/EF, K-Lyte, K-Vescent

potassium chloride
Apo-K*, Cena-K, Gen-K, K-8, K-10*, Kalium Durules*, Kaochlor S-F, Kaon-Cl, Kaon-Cl-10, Kato, Kay Ciel, K+ Care, KCL*, K-Dur, K-Ide, K-Lease, K-Long*, K-Lor, Klor-Con, Klorvess, Klotrix, K-Lyte/Cl Powder, K-Med 900*, K-Norm, K-Sol, K-Tab, Micro-K Extencaps, Micro-K 10 Extencaps, Potasalan, Rum-K, Slow-K, Ten-K

potassium gluconate

Pharmacologic classification: potassium supplement
Therapeutic classification: therapeutic agent for electrolyte balance
Pregnancy risk category C

How supplied
Available by prescription only
Tablets (effervescent): 20 mEq, 25 mEq, 50 mEq
Liquid: 15 mEq/15 ml, 20 mEq/15 ml, 30 mEq/15 ml, 40 mEq/15 ml
potassium acetate
Vials: 2 mEq/ml, 4 mEq/ml in 20-ml vials
potassium chloride
Tablets (sustained-release): 6.7 mEq, 8 mEq, 10 mEq, 20 mEq

Powder: 15 mEq/package, 20 mEq/package, and 25 mEq/package
potassium gluconate
Liquid: 15 mEq/15 ml, 20 mEq/15 ml

Indications, route, and dosage

Hypokalemia
Adults and children: 40- to 100-mEq tablets divided into two to four doses daily. Use I.V. potassium chloride when oral replacement is not feasible or when hypokalemia is life-threatening. Dosage up to 20 mEq/hour in concentration of 60 mEq/L or less. Further dose based on serum potassium determinations. Do not exceed total daily dose of 150 mEq (3 mEq/kg in children).

Further doses are based on serum potassium levels and blood pH. I.V. potassium replacement should be carried out only with ECG monitoring and frequent serum potassium determinations.

Prevention of hypokalemia
Adults and children: Initially, 20 mEq of potassium supplement P.O. daily, in divided doses. Adjust dosage p.r.n. based on serum potassium levels.

Potassium replacement
Adults and children: Potassium chloride should be diluted in a suitable I.V. solution (not more than 40 mEq/L) and administered at rate not exceeding 20 mEq/hour. Do not exceed total dosage of 400 mEq/day (3 mEq/kg/day or 40 mEq/m^2/day for children). I.V. potassium replacement should be carried out only with ECG monitoring and frequent serum potassium determinations.

Pharmacodynamics

Potassium replacement action: Potassium, the main cation in body tissue, is necessary for physiologic processes such as maintaining intracellular tonicity, maintaining a balance with sodium across cell membranes, transmitting nerve impulses, maintaining cellular metabolism, contracting cardiac and skeletal muscle, maintaining acid-base balance, and maintaining normal renal function.

Pharmacokinetics

- *Absorption:* Potassium is well absorbed from the GI tract. It should be taken with meals and sipped slowly over a 5- to 10-minute period to decrease irritation. Potassium bicarbonate does not correct hypochloremic alkalosis.
- *Distribution:* The normal serum levels of potassium range from 3.8 to 5 mEq/L. Plasma potassium concentrations up to 7.7 mEq/L may be normal in neonates. Up to 60 mEq/L of potassium may be found in gastric secretions and diarrhea fluid.
- *Metabolism:* None significant.
- *Excretion:* Potassium is excreted largely by the kidneys. Small amounts of potassium may be excreted via the skin and intestinal tract, but intestinal potassium usually is reabsorbed. A healthy patient on a potassium-free diet will excrete 40 to 50 mEq of potassium daily.

Contraindications and precautions

Contraindicated in patients with severe renal impairment with oliguria, anuria, or azotemia; in those with untreated Addison's disease; and in those with acute dehydration, heat cramps, hyperkalemia, hyperkalemic form of familial periodic paralysis, and conditions associated with extensive tissue breakdown.

Use cautiously in patients with cardiac or renal disease.

Interactions

When used concomitantly with potassium, *anticholinergics* that slow GI motility may increase the chance of GI irritation and ulceration.

Concomitant administration with *potassium-containing products* may cause hyperkalemia within 1 to 2 days. Potassium is not recommended in *digitalized* patients with severe or complete heart block because of potential for arrhythmias. Concomitant use of potassium with *potassium-sparing diuretics, ACE inhibitors (captopril),* or *salt substitutes containing potassium salts* can cause severe hyperkalemia.

Effects on diagnostic tests

None reported.

Adverse reactions

Signs of hyperkalemia
CNS: paresthesia of the extremities, listlessness, mental confusion, weakness or heaviness of legs, flaccid paralysis.
CV: hypotension, ***arrhythmias, cardiac arrest,*** heart block, ECG changes.
GI: nausea, vomiting, abdominal pain, diarrhea.
Respiratory: ***respiratory paralysis.***
Other: pain and redness at infusion site, fever, hyperkalemia.

Overdose and treatment

Clinical manifestations of overdose include increased serum potassium concentration and characteristic ECG changes, including tall peaked T waves, depression of ST segment, disappearance of P wave, prolonged QT interval, and widening and slurring of the QRS complex. Late clinical signs include weakness, paralysis of voluntary muscles, respiratory distress, and dysphagia. These may precede severe or fatal cardiac toxicity. Hyperkalemia produces symptoms paradoxically similar to those of hypokalemia.

Treatment of potassium overdose includes discontinuation of the potassium supplement and, if necessary, lavage of the GI tract. In patients with a potassium concentration greater then 6.5 mEq/L, supportive therapy may include the following interventions (with continuous ECG monitoring):

Infuse 40 to 160 mEq sodium bicarbonate I.V. over a 5-minute interval; repeat in 10 to 15 minutes if ECG abnormalities persist.

Infuse 300 to 500 ml of dextrose 10% to 25% over 1 hour. Insulin (5 to 10 units per 20 g of dextrose) should be added to the infusion or, ideally, administered as a separate injection.

Patients with absent P waves or broad QRS complex who are not receiving cardiotonic glycosides should immediately be given 0.5 g to 1 g of calcium gluconate or another calcium salt I.V. over a 2-minute period (with continuous ECG monitoring) to antagonize the cardiotoxic effect of the potassium. May be repeated in 1 to 2 minutes if ECG abnormalities persist.

To remove potassium from the body, use sodium polystyrene sulfonate resin, hemodialysis, or peritoneal dialysis. Administer potassium-free I.V. fluids when hyperkalemia is associated with water loss.

☑ Special considerations

- In patients receiving cardiac glycosides, removing potassium too rapidly may result in digitalis toxicity.
- Monitor serum potassium, BUN, and serum creatinine levels; pH; and intake and output.
- Do not give potassium during immediate postoperative period until urine flow is established.
- Give parenteral potassium by slow infusion only, never by I.V. push or I.M. Dilute I.V. potassium preparations with large volume of parenteral solutions.
- Give oral potassium supplements with extreme caution because its many forms deliver varying amounts of potassium. Patient may tolerate one product better than another.
- Potassium gluconate does not correct hypokalemic hypochloremic alkalosis.
- Enteric-coated tablets are not recommended because of the potential for GI bleeding and small-bowel ulcerations.
- Tablets in wax matrix sometimes lodge in esophagus and cause ulceration in cardiac patients who have esophageal compression due to enlarged left atrium. In such patients and in those with esophageal or GI stasis or obstruction, use liquid form.
- Often used orally with diuretics that cause potassium excretion. Potassium chloride most useful because diuretics waste chloride ions. Hypokalemic alkalosis treated best with potassium chloride.
- Monitor ECG, pH, serum potassium levels, and other electrolytes during therapy.
- Do not crush sustained-released potassium products.

Patient education

- Tell patient potassium is available only with a prescription because the wrong amount may cause severe reactions.
- Suggest diluting liquid potassium product in at least 4 to 8 oz (120 to 240 ml) of water; to take it after meals; and to sip liquid potassium slowly to minimize GI irritation.
- Tell patient to dissolve powder, soluble tablets, or granules completely in at least 4 oz (120 ml) of water or juice, and to allow fizzing to finish before drinking.
- Instruct patient not to crush or chew sustained-release capsules; contents of capsule can be opened and sprinkled onto applesauce or other soft food.
- Tell patient to stop taking drug immediately and report the following reactions: confusion; irregular heartbeat; numbness of feet, fingers or lips; shortness of breath; anxiety, excessive tiredness or weakness of legs; unexplained diarrhea; nausea and vomiting; stomach pain; or bloody or black stools. Such reactions are rare.
- Tell patient that expelling a whole tablet in the stool (sustained-release tablet) is normal. The body eliminates the shell after absorbing the potassium.
- Warn patient to avoid salt substitutes except when prescribed.

Pediatric use

- Use cautiously in pediatric patients.

Breast-feeding

- Potassium supplements pass into the breast milk. Safety in breast-feeding has not been established; therefore, use potassium only when the benefits to the breast-feeding woman outweigh the risk to the infant.

---

pralidoxime chloride (2-PAM chloride, 2-pyridine aldoxime methochloride)

Protopam Chloride

Pharmacologic classification: quaternary ammonium oxime
Therapeutic classification: antidote
Pregnancy risk category C

How supplied

Available by prescription only
Injection: 1 g/20 ml vial (without diluent or syringe); 1 g/20 ml vial with diluent, syringe, needle, alcohol swab (emergency kit); 600 mg/2 ml auto-injector, parenteral

Indications, route, and dosage

Organophosphate pesticide poisoning
Adults: 1 to 2 g I.V. in 100 ml of 0.9% NaCl over 15 to 30 minutes. May repeat in 1 hour if muscle weakness continues. For subconjunctival injection, give 0.1 to 0.2 ml of a 5% solution.
Children: 20 to 40 mg/kg I.V. in 100 ml of 0.9% NaCl over 15 to 30 minutes. May repeat in 1 hour if muscle weakness continues.

Drug is most effective when administered within 24 hours of exposure. It should be administered with atropine.

Anticholinesterase drug overdose
Adults: 1 to 2 g I.V. followed by increments of 250 mg q 5 minutes.

Pharmacodynamics

Antidote action: Pralidoxime reactivates cholinesterase that has been inactivated by phosphorylation due to exposure to an organophosphate pesticide or related compound. One of the few drugs that correct a biochemical lesion, pralidoxime acts by removing the phosphoryl group from the active site of the inhibited enzyme, freeing and reactivating acetylcholinesterase. It also directly reacts with and detoxifies the organophosphorus molecule and may also react with cholinesterase to protect it from inhibition.

Cholinesterase reactivation occurs primarily at the neuromuscular junction where pralidoxime exerts its most critical effect—reversal of respiratory paralysis or paralysis of other skeletal muscles. Reactivation also occurs at autonomic effector sites and, to a lesser degree, within the CNS. Pralidoxime is effective against nicotinic manifestations but it does not substantially influence muscarinic effects. Therefore, it is used in conjunction with atropine, which ameliorates muscarinic symptoms and directly blocks the effects of accumulation of excess acetylcholine at various sites including the respiratory center.

Pharmacokinetics

- *Absorption:* After I.V. administration, peak plasma levels are reached in 5 to 15 minutes; after I.M., in 10 to 20 minutes.
- *Distribution:* Drug is distributed throughout the extracellular water; it is not appreciably bound to plasma protein. It does not readily pass into the CNS. Distribution into breast milk is unknown. Therapeutic concentrations are achieved in the eye following subconjunctival injection.
- *Metabolism:* Exact mechanism is unknown, but hepatic metabolism is considered likely.
- *Excretion:* Drug is excreted rapidly in urine as unchanged drug and metabolite; 80% to 90% of I.V. or I.M. dose is excreted unchanged within 12 hours.

Contraindications and precautions

Contraindicated in patients with hypersensitivity to any component of product. Use cautiously in patients with myasthenia gravis.

Interactions

Concurrent use of *respiratory or CNS depressants, skeletal muscle relaxants*, or *drugs that lower the seizure threshold* should be avoided in patients with anticholinesterase poisoning. Therefore, avoid the use of *aminophylline, morphine, phenothiazines, reserpine, succinylcholine, theophylline,* and *other respiratory depressants* in patients receiving pralidoxime. Use *barbiturates* with caution to treat seizures because barbiturates are potentiated by anticholinesterase.

Effects on diagnostic tests

AST and ALT levels are elevated but return to normal in 2 weeks; transient elevation in CK levels.

Adverse reactions

CNS: dizziness, headache, drowsiness.
CV: tachycardia, hypertension.
EENT: blurred vision, diplopia, impaired accommodation.
GI: nausea.
Other: muscle weakness, hyperventilation, mild to moderate pain at injection site, transient elevation of liver enzymes.

Overdose and treatment

Clinical manifestations of overdose include dizziness, headache, blurred vision, diplopia, impaired accommodation, nausea, and tachycardia. However, these effects may also result from organophosphate toxicity or the use of atropine.

To treat, remove secretions and all contaminated clothing. Administer artificial respiration; maintain airway. Provide supportive therapy as needed, and monitor ECG. After ingested overdose, induce emesis if patient is fully alert. Perform gastric lavage with activated charcoal and sodium sulfate.

☑ Special considerations

- Assess vital signs and insert I.V. line. Use requires close medical supervision, and close observation of the patient for at least 24 hours.
- Reconstitute drug with 20 ml of sterile water for injection to provide a solution containing 50 mg/ml. For I.V. infusion, dilute calculated dose to a volume of 100 ml with 0.9% NaCl injection. Use within a few hours.
- Drug usually is administered by I.V. infusion over 15 to 30 minutes. Rapid administration has produced tachycardia, laryngospasm, muscle ridigity, and transient neuromuscular blockade. Hypertension may also occur, related to dose and rate of infusion; it may be treated by discontinuing the infusion or slowing the rate of infusion. Five mg of phentolamine I.V. quickly reverses pralidoxime-induced hypertension. Closely monitor blood pressure.
- In patients with pulmonary edema, or when I.V. infusion is not practical, or a more rapid effect is needed, drug may be given by slow I.V. injection over at least 5 minutes. It may also be given I.M. or S.C.
- Use reduced dosage in renally impaired patients.
- Institute treatment of organophosphate poisoning without waiting for laboratory test results. Draw blood for RBC and cholinesterase levels before giving pralidoxime. Begin pralidoxime and atropine therapy simultaneously. Give 2 to 6 mg of atropine I.V. (I.M. if patient is cyanotic) every 5 to 60 minutes in adults until muscarinic effects (dyspnea, cough, salivation, bronchopasm) subside. Repeat dosage if signs reappear. Maintain some degree of atropinism for at least 48 hours.
- Treatment is most effective when started within the first 24 hours, preferably within a few hours after poisoning. Even severe poisoning may be reversed if drug is given within 48 hours. Monitor effect of therapy by ECG because of possible heart block due to the anticholinesterase. Continued absorption of the anticholinesterase from the lower bowel constitutes new toxic exposure that may require additional doses of pralidoxime every 3 to 8 hours, or over several days.
- After dermal exposure, patient's clothing should be removed and hair and skin should be washed with sodium bicarbonate, soap, water, or alcohol as soon as possible. While cleaning patient, caregiver should wear gloves and protective clothing to avoid contamination. Patient may need a second washing.
- Drug is not effective in treating toxic exposure to phosphorus, inorganic phosphates, or organophosphates that do not have anticholinesterase activity.
- Give I.V. sodium thiopental or diazepam if seizures interfere with respiration.
- Subconjunctival injection is currently an unapproved method of administration but has been used to reverse adverse ocular effects resulting from systemic overdose or splashing of an organophosphate agent into the eye.

Patient education
- Warn patient that mild to moderate pain may occur 20 to 40 minutes after I.M. injection.

Pediatric use
- Safety has not been established.

Breast-feeding
- It is unknown if drug is distributed into breast milk.

pramipexole dihydrochloride
Mirapex

Pharmacologic classification: nonergot dopamine agonist
Therapeutic classification: antiparkinsonian
Pregnancy risk category C

How supplied
Available by prescription only
Tablets: 0.125 mg, 0.25 mg, 1 mg, 1.5 mg

Indications, route, and dosage
Treatment of idiopathic Parkinson's disease
Adults: Initially, 0.375 mg P.O. daily given in three divided doses; do not increase more than q 5 to 7 days. Increase dose by 0.75 mg in divided doses weekly until maximum dose of 1.5 mg t.i.d. is reached after 7 weeks of therapy. Maintenance dosing ranges from 1.5 to 4.5 mg daily administered in three divided doses.
✦ ***Dosage adjustment.*** In patients with impaired renal function and creatinine clearance of 35 to 59 ml/minute, initial dose is 0.125 mg P.O. b.i.d. and maintenance maximum dose is 1.5 mg b.i.d. For patients with creatinine clearance of 15 to 34 ml/minute, initial dose is 0.125 mg P.O. daily and maintenance maximum dose is 1.5 mg daily.

Pharmacodynamics
Antiparkinsonian action: Drug is thought to stimulate dopamine receptors in striatum; in animal studies, pramipexole influences striatal neuronal firing rates via activation of dopamine receptors in the striatum and the substantia nigra, the site of neurons that send projections to the striatum.

Pharmacokinetics
- *Absorption:* Rapidly absorbed, reaching peak concentrations in about 2 hours. Absolute bioavailability of drug is over 90%, suggesting that it is well absorbed and undergoes little presystemic metabolism. Food does not affect extent of absorption but time of maximum plasma concentration is increased by about 1 hour when drug is taken with meals.
- *Distribution:* Extensively distributed, with a volume of distribution of about 500 L. About 15% is bound to plasma proteins. Drug also distributes into RBCs. Terminal half-life is 8 to 12 hours; steady state is reached within 2 days of dosing.
- *Metabolism:* 90% of dose is excreted unchanged in urine.
- *Excretion:* Principally in the urine. Nonrenal routes may contribute to a small extent to elimination, although no metabolites have been identified in plasma or urine. Drug is secreted by the renal tubules, probably by the organic transport system.

Contraindications and precautions
Contraindicated in patients with hypersensitivity to drug or its components. Use with caution in patients who have renal impairment, such as the elderly or those patients with Parkinson's disease, because dosing may need to be adjusted.

Interactions
Concurrent administration with *levodopa* causes an increase in levodopa's maximum plasma concentrations. *Cimetidine* causes an increase in pramipexole's bioavailability and half-life.

Drugs eliminated via renal secretion (cimetidine, diltiazem, quinidine, quinine, ranitidine, triamterene, verapamil) decrease oral clearance of pramipexole by approximately 20%.

Dopamine antagonists (butyrophenones, metoclopramide, phenothiazines, thiothixenes) may diminish the effectiveness of pramipexole.

Effects on diagnostic tests
None reported.

Adverse reactions
CNS: *dizziness,* somnolence, *insomnia,* hallucinations, *confusion,* amnesia, hypesthesia, dystonia, akathisia, thought abnormalities, myoclonus, *asthenia, dyskinesia, extrapyramidal syndrome, dream abnormalities,* gait abnormalities, hypertonia, paranoid reaction, delusions, sleep disorders.
CV: chest pain, peripheral edema, *orthostatic hypotension.*
EENT: accommodation abnormalities, diplopia, dry mouth, rhinitis, vision abnormalities.
GI: anorexia, *constipation,* dysphagia, nausea.
GU: impotence, urinary frequency, urinary tract infection, urinary incontinence.
Respiratory: dyspnea, pneumonia.
Skin: skin disorders.
Other: general edema, malaise, fever, unevaluable reaction, arthritis, twitching, bursitis, decreased libido, myasthenia, *accidental injury.*

Overdose and treatment
No known antidote; if signs of CNS stimulation occur, a phenothiazine or other butyrophenone neuroleptic agent may be given. Management of overdose may require general supportive measures with gastric lavage, I.V. fluids, and ECG monitoring.

☑ Special considerations
- If drug needs to be discontinued, it should be done over a 1-week period.
- Drug may cause orthostatic hypotension, especially during dose escalation; monitor patient carefully.
- Neuroleptic malignant syndrome (elevated temperature, muscular rigidity, altered consciousness, and autonomic instability) without obvious cause has occurred in association with rapid dose re-

duction or withdrawal of or changes in antiparkinsonian therapy.
• Titrate dosage gradually. Increase dosage to achieve maximum therapeutic effect, balanced against the main adverse effects of dyskinesia, hallucinations, somnolence, and dry mouth.

Patient education
• Tell patient to take drug only as prescribed.
• Instruct patient not to rise rapidly after sitting or lying down because of risk of orthostatic hypotension.
• Caution patient not to drive a car or operate complex machinery until response to drug is known.
• Tell patient to use caution before taking drug with other CNS depressants.
• Advise patient to take drug with food if nausea develops.

Geriatric use
• Drug clearance decreases with age because half-life and clearance are about 40% longer and 30% lower, respectively, in patients age 65 or older.

Pediatric use
• Safety and efficacy in children have not been established.

Breast-feeding
• It is not known if drug is excreted in breast milk. Use with caution.

pravastatin sodium
Pravachol

Pharmacologic classification: HMG-CoA reductase inhibitor
Therapeutic classification: antilipemic
Pregnancy risk category X

How supplied
Available by prescription only
Tablets: 10 mg, 20 mg, 40 mg

Indications, route, and dosage
Reduction of low-density lipoprotein and total cholesterol levels in patients with primary hypercholesterolemia (types IIa and IIb), primary prevention of coronary events
Adults: Initially, 10 to 20 mg daily h.s. Adjust dosage q 4 weeks based on patient tolerance and response; maximum daily dosage is 40 mg. Most elderly patients respond to a daily dosage of 20 mg or less.

Pharmacodynamics
Antilipemic action: Pravastatin inhibits the enzyme 3-hydroxy-3-methylglutaryl-coenzyme A (HMG-CoA) reductase. This hepatic enzyme is an early (and rate limiting) step in the synthetic pathway of cholesterol.

Pharmacokinetics
• *Absorption:* Rapidly absorbed, with peak plasma levels in 1 to 1½ hours. Average oral absorption is 34%, with absolute bioavailability of 17%. Although food reduces bioavailability, drug effects are the same if drug is taken with or 1 hour before meals.
• *Distribution:* Plasma levels of drug are proportional to dose, but do not necessarily correlate perfectly with lipid-lowering effects. About 50% is bound to plasma proteins. Drug experiences extensive first-pass extraction, possibly because of an active transport system into hepatocytes.
• *Metabolism:* Drug is metabolized by the liver; at least six metabolites have been identified. Some are active.
• *Excretion:* Excreted by the liver and kidneys.

Contraindications and precautions
Contraindicated in patients with hypersensitivity to drug; in those with active liver disease or conditions that cause unexplained, persistent elevations of serum transaminase levels; in pregnant and breast-feeding patients; and in women of childbearing age unless there is no risk of pregnancy.

Use cautiously in patients who consume large quantities of alcohol or have history of liver disease.

Interactions
Concomitant use with *immunosuppressive agents* (such as *cyclosporine), fibric acid derivatives* (*clofibrate, gemfibrozil*), high doses *of niacin* (1 g or more *nicotinic acid* daily), and *erythromycin* may increase risk of rhabdomyolysis. Monitor patient closely if concomitant use can't be avoided.

Hepatotoxic drugs or *chronic alcohol abuse* may increase risk of hepatotoxicity. Concurrent use with *cholestyramine* or *colestipol* may decrease plasma levels of pravastatin. Administer pravastatin 1 hour before or 4 hours after these drugs.

Avoid concomitant use with *gemfibrozil* because it decreases protein-binding and urinary clearance of pravastatin.

Drugs that decrease levels or activity of endogenous steroids *(cimetidine, ketoconazole, spironolactone*) may increase risk of endocrine dysfunction. No intervention appears necessary; take complete drug history in patients who develop endocrine dysfunction.

Effects on diagnostic tests
AST, ALT, CK, alkaline phosphatase, and bilirubin levels are increased; thyroid function test is abnormal.

Adverse reactions
CNS: headache, dizziness, fatigue.
CV: chest pain.
EENT: rhinitis.
GI: vomiting, diarrhea, heartburn, abdominal pain, constipation, flatulence, nausea.
GU: renal failure secondary to myoglobinuria, urinary abnormality.
Respiratory: cough, influenza, common cold.
Skin: rash.
Other: flulike symptoms, myositis, myopathy, *localized muscle pain,* myalgia, photosensitivity, ***rhabdomyolysis.***

Overdose and treatment
No information available. Treat symptomatically.

☑ Special considerations

• Discontinue drug temporarily in patient with an acute condition that suggests a developing myopathy or in patient with risk factors that may predispose him to development of renal failure secondary to rhabdomyolysis (including severe acute infection; severe endocrine, metabolic, or electrolyte disorders; hypotension; major surgery; or uncontrolled seizures).
• Watch for signs of myositis. Rarely, myopathy and marked elevations of CK, possibly leading to rhabdomyolysis and renal failure secondary to myoglobinuria, have been reported.
• Initiate drug therapy only after diet and other nonpharmacologic therapies have proved ineffective. Patients should continue a cholesterol-lowering diet during therapy.
• Give drug in the evening, preferably at bedtime. Drug may be given without regard to meals.
• Dosage adjustments should be made about every 4 weeks. May reduce dosage if cholesterol levels fall below target range.

Patient education

• Teach patient appropriate dietary management (restricting total fat and cholesterol intake), weight control, and exercise. Explain importance of these interventions in controlling serum lipids.
• Because of drug's possible impact on liver function, advise patient to restrict alcohol intake.
• Tell patient to call if he experiences adverse reactions, particularly muscle aches and pains.
• Inform patient to take drug at bedtime.

Geriatric use

• Maximum effectiveness is usually evident with daily doses of 20 mg or less.

Pediatric use

• Safety and efficacy in children under age 18 have not been established.

Breast-feeding

• Drug is excreted in breast milk. Women should not breast-feed while taking pravastatin.

prazosin hydrochloride

Minipress

Pharmacologic classification: alpha-adrenergic blocker
Therapeutic classification: antihypertensive
Pregnancy risk category C

How supplied

Available by prescription only
Capsules: 1 mg, 2 mg, 5 mg

Indications, route, and dosage

Hypertension
Adults: Initially, 1 mg P.O. b.i.d. or t.i.d.; gradually increased to maximum of 20 mg daily. Usual maintenance dosage is 6 to 15 mg daily in divided doses. If other antihypertensive agents or diuretics are added to prazosin therapy, reduce dosage of prazosin to 1 or 2 mg t.i.d. and then gradually increase as necessary.

◊ ***Benign prostatic hyperplasia***
Adults: Initially, 2 mg P.O. b.i.d. Dosage may range from 1 to 9 mg/day.

Pharmacodynamics

Antihypertensive action: Prazosin selectively and competitively inhibits alpha-adrenergic receptors, causing arterial and venous dilation, reducing peripheral vascular resistance and blood pressure.

Hypertrophic action: Prazosin's alpha blockade in nonvascular smooth muscle causes relaxation, notably in prostatic tissue, thereby reducing urinary symptoms in men with benign prostatic hyperplasia.

Pharmacokinetics

• *Absorption:* Absorption from the GI tract is variable; antihypertensive effect begins in about 2 hours, peaking in 2 to 4 hours. Full antihypertensive effect may not occur for 4 to 6 weeks.
• *Distribution:* Prazosin is distributed throughout the body and is highly protein-bound (approximately 97%).
• *Metabolism:* Prazosin is metabolized extensively in the liver.
• *Excretion:* Over 90% of a given dose is excreted in feces via bile; remainder is excreted in urine. Plasma half-life is 2 to 4 hours. Antihypertensive effect lasts less than 24 hours.

Contraindications and precautions

No known contraindications. Use cautiously in patients receiving antihypertensive medications and in those with chronic renal failure.

Interactions

The hypotensive effects of prazosin may be increased when administered concurrently with *diuretics* or *other antihypertensive agents.*

Because prazosin is highly bound to plasma proteins, it may interact with other *highly protein-bound drugs.*

Effects on diagnostic tests

Prazosin alters results of screening tests for pheochromocytoma and causes increases in levels of the urinary metabolite of norepinephrine and vanillylmandelic acid; it may cause positive antinuclear antibody titer and liver function test abnormalities. A transient fall in leukocyte count and increased serum uric acid and BUN levels may also occur.

Adverse reactions

CNS: *dizziness,* headache, drowsiness, nervousness, paresthesia, weakness, *"first-dose syncope,"* depression.
CV: orthostatic hypotension, *palpitations.*
EENT: blurred vision, tinnitus, conjunctivitis, nasal congestion, epistaxis.
GI: vomiting, diarrhea, abdominal cramps, constipation, *nausea.*
GU: priapism, impotence, urinary frequency, incontinence.

Respiratory: dyspnea.
Other: arthralgia, myalgia, pruritus, edema, fever.

Overdose and treatment

Overdose is manifested by hypotension and drowsiness. After acute ingestion, empty stomach by induced emesis or gastric lavage, and give activated charcoal to reduce absorption. Further treatment is usually symptomatic and supportive. Prazosin is not dialyzable.

☑ Special considerations

Besides those relevant to all *alpha-adrenergic blockers,* consider the following recommendations.

- First-dose syncope—dizziness, light-headedness, and syncope—may occur within ½ to 1 hour after initial dose; it may be severe, with loss of consciousness, if initial dose exceeds 2 mg. Effect is transient and may be diminished by giving drug at bedtime, by limiting the initial dose of prazosin to 1 mg, by subsequently increasing the dosage gradually, and by introducing other antihypertensive agents into the patient's regimen cautiously; it is more common during febrile illness and more severe if patient has hyponatremia. Always increase dosage gradually and have patient sit or lie down if he experiences dizziness.
- Prazosin's effect is most pronounced on diastolic blood pressure.
- Drug has been used to treat vasospasm associated with Raynaud's syndrome. It also has been used with diuretics and cardiac glycosides to treat severe heart failure, to manage the signs and symptoms of pheochromocytoma preoperatively, and to treat ergotamine-induced peripheral ischemia.

Patient education

- Teach patient about his disease and therapy, and explain that he must take drug exactly as prescribed, even when feeling well; advise him never to discontinue drug suddenly because severe rebound hypertension may occur, and to promptly report malaise or unusual adverse effects.
- Tell patient to avoid hazardous activities that require mental alertness until tolerance develops to sedation, drowsiness, and other CNS effects; to avoid sudden position changes to minimize orthostatic hypotension; and to use ice chips, candy, or gum to relieve dry mouth.
- Warn patient to seek medical approval before taking OTC cold preparations.

Geriatric use

- Elderly patients may be more sensitive to hypotensive effects and may require lower doses because of altered drug metabolism.

Pediatric use

- Safety and efficacy in children have not been established; use only when potential benefit outweighs risk.

Breast-feeding

- Small amounts of prazosin are excreted in breast milk; an alternative feeding method is recommended during therapy.

prednisolone (systemic)

Delta-Cortef, Prelone

prednisolone acetate

Key-Pred-25, Predalone-50, Predate, Predcor-50

prednisolone acetate and prednisolone sodium phosphate

Predicort-RP

prednisolone sodium phosphate

Hydeltrasol, Key-Pred SP, Pediapred, Predate S

prednisolone tebutate

Hydeltra-T.B.A., Nor-Pred T.B.A., Predate TBA, Predcor-TBA

Pharmacologic classification: glucocorticoid, mineralocorticoid
Therapeutic classification: anti-inflammatory, immunosuppressant
Pregnancy risk category C

How supplied

Available by prescription only
prednisolone
Tablets: 5 mg
Syrup: 15 mg/5 ml
prednisolone acetate
Injection: 25 mg/ml, 50 mg/ml, 100 mg/ml suspension
prednisolone acetate and prednisolone sodium phosphate
Injection: 80 mg acetate and 20 mg sodium phosphate/ml suspension
prednisolone sodium phosphate
Oral liquid: 6.7 mg (5 mg base)/5 ml
Injection: 20 mg/ml solution
prednisolone tebutate
Injection: 20 mg/ml suspension

Indications, route, and dosage

Severe inflammation, modification of body's immune response to disease
Adults: 2.5 to 15 mg P.O. b.i.d., t.i.d., or q.i.d.
Children: 0.14 to 2 mg/kg or 4 to 6 mg/m^2 daily in divided doses.
prednisolone acetate
Adults: 2 to 30 mg I.M. q 12 hours.
prednisolone sodium phosphate
Adults: 2 to 30 mg I.M. or I.V. q 12 hours, or into joints, lesions and soft tissue, p.r.n.
prednisolone tebutate
Adults: 4 to 40 mg into joints and lesions, p.r.n.
prednisolone acetate and prednisolone sodium phosphate suspension
Adults: 0.25 to 1 ml into joints weekly, p.r.n.

Pharmacodynamics

Anti-inflammatory action: Prednisolone stimulates the synthesis of enzymes needed to decrease the inflammatory response. It suppresses the immune system by reducing activity and volume of the lymphatic system, thus producing lymphocytopenia (primarily of T-lymphocytes), decreasing immunoglobulin and complement concentrations, decreasing passage of immune complexes through basement membranes, and possibly by depressing reactivity of tissue to antigen-antibody interactions.

The mineralocorticoids regulate electrolyte homeostasis by acting renally at the distal tubules to enhance the reabsorption of sodium ions (and thus water) from the tubular fluid into the plasma and enhance the excretion of both potassium and hydrogen ions.

Prednisolone is an adrenocorticoid with both glucocorticoid and mineralocorticoid properties. It is a weak mineralocorticoid with only half the potency of hydrocortisone but is a more potent glucocorticoid, having four times the potency of equal weight of hydrocortisone. It is used primarily as an anti-inflammatory agent and an immunosuppressant. It is not used for mineralocorticoid replacement therapy because of the availability of more specific and potent agents.

Prednisolone may be administered orally. Prednisolone sodium phosphate is highly soluble, has a rapid onset and a short duration of action, and may be given I.M. or I.V. Prednisolone acetate and tebutate are suspensions that may be administered by intra-articular, intrasynovial, intrabursal, intralesional, or soft-tissue injection. They have a slow onset but a long duration of action.

Prednisolone sodium phosphate and prednisolone acetate is a combination product of the rapid-acting phosphate salt and the slightly soluble, slowly released acetate salt. This product provides rapid anti-inflammatory effects with a sustained duration of action. It is a suspension and should not be given I.V. It is particularly useful as an anti-inflammatory agent in intra-articular, intradermal, and intralesional injections.

Pharmacokinetics

- *Absorption:* Drug is absorbed readily after oral administration. After oral and I.V. administration, peak effects occur in about 1 to 2 hours. Acetate and tebutate suspensions for injection have a variable absorption rate over 24 to 48 hours, depending on whether they are injected into an intra-articular space or a muscle, and on the blood supply to that muscle. Systemic absorption occurs slowly after intra-articular injection.
- *Distribution:* Removed rapidly from the blood and distributed to muscle, liver, skin, intestines, and kidneys. Drug is extensively bound to plasma proteins (transcortin and albumin). Only the unbound portion is active. Adrenocorticoids are distributed into breast milk and through the placenta.
- *Metabolism:* Metabolized in the liver to inactive glucuronide and sulfate metabolites.
- *Excretion:* The inactive metabolites, and small amounts of unmetabolized drug, are excreted in urine. Insignificant quantities of drug are excreted in feces. Biologic half-life of prednisolone is 18 to 36 hours.

Contraindications and precautions

Contraindicated in patients with hypersensitivity to drug or its ingredients and systemic fungal infections.

Use cautiously in patients with a recent MI, GI ulcer, renal disease, hypertension, osteoporosis, diabetes mellitus, hypothyroidism, cirrhosis, diverticulitis, nonspecific ulcerative colitis, recent intestinal anastamoses, thromboembolic disorders, seizures, myasthenia gravis, heart failure, tuberculosis, ocular herpes simplex, emotional instability, or psychotic tendencies.

Interactions

When used concomitantly, prednisolone rarely may decrease the effects *of oral anticoagulants* by unknown mechanisms.

Glucocorticoids increase the metabolism of *isoniazid* and *salicylates*; they cause hyperglycemia, requiring dosage adjustment of *insulin* or *oral antidiabetic agents* in diabetic patients; and may enhance hypokalemia associated with *amphotericin B* or *diuretic* therapy. The hypokalemia may increase the risk of toxicity in patients concurrently receiving *cardiac glycosides.*

Barbiturates, phenytoin, and *rifampin* may cause decreased corticosteroid effects because of increased hepatic metabolism. *Antacids, cholestyramine,* and *colestipol* decrease prednisolone's effect by adsorbing the corticosteroid, decreasing the amount absorbed.

Concomitant use with *estrogens* may reduce the metabolism of prednisolone by increasing the concentration of transcortin. The half-life of the corticosteroid is then prolonged because of increased protein binding. Concomitant administration of ulcerogenic drugs such as *NSAIDs* may increase risk of GI ulceration.

Effects on diagnostic tests

Prednisolone suppresses reactions to skin tests; causes false-negative results in the nitroblue tetrazolium test for systemic bacterial infections; decreases ^{131}I uptake and protein-bound iodine concentrations in thyroid function tests; may increase glucose and cholesterol levels; may decrease serum potassium, calcium, thyroxine, and triiodothyronine levels; and may increase urine glucose and calcium levels.

Adverse reactions

Most adverse reactions to corticosteroids are dose- or duration-dependent.

CNS: *euphoria, insomnia,* psychotic behavior, pseudotumor cerebri, vertigo, headache, paresthesia, ***seizures.***

CV: ***heart failure, thromboembolism,*** hypertension, edema, ***arrhythmias,*** thrombophlebitis.

EENT: cataracts, glaucoma.

Endocrine: menstrual irregularities, cushingoid state (moonface, buffalo hump, central obesity).

GI: *peptic ulceration,* GI irritation, increased appetite, pancreatitis, nausea, vomiting.

Skin: delayed wound healing, acne, various skin eruptions.
Other: muscle weakness, osteoporosis, hirsutism, susceptibility to infections; hypokalemia, hyperglycemia, and carbohydrate intolerance; growth suppression in children; ***acute adrenal insufficiency may occur with increased stress (infection, surgery, or trauma) or abrupt withdrawal after long-term therapy.***

After abrupt withdrawal: rebound inflammation, fatigue, weakness, arthralgia, fever, dizziness, lethargy, depression, fainting, orthostatic hypotension, dyspnea, anorexia, hypoglycemia. ***After prolonged use, sudden withdrawal may be fatal.***

Overdose and treatment

Acute ingestion, even in massive doses, is rarely a clinical problem. Toxic signs and symptoms rarely occur if drug is used for less than 3 weeks, even at large dosage ranges. However, chronic use causes adverse physiologic effects, including suppression of the hypothalamic-pituitary-adrenal axis, cushingoid appearance, muscle weakness, and osteoporosis.

☑ Special considerations

Recommendations for use of prednisolone and for care and teaching of patients are the same as those for all *systemic adrenocorticoids.*

Pediatric use

- Chronic use of adrenocorticoids or corticotropin may suppress growth and maturation in children and adolescents.

prednisolone acetate (ophthalmic)

AK-Tate, Econopred Ophthalmic, Ocu-Pred-A, Predair A, Pred Forte, Pred Mild Ophthalmic

prednisolone sodium phosphate

AK-Pred, Inflamase Forte, Inflamase Mild Ophthalmic, I-Pred, Ocu-Pred, Predair

Pharmacologic classification: corticosteroid
Therapeutic classification: ophthalmic anti-inflammatory
Pregnancy risk category C

How supplied

Available by prescription only
prednisolone acetate
Suspension: 0.12%, 0.125%, 0.25%, 1%
prednisolone sodium phosphate
Solution: 0.125%, 0.5%, 1%

Indications, route, and dosage

Inflammation of palpebral and bulbar conjunctiva, cornea, and anterior segment of globe; corneal injury; graft rejection
Adults and children: Instill 1 or 2 drops in eye. In severe conditions, may be used hourly, tapering to discontinuation as inflammation subsides. In mild conditions, may be used four to six times daily.

Pharmacodynamics

Anti-inflammatory action: Corticosteroids stimulate the synthesis of enzymes needed to decrease the inflammatory response. Prednisolone, a synthetic corticosteroid, has about four times the anti-inflammatory potency of an equal weight of hydrocortisone. Prednisolone acetate is poorly soluble and therefore has a slower onset of action, but a longer duration of action, when applied in a liquid suspension. The sodium phosphate salt is highly soluble and has a rapid onset but short duration of action.

Pharmacokinetics

- *Absorption:* After ophthalmic administration, prednisolone is absorbed through the aqueous humor. Systemic absorption rarely occurs.
- *Distribution:* After ophthalmic application, prednisolone is distributed throughout the local tissue layers. Any drug that is absorbed into circulation is rapidly removed from the blood and distributed into muscle, liver, skin, intestines, and kidneys.
- *Metabolism:* After ophthalmic administration, corticosteroids are primarily metabolized locally. The small amount that is absorbed into systemic circulation is metabolized primarily in the liver to inactive compounds.
- *Excretion:* Inactive metabolites are excreted by the kidneys, primarily as glucuronides and sulfates, but also as unconjugated products. Small amounts of the metabolites are excreted in feces.

Contraindications and precautions

Contraindicated in patients with acute, untreated, purulent ocular infections; acute superficial herpes simplex (dendritic keratitis); vaccinia, varicella, or other viral or fungal eye diseases; or ocular tuberculosis. Use cautiously in patients with corneal abrasions that may be contaminated (especially with herpes).

Interactions

None reported.

Effects on diagnostic tests

None reported.

Adverse reactions

EENT: increased intraocular pressure; thinning of cornea, interference with corneal wound healing, increased susceptibility to viral or fungal corneal infection, corneal ulceration; with excessive or long-term use: discharge, discomfort, foreign body sensation, glaucoma exacerbation, cataracts, visual acuity and visual field defects, optic nerve damage.
Other: systemic effects and adrenal suppression with excessive or long-term use.

Overdose and treatment

No information available.

☑ Special considerations

- Shake suspension and check dosage before administering. Store in tightly covered container.

prednisone

Apo-Prednisone*, Deltasone, Meticorten, Orasone, Prednicen-M, Sterapred, Winpred*

Pharmacologic classification: adrenocorticoid

Therapeutic classification: anti-inflammatory, immunosuppressant

Pregnancy risk category C

How supplied

Available by prescription only

Tablets: 1 mg, 2.5 mg, 5 mg, 10 mg, 20 mg, 25 mg, 50 mg

Oral solution: 5 mg/ml; 5 mg/5 ml

Syrup: 5 mg/5 ml

Indications, route, and dosage

Severe inflammation, modification of body's immune response to disease

Adults: 5 to 60 mg P.O. daily in single dose or divided doses. (Maximum daily dose, 250 mg.) Maintenance dose given once daily or every other day. Dosage must be individualized.

Children: 0.14 mg/kg or 4 to 6 mg/m^2 P.O. daily in divided doses; alternatively, may use the following dosage schedule.

Children age 11 to 18: 20 mg P.O. q.i.d.

Children age 5 to 10: 15 mg P.O. q.i.d.

Children age 18 months to 4 years: 7.5 to 10 mg P.O. q.i.d.

Acute exacerbations of multiple sclerosis

Adults: 200 mg P.O. daily for 1 week, then 80 mg every other day for 1 month.

◊ ***Adjunct to anti-infective therapy in the treatment of moderate to severe* Pneumocystis carinii *pneumonia***

Adults or children over age 13 with AIDS: 40 mg P.O. b.i.d. for 5 days; then 40 mg. P.O. once daily for 5 days; then 20 mg P.O. once daily for 11 days (or until completion of the concurrent anti-infective regimen).

Pharmacodynamics

Immunosuppressant action: Prednisone stimulates the synthesis of enzymes needed to decrease the inflammatory response. It suppresses the immune system by reducing activity and volume of the lymphatic system, thus producing lymphocytopenia (primarily of T-lymphocytes), decreasing immunoglobulin and complement concentrations, decreasing passage of immune complexes through basement membranes, and possibly by depressing reactivity of tissue to antigen-antibody interactions.

Anti-inflammatory action: Prednisone is one of the intermediate-acting glucocorticoids, with greater glucocorticoid activity than cortisone and hydrocortisone, but less anti-inflammatory activity than betamethasone, dexamethasone, and paramethasone. Prednisone is about four to five times more potent as an anti-inflammatory agent than hydrocortisone, but it has only half the mineralocorticoid activity of an equal weight of hydrocortisone. Prednisone is the oral glucocorticoid of choice for anti-inflammatory or immunosuppressant effects.

For those patients who cannot swallow tablets, liquid forms are available. The oral concentrate (5 mg/ml) may be diluted in juice or another flavored diluent or mixed in semisolid food (such as applesauce) before administration.

Pharmacokinetics

- *Absorption:* Drug is absorbed readily after oral administration, with peak effects occuring in about 1 to 2 hours.
- *Distribution:* Distributed rapidly to muscle, liver, skin, intestines, and kidneys. Prednisone is extensively bound to plasma proteins (transcortin and albumin). Only the unbound portion is active. Adrenocorticoids are distributed into breast milk and through the placenta.
- *Metabolism:* Metabolized in the liver to the active metabolite prednisolone, which in turn is then metabolized to inactive glucuronide and sulfate metabolites.
- *Excretion:* The inactive metabolites and small amounts of unmetabolized drug are excreted by the kidneys. Insignificant quantities of drug are also excreted in feces. Biologic half-life of prednisone is 18 to 36 hours.

Contraindications and precautions

Contraindicated in patients with hypersensitivity to drug or systemic fungal infections.

Use cautiously in patients with GI ulcer, renal disease, hypertension, osteoporosis, diabetes mellitus, hypothyroidism, cirrhosis, diverticulitis, nonspecific ulcerative colitis, recent intestinal anastamoses, thromboembolic disorders, seizures, myasthenia gravis, heart failure, tuberculosis, ocular herpes simplex, emotional instability, and psychotic tendencies.

Interactions

Concomitant use of prednisone rarely may decrease the effects *of oral anticoagulants* by unknown mechanisms.

Prednisone increases the metabolism of *isoniazid* and *salicylates;* causes hyperglycemia, requiring dosage adjustment of *insulin* or *oral antidiabetic agents* in diabetic patients; and may enhance hypokalemia associated with *diuretic* or *amphotericin B* therapy. The hypokalemia may increase the risk of toxicity in patients concurrently receiving *cardiac glycosides.*

Barbiturates, phenytoin, and *rifampin* may cause decreased effects because of increased hepatic metabolism. *Antacids, cholestyramine, colestipol,* and decrease the effect of prednisone by adsorbing the corticosteroid, decreasing the amount absorbed.

Concomitant use with *estrogens* may reduce the metabolism of prednisone by increasing the concentration of transcortin. The half-life of prednisone is then prolonged because of increased protein binding.

Concomitant administration of *ulcerogenic drugs* such as *NSAIDs* may increase the risk of GI ulceration.

* Canada only

◊ Unlabeled clinical use

Effects on diagnostic tests
Prednisone suppresses reactions to skin tests; causes false-negative results in the nitroblue tetrazolium test for systemic bacterial infections; decreases ^{131}I uptake and protein-bound iodine concentrations in thyroid function tests; may increase glucose and cholesterol levels; may decrease serum potassium, calcium, thyroxine, and triiodothyronine levels; and may increase urine glucose and calcium levels.

Adverse reactions
Most adverse reactions to corticosteroids are dose- or duration-dependent.
CNS: *euphoria, insomnia,* psychotic behavior, pseudotumor cerebri, vertigo, headache, paresthesia, ***seizures.***
CV: hypertension, edema, ***arrhythmias,*** thrombophlebitis, ***thromboembolism, heart failure.***
EENT: cataracts, glaucoma.
Endocrine: menstrual irregularities, cushingoid state (moonface, buffalo hump, central obesity).
GI: *peptic ulceration,* GI irritation, increased appetite, pancreatitis, nausea, vomiting.
Skin: delayed wound healing, acne, various skin eruptions.
Other: muscle weakness, osteoporosis, hirsutism, susceptibility to infections; hypokalemia, hyperglycemia, and carbohydrate intolerance; growth suppression in children; ***acute adrenal insufficiency may occur with increased stress (infection, surgery, or trauma) or abrupt withdrawal after long-term therapy.***

After abrupt withdrawal: rebound inflammation, fatigue, weakness, arthralgia, fever, dizziness, lethargy, depression, fainting, orthostatic hypotension, dyspnea, anorexia, hypoglycemia. ***After prolonged use, sudden withdrawal may be fatal.***

Overdose and treatment
Acute ingestion, even in massive doses, is rarely a clinical problem. Toxic signs and symptoms rarely occur if drug is used for less than 3 weeks, even at large dosage ranges. However, chronic use causes adverse physiologic effects, including suppression of the hypothalamic-pituitary-adrenal axis, cushingoid appearance, muscle weakness, and osteoporosis.

☑ Special considerations
Recommendations for use of prednisone and for care and teaching of patients are the same as those for all *systemic adrenocorticoids.*

Pediatric use
- Chronic use of prednisone in drug or adolescents may delay growth and maturation.

primaquine phosphate

Pharmacologic classification: 8-aminoquinoline
Therapeutic classification: antimalarial
Pregnancy risk category C

How supplied
Available by prescription only
Tablets: 26.3 mg (15-mg base)

Indications, route, and dosage
Radical cure of relapsing vivax malaria, eliminating symptoms and infection completely, and prevention of relapse
Adults: 15 mg (base) P.O. daily for 14 days (26.3-mg tablet equals 15 mg of base), or 79 mg (45-mg base) once weekly for 8 weeks.
Children: 0.3 mg (base)/kg/day for 14 days, or 0.9 mg (base)/kg/day once weekly for 8 weeks.
◊ **Pneumocystis carinii *pneumonia***
Adults: 15 to 30 mg (base) P.O. daily.

Pharmacodynamics
Antimalarial action: Primaquine disrupts the parasitic mitochondria, thereby interrupting metabolic processes requiring energy.

Spectrum of activity includes preerythrocytic and exoerythrocytic forms of *Plasmodium falciparum, P. malariae, P. ovale,* and *P. vivax.* Nifurtimox (Lampit), an investigational agent available from the Centers for Disease Control and Prevention, is preferred for intracellular parasites.

Pharmacokinetics
- *Absorption:* Drug is well absorbed from the GI tract, with peak concentrations occurring at 2 to 6 hours.
- *Distribution:* Distributed widely into the liver, lungs, heart, brain, skeletal muscle, and other tissues.
- *Metabolism:* Primaquine is carboxylated rapidly in the liver.
- *Excretion:* Only a small amount of primaquine is excreted unchanged in urine. Plasma half-life is 4 to 10 hours.

Contraindications and precautions
Contraindicated in patients with systemic diseases in which granulocytopenia may develop (such as lupus erythematosus or rheumatoid arthritis) and in those taking bone marrow suppressants and potentially hemolytic drugs.

Use cautiously in patients with previous idiosyncratic reaction (manifested by hemolytic anemia, methemoglobinemia, or leukopenia) and in those with family or personal history of favism, erythrocytic G6PD deficiency, or nicotinamide adenine dinucleotide (NADH) methemoglobin reductase deficiency.

Interactions
Quinacrine may potentiate the toxic effects of primaquine. Concomitant use with *magnesium* and *aluminum salts* may decrease GI absorption.

Effects on diagnostic tests
Decreases or increases in WBC counts and decreases in RBC counts may occur during primaquine therapy. Methemoglobinemia may occur.

Adverse reactions
GI: nausea, vomiting, epigastric distress, abdominal cramps.

Hematologic: leukopenia, ***hemolytic anemia in G6PD deficiency,*** methemoglobinemia in NADH methemoglobin reductase deficiency.

Overdose and treatment

Signs and symptoms of overdose include abdominal distress, vomiting, CNS and CV disturbances, cyanosis, methemoglobinemia, leukocytosis, leukopenia, and anemia. Treatment is symptomatic.

☑ Special considerations

- Primaquine is often used with a fast-acting antimalarial, such as chloroquine.
- Before starting therapy, screen patients for possible G6PD deficiency.
- Light-skinned patients taking more than 30 mg daily, dark-skinned patients taking more than 15 mg daily, and patients with severe anemia or suspected sensitivity should have frequent blood studies and urine examinations. A sudden fall in hemoglobin concentrations or erythrocyte or leukocyte counts, or a marked darkening of the urine suggests impending hemolytic reaction.
- Perform periodic blood studies and urinalyses to monitor for impending hemolytic reactions.

Patient education

- Teach patient signs and symptoms of adverse reactions and to report them if they occur.
- Advise patient to check urine color at each voiding and to report if urine darkens, becomes tinged with red, or decreases in volume.
- Tell patient to take drug with meals to minimize gastric irritation. Do not take with antacids, which may decrease absorption.
- Advise patient to complete entire course of therapy.

Breast-feeding

- Safety has not been established.

primidone

Myidone, Mysoline, Sertan

Pharmacologic classification: barbiturate analogue
Therapeutic classification: anticonvulsant
Pregnancy risk category NR

How supplied

Available by prescription only
Tablets: 50 mg, 250 mg
Suspension: 250 mg/5 ml

Indications, route, and dosage

Generalized tonic-clonic seizures, focal seizures, complex-partial (psychomotor) seizures
Adults and children age 8 and over: 100 to 125 mg P.O. h.s. on days 1 to 3; 100 to 125 mg P.O. b.i.d. on days 4 to 6; 100 to 125 mg P.O. t.i.d. on days 7 to 9; and maintenance dose of 250 mg P.O. t.i.d. on day 10. May require up to 2 g/day.
Children under age 8: 50 mg P.O. h.s. on days 1 to 3; 50 mg P.O. b.i.d. on days 4 to 6; 100 mg P.O. t.i.d. on days 7 to 9; and maintenance dose of 125 to 250 mg P.O. t.i.d. on day 10.
Benign familial tremor (essential tremor)
Adults: 750 mg P.O. daily.

Pharmacodynamics

Anticonvulsant action: Primidone acts as a nonspecific CNS depressant used alone or with other anticonvulsants to control refractory tonic-clonic seizures and to treat psychomotor or focal seizures. Mechanism of action is unknown; some activity may be from phenobarbital, an active metabolite.

Pharmacokinetics

- *Absorption:* Primidone is absorbed readily from the GI tract; serum concentrations peak at about 3 hours. Phenobarbital appears in plasma after several days of continuous therapy; most laboratory assays detect both phenobarbital and primidone. Therapeutic levels are 5 to 12 mcg/ml for primidone and 10 to 30 mcg/ml for phenobarbital.
- *Distribution:* Primidone is distributed widely throughout the body.
- *Metabolism:* Primidone is metabolized slowly by the liver to phenylethylmalonamide (PEMA) and phenobarbital; PEMA is the major metabolite.
- *Excretion:* Primidone is excreted in urine; substantial amounts are excreted in breast milk.

Contraindications and precautions

Contraindicated in patients with phenobarbital hypersensitivity or porphyria.

Interactions

Alcohol and other *CNS depressants,* including *narcotic analgesics,* cause excessive depression in patients taking primidone. *Carbamazepine* and *phenytoin* may decrease effects of primidone and increase its conversion to phenobarbital; monitor serum levels to prevent toxicity. Coadministration of *acetazolamide* and *succinimides* may decrease concentrations of primidone.

Effects on diagnostic tests

Primidone may cause abnormalities in liver function test results.

Adverse reactions

CNS: *drowsiness, ataxia,* emotional disturbances, vertigo, hyperirritability, fatigue, paranoia.
EENT: *diplopia,* nystagmus.
GI: anorexia, nausea, vomiting.
GU: impotence, polyuria.
Hematologic: megaloblastic anemia, ***thrombocytopenia.***
Skin: morbilliform rash.

Overdose and treatment

Signs and symptoms of overdose resemble those of barbiturate intoxication; they include CNS and respiratory depression, areflexia, oliguria, tachycardia, hypotension, hypothermia, and coma. Shock may occur.

Treat overdose supportively: In conscious patient with intact gag reflex, induce emesis with ipecac; follow in 30 minutes with repeated doses of activated charcoal. Use lavage if emesis is not feasible. Alkalinization of urine and forced diuresis may hasten excretion. Hemodialysis may be necessary. Monitor vital signs and fluid and electrolyte balance.

☑ Special considerations

Besides those relevant to all *barbiturates,* consider the following recommendations.

- Perform a CBC and liver function tests every 6 months.
- Abrupt withdrawal of drug may cause status epilepticus; dosage should be reduced gradually.
- Barbiturates impair ability to perform tasks requiring mental alertness such as driving a car.

Patient education

- Explain rationale for therapy and the potential risks and benefits.
- Teach patient signs and symptoms of adverse reactions.
- Tell patient to avoid alcohol and other sedatives to prevent added CNS depression.
- Instruct patient not to discontinue drug or to alter dosage without medical approval.
- Explain that barbiturates may render oral contraceptives ineffective; advise patient to consider a different birth control method.
- Advise patient to avoid hazardous tasks that require mental alertness until degree of sedative effect is determined. Tell the patient that dizziness and incoordination are common at first but will disappear.
- Recommend that patient wear a medical identification bracelet or necklace identifying him as having a seizure disorder and listing drug.
- Tell patient to shake oral suspension well before use.

Geriatric use

- Reduce dose in elderly patients; many have decreased renal function.

Pediatric use

- Primidone may cause hyperexcitability in children under age 6.

Breast-feeding

- Considerable amounts of drug occur in breast milk; use an alternative feeding method during therapy.

probenecid

Benemid, Probalan

Pharmacologic classification: sulfonamide-derivative
Therapeutic classification: uricosuric
Pregnancy risk category NR

How supplied

Available by prescription only
Tablets: 500 mg

Indications, route, and dosage

Adjunct to penicillin therapy

Adults and children over age 14 or weighing over 110 lb (50 kg): 500 mg P.O. q.i.d.

Children age 2 to 14 or weighing under 110 lb: Initially, 25 mg/kg or 700 mg/m² daily, then 40 mg/kg or 1.2 g/m² divided q.i.d.

Single-dose penicillin treatment of gonorrhea

Adults: 1 g P.O. given together with penicillin treatment, or 1 g P.O. 30 minutes before I.M. dose of penicillin.

Hyperuricemia associated with gout

Adults: 250 mg P.O. b.i.d. for first week, then 500 mg b.i.d., to maximum of 2 to 3 g daily.

◊ ***To diagnose parkinsonian syndrome or mental depression***

Adults: 500 mg P.O. q 12 hours for five doses.

Pharmacodynamics

Uricosuric action: Probenecid competitively inhibits the active reabsorption of uric acid at the proximal convoluted tubule, thereby increasing urinary excretion of uric acid.

Adjunctive action in antibiotic therapy: Probenecid competitively inhibits secretion of weak organic acids, including penicillins, cephalosporins, and other beta-lactam antibiotics, thereby increasing serum concentrations of these drugs.

Pharmacokinetics

- *Absorption:* Drug is completely absorbed after oral administration; peak serum levels are reached at 2 to 4 hours.
- *Distribution:* Distributes throughout the body; drug is about 75% protein-bound. CSF levels are about 2% of serum levels.
- *Metabolism:* Drug is metabolized in the liver to active metabolites, with some uricosuric effect.
- *Excretion:* Drug and metabolites are excreted in urine; probenecid (but not metabolites) is actively reabsorbed.

Contraindications and precautions

Contraindicated in patients with hypersensitivity to drug, uric acid kidney stones, or blood dyscrasias; in acute gout attack; and in children under age 2 years. Use cautiously in patients with impaired renal function or peptic ulcer.

Interactions

Probenecid significantly increases or prolongs effects of *cephalosporins, penicillins,* and other *beta-lactam antibiotics, sulfonamides,* and possibly *ketamine* and *thiopental*; it enhances hypoglycemic effects of *chlorpropamide* and *other oral sulfonylureas,* and increases serum levels (thus increasing risk of toxicity) of *aminosalicylic acid, dapsone, methotrexate,* and *nitrofurantoin.*

Probenecid inhibits urinary excretion of weak organic acids; it impairs naturietic effects of *bumetanide, ethacrynic acid,* and *furosemide;* it also decreases excretion of *indomethacin* and *naproxen,* permitting use of lower doses.

Alcohol, diuretics, and *pyrazinamide* decrease uric acid levels of probenecid; increased doses of probenecid may be required. *Salicylates* inhibit the uricosuric effect of probenecid only in doses that achieve levels of 50 mcg/ml or more; occasional use of low-dose *aspirin* does not interfere.

Concurrent administration with *zidovudine* has shown increased bioavailability of zidovudine; cutaneous eruptions accompanied by systemic symptoms, including malaise, myalgia, or fever, have occurred.

Effects on diagnostic tests

Probenecid causes false-positive test results for urinary glucose with tests using cupric sulfate reagent (Benedict's reagent, Clinitest, and Fehling's test); perform tests with glucose oxidase reagent (Diastix, Chemstrip uG, or glucose enzymatic test strip) instead.

Adverse reactions

CNS: *headache,* dizziness.
GI: anorexia, nausea, vomiting, sore gums.
GU: urinary frequency, renal colic, nephrotic syndrome.
Hematologic: ***hemolytic anemia, aplastic anemia,*** anemia.
Skin: dermatitis, pruritus.
Other: flushing, fever, exacerbation of gout, ***hepatic necrosis,*** hypersensitivity reactions (including ***anaphylaxis***).

Overdose and treatment

Clinical signs and symptoms include nausea, copious vomiting, stupor, coma, and tonic-clonic seizures. Treat supportively, using mechanical ventilation if needed; induce emesis or use gastric lavage, as appropriate. Control seizures with I.V. phenobarbital and phenytoin.

☑ Special considerations

- When used for hyperuricemia associated with gout, probenecid has no analgesic or anti-inflammatory actions, and no effect on acute attacks; start therapy after attack subsides. Because drug may increase the frequency of acute attacks during the first 6 to 12 months of therapy, prophylactic doses of colchicine or an NSAID should be administered during the first 3 to 6 months of drug therapy.
- Monitor BUN and serum creatinine levels closely; drug is ineffective in patients with severe renal insufficiency.
- Monitor uric acid levels and adjust dose to the lowest dose that maintains normal uric acid levels.
- Give with food, milk, or prescribed antacids to lessen GI upset.
- Maintain adequate hydration with high fluid intake to prevent formation of uric acid stones. Also maintain alkalinization of urine.
- Drug has been used in the diagnosis of parkinsonian syndrome and mental depression.

Patient education

- Instruct patient not to discontinue drug without medical approval.
- Warn patient not to use drug for pain or inflammation and not to increase dose during gouty attack.
- Tell patient to drink 8 to 10 glasses of fluid daily and to take drug with food to minimize GI upset.
- Warn patient to avoid aspirin and other salicylates, which may antagonize probenecid's uricosuric effect.
- Caution diabetic patients to use glucose enzymatic test strip, Diastix, or Chemstrip uG for urine glucose testing.

Geriatric use

- Lower doses are indicated in elderly patients.

Pediatric use

- Drug is contraindicated in infants under age 2.

Breast-feeding

- It is unknown if drug occurs in breast milk. An alternative feeding method is recommended during therapy.

procainamide hydrochloride

Procanbid, Promine, Pronestyl, Pronestyl-SR

Pharmacologic classification: procaine derivative
Therapeutic classification: ventricular antiarrhythmic, supraventricular antiarrhythmic
Pregnancy risk category C

How supplied

Available by prescription only
Tablets: 250 mg, 375 mg, 500 mg
Tablets (extended-release): 500 mg, 1 g
Tablets (sustained-release): 250 mg, 500 mg, 750 mg
Capsules: 250 mg, 375 mg, 500 mg
Injection: 100 mg/ml, 500 mg/ml

Indications, route, and dosage

Symptomatic PVCs; life-threatening ventricular tachycardia; ◊ atrial fibrillation and flutter unresponsive to quinidine; ◊ paroxysmal atrial tachycardia

Adults: 50 to 100 mg q 5 minutes by slow I.V. push, no faster than 25 to 50 mg/minute, until arrhythmias disappear, adverse effects develop, or 500 mg has been given. When arrhythmias disappear, give continuous infusion of 1 to 6 mg/minute. Usual effective loading dose is 500 to 600 mg. If arrhythmias recur, repeat bolus as above and increase infusion rate. For I.M. administration, give 50 mg/kg divided q 3 to 6 hours; during surgery, 100 to 500 mg I.M. For oral therapy, initiate dosage at 50 mg/kg P.O. in divided doses q 3 hours until therapeutic levels are reached. Once patient is stable, may substitute sustained-release form q 6 hours or extended-release form at dose of 50 mg/kg in two divided doses q 12 hours.

◊ Loading dose to prevent atrial fibrillation or paroxysmal atrial tachycardia

Adults: 1 to 1.25 g P.O. If arrhythmias persist after 1 hour, give additional 750 mg. If no change occurs, give 500 mg to 1 g q 2 hours until arrhythmias disappear or adverse effects occur.

Loading dose to prevent ventricular tachycardia

Adults: 1 g P.O. Maintenance dosage is 50 mg/kg/day given at 3-hour intervals; average is 250 to 500 mg q 4 hours but may require 1 to 1.5 g q 4 to 6 hours.

◊ ***Treatment of malignant hyperthermia***

Adults: 200 to 900 mg I.V., followed by an infusion.

Pharmacodynamics

Antiarrhythmic action: A class IA antiarrhythmic agent, procainamide depresses phase 0 of the action potential. It is considered a myocardial depressant because it decreases myocardial excitability and conduction velocity and may depress myocardial contractility. It also possesses anticholinergic activity, which may modify its direct myocardial effects. In therapeutic doses, it reduces conduction velocity in the atria, ventricles, and His-Purkinje system. Its effectiveness in controlling atrial tachyarrhythmias stems from its ability to prolong the effective refractory period (ERP) and increase the action potential duration in the atria, ventricles, and His-Purkinje system. Because ERP prolongation exceeds action potential duration, tissue remains refractory even after returning to resting membrane potential (membrane-stabilizing effect).

Procainamide shortens the effective refractory period of the AV node. Drug's anticholinergic action also may increase AV node conductivity. Suppression of automaticity in the His-Purkinje system and ectopic pacemakers accounts for drug's effectiveness in treating ventricular premature beats. At therapeutic doses, procainamide prolongs the PR and QT intervals. (This effect may be used as an index of drug effectiveness and toxicity.) The QRS interval usually is not prolonged beyond normal range; the QT interval is not prolonged to the extent achieved with quinidine.

Procainamide exerts a peripheral vasodilatory effect; with I.V. administration, it may cause hypotension, which limits the administration rate and amount of drug deliverable.

Pharmacokinetics

• *Absorption:* Rate and extent of drug's absorption from the intestines vary; usually, 75% to 95% of an orally administered dose is absorbed. With administration of tablets and capsules, peak plasma levels occur in approximately 1 hour. Extended-release tablets are formulated to provide a sustained and relatively constant rate of release and absorption throughout the small intestine. After drug's release, extended wax matrix is not absorbed and may appear in feces after 15 minutes to 1 hour. With I.M. injection, onset of action occurs in about 10 to 30 minutes, with peak levels in about 1 hour.

• *Distribution:* Procainamide is distributed widely in most body tissues, including cerebrospinal fluid, liver, spleen, kidneys, lungs, muscles, brain, and heart. Only about 15% binds to plasma proteins. Usual therapeutic range for serum procainamide concentrations is 4 to 8 mcg/ml. Some experts suggest that a range of 10 to 30 mcg/ml for the sum of procainamide and N-acetyl procainamide (NAPA) serum concentrations are therapeutic.

• *Metabolism:* Procainamide is acetylated in the liver to form NAPA. Acetylation rate is determined genetically and affects NAPA formation. (NAPA also exerts antiarrhythmic activity.)

• *Excretion:* Procainamide and NAPA metabolite are excreted in the urine. Procainamide's half-life is about 2½ to 4¾ hours. NAPA's half-life is about 6 hours. In patients with heart failure or renal dysfunction, half-life increases; therefore, in such patients, dosage reduction is required to avoid toxicity.

Contraindications and precautions

Contraindicated in patients with hypersensitivity to procaine and related drugs; in those with complete, second-, or third-degree heart block in the absence of an artificial pacemaker; and in patients with myasthenia gravis or systemic lupus erythematosus. Also contraindicated in patients with atypical ventricular tachycardia (torsades de pointes) because procainamide may aggravate this condition.

Use cautiously in patients with ventricular tachycardia during coronary occlusion, heart failure or other conduction disturbances (bundle-branch heart block, sinus bradycardia, cardiac glycoside intoxication), impaired renal or hepatic function, preexisting blood dyscrasia, or bone marrow suppression.

Interactions

Concomitant use of procainamide with *neuromuscular blocking agents* (such as *decamethonium bromide, gallium triethiodide, metocurine iodide, pancuronium bromide, succinylcholine chloride,* and *tubocurarine chloride)* may potentiate the effects of the neuromuscular blocking agents. Concomitant use with *anticholinergic agents (atropine, diphenhydramine, tricyclic antidepressants*) may cause additive anticholinergic effects.

Concomitant use with *cholinergic agents (neostigmine, pyridostigmine*, which are used to treat myasthenia gravis) may negate the effects of these agents, requiring increased dosage.

Concomitant use with *antihypertensives* may cause additive hypotensive effects (most common with I.V. procainamide). Concomitant use with other *antiarrhythmics* may result in additive or antagonistic cardiac effects and with possible additive toxic effects. Concomitant use with *cimetidine* may result in impaired renal clearance of procainamide and NAPA, with elevated serum drug concentrations.

Effects on diagnostic tests

Procainamide will invalidate bentiromide test results; discontinue at least 3 days before bentiromide test. Procainamide may alter edrophonium test results; positive antinuclear antibody (ANA) titers, positive direct antiglobulin (Coombs') tests, and ECG changes may be seen. The physiologic effects of drug may result in decreased leukocytes and platelets, and increased bilirubin, LD, alkaline phosphatase, ALT, and AST.

Adverse reactions

CNS: hallucinations, confusion, ***seizures,*** depression, dizziness.
CV: *hypotension,* ***ventricular asystole,*** *bradycardia,* AV block, ***ventricular fibrillation*** (after parenteral use).
GI: nausea, vomiting, anorexia, diarrhea, bitter taste.
Hematologic: ***thrombocytopenia, neutropenia*** (especially with sustained-release forms), ***agranulocytosis, hemolytic anemia.***
Skin: *maculopapular rash, urticaria, pruritus, flushing, angioneurotic edema.*
Other: *fever, lupuslike syndrome* (especially after prolonged administration).

Overdose and treatment

Clinical effects of overdose include severe hypotension, widening QRS complex, junctional tachycardia, intraventricular conduction delay, ventricular fibrillation, oliguria, confusion and lethargy, and nausea and vomiting.

Treatment involves general supportive measures (including respiratory and CV support) with hemodynamic and ECG monitoring. After recent ingestion of oral form, gastric lavage, emesis, and activated charcoal may be used to decrease absorption. Phenylephrine or norepinephrine may be used to treat hypotension after adequate hydration has been ensured. Hemodialysis may be effective in removing procainamide and NAPA. A 1/6 M solution of sodium lactate may reduce procainamide's cardiotoxic effect.

☑ Special considerations

- In treating atrial fibrillation and flutter, ventricular rate may accelerate due to vagolytic effects on the AV node; to prevent this effect, a cardiac glycoside may be administered before procainamide therapy begins.
- Monitor patient receiving infusions at all times.
- Infusion pump or microdrip system and timer should be used to monitor infusion precisely.
- Monitor blood pressure and ECG continuously during I.V. administration. Watch for prolonged QT and QRS intervals (50% or greater widening), heart block, or increased arrhythmias. When these ECG signs appear, procainamide should be discontinued and the patient monitored closely.
- Monitor therapeutic serum levels of procainamide: 3 to 10 mcg/ml (most patients are controlled at 4 to 8 mcg/ml); may exhibit toxicity at levels greater than 16 mcg/ml). Monitor NAPA levels as well; some clinicians feel that procainamide and NAPA levels should be 10 to 30 mcg/ml.
- Baseline and periodic determinations of ANA titers, lupus erythematosus cell preparations, and CBCs may be indicated because procainamide therapy (usually long-term) has been associated with syndrome resembling systemic lupus erythematosus.
- For initial oral therapy, use conventional capsules and tablets; use extended-release tablets only for maintenance therapy.
- I.V. drug form is more likely to cause adverse cardiac effects, possibly resulting in severe hypotension.
- In prolonged use of oral form, perform ECGs occasionally to determine continued need for drug.

Geriatric use

- Elderly patients may require reduced dosage. Because of highly variable metabolism, monitoring of serum levels is recommended.

Pediatric use

- Manufacturer has not established dosage guidelines for pediatric patients. For treating arrhythmias, the suggested dosage is 40 to 60 mg/kg of standard tablets or capsules, P.O. daily, given in four to six divided doses; or 3 to 6 mg/kg I.V. over 5 minutes, followed by a drip of 0.02 to 0.08 mg/kg/minute.

Breast-feeding

- Because procainamide and NAPA are distributed into breast milk, an alternative feeding method is recommended for women receiving procainamide.

procarbazine hydrochloride

Matulane, Natulan*

Pharmacologic classification: antibiotic antineoplastic (cell cycle–phase specific, S phase)
Therapeutic classification: antineoplastic
Pregnancy risk category D

How supplied

Available by prescription only
Capsules: 50 mg

Indications, route, and dosage

Dosage and indications may vary. Check current literature for recommended protocol.

Hodgkin's disease, lymphomas, brain and lung cancer
Adults: 2 to 4 mg/kg/day P.O. in single or divided doses for the first week, followed by 4 to 6 mg/kg/day until response or toxicity occurs. Maintenance dosage is 1 to 2 mg/kg/day.
Children: 50 mg/m^2 daily P.O. for first week, then 100 mg/m^2 daily until response or toxicity occurs. Maintenance dosage is 50 mg/m^2 P.O. daily after bone marrow recovery.

Pharmacodynamics

Antineoplastic action: Exact mechanism of procarbazine's cytotoxic activity is unknown. Drug appears to have several sites of action; the result is inhibition of DNA, RNA, and protein synthesis. Procarbazine has also been reported to damage DNA directly and to inhibit the mitotic S phase of cell division.

Pharmacokinetics

- *Absorption:* Drug is rapidly and completely absorbed following oral administration.
- *Distribution:* Drug distributes widely into body tissues, with the highest concentrations found in the liver, kidneys, intestinal wall, and skin. Drug crosses the blood-brain barrier.

• *Metabolism:* Extensively metabolized in the liver. Some metabolites have cytotoxic activity.
• *Excretion:* Drug and its metabolites are excreted primarily in urine.

Contraindications and precautions
Contraindicated in patients hypersensitive to drug and in those with inadequate bone marrow reserve as shown by bone marrow aspiration. Use cautiously in patients with impaired renal or hepatic function.

Interactions
Concomitant use of procarbazine with *alcohol* can cause a disulfiram-like reaction. The mechanism of this interaction is poorly defined. Concomitant use with *CNS depressants* enhances CNS depression through an additive mechanism; concomitant use with *MAO inhibitors, selective serotonin reuptake inhibitors, sympathomimetics, tricyclic antidepressants,* or *tyramine-rich foods* can cause a hypertensive crisis, tremors, excitation, and cardiac palpitations through inhibition of MAO by procarbazine. Serum *digoxin* levels may be decreased. Concomitant use with *meperidine* may result in severe hypotension and death. Administration with *levodopa* may cause flushing and a significant rise in blood pressure.

Effects on diagnostic tests
None reported.

Adverse reactions
CNS: nervousness, depression, headache, dizziness, ***coma, seizures,*** insomnia, nightmares, paresthesia, neuropathy, *hallucinations,* confusion.
CV: hypotension, tachycardia, syncope.
EENT: retinal hemorrhage, nystagmus, photophobia.
GI: *nausea, vomiting,* anorexia, stomatitis, dry mouth, dysphagia, diarrhea, constipation.
GU: hematuria, urinary frequency, nocturia.
Hematologic: ***bleeding tendency, thrombocytopenia, leukopenia, anemia,*** hemolytic anemia.
Respiratory: ***pleural effusion,*** pneumonitis, cough.
Skin: dermatitis, pruritus, rash.
Other: reversible alopecia, allergic reactions, gynecomastia.

Overdose and treatment
Clinical manifestations of overdose include myalgia, arthralgia, fever, weakness, dermatitis, alopecia, paresthesia, hallucinations, tremors, seizures, coma, myelosuppression, nausea, and vomiting.

Treatment is usually supportive and includes transfusion of blood components, antiemetics, antipyretics, and appropriate antianxiety agents.

☑ Special considerations
• Nausea and vomiting may be decreased if drug is taken at bedtime and in divided doses.
• Procarbazine inhibits MAO. Use procarbazine cautiously with MAO inhibitors, tricyclic antidepressants and selective serotonin reuptake inhibitors, other drugs that interact with MAO inhibitors, or tyramine-rich foods.
• Use cautiously in inadequate bone marrow reserve, leukopenia, thrombocytopenia, anemia, and impaired hepatic or renal function.
• Observe for signs of bleeding.
• Store capsules in dry environment.

Patient education
• Emphasize importance of continuing medication despite nausea and vomiting.
• Advise patient to call immediately if vomiting occurs shortly after taking dose.
• Warn patient that drowsiness may occur, so patient should avoid hazardous activities that require alertness until drug's effect is established.
• Warn patient not to drink alcoholic beverages or tyramine-containing foods while taking drug.
• Instruct patient to stop medication and call immediately if disulfiram-like reaction occurs (chest pains, rapid or irregular heartbeat, severe headache, stiff neck).
• Tell patient to avoid exposure to people with infections.
• Warn patient to avoid prolonged sun exposure because photosensitivity occurs during therapy.
• Tell patient to call if a sore throat or fever or unusual bruising or bleeding occurs.

Pediatric use
• Severe reactions, such as tremors, seizures, and coma, have occurred after administration of procarbazine to children.

Breast-feeding
• It is not known if drug occurs in breast milk. However, because of potential for serious adverse reactions, mutagenicity, and carcinogenicity in the infant, breast-feeding is not recommended.

prochlorperazine
Compazine, Stemetil*

prochlorperazine edisylate
Compazine

prochlorperazine maleate
Compazine, Compazine Spansule, Stemetil*

Pharmacologic classification: phenothiazine (piperazine derivative)
Therapeutic classification: antipsychotic, antiemetic, antianxiety
Pregnancy risk category C

How supplied
Available by prescription only
prochlorperazine maleate
Tablets: 5 mg, 10 mg, 25 mg
prochlorperazine edisylate
Spansules (sustained-release): 10 mg, 15 mg, 30 mg
Syrup: 1 mg/ml
Injection: 5 mg/ml
Suppositories: 2.5 mg, 5 mg, 25 mg

Indications, route, and dosage

Preoperative nausea control

Adults: 5 to 10 mg I.M. 1 to 2 hours before induction of anesthesia, repeated once in 30 minutes if necessary; or 5 to 10 mg I.V. 15 to 30 minutes before induction of anesthesia, repeated once if necessary; or 20 mg/L D_5W and 0.9% NaCl solution by I.V. infusion, added to infusion 15 to 30 minutes before induction. Maximum parenteral dosage is 40 mg daily.

Severe nausea, vomiting

Adults: 5 to 10 mg P.O. t.i.d. or q.i.d.; or 15 mg of sustained-release form P.O. on arising; or 10 mg of sustained-release form P.O. q 12 hours; or 25 mg P.R. b.i.d.; or 5 to 10 mg I.M. injected deeply into upper outer quadrant of gluteal region. Repeat q 3 to 4 hours, p.r.n. May be given I.V. Maximum parenteral dosage, 40 mg daily.

Children weighing 39 to 86 lb (18 to 39 kg): 2.5 mg P.O. or rectally t.i.d.; or 5 mg P.O. or P.R. b.i.d.; or 0.132 mg/kg deep I.M. injection. (Control usually obtained with one dose.) Maximum dosage is 15 mg daily.

Children weighing 31 to 38 lb (14 to 17 kg): 2.5 mg P.O. or P.R. b.i.d. or t.i.d.; or 0.132 mg/kg deep I.M. injection. (Control usually is obtained with one dose.) Maximum dosage, 10 mg daily.

Children weighing 20 to 30 lb (9 to 14 kg): 2.5 mg P.O. or P.R. daily or b.i.d.; or 0.132 mg/kg deep I.M. injection. (Control usually is obtained with one dose.) Maximum dosage, 7.5 mg daily.

Anxiety

Adults: 5 mg P.O. t.i.d. or q.i.d.

Psychotic disorders

Adults: 5 to 10 mg P.O. or 10 to 20 mg I.M. t.i.d. or q.i.d.; up to 150 mg daily P.O. for hospitalized patients.

Pharmacodynamics

Antipsychotic action: Prochlorperazine is thought to exert its antipsychotic effects by postsynaptic blockade of CNS dopamine receptors, thus inhibiting dopamine-mediated effects.

Antiemetic action: Antiemetic effects are attributed to dopamine receptor blockade in the medullary chemoreceptor trigger zone.

Prochlorperazine has many other central and peripheral effects: It produces alpha and ganglionic blockade and counteracts histamine- and serotonin-mediated activity. Its most prevalent adverse reactions are extrapyramidal. It is used primarily as an antiemetic; it is ineffective against motion sickness.

Pharmacokinetics

- *Absorption:* Rate and extent of absorption vary with administration route: oral tablet absorption is erratic and variable, with onset of action ranging from ½ to 1 hour; oral concentrate absorption is more predictable. I.M. drug is absorbed rapidly.
- *Distribution:* Drug is distributed widely into the body, including breast milk. Drug is 91% to 99% protein-bound. Peak effect occurs at 2 to 4 hours; steady-state serum levels are achieved within 4 to 7 days.
- *Metabolism:* Metabolized extensively by the liver, but no active metabolites are formed; duration of action is about 3 to 4 hours and 10 to 12 hours for the extended-release form.
- *Excretion:* Mostly excreted in urine via the kidneys; some is excreted in feces via the biliary tract.

Contraindications and precautions

Contraindicated in patients hypersensitive to phenothiazines and in those with CNS depression including coma; during pediatric surgery; when using spinal or epidural anesthetic, adrenergic blockers, or ethanol; and in infants under age 2.

Use cautiously in patients with impaired CV function, glaucoma, seizure disorders; in those who have been exposed to extreme heat; and in children with acute illness.

Interactions

Concomitant use of prochlorperazine with *sympathomimetics*, including *epinephrine, phenylephrine, phenylpropanolamine*, and *ephedrine* (commonly found in nasal sprays), and with *appetite suppressants* may decrease their stimulatory and pressor effects and may cause epinephrine reversal (hypotensive response to epinephrine).

Prochlorperazine may inhibit blood pressure response *to centrally acting antihypertensive drugs*, such as *clonidine, guanabenz, guanadrel, guanethidine, methyldopa*, and *reserpine*. Additive effects are likely after concomitant use of prochlorperazine with *CNS depressants*, including *alcohol, barbiturates, narcotics, tranquilizers*, and *anesthetics (general, spinal, epidural), and parenteral magnesium sulfate* (oversedation, respiratory depression, and hypotension); *antiarrhythmic agents, disopyramide, procainamide*, and *quinidine* (increased incidence of arrhythmias and conduction defects); *atropine* and *other anticholinergic drugs*, including *antidepressants, antihistamines, MAO inhibitors, meperidine, phenothiazines*, and *antiparkinson agents* (oversedation, paralytic ileus, visual changes, and severe constipation); *nitrates* (hypotension); and *metrizamide* (increased risk of seizures).

Beta-blocking agents may inhibit prochlorperazine metabolism, increasing plasma levels and toxicity.

Concomitant use with *propylthiouracil* increases risk of agranulocytosis; concomitant use with *lithium* may result in severe neurologic toxicity with an encephalitis-like syndrome, and in decreased therapeutic response to prochlorperazine.

Pharmacokinetic alterations and subsequent decreased therapeutic response to prochlorperazine may follow concomitant use with *phenobarbital* (enhanced renal excretion); *aluminum-* and *magnesium-containing antacids* and *antidiarrheals* (decreased absorption); *caffeine*; or *heavy smoking* (increased metabolism).

Prochlorperazine may antagonize therapeutic effect of *bromocriptine* on prolactin secretion; it also may decrease the vasoconstricting effects of *high-dose dopamine* and may decrease effectiveness and increase toxicity of *levodopa* (by dopamine blockade). Prochlorperazine may inhibit metabolism and increase toxicity of *phenytoin*.

Effects on diagnostic tests

Prochlorperazine causes false-positive test results for urinary porphyrins, urobilinogen, amylase, and 5-hydroxyindoleacetic acid because of darkening of urine by metabolites; it also causes false-positive urine pregnancy results in tests using human chorionic gonadotropin as the indicator.

Prochlorperazine elevates test results for liver enzymes and protein-bound iodine and causes quinidine-like ECG effects.

Adverse reactions

CNS: *extrapyramidal reactions,* sedation, pseudoparkinsonism, EEG changes, dizziness.
CV: *orthostatic hypotension,* tachycardia, ECG changes.
EENT: *ocular changes, blurred vision.*
GI: *dry mouth, constipation,* ileus.
GU: *urine retention,* dark urine, menstrual irregularities, inhibited ejaculation.
Hematologic: *transient leukopenia,* ***agranulocytosis, thrombocytopenia, hemolytic anemia.***
Hepatic: *cholestatic jaundice.*
Skin: mild photosensitivity, allergic reactions, **exfoliative dermatitis.**
Other: hyperprolactinemia, gynecomastia, weight gain, increased appetite, hyperglycemia or hypoglycemia.

Overdose and treatment

CNS depression is characterized by deep, unarousable sleep and possible coma, hypotension or hypertension, extrapyramidal symptoms, dystonia, abnormal involuntary muscle movements, agitation, seizures, arrhythmias, ECG changes, hypothermia or hyperthermia, and autonomic nervous system dysfunction.

Treatment is symptomatic and supportive and includes maintaining vital signs, airway, stable body temperature, and fluid and electrolyte balance.

Do not induce vomiting: Drug inhibits cough reflex, and aspiration may occur. Use gastric lavage, then activated charcoal and NaCl cathartics; dialysis does not help. Regulate body temperature as needed. Treat hypotension with I.V. fluids: *Do not give epinephrine.* Treat seizures with parenteral diazepam or barbiturates; arrhythmias with parenteral phenytoin (1 mg/kg with rate titrated to blood pressure); and extrapyramidal reactions with benztropine or parenteral diphenhydramine 2 mg/kg/minute.

☑ Special considerations

Besides those relevant to all *phenothiazines,* consider the following recommendations.

- Liquid and injectable formulations may cause a rash after contact with skin.
- Drug may cause a pink to brown discoloration of urine.
- Drug is associated with a high incidence of extrapyramidal effects and, in institutionalized psychiatric patients, photosensitivity reactions; patient should avoid exposure to sunlight or heat lamps.
- Oral formulations may cause stomach upset. Administer with food or fluid.
- Dilute the concentrate in 2 to 4 oz (60 to 120 ml) of water. The suppository form should be stored in a cool place.
- Give I.V. dose slowly (5 mg/minute). I.M. injection may cause skin necrosis; take care to prevent extravasation. Do not mix with other medications in the syringe. Do not administer S.C.
- Administer I.M. injection deep into the upper outer quadrant of the buttock. Massaging the area after administration may prevent formation of abscesses.
- Solution for injection may be slightly discolored. Do not use if excessively discolored or if a precipitate is evident. Contact pharmacist.
- Monitor patient's blood pressure before and after parenteral administration.
- Do not give sustained-release form to children.
- Drug is ineffective in treating motion sickness.
- Chewing gum, hard candy, or ice may help relieve dry mouth.
- Protect the liquid formulation from light.

Patient education

- Explain risks of dystonic reactions and tardive dyskinesia. Tell patient to report abnormal body movements promptly.
- Tell patient to avoid sun exposure and to wear sunscreen when going outdoors to prevent photosensitivity reactions. (Note that heat lamps and tanning beds also may cause burning of the skin or skin discoloration.)
- Tell patient to avoid spilling the liquid form. Contact with skin may cause rash and irritation.
- Warn patient to avoid extremely hot or cold baths and exposure to temperature extremes, sunlamps, or tanning beds; drug may cause thermoregulatory changes.
- Advise patient to take drug exactly as prescribed, not to double doses after missing one, and not to share drug with others.
- Warn patient to avoid alcohol or take other medications that may cause excessive sedation.
- Tell patient to dilute the concentrate in water; explain the dropper technique of measuring dose; teach correct use of suppository.
- Tell patient that hard candy, chewing gum, or ice chips can alleviate dry mouth.
- Urge patient to store drug safely away from children.
- Inform patient that interactions are possible with many drugs. Warn him to seek medical approval before taking self-prescribed medication.
- Warn patient not to stop taking drug suddenly and to promptly report difficulty urinating, sore throat, dizziness, or fainting. Reassure patient that most reactions can be relieved by reducing dose.
- Caution patient to avoid hazardous activities that require alertness until drug's effect is established. Reassure patient that sedative effects subside and become tolerable in several weeks.

Geriatric use

- Elderly patients tend to require lower doses, titrated to individual effects. These patients are at greater risk for adverse reactions, especially tardive dyskinesia, other extrapyramidal effects, and hypotension.

Pediatric use

- Prochlorperazine is not recommended for patients under age 2 or weighing less than 20 lb (9 kg).

Breast-feeding

- Drug may enter breast milk and should be used with caution. Potential benefits to the mother should outweigh potential harm to the infant.

progesterone

Crinone, Gesterol 50, Progestasert

Pharmacologic classification: progestin
Therapeutic classification: progestin, contraceptive
Pregnancy risk category X

How supplied

Available by prescription only
Gel: 4% (45 mg), 8% (90 mg)
Injection: 25 mg, 50 mg, and 100 mg/ml (in oil); 25 mg and 50 mg/ml (aqueous)
Intrauterine device: 38 mg (with barium sulfate, dispersed in silicone fluid)

Indications, route, and dosage

Amenorrhea
Adults: 5 to 10 mg I.M. daily for 6 to 8 days. Or, for secondary amenorrhea, one application of 4% gel vaginally every other day up to a total of six doses. If no response, may use Crinone 8% every other day up to a total of six doses.

Dysfunctional uterine bleeding
Adults: 5 to 10 mg I.M. daily for 6 days. Alternatively, a single 50 to 100 mg I.M. dose.

Corpus luteum insufficiency
Adults: 12.5 mg I.M. initiated within several days of ovulation and continuing for 2 weeks. May continue for up to 11th week of gestation. Or, for infertility, one application of 8% gel vaginally, daily or twice daily. If pregnancy occurs, treatment may be continued until placental autonomy is achieved up to 10 to 12 weeks.

Contraception (as an intrauterine device [IUD])
Adults: Progestasert system inserted into uterine cavity; replaced after 1 year.

Pharmacodynamics

Contraceptive action: Progesterone suppresses ovulation, thickens cervical mucus, and induces sloughing of the endometrium.

Pharmacokinetics

- *Absorption:* Progesterone must be administered parenterally because it is inactivated by the liver after oral administration.
- *Distribution:* Little information available.
- *Metabolism:* Progesterone is reduced to pregnanediol in the liver, then conjugated with glucuronic acid. Plasma half-life of progesterone is short (several minutes).
- *Excretion:* Glucuronide-conjugated pregnanediol is excreted in urine.

Contraindications and precautions

Contraindicated in patients with thromboembolic disorders or cerebral apoplexy (or history of these conditions), hypersensitivity to drug, breast cancer, undiagnosed abnormal vaginal bleeding, severe hepatic disease, or missed abortion.

Use cautiously in patients with diabetes mellitus, seizures, migraines, cardiac or renal disease, asthma, or mental depression.

Interactions

Progesterone may cause amenorrhea or galactorrhea, thus interfering with the action of *bromocriptine.* Concurrent use of these drugs is not recommended. Use IUD with caution in patients receiving *anticoagulants.*

Effects on diagnostic tests

Pregnanediol excretion may decrease; serum alkaline phosphatase and amino acid levels may increase. Glucose tolerance has been shown to decrease in a small percentage of patients receiving drug.

Adverse reactions

CNS: depression, somnolence, headache (Crinone).
CV: thrombophlebitis, ***thromboembolism, CVA, pulmonary embolism,*** edema.
GI: nausea, constipation, diarrhea, vomiting (Crinone).
GU: breakthrough bleeding, dysmenorrhea, amenorrhea, cervical erosion, abnormal secretions, nocturia (Crinone).
Hepatic: cholestatic jaundice.
Skin: melasma, rash, acne, pruritus, pain at injection site
Other: breast tenderness, enlargement, or secretion.

Overdose and treatment

No information available.

☑ Special considerations

Besides those relevant to all *progestins,* consider the following recommendations.

- Parenteral form is for I.M. administration only. Inject deep into large muscle mass, preferably the gluteal muscle. Check sites for irritation.
- Large doses of progesterone may cause a moderate catabolic effect and a transient increase in sodium and chloride excretion.

Patient education

- Advise patient that withdrawal bleeding usually occurs 2 to 3 days after discontinuing drug.
- Instruct patient to call promptly if she suspects pregnancy while receiving progestin therapy.

For patient using Progestasert

- Inform patient that bleeding and cramping may occur for a few weeks after insertion.
- Advise patient to call if abnormal or excessive bleeding, severe cramping, abnormal vaginal discharge, fever, or flulike syndrome occurs.
- Teach patient how to check for proper placement of IUD.

• Tell patient with Progestasert IUD that the progesterone supply is depleted in 1 year and the device must be changed at that time. Pregnancy risk increases after 1 year if patient relies on progesterone-depleted device for contraception.
• Inform patient of adverse effects, including uterine perforation, increased risk of infection, pelvic inflammatory disease, ectopic pregnancy, abdominal cramping, increased menstrual flow, and expulsion of the device.

For patient using Crinone gel
• Inform patient not to use the gel concurrently with other local intravaginal therapy. If other local intravaginal therapy is used concurrently, there should be at least a 6 hour period before or after gel administration.

Breast-feeding
• Contraindicated in breast-feeding women.

promethazine hydrochloride
Anergan 25, Anergan 50, Histantil*, Pentazine, Phencen-50, Phenergan, Phenergan Fortis, Phenergan Plain, Phenoject-50, Promet, Prorex-25, Prorex-50, Prothazine, Prothazine Plain, V-Gan-25, V-Gan-50

Pharmacologic classification: phenothiazine derivative
Therapeutic classification: antiemetic antivertigo, antihistamine (H_1-receptor antagonist), preoperative, postoperative, or obstetric sedative and adjunct to analgesics
Pregnancy risk category NR

How supplied
Available by prescription only
Tablets: 12.5 mg, 25 mg, 50 mg
Syrup: 6.25 mg/5 ml, 10 mg/5 ml, 25 mg/5 ml
Suppositories: 12.5 mg, 25 mg, 50 mg
Injection: 25 mg/ml, 50 mg/ml

Indications, route, and dosage
Motion sickness
Adults: 25 mg P.O. b.i.d.
Children: 12.5 to 25 mg P.O., I.M., or P.R. b.i.d.
Nausea
Adults: 12.5 to 25 mg P.O., I.M., or P.R. q 4 to 6 hours, p.r.n.
Children: 0.25 to 0.5 mg/kg I.M. or P.R. q 4 to 6 hours, p.r.n.
Rhinitis, allergy symptoms
Adults: 12.5 to 25 mg P.O. before meals and h.s.; or 25 mg P.O. h.s.
Children: 6.25 to 12.5 mg P.O. t.i.d., or 25 mg P.O. or P.R. h.s.
Sedation
Adults: 25 to 50 mg P.O. or I.M. h.s. or p.r.n.
Children: 12.5 to 25 mg P.O., I.M., or P.R. h.s.
Routine preoperative or postoperative sedation or as an adjunct to analgesics
Adults: 25 to 50 mg I.M., I.V., or P.O.
Children: 12.5 to 25 mg I.M., I.V., or P.O.
Obstetric sedation
25 to 50 mg I.M. or I.V. in early stages of labor, and 25 to 75 mg after labor is established; repeat q 2 to 4 hours, p.r.n. Maximum daily dosage, 100 mg.

Pharmacodynamics
Antiemetic and antivertigo action: The central antimuscarinic actions of antihistamines probably are responsible for their antivertigo and antiemetic effects; promethazine also is believed to inhibit the medullary chemoreceptor trigger zone.

Antihistamine action: Promethazine competes with histamine for the H_1-receptor, thereby suppressing allergic rhinitis and urticaria; drug does not prevent the release of histamine.

Sedative action: CNS depressant mechanism of promethazine is unknown; phenothiazines probably cause sedation by reducing stimuli to the brainstem reticular system.

Pharmacokinetics
• *Absorption:* Promethazine is well absorbed from the GI tract. Onset begins 20 minutes after P.O., P.R., or I.M. administration and within 3 to 5 minutes after I.V. administration. Effects usually last 4 to 6 hours but may persist for 12 hours.
• *Distribution:* Drug is distributed widely throughout the body; it crosses the placenta.
• *Metabolism:* Metabolized in the liver.
• *Excretion:* Metabolites are excreted in urine and feces.

Contraindications and precautions
Contraindicated in patients with hypersensitivity to drug; in those with intestinal obstruction, prostatic hyperplasia, bladder neck obstruction, seizure disorders, coma, CNS depression, and stenosing peptic ulcerations; in newborns, premature neonates, and breast-feeding patients; and in acutely ill or dehydrated children.

Use cautiously in patients with asthma or cardiac, pulmonary, or hepatic disease.

Interactions
Do not give promethazine concomitantly with *epinephrine* because it may result in partial adrenergic blockade, producing further hypotension; or with *MAO inhibitors,* which interfere with the detoxification of antihistamines and phenothiazines and thus prolong and intensify their sedative and anticholinergic effects.

Additive CNS depression may occur when promethazine is given with *other antihistamines* or *CNS depressants,* such as *alcohol, antianxiety agents, barbiturates, sleeping aids,* and *tranquilizers.* Promethazine may block the antiparkinsonian action of *levodopa.*

Effects on diagnostic tests
Promethazine should be discontinued 4 days before diagnostic skin tests to avoid preventing, reducing, or masking test response. Promethazine may cause hyperglycemia and either false-positive or false-negative pregnancy test results. It also may interfere with blood grouping in the ABO system.

Adverse reactions
CNS: *sedation,* confusion, sleepiness, dizziness, disorientation, extrapyramidal symptoms, *drowsiness.*
CV: hypotension, hypertension.
EENT: blurred vision.
GI: nausea, vomiting, *dry mouth.*
GU: urine retention.
Hematologic: leukopenia, ***agranulocytosis, thrombocytopenia.***
Other: photosensitivity, rash.

Overdose and treatment
Clinical manifestations of overdose may include either CNS depression (sedation, reduced mental alertness, apnea, and CV collapse) or CNS stimulation (insomnia, hallucinations, tremors, or seizures). Atropine-like signs and symptoms, such as dry mouth, flushed skin, fixed and dilated pupils, and GI symptoms, are common, especially in children. Empty stomach by gastric lavage; do not induce vomiting. Treat hypotension with vasopressors, and control seizures with diazepam or phenytoin; correct acidosis and electrolyte imbalance. Urinary acidification promotes excretion of drug. *Do not give stimulants.*

☑ Special considerations
Besides those relevant to all *phenothiazines,* consider the following recommendations.
- Pronounced sedative effects may limit use in some ambulatory patients.
- The 50 mg/ml concentration is for I.M. use only; inject deep into large muscle mass. Do not administer drug S.C.; this may cause chemical irritation and necrosis. Drug may be administered I.V., in concentrations not to exceed 25 mg/ml and at a rate not to exceed 25 mg/minute; when using I.V. drip, wrap in aluminum foil to protect drug from light.
- Promethazine and meperidine (Demerol) may be mixed in the same syringe.

Patient education
- Warn patient about possible photosensitivity and ways to avoid it.
- When treating motion sickness, tell patient to take first dose 30 to 60 minutes before travel; on succeeding days, he should take dose upon arising and with evening meal.

Geriatric use
- Elderly patients are usually more sensitive to adverse effects of antihistamines and are especially likely to experience a greater degree of dizziness, sedation, hyperexcitability, dry mouth, and urine retention than younger patients. Symptoms usually respond to a decrease in medication dosage.

Pediatric use
- Use cautiously in children with respiratory dysfunction. Safety and efficacy in those younger than age 2 have not been established; do not give promethazine to infants under age 3 months.

Breast-feeding
- Antihistamines such as promethazine should not be used during breast-feeding. Many of these drugs are secreted in breast milk, exposing the infant to risks of unusual excitability, especially premature infants and other neonates, who may experience seizures.

propafenone hydrochloride
Rythmo

Pharmacologic classification: sodium channel antagonist
Therapeutic classification: antiarrhythmic
Pregnancy risk category C

How supplied
Available by prescription only
Tablets: 150 mg, 225 mg, 300 mg

Indications, route, and dosage
Suppression of documented life-threatening ventricular arrhythmias
Adults: Initially, 150 mg P.O. q 8 hours. Dosage may be increased to 225 mg q 8 hours after 3 or 4 days; if necessary, increase dosage to 300 mg q 8 hours. Maximum daily dosage, 900 mg.
✦ ***Dosage adjustment.*** Reduce dosage in patients with hepatic failure to 20% to 30% of usual dosage.

Pharmacodynamics
Antiarrhythmic action: Propafenone reduces the inward sodium current in myocardial cells and Purkinje fibers; it also has weak beta-adrenergic blocking effects. It slows the upstroke velocity of the action potential (phase 0 depolarization) and slows conduction in the AV node, His-Purkinje system, and intraventricular conduction system and prolongs the refractory period in the AV node.

Pharmacokinetics
- *Absorption:* Propafenone is well absorbed from the GI tract; absorption is not affected by food. Because of a significant first-pass effect, bioavailability is limited; however, it increases with dosage. Absolute bioavailability is 3.4% with the 150-mg tablet and 10.6% with the 300-mg tablet.
- *Distribution:* Peak plasma levels occur about 3½ hours after administration.
- *Metabolism:* Hepatic, with a significant first-pass effect. Two active metabolites have been identified: 5-hydroxypropafenone and N-depropylpropafenone. A few patients (10% of all patients and patients receiving quinidine) metabolize drug more slowly. Little (if any) 5-hydroxypropafenone is present in the plasma
- *Excretion:* Elimination half-life of drug is 2 to 10 hours in normal metabolizers (about 90% of patients); it can be as long as 10 to 32 hours in slow metabolizers.

Contraindications and precautions
Contraindicated in patients with hypersensitivity to drug and in those with severe or uncontrolled heart failure; cardiogenic shock; SA, AV, or intraventric-

ular disorders of impulse conduction in the absence of a pacemaker; bradycardia; marked hypotension; bronchospastic disorders; and electrolyte imbalance.

Use cautiously in patients with renal or hepatic failure or heart failure, and in those receiving other cardiac depressant drugs.

Interactions

Concurrent use of *quinidine* competitively inhibits one of the metabolic pathways for propafenone, thereby increasing its half-life, and is not recommended. *Cimetidine* may increase the plasma levels of propafenone. Monitor patients closely. Concurrent use of *local anesthetics* may increase the risk of CNS toxicity.

Propafenone causes a dose-related increase in plasma *digoxin* levels, ranging from 35% at 450 mg/day to 85% at 900 mg/day. Monitor plasma digoxin levels closely and adjust dosage of digoxin as necessary. In addition, propafenone may increase plasma levels of some *beta-adrenergic blocking agents*, including *metoprolol* and *propranolol*, and of *warfarin*, resulting in increased INR. Monitor appropriately.

Effects on diagnostic tests

Although drug may slow conduction and increase PR interval and QRS duration, ECG changes alone cannot be used to predict plasma concentration or drug efficacy.

Increased liver enzymes have been rarely reported (less than 0.2% of patients). Hematologic abnormalities have also been rarely reported (positive antinuclear antibody titer, decreased CBC, and altered electrolyte levels).

Adverse reactions

CNS: anxiety, ataxia, *dizziness*, drowsiness, fatigue, headache, insomnia, syncope, tremor.
CV: atrial fibrillation, bradycardia, bundle-branch block, angina, chest pain, edema, first-degree AV block, hypotension, increased QRS duration, intraventricular conduction delay, palpitations, ***heart failure, proarrhythmic events (ventricular tachycardia, PVCs, ventricular fibrillation).***
EENT: blurred vision.
GI: abdominal pain or cramps, constipation, diarrhea, dyspepsia, anorexia, flatulence, *nausea, vomiting,* dry mouth, unusual taste.
Respiratory: dyspnea.
Skin: rash.
Other: diaphoresis, joint pain.

Overdose and treatment

Symptoms usually develop within 3 hours of ingestion. Hypotension, somnolence, bradycardia, conduction disturbances, ventricular arrhythmias, and seizures have been reported. Provide supportive treatment and assist respirations as necessary. Rhythm and blood pressure may be controlled with dopamine and isoproterenol; seizures may respond to I.V. diazepam.

☑ Special considerations

- Propafenone pharmacokinetics are complex; studies have shown that a threefold increase in daily dosage (from 300 to 900 mg/day) may produce a tenfold increase in plasma levels. Dosage must be individualized for each patient.

Patient education

- Instruct patient to report signs and symptoms of infection, such as sore throat, chills, or fever.

Geriatric use

- In elderly patients and patients with substantial heart disease, increase dosage more gradually during the initial phase of treatment.

Breast-feeding

- It is not known if drug is excreted in breast milk. Because of potential for serious toxicity in the infant, consider alternative feeding methods during therapy.

propantheline bromide

Pro-Banthine, Propanthel*

Pharmacologic classification: anticholinergic
Therapeutic classification: antimuscarinic, GI antispasmodic
Pregnancy risk category C

How supplied

Available by prescription only
Tablets: 7.5 mg, 15 mg

Indications, route, and dosage

Adjunctive treatment of peptic ulcer, irritable bowel syndrome, and other GI disorders; to reduce duodenal motility during diagnostic radiologic procedures
Adults: 15 mg P.O. t.i.d. before meals, and 30 mg h.s. up to 60 mg q.i.d.
Elderly patients: 7.5 mg P.O. t.i.d. before meals.
Children: Antispasmodic dose 2 to 3 mg/kg/day P.O. divided q 4 hours to q 6 hours and h.s. Antisecretory dose 1.5 mg/kg/day P.O. divided q 6 hours to q 8 hours.

Pharmacodynamics

Anticholinergic action: Propantheline competitively blocks acetylcholine's actions at cholinergic neuroeffector sites, decreasing GI motility and inhibiting gastric acid secretion.

Pharmacokinetics

- *Absorption:* Only about 10% to 25% of propantheline is absorbed (absorption varies among patients).
- *Distribution:* Propantheline does not cross the blood-brain barrier; little else is known about its distribution.
- *Metabolism:* Drug appears to undergo considerable metabolism in the upper small intestine and liver.

• *Excretion:* Absorbed drug is excreted in urine as metabolites and unchanged drug.

Contraindications and precautions
Contraindicated in patients with angle-closure glaucoma, obstructive uropathy, obstructive disease of the GI tract, severe ulcerative colitis, myasthenia gravis, hypersensitivity to anticholinergics, paralytic ileus, intestinal atony, unstable CV status in acute hemorrhage, or toxic megacolon.

Use cautiously in patients with impaired renal or hepatic function, autonomic neuropathy, hyperthyroidism, coronary artery disease, arrhythmias, heart failure, hypertension, hiatal hernia associated with gastric reflux, or ulcerative colitis and in those living in a hot or humid environment.

Interactions
Concurrent administration of *antacids* decreases oral absorption of anticholinergics. Administer propantheline at least 1 hour before antacids. Concomitant administration of *drugs with anticholinergic effects* may cause additive toxicity.

Decreased GI absorption of many drugs has been reported after the use of anticholinergics *(ketoconazole, levodopa)*. Conversely, slowly dissolving *digoxin* tablets may yield higher serum digoxin levels when administered with anticholinergics.

Use cautiously with *oral potassium supplements* (especially *wax-matrix formulations*) because the incidence of potassium-induced GI ulcerations may be increased.

Propantheline may increase *atenolol* absorption, thereby enhancing atenolol's effects.

Effects on diagnostic tests
None reported.

Adverse reactions
CNS: headache, insomnia, drowsiness, dizziness, *confusion or excitement in elderly patients,* nervousness, weakness.
CV: *palpitations,* tachycardia.
EENT: *blurred vision,* mydriasis, increased intraocular pressure, cycloplegia, drying of salivary secretions.
GI: *dry mouth,* constipation, loss of taste, nausea, vomiting, paralytic ileus, bloated feeling.
GU: *urinary hesitancy, urine retention,* impotence.
Skin: urticaria, decreased sweating or possible anhidrosis, other dermal manifestations.
Other: allergic reactions ***(anaphylaxis).***

Note: Overdose may cause curare-like effects such as respiratory paralysis.

Overdose and treatment
Clinical manifestations of overdose include curare-like symptoms and such peripheral effects as headache; dilated, nonreactive pupils; blurred vision; flushed, hot, dry skin; dryness of mucous membranes; dysphagia; decreased or absent bowel sounds; urine retention; hyperthermia; tachycardia; hypertension; and increased respirations.

Treatment is primarily symptomatic and supportive, as needed. If the patient is alert, induce emesis (or use gastric lavage) and follow with an NaCl cathartic and activated charcoal to prevent further drug absorption. In severe cases, physostigmine may be administered to block propantheline's antimuscarinic effects. Give fluids, as needed, to treat shock. If urine retention develops, catheterization may be necessary.

☑ Special considerations
Besides those relevant to all *anticholinergics,* consider the following recommendations.
• Drug may be used with histamine-2 receptor to treat Zollinger-Ellison syndrome as an unlabeled use.
• Titrate drug until therapeutic effect is obtained or adverse effects become intolerable.

Patient education
• Instruct patient to swallow tablets whole rather than chewing or crushing them.

Geriatric use
• Administer drug cautiously to elderly patients. Lower doses are recommended.

Breast-feeding
• Drug may be excreted in breast milk, possibly resulting in infant toxicity. Do not use in breast-feeding women. Propantheline may decrease milk production.

proparacaine hydrochloride
Ak-Taine, Alcaine, Ophthaine, Ophthetic

Pharmacologic classification: local anesthetic
Therapeutic classification: local anesthetic
Pregnancy risk category C

How supplied
Available by prescription only
Ophthalmic solution: 0.5%

Indications, route, and dosage
Anesthesia for tonometry
Adults and children: Instill 1 or 2 drops of 0.5% solution in eye just before procedure.
Anesthesia for removal of foreign bodies or sutures from the eye
Adults and children: Instill 1 or 2 drops 2 to 3 minutes before procedure or q 5 to 10 minutes for one to three doses.
Anesthesia for cataract extraction, glaucoma surgery
Adults and children: Instill 1 drop of 0.5% solution in eye q 5 to 10 minutes for five to seven doses.

Pharmacodynamics
Anesthetic action: Produces anesthesia by preventing initiation and transmission of impulse at the nerve cell membrane.

Pharmacokinetics
• *Absorption:* Onset of action is within 20 seconds of instillation. Duration of action is 15 to 20 minutes.

- *Distribution:* Unknown.
- *Metabolism:* Unknown.
- *Excretion:* Unknown.

Contraindications and precautions
Contraindicated in patients with hypersensitivity to ester-type local anesthetics, para-aminobenzoic acid or its derivatives, or any other ingredient in the preparation. Use cautiously in patients with cardiac disease or hyperthyroidism.

Interactions
None reported.

Effects on diagnostic tests
None reported.

Adverse reactions
EENT: occasional conjunctival congestion or hemorrhage, transient pain, pupil dilation, cycloplegic effect, softening and erosion of the corneal epithelium, hyperallergenic corneal reaction.
Other: hypersensitivity, allergic contact dermatitis.

Note: Discontinue drug symptoms if hypersensitivity occurs.

Overdose and treatment
Clinical manifestations of overdose are extremely rare with ophthalmic administration. Clinical manifestations are CNS stimulation (such as alertness, agitation), followed by depression.

Ocular overexposure should be treated by irrigation with warm water for at least 15 minutes.

☑ Special considerations
- Proparacaine is the topical ophthalmic anesthetic of choice in diagnostic and minor surgical procedures.
- Drug is not for long-term use; may delay wound healing and may cause corneal opacification with accompanying loss of vision.
- Do not use discolored solution; store in tightly closed original container.
- Ophthaine brand packaging resembles that of Hemoccult in size and shape; check label carefully.

Patient education
- Warn patient not to rub or touch eye while cornea is anesthetized; this may cause corneal abrasion and greater discomfort when anesthesia wears off; advise use of a protective eye patch after procedures.
- Explain that corneal pain associated with an abrasion is relieved only temporarily by the application of proparacaine hydrochloride.
- Tell patient local irritation or stinging may occur several hours after instillation of proparacaine.
- Instruct patient to avoid contaminating the dropper and to replace cap after use.

Geriatric use
- Dosage may need to be reduced in elderly, debilitated patients.

propofol
Diprivan

Pharmacologic classification: phenol derivative
Therapeutic classification: anesthetic
Pregnancy risk category B

How supplied
Available by prescription only
Injection: 10 mg/ml in 20-ml ampules and 50-ml and 100-ml infusion vials

Indications, route, and dosage
Induction and maintenance of sedation in mechanically ventilated intensive care unit patients
Adults: Initially, 5 mcg/kg/minute I.V. for 5 minutes (0.3 mg/kg/hour). Subsequent increments of 5 to 10 mcg/kg/minute (0.3 to 0.6 mg/kg/hour) over 5 to 10 minutes until desired level of sedation is achieved. Maintenance rates of 5 to 50 mcg/kg/minute (0.3 to 3 mg/kg/hour) or higher may be required. Minimum amount necessary should be used. Lower dosages are required for patients over age 55.
Induction of anesthesia
Adults: Individualize doses based on patient's condition and age. Most patients classified as American Society of Anesthesiologists (ASA) Physical Status category (PS) I or II under age 55 require 2 to 2.5 mg/kg I.V. Drug is usually administered in a 40-mg bolus q 10 seconds until desired response is obtained.
Children age 3 and over: 2.5 to 3.5 mg/kg I.V. over 20 to 30 seconds.
Elderly, debilitated, or hypovolemic patients or patients in ASA PS III or IV: Half of the usual induction dose (20-mg bolus q 10 seconds).
Maintenance of anesthesia
Adults: May give as a variable rate infusion, titrated to clinical effect. Most patients may be maintained with 0.1 to 0.2 mg/kg/minute (6 to 12 mg/kg/hour).
Elderly, debilitated, or hypovolemic patients or patients in ASA PS III or IV: Half the usual maintenance dose (0.05 to 0.1 mg/kg/minute or 3 to 6 mg/kg/hour).
Children age 3 and over: 125 to 300 mcg/kg/minute I.V.

Pharmacodynamics
Anesthetic action: Propofol produces a dose-dependent CNS depression similar to benzodiazepines and barbiturates. However, it can be used to maintain anesthesia through careful titration of infusion rate.

Pharmacokinetics
- *Absorption:* Propofol must be administered I.V.
- *Distribution:* Drug has a terminal half-life of 1 to 3 days.
- *Metabolism:* Metabolized within liver and tissues. Metabolites are not fully characterized.

• *Excretion:* Drug is excreted through the kidneys. However, termination of drug action is probably caused by redistribution out of the CNS as well as metabolism.

Contraindications and precautions

Contraindicated in patients hypersensitive to propofol or components of the emulsion, including soybean oil, egg lecithin, and glycerol. Because drug is administered as an emulsion, administer with caution to patients with a disorder of lipid metabolism (such as pancreatitis, primary hyperlipoproteinemia, and diabetic hyperlipidemia). Use cautiously if patient is receiving lipids as part of a total parenteral nutrition infusion; I.V. lipid dose may need to be reduced. Use cautiously in elderly or debilitated patients and in those with circulatory disorders. Although the hemodynamic effects of drug can vary, its major effect in patients maintaining spontaneous ventilation is arterial hypotension (arterial pressure can decrease as much as 30%) with little or no change in heart rate and cardiac output. However, significant depression of cardiac output may occur in patients undergoing assisted or controlled positive pressure ventilation.

Do not use drug in obstetric anesthesia because safety to fetus has not been established. Also avoid in patients with increased intracranial pressure or impaired cerebral circulation because the reduction in systemic arterial pressure caused by drug may substantially reduce cerebral perfusion pressure.

Do not use drug in children under age 3 and in those in intensive care units or under monitored anesthesia care sedation.

Administer drug under direct medical supervision by persons familiar with airway management and the administration of I.V. anesthetics.

Interactions

Concomitant use of *inhalational anesthetics (enflurane, halothane, isoflurane)* or *supplemental anesthetics (nitrous oxide, opiates)* may be expected to enhance the anesthetic and CV actions of propofol. Use with *opiate analgesics* or *sedatives* may intensify the reduction of systolic, diastolic, mean arterial pressure, and cardiac output and may decrease induction dose requirements.

Do not mix propofol with other drugs or blood products. If it is to be diluted before infusion, use only D_5W and do not dilute to a concentration less than 2 mg/ml. After dilution, drug appears to be more stable in glass containers than plastic.

Effects on diagnostic tests

Drug may cause hyperlipidemia.

Adverse reactions

CNS: *movement,* headache, dizziness, twitching, clonic-myoclonic movement.
CV: *hypotension,* bradycardia, hypertension.
GI: nausea, vomiting, abdominal cramping.
Respiratory: ***apnea,*** cough, hiccups.
Skin: flushing.
Other: fever, discolored urine, *injection site burning or stinging, pain,* tingling or numbness, coldness.

Overdose and treatment

Specific information not available. However, treatment of overdosage may include support of respiration and administration of fluids, pressor agents, and anticholinergics as indicated.

☑ Special considerations

• Monitor patients receiving drug for signs of significant hypotension or bradycardia. Treatment may include increased rate of fluid administration, pressor agents, elevation of lower extremities, or atropine. Apnea may occur during induction and may persist for longer than 60 seconds. Ventilatory support may be required.
• Drug has no vagolytic activity. Premedication with anticholinergics, such as glycopyrrolate or atropine, may help manage potential increases in vagal tone caused by other drugs or surgical manipulations.
• When administered into a running I.V. catheter, emulsion is compatible with D_5W, lactated Ringer's injection, lactated Ringers and 5% dextrose injection, 5% dextrose and 0.45% NaCl injection, and 5% dextrose and 0.2% NaCl injection.
• Store emulsion above 40° F (4° C) and below 72° F (22° C). Refrigeration is not recommended.
• If used for sedation of mechanically ventilated patients, wake patient every 24 hours.
• Use strict aseptic technique when administering drug; discard unused drug after 12 hours.

Geriatric use

• Pharmacokinetics of propofol are not influenced by chronic hepatic cirrhosis, chronic renal failure, or gender.

Pediatric use

• Safe use in children has not been established.

Breast-feeding

• Because propofol is excreted in breast milk, it should not be used by breast-feeding women.

propoxyphene hydrochloride

Darvon, Dolene

propoxyphene napsylate

Darvon-N

Pharmacologic classification: opioid
Therapeutic classification: analgesic
Controlled substance schedule IV
Pregnancy risk category NR

How supplied

Available by prescription only
propoxyphene hydrochloride
Tablets: 65 mg
Capsules: 65 mg
propoxyphene napsylate
Tablets: 50 mg, 100 mg
Capsules: 50 mg, 100 mg
Suspension: 50 mg/5 ml

Indications, route, and dosage

Mild to moderate pain
Adults: 65 mg (hydrochloride) P.O. q 4 hours, p.r.n., or 100 mg (napsylate) P.O. q 4 hours, p.r.n.

Pharmacodynamics

Analgesic action: Propoxyphene exerts its analgesic effect via opiate agonist activity and alters the patient's response to painful stimuli, particularly mild to moderate pain.

Pharmacokinetics

- *Absorption:* After oral administration, drug is absorbed primarily in the upper small intestine. Equimolar doses of the hydrochloride and napsylate salts provide similar plasma concentrations. Onset of analgesia occurs in 20 to 60 minutes, and peak analgesic effects occur at 2 to 2½ hours.
- *Distribution:* Drug enters the CSF. It is assumed that it crosses the placental barrier; however, placental fluid and fetal blood concentrations have not been determined.
- *Metabolism:* Propoxyphene is degraded mainly in the liver; about one quarter of a dose is metabolized to norpropoxyphene, an active metabolite.
- *Excretion:* Drug is excreted in the urine. Duration of effect is 4 to 6 hours.

Contraindications and precautions

Contraindicated in patients with hypersensitivity to drug. Use cautiously in patients with impaired renal or hepatic function, emotional instability, or history of drug or alcohol abuse.

Interactions

Concomitant use with *carbamazepine* will increase carbamazepine's effects. (Monitor serum carbamazepine levels.) Propoxyphene may inhibit the metabolism of *antidepressants*, such as *doxepin*, necessitating a lower dose of antidepressant.

Reduced doses of propoxyphene are usually needed when given concomitantly with other *CNS depressants (narcotic analgesics, general anesthetics, antidepressants, antihistamines, barbiturates, benzodiazepines, muscle relaxants, phenothiazines, sedative-hypnotics)* to avoid potentiation of adverse effects (respiratory depression, sedation, hypotension).

Concurrent use with *cimetidine* may enhance respiratory and CNS depression, resulting in confusion, disorientation, apnea, or seizures. Ingestion of *alcohol* will significantly potentiate the CNS depressant effects of propoxyphene.

Use propoxyphene with caution with drugs that are highly metabolized in the liver *(digitoxin, phenytoin, rifampin)* because accumulation of either drug may occur. Withdrawal symptoms may result if used together.

Patients who become physically dependent on propoxyphene may experience acute withdrawal syndrome when given a single dose of an *antagonist.* Use with caution and monitor closely. Severe CV depression may result from concomitant use with *general anesthetics.*

Effects on diagnostic tests

Drug may cause false decrease in test for urinary steroid excretion.

Adverse reactions

CNS: *dizziness, sedation,* headache, euphoria, light-headedness, weakness, hallucinations.
GI: *nausea, vomiting,* constipation, abdominal pain.
Respiratory: ***respiratory depression.***
Other: psychological and physical dependence, abnormal liver function tests.

Overdose and treatment

The most common signs and symptoms of overdose are CNS depression, respiratory depression, and miosis (pinpoint pupils). Others include hypotension, bradycardia, hypothermia, shock, apnea, cardiopulmonary arrest, circulatory collapse, pulmonary edema, and seizures.

Drug is known to cause ECG changes (prolonged QRS complex) and nephrogenic diabetes insipidus in acute toxic doses. Death from an acute overdose is most likely to occur within the first hour. Signs and symptoms of overdose with propoxyphene combination products may include salicylism from aspirin or acetaminophen toxicity.

To treat an acute overdose, first establish adequate respiratory exchange via a patent airway and ventilation as needed; administer a narcotic antagonist (naloxone) to reverse respiratory depression. (Because the duration of action of drug is longer than naloxone, repeated dosing is necessary.) Do not give naloxone in the absence of clinically significant respiratory or CV depression. Monitor vital signs closely.

If patient presents within 2 hours of ingestion of an oral overdose, empty the stomach immediately by inducing emesis (ipecac syrup) or gastric lavage. Use caution to avoid risk of aspiration. Administer activated charcoal via nasogastric tube for further removal of drug in an oral overdose.

Provide symptomatic and supportive treatment (continued respiratory support, correction of fluid or electrolyte imbalance). Anticonvulsants may be needed; monitor laboratory parameters, vital signs, and neurologic status closely. Dialysis may be helpful in the treatment of overdose with propoxyphene combination products containing aspirin or acetaminophen.

☑ Special considerations

Besides those relevant to all *opioids,* consider the following recommendations.

- Propoxyphene may obscure the signs and symptoms of an acute abdominal condition or worsen gallbladder pain.
- Do not prescribe drug maintenance purposes in narcotic addiction.
- Propoxyphene can be considered a mild narcotic analgesic, but pain relief is equivalent to aspirin.

Patient education

- Warn patient not to exceed recommended dosage.
- Tell patient to avoid use of alcohol because it will cause additive CNS depressant effects.

- Warn patient of additive depressant effect that can occur if drug is prescribed for medical conditions requiring use of sedatives, tranquilizers, muscle relaxants, antidepressants, or other CNS-depressant drugs.
- Tell patient to take drug with food if GI upset occurs.

Geriatric use

- Lower doses are usually indicated for elderly patients because they may be more sensitive to the therapeutic and adverse effects of drug.

Breast-feeding

- Drug is excreted in breast milk; use with caution in breast-feeding women.

propranolol hydrochloride

Inderal, Inderal LA

Pharmacologic classification: beta-adrenergic blocker
Therapeutic classification: antihypertensive, antianginal, antiarrhythmic, adjunctive therapy of migraine, adjunctive therapy of MI
Pregnancy risk category C

How supplied

Available by prescription only
Tablets: 10 mg, 20 mg, 40 mg, 60 mg, 80 mg, 90 mg
Capsules (extended-release): 60 mg, 80 mg, 120 mg, 160 mg
Injection: 1 mg/ml
Solution: 4 mg/ml, 8 mg/ml, 20 mg/5 ml, 40 mg/5 ml, 80 mg/ml (concentrated)

Indications, route, and dosage

Hypertension
Adults: Initially, 80 mg P.O. daily in two to four divided doses or sustained-release form once daily. Increase at 3- to 7-day intervals to maximum daily dosage of 640 mg. Usual maintenance dosage is 160 to 480 mg daily.
◊ *Children:* 1 mg/kg P.O. daily (maximum daily dosage is 16 mg/kg).
Management of angina pectoris
Adults: 10 to 20 mg t.i.d. or q.i.d., or one 80-mg sustained-release capsule daily. Dosage may be increased at 7- to 10-day intervals. Average optimum dosage is 160 to 240 mg daily.
Supraventricular, ventricular, and atrial arrhythmias; tachyarrhythmias caused by excessive catecholamine action during anesthesia, hyperthyroidism, and pheochromocytoma
Adults: 1 to 3 mg I.V. diluted in 50 ml D_5W or 0.9% NaCl solution infused slowly, not to exceed 1 mg/minute. After 3 mg have been infused, another dose may be given in 2 minutes; subsequent doses no sooner than q 4 hours. Usual maintenance dosage is 10 to 30 mg P.O. t.i.d. or q.i.d.
Prevention of frequent, severe, uncontrollable, or disabling migraine or vascular headache
Adults: Initially, 80 mg daily in divided doses or one sustained-release capsule once daily. Usual maintenance dosage is 160 to 240 mg daily, divided t.i.d. or q.i.d.
To reduce mortality after MI
Adults: 180 to 240 mg P.O. daily in divided doses. Usually administered in three to four doses daily, beginning 5 to 21 days after infarct.
Hypertrophic subaortic stenosis
Adults: 10 to 20 mg P.O. t.i.d. or q.i.d. before meals and h.s.
Preoperative pheochromocytoma
Adults: 60 mg P.O. daily.
◊ ***Adjunctive treatment of anxiety***
Adults: 10 to 80 mg P.O. 1 hour before anxiety-provoking activity.
◊ ***Treatment of essential, familial, or senile movement tremors***
Adults: 40 mg P.O. b.i.d., as tolerated and needed.

Pharmacodynamics

Antihypertensive action: Exact mechanism of propranolol's antihypertensive effect is unknown; drug may reduce blood pressure by blocking adrenergic receptors (thus decreasing cardiac output), by decreasing sympathetic outflow from the CNS, and by suppressing renin release.

Antianginal action: Propranolol decreases myocardial oxygen consumption by blocking catecholamine access to beta-adrenergic receptors, thus relieving angina.

Antiarrhythmic action: Propranolol decreases heart rate and prevents exercise-induced increases in heart rate. It also decreases myocardial contractility, cardiac output, and SA and AV nodal conduction velocity.

Migraine prophylactic action: Migraine-preventive effect of propranolol is thought to result from inhibition of vasodilation.

MI prophylactic action: Exact mechanism by which propranolol decreases mortality after MI is unknown.

Pharmacokinetics

- *Absorption:* Drug is absorbed almost completely from the GI tract. Absorption is enhanced when given with food. Peak plasma concentrations occur 60 to 90 minutes after administration of regular-release tablets. After I.V. administration, peak concentrations occur in about 1 minute, with virtually immediate onset of action.
- *Distribution:* Distributed widely throughout the body; drug is more than 90% protein-bound.
- *Metabolism:* Hepatic metabolism is almost total; oral dosage form undergoes extensive first-pass metabolism.
- *Excretion:* Approximately 96% to 99% of a given dose of propranolol is excreted in urine as metabolites; remainder is excreted in feces as unchanged drug and metabolites. Biologic half-life is about 4 hours.

Contraindications and precautions

Contraindicated in patients with bronchial asthma, sinus bradycardia and heart block greater than first-degree, cardiogenic shock, and heart failure (unless failure is secondary to a tachyarrhythmia that can be treated with propranolol).

Use cautiously in the elderly; in patients with impaired renal or hepatic function, nonallergic bronchospastic diseases, diabetes mellitus, or thyrotoxicosis; and in those receiving other antihypertensive medications.

Interactions

Concomitant use of propranolol, a beta blocker, with *calcium channel blockers*, especially *I.V. verapamil*, may depress myocardial contractility or AV conduction. On rare occasions, the concomitant I.V. use of a beta blocker and *verapamil* has resulted in serious adverse reactions especially in patients with severe cardiomyopathy, heart failure, or recent MI. *Cimetidine* may decrease clearance of propranolol via inhibition of hepatic metabolism, and thus also enhance its beta-blocking effects. Propranolol may potentiate antihypertensive effects of other *antihypertensive agents*, especially *catecholamine-depleting agents* such as *reserpine*.

Propranolol may antagonize beta-adrenergic stimulating effects *of sympathomimetic agents* such as *isoproterenol* and of *MAO inhibitors;* use with *epinephrine* causes severe vasoconstriction.

Atropine, tricyclic antidepressants, and other drugs with *anticholinergic effects* may antagonize propranolol-induced bradycardia; *NSAIDs* may antagonize its hypotensive effects.

High doses of propranolol may potentiate neuromuscular blocking effect of *tubocurarine* and related compounds.

Concomitant use with *insulin* or *antidiabetic agents* can alter dosage requirements in previously stable diabetic patients.

Aluminum hydroxide antacid decreases GI absorption; ethanol slows the rate of absorption. *Phenytoin* and *rifampin* accelerate clearance of propranolol.

Effects on diagnostic tests

Propranolol may elevate serum transaminase, alkaline phosphatase, and LD levels and may elevate BUN levels in patients with severe heart disease.

Adverse reactions

CNS: *fatigue, lethargy,* vivid dreams, hallucinations, mental depression, light-headedness, insomnia.
CV: *bradycardia, hypotension,* ***heart failure,*** intermittent claudication, intensification of AV block.
GI: nausea, vomiting, diarrhea, abdominal cramping.
Respiratory: ***bronchospasm.***
Skin: rash.
Other: fever, ***agranulocytosis.***

Overdose and treatment

Clinical signs of overdose include severe hypotension, bradycardia, heart failure, and bronchospasm.

After acute ingestion, induce emesis or empty stomach by gastric lavage; follow with activated charcoal to reduce absorption, and administer symptomatic and supportive care. Treat bradycardia with atropine (0.25 to 1 mg); if no response, administer isoproterenol cautiously. Treat cardiac failure with cardiac glycosides and diuretics and hypotension with glucagon and/or vasopressors: epinephrine is preferred. Treat bronchospasm with isoproterenol and aminophylline.

☑ Special considerations

Besides those relevant to all *beta-adrenergic blockers*, consider the following recommendations.

- Propranolol also has been used to treat aggression and rage, stage fright, recurrent GI bleeding in cirrhotic patients, and menopausal symptoms.
- Never administer propranolol as an adjunct in treatment of pheochromocytoma unless patient has been pretreated with alpha-adrenergic blocking agents.
- Drug may mask signs of hypoglycemia.

Patient education

- Warn patient not to abruptly stop taking propranolol.
- Instruct patient on proper use, dosage, and potential adverse effects of propranolol.
- Tell patient to call before taking OTC drugs that may interact with propranolol, such as nasal decongestants or cold preparations.

Geriatric use

- Elderly patients may require lower maintenance doses of propranolol because of increased bioavailability or delayed metabolism; they also may experience enhanced adverse effects.

Pediatric use

- Safety and efficacy of propranolol in children have not been established; use only if potential benefit outweighs risk.

Breast-feeding

- Drug is distributed into breast milk; an alternative feeding method is recommended during therapy.

propylthiouracil (PTU)

Propyl-Thyracil*

Pharmacologic classification: thyroid hormone antagonist
Therapeutic classification: antihyperthyroid
Pregnancy risk category D

How supplied

Available by prescription only
Tablets: 50 mg

Indications, route, and dosage

Hyperthyroidism

Adults: 300 to 450 mg P.O. daily in divided doses. Continue until patient is euthyroid; then start maintenance dose of 100 mg daily to t.i.d.
Neonates and children: 5 to 7 mg/kg P.O. daily in divided doses q 8 hours. Alternatively, give according to age.
Children age 6 to 10: 50 to 150 mg P.O. daily in divided doses q 8 hours.

Children over age 10: 100 mg P.O. t.i.d. Continue until patient is euthyroid; then start maintenance dosage of 25 mg t.i.d. to 100 mg b.i.d.

Pharmacodynamics

Antithyroid action: Used to treat hyperthyroidism, PTU inhibits synthesis of thyroid hormone by interfering with the incorporation of iodine into thyroglobulin; it also inhibits the formation of iodothyronine. Besides blocking hormone synthesis, it also inhibits the peripheral deiodination of thyroxine to triiodothyronine (liothyronine). Clinical effects become evident only when the preformed hormone is depleted and circulating hormone levels decline.

As preparation for thyroidectomy, PTU inhibits synthesis of the thyroid hormone and causes a euthyroid state, reducing surgical problems during thyroidectomy; as a result, the mortality for a single-stage thyroidectomy is low. Iodide reduces the vascularity of the gland and makes it less friable.

Used in treating thyrotoxic crisis, PTU inhibits peripheral deiodination of thyroxine to triiodothyronine. Theoretically, it is preferred over methimazole in thyroid storm because of its peripheral action.

Pharmacokinetics

- *Absorption:* Drug is absorbed rapidly and readily (about 80%) from the GI tract. Peak levels occur at 1 to 1½ hours.
- *Distribution:* PTU appears to be concentrated in the thyroid gland. PTU readily crosses the placenta and is distributed into breast milk. It is 75% to 80% protein-bound.
- *Metabolism:* Metabolized rapidly in the liver.
- *Excretion:* About 35% of a dose is excreted in urine. Half-life is 1 to 2 hours in patients with normal renal function and 8½ hours in anuric patients.

Contraindications and precautions

Contraindicated in patients with hypersensitivity to drug and in breast-feeding patients. Use cautiously in pregnant patients.

Interactions

Concomitant use of PTU with *adrenocorticoids* or *corticotropin* may require a dosage adjustment of the steroid when thyroid status changes. Concomitant use *with bone marrow depressant agents* increases the risk of agranulocytosis; use with *hepatotoxic agents* increases the risk of hepatotoxicity; use with *iodinated glycerol, lithium,* or *potassium iodide* may potentiate hypothyroid effects.

Oral anticoagulants may be potentiated by the anti-vitamin K activity attributed to PTU.

Effects on diagnostic tests

PTU therapy alters selenomethionine levels and INR; it also alters AST, ALT, and LD levels, as well as liothyronine uptake.

Adverse reactions

CNS: headache, drowsiness, vertigo, paresthesia, neuritis, neuropathies, CNS stimulation, depression.
CV: vasculitis.
EENT: visual disturbances.
GI: diarrhea, *nausea, vomiting* (may be dose-related), epigastric distress, salivary gland enlargement, loss of taste.
GU: nephritis.
Hematologic: ***agranulocytosis, thrombocytopenia, aplastic anemia,*** leukopenia.
Hepatic: jaundice, ***hepatotoxicity.***
Skin: rash, urticaria, skin discoloration, pruritus, erythema nodosum, exfoliative dermatitis, lupus-like syndrome.
Other: arthralgia, myalgia, fever, lymphadenopathy; dose-related hypothyroidism (mental depression; hypoprothrombinemia and bleeding; cold intolerance; hard, nonpitting edema).

Overdose and treatment

Clinical manifestations of overdose include nausea, vomiting, epigastric distress, fever, headache, arthralgia, pruritus, edema, and pancytopenia.

Treatment includes withdrawal of drug in the presence of agranulocytosis, pancytopenia, hepatitis, fever, or exfoliative dermatitis. For depression of bone marrow, treatment may require antibiotics and transfusions of fresh whole blood. For hepatitis, treatment includes rest, adequate diet, and symptomatic support, including analgesics, gastric lavage, I.V. fluids, and mild sedation.

☑ Special considerations

- Best response occurs when drug is administered around the clock and given at the same time each day in respect to meals.
- A beta blocker, usually propranolol, commonly is given to manage the peripheral signs of hyperthyroidism, which are primarily cardiac-related (tachycardia).
- Observe for signs and symptoms of hypothyroidism (mental depression; cold intolerance; hard, nonpitting edema; hair loss).
- Discontinue drug if patient develops severe rash or enlarged cervical lymph nodes.

Patient education

- Warn patient to avoid using self-prescribed cough medicines; many contain iodine.
- Suggest taking drug with meals to reduce GI adverse effects.
- Instruct patient to store drug in a light-resistant container. Warn patient not to store medication in the bathroom; heat and humidity may cause drug to deteriorate.
- Tell patient to promptly report fever, sore throat, malaise, unusual bleeding, yellowing of eyes, nausea, or vomiting.
- Advise patient to have medical review of thyroid status before undergoing surgery (including dental surgery).
- Teach patient how to recognize the signs of hyperthyroidism and hypothyroidism and what to do if they occur.

Breast-feeding

- Because PTU is excreted in breast milk, avoid breast-feeding during treatment. However, if it is necessary, PTU is the preferred antithyroid agent.

protamine sulfate

Pharmacologic classification: antidote
Therapeutic classification: heparin antagonist
Pregnancy risk category C

How supplied
Available by prescription only
Injection: 10 mg/ml in 5-ml ampule, 25-ml ampule, 5-ml vial, 10-ml vial, 25-ml vial

Indications, route, and dosage
Heparin overdose
Adults and children: Dosage based on venous blood coagulation studies, usually 1 mg for each 90 units of heparin derived from lung tissue or 1 mg for each 115 units of heparin derived from intestinal mucosa. Give by slow I.V. injection over 1 to 3 minutes. Maximum dosage, 50 mg in any 10-minute period.

Pharmacodynamics
Heparin antagonism: Protamine has weak anticoagulant activity; however, when given in the presence of heparin, it forms a salt that neutralizes anticoagulant effects of both drugs.

Pharmacokinetics
- *Absorption:* Heparin-neutralizing effect of protamine occurs within 30 to 60 seconds.
- *Distribution:* Unknown.
- *Metabolism:* Fate of the heparin-protamine complex is unknown; however, it appears to be partially degraded, with release of some heparin.
- *Excretion:* Protamine's binding action lasts about 2 hours.

Contraindications and precautions
Contraindicated in patients with hypersensitivity to drug. Use cautiously after cardiac surgery.

Interactions
None significant.

Effects on diagnostic tests
Drug shortens heparin-prolonged partial thromboplastin time.

Adverse reactions
CV: fall in blood pressure, bradycardia, ***circulatory collapse.***
GI: nausea, vomiting.
Respiratory: dyspnea, ***pulmonary edema, acute pulmonary hypertension.***
Other: transitory flushing, feeling of warmth, ***anaphylaxis, anaphylactoid reactions,*** lassitude.

Overdose and treatment
Overdose may cause bleeding secondary to interaction with platelets and proteins including fibrinogen. Replace blood loss with blood transfusions or fresh frozen plasma. If hypotension occurs, consider treating with fluids, epinephrine, dobutamine, or dopamine.

☑ Special considerations
- Check for possible fish allergy.
- Do not mix protamine with any other medication.
- Reconstitute powder by adding 5 ml sterile water to 50-mg vial (25 ml to 250-mg vial); discard unused solution.
- Slow I.V. administration (over 1 to 3 minutes) decreases adverse effects; have antishock equipment available.
- Monitor patient continually, and check vital signs frequently; blood pressure may fall suddenly.
- Dosage is based on blood coagulation studies as well as on route of administration of heparin and time elapsed since heparin was administered.

Patient education
- Advise patient that he may experience transitory flushing or feel warm after I.V. administration.

pseudoephedrine hydrochloride

pseudoephedrine sulfate
Cenafed, Decofed, Efidac 24, Myfedrine, Novafed, PediaCare Infants' Decongestant Drops, Pseudogest, Sinufed Timecelles, Sudafed

Pharmacologic classification: adrenergic
Therapeutic classification: decongestant
Pregnancy risk category B

How supplied
Available without prescription
Oral solution: 7.5 mg/0.8 ml, 15 mg/5 ml, 30 mg/5 ml
Tablets: 30 mg, 60 mg
Tablets (extended-release): 120 mg, 240 mg
Capsules: 60 mg
Capsules (extended-release): 120 mg

Indications, route, and dosage
Nasal and eustachian tube decongestant
Adults and children age 12 and over: 60 mg P.O. q 4 to 6 hours. Maximum dosage, 240 mg daily, or 120 mg P.O. extended-release tablet q 12 hours.
Children age 6 to 11: Administer 30 mg P.O. q 4 to 6 hours. Maximum dosage, 120 mg daily.
Children age 2 to 5: 15 mg P.O. q 4 to 6 hours. Maximum dosage, 60 mg/day, or 4 mg/kg or 125 mg/m² P.O. divided q.i.d.

Pharmacodynamics
Decongestant action: Pseudoephedrine directly stimulates alpha-adrenergic receptors of respiratory mucosa to produce vasoconstriction; shrinkage of swollen nasal mucous membranes; reduction of tissue hyperemia, edema, and nasal congestion; an increase in airway (nasal) patency and drainage of sinus excretions; and opening of obstructed eustachian ostia. Relaxation of bronchial smooth muscle may result from direct stimulation of beta-adrenergic receptors. Mild CNS stimulation may also occur.

Pharmacokinetics
- *Absorption:* Nasal decongestion occurs within 30 minutes and persists 4 to 6 hours after oral dose of 60-mg tablet or oral solution. Effects persist 8 hours after 60-mg dose and up to 12 hours after 120-mg dose of extended-release form.
- *Distribution:* Widely distributed throughout the body.
- *Metabolism:* Drug is incompletely metabolized in liver by N-demethylation to inactive compounds.
- *Excretion:* 55% to 75% of a dose is excreted unchanged in urine; remainder is excreted as unchanged drug and metabolites.

Contraindications and precautions
Contraindicated in patients with severe hypertension or severe coronary artery disease; in those receiving MAO inhibitors; and in breast-feeding patients. Extended-release preparations are contraindicated in children under age 12.

Use cautiously in the elderly and in patients with hypertension, cardiac disease, diabetes, glaucoma, hyperthyroidism, or prostatic hyperplasia.

Interactions
Concomitant use with other *sympathomimetics* may produce additive effects and toxicity; with *methyldopa* and *reserpine,* may reduce their anithypertensive effects.

Beta blockers may increase pressor effects of pseudoephedrine. *Tricyclic antidepressants* may antagonize effects of pseudoephedrine. *MAO inhibitors* potentiate pressor effects of pseudoephedrine.

Effects on diagnostic tests
None reported.

Adverse reactions
CNS: *anxiety,* transient stimulation, tremor, dizziness, headache, insomnia, *nervousness.*
CV: ***arrhythmias,*** *palpitations,* tachycardia.
GI: anorexia, nausea, vomiting, dry mouth.
GU: difficulty urinating.
Respiratory: respiratory difficulties.
Skin: pallor.

Overdose and treatment
Clinical manifestations of overdose include exaggeration of common adverse reactions, particularly seizures, arrhythmias, and nausea and vomiting.

Treatment may include an emetic and gastric lavage within 4 hours of ingestion. Charcoal is effective only if administered within 1 hour, unless extended-release form was used. If renal function is adequate, forced diuresis will increase elimination. Do not force diuresis in severe overdose. Monitor vital signs, cardiac state, and electrolyte levels. I.V. propranolol may control cardiac toxicity; I.V. diazepam may be helpful to manage delirium or seizures; dilute potassium chloride solutions (I.V.) may be given for hypokalemia.

☑ Special considerations
Besides those relevant to all *adrenergics,* consider the following recommendations.
- Administer last daily dose several hours before bedtime to minimize insomnia.
- If symptoms persist longer than 5 days or fever is present, reevaluate therapy.
- Observe patient for complaints of headache or dizziness; monitor blood pressure.

Patient education
- If patient finds swallowing medication difficult, suggest opening capsules and mixing contents with applesauce, jelly, honey, or syrup. Mixture must be swallowed without chewing.
- Tell patient that dry mouth may occur and suggest using ice chips, sugarless gum, or hard candy for relief.
- Instruct patient to take missed dose if remembered within 1 hour. If beyond 1 hour, patient should skip and resume regular schedule and should not double dose.
- Tell patient to store drug away from heat and light (not in bathroom medicine cabinet) and safely out of reach of children.
- Caution patient that many OTC preparations may contain sympathomimetics, which can cause additive, hazardous reactions.
- Advise patient to take last dose at least 2 to 3 hours before bedtime to avoid insomnia.

Geriatric use
- Elderly patients may be sensitive to effects of drug; lower dose may be needed. Overdosage may cause hallucinations, CNS depression, seizures, and death in patients over age 60. Use extended-release preparations with caution in elderly patients.

Pediatric use
- Do not use extended-release form in patients under age 12.

Breast-feeding
- Because drug may occur in breast milk, avoid use in breast-feeding women; infant may be susceptible to drug effects.

psyllium
Cillium, Fiberall, Hydrocil Instant, Konsyl, Konsyl-D, Metamucil, Naturacil, Reguloid, Serutan, Siblin, Syllact, V-Lax

Pharmacologic classification: adsorbent
Therapeutic classification: bulk laxative
Pregnancy risk category C

How supplied
Available without a prescription
Powder: 3.3 g/tsp, 3.4 g/tsp, 3.5 g/tsp, 4.94 g/tsp
Poweder (effervescent): 3.4 g/packet, 3.7 g/packet
Granules: 2.5 g/tsp, 4.03 g/tsp
Chewable pieces: 1.7 g/piece
Wafers: 1.7 g/wafer, 3.4 g/wafer

Indications, route, and dosage
Constipation, bowel management, irritable bowel syndrome
Adults: 1 to 2 rounded tsp P.O. in full glass of liquid daily, b.i.d. or t.i.d., followed by second glass of

liquid; or 1 packet P.O. dissolved in water daily; or 2 wafers b.i.d., or t.i.d.
Children over age 6: 1 level tsp P.O. in ½ glass of liquid h.s.

Pharmacodynamics
Laxative action: Psyllium adsorbs water in the gut; it also serves as a source of indigestible fiber, increasing stool bulk and moisture, thus stimulating peristaltic activity and bowel evacuation.

Pharmacokinetics
- *Absorption:* None; onset of action varies from 12 hours to 3 days.
- *Distribution:* Psyllium is distributed locally in the gut.
- *Metabolism:* None.
- *Excretion:* Excreted in feces.

Contraindications and precautions
Contraindicated in patients with hypersensitivity to drug, abdominal pain, nausea, vomiting, or other symptoms of appendicitis and in those with intestinal obstruction or ulceration, disabling adhesions, or difficulty swallowing.

Interactions
Psyllium may adsorb oral medications, such as *anticoagulants, cardiac glycosides,* and *salicylates.*

Effects on diagnostic tests
None reported.

Adverse reactions
GI: nausea, vomiting, diarrhea (with excessive use); esophageal, gastric, small intestinal, and rectal obstruction when drug is taken in dry form; abdominal cramps, especially in severe constipation.

Overdose and treatment
No cases of overdose have been reported; probable clinical effects include abdominal pain and diarrhea.

☑ Special considerations
- Before administering drug, add at least 8 oz (240 ml) of water or juice and stir for a few seconds (improves drug's taste). Have patient drink mixture immediately to prevent it from congealing; then have him drink another glass of fluid.
- Separate administration of psyllium and oral anticoagulants, cardiac glycosides, and salicylates by at least 2 hours.
- Drug may reduce appetite if administered before meals.
- Psyllium and other bulk laxatives most closely mimic natural bowel function and do not cause laxative dependence; they are especially useful for patients with postpartum constipation or diverticular disease, for debilitated patients, for irritable bowel syndrome, and for chronic laxative users.
- Give diabetic patients a sugar- and sodium-free psyllium product.

Patient education
- Warn patient not to swallow drug in dry form; he should mix it with at least 8 oz (240 ml) of fluid, stir briefly, drink immediately (to prevent mixture from congealing), and follow it with another 8 oz of fluid.
- Explain that drug may reduce appetite if taken before meals; recommend taking drug 2 hours after meals and any other oral medication.
- Advise diabetic patients and those with restricted sodium or sugar intake to avoid psyllium products containing salt or sugar. Advise patients who must restrict phenylalanine intake to avoid psyllium products containing aspartame.

Breast-feeding
- Because drug is not absorbed, it presumably is safe for use in breast-feeding women.

pyrantel pamoate
Antiminth, Combantrin*, Pin-X, Reese's Pinworm

Pharmacologic classification: pyrimidine derivative
Therapeutic classification: anthelmintic
Pregnancy risk category C

How supplied
Available by prescription only
Oral suspension: 50 mg/ml

Indications, route, and dosage
Roundworm and pinworm infections
Adults and children over age 2: Single dose of 11 mg/kg P.O. Maximum dosage is 1 g. For pinworm infection, dosage should be repeated in 2 weeks.

Pharmacodynamics
Anthelmintic action: Pyrantel causes the release of acetylcholine and inhibits cholinesterases, paralyzing the worms. It is active against *Enterobius vermicularis, Ascaris lumbricoides, Ancylostoma duodenale, Necator americanus,* and *Trichostrongylus orientalis.*

Pharmacokinetics
- *Absorption:* Pyrantel pamoate is absorbed poorly; peak concentrations occur in 1 to 3 hours.
- *Distribution:* Little known.
- *Metabolism:* Small amount of absorbed drug is metabolized partially in the liver.
- *Excretion:* Over 50% of an oral dose is excreted unchanged in feces; about 7% is excreted in urine as unchanged drug or known metabolites.

Contraindications and precautions
Contraindicated in patients with hypersensitivity to drug and during pregnancy. Use cautiously in patients with hepatic dysfunction or severe malnutrition or anemia.

Interactions
Pyrantel pamoate antagonizes the effects of *piperazine.*

Effects on diagnostic tests
None reported.

Adverse reactions
CNS: headache, dizziness, drowsiness, insomnia.
GI: anorexia, nausea, vomiting, gastralgia, abdominal cramps, diarrhea, tenesmus.
Hepatic: transient elevation of AST.
Skin: rash.
Other: fever, weakness.

Overdose and treatment
Treatment of overdose is largely supportive, particularly of CV and respiratory functions. After recent ingestion (within 4 hours), empty stomach by induced emesis or gastric lavage. Follow with activated charcoal to decrease absorption. Osmotic cathartics may be helpful.

☑ Special considerations
- Shake suspension well before measuring, to ensure accurate dosage.
- Drug may be given with milk, fruit juice, or food.
- Laxatives, enemas, or dietary restrictions are unnecessary.
- Protect drug from light.
- Treat all family members.

Patient education
- Tell patient to wash perianal area daily and to change undergarments and bedclothes daily.
- To help prevent reinfection, instruct patient and family members in personal hygiene, including sanitary disposal of feces and hand washing and nail cleaning after defecation and before handling, preparing, or eating food.
- Explain routes of transmission and tell patient to encourage other household members and suspected contacts to be tested and, if necessary, treated.

Pediatric use
- Safety and efficacy for patients under age 2 have not been established.

Breast-feeding
- Safety has not been established.

pyrazinamide
PMS-Pyrazinamide*, Tebrazid*

Pharmacologic classification: synthetic pyrazine analogue of nicotinamide
Therapeutic classification: antituberculosis
Pregnancy risk category C

How supplied
Available by prescription only
Tablets: 500 mg

Indications, route, and dosage
Adjunctive treatment of tuberculosis (when primary and secondary antitubercular drugs cannot be used or have failed)

Adults: 15 to 30 mg/kg P.O. daily, in one or more doses. Maximum dosage is 3 g daily. Alternatively, a twice-weekly dose of 50 to 70 mg/kg (based on lean body weight) has been developed to promote patient compliance. Lower dosage is recommended in decreased renal function.

Pharmacodynamics
Antibiotic action: Mechanism of action is unknown; drug may be bactericidal or bacteriostatic depending on organism susceptibility and drug concentration at infection site. Pyrazinamide is active only against *Mycobacterium tuberculosis.* Pyrazinamide is considered adjunctive in tuberculosis therapy and is given with other drugs to prevent or delay development of resistance to pyrazinamide by *M. tuberculosis.*

Pharmacokinetics
- *Absorption:* Pyrazinamide is well absorbed after oral administration; peak serum levels occur 2 hours after an oral dose.
- *Distribution:* Distributed widely into body tissues and fluids, including lungs, liver, and CSF; drug is 50% protein-bound. It is not known if it crosses the placenta.
- *Metabolism:* Pyrazinamide is hydrolyzed in the liver; some hydrolysis occurs in stomach.
- *Excretion:* Excreted almost completely in urine by glomerular filtration. It is not known if drug is excreted in breast milk. Elimination half-life in adults is 9 to 10 hours. Half-life is prolonged in renal and hepatic impairment.

Contraindications and precautions
Contraindicated in patients with hypersensitivity to drug, severe hepatic disease, or acute gout. Use cautiously in patients with diabetes mellitus, renal failure, or gout.

Interactions
None reported.

Effects on diagnostic tests
Pyrazinamide may interfere with urine ketone determinations. Drug's systemic effects may temporarily decrease 17-ketosteroid levels; it may increase protein-bound iodine and urate levels and results of liver enzyme tests.

Adverse reactions
GI: anorexia, nausea, vomiting.
GU: dysuria.
Hematologic: sideroblastic anemia, ***thrombocytopenia.***
Skin: rash, urticaria, pruritus, photosensitivity.
Other: malaise, fever, porphyria, hyperuricemia and gout, interstitial nephritis, *arthralgia, myalgia,* ***hepatitis.***

Overdose and treatment
No specific recommendations are available. Treatment is supportive. After recent ingestion (4 hours or less), empty stomach by induced emesis or gastric lavage. Follow with activated charcoal to decrease absorption.

☑ Special considerations

- Monitor liver function, especially enzyme and bilirubin levels, and renal function, especially serum uric acid levels, before therapy and thereafter at 2- to 4-week intervals; observe patient for signs of liver damage or decreased renal function.
- In patients with diabetes mellitus, pyrazinamide therapy may hinder stabilization of serum glucose levels.
- In many cases, drug elevates serum uric acid levels. Although usually asymptomatic, a uricosuric agent, such as probenecid or allopurinol, may be necessary.
- Patients with concomitant infection HIV may require a longer course of treatment.

Patient education

- Explain disease process and rationale for long-term therapy.
- Teach signs and symptoms of hypersensitivity and other adverse reactions, and emphasize need to report them; urge patient to report unusual reactions, especially signs of gout.
- Be sure patient understands how and when to take drugs; urge patient to complete entire prescribed regimen, to comply with instructions for around-the-clock dosage, and to keep follow-up appointments.

Geriatric use

- Because elderly patients commonly have diminished renal function, which decreases drug excretion, pyrazinamide should be used with caution.

Pediatric use

- Drug is not recommended for use in children.

Breast-feeding

- Safety in breast-feeding women has not been established. Alternative feeding method is recommended during therapy.

pyridostigmine bromide

Mestinon, Regonol

Pharmacologic classification: cholinesterase inhibitor

Therapeutic classification: muscle stimulant

Pregnancy risk category NR

How supplied

Available by prescription only

Tablets: 60 mg

Tablets (sustained-release): 180 mg

Syrup: 60 mg/5 ml

Injection: 5 mg/ml in 2-ml ampule or 5-ml vial

Indications, route, and dosage

Reversal of the effects of nondepolarizing agents, curariform antagonist (postoperatively)

Adults: 10 to 20 mg I.V. preceded by atropine sulfate 0.6 to 1.2 mg I.V.

Myasthenia gravis

Adults: 60 to 180 mg P.O. b.i.d. or q.i.d. Usual dose 600 mg daily, but higher doses may be needed (up to 1,500 mg daily). Give 1/30 of oral dose I.M. or I.V. Adjust dosage based on patient response and tolerance of adverse effects. Sustained-release and rapid-release forms are often used together depending on patient's symptoms.

Children: 7 mg/kg/24 hours P.O. divided into five or six doses.

Neonates of myasthenic mothers: 0.05 to 0.15 mg/kg I.M.

Pharmacodynamics

Muscle stimulant action: Pyridostigmine blocks acetylcholine's hydrolysis by cholinesterase, resulting in acetylcholine accumulation at cholinergic synapses, increasing stimulation of cholinergic receptors at the myoneural junction.

Pharmacokinetics

- *Absorption:* Poorly absorbed from the GI tract. Onset of action usually occurs 30 to 45 minutes after oral administration, 2 to 5 minutes after I.V., and 15 minutes after I.M.
- *Distribution:* Little known; however, drug may cross the placenta, especially when administered in large doses.
- *Metabolism:* Exact metabolic fate is unknown. Duration of effect is usually 3 to 6 hours after oral dose and 2 to 3 hours after I.V. dose, depending on patient's physical and emotional status and disease severity. Pyridostigmine is hydrolyzed by cholinesterase.
- *Excretion:* Drug and metabolites are excreted in urine.

Contraindications and precautions

Contraindicated in patients with hypersensitivity to anticholinesterase agents and in those with mechanical obstruction of the intestine or urinary tract. Use cautiously in patients with bronchial asthma, bradycardia, and arrhythmias.

Interactions

Aminoglycoside antibiotics have a mild but definite nondepolarizing blocking action that may accentuate neuromuscular block.

Concomitant use with *procainamide or quinidine* may reverse pyridostigmine's cholinergic effect on muscle. *Corticosteroids* may decrease pyridostigmine's cholinergic effect; when corticosteroids are stopped, this effect may increase, possibly affecting muscle strength.

Concomitant use with *succinylcholine* may result in prolonged respiratory depression from plasma esterase inhibition, delaying succinylcholine hydrolysis. Concomitant use with *ganglionic blockers* may critically decrease blood pressure; effect is usually preceded by abdominal symptoms. *Magnesium* has a direct depressant effect on skeletal muscle and may antagonize pyridostigmine's beneficial effects.

Effects on diagnostic tests

None reported.

Adverse reactions
CNS: headache (with high doses), weakness.
CV: bradycardia, hypotension.
EENT: miosis.
GI: abdominal cramps, nausea, vomiting, diarrhea, excessive salivation, increased peristalsis.
Respiratory: ***bronchospasm, bronchoconstriction,*** increased bronchial secretions.
Skin: rash, diaphoresis.
Other: muscle cramps, muscle fasciculations, thrombophlebitis.

Overdose and treatment
Clinical effects of overdose include nausea, vomiting, diarrhea, blurred vision, miosis, excessive tearing, bronchospasm, increased bronchial secretions, hypotension, incoordination, excessive sweating, muscle weakness, cramps, fasciculations, paralysis, bradycardia or tachycardia, excessive salivation, and restlessness or agitation.

Support respiration; bronchial suctioning may be performed. Drug should be discontinued immediately. Atropine may be given to block pyridostigmine's muscarinic effects; however, it will not counter skeletal muscle paralysis. Avoid atropine overdose because it may lead to bronchial plug formation.

☑ Special considerations
- If muscle weakness is severe, determine if this effect stems from drug toxicity or exacerbation of myasthenia gravis. A test dose of edrophonium I.V. will aggravate drug-induced weakness but will temporarily relieve weakness that results from the disease.
- Avoid giving large doses to patients with decreased GI motility because toxicity may result once motility has been restored.
- Give drug with food or milk to reduce risk of muscarinic adverse effects.
- Atropine sulfate should always be readily available as an antagonist for the muscarinic effects of pyridostigmine.
- Stop all other cholinergic drugs during drug therapy to avoid additive toxicity.
- Patients may develop resistance to drug.

Patient education
- When drug is used in patient with myasthenia gravis, stress importance of taking drug exactly as ordered, on time, and in evenly spaced doses.
- If patient is taking sustained-release tablets, explain how these work and instruct him to take them at the same time each day and to swallow these tablets whole rather than crushing them.
- Teach patient how to evaluate muscle strength; instruct him to observe changes in muscle strength and to report muscle cramps, rash, or fatigue.

Breast-feeding
- It is not known if drug is excreted in breast milk. Because of the potential for serious adverse reactions in breast-fed infant, either breast-feeding or drug should be discontinued, taking into account the importance of drug to the mother.

pyridoxine hydrochloride (vitamin B_6)
Beesix, Nestrex

Pharmacologic classification: water-soluble vitamin
Therapeutic classification: nutritional supplement
Pregnancy risk category A (C if greater than RDA)

How supplied
Available by prescription only
Injection: 10-ml vial (100 mg/ml), 30-ml vial (100 mg/ml), 10-ml vial (100 mg/ml, with 1.5% benzyl alcohol), 30-ml vial (100 mg/ml, with 1.5% benzyl alcohol), 10-ml vial (100 mg/ml, with 0.5% chlorobutanol), 1-ml vial (100 mg/ml)

Available without a prescription
Tablets: 10 mg, 25 mg, 50 mg, 100 mg, 200 mg, 250 mg, 500 mg, 500 mg timed-release

Indications, route, and dosage
RDA
Neonates and infants to age 6 months: 0.3 mg daily.
Infants age 6 months to 1 year: 0.6 mg daily.
Children age 1 to 3: 1 mg daily.
Children age 4 to 6: 1.1 mg daily.
Children age 7 to 10: 1.4 mg daily.
Females age 11 to 14: 1.4 mg daily.
Females age 15 to 18: 1.5 mg daily.
Females age 19 and older: 1.6 mg daily.
Females during pregnancy: 2.2 mg daily.
Breast-feeding women: 2.1 mg daily.
Males age 11 to 14: 1.7 mg daily.
Males age 15 and over: 2 mg daily.
Dietary vitamin B_6 deficiency
Adults: 2.5 to 10 mg P.O., I.M., or I.V. daily for 3 weeks, then 2 to 5 mg daily as a supplement to a proper diet.
Children: 10 to 100 mg I.M., or I.V. to correct deficiency, then an adequate diet with supplementary RDA doses to prevent recurrence.
Seizures related to vitamin B_6 deficiency or dependency
Adults and children: 100 mg I.M. or I.V. in single dose.
Vitamin B_6–responsive anemias or dependency syndrome (inborn errors of metabolism)
Adults: 100 to 200 mg daily for 3 weeks then 2.5 to 100 mg daily until symptoms subside; then 50 mg daily for life.
Children: 100 mg I.M. or I.V., then 2 to 10 mg I.M. or 10 to 100 mg P.O. daily.
◊ ***Premenstrual syndrome***
Adults: 40 to 500 mg P.O., I.M., or I.V. daily.
◊ ***Hyperoxaluria type I***
Adults: 25 to 300 mg P.O., I.M., or I.V. daily.
Seizures secondary to isoniazid overdose
Adults and children: A dose of pyridoxine hydrochloride equal to the amount of isoniazid ingested is usually given; generally, 1 to 4 g I.V. initially and then 1 g I.M. q 30 minutes until the entire dose has been given.

Pharmacodynamics

Metabolic action: Natural vitamin B_6 contained in plant and animal foodstuffs is converted to physiologically active forms of vitamin B_6, pyridoxal phosphate, and pyridoxamine phosphate. Exogenous forms of the vitamin are metabolized in humans. Vitamin B_6 acts as a coenzyme in protein, carbohydrate, and fat metabolism and participates in the decarboxylation of amino acids in protein metabolism. Vitamin B_6 also helps convert tryptophan to niacin or serotonin as well as the deamination, transamination, and transulfuration of amino acids. Finally, vitamin B_6 is responsible for the breakdown of glycogen to glucose-1-phosphate in carbohydrate metabolism. The total adult body store consists of 16 to 27 mg of pyridoxine. The need for pyridoxine increases with the amount of protein in the diet.

Pharmacokinetics

- *Absorption:* After oral administration, pyridoxine and its substituents are absorbed readily from the GI tract. GI absorption may be diminished in patients with malabsorption syndromes or following gastric resection. Normal serum levels of pyridoxine are 30 to 80 ng/ml.
- *Distribution:* Pyridoxine is stored mainly in the liver. The total body store is approximately 16 to 27 mg. Pyridoxal and pyridoxal phosphate are the most common forms found in the blood and are highly protein-bound. Pyridoxal crosses the placenta; fetal plasma concentrations are five times greater than maternal plasma concentrations. After maternal intake of 2.5 to 5 mg/day of pyridoxine, the concentration of the vitamin in breast milk is approximately 240 ng/ml.
- *Metabolism:* Pyridoxine is degraded to 4-pyridoxic acid in the liver.
- *Excretion:* In erythrocytes, pyridoxine is converted to pyridoxal phosphate, and pyridoxamine is converted to pyridoxamine phosphate. The phosphorylated form of pyridoxine is transaminated to pyridoxal and pyridoxamine, which is phosphorylated rapidly. The conversion of pyridoxine phosphate to pyridoxal phosphate requires riboflavin. Biologic half-life is 15 to 20 days.

Contraindications and precautions

Contraindicated in patients hypersensitive to pyridoxine.

Interactions

Pyridoxine reverses the therapeutic effects of *levodopa* by accelerating peripheral metabolism. Concomitant use of pyridoxine with *phenobarbital* or *phenytoin* may cause a 50% decrease in serum concentrations of these *anticonvulsants. Cycloserine, hydralazine, isoniazid, oral contraceptives,* and *penicillamine* may increase pyridoxine requirements.

Effects on diagnostic tests

Pyridoxine therapy alters determinations for urobilinogen in the spot test using Ehrlich's reagent, resulting in a false-positive reaction.

Adverse reactions

CNS: paresthesia, unsteady gait, numbness, somnolence.

Overdose and treatment

Clinical manifestations of overdose include: ataxia and severe sensory neuropathy after chronic consumption of high daily doses of pyridoxine (2 to 6 g). These neurologic deficits usually resolve after pyridoxine is discontinued.

☑ Special considerations

- Prepare a dietary history. A single vitamin deficiency is unusual; lack of one vitamin often indicates a deficiency of others.
- Monitor protein intake; excessive protein intake increases pyridoxine requirements.
- A dosage of 25 mg/kg/day is well-tolerated. Adults consuming 200 mg/day for 33 days and on a normal dietary intake develop vitamin B_6 dependency.
- Do not mix with sodium bicarbonate in the same syringe.
- Patients receiving levodopa shouldn't take pyridoxine in dosages above 5 mg/day.
- To treat seizures and coma from isoniazid overdose, dosage equals dosage of isoniazid.
- Store in a tight, light-resistant container.
- Do not use injection solution if it contains precipitate. Slight darkening is acceptable.
- Pyridoxine is sometimes useful for treating nausea and vomiting during pregnancy.

Patient education

- Teach patient about dietary sources of vitamin B_6, such as yeast, wheat germ, liver, whole grain cereals, bananas, and legumes.

Pediatric use

- Safety and efficacy have not been established.
- The use of large doses of pyridoxine during pregnancy has been implicated in pyridoxine-dependency seizures in neonates.

Breast-feeding

- It is unknown if drug is excreted in breast milk. Use caution when administering to breast-feeding women. Pyridoxine may inhibit lactation by suppression of prolactin.

pyrimethamine

Daraprim

Pharmacologic classification: aminopyrimidine derivative (folic acid antagonist)
Therapeutic classification: antimalarial
Pregnancy risk category C

How supplied

Available by prescription only
Tablets: 25 mg

Indications, route, and dosage

Malaria prophylaxis and transmission control
Adults and children over age 10: 25 mg P.O. weekly.

Children age 4 to 10: 12.5 mg P.O. weekly.
Children under age 4: 6.25 mg P.O. weekly.

Dosage should be continued for all age-groups for at least 10 weeks after leaving endemic areas.

Acute attacks of malaria
Not recommended alone in nonimmune persons; use with faster-acting antimalarials, such as chloroquine, for 2 days to initiate transmission control and suppressive cure. For chloroquine-resistant strain, administer with sulfonamides, and possibly quinine.
Adults and children over age 15: 50 mg P.O. daily for 2 days.

Toxoplasmosis
Adults: 50 to 75 mg P.O. daily for 3 to 4 weeks, with sulfadiazine 2 to 8 g P.O. daily in three or four divided doses.
◊ *Children:* 1 mg/kg/day P.O. (maximum daily dosage, 25 mg) in divided doses q 12 hours for 3 days, then 1 mg/kg/day P.O. for 4 weeks. Administer with sulfadoxine 100 to 200 mg P.O. daily in divided doses.

◊ ***Isosporiasis***
Adults: 50 to 75 mg P.O. daily.

Pharmacodynamics
Antimalarial action: Pyrimethamine inhibits the reduction of dihydrofolate to tetrahydrofolate, thereby blocking folic acid metabolism needed for survival of susceptible organisms. This mechanism is distinct from sulfonamide-induced folic acid antagonism. Pyrimethamine is active against the asexual erythrocytic forms of susceptible plasmodia and against *Toxoplasma gondii.*

Pharmacokinetics
- *Absorption:* Well absorbed from the intestinal tract; peak serum concentrations occur within 2 hours.
- *Distribution:* Drug is distributed to the kidneys, liver, spleen, and lungs; it is approximately 80% bound to plasma proteins.
- *Metabolism:* Metabolized to several unidentified compounds.
- *Excretion:* Excreted in the urine and in breast milk; elimination half-life is 2 to 6 days. Its half-life is not changed in end-stage renal disease.

Contraindications and precautions
Contraindicated in patients with hypersensitivity to drug and in those with megaloblastic anemia caused by folic acid deficiency.

Use cautiously in patients with impaired renal or hepatic function, severe allergy or bronchial asthma, G6PD deficiency, or seizure disorders and in those following treatment with chloroquine.

Interactions
Pyrimethamine and *sulfonamides* act synergistically against some organisms because each inhibits folic acid synthesis at a different level.

Pyrimethamine and sulfadoxine combination should not be given concomitantly with other *sulfonamides* or with *co-trimoxazole* because of additive adverse effects. Concomitant use with *folic acid* and *para-aminobenzoic acid* reduces the antitoxoplasmic effects of pyrimethamine and may require higher dosage of the latter drug. Mild hepatotoxicity has been reported in patients receiving concomitant administration of *lorazepam.*

Effects on diagnostic tests
Drug therapy may decrease WBC, RBC, and platelet counts.

Adverse reactions
GI: anorexia, vomiting, atrophic glossitis.
Hematologic: ***aplastic anemia,*** megaloblastic anemia, leukopenia, ***thrombocytopenia, pancytopenia.***

Note: Adverse drug reactions related to sulfadiazine are similar to sulfonamides.

Overdose and treatment
Overdose is marked by anorexia, vomiting, and CNS stimulation, including seizures. Megaloblastic anemia, thrombocytopenia, leukopenia, glossitis, and crystalluria may also occur.

Treatment of overdose consists of gastric lavage followed by a cathartic; barbiturates may help to control seizures. Leucovorin (folinic acid) in a dosage of 5 to 15 mg/day P.O., I.M., or I.V. for 3 days or longer is used to restore decreased platelet or leukocyte counts.

☑ Special considerations
- No longer considered a first-line antimalarial agent. Other antimalarial drugs (mefloquine, chloroquine, sulfadoxine) are generally preferred.
- Give drug with meals to minimize GI distress.
- Monitor CBC, including platelet counts twice weekly.
- Monitor patient for signs of folate deficiency or bleeding when platelet count is low; if abnormalities appear, decrease dosage or discontinue drug. Leucovorin (folinic acid) may be prescribed to raise blood counts during reduced dosage or after drug is discontinued.
- Because severe reactions may occur, pyrimethamine with sulfadoxine should be given only to patients traveling to areas where chloroquine-resistant malaria is prevalent and only if traveler will be in such areas longer than 3 weeks.

Patient education
- Teach patient how to recognize signs and symptoms of adverse blood reactions and tell him to report them immediately. Teach emergency measures to control overt bleeding.
- Teach patient signs and symptoms of folate deficiency.
- Counsel patient about need to report adverse effects and to keep follow-up medical appointments.
- Tell patient to keep drug out of reach of children.

Pediatric use
- Use with caution in children.

Breast-feeding
- Pyrimethamine and sulfadoxine combination is contraindicated in breast-feeding women because it contains a sulfonamide.

quazepam
Doral

Pharmacologic classification: benzodiazepine
Therapeutic classification: hypnotic
Controlled substance schedule IV
Pregnancy risk category X

How supplied
Available by prescription only
Tablets: 7.5 mg, 15 mg

Indications, route, and dosage
Insomnia
Adults: 15 mg P.O. h.s. Some patients may respond to lower doses.

✦ ***Dosage adjustment.*** May need to decrease dosage to 7.5 mg P.O. h.s. after 2 days of therapy in some patients, especially the elderly.

Pharmacodynamics
Hypnotic action: Quazepam acts on the limbic system and thalamus of the CNS by binding to specific benzodiazepine receptors responsible for inducing sleep. Effects of drug appear to be mediated principally through the inhibitory neurotransmitter gamma-aminobutyric acid.

Pharmacokinetics
• *Absorption:* Drug is well absorbed from the GI tract. Peak plasma levels of about 15 ng/ml occur within 2 hours after administration of a 15-mg dose.
• *Distribution:* Distributed into most body tissues and fluids.
• *Metabolism:* Hepatic; two active metabolites have been identified (Z-oxoquazepam and N-desalkyl flurozepam).
• *Excretion:* 31% appears in the urine and 23% appears in the feces over a 5-day period. Only trace amounts of unchanged drug appear in the urine. Mean elimination half-life of parent drug and 2-oxoquazepam, a metabolite, is 39 hours; of N-desalkyl-2-oxoquazepam, 73 hours.

Contraindications and precautions
Contraindicated in patients with suspected or established sleep apnea or in those with hypersensitivity to drug or other benzodiazepines and during pregnancy. Use cautiously in the elderly and in patients with depression or renal, respiratory, or hepatic disease.

Interactions
Concomitant use with *alcohol, CNS depressants* including *antihistamines, opiate analgesics,* and *other benzodiazepines* causes increased CNS depression.

Effects on diagnostic tests
None reported.

Adverse reactions
CNS: *fatigue, dizziness, daytime drowsiness, headache.*
GI: dry mouth, dyspepsia.
Other: physical and psychological dependence.

Overdose and treatment
Although not specifically reported for quazepam, overdose with other benzodiazepines has produced somnolence, confusion, and coma.

General supportive measures, including gastric lavage and support of respirations, should be employed. Flumazenil, a specific benzodiazepine antagonist, may be useful. Metaraminol or levarterenol may be used to treat hypotension.

☑ Special considerations
• Prevent hoarding or self-overdosing by hospitalized patients who are depressed, suicidal, or known drug abusers.
• Avoid prolonged administration. In patients who have received prolonged therapy, avoid abrupt discontinuation of drug to prevent withdrawal symptoms.

Patient education
• Warn patient about possible excessive depressant effects that can occur with ingestion of alcohol. Additive effects can occur if alcohol is consumed on day after use of drug.
• Warn patient to avoid activities that require alertness such as driving a car until drug's effects on the CNS are known.
• Tell patient not to increase the dosage without medical approval and to call if drug is no longer effective.
• Advise female patient to call immediately if pregnancy is suspected.
• Inform patient that abrupt cessation of drug may cause withdrawal symptoms.

Geriatric use
• Elimination half-life of parent drug and metabolite 2-oxoquazepam are the same in elderly patients. However, elimination half-life of N-desalkyl-2-oxoquazepam is twice that of young adults.
• Elderly patients should have assistance with walking and other activities until the adverse CNS effects of drug are known.

Pediatric use
- Safety and efficacy in children under age 18 have not been established.

Breast-feeding
- Because drug and its metabolites are excreted in breast milk, breast-feeding is not recommended during therapy.

quetiapine fumarate
Seroquel

Pharmacologic classification: dibenzothiazepine derivative
Therapeutic classification: antipsychotic
Pregnancy risk category C

How supplied
Available by prescription only
Tablets: 25 mg, 100 mg, 200 mg

Indications, route, and dosage
Management of the manifestations of psychotic disorders
Adults: Initially, 25 mg P.O. b.i.d., with increases in increments of 25 to 50 mg b.i.d. or t.i.d. on days 2 and 3, as tolerated to a target dose range of 300 to 400 mg daily by day 4, divided into two or three doses. Further dosage adjustments, if indicated, should generally occur at intervals of not less than 2 days. Dosages can be increased or decreased by 25 to 50 mg b.i.d. Antipsychotic efficacy is generally in dosage range of 150 to 750 mg/day. Safety of doses above 800 mg/day has not been evaluated.
♦ ***Dosage adjustment.*** In elderly or debilitated patients or those who have hepatic impairment or a predisposition to hypotensive reactions, consider lower doses, slower titration, and careful monitoring during initial dosing period. No specific dosing recommendations are given.

Pharmacodynamics
Antipsychotic action: Exact mechanism of action is unknown. Quetiapine is a dibenzothiazepine derivative that is thought to exert antipsychotic activity through antagonism of dopamine type 2 (D_2) and serotonin type 2 ($5\text{-}HT_2$) receptors. Antagonism at serotonin $5\text{-}HT_{1A}$, D_1, H_1, and $alpha_1$- and $alpha_2$- adrenergic receptors may explain other effects.

Pharmacokinetics
- *Absorption:* Rapidly absorbed after oral administration. Peak plasma levels are reached in about 1.5 hours. Absorption is affected by food, with maximum concentration increasing 25% and bioavailability increasing 15%.
- *Distribution:* Apparent volume of distribution is 10 ±4 L/kg. Drug is 83% plasma-protein bound. Steady state levels are reached within 2 days.
- *Metabolism:* Extensively metabolized by the liver via sulfoxidation and oxidation. Cytochrome P-450 3A4 is the major isoenzyme involved.
- *Excretion:* Less than 1% of dose is excreted as unchanged drug. Approximately 73% is recovered in the urine and 20% in the feces. Mean terminal half-life is about 6 hours.

Contraindications and precautions
Contraindicated in patients hypersensitive to drug or its ingredients.

Use cautiously in patients with known CV or cerebrovascular disease or conditions that would predispose patient to hypotension; history of seizures or with conditions that potentially lower the seizure threshold; and in those at risk for aspiration pneumonia because of associated esophageal dysmotility and aspiration. Also use drug with caution in patients with conditions that may contribute to an elevation in core body temperature.

Interactions
Use cautiously in combination with *other centrally acting agents. Alcohol* may cause potentiated cognitive and motor effects; avoid use of alcohol during quetiapine therapy. Concomitant use of quetiapine with *antihypertensives* may potentiate the hypotensive effect of both drugs. Quetiapine may antagonize the effect of *levodopa* and *dopamine agonists.*

Phenytoin increases the mean oral clearance of quetiapine by fivefold. *Thioridazine* increases oral clearance of quetiapine by 65%. Multiple daily doses of *cimetidine* results in a 20% decrease in mean oral clearance of quetiapine. Use with caution when administering with a potent *cytochrome P-450 3A inhibitor (erythromycin, fluconazole, itraconazole, ketoconazole).* Mean oral clearance of *lorazepam* is reduced by 20% when coadministered with quetiapine.

Effects on diagnostic tests
None reported.

Adverse reactions
CNS: *dizziness, headache, somnolence,* hypertonia, dysarthria.
CV: orthostatic hypotension, tachycardia, palpitations, peripheral edema.
EENT: pharyngitis, rhinitis, ear pain.
GI: dry mouth, dyspepsia, abdominal pain, constipation, anorexia.
Hematologic: ***leukopenia.***
Metabolic: *weight gain.*
Respiratory: increased cough, dyspnea.
Skin: rash, diaphoresis.
Other: asthenia, back pain, fever, flulike syndrome.

Overdose and treatment
Usually, exaggeration of drug's pharmacologic effects is seen (drowsiness, sedation, tachycardia, hypotension). Hypokalemia and first-degree heart block may also occur.

For acute overdose, treatment includes establishing and maintaining an airway to ensure adequate oxygenation and ventilation. Consider gastric lavage and administration of activated charcoal or a laxative. Begin CV monitoring, including ECG monitoring, immediately. Avoid use of disopyramide, procainamide, quinidine, and bretylium if antiarrhythmic therapy is indicated. Administer I.V. fluids or sympathomimetic agents (not epinephrine or dopamine) to treat hypotension and circulatory collapse. For severe extrapyramidal symptoms, administer anticholinergic agents.

☑ Special considerations

- Examine the lens before therapy begins or shortly thereafter, and at 6-month intervals during chronic treatment for possible cataract formation.
- Know that a decrease in total and free T_4 may occur; this is usually not clinically significant. Although rare, some patients experience increased thyroid-stimulating hormone and require thyroid replacement.
- Know that increases in cholesterol and triglycerides have been observed.
- Be aware that asymptomatic, transient, and reversible increases in serum transaminases (primarily ALT) have been reported. These elevations usually occur within the first 3 weeks of therapy and promptly return to pretreatment levels with continued use.
- Neuroleptic malignant syndrome, a potentially fatal syndrome, has been reported with use of antipsychotic drugs. Clinical manifestations include hyperpyrexia, muscle rigidity, altered mental status, and evidence of autonomic instability. Carefully monitor at-risk patients.
- Use smallest effective dose for shortest duration to minimize risk of tardive dyskinesia.
- Closely supervise schizophrenic patient during drug therapy because of the inherent risk of a suicide attempt.

Patient education

- Advise patient of risk of orthostatic hypotension, especially during the 3 to 5-day period of initial dose titration and when dose is increased or treatment reinitiated.
- Tell patient to avoid becoming overheated or dehydrated.
- During initial dose titration period or dosage increases, warn patient to avoid activities that require mental alertness such as driving a car or operating hazardous machinery until CNS effects of drug are known.
- Advise patient to avoid alcohol while taking drug.
- Remind patient to have an initial eye examination at beginning of drug therapy and every 6 months during treatment period to monitor for cataract formation.
- Tell patient to call before taking other prescription or OTC drugs.
- Instruct female patient to call if pregnancy is being planned or is suspected. Advise her not to breast-feed during therapy.

Geriatric use

- There appears to be no difference in tolerability in patients age 65 or older. However, factors that may decrease pharmacokinetic clearance, increase pharmacodynamic response to the drug, or cause poorer tolerance or orthostasis should indicate use of a lower starting dose, slower titration, and careful monitoring during the initial dosing period.

Pediatric use

- Safety and effectiveness in children have not been established.

Breast-feeding

- Breast-feeding is not recommended during quetiapine therapy.

quinapril hydrochloride

Accupril

Pharmacologic classification: ACE inhibitor
Therapeutic classification: antihypertensive
Pregnancy risk category C (D second and third trimesters)

How supplied

Available by prescription only
Tablets: 5 mg, 10 mg, 20 mg, 40 mg

Indications, route, and dosage

Hypertension

Adults: Initially, 10 mg P.O. daily. Adjust dosage based on response at intervals of about 2 weeks. Most patients are controlled at 20, 40, or 80 mg daily, as a single dose or in two divided doses.

Hypertension in patients receiving diuretics, management of heart failure

Adults: Initially, 5 mg P.O. b.i.d. when added to diuretic and cardiac glycoside therapy. Adjust dosage weekly based on response. Usual dosage is 20 to 40 mg daily in two equally divided doses.

✦ ***Dosage adjustment.*** In adults with renal impairment, initial dose is 10 mg P.O. if creatinine clearance exceeds 60 ml/minute, 5 mg if it is 30 to 60 ml/minute, and 2.5 mg if it is 10 to 30 ml/minute. No dose recommendations are available for creatinine clearance below 10 ml/minute.

Pharmacodynamics

Antihypertensive action: Quinapril and its active metabolite, quinaprilat, inhibit ACE, preventing conversion of angiotensin I to angiotensin II, a potent vasoconstrictor. Reduced formation of angiotensin II decreases peripheral arterial resistance, decreases aldosterone secretion, reduces sodium and water retention, and lowers blood pressure. Quinapril also has antihypertensive activity in patients with low-renin hypertension.

Pharmacokinetics

- *Absorption:* At least 60% of drug is absorbed; peak plasma levels are seen within 1 hour. Rate and extent of absorption are decreased 25% to 30% when drug is administered during a high-fat meal.
- *Distribution:* About 97% of drug and active metabolite are bound to plasma proteins.

• *Metabolism:* About 38% of an oral dose is deesterified in the liver to quinaprilat, the active metabolite.
• *Excretion:* Primarily excreted in the urine; terminal elimination half-life is about 25 hours.

Contraindications and precautions

Contraindicated in patients with hypersensitivity to ACE inhibitors or history of angioedema related to treatment with an ACE inhibitor. Use cautiously in patients with impaired renal function.

Interactions

Potassium-sparing diuretics and *potassium supplements* may increase risk of hyperkalemia. Avoid concomitant use.

Increased serum *lithium* levels and lithium toxicity have been reported when used concurrently with ACE inhibitors.

Diuretics and *other antihypertensives* increase risk of excessive hypotension. Discontinue diuretic or lower dose of quinapril as needed.

Each tablet of quinapril contains magnesium carbonate and magnesium stearate. Concomitant administration of quinapril with *tetracycline* significantly impairs absorption of tetracycline.

Effects on diagnostic tests

None reported.

Adverse reactions

CNS: somnolence, vertigo, nervousness, headache, dizziness, fatigue, depression.
CV: palpitations, tachycardia, angina, hypertensive crisis, orthostatic hypotension, chest pain, *rhythm disturbances.*
GI: dry mouth, abdominal pain, constipation, vomiting, nausea, hemorrhage.
Hepatic: elevated liver enzymes.
Respiratory: *dry, persistent, tickling, nonproductive cough.*
Skin: pruritus, ***exfoliative dermatitis,*** *photosensitivity,* diaphoresis.
Other: ***angioedema,*** hyperkalemia, thrombocytopenia, agranulocytosis.

Overdose and treatment

No information is available regarding overdosage in humans. Animal studies suggest that the most likely symptom would be hypotension.

Peritoneal dialysis or hemodialysis would not be beneficial; no data are available to support use of certain physiologic maneuvers such as acidification of urine. Treat symptomatically. Infusions of 0.9% NaCl solution have been suggested to treat hypotension.

☑ Special considerations

• Blood pressure measurements should be made when drug levels are at their peak (2 to 6 hours after dosing) and at their trough (just before a dose) to verify adequate blood pressure control.
• Because concurrent administration with diuretics is associated with risk of excessive hypotension, diuretic therapy should be discontinued 2 to 3 days before start of quinapril, if possible. If quinapril alone does not adequately control blood pressure, a diuretic may be carefully added to the regimen.
• Like other ACE inhibitors, drug may cause a dry, persistent, tickling cough; it is reversible when therapy is discontinued.
• Assess renal and hepatic function before and periodically throughout therapy. Also monitor CBC and serum potassium levels.

Patient education

• Tell patient that drug should be taken on an empty stomach because meals, particularly high-fat meals, can impair absorption.
• Tell patient to immediately report signs or symptoms of angioedema: swelling of face, eyes, lips, tongue, or difficulty in breathing. If these occur, patient should stop taking drug and seek immediate medical attention.
• Warn patient that light-headedness may occur, especially during first few days of therapy. Tell him to arise slowly to minimize this effect and to report persistent or severe symptoms. If syncope (fainting) occurs, patient should stop taking drug and call immediately.
• Inadequate fluid intake, vomiting, diarrhea, and excessive perspiration can lead to light-headedness and syncope. Patient should take care in hot weather and during periods of exercise to avoid dehydration and overheating.
• Tell patient not to use sodium substitutes because they contain potassium and can cause hyperkalemia.
• Tell patient to report immediately signs or symptoms of infection (sore throat, fever) or of easy bruising or bleeding. Other ACE inhibitors have been associated with development of agranulocytosis and neutropenia.

Geriatric use

• Elderly patients have demonstrated higher peak plasma levels and slower elimination of drug; these changes were related to decreased renal function that often occurs in elderly patients. No overall differences in safety or efficacy have been seen in elderly patients.

Pediatric use

• Safety and efficacy in children have not been established.

Breast-feeding

• It is unknown if drug is excreted in breast milk. Use with caution in breast-feeding women.

quinidine gluconate
Quinaglute Dura-Tabs, Quinalan

quinidine polygalacturonate
Cardioquin

quinidine sulfate
Apo-Quinidine*, Quinidex Extentabs, Quinora

Pharmacologic classification: cinchona alkaloid
Therapeutic classification: ventricular antiarrhythmic, supraventricular antiarrhythmic, atrial antitachyarrhythmic
Pregnancy risk category C

How supplied
Available by prescription only
Tablets: 325 mg* (gluconate); 275 mg (polygalacturonate); 200 mg, 300 mg (sulfate); 300 mg (*extended-release,* sulfate); 324 mg (*extended-release,* gluconate)
Injection: 80 mg/ml (gluconate); 200 mg/ml (sulfate); 190 mg/ml (sulfate)*

Indications, route, and dosage
Atrial flutter or fibrillation
Adults: 200 mg (sulfate or equivalent base) P.O. q 2 to 3 hours for five to eight doses with subsequent daily increases until sinus rhythm is restored or toxic effects develop. Administer quinidine only after digitalization, to avoid increasing AV conduction. Maximum dosage, 3 to 4 g daily.

Maintenance dosage, 200 to 400 mg P.O. t.i.d. or q.i.d. or 600 mg P.O. q 8 to 12 hours daily (extended-release).
Paroxysmal supraventricular tachycardia
Adults: 400 to 600 mg (sulfate) P.O. q 2 to 3 hours until toxic effects develop or arrhythmia subsides.
Premature atrial contractions, PVCs, paroxysmal AV junctional rhythm or atrial or ventricular tachycardia, maintenance of cardioversion
Adults: Give test dose of 50 to 200 mg P.O. of sulfate (or 200 mg gluconate I.M.); then monitor vital signs before beginning therapy: 200 to 400 mg P.O. sulfate or equivalent base q 4 to 6 hours; or initially, 600 mg of gluconate I.M., then up to 400 mg q 2 hours, p.r.n.; or 800 mg I.V. gluconate diluted in 40 ml of D_5W, infused at 16 mg (1 ml)/minute. Alternatively, give 300 to 600 mg of sulfate (extended-release), or 324 to 648 mg of gluconate (extended-release), q 8 to 12 hours.
Children: Give test dose of 2 mg/kg, then 30 mg/kg/day P.O. or 900 mg/m^2/day P.O. in five divided doses.
◇ ***Malaria (when quinine dihydrochloride is unavailable)***
Adults: Administer quinidine gluconate by continuous I.V. infusion. Initial loading dose of 10 mg/kg diluted in 250 ml of 0.9% NaCl injection and infused over 1 to 2 hours, followed by a continuous maintenance infusion of 0.02 mg/kg/minute (20 mcg/kg/minute) for 72 hours or until parasitemia is reduced to less than 1% or oral therapy can be started; or 10 mg/kg quinidine sulfate P.O. q 8 hours for 5 to 7 days. Contact the Centers for Disease Control and Prevention (CDC) Malaria Branch for protocol instructions for recommendations at (707) 488-7760 (weekdays) or (707) 639-2888 (evenings, weekends, holidays), if using regimen.

Pharmacodynamics
Antiarrhythmic action: A class IA antiarrhythmic, quinidine depresses phase O of the action potential. It is considered a myocardial depressant because it decreases myocardial excitability and conduction velocity and may depress myocardial contractility.

It also exerts anticholinergic activity, which may modify its direct myocardial effects. In therapeutic doses, quinidine reduces conduction velocity in the atria, ventricles, and His-Purkinje system. It helps control atrial tachyarrhythmias by prolonging the effective refractory period (ERP) and increasing the action potential duration in the atria, ventricles, and His-Purkinje system. Because ERP prolongation exceeds action potential duration, tissue remains refractory even after returning to resting membrane potential (membrane-stabilizing effect). Quinidine shortens the effective refractory period of the AV node. Because quinidine's anticholinergic action also may increase AV node conductivity, a cardiac glycoside should be administered for atrial tachyarrhythmias before quinidine therapy begins, to prevent ventricular tachyarrhythmias. Quinidine also suppresses automaticity in the His-Purkinje system and ectopic pacemakers, making it useful in treating PVCs. At therapeutic doses, quinidine prolongs the QRS duration and QT interval; these ECG effects may be used as an index of drug effectiveness and toxicity.

Pharmacokinetics
- *Absorption:* Although all quinidine salts are well absorbed from the GI tract, individual serum drug levels vary greatly. Onset of action of quinidine sulfate is from 1 to 3 hours. For extended-release forms, onset of action may be slightly slower but duration of effect is longer because drug delivery system allows longer-than-usual dosing intervals. Peak plasma levels occur in 3 to 4 hours for quinidine gluconate and 6 hours for quinidine polygalacturonate.
- *Distribution:* Well distributed in all tissues except the brain. Drug concentrates in the heart, liver, kidneys, and skeletal muscle. Distribution volume decreases in patients with heart failure, possibly requiring reduction in maintenance dosage. About 80% of drug is bound to plasma proteins; the unbound (active) fraction may increase in patients with hypoalbuminemia from various causes, including hepatic insufficiency. Usual therapeutic serum levels depend on assay method and ranges as follows:

– Specific assay (enzyme multiplied immunoassay technique, high-performance liquid chromatography, fluorescence polarization): 2 to 5 mcg/ml
– Nonspecific assay (fluorometric): 4 to 8 mcg/ml.

• *Metabolism:* About 60% to 80% of drug is metabolized in the liver to two metabolites that may have some pharmacologic activity.
• *Excretion:* Approximately 10% to 30% of administered dose is excreted in the urine within 24 hours as unchanged drug. Urine acidification increases quinidine excretion; alkalinization decreases excretion. Most of an administered dose is eliminated in the urine as metabolites; elimination half-life ranges from 5 to 12 hours (usual half-life is about 6½ hours). Duration of effect ranges from 6 to 8 hours.

Contraindications and precautions

Contraindicated in patients with idiosyncrasy or hypersensitivity to quinidine or related cinchona derivatives, intraventricular conduction defects, cardiac glycoside toxicity when AV conduction is grossly impaired, abnormal rhythms due to escape mechanisms, and history of drug-induced torsades de pointes or QT syndrome.

Use cautiously in patients with impaired renal or hepatic function, asthma, muscle weakness, or infection accompanied by a fever because hypersensitivity reactions may be masked.

Interactions

Concomitant use of quinidine with *hypotensive agents* may cause additive hypotensive effects (mainly when administered I.V.); with *phenothiazines* or *reserpine,* it may cause additive cardiac depressant effects.

Concomitant use with *digitoxin* or *digoxin* may cause increased (possibly toxic) serum digoxin levels. (Some experts recommend a 50% reduction in digoxin dosage when quinidine therapy is initiated, with subsequent monitoring of serum concentrations.)

Concomitant use with *anticonvulsants* (such as *phenobarbital, phenytoin*) increases the rate of quinidine metabolism; this leads to decreased quinidine levels. Concomitant use with *coumarin* may potentiate coumarin's anticoagulant effect, possibly leading to hypoprothrombinemic hemorrhage.

When used concomitantly, *cholinergic agents* may fail to terminate paroxysmal supraventricular tachycardia because quinidine antagonizes cholinergics' vagal excitation effect on the atria and AV node. Also, quinidine's anticholinergic effects may negate the effects of such anticholinesterase drugs as *neostigmine* and *pyridostigmine*, when these agents are used to treat myasthenia gravis.

Concomitant use with *anticholinergic agents* may lead to additive anticholinergic effects. Concomitant use with *neuromuscular blocking agents* (such as *metocurine iodide, pancuronium bromide, succinylcholine chloride, tubocurarine chloride*) may potentiate anticholinergic effects. Use of quinidine should be avoided immediately after use of these agents; if quinidine must be used, respiratory support may be needed.

Concomitant use with *some antacids, thiazide diuretics,* and *sodium bicarbonate* may decrease quinidine elimination when urine pH increases, requiring close monitoring of therapy.

Concomitant use with *rifampin* may increase quinidine metabolism and decrease serum quinidine levels possibly necessitating dosage adjustment when rifampin therapy is initiated or discontinued.

Concomitant use with *nifedipine* may result in decreased quinidine levels. Concomitant use with *verapamil* may result in significant hypotension in some patients with hypertrophic cardiomyopathy.

Concomitant use with *other antiarrhythmic agents* (such as *amiodarone, lidocaine, phenytoin, procainamide, propranolol*) may cause additive or antagonistic cardiac effects and additive toxic effects. For example, concurrent use of quinidine and other antiarrhythmics that increase the QT interval may further prolong the QT interval and lead to torsades de pointes tachycardia.

Effects on diagnostic tests

None reported.

Adverse reactions

CNS: *vertigo, headache, light-headedness,* confusion, ataxia, depression, dementia.
CV: *PVCs,* ***ventricular tachycardia; atypical ventricular tachycardia (torsades de pointes);*** *hypotension;* ***complete AV block,*** *tachycardia; ECG changes (particularly widening of QRS complex, widened QT and PR intervals).*
EENT: *tinnitus,* excessive salivation, blurred vision, diplopia, photophobia.
GI: *diarrhea, nausea, vomiting,* anorexia, abdominal pain.
Hematologic: ***hemolytic anemia, thrombocytopenia, agranulocytosis.***
Hepatic: ***hepatotoxicity.***
Respiratory: acute asthmatic attack, ***respiratory arrest.***
Skin: rash, petechial hemorrhage of buccal mucosa, pruritus, urticaria, lupus erythematosus, photosensitivity.
Other: angioedema, *fever, cinchonism.*

Overdose and treatment

The most serious clinical effects of overdose include severe hypotension, ventricular arrhythmias (including torsades de pointes), and seizures. QRS complexes and QT and PR intervals may be prolonged, and ataxia, anuria, respiratory distress, irritability, and hallucinations may develop. If ingestion was recent, gastric lavage, emesis, and activated charcoal may be used to decrease absorption. Urine acidification may be used to help increase quinidine elimination.

Treatment involves general supportive measures (including CV and respiratory support) with hemodynamic and ECG monitoring. Metaraminol or norepinephrine may be used to reverse hypotension (after adequate hydration has been ensured). CNS depressants should be avoided because CNS depression may occur, possibly with seizures. Cardiac pacing may be necessary. Isoproterenol or ventricular pacing possibly may be used to treat torsades de pointes tachycardia.

I.V. infusion of 1/6 M sodium lactate solution reduces quinidine's cardiotoxic effect. Hemodialysis, although rarely warranted, also may be effective.

☑ Special considerations

- When drug is used to treat atrial tachyarrhythmias, ventricular rate may be accelerated from drug's anticholinergic effects on AV node. This can be prevented by previous treatment with a digitalis glycoside.
- Because conversion of chronic atrial fibrillation may be associated with embolism, anticoagulant should be administered for several weeks before quinidine therapy begins.
- Check apical pulse rate, blood pressure, and ECG tracing, before starting therapy.
- I.V. route should be used for acute arrhythmias only; it is generally avoided because of the potential for severe hypotension.
- Do not use discolored (brownish) quinidine solution.
- For maintenance, give only by oral or I.M. route. Dosage requirements vary. Some patients may require drug q 4 hours, others q 6 hours. Titrate dose by both clinical response and blood levels.
- When changing administration route, alter dosage to compensate for variations in quinidine base content.
- Decrease dosage in patients with heart failure and hepatic disease.
- Monitor ECG, especially when large doses of drug are being administered. Quinidine-induced cardiotoxicity is evidenced by conduction defects (50% widening of the QRS complex), ventricular tachycardia or flutter, frequent PVCs, and complete AV block. When these ECG signs appear, discontinue drug and monitor patient closely.
- Monitor liver function tests during first 4 to 8 weeks of therapy.
- Drug may increase toxicity of cardiac glycoside derivatives. Use cautiously in patients receiving cardiac glycosides. Monitor digoxin levels and expect to reduce dosage of cardiac glycoside derivatives (many clinicians recommend that digoxin dosage be reduced by 50% when quinidine therapy is initiated).
- GI adverse effects, especially diarrhea, are signs of toxicity. Check quinidine blood levels; suspect toxicity when they exceed 8 mcg/ml. GI symptoms may be minimized by giving drug with meals.
- Lidocaine may be effective in treating quinidine-induced arrhythmias because it increases AV conduction.
- Quinidine may cause hemolysis in patients with G6PD deficiency.
- Small amounts of quinidine are removed by hemodialysis; drug is not removed by peritoneal dialysis.
- Amount of quinidine in the various salt forms varies as shown below:
  - Gluconate: 62% quinidine (324 mg of gluconate, 202 mg sulfate)
  - Polygalacturonate: 60% quinidine (275 mg polygalacturonate, 166 mg sulfate)
  - Sulfate: 83% quinidine. The sulfate form is considered the standard dosage preparation.
- Quinidine gluconate is reported to be as or more active in vitro against *Plasmodium falciparum* than quinine dihydrochloride. Because the latter drug is only available through the CDC, quinidine gluconate may be useful in the treatment of severe malaria when delay of therapy may be life-threatening. The current CDC protocol involves follow-up treatment with either tetracycline or sulfadoxine and pyrimethamine.

Patient education

- Instruct patient to report rash, fever, unusual bleeding, bruising, ringing in ears, or visual disturbance.

Geriatric use

- Dosage reduction may be necessary in elderly patients. Because of highly variable metabolism, monitor serum levels.

Breast-feeding

- Because drug is excreted in breast milk, alternative feeding method is recommended during therapy with quinidine.

quinine sulfate

Pharmacologic classification: cinchona alkaloid
Therapeutic classification: antimalarial
Pregnancy risk category X

How supplied

Available by prescription
Tablets: 260 mg, 325 mg
Capsules: 200 mg, 300 mg, 325 mg

Indications, route, and dosage

Malaria (chloroquine-resistant)
Adults: 650 mg P.O. q 8 hours for 10 days, with 25 mg pyrimethamine q 12 hours for 3 days and with 500 mg sulfadiazine q.i.d. for 5 days.
Children: 25 mg/kg/day divided into three doses for 10 days.

Babesia microti *infections*
Adults: 650 mg P.O. q 6 to 8 hours for 7 days.
Children: 25 mg/kg/day divided into three doses for 7 days.

◊ ***Nocturnal recumbency leg muscle cramps***
Adults: 200 to 300 mg P.O. h.s. Discontinue if leg cramps do not occur after several days to determine if continued therapy is necessary.

Pharmacodynamics

Antimalarial action: Quinine intercalates into DNA, disrupting the parasite's replication and transcription; it also depresses its oxygen uptake and carbohydrate metabolism. It is active against the asexual erythrocytic forms of *Plasmodium falciparum, P. malariae, P. ovale,* and *P. vivax* and is used for chloroquine-resistant malaria.

Skeletal muscle relaxant effects: Quinine increases the refractory period, decreases excitability of the motor end plate, and affects calcium distribution within muscle fibers.

Pharmacokinetics

• *Absorption:* Almost completely absorbed; peak serum levels occur at 1 to 3 hours.
• *Distribution:* Distributed widely into the liver, lungs, kidneys, and spleen; CSF levels reach 2% to 5% of serum levels. Quinine is about 70% bound to plasma proteins and readily crosses the placenta.
• *Metabolism:* Quinine is metabolized in the liver.
• *Excretion:* Less than 5% of a single dose is excreted unchanged in the urine; small amounts of metabolites appear in the feces, gastric juice, bile, saliva, and breast milk. Half-life is 7 to 21 hours in healthy or convalescing persons; it is longer in patients with malaria. Urine acidification hastens elimination.

Contraindications and precautions

Contraindicated during pregnancy and in patients with known hypersensitivity to drug, G6PD deficiency, optic neuritis, tinnitus, or history of blackwater fever or thrombocytopenic purpura associated with previous quinine ingestion.

Use cautiously in patients with arrhythmias and in those taking sodium bicarbonate concomitantly.

Interactions

Quinine may increase plasma levels of *digitoxin* and *digoxin.* It may potentiate the effects of *neuromuscular blocking agents*, and it may potentiate the action of *warfarin* by depressing synthesis of vitamin K–dependent clotting factors.

Concomitant use of *aluminum-containing antacids* may delay or decrease absorption of quinine. Concomitant use of *acetazolamide* or *sodium bicarbonate* may increase concentration of quinine by decreasing urinary excretion.

Effects on diagnostic tests

Drug may decrease platelet and RBC counts. It also may cause hypoglycemia and false elevations of urinary catecholamines and may interfere with 17-hydroxycorticosteroid and 17-ketogenic steroid tests.

Adverse reactions

CNS: severe headache, apprehension, excitement, confusion, delirium, syncope, hypothermia, ***seizures*** (with toxic doses).
CV: hypotension, ***CV collapse*** (with overdosage or rapid I.V. administration), conduction disturbances.
EENT: altered color perception, photophobia, blurred vision, night blindness, amblyopia, scotoma, diplopia, mydriasis, optic atrophy, tinnitus, impaired hearing.
GI: epigastric distress, diarrhea, nausea, vomiting.
GU: renal tubular damage, anuria.
Hematologic: hemolytic anemia, ***thrombocytopenia, agranulocytosis,*** hypoprothrombinemia, thrombosis at infusion site.
Skin: rash, pruritus.
Other: asthma, flushing, fever, facial edema, dyspnea, vertigo, hypoglycemia.

Note: Discontinue drug if signs of hypersensitivity or toxicity occur.

Overdose and treatment

Signs and symptoms of overdose include tinnitus, vertigo, headache, fever, rash, CV effects, GI distress (including vomiting), blindness, apprehension, confusion, and seizures.

Treatment includes gastric lavage followed by supportive measures, which may include fluid and electrolyte replacement, artificial respiration, and stabilization of blood pressure and renal function.

Anaphylactic reactions may require epinephrine, corticosteroids, or antihistamines. Urinary acidification may increase elimination of drug but will also augment renal obstruction. Hemodialysis or hemoperfusion may be helpful. Vasodilator therapy or stellate blockage may relieve visual disturbances.

☑ Special considerations

• Administer quinine after meals to minimize gastric distress; do not crush tablets, as drug irritates gastric mucosa.
• Stop drug if signs of idiosyncrasy or toxicity occur.
• Serum concentrations of 10 mcg/ml or more may confirm toxicity as the cause of tinnitus or hearing loss.
• Quinine is no longer used for acute malarial attack by *P. vivax* or for suppression of malaria from resistant organisms.

Patient education

• Teach patient about adverse reactions and need to report these immediately—especially tinnitus and hearing impairment.
• Tell patient to avoid concomitant use of aluminum-containing antacids because these may alter drug absorption.
• Instruct patient to keep drug out of reach of children.

Geriatric use

• Use with caution in patients with conduction disturbances.

Breast-feeding

• Before drug is given to patient who is breast-feeding, evaluate the infant for possible G6PD deficiency.

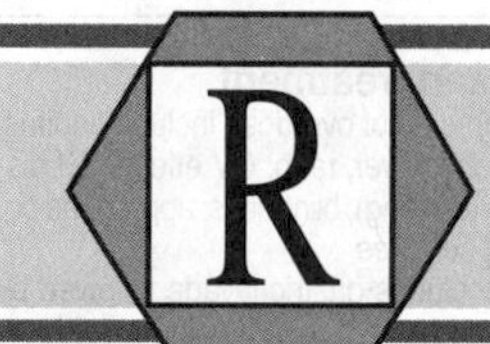

rabies immune globulin, human (RIG)

Hyperab, Imogam Rabies Immune Globulin

Pharmacologic classification: immune serum
Therapeutic classification: rabies prophylaxis
Pregnancy risk category C

How supplied
Available by prescription only
Injection: 150 IU/ml in 2-ml and 10-ml vials

Indications, route, and dosage
Rabies exposure
Adults and children: 20 IU/kg at time of first dose of rabies vaccine. Use half dose to infiltrate wound area. Give remainder I.M. (gluteal area preferred). Do not give rabies vaccine and RIG in same syringe or at same site.

Pharmacodynamics
Postexposure rabies prophylaxis: RIG provides passive immunity to rabies.

Pharmacokinetics
- *Absorption:* After slow I.M. absorption, rabies antibody appears in serum within 24 hours and peaks within 2 to 13 days.
- *Distribution:* RIG probably crosses the placenta and distributes into breast milk.
- *Metabolism:* No information available.
- *Excretion:* Serum half-life for rabies antibody titer is about 24 days.

Contraindications and precautions
Do not give repeated doses once vaccine treatment has been started. Use cautiously in patients with immunoglobulin A deficiency or history of prior systemic allergic reactions following administration of human immunoglobulin preparations and in those with known hypersensitivity to thimerosal.

Interactions
Concomitant use of drug with *corticosteroids* and *immunosuppressant agents* may interfere with the immune response to RIG. Whenever possible, avoid using these agents during the postexposure immunization period. Because antirabies serum may partially suppress the antibody response to rabies vaccine, use only the recommended dose of antirabies vaccine. Also, RIG may interfere with the immune response to *live virus vaccine*, such as *measles, mumps, and rubella.* Do not administer live virus vaccines within 3 months after administration of RIG.

Effects on diagnostic tests
None reported.

Adverse reactions
Skin: ***rash,*** pain, redness, induration at injection site.
Other: slight fever, ***anaphylaxis, angioedema, nephrotic syndrome.***

Overdose and treatment
No information available.

☑ Special considerations
- Obtain a thorough history of the animal bite, allergies, and reactions to immunizations.
- Epinephrine solution 1:1,000 should be available to treat allergic reactions.
- Repeated doses of RIG should not be given after rabies vaccine is started.
- Do not administer more than 5 ml I.M. at one injection site; divide I.M. doses exceeding 5 ml and administer them at different sites.
- Do not confuse drug with rabies vaccine, which is a suspension of attenuated or killed microorganisms used to confer active immunity. These two drugs are commonly given together prophylactically after exposure to known or suspected rabid animals.
- Because rabies can be fatal if untreated, use of RIG during pregnancy appears justified. No fetal risk from RIG use has been reported to date.
- Ask patient when he received his last tetanus immunization; a booster may be indicated.
- Patients previously immunized with a tissue culture-derived rabies vaccine and those who have confirmed adequate rabies antibody titers should receive only the vaccine.
- RIG has not been associated with an increased frequency of AIDS. The immune globulin is devoid of HIV. Immune globulin recipients do not develop antibodies to HIV.
- Store between 36° to 46° F (2° to 8° C). Do not freeze.

Patient education
- Explain that the body needs about 1 week to develop immunity to rabies after vaccine is administered. Therefore, patients receive RIG to provide antibodies in their blood for immediate protection against rabies.
- Reactions to antirabies serum may occur up to 12 days after product is administered. Encourage patient to report skin changes, difficulty breathing, or headache.

• Tell patient that local pain, swelling, and tenderness at injection site may occur. Recommend acetaminophen to alleviate these minor effects.

Breast-feeding

• Safety in breast-feeding women has not been established. RIG probably distributes into breast milk. An alternative feeding method is recommended.

rabies vaccine, adsorbed

Pharmacologic classification: vaccine
Therapeutic classification: viral vaccine
Pregnancy risk category C

How supplied

Available by prescription only
Injection: 1 ml single-dose vial

Indications, route, and dosage

Preexposure prophylaxis rabies immunization for persons in high-risk groups
Adults and children: 1 ml I.M. at 0, 7, and 21 or 28 days for a total of three injections. Patients at increased risk for rabies should be checked q 6 months and given a booster vaccination, 1 ml I.M., p.r.n. to maintain adequate serum titer.
Postexposure rabies prophylaxis
Adults and children not previously vaccinated against rabies: 20 IU/kg of human rabies immune globulin (HRIG) I.M. and five 1-ml injections of rabies vaccine, adsorbed, I.M. given one each on days 0, 3, 7, 14, and 28.
Adults and children previously vaccinated against rabies: Two 1-ml injections of rabies vaccine, adsorbed, I.M. given one each on days 0 and 3. HRIG should not be given.

Pharmacodynamics

Vaccine action: Promotes active immunity to rabies.

Pharmacokinetics

• *Absorption:* Antibodies can be detected consistently in serum samples about 2 weeks after last injection in series. People at high risk should be retested for rabies antibody titer every 6 months.
• *Distribution:* No information available.
• *Metabolism:* No information available.
• *Excretion:* No information available.

Contraindications and precautions

Contraindicated in patients who have experienced life-threatening allergic reactions to previous injections of vaccine or its components, including thimerosal. Use cautiously in patients with history of nonlife-threatening allergic reactions to previous injections of vaccine or hypersensitivity to monkey proteins.

Interactions

Antimalarial drugs, corticosteroids, and *immunosuppressive agents* decrease response to rabies vaccine. Avoid concomitant use.

Effects on diagnostic tests

None reported.

Adverse reactions

CNS: *headache, dizziness.*
Other: ***anaphylaxis,*** aching of injected muscle, *fatigue, myalgia, nausea, slight fever, abdominal pain,* serum sickness–like reactions; transient pain, erythema, swelling, itching, mild inflammatory reaction (at injection site).

Overdose and treatment

No information available.

☑ Special considerations

• Keep epinephrine 1:1,000 readily available to treat an anaphylactoid reaction.
• Administer I.M. into deltoid region in adults and older children; midanterolateral aspect of the thigh is acceptable for younger children. Vaccine should not be used by intradermal route. Do not inject vaccine in close approximation to a peripheral nerve or in adipose and subcutaneous tissue.
• Vaccine is normally a light pink color because of presence of phenol red in the suspension.
• Preexposure immunization should be delayed in patient with acute intercurrent illness.
• If patient experiences a serious adverse reaction to the vaccine, report him promptly to the manufacturer: Michigan Department of Public Health, (517) 335-8050 during working hours or (517) 335-9030 at other times.

Patient education

• Tell patient what to expect after vaccination: pain, swelling and itching at injection site, headache, stomach upset, or fever.
• Recommend acetaminophen to alleviate headache, fever, and muscle aches.

Pediatric use

• Use caution when administering vaccine to children because of limited experience with the use of the vaccine in children.

rabies vaccine, human diploid cell (HDCV)

Imovax Rabies I.D. Vaccine (inactivated whole virus), Imovax Rabies Vaccine

Pharmacologic classification: vaccine
Therapeutic classification: viral vaccine
Pregnancy risk category C

How supplied

Available by prescription only
Intramuscular injection: 2.5 IU of rabies antigen/ml, in single-dose vial with diluent
Intradermal injection: 0.25 IU rabies antigen per dose

Indications, route, and dosage

Preexposure prophylaxis immunization for persons in high-risk groups
Adults and children: Three 0.1-ml injections intra-

dermally or three 1-ml injections I.M. Give first dose on day 0 (the first day vaccination), second dose on day 7, and third dose on either day 21 or 28.
Booster: Persons exposed to rabies virus at their workplace should have antibody titers checked q 6 months. Those persons with continued risk of exposure should have antibody titers checked q 2 years. When the titers are inadequate, administer a booster dose.

Primary postexposure dosage
Five 1-ml doses I.M. on each of days 3, 7, 14, and 28 (in conjunction with rabies immune globulin on day 0). A sixth dose may be given on day 90. For patients who previously received the full HDCV vaccination regimen or who have demonstrated rabies antibody, administer two 1-ml doses I.M. Give first dose on day 0 and the second 3 days later. Rabies immune globulin should not be given.

Pharmacodynamics
Rabies prophylaxis: Vaccine promotes active immunity to rabies.

Pharmacokinetics
- *Absorption:* After intradermal injection, rabies antibodies appear in the serum within 7 to 10 days and peak at 30 to 60 days. Vaccine-induced immunity persists for about 1 year.
- *Distribution:* No information available.
- *Metabolism:* No information available.
- *Excretion:* No information available.

Contraindications and precautions
No contraindications reported for persons after exposure. An acute febrile illness contraindicates use of vaccine for persons previously exposed. Use cautiously in patients with history of hypersensitivity.

Interactions
Concomitant use of rabies vaccine with *corticosteroids* or *immunosuppressants* may interfere with the development of active immunity to rabies vaccine. Avoid its use in this situation whenever possible.

Effects on diagnostic tests
None reported.

Adverse reactions
CNS: *headache,* dizziness.
Other: abdominal pain, ***anaphylaxis,*** diarrhea, *fatigue, fever,* muscle aches, *nausea, serum sickness; pain, erythema, swelling, itching* (at injection site).

Overdose and treatment
No information available.

☑ Special considerations
- Intradermal form is for preexposure use only.
- Obtain a thorough history of allergies, especially to antibiotics, and of reactions to immunizations.
- Epinephrine solution 1:1,000 should be available to treat allergic reactions.
- I.M. injections should be made in the deltoid or upper outer quadrant of the gluteus muscle in adults and children. In infants and small children, use the midlateral aspect of the thigh.
- Reconstitute with diluent provided. Gently shake vial until vaccine is completely dissolved.
- Store vaccine at 36° to 46° F (2° to 8° C). Do not freeze.

Patient education
- Tell patient that pain, swelling, and itching at injection site as well as headache, stomach upset, or fever may occur after vaccination.
- Recommend acetaminophen to alleviate headache, fever, and muscle aches.

Breast-feeding
- It is not known if HDCV distributes into breast milk or if transmission to breast-feeding infant presents risk. Breast-feeding women should choose an alternative feeding method.

raloxifene hydrochloride
Evista

Pharmacologic classification: selective estrogen receptor modulator (SERM)
Therapeutic classification: antiosteoporotic
Pregnancy risk category X

How supplied
Available by prescription only
Tablets: 60 mg

Indications, route, and dosage
Prevention of osteoporosis in postmenopausal women
Adults: 60 mg P.O. daily.

Pharmacodynamics
Antiosteoporotic action: Decreases bone turnover and reduces bone resorption. These effects are manifested as reductions in serum and urine levels of bone turnover markers and increases in bone mineral density. Raloxifene's biologic actions are mediated through binding to estrogen receptors resulting in differential expression of multiple estrogen-regulated genes in different tissues.

Pharmacokinetics
- *Absorption:* Rapidly absorbed. Peak levels depend upon systemic interconversion and enterohepatic cycling of drug and its metabolites. Following oral administration, approximately 60% of raloxifene is absorbed. Due to extensive presystemic glucuronide conjugation, absolute bioavailability is 2%.
- *Distribution:* Apparent volume of distribution is 2,348 L/kg and does not depend on dose administered. Drug is highly bound to plasma proteins, both albumin and alpha-1 acid glycoprotein, but it does not appear to interact with the binding of warfarin, phenytoin, or tamoxifen to plasma proteins.
- *Metabolism:* Undergoes extensive first-pass metabolism to glucuronide conjugates.
- *Excretion:* Primarily excreted in the feces with less than 6% of dose eliminated as glucuronide

conjugates in the urine. Less than 0.2% of the dose is excreted unchanged in the urine.

Contraindications and precautions

Contraindicated in patients hypersensitive to drug or constituents of tablet. Also contraindicated in pregnant women or those planning pregnancy and in women with past history of or currently active venous thromboembolic events including pulmonary embolism, retinal vein thrombosis, and deep vein thrombosis. Concomitant use of raloxifene with hormone replacement therapy or systemic estrogen has not been evaluated and, therefore, is not recommended. Use with caution in patients with severe hepatic impairment.

Interactions

Cholestyramine causes a significant reduction in absorption of raloxifene; do not use these drugs concomitantly. Coadministration with *warfarin* causes a decrease in PT; monitor PT and INR. Although raloxifene is highly protein-bound, there appears to be no effect on the pharmacokinetics of *digoxin, phenytoin, tamoxifen,* or *warfarin.* However, use caution when administering raloxifene with *other highly protein-bound drugs (clofibrate, diazepam, diazoxide, ibuprofen, indomethacin, naproxen*).

Effect on diagnostic tests

Drug therapy causes increased apolipoprotein A1 and reduced serum total cholesterol, low-density lipoprotein cholesterol, fibrinogen, apolipoprotein B, and lipoprotein (a). Raloxifene modestly increases hormone-binding globulin concentrations. There were small decreases in serum total calcium, inorganic phosphate, total protein, albumin, and platelet count.

Adverse reactions

CNS: depression, insomnia, migraine.
CV: chest pain.
EENT: *sinusitis,* pharyngitis, laryngitis.
GI: nausea, dyspepsia, vomiting, flatulance, GI disorder, gastroenteritis, abdominal pain.
GU: vaginitis, urinary tract infection, cystitis, leukorrhea, endometrial disorder, *hot flashes,* vaginal bleeding, breast pain.
Metabolic: weight gain.
Musculoskeletal: *arthralgia,* myalgia, arthritis, leg cramps.
Respiratory: increased cough, pneumonia.
Skin: rash, sweating.
Other: *infection, flu syndrome,* fever, peripheral edema.

Overdose and treatment

There have been no reports of overdose in humans. No specific antidote for raloxifene overdose exists. In one study, a dose of 600 mg/day was safely tolerated.

☑ Special considerations

- The greatest risk for thromboembolic events (deep vein thrombosis, pulmonary embolism, retinal vein thrombosis) occurs during first 4 months of treatment.
- Discontinue drug at least 72 hours before prolonged immobilization.
- Endometrial proliferation has not been associated with drug use. Evaluate unexplained uterine bleeding.
- No association between breast enlargement, breast pain, or an increased risk of breast cancer has been shown. Evaluate breast abnormalities that occur during treatment.
- A decrease in total and low-density lipoprotein cholesterol by 6% and 11% respectively has been reported. No effect on high-density lipoprotein or triglycerides has been shown.
- There are no data to support drug use in premenopausal women; avoid use in this population.
- Safety and efficacy have not been evaluated in men.
- Effect on bone mineral density beyond 2 years of drug treatment is not known.

Patient education

- Tell patient to avoid long periods of restricted movement (such as during traveling) because of an increased risk of venous thromboembolic events (such as deep vein thrombosis and pulmonary embolism).
- Inform patient that hot flashes or flushing may occur and do not disappear with drug use.
- Tell patient to take supplemental calcium and vitamin D if dietary intake is inadequate.
- Encourage patient to perform weight-bearing exercises. Also advise her to stop alcohol consumption and smoking.
- Tell patient that drug may be taken without regard for food.

Geriatric use

- No age-related differences have been observed in patients age 42 to 84.

Pediatric use

- Drug has not been evaluated in children; do not use in this population.

Breast-feeding

- It is unknown if drug occurs in breast milk. Do not use in breast-feeding patients.

ramipril

Altace

Pharmacologic classification: ACE inhibitor
Therapeutic classification: antihypertensive
Pregnancy risk category C (D, second and third trimesters)

How supplied

Available by prescription only
Capsules: 1.25 mg, 2.5 mg, 5 mg, 10 mg

Indications, route, and dosage

Treatment of hypertension either alone or in combination with thiazide diuretics
Adults: Initially, 2.5 mg P.O. daily in patients not re-

ceiving concomitant diuretic therapy. Adjust dose based on blood pressure response. Usual maintenance dosage is 2.5 to 20 mg daily as a single dose or in two equal doses.

In patients receiving diuretic therapy, symptomatic hypotension may occur. To minimize this, discontinue diuretic, if possible, 2 to 3 days before starting ramipril. When this is not possible, initial dose of ramipril should be 1.25 mg.

✦ ***Dosage adjustment.*** In renally impaired patients with creatinine clearance below 40 ml/minute (serum creatinine above 2.5 mg/dl), recommended initial dose is 1.25 mg daily, titrated upward to maximum dose of 5 mg based on blood pressure response.

Heart failure post-MI

Adults: Initially, 2.5 mg P.O. b.i.d. Titrate to target dose of 5 mg P.O. b.i.d.

Pharmacodynamics

Antihypertensive action: Ramipril and its active metabolite, ramiprilat, inhibit ACE, preventing conversion of angiotensin I to angiotensin II, a potent vasoconstrictor. Reduced formation of angiotensin II decreases peripheral arterial resistance and, in turn, decreases aldosterone secretion, reduces sodium and water retention, and lowers blood pressure. Ramipril also has antihypertensive activity in patients with low-renin hypertension.

Pharmacokinetics

- *Absorption:* 50% to 60% is absorbed after oral administration with peak concentrations reached within 1 hour. Peak plasma levels of ramiprilat are achieved in 2 to 4 hours.
- *Distribution:* Ramipril is 73% serum protein-bound; ramiprilat, 56%.
- *Metabolism:* Ramipril is almost completely metabolized to ramiprilat, which has six times more ACE inhibitory effects than parent drug.
- *Excretion:* 60% is excreted in urine; 40% in feces. Less than 2% of administered dose is excreted in urine as unchanged drug.

Contraindications and precautions

Contraindicated in patients with hypersensitivity to ACE inhibitors or history of angioedema related to treatment with an ACE inhibitor. Use cautiously in patients with impaired renal function.

Interactions

Concurrent use of *potassium-sparing diuretics* or *potassium supplements* may result in hyperkalemia. Increased serum *lithium* levels and lithium toxicity have been reported with concomitant use. Excessive hypotension may result with concomitant use of *diuretics;* discontinue diuretic or lower dosage of ramipril as needed.

Effects on diagnostic tests

Transient increases in BUN and creatinine levels, decreases in hemoglobin levels and hematocrit, and elevations of liver enzymes, serum bilirubin, uric acid, and blood glucose levels have been reported.

Adverse reactions

CNS: asthenia, dizziness, fatigue, headache, malaise, light-headedness, anxiety, amnesia, ***seizures,*** depression, insomnia, nervousness, neuralgia, neuropathy, paresthesia, somnolence, tremor, vertigo.
CV: orthostatic hypotension, syncope, angina, ***arrhythmias, MI,*** chest pain, palpitations.
EENT: epistaxis, tinnitus.
GI: nausea, vomiting, abdominal pain, anorexia, constipation, diarrhea, dyspepsia, dry mouth, gastroenteritis, ***hepatitis.***
GU: impotence.
Respiratory: *dry, persistent, tickling, nonproductive cough;* dyspnea.
Skin: hypersensitivity reactions, rash, dermatitis, pruritus, photosensitivity.
Other: ***angioedema,*** edema, hyperkalemia, increased diaphoresis, weight gain, arthralgia, arthritis, myalgia, hemolytic anemia, ***pancytopenia, neutropenia, thrombocytopenia.***

Overdose and treatment

The most common manifestation is expected to be hypotension. No cases of overdose have been reported; specific management of ramipril overdose has not been established. Provide supportive care.

☑ Special considerations

- Diuretic therapy should be discontinued 2 to 3 days before starting ramipril therapy, if possible, to decrease potential for excessive hypotensive response.
- Like other ACE inhibitors, ramipril may cause a dry, persistent, tickling, nonproductive cough, which is reversible when drug is stopped.
- Assess renal and hepatic function before and periodically throughout therapy.
- Monitor serum potassium levels.

Patient education

- Tell patient to report signs or symptoms of angioedema immediately: swelling of face, eyes, lips or tongue or difficulty in breathing. Tell him to stop taking drug and seek medical attention.
- Warn patient that light-headedness can occur, especially during first few days of therapy. Tell him to change positions slowly to reduce hypotensive effect and to report these symptoms. If syncope (fainting) occurs, instruct patient to stop drug and call immediately.
- Warn patient that inadequate fluid intake, vomiting, diarrhea, or excessive perspiration can lead to light-headedness and syncope. Advise caution in excessive heat and during exercise.
- Tell patient to avoid using sodium substitutes containing potassium unless instructed.
- Tell patient to report immediately signs of infection, such as sore throat or fever.

Geriatric use

- No age-related differences in safety or efficacy have been observed.

Pediatric use

- Safety and efficacy have not been established.

Breast-feeding
• Drug should not be administered to breast-feeding women.

ranitidine
Zantac, Zantac 75, Zantac EFFERdose, Zantac Geldose

Pharmacologic classification: H_2-receptor antagonist
Therapeutic classification: antiulcer
Pregnancy risk category B

How supplied
Available by prescription only
Tablets: 150 mg, 300 mg
Tablets (effervescent): 150 mg
Capsules: 150 mg, 300 mg
Granules (effervescent): 150 mg
Injection: 25 mg/ml
Injection (premixed): 50 mg/50 ml, 50 mg/100 ml
Syrup: 15 mg/ml

Available without a prescription
Tablets: 75 mg

Indications, route, and dosage
Duodenal and gastric ulcer (short-term treatment); pathologic hypersecretory conditions such as Zollinger-Ellison syndrome
Adults: 150 mg P.O. b.i.d. or 300 mg h.s. Doses up to 6 g/day may be given in patients with Zollinger-Ellison syndrome. May give drug parenterally: 50 mg I.V. or I.M. q 6 to 8 hours.
Maintenance therapy in duodenal ulcer
Adults: 150 mg P.O. h.s.
Prophylaxis of stress ulcer
Adults: Continuous I.V. infusion of 150 mg in 250 ml compatible solution delivered at a rate of 6.25 mg/ hour using an infusion pump.
Gastroesophageal reflux disease
Adults: 150 mg P.O. b.i.d.
Erosive esophagitis
Adults: 150 mg or 10 ml (2 teaspoonfuls equivalent to 150 mg of ranitidine) P.O. q.i.d.
Self-medication for relief of occasional heartburn, acid indigestion, and sour stomach
Adults and adolescents age 12 and older: 75 mg once or twice daily; maximum dose, 150 mg in 24 hours.

Pharmacodynamics
Antiulcer action: Ranitidine competitively inhibits histamine's action at H_2-receptors in gastric parietal cells. This reduces basal and nocturnal gastric acid secretion as well as that caused by histamine, food, amino acids, insulin, and pentagastrin.

Pharmacokinetics
• *Absorption:* Approximately 50% to 60% of an oral dose is absorbed; food does not significantly affect absorption. After I.M. injection, drug is absorbed rapidly from parenteral sites.
• *Distribution:* Distributed to many body tissues and appears in CSF and breast milk. Drug is about 10% to 19% protein-bound.
• *Metabolism:* Drug is metabolized in the liver.
• *Excretion:* Drug is excreted in urine and feces. Half-life is 2 to 3 hours.

Contraindications and precautions
Contraindicated in patients hypersensitive to drug or in those with history of acute porphyria. Use cautiously in patients with impaired renal or hepatic function.

Interactions
Antacids decrease ranitidine absorption; separate drugs by at least 1 hour. Concomitant use decreases absorption of *diazepam.*

Use with *glipizide* may increase hypoglycemic effect; dosage adjustment of glipizide may be necessary. Drug may decrease renal clearance of *procainamide* and may interfere with clearance of *warfarin.*

Effects on diagnostic tests
Drug may cause false-positive results in urine protein tests using Multistix. Drug may increase serum creatinine, LD, alkaline phosphatase, AST, ALT, and total bilirubin levels. It may decrease WBC, RBC, and platelet counts.

Adverse reactions
CNS: malaise, vertigo.
EENT: blurred vision.
Hematologic: reversible leukopenia, ***pancytopenia, granulocytopenia, thrombocytopenia.***
Hepatic: elevated liver enzymes, jaundice.
Other: burning, itching (at injection site); ***anaphylaxis;*** angioneurotic edema.

Overdose and treatment
No cases of overdose have been reported. However, treatment would involve emesis or gastric lavage and supportive measures as needed. Drug is removed by hemodialysis.

☑ Special considerations
• When administering I.V. push, dilute to a total volume of 20 ml and inject over 5 minutes. No dilution necessary when administering I.M. Drug may also be administered by intermittent I.V. infusion. Dilute 50 mg ranitidine in 100 ml of D_5W and infuse over 15 to 20 minutes.
• Dosage adjustment may be required in patients with impaired renal function.
• Dialysis removes ranitidine; administer drug after treatment.

Patient education
• Instruct patient to take drug as directed, even after pain subsides, to ensure proper healing.
• If patient is taking a single daily dose, advise him to take it at bedtime.
• Instruct patient not to take OTC preparations continuously for longer than 2 weeks without medical supervision.

• Tell patient to swallow oral medication whole with water; do not chew.

Geriatric use
• Elderly patients may experience more adverse reactions because of reduced renal clearance. Debilitated patients may experience reversible confusion, agitation, depression, and hallucinations.

Breast-feeding
• Drug is excreted in breast milk; use cautiously in breast-feeding women.

ranitidine bismuth citrate
Tritec

Pharmacologic classification: H_2-receptor antagonist, antimicrobial
Therapeutic classification: antiulcer
Pregnancy risk category C

How supplied
Available by prescription only
Tablets: 400 mg

Indications, route, and dosage
In combination with clarithromycin for treatment of active duodenal ulcer associated with* Heliobacter pylori *infection
Adults: 400 mg P.O. b.i.d for 28 days in conjunction with clarithromycin 500 mg P.O. t.i.d for first 14 days.

Pharmacodynamics
Antiulcer activity: Ranitidine reduces gastric acid secretion by competitively inhibiting histamine at the H_2-receptor of the gastric parietal cells. Bismuth is a topical agent that disrupts the integrity of bacterial cell walls, prevents adhesion of *H. pylori* to gastric epithelium, decreases the development of resistance, and inhibits *H. pylori's* urease, phospholipase and proteolytic activity.

Pharmacokinetics
• *Absorption:* Drug dissociates to ranitidine and bismuth following ingestion. Mean peak plasma levels of ranitidine occur within ½ to 5 hours. Oral bioavailability of bismuth is variable, with mean peak plasma levels occurring 15 to 60 minutes after a 400-mg dose.
• *Distribution:* Volume of distribution of ranitidine is 1.7 L/kg. Ranitidine and bismuth are 15% and 98% protein-bound, respectively.
• *Metabolism:* Metabolized by the liver. It is not known if bismuth undergoes biotransformation.
• *Excretion:* Ranitidine is primarily eliminated by the kidney. Elimination half-life of ranitidine is approximately 3 hours. Bismuth is excreted primarily in feces. Bismuth also undergoes minor excretion in the bile and urine. Terminal elimination half-life of bismuth is 11 to 28 days.

Contraindications and precautions
Contraindicated in patients with known hypersensitivity to drug or its components.

Interactions
Coadministration with *high-dose antacids* (170 mEq) may decrease plasma concentration of ranitidine and bismuth. Concomitant use may decrease *diazepam* absorption; therefore, stagger administration times. Ranitidine may increase the hypoglycemic effects of *glipizide*. Ranitidine may increase plasma levels of *procainamide*. Concomitant use may increase *warfarin's* hypoprothrombinemic effects. Ranitidine bismuth citrate in combination with *clarithromycin* should not be used in patients with history of acute porphyria. This combination is not recommended in patients with creatinine clearance below 25 ml/minute.

Effects on diagnostic tests
Drug may cause false-positive results in urine protein tests using Multistix; test with sulfosalicylic acid if necessary.

Adverse reactions
CNS: headache.
GI: constipation, diarrhea.

Overdose and treatment
There has been limited experience with overdosage. If overdose occurs, take measures to remove unabsorbed drug from GI tract. Monitor symptoms and use other supportive measures if necessary.

☑ Special considerations
• Drug should not be prescribed alone for treatment of active duodenal ulcers.
• If drug therapy in combination with clarithromycin is not successful, patient is considered to have clarithromycin-resistant *H. pylori* and should not be retreated with another regimen containing clarithromycin.
• Dialysis removes ranitidine; administer drug after treatment.

Patient education
• Inform patient that drug may be administered without regard to food.
• Instruct patient to take drug as directed, even after pain has subsided.
• Tell patient that it is important to take clarithromycin with drug for specified length of time.
• Inform patient that a temporary and harmless darkening of the tongue or stool may occur with drug use.

Geriatric use
• Serum drug levels may be increased in elderly patients.

Pediatric use
• Safety and efficacy have not been established in children.

Breast-feeding
• Ranitidine has been shown to be excreted in breast milk; use caution when administering product to breast-feeding women

remifentanil hydrochloride

Ultiva

Pharmacologic classification: mu-opioid agonist
Therapeutic classification: analgesic, anesthetic
Controlled substance schedule II
Pregnancy risk category C

How supplied

Available by prescription only
Injection: 1 mg/3 ml, 2 mg/5 ml, 5 mg/10 ml vials

Indications, route, and dosage

Induction of anesthesia through intubation
Adults: 0.5 to 1 mcg/kg/minute with hypnotic or volatile agent; may load with 1 mcg/kg over 30 to 60 seconds if endotracheal intubation is to occur less than 8 minutes after start of remifentanil infusion.
Maintenance of anesthesia
Adults: 0.25 to 0.4 mcg/kg/minute, based on concurrent anesthetic modalities (nitrous oxide, isoflurane, propofol). Increase doses by 25% to 100% and decrease by 25% to 50% q 2 to 5 minutes p.r.n. If rate exceeds 1 mcg/kg/minute, consider increases in concomitant anesthetic agents. May supplement with 1 mcg/kg boluses over 30 to 60 seconds q 2 to 5 minutes p.r.n.
Continuation as analgesic immediately postoperatively
Adults: 0.1 mcg/kg/minute, followed by infusion rate of 0.025 to 0.2 mcg/kg/minute. Adjust rate by 0.025-mcg/kg/minute increments q 5 minutes. Rates over 0.2 mcg/kg/minute are associated with respiratory depression (under 8 breaths/minute).
Dosing for monitored anesthesia care
Adults: As single I.V. dose: administer 0.5 to 1 mcg/kg over 30 to 60 seconds starting 90 seconds before placement of local or regional anesthetic. Decrease dose by 50% if given with 2 mg midazolam.

As continuous I.V. infusion: 0.1 mcg/kg/minute beginning 5 minutes before local anesthetic given; after placement of local anesthetic, adjust rate to 0.05 mcg/kg/minute. Adjust rate by 0.025 mcg/kg/minute q 5 minutes p.r.n. Rates over 0.2 mcg/kg/minute are associated with respiratory depression (less than 8 breaths/minute). Decrease dose by 50% if given with 2 mg midazolam. Bolus doses administered simultaneously with continuously infusing remifentanil to spontaneously breathing patients are not recommended.

✦ ***Dosage adjustment.*** In obese patients, base starting dose on ideal body weight (IBW) (over 30% over IBW).

In patients over age 65, decrease starting dose by 50%. Cautiously titrate to effect.

Pharmacodynamics

Analgesic action: Drug binds to mu-opiate receptors throughout the CNS, resulting in analgesia.

Pharmacokinetics

• *Absorption:* After I.V. administration, drug is rapidly absorbed. Blood concentration decreases 50% in 3 to 6 minutes after a 1-minute infusion because of rapid distribution and elimination processes, which are independent of drug administration.
• *Distribution:* Initially, throughout the blood and rapidly perfused tissues; then subsequently distributes into peripheral tissues. Drug is approximately 70% bound to plasma proteins of which two-thirds is bound to alpha$_1$-acid-glycoprotein.
• *Metabolism.* Rapidly metabolized by hydrolysis via blood and tissue esterases, resulting in an inactive carboxylic acid metabolite. Drug is not metabolized by plasma cholinesterase and is not appreciably metabolized by the liver or lungs.
• *Excretion:* After hydrolysis, inactive metabolite is excreted by the kidneys with an elimination half-life of approximately 90 minutes. Clearance of active drug is high; elimination half-life of 3 to 10 minutes.

Contraindications and precautions

Do not use via epidural or intrathecal routes because of presence of glycine in preparation. Contraindicated in patients with known hypersensitivity to fentanyl analogues.

Interactions

Inhaled anesthetics, hypnotics, and *benzodiazepines* produce a synergistic effect.

Effects on diagnostic tests

None reported.

Adverse reactions

CNS: agitation, chills, dizziness, *headache.*
CV: ***bradycardia***, hypertension, *hypotension*, tachycardia.
EENT: visual disturbances.
GI: *nausea, vomiting.*
Musculoskeletal: *muscle rigidity.*
Respiratory: ***apnea***, *hypoxia, respiratory depression.*
Skin: flushing, pain at injection site, *pruritus.*
Other: chills, fever, postoperative pain, shivering, sweating, warm sensation.

Overdose and treatment

Clinical signs of overdose include apnea, chest wall rigidity, hypoxemia, hypotension, seizures, or bradycardia. If these signs occur, discontinue drug, maintain patent airway, initiate assisted or controlled ventilation with oxygen, and maintain CV function. Administer a neuromuscular blocker or opioid antagonist if decreased respiration is associated with muscle rigidity. Administer I.V. fluids and vasopressors for hypotension and glycopyrrolate or atropine for bradycardia. Naloxone may be used to manage severe respiratory depression. Use other supportive measures as needed.

☑ Special considerations

• Monitor vital signs and oxygenation continually throughout drug administration.
• Do not use as a single agent in general anesthesia.

• If respiratory depression in a spontaneously breathing patient, decrease infusion rate by 50% or temporarily discontinue infusion.
• If skeletal muscle rigidity occurs in a spontaneously breathing patient, stop or decrease rate of infusion.
• Effects of long-term (over 16 hours) use in intensive care settings is not known.
• Bradycardia has been reported and is responsive to ephedrine, atropine, and glycopyrrolate.
• If hypotension occurs, treat by decreasing administration rate, I.V. fluids, or catecholamine administration.
• Continuous infusions of drug must be administered by infusion device; I.V. bolus administration should be used only during maintenance of general anesthesia. In nonintubated patients, single doses should be administered over 30 to 60 seconds. Interruption of drug infusion results in rapid reversal (no residual opioid effects within 5 to 10 minutes of infusion discontinuation) of effects; adequate postoperative anesthesia should first be established. Upon discontinuation of drug, I.V. tubing should be cleared to avoid inadvertent administration of drug at a later time.
• Drug should not be used outside the monitored anesthesia care setting.
• Drug is incompatible with blood products; do not mix with lactated Ringer's solution or dextrose 5% lactated Ringer's solutions, but can coadminister with the above two diluents into a running I.V. administration set.
• Obtain history from patient regarding previous adverse anesthesia reactions in patient or patient's family.

Patient education
• Reassure patient that appropriate monitoring will occur during anesthesia administration.

Geriatric use
• Decrease initial doses by 50% in the elderly and titrate to desired effect.

Pediatric use
• Use in children under age 2 has not been studied.

Breast-feeding
• Because fentanyl analogues are excreted in breast milk, use with caution in breast-feeding women.

repaglinide
Prandin

Pharmacologic classification: meglitinide
Therapeutic classification: antidiabetic
Pregnancy risk category C

How supplied
Available by prescription only
Tablets: 0.5 mg, 1 mg, 2 mg

Indications, route and dosage
Adjunct to diet and exercise in lowering blood glucose in patients with type 2 diabetes mellitus whose hyperglycemia cannot be controlled by diet and exercise alone
Adults: For patients not previously treated or whose HbA_{1c} is below 8%, starting dose is 0.5 mg P.O. with each meal given 15 minutes before meal; however, time may vary from immediately before to as long as 30 minutes before meal. For patients previously treated with glucose-lowering drugs and whose HbA_{1c} is 8% or more, initial dosage is 1 to 2 mg P.O. with each meal. Recommended dosage range is 0.5 to 4 mg with meals b.i.d., t.i.d., or q.i.d. Maximum daily dosage is 16 mg.

Dosage should be determined by blood glucose response. May double dosage up to 4 mg with each meal until satisfactory blood glucose response is achieved. At least 1 week should elapse between dosage adjustments to assess response to each dose.

Metformin may be added if repaglinide monotherapy is inadequate.

Pharmacodynamics
Antidiabetic action: Stimulates the release of insulin from the beta cells in the pancreas. Repaglinide closes ATP-dependent potassium channels in the beta cell membrane which causes depolarization of the B-cell and opening of the calcium channels. The increased calcium influx induces insulin secretion; the overall effect is to lower the blood glucose level.

Pharmacokinetics
• *Absorption:* Rapidly and completely absorbed with oral administration; peak plasma levels occur within 1 hour.
• *Distribution:* Mean volume of distribution after I.V. administration is 31 L; protein binding to albumin exceeds 98%.
• *Metabolism:* Drug is completely metabolized by oxidative biotransformation and conjugation with glucuronic acid. The P-450 isoenzyme system (specifically CYP 3A4) has also been shown to be involved in N-dealkylation of repaglinide. All metabolites are inactive and do not contribute to the blood glucose-lowering effect.
• *Excretion:* Approximately 90% of dose occurs in the feces as metabolites. Approximately 8% of a dose is recovered in the urine as metabolites and less than 0.1% as parent drug. Half-life is about 1 hour.

Contraindications and precautions
Contraindicated in patients with hypersensitivity to drug or its inactive ingredients and in those with insulin-dependent diabetes mellitus or ketoacidosis. Use cautiously in patients with hepatic insufficiency in whom reduced metabolism could cause elevated blood levels of repaglinide and hypoglycemia.

Interactions
Repaglinide metabolism may be inhibited by *erythromycin, ketoconazole, miconazole,* and similar *inhibitors of the P-450 cytochrome system 3A4. In-*

ducers of the P-450 cytochrome system 3A4, such as *barbiturates, carbamazepine, rifampin,* and *troglitazone* may increase the metabolism of repaglinide. *NSAIDs and others drugs that are highly protein bound, beta-adrenergic blocking agents, chloramphenicol, coumarins, MAO inhibitors, probenecid, salicylates,* and *sulfonamides* may potentiate the hypoglycemic action of repaglinide. *Thiazides and other diuretics, calcium channel blockers, corticosteroids, estrogens, isoniazid, nicotinic acid, oral contraceptives, phenothiazines, phenytoin, sympathomimetics,* and *thyroid products* may produce hyperglycemia resulting in a loss of glycemic control.

Effects on diagnostic tests
None reported.

Adverse reactions
CNS: *headache.*
CV: chest pain, angina.
EENT: tooth disorder, rhinitis.
GI: nausea, diarrhea, constipation, vomiting, dyspepsia.
GU: urinary tract infection.
Metabolic: HYPOGLYCEMIA.
Musculoskeletal: arthralgia, back pain.
Respiratory: bronchitis, sinusitis, *upper respiratory infection.*

Overdose and treatment
Overdosage is associated with few adverse effects other than those associated with the intended effect of lowering blood glucose. Treat hypoglycemic symptoms without loss of consciousness or neurologic findings aggressively with oral glucose and dosage or meal pattern adjustments. Monitor patient closely for minimum of 24 to 48 hours because hypoglycemia may reoccur after apparent clinical recovery. Treat severe hypoglycemic reactions with coma, seizure, or other neurologic impairment immediately with I.V. dextrose 50% solution followed by a continuous infusion of glucose 10% solution. Careful blood sugar monitoring must occur.

☑ Special considerations
- Know that administration of other oral antidiabetic agents has been reported to be associated with increased CV mortality compared with diet treatment alone. Although not specifically evaluated for repaglinide, this warning may also apply.
- Loss of glycemic control can occur during stress, such as fever, trauma, infection, or surgery. If this occurs, discontinue drug and administer insulin.
- Be aware that hypoglycemia may be difficult to recognize in the elderly and in patients taking beta-adrenergic blocking drugs.
- Use caution when increasing drug dosage in patients with impaired renal function or renal failure requiring dialysis.
- Monitor patient's blood glucose periodically to determine minimum effective dose.

Patient education
- Instruct patient on importance of diet and exercise in combination with drug therapy.
- Discuss symptoms of hypoglycemia with patient and family.
- Monitor long-term efficacy by measuring HbA_{1c} levels every 3 months.
- Tell patient to take drug before meals, usually 15 minutes before start of meal; however, time can vary from immediately preceding meal to up to 30 minutes before meal.
- Tell patient that if a meal is skipped or an extra meal added, he should skip the dose or add an extra dose of drug for that meal.

Geriatric use
- In clinical studies there was no increase in the frequency or severity of hypoglycemia in older patients.

Pediatric use
- No studies have been performed in pediatric patients to determine safety and efficacy.

Breast-feeding
- Although it is not known if drug occurs in breast milk, animal studies have indicated excretion similar to other glucose-lowering agents. Because the potential for hypoglycemia in a breast-fed infant exists, a decision should be made as to whether to discontinue drug or breast-feeding.

respiratory syncytial virus immune globulin intravenous, human (RSV-IGIV)
RespiGam

Pharmacologic classification: immunoglobulin G
Therapeutic classification: immune serum
Pregnancy risk category C

How supplied
Available by prescription only
Injection: 2,500 mg (± 500 mg) in a 50-ml single-use vial

Indications, route, and dosage
Prevention of serious lower respiratory tract infection caused by RSV in children with bronchopulmonary dysplasia (BPD) or history of premature birth (35 weeks' gestation or less)
Premature neonates and infants under age 2: 1.5 ml/kg/hour I.V. for 15 minutes. If clinical condition allows, increase rate to 3 ml/kg/hour for 15 minutes, and then again to 6 ml/kg/hour until end of infusion once monthly. Maximum recommended total dosage per monthly infusion, 750 mg/kg.

Pharmacodynamics
Immune serum effect: RSV-IGIV provides passive immunity to RSV.

Pharmacokinetics
- *Absorption:* No information available.
- *Distribution:* No information available.
- *Metabolism:* No information available.

• *Excretion:* Little information available. Mean half-life of serum RSV-neutralizing antibodies after drug infusion is 22 to 28 days.

Contraindications and precautions
Contraindicated in patients with history of severe hypersensitivity to drug or other human immunoglobulins.

Interactions
Live-virus vaccines, such as *mumps, rubella*, and especially *measles*, may interfere with response. If such vaccines are given during or within 10 months after RSV-IGIV, reimmunization is recommended, if appropriate.

Effects on diagnostic tests
None reported.

Adverse reactions
CNS: dizziness, anxiety.
CV: fluid overload, tachycardia, hypertension, palpitations, chest tightness.
GI: vomiting, diarrhea, gastroenteritis, abdominal cramps.
Respiratory: respiratory distress, wheezing, crackles, hypoxia, tachypnea, dyspnea.
Skin: rash, flushing, pruritus.
Other: fever, inflammation at injection site, overdose effect, myalgia, arthralgia, hypersensitivity reactions including anaphylaxis.

Overdose and treatment
No information available.

☑ Special considerations
• Administer first dose of drug before beginning of RSV season; then subsequent doses given monthly throughout RSV season to maintain protection. Children infected with RSV should continue to receive monthly doses of drug for rest of RSV season.
• Drug does not contain a preservative. Single-use vial should be entered only once for administration purposes and infusion should begin within 6 hours and completed within 12 hours after single-use vial is entered. Do not use if solution is turbid. Administer through an I.V. line using a constant infusion pump. Predilution of drug before infusion is not advised. Although filters are not needed, an in-line filter with pore size over 15 micrometers may be used for infusion. Give drug separately from other drugs.
• Adhere to infusion rate guidelines; most adverse reactions may be due to administration rate. In very ill children with BPD, slower rates may be needed.
• Assess patient's cardiopulmonary status and vital signs before infusion, before each rate increase, and thereafter at 30-minute intervals until 30 minutes following end of infusion.
• Monitor children receiving drug closely for signs of fluid overload. Children with BPD may be at higher risk. Keep a loop diuretic, such as furosemide or bumetanide, available for treatment of fluid overload.
• If patient develops hypotension or anaphylaxis or if severe allergic reaction occurs, discontinue infusion and administer epinephrine (1:1,000).
• Patients with selective immunoglobulin A (IgA) deficiency may develop antibodies to IgA and have anaphylactic or allergic reactions to subsequent administration of blood products containing IgA, including RSV-IGIV. Monitor such patients closely during subsequent RSV-IGIV administration.

Pediatric use
• Children with clinically apparent fluid overload should not receive drug. Safety and efficacy of drug in children with congenital heart disease have not been established. In clinical trials, children receiving drug who also had congenital heart disease, especially those with right to left shunts, had an increased frequency of cardiac surgery and a greater frequency of severe and life-threatening adverse events associated with cardiac surgery.

reteplase, recombinant
Retavase

Pharmacologic classification: tissue-plasminogen activator
Therapeutic classification: thrombolytic enzyme
Pregnancy risk category C

How supplied
Available by prescription only
Injection: 10.8 units (18.8 mg)/vial (Supplied in kit with components for reconstitution and administration of two single-use vials.)

Indications, route, and dosage
Management of acute MI
Adults: Double-bolus injection of 10 + 10 units. Give each bolus I.V. over 2 minutes. If no complications occur after first bolus, such as serious bleeding or anaphylactoid reactions, give second bolus 30 minutes after start of first bolus. Initiate treatment soon after onset of symptoms of acute MI. There is no experience of repeat courses with reteplase.

Pharmacodynamics
Thrombolytic action: Drug catalyzes the cleavage of plasminogen to generate plasmin, which leads to fibrinolysis.

Pharmacokinetics
• *Absorption:* Given I.V.
• *Distribution:* Cleared from the plasma at a rate of 250 to 450 ml/minute.
• *Metabolism:* Primarily by the liver and kidney.
• *Excretion:* Plasma half-life is 13 to 16 minutes.

Contraindications and precautions
Contraindicated in patients with active internal bleeding, known bleeding diathesis, history of CVA, recent intracranial or intraspinal surgery or trauma, severe uncontrolled hypertension, intracranial neoplasm, arteriovenous malformation, or aneurysm.

Use cautiously in patients with recent (within 10 days) major surgery, obstetric delivery, organ biopsy, or trauma; previous puncture of noncompressible vessels; cerebrovascular disease; recent GI or

GU bleeding; hypertension (systolic pressure 180 mm Hg or more or diastolic pressure 110 mm Hg or more); likelihood of left-sided heart thrombus; subacute bacterial endocarditis; acute pericarditis; hemostatic defects; diabetic hemorrhagic retinopathy; septic thrombophlebitis; other conditions in which bleeding would be difficult to manage; pregnancy; and in patients age 75 or older.

Interactions

Heparin, oral anticoagulants, vitamin K antagonists, and *platelet inhibitors (abciximab, aspirin,* and *dipyridamole*) may increase risk of bleeding. Use together cautiously.

Effects on diagnostic tests

Drug may alter coagulation studies; it remains active in vitro and can lead to degradation of fibrinogen in sample. Collect blood samples in the presence of PPACK (chloromethylketone) at 2-micromolar concentrations.

Adverse reactions

CNS: ***intracranial hemorrhage.***
CV: ***arrhythmias, cholesterol embolization.***
GI: *GI hemorrhage.*
GU: hematuria.
Hematologic: *anemia,* ***bleeding tendency.***
Other: *bleeding* (at puncture site), ***hemorrhage.***

Overdose and treatment

No information available. Monitor for increased bleeding.

☑ Special considerations

- Carefully monitor ECG during treatment. Coronary thrombolysis may result in arrhythmias associated with reperfusion. Be prepared to treat bradycardia or ventricular irritability.
- Monitor for bleeding. Avoid I.M. injections, invasive procedures, and nonessential handling of patient. Bleeding is the most common adverse reaction and may occur internally or at external puncture sites. If local measures do not control serious bleeding, discontinue concomitant anticoagulation therapy. Withhold second bolus of reteplase.
- Drug is administered I.V. as a double-bolus injection. If bleeding or anaphylactoid reactions occur after first bolus; second bolus may be withheld.
- Reconstitute drug according to manufacturer's instructions using items provided in the kit.
- Do not administer drug with other I.V. medications through same I.V. line. Heparin and reteplase are incompatible in solution.
- Be aware that potency is expressed in terms of units specific for reteplase and not comparable to other thrombolytic agents.
- Avoid use of noncompressible pressure sites during therapy. If an arterial puncture is needed, an upper extremity vessel should be used. Apply pressure for at least 30 minutes; then apply a pressure dressing. Check site frequently.

Patient education

- Explain to patient and family about use and administration of reteplase.
- Tell patient to report adverse reactions such as signs and symptoms of bleeding or allergic reaction immediately.
- Advise patient about proper dental care to avoid excessive gum trauma.

Geriatric use

- Use cautiously in elderly patients. Risk of intracranial hemorrhage increases with age.

Pediatric use

- Safety and efficacy have not been established.

Breast-feeding

- It is not known if drug is excreted in the breast milk. Exercise caution if administered.

Rh_o (D) immune globulin, human

Gamulin Rh, HypRho-D, RhoGAM

Rh_o (D) immune globulin, micro-dose

HypRho-D Mini-Dose, MICRhoGAM, Mini-Gamulin Rh

Pharmacologic classification: immune serum
Therapeutic classification: anti-Rh_o (D)–positive prophylaxis
Pregnancy risk category C

How supplied

Available by prescription only
Injection: 300 mcg of Rh_o (D) immune globulin/vial (standard dose); 50 mcg of Rh_o (D) immune globulin/vial (microdose)

Indications, route, and dosage

Rh-positive exposure (full-term pregnancy or termination of pregnancy beyond 13 weeks' gestation), threatened abortion

Women: Administer 1 vial I.M. for each 15 ml of estimated fetal packed RBC volume entering patient's blood, as determined by a modified Kleihauer-Betke technique to determine fetal packed RBC volume. Usual (standard) dose after delivery of full-term infant is 1 vial; it must be given within 72 hours after delivery or miscarriage.

If Rh_o (D) immune globulin is indicated before delivery, administer 1 vial (standard dose) at approximately 28 weeks' gestation and give a second vial within 72 hours of delivery.

Transfusion accidents

Premenopausal women: Consult blood bank or transfusion unit at once. The number of vials (standard dose) to administer is calculated via the following formula:

$$\text{Number of vials} = \frac{\text{volume of whole blood transfused} \times \text{donor unit hematocrit}}{15}$$

Dose must be given within 72 hours.

Termination of pregnancy (spontaneous or induced abortion or ectopic pregnancy) up to and including 12 weeks' gestation
Women: 1 vial of microdose immune globulin I.M.; ideally, given within 3 hours but may give up to 72 hours after abortion or miscarriage.
Amniocentesis or abdominal trauma during pregnancy
Women: Dosage varies, based on extent of estimated fetomaternal hemorrhage.

Pharmacodynamics
Rh reaction prophylaxis: Rh_o (D) immune globulin suppresses the active antibody response and formation of anti-Rh_o (D) in Rh_o (D)-negative or D_u-negative individuals exposed to Rh-positive blood. It provides passive immunity to women exposed to Rh_o-positive fetal blood during pregnancy. It prevents formation of maternal antibodies (active immunity), which prevents hemolytic disease of the Rh-positive newborn in a subsequent pregnancy.

Pharmacokinetics
- *Absorption:* No information available.
- *Distribution:* No information available.
- *Metabolism:* No information available.
- *Excretion:* No information available.

Contraindications and precautions
Contraindicated in Rh (D)-positive or D-positive patients and those previously immunized to Rh (D) blood factor. Also contraindicated in patients with anaphylactic or severe systemic reaction to human globulin. Use with extreme caution in patients with immunoglobulin A deficiency due to increased risk of an anaphylactic reaction.

Interactions
Rh_o (D) immune globulin may interfere with the immune response to *live virus vaccines*, for example, those for *measles, mumps*, and *rubella*. Do not administer live virus vaccines within 3 months after administration of Rh_o (D) immune globulin. If postpartum women receive both Rh_o (D) immune globulin and rubella virus vaccine within a 3-month period, serologic tests should be performed 6 to 8 weeks after vaccination to confirm seroconversion.

Effects on diagnostic tests
None reported.

Adverse reactions
Other: discomfort (at injection site), slight fever.

Overdose and treatment
No information available.

☑ Special considerations
- Obtain a thorough history of allergies and reactions to immunizations.
- Have epinephrine solution 1:1,000 available.
- Immediately after delivery, send a sample of the infant's cord blood to laboratory for typing and cross matching and direct antiglobulin test. Infant must be Rh_o (D)-positive or D_u-positive. Confirm that mother is Rh_o (D)-negative and D_u-negative.
- For best results, Rh_o (D) immune globulin must be administered within 72 hours of Rh-incompatible delivery, spontaneous or induced abortion, or transfusion.
- The microdose formulation is recommended for use after every spontaneous or induced abortion up to and including 12 weeks' gestation unless mother is Rh_o (D)-positive or D_u-positive, she has Rh antibodies, or father or fetus is Rh-negative.
- Administer I.M. in the anterolateral aspect of the upper thigh and deltoid muscle. Do not give I.V.
- Rh_o (D) immune globulin has not been associated with an increased frequency of acquired immunodeficiency syndrome. The immune globulin is devoid of HIV. Immune globulin recipients do not develop antibodies to HIV.
- Store product between 36° and 46° F (2° and 8° C). Do not freeze.

Patient education
- Inform patient that she is receiving this product because her blood has been exposed to the Rh-positive factor. Tell the postpartum patient that her body will naturally develop antibodies to destroy this factor, which could threaten future Rh-positive pregnancies.
- Tell patient there is no known risk of HIV infection after receiving product.
- Tell patient local pain, swelling, and tenderness at injection site may occur after vaccination. Recommend acetaminophen to ease minor discomfort.
- Tell patient to report headache, skin changes, or difficulty breathing.

Breast-feeding
- Immune globulins occur in breast milk. Safety in breast-feeding women has not been established.

ribavirin
Virazole

Pharmacologic classification: synthetic nucleoside
Therapeutic classification: antiviral
Pregnancy risk category X

How supplied
Available by prescription only
Powder to be reconstituted for inhalation: 6 g in 100-ml glass vial

Indications, route, and dosage
Treatment of hospitalized infants and young children infected by respiratory syncytial virus (RSV)
Infants and young children: Solution in concentration of 20 mg/ml delivered via the Viratek Small Particle Aerosol Generator (SPAG-2) results in a mist with a concentration of 190 mcg/L. Treatment is carried out for 12 to 18 hours/day for at least 3, and no more than 7, days with a flow rate of 12.5 L of mist per minute.

For ventilated patients, use same dose with a pressure- or volume-cycled ventilator in conjunction with SPAG-2. Patient should be suctioned q 1 to 2 hours and pulmonary pressures checked q 2 to 4 hours.

Pharmacodynamics

Antiviral action: Drug action probably involves inhibition of RNA and DNA synthesis, inhibition of RNA polymerase, and interference with completion of viral polypeptide coat.

Pharmacokinetics

- *Absorption:* Some ribavirin is absorbed systemically.
- *Distribution:* Ribavirin concentrates in bronchial secretions; plasma levels are subtherapeutic for plaque inhibition.
- *Metabolism:* Ribavirin is metabolized to 1,2,4-triazole-3-carboxamide (deribosylated ribavirin).
- *Excretion:* Mostly excreted renally. First phase of plasma half-life is 9½ hours; second phase has extended half-life of 40 hours (from slow drug release from RBC binding sites).

Contraindications and precautions

Contraindicated in patients with hypersensitivity to drug and in women who are or may become pregnant during treatment.

Interactions

None reported.

Effects on diagnostic tests

None reported.

Adverse reactions

CV: ***cardiac arrest,*** hypotension.
EENT: conjunctivitis.
Hematologic: anemia, reticulocytosis.
Respiratory: worsening respiratory state, ***apnea,*** bacterial pneumonia, pneumothorax, ***bronchospasm.***
Other: rash, erythema of eyelids.

Overdose and treatment

No information available for human overdosage; high doses in animals have produced GI symptoms.

☑ Special considerations

- Ribavirin aerosol is indicated only for lower respiratory tract infection caused by RSV. (Although treatment may begin before test results are available, RSV infection must eventually be confirmed.)
- Administer ribavirin aerosol only by SPAG-2. Do not use other aerosol-generating devices.
- To prepare drug, reconstitute solution with USP sterile water for injection or inhalation, then transfer aseptically to sterile 500-ml Erlenmeyer flask. Dilute further with sterile water to 300 ml to yield final concentration of 20 mg/ml. Solution remains stable for 24 hours at room temperature.
- Do not use bacteriostatic water (or any other water containing antimicrobial agent) to reconstitute drug.
- Discard unused solution in SPAG-2 unit before adding newly reconstituted solution. Solution should be changed at least every 24 hours.
- Monitor ventilator-dependent patients carefully because drug may precipitate in ventilatory apparatus. Change heated wire connective tubing and bacteria filters in series in expiratory limb of the system frequently (such as every 4 hours).
- Drug is most useful for infants with most severe RSV form—typically premature infants and those with underlying disorders such as cardiopulmonary disease. (Most other infants and children with RSV infection do not require treatment because disease is self-limiting.)
- Drug therapy must be accompanied by appropriate respiratory and fluid therapy.

riboflavin (vitamin B_2)

Pharmacologic classification: water-soluble vitamin
Therapeutic classification: vitamin B complex vitamin
Pregnancy risk category A (C if more than the RDA)

How supplied

Available without a prescription, as appropriate
Tablets: 10 mg, 25 mg, 50 mg, 100 mg, 250 mg

Indications, route, and dosage

Riboflavin deficiency or adjunct to thiamine treatment for polyneuritis or cheilosis secondary to pellagra
Adults and adolescents over age 12: 5 to 30 mg P.O. daily, depending on severity.
Children under age 12: 3 to 10 mg P.O. daily, depending on severity.
Microcytic anemia associated with splenomegaly and glutathione reductase deficiency
Adults: 10 mg P.O. daily for 10 days.
Dietary supplementation
Adults: 1 to 4 mg P.O. daily. For maintenance, increase nutritional intake and supplement with vitamin B complex.

Pharmacodynamics

Metabolic action: Riboflavin, a coenzyme, functions in the forms of flavin adenine dinucleotide (FAD) and flavin mononucleotide (FMN) and plays a vital metabolic role in numerous tissue respiration systems. FAD and FMN act as hydrogen-carrier molecules for several flavoproteins involved in intermediary metabolism. Riboflavin is also directly involved in maintaining erythrocyte integrity.

Riboflavin deficiency causes a clinical syndrome with the following symptoms: cheilosis, angular stomatitis, glossitis, keratitis, scrotal skin changes, ocular changes, and seborrheic dermatitis. In severe deficiency, normochromic, normocytic anemia and neuropathy may occur. Clinical signs may become evident after 3 to 8 months of inadequate riboflavin intake. Administration of riboflavin reverses signs of deficiency. Riboflavin deficiency rarely occurs alone and is commonly associated with deficiency of other B vitamins and protein.

Pharmacokinetics

• *Absorption:* Although riboflavin is absorbed readily from the GI tract, extent of absorption is limited. Absorption occurs at a specialized segment of the mucosa; drug absorption is limited by duration of drug's contact with this area. Before being absorbed, riboflavin-5-phosphate is rapidly dephosphorylated in the GI lumen. GI absorption increases when drug is administered with food and decreases when hepatitis, cirrhosis, biliary obstruction, or probenecid administration is present.
• *Distribution:* FAD and FMN are distributed widely to body tissues. Free riboflavin is present in the retina. Riboflavin is stored in limited amounts in the liver, spleen, kidneys, and heart, mainly in the form of FAD. FAD and FMN are approximately 60% protein-bound in blood. Drug crosses the placenta, and breast milk contains about 400 ng/ml.
• *Metabolism:* Drug is metabolized in the liver.
• *Excretion:* After a single oral dose, biologic half-life is about 66 to 84 minutes in healthy individuals. Drug is metabolized to FMN in erythrocytes, GI mucosal cells, and the liver; FMN is converted to FAD in the liver. Approximately 9% of drug is excreted unchanged in the urine after normal ingestion. Excretion involves renal tubular secretion and glomerular filtration. Amount renally excreted unchanged is directly proportional to the dose. Drug removal by hemodialysis is slower than by natural renal excretion.

Contraindications and precautions

No known contraindications.

Interactions

Concomitant use of riboflavin with *propantheline bromide* delays absorption rate of riboflavin but increases total amount absorbed. If patient is using *oral contraceptives*, riboflavin's dose may need to be increased. *Alcohol* impairs intestinal absorption of riboflavin.

Effects on diagnostic tests

Riboflavin therapy alters urinalysis based on spectrophotometry or color reactions. Large doses of drug result in bright yellow urine. Riboflavin produces fluorescent substances in urine and plasma, which can falsely elevate fluorometric determinations of catecholamines and urobilinogen.

Adverse reactions

GU: bright yellow urine (with high doses).

Overdose and treatment

No information available.

☑ Special considerations

• RDA of riboflavin is 0.4 to 1.8 mg/day in children, 1.2 to 1.7 mg/day in adults, and 1.6 to 1.8 mg/day in pregnant and breast-feeding women.
• Give oral preparation of riboflavin with food to increase absorption.
• Obtain dietary history because other vitamin deficiencies may coexist.

Patient education

• Inform patient that riboflavin may cause a yellow discoloration of the urine.
• Teach patient about good dietary sources of riboflavin, such as whole grain cereals and green vegetables. Liver, kidney, heart, eggs, and dairy products are also dietary sources but may not be appropriate, based on patient's serum cholesterol and triglyceride levels.
• Tell patient to store riboflavin in a tight, light-resistant container.

Breast-feeding

• Drug crosses the placenta; during pregnancy and lactation, riboflavin requirements are increased. Increased food intake during this time usually provides adequate amounts of the vitamin. The National Research Council recommends daily intake of 1.8 mg/day during first 6 months of breast-feeding.

rifabutin

Mycobutin

Pharmacologic classification: semisynthetic ansamycin
Therapeutic classification: antibiotic
Pregnancy risk category B

How supplied

Available by prescription only
Capsules: 150 mg

Indications, route, and dosage

Prevention of disseminated* Mycobacterium avium *complex (MAC) disease in patients with advanced HIV infection
Adults: 300 mg P.O. daily as a single dose or divided b.i.d. with food.

Pharmacodynamics

Antibiotic action: Rifabutin inhibits DNA-dependent RNA polymerase in susceptible strains of *Escherichia coli* and *Bacillus subtilis,* but not in mammalian cells. It is not known whether rifabutin inhibits this enzyme in *M. avium* or in *M. intracellulare,* which compose MAC.

Pharmacokinetics

• *Absorption:* Drug is readily absorbed from the GI tract. Plasma levels peak 2 to 4 hours after an oral dose.
• *Distribution:* Because of its high lipophilicity, rifabutin demonstrates a high propensity for distribution and intracellular tissue uptake. About 85% of drug is bound in a concentration-independent manner to plasma proteins.
• *Metabolism:* Metabolized in the liver to five identified metabolites. The 25-0-desacetyl metabolite has an activity equal to parent drug and contributes up to 10% of total antimicrobial activity.
• *Excretion:* Less than 10% of rifabutin is excreted in urine as unchanged drug. Approximately 53% of the oral dose is excreted in urine, primarily as metabolites. About 30% is excreted in feces.

Contraindications and precautions
Contraindicated in patients with hypersensitivity to drug or other rifamycin derivatives (such as rifampin) and in patients with active tuberculosis because single-agent therapy with rifabutin increases the risk of inducing bacterial resistance to both rifabutin and rifampin.

Use cautiously in patients with preexisting neutropenia and thrombocytopenia.

Interactions
Rifabutin may decrease the serum levels of *zidovudine*, although it does not affect zidovudine's inhibition of HIV. Because rifabutin has liver enzyme-inducing properties, it may lower serum levels of many other drugs as well. Although dosage adjustments may be necessary, further study is needed. Rifabutin decreases the effectiveness of *oral contraceptives*. Instruct patient to use nonhormonal forms of birth control.

Effects on diagnostic tests
None reported.

Adverse reactions
GI: dyspepsia, eructation, flatulence, diarrhea, nausea, vomiting, abdominal pain, altered taste.
GU: *discolored urine* (brown-orange).
Hematologic: NEUTROPENIA, LEUKOPENIA, ***thrombocytopenia,*** eosinophilia.
Skin: *rash.*
Other: fever, myalgia, headache, insomnia.

Overdose and treatment
Although there is no experience in the treatment of drug overdose, clinical experience with rifamycins suggests that gastric lavage to evacuate gastric contents (within a few hours of overdose), followed by instillation of an activated charcoal slurry into the stomach, may help absorb any remaining drug from the GI tract. Hemodialysis or forced diuresis is not expected to enhance systemic elimination of unchanged rifabutin.

☑ Special considerations
- Evaluate patient who develops complaints consistent with active tuberculosis during rifabutin prophylaxis immediately, so that active disease may be given an effective combination regimen of antituberculosis medications. Administration of single-agent rifabutin to patients with active tuberculosis likely leads to development of tuberculosis that is resistant to rifabutin and rifampin.
- Because rifabutin may be associated with neutropenia, and more rarely thrombocytopenia, consider obtaining hematologic studies periodically in patients receiving rifabutin prophylaxis.
- High-fat meals slow rate but not extent of drug absorption.

Patient education
- Inform female patient using oral contraceptives that drug may decrease their effectiveness. Recommend that she use a nonhormonal form of birth control during drug therapy.
- Tell patient with swallowing difficulty to mix drug with soft foods such as applesauce.
- Advise patient with nausea, vomiting, or other GI upset to take drug with food, in two divided doses.
- Warn patient that urine and other body fluids may become discolored (brown-orange). Clothes and soft contact lenses may become permanently discolored.

Pediatric use
- Although safety and effectiveness in children have not been fully established, several studies indicate that drug may be helpful in children at maximum daily dose of 5 mg/kg.

Breast-feeding
- It is not known if drug is excreted in breast milk. Because of potential for serious adverse effects in breast-fed infants, either the breast-feeding or drug should be discontinued, depending on importance of drug to mother.

---

rifampin
Rifadin, Rimactane

Pharmacologic classification: semisynthetic rifamycin B derivative (macrocyclic antibiotic)
Therapeutic classification: antituberculosis
Pregnancy risk category C

How supplied
Available by prescription only
Capsules: 150 mg, 300 mg
Injection: 600 mg/vial

Indications, route, and dosage
Primary treatment in pulmonary tuberculosis
Adults: 600 mg P.O. or I.V. daily as a single dose (give P.O. dose 1 hour before or 2 hours after meals).
Children: 10 to 20 mg/kg P.O. or I.V. daily as a single dose (give P.O. dose 1 hour before or 2 hours after meals). Maximum daily dosage, 600 mg. Concomitant administration of other effective antitubercular drugs is recommended. Treatment usually lasts 6 to 9 months.
Asymptomatic meningococcal carriers
Adults: 600 mg P.O. b.i.d. for 2 days.
Infants and children over age 1 month: 10 mg/kg P.O. b.i.d. for 2 days.
Neonates under age 1 month: 5 mg/kg P.O. b.i.d. for 2 days.
✦ ***Dosage adjustment.*** Reduce dosage in patients with hepatic dysfunction.
Prophylaxis of* Haemophilus influenzae *type B
Adults and children: 20 mg/kg (up to 600 mg) once daily for 4 consecutive days.
◊ ***Leprosy***
Adults: 600 mg P.O. once monthly, usually used in combination with other agents.

Pharmacodynamics
Antibiotic action: Rifampin impairs RNA synthesis by inhibiting DNA-dependent RNA polymerase. Rifampin may be bacteriostatic or bactericidal, de-

pending on organism susceptibility and drug concentration at infection site.

Rifampin acts against *Mycobacterium tuberculosis, M. bovis, M. marinum, M. kansasii,* some strains of *M. fortuitum, M. avium,* and *M. avium-intracellulare,* and many gram-positive and some gram-negative bacteria. Resistance to rifampin by *M. tuberculosis* can develop rapidly; rifampin is usually given with other antituberculosis drugs to prevent or delay resistance.

Pharmacokinetics

- *Absorption:* Drug is absorbed completely from the GI tract after oral administration; peak serum concentrations occur 1 to 4 hours after ingestion. Food delays absorption.
- *Distribution:* Rifampin is distributed widely into body tissues and fluids, including ascitic, pleural, seminal, and cerebrospinal fluids, tears, and saliva; and into liver, prostate, lungs, and bone. Drug crosses the placenta; it is 84% to 91% protein-bound.
- *Metabolism:* Drug is metabolized extensively in the liver by deacetylation. It undergoes interohepatic circulation.
- *Excretion:* Rifampin undergoes enterohepatic circulation, and drug and metabolite are excreted primarily in bile; drug, but not metabolite, is reabsorbed. From 6% to 30% of rifampin and metabolite appear unchanged in urine in 24 hours; about 60% is excreted in feces. Some drug is excreted in breast milk. Plasma half-life in adults is 1½ to 5 hours; serum levels rise in obstructive jaundice. Dosage adjustment is not necessary for patients with renal failure. Rifampin is not removed by either hemodialysis or peritoneal dialysis.

Contraindications and precautions

Contraindicated in patients with hypersensitivity to drug. Use cautiously in patients with hepatic disease.

Interactions

Rifampin-induced enzyme activity may accelerate metabolic conversion of *isoniazid* to hepatotoxic metabolites, increasing hazard of isoniazid hepatotoxicity.

Concomitant use of *para-aminosalicylate* may decrease oral absorption of rifampin, lowering serum concentrations; administer drugs 8 to 12 hours apart. Rifampin-induced hepatic microsomal enzymes inactivate the following drugs: *anticoagulants, barbiturates, beta blockers, chloramphenicol, clofibrate, corticosteroids, cyclosporine, cardiac glycoside derivatives, dapsone, disopyramide, estrogens, methadone, oral contraceptives, oral sulfonylureas, phenytoin, quinidine, tocainide,* and *verapamil;* decreased serum concentrations of those drugs require dosage adjustments.

Daily use of *alcohol* while using rifampin may increase risk of hepatotoxicity.

Effects on diagnostic tests

Rifampin alters standard serum folate and vitamin B_{12} assays. Drug's systemic effects may cause asymptomatic elevation of liver function tests (14%) and serum uric acid.

Rifampin may cause temporary retention of sulfobromophthalein in the liver excretion test; it may also interfere with contrast material in gallbladder studies and urinalysis based on spectrophotometry.

Adverse reactions

CNS: headache, fatigue, drowsiness, behavioral changes, dizziness, mental confusion, generalized numbness.
GI: epigastric distress, anorexia, nausea, vomiting, abdominal pain, diarrhea, flatulence, sore mouth and tongue, pseudomembranous colitis, pancreatitis.
GU: hemoglobinuria, hematuria, ***acute renal failure.***
Hematologic: eosinophilia, ***thrombocytopenia,*** transient leukopenia, hemolytic anemia.
Hepatic: ***hepatotoxicity,*** *transient abnormalities in liver function tests.*
Skin: pruritus, urticaria, rash.
Other: flulike syndrome, discoloration of body fluids, hyperuricemia, shortness of breath, wheezing, ***shock,*** ataxia, osteomalacia, visual disturbances, exudative conjunctivitis, porphyria exacerbation, menstrual disturbances.

Overdose and treatment

Signs of overdose include lethargy, nausea, and vomiting; hepatotoxicity from massive overdose includes hepatomegaly, jaundice, elevated liver function studies and bilirubin levels, and loss of consciousness. Red-orange discoloration of the skin, urine, sweat, saliva, tears, and feces may occur.

Treat by gastric lavage, followed by activated charcoal; if necessary, force diuresis. Perform bile drainage if hepatic dysfunction persists beyond 24 to 48 hours.

☑ Special considerations

- Give drug 1 hour before or 2 hours after meals for maximum absorption; capsule contents may be mixed with food or fluid to enhance swallowing.
- Obtain specimens for culture and sensitivity testing before giving first dose but do not delay therapy; repeat periodically to detect drug resistance.
- Observe patient for adverse reactions and monitor hematologic, renal and liver function studies, and serum electrolytes to minimize toxicity. Watch for signs and symptoms of hepatic impairment (anorexia, fatigue, malaise, jaundice, dark urine, liver tenderness).
- Increased liver enzyme activity inactivates certain drugs (especially warfarin, corticosteroids, and oral hypoglycemics), requiring dosage adjustments.
- Reconstituted solution is stable for 24 hours at room temperature. Infusion solutions of 100 to 500 ml should be used within 4 hours.

Patient education

- Explain disease process and rationale for long-term therapy.
- Teach signs and symptoms of hypersensitivity and other adverse reactions, and emphasize need to call if these occur; urge patient to report *any* unusual reactions.

• Tell patient to take rifampin on an empty stomach, at least 1 hour before or 2 hours after a meal. If GI irritation occurs, patient may need to take drug with food.
• Urge patient to comply with prescribed regimen, not to miss doses, and not to discontinue drug without medical approval. Explain importance of follow-up appointments.
• Encourage patient to report promptly any flulike signs or symptoms, weakness, sore throat, loss of appetite, unusual bruising, rash, itching, tea-colored urine, clay-colored stools, or yellow discoloration of eyes or skin.
• Explain that drug turns all body fluids red-orange color; advise patient of possible permanent stains on clothes and soft contact lenses.
• Advise oral contraceptive users to substitute other methods; rifampin inactivates such drugs and may alter menstrual patterns.

Geriatric use
• Usual dose in elderly and debilitated patients is 10 mg/kg once daily.

Pediatric use
• Safety in children under age 5 has not been established.

Breast-feeding
• Drug may be excreted in breast milk. Use with caution in breast-feeding women.

riluzole
Rilutek

Pharmacologic classification: benzothiazole
Therapeutic classification: neuroprotector
Pregnancy risk category C

How supplied
Available by prescription only
Tablets: 50 mg

Indications, route, and dosage
Amyotrophic lateral sclerosis (ALS)
Adults: 50 mg P.O. q 12 hours on an empty stomach.

Pharmacodynamics
Neuroprotector action: It is not known how riluzole improves signs and symptoms of ALS.

Pharmacokinetics
• *Absorption:* Well absorbed from GI tract (about 90%) with average absolute oral bioavailability of about 60%. A high-fat meal decreases absorption.
• *Distribution:* Riluzole is 96% protein-bound.
• *Metabolism:* Extensively metabolized in the liver to six major and several minor metabolites, not all of which have been identified.
• *Excretion:* Drug is excreted primarily in urine and a small amount in feces. Half-life is 12 hours with repeated doses.

Contraindications and precautions
Contraindicated in patients with history of severe hypersensitivity reactions to drug or components in its tablets.

Use cautiously in patients with hepatic or renal dysfunction and in the elderly. Also use cautiously in females and Japanese patients who may possess a lower metabolic capacity to eliminate drug compared with males and white subjects, respectively.

Interactions
There have been no clinical studies designed to evaluate the interaction of riluzole with other drugs. As with all drugs, the potential for interaction by several mechanisms is a possibility and requires close monitoring of patients who are receiving concomitant drug therapy. In particular, use caution when administering potentially hepatotoxic drugs, such as *allopurinol, methyldopa,* or *sulfasalazine,* concomitantly.

Effects on diagnostic tests
None reported.

Adverse reactions
CNS: headache, aggravation reaction, hypertonia, depression, dizziness, insomnia, somnolence, vertigo, circumoral paresthesia.
CV: hypertension, tachycardia, palpitation, orthostatic hypotension.
GI: abdominal pain, *nausea,* vomiting, dyspepsia, anorexia, diarrhea, flatulence, stomatitis, tooth disorder, oral moniliasis.
GU: urinary tract infection, dysuria.
Respiratory: *decreased lung function,* rhinitis, increased cough, sinusitis.
Skin: pruritus, eczema, alopecia, exfoliative dermatitis.
Other: *asthenia,* back pain, malaise, dry mouth, phlebitis, weight loss, peripheral edema, arthralgia.

Overdose and treatment
No information available. In the event of an overdose, discontinue therapy immediately and implement supportive measures.

☑ Special considerations
• Baseline elevations in liver function studies (especially elevated bilirubin) should preclude use of riluzole. Perform liver function studies periodically during therapy. In many patients, drug may cause serum aminotransferase elevations; discontinue drug if levels exceed 10 times upper limit of normal range or if clinical jaundice develops.
• Give drug at least 1 hour before, or 2 hours after, a meal to avoid a food-related decrease in bioavailability.

Patient education
• Tell patient or caregiver that drug must be taken regularly and at the same time each day. If a dose is missed, tell patient to take the next tablet as originally planned.

• Instruct patient to report febrile illness because the patient's WBC count should be checked.
• Warn patient to avoid hazardous activities until CNS effects of drug are known.
• Advise patient to avoid excessive alcohol intake while taking drug.
• Tell patient to store drug at room temperature and protect it from bright light.
• Stress importance of keeping drug out of reach of children.

Geriatric use
• Age-related decreased renal and hepatic function may cause a decrease in clearance of riluzole; administer drug cautiously to this age-group.

Pediatric use
• Safety and effectiveness in children have not been established.

Breast-feeding
• It is not known if drug is excreted in breast milk. Because of potential for serious adverse reactions in breast-fed infants, use of drug in breast-feeding patients is not recommended.

rimantadine hydrochloride
Flumadine

Pharmacologic classification: adamantine
Therapeutic classification: antiviral
Pregnancy risk category C

How supplied
Available by prescription only
Tablets: 100 mg
Syrup: 50 mg/5 ml

Indications, route, and dosage
Prophylaxis against influenza A virus
Adults and children age 10 and older: 100 mg P.O. b.i.d.; for patients with severe hepatic dysfunction or renal failure (creatinine clearance 10 ml/minute or less) and for elderly nursing home patients, a dose reduction to 100 mg P.O. daily is recommended.
Children under age 10: 5 mg/kg P.O. once daily. Maximum dosage, 150 mg.
Treatment of illness caused by various strains of influenza A virus
Adults: 100 mg P.O. b.i.d. for 7 days from initial onset of symptoms; for patients with severe hepatic dysfunction or renal failure (creatinine clearance 10 ml/minute or less) and for elderly nursing home patients, a dose reduction to 100 mg P.O. daily is recommended.

Note: If seizures develop, discontinue rimantadine.

Pharmacodynamics
Antiviral action: Rimantadine's mechanism of action is not fully understood. It appears to exert its inhibitory effect early in the viral replicative cycle, possibly inhibiting the uncoating of the virus. Genetic studies suggest that a virus protein specified by the virion M^2 gene plays an important role in the susceptibility of influenza A virus to inhibition by rimantadine.

Pharmacokinetics
• *Absorption:* Tablet and syrup formulations are equally absorbed after oral administration. The time to peak concentration is about 6 hours in an otherwise healthy adult.
• *Distribution:* Plasma protein binding is about 40% for rimantadine.
• *Metabolism:* Drug is extensively metabolized in the liver.
• *Excretion:* Less than 25% of rimantadine is excreted in urine as unchanged drug. Elimination half-life of drug is approximately 25.4 to 32 hours. Hemodialysis does not contribute to drug clearance.

Contraindications and precautions
Contraindicated in patients with hypersensitivity to drug or *amantadine.* Use cautiously during pregnancy and in patients with impaired renal or hepatic function or seizure disorders (especially epilepsy).

Interactions
Coadministration with *acetaminophen* reduced peak concentration and area-under-the-curve values for rimantadine by 11%; coadministration with *aspirin* reduced the values by 10%. Monitor the effectiveness of rimantadine.

Cimetidine may decrease total rimantadine clearance by about 16%. Monitor the patient for adverse effects associated with rimantadine use.

Effects on diagnostic tests
None reported.

Adverse reactions
CNS: insomnia, headache, dizziness, nervousness, fatigue, asthenia.
GI: nausea, vomiting, anorexia, dry mouth, abdominal pain.

Overdose and treatment
Information specific to rimantadine overdose is not available. As with any overdose, administer supportive therapy as indicated. Overdoses of a related drug, amantadine, have been reported, with reactions ranging from agitation to hallucinations, cardiac arrhythmia, and death. Administration of I.V. physostigmine (1 to 2 mg in adults and 0.5 mg in children; repeated as needed but not to exceed 2 mg/hour) has been reported anecdotally to benefit patients with CNS effects from overdose of amantadine.

☑ Special considerations
• For illnesses associated with various strains of influenza A, treatment should begin as soon as possible (preferably within 48 hours after onset of signs and symptoms) to reduce duration of fever and systematic symptoms.
• Because of risk of drug metabolites accumulation during multiple dosing, monitor patient with any

degree of renal insufficiency for adverse effects, and adjust dosage as necessary.
• An increased incidence of seizures has been observed in some patients with history of seizures who were not taking anticonvulsant medication during rimantadine therapy. If seizures develop, discontinue drug.
• Influenza A–resistant strains can emerge during therapy. Patients taking drug may still be able to spread the disease.

Patient education
• Tell patient to take drug several hours before bedtime to prevent insomnia.
• Inform patient that taking drug does not prevent him from spreading the disease and that he should limit contact with others until fully recovered.
• Warn patient that drug may cause adverse CNS effects; he should not drive or perform activities that require mental alertness until these effects are known.
• Tell patient with history of epilepsy to stop taking drug and call if seizure activity occurs.

Geriatric use
• Adverse reactions associated with drug occur more frequently in elderly patients than general population. Monitor these patients closely.

Pediatric use
• Drug is recommended for prophylaxis of influenza A. Safety and effectiveness of drug in treating symptomatic influenza infection in children have not been established. Prophylaxis studies with rimantadine have not been performed in those under age 1.

Breast-feeding
• Drug should not be administered to breast-feeding women because of the potential adverse effects to the infant.

rimexolone
Vexol

Pharmacologic classification: ophthalmic steroid
Therapeutic classification: anti-inflammatory
Pregnancy risk category C

How supplied
Available by prescription only
Ophthalmic suspension: 1%

Indications, route, and dosage
Postoperative inflammation following ocular surgery
Adults: Instill 1 to 2 drops into the conjunctival sac of the affected eye q.i.d. beginning 24 hours after surgery and continuing throughout first 2 weeks after surgery.
Anterior uveitis
Adults: Instill 1 to 2 drops into the conjunctival sac of the affected eye hourly during waking hours for first week, 1 drop q 2 hours during waking hours of second week, and then taper dosage until uveitis is resolved.

Pharmacodynamics
Anti-inflammatory action: Exact mechanism of action is unknown, although rimexolone is a corticosteroid that inhibits edema, cellular infiltration, capillary dilation, fibroblastic proliferation, deposition of collagen, and scar formation associated with inflammation.

Pharmacokinetics
• *Absorption:* No information available.
• *Distribution:* No information available.
• *Metabolism:* No information available.
• *Excretion:* No information available.

Contraindications and precautions
Contraindicated in patients with hypersensitivity to any component of drug; epithelial herpes simplex keratitis; vaccinia, varicella, and most other viral diseases of the cornea and conjunctiva; mycobacterial infection of the eye; fungal diseases of the eye; and acute purulent untreated infections that may be masked or enhanced by presence of a steroid.

Interactions
None reported.

Effects on diagnostic tests
None reported.

Adverse reactions
EENT: *blurred vision, discharge, ocular pain or discomfort, increased intraocular pressure, foreign body sensation, ocular hyperemia, ocular pruritus,* sticky sensation, increased fibrin, dry eye, conjunctival edema, corneal staining, keratitis, tearing, photophobia, edema, irritation, corneal ulcer, browache, lid margin crusting, corneal edema, infiltrate, corneal erosion.
Other: headache, hypotension, rhinitis, pharyngitis, and taste perversion.

Overdose and treatment
No information available.

☑ Special considerations
• Patients receiving drug should have their intraocular pressure checked frequently.
• Fungal infections of the cornea are particularly prone to develop coincidentally with long-term corticosteroid application.

Patient education
• Teach patient how to instill drops. Advise him to shake the dispenser well before using, and to wash hands before and after instilling suspension; warn against touching the dropper or tip to eye or surrounding tissue.
• Advise patient to apply light finger pressure on lacrimal sac for 1 minute after instillation.
• Stress importance of compliance with recommended therapy.

- Warn patient not to use leftover medication for a new eye inflammation because this may cause serious problems.
- Remind patient to discard drug when it is no longer needed.

Pediatric use
- Safety and effectiveness in children have not been established.

Breast-feeding
- It is not known if drug is excreted into breast milk. Use of drug in breast-feeding women is not recommended.

Ringer's injection

Pharmacologic classification: electrolyte solution
Therapeutic classification: electrolyte and fluid replenishment
Pregnancy risk category C

How supplied
Available by prescription only
Injection: 250 ml, 500 ml, 1,000 ml

Indications, route, and dosage
Fluid and electrolyte replacement
Adults and children: Dose highly individualized according to patient's size and clinical condition.

Pharmacodynamics
Fluid and electrolyte replacement: Ringer's injection replaces fluid and supplies important electrolytes: sodium 147 mEq/L, potassium 4 mEq/L, calcium 4.5 mEq/L, and chloride 155.5 mEq/L. However, clinically, the addition of potassium and calcium only slightly increases the therapeutic value of an isotonic sodium chloride solution. Neither potassium nor calcium is present in sufficient concentration in Ringer's injection to correct a deficit of these ions adequately. Large volumes of Ringer's injection usually cause minimal distortion of cation composition of the extracellular fluid. The solution may alter the acid-base balance.

Pharmacokinetics
- *Absorption:* Given by direct I.V. infusion.
- *Distribution:* Widely distributed.
- *Metabolism:* None significant.
- *Excretion:* Excreted primarily in urine.

Contraindications and precautions
Contraindicated in patients with renal failure, except as emergency volume expander. Use cautiously in patients with heart failure, circulatory insufficiency, renal dysfunction, hypoproteinemia, and pulmonary edema.

Interactions
Several drugs as well as *packed RBCs* are incompatible with Ringer's solution. Consult specialized references for further information.

Effects on diagnostic tests
None reported.

Adverse reactions
CV: fluid overload.

Overdose and treatment
If overinfusion occurs, stopping infusion is usually sufficient treatment. In some cases, a loop diuretic such as furosemide may be necessary to increase the rate of fluid and electrolyte elimination. Dialysis may be needed in renal failure.

☑ Special considerations
- Monitor for acid-base imbalance when large volume of solution is infused. Ringer's injection is a colorless, odorless solution with a salty taste and a pH between 5.0 and 7.5.

Patient education
- Explain need for I.V. therapy.
- Tell patient to report adverse reactions at once.

Ringer's injection, lactated

Pharmacologic classification: electrolyte-carbohydrate solution
Therapeutic classification: electrolyte and fluid replenishment
Pregnancy risk category C

How supplied
Available by prescription only
Injection: 150 ml, 250 ml, 500 ml, 1,000 ml

Indications, route, and dosage
Fluid and electrolyte replacement
Adults and children: Dose highly individualized. Solution approximates the contents of the blood more closely than Ringer's injection does; however, additional electrolytes may have to be added to meet the patient's needs. Specific formulations of I.V. solutions are generally preferred to this premixed formulation.

Pharmacodynamics
Fluid and electrolyte replacement: Lactated Ringer's injection replaces fluid and supplies important electrolytes: sodium 130 mEq/L, potassium 4 mEq/L, calcium 3 mEq/L, chloride 109.7 mEq/L, and lactate 28 mEq/L. However, clinically, the addition of potassium and calcium only slightly increases the therapeutic value of an isotonic sodium chloride solution. Neither potassium nor calcium is present in sufficient concentration in lactated Ringer's injection to correct a deficit of these ions. Large volumes of lactated Ringer's injection usually cause minimal distortion of cation composition of the extracellular fluid. The solution may alter the acid-base balance.

Lactated Ringer's injection may be used for its alkalinizing effect because the lactate is ultimately metabolized to bicarbonate. In persons with normal cellular oxidative activity, the alkalinizing effect will be fully realized in 1 to 2 hours.

Pharmacokinetics
• *Absorption:* Given by direct I.V. infusion.
• *Distribution:* Distributed widely.
• *Metabolism:* None significant for electrolytes. Lactate is oxidized to bicarbonate.
• *Excretion:* Lactated Ringer's injection is excreted primarily in urine.

Contraindications and precautions
Contraindicated in patients with renal failure, except as emergency volume expander. Use cautiously in patients with heart failure, circulatory insufficiency, renal dysfunction, hypoproteinemia, and pulmonary edema.

Interactions
Several drugs as well as *packed RBCs* are incompatible with lactated Ringer's injection. Consult specialized references for further information.

Effects on diagnostic tests
None reported.

Adverse reactions
CV: fluid overload.

Overdose and treatment
If overinfusion occurs, stopping infusion is usually sufficient treatment. Dialysis may be needed in renal failure. Monitor blood acid-base balance.

☑ Special considerations
• Solution is colorless and odorless with a salty taste and a pH between 6 and 7.5. The absence of bicarbonate from the solution stabilizes the calcium, which may precipitate as calcium bicarbonate. It contains no antibacterial agent.
• Monitor for acid-base imbalance when large volume of solution is infused.

Patient education
• Explain need for I.V. therapy.
• Tell patient to report adverse reactions at once.

risperidone
Risperdal

Pharmacologic classification: benzisoxazole derivative
Therapeutic classification: antipsychotic
Pregnancy risk category C

How supplied
Available by prescription only
Tablets: 1 mg, 2 mg, 3 mg, 4 mg

Indications, route, and dosage
Psychosis
Adults: Initially, 1 mg P.O. b.i.d. Increase in increments of 1 mg b.i.d. on day 2 and 3 of treatment to a target dose of 3 mg b.i.d. Wait at least 1 week before adjusting dosage further. Doses above 6 mg/day were not found to be more effective than lower doses and were associated with more extrapyramidal effects.

✦ ***Dosage adjustment.*** Elderly or debilitated patients, hypotensive patients, or patients with severe renal or hepatic impairment should initially receive 0.5 mg P.O b.i.d. Increase dosage in increments of 0.5 mg b.i.d. on second and third day of treatment to target dosage of 1.5 mg P.O. b.i.d. Wait at least 1 week before increasing dosage further.

Pharmacodynamics
Antipsychotic action: Risperidone's exact mechanism of action is unknown. Its antipsychotic activity may be mediated through a combination of dopamine type 2 (D_2) and serotonin type 2 ($5\text{-}HT_2$) antagonism. Antagonism at receptors other than D_2 and $5\text{-}HT_2$ may explain other effects of drug.

Pharmacokinetics
• *Absorption:* Drug is well absorbed after oral administration. Absolute oral bioavailability is 70%. Food does not affect rate or extent of absorption.
• *Distribution:* Plasma protein binding is about 90% for drug and 77% for its major active metabolite, 9-hydroxyrisperidone.
• *Metabolism:* Drug is extensively metabolized in the liver to 9-hydroxyrisperidone, which is the predominant circulating species and appears approximately equi-effective with risperidone with respect to receptor binding activity. (About 6% to 8% of whites and a low percentage of Asians show little or no receptor binding activity and are "poor metabolizers").
• *Excretion:* Metabolite is excreted by the kidney. Clearance of drug and its metabolite is reduced in renally impaired patients.

Contraindications and precautions
Contraindicated in patients hypersensitive to drug and in breast-feeding patients. Use cautiously in patients with prolonged QT interval, CV disease, cerebrovascular disease, dehydration, hypovolemia, history of seizures, or exposure to extreme heat or conditions that could affect metabolism or hemodynamic responses.

Interactions
Carbamazepine may increase the clearance of risperidone, thereby decreasing the latter drug's effectiveness; monitor the patient closely. *Clozapine* may decrease the clearance of risperidone, increasing the risk of toxicity; monitor the patient closely. *Ethanol* and other *CNS depressants* may cause additive CNS depression when administered concomitantly; administer these drugs together with caution. Because of risperidone's potential for inducing hypotension, it may enhance the effects of certain *antihypertensive agents.* Risperidone may antagonize the effects of *levodopa* and *dopamine agonists.*

Effects on diagnostic tests
Risperidone may increase serum prolactin levels.

Adverse reactions
CNS: *somnolence, extrapyramidal symptoms, headache, insomnia, agitation, anxiety,* tardive dyskinesia, aggressiveness.

CV: tachycardia, chest pain, orthostatic hypotension, prolonged QT interval.
EENT: *rhinitis,* sinusitis, pharyngitis, abnormal vision.
GI: *constipation, nausea, vomiting, dyspepsia.*
Respiratory: coughing, upper respiratory infection.
Skin: rash, dry skin, photosensitivity.
Other: arthralgia, back pain, fever, ***neuroleptic malignant syndrome*** (rare).

Overdose and treatment

Signs and symptoms of overdosage result from an exaggeration of risperidone's known pharmacologic effects (drowsiness and sedation, tachycardia and hypotension, and extrapyramidal symptoms). Hyponatremia, hypokalemia, prolonged QT, widened QRS, and seizures also have been reported.

There is no specific antidote to risperidone overdosage; appropriate supportive measures should be instituted. Gastric lavage (after intubation, if patient is unconscious) and administration of activated charcoal with a laxative should be considered. CV monitoring is essential to detect possible arrhythmias. If antiarrhythmic therapy is administered, disopyramide, procainamide, and quinidine carry a theoretical hazard of QT-prolonging effects that might be additive to those of risperidone. Similarly, alpha-blocking properties of bretylium may be expected to be additive to those of risperidone, resulting in problematic hypotension.

☑ Special considerations

- Risperidone and 9-hydroxyrisperidone appear to lengthen the QT interval in some patients, although there is no average increase in treated patients, even at 12 to 16 mg/day (well above recommended dose). Other drugs that prolong the QT interval have been associated with torsades de pointes, a life-threatening arrhythmia. Bradycardia, electrolyte imbalance, concomitant use with other drugs that prolong the QT interval, or congenital prolongation of the QT interval can increase risk for occurrence of this arrhythmia.
- Drug has an antiemetic effect in animals; this may occur in humans, masking signs and symptoms of overdosage or of such conditions as intestinal obstruction, Reye's syndrome, and brain tumor.
- Tardive dyskinesia may occur after prolonged risperidone therapy. It may not appear until months or years later and may disappear spontaneously or persist for life despite discontinuation of drug.
- Neuroleptic malignant syndrome is rare, but in many cases fatal. It is not necessarily related to length of drug use or type of neuroleptic. Monitor patient closely for symptoms, including hyperpyrexia, muscle rigidity, altered mental status, irregular pulse, alteration in blood pressure, and diaphoresis.
- When restarting drug therapy for patients who have been off drug, follow initial 3-day dose initiation schedule.
- When switching patient from another antipsychotic agent to risperidone, immediately discontinue other antipsychotic agent on initiation of risperidone therapy when medically appropriate.

Patient education

- Advise patient to rise slowly from a recumbent or seated position to minimize light-headedness.
- Warn patient not to operate hazardous machinery, including driving a car, until drug's effects are known.
- Tell female patient to call if pregnancy is being planned or is suspected.
- Tell patient to call before taking new medications, including OTC drugs, because of potential for interactions.
- Advise patient to avoid alcohol during drug therapy.

Geriatric use

- A lower starting dose is recommended for elderly patients because they have decreased pharmacokinetic clearance; a greater incidence of hepatic, renal, or cardiac dysfunction; and a greater tendency toward postural hypotension.

Pediatric use

- Safety and effectiveness in children have not been established.

Breast-feeding

- Breast-feeding should be discontinued in patient receiving drug.

ritodrine hydrochloride

Yutopar

Pharmacologic classification: beta-receptor agonist
Therapeutic classification: adjunct in suppression of preterm labor
Pregnancy risk category B

How supplied

Available by prescription only
Injection (ampule): 10 mg/ml, 15 mg/ml
Injection (premixed): 0.3 mg/ml

Indications, route, and dosage

Management of preterm labor
Adults: Initially, 0.05 mg/minute I.V. infusion; increase q 10 minutes p.r.n. or until maternal heart rate is 130 beats/minute, in 0.05-mg increments to effective dose (usually, 0.15 to 0.35 mg/minute). Continue for at least 12 hours after uterine contractions cease. Dose should not exceed 0.35 mg/minute. Initiate oral 10 mg 30 minutes before I.V. infusion is discontinued, then 10 mg q 2 hours for 24 hours. Maintenance dose of 10 to 20 mg P.O. q 4 to 6 hours until term or until medical judgement dictates.

Pharmacodynamics

Tocolytic action: Ritodrine is a beta-receptor agonist that exerts a preferential effect on beta$_2$-adrenergic receptors (such as uterine smooth muscle). Stimulation of the beta$_2$-receptors inhibits contractility of the uterine smooth muscle. Ritodrine also may act to affect directly the interaction between actin and myosin in muscle to decrease the intensity and frequency of contractions.

Pharmacokinetics

- *Absorption:* Drug is 100% absorbed by I.V. route.
- *Distribution:* Peak ritodrine serum levels are 32 to 50 ng/ml after an I.V. infusion of 60 minutes. I.V. dose has a distribution half-life of 6 to 9 minutes.
- *Metabolism:* Drug is metabolized in the liver, primarily to inactive sulfate and glucuronide conjugates.
- *Excretion:* About 70% to 90% of I.V. dose is excreted in urine in 10 to 12 hours as unchanged drug and its conjugates. Drug can be removed by dialysis.

Contraindications and precautions

Contraindicated in pregnant women before 20th week of pregnancy and in women with antepartum hemorrhage, eclampsia, intrauterine fetal death, chorioamnionitis, maternal cardiac disease, pulmonary hypertension, maternal hyperthyroidism, or uncontrolled maternal diabetes mellitus. Also contraindicated in patients hypersensitive to drug or with preexisting maternal medical conditions that would seriously be affected by the known pharmacologic properties of drug, such as hypovolemia, pheochromocytoma, or uncontrolled hypertension.

Use cautiously in patients with sulfite allergies.

Interactions

Concomitant use of ritodrine with *corticosteroids* may produce additive diabetogenic effects, pulmonary edema, and possibly death in mother. Discontinue drugs if pulmonary edema occurs. Monitor patient closely during concurrent use.

Concomitant use with *beta blockers* (*propranolol*) may inhibit ritodrine's action. Avoid concurrent administration. Use with *sympathomimetic amines* may produce an additive effect (especially CV). Use together with caution.

Concurrent use with *diazoxide, magnesium sulfate,* or *meperidine* may potentiate CV effects. Use with atropine may worsen hypertension.

Effects on diagnostic tests

I.V. administration of ritodrine elevates the plasma insulin and glucose levels and decreases plasma potassium concentrations (values usually return to normal within 24 hours after drug is stopped).

Adverse reactions

CNS: nervousness; anxiety, *headache,* emotional upset, malaise (with I.V. administration); *tremor* (with oral administration).
CV: *palpitation; dose-related alterations in blood pressure, tachycardia,* ***pulmonary edema*** (with I.V. administration).
GI: *nausea, vomiting.*
Hematologic: leukopenia, ***agranulocytosis.***
Skin: rash.
Other: *erythema, hyperglycemia,* hypokalemia, *anaphylactic shock.*

Overdose and treatment

Overdose produces signs and symptoms similar to those of excessive beta-adrenergic stimulation (maternal and fetal tachycardia, palpitations, cardiac arrhythmia, hypotension, nervousness, tremor, nausea, and vomiting).

Treat I.V. overdose by stopping infusion and administering appropriate beta-adrenergic blocking agent (such as propranolol) as an antidote. Treat oral overdose by emptying stomach and administering activated charcoal. Subsequent treatment is supportive and symptomatic.

☑ Special considerations

- Because CV responses are common, especially during I.V. administration, CV effects—including maternal pulse rate and blood pressure and fetal heart rate—must be closely monitored. A maternal tachycardia of over 140 beats/minute or persistent respiratory rate of over 20 breaths/minute may be signs of impending pulmonary edema.
- Monitor blood glucose concentrations during ritodrine infusions, especially in mothers predisposed to diabetes mellitus.
- Discontinue drug if pulmonary edema occurs.
- Monitor amount of I.V. fluid administered, to prevent circulatory overload.
- Do not use drug I.V. if solution is discolored or contains a precipitate. Do not use more than 48 hours after preparation.
- Control infusion rate by use of a microdrip chamber I.V. infusion set or an infusion control device.
- Prepare I.V. solution by diluting 150 mg ritodrine in 500 ml of D_5W to produce a solution containing 300 mcg (0.3 mg) of ritodrine per milliliter. Use of NaCl diluents (0.9% NaCl, Ringer's solution, and Hartmann's solution) should be reserved for cases in which dextrose solution is medically undesirable due to increased probability of pulmonary edema.
- Place patient in left lateral recumbent position to reduce risk of hypotension.
- Drug may uncover previously unknown cardiac pathology. Sinus bradycardia may follow drug withdrawal.
- Maternal tachycardia or decreased diastolic blood pressure usually reverses with a dosage reduction but requires discontinuation of drug in 1% of patients.

Patient education

- Advise patient to adhere to scheduled follow-up appointments and to report adverse reactions promptly.

---

ritonavir

Norvir

Pharmacologic classification: HIV protease inhibitor
Therapeutic classification: antiviral
Pregnancy risk category B

How supplied

Available by prescription only
Capsules: 100 mg
Oral solution: 80 mg/ml

Indications, route, and dosage

Treatment of HIV infection when antiretroviral therapy is warranted

Adults: 600 mg P.O. b.i.d. with meals. If nausea occurs, increased dosage may provide some relief: 300 mg b.i.d. for 1 day, 400 mg b.i.d. for 2 days, 500 mg b.i.d. for 1 day, and then 600 mg b.i.d. thereafter.

Pharmacodynamics

Antiviral action: Ritonavir is a HIV protease inhibitor. HIV protease is an enzyme required for the proteolytic cleavage of the viral polyprotein precursors into the individual functional proteins found in infectious HIV. Ritonavir binds to the protease active site and inhibits the activity of the enzyme. This inhibition prevents cleavage of the viral polyproteins, resulting in the formation of immature noninfectious viral particles.

Pharmacokinetics

- *Absorption:* Drug is absorbed better when taken with food; its absolute bioavailability has not been determined.
- *Distribution:* Ritonavir is 98% to 99% bound to plasma proteins.
- *Metabolism:* Metabolized in the liver; P-450 3A (CYP3A) is the major isoform involved in ritonavir metabolism.
- *Excretion:* Drug is primarily excreted in feces, although a small amount has been found in the urine. Half-life is 3 to 5 hours.

Contraindications and precautions

Contraindicated in patients with hypersensitivity to any components of drug. Use cautiously in patients with hepatic insufficiency.

Interactions

Do not administer drug concurrently with *amiodarone, astemizole, bepridil, bupropion, cisapride, clozapine, encainide, flecainide, meperidine, piroxicam, propafenone, propoxyphene, quinidine,* and *rifabutin,* because ritonavir is expected to produce large increases in the plasma concentrations of these drugs, thus increasing the patient's risk of arrhythmias, hematologic abnormalities, seizures, or other potentially serious adverse effects.

Coadministration of ritonavir is also likely to produce large increases in *alprazolam, clorazepate, diazepam, estazolam, flurazepam, midazolam, triazolam,* and *zolpidem.* Because of the potential for extreme sedation and respiratory depression from these agents, they should not be co-administered with ritonavir.

Agents that increase CYP3A activity (for example, *carbamazepine, dexamethasone, phenytoin, rifabutin, rifampin, phenobarbital*) would be expected to increase the clearance of ritonavir resulting in decreased ritonavir plasma concentrations.

Tobacco use is associated with an 18% decrease in the area under the curve of ritonavir. Ritonavir may increase the activity of *glucuronosyltransferases*; thus, loss of therapeutic effects from directly *glucuronidated agents* during ritonavir therapy may signify need for dosage alteration of these agents. Concomitant use of any of these agents with ritonavir should also be accompanied by therapeutic drug concentration monitoring and increased monitoring of therapeutic and adverse effects, especially for agents with narrow therapeutic margins, such as *oral anticoagulants* or *immunosuppressants.* A dosage reduction greater than 50% may be required for those agents extensively metabolized by CYP3A.

Patients with impaired renal function receiving *clarithromycin* concomitantly with ritonavir require a 50% reduction in their clarithromycin if creatinine clearance is 30 to 60 ml/minute and a 75% reduction if it is below 30 ml/minute. Concomitant administration of *desipramine* may require a dosage adjustment when administered with ritonavir. Ritonavir formulations contain alcohol that can produce reactions when co-administered with *disulfiram* or *other drugs that produce disulfiram-like reactions* such as *metronidazole.*

Concomitant therapy with *oral contraceptives* may require a dosage increase in the oral contraceptive or alternate contraceptive measures. Increased dosage of *theophylline* may be required when coadministered with ritonavir.

Effects on diagnostic tests

Ritonavir may cause alterations in triglycerides, AST, ALT, gamma-glutamyltransferase, CK, and uric acid levels.

Adverse reactions

CNS: *asthenia,* headache, malaise, circumoral paresthesia, dizziness, insomnia, paresthesia, peripheral paresthesia, somnolence, thinking abnormality, *taste perversion,* migraine headache, syncope, abnormal dreams, abnormal gait, agitation, amnesia, anxiety, aphasia, ataxia, confusion, depression, diplopia, emotional lability, euphoria, ***generalized tonic-clonic seizure,*** hallucinations, hyperesthesia, incoordination, decreased libido, nervousness, neuralgia, neuropathy, paralysis, peripheral neuropathy, peripheral sensory neuropathy, personality disorder, tremor, vertigo.

CV: vasodilation, hemorrhage, hypertension, palpation, peripheral vascular disorder, orthostatic hypotension, tachycardia.

EENT: abnormal electrooculogram, abnormal electroretinogram, abnormal vision, amblyopia, blurred vision, blepharitis, epistaxis, ear pain, eye pain, hearing impairment, hiccup, increased cerumen, iritis, parosmia, pharyngitis, photophobia, rhinitis, taste loss, tinnitus, uveitis, visual field defect.

GI: abdominal pain, anorexia, constipation, *diarrhea, nausea, vomiting,* dyspepsia, flatulence, enlarged abdomen, abnormal stools, bloody diarrhea, cheilitis, cholangitis, colitis, dry mouth, dysphagia, eructation, esophagitis, gastritis, gastroenteritis, GI disorder, GI hemorrhage, gingivitis, hepatitis, hepatomegaly, ileitis, liver damage, liver function tests abnormality, mouth ulcer, oral moniliasis, pancreatitis, periodontal abscess, rectal disorder, tenesmus, thirst.

GU: kidney pain, dysuria, hematuria, impotence, kidney calculus, kidney failure, nocturia, penis dis-

order, polyuria, pyelonephritis, urethritis, urine retention, urinary frequency.
Hematologic: anemia, ecchymosis, leukopenia, lymphadenopathy, lymphocytosis, ***thrombocytopenia.***
Metabolic: altered hormonal levels, diabetes mellitus, avitaminosis, glycosuria, gout, hypercholesteremia.
Musculoskeletal: arthralgia, arthrosis, joint disorder, muscle cramps, muscle weakness, myalgia, myositis, and twitching.
Respiratory: asthma, dyspnea, hypoventilation, increased cough, interstitial pneumonia, lung disorder.
Skin: rash, sweating, photosensitivity reaction, acne, contact dermatitis, dry skin, eczema, folliculitis, maculopapular rash, molluscum contagiosum, pruritus, psoriasis, seborrhea, urticaria, vesiculobullous rash.
Other: fever, local throat irritation, increased CK level, hyperlipidemia, allergic reaction, back pain, cachexia, chest pain, chills, facial edema, facial pain, flu syndrome, hypothermia, neck pain, neck rigidity, pain (unspecified, substernal chest pain, peripheral edema, dehydration, edema).

Overdose and treatment

Information is limited to one patient who reported paresthesia, which resolved after the dose was decreased. Treatment consists of general supportive measures. Emesis or gastric lavage may be used as well as activated charcoal. Dialysis is not likely to be beneficial.

☑ Special considerations

- Drug may be administered alone or in combination with nucleoside analogues.
- GI tolerance may be improved in patients initiating combination regimens with ritonavir and nucleosides by initiating ritonavir alone and subsequently adding nucleosides before completing 2 weeks of ritonavir monotherapy.

Patient education

- Inform patient that drug is not a cure for HIV infection. He may continue to develop opportunistic infections and other complications associated with HIV infection. Drug has also not been shown to reduce risk of transmitting HIV to others through sexual contact or blood contamination.
- Caution patient not to adjust dosage or discontinue ritonavir therapy without medical approval.
- Tell patient that he may improve taste of oral solution by mixing with chocolate milk, Ensure, or Advera within 1 hour of dosing.
- Instruct patient to take drug with meals to improve absorption.
- Tell patient that if a dose is missed, he should take the next dose as soon as possible. However, if a dose is skipped, he should not double the next dose.
- Advise patient to report use of other medications, including OTC drugs, because of drug interactions.

Pediatric use

- Safety and effectiveness in children under age 12 have not been established.

Breast-feeding

- It is not known if ritonavir is excreted in breast milk. However, HIV-positive women should not breast-feed to prevent transmission of infection.

rituximab

Rituxan

Pharmacologic classification: monoclonal antibody
Therapeutic classification: antineoplastic
Pregnancy risk factor C

How supplied

Available by prescription only
Injection: 10 mg/ml; 10 ml, 50 ml single-use vials

Indications, route & dosage

Treatment of patients with relapsed or refractory low-grade or follicular, CD20 positive, B-cell nonHodgkin's lymphoma
Adults: 375 mg/m^2 I.V. infusion once weekly for four doses (days 1, 8, 15, 22). Initial infusion should be started at 50 mg/hour. If hypersensitivity or infusion-related events do not occur, increase rate 50 mg/hour q 30 minutes to maximum of 400 mg/hour. Administer subsequent infusions at initial rate of 100 mg/hour and increase by increments of 100 mg/hour at 30-minute intervals, to maximum of 400 mg/hour as tolerated.

Pharmacodynamics

Antineoplastic action: A murine/human monoclonal antibody directed against CD20 antigen found on the surface of normal and malignant B-lymphocytes. CD20 regulates early steps in cell cycle initiation and differentiation processes. Binding to this antigen mediates the lysis of the B cells.

Pharmacokinetics

- *Absorption:* No information available.
- *Distribution:* No information available.
- *Metabolism:* No information available.
- *Excretion:* No information available.

Contraindications and precautions

Contraindicated in patients with known type I hypersensitivity or anaphylactic reactions to murine proteins or to any component of drug.

Patients with preexisting cardiac conditions, including arrhythmias and angina, could have recurrences during drug therapy and should be monitored throughout infusion period.

Interactions

None reported.

Effects on diagnostic tests

None reported.

Adverse reactions

CNS: dizziness, *asthenia, headache,* fatigue, paresthesia, malaise, agitation, insomnia, hypesthesia, hypertonia, nervousness, anxiety.
CV: *hypotension,* ***arrhythmias,*** hypertension, peripheral edema, chest pain, tachycardia, orthostatic hypotension, bradycardia.
EENT: sore throat, rhinitis, sinusitis, lacrimation disorder, conjunctivitis.
GI: *nausea,* vomiting, abdominal pain or enlargement, diarrhea, dyspepsia, anorexia, increased lactate dehydrogenase, taste perversion.
Hematologic: LEUKOPENIA, ***thrombocytopenia, neutropenia,*** anemia.
Musculoskeletal: arthralgia, myalgia.
Respiratory: ***bronchospasm,*** dyspnea, cough increase, bronchitis.
Skin: *pruritus, rash,* urticaria, flushing.
Other: ANGIOEDEMA, *fever, chills, rigor,* back pain, pain, hyperglycemia, hypocalcemia, pain at injection site, tumor pain.

Overdose and treatment

No information available.

☑ Special considerations

- Drug must be given as I.V. infusion; do not give as an I.V. push or bolus. Drug may be diluted to a final concentration of 1 to 4 mg/ml in 0.9% NaCl solution or D_5W.
- Consider premedicating patient with acetaminophen and diphenhydramine before each infusion as hypersensitivity reactions may occur.
- Monitor patient closely for signs and symptoms of hypersensitivity reaction.
- Hypotension, bronchospasm, and angioedema have occurred as part of an infusion-related symptom complex. Have medications such as epinephrine, diphenhydramine, and corticosteroids available to immediately treat such a reaction. Monitor patient's blood pressure closely during infusion. If an infusion-related symptom complex occurs, discontinue infusion and restart at a 50% rate reduction when symptoms resolve. Recommended symptom treatment includes acetaminophen, diphenhydramine; bronchodilators or I.V. saline may be indicated. In most cases, patients have been able to proceed with a full course of drug therapy.
- Perform cardiac monitoring during and after subsequent drug infusions in patients who develop clinically significant infusion-related symptoms.
- Discontinue infusion if serious or life-threatening cardiac arrhythmias occur.
- Human anti-murine antibody (HAMA) and human antichimeric antibody (HACA) have been detected in less than 1% of patients in clinical trials. If HAMA or HACA titers develop, patient may develop allergic or hypersensitivity reactions to drug or other murine or chimeric monoclonal antibody preparations.
- Immunization safety or efficacy during drug therapy has not been studied.
- Obtain CBCs at regular intervals and more frequently in patients who develop cytopenias.
- Because transient hypotension may occur during infusion, consider withholding antihypertensive medications 12 hours before infusion.

Patient education

- Tell patient to report symptoms during and after infusion.
- Advise patient to inform primary health care provider of history of cardiac problems.
- Instruct patient not to receive any vaccinations (especially live viral vaccines) during drug therapy unless approved by primary health care provider.
- Inform patient that frequent CBCs may be necessary.

Pediatric use

- Safety and effectiveness in children have not been established.

Breast-feeding

- It is unknown if drug occurs in breast milk. Because other antibodies can occur, advise patient to stop breast-feeding until circulation levels of drug are undetectable.

rocuronium bromide

Zemuron

Pharmacologic classification: nondepolarizing neuromuscular blocker
Therapeutic classification: skeletal muscle relaxant
Pregnancy risk category B

How supplied

Injection: 10 mg/ml

Indications, route, and dosage

Adjunct to general anesthesia, facilitation of endotracheal intubation, or skeletal muscle relaxation during surgery or mechanical ventilation

Adults and children age 3 months or older: Initially, 0.6 to 1.2 mg/kg I.V. bolus. In most patients, tracheal intubation may be performed within 2 minutes; muscle paralysis should last about 31 minutes. Maintenance dosage of 0.1 mg/kg should provide an additional 12 minutes of muscle relaxation (0.15 mg/kg will add 17 minutes; 0.2 mg/kg will add 24 minutes).

Note: Dosage depends on anesthetic used, individual needs, and response. Dosages are representative and must be adjusted.

Pharmacodynamics

Skeletal muscle relaxation action: Rocuronium acts by competing for cholinergic receptors at the motor end plate. This action is antagonized by acetylcholinesterase inhibitors, such as neostigmine and edrophonium.

Pharmacokinetics

- *Absorption:* Not applicable with I.V. administration.

• *Distribution:* Rapid distribution half-life is 1 to 2 minutes; slower distribution half-life is 14 to 18 minutes. Drug is approximately 30% bound to plasma proteins.
• *Metabolism:* Information not available, but hepatic clearance could be significant. The rocuronium analogue 17-desacetyl-rocuronium, a metabolite, has rarely been observed in plasma or urine.
• *Excretion:* Approximately 33% of administered dose recovered in the urine within 24 hours.

Contraindications and precautions

Contraindicated in patients with hypersensitivity to bromides. Use cautiously in patients with hepatic disease, severe obesity, bronchogenic carcinoma, electrolyte disturbances, neuromuscular disease, or altered circulation time caused by CV, age, or edematous states.

Interactions

Enflurane and *isoflurane* may prolong duration of action of initial and maintenance doses of rocuronium and decrease the average infusion requirement of rocuronium by 40% compared with opioid, nitrous oxide, oxygen anesthesia. Patients chronically receiving *anticonvulsant therapy*, such as *carbamazepine* or *phenytoin*, may develop a form of diminished magnitude of neuromuscular block or shortened clinical duration. Drugs that may enhance the neuromuscular blocking action of rocuronium include *antibiotics*, such as *aminoglycosides, bacitracin, colistimethate sodium, colistin, polymyxins, tetracylines,* and *vancomycin*. An injection of *quinidine* during recovery from rocuronium may cause recurrent paralysis.

Effects on diagnostic tests

None reported.

Adverse reactions

CV: tachycardia, abnormal ECG, ***arrhythmias*** (rare), transient hypotension, hypertension.
GI: nausea, vomiting.
Respiratory: asthma.
Skin: rash, edema, pruritus.
Other: hiccups.

Overdose and treatment

No cases of rocuronium overdose have been reported. Overdosage with neuromuscular blocking agents may result in neuromuscular block beyond the time needed for surgery and anesthesia. Primary treatment is maintenance of a patent airway and controlled ventilation until patient recovers normal neuromuscular function. After initial evidence of such recovery is observed, further recovery may be facilitated by administration of an anticholinesterase agent (such as neostigmine or edrophonium) in conjunction with an appropriate anticholinergic agent.

☑ Special considerations

• Drug should be used only by personnel experienced in airway management.
• Keep airway clear. Have emergency respiratory support equipment (endotracheal equipment, ventilator, oxygen, atropine, edrophonium, epinephrine, and neostigmine) available.
• Neuromuscular blockers do not obtund consciousness or alter the pain threshold. Patients should receive sedatives or general anesthetics before neuromuscular blockers are administered.
• Drug is well tolerated in patients with renal failure.
• In obese patients, initial dose should be based on patient's actual body weight.
• A peripheral nerve stimulator should be used to measure neuromuscular function during drug administration to monitor drug effect, determine need for additional doses, and confirm recovery from neuromuscular block. Once spontaneous recovery starts, drug-induced neuromuscular blockade may be reversed with an anticholinesterase agent.
• Drug, which has an acid pH, should not be mixed with alkaline solutions (such as barbiturate solutions) in same syringe or administered simultaneously during I.V. infusion through same needle.
• Store reconstituted solution in refrigerator. Discard after 24 hours.

Pediatric use

• Use of rocuronium in children under age 3 months has not been studied.

ropinirole hydrochloride

Requip

Pharmacologic classification: nonergoline dopamine agonist
Therapeutic classification: antiparkinsonian
Pregnancy risk category C

How supplied

Available by prescription only
Tablets: 0.25 mg, 0.5 mg, 1 mg, 2 mg, 5 mg

Indications, route and dosage

Treatment of signs and symptoms of idiopathic Parkinson's disease
Adults: Initially, 0.25 mg P.O. t.i.d. Based on patient response, dosage should then be titrated at weekly intervals: 0.5 mg t.i.d. after week 1, 0.75 mg t.i.d. after week 2, and 1 mg t.i.d. after week 3. After week 4, dosage may be increased by 1.5 mg/day on a weekly basis up to a dose of 9 mg/day and then increased weekly by up to 3 mg/day to maximum dose of 24 mg/day.

Pharmacodynamics

Antiparkinsonian action: Exact mechanism of action is unknown. Ropinirole is a nonergoline dopamine agonist thought to stimulate postsynaptic dopamine D_2 receptors within the caudate-putamen in the brain.

Pharmacokinetics

• *Absorption:* Rapidly absorbed reaching peak concentration in approximately 1 to 2 hours. Absolute bioavailability is 55%.

• *Distribution:* Widely distributed throughout the body, with an apparent volume of distribution of 7.5 L/kg. Up to 40% is bound to plasma proteins.
• *Metabolism:* Extensively metabolized by cytochrome P-450 CYP1A2 isoenzyme to inactive metabolites.
• *Excretion:* Less than 10% of the administered dose is excreted unchanged in the urine. Elimination half-life is 6 hours.

Contraindications and precautions

Contraindicated in patients with known hypersensitivity to drug or its components. Use cautiously in patients with severe renal or hepatic impairment.

Interactions

CNS depressants (antidepressants, antipsychotics, benzodiazepines) increase CNS effects. Use cautiously. *Estrogens* reduce clearance of ropinirole. Adjust ropinirole dose if estrogens are started or stopped during ropinirole treatment.

Inhibitors or substrates of cytochrome P-450 CYP1A2 (ciprofloxacin, fluvoxamine, mexiletine, norfloxacin) alter clearance. Dosage adjustment of ropinirole may be required.

Ciprofloxacin causes an increase in ropinirole concentrations when coadministered. *Dopamine antagonists (butyrophenones, metoclopramide, phenothiazines, thioxanthenes)* may decrease the effectiveness of ropinirole when administered concomitantly. *Smoking* may increase clearance of ropinirole. Monitor closely.

Effects on diagnostic tests

None reported.

Adverse reactions

Early Parkinson's disease (without levodopa)—
CNS: asthenia, hallucinations, *dizziness,* aggravated Parkinson's disease, *somnolence, fatigue,* headache, confusion, hyperkinesia, hypesthesia, vertigo, amnesia, impaired concentration, malaise.
CV: orthostatic hypotension, orthostatic symptoms, hypertension, *syncope,* edema, chest pain, extrasystoles, ***atrial fibrillation,*** palpitation, tachycardia.
EENT: pharyngitis, dry mouth, abnormal vision, eye abnormality, xerophthalmia, rhinitis, sinusitis.
GI: *nausea, vomiting, dyspepsia,* flatulence, abdominal pain, anorexia, abdominal pain.
GU: urinary tract infection, impotence.
Respiratory: bronchitis; dyspnea.
Skin: flushing, increased sweating.
Other: *viral infection,* pain, yawning, peripheral ischemia.
Advanced Parkinson's disease (with levodopa)—
CNS: *dizziness,* aggravated parkinsonism, *somnolence, headache,* insomnia, *hallucinations,* abnormal dreaming, confusion, tremor, *dyskinesia,* anxiety, nervousness, amnesia, hypokinesia, paresthesia, paresis.
CV: hypotension, syncope.
EENT: diplopia, dry mouth.
GI: *nausea,* abdominal pain, vomiting, constipation, diarrhea, dysphagia, flatulence, increased saliva.
GU: urinary tract infection, pyuria, urinary incontinence.
Hematologic: anemia.
Metabolic: weight decrease.
Musculoskeletal: arthralgia, arthritis.
Respiratory: upper respiratory infection, dyspnea.
Skin: increased sweating.
Other: injury, *falls,* viral infection, increased drug level, pain.

Overdose and treatment

There are reports of 10 patients ingesting more than 24 mg/day. Symptoms of overdosage include mild or facial dyskinesia, agitation, increased dyskinesia, grogginess, sedation, orthostatic hypotension, chest pain, confusion, vomiting, and nausea. Treatment involves general supportive measures and removal of unabsorbed drug.

☑ Special considerations

• Dosage adjustment is not needed in patients with mild to moderate renal impairment.
• Titrate drug with caution in patients with severe renal or hepatic impairment.
• Drug may cause increased alkaline phosphatase and BUN levels.
• Although not reported with ropinirole, a symptom complex resembling neuroleptic malignant syndrome (elevated temperature, muscular rigidity, altered consciousness, and autonomic instability) has been reported with rapid dose reduction or withdrawal of antiparkinsonian agents. If this occurs, stop drug gradually over 7 days and reduce frequency of administration to twice daily for 4 days and then once daily over the remaining 3 days.
• Symptomatic hypotension may occur due to dopamine agonists impairment of systemic regulation of blood pressure. Monitor patient carefully for orthostatic hypotension, especially during dose escalation.
• Syncope, with or without bradycardia, has been reported. Monitor patient carefully, especially after 4 weeks of initiation of therapy and with dosage increases.
• Know that other adverse events reported with dopaminergic therapy may occur with ropinirole; these include withdrawal emergent hyperpyrexia and confusion, and fibrotic complications.
• Ropinirole can potentiate the dopaminergic adverse effects of levodopa and may cause or exacerbate existing dyskinesia. If this occurs, the dose of levodopa may need to be decreased.

Patient education

• Inform patient to take drug with food to reduce nausea.
• Advise patient that hallucinations may occur. Elderly patients are at greater risk than younger patients with Parkinson's disease.
• Instruct patient to rise slowly after sitting or lying down because of risk of postural hypotension, which may occur during initial therapy or after a dosage increase.
• Advise patient to use caution when driving or operating machinery until CNS effects of drug are known.

• Advise patient to avoid alcohol and other CNS depressants.
• Tell female patient to notify primary health care provider if pregnancy is suspected or is being planned; also to inform primary health care provider if she is breast-feeding.

Geriatric use
• Dosage adjustments are not necessary.

Pediatric use
• Safety and effectiveness in children have not been established.

Breast-feeding
• Drug inhibits prolactin secretion in humans and could potentially inhibit lactation. It is not known if drug is excreted in breast milk. A decision should be made whether to discontinue the drug or breast-feeding, taking into account the importance of drug to the mother.

ropivacaine hydrochloride
Naropin

Pharmacologic classification: aminoamide
Therapeutic classification: local anesthetic
Pregnancy risk category B

How supplied
Available by prescription only
E-Z off single-dose vials: 7.5 mg/ml, 10 mg/ml in 10-ml vials
Single-dose vials: 2 mg/ml, 7.5 mg/ml, 10 mg/ml in 20-ml vials; 5 mg/ml in 30-ml vials
Single-dose ampules: 2 mg/ml, 7.5 mg/ml, 10 mg/ml in 20-ml ampules; 5 mg/ml in 30-ml ampules
Infusion bottles: 2 mg/ml in 100-ml and 200-ml bottles
Sterile-pak single-dose vials: 2 mg/ml, 7.5 mg/ml, 10 mg/ml in 20-ml vials; 5 mg/ml in 30-ml vials

Indications, route, and dosage
Surgical anesthesia
Adults: Lumbar epidural administration in surgery: 75 to 200 mg doses (duration, 2 to 6 hours). Lumbar epidural administration for cesarean section: 100 to 150 mg (duration, 2 to 4 hours). Thoracic epidural administration: 25 to 75 mg doses to establish block for postoperative pain relief. Major nerve block (for example, brachial plexus block): 175 to 250 mg (duration, 5 to 8 hours). Field block (such as minor nerve blocks and infiltration): 5 to 200 mg (duration, 2 to 6 hours).
Labor pain management
Adults: Lumbar epidural administration: initially, 20 to 40 mg (duration, 0.5 to 1.5 hours), then 12 to 28 mg/hour as continuous infusion or 20 to 30 mg/hour as incremental "top-up" injections.
Postoperative pain management
Adults: Lumbar epidural administration: 12 to 20 mg/hour as continuous infusion. Thoracic epidural administration: 8 to 16 mg/hour as continuous infusion. For infiltration (minor nerve block): 2 to 200 mg (duration, 2 to 6 hours).

Pharmacodynamics
Anesthetic action: Drug blocks the generation and conduction of nerve impulses, presumably by increasing the threshold for electrical excitation in the nerve by slowing the propagation of the nerve impulse and by reducing the rate of the action potential. Generally, progression of anesthesia is related to the diameter, myelination and conduction velocity of affected nerve fibers. Clinically, the order of loss of nerve function is as follows: pain, temperature, touch, proprioception, and skeletal muscle tone.

Pharmacokinetics
• *Absorption:* Absorption depends on total dose and concentration of administered drug, route of administration, patient's hemodynamic or circulatory condition, and vascularity of administration site. From the epidural space, drug shows complete and biphasic absorption; mean half-lives of two phases are 14 minutes and 4.2 hours, respectively. The slow absorption is a rate-limiting factor in elimination of drug. Terminal half-life is longer after epidural than after I.V. administration.
• *Distribution:* After intravascular infusion, drug has steady-state volume of distribution of 41 ± 7 L. Drug is 94% protein-bound, mainly to alpha$_1$ acid glycoprotein. An increase in total plasma concentrations during continuous epidural infusion has been observed, secondary to a postoperative increase in alpha$_1$ acid glycoprotein.
• *Metabolism:* Extensively metabolized in the liver, via cytochrome P-4501A to 3-hydroxy ropivacaine. Approximately 37% of dose is excreted in the urine as free drug and as a conjugated metabolites. Urinary excretion of metabolites accounts for only 3% of dose.
• *Excretion:* Primarily by the kidney; 86% of the dose is excreted in the urine after I.V. administration of which only 1% relates to unchanged drug.

Contraindications and precautions
Contraindicated in patients with known hypersensitivity to drug or local anesthetics of amide type.

Use with caution in debilitated, elderly, and acutely ill patients because accumulation may result. Also use cautiously in patients with hypotension, hypovolemia, impaired CV function, or heart block and in those with hepatic disease, especially repeat doses of drug.

Interactions
Amide-type anesthetics effects are additive if given with ropivacaine. Use with caution. Concomitant use with *fluvoxamine, imipramine, theophylline,* and *verapamil* may result in competitive inhibition of ropivacaine. Use with caution.

Effects on diagnostic tests
None reported.

Adverse reactions

CNS: anxiety, dizziness, headache, hypoesthesia, pain, paresthesia.
CV: *bradycardia*, chest pain, *hypotension*, hypertension, tachycardia.
GI: *nausea*, neonatal vomiting, vomiting.
GU: oliguria, urine retention.
Hematologic: anemia.
Hepatic: neonatal jaundice.
Respiratory: ***neonatal tachypnea, respiratory distress.***
Skin: pruritus.
Other: back pain, FETAL BRADYCARDIA, ***fetal tachycardia***, FETAL DISTRESS, fever, neonatal fever, postoperative complications, rigors.

Overdose and treatment

Treatment should be supportive and symptomatic. Discontinue drug. In case of unintentional subarachnoid injection of drug, establish a patent airway and administer 100% oxygen. This may prevent seizures if they have not already occurred. Administer medication to control seizures as needed.

☑ Special considerations

- Do not inject drug rapidly. Have emergency equipment and personnel immediately available.
- Drug should only be used by personnel familiar with use of drug.
- Increase doses in incremental steps.
- Do not use in emergency situations where a rapid onset of surgical anesthesia is necessary. Drug should not be used for production of obstetric paracervical block anesthesia, retrobulbar block, or spinal anesthesia (subarachnoid block) because of insufficient data to support use. I.V. regional anesthesia (bier block) should not be performed because of lack of clinical experience and risk of obtaining toxic blood levels of ropivacaine.
- To reduce risk of potentially serious adverse reactions, attempts should be made to optimize patient who may be at risk, such as those with complete heart block, and hepatic or renal impairment.
- Use an adequate test dose (3 to 5 ml of short-acting local anesthetic solution containing epinephrine) before induction of complete block.
- Early signs of CNS toxicity include restlessness, anxiety, incoherent speech, light-headedness, numbness and tingling of mouth and lips, metallic taste, tinnitus, dizziness, blurred vision, tremors, twitching, depression, or drowsiness.
- Do not use drug in ophthalmic surgery.

Patient education

- Tell patient that he may experience a temporary loss of sensation and motor activity in the anesthetized body part following proper administration of lumbar epidural anesthesia. Also explain adverse reactions that may occur.

Pediatric use

- Drug is not recommended in children under age 12.

Breast-feeding

- Excretion of drug in breast milk has not been studied; use with caution.

rubella and mumps virus vaccine, live

Biavax II

Pharmacologic classification: vaccine
Therapeutic classification: viral vaccine
Pregnancy risk category C

How supplied

Available by prescription only
Injection: single-dose vial containing not less than 1,000 $TCID_{50}$ (tissue culture infective doses) of the Wistar RA 27/3 rubella virus (propagated in human diploid cell culture) and not less than 20,000 $TCID_{50}$ of the Jeryl Lynn mumps strain (grown in chick embryo cell culture)

Indications, route, and dosage

Rubella (German measles) and mumps immunization
Adults and children over age 1: 1 vial (0.5 ml) S.C. in outer aspect of the upper arm.

Pharmacodynamics

Live rubella and mumps prophylaxis: Vaccine promotes active immunity to rubella and mumps by inducing production of antibodies.

Pharmacokinetics

- *Absorption:* Antibodies are usually detectable within 2 to 6 weeks; duration of vaccine-induced immunity is expected to be lifelong.
- *Distribution:* No information available.
- *Metabolism:* No information available.
- *Excretion:* No information available.

Contraindications and precautions

Contraindicated in pregnant or immunosuppressed patients; in those with cancer, blood dyscrasia, gamma globulin disorders, fever, active untreated tuberculosis, or history of anaphylaxis or anaphylactoid reactions to neomycin or eggs; and in those receiving corticosteroids (except those receiving corticosteroids as replacement therapy) or radiation therapy.

Interactions

Concomitant use of rubella and mumps vaccine with *immune serum globulin* or transfusions of *blood and blood products* may impair the immune response to the vaccine. Defer vaccination for 3 months in these situations. The administration of *immunosuppressive agents* may interfere with the response to vaccine.

Effects on diagnostic tests

Rubella and mumps vaccine temporarily may decrease the response to tuberculin skin testing. Should a tuberculin skin test be necessary, administer it either before or simultaneously with rubella and mumps vaccine.

Adverse reactions

Other: polyneuritis, rash, thrombocytopenic purpura, urticaria, fever, diarrhea, arthritis, arthralgia, ***anaphylaxis,*** lymphadenopathy; pain, erythema, induration (at injection site).

Overdose and treatment

No information available.

☑ Special considerations

- Obtain a thorough history of allergies (especially to antibiotics, eggs, chicken, or chicken feathers) and of reactions to immunizations.
- Perform skin testing first to assess vaccine sensitivity (against a control of 0.9% NaCl solution in the opposite arm) in patients with history of anaphylactoid reactions to egg ingestion. Administer intradermal or scratch test with a 1:10 dilution. Read results after 5 to 30 minutes. Positive reaction is a wheal with or without pseudopodia and surrounding erythema.
- Epinephrine solution 1:1,000 should be available to treat allergic reactions.
- Rubella and mumps vaccine should not be given less than 1 month before or after immunization with other live virus vaccines—except for monovalent or trivalent live poliovirus vaccine or live, attenuated measles virus vaccine, which may be administered simultaneously.
- Use only the diluent supplied. Discard reconstituted vaccine after 8 hours.
- Inject S.C. (not I.M.) into the outer aspect of the upper arm.
- Revaccination or booster is not required if patient was previously vaccinated at age 1 or older; however, there is no conclusive evidence of an increased risk of adverse reactions for persons who are already immune when vaccinated.
- Women who have rubella antibody titers of 1:8 or greater (by hemagglutination inhibition) need not be vaccinated with the rubella vaccine component.
- Vaccine will not offer protection when given after exposure to natural rubella or mumps, but there is no evidence that it would be harmful.
- Although rubella vaccine administration should be deferred in patients with febrile illness, it may be administered to susceptible children with mild illness such as upper respiratory infection.
- According to Centers for Disease Control and Prevention recommendations, measles, mumps, and rubella is the preferred vaccine.
- Women who are not immune to rubella are at risk of congenital rubella injury to the fetus if exposed to it during pregnancy.
- Store vaccine at 36° to 46° F (2° to 8° C) and protect from light. Solution may be used if red, pink, or yellow, but it must be clear.

Patient education

- Tell patient that tingling sensations in the extremities or joint aches and pains that may resemble arthritis, may occur beginning several days to several weeks after vaccination. These symptoms usually resolve within 1 week. Pain and inflammation at injection site and low-grade fever, rash, or breathing difficulties may also occur. Encourage patient to report distressing adverse reactions.
- Recommend acetaminophen to relieve fever or other minor discomfort.
- Tell female patients of childbearing age to avoid pregnancy for 3 months after immunization. Provide contraceptive information if necessary.

Pediatric use

- Live rubella and mumps virus vaccine is not recommended for children under age 1 because retained maternal antibodies may interfere with immune response.

Breast-feeding

- Some reports have demonstrated transfer of rubella virus or virus antigen into breast milk in approximately 68% of patients. Few adverse effects have been associated with breast-feeding after immunization with rubella-containing vaccines. Therefore, use caution when administering vaccine to breast-feeding patients.

rubella virus vaccine, live

Meruvax II

Pharmacologic classification: vaccine
Therapeutic classification: viral vaccine
Pregnancy risk category C

How supplied

Available by prescription only
Injection: single-dose vial containing not less than 1,000 $TCID_{50}$ (tissue culture infective doses) of the Wistar RA 27/3 strain of rubella virus propagated in human diploid cell culture

Indications, route, and dosage

Rubella (German measles) immunization
Adults and children over age 1: 1 vial (0.5 ml) S.C.

Pharmacodynamics

Rubella prophylaxis: Vaccine promotes active immunity to rubella by inducing production of antibodies.

Pharmacokinetics

- *Absorption:* Antibodies are usually detectable 2 to 6 weeks after injection; duration of vaccine-induced immunity is expected to be lifelong.
- *Distribution:* No information available.
- *Metabolism:* No information available.
- *Excretion:* No information available.

Contraindications and precautions

Contraindicated in pregnant or immunosuppressed patients; in those with cancer, blood dyscrasia, gamma globulin disorders, fever, active untreated tuberculosis, or history of hypersensitivity to neomycin; and in patients receiving corticosteroid (except those receiving corticosteroids as replacement therapy) or radiation therapy.

Interactions

Concomitant use of rubella vaccine with *immune serum globulin* or transfusions of *blood and blood products* may impair the immune response to the vaccine. If possible, defer vaccination for 3 months in these situations.

Effects on diagnostic tests

Rubella vaccine may temporarily decrease response to *tuberculin skin testing.* If a tuberculin test is necessary, administer it either before, simultaneously with, or at least 8 weeks after rubella vaccine.

Adverse reactions

Other: polyneuritis, rash, thrombocytopenic purpura, urticaria, arthralgia, malaise, headache, sore throat, fever, arthritis, ***anaphylaxis,*** lymphadenopathy; pain, erythema, induration (at injection site).

Overdose and treatment

No information available.

☑ Special considerations

- Obtain a thorough history of allergies, especially to antibiotics, and of reactions to immunizations.
- Epinephrine solution 1:1,000 should be available to treat allergic reactions.
- Do not give rubella vaccine less than 1 month before or after immunization with other live virus vaccines—except for monovalent or trivalent live poliovirus vaccine; live, attenuated measles virus vaccine; or live mumps virus vaccine, which may be administered simultaneously.
- Do not inject I.M. Inject S.C. into the outer aspect of the upper arm.
- Use only diluent supplied. Discard 8 hours after reconstituting.
- Store vaccine at 36° to 46° F (2° to 8° C), and protect from light. Solution may be used if red, pink, or yellow, but it must be clear.
- Vaccine will not offer protection when given after exposure to natural rubella, although there is no evidence that it would be harmful.
- Revaccination or booster dose is required if patient was previously vaccinated under age 1. The Advisory Committee on Immunization Practices and the American Academy of Pediatrics currently recommend that a second dose be routinely given at age 4 to 6 or 11 to 12. It may be given at any other time provided at least 1 month has elapsed since the first dose. There is no conclusive evidence of an increased risk of adverse reactions for persons who are already immune when revaccinated.
- Although rubella vaccine administration should be deferred in patients with febrile illness, it may be administered to susceptible children with mild illnesses such as upper respiratory infection.
- Women who are not immune to rubella are at risk of congenital rubella injury to the fetus if exposed to rubella during pregnancy.
- Women who have rubella antibody titers of 1:8 or greater (by hemagglutination inhibition) need not be vaccinated with rubella virus vaccine.

Patient education

- Tell patient to expect tingling sensations in the extremities or joint aches and pains that may resemble arthritis, to occur beginning several days to several weeks after vaccination. The symptoms usually resolve within 1 week. Pain and inflammation at injection site and low-grade fever, rash, or breathing difficulties may also occur. Encourage patient to report distressing reactions.
- Recommend acetaminophen to relieve fever or other minor discomfort after vaccination.
- Tell women of childbearing age to avoid pregnancy for 3 months after rubella immunization. Provide contraceptive information if necessary.

Pediatric use

- Live, attenuated rubella virus vaccine is not recommended for children under age 1 because retained maternal antibodies may impair immune response.

Breast-feeding

- Although early studies failed to show evidence of attenuated rubella virus in breast milk, subsequent reports showed transfer of rubella virus or virus antigen into breast milk in approximately 68% of patients. Few adverse effects have been associated with breast-feeding after immunization with rubella-containing vaccines. Risk-benefit ratio suggests that breast-feeding women may be immunized if necessary.

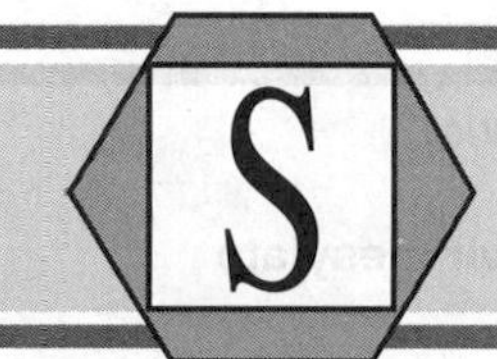

salmeterol xinafoate

Serevent

Pharmacologic classification: selective beta$_2$-adrenergic stimulating agonist
Therapeutic classification: bronchodilator
Pregnancy risk category C

How supplied

Available by prescription only
Inhalation aerosol: 25 mcg per activation in 6.5-g canister (60 activations), 25 mcg per activation in 13-g canister (120 activations)

Indications, route, and dosage

Long-term maintenance treatment of asthma; prevention of bronchospasm in patients with nocturnal asthma or reversible obstructive airway disease who require regular treatment with short-acting beta agonists

Adults and children over age 12: Two inhalations b.i.d. in the morning and evening.

Prevention of exercise-induced bronchospasm

Adults and children over age 12: Two inhalations at least 30 to 60 minutes before exercise.

Note: Paradoxical bronchospasms (which can be life-threatening) have been reported after use of salmeterol. If they occur, salmeterol should be discontinued immediately and alternative therapy instituted.

◊ ***COPD or emphysema***

Adults and children over age 12: Single oral inhalation of 42 to 63 mcg.

Pharmacodynamics

Bronchodilator action: Salmeterol selectively stimulates beta$_2$-adrenergic receptors, resulting in bronchodilation. Drug also blocks the release of histamine from mast cells lining the respiratory tract, which produces vasodilation and increases ciliary motility.

Pharmacokinetics

- *Absorption:* Because of the low therapeutic dose, systemic levels of salmeterol are low or undetectable after inhalation of recommended doses.
- *Distribution:* Drug is highly bound to human plasma proteins (94% to 99%).
- *Metabolism:* Drug is extensively metabolized by hydroxylation.
- *Excretion:* Excreted primarily in the feces.

Contraindications and precautions

Contraindicated in patients with hypersensitivity to drug or its formulation. Use cautiously in patients with coronary insufficiency, arrhythmias, hypertension, other CV disorders, thyrotoxicosis, or seizure disorders and in those unusually responsive to sympathomimetics.

Interactions

Concomitant administration with *beta-adrenergic agonists, theophylline,* or other *methylxanthines* may result in possible adverse cardiac effects with excessive use of salmeterol. Monitor the patient closely.

Concomitant use with *MAO inhibitors* or *tricyclic antidepressants* carries a risk of severe adverse CV effects. Avoid use of salmeterol within 14 days of MAO therapy.

Effects on diagnostic tests

None reported.

Adverse reactions

CNS: *headache,* sinus headache, tremor, nervousness, giddiness.
CV: tachycardia, palpitations, ***ventricular arrhythmias.***
EENT: *upper respiratory infection, nasopharyngitis,* nasal cavity or sinus disorder.
GI: nausea, vomiting, diarrhea, heartburn.
Respiratory: cough, lower respiratory infection, ***bronchospasm.***
Other: hypersensitivity reactions (rash, urticaria), joint and back pain, myalgia.

Overdose and treatment

Overdose may result in exaggerated pharmacologic adverse effects associated with beta-adrenoceptor agonists: tachycardia, arrhythmia, tremor, headache, and muscle cramps. Overdose can lead to clinically significant prolongation of the QT interval, which can produce ventricular arrhythmias. Cardiac arrest and death may be associated with abuse of salmeterol. Other signs of overdose may include hypokalemia and hyperglycemia.

In these cases, therapy with salmeterol and all beta-adrenergic-stimulant drugs should be stopped, supportive therapy should be provided, and judicious use of a beta-adrenergic blocking agent should be considered, bearing in mind the possibility that such agents can produce bronchospasm. Cardiac monitoring is recommended in cases of salmeterol overdose. Dialysis is not appropriate treatment.

☑ Special considerations

- Do not use drug in patients whose asthma can be managed by occasional use of a short-acting, inhaled beta$_2$-agonist such as albuterol.
- Salmeterol inhalation should not be used more than twice daily (morning and evening) at the recommended dose. Provide patient with a short-acting

inhaled $beta_2$-agonist for treatment of symptoms that occur despite regular twice-daily use of salmeterol.

- Patients who are taking a short-acting inhaled $beta_2$-agonist daily should be advised to use it only as needed if they develop asthma symptoms while taking salmeterol.
- Salmeterol is not a substitute for oral or inhaled corticosteroids.
- Patients receiving drug twice daily should not use additional doses for prevention of exercise-induced bronchospasm.

Patient education

- Instruct patient on the proper use of the salmeterol inhalation device and tell him to review the illustrated instructions in the package insert.
- Remind patient to shake the container well before using.
- Remind patient to take drug at approximately 12-hour intervals for optimum effect and to take it even when he is feeling better.
- Inform patient that drug is not meant to relieve acute asthmatic symptoms. Instead, acute symptoms should be treated with an inhaled, short-acting bronchodilator that has been prescribed for symptomatic relief.
- Tell patient to call if the short-acting agonist no longer provides sufficient relief or if more than four inhalations are being used daily. This may be a sign that asthma symptoms are worsening.
- Instruct patient already receiving short-acting $beta_2$-agonist to discontinue the regular daily-dosing regimen for drug and to use the short-acting agent only if asthma symptoms are experienced while taking salmeterol.
- Tell patient taking an inhaled corticosteroid to continue to use it regularly. Warn patient not to take other medications without medical approval.
- If drug is being used to prevent exercise-induced bronchospasm, tell patient to take it 30 to 60 minutes before exercise.

Geriatric use

- As with other $beta_2$-agonists, use with extreme caution when using drug in elderly patients who have concomitant CV disease that could be adversely affected by this class of drugs.

Pediatric use

- Safety and effectiveness in children under age 12 have not been established.

Breast-feeding

- Use caution when administering drug to a breast-feeding woman because it is not known if drug is distributed to breast milk.

saquinavir
Fortovase

saquinavir mesylate
Invirase

Pharmacologic classification: HIV-1 and HIV-2 proteinase inhibitor
Therapeutic classification: antiviral
Pregnancy risk category B

How supplied

Available by prescription only
saquinavir
Capsules (soft gelatin): 200 mg
saquinavir mesylate
Capsules (hard gelatin): 200 mg

Indications, route, and dosage

Adjunct treatment of advanced HIV infection in selected patients

Adults: 600 mg (Invirase, three 200-mg capsules) P.O. t.i.d. taken within 2 hours after a full meal and in combination with a nucleoside analogue such as zalcitabine at a dosage of 0.75 mg P.O. t.i.d. or 200 mg zidovudine P.O. t.i.d. Or, 1,200 mg (Fortovase, six 200-mg capsules) t.i.d. within 2 hours after a full meal in combination with a nucleoside analogue.

✦ ***Dosage adjustment.*** For toxicities that may occur with saquinavir or saquinavir mesylate, interrupt drug therapy. In combination therapy with nucleoside analogues, dosage adjustments of the nucleoside analogue should be based on the known toxicity profile of specific drug.

Pharmacodynamics

Antiviral action: Saquinavir inhibits the activity of HIV protease and prevents the cleavage of HIV polyproteins, which are essential for the maturation of HIV.

Pharmacokinetics

- *Absorption:* Saquinavir is poorly absorbed from the GI tract. Higher saquinavir concentrations are achieved with Fortovase compared with Invirase. (Fortovase has a relative bioavailability of 331% of Invirase.)
- *Distribution:* Saquinavir is approximately 98% bound to plasma proteins.
- *Metabolism:* Saquinavir is rapidly metabolized.
- *Excretion:* Saquinavir is excreted mainly in feces.

Contraindications and precautions

Contraindicated in patients with hypersensitivity to drug or the components contained in the capsule. Safety of drug has not been established in pregnant women.

Interactions

Rifabutin and *rifampin* reduce the steady state concentration of saquinavir. Use together cautiously. Concomitant use with *astemizole* or *cisapride* may cause serious CV events; avoid use with these drugs.

Effects on diagnostic tests
None reported.

Adverse reactions
CNS: paresthesia, headache.
GI: diarrhea, ulcerated buccal mucosa, abdominal pain, nausea, increased liver function tests (rare).
Respiratory: bronchitis, dyspnea, hemoptysis, pharyngitis, rhinitis, upper respiratory tract disorder, cough, epistaxis.
Other: asthenia, rash, musculoskeletal pain.

Overdose and treatment
Limited information available. One patient in clinical studies ingested 8 g as a single dose without showing evidence of acute toxicity. Emesis was induced in the patient within 2 to 4 hours after ingestion.

☑ Special considerations
- Evaluate CBC, platelets, electrolytes, uric acid, liver enzymes, and bilirubin before therapy is begun and then at appropriate intervals during therapy.
- If a serious or severe toxicity occurs during treatment, discontinue drug until the cause is identified or the toxicity resolves. Dosage modification is not needed when drug is resumed.
- Know that Invirase will be phased out and replaced by Fortovase. Be aware of the dosing differences.

Patient education
- Inform patient that drug should be taken within 2 hours following a full meal.
- Tell patient to report adverse reactions.
- Inform patient that drug is usually administered together with other AIDS-related antiviral agents.
- Tell patient to use Fortovase within 3 months when stored at room temperature or refer to expiration date on the label if capsules are refrigerated.

Pediatric use
- Safety and effectiveness in children under age 16 have not been established.

Breast-feeding
- Although safety has not been established in breast-feeding women, women with HIV infection should not breast-feed to avoid transmitting virus to infant.

sargramostim (granulocyte macrophage-colony stimulating factor, GM-CSF)
Leukine

Pharmacologic classification: biologic response modifier
Therapeutic classification: colony stimulating factor
Pregnancy risk category C

How supplied
Available by prescription only
Injection (preservative-free): 250 mcg, 500 mcg (as lyophilized powder) in single-dose vials

Indications, route, and dosage
Acceleration of hematopoietic reconstitution after autologous bone marrow transplantation in patients with malignant lymphoma, acute lymphoblastic leukemia, or Hodgkin's disease
Adults: 250 mcg/m^2 daily for 21 consecutive days given as a 2-hour I.V. infusion daily, beginning 2 to 4 hours after the bone marrow transplant. Do not administer within 24 hours of last dose of chemotherapy or within 12 hours after last dose of radiotherapy because of potential sensitivity of rapidly dividing progenitor cells to cytotoxic chemotherapeutic or radiologic therapies.
✦ ***Dosage adjustment.*** Reduce dosage by half or temporarily discontinue if severe adverse reactions occur. Therapy may be resumed when reaction abates. If blast cells appear or increase to 10% or more of the WBC count or if progression of the underlying disease occurs, discontinue therapy. If absolute neutrophil count is more than 20,000 cells/mm^3 or if WBC counts are more than 50,000 cells/mm^3, therapy should be discontinued temporarily or the dose reduced by half.
Bone marrow transplantation failure or engraftment delay
Adults: 250 mcg/m^2 daily for 14 days as a 2-hour I.V. infusion. Same course may be repeated after 7 days off therapy if engraftment has not occurred. Third course of 500 mcg/m^2 daily for 14 days may be given after another 7 days off therapy if engraftment has not occurred.
Acute myelogenous leukemia
Adults: 250 mcg/m^2 daily by I.V. infusion over 4 hours. Start therapy about day 11 or 4 days following completion of induction therapy. Use only if bone marrow is hypoplastic (fewer than 5% blasts on day 10). Continue until absolute neutrophil count exceeds 1,500/mm^3 for 3 consecutive days or for a maximum of 42 days.
◊ ***Myelodysplastic syndromes***
Adults: 15 to 500 mcg/m^2 daily by I.V. infusion over 1 to 12 hours.
◊ ***Aplastic anemia***
Adults: 15 to 480 mcg/m^2 daily by I.V. infusion over 1 to 12 hours.

Pharmacodynamics
Immunostimulant action: Sargramostim is a 127-amino acid glycoprotein manufactured by recombinant DNA technology in a yeast expression system. It differs from the natural human granulocyte-macrophage colony stimulating factor by substitution of leucine for arginine at position 23. The carbohydrate moiety may also be different. Sargramostim induces cellular responses by binding to specific receptors on cell surfaces of target cells. Blood counts return to normal or baseline levels within 2 to 10 days after stopping treatment.

Pharmacokinetics
- *Absorption:* Blood levels are detected within 5 minutes after S.C. administration; peak levels, within 2 hours.
- *Distribution:* Bound to specific receptors on target cells.
- *Metabolism:* Undetermined.

• *Excretion:* Unknown.

Contraindications and precautions

Contraindicated in patients with excessive leukemic myeloid blasts in bone marrow or peripheral blood and in those with hypersensitivity to drug or its components or to yeast-derived products. Also contraindicated for concomitant use with chemotherapy or radiotherapy.

Use cautiously in patients with impaired renal or hepatic function, preexisting cardiac disease or fluid retention, hypoxia, pulmonary infiltrates, or heart failure.

Interactions

Corticosteroids and *lithium* should be used with caution because they may potentiate the myeloproliferative effects of sargramostim.

Effects on diagnostic tests

None reported. Because hematopoiesis is stimulated, effects on CBC and differential blood counts will be noted.

Adverse reactions

CNS: *malaise, CNS disorders, asthenia.*
CV: *blood dyscrasias, edema,* hemorrhage, supraventricular arrhythmia, pericardial effusion.
GI: *nausea, vomiting, diarrhea, anorexia, hemorrhage, GI disorders, stomatitis.*
GU: *urinary tract disorder,* abnormal kidney function.
Hepatic: *liver damage.*
Respiratory: *dyspnea, lung disorders,* pleural effusion.
Skin: *alopecia, rash.*
Other: *fever, mucous membrane disorder, bone pain, peripheral edema, sepsis.*

Overdose and treatment

Doses up to 16 times the recommended dose have been administered with the following reversible adverse reactions: WBC counts up to 200,000/mm^3, dyspnea, malaise, nausea, fever, rash, sinus tachycardia, headache, and chills. The maximum dose that can be administered safely has yet to be determined. If overdose is suspected, monitor WBC count increase and respiratory symptoms.

☑ Special considerations

• Stimulation of marrow precursors may result in rapid elevation of WBC count; biweekly monitoring of CBC count with differential, including examination for blast cells, is recommended.
• Transient rash and local injection site reactions may occur; no serious allergic or anaphylactic reactions have been reported.
• Drug can act as a growth factor for any tumor type, particularly myeloid malignancies.
• Unlabeled indications include use to increase WBC counts in patients with myelodysplastic syndromes and in patients with AIDS on zidovudine; to decrease nadir of leukopenia secondary to myelosuppressive chemotherapy; to decrease myelosuppression in preleukemic patients; to correct neutropenia in patients with aplastic anemia; and to decrease transplant-associated organ system damage, particularly of the liver and kidneys.
• Drug is effective in accelerating myeloid recovery in patients receiving bone marrow purged from monoclonal antibodies.
• The effect of drug may be limited in patients who have received extensive radiotherapy to hematopoietic sites for treatment of primary disease in the abdomen or chest or have been exposed to multiple agents (alkylating agents, anthracycline antibiotics, antimetabolites) before autologous bone marrow transplant.
• Refrigerate the sterile powder, reconstituted solution, and diluted solution for injection. Do not freeze or shake. Do not use after expiration date.
• To prepare, reconstitute with 1 ml sterile water for injection. Do not reenter or reuse the single-dose vial. Discard unused portion. Direct stream of sterile water against side of vial and *gently swirl* contents to minimize foaming. Avoid excessive or vigorous agitation or shaking. Dilute in 0.9% NaCl. If final concentration is below 10 mcg/ml, add albumin (human) at a final concentration of 0.1% to the NaCl *before* addition of sargramostim to prevent adsorption to components of the delivery system. For a final concentration of 0.1% human albumin, add 1 mg human albumin/ml 0.9% NaCl. Administer as soon as possible after admixture, because sargramostim has no preservative, and within 6 hours of reconstitution or dilution. Do not add other medications to infusion solution without compatibility and stability data. Discard unused solution after 6 hours. Do not infuse drug using an in-line membrane filter because absorption of drug could occur.

Pediatric use

• Safety and efficacy have not been established; however, available data suggest that no differences in toxicity exist. The type and frequency of adverse reactions were comparable with those seen in adults.

Breast-feeding

• It is unknown if drug is excreted in breast milk; use with caution.

scopolamine hydrobromide

Isopto Hyoscine

Pharmacologic classification: anticholinergic
Therapeutic classification: antimuscarinic, cycloplegic mydriatic
Pregnancy risk category C

How supplied

Available by prescription only
Injection: 0.3 and 1 mg/ml in 1-ml vials and ampules; 0.4 mg/ml, 0.86 mg/ml in 0.5-ml ampules
Ophthalmic solution: 0.25%

Indications, route, and dosage

Antimuscarinic; adjunct to anesthesia; prevention of nausea and vomiting
Adults: 0.3 to 0.6 mg I.M., S.C., or I.V. (after dilution with sterile water for injection) as a single dose.

Children: 0.006 mg/kg I.M., S.C., or I.V. (after dilution with sterile water for injection) as a single daily dose; maximum dose, 0.3 mg.
Cycloplegic refraction
Adults: 1 to 2 drops 0.25% solution in eye 1 hour before refraction.
Children: 1 drop 0.25% solution b.i.d. for 2 days before refraction.
Iritis, uveitis
Adults: 1 to 2 drops of 0.25% solution daily or up to t.i.d.
Children: 1 drop of 0.25% solution up to t.i.d.

Pharmacodynamics
Antimuscarinic action: Scopolamine inhibits the muscarinic actions of acetylcholine on autonomic effectors, resulting in decreased secretions and GI motility; it also blocks vagal inhibition of the SA node.

Mydriatic action: Scopolamine competitively blocks acetylcholine at cholinergic neuroeffector sites, antagonizing the effects of acetylcholine on the sphincter muscle and ciliary body, thereby producing mydriasis and cycloplegia; these effects are used to produce cycloplegic refraction and pupil dilation to treat preoperative and postoperative iridocyclitis.

Pharmacokinetics
- *Absorption:* Rapidly absorbed when administered I.M. or S.C.; effects occur 15 to 30 minutes after I.M. or S.C. administration. Systemic drug absorption may occur from drug passage through the nasolacrimal duct. Ophthalmic mydriatic effect peaks at 20 to 30 minutes after administration; cycloplegic effects peak 30 to 60 minutes after administration.
- *Distribution:* Distributed widely throughout body tissues. Drug crosses the placenta and probably the blood-brain barrier.
- *Metabolism:* Drug is probably metabolized completely in the liver; however, its exact metabolic fate is unknown. Mydriatic and cycloplegic effects persist for 3 to 7 days.
- *Excretion:* Scopolamine is probably excreted in urine as metabolites.

Contraindications and precautions
Systemic form is contraindicated in patients with angle-closure glaucoma, obstructive uropathy, obstructive disease of the GI tract, asthma, chronic pulmonary disease, myasthenia gravis, paralytic ileus, intestinal atony, unstable CV status in acute hemorrhage, or toxic megacolon. Ophthalmic form is contraindicated in patients with shallow anterior chamber and angle-closure glaucoma or hypersensitivity to drug.

Use systemic form cautiously in patients with autonomic neuropathy, hyperthyroidism, coronary artery disease, arrhythmias, heart failure, hypertension, hiatal hernia associated with reflux esophagitis, hepatic or renal disease, or ulcerative colitis; in children under age 6; or in patients in a hot or humid environment. Use ophthalmic form cautiously in the elderly, in infants and children, and in those with cardiac disease.

Interactions
Concomitant use of scopolamine with *CNS depressants (alcohol, sedative-hypnotics, tranquilizers)* may increase CNS depression. Concomitant administration of *drugs with anticholinergic effects* may cause additive toxicity.

Decreased GI absorption of many drugs has been reported after the use of *anticholinergics* (for example, *ketoconazole, levodopa)*. Conversely, *slowly dissolving digoxin tablets* may yield higher serum digoxin levels when administered with anticholinergics. Use cautiously with *oral potassium supplements* (especially *wax-matrix formulations*) because the incidence of potassium-induced GI ulcerations may be increased.

Effects on diagnostic tests
None reported.

Adverse reactions
CNS: disorientation, restlessness, irritability, dizziness, drowsiness, headache, confusion, hallucinations, delirium.
CV: tachycardia; palpitations, paradoxical bradycardia (with systemic form).
EENT: blurred vision, photophobia, increased intraocular pressure; dilated pupils, difficulty swallowing (with systemic form); ocular congestion (with prolonged use), conjunctivitis, eye dryness, transient stinging and burning, edema (with ophthalmic form).
GI: dry mouth; *constipation, nausea, vomiting, epigastric distress* (with systemic form).
GU: urinary hesitancy, urine retention (with systemic form).
Respiratory: bronchial plugging, depressed respirations (with systemic form).
Skin: rash, flushing (with systemic form); dryness or contact dermatitis (with ophthalmic form).
Other: fever (with systemic form).

Adverse reactions may be caused by pending atropine-like toxicity and are dose-related. Individual tolerance varies greatly.

Many adverse reactions (such as dry mouth, constipation) are an expected extension of drug's pharmacologic activity.

Overdose and treatment
Clinical effects of overdose include excitability, seizures, CNS stimulation followed by depression, and such psychotic symptoms as disorientation, confusion, hallucinations, delusions, anxiety, agitation, and restlessness. Peripheral effects include dilated, nonreactive pupils; blurred vision; flushed, hot, dry skin; dryness of mucous membranes; dysphagia; decreased or absent bowel sounds; urine retention; hyperthermia; tachycardia; hypertension; and increased respiration.

Treatment is primarily symptomatic and supportive, as needed. Maintain patent airway. If patient is awake and alert, induce emesis (or use gastric lavage) and follow with a sodium chloride cathartic and activated charcoal to prevent further drug absorption. In severe life-threatening cases, physostigmine may be administered to block the antimuscarinic effects of scopolamine. Give fluids, as needed, to treat shock; diazepam to control psychotic symptoms; and pilocarpine (instilled into the eyes) to relieve mydriasis. If urine retention develops, catheterization may be necessary.

☑ Special considerations

Besides those relevant to all *anticholinergics,* consider the following recommendations.
- Therapeutic doses may produce amnesia, drowsiness, and euphoria (desired effects for use as an adjunct to anesthesia). As necessary, reorient patient.
- Some patients (especially the elderly) may experience transient excitement or disorientation.

Ophthalmic
- Apply pressure to the lacrimal sac for 1 minute after instillation to reduce the risk of systemic drug absorption.
- Have patient lie down, tilt head back, or look at ceiling to aid instillation.

Patient education

Ophthalmic
- Instruct patient to apply pressure to bridge of nose for about 1 minute after instillation.
- Advise patient not to close eyes tightly or blink for about 1 minute after instillation.

Geriatric use
- Use caution when administering drug to elderly patients. Lower doses are indicated.

Pediatric use
- Use ophthalmic form cautiously, if at all, in infants and small children.

Breast-feeding
- Drug may occur in breast milk, possibly resulting in infant toxicity. Avoid use of drug in breast-feeding women because it may decrease milk production.

secobarbital sodium

Novosecobarb*, Seconal

Pharmacologic classification: barbiturate
Therapeutic classification: sedative-hypnotic, anticonvulsant
Controlled substance schedule II
Pregnancy risk category D

How supplied

Available by prescription only
Capsules: 50 mg, 100 mg
Injection: 50 mg/ml in 2-ml disposable syringe

Indications, route, and dosage

Preoperative sedation
Adults: 200 to 300 mg P.O. 1 to 2 hours before surgery or 1 mg/kg I.M. 15 minutes before procedure.
Children: 2 to 6 mg/kg P.O. (maximum dose, 100 mg) or 4 to 5 mg/kg I.M.

Insomnia
Adults: 100 mg P.O., 100 to 200 mg I.M., or 50 to 250 mg I.V.

Status epilepticus
Adults: 250 to 350 mg I.M. or I.V.
Children: 15 to 20 mg/kg I.V. over 15 minutes.

Note: No more than 250 mg (5 ml) should be injected in any one site.

Pharmacodynamics

Sedative-hypnotic action: Secobarbital acts throughout the CNS as a nonselective depressant with a rapid onset of action and short duration of action. Particularly sensitive to this drug is the reticular activating system, which controls CNS arousal. Secobarbital decreases both presynaptic and postsynaptic membrane excitability by facilitating the action of gamma-aminobutyric acid. The exact cellular site and mechanisms of action are unknown.

Pharmacokinetics

- *Absorption:* After oral administration, 90% of secobarbital is absorbed rapidly. After rectal administration, secobarbital is nearly 100% absorbed. Peak serum concentration after oral or rectal administration occurs between 2 and 4 hours. Onset of action is rapid, occurring within 15 minutes when administered orally. Peak effects are seen 15 to 30 minutes after oral and rectal administration, 7 to 10 minutes after I.M. administration, and 1 to 3 minutes after I.V. administration. Concentrations of 1 to 5 mcg/ml are needed to produce sedation; 5 to 15 mcg/ml are needed for hypnosis. Hypnosis lasts for 1 to 4 hours after oral doses of 100 to 150 mg.
- *Distribution:* Distributed rapidly throughout body tissues and fluids; approximately 30% to 45% is protein-bound.
- *Metabolism:* Drug is oxidized in the liver to inactive metabolites. Duration of action is 3 to 4 hours.
- *Excretion:* 95% of a dose is eliminated as glucuronide conjugates and other metabolites in urine. Drug has an elimination half-life of about 30 hours.

Contraindications and precautions

Contraindicated in patients with respiratory disease in which dyspnea or obstruction is evident, or there is hypersensitivity to barbiturates or porphyria. Use cautiously in patients with acute or chronic pain, depression, suicidal tendencies, history of drug abuse, or impaired hepatic or renal function.

Interactions

Secobarbital may add to or potentiate CNS and respiratory depressant effects of other *sedative-hypnotics, alcohol, antidepressants, antihistamines, narcotics,* and *tranquilizers.*

Secobarbital enhances the enzymatic degradation of *warfarin* and other *oral anticoagulants;* patients may require increased doses of the anticoagulant. Drug also enhances hepatic metabolism of some drugs, including *digitoxin* (not digoxin), *corticosteroids, oral contraceptives* and other *estrogens, theophylline* and other *xanthines,* and *doxycycline.* Secobarbital impairs the effectiveness of *griseofulvin* by decreasing absorption from the GI tract.

Disulfiram, MAO inhibitors, and *valproic acid* decrease the metabolism of secobarbital and can increase its toxicity. *Rifampin* may decrease secobarbital levels by increasing metabolism.

Effects on diagnostic tests
Secobarbital may cause a false-positive phentolamine test. The physiologic effects of the drug may impair the absorption of cyanocobalamin C57; it may decrease serum bilirubin concentrations in neonates, epileptic patients, and in patients with congenital nonhemolytic unconjugated hyperbilirubinemia. EEG patterns show a change in low-voltage, fast activity; changes persist for a time after discontinuation of therapy.

Adverse reactions
CNS: *drowsiness, lethargy, hangover,* paradoxical excitement in elderly patients, somnolence.
CV: hypotension (with I.V. use).
GI: nausea, vomiting.
Hematologic: exacerbation of porphyria.
Respiratory: ***respiratory depression.***
Skin: rash, urticaria, ***Stevens-Johnson syndrome,*** tissue reactions, injection-site pain.
Other: ***angioedema,*** physical and psychological dependence.

Overdose and treatment
Clinical manifestations of overdose include unsteady gait, slurred speech, sustained nystagmus, somnolence, confusion, respiratory depression, pulmonary edema, areflexia, and coma. Typical shock syndrome with tachycardia and hypotension, jaundice, hypothermia followed by fever, and oliguria may occur.

Maintain and support ventilation and pulmonary function as necessary; support cardiac function and circulation with vasopressors and I.V. fluids as needed. If patient is conscious and gag reflex is intact, induce emesis (if ingestion was recent) by administering ipecac syrup. If emesis is contraindicated, perform gastric lavage while a cuffed endotracheal tube is in place to prevent aspiration. Follow with administration of activated charcoal or sodium chloride cathartic. Measure intake and output, vital signs, and laboratory parameters; maintain body temperature. Patient should be rolled from side to side every 30 minutes to avoid pulmonary congestion.

Alkalinization of urine may be helpful in removing drug from the body; hemodialysis may be useful in severe overdose.

☑ Special considerations
Besides those relevant to all *barbiturates,* consider the following recommendations.
- Use I.V. route of administration only in emergencies or when other routes are unavailable.
- Dilute secobarbital injection with sterile water for injection solution, 0.9% NaCl injection, or Ringer's injection solution. Total I.V. dose should not exceed 500 mg. Do not use if solution is discolored or if a precipitate forms.
- Avoid I.V. administration at a rate greater than 50 mg/15 seconds to prevent hypotension and respiratory depression. Have emergency resuscitative equipment on hand.
- Administer I.M. dose deep into large muscle mass to prevent tissue injury.
- Secobarbital sodium injection, diluted with lukewarm tap water to a concentration of 10 to 15 mg/ml, may be administered rectally in children. A cleansing enema should be administered before secobarbital enema.
- Monitor hepatic and renal studies frequently to prevent possible toxicity.

Patient education
- Emphasize danger of combining drug with alcohol. An excessive depressive effect is possible even if drug is taken the evening before ingestion of alcohol.

Geriatric use
- Elderly patients are more susceptible to drug's effects and usually require lower doses. Confusion, disorientation, and excitability may occur in elderly patients.

Pediatric use
- Drug may cause paradoxical excitement in children; use cautiously.

Breast-feeding
- Because drug enters breast milk, do not administer to breast-feeding women.

selegiline hydrochloride (L-deprenyl hydrochloride)
Eldepryl

Pharmacologic classification: MAO inhibitor
Therapeutic classification: antiparkinsonian
Pregnancy risk category C

How supplied
Available by prescription only
Capsules: 5 mg

Indications, route, and dosage
Adjunctive treatment to carbidopa-levodopa in the management of symptoms associated with Parkinson's disease
Adults: 10 mg P.O. daily, taken as 5 mg at breakfast and 5 mg at lunch. After 2 or 3 days of therapy, begin gradual decrease of carbidopa-levodopa dosage.

Pharmacodynamics
Antiparkinsonian action: Probably acts by selectively inhibiting MAO type B (found mostly in the brain). At higher-than-recommended doses, it is a nonselective inhibitor of MAO, including MAO type A found in the GI tract. It may also directly increase dopaminergic activity by decreasing the reuptake of dopamine into nerve cells. It has pharmacologically active metabolites (amphetamine and methamphetamine) that may contribute to this effect.

Pharmacokinetics

• *Absorption:* Drug is rapidly absorbed; about 73% of dose is absorbed.
• *Distribution:* After a single dose, plasma levels are below detectable levels (less than 10 ng/ml).
• *Metabolism:* Three metabolites have been detected in the serum and urine: N-desmethyldeprenyl, amphetamine, and methamphetamine.
• *Excretion:* 45% of drug appears as a metabolite in the urine after 48 hours.

Contraindications and precautions

Contraindicated in patients with hypersensitivity to drug and in those receiving meperidine and other opioids.

Interactions

Concomitant use with *adrenergic agents* may increase the pressor response, particularly in patients who have taken an overdose of selegiline. Contraindicated for use with *meperidine* because fatal interactions have been reported.

Effects on diagnostic tests

None reported.

Adverse reactions

CNS: *dizziness,* increased tremor, chorea, loss of balance, restlessness, increased bradykinesia, facial grimacing, stiff neck, dyskinesia, involuntary movements, twitching, increased apraxia, behavioral changes, fatigue, headache, confusion, hallucinations, vivid dreams, anxiety, insomnia, lethargy.
CV: orthostatic hypotension, hypertension, hypotension, ***arrhythmias,*** palpitations, new or increased anginal pain, tachycardia, peripheral edema, syncope.
EENT: blepharospasm.
GI: dry mouth, *nausea,* vomiting, constipation, weight loss, abdominal pain, anorexia or poor appetite, dysphagia, diarrhea, heartburn.
GU: slow urination, transient nocturia, prostatic hyperplasia, urinary hesitancy, urinary frequency, urine retention, sexual dysfunction.
Skin: rash, hair loss.
Other: malaise, diaphoresis.

Overdose and treatment

Limited experience with overdosage suggests that symptoms may include hypotension and psychomotor agitation. Because selegiline becomes a nonselective MAO inhibitor in high doses, consider the possibility of symptoms of MAO inhibitor poisoning: drowsiness, dizziness, hyperactivity, agitation, seizures, coma, hypertension, hypotension, cardiac conduction disturbances, and CV collapse. These symptoms may not develop immediately after ingestion (delays of 12 hours or more are possible).

Provide supportive treatment and closely monitor the patient for worsening of symptoms. Emesis or lavage may be helpful in the early stages of overdose treatment. Avoid phenothiazine derivatives and CNS stimulants; adrenergic agents may provoke an exaggerated response. Diazepam may be useful in treating seizures.

☑ Special considerations

• In some patients who experience an increase of adverse reactions associated with levodopa (including muscle twitches), reduction of carbidopa-levodopa is necessary. Most of these patients require a carbidopa-levodopa dosage reduction of 10% to 30%.

Patient education

• Advise patient not to take more than 10 mg daily. There is no evidence that higher dosage improves efficacy and it may increase adverse reactions.
• Warn patient to move about cautiously at the start of therapy because dizziness may occur, which can cause falls.
• Because drug is an MAO inhibitor, tell patient about the possibility of an interaction with tyramine-containing foods. Tell patient to immediately report signs or symptoms of hypertension, including severe headache. Reportedly, however, this interaction does not occur at the recommended dosage; at 10 mg daily, drug inhibits only MAO type B. Therefore, dietary restrictions appear unnecessary, provided that patient does not exceed the recommended dose.
• Emphasize danger of combining drug with alcohol. An excessive depressant effect is possible even if drug is taken the evening before ingestion of alcohol.

Breast-feeding

• It is not known if drug is excreted in breast milk. Use with caution in breast-feeding women.

senna

Black-Draught, Fletcher's Castoria, Gentlax S, Nytilax, Senexon, Senokot, Senolax, X-Prep

Pharmacologic classification: anthraquinone derivative
Therapeutic classification: stimulant laxative
Pregnancy risk category C

How supplied

Available without a prescription
Tablets: 187 mg, 217 mg, 374 mg, 600 mg
Granules: 326 mg/tsp, 1.65 g/½ tsp
Liquid: 33.3 mg/ml
Suppositories: 652 mg
Syrup: 218 mg/5 ml

Indications, route, and dosage

Acute constipation, preparation for bowel examination
Black-Draught
Adults: 2 tablets or ¼ to ½ level tsp of granules mixed with water. Not recommended for children.
Other preparations
Adults and children age 12 and over: Usual dose is 2 tablets, 1 tsp of granules dissolved in water, 1 suppository, or 10 to 15 ml syrup h.s. Maximum dosage varies with preparation used.

Children age 6 to 11: 1 tablet, ½ tsp of granules dissolved in water, ½ suppository h.s., or 5 to 10 ml syrup. Maximum dosage is 2 tablets b.i.d. or 1 tsp of granules b.i.d.
Children age 2 to 5: ½ tablet, ¼ tsp of granules dissolved in water. Maximum dosage is 1 tablet b.i.d. or ½ tsp of granules b.i.d.
Children age 1 to 5: 2.5 to 5 ml syrup h.s.
Children age 1 to 12 months: 1.25 to 2.5 ml syrup h.s.

Pharmacodynamics
Laxative action: Senna has a local irritant effect on the colon, which promotes peristalsis and bowel evacuation. It also enhances intestinal fluid accumulation, thereby increasing the stool's moisture content.

Pharmacokinetics
- *Absorption:* Senna is absorbed minimally. With oral administration, laxative effect occurs in 6 to 10 hours; with suppository administration, laxative effect occurs in 30 minutes to 2 hours.
- *Distribution:* Senna may be distributed in bile, saliva, the colonic mucosa, and breast milk.
- *Metabolism:* Absorbed portion is metabolized in the liver.
- *Excretion:* Unabsorbed senna is excreted mainly in feces; absorbed drug is excreted in urine and feces.

Contraindications and precautions
Contraindicated in patients with ulcerative bowel lesions; nausea, vomiting, abdominal pain, or other symptoms of appendicitis or acute surgical abdomen; fecal impaction; or intestinal obstruction or perforation.

Interactions
None reported.

Effects on diagnostic tests
In the phenolsulfonphthalein excretion test, senna may turn urine pink to red, red to violet, or red to brown.

Adverse reactions
GI: *nausea,* vomiting, diarrhea, loss of normal bowel function with excessive use, *abdominal cramps* (especially in severe constipation), malabsorption of nutrients, "cathartic colon" (syndrome resembling ulcerative colitis radiologically) with chronic misuse, possible constipation after catharsis, yellow or yellow-green cast to feces, diarrhea in breast-feeding infants of mothers receiving senna, darkened pigmentation of rectal mucosa with long-term use (usually reversible within 4 to 12 months after stopping drug), laxative dependence with excessive use.
GU: red-pink discoloration in alkaline urine; yellow-brown color to acidic urine.
Other: protein-losing enteropathy, electrolyte imbalance (such as hypokalemia).

Overdose and treatment
No information available.

☑ Special considerations
- Protect drug from excessive heat or light.

Patient education
- Warn patient that drug may turn urine pink, red, violet, or brown, depending on urinary pH.
- Instruct patient that laxative use should not exceed 1 week. Excessive use may result in dependence or electrolyte imbalance.
- Tell patient that bowel movement may have a yellow or yellow-green cast.

Geriatric use
- Elderly persons often overuse laxatives and may be more prone to laxative dependency.

Pediatric use
- Senna and other stimulant laxatives usually are not used in children.

Breast-feeding
- Senna enters breast milk; diarrhea has been reported in breast-feeding infants.

sertraline hydrochloride
Zoloft

Pharmacologic classification: serotonin uptake inhibitor
Therapeutic classification: antidepressant
Pregnancy risk category B

How supplied
Available by prescription only
Tablets: 50 mg, 100 mg

Indications, route, and dosage
Depression, obsessive-compulsive disorder
Adults: 50 mg P.O. daily. Adjust dosage as needed and tolerated; clinical trials involved dosage of 50 to 200 mg daily. Dosage adjustments should be made at intervals of no less than 1 week.
✦ ***Dosage adjustment.*** A lower or less frequent dosage should be used in patients with hepatic impairment. Particular care should be used in patients with renal failure.

Pharmacodynamics
Antidepressant action: Sertraline probably acts by blocking the reuptake of serotonin (5-hydroxytryptamine; 5-HT) into presynaptic neurons in the CNS, prolonging the action of 5-HT.

Pharmacokinetics
- *Absorption:* Well absorbed after oral administration; absorption rate and extent are enhanced when taken with food. Peak serum levels occur between 4.5 and 8.4 hours after a dose.
- *Distribution:* In vitro studies indicate that drug is highly protein-bound (more than 98%).
- *Metabolism:* Metabolism is probably hepatic; drug undergoes significant first-pass metabolism. N-desmethylsertraline is substantially less active than the parent compound.

• *Excretion:* Drug is excreted mostly as metabolites in the urine and feces. Mean elimination half-life is 26 hours. Steady-state levels are reached within 1 week of daily dosing in young, healthy patients.

Contraindications and precautions
Contraindicated in patients receiving MAO inhibitors. Use cautiously in patients at risk for suicide and in those with seizure disorders, major affective disorder, or diseases or conditions that affect metabolism or hemodynamic responses.

Interactions
Clearance of *diazepam* and *tolbutamide* is decreased by sertraline. Clinical significance is unknown; however, monitor patient for increased drug effects.

Concomitant use with *MAO inhibitors* may cause serious mental status changes, hyperthermia, autonomic instability, rapid fluctuations of vital signs, delirium, coma, and death. Do not administer within 14 days after discontinuing an *MAO inhibitor.* Allow 14 days after discontinuing sertraline before starting an MAO inhibitor.

Warfarin and other *highly protein-bound drugs* may cause interactions, increasing the plasma levels of sertraline or the other highly bound drug. Small (8%) increases in PT have occurred with concomitant use of warfarin. Monitor closely.

In one study, *cimetidine* increased sertraline bioavailability, peak plasma concentrations, and half-life. Clinical significance is unknown.

Effects on diagnostic tests
Minor changes in several laboratory values have occurred in patients taking sertraline. Elevated serum transaminase levels (AST, ALT) have occurred, usually within the first 9 weeks of therapy; values returned to normal after discontinuing drug. Minor increases in serum cholesterol and triglycerides and minor decreases in uric acid have been seen. Clinical significance is unknown.

Adverse reactions
CNS: *headache, tremor, dizziness, insomnia, somnolence,* paresthesia, hypoesthesia, *fatigue,* nervousness, anxiety, agitation, hypertonia, twitching, confusion.
CV: palpitations, chest pain, hot flashes.
GI: *dry mouth, nausea, diarrhea, loose stools, dyspepsia,* vomiting, constipation, thirst, flatulence, anorexia, abdominal pain, increased appetite.
GU: *male sexual dysfunction,* polyuria, nocturia, dysuria.
Skin: rash, pruritus.
Other: *diaphoresis,* myalgia.

Overdose and treatment
Clinical experience with sertraline overdosage is limited. Treatment is supportive. Establish an airway and maintain adequate ventilation. Because recent studies question the value of forced emesis or lavage, consider the use of activated charcoal in sorbitol to bind drug in the GI tract.

There is no specific antidote for sertraline. Monitor vital signs closely. Because drug has a large volume of distribution, hemodialysis, peritoneal dialysis, or forced diuresis probably is not useful.

☑ Special considerations
• Patients who respond during the first 8 weeks of therapy will probably continue to respond to drug, although there are limited studies of drug in depressed patients for periods longer than 16 weeks. If patients are continued on drug for prolonged therapy, periodically monitor the effectiveness of drug. It is unknown if periodic dosage adjustments are necessary to maintain effectiveness.
• Drug may activate mania or hypomania in patients with cyclic disorders.

Patient education
• Tell patient to take drug once daily, either in the morning or evening, with or without food.
• Advise patient to avoid use of alcohol while taking drug and to call before taking OTC medications.
• Although problems have not been reported to date, advise patient to use caution when performing hazardous tasks that require alertness, such as driving and operating heavy machinery. Drugs that influence the CNS may impair judgment.

Geriatric use
• Plasma clearance of drug is slower in elderly patients. Studies indicate that it may take 2 to 3 weeks of daily dosing before steady-state levels are reached.

Pediatric use
• Safety and efficacy have not been established.

Breast-feeding
• It is unknown if drug is excreted in breast milk. Use with caution in breast-feeding women.

sevoflurane
Ultane

Pharmacologic classification: halogenated (fluorinated) ether general anesthetic
Therapeutic classification: volatile general anesthetic
Pregnancy risk category B

How supplied
Available by prescription only
Volatile liquid for inhalation: 250-ml amber-colored bottles

Indications, route, and dosage
Induction and maintenance of general anesthesia
Adults and children: Surgical levels of anesthesia can usually be achieved with 0.5% to 3% sevoflurane with or without concomitant use of nitrous oxide. Administration of general anesthesia is individualized based on patient's response.

Minimum alveolar concentration (MAC) values for adults and pediatric patients vary according to age.

Patient age	Sevoflurane in oxygen	Sevoflurane in 65% N_2O/35% O_2
0 to 1 months	3.3%	-
1 to < 6 months	3%	-
6 months to < 3 years	2.8%	2%
3 to 12 years	2.5%	-
25 years	2.6%	1.4%
40 years	2.1%	1.1%
60 years	1.7%	0.9%
80 years	1.4%	0.7%

*In pediatric patients age 3 to < 5 years, 60% N_2O/40% O_2 was used.

Pharmacodynamics
Anesthetic action: Changes in depth of sevoflurane anesthesia rapidly follow changes in inspired concentration. Because of its low blood solubility, induction and emergence from anesthesia are more rapid with sevoflurane than with isoflurane or halothane.

Pharmacokinetics
• *Absorption:* Drug has a low solubility in blood; therefore, induction of anesthesia is faster than with isoflurane and halothane. There is a rapid rate of increase in the alveolar (end-tidal) concentration toward the inspired concentration during induction.
• *Distribution:* Uptake and distribution are faster with sevoflurane than with isoflurane and halothane, and similar to desflurane.
• *Metabolism:* Metabolized in the liver by cytochrome P-450 2E1 to hexafluoroisopropanol with release of inorganic fluoride and carbon dioxide. Major metabolite is rapidly conjugated with glucuronic acid and eliminated in the urine. Metabolism is inducible by chronic exposure to isoniazid and ethanol but not by barbiturates.
• *Excretion:* Low blood solubility facilitates rapid and extensive elimination via the lungs. Rate of elimination is similar to desflurane but faster than halothane or isoflurane. Up to 3.5% is eliminated in the urine as inorganic fluoride.

Contraindications and precautions
Contraindicated in patients with known history of sensitivity to drug or other halogenated agents. Use cautiously in patients with renal impairment or mild to moderate hepatic impairment.

Interactions
Benzodiazepines and *opioids* may decrease MAC of sevoflurane. *Nitrous oxide* (50%) decreases the anesthetic requirement for sevoflurane by 50% in adults and approximately 25% in children. Sevoflurane increases the intensity and duration of neuromuscular blockade induced by *nondepolarizing muscle relaxants;* adjust dosages.

Effects on diagnostic tests
Occasional cases of transient changes in postoperative hepatic function tests have been reported. Serum fluoride levels increase with duration and concentration of exposure to sevoflurane. Transient elevations in glucose, liver function tests, and WBC count may occur (as with other anesthetic agents).

Adverse reactions
CNS: *agitation,* dizziness, headache, somnolence.
CV: bradycardia, *hypotension,* hypertension, tachycardia.
GI: increased salivation, *nausea, vomiting.*
Respiratory: ***airway obstruction, apnea,*** breath-holding, *increased cough,* ***laryngospasm.***
Other: fever, hypothermia, shivering.

Overdose and treatment
In the event of possible or actual overdosage, discontinue administration of sevoflurane; maintain a patent airway; initiate assisted or controlled ventilation with oxygen and maintain adequate CV function.

☑ Special considerations
• Drug has a nonpungent odor that does not cause respiratory irritability; it is suitable for mask induction.
• Concentration of drug being delivered from a vaporizer calibrated for sevoflurane should be known.
• MAC of sevoflurane in oxygen for patients age 40 is 2.1%; MAC decreases with age.
• Obtain renal function studies before administering anesthesia.
• Ask patient about patient or family history of adverse reactions to anesthesia.
• Drug can cause malignant hyperthermia, which is signaled by hypercapnia, muscle rigidity, tachycardia, tachypnea, cyanosis, arrhythmias, and unstable blood pressure. Treatment includes discontinuation of triggering agents, administration of I.V. dantrolene sodium, and providing supportive therapy. Monitor urine flow because renal failure may occur in the late stages of malignant hyperthermia.
• Increasing the concentration of sevoflurane during maintenance produces dose-dependent decreases in blood pressure, which may be seen more rapidly than with other volatile anesthetics. Excessive decreases in blood pressure or respiratory depression can be corrected by decreasing the inspired concentration of sevoflurane.
• Ask patient about previous adverse experiences or reactions to general anesthetics.

Patient education
• Reassure patient about receiving general anesthesia.

Geriatric use
• Decrease dose of drug with increasing age.

Breast-feeding
• Concentrations of sevoflurane in breast milk are probably insignificant 24 hours after discontinuation of anesthesia and may be less than other volatile

anesthetics because of rapid washout and poor solubility.

sibutramine hydrochloride monohydrate
Meridia

Pharmacologic classification: norepinephrine, serotonin, and dopamine reuptake inhibitor
Therapeutic classification: antiobesity
Controlled substance schedule IV
Pregnancy risk category C

How supplied
Available by prescription only
Capsules: 5 mg, 10 mg, 15 mg

Indications, route, and dosage
Management of obesity, including weight loss and maintenance of weight loss; should be used in conjunction with a reduced-calorie diet
Adults: 10 mg P.O. once daily with or without food. May increase dose to 15 mg daily after 4 weeks if there is inadequate weight loss. Patients who do not tolerate the 10-mg dose may receive 5 mg daily. Doses above 15 mg daily are not recommended.

Pharmacodynamics
Antiobesity action: Sibutramine produces its therapeutic effects by inhibiting the reuptake of norepinephrine, serotonin, and dopamine.

Pharmacokinetics
• *Absorption:* Rapidly absorbed from the GI tract. Peak plasma concentrations of mono- and didesmethyl metabolites M_1 and M_2 are reached within 3 to 4 hours. On average, at least 77% of a single oral dose of sibutramine is absorbed.
• *Distribution:* Extensive distribution into tissues, especially the liver and kidney with relatively low transfer to the fetus. In vitro, sibutramine, M_1, and M_2 are extensively bound (97%, 94%, and 94%, respectively) to human plasma proteins.
• *Metabolism:* Drug undergoes extensive first-pass metabolism by the cytochrome P-450 3A4 isoenzyme to active desmethyl metabolites M_1 and M_2; elimination half-lives of M_1 and M_2 are 14 and 16 hours, respectively.
• *Excretion:* About 77% of a single oral dose is excreted in the urine.

Contraindications and precautions
Contraindicated in patients taking MAO inhibitors or other centrally acting appetite-suppressant drugs. Also contraindicated in patients with known hypersensitivity to drug or its inactive ingredients and in those with anorexia nervosa.

Do not use drug in patients with history of coronary artery disease, heart failure, arrhythmias, stroke, severe renal failure, hepatic dysfunction, or a history of seizures.

Use cautiously in patients with narrow angle glaucoma.

Interactions
CNS depressants may enhance CNS depression. *Dextromethorphan, dihydroergotamine, fentanyl, fluoxetine, fluvoxamine, lithium, MAO inhibitors, meperidine, paroxetine, pentazocine, sertraline, sumatriptan, tryptophan,* and *venlafaxine* may cause hyperthermia, tachycardia, and loss of consciousness. Avoid concomitant use.

Concomitant use of *ephedrine, phenylpropanolamine,* or *pseudoephedrine* may increase blood pressure or heart rate. Monitor patient carefully. May need reduced dosage of sibutramine when given concurrently with *drugs that inhibit cytochrome P-450 3A4 metabolism (erythromycin, ketoconazole).*

Effects on diagnostic tests
Drug may cause elevated liver function tests.

Adverse reactions
CNS: *headache, insomnia,* dizziness, nervousness, anxiety, depression, paresthesia, somnolence, CNS stimulation, emotional lability, migraine.
CV: tachycardia, vasodilation, hypertension, palpitation, chest pain.
EENT: thirst, *dry mouth, rhinitis, pharyngitis,* laryngitis, sinusitis, taste perversion, ear disorder, ear pain.
GI: *anorexia, constipation,* increased appetite, nausea, dyspepsia, gastritis, vomiting, abdominal pain, rectal disorder.
GU: dysmenorrhea, urinary tract infection, vaginal monilia, metrorrhagia.
Musculoskeletal: arthralgia, myalgia, tenosynovitis, joint disorder, neck or back pain.
Respiratory: cough increase, laryngitis.
Skin: rash, sweating, herpes simplex, acne.
Other: flu syndrome, asthenia, neck pain, *allergic reaction,* generalized edema.

Overdose and treatment
There is no specific antidote to sibutramine. Treatment should consist of general measures used in the management of overdosage: Establish an airway, monitor cardiac and vital signs, and institute general symptomatic and supportive measures. Cautious use of beta blockers may be indicated to control elevated blood pressure or tachycardia. The benefits of forced diuresis and hemodialysis are unknown.

☑ Special considerations
• Drug is recommended for obese patients with an initial body mass index of 30 kg/m^2 or more or 27 kg/m^2 or more in the presence of other risk factors (such as hypertension, diabetes, or dyslipidemia).
• Rule out organic causes of obesity before starting therapy.
• Measure blood pressure and heart rate before starting therapy, with dosage changes, and at regular intervals during therapy because drug is known to increase both blood pressure and heart rate.
• Know that at least 2 weeks should elapse between stopping an MAO inhibitor and starting sibutramine, and vice versa.

• Weight loss can precipitate or exacerbate gallstone formation.
• Although not reported with sibutramine, some centrally acting weight-loss agents have been associated with a rare but fatal condition known as primary pulmonary hypertension.
• If a patient has not lost at least 4 lbs in the first 4 weeks of treatment, reevaluate therapy to consider dosage increase or discontinuation of drug.

Patient education
• Advise patient to read the package insert before starting therapy and to review again each time the prescription is renewed.
• Instruct patient to report rash, hives, or other allergic reactions immediately.
• Inform patient to inform health care provider of other prescription or OTC drugs being taken, especially other weight-reducing agents, decongestants, antidepressants, cough suppressants, lithium, dihydroergotamine, sumatriptan, or tryptophan, as there is a potential for drug interactions.
• Suggest that blood pressure and heart rate be monitored regularly. Emphasize importance of regular follow-up visits with health care provider.
• Advise patient to use drug with a reduced-calorie diet.

Geriatric use
• Dose selection for an elderly patient should be cautious, reflecting the greater frequency of decreased hepatic, renal, or cardiac function, and of concomitant disease or other drug therapy.

Pediatric use
• Safety and efficacy in children under age 16 have not been established.

Breast-feeding
• It is not known if drug or its metabolites are excreted in breast milk. Avoid use of drug in breast-feeding women. Tell patient to inform health care provider if she is breast-feeding.

sildenafil citrate
Viagra

Pharmacologic classification: selective inhibitor of cyclic guanosine monophosphate-specific phosphodiesterase type 5
Therapeutic classification: therapy for erectile dysfunction
Pregnancy risk category B

How supplied
Available by prescription only
Tablets: 25 mg, 50 mg, 100 mg

Indications, route, and dosage
Treatment of erectile dysfunction
Adults: 50 mg P.O. as a single dose p.r.n. 1 hour before sexual activity. However, may take drug 30 minutes to 4 hours before sexual activity. Based on effectiveness and tolerance by patient, may increase dose to maximum single dose of 100 mg or decrease dose to 25 mg. A maximum recommended dosing frequency is once daily.
✦ ***Dosage adjustment.*** In the elderly, patients with hepatic or severe renal impairment, and those concurrently taking potent cytochrome P-450 3A4 inhibitors, consider starting dose of 25 mg.

Pharmacodynamics
Erectile action: Sildenafil has no direct relaxant effect on isolated human corpus cavernosum, but enhances the effect of nitric oxide (NO) by inhibiting phosphodiesterase type 5 (PDE5), which is responsible for degradation of cyclic guanosine monophosphate (cGMP) in the corpus cavernosum. When sexual stimulation causes local release of NO, inhibition of PDE5 by sildenafil causes increased levels of cGMP in the corpus cavernosum, resulting in smooth muscle relaxation and inflow of blood to the corpus cavernosum.

Pharmacokinetics
• *Absorption:* Rapidly absorbed after oral administration. Peak plasma levels are reached in ½ to 2 hours (median, 1 hour); a high-fat meal delays the rate of absorption by 1 hour and reduces peak levels by one-third. Absolute bioavailability is 40%.
• *Distribution:* Occurs widely in body tissues; mean volume of distribution is 105 L. Drug and its major active metabolite are 96% plasma protein-bound. Protein binding is independent of drug levels.
• *Metabolism:* The primary pathway for sildenafil elimination is metabolism by the CYP 3A4 and CYP 2C9 hepatic microsomal isoenzymes. N-desmethylation converts sildenafil into the major circulating metabolite, which accounts for about 20% of sildenafil's pharmacologic effects.
• *Excretion:* Approximately 80% of an oral dose is excreted in the feces; about 13% excreted in urine.

Contraindications and precautions
Contraindicated in patients also using organic nitrates and in those with known hypersensitivity to drug or its components. Use with caution in patients who have suffered an MI, stroke, or life-threatening arrhythmias within the last 6 months; have a history of heart failure, coronary artery disease, uncontrolled high or low blood pressure, anatomic deformation of the penis; and in those predisposed to priapism (sickle cell anemia, multiple myeloma, leukemia), retinitis pigmentosa, bleeding disorders, or active peptic ulcers.

Interactions
Inhibitors of cytochrome P-450 isoforms 3A4 (cimetidine, erythromycin, itraconazole, ketoconazole) may reduce the clearance of sildenafil. *Rifampin,* a CYP 3A4 inducer, is expected to reduce sildenafil plasma levels. Sildenafil enhances the hypotensive effects of *nitrates.*

Effects on diagnostic tests
None reported.

Adverse reactions
CNS: *headache,* dizziness.
CV: *flushing.*

EENT: nasal congestion, abnormal vision (photophobia, color blindness).
GI: dyspepsia, diarrhea.
GU: urinary tract infection.
Skin: rash.

Overdose and treatment

In studies in healthy volunteers, doses up to 800 mg produced adverse events similar to those seen at lower doses, but at an increased rate. Standard supportive measures should be used to treat overdose. Because of sildenafil's high protein binding, renal dialysis is not expected to increase clearance.

☑ Special considerations

- Because cardiac risk is associated with sexual activity, evaluate patient's CV status before initiating therapy.
- Because drug appears to have favorable teratogenic, embryotoxic, and fetotoxic profiles, and is not readily distributed into semen, the drug would not be expected to be harmful to pregnant women.

Patient education

- Advise patient to take drug after a high-fat meal to decrease its effects.
- Inform patient that drug does not offer protection against sexually transmitted diseases and that he should use protective measures to prevent infection.
- Instruct patient not to take drug concurrently with nitrates.
- Tell patient to notify health care provider of visual changes.
- Advise patient that drug has no effect in the absence of sexual stimulation.
- Urge patient to seek immediate medical assistance if erection lasts longer than 4 hours.

Geriatric use

- Reduced drug clearance is seen in healthy elderly volunteers age 65 or older. This reduction results in plasma concentrations approximately 40% greater than those in younger subjects.

Pediatric use

- Drug should not be used in children or newborns.

Breast-feeding

- Drug is not indicated for use in women.

silver nitrate

Silver Nitrate

Pharmacologic classification: heavy metal (silver compound)
Therapeutic classification: ophthalmic antiseptic; topical cauterizing
Pregnancy risk category C

How supplied

Available by prescription only
Ophthalmic solution: 1%
Topical ointment: 10%
Topical solution: 10%, 25%, 50%

Indications, route, and dosage

Prevention of gonorrheal ophthalmia neonatorum

Neonates: Clean lids thoroughly; instill 2 drops of 1% solution into lower conjunctival sac of each eye and ensure that solution contacts the entire conjunctival sac for 30 seconds or longer.

To treat indolent wounds, destroy exuberant granulations, freshen the edges of ulcers and fissures, provide styptic action, and treat vesicular bullous or aphthous lesions

Adults: Apply ointment on a pad to lesion for 5 days; or a cotton applicator dipped in solution to affected area two to three times a week for 2 to 3 weeks.

Pharmacodynamics

Antiseptic action: Liberated silver ions precipitate bacterial proteins, resulting in germicidal activity. Drug is effective mainly in preventing gonorrheal ophthalmia neonatorum.

Cauterizing action: Denatures protein, producing a caustic or corrosive effect.

Pharmacokinetics

- *Absorption:* Silver nitrate is not readily absorbed from mucous membranes or other tissues.
- *Distribution:* Unknown.
- *Metabolism:* Unknown.
- *Excretion:* Unknown.

Contraindications and precautions

None reported.

Interactions

Silver nitrate is incompatible with *alkalies, benzalkonium chloride, halogenated acids* or *salts, phosphates,* and *thimerosal.*

Effects on diagnostic tests

None reported.

Adverse reactions

EENT: periorbital edema, temporary staining of lids and surrounding tissue, *conjunctivitis.*

Overdose and treatment

Clinical manifestations of overdose are extremely rare with ophthalmic use.

Toxicity is highly dependent on the concentration of silver nitrate and extent of exposure. Oral overdose is treated by dilution with 4 to 8 oz (120 to 240 ml) of water. To remove the chemical, administer NaCl (10 g/L) by lavage to precipitate silver chloride. Activated charcoal or a cathartic can be used. Treat eye overexposure initially by irrigation with tepid water for at least 15 minutes. Treat dermal overexposure by washing with soap and water twice. Dizziness, seizures, mucous membrane irritation, nausea, vomiting, stomach ache and diarrhea, methemoglobinemia, dermatitis, rash, and hypochloremia with associated hyponatremia may occur. Treat seizures with diazepam. Depending on the extent of exposure, evaluate for methemoglobinemia; treat with methylene blue.

☑ Special considerations
- Silver nitrate is bacteriostatic, germicidal, and astringent.
- Do not use repeatedly.
- If solution stronger than 1% is accidentally used in eye, promptly irrigate with isotonic NaCl to prevent eye irritation.
- Handle drug carefully; solution may stain skin and utensils.
- Instillation may be briefly delayed to allow neonate to bond with mother; however, application should occur within 1 hour after delivery. Most states require instillation by law at birth; do not irrigate eyes after instillation. Store wax ampules away from light and heat.
- Do not use solution if it is discolored or contains a precipitate.
- Topical use of solutions above 1% concentration may cause burns. Avoid contact with skin and eyes. If accidental contact with skin occurs, flush with water for at least 15 minutes; for accidental contact with eyes, irrigate with sterile water or 0.9% NaCl immediately.
- Moisten silver nitrate pencils with water before use.
- In low concentrations (0.125% to 0.5%) as a wet dressing, silver nitrate is used as a local anti-infective to treat burns and skin wounds or ulcers.
- Drug may be painful when administered topically in higher concentrations.

Patient education
- Explain that preparations may stain skin and clothing. Teach parents that silver nitrate may discolor neonate's eyelids temporarily.
- Inform parents that instillation at birth is required by law in most states.

silver sulfadiazine
Silvadene, SSD AF, SSD Cream, Thermazene

Pharmacologic classification: synthetic anti-infective
Therapeutic classification: topical antibacterial
Pregnancy risk category B

How supplied
Available by prescription only
Cream: 1%

Indications, route, and dosage
Adjunct in the prevention and treatment of wound infection for second- and third-degree burns
Adults and children: Apply 1/16″ (16 mm) thickness of ointment to cleansed and debrided burn wound once or twice daily. Reapply if accidentally removed.

Pharmacodynamics
Antibacterial action: Acts on bacterial cell membrane and bacterial cell wall. Silver sulfadiazine has a broad spectrum of activity, including against gram-negative and gram-positive organisms.

Pharmacokinetics
- *Absorption:* Limited with topical use.
- *Distribution:* None.
- *Metabolism:* None.
- *Excretion:* Silver sulfadiazine is excreted in the urine.

Contraindications and precautions
Contraindicated in premature and full-term neonates during first 2 months of life. Drug may increase possibility of kernicterus. Also contraindicated in patients with hypersensitivity to drug or in pregnant women at or near term. Use cautiously in patients with sulfonamide sensitivity.

Interactions
Collagenase, papain, and *sutilains* may be inactivated if used concurrently.

Effects on diagnostic tests
If used on extensive areas of body surface, systemic absorption may result in a decreased neutrophil count, indicating a reversible leukopenia.

Adverse reactions
Hematologic: LEUKOPENIA.
Skin: pain, burning, rash, pruritus, skin necrosis, erythema multiforme, skin discoloration.

Overdose and treatment
To treat local overapplication, discontinue drug and clean area thoroughly.

☑ Special considerations
- Avoid drug contact with eyes and mucous membranes.
- Apply drug with a sterile gloved hand. The burned area should be covered with cream at all times.
- Daily bathing is an aid in debridement of burn wounds.
- Continue treatment until site is healed or is ready for skin grafting.
- Monitor for signs of fungal superinfection.
- Delayed eschar separation may result when drug is used.
- Monitor CBCs, serum sulfadiazine levels, and urine for crystalluria and calculi formation.

Patient education
- Teach patient about wound care.
- Advise patient that silver sulfadiazine does not stain the skin.
- Teach patient proper application.
- Warn patient of potential photosensitivity.

Pediatric use
- Silver sulfadiazine is contraindicated in premature infants or infants under age 2 months.

Breast-feeding
- Avoid breast-feeding during and for several days after drug therapy.

...icone

...s-X, Mylicon, Phazyme

Pharmacologic classification: dispersant
Therapeutic classification: antiflatulent
Pregnancy risk category C

How supplied

Available without a prescription
Tablets (delayed-release; enteric-coated core): 60 mg, 95 mg
Tablets (chewable): 40 mg, 80 mg, 125 mg
Capsules: 125 mg
Drops: 40 mg/0.6 ml

Indications, route, and dosage

Flatulence, functional gastric bloating
Adults and children over age 12: 40 to 125 mg P.O. after each meal and h.s.
Children age 2 to 12: 40 mg (drops) P.O. q.i.d.
Children under age 2: 20 mg (drops) P.O. q.i.d., up to 240 mg/day.

Pharmacodynamics

Antiflatulent action: Simethicone acts as a defoaming agent by decreasing the surface tension of gas bubbles, thereby preventing the formation of mucus-coated gas bubbles.

Pharmacokinetics

- *Absorption:* None.
- *Distribution:* None.
- *Metabolism:* None.
- *Excretion:* Simethicone is excreted in feces.

Contraindications and precautions

Contraindicated in patients hypersensitive to drug.

Interactions

Simethicone may decrease the effectiveness of *alginic acid.*

Effects on diagnostic tests

None reported.

Adverse reactions

GI: expulsion of excessive liberated gas as belching, rectal flatus.

Overdose and treatment

No information available.

☑ Special considerations

- Simethicone is found in many combination antacid products.

Patient education

- Tell patient to chew tablets thoroughly or to shake suspension well before using.

Pediatric use

- Simethicone is not recommended as treatment for infant colic; it has limited use in children.

simvastatin

Zocor

Pharmacologic classification: HMG-CoA reductase inhibitor
Therapeutic classification: antilipemic, cholesterol-lowering
Pregnancy risk category X

How supplied

Available by prescription only
Tablets: 5 mg, 10 mg, 20 mg, 40 mg

Indications, route, and dosage

Reduction of low-density lipoprotein (LDL) and total cholesterol levels in patients with primary hypercholesterolemia (types IIa and IIb)
Adults: Initially, 5 to 10 mg daily in the evening. Adjust dosage q 4 weeks based on patient tolerance and response; maximum daily dosage, 40 mg. Maximum daily dosage for elderly patients, 20 mg.
✦ ***Dosage adjustment.*** For patients receiving immunosuppressants, start with 5 mg/day; maximum daily dosage, 10 mg. For patients with mild to moderate renal insufficiency, give usual daily dose; in those with severe renal impairment, start therapy with 5 mg P.O. daily and closely monitor patient.

Pharmacodynamics

Antilipemic action: Simvastatin inhibits the enzyme 3-hydroxy-3-methylglutaryl-coenzyme A (HMG-CoA) reductase. This hepatic enzyme is an early (and rate limiting) step in the synthetic pathway of cholesterol.

Pharmacokinetics

- *Absorption:* Drug is readily absorbed; however, extensive hepatic extraction limits the plasma availability of active inhibitors to 5% of a dose or less. Individual absorption varies considerably.
- *Distribution:* Parent drug and active metabolites are more than 95% bound to plasma proteins.
- *Metabolism:* Hydrolysis occurs in the plasma; at least three major metabolites have been identified.
- *Excretion:* Excretion is primarily in bile.

Contraindications and precautions

Contraindicated in patients with hypersensitivity to drug and in those with active hepatic disease or conditions that cause unexplained persistent elevations of serum transaminase; in pregnant and breast-feeding patients; and in women of childbearing age unless there is no risk of pregnancy.

Use cautiously in patients with history of liver disease or who consume excessive amounts of alcohol.

Interactions

Concomitant use with *immunosuppressive agents* (such as *cyclosporine*), *fibric acid derivatives* (such as *clofibrate, gemfibrozil),* high doses of *niacin* (*nicotinic acid;* 1 g or more daily), or *erythromycin* may increase risk of rhabdomyolysis. Monitor patient closely if concomitant use cannot be avoided.

Limit daily dosage of simvastatin to 10 mg if patient must take *cyclosporine.*

Patients taking *hepatotoxic drugs* and those who *chronically abuse alcohol* may be at increased risk for hepatotoxicity. Simvastatin may slightly elevate *digoxin* levels. Closely monitor plasma digoxin levels at the start of simvastatin therapy.

Simvastatin may slightly enhance the anticoagulant effect of *warfarin.* Monitor PT at the start of therapy and during dosage adjustment.

Drugs that decrease the levels or activity of *endogenous steroids* (such as *cimetidine, ketoconazole, spironolactone*) may increase the risk of development of endocrine dysfunction. No intervention appears necessary; obtain complete drug history in patients in whom endocrine dysfunction develops.

Effects on diagnostic tests

As an expected pharmacologic effect, simvastatin reduces total plasma cholesterol, very low-density lipoprotein, and LDL and may variably increase high-density lipoprotein (HDL). The ratios of total cholesterol to HDL, total cholesterol to LDL, and LDL to HDL are reduced. Modest decreases in triglycerides may also occur.

Toxic effects of drug may be evident by marked, persistent elevations of serum transaminases. During clinical trials, about 5% of patients had asymptomatic, marked elevations in the noncardiac fraction of CK.

Adverse reactions

CNS: headache, asthenia.
GI: abdominal pain, constipation, diarrhea, dyspepsia, flatulence, nausea, vomiting.
Hepatic: elevated liver enzymes.
Respiratory: upper respiratory tract infection.

Overdose and treatment

There has been no experience with simvastatin overdosage in humans. No specific antidote is known. Treat symptomatically.

☑ Special considerations

- Dosage adjustments should be made about every 4 weeks. If the cholesterol levels decrease below the target range, dosage may be reduced.
- Perform liver function tests frequently at the start of therapy and periodically thereafter.
- Initiate simvastatin only after diet and other nonpharmacologic therapies have proved ineffective. Patient should continue a cholesterol-lowering diet during therapy.

Patient education

- Tell patient that drug should be taken in the evening and may be taken without regard to meals.
- Because of the possible impact of drug on liver function, advise patient to restrict alcohol intake.
- Tell patient to report adverse reactions, particularly muscle aches and pains.
- Explain importance of controlling serum lipids to CV health. Teach appropriate dietary management (restricting total fat and cholesterol intake), weight control, and exercise.

Geriatric use

- Most elderly patients respond to daily dosage of 20 mg or less.

Pediatric use

- Safety and efficacy have not been established.

Breast-feeding

- It is unknown if drug occurs in breast milk. Because of the risk to infants, breast-feeding should be avoided during therapy.

sodium bicarbonate

Bell/ans, Neut, Soda Mint

Pharmacologic classification: alkalinizing
Therapeutic classification: systemic and urinary alkalinizer, systemic hydrogen ion buffer, oral antacid
Pregnancy risk category C

How supplied

Available by prescription only
Injection: 4% (2.4 mEq/5 ml), 4.2% (5 mEq/10 ml), 5% (297.5 mEq/500 ml), 7.5% (8.92 mEq/10 ml and 44.6 mEq/50 ml), 8.4% (10 mEq/10 ml and 50 mEq/50 ml)

Available without a prescription
Tablets: 325 mg, 500 mg, 520 mg, 650 mg

Indications, route, and dosage

Adjunct to advanced cardiac life support

Adults and children over age 2: Although no longer routinely recommended, inject either 300 to 500 ml of a 5% solution or 200 to 300 mEq of a 7.5% or 8.4% solution as rapidly as possible. Base further doses on subsequent blood gas values.

Children age 2 or younger: 1 mEq/kg I.V. bolus of a 4.2% solution. Dose may be repeated q 10 minutes depending on blood gas values. Do not exceed daily dosage of 8 mEq/kg.

Metabolic acidosis

Adults and children: Dose depends on blood carbon dioxide content, pH, and patient's clinical condition. Generally, administer 90 to 180 mEq/L I.V. during first hour, then adjust p.r.n.

Urinary alkalization

Adults: 325 mg to 2 g P.O., up to q.i.d. Do not exceed 17 g in patients under age 60 or 8 g in patients over age 60.

Children: 1 to 10 mEq (84 to 840 mg)/kg daily.

Antacid

Adults: 300 mg to 2 g P.O. one to four times daily.

Pharmacodynamics

Alkalizing buffering action: Sodium bicarbonate is an alkalinizing agent that dissociates to provide bicarbonate ion. Bicarbonate in excess of that needed to buffer hydrogen ions causes systemic alkalinization and, when excreted, urinary alkalinization as well.

Oral antacid action: Taken orally, sodium bicarbonate neutralizes stomach acid by the above mechanism.

Pharmacokinetics
• *Absorption:* Sodium bicarbonate is well absorbed after oral administration as sodium ion and bicarbonate.
• *Distribution:* Bicarbonate occurs naturally and is confined to the systemic circulation.
• *Metabolism:* None.
• *Excretion:* Bicarbonate is filtered and reabsorbed by the kidney; less than 1% of filtered bicarbonate is excreted.

Contraindications and precautions
Contraindicated in patients with metabolic or respiratory alkalosis; in those who are losing chlorides by vomiting or from continuous GI suction; in those receiving diuretics known to produce hypochloremic alkalosis; and in patients with hypocalcemia in which alkalosis may produce tetany, hypertension, seizures, or heart failure. Orally administered sodium bicarbonate is contraindicated in patients with acute ingestion of strong mineral acids.

Use with extreme caution in patients with heart failure, renal insufficiency, or other edematous or sodium-retaining conditions.

Interactions
If urinary alkalinization occurs, sodium bicarbonate increases half-life of *amphetamines, ephedrine, pseudoephedrine,* and *quinidine,* and it increases urinary excretion of *chlorpropamide, lithium, salicylates,* and *tetracyclines.* Use with *corticosteroids* may increase sodium retention.

Effects on diagnostic tests
Sodium bicarbonate therapy may alter serum electrolyte levels and may increase serum lactate levels.

Adverse reactions
GI: gastric distention, belching, flatulence.
Other: local pain and irritation at injection site, ***metabolic alkalosis,*** hypernatremia, hyperosmolarity (with overdose).

Overdose and treatment
Clinical signs of overdose include depressed consciousness and obtundation from hypernatremia, tetany from hypocalcemia, arrhythmias from hypokalemia, and seizures from alkalosis. Correct fluid, electrolyte, and pH abnormalities. Monitor vital signs and fluid and electrolytes closely.

☑ Special considerations
• Monitor vital signs regularly; when drug is used as urinary alkalinizer, monitor urine pH.
• Avoid extravasation of I.V. solutions. Addition of calcium salts may cause precipitate; bicarbonate may inactivate catecholamines in solution (epinephrine, phenylephrine, and dopamine).
• Discourage use as an oral antacid because of hazardous excessive systemic absorption.
• Assess patient for milk-alkali syndrome if drug use is long-term.
• Drug may be used as an adjunct to treat hyperkalemia (with dextrose and insulin).

Patient education
• Advise patient to avoid chronic use as oral antacid, and recommend nonabsorbable antacids.
• If patient takes an oral dosage form, tell patient to take drug 1 hour before or 2 hours after taking enteric-coated medications because drug may cause enteric-coated products to dissolve in the stomach.

Geriatric use
• Elderly patients with heart failure or other fluid-retaining conditions are at greater risk for increased fluid retention; therefore, use drug with caution.

Pediatric use
• Avoid rapid infusion (10 ml/minute) of hypertonic solutions in children under age 2.

Breast-feeding
• It is not known if sodium bicarbonate occurs in breast milk. Use cautiously when administering to breast-feeding women.

sodium chloride (NaCl)

Pharmacologic classification: electrolyte
Therapeutic classification: sodium and chloride replacement
Pregnancy risk category C

How supplied
Available by prescription only
Injection: 0.45% NaCl 25 ml, 50 ml, 150 ml, 250 ml, 500 ml, 1,000 ml; 0.9% NaCl 2 ml, 3 ml, 5 ml, 10 ml, 20 ml, 25 ml, 30 ml, 50 ml, 100 ml, 150 ml, 250 ml, 500 ml, 1,000 ml; 3% NaCl 500 ml; 5% NaCl 500 ml

Available without a prescription
Tablets: 650 mg, 1 g
Tablets (slow-release): 600 mg

Indications, route, and dosage
Water and electrolyte replacement in hyponatremia from electrolyte loss or severe NaCl depletion
Adults and children: Treatment is highly individualized based on frequent laboratory values and clinical picture. See manufacturer's recommendations for P.O. dosing.

Pharmacodynamics
Electrolyte replacement: Sodium chloride solution replaces deficiencies of the sodium and chloride ions in the blood plasma.

Pharmacokinetics
• *Absorption:* Oral and parenteral NaCl are absorbed readily.
• *Distribution:* NaCl is distributed widely.
• *Metabolism:* None significant.
• *Excretion:* Sodium and chloride are eliminated primarily in urine, but also in the sweat, tears, and saliva.

Contraindications and precautions

Contraindicated in patients with conditions in which sodium and chloride administration is detrimental. NaCl 3% and 5% injections are contraindicated in patients with increased, normal, or only slightly decreased serum electrolyte concentrations.

Use cautiously in patients with heart failure, renal dysfunction, circulatory insufficiency, or hypoproteinemia and in elderly or postoperative patients.

Interactions

None reported.

Effects on diagnostic tests

None reported.

Adverse reactions

CV: aggravation of heart failure; edema (if given too rapidly or in excess).
Respiratory: ***pulmonary edema*** (if given too rapidly or in excess).
Other: hypernatremia and aggravation of existing metabolic acidosis (with excessive infusion); serious electrolyte disturbances, loss of potassium; local tenderness, abscess, tissue necrosis at injection site; thrombophlebitis.

Overdose and treatment

NaCl overdose causes serious electrolyte disturbances. Oral ingestion of large quantities irritates the GI mucosa and may cause nausea and vomiting, diarrhea, and abdominal cramps.

Treatment of oral overdose consists of emptying the stomach, giving magnesium sulfate as a cathartic, and supportive therapy. Provide airway and ventilation if necessary. Excessive I.V. administration requires discontinuation of NaCl infusion.

☑ Special considerations

- Use concentrated solutions (3% and 5%) only for correcting severe sodium deficits (sodium level below 120 mEq/ml). The solutions should be infused very slowly and with caution to avoid pulmonary edema. Observe patient constantly.
- Concentrated solutions (3.5 and 4 mEq/ml) are available for addition to parenteral nutrition solutions.
- Monitor changes in fluid balance, serum electrolyte disturbances, and acid-base imbalances.
- Monitor for hypokalemia with administration of potassium-free solutions.
- 0.9% NaCl may be used in managing extreme dilution of hyponatremia and hypochloremia resulting from administration of sodium-free fluids during fluid and electrolyte therapy, and in managing extreme dilution of extracellular fluid after excessive water intake (for example, after multiple enemas).

sodium fluoride

ACT, Fluorigard, Fluorinse, Fluoritab, Flura-Drops, Flura-Loz, Karidium, Karigel, Karigel-N, Listermint with Fluoride, Luride, Luride Lozi-Tabs, Luride-SF Lozi-Tabs, Pediaflor, Phos-Flur, Point-Two, Prevident, Thera-Flur, Thera-Flur-N

Pharmacologic classification: trace mineral
Therapeutic classification: dental caries prophylactic
Pregnancy risk category C

How supplied

Available by prescription only
Tablets: 1 mg (sugar-free)
Tablets (chewable): 0.5 mg, 1 mg (sugar-free)
Drops: 0.125 mg/drop (30 ml), 0.125 mg/drop (60 ml, sugar-free), 0.25 mg/drop (19 ml), 0.25 mg/drop (24 ml, sugar-free), 0.5 mg/ml (50 ml)
Rinse: 0.09% (240 ml, 480 ml), 0.09% (480 ml, sugar-free)
Gel: 0.1% (65 g, 105 g, 122 g), 0.5% (24 g, 30 g, 60 g, 120 g, 130 g, 250 g), 1.23% (480 ml)
Gel drops: 0.5% (24 ml)

Available without a prescription
Rinse: 0.01% (180 ml, 300 ml, 360 ml, 480 ml, 540 ml, 720 ml, 960 ml, 1,740 ml); 0.02% (90 ml, 180 ml, 300 ml, 360 ml, 480 ml)
Gel: 0.1% (60 g, 120 g)

Indications, route, and dosage

Aid in the prevention of dental caries
Oral
Children age 6 months to 3 years: 0.25 mg daily.
Children age 3 to 6: 0.5 mg daily.
Children age 6 to 16: 1 mg daily.
✦ ***Dosage adjustment.*** If fluoride in the drinking water is below 0.3 ppm, use dosage listed; if fluoride content is 0.3 to 0.7 ppm, use one half of dosage; if fluoride content exceeds 0.7 ppm, do not use.
Topical
Adults and children over age 12: 10 ml of 0.09% (0.2% fluoride ion) rinse. Use once daily after thoroughly brushing teeth and rinsing mouth. Rinse around and between teeth for 1 minute, then spit out.
Children age 6 to 12: 5 ml of 0.09% (0.2% fluoride ion) solution.

Pharmacodynamics

Dental caries prophylactic action: Sodium fluoride acts systemically before tooth eruption and topically afterward by increasing tooth resistance to acid dissolution, by promoting remineralization, and by inhibiting the cariogenic microbial process. Acidulation provides greater topical fluoride uptake by dental enamel than neutral solutions. When topical fluoride is applied to hypersensitive exposed dentin, the formation of insoluble materials within the dentinal tubules blocks transmission of painful stimuli.

Pharmacokinetics

• *Absorption:* Absorbed readily and almost completely from the GI tract. A large amount of an oral dose may be absorbed in the stomach; rate of absorption may depend on the gastric pH. Oral fluoride absorption may be decreased by simultaneous ingestion of aluminum or magnesium hydroxide. Simultaneous ingestion of calcium also may decrease absorption of large doses. Normal total plasma fluoride concentrations range from 0.14 to 0.19 mcg/ml.
• *Distribution:* Sodium fluoride is stored in bones and developing teeth after absorption. Skeletal tissue also has a high storage capacity for fluoride ions. Because of the storage-mobilization mechanism in skeletal tissue, a constant fluoride supply may be provided. Although teeth have a small mass, they also serve as storage sites. Fluoride deposited in teeth is not released readily. Fluoride has been found in all organs and tissues with a low accumulation in noncalcified tissues. Fluoride is distributed into sweat, tears, hair, and saliva. Fluoride crosses the placenta and is distributed into breast milk. Fluoride concentrations in milk range from approximately 0.05 to 0.13 ppm and remain fairly constant.
• *Metabolism:* None.
• *Excretion:* Fluoride is excreted rapidly, mainly in the urine. About 90% of fluoride is filtered by the glomerulus and reabsorbed by the renal tubules.

Contraindications and precautions

Contraindicated in patients hypersensitive to fluoride or when intake from drinking water exceeds 0.6 ppm.

Interactions

Incompatibility of systemic fluoride with *dairy foods* has reportedly caused calcium fluoride formation.

Concomitant use with *magnesium* or *aluminum hydroxide* may impair the absorption of sodium fluoride.

Effects on diagnostic tests

None reported.

Adverse reactions

CNS: headache, weakness.
GI: gastric distress.
Skin: hypersensitivity reactions (atopic dermatitis, eczema, urticaria).
Other: staining of teeth.

Overdose and treatment

In children, acute ingestion of 10 to 20 mg of sodium fluoride may cause excessive salivation and GI disturbances; 500 mg may be fatal. GI disturbances include salivation, nausea, abdominal pain, vomiting, and diarrhea. CNS disturbances include CNS irritability, paresthesias, tetany, hyperactive reflexes, seizures, and respiratory or cardiac failure (from the calcium-binding effect of fluoride). Hypoglycemia and hypocalcemia are frequent laboratory findings.

By using gastric lavage with 1% to 5% calcium chloride solution, the fluoride may be precipitated. Administer glucose I.V. in NaCl solution; parenteral calcium administration may be indicated for tetany. Adequate urine output should be maintained.

☑ Special considerations

• Recommended doses are currently under study. Some evidence suggests that considerably less fluoride is needed for adequate supplementation.
• Review dietary history with the family. A diet that includes large amounts of fish, mineral water, and tea provides approximately 5 mg/day of fluoride.
• Fluoride supplementation must be continuous from infancy to age 14 to be effective.
• Tablets can be dissolved in the mouth, chewed, swallowed whole, added to drinking water or fruit juice, or added to water in infant formula or other foods.
• Drops may be administered orally undiluted or added to fluids or food.
• Sodium fluoride may be preferred to stannous fluoride to avoid staining tooth surfaces. Neutral sodium fluoride may also be preferred to acidulated fluoride to avoid dulling of porcelain and ceramic restorations.
• Prolonged intake of drinking water containing a fluoride ion concentration of 0.4 to 0.8 ppm may result in increased density of bone mineral and fluoride osteosclerosis.
• An oral sodium fluoride dose of 40 to 65 mg/day has resulted in adverse rheumatic effects.
• Drug is used investigationally to treat osteoporosis.

Patient education

• Tell patient that sodium fluoride tablets and drops should be taken with meals. Because milk and other dairy products may decrease the absorption of sodium fluoride tablets, tell patient to avoid simultaneous ingestion.
• Advise patient that rinse and gel are most effective if used immediately after brushing or flossing and when taken just before retiring to bed.
• Tell patient to expectorate (and not swallow) excess liquid or gel.
• Warn patient not to eat, drink, or rinse mouth for 15 to 30 minutes after application. Tell patient to use a plastic container—not glass—to dilute drops or rinse, because the fluoride interacts with glass.
• Encourage patient to notify dentist if mottling of teeth occurs.
• Advise patient that if there is a change in water supply or if the patient moves to another area, then a dentist should be contacted because excessive fluoride causes mottled tooth enamel. If patient uses a private well, the water should be tested for fluoride.
• Warn parents to treat fluoride tablets as a drug and to keep them away from children.

Pediatric use

• Young children usually cannot perform the rinse process necessary with oral solutions.
• Because prolonged ingestion or improper techniques may result in dental fluorosis and osseous changes, the dosage must be carefully adjusted according to the amount of fluoride ion in drinking water.

Breast-feeding
• Very little sodium fluoride is distributed into breast milk. The fluoride concentrations in breast milk increase only when daily intake exceeds 1.5 mg.

sodium lactate

Pharmacologic classification: alkalinizer
Therapeutic classification: systemic alkalizer
Pregnancy risk category C

How supplied
Available by prescription only
Injection: 1/6 M solution
Injection for preparations of I.V. admixtures: 5 mEq/ml

Indications, route, and dosage
To alkalinize urine
Adults: 30 ml of a 1/6 M solution/kg of body weight given in divided doses over 24 hours P.O.
Mild to moderate metabolic acidosis
Adults and children: Dosage is highly individualized and depends on the severity of acidosis; patient's age, weight, and clinical condition; and laboratory determinants. Use the following formula to determine dosage for administration by I.V. infusion.

$$\text{Dose in ml of 1/6 M solution} = (60 - \text{plasma } CO_2) \times (0.8 \times \text{body weight in lb})$$

Pharmacodynamics
Alkalizing action: Sodium lactate is metabolized in the liver, producing bicarbonate, the primary extracellular alkalotic buffer for the body's acid-base system, and glycogen. The simultaneous removal of lactate and hydrogen ion during metabolism also produces alkalinization.

Pharmacokinetics
• *Absorption:* Not applicable.
• *Distribution:* Lactate ion occurs naturally throughout the human body.
• *Metabolism:* Lactate is metabolized in the liver to glycogen.
• *Excretion:* None.

Contraindications and precautions
Contraindicated in patients with hypernatremia, lactic acidosis, or conditions in which sodium administration is detrimental. Use extreme caution in patients with metabolic or respiratory alkalosis, severe renal or hepatic disease, shock, hypoxia, or beriberi.

Interactions
None reported.

Effects on diagnostic tests
None reported.

Adverse reactions
Other: fever, infection or thrombophlebitis at injection site; ***metabolic alkalosis,*** hypernatremia, hyperosmolarity (with overdose).

Overdose and treatment
Clinical manifestations of overdose include tetany from hypocalcemia, seizures from alkalosis, and arrhythmias from hypokalemia. Correct fluid, electrolyte, and pH abnormalities. Monitor vital signs and fluid status closely.

☑ Special considerations
• Assess electrolyte, fluid, and acid-base status throughout infusion to prevent alkalosis.
• Monitor injection site for infiltration or extravasation or both.
• Drug should not be used to treat severe metabolic acidosis because the production of bicarbonate from lactate may take 1 to 2 hours.
• I.V. infusion rate should not exceed 300 ml/hour.
• Sodium lactate is physically incompatible with sodium bicarbonate solutions.

Geriatric use
• Use cautiously in elderly patients with heart failure and other fluid- and sodium-retaining states.

Pediatric use
• Drug is safe to use in children; lower doses are usually indicated.

Breast-feeding
• Safety in breast-feeding women is unknown.

sodium phosphates (sodium phosphate and sodium biphosphate)
Fleet Phospho-soda

Pharmacologic classification: acid salt
Therapeutic classification: NaCl laxative
Pregnancy risk category C

How supplied
Available without a prescription
Solution: 18 g sodium phosphate and 48 g sodium biphosphate/100 ml

Indications, route, and dosage
Constipation
Adults: 20 to 30 ml solution mixed with 4 oz (120 ml) cold water.
Children age 10 to 12: 10 ml solution mixed with 4 oz cold water.
Children age 5 to 10: 5 ml solution mixed with 4 oz cold water.
Purgative action
Adults: 45 ml solution mixed with 4 oz cold water.

Pharmacodynamics
Laxative action: Sodium phosphate and sodium biphosphate exert an osmotic effect in the small intestine by drawing water into the intestinal lumen,

producing distention that promotes peristalsis and bowel evacuation.

Pharmacokinetics

• *Absorption:* About 1% to 20% of an oral dose of sodium and phosphate is absorbed. With oral administration, action begins in 3 to 6 hours.
• *Distribution:* Unknown.
• *Metabolism:* Unknown.
• *Excretion:* Unknown; probably in feces and urine.

Contraindications and precautions

Contraindicated in patients with abdominal pain, nausea, vomiting, or other symptoms of appendicitis or acute surgical abdomen; intestinal obstruction or perforation; edema; heart failure; megacolon; or impaired renal function and in patients on sodium-restricted diets. Use cautiously in patients with large hemorrhoids or anal excoriations.

Interactions

Concomitant administration of drug with *antacids* may cause inactivation of both.

Effects on diagnostic tests

None reported.

Adverse reactions

GI: *abdominal cramping.*
Other: fluid and electrolyte disturbances (hypernatremia, hyperphosphatemia) with daily use; laxative dependence with long-term or excessive use.

Overdose and treatment

No information available; probable clinical effects include abdominal pain and diarrhea.

☑ Special considerations

• Dilute drug with water before giving orally (add 30 ml of drug to 120 ml of water). Follow drug administration with full glass of water.
• Monitor serum electrolyte levels; when drug is given as NaCl laxative, up to 10% of sodium content may be absorbed.
• Drug is not routinely used to treat constipation but is commonly used to evacuate the bowel.

Patient education

• Instruct patient on how to mix the drug and on dosage schedule.
• Warn patient that frequent or prolonged use of drug may lead to laxative dependence.

sodium polystyrene sulfonate

Kayexalate, SPS

Pharmacologic classification: cation-exchange resin
Therapeutic classification: potassium-removing resin
Pregnancy risk category C

How supplied

Available by prescription only
Oral powder: 1.25 g/5 ml suspension
Powder for oral or rectal administration: 453.6 g in 1-lb jar
Rectal administration: 1.25 g/5 ml, 15 g/60 ml suspension

Indications, route, and dosage

Hyperkalemia
Adults: 15 g P.O. daily to q.i.d. in water or sorbitol. Alternatively, give 30 to 50 g q.i.d. or q 6 hours as a retention enema.

Pharmacodynamics

Potassium-removing action: Sodium polystyrene sulfonate is a cation-exchange resin that releases sodium in exchange for other cations in the GI tract. High levels of potassium ion are found in the large intestine and therefore are exchanged and eliminated.

Pharmacokinetics

• *Absorption:* Sodium polystyrene sulfonate is not absorbed. The onset of action varies from hours to days.
• *Distribution:* None.
• *Metabolism:* None.
• *Excretion:* Drug is excreted unchanged in feces.

Contraindications and precautions

Contraindicated in patients with hypokalemia or hypersensitivity to drug. Use cautiously in patients with marked edema or severe heart failure or hypertension.

Interactions

When used concomitantly, *magnesium-* and *calcium-containing antacids* are bound by the resin, possibly causing metabolic alkalosis in patients with renal impairment. Toxic effects of *cardiac glycosides* are exaggerated by hypokalemia, even when serum digoxin concentrations are in the normal range.

Effects on diagnostic tests

Sodium polystyrene sulfonate therapy may alter serum magnesium and calcium levels.

Adverse reactions

GI: *constipation,* fecal impaction (in elderly patients), anorexia, gastric irritation, nausea, vomiting, *diarrhea* (with sorbitol emulsions).
Other: ***hypokalemia,*** hypocalcemia, sodium retention.

Overdose and treatment

Clinical manifestations of overdose include signs and symptoms of hypokalemia (irritability, confusion, arrhythmias, ECG changes, severe muscle weakness, and sometimes paralysis) and digitalis toxicity in digitalized patients. Drug may be discontinued or dose lowered when serum potassium level falls to the 4 to 5 mEq/L range.

☑ Special considerations

• For oral administration: mix resin only with water or sorbitol; never mix with orange juice (high potassium content).

• Chill oral suspension to increase palatability; do not heat because that inactivates resin.
• Rectal route is recommended when vomiting, P.O. restrictions, or upper GI tract problems are present.
• Fecal impaction can be prevented in elderly patients by administering resin rectally. Cleaning enema should precede rectal administration.
• For rectal administration, mix polystyrene resin only with water and sorbitol for rectal use. Do not use other vehicles (that is, mineral oil) for rectal administration, to prevent impactions. Ion exchange requires aqueous medium. Sorbitol content prevents impaction. Prepare rectal dose at room temperature. Stir emulsion gently during administration.
• Monitor serum potassium at least once daily. Watch for other signs of hypokalemia.
• Monitor for symptoms of other electrolyte deficiencies (magnesium, calcium) because drug is nonselective. Monitor serum calcium determination in patients receiving sodium polystyrene therapy for more than 3 days. Supplementary calcium may be needed.
• Constipation is more likely to occur when drug is given with concurrent phosphate binders (such as aluminum hydroxide). Monitor patient's bowel habits.
• If hyperkalemia is severe, more drastic modalities should be added; for example, dextrose 50% with regular insulin I.V. push. Do not depend solely on polystyrene resin to lower serum potassium levels in severe hyperkalemia.

Patient education
• Instruct patient in the importance of following a prescribed low-potassium diet.
• Explain necessity of retaining enema to patient. Retention for 6 to 10 hours is ideal, but 30 to 60 minutes is acceptable.

Geriatric use
• Fecal impaction is more likely in elderly patients.

Pediatric use
• Adjust dosage based upon a calculation of 1 mEq of potassium bound for each 1 g of resin.

somatrem
Protropin

Pharmacologic classification: anterior pituitary hormone
Therapeutic classification: human growth hormone
Pregnancy risk category C

How supplied
Available by prescription only
Injectable lyophilized powder: 5 mg (15 IU)/vial, 10 mg (30 IU)/vial

Indications, route, and dosage
Long-term treatment of growth failure from lack of adequate endogenous growth hormone secretion
Children (prepuberty): A weekly dosage of 0.3 mg/kg divided into daily I.M. or S.C. injection. Some clinicians administer up to 0.1 mg/kg three times weekly. A weekly dose of 0.3 mg/kg should not be exceeded.

Pharmacodynamics
Growth-stimulating action: Somatrem is a purified polypeptide hormone of recombinant DNA origin containing a sequence of 192 amino acids identical to the naturally occurring human growth hormone (plus methionine). Somatrem stimulates growth of linear bone, skeletal muscle, and organs and increases RBC mass by stimulating erythropoietin. Most actions are mediated through somatomedins (liver-synthesized hormones).

Pharmacokinetics
• *Absorption:* Somatrem is given by I.M. or S.C. injection.
• *Distribution:* Not fully understood.
• *Metabolism:* Approximately 90% of a dose is metabolized in the liver.
• *Excretion:* Approximately 0.1% of a dose is excreted in urine unchanged. Half-life is 20 to 30 minutes; however, its tissue effects are long-lasting.

Contraindications and precautions
Contraindicated in patients with epiphyseal closure, active neoplasia, or hypersensitivity to benzyl alcohol. Use cautiously in patients with hypothyroidism and in those whose growth hormone deficiency is caused by an intracranial lesion.

Interactions
Concomitant use of somatrem with *adrenocorticoids, corticotropin,* or *glucocorticoids* may inhibit growth response. Concomitant use of somatrem with *anabolic steroids, androgens, estrogens,* or *thyroid hormones* may accelerate epiphyseal maturation.

Effects on diagnostic tests
Somatrem therapy alters glucose tolerance test (reduced with high doses) and total protein and thyroid function tests (thyroxine-binding capacity and ^{131}I uptake may be decreased).

Adverse reactions
Other: hypothyroidism, hyperglycemia, ***antibodies to growth hormone.***

Overdose and treatment
Clinical manifestations of overdose include gigantism in children and acromegalic features, organ enlargement, diabetes mellitus, atherosclerosis, and hypertension in patients who are not growth hormone deficient. The drug should be discontinued in such situations.

☑ Special considerations
• To prepare the solution, inject the bacteriostatic water for injection (supplied) into the vial containing the drug. Then swirl the vial with a gentle rotary motion until the contents are completely dissolved. *Do not shake the vial.*

• After reconstitution, vial solution should be clear. Do not inject if the solution is cloudy or contains particles.
• Store reconstituted vial in refrigerator; it must be used within 14 days.
• Be sure to check the expiration date.
• Observe patient for signs of glucose intolerance.
• Monitor thyroid function tests for development of hypothyroidism.

Patient education
• Emphasize to parents the importance of regular follow-up visits.
• Advise parents to seek medical approval before administering other medications.

somatropin
Humatrope, Nutropin

Pharmacologic classification: anterior pituitary hormone
Therapeutic classification: purified growth hormone (GH)
Pregnancy risk category C

How supplied
Available by prescription only
Injection: 10 mg (30 IU)/2-ml vial
Powder for injection: 5 mg (15 IU)/vial with 5-ml diluent

Indications, route, and dosage
Long-term treatment of growth failure in children with inadequate secretion of endogenous GH
Children: Administer up to 0.06 mg/kg of body weight of Humatrope S.C. or I.M. three times weekly or 0.30 mg/kg of body weight of Nutropin S.C. weekly in daily divided doses.
Growth failure in children associated with chronic renal insufficiency up to time of renal transplantation
Children: Administer 0.35 mg/kg of body weight of Nutropin S.C. weekly in daily divided doses.

Pharmacodynamics
Growth-stimulating action: Somatropin is a purified GH of recombinant DNA origin that stimulates skeletal, linear bone, muscle, and organ growth.

Pharmacokinetics
• *Absorption:* Drug is absorbed from the injection site in a similar fashion as somatrem (human GH).
• *Distribution:* Somatropin localizes to highly perfused organs, notably the liver and kidney.
• *Metabolism:* Metabolized in the liver.
• *Excretion:* Drug is returned to the systemic circulation as amino acids.

Contraindications and precautions
Contraindicated in patients with closed epiphyses or an active underlying intracranial lesion. Humatrope should not be reconstituted with the supplied diluent for patients with known sensitivity to either m-cresol or glycerin.

Use cautiously in children with hypothyroidism and in those whose GH deficiency results from an intracranial lesion; these children should be examined frequently for progression or recurrence of underlying disease.

Interactions
None reported.

Effects on diagnostic tests
Serum levels of inorganic phosphorus, alkaline phosphatase, and parathyroid hormone may increase with somatropin therapy. Laboratory measurements of thyroid hormone may also change.

Adverse reactions
CNS: headache, weakness.
CV: mild, transient edema.
Hematologic: ***leukemia.***
Metabolic: mild hyperglycemia, hypothyroidism.
Other: injection site pain, localized muscle pain, antibody formation to GH.

Overdose and treatment
Long-term overdosage may result in signs and symptoms of gigantism or acromegaly consistent with the known effects of excess human GH.

☑ Special considerations
• To prepare solution, inject the supplied diluent into the vial containing the drug by aiming the stream of the liquid against the glass wall of the vial. Swirl the vial with a gentle rotary motion until the contents are completely dissolved. *Do not shake the vial.*
• After reconstitution, vial solution should be clear. Do not use if it is cloudy or contains particles.
• Store reconstituted vial in refrigerator; use within 14 days.
• If sensitivity to diluent occurs, vial may be reconstituted with sterile water for injection. When drug is reconstituted in this manner, use only one reconstituted dose per vial and refrigerate the solution if it is not used immediately after reconstitution. Use reconstituted dose within 24 hours, and discard unused portion.
• Monitor child's height regularly. Regular monitoring of blood and radiologic studies is also necessary.
• Monitor patient's blood glucose levels regularly because GH may induce a state of insulin resistance.
• Excessive glucocorticoid therapy inhibits the growth-promoting effect of somatropin. Adjust glucocorticoid replacement dose in patients with a coexisting corticotropin deficiency to avoid an inhibitory effect on growth.
• Periodically monitor thyroid function tests for hypothyroidism, which may require treatment with a thyroid hormone.

Patient education
• Inform parents that children with endocrine disorders including GH deficiency are more likely to develop slipped capital epiphyses. Tell them to call if they notice a limp in their child.

sotalol

Betapace

Pharmacologic classification: beta-adrenergic blocker
Therapeutic classification: antiarrhythmic
Pregnancy risk category B

How supplied

Available by prescription only
Tablets: 80 mg, 120 mg, 160 mg, 240 mg

Indications, route, and dosage

Documented, life-threatening ventricular arrhythmias

Adults: Initially, 80 mg P.O. b.i.d. Increase dosage q 2 to 3 days as needed and tolerated. Most patients respond to daily dosage of 160 to 320 mg. A few patients with refractory arrhythmias have received as much as 640 mg daily.

✦ ***Dosage adjustment.*** For adults with renal failure and creatinine clearance above 60 ml/minute, no adjustment in dosage interval is necessary. If creatinine clearance is 30 to 60 ml/minute, give q 24 hours; 10 to 30 ml/minute, q 36 to 48 hours; and if it is less than 10 ml/minute, individualize dosage.

Pharmacodynamics

Antiarrhythmic action: Sotalol is a nonselective beta-adrenergic blocker that depresses sinus heart rate, slows AV conduction, increases AV nodal refractoriness, prolongs the refractory period of atrial and ventricular muscle and AV accessory pathways in anterograde and retrograde directions, decreases cardiac output, and lowers systolic and diastolic blood pressure.

Pharmacokinetics

- *Absorption:* Well absorbed after oral administration, with a bioavailability of 90% to 100%. After oral administration, peak plasma concentrations are reached in 2.5 to 4 hours and steady-state plasma concentrations are attained in 2 to 3 days (after 5 to 6 doses when administered twice daily).
- *Distribution:* Sotalol does not bind to plasma proteins and crosses the blood-brain barrier poorly.
- *Metabolism:* Sotalol is not metabolized.
- *Excretion:* Drug is excreted primarily in the urine unchanged.

Contraindications and precautions

Contraindicated in patients with hypersensitivity to drug, severe sinus node dysfunction, sinus bradycardia, second- and third-degree AV block in the absence of an artificial pacemaker, congenital or acquired long QT syndrome, cardiogenic shock, uncontrolled heart failure, and bronchial asthma.

Use cautiously in patients with impaired renal function or diabetes mellitus.

Interactions

Antiarrhythmic agents cause additive effects when administered with sotalol. Concomitant use should be avoided. *Catecholamine-depleting drugs,* such as *guanethidine* and *reserpine,* enhance the hypotensive effects of sotalol. Monitor the patient closely. *Calcium channel antagonists* enhance myocardial depression and should not be given concomitantly with sotalol. Sotalol may enhance the rebound hypertensive effect seen after withdrawal of *clonidine.* Discontinue sotalol several days before withdrawing *clonidine.* Sotalol may require dosage adjustments with *insulin* or *oral antidiabetic agents* because it may increase blood glucose levels. It also may mask symptoms of hypoglycemia.

Effects on diagnostic tests

Sotalol may increase blood glucose and liver enzyme levels.

Adverse reactions

CNS: *asthenia, light-headedness, headache, dizziness, weakness, fatigue,* sleep problems.
CV: *bradycardia, palpitations, chest pain,* ***arrhythmias, heart failure, AV block, proarrhythmic events (ventricular tachycardia, PVCs, ventricular fibrillation),*** edema, ECG abnormalities, hypotension.
GI: *nausea, vomiting,* diarrhea, dyspepsia.
Respiratory: *dyspnea,* ***bronchospasm.***

Overdose and treatment

The most common signs of overdosage are bradycardia, heart failure, hypotension, bronchospasm, and hypoglycemia. If overdosage occurs, sotalol should be discontinued and the patient observed closely. Because of the lack of protein binding, hemodialysis is useful in reducing sotalol plasma concentrations. Patients should be carefully observed until QT intervals are normalized.

Atropine, another anticholinergic drug, a beta-adrenergic agonist, or transvenous cardiac pacing may also be used to treat bradycardia; transvenous cardiac pacing to treat second- or third-degree heart block; epinephrine to treat hypotension (depending on associated factors); aminophylline or an aerosol beta$_2$-receptor stimulant to treat bronchospasm; and DC cardioversion, transvenous cardiac pacing, epinephrine, or magnesium sulfate to treat torsades de pointes.

☑ Special considerations

- Make dosage adjustments slowly, allowing 2 to 3 days between dosage increments for adequate monitoring of QT intervals and for drug plasma levels to reach steady state.
- Because proarrhythmic events, such as sustained ventricular tachycardia or ventricular fibrillation, may occur at start of therapy and during dosage adjustments, patient should be hospitalized. Facilities and personnel should be available for cardiac rhythm monitoring and ECG interpretation.
- Although patients receiving I.V. lidocaine have begun sotalol therapy without ill effect, other antiarrhythmic drugs should be withdrawn before sotalol therapy begins. Sotalol therapy typically is delayed until two or three half-lives of the withdrawn drug have elapsed. After withdrawal of amiodarone, sotalol should not be administered until the QT interval normalizes.

• Monitor serum electrolytes regularly, especially if patient is receiving diuretics. Electrolyte imbalances, such as hypokalemia or hypomagnesemia, may enhance QT prolongation and increase risk of serious arrhythmias, such as torsades de pointes.

Patient education

• Explain importance of taking sotalol as prescribed, even when he is feeling well.
• Caution patient not to stop drug suddenly.

Pediatric use

• Safety and effectiveness in children have not been established.

Breast-feeding

• Because drug may occur in breast milk, either breast-feeding or sotalol may be discontinued depending on importance of drug to patient's health.

sparfloxacin

Zagam

Pharmacologic classification: fluorinated quinolone
Therapeutic classification: broad-spectrum antibacterial
Pregnancy risk category C

How supplied

Available by prescription only
Tablets: 200 mg

Indications, route, and dosage

***Acute bacterial exacerbation of chronic bronchitis caused by* Staphylococcus aureus, Streptococcus pneumoniae, Chlamydia pneumoniae, Enterobacter cloacae, Klebsiella pneumoniae, Moraxella catarrhalis, Haemophilus influenzae, *or* H. parainfluenzae**

Adults over age 18: 400 mg P.O. on first day as a loading dose, then 200 mg daily for total of 10 days of therapy (total, 11 tablets).

***Community-acquired pneumonia caused* by S. pneumoniae, M. catarrhalis, H. influenzae, H. parainfluenzae, C. pneumoniae, *or* Mycoplasma pneumoniae**

Adults over age 18: 400 mg P.O. on first day as a loading dose, then 200 mg daily for total of 10 days of therapy (total, 11 tablets).

✦ ***Dosage adjustment.*** In patients with renal impairment, if creatinine clearance is below 50 ml/minute, give a loading dose of 400 mg P.O.; thereafter, 200 mg P.O. q 48 hours for a total of 9 days of therapy (total, six tablets).

Pharmacodynamics

Antibactericidal action: Inhibits bacterial DNA gyrase and prevents DNA replication, transcription, repair, and deactivation in susceptible bacteria.

Pharmacokinetics

• *Absorption:* Well absorbed following oral administration with an absolute bioavailability of 92%. Maximum plasma concentrations are achieved 3 to 6 hours after dosing.
• *Distribution:* Volume of distribution is approximately 3.9 L/kg, indicating distribution well into the tissues. Concentration of drug in respiratory tissues at 2 to 6 hours following dosing is approximately three to six times greater than plasma.
• *Metabolism:* Drug is metabolized by the liver, primarily by phase II glucuronidation. Its metabolism does not interfere with or use the cytochrome P-450 system.
• *Excretion:* Excreted in both the urine (50%) and feces (50%). Terminal elimination half-life varies between 16 and 30 hours; mean, 20 hours.

Contraindications and precautions

Contraindicated in patients with history of hypersensitivity or photosensitivity reactions to drugs and those who cannot stay out of the sun. Do not use in patients with cardiac conditions that predispose them to arrhythmias.

Use with caution in patients with known or suspected CNS disorders, such as seizures, toxic psychoses, or tremors.

Interactions

Antacids containing aluminum or magnesium, iron salts, zinc, or sucralfate may interfere with GI absorption of sparfloxacin. Administer at least 4 hours apart. *Drugs that prolong the QTc interval and may cause torsades de pointes* (including *amiodarone, bepridil, disopyramide, class Ia antiarrythmics [procainamide, quinidine], class III drugs [sotalol]*) are contraindicated in these patients. Other *QTc-prolonging drugs* include *astemizole, cisapride, erythromycin, pentamidine, tricyclic antidepressants,* and *some antipsychotics* including *phenothiazines.*

Effects on diagnostic tests

Drug may produce false-negative culture results for *Mycobacterium tuberculosis* and elevations in ALT and AST levels and WBC count.

Adverse reactions

CNS: asthenia, dizziness, headache, insomnia, seizures, somnolence.
CV: *QT interval prolongation,* vasodilatation.
EENT: dry mouth, taste perversion.
GI: abdominal pain, diarrhea, dyspepsia, flatulence, nausea, pseudomembranous colitis, vomiting.
GU: vaginal moniliasis.
Musculoskeletal: tendon rupture.
Skin: photosensitivity, pruritus, rash.
Other: hypersensitivity reactions.

Overdose and treatment

If overdose is suspected, have patient avoid sunlight exposure for 5 days. Monitor ECG for possible QTc prolongation. It is not known if drug is dialyzable.

☑ Special considerations

• Because moderate to severe phototoxic reactions have occurred, avoid exposure to the sun, bright natural light, or ultraviolet light during therapy and for 5 days after therapy.

Patient education
- Inform patient that drug may be taken with food, milk, or products that contain caffeine.
- Tell patient to take drug as prescribed, even if symptoms disappear.
- Advise patient to take drug with plenty of fluids and to avoid antacids, sucralfate, and products containing iron or zinc for at least 4 hours after each dose.
- Warn patient to avoid hazardous tasks until adverse CNS effects of drug are known.
- Advise patient to avoid direct, indirect, and artificial ultraviolet light, even with sunscreen on, during treatment and for 5 days after treatment. Patient should stop drug and call if signs or symptoms of phototoxicity (skin burning, redness, swelling, blisters, rash, itching) occur.
- Tell patient to discontinue drug and report pain or inflammation; tendon rupture can occur with drug. Tell patient to rest and refrain from exercise until a diagnosis is made.
- Instruct patient to drink fluids liberally.

Geriatric use
- Drug's pharmacokinetics are not altered in the elderly with normal renal function.

Pediatric use
- Safety and effectiveness of children and adolescents under age 18 have not been established. Quinolones, including sparfloxacin, cause arthropathy and osteochondrosis in juvenile animals of several species.

Breast-feeding
- Because drug is excreted in breast milk, discontinue breast-feeding or drug.

spectinomycin hydrochloride
Trobicin

Pharmacologic classification: aminocyclitol
Therapeutic classification: antibiotic
Pregnancy risk category NR

How supplied
Available by prescription only
Injection: 2-g vial with 3.2-ml diluent; 4-g vial with 6.2-ml diluent

Indications, route, and dosage
Uncomplicated gonorrhea in patients who are hypersensitive to penicillins or cephalosporins
Adults: 2 to 4 g I.M. single dose injected deeply into upper outer quadrant of the buttocks (4-g dose should be divided into two sites).
◇ ***Disseminated gonorrhea***
Adults: 2 g I.M. b.i.d. for 3 to 7 days. Inject deeply into upper outer quadrant of the buttocks.

Pharmacodynamics
Antibacterial action: Bacteriostatic effect results from binding of drug to 30S ribosomal subunits, thus inhibiting protein synthesis. Although drug is effective against many gram-positive and gram-negative organisms, it is used mostly against penicillin-resistant *Neisseria gonorrhoeae.*

Pharmacokinetics
- *Absorption:* Drug is not absorbed orally. I.M. injection results in rapid absorption; peak concentrations occur in 1 and 2 hours for 2-g and 4-g doses, respectively.
- *Distribution:* Unknown.
- *Metabolism:* Unknown.
- *Excretion:* Most of dose is excreted unchanged in the urine. Elimination half-life ranges from 1 to 3 hours. Drug dosage is unchanged in renal failure.

Contraindications and precautions
Contraindicated in patients with hypersensitivity to drug.

Interactions
None reported.

Effects on diagnostic tests
BUN, AST, and serum alkaline phosphatase levels increase, and hemoglobin, hematocrit, and creatinine clearance levels decrease during spectinomycin therapy.

Adverse reactions
CNS: insomnia, dizziness.
GI: nausea.
GU: decreased urine output and creatinine clearance, increased BUN.
Hematologic: decreased hemoglobin and hematocrit levels.
Skin: urticaria.
Other: fever, chills (may mask or delay symptoms of incubating syphilis), transient increases in liver enzymes, pain at injection site.

Overdose and treatment
No information available.

☑ Special considerations
- Obtain specimen for culture and sensitivity tests before starting therapy.
- Drug is usually reserved for patients with penicillin-resistant gonorrhea strains or for whom other drugs are contraindicated. Ceftriaxone is considered drug of choice for uncomplicated gonorrhea.
- To prepare drug, add supplied diluent to vial and shake until completely dissolved. Use reconstituted solution within 24 hours.
- Inject deep I.M. into upper outer quadrant of gluteal muscle. Give 2-g dose at single site; divide 4-g dose into two equal injections and give at two sites.
- Drug is ineffective against syphilis and may mask symptoms of incubating syphilis infection; it is also not effective in pharyngeal gonococcal infections.
- Lack of response to drug usually results from reinfection.

Patient education
- Tell patient that sexual partners must be treated.

Pediatric use

• Because its safety in infants and children has not been established, drug is not first choice in treatment of these patients. A single dose of 40 mg/kg is recommended by the Centers for Disease Control and Prevention.

Breast-feeding

• Because researchers do not know if drug is excreted in breast milk, an alternative feeding method is recommended during therapy.

spironolactone

Aldactone

Pharmacologic classification: potassium-sparing diuretic
Therapeutic classification: management of edema; antihypertensive; diagnosis of primary hyperaldosteronism; treatment of diuretic-induced hypokalemia
Pregnancy risk category NR

How supplied

Available by prescription only
Tablets: 25 mg, 50 mg, 100 mg

Indications, route, and dosage

Edema
Adults: 25 to 200 mg P.O. daily in divided doses.
Children: Initially, 3.3 mg/kg or 60 mg/m^2 P.O. daily in divided doses.
Hypertension
Adults: 50 to 100 mg P.O. daily in divided doses.
Diuretic-induced hypokalemia
Adults: 25 to 100 mg P.O. daily when oral potassium supplements are considered inappropriate.
Detection of primary hyperaldosteronism
Adults: 400 mg P.O. daily for 4 days (short test) or for 3 to 4 weeks (long test). If hypokalemia and hypertension are corrected, a presumptive diagnosis of primary hyperaldosteronism is made.
◊ ***Hirsutism***
Adults: 50 to 200 mg P.O. daily.
◊ ***Premenstrual syndrome***
Adults: 25 mg q.i.d. P.O. on day 14 of menstrual cycle.
◊ ***To decrease risk of metrorrhagia***
Adults: 50 mg b.i.d. P.O. on days 4 through 21 of menstrual cycle.
◊ ***Acne vulgaris***
Adults: 100 mg P.O. daily.

Pharmacodynamics

Diuretic and potassium-sparing action: Spironolactone competitively inhibits aldosterone effects on the distal renal tubules, increasing sodium and water excretion and decreasing potassium excretion.

Spironolactone is used to treat edema associated with excessive aldosterone secretion, such as that associated with hepatic cirrhosis, nephrotic syndrome, and heart failure. It is also used to treat diuretic-induced hypokalemia.

Antihypertensive action: The mechanism of action is unknown; spironolactone may block the effect of aldosterone on arteriolar smooth muscle.

Diagnosis of primary hyperaldosteronism: Spironolactone inhibits the effects of aldosterone; therefore, correction of hypokalemia and hypertension is presumptive evidence of primary hyperaldosteronism.

Pharmacokinetics

• *Absorption:* About 90% of drug is absorbed after oral administration. Onset of action is gradual; maximum effect occurs on third day of therapy.
• *Distribution:* Drug and its major metabolite, canrenone, are more than 90% plasma protein-bound.
• *Metabolism:* Rapidly and extensively metabolized to canrenone.
• *Excretion:* Canrenone and other metabolites are excreted primarily in urine, and a small amount is excreted in feces via the biliary tract; half-life of canrenone is 13 to 24 hours. Half-life of parent compound is 1 to 2 hours.

Contraindications and precautions

Contraindicated in patients with anuria, acute or progressive renal insufficiency, or hyperkalemia. Use cautiously in patients with impaired renal function, hepatic disease, or fluid and electrolyte imbalances.

Interactions

Spironolactone may potentiate the hypotensive effects of *other antihypertensive agents;* this may be used to therapeutic advantage.

Spironolactone increases the risk of hyperkalemia when administered with *other potassium-sparing diuretics, ACE inhibitors, potassium supplements, potassium-containing medications (parenteral penicillin G),* or *salt substitutes.*

NSAIDs, such as *ibuprofen* or *indomethacin,* may impair renal function and thus affect potassium excretion. *Aspirin* may slightly decrease the clinical response to spironolactone.

Effects on diagnostic tests

Spironolactone therapy alters fluorometric determinations of plasma and urinary 17-hydroxycorticosteroid levels and may cause false elevations on radioimmunoassay of serum digoxin.

Adverse reactions

CNS: headache, drowsiness, lethargy, confusion, ataxia.
GI: diarrhea, gastric bleeding, ulceration, cramping, gastritis, vomiting.
Skin: urticaria, maculopapular eruptions.
Other: ***hyperkalemia, agranulocytosis,*** dehydration, hyponatremia, transient elevation in BUN, metabolic acidosis, inability to maintain erection, hirsutism, gynecomastia, breast soreness and menstrual disturbances in women, drug fever.

Overdose and treatment

Clinical signs of overdose are consistent with dehydration and electrolyte disturbance.

Treatment is supportive and symptomatic. In acute ingestion, empty stomach by emesis or lavage. In severe hyperkalemia (over 6.5 mEq/L), reduce serum potassium levels with I.V. sodium bicarbonate or glucose with insulin. A cation exchange resin, sodium polystyrene sulfonate (Kayexalate), given orally or as a retention enema, may also reduce serum potassium levels.

☑ Special considerations

Besides those relevant to all *potassium-sparing diuretics,* consider the following recommendations.
- Give drug with meals to enhance absorption.
- Diuretic effect may be delayed 2 to 3 days if drug is used alone; maximum antihypertensive effect may be delayed 2 to 3 weeks.
- Protect drug from light.
- Adverse reactions are related to dosage levels and duration of therapy and usually disappear with withdrawal of drug; however, gynecomastia may persist.
- Spironolactone is antiandrogenic and has been used to treat hirsutism in dosages of 200 mg/day.
- Avoid unnecessary use of drug. Drug has been shown to induce tumors in laboratory animals.

Patient education

- Explain that maximal diuresis may not occur until day 3 of therapy and that diuresis may continue for 2 to 3 days after drug is withdrawn.
- Instruct patient to report mental confusion or lethargy immediately.
- Explain that adverse reactions usually disappear after drug is discontinued; gynecomastia, however, may persist.
- Caution patient to avoid such hazardous activities as driving until response to drug is known.

Geriatric use

- Elderly patients are more susceptible to diuretic effects and may require lower doses to prevent excessive diuresis.

Pediatric use

- When administering drug to children, crush tablets and administer them in cherry syrup as an oral suspension.

Breast-feeding

- Spironolactone's safety during breast-feeding has not been established. Canrenone, a metabolite, is distributed into breast milk. Alternative feeding method is recommended during therapy with spironolactone.

stavudine (d4T)

Zerit

Pharmacologic classification: synthetic thymidine nucleoside analogue
Therapeutic classification: antiviral
Pregnancy risk category C

How supplied

Available by prescription only
Capsules: 15 mg, 20 mg, 30 mg, 40 mg

Indications, route, and dosage

Treatment of patients HIV infection who have received prolonged prior zidovudine therapy
Adults: For patients weighing 132 lb (60 kg) or more, 40 mg P.O. q 12 hours; for patients weighing below 132 lb, 30 mg P.O. q 12 hours.
✦ ***Dosage adjustment.*** Refer to dosing chart below for patients with renal impairment.

Creatinine clearance (ml/min)	Dosage for patients weighing ≥ 60 kg	Dosage for patients weighing < 60 kg
> 50	40 mg q 12 hr	30 mg q 12 hr
26 to 50	20 mg q 12 hr	15 mg q 12 hr
10 to 25	20 mg q 24 hr	15 mg q 24 hr

Pharmacodynamics

Antiviral action: Stavudine is phosphorylated by cellular kinases to stavudine triphosphate, which exerts antiviral activity. Stavudine triphosphate inhibits HIV replication by two known mechanisms. First, it inhibits HIV reverse transcriptase by competing with the natural substrate deoxythymidine triphosphate. Second, it inhibits viral DNA synthesis by causing DNA chain termination because stavudine lacks the 3″-hydroxyl group necessary for DNA elongation. Stavudine triphosphate also inhibits cellular DNA polymerase beta and gamma and markedly reduces mitochondrial DNA synthesis.

Pharmacokinetics

- *Absorption:* Rapidly absorbed with a mean absolute bioavailability of 86.4%. Peak plasma concentrations occur in 1 hour or less.
- *Distribution:* Mean volume of distribution is 58 L, suggesting distribution into extravascular space. Drug is distributed equally between RBCs and plasma. It binds poorly to plasma proteins.
- *Metabolism:* Not clearly defined in humans.
- *Excretion:* Renal elimination accounts for approximately 40% of overall clearance, regardless of administration route; there is active tubular secretion in addition to glomerular filtration.

Contraindications and precautions

Contraindicated in patients with hypersensitivity to drug. Use cautiously in patients with impaired renal function or history of peripheral neuropathy and in pregnant women.

Interactions

None significant.

Effects on diagnostic tests

Stavudine may cause a mild to moderate increase in AST and ALT levels.

Adverse reactions

CNS: *peripheral neuropathy, headache, malaise, insomnia, anxiety, depression, nervousness,* dizziness.
CV: chest pain.
GI: *abdominal pain, diarrhea, nausea, vomiting, anorexia,* dyspepsia, constipation, weight loss.
Hematologic: ***neutropenia, thrombocytopenia,*** anemia.
Skin: *rash, diaphoresis, pruritus,* maculopapular rash.
Other: *myalgia, hepatotoxicity, chills, fever, asthenia, back pain, arthralgia, dyspnea,* conjunctivitis.

Overdose and treatment

Experience with adults who had received 12 to 24 times the recommended daily dosage revealed no acute toxicity. Complications of chronic overdosage include peripheral neuropathy and hepatic toxicity. It is not known if drug is eliminated by peritoneal dialysis or hemodialysis.

☑ Special considerations

- Monitor patient for development of peripheral neuropathy, usually characterized by numbness, tingling, or pain in the feet or hands. If symptoms develop, interrupt drug therapy. Symptoms may resolve if therapy is withdrawn promptly. Sometimes symptoms may worsen temporarily after drug discontinuation. If symptoms resolve completely, resume treatment using the following dosage schedule: patients weighing 132 lb or more should receive 20 mg twice daily; patients weighing less than 132 lb should receive 15 mg twice daily. Manage clinically significant elevations of hepatic transaminase levels in same way.

Patient education

- Inform patient that stavudine is not a cure for HIV infection and that the patient may continue to acquire illnesses associated with AIDS or AIDS-related complex, including opportunistic infections.
- Inform patient that drug does not reduce risk of transmitting HIV to others through sexual contact or blood contamination.
- Instruct patient to report signs of peripheral neuropathy, such as tingling, burning, pain, or numbness in the hands or feet, because dosage adjustments may be necessary. Counsel patient that this toxicity occurs with greater frequency in patients with history of peripheral neuropathy. Also advise patient not to use other medications, including OTC preparations, without calling first; some drugs can exacerbate peripheral neuropathy.
- Explain that long-term effects of drug are currently unknown.

Pediatric use

- Safety and effectiveness of drug for treatment of HIV in children have not been established.

Breast-feeding

- It is not known if drug occurs in breast milk. Because of the potential for adverse reactions from stavudine in breast-fed infants, discontinue breast-feeding during therapy.

streptokinase

Kabikinase, Streptase

Pharmacologic classification: plasminogen activator
Therapeutic classification: thrombolytic enzyme
Pregnancy risk category C

How supplied

Available by prescription only
Injection: 250,000 IU, 600,000 IU, 750,000 IU, 1,500,000 IU in vials for reconstitution

Indications, route, and dosage

Lysis of coronary artery thrombi after acute MI
Adults: 1,500,000 IU by I.V. infusion over 60 minutes; intracoronary loading dose of 20,000 IU via coronary catheter, followed by a maintenance dose of 2,000 IU/minute for 60 minutes as an infusion.
Arteriovenous cannula occlusion
Adults: 250,000 IU in 2 ml I.V. solution by I.V. infusion pump into each occluded limb of the cannula over 25 to 35 minutes. Clamp off cannula for 2 hours, then aspirate contents of cannula, flush with NaCl solution, and reconnect.
Venous thrombosis, pulmonary embolism, and arterial thrombosis and embolism
Adults: Loading dose of 250,000 IU I.V. infusion over 30 minutes. Sustaining dose: 100,000 IU/hour I.V. infusion for 72 hours for deep vein thrombosis and 100,000 IU/hour over 24 hours by I.V. infusion pump for pulmonary embolism.

Pharmacodynamics

Thrombolytic action: Streptokinase promotes thrombolysis by activating plasminogen in two steps. First, plasminogen and streptokinase form a complex, exposing plasminogen-activating site, and second, cleavage of peptide bond converts plasminogen to plasmin.

In treatment of acute MI, streptokinase prevents primary or secondary thrombus formation in microcirculation surrounding the necrotic area.

Pharmacokinetics

- *Absorption:* Plasminogen activation begins promptly after infusion or instillation of streptokinase; adequate activation of fibrinolytic system occurs in 3 to 4 hours.
- *Distribution:* Streptokinase does not cross placenta, but antibodies do.
- *Metabolism:* Insignificant.
- *Excretion:* Streptokinase is removed from circulation by antibodies and reticuloendothelial system. Half-life is biphasic; initially it is 18 minutes (from antibody action) and then extends up to 83 minutes. Anticoagulant effect may persist for 12 to 24 hours after infusion is discontinued.

Contraindications and precautions

Contraindicated in patients with ulcerative wounds, active internal bleeding, and recent CVA; recent trauma with possible internal injuries; visceral or intracranial malignant neoplasms; ulcerative colitis; diverticulitis; severe hypertension; acute or chronic hepatic or renal insufficiency; uncontrolled hypocoagulation; chronic pulmonary disease with cavitation; subacute bacterial endocarditis or rheumatic valvular disease; or recent cerebral embolism, thrombosis, or hemorrhage.

Also contraindicated within 10 days after intra-arterial diagnostic procedure or any surgery, including liver or kidney biopsy, lumbar puncture, thoracentesis, paracentesis, or extensive or multiple cutdowns. I.M. injections and other invasive procedures are contraindicated during streptokinase therapy.

Use cautiously in patients with arterial embolism that originates from the left side of the heart.

Interactions

Concomitant use with *anticoagulants* may cause hemorrhage. It may also be necessary to reverse effects of oral anticoagulants before beginning therapy. Concomitant use with *aspirin, indomethacin, phenylbutazone*, or other *drugs affecting platelet activity* increases risk of bleeding. *Aminocaproic acid* inhibits streptokinase-induced activation of plasminogen.

Effects on diagnostic tests

Streptokinase increases thrombin time, activated partial thromboplastin time, and PT; drug sometimes moderately decreases hematocrit.

Adverse reactions

CNS: polyradiculoneuropathy, headache.
CV: ***reperfusion arrhythmias,*** *hypotension,* vasculitis.
EENT: periorbital edema.
GI: nausea.
Hematologic: ***bleeding.***
Respiratory: minor breathing difficulty, ***bronchospasm.***
Skin: urticaria, pruritus, flushing.
Other: phlebitis at injection site, hypersensitivity reactions ***(anaphylaxis),*** delayed hypersensitivity reactions (interstitial nephritis, serum sickness-like reactions), musculoskeletal pain, ***angioedema,*** *fever.*

Overdose and treatment

Clinical manifestations of overdose include signs of potentially serious bleeding: bleeding gums, epistaxis, hematoma, spontaneous ecchymoses, oozing at catheter site, increased pulse, and pain from internal bleeding. Discontinue drug and restart when bleeding stops.

☑ Special considerations

Besides those relevant to all *thrombolytic enzymes,* consider the following recommendations.

- Reconstitute vial with 5 ml 0.9% NaCl injection, and further dilute to 45 ml; roll gently to mix. *Do not shake.* Use immediately; refrigerate remainder and discard after 8 hours. Store powder at room temperature.
- Rate of I.V. infusion depends on thrombin time and streptokinase resistance; higher loading dose may be necessary in patients with recent streptococcal infection or recent treatment with streptokinase, to compensate for antibody drug neutralization.
- Do not discontinue therapy for minor allergic reactions that can be treated with antihistamines or corticosteroids; about one third of patients experience a slight temperature elevation, and some have chills. Symptomatic treatment with acetaminophen (but not aspirin or other salicylates) is indicated if temperature reaches 104° F (40° C). Patients may be pretreated with corticosteroids, repeating doses during therapy, to minimize pyrogenic or allergic reactions.
- If minor bleeding can be controlled by local pressure, do not decrease dose so that more plasminogen is available for conversion to plasmin.
- Antibodies to streptokinase can persist for 3 to 6 months or longer after the initial dose; if further thrombolytic therapy is needed, consider urokinase.

Geriatric use

- Patients age 75 or older have a greater risk of cerebral hemorrhage, because they are likely to have preexisting cerebrovascular disease.

Pediatric use

- Safety and effectiveness in children have not been established.

streptomycin sulfate

Pharmacologic classification: aminoglycoside
Therapeutic classification: antibiotic
Pregnancy risk category D

How supplied

Available by prescription only
Injection: 400 mg/ml

Indications, route, and dosage

Primary and adjunctive treatment in tuberculosis

Adults with normal renal function: 1 g or 15 mg/kg I.M. daily for 2 to 3 months, then 1 g two or three times weekly. Inject deeply into upper outer quadrant of buttocks or midlateral thigh. Maximum daily dose, 1 g.

Children with normal renal function: 20 to 40 mg/kg I.M. daily in divided doses injected deeply into large muscle mass, preferably in the midlateral muscles of the thigh. Give concurrently with other antitubercular agents, but *not* with capreomycin, and continue until sputum specimen becomes negative. Maximum daily dose, 1 g.

Enterococcal endocarditis

Adults: 1 g I.M. q 12 hours for 2 weeks, then 500 mg I.M. q 12 hours for 4 weeks with penicillin.

Tularemia

Adults: 1 to 2 g I.M. daily in divided doses injected deep into upper outer quadrant of buttocks. Continue until patient is afebrile for 5 to 7 days.

Plague

Adults: 2 g I.M. daily in divided doses injected deep into upper outer quadrant of buttocks for a minimum of 10 days.

◇**Mycobacterium avium**
Adults: 11 to 13 mg/kg/24 hours I.V. or 15 mg/kg/day I.M.

✦ ***Dosage adjustment.*** In adults and children with renal failure, initial dosage is same as for those with normal renal function. Subsequent doses and frequency determined by renal function study results and blood serum concentrations; peak serum levels should not exceed 20 to 25 mcg/ml, and trough levels should be 5 mcg/ml or less. Patients with a creatinine clearance over 50 ml/minute usually can tolerate drug daily; if creatinine clearance is 10 to 50 ml/minute, increase administration interval to q 24 to 72 hours. Patients with a creatinine clearance under 10 ml/minute may require 72 to 96 hours between doses.

Pharmacodynamics

Antibiotic action: Streptomycin is bactericidal; it binds directly to the 30S ribosomal subunit, thus inhibiting bacterial protein synthesis. Its spectrum of activity includes many aerobic gram-negative organisms and some aerobic gram-positive organisms. Streptomycin is generally less active against many gram-negative organisms than is tobramycin, gentamicin, amikacin, or netilmicin. Streptomycin is also active against *Mycobacterium* and *Brucella.*

Pharmacokinetics

- *Absorption:* Absorbed poorly after oral administration and usually is given parenterally; peak serum concentrations occur 1 to 2 hours after I.M. administration.
- *Distribution:* Widely distributed after parenteral administration; intraocular penetration is poor. CSF penetration is low, even in patients with inflamed meninges. Streptomycin crosses the placenta; it is 36% protein-bound.
- *Metabolism:* Not metabolized.
- *Excretion:* Drug is excreted primarily in urine by glomerular filtration; small amounts may be excreted in bile and breast milk. Elimination half-life in adults is 2 to 3 hours. In severe renal damage, half-life may extend to 110 hours.

Contraindications and precautions

Contraindicated in patients with hypersensitivity to drug or other aminoglycosides and in those with labyrinthine disease. Never administer I.V. Use cautiously in patients with impaired renal function or neuromuscular disorders and in the elderly.

Interactions

Concomitant use with the following drugs may increase the hazard of nephrotoxicity, ototoxicity, and neurotoxicity: *amphotericin B, capreomycin, cephalosporins, cisplatin, methoxyflurane, polymyxin B, vancomycin,* and other *aminoglycosides.* Hazard of ototoxicity is also increased during use with *bumetanide, ethacrynic acid, furosemide, mannitol,* or *urea. Dimenhydrinate* and other *antiemetic* and *antivertigo* drugs may mask streptomycin-induced ototoxicity.

Concomitant use with *penicillins* results in synergistic bactericidal effect against *Pseudomonas aeruginosa, Escherichia coli, Klebsiella, Citrobacter, Enterobacter, Serratia,* and *Proteus mirabilis;* however, the drugs are physically and chemically incompatible and are inactivated when mixed or given together. In vivo inactivation has been reported when aminoglycosides and *penicillins* are used concomitantly.

Streptomycin may potentiate neuromuscular blockade from *general anesthetics* or *neuromuscular blocking agents* such as *succinylcholine* and *tubocurarine.*

Effects on diagnostic tests

Streptomycin may cause false-positive reaction in copper sulfate test for urine glucose (Benedict's reagent or Clinitest).

Streptomycin-induced nephrotoxicity may elevate levels of BUN, nonprotein nitrogen, or serum creatinine levels and increase urinary excretion of casts.

Adverse reactions

CNS: ***neuromuscular blockade.***
EENT: *ototoxicity.*
GI: vomiting, nausea.
GU: some nephrotoxicity (not as frequently as with other aminoglycosides).
Hematologic: eosinophilia, leukopenia, ***thrombocytopenia.***
Respiratory: ***apnea.***
Skin: ***exfoliative dermatitis.***
Other: hypersensitivity reactions (rash, fever, urticaria, angioedema), ***anaphylaxis.***

Overdose and treatment

Clinical signs of overdose include ototoxicity, nephrotoxicity, and neuromuscular toxicity. Remove drug by hemodialysis or peritoneal dialysis. Treatment with calcium salts or anticholinesterases reverses neuromuscular blockade.

☑ Special considerations

Besides those relevant to all *aminoglycosides,* consider the following recommendations.

- Protect hands when preparing drug; drug irritates skin.
- In primary tuberculosis therapy, discontinue streptomycin when sputum culture is negative.
- Because streptomycin is dialyzable, patients undergoing hemodialysis may need dosage adjustments.

streptozocin

Zanosar

Pharmacologic classification: antibiotic antineoplastic nitrosourea (cell cycle–phase nonspecific)
Therapeutic classification: antineoplastic
Pregnancy risk category C

How supplied

Available by prescription only
Injection: 1-g vials

Indications, route, and dosage

Dosage and indications may vary. Check current literature for recommended protocol.

Metastatic islet cell carcinoma of the pancreas

Adults and children: 500 mg/m^2 I.V. for 5 consecutive days q 6 weeks until maximum benefit or toxicity is observed. Alternatively, 1,000 mg/m^2 at weekly intervals for first 2 weeks; may be increased to a maximum single dose of 1,500 mg/m^2. Usual course of therapy is 4 to 6 weeks.

✦ ***Dosage adjustment.*** In patients with impaired renal function, give 75% of dose if creatinine clearance is 10 to 50 ml/minute and 50% of dose if it is less than 10 ml/minute.

Pharmacodynamics

Antineoplastic action: Streptozocin exerts its cytotoxic activity by selectively inhibiting DNA synthesis. The drug also causes cross-linking of DNA strands through an alkylation mechanism.

Pharmacokinetics

- *Absorption:* Streptozocin is not active orally; it must be given I.V.
- *Distribution:* After an I.V. dose, drug and its metabolites distribute mainly into the liver, kidneys, intestines, and pancreas. Drug has not been shown to cross the blood-brain barrier; however, its metabolites achieve concentrations in the CSF equivalent to the concentration in the plasma.
- *Metabolism:* Extensively metabolized in the liver and kidneys.
- *Excretion:* Elimination of drug from the plasma is biphasic, with an initial half-life of 5 minutes and a terminal phase half-life of 35 to 40 minutes. Plasma half-life of metabolites is longer than parent drug. Drug and its metabolites are excreted primarily in urine and a small amount of dose may also be excreted in expired air.

Contraindications and precautions

No known contraindications. Use cautiously in patients with preexisting renal and hepatic disease.

Interactions

When used concomitantly, other *nephrotoxic drugs* may potentiate the nephrotoxicity caused by streptozocin. Concomitant use with *doxorubicin* prolongs the elimination half-life of *doxorubicin* and necessitates reduced dosage of *doxorubicin.* Concurrent use with *phenytoin* may decrease the effects of streptozocin on the pancreas.

Effects on diagnostic tests

Drug therapy may decrease serum albumin and increase liver function test values; these increases are a sign of hepatotoxicity. BUN and serum creatinine levels may be increased, indicating nephrotoxicity. Drug may decrease blood glucose levels because of a sudden release of insulin.

Adverse reactions

CNS: confusion, lethargy, depression.
GI: *nausea, vomiting,* diarrhea.
GU: *renal toxicity* (evidenced by azotemia, glycosuria, and renal tubular acidosis), mild proteinuria.
Hematologic: ***anemia, leukopenia, thrombocytopenia.***
Hepatic: elevated liver enzyme levels, jaundice, *liver dysfunction.*
Other: hyperglycemia, hypoglycemia, diabetes mellitus.

Overdose and treatment

Clinical manifestations of overdose include myelosuppression, nausea, and vomiting.

Treatment is usually supportive and includes transfusion of blood components and antiemetics.

☑ Special considerations

- To reconstitute drug, use 9.5 ml of 0.9% NaCl injection to yield a concentration of 100 mg/ml.
- Drug should be used within 12 hours of reconstitution. Reconstituted solution is a golden color that changes to dark brown upon decomposition.
- Product contains no preservatives and is not intended as a multiple-dose vial.
- Drug may be administered by rapid I.V. push injection.
- Drug may be further diluted in 10 to 200 ml of D_5W to infuse over 10 to 15 minutes. It can also be infused over 6 hours.
- Gloves should be worn to protect the skin from contact during preparation or administration. If contact occurs, wash solution off immediately with soap and water. Follow recommended procedures for the safe preparation, administration, and disposal of chemotherapeutic agents.
- Extravasation may cause ulceration and tissue necrosis.
- Keep dextrose 50% at bedside because of risk of hypoglycemia from sudden release of insulin.
- Nausea and vomiting occur in almost all patients within 1 to 4 hours. Make sure patient is being treated with an antiemetic.
- Mild proteinuria is one of the first signs of renal toxicity and may necessitate dosage reduction.
- Test urine regularly for protein and glucose.
- Monitor CBC and liver function studies at least weekly.
- Renal toxicity resulting from therapy is dose related and cumulative. Monitor renal function before and after each course of therapy. Obtain urinalysis, BUN levels, and creatinine clearance before therapy and at least weekly during drug administration. Continue weekly monitoring for 4 weeks after each course.
- Drug has also been used in the treatment of colon cancer, pancreatic adenocarcinoma, and carcinoid tumors. These uses are unlabeled and dosing schedules and protocols vary.

Patient education

- Encourage adequate fluid intake to increase urine output and reduce potential for renal toxicity.
- Remind diabetic patients that intensive monitoring of blood glucose levels is necessary.
- Tell patient to report symptoms of anemia, infection, or bleeding immediately.
- Warn patient that he may bruise easily because of drug's effect on blood count.

Breast-feeding
• It is not known if drug occurs in breast milk. However, because of the potential for serious adverse reactions, mutagenicity, and carcinogenicity in the infant, breast-feeding is not recommended.

strontium-89 chloride
Metastron

Pharmacologic classification: radioisotope
Therapeutic classification: radioisotope for metastatic bone pain
Pregnancy risk category D

How supplied
Available by prescription only
Injection: 10.9 to 22.6 mg/ml in 10-ml vial

Indications, route, and dosage
Relief of metastatic bone pain
Adults: 148 MBq, 4 mCi administered by slow I.V. injection (1 to 2 minutes). Alternatively, a dose of 1.5 to 2.2 MBq/kg, 40 to 60 mcCi/kg may be used. Do not repeat dose for at least 90 days.

Pharmacodynamics
Analgesic action: Strontium-89 chloride selectively irradiates sites of primary metastatic bone involvement with minimal irradiation of soft tissues distant from the bone lesions.

Pharmacokinetics
• *Absorption:* Rapidly cleared from the blood and selectively localized in bone mineral.
• *Distribution:* Uptake of strontium-89 by bone occurs preferentially in sites of active osteogenesis; thus, primary bone tumors and areas of metastatic involvement (blastic lesions) can accumulate significantly greater concentrations of strontium-89 than surrounding normal bone.
• *Metabolism:* Strontium-89 decays by beta emission with a physical half-life of 50.5 days.
• *Excretion:* Excretion pathways are two thirds urinary and one third fecal in patients with bone metastases. Urine excretion, which is higher in people without bone lesions, is greatest in the first 2 days after injection.

Contraindications and precautions
Contraindicated in pregnant patients. Use cautiously in patients with platelet counts below 60,000/mm^3 or WBC counts below 2,400/mm^3.

Interactions
None reported.

Effects on diagnostic tests
None reported.

Adverse reactions
CV: cutaneous flushing with rapid injection.
Hematologic: ***bone marrow suppression.***
Other: transient increase in pain ("flare" reaction).

Overdose and treatment
No information available.

☑ Special considerations
• Measure patient dose by a suitable radioactivity calibration system immediately before administration.
• Bone marrow toxicity is to be expected after administration, particularly involving WBCs and platelets. The extent of toxicity varies. Monitor patient's peripheral blood cell counts at least once every other week. Typically, platelet count is depressed by about 30% compared with preadministration levels. The nadir of platelet depression in most patients is between 12 and 16 weeks after administration of strontium-89. WBCs are usually depressed to a varying extent compared with preadministration levels. Therefore, recovery occurs slowly, typically reaching preadministration levels 6 months after treatment unless patient's disease or additional therapy intervenes.
• In considering repeat administration, carefully evaluate patient's hematologic response to initial dose, current platelet level, and other evidence of marrow depletion. Repeat doses are generally not recommended at intervals of less than 90 days.
• Verify dose and patient before administration because strontium-89 delivers a relatively high dose of radioactivity.
• Strontium-89 is a potential carcinogen; restrict use to patients with well-documented metastatic bone disease.
• Like other radioactive drugs, strontium-89 requires careful handling and appropriate safety measures to minimize radiation to clinical personnel.
• Because of delayed onset of pain relief (typically 7 to 20 days after injection), use in patients with very short life expectancy is not recommended.
• Avoid administering strontium-89 too rapidly; a calcium-like flushing sensation can occur if the injection takes less than 30 seconds to administer.
• Take special precautions, such as urinary catheterization, after administration to incontinent patients to minimize risk of radioactive contamination of clothing, bed linen, and patient's environment.

Patient education
• Advise women of childbearing age to avoid pregnancy because strontium-89 may cause fetal harm.
• Inform patient that pain relief usually occurs from 7 to 20 days after injection and lasts for several months.
• Explain that a slight increase in pain 2 to 3 days after injection is normal. A temporary increase in the dose of pain medication may be recommended until the pain subsides.
• Tell patient that routine blood tests may be required periodically.
• Advise patient to inform anyone providing medical treatment that he has received strontium-89.
• Instruct patient to take radiation precautions for 1 week after injection of strontium-89 because it will be present in the blood and urine.

Pediatric use
- Safety and effectiveness in children under age 18 have not been established.

Breast-feeding
- It is not known if strontium-89 is excreted in breast milk. Therefore, breast-feeding should be discontinued by patient about to receive drug.

succimer
Chemet

Pharmacologic classification: heavy metal
Therapeutic classification: chelating agent
Pregnancy risk category C

How supplied
Available by prescription only
Capsules: 100 mg

Indications, route, and dosage
Treatment of lead poisoning in children with blood lead levels above 45 mcg/dl
Children: Initially, 10 mg/kg or 350 mg/m² P.O. q 8 hours for 5 days. Higher starting doses are not recommended. Frequency of administration may be reduced to 10 mg/kg or 350 mg/m² q 12 hours for an additional 2 weeks of therapy. A course of treatment lasts 19 days and repeated courses may be necessary if indicated by weekly monitoring of blood lead levels. A minimum of 2 weeks between courses is recommended unless blood lead concentrations mandate more prompt action.
✦ ***Dosage adjustment.*** Dose is to be administered q 8 hours for 5 days, followed by same dose q 12 hours for 14 days.

PEDIATRIC DOSING CHART

Weight (lb)	Weight (kg)	Dose (mg)	No. of Capsules
18 to 35	8 to 15	100	1
36 to 55	16 to 23	200	2
56 to 75	24 to 34	300	3
76 to 100	35 to 45	400	4
> 100	> 45	500	5

Pharmacodynamics
Antidote action: Succimer forms water-soluble chelates and increases the urinary excretion of lead.

Pharmacokinetics
- *Absorption:* Rapid but variable absorption after oral administration; peak blood levels in 1 to 2 hours.
- *Distribution:* Unknown.
- *Metabolism:* Rapidly and extensively metabolized.
- *Excretion:* 39% in feces as nonabsorbed drug; 9%, in urine; 1%, as carbon dioxide from the lungs. Approximately 90% of absorbed drug is excreted in urine.

Contraindications and precautions
Contraindicated in patients with hypersensitivity to drug. Use cautiously in patients with impaired renal function.

Interactions
Concurrent administration of succimer with *other chelating agents* is not recommended.

Effects on diagnostic tests
False-positive results for ketones in urine using nitroprusside reagents (Ketostix) and false decreased levels of serum uric acid and CK have been reported. Transient mild elevations of serum transaminase levels have also been observed.

Adverse reactions
CNS: *drowsiness, dizziness, sensory motor neuropathy, sleepiness, paresthesia, headache.*
CV: ***arrhythmias.***
EENT: plugged ears, cloudy film in eyes, otitis media, watery eyes, sore throat, rhinorrhea, nasal congestion.
GI: *nausea, vomiting, diarrhea, loss of appetite, abdominal cramps, hemorrhoidal symptoms, metallic taste in mouth, loose stools.*
GU: decreased urination, difficult urination, proteinuria.
Hematologic: increased platelet count, intermittent eosinophilia.
Respiratory: cough, head cold.
Skin: papular rash, herpetic rash, mucocutaneous eruptions, pruritus.
Other: *leg, kneecap, back, stomach, rib, or flank pain; flu-like symptoms;* moniliasis; *elevated serum AST, ALT, alkaline phosphatase, or cholesterol levels.*

Overdose and treatment
No cases of overdose have been reported. In cases of acute overdose, induce vomiting with ipecac syrup or perform gastric lavage, followed by administration of activated charcoal slurry and appropriate supportive therapy.

☑ Special considerations
- Identification and abatement of lead sources in child's environment are critical to successful therapy. Chelation therapy is not a substitute for preventing further exposure and should not be used to permit continued exposure.
- Patients who have received ethylenediaminetetraacetic acid, with or without dimercaprol, may use succimer as subsequent therapy after an interval of 4 weeks. Use with other chelating agents concurrently is not recommended.
- Monitor serum transaminase levels before and at least weekly during therapy. Patients with a history of hepatic disease should be monitored more closely.
- Consider the possibility of allergic or other mucocutaneous reactions each time drug is used, including the initial course.

• Elevated blood lead levels and associated symptoms may return rapidly after drug is discontinued because of redistribution of lead from bone to soft tissues and blood. Monitor patients at least once weekly for rebound blood lead levels.
• The severity of lead intoxication should be used as a guide for more frequent blood lead monitoring. This is measured by the initial blood lead level and the rate and degree of rebound of blood lead.
• Drug is not indicated for prophylaxis of lead poisoning.

Patient education
• Instruct parents to maintain adequate fluid intake.
• Tell parents to report rash.
• Urge parents to identify and remove source of lead in environment.
• Tell parents to store capsules at room temperature, out of children's reach.

Pediatric use
• For young children who cannot swallow capsules, succimer capsule may be opened and sprinkled on a small amount of soft food or medicated beads from the capsules may be poured onto a spoon for administration and followed with a fruit drink.

succinylcholine chloride (suxamethonium chloride)
Anectine, Anectine Flo-Pack, Quelicin, Sucostrin

Pharmacologic classification: depolarizing neuromuscular blocker
Therapeutic classification: skeletal muscle relaxant
Pregnancy risk category C

How supplied
Available by prescription only
Injection: 20 mg/ml, 50 mg/ml, 100 mg/ml (parenteral); 500 mg, 1 g (sterile for I.V. infusion)
Powder for injection: 100 mg

Indications, route, and dosage
To induce skeletal muscle relaxation; facilitate intubation, ventilation, or orthopedic manipulations; and lessen muscle contractions in induced seizures
Dosage depends on the anesthetic used, patient's needs, and response. Doses are representative and must be adjusted. Paralysis is induced after inducing hypnosis with thiopental or other appropriate agent.
Adults: For short procedures, 0.6 mg/kg (range, 0.3 to 1.1 mg/kg) I.V. over 10 to 30 seconds; additional doses may be given if needed. For long procedures, 2.5 mg/minute (range, 0.5 to 10 mg/minute) continuous I.V. infusion, or alternatively, 0.3 to 1.1 mg/kg by intermittent I.V injection, followed by additional doses of 0.04 to 0.07 mg/kg p.r.n.
Children: Administer 2 mg/kg I.V. for infants; for older children and adolescents, give 1 mg/kg I.V. or 3 to 4 mg/kg I.M. (do not exceed 150 mg).

Pharmacodynamics
Skeletal muscle relaxant action: Similar to acetylcholine (ACh), succinylcholine produces depolarization of the motor end-plate at the myoneural junction. Drug has a high affinity for ACh receptor sites and is resistant to acetylcholinesterase, thus producing a more prolonged depolarization at the motor end-plate. It also possesses histamine-releasing properties and reportedly stimulates the cardiac vagus and sympathetic ganglia.

A transient increase in intraocular pressure occurs immediately after injection and may persist after the onset of complete paralysis.

Pharmacokinetics
• *Absorption:* After I.V. administration, drug has a rapid onset of action (30 seconds), reaches its peak within 1 minute, and persists for 2 to 3 minutes, gradually dissipating within 10 minutes. After I.M. administration, onset occurs within 2 to 3 minutes and persists for 10 to 30 minutes.
• *Distribution:* After I.V. administration, drug is distributed in extracellular fluid and rapidly reaches its site of action. It crosses the placenta.
• *Metabolism:* Occurs rapidly by plasma pseudocholinesterase.
• *Excretion:* About 10% is excreted unchanged in urine.

Contraindications and precautions
Contraindicated in patients with hypersensitivity to drug and in those with abnormally low plasma pseudocholinesterase, angle-closure glaucoma, malignant hyperthermia, or penetrating eye injuries.

Use cautiously in elderly or debilitated patients; in those receiving quinidine or cardiac glycoside therapy; in those undergoing a cesarean section; and in patients with respiratory depression, severe burns or trauma, electrolyte imbalances, hyperkalemia, paraplegia, spinal neuraxis injury, CVA, degenerative or dystrophic neuromuscular disease, myasthenia gravis, myasthenic syndrome of lung or bronchiogenic cancer, dehydration, thyroid disorders, collagen diseases, porphyria, fractures, muscle spasms, eye surgery, pheochromocytoma, or impaired renal, pulmonary, or hepatic function.

Interactions
Concomitant use with *aminoglycoside antibiotics* (including *amikacin, gentamicin, kanamycin, neomycin, streptomycin), polymyxin antibiotics (colistin, polymyxin B sulfate), clindamycin, lincomycin, general anesthetics, local anesthetics, antimalarial agents, cholinesterase inhibitors (demecarium, echothiophate, isoflurane), cyclophosphamide, oral contraceptives, nondepolarizing neuromuscular blocking agents, parenteral magnesium salts, lithium, phenelzine, quinidine, quinine, pancuronium, phenothiazines, thiotepa,* and exposure to *neurotoxic insecticides* enhance or prolong succinylcholine's neuromuscular blocking effects. Use these drugs cautiously during surgical and postoperative periods.

Concomitant use with *cardiac glycosides* produces possible arrhythmias. Use together cautiously.

Effects on diagnostic tests
Use of succinylcholine may increase serum potassium concentrations.

Adverse reactions
CV: bradycardia, tachycardia, hypertension, hypotension, ***arrhythmias,*** flushing, ***cardiac arrest.***
EENT: increased intraocular pressure.
Respiratory: ***prolonged respiratory depression, apnea,*** bronchostriction.
Other: ***malignant hyperthermia,*** muscle fasciculation, *postoperative muscle pain,* myoglobinemia, allergic or idiosyncratic hypersensitivity reactions ***(anaphylaxis).***

Overdose and treatment
Clinical manifestations of overdose include apnea or prolonged muscle paralysis, which may be treated with controlled respiration. Use a peripheral nerve stimulator to monitor effects and degree of blockade.

☑ Special considerations
- Succinylcholine is drug of choice for short procedures (less than 3 minutes) and for orthopedic manipulations; use cautiously in fractures or dislocations.
- Duration of action is prolonged to 20 minutes with continuous I.V. infusion or when given with hexafluorenium bromide.
- Some clinicians advocate pretreating adult patients with tubocurarine (3 to 6 mg) to minimize muscle fasciculations.
- Repeated fractional doses of succinylcholine alone are not advised; they may cause reduced response or prolonged apnea.
- Monitor baseline electrolyte determinations and vital signs (check respirations every 5 to 10 minutes during infusion).
- Keep airway clear. Have emergency respiratory support (endotracheal equipment, ventilator, oxygen, atropine, neostigmine) on hand.
- Store injectable form in refrigerator. Store powder form at room temperature and keep tightly closed. Use immediately after reconstitution.
- Do not mix drug with alkaline solutions (thiopental, sodium bicarbonate, barbiturates).
- Administration requires direct medical supervision by trained anesthesia personnel.
- Usually administered I.V., succinylcholine may be administered I.M. if suitable vein is inaccessible. Give deep I.M., preferably high into the deltoid muscle.
- Tachyphylaxis may occur.

Patient education
- Reassure patient that postoperative stiffness is normal and will soon subside. Monitor for residual muscle weakness.

Geriatric use
- Use with caution in elderly patients.

Breast-feeding
- Use cautiously in breast-feeding patients because it is unknown if drug occurs in breast milk.

sucralfate
Carafate

Pharmacologic classification: pepsin inhibitor
Therapeutic classification: antiulcer
Pregnancy risk category B

How supplied
Available by prescription only
Tablets: 1 g
Suspension: 1 g/10 ml

Indications, route, and dosage
Short-term (up to 8 weeks) treatment of duodenal ulcer, ◊ aspirin-induced gastric erosion
Adults: 1 g P.O. q.i.d. 1 hour before meals and h.s.
Maintenance therapy of duodenal ulcer
Adults: 1 g P.O. b.i.d.

Pharmacodynamics
Antiulcer action: Sucralfate has a unique mechanism of action. It adheres to proteins at the ulcer site, forming a protective coating against gastric acid, pepsin, and bile salts. It also inhibits pepsin, exhibits a cytoprotective effect, and forms a viscous, adhesive barrier on the surface of the intact intestinal mucosa and stomach.

Pharmacokinetics
- *Absorption:* Only about 3% to 5% of a dose is absorbed. Drug activity is not related to the amount absorbed.
- *Distribution:* Sucralfate acts locally, at the ulcer site. Absorbed drug is distributed to many body tissues, including the liver and kidneys.
- *Metabolism:* None.
- *Excretion:* About 90% of a dose is excreted in feces; absorbed drug is excreted unchanged in urine. Duration of effect is 6 hours.

Contraindications and precautions
No known contraindications. Use cautiously in patients with chronic renal failure.

Interactions
Sucralfate decreases absorption of *cimetidine, digoxin, phenytoin, quinidine, quinolones, ranitidine, tetracycline, theophylline,* and *fat-soluble vitamins A, D, E, and K. Antacids* may decrease binding of drug to gastroduodenal mucosa, impairing effectiveness. Separate dosing of sucralfate and antacids by 30 minutes.

Effects on diagnostic tests
None reported.

Adverse reactions
CNS: dizziness, sleepiness, headache, vertigo.
GI: *constipation,* nausea, gastric discomfort, diarrhea, bezoar formation, vomiting, flatulence, dry mouth, indigestion.
Skin: rash, pruritus.
Other: back pain.

Overdose and treatment
No information available.

☑ Special considerations
- Sucralfate may inhibit absorption of other drugs. Schedule other medications 2 hours before or after sucralfate.
- Drug is poorly water-soluble. For administration by nasogastric tube, have pharmacist prepare water-sorbitol suspension of sucralfate. Alternatively, place tablet in 60-ml syringe; add 20 ml water. Let stand with tip up for about 5 minutes, occasionally shaking gently. The resultant suspension may be administered from the syringe. After administration, tube should be flushed several times to ensure that the patient receives the entire dose.
- Patients who have difficulty swallowing tablet may place it in 15 to 30 ml of water at room temperature, allow it to disintegrate, and then ingest the resulting suspension. This is particularly useful for patients with esophagitis and painful swallowing.
- Monitor patient for constipation.
- Therapy exceeding 8 weeks is not recommended.
- Some experts believe that 2 g given b.i.d. is as effective as the standard regimen.
- Drug treats ulcers as effectively as H_2-receptor antagonists.

Patient education
- Remind patient to take drug on an empty stomach and to take sucralfate at least 1 hour before meals.
- Advise patient to continue taking drug as directed, even after pain begins to subside, to ensure adequate healing.
- Tell patient that he may take an antacid 30 minutes before or 2 hours after sucralfate.
- Warn patient not to take drug for more than 8 weeks.

Breast-feeding
- The risks to breast-feeding infants must be weighed against benefits.

sufentanil citrate
Sufenta

Pharmacologic classification: opioid
Therapeutic classification: analgesic, adjunct to anesthesia, anesthetic
Controlled substance schedule II
Pregnancy risk category C

How supplied
Available by prescription only
Injection: 50 mcg/ml

Indications, route, and dosage
Adjunct to general anesthetic
Adults: 1 to 8 mcg/kg I.V. administered with nitrous oxide and oxygen. Maintenance dose, 10 to 50 mcg.
Primary anesthetic
Adults: 8 to 30 mcg/kg I.V. administered with 100% oxygen and a muscle relaxant. Maintenance dose, 25 to 50 mcg.
Children: 10 to 25 mcg/kg I.V. administered with 100% oxygen and a muscle relaxant. Maintenance dose, up to 25 to 50 mcg.

Pharmacodynamics
Analgesic action: Sufentanil has a high affinity for the opiate receptors with an agonistic effect to provide analgesia. It is also used as an adjunct to anesthesia or as a primary anesthetic because of its potent CNS depressant effects.

Pharmacokinetics
- *Absorption:* After I.V. administration, sufentanil has a more rapid onset of action (1½ to 3 minutes) than does morphine or fentanyl.
- *Distribution:* Drug is highly lipophilic and is rapidly and extensively distributed in animals. It is highly protein-bound (greater than 90%) and redistributed rapidly.
- *Metabolism:* Appears to be metabolized mainly in the liver and small intestine. Relatively little accumulation occurs. Drug has an elimination half-life of about 2.5 hours.
- *Excretion:* Drug and its metabolites are excreted primarily in urine.

Contraindications and precautions
Contraindicated in patients with hypersensitivity to drug. Use cautiously in elderly or debilitated patients and in those with decreased respiratory reserve, head injuries, or renal, pulmonary, or hepatic disease.

Interactions
Concomitant use with other *CNS depressants (alcohol, antihistamines, barbiturates, benzodiazepines, general anesthetics, muscle relaxants, narcotic analgesics, phenothiazines, sedative-hypnotics, tricyclic antidepressants)* potentiates respiratory and CNS depression, sedation, and hypotensive effects of the drug. Concomitant use with *cimetidine* may also increase respiratory and CNS depression, causing confusion, disorientation, apnea, or seizures. Reduced dosage of sufentanil is usually necessary.

Drug accumulation and enhanced effects may result from concomitant use with other *drugs that are extensively metabolized in the liver (digitoxin, phenytoin, rifampin);* combined use with *anticholinergics* may cause paralytic ileus.

Patients who become physically dependent on drug may experience acute withdrawal syndrome if given high doses of a narcotic agonist-antagonist or a single dose of an antagonist.

Severe CV depression may result from the concomitant use of sufentanil with *general anesthetics.* If *beta blockers* have been used preoperatively, decrease dose of sufentanil. *Nitrous oxide* may produce CV depression when given with high doses of sufentanil.

The vagolytic effects of *pancuronium* may produce a dose-dependent elevation in heart rate during sufentanil and oxygen anesthesia; use moderate doses of *pancuronium* or a less vagolytic neuromuscular blocking agent; the vagolytic effect of pancuronium may be reduced in patients administered nitrous oxide with sufentanil.

Sufentanil may produce muscle rigidity involving all the skeletal muscles (incidence and severity are dose-related). Choose a neuromuscular blocking agent appropriate for the patient's CV status.

Effects on diagnostic tests

Sufentanil may increase plasma amylase and lipase and serum prolactin levels.

Adverse reactions

CNS: chills, somnolence.
CV: *hypotension, bradycardia,* hypertension, ***arrhythmias,*** tachycardia.
GI: nausea, vomiting.
Respiratory: ***chest wall rigidity, apnea, bronchospasm.***
Skin: *pruritus,* erythema.
Other: intraoperative muscle movement.

Overdose and treatment

There is no clinical experience with acute overdose of sufentanil, but signs and symptoms are expected to be similar to those occurring with other opioids, with less CV toxicity. The most common signs and symptoms of acute opiate overdose are CNS depression, respiratory depression, and miosis (pinpoint pupils). Other acute toxic effects include hypotension, bradycardia, hypothermia, shock, apnea, cardiopulmonary arrest, circulatory collapse, pulmonary edema, and seizures.

To treat acute overdose, establish adequate respiratory exchange via a patent airway and ventilation as needed; administer a narcotic antagonist (naloxone) to reverse respiratory depression. (Because the duration of action of sufentanil is longer than that of naloxone, repeated naloxone dosing is necessary.) Do not give naloxone unless the patient has clinically significant respiratory or CV depression. Monitor vital signs closely.

Provide symptomatic and supportive treatment (continued respiratory support, correction of fluid or electrolyte imbalance). Monitor laboratory parameters, vital signs, and neurologic status closely.

☑ Special considerations

Besides those relevant to all *opioids,* consider the following recommendations.

- Sufentanil should only be administered by persons specifically trained in the use of I.V. anesthetics.
- When used at doses exceeding 8 mcg/kg, postoperative mechanical ventilation and observation are essential because of extended postoperative respiratory depression.
- Compared with fentanyl, sufentanil has a more rapid onset and shorter duration of action.
- High doses can produce muscle rigidity. This effect can be reversed by administration of neuromuscular blocking agents.
- In patients weighing more than 20% above ideal body weight, determine dosage based on ideal body weight.

Geriatric use

- Lower doses are usually indicated for elderly patients, who may be more sensitive to the therapeutic and adverse effects of drug.

Pediatric use

- Safety and efficacy in children under age 2 have been documented in only a limited number of patients (who were undergoing CV surgery).

sulconazole nitrate

Exelderm

Pharmacologic classification: imidazole derivative
Therapeutic classification: antifungal
Pregnancy risk category C

How supplied

Available by prescription only
Cream: 1%
Topical solution: 1%

Indications, route, and dosage

***Treatment of tinea cruris, tinea corporis, and tinea pedis caused by* Trichophyton mentagrophytes, Epidermophyton floccosum, *and* Microsporum canis; *treatment of tinea versicolor caused by* Malassezia furfur**

Adults: Massage a small amount of solution or cream into affected area daily to b.i.d. except in tinea pedis, where administration should be b.i.d.

Pharmacodynamics

Antifungal action: Mechanism is unknown. Drug is an imidazole derivative that inhibits the growth of both fungi and yeast.

Pharmacokinetics

- *Absorption:* No information available.
- *Distribution:* No information available.
- *Metabolism:* No information available.
- *Excretion:* No information available.

Contraindications and precautions

Contraindicated in patients hypersensitive to any component of drug.

Interactions

None reported.

Effects on diagnostic tests

None reported.

Adverse reactions

Skin: pruritus, burning, stinging, redness.

Overdose and treatment

No information available.

☑ Special considerations

- Clinical improvement usually is noted within 1 week, with symptomatic relief in just a few days. Treatment for tinea corporis, cruris, or versicolor should continue for 3 weeks and tinea pedis for 4 weeks. If there is no improvement after 4 weeks, diagnosis should be reconsidered. Efficacy of solution has not been proven in tinea pedis (athlete's foot).

Patient education
- Inform patient to discontinue drug and call if irritation develops during treatment.
- Explain that therapy should continue for the full course to prevent recurrence.
- Tell patient to avoid drug contact with the eyes and to wash hands thoroughly after applying.

Breast-feeding
- It is not known whether drug appears in breast milk. Use with caution in breast-feeding women.

sulfacetamide sodium
AK-Sulf Ointment, Bleph-10, Cetamide, Isopto Cetamide, Ocusulf-10, Sodium Sulamyd, Sulf-10, Sulfair 15, Sulfex*, Sulten-10

Pharmacologic classification: sulfonamide
Therapeutic classification: antibiotic
Pregnancy risk category C

How supplied
Available by prescription only
Ophthalmic solution: 10%, 15%, 30%
Ophthalmic ointment: 10%

Indications, route, and dosage
Inclusion conjunctivitis, corneal ulcers, trachoma, prophylaxis to ocular infection
Adults and children: Instill 1 or 2 drops of 10% solution into lower conjunctival sac q 2 to 3 hours during day, less often at night; or instill 1 or 2 drops of 15% solution into lower conjunctival sac q 1 to 2 hours initially, increasing interval as condition responds; or instill 1 drop of 30% solution into lower conjunctival sac q 2 hours. Instill ½″ to 1″ of 10% ointment into conjunctival sac q.i.d. and h.s. Ointment may be used at night along with drops during the day. Usual duration of treatment is 7 to 10 days.

Pharmacodynamics
Antibiotic action: Sulfonamides act by inhibiting the uptake of para-aminobenzoic acid, which is required in the synthesis of folic acid needed for bacterial growth.

Pharmacokinetics
- *Absorption:* Drug is not readily absorbed from mucous membranes.
- *Distribution:* Unknown.
- *Metabolism:* Unknown.
- *Excretion:* Unknown.

Contraindications and precautions
Contraindicated in patients hypersensitive to sulfonamides and in children under age 2 months.

Interactions
Tetracaine or other *local anesthetics* that are *para-aminobenzoic acid derivatives* may decrease the antibacterial activity of sulfacetamide. Concomitant use of *silver preparations* or *gentamicin sulfate ophthalmic solution* is not recommended.

Sulfonamides are inactivated by *para-aminobenzoic acid* present in purulent exudates.

Effects on diagnostic tests
None reported.

Adverse reactions
EENT: slowed corneal wound healing (ointment), pain (on instillation of eyedrops), headache or brow pain, photophobia, periorbital edema.
Hematologic: ***agranulocytosis, aplastic anemia.***
Hepatic: ***fulminant hepatic necrosis.***
Other: hypersensitivity reactions (including itching or burning), overgrowth of nonsusceptible organisms, ***Stevens-Johnson syndrome.***

Overdose and treatment
No information available.

☑ Special considerations
- Drug has largely been replaced by antibiotics for treating major infections, but it is still used in minor ocular infections.
- Purulent exudate interferes with sulfacetamide action; remove as much as possible from lids before instilling sulfacetamide.
- Store in tightly closed, light-resistant container away from heat and light; do not use discolored (dark brown) solution.

Patient education
- Warn patient that eyedrops may burn slightly.
- Caution patient against touching tip of tube or dropper to eye or surrounding tissue.
- Teach patient how to instill drops correctly.
- Tell patient to watch for signs of sensitivity, such as itching lids or constant burning, and to report them immediately.
- Tell patient to avoid sharing washcloths and towels with family members.
- Advise patient to wait for 10 minutes before using another eye preparation.

Pediatric use
- Use of drug in children under age 2 months is not recommended.

Breast-feeding
- Although orally ingested sulfonamides have been reported to be excreted in low concentrations in breast milk, no data are available concerning ophthalmic sulfacetamide.

sulfadiazine

Pharmacologic classification: sulfonamide
Therapeutic classification: antibiotic
Pregnancy risk category NR

How supplied

Available by prescription only
Tablets: 500 mg

Indications, route, and dosage

Urinary tract infection
Adults: Initially, 2 to 4 g P.O.; then 4 to 8 g/day in four to six divided doses.
Children age 2 months or older: Initially, 75 mg/kg or 2 g/m² P.O.; then 120 mg/kg/day P.O. in four to six divided doses. Maximum daily dosage, 6 g.
Rheumatic fever prophylaxis, as an alternative to penicillin
Children weighing over 66 lb (30 kg): 1 g P.O. daily.
Children weighing under 66 lb: 500 mg P.O. daily.
Adjunctive treatment in toxoplasmosis
Adults: 2 to 8 g daily P.O. in divided doses q 6 hours for 3 to 4 weeks and up to 6 months or longer in patients with AIDS; given with pyrimethamine 25 mg P.O. daily.
Children: 100 to 200 mg/kg P.O. daily in divided doses q 6 hours for 3 to 4 weeks; given with pyrimethamine 2 mg/kg daily for 3 days, then 1 mg/kg daily for 3 to 4 weeks.
Uncomplicated attacks of malaria
Adults: 500 mg P.O. q.i.d. for 5 days.
Children: 25 to 50 mg/kg P.O. q.i.d. for 5 days.
Nocardiasis
Adults: 4 to 8 g P.O. daily in divided doses q 6 hours for 6 weeks.
Asymptomatic meningococcal carrier
Adults: 1 g P.O. b.i.d. for 2 days.
Children age 1 to 12: 500 mg P.O. b.i.d. for 2 days.
Children age 2 to 12 months: 500 mg P.O. daily for 2 days.

Pharmacodynamics

Antibacterial action: Sulfadiazine is bacteriostatic. It inhibits formation of tetrahydrofolic acid from para-aminobenzoic acid (PABA), thus preventing bacterial cell synthesis of folic acid.

Sulfadiazine is active against many gram-positive bacteria, *Chlamydia trachomatis,* many Enterobacteriaceae, and some strains of *Toxoplasma gondii* and *Plasmodium falciparum.*

Pharmacokinetics

- *Absorption:* Drug is absorbed from the GI tract after oral administration; peak serum levels occur at 2 hours.
- *Distribution:* Distributed widely into most body tissues and fluids, including synovial, pleural, amniotic, prostatic, peritoneal, and seminal fluids; CSF penetration is poor. Drug crosses the placenta; it is 32% to 56% protein-bound.
- *Metabolism:* Metabolized partially in the liver.
- *Excretion:* Both unchanged drug and metabolites are excreted primarily in urine by glomerular filtration and, to a lesser extent, renal tubular secretion; some drug is excreted in breast milk. Urine solubility of unchanged drug increases as urine pH increases.

Contraindications and precautions

Contraindicated in patients with hypersensitivity to sulfonamides, in those with porphyria, in infants under age 2 months (except in congenital toxoplasmosis), in pregnant women at term, and during breast-feeding.

Use cautiously in patients with impaired renal or hepatic function, bronchial asthma, multiple allergies, G6PD deficiency, or blood dyscrasia.

Interactions

Sulfadiazine may inhibit hepatic metabolism of *oral anticoagulants,* displacing them from binding sites and enhancing anticoagulant effects.

Concomitant use with *PABA* antagonizes effects of sulfonamides; with *oral antidiabetic agents (sulfonylureas)* enhances their hypoglycemic effects, probably by displacing *sulfonylureas* from protein-binding sites; with either *trimethoprim* or *pyrimethamine* (*folic acid antagonists* with different mechanisms of action) results in synergistic antibacterial effects and delays or prevents bacterial resistance.

Effects on diagnostic tests

Sulfadiazine alters urine glucose tests using cupric sulfate (Benedict's reagent or Clinitest). Sulfadiazine may elevate liver function test results; it may decrease serum levels of erythrocytes, platelets, or leukocytes. It may elevate serum creatinine.

Adverse reactions

CNS: headache, mental depression, ***seizures,*** hallucinations.
GI: *nausea, vomiting, diarrhea,* abdominal pain, anorexia, stomatitis.
GU: *toxic nephrosis* with oliguria and anuria, crystalluria, hematuria.
Hematologic: ***agranulocytosis, aplastic anemia, hemolytic anemia, thrombocytopenia,*** megaloblastic anemia, leukopenia.
Skin: ***erythema multiforme (Stevens-Johnson syndrome),*** generalized skin eruption, ***epidermal necrolysis, exfoliative dermatitis,*** photosensitivity, urticaria, pruritus.
Other: hypersensitivity reactions (*serum sickness, drug fever,* ***anaphylaxis***), jaundice, local irritation, extravasation.

Overdose and treatment

Clinical signs of overdose include dizziness, drowsiness, headache, unconsciousness, anorexia, abdominal pain, nausea, and vomiting. More severe complications, including hemolytic anemia, agranulocytosis, dermatitis, acidosis, sensitivity reactions, and jaundice, may be fatal.

Treatment includes gastric lavage if ingestion has occurred within the preceding 4 hours followed by correction of acidosis, forced fluids, and urinary alkalinization to enhance solubility and excretion. Treatment of renal failure as well as transfusion of appropriate blood products (in severe hematologic toxicity) may be required.

☑ Special considerations

Besides those relevant to all *sulfonamides,* consider the following recommendation.

- Sulfadiazine is a less soluble sulfonamide; therefore, it is more likely to cause crystalluria. Avoid concomitant use of urine acidifiers and ensure adequate fluid intake. If adequate fluid intake cannot be ensured, recommend sodium bicarbonate to reduce risk of crystalluria.

Pediatric use
- Contraindicated in children under age 2 months.

Breast-feeding
- Drug is excreted in breast milk and should not be used in breast-feeding women.

sulfamethoxazole
Gantanol

Pharmacologic classification: sulfonamide
Therapeutic classification: antibiotic
Pregnancy risk category C

How supplied
Available by prescription only
Tablets: 500 mg
Suspension: 500 mg/5 ml

Indications, route, and dosage
Urinary tract and systemic infections
Adults: Initially, 2 g P.O.; then 1 g P.O. b.i.d., up to t.i.d. for severe infections.
Children and infants over age 2 months: Initially, 50 to 60 mg/kg P.O., then 25 to 30 mg/kg b.i.d. Maximum dosage should not exceed 75 mg/kg daily.
Lymphogranuloma venereum (genital, inguinal, or anorectal infection)
Adults: 1 g P.O. b.i.d. for 21 days.

Pharmacodynamics
Antibacterial action: Sulfamethoxazole is bacteriostatic. It acts by inhibiting formation of tetrahydrofolic acid from para-aminobenzoic acid (PABA), thus preventing bacterial cell synthesis of folic acid.

Spectrum of action includes some gram-positive bacteria, *Chlamydia trachomatis,* many Enterobacteriaceae, and some strains of *Toxoplasma* and *Plasmodium.*

Pharmacokinetics
- *Absorption:* Absorbed from the GI tract after oral administration; peak serum levels occur at 3 to 4 hours.
- *Distribution:* Drug is distributed widely into most body tissues and fluids, including cerebrospinal, synovial, pleural, amniotic, prostatic, peritoneal, and seminal fluids. Sulfamethoxazole crosses the placenta; it is 50% to 70% protein-bound.
- *Metabolism:* Metabolized partially in the liver.
- *Excretion:* Both unchanged drug and metabolites are excreted primarily in urine by glomerular filtration and, to a lesser extent, renal tubular secretion; some drug is excreted in breast milk. Urinary solubility of unchanged drug increases as urine pH increases. Elimination half-life in patients with normal renal function is 7 to 12 hours.

Contraindications and precautions
Contraindicated in patients with porphyria or hypersensitivity to sulfonamides, in infants under age 2 months (except in congenital toxoplasmosis), in pregnant women at term, and during breast-feeding. Use cautiously in patients with renal or hepatic impairment, bronchial asthma, severe allergies, G6PD deficiency, or blood dyscrasia.

Interactions
Sulfamethoxazole may inhibit hepatic metabolism of *oral anticoagulants,* displacing them from binding sites and enhancing anticoagulant effects. Concomitant use with *PABA* antagonizes sulfonamide effects; with *oral antidiabetic agents (sulfonylureas)* enhances their hypoglycemic effects, probably by displacing sulfonylureas from protein-binding sites; and with either *trimethoprim* or *pyrimethamine (folic acid antagonists* with different mechanisms of action*)* results in synergistic antibacterial effects and delays or prevents bacterial resistance.

Effects on diagnostic tests
Sulfamethoxazole alters results of urine glucose tests using cupric sulfate (Benedict's reagent or Clinitest).

Sulfamethoxazole may elevate liver function test results; it may decrease serum levels of erythrocytes, platelets, or leukocytes.

Adverse reactions
CNS: headache, mental depression, ***seizures,*** hallucinations, aseptic meningitis, tinnitus, apathy.
GI: *nausea, vomiting, diarrhea,* abdominal pain, anorexia, stomatitis, pancreatitis, pseudomembranous colitis.
GU: *toxic nephrosis with oliguria and anuria,* crystalluria, hematuria, interstitial nephritis.
Hematologic: ***agranulocytosis, hemolytic anemia, aplastic anemia,*** megaloblastic anemia, ***thrombocytopenia,*** leukopenia.
Skin: ***erythema multiforme (Stevens-Johnson syndrome),*** generalized skin eruption, ***epidermal necrolysis, exfoliative dermatitis,*** photosensitivity, urticaria, pruritus.
Other: hypersensitivity reactions *(serum sickness, drug fever,* ***anaphylaxis****), jaundice.*

Overdose and treatment
Clinical signs of overdose include dizziness, drowsiness, headache, unconsciousness, anorexia, abdominal pain, nausea, and vomiting. More severe complications, including hemolytic anemia, agranulocytosis, dermatitis, acidosis, sensitivity reactions, and jaundice, may be fatal.

Treat by gastric lavage, if ingestion has occurred within the preceding 4 hours, followed by correction of acidosis, forced fluids, and I.V. fluids if urine output is low and renal function is normal. Treatment of renal failure and transfusion of appropriate blood products (in severe hematologic toxicity) may be required.

☑ Special considerations
Recommendations for administration, preparation and storage, and care and teaching of the patient

during therapy with sulfamethoxazole are those common to all *sulfonamides.*

Pediatric use

- Sulfamethoxazole is contraindicated in children under age 2 months.

Breast-feeding

- Sulfamethoxazole is excreted in breast milk and should not be administered to breast-feeding women.

sulfasalazine

Azulfidine, Azulfidine En-tabs

Pharmacologic classification: sulfonamide
Therapeutic classification: antibiotic
Pregnancy risk category B

How supplied

Available by prescription only
Tablets (with or without enteric coating): 500 mg
Suspension: 250 mg/5 ml

Indications, route, and dosage

Mild to moderate ulcerative colitis, adjunctive therapy in severe ulcerative colitis

Adults: Initially, 3 to 4 g P.O. daily in evenly divided doses. Maintenance dose is 2 g P.O. daily in divided doses q 6 hours. May need to start with 1 to 2 g initially, with a gradual increase in dose to minimize adverse reactions.

Children over age 2: Initially, 40 to 60 mg/kg P.O. daily, divided into three to six doses; then 30 mg/kg daily in four doses. Maximum daily dosage, 2 g. May need to start at lower dose if GI intolerance occurs.

Pharmacodynamics

Antibacterial action: Exact mechanism of action of drug in ulcerative colitis is unknown; it is believed to be a prodrug metabolized by intestinal flora in the colon. One metabolite (5-aminosalicylic acid or mesalamine) is responsible for the anti-inflammatory effect; the other metabolite (sulfapyridine) may be responsible for antibacterial action and for some adverse effects.

Pharmacokinetics

- *Absorption:* Poorly from the GI tract after oral administration; 70% to 90% is transported to the colon where intestinal flora metabolize drug to its active ingredients, sulfapyridine (antibacterial) and 5-aminosalicylic acid (anti-inflammatory), which exert their effects locally. Sulfapyridine is absorbed from the colon, but only a small portion of 5-aminosalicylic acid is absorbed.
- *Distribution:* Human data on sulfasalazine distribution is lacking; animal studies have identified drug and metabolites in sera, liver, and intestinal walls. Parent drug and both metabolites cross the placenta.
- *Metabolism:* Sulfasalazine is cleaved by intestinal flora in the colon.
- *Excretion:* Systemically absorbed sulfasalazine is excreted chiefly in urine; some parent drug and metabolites are excreted in breast milk. Plasma half-life is about 6 to 8 hours.

Contraindications and precautions

Contraindicated in patients with known hypersensitivity to salicylates or sulfonamides or to other drugs containing sulfur (such as thiazides, furosemide, or oral sulfonylureas); in those with porphyria or severe renal or hepatic dysfunction; during pregnancy and at term; in breast-feeding patients; and in infants and children under age 2. Sulfasalazine is also contraindicated in patients with intestinal or urinary tract obstructions because of the risk of local GI irritation and crystalluria.

Use cautiously in patients with mild to moderate renal or hepatic dysfunction, severe allergies, asthma, blood dyscrasia, or G6PD deficiency.

Interactions

Sulfasalazine may inhibit hepatic metabolism of *oral anticoagulants,* displacing them from binding sites and enhancing anticoagulant effects.

Concomitant use with *oral antidiabetic agents (sulfonylureas)* enhances hypoglycemic effects, probably by displacing *sulfonylureas* from protein-binding sites.

Sulfasalazine may reduce GI absorption of *digoxin* and *folic acid.* Concomitant use of *urine acidifying agents (ammonium chloride, ascorbic acid)* decreases urine pH and sulfonamide solubility, thus increasing risk of crystalluria. Concomitant use with *antibiotics that alter intestinal flora* may interfere with conversion of sulfasalazine to sulfapyridine and 5-aminosalicylic acid, decreasing its effectiveness.

Concomitant use of *antacids* may cause premature dissolution of enteric-coated tablets (which are designed to dissolve in the intestines), thus increasing systemic absorption and hazard of toxicity.

Effects on diagnostic tests

Sulfasalazine alters results of urine glucose tests using cupric sulfate (Benedict's reagent or Clinitest).

Sulfasalazine may elevate liver function test results; it may decrease serum levels of erythrocytes, platelets, or leukocytes.

Adverse reactions

CNS: headache, mental depression, ***seizures,*** hallucinations, tinnitus.
GI: *nausea, vomiting, diarrhea, abdominal pain, anorexia,* stomatitis.
GU: toxic nephrosis with oliguria and anuria, crystalluria, hematuria, oligospermia, infertility.
Hematologic: ***agranulocytosis, aplastic anemia,*** megaloblastic anemia, ***thrombocytopenia,*** leukopenia, hemolytic anemia.
Hepatic: jaundice.
Skin: ***erythema multiforme (Stevens-Johnson syndrome),*** generalized skin eruption, ***epidermal necrolysis, exfoliative dermatitis,*** photosensitivity, urticaria, pruritus.
Other: ***hypersensitivity reactions,*** serum sickness, drug fever, ***anaphylaxis,*** bacterial and fungal superinfection.

Note: Drug should be discontinued if signs of toxicity or hypersensitivity occur; if hematologic abnormalities are accompanied by sore throat, pallor, fever, jaundice, purpura, or weakness; if crystalluria is accompanied by renal colic, hematuria, oliguria, proteinuria, urinary obstruction, urolithiasis, increased BUN levels, or anuria; if severe diarrhea indicates pseudomembranous colitis; or if severe nausea, vomiting, or diarrhea persists.

Overdose and treatment

Clinical signs of overdose include dizziness, drowsiness, headache, unconsciousness, anorexia, abdominal pain, nausea, and vomiting. More severe complications, including hemolytic anemia, agranulocytosis, dermatitis, acidosis, sensitivity reactions, and jaundice, may be fatal.

Treat by gastric lavage, if ingestion has occurred within the preceding 4 hours, followed by correction of acidosis, forced fluids, and urinary alkalinization to enhance solubility and excretion. Treatment of renal failure and transfusion of appropriate blood products (in severe hematologic toxicity) may be required.

☑ Special considerations

Besides those relevant to all *sulfonamides,* consider the following recommendations.

- Most adverse effects involve the GI tract; minimize reactions and facilitate absorption by spacing doses evenly and administering drug after food.
- Drug colors urine orange-yellow; may also color patient's skin orange-yellow.
- Do not administer antacids concomitantly with enteric-coated sulfasalazine; they may alter absorption.

Patient education

- Tell patient that sulfasalazine normally turns urine orange-yellow. Warn him that skin may also turn orange-yellow and that drug may permanently stain soft contact lenses yellow.
- Advise patient not to take antacids simultaneously with sulfasalazine.
- Advise patient to take drug after meals to reduce GI distress and to facilitate passage into intestines.
- Tell patient to avoid prolonged exposure to sunlight because photosensitivity may occur and to wear protective clothing and sunscreen.

Pediatric use

- Contraindicated in patients under age 2 months.

Breast-feeding

- Drug occurs in breast milk; use with caution.

sulfinpyrazone

Anturane

Pharmacologic classification: uricosuric
Therapeutic classification: renal tubular-blocking agent, platelet aggregation inhibitor
Pregnancy risk category NR

How supplied

Available by prescription only
Tablets: 100 mg
Capsules: 200 mg

Indications, route, and dosage

Chronic gouty arthritis and intermittent gouty arthritis, or hyperuricemia associated with gout

Adults: Initially, 200 to 400 mg P.O. daily in two divided doses, gradually increasing to maintenance dosage in 1 week. Maintenance dosage is 400 mg P.O. daily in two divided doses; may increase to 800 mg daily or decrease to 200 mg daily.

◊ ***Prophylaxis of thromboembolic disorders, including angina, MI, and transient (cerebral) ischemic attacks, and in patients with prosthetic heart valves***

Adults: 600 to 800 mg daily in divided doses to decrease platelet aggregation.

Pharmacodynamics

Uricosuric action: Sulfinpyrazone competitively inhibits renal tubule reabsorption of uric acid. Sulfinpyrazone inhibits adenosine diphosphate and 5-HT, resulting in decreased platelet adhesiveness and increased platelet survival time.

Pharmacokinetics

- *Absorption:* Drug is absorbed completely after oral administration; peak plasma levels occur in 2 hours. Effects usually last 4 to 6 hours but may persist up to 10 hours.
- *Distribution:* Sulfinpyrazone is 98% to 99% protein-bound.
- *Metabolism:* Metabolized rapidly in the liver.
- *Excretion:* Drug and its metabolites are eliminated in urine; about 50% is excreted unchanged.

Contraindications and precautions

Contraindicated in patients with hypersensitivity to pyrazolone derivatives (including oxyphenbutazone and phenylbutazone), blood dyscrasia, active peptic ulcer, or symptoms of GI inflammation or ulceration. Use cautiously in patients with healed peptic ulcer and during pregnancy.

Interactions

Sulfinpyrazone decreases renal tubular secretion of *penicillin, other beta-lactam antibiotics, nitrofurantoin,* and *sulfonylureas.* Reduced excretion of *nitrofurantoin* decreases the efficacy of sulfinpyrazone in urinary tract infections and increases systemic toxicity; decreased excretion of sulfonylureas may cause hypoglycemia. Sulfinpyrazone may potentiate effects of *oral antidiabetic agents,* such as *sulfonylureas.*

Sulfinpyrazone decreases the metabolism of *warfarin,* enhancing its hypoprothrombinemic effect and the risk of bleeding; increased bleeding in these patients also may result from the antiplatelet effect of sulfinpyrazone.

Most *alcohol, diazoxide, diuretics,* and *pyrazinamide* increase serum uric acid and thus increase sulfinpyrazone dosage requirements.

Salicylates block the uricosuric effects of sulfinpyrazone only in high doses; small occasional doses usually do not interact significantly.

Cholestyramine decreases absorption of sulfinpyrazone; sulfinpyrazone should be taken 1 hour before or 4 to 6 hours after cholestyramine. *Probenecid* inhibits renal excretion of sulfinpyrazone.

Effects on diagnostic tests
Drug decreases urinary excretion of aminohippuric acid and phenolsulfonphthalein and may alter renal function test results.

Adverse reactions
GI: *nausea, dyspepsia,* epigastric pain, reactivation of peptic ulcerations.
Hematologic: ***blood dyscrasia*** (such as anemia, leukopenia, ***agranulocytosis, thrombocytopenia, aplastic anemia***).
Respiratory: bronchoconstriction in patients with aspirin-induced asthma.
Skin: rash.

Overdose and treatment
Clinical signs of overdose include nausea, vomiting, epigastric pain, ataxia, labored breathing, seizures, and coma. Treat supportively; induce emesis or use gastric lavage as appropriate. Treat seizures with diazepam or phenytoin or both.

☑ Special considerations
- Drug does not accumulate and tolerance to it does not develop; it is suitable for long-term use.
- Drug has no analgesic or anti-inflammatory actions.
- Drug may not be effective and should be avoided when creatinine clearance is less than 50 ml/minute.
- Monitor renal function and CBC routinely.
- Monitor serum uric acid levels and adjust dosage accordingly.
- Give with food, milk, or prescribed antacids to lessen GI upset.
- Sulfinpyrazone is used investigationally to increase platelet survival time, to treat thromboembolic phenomena, and to prevent MI recurrence.
- Maintain adequate hydration with high fluid intake to prevent formation of uric acid kidney stones.

Patient education
- Explain that gouty attacks may increase during first 6 to 12 months of therapy; patient should not discontinue drug without medical approval.
- Encourage patient to comply with dosage regimen and to keep scheduled follow-up visits.
- Tell patient to drink 8 to 10 glasses of fluid each day and to take drug with food to minimize GI upset; warn patient to avoid alcoholic beverages, which decrease the therapeutic effect of sulfinpyrazone.

Geriatric use
- Elderly patients are more likely to have glomerular filtration rates below 50 ml/minute; sulfinpyrazone may be ineffective.

Breast-feeding
- Safety has not been established. An alternative feeding method is recommended during therapy.

sulfisoxazole
Gantrisin

sulfisoxazole diolamine
Gantrisin (Ophthalmic Solution)

Pharmacologic classification: sulfonamide
Therapeutic classification: antibiotic
Pregnancy risk category C

How supplied
Available by prescription only
Tablets: 500 mg
Liquid: 500 mg/5 ml
Ophthalmic solution: 4%

Indications, route, and dosage
Urinary tract and systemic infections
Adults: Initially, 2 to 4 g P.O. then 4 to 8 g P.O. daily in divided doses q 4 to 6 hours.
Children and infants over age 2 months: Initially, 75 mg/kg P.O., then 150 mg/kg (or 4 g/m^2) P.O. daily in divided doses q 4 to 6 hours. Maximum dose should not exceed 6 g/24 hours.
Lymphogranuloma venereum (genital, inguinal, or anorectal infection)
Adults: 500 mg to 1 g q.i.d. for 3 weeks.
Conjunctivitis, corneal ulcer, superficial ocular infections; adjunct in systemic treatment of trachoma
Adults: Instill 1 to 2 drops in the lower conjuctival sac of affected eye daily q 1 to 4 hours.

Pharmacodynamics
Antibacterial action: Sulfisoxazole is bacteriostatic. It acts by inhibiting formation of tetrahydrofolic acid from para-aminobenzoic acid (PABA), thus preventing bacterial cell synthesis of folic acid. It acts synergistically with folic acid antagonists such as trimethoprim, which block folic acid synthesis at a later stage, thus delaying or preventing bacterial resistance.

Sulfisoxazole is active against some gram-positive bacteria, *Chlamydia trachomatis,* many Enterobacteriaceae, and some strains of *Toxoplasma* and *Plasmodium.*

Pharmacokinetics
- *Absorption:* Drug is absorbed readily from the GI tract after oral administration; peak serum levels occur at 2 to 4 hours.
- *Distribution:* Distributed into extracellular compartments; CSF penetration is 8% to 57% of blood concentrations in uninflamed meninges. Sulfisoxazole crosses the placenta; it is 85% protein-bound.
- *Metabolism:* Drug is metabolized partially in the liver.
- *Excretion:* Both unchanged drug and metabolites are excreted primarily in urine by glomerular filtration and, to a lesser extent, renal tubular secretion; some drug is excreted in breast milk. Urinary sol-

ubility of unchanged drug increases as urine pH increases. Plasma half-life in patients with normal renal function is about 4½ to 8 hours.

Contraindications and precautions
Contraindicated in patients with hypersensitivity to sulfonamines, in infants under age 2 months (except in congenital toxoplasmosis [with oral form only]), in pregnant women at term, and during breast-feeding.

Use oral form cautiously in patients with impaired renal or hepatic function, severe allergies, bronchial asthma, or G6PD deficiency. Use ophthalmic form cautiously in patients with severely dry eyes.

Interactions
Sulfisoxazole may inhibit hepatic metabolism of *oral anticoagulants,* displacing them from binding sites and exaggerating anticoagulant effects. Concomitant use with *PABA* antagonizes effects of sulfonamides; with *oral antidiabetic agents (sulfonylureas)* enhances hypoglycemic effects, probably by displacing sulfonylureas from protein-binding sites; with either *trimethoprim* or *pyrimethamine (folic acid antagonists* with different mechanisms of action) results in synergistic antibacterial effects and delays or prevents bacterial resistance.

Concomitant use of *urine acidifying agents (ammonium chloride, ascorbic acid)* decreases urine pH and sulfonamide solubility, thus increasing risk of crystalluria.

Effects on diagnostic tests
Sulfisoxazole alters results of urine glucose tests using cupric sulfate (Benedict's reagent or Clinitest).

Drug may elevate liver function test results; it may decrease serum levels of erythrocytes, platelets, or leukocytes.

Adverse reactions
CNS: headache; mental depression, hallucinations, ***seizures*** (with oral administration).
CV: tachycardia, palpitations, syncope, cyanosis (with oral administration).
EENT: *ocular irritation, itching, chemosis, periorbital edema* (with ophthalmic form).
GI: *nausea, vomiting, diarrhea,* abdominal pain, anorexia, stomatitis, ***hepatitis,*** pseudomembranous colitis (with oral administration).
GU: *toxic nephrosis with oliguria and anuria, acute renal failure,* crystalluria, hematuria (with oral administration).
Hematologic: ***agranulocytosis, aplastic anemia, thrombocytopenia, hemolytic anemia,*** megaloblastic anemia, leukopenia (with oral administration).
Skin: ***erythema multiforme, epidermal necrolysis, exfoliative dermatitis,*** *generalized skin eruption,* photosensitivity, urticaria, pruritus (with oral administration).
Other: hypersensitivity reactions (*serum sickness, drug fever,* ***anaphylaxis***), jaundice (with oral administration); ***Stevens-Johnson syndrome,*** overgrowth of nonsusceptible organisms (with ophthalmic form).

Overdose and treatment
Clinical signs of overdose include dizziness, drowsiness, headache, unconsciousness, anorexia, abdominal pain, nausea, and vomiting. More severe complications, including hemolytic anemia, agranulocytosis, dermatitis, acidosis, sensitivity reactions, and jaundice, may be fatal.

Treatment requires gastric lavage, if ingestion has occurred within the preceding 4 hours, followed by correction of acidosis, and forced fluids and urinary alkalinization to enhance solubility and excretion. Treatment of renal failure and transfusion of appropriate blood products (in severe hematologic toxicity) may be required.

☑ Special considerations
Besides those relevant to all *sulfonamides,* consider the following recommendation.
- Sulfisoxazole-pyrimethamine is used to treat toxoplasmosis.

Patient education
- Tell patient to drink 8 oz (240 ml) of water with each oral dose and to take drug on an empty stomach.
- Tell patient to complete prescribed medication.
- Teach patient how to use ophthalmic preparations. Warn patient not to touch tip of dropper or tube to any surface.
- Warn patient that ophthalmic solution may cause blurred vision immediately after application. Tell patient to gently close eyes and keep closed for 1 to 2 minutes.
- Tell patient to avoid prolonged exposure to sunlight because photosensitivity may occur and to wear protective clothing and sunscreen.

Pediatric use
- Contraindicated in children under age 2 months.

Breast-feeding
- Drug occurs in breast milk and should not be administered to breast-feeding women.

sulindac
Clinoril

Pharmacologic classification: NSAID
Therapeutic classification: nonnarcotic analgesic, antipyretic, anti-inflammatory
Pregnancy risk category NR

How supplied
Available by prescription only
Tablets: 150 mg, 200 mg

Indications, route, and dosage
Osteoarthritis, rheumatoid arthritis, ankylosing spondylitis
Adults: 150 mg P.O. b.i.d. initially; may increase to 200 mg P.O. b.i.d.
Acute subacromial bursitis or supraspinatus tendinitis, acute gouty arthritis
Adults: 200 mg P.O. b.i.d. for 7 to 14 days. Dose may be reduced as symptoms subside.

Pharmacodynamics

Analgesic, antipyretic, and anti-inflammatory actions: Mechanisms of action are unknown but are thought to inhibit prostaglandin synthesis.

Pharmacokinetics

- *Absorption:* Rapidly and completely absorbed from the GI tract.
- *Distribution:* Drug is highly protein-bound.
- *Metabolism:* Sulindac is inactive and is metabolized hepatically to the active sulfide metabolite.
- *Excretion:* Excreted in urine. Half-life of parent drug is about 8 hours; half-life of active metabolite is about 16 hours.

Contraindications and precautions

Contraindicated in patients with hypersensitivity to drug or in whom acute asthmatic attacks, urticaria, or rhinitis is precipitated by use of aspirin or NSAIDs. Avoid use during pregnancy.

Use cautiously in patients with history of ulcer or GI bleeding, renal dysfunction, compromised cardiac function, hypertension, or conditions predisposing to fluid retention.

Interactions

When used concomitantly, *anticoagulants* and *thrombolytic drugs* may be potentiated by the platelet-inhibiting effect of sulindac. Concomitant use of sulindac with *highly protein-bound drugs (phenytoin, sulfonylureas, warfarin)* may cause displacement of either drug, and adverse effects. Monitor therapy closely for both drugs. Concomitant use with other *GI-irritating drugs (antibiotics, NSAIDs, steroids)* may potentiate the adverse GI effects of sulindac. Use together with caution.

Antacids and *food* delay and decrease the absorption of sulindac. NSAIDs are known to decrease renal clearance of *lithium carbonate,* thus increasing lithium serum levels and risks of adverse effects. *Dimethyl sulfoxide* may interact with sulindac, causing decreased plasma levels of the active sulfide metabolite. Peripheral neuropathies have also been reported with this combination. *Diflunisal* and *aspirin* are known to cause decreased plasma levels of the active sulfide metabolite. *Probenecid* increases plasma levels of sulindac and its inactive sulfane metabolite; sulindac may decrease the uricosuric effect of *probenecid.*

Effects on diagnostic tests

The physiologic effect of the drug may result in increased bleeding time; increased BUN, serum creatinine, and potassium levels; and increased serum alkaline phosphatase and serum transaminase concentrations.

Adverse reactions

CNS: dizziness, headache, nervousness, psychosis.
CV: hypertension, ***heart failure,*** palpitations.
EENT: tinnitus, transient visual disturbances.
GI: *epigastric distress,* ***peptic ulceration, GI bleeding, pancreatitis,*** occult blood loss, nausea, constipation, dyspepsia, flatulence, anorexia, vomiting, diarrhea.
GU: interstitial nephritis, ***nephrotic syndrome, renal failure.***
Hematologic: prolonged bleeding time, ***aplastic anemia, thrombocytopenia, agranulocytosis, neutropenia,*** hemolytic anemia.
Skin: *rash,* pruritus.
Other: edema, drug fever, ***anaphylaxis, hypersensitivity syndrome,*** angioedema.

Overdose and treatment

Clinical manifestations of overdose include dizziness, drowsiness, mental confusion, disorientation, lethargy, paresthesias, numbness, vomiting, gastric irritation, nausea, abdominal pain, headache, stupor, coma, and hypotension.

To treat overdose of sulindac, empty stomach immediately by inducing emesis with ipecac syrup or by gastric lavage. Administer activated charcoal via nasogastric tube. Provide symptomatic and supportive measures (respiratory support and correction of fluid and electrolyte imbalances). Dialysis is thought to be of minimal value because sulindac is highly protein-bound. Monitor laboratory parameters and vital signs closely.

☑ Special considerations

Besides those relevant to all *NSAIDs,* consider the following recommendations.

- Sulindac may be the safest NSAID for patients with mild renal impairment. It may also be less likely to cause further renal toxicity.
- Assess cardiopulmonary status frequently. Monitor vital signs, especially heart rate and blood pressure, to detect abnormalities.
- Assess fluid balance status. Monitor intake and output and daily weight. Observe for presence and amount of edema.
- Impose safety measures to prevent injury, such as using raised side rails and supervised ambulation.
- Symptomatic improvement may take 7 days or longer. Evaluate patient's response as evidenced by a reduction in symptoms.

Patient education

- Caution patient to avoid use of OTC medications unless medically approved.
- Teach patient how to recognize signs and symptoms of possible adverse reactions; instruct patient to report such adverse reactions.
- Instruct patient to check weight two or three times weekly and to report weight gain of 3 lb (1.4 kg) or more within 1 week.
- Because drug causes sodium retention, advise patient to report edema and to have blood pressure checked routinely.
- Instruct patient in safety measures; advise him to avoid hazardous activities that require alertness until CNS effects of drug are known.

Geriatric use

- Patients over age 60 are more sensitive to the adverse effects of sulindac. Use with caution.
- Because of its effect on renal prostaglandins, drug may cause fluid retention and edema. This

may be significant in elderly patients and those with heart failure.

Pediatric use

- Safety of long-term drug use in children has not been established.

Breast-feeding

- Safe use of sulindac during breast-feeding has not been established. Avoid use of drug in breast-feeding women.

sumatriptan succinate

Imitrex

Pharmacologic classification: selective 5-hydroxytryptamine ($5HT_1$)-receptor agonist
Therapeutic classification: antimigraine
Pregnancy risk category C

How supplied

Available by prescription only
Tablets: 25 mg, 50 mg
Injection: 12 mg/ml (0.5 ml in 1-ml prefilled syringe), 6-mg single-dose (0.5 ml in 2 ml) vial, and self-dose system kit
Nasal spray: 5 mg, 20 mg unit dose nasal spray device

Indications, route, and dosage

Acute migraine attacks (with or without aura)
Adults: 6 mg S.C. Maximum recommended dosage is two 6-mg injections in 24 hours, separated by at least 1 hour, or 25 to 100 mg P.O. initially. If response is not achieved in 2 hours, may give second dose of 25 to 100 mg. Additional doses may be used in at least 2-hour intervals. Maximum daily dosage, 300 mg.

For nasal spray, administer single dose of 5 mg, 10 mg, or 20 mg once in one nostril; may repeat once after 2 hours under health care provider guidance for maximum daily dose of 40 mg. (A 10-mg dose may be achieved by the administration of a single 5-mg dose in each nostril).

Pharmacodynamics

Antimigraine action: Sumatriptan selectively binds to a $5\text{-}HT_1$ receptor subtype found in the basilar artery and vasculature of dura mater, where it presumably exerts its antimigraine effect. In these tissues, sumatriptan activates the receptor to cause vasoconstriction, an action in humans correlating with the relief of migraine.

Pharmacokinetics

- *Absorption:* Bioavailability via S.C. injection is 97% of that obtained via I.V. injection. Peak concentration after S.C. injection of sumatriptan occurs in approximately 12 minutes.
- *Distribution:* Drug has a low protein-binding capacity (approximately 14% to 21%).
- *Metabolism:* Approximately 80% of drug is metabolized in the liver, primarily to an inactive indoleacetic acid metabolite.
- *Excretion:* Excreted primarily in urine, partly (20%) as unchanged drug and partly as the indoleacetic acid metabolite. Elimination half-life is about 2 hours.

Contraindications and precautions

Contraindicated in patients with hypersensitivity to drug; in those with uncontrolled hypertension, ischemic heart disease (such as angina pectoris, Prinzmetal's angina, history of MI, or documented silent ischemia), or hemiplegic or basilar migraine; within 14 days of MAO therapy; and in patients taking ergotamine.

Use cautiously in patients who may be at risk for coronary artery disease (CAD) (such as postmenopausal women or male patients over age 40) or those with risk factors such as hypertension, hypercholesterolemia, obesity, diabetes, smoking, or family history. Use cautiously in women of childbearing age and during pregnancy.

Interactions

Ergot and *ergot derivatives* prolong vasospastic effects when given concurrently with sumatriptan. These drugs should not be used within 24 hours of sumatriptan therapy.

Effects on diagnostic tests

None reported.

Adverse reactions

CNS: *dizziness, vertigo,* drowsiness, headache, anxiety, malaise, fatigue.
CV: ***atrial fibrillation, ventricular fibrillation, ventricular tachycardia, MI,*** *ECG changes such as ischemic ST-segment elevation* (rare).
EENT: discomfort of throat, nasal cavity or sinus, mouth, jaw, or tongue; altered vision.
GI: abdominal discomfort, dysphagia.
Skin: flushing.
Other: *tingling; warm or hot sensation; burning sensation; heaviness, pressure or tightness;* anxious feeling; tight feeling in head; cold sensation; pressure or tightness in chest; myalgia; muscle cramps; diaphoresis; neck pain; *injection site reaction.*

Overdose and treatment

No specific information available. However, it would be expected to cause seizures, tremor, inactivity, erythema of the extremities, reduced respiratory rate, cyanosis, ataxia, mydriasis, injection site reactions, and paralysis. Continue monitoring of patient while signs and symptoms persist and for at least 10 hours thereafter. Effect of hemodialysis or peritoneal dialysis on serum concentrations of sumatriptan is unknown.

☑ Special considerations

- Do not use drug for management of hemiplegic or basilar migraine. Safety and effectiveness also have not been established for cluster headache, which occurs in an older, predominantly male population.
- Do not give drug I.V. because coronary vasospasm may occur.

• Nasal spray is generally well tolerated, however adverse reactions seen with the other forms of the drug can still occur.
• Clinical data on sumatriptan injection include rare reports of serious or life-threatening arrhythmias, such as atrial and ventricular fibrillation, ventricular tachycardia, MI, and marked ischemic ST elevations. Data also include rare, but more frequent, reports of chest and arm discomfort thought to represent angina pectoris. Because such coronary events can occur, consider administering first dose in an outpatient setting to patients in whom unrecognized coronary artery disease (CAD) is comparatively likely (postmenopausal women; males over age 40; and patients with risk factors for CAD, such as hypertension, hypercholesterolemia, obesity, diabetes, smoking, and strong family history of CAD).
• Patient response to nasal spray may be varied. The choice of dose should be made individually, weighing the possible benefit of the 20-mg dose with the potential for a greater risk of adverse events.

Patient education
• Tell patient that drug may be given at any time during a migraine attack, but preferably as soon as symptoms begin. A second injection may be given if symptoms recur. Tell patient not to use more than two injections in 24 hours and to allow at least 1 hour between doses. Pain or redness at the injection site may occur but usually lasts less than 1 hour.
• Explain that drug is intended to relieve migraine, not to prevent or reduce the number of attacks.
• Tell patient not to use a second nasal spray dose if there was no response to the initial dose unless the health care provider is first contacted.
• Explain that drug is available in a spring-loaded injector system that facilitates self-administration. Review detailed information with patient. Be sure he understands how to load the injector, administer the injection, and dispose of the used syringes.
• Tell pregnant patient or one who intends to become pregnant during therapy to consult health care provider and discuss risks and benefits of drug use.
• Tell patient who feels persistent or severe chest pain to call immediately. Tell patient who experiences pain or tightness in the throat, wheezing, heart throbbing, rash, lumps, hives, or swollen eyelids, face, or lips to stop using the drug and call at once.

Pediatric use
• Safety and efficacy have not been established.

Breast-feeding
• Drug is excreted in breast milk. Use caution when administrating to breast-feeding women.

suprofen
Profenal

Pharmacologic classification: phenylalkanoic acid derivative; NSAID
Therapeutic classification: ophthalmic anti-inflammatory
Pregnancy risk category C

How supplied
Available by prescription only
Ophthalmic solution: 1%

Indications, route, and dosage
Inhibition of intraoperative miosis
Adults: Instill 2 drops into the conjunctival sac q 4 hours the day before surgery. On the day of surgery, instill 2 drops 3 hours, 2 hours, and 1 hour before surgery.

Pharmacodynamics
Anti-inflammatory action: Suprofen inhibits the action of cyclo-oxygenase, an enzyme responsible for the synthesis of prostaglandins. Prostaglandins are mediators of the inflammatory response and also cause miosis.

Pharmacokinetics
• *Absorption:* Some drug is absorbed systemically.
• *Distribution:* Unknown.
• *Metabolism:* Unknown.
• *Excretion:* Unknown.

Contraindications and precautions
Contraindicated in patients hypersensitive to any component of the formulation and in those with epithelial herpes simplex keratitis. Use cautiously in patients with bleeding disorders or sensitivity to NSAIDs or aspirin.

Interactions
Acetylcholine and *carbachol* may be ineffective in patients given suprofen.

Effects on diagnostic tests
None reported.

Adverse reactions
EENT: *transient stinging and burning on instillation,* discomfort, itching, redness, iritis, pain, chemosis, photophobia, irritation, punctate epithelial staining.

Overdose and treatment
Overdosage usually does not cause symptoms. Oral ingestion of drug may be treated by giving fluids to dilute.

☑ Special considerations
• Store away from heat in a dark, tightly closed container; protect drug from freezing.

Patient education
• Teach patient not to touch dropper to eye.
• Advise patient to discard drug when no longer needed.

Pediatric use
• Safety and efficacy have not been established.

Breast-feeding
• After systemic administration, drug is excreted in breast milk. Because of the risk of serious adverse effects to the infant, do not administer to breast-feeding women.

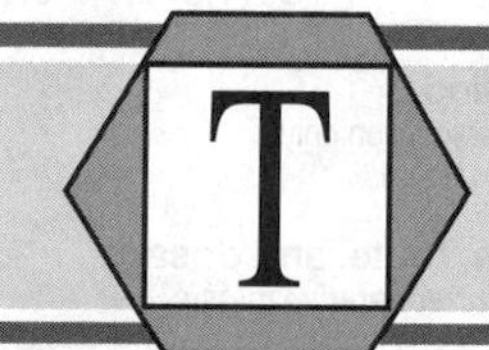

tacrine hydrochloride

Cognex

Pharmacologic classification: centrally acting reversible cholinesterase inhibitor
Therapeutic classification: psychotherapeutic agent (for Alzheimer's disease)
Pregnancy risk category C

How supplied

Available by prescription only
Capsules: 10 mg, 20 mg, 30 mg, 40 mg

Indications, route, and dosage

Mild to moderate dementia of the Alzheimer's type

Adults: Initially, 10 mg P.O. q.i.d. Maintain dose for at least 6 weeks, with every-other-week monitoring of transaminase levels. If patient tolerates treatment and transaminase levels remain normal, increase to 20 mg P.O. q.i.d. After 6 weeks, titrate dosage to 30 mg P.O. q.i.d. If still tolerated, increase to 40 mg P.O. q.i.d. after another 6 weeks.

✦ ***Dosage adjustment.*** In patients with ALT level two to three times upper limit of normal, monitor ALT level weekly. If ALT level is three to five times the upper normal limit, reduce daily dose by 40 mg/day and monitor ALT level weekly. Resume dose titration and every-other-week monitoring when ALT level returns to normal. If ALT level is above five times upper normal limit, stop treatment and monitor ALT level. Monitor for signs and symptoms associated with hepatitis. Rechallenge when ALT level is normal and monitor weekly.

Pharmacodynamics

Psychotherapeutic action: Tacrine presumably slows degradation of acetylcholine released by still-intact cholinergic neurons, thereby elevating acetylcholine concentrations in the cerebral cortex. If this theory is correct, the effects of tacrine may lessen as the disease process advances and fewer cholinergic neurons remain functionally intact. No evidence suggests that tacrine alters the course of the underlying dementia.

Pharmacokinetics

- *Absorption:* Rapidly absorbed after oral administration; maximum plasma concentrations occur within 1 to 2 hours. Absolute bioavailability of tacrine is approximately 17%. Food reduces tacrine bioavailability by approximately 30% to 40%; however, there is no food effect if tacrine is administered at least 1 hour before meals.
- *Distribution:* Drug is about 55% bound to plasma proteins.
- *Metabolism:* Tacrine undergoes first-pass metabolism, which is dose dependent. It is extensively metabolized by the cytochrome P-450 system to multiple metabolites, not all of which have been identified.
- *Excretion:* Elimination half-life is approximately 2 to 4 hours.

Contraindications and precautions

Contraindicated in patients hypersensitive to drug or acridine derivatives. Also contraindicated in patients in whom tacrine-related jaundice, which has been confirmed with an elevated total bilirubin level of more than 3 mg/dl, has previously developed.

Use cautiously in patients with sick sinus syndrome, bradycardia, history of hepatic disease, renal disease, Parkinson's disease, asthma, prostatic hyperplasia, or other urinary outflow impairment and in those at risk for peptic ulcer.

Interactions

Because of its mechanism of action, tacrine has the potential to interfere with the activity of *anticholinergic medications.* A synergistic effect is expected when tacrine is given concurrently with *cholinesterase inhibitors, succinylcholine,* or *cholinergic agonists* such as *bethanechol.* Coadministration of tacrine with *theophylline* increases theophylline elimination half-life and average plasma concentrations. Therefore, monitoring of plasma theophylline concentrations and appropriate reduction of theophylline dose are recommended.

Drug interactions may occur with coadministration with agents that undergo extensive metabolism via *cytochrome P-450.* Concurrent use with *cimetidine* increases the plasma concentration of tacrine. Concurrent use of *NSAIDs* may contribute to GI irritation and gastric bleeding.

Effects on diagnostic tests

Tacrine may cause significant abnormalities in serum transaminase (ALT, AST), bilirubin, and gamma-glutamyl transpeptidase levels.

Adverse reactions

CNS: agitation, ataxia, insomnia, abnormal thinking, somnolence, depression, anxiety, *headache, dizziness,* fatigue, confusion, seizures.
CV: bradycardia, hypertension, palpitations.
GI: *nausea, vomiting, diarrhea,* dyspepsia, loose stools, changes in stool color, anorexia, abdominal pain, flatulence, constipation.
Respiratory: rhinitis, upper respiratory tract infection, cough.
Skin: rash, jaundice, facial flushing.

Other: *elevations in transaminases* (especially ALT), myalgia, chest pain, weight loss, increased sweating.

Overdose and treatment

Overdosage with cholinesterase inhibitors can cause a cholinergic crisis characterized by severe nausea, vomiting, salivation, sweating, bradycardia, hypotension, and seizures. Increasing muscle weakness may occur and can result in death if respiratory muscles are involved. As in any overdose, use general supportive measures. Tertiary anticholinergics such as atropine may be used as an antidote for tacrine overdosage. I.V. atropine sulfate titrated to effect is recommended (initial dose of 1 to 2 mg I.V., with subsequent doses based on clinical response). It is not known whether tacrine or its metabolites can be eliminated by dialysis.

☑ Special considerations

- Tacrine as a cholinesterase inhibitor is likely to exaggerate succinylcholine-type muscle relaxation during anesthesia.
- Because of its cholinomimetic action, drug may have vagotonic effects on the heart rate (such as bradycardia), which may be particularly important to patients with sick sinus syndrome.
- Monitor serum ALT levels weekly for first 18 weeks of therapy. With moderately elevated levels after 18 weeks (twice the upper limit of normal), continue weekly monitoring. If no problems are detected, decrease frequency to once every 3 months. With each dosage increase, resume weekly monitoring for at least 6 weeks. The incidence of transaminase elevations is higher among females. There are no other known predictors of risk of hepatocellular injury.
- Rate of dose escalation may be slowed if patient is intolerant to the recommended titration schedule. However, do not accelerate the dose incrementation plan.
- If drug is discontinued for 4 weeks or more, restart full dose titration and monitoring schedule.
- Cognitive function can worsen after abrupt discontinuation of tacrine or after a reduction in total daily dose of 80 mg/day or more.

Patient education

- Tell patient and caregiver that drug should be taken between meals when possible. However, if GI upset occurs, drug may be taken with meals but may reduce plasma levels.
- Inform patient and family that drug does not alter the underlying degenerative disease but can alleviate symptoms. Effectiveness of therapy depends on drug administration at regular intervals.
- Remind caregiver that dosage titration is an integral part of the safe use of drug. Abrupt discontinuation or a large reduction in daily dosage (80 mg/day or more) may precipitate behavioral disturbances and a decline in cognitive function.
- Advise patient and caregiver to report significant adverse effects or changes in status immediately.

tacrolimus (FK506)

Prograf

Pharmacologic classification: bacteria-derived macrolide
Therapeutic classification: immunosuppressant
Pregnancy risk category C

How supplied

Available by prescription only
Capsules: 1 mg, 5 mg
Injection: 5 mg/ml

Indications, route, and dosage

Organ liver rejection prophylaxis

Adults: Initially, 0.05 to 0.1 mg/kg/day as a continuous I.V. infusion or, if tolerated, 0.15 to 0.3 mg/kg/day P.O. given no sooner than 6 hours after transplantation. I.V. route should be maintained only until patient can tolerate oral administration (usually within 2 to 3 days); then give 0.15 to 0.3 mg/kg/day P.O. in two divided doses q 12 hours, beginning 8 to 12 hours after discontinuing infusion.
Children: 0.1 mg/kg/day I.V. or 0.3 mg/kg/day P.O. given no sooner than 6 hours after transplantation. I.V. route should be maintained only until patient can tolerate oral administration (usually within 2 to 3 days); then give 0.3 mg/kg/day P.O. in two divided doses q 12 hours, beginning 8 to 12 hours after discontinuing infusion.

Note: Tacrolimus therapy is usually delayed 48 hours or longer in patients with postoperative oliguria.

Pharmacodynamics

Immunosuppressant action: Tacrolimus inhibits T-lymphocyte activation, although the exact mechanism of action is unknown. Evidence suggests that drug binds to an intracellular protein, FKBP-12. A complex of tacrolimus-FKBP-12, calcium, calmodulin, and calcineurin then forms, inhibiting the phosphatase activity of calcineurin. This effect may prevent the generation of nuclear factor of activated T-cells, a nuclear component thought to initiate gene transcription for the formation of lymphocyte activation and, therefore, to cause immunosuppression.

Pharmacokinetics

- *Absorption:* Absorption of oral tacrolimus from the GI tract varies. Absorption half-life in liver transplant patients is approximately 5.7 hours. Peak concentration levels in blood and plasma are achieved in 1.5 to 3.5 hours. Food reduces the absorption and bioavailability of tacrolimus.
- *Distribution:* Drug is bound to proteins, mainly albumin and alpha$_1$-acid glycoprotein, and is highly bound to erythrocytes. Protein binding is between 75% and 99%. Distribution of drug between whole blood and plasma depends on several factors, such as hematocrit, temperature of separation of plasma, drug concentration, and plasma protein concentration.

• *Metabolism:* Extensively metabolized by the mixed-function oxidase system, primarily cytochrome P-450.
• *Excretion:* Less than 1% of the administered dose is excreted unchanged in urine. Ten possible metabolites have been identified in human plasma. Two metabolites, a demethylated and a double demethylated tacrolimus, were shown to retain 10% and 7%, respectively, of the inhibitory effect of tacrolimus on T-lymphocyte activation.

Contraindications and precautions
Contraindicated in patients with hypersensitivity to drug. I.V. form is contraindicated in those who are hypersensitive to castor oil derivatives. Use cautiously in patients with impaired renal or hepatic function.

Interactions
Concomitant administration of tacrolimus with other *nephrotoxic agents (aminoglycosides, amphotericin B, cisplatin, cyclosporine)* increases risk of nephrotoxicity. In particular, concomitant use of tacrolimus and *cyclosporine* should be avoided; discontinue one at least 24 hours before initiating the other. With elevated tacrolimus or cyclosporine concentrations, further dosing with the other drug is usually delayed.

Tacrolimus should not be administered with other *immunosuppressive agents except adrenal corticosteroids* because of increased susceptibility to infection.

Antifungals, bromocriptine, calcium channel blocking agents, cimetidine, clarithromycin, danazol, diltiazem, erythromycin, methylprednisolone, and *metoclopramide* may interfere with tacrolimus metabolism, requiring a reduced tacrolimus dosage.

Carbamazepine, phenobarbital, phenytoin, and *rifamycins* may decrease tacrolimus blood levels, requiring an increased tacrolimus dosage.

Avoid use of *live vaccines* (such as *measles, mumps, rubella, oral polio, BCG, yellow fever, TY 21a typhoid*) during treatment with tacrolimus.

Effects on diagnostic tests
None reported.

Adverse reactions
CNS: *headache, tremor, insomnia, paresthesia.*
CV: *hypertension, peripheral edema.*
GI: *diarrhea, nausea, constipation, abnormal liver function test, anorexia, vomiting, abdominal pain.*
GU: *abnormal renal function, increased creatinine or BUN levels, urinary tract infection, oliguria.*
Hematologic: *anemia, leukocytosis,* THROMBOCYTOPENIA.
Metabolic: *hyperkalemia, hypokalemia, hyperglycemia, hypomagnesemia.*
Respiratory: *pleural effusion, atelectasis, dyspnea.*
Skin: *pruritus, rash.*
Other: *pain, fever, asthenia, back pain, ascites,* ***anaphylaxis.***

Overdose and treatment
There is minimal experience with overdosage. In patients who have received inadvertent overdosage of tacrolimus, no adverse reactions different from those reported in patients receiving therapeutic doses have been described. Follow general supportive measures and systemic treatment in all cases of overdosage. Based on poor aqueous solubility and extensive erythrocyte and plasma protein binding, tacrolimus is probably not dialyzable to a significant extent.

☑ Special considerations
• Give adult patients doses at lower end of dosing range. Titrate dosing based on clinical assessment of rejection and tolerance. Lower dosages may be sufficient as maintenance therapy. Tacrolimus should be used concomitantly with adrenal corticosteroids in early post-transplant period.
• Because of risk of anaphylaxis, reserve injection for patients unable to take capsules.
• Drug is being investigated for use in kidney, bone marrow, cardiac, pancreas, pancreatic island cell, and small bowel transplantation. It also may be used to treat autoimmune disease and severe recalcitrant psoriasis.
• Closely monitor patient with impaired renal function; dosage may need to be reduced. In patients with persistent elevations of serum creatinine who are unresponsive to dosage adjustments, consider changing to another immunosuppressive therapy. Also closely monitor patient experiencing post-transplant hepatic impairment because of increased risk of renal insufficiency related to high whole-blood levels of tacrolimus. Dosage adjustments may be necessary.
• Because of risk of hyperkalemia (mild to severe hyperkalemia has been noted in 10% to 44% of liver transplant recipients given tacrolimus), monitor serum potassium levels and do not use potassium-sparing diuretics.
• Patients receiving tacrolimus are at increased risk for developing lymphomas and other malignancies, particularly of the skin. The risk appears to be related to intensity and duration of immunosuppression, rather than to use of any specific agent.
• A lymphoproliferative disorder (LPD) related to Epstein-Barr virus (EBV) has been reported in immunosuppressed organ transplant recipients. The risk of LPD appears greatest in young children who are at risk for primary EBV infection while immunosuppressed or who are switched to tacrolimus after long-term immunosuppression therapy.
• Antihypertensive therapy may be required to control blood pressure elevations associated with drug use. Likewise, therapy may be required to control blood glucose elevations associated with drug use.
• Most study centers have found monitoring of drug blood concentration helpful in patient management. Even though no fixed relationship has been established, such blood monitoring may assist in the clinical evaluation of rejection and toxicity, dosage adjustments, and assessment of compliance.
• Dilute I.V. form with 0.9% NaCl injection or 5% dextrose injection to a concentration between 0.004 and 0.02 mg/ml before use.
• Continuously observe patients receiving drug I.V. for at least 30 minutes after the start of infusion and frequently thereafter. Stop infusion if signs or symp-

toms of anaphylaxis occur. Have an aqueous solution of epinephrine 1:1,000 and a source of oxygen available at the patient's bedside.
- Store diluted infusion solution in glass or polyethylene container and discard after 24 hours. Do not store in a polyvinyl chloride container because of decreased stability and the potential for extraction of phthalates.

Patient education
- Tell patient to take capsules on an empty stomach because food affects drug absorption.
- Inform patient of need for repeated laboratory tests during therapy to monitor for adverse reactions and drug effectiveness.
- Advise female patient of childbearing age to consult doctor if she becomes pregnant or plans to do so.

Pediatric use
- Children without preexisting renal or hepatic dysfunction have required and tolerated higher doses than adults to achieve similar blood concentrations. Pediatric patients should receive the high end of the recommended adult I.V. and oral dosing ranges (0.1 mg/kg/day I.V. and 0.3 mg/kg/day P.O.). Dose adjustments may be required.

Breast-feeding
- Because drug occurs in breast milk, women receiving tacrolimus should avoid breast-feeding.

tamoxifen citrate
Nolvadex, Nolvadex-D*, Tamofen*

Pharmacologic classification: nonsteroidal antiestrogen
Therapeutic classification: antineoplastic
Pregnancy risk category D

How supplied
Available by prescription only
Tablets: 10 mg, 20 mg
Tablets (enteric coated): 20 mg*

Indications, route, and dosage
Dosage and indications may vary. Check current literature for recommended protocol.

Advanced breast cancer (men and postmenopausal women)
Adults: 10 to 20 mg P.O. b.i.d.

Adjunct treatment for breast cancer
Adults: 10 mg P.O. b.i.d. to t.i.d. for no more than 2 years.

◊ ***Mastalgia***
Adults: 10 mg P.O. daily for 4 months.

◊ ***Stimulate ovulation***
Adults: 5 to 40 mg P.O. b.i.d. for 4 days.

Pharmacodynamics
Antineoplastic action: Exact mechanism of action is unclear. Tamoxifen may exert its cytotoxic action by blocking estrogen receptors within tumor cells that require estrogen to thrive. The estrogen receptor-tamoxifen complex may be translocated into the nucleus of the tumor cell, where it inhibits DNA synthesis.

Pharmacokinetics
- *Absorption:* Drug appears to be well absorbed across the GI tract after oral administration. Steady state serum concentrations are generally attained after 3 to 4 weeks.
- *Distribution:* Distribution of drug and its metabolites into body tissues and fluids has not been fully established.
- *Metabolism:* Metabolized extensively in the liver to several metabolites.
- *Excretion:* Excreted primarily in feces, mostly as metabolites. Drug has a distribution phase half-life of 7 to 14 hours. Secondary peak plasma levels occur 4 days after a dose, probably because of enterohepatic circulation. Half-life of the terminal elimination phase is more than 7 days.

Contraindications and precautions
Contraindicated in patients hypersensitive to drug and during pregnancy. Use cautiously in patients with existing leukopenia or thrombocytopenia.

Interactions
Concurrent use of *coumadin* may result in a significant increase in anticoagulation effect. Coadministration with *cytotoxic agents* has shown an increase in thromboembolic events. Concomitant use with *estrogens* may interfere with the therapeutic effect of drug.

Effects on diagnostic tests
Drug therapy may increase concentrations of serum calcium. This effect usually occurs in patients with bone metastases. Serum triglycerides and cholesterol may be increased. Thyroxine and hepatic enzymes may be increased. Variations on karyopyknotic index in vaginal smears and various degrees of estrogen effect on Papanicolaou smears have been seen in some postmenopausal patients.

Adverse reactions
GI: *nausea, vomiting, diarrhea.*
GU: *vaginal discharge* and bleeding, *irregular menses, increased BUN, amenorrhea.*
Hematologic: transient decrease in WBC or platelet count, leukopenia, ***thrombocytopenia.***
Skin: *skin changes.*
Other: temporary bone or tumor pain, *hot flashes,* brief exacerbation of pain from osseous metastases, *weight gain or loss, fluid retention.*

Overdose and treatment
Acute overdosage in humans has not been reported. No specific treatment is known. Treatment should include supportive measures.

☑ Special considerations
- Initial adverse reactions (increased bone pain) may be associated with a good tumor response shortly after starting tamoxifen therapy.
- Analgesics are indicated to relieve pain.

• Adverse reactions are usually minor and well tolerated. They can usually be controlled by dosage reduction.
• Clotting factor abnormalities may occur with prolonged tamoxifen therapy at usual dosages.
• Monitor WBC and platelet counts and periodic liver function tests.
• Monitor serum calcium levels; hypercalcemia may occur during initial therapy in patients with bone metastases.
• Tamoxifen acts as an antiestrogen. Best results occur in patients with positive estrogen receptors.
• Drug is also used to treat breast cancer in males and advanced ovarian cancer in women.

Patient education

• Emphasize importance of continuing drug despite occurrence of nausea and vomiting.
• Tell patient to promptly report vomiting if it occurs shortly after a dose is taken.
• Reassure patient that acute exacerbation of bone pain during tamoxifen therapy usually indicates drug will produce good response.
• Stress importance of swallowing enteric-coated tablets without crushing or breaking them.
• Advise women to avoid becoming pregnant during drug therapy. Also recommend barrier or nonhormonal contraceptive measures for sexually active patients during treatment period.

Breast-feeding

• It is not known if drug occurs in breast milk. However, because of the potential for serious adverse reactions and carcinogenicity in the infant, breast-feeding is not recommended.

tamsulosin hydrochloride

Flomax

Pharmacologic classification: alpha$_{1A}$-antagonist
Therapeutic classification: benign prostatic hyperplasia (BPH) agent
Pregnancy risk category B

How supplied

Available by prescription only
Capsules: 0.4 mg

Indications, route, and dosage

BPH

Adult men: 0.4 mg P.O. once daily, administered 30 minutes after same meal each day. For those who fail to respond after 2 to 4 weeks, increase dose to 0.8 mg P.O. once daily. If either dosing regimen is interrupted for several days, restart therapy with the 0.4-mg once-daily dose.

Pharmacodynamics

Anti-BPH action: Drug selectively blocks alpha$_1$-receptors in the prostate, leading to relaxation of smooth muscles in the bladder neck and prostate, improving urine flow, and reducing BPH symptoms.

Pharmacokinetics

• *Absorption:* Essentially complete following oral administration under fasting conditions. Steady state is achieved by day 5 of once-daily dosing. Maximum concentrations are achieved 4 to 5 hours under fasting conditions and 6 to 7 hours when administered with food.
• *Distribution:* Studies suggest distribution into extracellular fluids and most tissues, including kidney, prostate, gallbladder, heart, aorta, and brown fat, with minimal distribution into brain, spinal cord, and testes. Drug is extensively bound to plasma proteins but is not thought to affect other highly bound drugs.
• *Metabolism:* Metabolized by cytochrome P-450 in the liver, with less than 10% excreted unchanged; however, pharmacokinetic profile of metabolites has not been established. Drug's metabolites undergo extensive conjugation to glucuronide or sulfate prior to renal excretion.
• *Excretion:* Primarily in the urine (76%); approximately 21% excreted in feces. Elimination half-life is 5 to 7 hours, with apparent half-life from 9 to 15 hours secondary to rate-controlled absorption pharmacokinetics.

Contraindications and precautions

Contraindicated in patients with hypersensitivity to drug or its components.

Interactions

Alpha-adrenergic blocking agents are presumed to interact with drug; do not use together. *Cimetidine* decreases clearance of tamsulosin; use together with caution, particularly if tamsulosin dose is over 0.4 mg. Studies with *warfarin* are inconclusive; use together with caution. Use drug cautiously with *cytochrome P-450 metabolized drugs.*

Effects on diagnostic tests

None reported.

Adverse reactions

CNS: *dizziness, headache,* insomnia, somnolence.
CV: chest pain, syncope.
EENT: amblyopia, pharyngitis, *rhinitis,* sinusitis.
GI: diarrhea, nausea.
GU: abnormal ejaculation, decrease in libido.
Respiratory: increased cough.
Other: asthenia, back pain, *infection,* tooth disorder.

Overdose and treatment

Can lead to hypotension; support CV system. Keep patient in supine position; administer I.V. fluids if necessary. Initiate vasopressors if needed and monitor renal function, supporting as needed. Dialysis in unlikely to be beneficial.

☑ Special considerations

• Monitor patient for decreased blood pressure.
• Symptoms of BPH and carcinoma of the prostate are similar; rule out carcinoma prior to initiating therapy with tamsulosin.
• If treatment is interrupted for several days or more, restart therapy at 1 capsule daily.

Patient education
- Instruct patient not to crush, chew, or open capsules.
- Tell patient to get up slowly from chair or bed during initiation of therapy.
- Instruct patient not to drive or perform hazardous tasks during initiation if therapy and for 12 hours following the initial dose or changes in dose until response can be monitored.
- Tell patient to take drug approximately 30 minutes following same meal each day.
- Caution patient to avoid situations where injury could occur due to syncope.

Pediatric use
- Drug is not indicated for use in children.

Breast-feeding
- Drug is not indicated for use in women.

temazepam
Restoril

Pharmacologic classification: benzodiazepine
Therapeutic classification: sedative-hypnotic
Controlled substance schedule IV
Pregnancy risk category X

How supplied
Available by prescription only
Capsules: 7.5 mg, 15 mg, 30 mg

Indications, route, and dosage
Insomnia
Adults: 7.5 to 30 mg P.O. 30 minutes before bedtime.
✦ ***Dosage adjustment.*** In adults over age 65, 7.5 mg P.O. h.s.

Pharmacodynamics
Sedative-hypnotic action: Temazepam depresses the CNS at the limbic and subcortical levels of the brain. It produces a sedative-hypnotic effect by potentiating the effect of the neurotransmitter gamma-aminobutyric acid on its receptor in the ascending reticular activating system, which increases inhibition and blocks both cortical and limbic arousal.

Pharmacokinetics
- *Absorption:* When administered orally, drug is well absorbed through the GI tract. Peak levels occur in 1.2 to 1.6 hours (mean 1.5 hours). Onset of action occurs at 30 to 60 minutes.
- *Distribution:* Widely distributed throughout the body. Drug is 96% protein-bound.
- *Metabolism:* Drug is metabolized in the liver primarily to inactive metabolites.
- *Excretion:* Metabolites are excreted in urine as glucuronide conjugates. Half-life of drug ranges between 4 and 20 hours.

Contraindications and precautions
Contraindicated in patients with hypersensitivity to drug or other benzodiazepines and during pregnancy. Use cautiously in patients with impaired renal or hepatic function, chronic pulmonary insufficiency, severe or latent mental depression, suicidal tendencies, or history of drug abuse.

Interactions
Temazepam potentiates the CNS depressant effects of *alcohol, antidepressants, antihistamines, barbiturates, general anesthetics, MAO inhibitors, narcotics,* and *phenothiazines.*

Heavy smoking accelerates temazepam metabolism, thus lowering clinical effectiveness. Benzodiazepines block the therapeutic effects of *levodopa.* Temazepam may decrease plasma levels of *haloperidol.*

Effects on diagnostic tests
Temazepam therapy may increase liver function test results. Minor changes in EEG patterns, usually low-voltage, fast activity, may occur during and after temazepam therapy.

Adverse reactions
CNS: *drowsiness, dizziness, lethargy,* disturbed coordination, daytime sedation, confusion, nightmares, vertigo, euphoria, weakness, headache, fatigue, nervousness, anxiety, depression.
EENT: blurred vision.
GI: diarrhea, nausea, dry mouth.
Other: physical and psychological dependence.

Overdose and treatment
Clinical manifestations of overdose include somnolence, confusion, hypoactive or absent reflexes, dyspnea, labored breathing, hypotension, bradycardia, slurred speech, unsteady gait or impaired coordination and, ultimately, coma.

Support blood pressure and respiration until drug effects subside; monitor vital signs. Mechanical ventilatory assistance via endotracheal tube may be required to maintain a patent airway and support adequate oxygenation. Flumazenil, a specific benzodiazepine antagonist, may be useful. Use I.V. fluids and vasopressors, such as dopamine and phenylephrine, to treat hypotension as needed. If patient is conscious, induce emesis. Use gastric lavage if ingestion was recent, but only if an endotracheal tube is present to prevent aspiration. After emesis or lavage, administer activated charcoal with a cathartic as a single dose. Do not use barbiturates if excitation occurs. Dialysis is of limited value.

☑ Special considerations
Besides those relevant to all *benzodiazepines,* consider the following recommendations.
- Evaluate patient for cause of insomnia, which is commonly a symptom of an underlying disorder such as depression.
- Drug is useful for patients who have difficulty falling asleep or who awaken frequently in the night.
- Prolonged use is not recommended; however, drug has proven effective for up to 4 weeks of continuous use.
- Remove all potential safety hazards such as cigarettes from patient's reach.

• Impose safety measures, such as call bell within reach and side rails raised, to prevent possible injury.
• Monitor hepatic function studies to prevent toxicity; lower doses are indicated in patients with hepatic dysfunction.
• After long-term use, abrupt withdrawal should be avoided and a gradual tapering dose schedule followed.
• Store drug in a cool, dry place away from light.

Patient education
• Instruct patient to seek medical approval before making changes in medication regimen.
• As necessary, teach patient safety measures to prevent injury, such as gradual position changes and supervised ambulation.
• Inform patient of the risk for physical and psychological dependence with chronic use.
• Advise female patient to call immediately if pregnancy is suspected.
• Emphasize potential for excessive CNS depression if drug is taken with alcohol.
• Tell patient that rebound insomnia may occur after stopping drug.

Geriatric use
• Elderly patients are more susceptible to the CNS depressant effects of temazepam. Use with caution.
• Lower doses are usually effective in elderly patients because of decreased elimination.
• Elderly patients who receive drug require supervision with ambulation and activities of daily living during initiation of therapy or after an increase in dose.

Pediatric use
• Safe use in patients under age 18 has not been established.

Breast-feeding
• Temazepam is excreted in breast milk. A breast-fed infant may become sedated, have feeding difficulties, or lose weight. Avoid use in breast-feeding women.

teniposide (VM-26)
Vumon

Pharmacologic classification: podophyllotoxin (cell cycle-phase specific, G_2 and late S phase)
Therapeutic classification: antineoplastic
Pregnancy risk category D

How supplied
Available by prescription only
Injection: 50 mg/5 ml ampules

Indications, route, and dosage
Dosage and indications may vary. Check current literature for recommended protocol.
Acute lymphoblastic leukemia induction therapy in childhood
Children: Optimum dosage has not been established. One protocol reported by manufacturer is 165 mg/m² I.V. teniposide with cytarabine 300 mg/m² I.V. twice weekly for eight or nine doses.

Pharmacodynamics
Antineoplastic action: Teniposide causes single- and double-stranded breaks in DNA and DNA protein cross-links, thus preventing cells from entering mitosis.

Pharmacokinetics
• *Absorption:* Teniposide is not administered orally.
• *Distribution:* Drug is highly bound to plasma proteins. Teniposide crosses the blood-brain barrier to a limited extent.
• *Metabolism:* Metabolized extensively in the liver.
• *Excretion:* Approximately 40% of a dose is eliminated through the kidneys as unchanged drug or metabolites. Terminal half-life of drug is 5 hours.

Contraindications and precautions
Contraindicated in patients hypersensitive to drug or to polyoxyethylated castor oil, an injection vehicle.

Interactions
Teniposide may increase the effects of *methotrexate. Sodium salicylate, sulfamethizole,* and *tolbutamide* may displace teniposide from protein-binding sites, causing a potentiation of toxicity.

Effects on diagnostic tests
Teniposide therapy may increase blood and urine concentrations of uric acid.

Adverse reactions
CV: hypotension from rapid infusion.
GI: *nausea, vomiting, mucositis, diarrhea.*
Hematologic: LEUKOPENIA, NEUTROPENIA, THROMBOCYTOPENIA, MYELOSUPPRESSION (dose-limiting), *anemia.*
Skin: rash.
Other: alopecia (rare), ***anaphylaxis*** (rare), *infection,* bleeding, hypersensitivity reactions (chills, fever, urticaria, tachycardia, ***bronchospasm,*** dyspnea, hypotension, flushing); *phlebitis and extravasation* (at injection site).

Overdose and treatment
Clinical manifestations of overdose include myelosuppression, nausea, and vomiting.

Treatment is usually supportive and includes transfusion of blood components, antiemetics, and antibiotics for infections that may develop.

☑ Special considerations
• Dilute with 5% dextrose injection USP or 0.9% NaCl injection USP to give final teniposide concentrations of 0.1 mg/ml, 0.2 mg/ml, 0.4 mg/ml, or 1 mg/ml.
• Solutions containing concentrations of 0.1 mg/ml, 0.2 mg/ml, or 0.4 mg/ml are stable at room temperature for 24 hours. Solutions with a final concentration of 1 mg/ml should be administered within 4 hours of preparation.

- Do not administer drug through a membrane-type in-line filter because the diluent may dissolve the filter.
- Administer I.V. infusion over 30 to 60 minutes to prevent hypotension. Avoid I.V. push because of increased risk of hypotension.
- Use glass or polyolefin plastic bags or containers for infusion. Do not use polyvinyl chloride containers.
- Dosage should be decreased in patients with renal or hepatic insufficiency and in patients with Down syndrome.
- Monitor for chemical phlebitis at injection site.
- Have diphenhydramine, hydrocortisone, epinephrine, and oral airway available in case of an anaphylactic reaction.
- Monitor blood pressure before infusion and at 30-minute intervals during infusion. If systolic blood pressure decreases below 90 mm Hg, stop infusion.
- Monitor CBC. Observe patient for signs of bone marrow depression.

Patient education

- Encourage adequate fluid intake to increase urine output and facilitate excretion of uric acid.
- Tell patient to avoid exposure to people with infections.
- Advise patient that hair should grow back after treatment is discontinued.
- Tell patient to call promptly if a sore throat or fever develop or if unusual bruising or bleeding occur.

Breast-feeding

- It is not known if drug occurs in breast milk. However, because of the risk of serious adverse reactions, mutagenicity, and carcinogenicity in the infant, breast-feeding is not recommended.

terazosin hydrochloride

Hytrin

Pharmacologic classification: selective $alpha_1$ blocker
Therapeutic classification: antihypertensive
Pregnancy risk category C

How supplied

Available by prescription only
Tablets: 1 mg, 2 mg, 5 mg, 10 mg

Indications, route, and dosage

Mild to moderate hypertension

Adults: Initially, 1 mg h.s. Adjust dose and schedule according to patient response. Recommended range, 1 to 5 mg daily or divided b.i.d.

If therapy is discontinued for several days or longer, reinstitute using the initial dosing regimen of 1 mg h.s. Slowly increase dose until desired blood pressure is attained. Doses over 20 mg do not appear to further affect blood pressure.

Benign prostatic hyperplasia

Adults: Initially, 1 mg h.s. Dosage may be adjusted upward based on patient response. Increase in a stepwise manner to 2 mg, 5 mg, and 10 mg. A daily dose of 10 mg may be required.

Pharmacodynamics

Antihypertensive action: Terazosin reduces blood pressure by selectively inhibiting $alpha_1$ receptors in vascular smooth muscle and thus reducing peripheral vascular resistance. Due to its selectivity for $alpha_1$ receptors, heart rate increases minimally. Significant decreases in serum cholesterol, low-density lipoprotein, and very-low-density lipoprotein cholesterol fractions occur during therapy; the significance of these changes is unknown, as is the mechanism by which they occur.

Terazosin administration does not significantly alter potassium or glucose levels; it has been used successfully with diuretics, beta blockers, and a combination of other antihypertensive regimens.

Hypertrophic action: Alpha-blockade in nonvascular smooth muscle causes relaxation, notably in prostatic tissue, thereby reducing urinary symptoms in men with benign prostatic hyperplasia.

Pharmacokinetics

- *Absorption:* Rapidly absorbed after oral administration, reaching peak plasma concentrations in 1 to 2 hours. Approximately 90% of oral dose is bioavailable; ingestion of food does not appear to alter bioavailability.
- *Distribution:* About 90% to 94% is plasma protein-bound.
- *Metabolism:* Drug is metabolized in the liver. The pharmacokinetics of terazosin do not appear to be affected by hypertension, heart failure, or age.
- *Excretion:* About 40% is excreted in urine, 60% in feces, mostly as metabolites. Up to 30% may be excreted unchanged. Elimination half-life is approximately 12 hours.

Contraindications and precautions

Contraindicated in patients with hypersensitivity to drug.

Interactions

Use caution when administering terazosin concomitantly with *other antihypertensive agents.* When adding a *diuretic* or another antihypertensive agent, dosage reduction and retitration may be necessary.

Effects on diagnostic tests

Terazosin therapy causes small but significant decreases in hematocrit, WBC count, and hemoglobin, total protein, and albumin levels; the magnitude of these decreases has not been shown to worsen with time, suggesting the possibility of hemodilution.

Adverse reactions

CNS: *asthenia, dizziness, headache,* nervousness, paresthesia, somnolence.
CV: *palpitations, peripheral edema,* orthostatic hypotension, tachycardia, syncope.
EENT: *nasal congestion,* sinusitis, blurred vision.
GI: *nausea.*
GU: impotence.
Respiratory: dyspnea.
Other: back pain, muscle pain.

Overdose and treatment
Clinical signs of overdose are exaggerated adverse reactions, particularly hypotension and shock. In case of overdose, treatment is symptomatic and supportive. Dialysis may not be helpful because drug is highly protein-bound.

☑ Special considerations
Besides those relevant to all *alpha-adrenergic blockers,* consider the following recommendation.
- Terazosin can cause marked hypotension, especially postural hypotension, and syncope with the first dose or during the first few days of therapy. A similar response occurs if therapy is interrupted for more than a few doses.

Patient education
- Instruct patient to take first dose at bedtime.
- Warn patient to avoid hazardous tasks that require alertness for 12 hours after first dose, when dose is first increased, or when restarting dose after interruption of therapy.
- Caution patient to rise carefully and slowly from sitting and supine positions and to report dizziness, light-headedness, or palpitations. Dosage adjustment may be necessary.

terbinafine hydrochloride
Lamisil

Pharmacologic classification: synthetic allylamine derivative
Therapeutic classification: antifungal
Pregnancy risk category B

How supplied
Available by prescription only
Cream: 1% in 15-g and 30-g containers
Tablets: 250 mg

Indications, route, and dosage
***Interdigital tinea pedis (athlete's foot), tinea cruris (jock itch), or tinea corporis (ringworm) caused by* Epidermophyton floccosum, Trichophyton mentagrophytes, *or* T. rubrum**
Adults and children over age 12: For interdigital tinea pedis, apply to cover the affected and immediately surrounding areas b.i.d. until clinical signs and symptoms are significantly improved (for most patients this occurs by day 7 of drug therapy); for tinea cruris or tinea corporis, apply to cover the affected and immediately surrounding areas once or twice daily until clinical signs and symptoms are significantly improved (for most patients this occurs by day 7 of drug therapy). Treatment should not exceed 4 weeks.

Note: If irritation or sensitivity develops, discontinue treatment and institute appropriate therapy.

Onychomycosis of fingernails or toenails caused by dermatophytes (tinea unguium)
Adults and adolescents over age 12: For treatment of fingernails, give 250 mg/day P.O. for 6 weeks; for toenails, give 250 mg/day P.O. for 12 weeks.

Pharmacodynamics
Antifungal action: Terbinafine exerts its antifungal effect by inhibiting squalene epoxidase, a key enzyme in sterol biosynthesis in fungi. This action results in a deficiency in ergosterol and a corresponding accumulation of squalene within the fungal cell and causes fungal cell death.

Pharmacokinetics
Topical
- *Absorption:* Systemic absorption of terbinafine is highly variable.
- *Distribution:* No information available.
- *Metabolism:* No information available.
- *Excretion:* Approximately 75% of cutaneously absorbed terbinafine is eliminated in the urine, predominantly as metabolites.

Oral
- *Absorption:* More than 70% of drug is absorbed; food enhances absorption. Peak plasma concentration is 1 mcg/ml within 2 hours of first dose.
- *Distribution:* Drug is distributed to serum and skin. Plasma half-life is about 36 hours; half-life in tissue is 200 to 400 hours. More than 99% of drug is bound to plasma proteins.
- *Metabolism:* First-pass metabolism is about 40%.
- *Excretion:* About 70% of the administered dose is eliminated in urine; clearance is decreased by 50% in patients with hepatic cirrhosis and impaired renal function.

Contraindications and precautions
Contraindicated in patients hypersensitive to drug. Oral form is also contraindicated in patients with preexisting hepatic disease or impaired renal function (creatinine clearance of 50 ml/minute or less) and during pregnancy.

Interactions
None reported for topical form.

For oral form, concomitant administration of *I.V. caffeine* decreases clearance of caffeine by 19%. Concurrent administration with *cyclosporine* increases cyclosporine clearance by 15%. *Rifampin* increases clearance of terbinafine by 100%, whereas *cimetidine* decreases terbinafine clearance by 33%.

Effects on diagnostic tests
Drug may cause liver enzyme abnormalities at least twice the upper limit of normal range.

Adverse reactions
GI: diarrhea, dyspepsia, abdominal pain, nausea, flatulence.
Skin: ***Stevens-Johnson syndrome,*** irritation, burning, pruritus, dryness.
Other: liver enzyme abnormalities, taste disturbances, visual disturbances, *headache.*

Overdose and treatment
Acute overdosage with topical application is unlikely because of the limited absorption of topically applied drug and would not be expected to lead to a life-threatening situation.

☑ Special considerations

- Topical form of drug is for topical use only; it is not for oral, ophthalmic, or intravaginal use.
- Diagnosis should be confirmed either by direct microscopic examination of scrapings from infected tissue mounted in a solution of potassium hydroxide or by culture.

For topical form

- Know that duration of drug therapy should be for a minimum of 1 week and should not exceed 4 weeks.
- Many patients treated with shorter durations of therapy (1 to 2 weeks) continue to improve during the 2 to 4 weeks after drug therapy has been completed. As a consequence, patients should not be considered therapeutic failures until they have been observed for a period of 2 to 4 weeks off therapy. If successful outcome is not achieved during the post-treatment observation period, review the diagnosis.
- Monitor patient for irritation or sensitivity to drug. Discontinue therapy if present and institute appropriate treatment measures.

For oral form

- Perform liver function tests for patients receiving oral treatment for more than 6 weeks.

Patient education

- Advise patient to use drug as directed and to avoid contact with the eyes, nose, mouth, or other mucous membranes.
- Stress importance of using drug for recommended treatment time.
- Tell patient to call if the area of application shows signs or symptoms of increased irritation or possible sensitization (redness, itching, burning, blistering, swelling, or oozing).
- Instruct patient *not* to use occlusive dressings unless directed.

Pediatric use

- Safety and efficacy in children under age 12 have not been established.

Breast-feeding

- Drug occurs in breast milk. A decision to either discontinue breast-feeding or drug, taking into account the importance of drug to the mother, must be made. Women who are breast-feeding should avoid application of terbinafine cream to the breast.

terbutaline sulfate

Brethaire, Brethine, Bricanyl

Pharmacologic classification: adrenergic (beta$_2$ agonist)
Therapeutic classification: bronchodilator, premature labor inhibitor (tocolytic)
Pregnancy risk category B

How supplied

Available by prescription only
Tablets: 2.5 mg, 5 mg
Aerosol inhaler: 200 mcg/metered spray
Injection: 1 mg/ml parenteral

Indications, route, and dosage

Relief of bronchospasm in patients with reversible obstructive airway disease

Adults and adolescents age 15 or older: Administer 5 mg P.O. t.i.d. at 6-hour intervals. Maximum daily dose, 15 mg. Alternatively, 0.25 mg S.C. may be repeated in 15 to 30 minutes; maximum, 0.5 mg q 4 hours. Alternatively, 2 inhalations may be given q 4 to 6 hours with 1 minute between inhalations.
Adolescents age 12 to 15: 2.5 mg P.O. t.i.d. Maximum daily dose, 7.5 mg. Alternatively, 2 inhalations may be given q 4 to 6 hours with 1 minute between inhalations.

◇ ***Premature labor***

Adults: Initially, 10 mcg/minute I.V. Titrate to maximum dose of 80 mcg/minute. Maintain I.V. dosage at minimum effective dose for 4 hours. Maintenance therapy until term is 2.5 mg P.O. q 4 to 6 hours.

Pharmacodynamics

Bronchodilator action: Terbutaline acts directly on beta$_2$-adrenergic receptors to relax bronchial smooth muscle, relieving bronchospasm and reducing airway resistance. Cardiac and CNS stimulation may occur with high doses.

Tocolytic action: When used in premature labor, terbutaline relaxes uterine smooth muscle, which inhibits uterine contractions.

Pharmacokinetics

- *Absorption:* 33% to 50% of an oral dose is absorbed through the GI tract. Onset of action occurs within 30 minutes, peaks within 2 to 3 hours, and persists for 4 to 8 hours. After S.C. injection, onset occurs within 15 minutes, peaks within 30 to 60 minutes, and persists for 1½ to 4 hours. After oral inhalation, onset of action occurs within 5 to 30 minutes, peaks within 1 to 2 hours, and persists for 3 to 4 hours.
- *Distribution:* Widely distributed throughout the body.
- *Metabolism:* Partially metabolized in liver to inactive compounds.
- *Excretion:* After parenteral administration, 60% is excreted unchanged in urine, 3% in feces via bile, and the remainder in urine as metabolites. After oral administration, most drug is excreted as metabolites.

Contraindications and precautions

Contraindicated in patients with hypersensitivity to drug or sympathomimetic amines. Use cautiously in patients with CV disorders, hyperthyroidism, diabetes, or seizure disorders.

Interactions

When used concomitantly with *other sympathomimetics,* terbutaline may potentiate adverse CV effects of the other drugs; however, as an aerosol *bronchodilator* (*adrenergic stimulator* type), concomitant use may relieve acute bronchospasm in patients on long-term oral terbutaline therapy.

Beta blockers may antagonize bronchodilating effects of terbutaline. Use of *MAO inhibitors* within 14 days of terbutaline or the concomitant use of *tricyclic antidepressants* may potentiate effects of terbutaline on the vascular system.

Effects on diagnostic tests
Terbutaline may reduce the sensitivity of spirometry for diagnosis of bronchospasm.

Adverse reactions
CNS: *nervousness, tremor, drowsiness, dizziness, headache,* weakness.
CV: *palpitations,* tachycardia, ***arrhythmias,*** flushing.
EENT: dry and irritated nose and throat (with inhaled form).
GI: *vomiting, nausea,* heartburn.
Respiratory: ***paradoxical bronchospasm with prolonged usage,*** dyspnea.
Other: hypokalemia (with high doses), diaphoresis.

Overdose and treatment
Clinical manifestations of overdose include exaggeration of common adverse reactions, particularly arrhythmias, seizures, nausea, and vomiting. Treatment requires supportive measures. If patient is conscious and ingestion was recent, induce emesis and follow with gastric lavage. If patient is comatose, after endotracheal tube is in place with cuff inflated, perform gastric lavage; then administer activated charcoal to reduce drug absorption. Maintain adequate airway, provide cardiac and respiratory support, and monitor vital signs closely.

☑ Special considerations
Besides those relevant to all *adrenergics,* consider the following recommendations.
- Store injection solution away from light. Do not use if discolored.
- Double-check dosage: oral is 2.5 mg, whereas S.C. is 0.25 mg. A decimal error can be fatal.
- Give S.C. injection in lateral deltoid area.
- CV effects are more likely with S.C. route and when patient has arrhythmias. Check pulse rate and blood pressure before each dose and monitor for changes from baseline.
- Most adverse reactions are transient; however, tachycardia may persist for a relatively long time.
- Patient may use tablets and aerosol concomitantly. Carefully monitor patient for toxicity.
- Aerosol terbutaline produces minimal cardiac stimulation and tremors.
- When drug is used for tocolytic therapy, monitor patient for CV effects, including tachycardia, for 12 hours after discontinuation of drug. Monitor intake and output; fluid restriction may be necessary. Muscle tremor is common but may subside with continued use.
- Monitor neonate for hypoglycemia if the mother used terbutaline during pregnancy.

Patient education
- Instruct patient taking oral terbutaline on how to take pulse rate and to report if pulse varies significantly from baseline.
- Instruct patient to avoid simultaneous administration with adrenocorticoid aerosol. Separate administration time by 15 minutes.
- Demonstrate and give patient instructions on proper use of inhaler: Shake canister thoroughly to activate; place mouthpiece well into mouth, aimed at back of throat. Close lips and teeth around mouthpiece. Exhale through nose as completely as possible, then inhale through mouth slowly and deeply while actuating the nebulizer to release dose. Hold breath 10 seconds (count "1-100, 2-100, 3-100," up to "10-100"); remove mouthpiece and then exhale slowly.
- Warn patient not to puncture aerosol terbutaline container. Contents are under pressure. Instruct the patient not to store the container near heat or open flame or to expose it to temperatures of more than 120° F (49° C), which may burst the container. Tell patient that cans should not be discarded into a fire or incinerator and that they should be stored out of children's reach.
- Advise patient to take a missed dose within 1 hour. After 1 hour, patient should skip the dose and resume regular schedule. Patient should not double dose.
- Instruct patient to use terbutaline only as directed. If drug produces no relief or if condition worsens, he should call promptly.
- Warn patient not to use OTC drugs without medical approval. Many cold and allergy remedies contain a sympathomimetic agent that may be harmful when combined with terbutaline.
- Advise patient to report decreased effectiveness. Excessive or prolonged use of aerosol form can lead to tolerance.

Geriatric use
- Elderly patients are more sensitive to the effects of terbutaline; a lower dose may be required.

Pediatric use
- Drug is not recommended for use in children under age 12.

Breast-feeding
- Drug is distributed into breast milk in minute amounts. Use cautiously in breast-feeding women.

terconazole
Terazol 3, Terazol 7

Pharmacologic classification: triazole derivative
Therapeutic classification: antifungal
Pregnancy risk category C

How supplied
Available by prescription only
Vaginal cream: 0.4% in 45-g tube, 0.8% in 20-g tube with applicator
Vaginal suppositories: 80 mg

Indications, route, and dosage
Local treatment of vulvovaginal candidiasis (moniliasis)
Adults: 0.4%: 1 full applicator (5 g) intravaginally once daily h.s. for 7 consecutive days. 0.8%: 1 full applicator (5 g) intravaginally once daily h.s. for 3 consecutive days. Alternatively, insert 1 suppository vaginally h.s. for 3 consecutive days.

Pharmacodynamics
Exact mechanism of action is unknown. Terconazole may disrupt fungal cell membrane permeability.

Pharmacokinetics
- *Absorption:* Minimal; absorption may range from 5% to 16%.
- *Distribution:* Effect is mainly local.
- *Metabolism:* Drug is metabolized mainly by oxidative *N*- and *O*-dealkylation, dioxolane ring cleavage, and conjugation pathways.
- *Excretion:* Following oral administration of terconazole, 32% to 56% of dose is excreted in urine and 47% to 52% is excreted in feces within 24 hours.

Contraindications and precautions
Contraindicated in patients with known sensitivity to terconazole or any inactive ingredients in drug.

Interactions
None reported.

Effects on diagnostic tests
None reported.

Adverse reactions
CNS: *headache.*
GU: dysmenorrhea, pain of the female genitalia, vulvovaginal burning.
Skin: irritation, *pruritus,* photosensitivity.
Other: fever, chills, body aches.

Overdose and treatment
No information available.

☑ Special considerations
- Drug is only effective against vulvovaginitis caused by *Candida.* Diagnosis should be confirmed by cultures or potassium hydroxide smears.
- A persistent infection may be caused by reinfection. Evaluate patient for possible sources.
- Intractable candidiasis may be a sign of diabetes mellitus. Perform blood and urine glucose determinations to rule out undiagnosed diabetes mellitus.

Patient education
- Instruct patient to insert cream high into the vagina.
- Tell patient to complete full course of therapy and to use it continuously, even during menstrual period. The therapeutic effect of terconazole is not affected by menstruation.
- Inform patient to report if drug causes burning or irritation.
- Advise patient to refrain from sexual intercourse or suggest partner use a condom to avoid reinfection.
- Advise patient to use a sanitary napkin to prevent staining of clothing.

Breast-feeding
- Safety is not established. Breast-feeding is not recommended during therapy with terconazole.

testolactone
Teslac

Pharmacologic classification: androgen
Therapeutic classification: antineoplastic
Pregnancy risk category C

How supplied
Available by prescription only
Tablets: 50 mg

Indications, route, and dosage
Dosage and indications may vary. Check current literature for recommended protocol.
Advanced postmenopausal breast cancer
Adults: 250 mg P.O. q.i.d.

Pharmacodynamics
Antineoplastic action: Exact mechanism of action is unclear. Cytotoxic activity may result from depressed ovarian function that follows inhibition of pituitary gonadotropin synthesis or prevention of steroid action on tumor cell, which the cell requires for survival.

Pharmacokinetics
- *Absorption:* Drug is well absorbed across the GI tract after oral administration.
- *Distribution:* Widely distributed into total body water.
- *Metabolism:* Extensively metabolized in the liver.
- *Excretion:* Drug and its metabolites are excreted primarily in urine.

Contraindications and precautions
Contraindicated in patients hypersensitive to drug and in men with breast cancer.

Interactions
Concomitant administration with *oral anticoagulants* results in excessive anticoagulation.

Effects on diagnostic tests
Testolactone therapy may increase concentrations of serum calcium, urinary creatinine, and urinary 17-ketosteroids. Estradiol levels measured by radioimmunoassay may be decreased.

Adverse reactions
CNS: paresthesia, peripheral neuropathy.
CV: increased blood pressure, edema.
GI: nausea, vomiting, diarrhea, anorexia, glossitis.
Other: alopecia, erythema.

Overdose and treatment
No information available.

☑ Special considerations
- Adequate trial is 3 months. Reassure patient that therapeutic response is not immediate.
- Monitor fluids and electrolytes, especially calcium levels.

- Immobilized patients are prone to hypercalcemia. Exercise may prevent it. Force fluids to aid calcium excretion.
- Treat hypercalcemia with generous hydration; obtain calcium levels before and during therapy.
- Higher-than-recommended doses do not increase incidence of remission.
- Drug does not cause virilization when used at recommended doses.

Patient education
- Emphasize importance of continuing medication despite nausea and vomiting.
- Tell patient to call promptly if vomiting occurs shortly after a dose is taken.
- Advise patient to use contraceptive measures during treatment period.

Breast-feeding
- It is not known if drug occurs in breast milk. However, because of the risk of serious adverse reactions in the infant, breast-feeding is not recommended.

testosterone
Histerone 100, Malogen in Oil*, Tesamone, Testandro, Testaqua, Testoject-50

testosterone cypionate
depAndro 100, depAndro 200, Depotest 100, Depotest 200, Depo-Testosterone, Duratest-100, Duratest-200, T-Cypionate, Testred Cypionate 200, Virilon IM

testosterone enanthate
Andro L.A. 200, Andropository 200, Delatestryl, Durathate-200, Everone 200, Testrin-P.A.

testosterone propionate
Malogen in Oil*, Testex

Pharmacologic classification: androgen
Therapeutic classification: androgen replacement, antineoplastic
Controlled substance schedule III
Pregnancy risk category X

How supplied
Available by prescription only
testosterone
Injection (aqueous suspension): 25 mg/ml, 50 mg/ml, 100 mg/ml
testosterone cypionate (in oil)
Injection: 100 mg/ml, 200 mg/ml
testosterone enanthate (in oil)
Injection: 100 mg/ml, 200 mg/ml
testosterone propionate (in oil)
Injection: 50 mg/ml, 100 mg/ml

Indications, route, and dosage
Male hypogonadism
testosterone or testosterone propionate
Adults: 10 to 25 mg I.M. two or three times weekly.
testosterone cypionate or enanthate
Adults: 50 to 400 mg I.M. q 2 to 4 weeks.
Delayed puberty in males
testosterone or testosterone propionate
Children: 25 to 50 mg I.M. two or three times weekly for up to 6 months.
testosterone cypionate or enanthate
Children: 50 to 200 mg I.M. q 2 to 4 weeks for up to 6 months.
Postpartum breast pain and engorgement
testosterone or testosterone propionate
Adults: 25 to 50 mg I.M. daily for 3 to 4 days.
Inoperable breast cancer
testosterone propionate
Adults: 50 to 100 mg I.M. three times weekly.
testosterone cypionate or enanthate
Adults: 200 to 400 mg I.M. q 2 to 4 weeks.
testosterone
Adults: 100 mg I.M. three times weekly.
Postpubertal cryptorchidism
testosterone or testosterone propionate
Adults: 10 to 25 mg I.M. two or three times weekly.
Growth stimulation in Turner's syndrome
testosterone propionate
Adults: 40 to 50 mg/m^2 I.M. once monthly for 6 months.

Pharmacodynamics
Androgenic action: Testosterone is the endogenous androgen that stimulates receptors in androgen-responsive organs and tissues to promote growth and development of male sexual organs and secondary sexual characteristics.

Antineoplastic action: Testosterone exerts inhibitory, antiestrogenic effects on hormone-responsive breast tumors and metastases.

Pharmacokinetics
- *Absorption:* Testosterone and its esters must be administered parenterally because they are inactivated rapidly by the liver when given orally. The onset of action of cypionate and enanthate esters of testosterone is somewhat slower than that of testosterone itself.
- *Distribution:* Drug is normally 98% to 99% plasma protein-bound, primarily to the testosterone-estradiol binding globulin.
- *Metabolism:* Metabolized to several 17-ketosteroids by two main pathways in the liver. A large portion of these metabolites then form glucuronide and sulfate conjugates. Plasma half-life of testosterone ranges from 10 to 100 minutes. The cypionate and enanthate esters of testosterone have longer durations of action than testosterone.
- *Excretion:* Very little unchanged testosterone appears in urine or feces. Approximately 90% of metabolized testosterone is excreted in urine in the form of sulfate and glucuronide conjugates.

Contraindications and precautions
Contraindicated in men with breast or prostate cancer; in patients with hypercalcemia or cardiac, hepatic, or renal decompensation; during pregnancy; and in breast-feeding women. Use cautiously in the elderly and in women of childbearing age.

Interactions

In patients with diabetes, decreased blood glucose levels may require adjustment of *insulin* or *oral antidiabetic drug* dosage.

Testosterone may potentiate the effects of *warfarin-type anticoagulants*, prolonging PT. Concurrent administration with *oxyphenbutazone* may increase serum oxyphenbutazone concentrations.

Effects on diagnostic tests

Testosterone may cause abnormal results of glucose tolerance tests. Thyroid function test results (protein-bound iodine, ^{131}I uptake, thyroid-binding capacity) and serum 17-ketosteroid levels may decrease. Liver function test results, PT (especially in patients on anticoagulant therapy), and serum creatinine levels may be elevated. Because of the anabolic activity of testosterone, increases may occur in serum sodium, potassium, calcium, phosphate, and cholesterol levels.

Adverse reactions

CNS: headache, anxiety, depression, paresthesia, sleep apnea syndrome.
CV: edema.
GI: nausea.
GU: hypoestrogenic effects in women (flushing; diaphoresis; vaginitis, including itching, drying, and burning; vaginal bleeding; menstrual irregularities); excessive hormonal effects in men (prepubertal—premature epiphyseal closure, *acne,* priapism, *growth of body and facial hair,* phallic enlargement; postpubertal—testicular atrophy, oligospermia, decreased ejaculatory volume, impotence, gynecomastia, epididymitis).
Hepatic: reversible jaundice, cholestatic hepatitis, abnormal liver enzyme levels.
Skin: pain and induration at injection site, local edema, hypersensitivity manifestations.
Other: hypercalcemia; polycythemia; suppression of clotting factors; androgenic effects in women (*acne, edema, oily skin, weight gain, hirsutism, hoarseness,* clitoral enlargement, deepening voice, decreased or increased libido).

Overdose and treatment

No information available.

☑ Special considerations

Besides those relevant to all *androgens,* consider the following recommendations.

- When used to treat male hypogonadism, initiate therapy with full therapeutic doses and taper according to patient tolerance and response. Administering long-acting esters (enanthate or cypionate) at intervals greater than every 2 to 3 weeks may cause hormone levels to fall below those found in normal adults.
- Carefully observe female patients for signs of excessive virilization. If possible, discontinue therapy at first sign of virilization because some adverse effects (deepening of voice, clitoral enlargement) are irreversible. Patients with metastatic breast cancer should have regular determinations of serum calcium levels to avoid serious hypercalcemia.
- Inject deeply I.M., preferably into a large muscle mass such as the upper outer quadrant of the gluteal muscle.
- Testosterone enanthate has been used for postmenopausal osteoporosis and to stimulate erythropoiesis.
- Solutions of long-acting esters (enanthate and cypionate) may become cloudy if a wet needle is used to draw up the solution. This does not affect potency.
- Warm (to room temperature) and shake vial to help redissolve crystals that have formed after storage.

Patient education

- Explain to female patient that virilization may occur. Tell patient to report androgenic effects immediately. Stopping drug prevents further androgenic changes but probably will not reverse those already present.
- Tell female patient to report menstrual irregularities; drug may be discontinued pending determination of the cause.
- Inform male patient to report too frequent or persistent penile erections.
- Advise patient to report persistent GI distress, diarrhea, or the onset of jaundice.

Geriatric use

- Observe elderly male patients for prostatic hyperplasia. Development of symptomatic prostatic hyperplasia or prostatic carcinoma mandates the discontinuation of drug.

Pediatric use

- Use with extreme caution in children to avoid precocious puberty and premature closure of the epiphyses. Obtain X-ray examinations every 6 months to assess skeletal maturation.

Breast-feeding

- Distribution into breast milk is unknown. An alternative feeding method is recommended because of potential for severe adverse effects of androgens on the infant.

testosterone transdermal system

Androderm, Testoderm

Pharmacologic classification: androgen
Therapeutic classification: androgen replacement
Controlled substance schedule III
Pregnancy risk category X

How supplied

Available by prescription only
Transdermal system: 2.5 mg/day, 4 mg/day, 6 mg/day

Indications, route, and dosage

Primary or hypogonadotropic hypogonadism
Testoderm
Adult men age 18 and older: Apply one 6-mg/day

patch to scrotal area daily for 22 to 24 hours. If scrotal area is too small for 6-mg/day patch, start therapy with 4-mg/day patch.

Androderm

Adult men age 18 and older: Two systems applied nightly for 24 hours, providing a total dose of 5 mg/day. Apply on dry area of skin on back, abdomen, upper arms, or thighs. Do *not* apply to scrotum.

Note: Discontinue testosterone transdermal system if edema occurs.

Pharmacodynamics

Androgenic action: Testosterone transdermal system releases testosterone, the endogenous androgen that stimulates receptors in androgen-responsive organs and tissues to promote growth and development of male sex organs and secondary sex characteristics.

Pharmacokinetics

- *Absorption:* After placement of a testosterone transdermal system on scrotal skin, serum testosterone concentration increases to a maximum in 2 to 4 hours and returns toward baseline within approximately 2 hours after system removal. Following application to nonscrotal skin, testosterone is absorbed during the 24-hour dosing period. Daily application of two Androderm systems at bedtime results in a serum testosterone concentration profile that mimics the normal circadian variation observed in healthy young men.
- *Distribution:* Circulating testosterone is chiefly bound in the serum to sex hormone–binding globulin and albumin.
- *Metabolism:* Testosterone is metabolized to various 17-ketosteroids through two different pathways; the major active metabolites are estradiol and dihydrotestosterone.
- *Excretion:* Little unchanged testosterone appears in urine or feces.

Contraindications and precautions

Contraindicated in patients hypersensitive to drug, in women, and in men with known or suspected breast or prostate cancer. Use cautiously in patients with preexisting renal, cardiac, or hepatic disease and in elderly men.

Interactions

In diabetic patients, testosterone transdermal system may decrease blood glucose levels and, therefore, requirements for *antidiabetic agents* such as *insulin.* C-17 substituted derivatives of testosterone have reportedly decreased the anticoagulant requirements of patients receiving *oral anticoagulants.* Patients receiving oral anticoagulant therapy require close monitoring, especially when testosterone transdermal system is started or stopped. Concurrent administration of *oxyphenbutazone* and testosterone transdermal system may result in elevated serum levels of oxyphenbutazone.

Effects on diagnostic tests

Androgens such as testosterone may decrease levels of thyroxin-binding globulin, resulting in decreased total T_4 serum levels and increased resin uptake of T_3 and T_4.

Adverse reactions

CNS: ***CVA.***
GU: *gynecomastia,* prostatitis, urinary tract infection, breast tenderness.
Skin: acne, *pruritus.*
Other: discomfort, irritation.

Overdose and treatment

Testosterone levels of up to 11,400 ng/dl have been implicated in CVA. No other information is available.

☑ Special considerations

- Testoderm form of testosterone transdermal system does not produce adequate serum testosterone concentration if applied to nongenital skin.
- Edema with or without heart failure may be a serious complication in patients with preexisting cardiac, renal, or hepatic disease. In addition to discontinuation of testosterone transdermal system, diuretic therapy may be required.
- Gynecomastia commonly develops and occasionally persists in patients receiving treatment for hypogonadism.
- Topical adverse reactions decrease with duration of use.
- Check hemoglobin levels and hematocrit periodically (to detect polycythemia) in patients on long-term androgen therapy.
- Check liver function, prostatic acid phosphatase, prostatic specific antigen, cholesterol, and high-density lipoproteins periodically.
- After 3 to 4 weeks of daily system use in patients receiving Testoderm, draw blood 2 to 4 hours after system application for determination of serum total testosterone. For patients receiving Androderm, monitor serum testosterone the morning following regular evening application. Because of variability in analytical values among diagnostic laboratories, this laboratory work and later analyses for assessing the effect of testosterone transdermal system should be performed at the same laboratory.
- If patient has not achieved desired results within 8 weeks, another form of testosterone replacement therapy should be considered.
- Store testosterone transdermal system at room temperature.

Patient education

- Show patient how to use testosterone transdermal system. For Testoderm, tell him to place system on clean, dry scrotal skin. Scrotal hair should be dry-shaved for optimal skin contact. Chemical depilatories should not be used. For Androderm, tell patient to apply patches to clean, dry designated areas.
- Tell patient to wear the Testoderm transdermal system 22 to 24 hours daily. Tell patient to wear Androderm 24 hours daily and to rotate the site, allowing 7 days between applications to the same site.
- Instruct patient to report if nausea, vomiting, skin color changes, ankle edema, too-frequent or persistent penile erections occur.

• Inform patient that topical testosterone preparations used by men have caused virilization in female partners. Changes in body hair distribution or significant increase in acne of the female partner should be reported.

Geriatric use
• Geriatric patients treated with androgens may be at increased risk for development of prostatic hyperplasia and prostatic carcinoma. Cautious use of testosterone transdermal system is required in this age-group.

Pediatric use
• Testosterone transdermal system has not been evaluated clinically in males under age 18.

Breast-feeding
• Do not use in women.

tetanus immune globulin, human (TIG)
Hyper-Tet

Pharmacologic classification: immune serum
Therapeutic classification: tetanus prophylaxis
Pregnancy risk category C

How supplied
Available by prescription only
Injection: 250 units/ml in 1 ml vial or syringe

Indications, route, and dosage
Tetanus prophylactic dose
Adults and children over age 7: 250 units I.M.
Children under age 7: 4 units/kg I.M.
Tetanus treatment
Adults: Single doses of 3,000 to 6,000 units I.M. have been used. Optimal dosage schedules are not established. Do not give at same site as toxoid.
Children: Single doses of 500 to 3,000 units I.M. have been used.

Pharmacodynamics
Antitetanus action: TIG provides passive immunity to tetanus. Antibodies remain at effective levels for 3 weeks or longer. TIG protects the patient for the incubation period of most tetanus cases.

Pharmacokinetics
• *Absorption:* Slow.
• *Distribution:* No information available.
• *Metabolism:* No information available.
• *Excretion:* Serum half-life of TIG is approximately 28 days.

Contraindications and precautions
Contraindicated in patients with thrombocytopenia or any coagulation disorder that contraindicates I.M. injection unless potential benefits outweigh risks. Contraindicated for use in patients with hypersensitivity to thimerosal or TIG. Not recommended for use in immunoglobulin A deficiency. Do not give I.V.

Interactions
None reported.

Effects on diagnostic tests
None reported.

Adverse reactions
Other: slight fever, hypersensitivity reactions, ***anaphylaxis,*** angioedema, nephrotic syndrome, pain, stiffness, erythema at injection site.

Overdose and treatment
No information available.

☑ Special considerations
• Obtain a thorough history of injury, tetanus immunizations, last tetanus toxoid injection, allergies, and reactions to immunizations.
• Have epinephrine solution 1:1,000 available to treat allergic reactions.
• For wound management, use TIG for prophylaxis in patients with dirty wounds if patient has had fewer than three previous tetanus toxoid injections or if the immunization history is unknown or uncertain.
• Thoroughly clean and remove all foreign matter and necrotic tissue from wound.
• Give tetanus antitoxin when TIG is not available.
• Do not confuse drug with tetanus toxoid, which should be given at the same time (but at different sites) to produce active immunization.
• Administer I.M. in the deltoid muscle for adults and in the anterolateral thigh for infants and small children. Do not inject I.V.
• Tetanus increases risks of severe morbidity and mortality in both mother and fetus if untreated. No fetal risk from the use of immune globulin has been reported to date.
• TIG has not been associated with an increase AIDS cases. The immune globulin is devoid of HIV. Immune globulin recipients do not develop antibodies to HIV.
• Store TIG between 36° and 46° F (2° and 8° C). Do not freeze.

Patient education
• Tell patient that available data indicate that TIG administration does not cause AIDS or hepatitis.
• Inform patient that he may experience some local pain, swelling, and tenderness at the injection site. Recommend acetaminophen to alleviate these minor effects.
• Encourage patient to report headache, skin changes, or difficulty breathing.

Breast-feeding
• It is unknown if TIG is distributed into breast milk. Use with caution in breast-feeding women.

tetanus toxoid, adsorbed
tetanus toxoid, fluid

Pharmacologic classification: toxoid
Therapeutic classification: tetanus prophylaxis
Pregnancy risk category C

How supplied
Available by prescription only
Adsorbed toxoid
Injection: 5 to 10 Lf units of inactivated tetanus/ 0.5-ml dose, in 0.5-ml syringes and 5-ml vials
Fluid toxoid
Injection: 4 to 5 Lf units of inactivated tetanus/ 0.5-ml dose, in 0.5-ml syringes and 7.5-ml vials

Indications, route, and dosage
Primary immunization (adsorbed formulation)
Adults and children age 1 and older: 0.5 ml I.M. 4 to 8 weeks apart for two doses, then a third dose 6 to 12 months after the second dose.
Children age 2 to 12 months: 0.5 ml I.M. 4 to 8 weeks apart for three doses, followed by a fourth dose of 0.5 ml, 6 to 12 months after the third dose. Booster dosage, 0.5 ml I.M. q 5 to 10 years.
Primary immunization (fluid formulation)
Adults and children: 0.5 ml I.M. or S.C. 4 to 8 weeks apart for three doses, then a fourth dose 6 to 12 months after the third dose. Booster dosage, 0.5 ml I.M. or S.C. q 10 years.

Pharmacodynamics
Tetanus prophylaxis action: Tetanus toxoid promotes active immunity by inducing production of tetanus antitoxin.

Pharmacokinetics
- *Absorption:* Slow. Fluid formulation provides quicker booster effect.
- *Distribution:* Unknown.
- *Metabolism:* Unknown.
- *Excretion:* Unknown. Active immunity usually persists for 10 years. Adsorbed tetanus toxoid usually produces more persistent antitoxin titers than fluid tetanus toxoid.

Contraindications and precautions
Contraindicated in immunosuppressed patients and in those with immunoglobulin abnormalities or severe hypersensitivity or neurologic reactions to the toxoid or its ingredients such as thimerosal.

Also contraindicated in patients with thrombocytopenia or any coagulation disorder that would contraindicate I.M. injection unless the potential benefits outweigh the risks. Vaccination should be deferred in patients with acute illness and during polio outbreaks, except in emergencies.

Use absorbed form cautiously in infants or children with cerebral damage, neurologic disorders, or history of febrile seizures.

Interactions
Concomitant use with *chloramphenicol, corticosteroids,* or *immunosuppressants* theoretically may impair the immune response to tetanus toxoid. Avoid elective immunization under these circumstances.

Effects on diagnostic tests
None reported.

Adverse reactions
Skin: urticaria, pruritus, erythema, induration, nodule (at injection site).
Other: tachycardia, hypotension, slight fever, chills, malaise, aches and pains, flushing, ***anaphylaxis.***

Overdose and treatment
No information available.

☑ Special considerations
- Obtain a thorough history of allergies and reactions to immunizations.
- Have epinephrine 1:1,000 solution available to treat allergic reactions.
- Determine tetanus immunization status and date of last tetanus immunization.
- The preferred I.M. injection site is the deltoid or midlateral thigh in adults and children and the midlateral thigh in infants.
- Preferably, tetanus immunization should be completed and maintained using multiple antigen preparations appropriate for patient's age, such as DTP, DT, or Td.
- Shake vial vigorously to ensure a uniform suspension before withdrawing the dose.
- Do not confuse drug with tetanus immune globulin.
- These toxoids are used to prevent, not treat, tetanus infections.
- Store at 36° to 46° F (2° to 8° C). Do not freeze.

Patient education
- Tell patient what to expect after immunization: discomfort at the injection site and a nodule that may develop there and persist for several weeks. They also may develop fever, general malaise, or body aches and pains. Recommend acetaminophen to alleviate these effects.
- Instruct patient not to use hot or cold compresses at the injection site because this may increase the severity of the local reaction.
- Encourage patient to report distressing adverse reactions.
- Tell patient that immunization requires a series of injections. Stress the importance of keeping scheduled appointments for subsequent doses.

Breast-feeding
- It is unknown if tetanus toxoid occurs in breast milk. Use with caution in breast-feeding women.

tetracycline hydrochloride

Novotetra*, Panmycin, Robitet, Sumycin, Tetralan*, Topicycline

Pharmacologic classification: tetracycline
Therapeutic classification: antibiotic
Pregnancy risk category D (B for topical form)

How supplied

Available by prescription only
Capsules: 100 mg, 250 mg, 500 mg
Tablets: 250 mg, 500 mg
Suspension: 125 mg/5 ml
Topical solution: 2.2 mg/ml

Available without a prescription
Topical ointment: 3% *

Indications, route, and dosage

Infections caused by sensitive organisms
Adults: 1 to 2 g P.O. divided into two to four doses.
Children over age 8: 25 to 50 mg/kg P.O. daily, divided into two to four doses.
***Uncomplicated urethral, endocervical, or rectal infection caused by* Chlamydia trachomatis**
Adults: 500 mg P.O. q.i.d. for at least 7 days.
Brucellosis
Adults: 500 mg P.O. q 6 hours for 3 weeks with streptomycin 1 g I.M. q 12 hours week 1 and daily week 2.
Gonorrhea in patients sensitive to penicillin
Adults: Initially, 1.5 g P.O.; then 500 mg q 6 hours for 4 days.
Syphilis in nonpregnant patients sensitive to penicillin
Adults: 500 mg P.O. q.i.d. for 14 days.
Acne
Adults and adolescents: Initially, 500 to 1,000 mg P.O. divided q.i.d.; then 125 to 500 mg P.O. daily or every other day, apply topical ointment generously to affected areas b.i.d. until skin is thoroughly wet.
◊ ***Lyme disease***
Adults: 250 to 500 mg P.O. q.i.d. for 10 to 30 days.
◊ ***Acute transmitted epididymitis (children over age 9);*** ◊ ***pelvic inflammatory disease;*** ◊ **Helicobacter pylori *(all above indications use tetracycline as adjunctive therapy)***
Adults: 500 mg P.O. q.i.d. for 10 to 14 days.
Infection prophylaxis in minor skin abrasions and treatment of superficial infections caused by susceptible organisms
Adults and children: Apply topical ointment to infected area one to five times daily.

Pharmacodynamics

Antibacterial action: Tetracycline is bacteriostatic; it binds reversibly to ribosomal subunits, thus inhibiting bacterial protein synthesis. Its spectrum of action includes many gram-negative and gram-positive organisms, *Mycoplasma, Rickettsia, Chlamydia,* and spirochetes.

It is useful against brucellosis, glanders, mycoplasma pneumonia infections (some clinicians prefer erythromycin), leptospirosis, early stages of Lyme disease, rickettsial infections (such as Rocky Mountain spotted fever, Q fever, and typhus fever), and chlamydial infections. It is an alternative to penicillin for *Neisseria gonorrhoeae,* but because of a high level of resistance in the United States, other alternative agents should be considered.

Pharmacokinetics

- *Absorption:* Tetracycline is 75% to 80% absorbed after oral administration; peak serum levels occur at 2 to 4 hours. Food or milk products significantly reduce oral absorption.
- *Distribution:* Widely distributed into body tissues and fluids, including synovial, pleural, prostatic, and seminal fluids, bronchial secretions, saliva, and aqueous humor; CSF penetration is poor. Tetracycline crosses the placenta; it is 20% to 67% protein-bound.
- *Metabolism:* Tetracycline is not metabolized.
- *Excretion:* Drug is excreted primarily unchanged in urine by glomerular filtration; plasma half-life is 6 to 12 hours in adults with normal renal function. Some drug is excreted in breast milk. Only minimal amounts of tetracycline are removed by hemodialysis or peritoneal dialysis.

Contraindications and precautions

Contraindicated in patients with hypersensitivity to tetracyclines. Use cautiously in patients with impaired renal or hepatic function. Use oral form cautiously during last half of pregnancy and in children under age 8.

Interactions

Tetracycline absorption may be decreased by *antacids containing aluminum, calcium,* or *magnesium; laxatives containing magnesium* because of chelation; *food* and *dairy products; oral iron;* and *sodium bicarbonate.*

Tetracycline may antagonize bactericidal effects of *penicillin,* inhibiting cell growth from bacteriostatic action; administer penicillin 2 to 3 hours before tetracycline.

Concomitant use of tetracycline increases the risk of nephrotoxicity from *methoxyflurane.*

Coadministration with *oral contraceptives* may decrease their effectiveness. *Cimetidine* may decrease the GI absorption of tetracycline.

Concomitant use of tetracycline necessitates lowered dosage of *oral anticoagulants* because of enhanced effects and lowered dosage of digoxin because of increased bioavailability.

Effects on diagnostic tests

Tetracycline causes false-negative results in urine tests using glucose oxidase reagent (Diastix, Chemstrip uG, or glucose enzymatic test strip) and false elevations in fluorometric tests for urinary catecholamines.

Tetracycline may elevate BUN levels in patients with decreased renal function.

Adverse reactions

Unless otherwise noted, the following adverse reactions refer to oral form of drug.

* Canada only

◊ Unlabeled clinical use

CNS: dizziness, headache, ***intracranial hypertension (pseudotumor cerebri).***
CV: pericarditis.
EENT: sore throat, glossitis, dysphagia.
GI: anorexia, *epigastric distress, nausea,* vomiting, *diarrhea,* esophagitis, oral candidiasis, stomatitis, enterocolitis, inflammatory lesions in anogenital region.
Hematologic: neutropenia, eosinophilia.
Skin: *candidal superinfection, maculopapular and erythematous rashes, urticaria, photosensitivity, increased pigmentation;* temporary stinging or burning on application; slight yellowing of treated skin, especially in patients with light complexions; severe dermatitis (with topical administration).
Other: hypersensitivity reactions, elevated liver enzymes, *increased BUN levels, permanent discoloration of teeth, enamel defects, and retardation of bone growth if used in children under age 8.*

Overdose and treatment
Clinical signs of overdose are usually limited to GI tract; give antacids or empty stomach by gastric lavage if ingestion occurs within the preceding 4 hours.

☑ Special considerations
Besides those relevant to all *tetracyclines,* consider the following recommendations.
Topical use
- Discontinue use if condition stays the same or worsens.
- To control the rate of flow, increase or decrease pressure of applicator against skin.
- Avoid contact with eyes, nose, and mouth.
- Solution should be used within 2 months.

Patient education
- Warn patient to avoid sharing washcloths and towels with family members when using topical form.
- Instruct patient to take drug 1 hour before or 2 hours after meals or drinking milk.
- Tell patient not to share medication with others.
- Inform patient using topical form that she may continue normal use of cosmetics.
- Explain that floating plug in bottle of topical tetracycline is an inert and harmless result of proper reconstitution of the preparation and should not be removed.
- Tell patient that stinging may occur with topical use but resolves quickly and that drug may stain clothing.
- Warn patient to avoid prolonged exposure to sunlight.
- Tell patient to report persistent nausea and/or vomiting or yellowing of skin or eyes.

Pediatric use
- Do not use in children under age 8.

Breast-feeding
- Because drug is excreted in breast milk, do not use in breast-feeding women.

tetrahydrozoline hydrochloride
Collyrium Fresh Eye Drops, Eyesine, Murine Plus, Optigene 3, Tetrasine, Tyzine, Tyzine Pediatric, Visine

Pharmacologic classification: sympathomimetic
Therapeutic classification: vasoconstrictor, decongestant
Pregnancy risk category C

How supplied
Available by prescription only
Nasal solution: 0.05%, 0.1%
Available without a prescription
Ophthalmic solution: 0.05%

Indications, route, and dosage
Nasal congestion
Adults and children over age 6: Apply 2 to 4 drops or sprays of 0.1% nasal solution to nasal mucosa q 4 to 6 hours, p.r.n.
Children age 2 to 6: Apply 2 or 3 drops of 0.05% solution to nasal mucosa q 4 to 6 hours, p.r.n.
Conjunctival congestion
Adults: 1 or 2 drops of ophthalmic solution in each eye b.i.d. to q.i.d.

Pharmacodynamics
Decongestant action: In ocular use, vasoconstriction is produced by local adrenergic action on the blood vessels of the conjunctiva. After nasal application, drug acts on alpha-adrenergic receptors in nasal mucosa to produce constriction, thereby decreasing blood flow and nasal congestion.

Pharmacokinetics
- *Absorption:* Unknown.
- *Distribution:* Unknown.
- *Metabolism:* Unknown.
- *Excretion:* Unknown.

Contraindications and precautions
Contraindicated in patients hypersensitive to drug or its components and in those with angle-closure glaucoma or other serious eye diseases. Nasal solution is contraindicated in those under age 2; 0.1% solution is contraindicated in those under age 6.

Use cautiously in patients with hyperthyroidism, hypertension, and diabetes mellitus. Also, use ophthalmic form cautiously in patients with cardiac disease.

Interactions
When used concomitantly with *MAO inhibitors,* tetrahydrozoline may cause an increased adrenergic response and hypertensive crisis.

Effects on diagnostic tests
None reported.

Adverse reactions
CNS: headache, drowsiness, insomnia, dizziness, tremor (with ophthalmic form).

CV: *arrhythmias* (with ophthalmic form), tachycardia, palpitations.
EENT: transient eye stinging, pupillary dilation, increased intraocular pressure, keratitis, lacrimation, eye irritation (with ophthalmic form); transient burning, stinging; sneezing, rebound nasal congestion with excessive or long-term use (with nasal form).

Overdose and treatment

Clinical manifestations of accidental overdose include bradycardia, decreased body temperature, shocklike hypotension, apnea, drowsiness, CNS depression, and coma.

Because of rapid onset of sedation, emesis is not recommended unless induced early.

Activated charcoal or gastric lavage may be used initially. Monitor vital signs and ECG. Treat seizures with I.V. diazepam.

☑ Special considerations

- Excessive use of either preparation may cause rebound effect.
- Drug should not be used for more than 3 to 4 days.

Patient education

- Teach patient how to instill ophthalmic or nasal medication and tell him not to share drug with other family members.
- Advise patient not to exceed recommended dosage and to use drug only when needed.
- Tell patient to remove contact lenses before using drug.

Geriatric use

- Do not use in elderly patients to treat redness and inflammation, which may represent more serious eye conditions.
- Use in glaucoma requires close medical supervision.

Pediatric use

- The 0.1% nasal solution is contraindicated in children under age 6. All use is contraindicated in those under age 2.

theophylline

Accurbron, Aerolate, Aquaphyllin, Asmalix, Bronkodyl, Constant-T, Elixophyllin, Lanophyllin, Quibron-T, Respbid, Slo-bid Gyrocaps, Slo-Phyllin, Sustaire, Theobid Duracaps, Theochron, Theoclear-80, Theo-Dur, Theolair, Theo-Sav, Theo-24, Theospan-SR, Theostat-80, Theovent, Theo-X, T-Phyl, Uniphyl

Pharmacologic classification: xanthine derivative
Therapeutic classification: bronchodilator
Pregnancy risk category C

How supplied

Available by prescription only
Capsules: 100 mg, 200 mg
Capsules (extended-release): 50 mg, 60 mg, 65 mg, 75 mg, 100 mg, 125 mg, 130 mg, 200 mg, 250 mg, 260 mg, 300 mg
Tablets: 100 mg, 125 mg, 200 mg, 250 mg, 300 mg
Tablets (extended-release): 100 mg, 200 mg, 250 mg, 300 mg, 400 mg, 450 mg, 500 mg
Elixir: 50 mg/5 ml, 80 mg/15 ml
Syrup: 50 mg/5 ml, 80 mg/15 ml, 150 mg/15 ml
Dextrose 5% injection: 200 mg in 50 ml or 100 ml; 400 mg in 100 ml, 250 ml, 500 ml, or 1,000 ml; 800 mg in 500 ml or 1,000 ml

Indications, route, and dosage

Symptomatic relief of bronchospasm in patients not currently receiving theophylline who require rapid relief of acute symptoms
Loading dose: 6 mg/kg anhydrous theophylline, then:
Adults (nonsmokers): 3 mg/kg q 6 hours for two doses; then 3 mg/kg q 8 hours.
Older adults with cor pulmonale: 2 mg/kg q 6 hours for two doses; then 2 mg/kg q 8 hours.
Adults with heart failure: 2 mg/kg q 8 hours for two doses; then 1 to 2 mg/kg q 12 hours.
Children and adolescents age 9 to 16 and young adult smokers: 3 mg/kg q 4 hours for three doses; then 3 mg/kg q 6 hours.
Neonates and children age 6 months to 9 years: 4 mg/kg q 4 hours for three doses; then 4 mg/kg q 6 hours.
◊ *Neonates and infants under age 6 months:* Dosage is highly individualized. It is recommended that serum theophylline concentrations be maintained below 10 mcg/ml in neonates and below 20 mcg/ml in older infants.
Loading dose: 1 mg/kg for each 2 mcg/ml increase in theophylline concentration, then:
Infants age 8 weeks to 6 months: 1 to 3 mg/kg q 6 hours.
Infants age 4 to 8 weeks: 1 to 2 mg/kg q 8 hours.
Neonates up to age 4 weeks: 1 to 2 mg/kg q 12 hours.
Premature neonates (less than 40 weeks' gestational age): 1 mg/kg q 12 hours.
Parenteral theophylline for patients not currently receiving theophylline
Loading dose: 4.7 mg/kg (equivalent to 6 mg/kg anhydrous aminophylline) I.V. slowly; then maintenance infusion.
Adults (nonsmokers): 0.55 mg/kg/hour (equivalent to 0.7 mg/kg/hour anhydrous aminophylline) for 12 hours, then 0.39 mg/kg/hour (equivalent to 0.5 mg/kg/hour anhydrous aminophylline).
Older adults with cor pulmonale: 0.47 mg/kg/hour (equivalent to 0.6 mg/kg/hour anhydrous aminophylline) for 12 hours; then 0.24 mg/kg/hour (equivalent to 0.3 mg/kg/hour anhydrous aminophylline).
Adults with heart failure or liver disease: 0.39 mg/kg/hour (equivalent to 0.5 mg/kg/hour anhydrous aminophylline) for 12 hours; then 0.08 to 0.16 mg/kg/hour (equivalent to 0.1 to 0.2 mg/kg/hour anhydrous aminophylline).
Children age 9 to 16: 0.79 mg/kg/hour (equivalent to 1 mg/kg/hour anhydrous aminophylline) for 12 hours; then 0.63 mg/kg/hour (equivalent to 0.8 mg/kg/hour anhydrous aminophylline).

Infants and children age 6 months to 9 years: 0.95 mg/kg/hour (equivalent to 1.2 mg/kg/hour anhydrous aminophylline) for 12 hours; then 0.79 mg/kg/hour (equivalent to 1 mg/kg/hour anhydrous aminophylline).

Switch to oral theophylline as soon as patient shows adequate improvement.

Symptomatic relief of bronchospasm in patients currently receiving theophylline
Adults and children: Each 0.5 mg/kg I.V. or P.O. (loading dose) increases plasma levels by 1 mcg/ml. Ideally, dose is based on current theophylline level and lean body weight. In emergency situations, may use a 2.5 mg/kg P.O. dose of rapidly absorbed form if no obvious signs of theophylline toxicity are present.

Prophylaxis of bronchial asthma, bronchospasm of chronic bronchitis, and emphysema
Adults and children: Using rapidly absorbed dosage forms, initial dosage is 16 mg/kg or 400 mg P.O. daily (whichever is less) divided q 6 to 8 hours; dosage may be increased in approximate increments of 25% at 2- to 3-day intervals. Using extended-release dosage forms, initial dose is 12 mg/kg or 400 mg P.O. daily (whichever is less) divided q 8 to 12 hours; dosage may be increased, if tolerated, by 2 to 3 mg/kg daily at 3-day intervals. Regardless of dosage form used, dosage may be increased, if tolerated, up to the following maximum daily doses, without measurements of serum theophylline concentration.
Adults and adolescents age 16 and older: 13 mg/kg P.O. or 900 mg P.O. daily in divided doses.
Adolescents age 12 to 16: 18 mg/kg P.O. daily in divided doses.
Children age 9 to 12: 20 mg/kg P.O. daily in divided doses.
Children under age 9: 24 mg/kg P.O. daily in divided doses.

Note: Dosage individualization is required. Use peak plasma and trough levels to estimate dose. Therapeutic range is 10 to 20 mcg/ml. All doses are based on theophylline anhydrous and lean body weight.

◇ Cystic fibrosis
Infants: 10 to 20 mg/kg I.V. daily.

◇ Promotion of diuresis; ◇ treatment of Cheyne-Stokes respirations; ◇ paroxysmal nocturnal dyspnea
Adults: 200 to 400 mg I.V. bolus (single dose).

Pharmacodynamics

Bronchodilator action: Drug may act by inhibiting phosphodiesterase, elevating cellular cyclic AMP levels, or antagonizing adenosine receptors in the bronchi, resulting in relaxation of the smooth muscle.

Drug also increases sensitivity of the medullary respiratory center to carbon dioxide, to reduce apneic episodes. It prevents muscle fatigue, especially that of the diaphragm. It also causes diuresis and cardiac and CNS stimulation.

Pharmacokinetics

- *Absorption:* Drug is well absorbed. Rate and onset of action depend on the dosage form; food may further alter rate of absorption, especially of some extended-release preparations.
- *Distribution:* Distributed throughout the extracellular fluids; equilibrium between fluid and tissues occurs within 1 hour of an I.V. loading dose. Therapeutic plasma levels are 10 to 20 mcg/ml, but many patients respond to lower levels.
- *Metabolism:* Theophylline is metabolized in the liver to inactive compounds. Half-life is 7 to 9 hours in adults, 4 to 5 hours in smokers, 20 to 30 hours in premature infants, and 3 to 5 hours in children.
- *Excretion:* About 10% of dose is excreted in urine unchanged. Other metabolites include 1,3 dimethyluric acid, 1 methyluric acid, and 3-methylxanthine.

Contraindications and precautions

Contraindicated in patients with hypersensitivity to xanthine compounds (caffeine, theobromine) and in those with active peptic ulcer and seizure disorders.

Use cautiously in the elderly; in neonates, infants under age 1, and young children; and in patients with COPD, cardiac failure, cor pulmonale, renal or hepatic disease, peptic ulcer, hyperthyroidism, diabetes mellitus, glaucoma, severe hypoxemia, hypertension, compromised cardiac or circulatory function, angina, acute MI, or sulfite sensitivity.

Interactions

When used concomitantly, theophylline increases the excretion of *lithium.* Also, *allopurinol (high dose), calcium channel blockers, cimetidine, corticosteroids, erythromycin, interferon, mexiletine, oral contraceptives, propranolol, quinolones,* and *troleandomycin* may cause an increase in serum concentrations of theophylline by decreasing the hepatic clearance. *Rifampin* may decrease serum theophylline levels by increasing hepatic clearance of theophylline.

Barbiturates and *phenytoin* enhance hepatic metabolism of theophylline, decreasing plasma levels. *Beta-adrenergic blockers* exert an antagonistic pharmacologic effect. *Charcoal* and *ketoconazole* may decrease theophylline levels. *Carbamazapine, isoniazid,* and *loop diuretics* may increase or decrease theophylline levels.

Effects on diagnostic tests

Theophylline increases plasma-free fatty acids and urinary catecholamines. Depending on assay used, theophylline levels may be falsely elevated in the presence of furosemide, phenylbutazone, probenecid, theobromine, caffeine, tea, chocolate, cola beverages, and acetaminophen.

Adverse reactions

CNS: *restlessness, dizziness, insomnia,* headache, irritability, ***seizures,*** muscle twitching.
CV: *palpitations, sinus tachycardia,* extrasystoles, flushing, marked hypotension, ***arrhythmias.***
GI: *nausea, vomiting,* diarrhea, epigastric pain.
Respiratory: tachypnea, ***respiratory arrest.***

Overdose and treatment
Clinical manifestations of overdose include nausea, vomiting, insomnia, irritability, tachycardia, extrasystoles, tachypnea, or tonic-clonic seizures. The onset of toxicity may be sudden and severe, with arrhythmias and seizures as the first signs. Induce emesis except in convulsing patients, then use activated charcoal and cathartics. Treat arrhythmias with lidocaine and seizures with I.V. diazepam; support respiratory and CV systems.

☑ Special considerations
- Do not crush extended-release tablets. Some capsules are formulated to be opened and sprinkled on food.
- Monitor vital signs and observe for signs and symptoms of toxicity.
- Obtain serum theophylline measurements in patients receiving long-term therapy. Ideal levels are between 10 and 20 mcg/ml, although some patients may respond adequately with lower serum levels. Check every 6 months. If levels are less than 10 mcg/ml, increase dose by about 25% each day. If levels are 20 to 25 mcg/ml, decrease dose by about 10% each day. If levels are 25 to 30 mcg/ml, skip next dose and decrease by 25% each day. If levels are more than 30 mcg/ml, skip next two doses and decrease by 50% each day. Repeat serum level determination.

Patient education
- Instruct patient regarding medications and dosage schedule; if a dose is missed, he should take it as soon as possible, but doses should not be doubled.
- Advise patient to take drug at regular intervals as instructed, around the clock.
- Inform patient of adverse effects and possible signs of toxicity.
- Tell patient to avoid excessive use of xanthine-containing foods and caffeine-containing beverages.
- Warn elderly patient of dizziness, a common reaction at start of therapy.
- Tell patient to take drug with food if GI upset occurs with liquid preparations or nonsustained release forms.
- Instruct patient to continue to use the same brand of theophylline.

Pediatric use
- Use with caution in neonates. Children usually require higher doses (on a mg/kg basis) than adults. Maximum recommended doses are 24 mg/kg/day in children under age 9; 20 mg/kg/day in children age 9 to 12; 18 mg/kg/day in adolescents age 12 to 16; 13 mg/kg/day or 900 mg (whichever is less) in adolescents and adults age 16 or older.

Breast-feeding
- Drug is excreted in breast milk and may cause irritability, insomnia, or fretfulness in the breast-fed infant. Therefore, a decision must be made to either stop breast-feeding or stop drug therapy.

thiabendazole
Mintezol

Pharmacologic classification: benzimidazole
Therapeutic classification: anthelmintic
Pregnancy risk category C

How supplied
Available by prescription only
Tablets (chewable): 500 mg
Oral suspension: 500 mg/5 ml

Indications, route, and dosage
Systemic infections with pinworm, roundworm, threadworm, whipworm, visceral larva migrans, trichinosis
Adults and children weighing between 30 and 154 lb (14 and 70 kg): 25 mg/kg P.O. q 12 hours for 2 successive days.
Adults and children weighing over 154 lb: 1.5 g q 12 hours for 2 successive days. Maximum dosage, 3 g daily.
Trichinosis—Two doses daily for 2 to 4 successive days.
Visceral larva migran—Two doses daily for 7 successive days.
Cutaneous infestations with larva migrans (creeping eruption)
Adults and children: 25 mg/kg P.O. b.i.d. for 2 to 5 days. Maximum dosage, 3 g daily. If lesions persist after 2 days, repeat course.
◊ ***Dracunculiasis;*** ◊ ***infections caused by* Angiostrongylus costaricensis**
Adults: 25 to 37.5 mg/kg P.O. b.i.d. (25 mg t.i.d. for *A. costaricensis*) for 3 successive days.
◊ ***Capillariasis***
Adults: 25 mg/kg P.O. q 12 hours for 30 days.

Pharmacodynamics
Anthelmintic action: Thiabendazole kills susceptible helminths by inhibiting fumarate reductase. It is drug of choice for *Strongyloides stercoralis* (threadworm) infections and may be useful in disseminated strongyloidiasis. It is also preferred for oral and topical therapy of *Ancylostoma braziliense, Toxocara canis,* and *T. cati.* It has shown activity in certain other nematode infections, but other agents are preferred for the treatment of ascariasis, trichuriasis, uncinariasis, and enterobiasis.

Pharmacokinetics
- *Absorption:* Drug is absorbed readily; peak serum concentrations occur at 1 to 2 hours.
- *Distribution:* Little is known about the distribution of thiabendazole.
- *Metabolism:* Drug is metabolized almost completely by hydroxylation and conjugation.
- *Excretion:* Approximately 90% of dose is excreted in urine as metabolites within 48 hours; about 5% is excreted in feces.

Contraindications and precautions
Contraindicated in patients with hypersensitivity to drug. Use cautiously in patients with renal or he-

patic dysfunction, severe malnutrition, or anemia and in those who are vomiting.

Interactions
Drug may inhibit the metabolism of *aminophylline;* concomitant use elevates theophylline levels.

Effects on diagnostic tests
Transient elevations of AST levels have been reported. Glucose levels may be increased.

Adverse reactions
CNS: impaired mental alertness, impaired coordination, numbness, seizures, *drowsiness, fatigue, headache,* giddiness, dizziness.
CV: *hypotension.*
EENT: tinnitus, blurry or yellow vision, dry mouth and eyes, xanthopsia.
GI: *anorexia, nausea, vomiting,* diarrhea, epigastric distress, cholestasis.
GU: hematuria, enuresis, crystalluria, malodorous urine.
Hematologic: leukopenia.
Hepatic: ***jaundice, parenchymal liver damage.***
Skin: *rash, pruritus,* ***erythema multiforme, Stevens-Johnson syndrome.***
Other: lymphadenopathy, fever, flushing, chills, hyperglycemia, ***angioedema, anaphylaxis.***

Overdose and treatment
Signs of overdose may include visual disturbances and altered mental status. Treatment includes induced emesis or gastric lavage if ingested within 4 hours, followed by supportive and symptomatic treatment.

☑ Special considerations
- Give drug after meals; shake suspension well to ensure accurate dosages.
- Drug may be given with milk, fruit juice, or food.
- Laxatives, enemas, and dietary restrictions are unnecessary.
- Assess patient and review laboratory reports for signs of anemia, dehydration, or malnutrition before starting therapy.
- Monitor patient for adverse reactions, which usually occur 3 to 4 hours after drug is administered. Adverse effects are usually mild and related to dosage and duration of therapy.

Patient education
- Warn patient that drug causes drowsiness or dizziness. Tell him to avoid driving or other hazardous activities during therapy.
- Teach patient the signs of hypersensitivity and to call immediately if they occur.
- Tell patient to wash perianal area daily and to change undergarments and bedclothes daily.
- To help prevent reinfection, instruct patient and family members in personal hygiene, including sanitary disposal of feces and hand washing and nail cleaning after defecation and before handling, preparing, or eating food.
- Explain routes of transmission, and encourage other household members and suspected contacts to be tested and, if necessary, treated.

Breast-feeding
- Safety has not been established.

thiamine hydrochloride (vitamin B_1)
Biamine, Thiamilate

Pharmacologic classification: water-soluble vitamin
Therapeutic classification: nutritional supplement
Pregnancy risk category A (C if more than RDA)

How supplied
Available by prescription only
Injection: 1-ml ampules (100 mg/ml), 1-ml vials (100 mg/ml), 2-ml vials (100 mg/ml), 10-ml vials (100 mg/ml), 30-ml vials (100 mg/ml), 30-ml vials (200 mg/ml), 30-ml vials (100 mg/ml, with 0.5% chlorobutanol)

Available without a prescription
Tablets: 5 mg, 10 mg, 25 mg, 50 mg, 100 mg, 250 mg, 500 mg
Tablets (enteric-coated): 20 mg

Indications, route, and dosage
Beriberi
Adults: 10 to 20 mg I.M., depending on severity (can receive up to 100 mg I.M. or I.V. for severe cases), t.i.d. for 2 weeks, followed by dietary correction and multivitamin supplement containing 5 to 30 mg thiamine daily in single or three divided doses for 1 month.
Children: 10 to 25 mg, depending on severity, I.M. daily for several weeks with adequate dietary intake.
Anemia secondary to thiamine deficiency; polyneuritis secondary to alcoholism, pregnancy, or pellagra
Adults and children: P.O. dosage is based on RDA for age-group.
Wernicke's encephalopathy
Adults: Initially, 100 mg I.V., followed by 50 to 100 mg I.M. or I.V. daily.
"Wet beriberi" with myocardial failure
Adults and children: 10 to 30 mg I.V. for emergency treatment.

Pharmacodynamics
Metabolic action: Exogenous thiamine is required for carbohydrate metabolism. Thiamine combines with ATP to form thiamine pyrophosphate, a coenzyme in carbohydrate metabolism and transketolation reactions. This coenzyme is also necessary in the hexose monophosphate shunt during pentose utilization. One sign of thiamine deficiency is an increase in pyruvic acid. The body's need for thiamine is greater when the carbohydrate content of the diet is high. Within 3 weeks of total absence of dietary thiamine, significant vitamin depletion can occur. Thiamine deficiency can cause beriberi.

Pharmacokinetics

- *Absorption:* Absorbed readily after oral administration of small doses; after oral administration of a large dose, the total amount absorbed is limited to 4 to 8 mg. In alcoholics and in patients with cirrhosis or malabsorption, GI absorption of thiamine is decreased. When given with meals, drug's GI rate of absorption decreases, but total absorption remains the same. After I.M. administration, drug is absorbed rapidly and completely.
- *Distribution:* Distributed widely into body tissues. When intake exceeds the minimal requirements, tissue stores become saturated. About 100 to 200 mcg/day of thiamine is distributed into the milk of breast-feeding women on a normal diet.
- *Metabolism:* Thiamine is metabolized in the liver.
- *Excretion:* Excess thiamine is excreted in the urine. After administration of large doses (more than 10 mg), both unchanged thiamine and metabolites are excreted in urine after tissue stores become saturated.

Contraindications and precautions

Contraindicated in patients hypersensitive to thiamine products.

Interactions

Concomitant use of thiamine with *neuromuscular blocking agents* may enhance the effects of the latter.

Thiamine may not be used in combination with *alkaline solutions (carbonates, citrates, bicarbonates);* thiamine is unstable in *neutral* or *alkaline solutions.*

Effects on diagnostic tests

Drug therapy may produce false-positive results in the phosphotungstate method for determination of uric acid and in the urine spot tests with Ehrlich's reagent for urobilinogen.

Large doses of thiamine interfere with the Schack and Waxler spectrophotometric determination of serum theophylline concentrations.

Adverse reactions

CNS: restlessness.
CV: ***angioedema, CV collapse,*** cyanosis.
EENT: tightness of throat (allergic reaction).
GI: nausea, hemorrhage.
Respiratory: pulmonary edema.
Skin: feeling of warmth, pruritus, urticaria, diaphoresis.
Other: weakness; tenderness and induration following I.M. administration.

Overdose and treatment

Very large doses of thiamine administered parenterally may produce neuromuscular and ganglionic blockade and neurologic symptoms. Treatment is supportive.

☑ Special considerations

- The RDA of thiamine is as follows:

Neonates and infants up to age 6 months: 0.3 mg daily.
Infants age 6 months to 1 year: 0.4 mg daily.
Children age 1 to 3: 0.7 mg daily.
Children age 4 to 6: 0.9 mg daily.
Childen age 7 to 10: 1 mg daily.
Males age 11 to 14: 1.3 mg daily.
Males age 15 to 50: 1.5 mg daily.
Males age 51 and over: 1.2 mg daily.
Females age 11 to 50: 1.1 mg daily.
Females age 51 and over: 1 mg daily.
Pregnant women: 1.5 mg daily.
Breast-feeding women: 1.6 mg daily.

- Give intradermal skin test before I.V. thiamine administration if sensitivity is suspected because anaphylaxis can occur. Keep epinephrine available when administering large parenteral doses.
- I.M. injection may be painful. Rotate injection sites and apply cold compresses to ease discomfort.
- Accurate dietary history is important during vitamin replacement therapy. Help patient develop a practical plan for adequate nutrition.
- Total absence of dietary thiamine can produce a deficiency state in about 3 weeks.
- Subclinical deficiency of thiamine or other B vitamins is common in patients who are poor, chronic alcoholics, or pregnant or who follow fad diets.
- Store thiamine in light-resistant, nonmetallic container.

Patient education

- Inform patient about dietary sources of thiamine, such as yeast, pork, beef, liver, whole grains, peas, and beans.

Breast-feeding

- Thiamine (in amounts that do not exceed the RDA) is safe to use in breast-feeding women. It is secreted into breast milk and fulfills a nutritional requirement of the infant.

thioguanine (6-thioguanine, 6-TG)

Lanvis*

Pharmacologic classification: antimetabolite (cell cycle-phase specific, S phase)
Therapeutic classification: antineoplastic
Pregnancy risk category D

How supplied

Available by prescription only
Tablets (scored): 40 mg

Indications, route, and dosage

Dosage and indications may vary. Check current literature for recommended protocol.

Acute nonlymphocytic leukemias

Adults and children: Initially, 2 mg/kg/day P.O. (usually calculated to nearest 20 mg); then, if no toxic effects occur, increase dose gradually over 3 to 4 weeks to 3 mg/kg/day. Maintenance dosage, 2 to 3 mg/kg/day P.O.

Pharmacodynamics
Antineoplastic action: Thioguanine requires conversion intracellularly to its active form to exert its cytotoxic activity. Acting as a false metabolite, thioguanine inhibits purine synthesis. Cross-resistance exists between mercaptopurine and thioguanine.

Pharmacokinetics
• *Absorption:* After an oral dose, absorption is incomplete and variable. The average bioavailability is 30%.
• *Distribution:* Drug distributes well into bone marrow cells. It does not cross the blood-brain barrier to any appreciable extent.
• *Metabolism:* Extensively metabolized to a less active form in the liver and other tissues.
• *Excretion:* Plasma concentrations of thioguanine decrease in a biphasic manner, with a half-life of 15 minutes in the initial phase and 11 hours in the terminal phase. Drug is excreted in the urine, mainly as metabolites.

Contraindications and precautions
Contraindicated in patients whose disease has shown resistance to drug and in those who have a known hypersensitivity to drug or mercaptopurine. Use cautiously in patients with renal or hepatic dysfunction.

Interactions
None reported.

Effects on diagnostic tests
Drug therapy may increase blood and urine levels of uric acid.

Adverse reactions
GI: nausea, vomiting, stomatitis, diarrhea, anorexia.
Hematologic: ***leukopenia, anemia, thrombocytopenia*** (occurs slowly over 2 to 4 weeks).
Hepatic: ***hepatotoxicity,*** jaundice.
Other: hyperuricemia, rash.

Overdose and treatment
Clinical manifestations of overdose include myelosuppression, nausea, vomiting, malaise, hypertension, and diaphoresis.

Treatment is usually supportive and includes transfusion of blood components and antiemetics. Induction of emesis may be helpful if performed soon after ingestion.

☑ Special considerations
• Total daily dosage can be given at one time.
• Give dose between meals to facilitate complete absorption.
• Dose modification may be required in renal or hepatic dysfunction.
• Monitor serum uric acid levels. Use oral hydration to prevent uric acid nephropathy. Alkalinize urine if serum uric acid levels are elevated.
• Monitor liver function tests. Stop drug if hepatotoxicity or hepatic tenderness occurs. Watch for jaundice, which may reverse if drug is stopped promptly.
• Conduct CBC daily during induction, then weekly during maintenance therapy.
• Drug is sometimes ordered as 6-thioguanine.
• Avoid all I.M. injections when platelet count is less than 100,000/mm^3.

Patient education
• Emphasize importance of continuing medication despite occurrence of nausea and vomiting.
• Tell patient to report promptly if vomiting occurs shortly after a dose is taken.
• Advise avoiding exposure to people with infections and tell patient to call immediately if signs of infection or unusual bleeding occur.
• Encourage adequate fluid intake to increase urine output and facilitate excretion of uric acid.
• Advise patient to use reliable contraceptive measures during therapy.

Breast-feeding
• It is not known if drug occurs in breast milk. However, because of risk of serious adverse reactions, mutagenicity, and carcinogenicity in the infant, breast-feeding is not recommended.

thiopental sodium
Pentothal

Pharmacologic classification: barbiturate
Therapeutic classification: anesthetic
Controlled substance schedule III
Pregnancy risk category C

How supplied
Available by prescription only
Injection: 250-mg (2.5%), 400-mg (2% or 2.5%), 500-mg (2.5%) syringes; 500-mg (2.5%), 1-g (2.5%), 2.5-g (2.5%), 5-g (2.5%), 1-g (2%), 2.5-g (2%), 5-g (2%) kits
Rectal suspension: 2-g disposable syringe (400 mg/g of suspension)

Indications, route, and dosage
General anesthetic for short-term procedures
Adults and children: 2 to 4 ml 2.5% solution (50 to 100 mg) administered I.V. for induction and repeated as a maintenance dose; however, dosage is individualized.
Convulsive states following anesthesia
Adults: 50 to 125 mg (2 to 5 ml 2.5% solution) I.V.
Basal anesthesia by rectal administration
Adults and children: Administer 30 mg/kg P.R.

Pharmacodynamics
Anesthetic action: Thiopental produces anesthesia by direct depression of the polysynaptic midbrain reticular activating system. Thiopental decreases presynaptic (via decreased neurotransmitter release) and postsynaptic excitation. These effects may be subsequent to increased gamma-aminobutyric acid (GABA) levels, enhancement of GABA effects, or a direct effect on GABA receptor sites.

Pharmacokinetics

• *Absorption:* Thiopental I.V. produces peak brain concentrations in 10 to 20 seconds. Depth of anesthesia may increase for up to 40 seconds. Consciousness returns in 20 to 30 minutes.
• *Distribution:* Drug distributes throughout the body; highest initial concentration occurs in vascular areas of the brain, primarily gray matter; drug is 80% protein-bound. Redistribution of drug is primarily responsible for its short duration of action.
• *Metabolism:* Drug is metabolized extensively but slowly in the liver.
• *Excretion:* Unchanged thiopental is not excreted in significant amounts; duration of action depends on tissue redistribution.

Contraindications and precautions

Contraindicated in patients with acute intermittent or variegate porphyria but not in other porphyrias; in those with known hypersensitivity to drug; and whenever general anesthesia is contraindicated. Do not use rectal form in patients with ulcerative, bleeding rectal lesions, or neoplasms of the lower bowel or in those undergoing rectal surgery.

Use cautiously in patients with respiratory, cardiac, circulatory, renal, or hepatic dysfunction; severe anemia; shock; myxedema; and status asthmaticus (use *extreme* caution) because drug may worsen these conditions. Also use cautiously in patients with hypotension, Addison's disease, myasthenia gravis, or increased intracranial pressure and in breast-feeding patients.

Interactions

Drug may potentiate or add to the CNS depressant effects of *alcohol, antihistamines, benzodiazepines, hypnotics, narcotics, phenothiazines,* and *sedatives.*

Effects on diagnostic tests

Thiopental causes dose-dependent alteration in EEG patterns.

Adverse reactions

CNS: anxiety, restlessness, retrograde amnesia, prolonged somnolence.
CV: thrombophlebitis, hypotension, tachycardia, peripheral vascular collapse, ***myocardial depression, arrhythmias.***
GI: nausea and vomiting, abdominal pain; diarrhea, cramping, rectal bleeding (with rectal form).
Respiratory: *respiratory depression, apnea,* laryngospasm, ***bronchospasm.***
Other: pain, swelling, ulceration, necrosis on extravasation (unlikely at concentrations less than 2.5%), gangrene after intra-arterial injection, allergic reactions, hiccups, coughing, sneezing, shivering, local irritation.

Note: Drug should be discontinued if peripheral vascular collapse, respiratory arrest, or hypersensitivity occurs.

Overdose and treatment

Clinical signs of overdose include respiratory depression, respiratory arrest, hypotension, and shock. Treat supportively, using mechanical ventilation if needed; give I.V. fluids or vasopressors (dopamine, phenylephrine) for hypotension. Monitor vital signs closely.

☑ Special considerations

• Solutions of succinylcholine, tubocurarine, or atropine should not be mixed with thiopental but can be given to the patient concomitantly.
• A small test dose (25 to 75 mg) may be administered to assess tolerance or unusual sensitivity.

Geriatric use

• Lower doses may be indicated.

Pediatric use

• Use cautiously.

thioridazine

Mellaril-S

thioridazine hydrochloride

Apo-Thioridazine*, Mellaril, Novo-Ridazine*, PMS Thioridazine*

Pharmacologic classification: phenothiazine (piperidine derivative)
Therapeutic classification: antipsychotic
Pregnancy risk category C

How supplied

Available by prescription only
Tablets: 10 mg, 15 mg, 25 mg, 50 mg, 100 mg, 150 mg, 200 mg
Oral concentrate: 30 mg/ml, 100 mg/ml (3% to 4.2% alcohol)
Suspension: 25 mg/5 ml, 100 mg/5 ml

Indications, route, and dosage

Psychosis
Adults: Initially, 50 to 100 mg P.O. t.i.d., with gradual increments up to 800 mg daily in divided doses, if needed. Dosage varies.
Dysthymic disorder (neurotic depression), dementia in geriatric patients, behavioral problems in children
Adults: Initially, 25 mg P.O. t.i.d. Maintenance dosage is 20 to 200 mg daily.
Children over age 2: Usually, 0.5 to 3 mg/kg/day P.O. in divided doses. Give 10 mg b.i.d. or t.i.d. to children with moderate disorders and 25 mg b.i.d. or t.i.d. to hospitalized children.

Pharmacodynamics

Antipsychotic action: Thioridazine is thought to exert its antipsychotic effects by postsynaptic blockade of CNS dopamine receptors, thereby inhibiting dopamine-mediated effects.

Thioridazine has many other central and peripheral effects: It produces both alpha and ganglionic blockade and counteracts histamine- and serotonin-mediated activity. Its most prevalent adverse reactions are antimuscarinic and sedative; it causes fewer extrapyramidal effects than other antipsychotics.

Pharmacokinetics

• *Absorption:* Rate and extent of absorption vary with administration route. Oral tablet absorption is erratic and variable, with onset ranging from ½ to 1 hour. Oral concentrates and suspensions are much more predictable.
• *Distribution:* Distributed widely into the body, including breast milk. Peak effects occur at 2 to 4 hours; steady state serum level is achieved within 4 to 7 days. Drug is 91% to 99% protein-bound.
• *Metabolism:* Drug is metabolized extensively by the liver and forms the active metabolite mesoridazine; duration of action is 4 to 6 hours.
• *Excretion:* Mostly excreted as metabolites in urine; some excreted in feces via the biliary tract.

Contraindications and precautions

Contraindicated in patients with hypersensitivity to drug or in those experiencing coma, CNS depression, or severe hypertensive or hypotensive cardiac disease.

Use cautiously in elderly or debilitated patients and in those with hepatic or CV disease, respiratory or seizure disorders, hypocalcemia, severe reactions to insulin or electroconvulsive therapy, and exposure to extreme cold or heat or to organophosphate insecticides.

Interactions

Concomitant use of thioridazine with *sympathomimetics*, including *epinephrine, phenylephrine, phenylpropanolamine*, and *ephedrine* (commonly found in nasal sprays) and with *appetite suppressants* may decrease their stimulatory and pressor effects. Thioridazine may cause *epinephrine reversal.*

Thioridazine may inhibit blood pressure response to *centrally acting antihypertensive drugs,* such as *clonidine, guanabenz, guanadrel, guanethidine, methyldopa,* and *reserpine.* Additive effects are likely after concomitant use of thioridazine with *CNS depressants,* including *alcohol, analgesics, barbiturates, narcotics, tranquilizers, anesthetics (general, spinal,* or *epidural),* and *parenteral magnesium sulfate* (oversedation, respiratory depression, and hypotension); *antiarrhythmic agents,* including *quinidine, disopyramide,* and *procainamide* (increased incidence of arrhythmias and conduction defects); *atropine* and other *anticholinergic drugs,* including *antidepressants, antihistamines, MAO inhibitors, meperidine, phenothiazines,* and *antiparkinsonian agents* (oversedation, paralytic ileus, visual changes, and severe constipation); *nitrates* (hypotension); and *metrizamide* (increased risk of seizures).

Beta-blocking agents may inhibit thioridazine metabolism, increasing plasma levels and toxicity. Concomitant use with *propylthiouracil* increases risk of agranulocytosis; concomitant use with *lithium* may result in severe neurologic toxicity with an encephalitis-like syndrome and in decreased therapeutic response to thioridazine.

Pharmacokinetic alterations and subsequent decreased therapeutic response to thioridazine may follow concomitant use with phenobarbital (enhanced renal excretion); *aluminum-* and *magnesium-containing antacids* and *antidiarrheals* (decreased absorption); *caffeine;* or *heavy smoking* (increased metabolism).

Thioridazine may antagonize therapeutic effect of *bromocriptine* on prolactin secretion; it also may decrease the vasoconstricting effects of *high-dose dopamine* and may decrease effectiveness and increase toxicity of levodopa (by dopamine blockade). Thioridazine may inhibit metabolism and increase toxicity of *phenytoin.*

Effects on diagnostic tests

Thioridazine causes false-positive test results for urinary porphyrins, urobilinogen, amylase, and 5-hydroxyindoleacetic acid because of darkening of urine by metabolites; it also causes false-positive urine pregnancy results in tests using human chorionic gonadotropin as the indicator.

Thioridazine elevates test results for liver enzymes and protein-bound iodine and causes quinidine-like effects on ECG.

Adverse reactions

CNS: extrapyramidal reactions (low incidence), *tardive dyskinesia, sedation* (high incidence), EEG changes, dizziness.
CV: *orthostatic hypotension,* tachycardia, ECG changes.
EENT: *ocular changes, blurred vision,* retinitis pigmentosa.
GI: *dry mouth, constipation.*
GU: *urine retention,* dark urine, menstrual irregularities, gynecomastia, inhibited ejaculation.
Hematologic: transient leukopenia, ***agranulocytosis,*** hyperprolactinemia.
Hepatic: cholestatic jaundice.
Skin: *mild photosensitivity,* allergic reactions.
Other: weight gain; increased appetite; ***neuroleptic malignant syndrome*** (rare).

After abrupt withdrawal of long-term therapy: gastritis, nausea, vomiting, dizziness, tremor, feeling of warmth or cold, diaphoresis, tachycardia, headache, insomnia.

Overdose and treatment

CNS depression is characterized by deep, unarousable sleep and possible coma, hypotension or hypertension, extrapyramidal symptoms, abnormal involuntary muscle movements, agitation, seizures, arrhythmias, ECG changes, hypothermia or hyperthermia, and autonomic nervous system dysfunction.

Treatment is symptomatic and supportive and includes maintaining vital signs, airway, stable body temperature, and fluid and electrolyte balance.

Do not induce vomiting: Drug inhibits cough reflex, and aspiration may occur. Use gastric lavage, then activated charcoal and sodium chloride cathartics; dialysis does not help. Regulate body temperature as needed. Treat hypotension with I.V. fluids: *Do not give epinephrine.* Treat seizures with parenteral diazepam or barbiturates; arrhythmias with parenteral phenytoin (1 mg/kg with rate titrated to blood pressure); and extrapyramidal reactions with benztropine at 1 to 2 mg or parenteral diphenhydramine at 10 to 50 mg. Contact local or regional poison information center for specific instructions.

☑ Special considerations

Besides those relevant to all *phenothiazines,* consider the following recommendations.
- Doses above 300 mg/day are usually reserved for adults with severe psychosis. Do *not* exceed 800 mg daily because of ophthalmic toxicity.
- Liquid formulations may cause a rash if skin contact occurs.
- Drug can cause pink to brown discoloration of patient's urine.
- Thioridazine is associated with a high incidence of sedation, anticholinergic effects, orthostatic hypotension, photosensitivity reactions, and delayed or absent ejaculation. It has the lowest potential for extrapyramidal reactions of all phenothiazines.
- Oral formulations may cause stomach upset. Administer with food or fluid.
- Check patient regularly for abnormal body movements (at least once every 6 months).
- Concentrate must be diluted in 2 to 4 oz (60 to 120 ml) of liquid, preferably water, carbonated drinks, fruit juice, tomato juice, milk, or pudding.
- All liquid formulations must be protected from light.

Patient education
- Explain risks of dystonic reactions and tardive dyskinesia, and tell patient to report abnormal body movements.
- Tell patient to avoid sun exposure and to wear sunscreen when going outdoors to prevent photosensitivity reactions. (Heat lamps and tanning beds also may cause burning of the skin or skin discoloration.)
- Warn patient not to spill the liquid on the skin; rash and irritation may result.
- Warn patient to avoid extremely hot or cold baths or exposure to temperature extremes, sunlamps, or tanning beds; drug may cause thermoregulatory changes.
- Advise patient to take drug exactly as prescribed and not to double doses for doses that are missed.
- Explain that many drug interactions are possible. Patient should seek medical approval before taking *any* self-prescribed medication.
- Tell patient not to stop taking drug suddenly; most adverse reactions may be relieved by dosage reduction. However, patient should call promptly if difficulty urinating, sore throat, dizziness or fainting, or if visual changes develop.
- Warn patient to avoid hazardous activities that require alertness until the effect of drug is established. Reassure patient that excessive sedation usually subsides after several weeks.
- Tell patient not to drink alcohol or take other medications that may cause excessive sedation.
- Advise patient to maintain adequate hydration.
- Explain which fluids are appropriate for diluting the concentrate and the dropper technique of measuring dose.
- Suggest sugarless gum or candy, ice chips, or artificial saliva to relieve dry mouth.
- Tell patient to store drug safely away from children.

Geriatric use
- Elderly patients tend to require lower dosages, titrated to individual response. Such patients also are more likely to develop adverse reactions, especially tardive dyskinesia and other extrapyramidal effects.

Pediatric use
- Drug is not recommended for patients under age 2. For patients over age 2, dosage is 1 mg/kg/day in divided doses.

Breast-feeding
- Thioridazine may enter breast milk. Potential benefits to the mother should outweigh the potential harm to the infant.

---

thiotepa
Thioplex

Pharmacologic classification: alkylating (cell cycle-phase nonspecific)
Therapeutic classification: antineoplastic
Pregnancy risk category D

How supplied
Available by prescription only
Injection: 15-mg vials

Indications, route, and dosage
Dosage and indications may vary. Check current literature for recommended protocol.

Breast and ovarian cancer, Hodgkin's disease, lymphomas
Adults and adolescents age 12 and over: 0.2 mg/kg I.V. daily for 4 to 5 days, repeated q 2 to 4 weeks; or 0.3 to 0.4 mg/kg I.V. q 1 to 4 weeks.

Bladder tumor
Adults and adolescents age 12 and over: 60 mg in 30 to 60 ml of 0.9% NaCl solution (thiotepa in distilled water) instilled in bladder once weekly for 4 weeks.

Neoplastic effusions
Adults and adolescents age 12 and over: 0.6 to 0.8 mg/kg intracavity or intratumor q 1 to 4 weeks.

◊ ***Malignant meningeal neoplasm***
Adults: 1 to 10 mg/m^2 intrathecally, once to twice weekly.

Pharmacodynamics
Antineoplastic action: Thiotepa exerts its cytotoxic activity as an alkylating agent, cross-linking strands of DNA and RNA and inhibiting protein synthesis, resulting in cell death.

Pharmacokinetics
- *Absorption:* Incomplete absorption across the GI tract; absorption from the bladder is variable, ranging from 10% to 100% of an instilled dose. Absorption is increased by certain pathologic conditions. I.M. and pleural membrane absorption of thiotepa is also variable.
- *Distribution:* It is not known if drug or its metabolites are distributed into breast milk.

- *Metabolism:* Thiotepa is metabolized extensively in the liver.
- *Excretion:* Drug and its metabolites are excreted in urine.

Contraindications and precautions
Contraindicated in patients with hypersensitivity to drug and in those with severe bone marrow, hepatic, or renal dysfunction. Use cautiously in patients with impaired renal or hepatic function or bone marrow suppression.

Interactions
When used concomitantly, thiotepa may cause prolonged respirations and apnea in patients receiving *succinylcholine.* Thiotepa appears to inhibit the activity of *pseudocholinesterase,* the enzyme that deactivates succinylcholine. Use succinylcholine with extreme caution in patients receiving thiotepa.

Effects on diagnostic tests
Thiotepa therapy may increase blood and urine levels of uric acid and decrease plasma pseudocholinesterase concentrations.

Adverse reactions
CNS: headache, dizziness, blurred vision, fatigue, weakness.
EENT: laryngeal edema, conjunctivitis.
GI: *nausea, vomiting,* abdominal pain, anorexia.
GU: amenorrhea, decreased spermatogenesis, dysuria, urine retention, hemorrhagic cystitis.
Hematologic: ***leukopenia*** (begins within 5 to 10 days), ***thrombocytopenia, neutropenia, anemia.***
Respiratory: asthma.
Skin: hives, rash, dermatitis.
Other: fever, alopecia, hypersensitivity, ***anaphylactic shock.***

Overdose and treatment
Clinical manifestations of overdose include nausea, vomiting, and precipitation of uric acid in the renal tubules.

Treatment is usually supportive and includes transfusion of blood components, antiemetics, hydration, and allopurinol.

☑ Special considerations
- To reconstitute drug, use 1.5 ml of sterile water for injection to yield a concentration of 10 mg/ml. The solution is clear to slightly opaque.
- Use only sterile water for injection to reconstitute. Refrigerated solution is stable for 8 hours.
- Refrigerate dry powder; protect from light.
- Drug can be given by all parenteral routes, including direct injection into the tumor.
- Stop drug or decrease dosage if WBC count decreases below 4,000/mm³ or if platelet count decreases below 150,000/mm³.
- Drug may be mixed with procaine 2% or epinephrine 1:1,000, or both, for local use.
- Drug may be further diluted to larger volumes with 0.9% NaCl solution, D_5W, or lactated Ringer's solution for administration by I.V. infusion, intracavitary injection, or perfusion therapy.
- Withhold fluids for 8 to 10 hours before bladder instillation. Instill 60 ml of drug into bladder by catheter; ask patient to retain solution for 2 hours. Volume may be reduced to 30 ml if discomfort is too great. Reposition patient every 15 minutes for maximum area contact.
- To prevent hyperuricemia with resulting uric acid nephropathy, allopurinol may be given; keep patient well hydrated. Monitor uric acid.
- Monitor CBC weekly for at least 3 weeks after last dose. Warn patient to report even mild infections.
- Avoid all I.M. injections when platelet count is less than 100,000/mm³.
- Use anticoagulants and aspirin products cautiously. Watch closely for signs of bleeding.
- Toxicity may be delayed and prolonged because drug binds to tissues and stays in body several hours.

Patient education
- Encourage patient to maintain an adequate fluid intake to facilitate the excretion of uric acid.
- Instruct patient to avoid OTC products containing aspirin.
- Tell patient to avoid exposure to people with infections.
- Advise patient that hair should grow back after therapy has ended.
- Tell patient to report sore throat, fever, or unusual bruising or bleeding.

Breast-feeding
- It is not known if drug occurs in breast milk. However, because of risk of serious adverse reactions, mutagenicity, and carcinogenicity in the infant, breast-feeding is not recommended.

thiothixene

thiothixene hydrochloride
Navane

Pharmacologic classification: thioxanthene
Therapeutic classification: antipsychotic
Pregnancy risk category C

How supplied
Available by prescription only
Capsules: 1 mg, 2 mg, 5 mg, 10 mg, 20 mg
Oral concentrate: 5 mg/ml (7% alcohol)
Injection: 2 mg/ml, 5 mg/ml

Indications, route, and dosage
Acute agitation
Adults: 4 mg I.M. b.i.d. to q.i.d.; maximum dosage, 30 mg I.M. daily. Change to P.O. form as soon as possible; I.M. dosage form is irritating.
Mild to moderate psychosis
Adults: Initially, 2 mg P.O. t.i.d.; may increase gradually to 15 mg daily.
Severe psychosis
Adults: Initially, 5 mg P.O. b.i.d.; may increase gradually to 20 to 30 mg daily. Maximum recommended daily dosage, 60 mg.

Pharmacodynamics

Antipsychotic action: Thiothixene is thought to exert its antipsychotic effects by postsynaptic blockade of CNS dopamine receptors, thereby inhibiting dopamine-mediated effects.

Thiothixene has many other central and peripheral effects; it also acts as an alpha-blocking agent. Its most prominent adverse reactions are extrapyramidal.

Pharmacokinetics

- *Absorption:* Absorption is rapid; I.M. onset of action is 10 to 30 minutes.
- *Distribution:* Widely distributed into the body. Peak effects occur at 1 to 6 hours after I.M. administration; drug is 91% to 99% protein-bound.
- *Metabolism:* Thiothixene is metabolized in the liver.
- *Excretion:* Mostly excreted as parent drug in feces via the biliary tract.

Contraindications and precautions

Contraindicated in patients with hypersensitivity to drug and in those experiencing circulatory collapse, coma, CNS depression, or blood dyscrasia.

Use cautiously in elderly or debilitated patients; in those with history of seizure disorders, CV disease, heat exposure, glaucoma, or prostatic hyperplasia; and in those in a state of alcohol withdrawal.

Interactions

Concomitant use of thiothixene with *sympathomimetics,* including *epinephrine, phenylephrine, phenylpropanolamine,* and *ephedrine* (commonly found in nasal sprays), and with *appetite suppressants* may decrease their stimulatory and pressor effects. Thiothixene may cause *epinephrine* reversal; patients taking thiothixene may experience a decrease in blood pressure when *epinephrine* is used as a pressor agent.

Thiothixene may inhibit blood pressure response to *centrally acting antihypertensive drugs,* such as *clonidine, guanabenz, guanadrel, guanethidine, methyldopa,* and *reserpine.* Additive effects are likely after concomitant use of thiothixene with *CNS depressants,* including *alcohol, analgesics, barbiturates, narcotics, tranquilizers, anesthetics (general, spinal,* or *epidural),* and *parenteral magnesium sulfate* (oversedation, respiratory depression, and hypotension); *antiarrhythmic agents, including disopyramide, quinidine,* and *procainamide* (increased incidence of arrhythmias and conduction defects); *atropine* and other *anticholinergic drugs,* including *antidepressants, antihistamines, MAO inhibitors, meperidine, phenothiazines,* and *antiparkinsonian agents* (oversedation, paralytic ileus, visual changes, and severe constipation); *nitrates* (hypotension); and *metrizamide* (increased risk of seizures).

Beta-blocking agents may inhibit thiothixene metabolism, increasing plasma levels and toxicity.

Concomitant use with *propylthiouracil* increases risk of agranulocytosis; concomitant use with *lithium* may result in severe neurologic toxicity with an encephalitis-like syndrome and in decreased therapeutic response to thiothixene.

Pharmacokinetic alterations and subsequent decreased therapeutic response to thiothixene may follow concomitant use with *phenobarbital* (enhanced renal excretion); *aluminum-* and *magnesium-containing antacids* and *antidiarrheals* (decreased absorption); *caffeine;* or *heavy smoking* (increased metabolism).

Thiothixene may antagonize therapeutic effect of *bromocriptine* on prolactin secretion; it may also decrease the vasoconstricting effects of *high-dose dopamine* and may decrease effectiveness and increase toxicity of *levodopa* (by dopamine blockade). Thiothixene may inhibit metabolism and increase toxicity of *phenytoin.*

Effects on diagnostic tests

Drug causes false-positive test results for urinary porphyrins, urobilinogen, amylase, and 5-hydroxyindoleacetic acid because of darkening of urine by metabolites; it also causes false-positive urine pregnancy results in tests using human chorionic gonadotropin as the indicator.

Thiothixene elevates test results for liver enzymes and protein-bound iodine and causes quinidine-like effects on the ECG.

Adverse reactions

CNS: *extrapyramidal reactions,* drowsiness, restlessness, agitation, insomnia, *tardive dyskinesia,* sedation, pseudoparkinsonism, EEG changes, dizziness.
CV: *hypotension,* tachycardia, ECG changes.
EENT: ocular changes, *blurred vision,* nasal congestion.
GI: *dry mouth, constipation.*
GU: *urine retention,* menstrual irregularities, gynecomastia, inhibited ejaculation.
Hematologic: transient leukopenia, leukocytosis, ***agranulocytosis.***
Hepatic: jaundice.
Skin: *mild photosensitivity,* allergic reactions, pain at I.M. injection site, sterile abscess.
Other: weight gain, ***neuroleptic malignant syndrome.***

After abrupt withdrawal of long-term therapy: gastritis, nausea, vomiting, dizziness, tremor, feeling of warmth or cold, diaphoresis, tachycardia, headache, insomnia.

Overdose and treatment

CNS depression is characterized by deep, unarousable sleep and possible coma, hypotension or hypertension, extrapyramidal symptoms, abnormal involuntary muscle movements, agitation, seizures, arrhythmias, ECG changes, hypothermia or hyperthermia, and autonomic nervous system dysfunction.

Treatment is symptomatic and supportive and includes maintaining vital signs, airway, stable body temperature, and fluid and electrolyte balance.

Do not induce vomiting: Drug inhibits cough reflex, and aspiration may occur. Use gastric lavage, then activated charcoal and sodium chloride cathartics; dialysis does not help. Regulate body temperature as needed. Treat hypotension with I.V. fluids: *Do not give epinephrine.* Seizures may be treated with parenteral diazepam or barbiturates; arrhythmias with parenteral phenytoin (1 mg/kg with rate titrated to blood pressure); and extrapyramidal reactions with benztropine at 1 to 2 mg or parenteral diphenhydramine at 10 to 50 mg.

☑ Special considerations

- Liquid and injectable formulations may cause a rash if skin contact occurs.
- Drug is associated with a high incidence of extrapyramidal effects.
- Because stomach upset may occur, administer oral form with food or fluid.
- Check patient regularly for abnormal body movements (at least once every 6 months).
- Dilute the concentrate in 2 to 4 oz (60 to 120 ml) of liquid, preferably water, carbonated drinks, fruit juice, tomato juice, milk, or pudding.
- Photosensitivity reactions may occur; patient should avoid exposure to sunlight or heat lamps.
- Administer I.M. injection deep into upper outer quadrant of the buttock. Massaging the area after administration may prevent formation of abscesses. I.M. injection may cause skin necrosis; do not extravasate, or give drug I.V.
- Solution for injection may be slightly discolored. Do not use if excessively discolored or if a precipitate is evident. Contact pharmacist.
- Monitor blood pressure before and after parenteral administration.
- Shake concentrate before administration.
- Patient may chew sugarless gum, hard candy, or ice to help relieve dry mouth.
- Drug is stable after reconstitution for 48 hours at room temperature.
- Protect liquid formulation from light.

Patient education

- Explain risks of dystonic reactions and tardive dyskinesia, and tell patient to report abnormal body movements.
- Tell patient to avoid sun exposure and to wear sunscreen when going outdoors to prevent photosensitivity reactions. (Heat lamps and tanning beds also may cause burning of the skin or skin discoloration.)
- Instruct patient not to spill the liquid on skin. Contact with skin may cause rash and irritation.
- Warn patient to avoid extremely hot or cold baths or exposure to temperature extremes, sunlamps, or tanning beds; drug may cause thermoregulatory changes.
- Tell patient to take drug exactly as prescribed, not to double doses for missed doses, and not to share drug with others.
- Explain that many drug interactions are possible. He should seek medical approval before taking *any* self-prescribed medication.
- Tell patient not to stop taking drug suddenly; most adverse reactions may be relieved by reducing the dosage. However, patient should call if difficulty urinating, sore throat, dizziness, or fainting develops.
- Warn patient against hazardous activities that require alertness until effect of drug is established. Reassure patient that sedation usually subsides after several weeks.
- Tell patient not to drink alcohol or take other medications that may cause excessive sedation.
- Explain which fluids are appropriate for diluting the concentrate and the dropper technique of measuring dose.
- Recommend sugarless hard candy, chewing gum, or ice to alleviate dry mouth.
- Tell patient to shake concentrate before administration.
- Instruct patient to store drug away from children.

Geriatric use

- Elderly patients tend to require lower dosages, titrated to individual response. Adverse reactions are more likely to develop in such patients, especially tardive dyskinesia and other extrapyramidal effects.

Pediatric use

- Drug is not recommended for children under age 12.

thrombin

Thrombinar, Thrombin-JMI, Thrombogen, Thrombostat

Pharmacologic classification: enzyme
Therapeutic classification: topical hemostatic
Pregnancy risk category C

How supplied

Available by prescription only
Powder: 1,000-, 5,000-, 10,000-, 20,000-, and 50,000-unit vials
Kit: 5,000, 10,000, 20,000 units with sprayer assembly

Indications, route, and dosage

Bleeding from parenchyma, cancellous bone, dental sockets, during nasal and laryngeal surgery, and in plastic surgery and skin-graft-ing procedures

Adults: Apply 100 units/ml of sterile isotonic NaCl solution or sterile distilled water to area where clotting is needed (or apply dry powder in bone surgery); in major bleeding, apply 1,000 to 2,000 units/ml sterile isotonic NaCl solution. Sponge blood from area before application, but avoid sponging area after application.

Pharmacodynamics

Hemostatic action: Thrombin catalyzes the conversion of fibrinogen to fibrin, one of the last stages of clot formation.

Pharmacokinetics

Not applicable.

Contraindications and precautions

Contraindicated in patients with hypersensitivity to thrombin or to bovine products. *Do not inject throm-*

bin or allow it to enter large blood vessels; death may result from severe intravascular clotting.

Interactions
None significant.

Effects on diagnostic tests
None reported.

Adverse reactions
Other: hypersensitivity, fever, ***intravascular clotting*** (could cause death if thrombin enters large vessels).

Overdose and treatment
No information available.

☑ Special considerations
- Thrombostat can be stored at room temperature 59° to 86° F (15° to 30° C). Thrombinar and Thrombin-JMI must be refrigerated at 36° to 46° F (2° to 8° C). Thrombogen must be used immediately upon reconstitution. If necessary, it can be refrigerated at 36° to 46° F for up to 3 hours. Thrombin may be used with absorbable gelatin sponge, but not oxidized cellulose; check label before using.
- Obtain patient history of reactions to thrombin or bovine products.
- Observe patient for hypersensitivity reaction after administering.
- Contents of a 5,000-unit vial dissolved in 5 ml NaCl solution are capable of clotting an equal volume of blood in less than 1 second, or 1,000 ml in less than 1 minute.

Patient education
- Advise patient taking drug for GI hemorrhage to drink all prescribed milk and milk-thrombin solution.

Pediatric use
- Safety has not been established for children.

thyroid, desiccated
Armour Thyroid, S-P-T, Thyrar, Thyroid Strong, Thyroid USP, Westhroid

Pharmacologic classification: thyroid hormone
Therapeutic classification: thyroid
Pregnancy risk category A

How supplied
Available by prescription only
Tablets: 15 mg, 30 mg, 60 mg, 90 mg, 120 mg, 180 mg, 240 mg, 300 mg (Armour Thyroid)
Tablets (bovine): 30 mg, 60 mg, 120 mg (Thyrar)
Tablets (enteric-coated): 60 mg, 120 mg
Thyroid strong tablets (contain 0.3% iodine): 32.5 mg, 65 mg, 130 mg, 200 mg
Capsules (pork): 60 mg, 120 mg, 180 mg, 300 mg (S-P-T, suspended in soybean oil)

Indications, route, and dosage
Adult hypothyroidism
Adults: Initially, 30 mg P.O. daily, increased by 15 mg q 14 to 30 days depending on disease severity until desired response is achieved. Usual maintenance dosage is 60 to 180 mg P.O. daily as a single dose.
Congenital hypothyroidism
Children over age 12: Dosage may approach adult dosage (60 to 180 mg daily), depending on response.
Children age 6 to 12: 60 to 90 mg P.O. daily.
Children age 1 to 5: 45 to 60 mg P.O. daily.
Infants age 6 to 12 months: 30 to 45 mg P.O. daily.
Neonates and infants age 0 to 6 months: 15 to 30 mg P.O. daily.

Note: Thyroid Strong is 50% stronger than thyroid USP. Each grain is equivalent to 1½ grains of thyroid USP.

Pharmacodynamics
Thyrotropic action: Thyroid USP affects protein and carbohydrate metabolism, promotes gluconeogenesis, increases the utilization and mobilization of glycogen stores, stimulates protein synthesis, and regulates cell growth and differentiation. The major effect of thyroid is to increase the metabolic rate of tissue.

Pharmacokinetics
- *Absorption:* Thyroid USP is absorbed from the GI tract.
- *Distribution:* Not fully understood. Thyroid USP is highly protein-bound.
- *Metabolism:* Not fully understood.
- *Excretion:* Not fully understood.

Contraindications and precautions
Contraindicated in patients with hypersensitivity to drug, acute MI uncomplicated by hypothyroidism, untreated thyrotoxicosis, or uncorrected adrenal insufficiency. Use cautiously in the elderly and in patients with angina pectoris, hypertension, other CV disorders, renal insufficiency, or ischemia.

Interactions
Concomitant use of thyroid USP with *adrenocorticoids* or *corticotropin* causes changes in thyroid status, and changes in thyroid dosages may require adrenocorticoid or corticotropin dosage changes as well. Concomitant use with *anticoagulants* may alter anticoagulant effect; an increased thyroid USP dosage may necessitate a lower anticoagulant dose.

Use with *tricyclic antidepressants* or *sympathomimetics* may increase the effects of these medications or of thyroid USP, possibly leading to coronary insufficiency or arrhythmias. Use with *oral antidiabetic agents* or *insulin* may affect dosage requirements of these agents. *Estrogens,* which increase serum thyroxine-binding globulin levels, increase thyroid USP requirements.

Hepatic enzyme inducers (such as *phenytoin*) may increase hepatic degradation of *levothyroxine,* causing increased dosage requirements of levothyroxine. Concomitant use with *somatrem* may accelerate epiphyseal maturation. *I.V. phenytoin* may release free thyroid from thyroglobulin. *Cholestyramine* and *colestipol* may decrease absorption.

Effects on diagnostic tests

Thyroid USP therapy alters ^{131}I thyroid uptake, protein-bound iodine levels, and liothyronine uptake.

Adverse reactions

CNS: *nervousness, insomnia,* tremor, headache.
CV: *tachycardia,* ***arrhythmias, cardiac decompensation and collapse,*** angina pectoris.
GI: diarrhea, vomiting.
Other: weight loss, heat intolerance, diaphoresis, accelerated rate of bone maturation in infants and children, menstrual irregularities, allergic skin reactions.

Overdose and treatment

Clinical manifestations of overdose include signs and symptoms of hyperthyroidism, including weight loss, increased appetite, palpitations, nervousness, diarrhea, abdominal cramps, sweating, tachycardia, increased pulse and blood pressure, angina, arrhythmias, tremor, headache, insomnia, heat intolerance, fever, and menstrual irregularities.

Treatment of acute overdose requires reduction of GI absorption and efforts to counteract central and peripheral effects, primarily sympathetic activity. Use gastric lavage or induce emesis (followed with activated charcoal, if less than 4 hours after ingestion). If the patient is comatose or is having seizures, inflate cuff on endotracheal tube to prevent aspiration. Treatment may include oxygen and artificial ventilation to support respiration. It also should include appropriate measures to treat heart failure and control fever, hypoglycemia, and fluid loss. Propranolol may be used to combat many of the effects of increased sympathetic activity. Thyroid USP therapy should be withdrawn gradually over 2 to 6 days, then resumed at a lower dose.

☑ Special considerations

Besides those relevant to all *thyroid hormones,* consider the following recommendations.

- Levothyroxine is considered drug of choice for thyroid hormone supplementation.
- Commercial preparations may have variable hormonal content and produce fluctuating liothyronine and levothyroxine levels. Because of this variability, the use of thyroid has decreased considerably.
- Monitor patient's pulse rate and blood pressure. Thyroid may exert a greater incidence of CV adverse effects.
- In children, sleeping pulse rate and basal morning temperature are guides to treatment.
- Enteric-coated tablets give unreliable absorption.
- Digoxin levels should be monitored closely as patient becomes euthyroid.

Patient education

- Encourage patient to take daily dose at the same time each day, preferably in the morning to avoid insomnia.
- Advise patient to call if headache, diarrhea, nervousness, excessive sweating, heat intolerance, chest pain, increased pulse rate, or palpitations occur.
- Tell patient not to store drug in warm, humid areas such as the bathroom to prevent deterioration.
- Warn patient not to switch brands or dose.

Geriatric use

- Elderly patients are more sensitive to thyroid effects. In patients over age 60, initial dosage should be 25% lower than usual recommended dosage.

Pediatric use

- Partial hair loss may occur during the first few months of therapy. Reassure child and parents that this is temporary.

Breast-feeding

- Minimal amounts of drug are excreted in breast milk. Use with caution in breast-feeding women.

thyrotropin (thyroid stimulating hormone, TSH)

Thytropar

Pharmacologic classification: anterior pituitary hormone
Therapeutic classification: thyrotropic hormone
Pregnancy risk category C

How supplied

Available by prescription only
Powder for injection: 10 units (IU)/vial

Indications, route, and dosage

Diagnosis of thyroid cancer remnant with ^{131}I ***after surgery***
Adults and children: 10 IU I.M. or S.C. for 3 to 7 days.
Differential diagnosis of primary and secondary hypothyroidism
Adults and children: 10 IU I.M. or S.C. for 1 to 3 days.
In protein-bound iodine or ^{131}I ***uptake determinations for differential diagnosis of subclinical hypothyroidism or low thyroid reserve***
Adults and children: 10 IU I.M. or S.C.
Therapy for thyroid carcinoma (local or metastatic) with ^{131}I
Adults and children: 10 IU I.M. or S.C. for 3 to 8 days.
To determine thyroid status of patient receiving thyroid
Adults and children: 10 IU I.M. or S.C. for 1 to 3 days.

Pharmacodynamics

Thyrotropic action: Thyrotropin produces increased uptake of iodine by the thyroid and increased formation and release of thyroid hormone.

Pharmacokinetics

- *Absorption:* Onset occurs within minutes after injection.
- *Distribution:* Concentrated primarily in the thyroid gland.
- *Metabolism:* Not fully understood.
- *Excretion:* Excreted rapidly in the urine.

Contraindications and precautions

Contraindicated in patients with hypersensitivity to drug, coronary thrombosis, or untreated Addison's disease. Use cautiously in patients with angina pectoris, heart failure, hypopituitarism, and adrenocortical suppression.

Interactions

None reported.

Effects on diagnostic tests

Thyrotropin therapy alters ^{131}I thyroid uptake.

Adverse reactions

CNS: headache, fever.
CV: *tachycardia,* hypotension.
GI: nausea, vomiting.
Other: thyroid hyperplasia (with large doses), hypersensitivity reactions (postinjection flare, urticaria, ***anaphylaxis***).

Overdose and treatment

Clinical manifestations of overdose include headache, irritability, nervousness, sweating, tachycardia, increased GI motility, and menstrual irregularities. Angina or heart failure may be aggravated. Shock may develop.

Treatment includes administering propranolol (or another beta blocker) to treat adrenergic effects of hyperthyroidism. Recommended adult dosage of propranolol is 1 mg/dose over at least 1 minute, repeated every 2 to 5 minutes (to a maximum of 5 mg). Dosage in children is 0.01 to 0.1 mg/kg over 10 minutes (to a maximum of 1 mg). Monitor blood pressure and cardiac function. Exchange transfusions may be beneficial in acute overdose. Diuresis and dialysis are not effective.

☑ Special considerations

Besides those relevant to all *thyroid hormones,* consider the following recommendations.
- Thyrotropin may cause thyroid hyperplasia.
- Three-day dosage schedule may be used in long-standing pituitary myxedema or with prolonged use of thyroid medication.

Patient education

- Warn patient to report the following reactions: itching, redness, or swelling at injection site; rash; tightness of throat or wheezing; chest pain; irritability; nervousness; rapid heartbeat; shortness of breath; or unusual sweating.

tiagabine hydrochloride

Gabitril

Pharmacologic classification: gamma aminobutyric acid (GABA) enhancer
Therapeutic classification: anticonvulsant
Pregnancy risk category C

How supplied

Available by prescription only
Tablets: 4 mg, 12 mg, 16 mg, 20 mg

Indications, route, and dosage

Adjunctive therapy in the treatment of partial seizures

Adults: Initially, 4 mg P.O. once daily. May increase total daily dose by 4 to 8 mg at weekly intervals until clinical response occurs or up to maximum of 56 mg/day. Give total daily dose in divided doses b.i.d. to q.i.d.

Adolescents age 12 to 18: Initially, 4 mg P.O. once daily. May increase total daily dose by 4 mg beginning of week 2 and thereafter by 4 to 8 mg/week at weekly intervals until clinical response is seen or up to maximum of 32 mg/day. Give total daily dose in divided doses b.i.d. to q.i.d.

✦ ***Dosage adjustment.*** In patients with impaired liver function, initial and maintenance doses or longer dosing intervals may be reduced.

Pharmacodynamics

Anticonvulsant action: Exact mechanism unknown. Tiagabine is thought to act by enhancing the activity of GABA, the major inhibitory neurotransmitter in the CNS. It binds to recognition sites associated with the GABA uptake carrier and may thus permit more GABA to be available for binding to receptors on postsynaptic cells.

Pharmacokinetics

- *Absorption:* Drug is rapidly and nearly completely absorbed (over 95%). Peak plasma levels occur 45 minutes following an oral dose in the fasting state. Absolute bioavailability is about 90%.
- *Distribution:* About 96% is bound to human plasma proteins, mainly to serum albumin and alpha-1 acid glycoprotein.
- *Metabolism:* Likely to be metabolized by the cytochrome P-450 3A isoenzymes.
- *Excretion:* Approximately 2% is excreted unchanged, with 25% and 63% of dose excreted into the urine and feces, respectively.

Contraindications and precautions

Contraindicated in patients with hypersensitivity to drug or its ingredients. Use cautiously in breast-feeding patients.

Interactions

Carbamazepine, phenobarbital, and *phenytoin* increase tiagabine clearance. Tiagabine enhances the effects of *CNS depressants* and *alcohol.* Tiagabine causes a slight decrease in *valproate* concentration.

Effects on diagnostic tests

None reported.

Adverse reactions

CNS: *dizziness, asthenia, somnolence, nervousness,* tremor, difficulty with concentration and attention, insomnia, ataxia, confusion, speech disorder, difficulty with memory, paresthesia, depression, emotional lability, abnormal gait, hostility, language problems, agitation.
CV: vasodilation.
EENT: amblyopia, nystagmus, pharyngitis.

GI: abdominal pain, *nausea,* diarrhea, vomiting, increased appetite, mouth ulceration.
GU: urinary tract infection.
Musculoskeletal: myalgia, myasthenia.
Respiratory: increased cough.
Skin: rash, pruritus.
Other: "flulike" syndrome.

Overdose and treatment

The most common symptoms reported after an overdose include somnolence, impaired consciousness, impaired speech, agitation, confusion, speech difficulty, hostility, depression, weakness, and myoclonus. There is no specific antidote for tiagabine. If indicated, elimination of unabsorbed drug should be achieved by emesis or gastric lavage. Observe usual precautions to maintain the airway, and provide general supportive care.

☑ Special considerations

- Never withdraw drug suddenly because seizure frequency may increase. Withdraw tiagabine gradually unless safety concerns require a more rapid withdrawal.
- A therapeutic range for plasma drug concentrations has not been established.
- Because of the potential for pharmacokinetic interactions between tiagabine and drugs that induce or inhibit hepatic metabolizing enzymes, obtain plasma levels of tiagabine before and after changes are made in the therapeutic regimen.
- Status epilepticus and sudden unexpected death in epilepsy have occurred in patients receiving tiagabine. Patients who are not receiving at least one concomitant enzyme-inducing antiepilepsy drug at the time of tiagabine initiation may require lower doses or a slower dose titration.

Patient education

- Advise patient to take drug only as prescribed.
- Tell patient to take tiagabine with food.
- Warn patient that drug may cause dizziness, somnolence, and other symptoms and signs of CNS depression. Advise patient to avoid driving and other potentially hazardous activities that require mental alertness until drug's CNS effects are known.
- Tell female patient to call health care provider if pregnancy is being planned or suspected.
- Tell female patient to inform health care provider if she is planning to breast-feed because drug may be excreted in breast milk.

Geriatric use

- Because few patients over age 65 were exposed to drug during its clinical evaluation, safety or effectiveness in this age group is not clear.

Pediatric use

- Drug has not been investigated in adequate and well-controlled trials in patients under age 12.

Breast-feeding

- Studies in rats have shown that tiagabine and its metabolites are excreted in breast milk. Use in breast-feeding women only if the benefits clearly outweigh the risks.

ticarcillin disodium

Ticar

Pharmacologic classification: extended-spectrum penicillin, alpha-carboxypenicillin
Therapeutic classification: antibiotic
Pregnancy risk category B

How supplied

Available by prescription only
Injection: 1 g, 3 g, 6 g
Pharmacy bulk package: 20 g, 30 g
I.V. infusion: 3 g

Indications, route, and dosage

Serious infections caused by susceptible organisms
Adults: 200 to 300 mg/kg I.V. daily, divided into doses given q 4 or 6 hours.
Children weighing below 88 lb (40 kg): 200 to 300 mg/kg I.V. daily, divided into doses given q 4 to 6 hours.
Neonates weighing over 4.4 lb (2 kg): 225 to 300 mg/kg/day, divided into doses given q 8 hours.
Neonates weighing below 4.4 lb: 150 to 225 mg/kg/day, divided into doses given q 8 to 12 hours.
Urinary tract infection
Adults: For patients with complicated infection, give 150 to 200 mg/kg I.V. daily, divided into doses q 4 to 6 hours; for treating uncomplicated infections, give 1 g I.V. or I.M. q 6 hours.
✦ ***Dosage adjustment.*** In patients with renal failure, refer to following dosing chart.

Creatinine clearance (ml/min)	Dosage in adults
> 60	3 g I.V. q 4 hr
30 to 60	2 g I.V. q 4 hr
10 to 30	2 g I.V. q 8 hr
< 10	2 g I.V. q 12 hr or 1 g I.M. q 6 hr
< 10 with hepatic failure	2 g I.V. q 24 hr or 1 g I.M. q 12 hr
Patients on hemodialysis	2 g I.V. q 12 hr with 3 g I.V. after each treatment
Patients on peritoneal dialysis	3 g I.V. q 12 hr

Pharmacodynamics

Antibiotic action: Ticarcillin is bactericidal; it adheres to bacterial penicillin-binding proteins, thus inhibiting bacterial cell wall synthesis. Extended-spectrum penicillins are more resistant to inactivation by certain beta-lactamases, especially those produced by gram-negative organisms, but are still liable to inactivation by certain others.

Spectrum of activity includes many gram-negative aerobic and anaerobic bacilli, many gram-positive and gram-negative aerobic cocci, and some gram-positive aerobic and anaerobic bacilli. Drug may be effective against some strains of carbenicillin-resistant gram-negative bacilli.

In many cases, ticarcillin is more active (by weight) against *Pseudomonas aeruginosa* than is carbenicillin. Its primary use is in combination with an aminoglycoside to treat *P. aeruginosa* infections.

When ticarcillin is used alone, resistance develops rapidly. It is almost always used with other antibiotics (such as aminoglycosides).

Pharmacokinetics

• *Absorption:* Peak plasma concentrations occur 30 to 75 minutes after an I.M. dose. Approximately 86% of the dose is absorbed.
• *Distribution:* Ticarcillin disodium is distributed widely. It penetrates minimally into CSF with uninflamed meninges. Ticarcillin crosses the placenta; it is 45% to 65% protein-bound.
• *Metabolism:* About 13% of a dose is metabolized by hydrolysis to inactive compounds.
• *Excretion:* Excreted primarily (80% to 93%) in urine by renal tubular secretion and glomerular filtration; also excreted in bile and breast milk. Elimination half-life in adults is about 1 hour; in severe renal impairment, half-life is extended to about 3 hours. Drug is removed by hemodialysis but not by peritoneal dialysis.

Contraindications and precautions

Contraindicated in patients with hypersensitivity to drug or other penicillins. Use cautiously in patients with other drug allergies, especially to cephalosporins, impaired renal function, hemorrhagic conditions, hypokalemia, and sodium restrictions.

Interactions

Concomitant use with *aminoglycoside antibiotics* results in synergistic bactericidal effects against *P. aeruginosa, Escherichia coli, Klebsiella, Citrobacter, Enterobacter, Serratia,* and *Proteus mirabilis.* However, drugs are physically and chemically incompatible and are inactivated when mixed or given together.

Concomitant use of ticarcillin (and other extended-spectrum penicillins) with *clavulanic acid* also produces a synergistic bactericidal effect against certain beta-lactamase–producing bacteria.

Probenecid blocks renal tubular secretion of ticarcillin, raising serum concentrations of ticarcillin.

Large doses of penicillins may interfere with renal tubular secretion of *methotrexate,* thus delaying elimination and elevating serum concentrations of methotrexate.

Effects on diagnostic tests

Ticarcillin alters tests for urinary or serum proteins; it interferes with turbidimetric methods that use sulfosalicylic acid, trichloroacetic acid, acetic acid, or nitric acid. Ticarcillin does not interfere with tests using bromophenol blue (Albustix, Albutest, MultiStix).

Drug may falsely decrease serum aminoglycoside concentrations. Systemic effects of drug may cause positive Coombs' test, hypokalemia and hypernatremia, and may prolong PT; it may also cause transient elevations in liver function studies and transient reductions in RBC, WBC, and platelet counts.

Adverse reactions

CNS: ***seizures,*** neuromuscular excitability.
GI: nausea, diarrhea, vomiting, pseudomembranous colitis.
Hematologic: leukopenia, ***neutropenia,*** eosinophilia, ***thrombocytopenia,*** hemolytic anemia.
Other: hypersensitivity reactions (rash, pruritus, urticaria, chills, fever, edema, ***anaphylaxis***), overgrowth of nonsusceptible organisms, hypokalemia, pain at injection site, vein irritation, phlebitis.

Overdose and treatment

Clinical signs of overdose include neuromuscular hypersensitivity or seizures resulting from CNS irritation by high drug concentrations. Ticarcillin can be removed by hemodialysis.

☑ Special considerations

Besides those relevant to all *penicillins,* consider the following recommendations.

• Ticarcillin is almost always used with another antibiotic such as an aminoglycoside in life-threatening situations.
• Ticarcillin contains 5.2 mEq of sodium per gram of drug. Use with caution in patients who require sodium restriction.
• Monitor serum electrolytes to prevent hypokalemia and hypernatremia.
• Monitor neurologic status. High concentrations may cause seizures.
• Check CBC, differential, PT, and partial thromboplastin time. Drug may cause thrombocytopenia. Watch for signs of bleeding.
• Because drug is dialyzable, patients undergoing hemodialysis may need dosage adjustments.

Geriatric use

• Half-life may be prolonged in elderly patients because of impaired renal function.

Pediatric use

• Ticarcillin reconstituted for I.M. use with bacteriostatic water for injection containing benzyl alcohol should not be used in neonates because of potential for toxicity.

Breast-feeding

• Drug is excreted in breast milk; use cautiously in breast-feeding women.

ticarcillin disodium/ clavulanate potassium

Timentin

Pharmacologic classification: extended-spectrum penicillin, beta-lactamase inhibitor
Therapeutic classification: antibiotic
Pregnancy risk category B

How supplied

Available by prescription only
Injection: 3 g ticarcillin and 100 mg clavulanic acid

Indications, route, and dosage

Infections of the lower respiratory tract, urinary tract, bones and joints, skin and skin structure, and septicemia when caused by susceptible organisms

Adults: 3.1 g (contains 3 g ticarcillin and 0.1 g clavulanate potassium) diluted in 50 to 100 ml D_5W, NaCl, or lactated Ringer's injection and administered by I.V. infusion over 30 minutes q 4 to 6 hours.

✦ ***Dosage adjustment.*** In patients with renal failure, loading dose is 3.1 g (3 g ticarcillin with 100 mg clavulanate).

Creatinine clearance (ml/min)	Dosage in adults
> 60	3.1 g I.V. q 4 hr
30 to 60	2 g I.V. q 4 hr
10 to 30	2 g I.V. q 8 hr
< 10	2 g I.V. q 12 hr
< 10 with hepatic failure	2 g I.V. q 24 hr
Patients on hemodialysis	2 g I.V. q 12 hr, then 3.1 g after treatment
Patients on peritoneal dialysis	3.1 g I.V. q 12 hr

Pharmacodynamics

Antibiotic action: Ticarcillin is bactericidal; it adheres to bacterial penicillin-binding proteins, thus inhibiting bacterial cell wall synthesis. Extended-spectrum penicillins are more resistant to inactivation by certain beta-lactamases, especially those produced by gram-negative organisms, but are still liable to inactivation by certain others.

Clavulanic acid has only weak antibacterial activity and does not affect the action of ticarcillin. However, clavulanic acid has a beta-lactam ring and is structurally similar to penicillin and cephalosporins; it binds irreversibly with certain beta-lactamases, preventing inactivation of ticarcillin and broadening its bactericidal spectrum.

Spectrum of activity of ticarcillin includes many gram-negative aerobic and anaerobic bacilli, many gram-positive and gram-negative aerobic cocci, and some gram-positive aerobic and anaerobic bacilli. The combination of ticarcillin and clavulanate potassium is also effective against many beta-lactamase–producing strains, including *Staphylococcus aureus, Haemophilus influenzae, Neisseria gonorrhoeae, Escherichia coli, Klebsiella, Providencia,* and *Bacteroides fragilis,* but not *Pseudomonas aeruginosa.*

Pharmacokinetics

• *Absorption:* Ticarcillin disodium/calvulanate potassium is only administered I.V.; peak plasma concentration occurs immediately after infusion is complete.

• *Distribution:* Ticarcillin disodium is distributed widely. It penetrates minimally into CSF with uninflamed meninges; clavulanic acid penetrates into pleural fluid, lungs, and peritoneal fluid. Ticarcillin sodium achieves high concentrations in urine. Protein-binding is 45% to 65% for ticarcillin and 22% to 30% for clavulanic acid; both cross the placenta.

• *Metabolism:* About 13% of a ticarcillin dose is metabolized by hydrolysis to inactive compounds; clavulanic acid is thought to undergo extensive metabolism, but its fate is as yet unknown.

• *Excretion:* Ticarcillin is excreted primarily (83% to 90%) in urine by renal tubular secretion and glomerular filtration; it is also excreted in bile and in breast milk. Metabolites of clavulanate are excreted in urine by glomerular filtration and in breast milk. Elimination half-life of ticarcillin in adults is about 1 hour and that of clavulanate is about 1 hour; in severe renal impairment, half-life of ticarcillin is extended to about 8 hours and that of clavulanate to about 3 hours. Both drugs are removed by hemodialysis but only slightly by peritoneal dialysis.

Contraindications and precautions

Contraindicated in patients with hypersensitivity to drug or other penicillins. Use cautiously in patients with other drug allergies, especially to cephalosporins, impaired renal function, hemorrhagic conditions, hypokalemia, or sodium restrictions.

Interactions

Concomitant use of ticarcillin and clavulanate potassium with *aminoglycoside antibiotics* results in synergistic bactericidal effects against *Pseudomonas aeruginosa, Escherichia coli, Klebsiella, Citrobacter, Enterobacter, Serratia,* and *Proteus mirabilis.* However, drugs are physically and chemically incompatible and are inactivated when mixed or given together. In vivo inactivation has been reported when *aminoglycosides* and extended-spectrum penicillins are used concomitantly.

Probenecid blocks tubular secretion of ticarcillin, elevating its serum concentration; it has no effect on clavulanate.

Large doses of penicillin may interfere with renal tubular secretion of *methotrexate,* thus delaying elimination and elevating serum concentrations of methotrexate.

Effects on diagnostic tests

Ticarcillin disodium/clavulanate potassium alters tests for urinary or serum proteins; it interferes with turbidimetric methods that use sulfosalicylic acid, trichloroacetic acid, acetic acid, or nitric acid. Ticarcillin disodium/clavulanate potassium does not interfere with tests using bromophenol blue (Albustix, Albutest, MultiStix). It may falsely decrease serum aminoglycoside concentration.

Systemic effects of ticarcillin disodium/clavulanate potassium may cause positive Coombs' test, hypokalemia, and hypernatremia and may prolong PT; it may also cause transient elevations in liver function studies and transient reductions in RBC, WBC, and platelet counts.

Adverse reactions

CNS: ***seizures,*** neuromuscular excitability, headache, giddiness.

GI: nausea, diarrhea, stomatitis, vomiting, epigastric pain, flatulence, pseudomembranous colitis, taste and smell disturbances.
Hematologic: leukopenia, ***neutropenia,*** eosinophilia, ***thrombocytopenia,*** hemolytic anemia, anemia.
Other: hypersensitivity reactions (rash, pruritus, urticaria, chills, fever, edema, ***anaphylaxis***), overgrowth of nonsusceptible organisms, hypokalemia, pain at injection site, vein irritation, phlebitis.

Overdose and treatment

Clinical signs of overdose include neuromuscular hypersensitivity or seizures; ticarcillin and clavulanate potassium can be removed by hemodialysis.

☑ Special considerations

Besides those relevant to all *penicillins,* consider the following recommendations.

- Ticarcillin disodium/clavulanate potassium is almost always used with another antibiotic such as an aminoglycoside in life-threatening situations.
- Administer aminogylcosides 1 hour before or after administration of ticarcillin disodium/clavulanate potassium.
- Ticarcillin contains 5.2 mEq of sodium per gram of drug. Use with caution in patients with sodium restriction.
- Monitor serum electrolytes. Observe for signs of hypernatremia and hypokalemia.
- Monitor neurologic status. High blood levels may cause seizures.
- Because ticarcillin disodium/clavulanate potassium is dialyzable, patients undergoing hemodialysis may need dosage adjustments.

Geriatric use

- Half-life may be prolonged in elderly patients because of impaired renal function.

Breast-feeding

- Ticarcillin and clavulanate potassium are excreted in breast milk; use with caution in breast-feeding women.

ticlopidine hydrochloride

Ticlid

Pharmacologic classification: platelet aggregation inhibitor
Therapeutic classification: antithrombotic
Pregnancy risk category B

How supplied

Available by prescription only
Tablets (film-coated): 250 mg

Indications, route, and dosage

Reduction of risk of thrombotic stroke in patients with history of stroke, in those who have experienced stroke precursors, or in those who are intolerant to aspirin therapy
Adults: 250 mg P.O. b.i.d. with meals.

Pharmacodynamics

Antithrombotic action: Ticlopidine blocks adenosine diphosphate–induced platelet-fibrinogen and platelet-platelet binding, which is different from any other antiplatelet drug.

Pharmacokinetics

- *Absorption:* Rapidly and extensively (over 80%) absorbed after oral administration; peak plasma levels occur within 2 hours. Absorption is enhanced by food.
- *Distribution:* Drug is 98% bound to serum proteins and lipoproteins.
- *Metabolism:* Drug is extensively metabolized by the liver. Over 20 metabolites have been identified; it is unknown if parent drug or active metabolites are responsible for pharmacologic activity.
- *Excretion:* 60% of drug is excreted in urine and 23% in feces; only trace amounts of intact drug are found in urine.

Contraindications and precautions

Contraindicated in patients with hypersensitivity to drug, hematopoietic disorders (such as neutropenia, thrombocytopenia, or disorders of hemostasis), active pathologic bleeding from peptic ulceration or active intracranial bleeding, or severely impaired hepatic function.

Interactions

Use with *theophylline* causes decreased theophylline clearance and increased risk of toxicity; monitor closely and adjust theophylline dosage as indicated. Concurrent use with *antacids* decreases plasma levels of ticlopidine; separate administration times by at least 2 hours. Use with *aspirin* potentiates effects of aspirin on platelets; avoid concomitant use. *Cimetidine* decreases clearance of ticlopidine and increases risk of toxicity; avoid concomitant use. Use with *digoxin* causes slightly decreased serum digoxin levels; monitor serum digoxin levels.

Effects on diagnostic tests

Pharmacologic effects of drug result in prolonged bleeding time. Toxic effects are evident in a decreased neutrophil or platelet count and elevated liver function tests. A positive antinuclear antibody titer has been reported rarely.

Adverse reactions

CNS: dizziness, ***intracerebral bleeding,*** peripheral neuropathy.
CV: vasculitis.
EENT: epistaxis, conjunctival hemorrhage.
GI: *diarrhea, nausea, dyspepsia, abdominal pain,* anorexia, vomiting, flatulence, bleeding, light-colored stools.
GU: hematuria, ***nephrotic syndrome,*** dark-colored urine.
Hematologic: ***neutropenia, pancytopenia, agranulocytosis, immune thrombocytopenia.***
Hepatic: hepatitis, cholestatic jaundice, abnormal liver function tests.
Respiratory: ***allergic pneumonitis.***

Skin: *rash,* pruritus, ecchymoses, maculopapular rash, urticaria, ***thrombocytopenic purpura.***
Other: hypersensitivity reactions, postoperative bleeding, systemic lupus erythematosus, ***serum sickness, hyponatremia,*** arthropathy, myositis, *increased serum cholesterol levels.*

Overdose and treatment

Only one case of overdosage has been reported. The patient, who ingested over 6 g of drug, showed increased bleeding time and increased ALT levels. The patient recovered with supportive therapy alone.

☑ Special considerations

• If drug is being substituted for a fibrinolytic or anticoagulant drug, discontinue previous agent before starting ticlopidine therapy.
• If necessary, methylprednisolone 20 mg I.V. has been shown to normalize the bleeding time within 2 hours. Platelet transfusions may also be necessary.
• Monitor CBC and WBC differential every 2 weeks for the first 3 months of therapy. Severe hematologic adverse events can occur with ticlopidine.
• After the first 3 months of therapy, perform CBC and WBC differential determinations in patients showing signs of infection.
• Perform baseline liver function tests and repeat whenever liver dysfunction is suspected. Monitor closely, especially during the first 4 months of treatment.
• Drug has been used investigationally for many conditions, including intermittent claudication, chronic arterial occlusion, subarachnoid hemorrhage, primary glomerulonephritis, and sickle cell disease. When used preoperatively, it may decrease incidence of graft occlusion in patients receiving coronary artery bypass grafts and reduce severity of decreased platelet count in patients receiving extracorporeal hemoperfusion during open heart surgery.

Patient education

• Inform patient that an information leaflet is available that discusses safe use of drug.
• Tell patient to take drug with meals because food substantially increases bioavailability and improves GI tolerance.
• Instruct patient scheduled for elective surgery to notify his prescribing health care provider and be prepared to discontinue drug 10 to 14 days before procedure.
• Be sure that patient understands the need to report for regular blood tests. Neutropenia can result in an increased risk of infection. Tell patient to report signs and symptoms of infection, such as fever, chills, or sore throat, immediately.
• Tell patient to immediately report yellow skin or sclera, severe or persistent diarrhea, rash, subcutaneous bleeding, light-colored stools, or dark urine.
• Emphasize that drug prolongs bleeding time. Tell patient to report unusual bleeding and to inform dentists and other health care providers that he is taking ticlopidine.
• Warn patient to avoid aspirin and aspirin-containing products, which may also prolong bleeding. Instruct him to call before taking OTC medications because many contain aspirin.

Pediatric use

• Safety and efficacy in children under age 18 have not been established.

Breast-feeding

• Although drug has been found in breast milk in animals, it is unknown if it is excreted in human milk. Breast-feeding is not recommended.

tiludronate disodium

Skelid

Pharmacologic classification: bisphosphonate analogue
Therapeutic classification: antihypercalcemic
Pregnancy risk category C

How supplied

Available by prescription only
Tablets: 200 mg

Indications, route, and dosage

Paget's disease
Adults: 400 mg P.O. once daily taken with 6 to 8 oz (180 to 240 ml) of water for 3 months, given 2 hours before or after meals.

Pharmacodynamics

Antihypercalcemic action: Tiludronate is thought to suppress bone resorption by reducing osteoclastic activity. Appears to inhibit osteoclasts through the following mechanisms: disruption of the cytoskeletal ring structure, possibly by inhibiting protein-tyrosine-phosphatase, thus leading to detachment of osteoclasts from the bone surface; and the inhibition of the osteoclastic proton pump.

Pharmacokinetics

• *Absorption:* Bioavailability of drug on an empty stomach is 8%. Food and beverages other than water can reduce bioavailability by up to 90%.
• *Distribution:* Drug is widely distributed in bone and soft tissue. Protein binding is approximately 90% (mainly albumin).
• *Metabolism:* Tiludronate does not appear to be metabolized.
• *Excretion:* Principally in the urine. Mean plasma half-life, 150 hours.

Contraindications and precautions

Contraindicated in patients with known hypersensitivity to any component of drug and in patients with creatinine clearance below 30 ml/minute. Use cautiously in patients with upper GI disease, such as dysphagia, esophagitis, esophageal ulcer, or gastric ulcer.

Interactions

Calcium supplements, aluminum antacids, and *magnesium antacids* may dramatically reduce bioavailability of tiludronate 80%, 60%, and 60%, respectively, when administered 1 hour before tiludronate. *Aspirin* may decrease bioavailability by up to 50% when taken 2 hours after tiludronate. *Indomethacin* may also increase bioavailability of tiludronate.

Effects on diagnostic tests
None reported.

Adverse reactions
CNS: anxiety, dizziness, headache, insomnia, involuntary muscle contractions, paresthesia, somnolence, vertigo.
CV: chest pain, hypertension.
EENT: cataracts, conjunctivitis, glaucoma, pharyngitis, sinusitis, rhinitis.
Endocrine: hyperparathyroidism.
GI: anorexia, constipation, diarrhea, dry mouth, dyspepsia, flatulence, gastritis, nausea, tooth disorder, vomiting.
Metabolic: vitamin D deficiency.
Respiratory: bronchitis, coughing, crackles.
Skin: pruritus.
Other: arthralgia, arthrosis, edema, back pain, sweating, *whole body pain.*

Overdose and treatment
No specific information is available. Use standard treatment for hypocalcemia or renal insufficiency, if they occur. Dialysis is not beneficial.

☑ Special considerations
- Drug should be used in patients with Paget's disease who have serum alkaline phosphatase level at least twice the upper limit of normal or who are symptomatic or at risk for future complications of disease.
- Administer drug for 3 months to assess response.
- Hypocalcemia and other disturbances of mineral metabolism (such as vitamin D deficiency) should be corrected prior to initiating therapy.

Patient education
- Tell patient to take drug with 6 to 8 oz (180 to 240 ml) of water.
- Instruct patient that drug should not be taken within 2 hours of food.
- Advise patient to maintain adequate vitamin D and calcium intake.
- Inform patient that calcium supplements, aspirin, and indomethacin should not be taken within 2 hours before or after tiludronate.
- Tell patient that aluminum and magnesium containing antacids can be taken 2 hours after taking tiludronate.

Geriatric use
- Plasma concentrations may be higher in the elderly. However, dosage adjustment is not necessary.

Pediatric use
- Safety and effectiveness have not been established.

Breast-feeding
- It is not known if drug is excreted in breast milk. Therefore, use cautiously in breast-feeding women.

timolol maleate
Blocadren, Timoptic, Timoptic-XE

Pharmacologic classification: beta-adrenergic blocker
Therapeutic classification: antihypertensive, adjunct in MI, antiglaucoma
Pregnancy risk category C

How supplied
Available by prescription only
Tablets: 5 mg, 10 mg, 20 mg
Ophthalmic gel: 0.25%, 0.5%
Ophthalmic solution: 0.25%, 0.5%

Indications, route, and dosage
Hypertension
Adults: Initially, 10 mg P.O. b.i.d. Usual maintenance dosage, 20 to 40 mg/day. Maximum dosage, 60 mg/day.
Reduction of risk of CV mortality and reinfarction after MI
Adults: 10 mg P.O. b.i.d. initiated within 1 to 4 weeks after infarction.
◊ ***Angina***
Adults: 15 to 45 mg P.O. daily given in three divided doses.
Glaucoma
Adults: 1 drop of 0.25% or 0.5% solution to the conjunctiva once or twice daily; or 1 drop of 0.25% or 0.5% gel to the conjunctiva once daily.
◊ ***Migraine headache***
Adults: 10 mg P.O. daily b.i.d., then increase up to 20 mg; or 30-mg dose (10 mg P.O. in the morning and 20 mg P.O. in the evening).

Pharmacodynamics
Antihypertensive action: Exact mechanism of antihypertensive effect of timolol is unknown. Timolol may reduce blood pressure by blocking adrenergic receptors (thus decreasing cardiac output), by decreasing sympathetic outflow from the CNS, and by suppressing renin release.

MI prophylactic action: Exact mechanism by which timolol decreases mortality after MI is unknown. Timolol produces a negative chronotropic and inotropic activity. This decrease in heart rate and myocardial contractility results in reduced myocardial oxygen consumption.

Antiglaucoma action: Beta-blocking action of timolol decreases the production of aqueous humor, thereby decreasing intraocular pressure.

Pharmacokinetics
- *Absorption:* About 90% of an oral dose of timolol is absorbed from the GI tract; peak plasma concentration occurs in 1 to 2 hours.
- *Distribution:* After oral administration, timolol is distributed throughout the body; depending on assay method, drug is 10% to 60% protein-bound.

• *Metabolism:* About 80% of a given dose of timolol is metabolized in the liver to inactive metabolites.
• *Excretion:* Drug and its metabolites are excreted primarily in urine; half-life is approximately 4 hours. After topical application to the eye, effects of timolol last up to 24 hours.

Contraindications and precautions
Contraindicated in patients with bronchial asthma, severe COPD, sinus bradycardia and heart block greater than first degree, cardiogenic shock, heart failure, or hypersensitivity to drug.

Use cautiously in patients with diabetes, hyperthyroidism, or respiratory disease (especially nonallergic bronchospasm or emphysema). Use oral form cautiously in patients with compensated heart failure and hepatic or renal disease. Use ophthalmic form cautiously in patients with cerebrovascular insufficiency.

Interactions
When used as an antihypertensive, timolol may potentiate antihypertensive effects of *other antihypertensive agents*; its antihypertensive effects may be antagonized by *NSAIDs*. Patients receiving ophthalmic or oral timolol may experience excessive hypotension when administered *general anesthetics* or *fentanyl*. Timolol may antagonize the effects of *xanthines* or *beta-adrenergic stimulants*. arrhythmias may occur if used with *calcium channel blocking agents* or *cardiac glycosides*. Timolol may increase the plasma concentration of *phenothiazines*.

Effects on diagnostic tests
Drug may slightly increase BUN, serum potassium, uric acid, and blood glucose levels and may slightly lower hemoglobin levels and hematocrit.

Adverse reactions
CNS: fatigue, lethargy, dizziness; depression, hallucinations, confusion (with ophthalmic form).
CV: ***arrhythmias,*** bradycardia, hypotension, ***heart failure;*** peripheral vascular disease, pulmonary edema (with oral administration); ***CVA, cardiac arrest,*** heart block, palpitations (with ophthalmic form).
EENT: minor eye irritation, decreased corneal sensitivity with long-term use, conjunctivitis, blepharitis, keratitis, visual disturbances, diplopia, ptosis (with ophthalmic form).
GI: nausea, vomiting, diarrhea (with oral administration).
Respiratory: dyspnea, ***bronchospasm,*** increased airway resistance (with oral administration); ***asthmatic attacks in patients with history of asthma*** (with ophthalmic form).
Skin: pruritus (with oral administration).

Overdose and treatment
Clinical signs of overdose include severe hypotension, bradycardia, heart failure, and bronchospasm.

After acute ingestion, empty stomach by induced emesis or gastric lavage and give activated charcoal to reduce absorption. Subsequent treatment is usually symptomatic and supportive.

☑ Special considerations
Besides those relevant to all *beta-adrenergic blocking agents,* consider the following recommendations.
• Dosage adjustment may be necessary for a patient with renal or hepatic impairment.
• Although controversial, drug may need to be discontinued 48 hours before surgery in patients receiving ophthalmic timolol because systemic absorption occurs.

Patient education
• For ophthalmic form of timolol, teach patient proper method of eyedrop administration. Warn patient not to touch dropper to eye or surrounding tissue; lightly press lacrimal sac with finger after administration to decrease systemic absorption.
• Instruct patient to invert ophthalmic gel container once before each use.
• Instruct patient to administer other ophthalmic drugs at least 10 minutes before the ophthalmic gel.

Geriatric use
• Elderly patients may require lower oral maintenance dosages of timolol because of increased bioavailability or delayed metabolism; they also may experience enhanced adverse effects. Use cautiously because half-life may be prolonged in elderly patients.

Pediatric use
• Safety and efficacy in children have not been established; use only if potential benefit outweighs risk.

Breast-feeding
• Timolol is distributed into breast milk. Because of the potential for serious adverse reactions in breast-fed infants, an alternative feeding method is recommended during therapy.

tioconazole
Vagistat-1

Pharmacologic classification: imidazole derivative
Therapeutic classification: antifungal
Pregnancy risk category C

How supplied
Available by prescription only
Vaginal ointment: 6.5%

Indications, route, and dosage
Treatment of vulvovaginal candidiasis
Adults: Insert 1 full applicator (about 4.6 g) intravaginally h.s. as a single dose.

Pharmacodynamics
Antifungal action: Tioconazole is a fungicidal imidazole that alters cell wall permeability.

Pharmacokinetics
• *Absorption:* Negligible.
• *Distribution:* Unknown.

- *Metabolism:* Unknown.
- *Excretion:* Unknown.

Contraindications and precautions
Contraindicated in patients hypersensitive to drug or other imidazole antifungal agents (miconazole, ketoconazole) and in breast-feeding women.

Interactions
None reported.

Effects on diagnostic tests
None reported.

Adverse reactions
GU: *burning, pruritus,* discharge, vaginal pain, dysuria, dyspareunia, vulvar edema, irritation.

Overdose and treatment
No information available.

☑ Special considerations
- Because drug is useful only for candidal vulvovaginitis, the diagnosis should be confirmed by potassium hydroxide smears or cultures before treatment with tioconazole.

Patient education
- Review correct use of drug with patient. She should insert drug high into the vagina. Detailed instructions for the patient are available with the product.
- Tell patient to avoid sexual intercourse during therapy or advise partner to use a condom to prevent reinfection.
- Warn patient to open applicator just before using product to avoid contamination.
- Tell patient to watch for and report irritation or sensitivity.
- Emphasize need for patient to continue therapy for the full course, even if symptoms have improved, and during menstrual period.
- Advise patient to use a sanitary napkin to avoid staining of clothing.

Breast-feeding
- Instruct patient to temporarily stop breast-feeding during therapy.

tiopronin
Thiola

Pharmacologic classification: thiol compound
Therapeutic classification: cystine-solubilizing agent
Pregnancy risk category C

How supplied
Available by prescription only
Tablets: 100 mg

Indications, route, and dosage
Prevention of urinary cystine stone formation in patients with severe homozygous cystinuria (urinary cystine excretion exceeding 500 mg daily) that is unresponsive to other therapies
Adults: 800 mg P.O. daily, divided t.i.d. initially, then adjust dosage to control urinary cystine levels. Usual dosage is 1,000 mg daily in divided doses.
Children age 9 and over: 15 mg/kg P.O. daily, divided t.i.d.

Give 1 hour before or 2 hours after meals.

Pharmacodynamics
Cystine solubilizing action: Tiopronin undergoes a thiol-disulfide exchange with cystine in the urine. This complex is water soluble, increases cystine solubility, and prevents the formation of urinary cystine stones.

Pharmacokinetics
- *Absorption:* Rapidly absorbed after oral administration.
- *Distribution:* Not fully characterized.
- *Metabolism:* Not fully characterized.
- *Excretion:* Up to 48% of dose appears in urine after 4 hours; 78% after 3 days.

Contraindications and precautions
Contraindicated in patients with history of agranulocytosis, aplastic anemia, or thrombocytopenia.

Interactions
None reported.

Effects on diagnostic tests
None reported.

Adverse reactions
GI: hypogeusia.
Skin: rash, pruritus, wrinkling, friability.
Other: drug fever, lupus erythematosus-like reaction.

Overdose and treatment
No information available.

☑ Special considerations
- Dosage is usually adjusted to keep urinary cystine levels below 250 mg/L.
- Attempt conservative measures to treat cystinuria before administering drug. Patients should drink at least 3 L of fluid daily, including at least two 8-oz (240 ml) glasses of water at each meal and at bedtime. Patient's urine output should be at least 2 L daily, and urine pH should be at least 6.5. Excessive alkalization of urine may precipitate calcium stones. Urine pH should not exceed 7.
- Penicillamine has been used for cystinuria therapy, although patients may not tolerate it well. Studies indicate that about two thirds of patients who cannot tolerate penicillamine will tolerate tiopronin.
- Several clinical tests are recommended at 3- to 6-month intervals during treatment, including CBC, platelet counts, hemoglobin, serum albumin, liver function tests, 24-hour urinary protein, and routine urinalysis.
- Monitor urinary cystine frequently during first 6 months of treatment (to assess dosage level) and then at least every 6 months.

• An annual abdominal X-ray is advised to assess for presence of stones.

Patient education

• Tell patient to report signs or symptoms of hematologic abnormalities, including fever, sore throat, bleeding or bruising, or chills. Blood dyscrasias have been reported in patients receiving other drugs for cystinuria.
• Instruct patient to take drug at least 1 hour before or 2 hours after meals, if possible.
• Tell patient to report taste alterations. Hypogeusia may develop as a result of trace metal chelation by drug.

Pediatric use

• Safety and effectiveness in children under age 9 have not been established.

Breast-feeding

• Breast-feeding is not recommended. Drug may be excreted in breast milk, and it may be hazardous to neonates and infants.

tobramycin

tobramycin ophthalmic
Tobrex

tobramycin sulfate
Nebcin

tobramycin solution for inhalation
TOBI

Pharmacologic classification: aminoglycoside
Therapeutic classification: antibiotic
Pregnancy risk category D

How supplied

Available by prescription only
Injection: 40 mg/ml, 10 mg/ml (pediatric)
Ophthalmic solution: 0.3%
Ophthalmic ointment: 0.3%
Nebulizer solution for inhalation: single-use 5 ml (300 mg) ampule

Indications, route, and dosage

***Serious infections caused by sensitive* Escherichia coli, Proteus, Klebsiella, Enterobacter, Serratia, Staphylococcus aureus, Pseudomonas, Citrobacter, *or* Providencia**
Adults and children with normal renal function: 3 mg/kg I.M. or I.V. daily, divided q 8 hours. Up to 5 mg/kg I.M. or I.V. daily, divided q 6 to 8 hours for life-threatening infections.
Neonates under age 1 week: Up to 4 mg/kg I.M. or I.V. daily, divided q 12 hours. For I.V. use, dilute in 50 to 100 ml 0.9% NaCl solution or D_5W for adults and in less volume for children. Infuse over 20 to 60 minutes.
✦ ***Dosage adjustment.*** In patients with impaired renal function, initial dosage is same as for those with normal renal function. Subsequent doses and frequency are determined by renal function study results and blood levels; keep peak serum concentrations between 4 and 10 mcg/ml and trough serum concentrations between 1 and 2 mcg/ml. Several methods have been used to calculate dosage in renal failure.

After a 1 mg/kg loading dose, adjust subsequent dosage by reducing doses administered at 8-hour intervals or by prolonging the interval between normal doses. Both of these methods are useful when serum levels of tobramycin cannot be measured directly. They are based on either creatinine clearance (preferred) or serum creatinine because these values correlate with drug's half-life.

To calculate reduced dosage for 8-hour intervals, use available nomograms; or, if patient's steady state serum creatinine values are known, divide the normally recommended dose by patient's serum creatinine value. To determine frequency in hours for normal dosage (if creatinine clearance rate is not available), divide the normal dose by patient's serum creatinine value. Dosage schedules derived from either method require careful clinical and laboratory observations of patient and should be adjusted as appropriate. These methods of calculation may be misleading in elderly patients and in those with severe wasting; neither should be used when dialysis is performed.

Hemodialysis removes 50% to 75% of a dose in 6 hours. In anephric patients maintained by dialysis, 1.5 to 2 mg/kg after each dialysis usually maintains therapeutic, nontoxic serum levels. Patients receiving peritoneal dialysis twice a week should receive a 1.5 to 2 mg/kg loading dose followed by 1 mg/kg q 3 days. Those receiving dialysis q 2 days should receive a 1.5 mg/kg loading dose after first dialysis and 0.75 mg/kg after each subsequent dialysis.

◇ **Intrathecally or intraventricularly**
Adults: 3 to 8 mg q 18 to 48 hours.

***Management of cystic fibrosis patients with* P. aeruginosa**
Adults and children over age 6: 1 single use ampule (300 mg) administered by inhalation q 12 hours for 28 days, then off for 28 days, then on for 28 days as advised by health care provider. There is no dosage adjustment for age or renal failure.

Treatment of external ocular infection caused by susceptible gram-negative bacteria
Adults and children: In mild to moderate infections, instill 1 or 2 drops into affected eye q 4 to 6 hours. In severe infections, instill 2 drops into the affected eye hourly or apply a small amount of ointment into conjunctival sac t.i.d. or q.i.d.

Pharmacodynamics

Antibiotic action: Tobramycin is bactericidal; it binds directly to the 30S ribosomal subunit, thereby inhibiting bacterial protein synthesis. Its spectrum of activity includes many aerobic gram-negative organisms, including most strains of *P. aeruginosa* and some aerobic gram-positive organisms. Tobramycin may act against some bacterial strains resistant to other aminoglycosides; many strains resistant to tobramycin are susceptible to amikacin, gentamicin, or netilmicin.

Pharmacokinetics

- *Absorption:* Drug is absorbed poorly after oral administration and usually is given parenterally; peak serum concentrations occur 30 to 90 minutes after I.M. administration. Inhaled drug remains concentrated in the airway, with serum concentration after 20 weeks of therapy being 1.05 µg/ml 1 hour after dosing.
- *Distribution:* Drug is distributed widely after parenteral administration; intraocular penetration is poor. CSF penetration is low, even in patients with inflamed meninges. Protein binding is minimal; tobramycin crosses the placenta. Inhaled drug remains primarily concentrated in the airway.
- *Metabolism:* Not metabolized.
- *Excretion:* Excreted primarily in urine by glomerular filtration; small amounts may be excreted in bile and breast milk. Elimination half-life in adults, 2 to 3 hours. In severe renal damage, half-life may extend to 24 to 60 hours. With inhalation use, unabsorbed tobramycin is probably eliminated in the sputum.

Contraindications and precautions

Contraindicated in patients with hypersensitivity to drug or other aminoglycosides. Use injectable form cautiously in patients with impaired renal function or neuromuscular disorders and in the elderly.

Interactions

Concomitant use with the following drugs may increase the hazard of nephrotoxicity, ototoxicity, and neurotoxicity: *methoxyflurane, polymyxin B, vancomycin, capreomycin, cisplatin, cephalosporins, amphotericin B,* and *other aminoglycosides*; hazard of ototoxicity is also increased during use with *bumetanide, ethacrynic acid, furosemide, mannitol,* or *urea. Dimenhydrinate* and other *antiemetic* and *antivertigo drugs* may mask tobramycin-induced ototoxicity.

Concomitant use with some *penicillins* results in a synergistic bactericidal effect against *P. aeruginosa, E. coli, Klebsiella, Citrobacter, Enterobacter, Serratia,* and *Proteus mirabilis.* However, drugs are physically and chemically incompatible and are inactivated when mixed or given together. In vivo inactivation has been reported when *aminoglycosides* and *penicillins* are used concomitantly.

Tobramycin may potentiate neuromuscular blockade from *general anesthetics* or *neuromuscular blocking agents,* such as *succinylcholine* and *tubocurarine.*

Effects on diagnostic tests

Tobramycin may elevate BUN, nonprotein nitrogen, or serum creatinine levels and increase urinary excretion of casts.

Adverse reactions

CNS: headache, lethargy, confusion, disorientation (with injectable form).
EENT: *ototoxicity* (with injectable form); blurred vision (with ophthalmic ointment); burning or stinging on instillation, lid itching or swelling, conjunctival erythema (with ophthalmic administration).
GI: vomiting, nausea, diarrhea (with injectable form).
GU: *nephrotoxicity* (with injectable form).
Hematologic: anemia, eosinophilia, leukopenia, ***thrombocytopenia, granulocytopenia*** (with injectable form).
Respiratory: ***bronchospasm*** (with inhalation form).
Skin: rash, urticaria, pruritus (with injectable form).
Other: fever, hypersensitivity reactions, overgrowth of nonsusceptible organisms (with ophthalmic administration).

Overdose and treatment

Clinical signs of overdose include ototoxicity, nephrotoxicity, and neuromuscular toxicity. Remove drug by hemodialysis or peritoneal dialysis. Treatment with calcium salts or anticholinesterases reverses neuromuscular blockade.

☑ Special considerations

Besides those relevant to all *aminoglycosides,* consider the following recommendations.

- For I.V. administration, the usual volume of diluent (0.9% NaCl injection or 5% dextrose injection) for adult doses is 50 to 100 ml. For children, the volume should be proportionately less. Infusion should be over 20 to 60 minutes.
- Do not premix tobramycin with other drugs; administer separately at least 1 hour apart.
- Discontinue ophthalmic preparation if keratitis, erythema, lacrimation, edema, or lid itching occurs.
- Because tobramycin is dialyzable, patients undergoing hemodialysis may need dosage adjustments.
- Inhalation form of tobramycin is an orphan drug used specifically for management of cystic fibrosis patients with *P. aeruginosa.*

Patient education

- Advise patient that inhalation doses should be taken as close to 12 hours apart as possible and no less than 6 hours apart.
- Teach patient how to use and maintain nebulizer.

tocainide hydrochloride

Tonocard

Pharmacologic classification: local anesthetic (amide type)
Therapeutic classification: ventricular antiarrhythmic
Pregnancy risk category C

How supplied

Available by prescription only
Tablets: 400 mg, 600 mg

Indications, route, and dosage

Suppression of symptomatic ventricular arrhythmias, including frequent premature ventricular tachycardia
Dosage must be individualized based on antiarrhythmic response and tolerance.

Adults: Initially, 400 mg P.O. q 8 hours. Usual dosage is between 1,200 and 1,800 mg/day, divided into three doses.
✦ ***Dosage adjustment.*** Patients with impaired renal or hepatic function may be adequately treated with less than 1,200 mg/day.
◊ ***Myotonic dystrophy***
Adults: 800 to 1,200 mg P.O. daily.
◊ ***Trigeminal neuralgia***
Adults: 20 mg/kg/day P.O. t.i.d.

Pharmacodynamics

Antiarrhythmic action: Tocainide is structurally similar to lidocaine and possesses similar electrophysiologic and hemodynamic effects. A class IB antiarrhythmic, it suppresses automaticity and shortens the effective refractory period and action potential duration of His-Purkinje fibers and suppresses spontaneous ventricular depolarization during diastole. Conductive atrial tissue and AV conduction are not affected significantly at therapeutic concentrations. Unlike quinidine and procainamide, tocainide does not significantly alter hemodynamics when administered in usual doses. Tocainide exerts its effects on the conduction system, causing inhibition of reentry mechanisms and cessation of ventricular arrhythmias; these effects may be more pronounced in ischemic tissue. Tocainide does not cause a significant negative inotropic effect. Its direct cardiac effects are less potent than those of lidocaine.

Pharmacokinetics

- *Absorption:* Rapidly and completely absorbed from the GI tract; unlike lidocaine, it undergoes negligible first-pass effect in the liver. Peak serum levels occur in 30 minutes to 2 hours after oral administration. Bioavailability is nearly 100%.
- *Distribution:* Tocainide's distribution is only partially known. However, it appears to be distributed widely and apparently crosses the blood-brain barrier and placenta in animals (however, it is less lipophilic than lidocaine). Only about 10% to 20% of the drug is bound to plasma protein.
- *Metabolism:* Metabolized apparently in the liver to inactive metabolites.
- *Excretion:* Excreted in the urine as unchanged drug and inactive metabolites. About 30% to 50% of an orally administered dose is excreted in the urine as metabolites. Elimination half-life is approximately 11 to 23 hours, with an initial biphasic plasma concentration decline similar to that of lidocaine's. Half-life may be prolonged in patients with renal or hepatic insufficiency. Urine alkalinization may substantially decrease the amount of unchanged drug excreted in the urine.

Contraindications and precautions

Contraindicated in patients with hypersensitivity to lidocaine or other amide-type local anesthetics and in those with second- or third-degree AV block in the absence of an artificial pacemaker. Use cautiously in patients with heart failure, diminished cardiac reserve, or impaired renal or hepatic function.

Interactions

When used concomitantly with *other antiarrhythmics,* tocainide may cause additive, synergistic, or antagonistic effects. (Concomitant use with *lidocaine* may cause CNS toxicity.) Concomitant use with *metoprolol* may cause additive effects on cardiac index, left ventricular function, and pulmonary wedge pressure, necessitating monitoring for decreased myocardial contractility and bradycardia. *Rifampin* and *cimetidine* may decrease elimination half-life and bioavailability of tocainide. Allopurinal will increase the effects of this drug.

Effects on diagnostic tests

Drug may cause abnormal liver function tests, especially during early stages of therapy.

Adverse reactions

CNS: *light-headedness, tremor,* paresthesia, *dizziness, vertigo,* drowsiness, fatigue, confusion, headache.
CV: hypotension, ***new or worsened arrhythmias, heart failure,*** bradycardia, palpitations.
EENT: blurred vision, tinnitus.
GI: *nausea, vomiting,* diarrhea, anorexia.
Hematologic: ***blood dyscrasia.***
Hepatic: hepatitis.
Respiratory: ***respiratory arrest, pulmonary fibrosis, pneumonitis, pulmonary edema.***
Skin: rash, diaphoresis.

Overdose and treatment

Clinical effects of overdose include extensions of common adverse reactions, particularly those associated with the CNS or GI tract.

Treatment generally involves symptomatic and supportive care. In acute overdose, gastric emptying should be performed via emesis induction or gastric lavage. Respiratory depression necessitates immediate attention and maintenance of a patent airway with ventilatory assistance, if required. Seizures may be treated with small incremental doses of a benzodiazepine, such as diazepam or a short or ultrashort-acting barbiturate, such as pentobarbital or thiopental.

☑ Special considerations

- Use cautiously, and with lower doses, in patients with hepatic or renal impairment.
- Monitor blood levels; therapeutic levels range from 4 to 10 mcg/ml.
- Monitor periodic blood counts.
- Observe patient for tremors—a possible sign that maximum safe dosage has been reached.
- Adverse effects tend to be frequent and problematic.
- Drug is considered an oral lidocaine and may be used to ease transition from I.V. lidocaine to oral antiarrhythmic therapy.

Patient education

- Instruct patient to report unusual bleeding or bruising, signs or symptoms of infection (such as fever, sore throat, stomatitis, or chills) or pulmonary symptoms (such as cough, wheezing, or exertional dyspnea).

• Tell patient he may take tocainide with food to lessen GI upset.

Geriatric use
• Use with caution in elderly patients; increased serum drug levels and toxicity are more likely. Monitor carefully.
• Elderly patients are more likely to experience dizziness and should have assistance while walking.

Breast-feeding
• Safety has not been established. Alternative feeding method is recommended during therapy with tocainide.

tolazoline hydrochloride
Priscoline

Pharmacologic classification: peripheral vasodilator, alpha-adrenergic blocker
Therapeutic classification: antihypertensive
Pregnancy risk category C

How supplied
Available by prescription only
Injection: 25 mg/ml in 10-ml vials

Indications, route, and dosage
Persistent pulmonary vasoconstriction and hypertension of the newborn (persistent fetal circulation)
Neonates: Initially, 1 to 2 mg/kg I.V. via a scalp vein over 10 minutes, followed by an I.V. infusion of 1 to 2 mg/kg/hour.
◊ ***Peripheral vasospastic disorders***
Adults: 10 to 50 mg S.C., I.M., or I.V. q.i.d.
◊ ***To improve visualization of vasculature***
Adults: 12.5 to 50 mg intra-arterially before angiography.

Pharmacodynamics
Antihypertensive action: Tolazoline, by direct relaxation of vascular smooth muscle, causes peripheral vasodilation and decreased peripheral resistance. Tolazoline inhibits responses to adrenergic stimuli by competitively blocking alpha-adrenergic receptors; however, at usual doses, this effect is relatively transient and incomplete.

Pharmacokinetics
• *Absorption:* Drug is absorbed rapidly and almost completely after parenteral administration.
• *Distribution:* Tolazoline concentrates primarily in kidneys and liver.
• *Metabolism:* None.
• *Excretion:* Excreted in urine, primarily as unchanged drug; half-life is inversely related to urine output and can range from 1.5 to 41 hours.

Contraindications and precautions
Contraindicated in neonates with hypersensitivity to drug. Use cautiously in patients with known or suspected mitral stenosis.

Interactions
Tolazoline may cause a disulfiram-type reaction after *alcohol* ingestion because of the accumulation of *acetaldehyde*.

Concomitant use with *epinephrine* or *norepinephrine* may cause "epinephrine reversal"—a paradoxical decrease in blood pressure followed by exaggerated rebound hypertension.

Effects on diagnostic tests
None reported.

Adverse reactions
CV: ***arrhythmias,*** pain, *hypertension, flushing, hypotension,* tachycardia.
GI: *nausea, vomiting, diarrhea,* ***GI hemorrhage.***
GU: edema, oliguria, hematuria.
Hematologic: leukopenia, ***thrombocytopenia.***
Respiratory: ***pulmonary hemorrhage.***
Skin: increased pilomotor activity with tingling and chilliness, rash.

Overdose and treatment
Clinical manifestations of overdose include flushing, hypotension, and shock.

Treat overdose symptomatically and supportively; if vasopressor is necessary, use ephedrine, which has both central and peripheral actions. Avoid epinephrine or norepinephrine because epinephrine reversal may occur from the alpha-blocking effects of tolazoline.

☑ Special considerations
• Keeping patient warm increases the effect of drug.
• Monitor blood pH for acidosis, which may reduce the effect of drug.
• Drug has been used in adults as a provocative test for glaucoma, intra-arterially to improve vascular visualization during angiography, as a diagnostic agent to distinguish between vasospastic or obstructive components of occlusive peripheral vascular disease, and as adjunctive therapy in the treatment of peripheral vascular disorders.

Patient education
• Advise patient's family of treatment required.

Pediatric use
• Drug is indicated for neonatal hypertension and pulmonary vasoconstriction.
• Pretreatment of infants with antacids may prevent GI bleeding.

tolcapone
Tasmar

Pharmacologic classification: catechol-O-methyltransferase (COMT) inhibitor
Therapeutic classification: antiparkinsonian
Pregnancy risk category C

How supplied
Available by prescription only
Tablets: 100 mg, 200 mg

Indications, route, and dosage

Adjunct to levodopa and carbidopa for treatment of signs and symptoms of idiopathic Parkinson's disease

Adults: Initial dosing is 100 mg (preferred) or 200 mg P.O. t.i.d. If initiating treatment with 200 mg t.i.d. and dyskinesias occur then a decrease in dosage of levodopa may be necessary. Maximum daily dose is 600 mg. The first dose of the day of tolcapone should always be taken with the first dose of the day of levodopa/carbidopa.

✦ ***Dosage adjustment.*** Do not exceed 100 mg t.i.d. in patients with severe renal dysfunction.

Pharmacodynamics

Antiparkinsonian action: Exact mechanism unknown. Thought to reversibly inhibit human erythrocyte COMT when given with levodopa/carbidopa, resulting in a decrease in clearance of levodopa and a twofold increase in the bioavailability of levodopa. Decrease in levodopa clearance prolongs its elimination half-life from 2 to 3½ hours.

Pharmacokinetics

- *Absorption:* Drug is rapidly absorbed and reaches peak plasma levels within 2 hours. After oral administration, absolute bioavailability is 65%. Onset of effect occurs following administration of first dose. Absorption decreases when given 1 hour before or 2 hours after food; however, drug can be administered without regard to meals.
- *Distribution:* Highly bound to plasma proteins (over 99.9%), primarily to albumin. The steady-state volume of distribution is small.
- *Metabolism:* Completely metabolized, mainly by glucuronidation.
- *Excretion:* Only 0.5% of dose is found unchanged in the urine. Tolcapone is a low extraction ratio drug with a systemic clearance of 7 L/hour. Elimination half-life, 2 to 3 hours. Dialysis may not be helpful.

Contraindications and precautions

Contraindicated in patients with hypersensitivity to drug, patients with liver disease or those with elevated ALT or AST values, those who were withdrawn from tolcapone because of evidence of drug-induced hepatocellular injury or patients with history of nontraumatic rhabdomyolysis or hyperpyrexia and confusion possibly related to drug. Use cautiously in patients with Parkinson's disease because syncope and orthostatic hypotension may worsen.

Interactions

Administer *desipramine* cautiously with tolcapone because of an increased incidence of adverse effects. Although there is a risk for interactions with *cytochrome substrates 3A4 and 2A6,* they have not been reported. MAO and COMT are two enzyme systems involved in the metabolism of catecholamines. Therefore, it is possible that the combination of tolcapone and *nonselective MAO inhibitors (phenelzine, tranylcypromine)* could result in inhibition of these pathways. Avoid concomitant use of tolcapone and *MAO inhibitors* because it may lead to hypertensive crisis. There does not appear to be an interaction between tolcapone and selective MAO-B inhibitors *(selegiline).*

Effects on diagnostic tests

None reported.

Adverse reactions

CNS: *dyskinesia, sleep disorder, dystonia, excessive dreaming, somnolence, dizziness, confusion, headache, hallucinations,* hyperkinesia, fatigue, falling, syncope, balance loss, depression, tremor, speech disorder, paresthesia.
CV: *orthostatic complaints,* chest pain, chest discomfort, palpitation, hypotension.
EENT: pharyngitis, tinnitus.
GI: *nausea, anorexia, diarrhea,* flatulence, *vomiting,* constipation, abdominal pain, dyspepsia, dry mouth.
GU: urinary tract infection, urine discoloration, hematuria, urinary incontinence, impotence.
Hematologic: ***liver failure.***
Musculoskeletal: *muscle cramps,* myalgia, stiffness, arthritis, neck pain.
Respiratory: bronchitis, dyspnea, upper respiratory infections.
Skin: increased sweating, rash.

Overdose and treatment

The highest dose administered to humans is 800 mg t.i.d. The adverse effects observed were nausea, vomiting, and dizziness. Management includes hospitalization and supportive care if indicated.

☑ Special considerations

- Due to risk of potentially fatal, acute fulminant liver failure, use drug only in patients on levodopa and carbidopa who do not respond to or who are not suitable candidates for other adjunctive therapies.
- Use drug only after patient has provided written informed consent.
- Diarrhea occurs commonly in patients treated with tolcapone. It may occur 2 weeks after therapy begins or after 6 to 12 weeks. Although it usually resolves with discontinuation of drug.
- Dosage adjustments are not necessary in patients with mild to moderate renal dysfunction; however, use caution if patient has severe renal impairment.
- Because of risk of liver toxicity, monitor liver function tests. Stop drug if patient shows no benefit within 3 months. Also, stop drug if test results are elevated or if patient appears jaundiced.
- Do not treat patient concomitantly with a nonselective MAO inhibitor.

Patient education

- Advise patient to take drug exactly as prescribed.
- Tell patient to report signs of liver injury immediately.
- Warn patient about risk of orthostatic hypotension; tell them to use caution when rising from a seated or recumbent position.
- Caution patient to avoid hazardous activities until CNS effects of drug are known.
- Tell patient that nausea may occur upon initiation of therapy.

• Advise patient about risk of increased dyskinesia or dystonia.
• Inform patient that hallucinations may occur.
• Tell patient to report if pregnancy is being planned or suspected during therapy.

Pediatric use

• There is no identified potential use of drug in pediatric patients.

Breast-feeding

• Because of the possibility that tolcapone may be excreted in human breast milk, use caution when administering drug to breast-feeding women.

tolterodine tartrate

Detrol

Pharmacologic classification: muscarinic receptor antagonist
Therapeutic classification: anticholinergic agent
Pregnancy risk category C

How supplied

Available by prescription only
Tablets: 1 mg, 2 mg

Indications, route, and dosage

Treatment of patients with overactive bladder with symptoms of urinary frequency, urgency, or urge incontinence
Adults: Initial dosage is 2 mg P.O. b.i.d. May lower to 1 mg b.i.d. based on patient response and tolerance.
✦ ***Dosage adjustment.*** In patients with significantly reduced hepatic function or who are currently taking a drug that inhibits the cytochrome P-450 3A4 isoenzyme system, recommended dose is 1 mg b.i.d.

Pharmacodynamics

Anticholinergic action: Tolterodine is a competitive muscarinic receptor antagonist. Both urinary bladder contraction and salivation are mediated via cholinergic muscarinic receptors.

Pharmacokinetics

• *Absorption:* Well absorbed with approximately 77% bioavailability. Peak serum levels occur within 1 to 2 hours after administration. Food increases bioavailability by 53%.
• *Distribution:* Volume of distribution is approximately 113 L. Tolterodine is highly protein bound.
• *Metabolism:* Drug is extensively metabolized by the liver primarily by oxidation by the cytochrome P-450 2D6 pathway and leads to the formation of a pharmacologically active 5-hydroxymethyl metabolite.
• *Excretion:* Most of an administered dose is recovered in the urine and the rest in feces. Less than 1% of a dose is recovered as unchanged tolterodine and 5% to 14% is recovered as the active 5-hydroxymethyl metabolite. Half-life of drug is 1.9 to 3.7 hours.

Contraindications and precautions

Contraindicated in patients with urine or gastric retention and uncontrolled narrow-angle glaucoma. Also contraindicated in patients hypersensitive to tolterodine or its ingredients. Use with caution in patients with significantly reduced hepatic or renal function.

Interactions

Fluoxetine, a selective serotonin reuptake inhibitor and a potent inhibitor of cytochrome P-450 2D6, has been observed to significantly inhibit the metabolism of tolterodine in rapid metabolizers. No dosage adjustment is required.

Although patients concomitantly receiving *cytochrome P-450 3A4 inhibitors* such as *macrolide antibiotics (clarithromycin, erythromycin) or antifungal agents (itraconazole, ketoconazole, miconazole)* have not been studied, doses of tolterodine above 1 mg b.i.d. should not be given.

Effects on diagnostic tests

None reported.

Adverse reactions

CNS: paresthesia, vertigo, dizziness, *headache*, nervousness, somnolence, fatigue.
CV: hypertension, chest pain.
EENT: abnormal vision (including accommodation), xerophthalmia, pharyngitis, rhinitis, sinusitis.
GI: *dry mouth*, abdominal pain, constipation, diarrhea, dyspepsia, flatulence, nausea, vomiting.
GU: dysuria, micturition frequency, urine retention, urinary tract infection.
Musculoskeletal: arthalgia, back pain.
Respiratory: bronchitis, coughing, upper respiratory infection.
Skin: pruritis, rash, erythema, dry skin.
Other: flulike symptoms, weight gain.

Overdose and treatment

Overdoses can potentially result in severe central anticholinergic effects and should be treated accordingly. Perform ECG monitoring if an overdose occurs.

☑ Special considerations

• Food increases the absorption of tolterodine, but no dosage adjustment is needed.
• Dry mouth is the most frequently reported adverse event.

Patient education

• Inform patient that antimuscarinic agents such as tolterodine may produce blurred vision.
• Caution patient to avoid hazardous activities until drug's effects are known.

Geriatric use

• No overall differences in safety have been observed between older and younger patients.

Pediatric use

• Safety and effectiveness in pediatric patients have not been established.

Breast-feeding
• Excretion in human breast milk is unknown. Do not use drug during breast-feeding.

topiramate
Topamax

Pharmacologic classification: sulfamate-substituted monosaccharide
Therapeutic classification: antiepileptic
Pregnancy risk category C

How supplied
Available by prescription only
Tablets: 25, 100, 200 mg

Indications, route, and dosage
Adjunctive therapy of partial onset seizures
Adults: Titrate up to maximum daily dose of 400 mg in two divided doses. Titration schedule is as follows:

Week	A.M. dose	P.M. dose
1	None	50 mg
2	50 mg	50 mg
3	50 mg	100 mg
4	100 mg	100 mg
5	100 mg	150 mg
6	150 mg	150 mg
7	150 mg	200 mg
8	200 mg	200 mg

✦ ***Dosage adjustment.*** In patients with moderate to severe renal impairment, reduce dosage by 50%. A supplemental dose may be required during hemodialysis.

Pharmacodynamics
Antiepileptic action: Mechanism of action is unknown. Drug is thought to block action potential, suggestive of a state-dependant sodium channel blocking action. Drug may increase the frequency at which gamma-aminobutyric acid (GABA) activates $GABA_A$ receptors, as well as enhances the ability of GABA to induce a flux of chloride ions into neurons, suggesting that topiramate potentiates the activity of the inhibitory neurotransmitter. Drug may also antagonize the ability of kainate to activate the kainate/AMPA subtype of excitatory amino acid (glutamate) receptor. Topiramate also has weak carbonic anhydrase inhibitor activity, which is unrelated to its antiepileptic properties.

Pharmacokinetics
• *Absorption:* Rapid, with peak plasma concentrations occurring at approximately 2 hours following 400-mg oral dose. Relative bioavailability of drug is approximately 80% compared with a solution and is not affected by food.
• *Distribution:* Plasma concentrations increase proportionately with dose; mean elimination half-life is 21 hours. Steady state is reached in 4 days in patients with normal renal function. Drug is 13% to 17% bound to plasma proteins.
• *Metabolism:* Not extensively metabolized.
• *Excretion:* Primarily eliminated unchanged in the urine (approximately 70% of an administered dose).

Contraindications and precautions
Contraindicated in patients with history of hypersensitivity to any component of the preparation. Use cautiously in patients with hepatic impairment because drug clearance may be decreased.

Interactions
Concomitant use of *phenytoin* or *carbamazepine* with topiramate caused topiramate levels to be decreased. *Valproic acid, phenobarbital,* and *primidone* were either unevaluated or had minimal effects on topiramate concentrations. Topiramate increased *phenytoin* concentrations.

Although *CNS depressants* have not been evaluated, due to the risk of topiramate-induced CNS depression and other adverse cognitive and neuropsychiatric events, use with caution. Efficacy of *oral contraceptives* may be compromised by topiramate; tell patient to report changes in bleeding patterns. Concomitant use of *carbonic anhydrase inhibitors (acetazolamide, dichlorphenamide)* may increase the risk of renal stone formation; avoid use of both agents.

Effects on diagnostic tests
None reported.

Adverse reactions
CNS: abnormal coordination; agitation; apathy; asthenia; *ataxia; confusion;* depression; difficulty with concentration, attention, language, or memory; *dizziness;* emotional liability; euphoria; ***generalized tonic-clonic seizures;*** hallucination; hyperkinesia; hypertonia; hypoaesthesia; hypokinesia; insomnia; mood problems; *nervousness; nystagmus; paresthesia;* personality disorder; *psychomotor slowing;* psychosis; *somnolence; speech disorders;* stupor; suicidal attempts; *tremor,* vertigo.
CV: chest pain, palpitations.
EENT: *abnormal vision,* conjunctivitis, *diplopia,* eye pain, hearing or vestibular problems, pharyngitis, sinusitis, taste perversion, tinnitus.
GI: abdominal pain, anorexia, constipation, diarrhea, dry mouth, dyspepsia, flatulence, gastroenteritis, gingivitis, *nausea,* vomiting.
GU: amenorrhea, dysuria, dysmenorrhea, hematuria, impotence, intermenstrual bleeding, menstrual disorder, menorrhagia, micturition frequency, renal calculus, urinary incontinence, urinary tract infection, vaginitis.
Hematologic: anemia, epistaxis, leukopenia.
Metabolic: increased or decreased weight.
Respiratory: bronchitis, coughing, dyspnea, *upper respiratory infection.*
Skin: acne, alopecia, aggressive reaction, increased sweating, pruritus, rash.
Other: back pain, body odor, edema, *fatigue,* fever, flulike symptoms, hot flashes, leg pain, leukorrhea, malaise, myalgia, rigors.

Overdose and treatment
In acute overdose after recent ingestion, institute gastric lavage or emesis. Activated charcoal is not recommended. Institute supportive treatment. Hemodialysis is an effective means of removing drug.

☑ Special considerations
- Carefully review dosing schedule with patient to avoid under- or overmedication.
- If necessary, withdraw antiepileptic drugs (including drug) gradually to minimize risk of increased seizure activity.

Patient education
- Tell patient to maintain adequate fluid intake during therapy because of potential to form renal stones.
- Advise patient to avoid hazardous activities until drug's effects are known.

Geriatric use
- No age-related differences or adverse effects were seen in the elderly; however, age-related renal abnormalities should be considered.

Pediatric use
- Safety and effectiveness in children have not been established.

Breast-feeding
- It is not known if drug is excreted in breast milk; use with caution.

topotecan hydrochloride
Hycamtin

Pharmacologic classification: semisynthetic camptothecin derivative
Therapeutic classification: antineoplastic
Pregnancy risk category D

How supplied
Available by prescription only
Injection: 4-mg single-dose vial

Indications, route, and dosage
Metastatic carcinoma of the ovary after failure of initial or subsequent chemotherapy
Adults: 1.5 mg/m²/day as an I.V. infusion given over 30 minutes for 5 consecutive days, starting on day 1 of a 21-day cycle. Minimum of four cycles should be given.
✦ ***Dosage adjustment.*** In adults with renal impairment and creatinine clearance of 20 to 39 ml/minute, adjust dosage to 0.75 mg/m². In patients with mild renal impairment (creatinine clearance, 40 to 60 ml/minute), adjustment is not required. There are insufficient data available for a dosage recommendation for patients with creatinine clearance under 20 ml/minute.

Pharmacodynamics
Antineoplastic action: Topotecan relieves torsional strain in DNA by inducing reversible single-strand breaks. It binds to the topoisomerase I-DNA complex and prevents religation of these single-strand breaks. The cytotoxicity of topotecan is thought to be due to double-strand DNA damage produced during DNA synthesis when replication enzymes interact with the ternary complex formed by topotecan, topoisomerase I, and DNA.

Pharmacokinetics
- *Absorption:* Drug is given only I.V.
- *Distribution:* About 35% is bound to plasma protein.
- *Metabolism:* Topotecan undergoes a reversible pH-dependent hydrolysis of its lactone moiety; it is the lactone form that is pharmacologically active.
- *Excretion:* About 30% of drug is excreted in the urine. Terminal half-life is 2 to 3 hours.

Contraindications and precautions
Contraindicated in patients hypersensitive to drug or its components, in those with severe bone marrow depression, and in pregnant or breast-feeding women.

Interactions
Concomitant administration of *granulocyte-colony stimulating factor (G-CSF)* can prolong the duration of neutropenia; therefore, if G-CSF is to be used, do not initiate until day 6 of the course of therapy, 24 hours after completion of treatment with topotecan. Myelosuppression is more severe when topotecan is given in combination with *cisplatin.* Use both drugs with extreme caution.

Effects on diagnostic tests
None reported.

Adverse reactions
CNS: *fatigue, asthenia, headache,* paresthesia.
GI: *nausea, vomiting, diarrhea, constipation, abdominal pain, stomatitis, anorexia.*
Hematologic: ***neutropenia, leukopenia, thrombocytopenia,*** *anemia.*
Hepatic: transient elevations of liver enzymes.
Respiratory: *dyspnea.*
Skin: *alopecia.*
Other: ***sepsis,*** fever.

Overdose and treatment
The primary adverse effect associated with topotecan overdose is thought to be bone marrow suppression. Treatment should be supportive. There is no known antidote.

☑ Special considerations
- Before administration of the first course, baseline neutrophil count should exceed 1,500 cells/mm³ and a platelet count over 100,000 cells/mm³.
- Prepare drug under a vertical laminar flow hood wearing gloves and protective clothing. If drug solution contacts the skin, wash the skin immediately and thoroughly with soap and water. If mucous membranes are affected, flush areas thoroughly with water.
- Reconstitute each 4-mg vial with 4 ml sterile water for injection. Then dilute appropriate volume of reconstituted solution in either 0.9% NaCl or D_5W before use.

• Because the lyophilized dosage form contains no antibacterial preservative, use reconstituted product immediately.
• Protect unopened vials of drug from light. Reconstituted vials are stable at about 68° to 77° F (20° to 25° C) and ambient lighting conditions for 24 hours.
• Bone marrow suppression (primarily neutropenia) is the dose-limiting toxicity of topotecan. The nadir occurs at about 11 days. If severe neutropenia occurs during therapy, reduce dose by 0.25 mg/m² for subsequent courses. Alternatively, administer G-CSF after the subsequent course (before dose is reduced) starting from day 6 (24 hours after completion of topotecan administration). Neutropenia is not cumulative over time.
• The nadir for thrombocytopenia is about 5 days, platelets is 15 days, and anemia is 15 days. Blood or platelet (or both) transfusions may be necessary.
• Frequent monitoring of peripheral blood cell counts is necessary. Do not give patients subsequent courses of topotecan until neutrophil counts exceed 1,000 cells/mm³, platelet counts are over 100,000 cells/mm³, and hemoglobin levels are 9 mg/dl (with transfusion if needed).
• Inadvertent extravasation with topotecan has been associated with only mild local reactions, such as erythema and bruising.

Pediatric use
• Safety and effectiveness in children have not been established.

Breast-feeding
• Because it is not known whether drug is excreted in breast milk, avoid use of drug in breast-feeding women.

toremifene citrate
Fareston

Pharmacologic classification: nonsteroidal antiestrogen
Therapeutic classification: antineoplastic
Pregnancy risk category D

How supplied
Available by prescription only
Tablets: 60 mg

Indications, route, and dosage
For treatment of metastatic breast cancer in postmenopausal women with estrogen-receptor positive or unknown tumors
Adults: 60 mg P.O. once daily. Treatment is usually continued until disease progression is observed.

Pharmacodynamics
Antineoplastic action: Toremifene is a nonsteroidal triphenylethylene derivative that exerts its antitumor effect by competing with estrogen for binding sites in the tumor. This blocks the growth-stimulating effects of endogenous estrogen in the tumor, causing an antiestrogenic effect.

Pharmacokinetics
• *Absorption:* Well absorbed after oral administration and not influenced by food. Peak plasma concentrations are obtained within 3 hours. Steady-state concentrations are reached in about 4 to 6 weeks.
• *Distribution:* Apparent volume of distribution is 580 L; drug binds extensively (over 99.5%) to serum proteins, mainly albumin.
• *Metabolism:* Extensively metabolized, mainly by CYP 3A4, to N-demethyltoremifene, which is also antiestrogenic but with weak in vivo antitumor potency. Elimination half-life is about 5 days.
• *Excretion:* Eliminated in the feces, with about 10% excreted unchanged in the urine. Elimination is slow due to enterohepatic circulation.

Contraindications and precautions
Contraindicated in patients with known hypersensitivity to drug. Avoid use in patients with history of thromboembolic diseases. Do not use drug long-term in patients with preexisting endometrial hyperplasia.

Interactions
Drugs that decrease renal calcium excretion (such as *thiazide diuretics)* increase the risk of hypercalcemia. Monitor calcium levels closely. *Coumarin-like anticoagulants* (such as *warfarin)* given concomitantly with toremifene may further prolong PT and INR. Monitor PT and INR closely. *Cytochrome P-450 3A4 enzyme inducers* (such as *carbamazepine, phenobarbital, phenytoin)* increase the rate of toremifene metabolism. *Cytochrome P-450 3A4-6 enzyme inhibitors* (*erythromycin, ketoconazole)* decrease toremifene metabolism.

Effects on diagnostic tests
None reported.

Adverse reactions
CNS: dizziness, fatigue, depression.
CV: edema, ***thromboembolism, heart failure, MI, pulmonary embolism.***
EENT: visual disturbances, glaucoma, ocular changes (such as dry eyes), *cataracts, abnormal visual fields.*
GI: *nausea,* vomiting.
GU: *vaginal discharge,* vaginal bleeding.
Hepatic: *elevated levels of AST, alkaline phosphatase,* and bilirubin.
Metabolic: hypercalcemia.
Skin: *sweating.*
Other: *hot flashes.*

Overdose and treatment
Theoretically, overdose may be manifested as an increase of antiestrogenic effects (hot flashes), estrogenic effects (vaginal bleeding), or nervous system disorders (vertigo, dizziness, ataxia, and nausea). There is no specific antidote; treatment is symptomatic.

☑ Special considerations
• Drug causes fetal harm when given to pregnant women. If used during pregnancy, or if the patient becomes pregnant while receiving toremifene, coun-

sel her of potential hazard to the fetus or risk of pregnancy loss.
- Obtain periodic CBC, calcium levels, and liver function tests.
- Monitor calcium levels closely for first weeks of treatment in patients with bone metastases because of increased risk of hypercalcemia and tumor flare.

Patient education
- Instruct patient to take drug exactly as prescribed.
- Warn patient not to discontinue therapy without consulting with health care provider.
- Inform patient to report vaginal bleeding and other adverse effects.
- Warn patient that a disease flare-up may occur during first weeks of therapy. Reassure her that this does not indicate treatment failure.
- Advise patient to report leg or chest pain, severe headache, visual changes, or dyspnea.
- Inform patient with bone metastases of the signs and symptoms of hypercalcemia and instruct her to notify her health care provider if they occur.

Geriatric use
- No significant age-related differences in toremifene effectiveness or safety were noted.

Pediatric use
- There is no indication for the use of toremifene in pediatric patients.

Breast-feeding
- Toremifene's presence in human breast milk is not known.

torsemide
Demadex

Pharmacologic classification: loop diuretic
Therapeutic classification: diuretic/antihypertensive
Pregnancy risk category B

How supplied
Available by prescription only
Tablets: 5 mg, 10 mg, 20 mg, 100 mg
Solution: 2-ml ampule (10 mg/ml), 5-ml ampule (10 mg/ml)

Indications, route, and dosage
Diuresis in patients with heart failure
Adults: Initially, 10 to 20 mg P.O. or I.V. once daily. If response is inadequate, double the dose until response is obtained. Maximum dosage, 200 mg daily.
Diuresis in patients with chronic renal failure
Adults: Initially, 20 mg P.O. or I.V. once daily. If response is inadequate, double the dose until response is obtained. Maximum dosage, 200 mg daily.
Diuresis in patients with hepatic cirrhosis
Adults: Initially, 5 to 10 mg P.O. or I.V. once daily with an aldosterone antagonist or a potassium-sparing diuretic. If response is inadequate, double the dose until response is obtained. Maximum dosage, 40 mg daily.
Hypertension
Adults: Initially, 5 mg P.O. daily. Increase to 10 mg once daily in 4 to 6 weeks if needed and tolerated. If response is still inadequate, add another antihypertensive agent.

Note: If fluid and electrolyte imbalances occur, torsemide should be discontinued until the imbalances are corrected. Drug may then be restarted at a lower dose.

Pharmacodynamics
Diuretic/antihypertensive actions: Loop diuretics such as torsemide enhance excretion of sodium, chloride, and water by acting on the ascending portion of the loop of Henle. Torsemide does not significantly alter glomerular filtration rate, renal plasma flow, or acid-base balance.

Pharmacokinetics
- *Absorption:* Drug is absorbed with little first-pass metabolism, and the serum concentration reaches its peak within 1 hour after oral administration.
- *Distribution:* Volume of distribution is 12 to 15 L in healthy patients and in those with mild to moderate renal failure or heart failure. In patients with hepatic cirrhosis, volume of distribution is approximately doubled. Torsemide is extensively bound (97% to 99%) to plasma protein.
- *Metabolism:* Drug is metabolized in the liver to an inactive major metabolite and to two lesser metabolites that have some diuretic activity; for practical purposes, metabolism terminates action of drug. Duration of action is 6 to 8 hours after oral or I.V. use.
- *Excretion:* From 22% to 34% of dose is excreted unchanged in urine via active secretion of drug by the proximal tubules.

Contraindications and precautions
Contraindicated in patients with anuria or hypersensitivity to drug or other sulfonylurea derivatives. Use cautiously in patients with hepatic disease and associated cirrhosis and ascites.

Interactions
Cholestyramine may decrease torsemide absorption; administration times should be separated by at least 3 hours. Torsemide reduces the excretion of *salicylates,* possibly leading to salicylate toxicity; concomitant use should be avoided. *Probenecid* decreases the diuretic effect of torsemide, and *indomethacin* decreases the diuretic effect in sodium-restricted patients; concomitant use of these agents should be avoided. Torsemide may increase the risk of *lithium toxicity.* Auditory toxicity also appears to increase with concurrent use of *ototoxic drugs* such as *aminoglycosides.*

Renal dysfunction may occur when torsemide and *NSAIDs* are administered concomitantly. These agents should be used together with caution. *Digoxin* decreases torsemide clearance, whereas torsemide decreases the renal clearance of *spironolactone.* However, no dosage adjustments are necessary.

Effects on diagnostic tests
Torsemide therapy alters electrolyte balance and renal function tests. It also may mildly affect glucose, serum lipid, and alkaline phosphatase levels and CBC and platelet counts.

Adverse reactions
CNS: dizziness, headache, nervousness, insomnia, syncope.
CV: ECG abnormalities, chest pain, edema.
EENT: rhinitis, cough, sore throat.
GI: diarrhea, constipation, nausea, dyspepsia.
GU: *excessive urination.*
Other: asthenia, arthralgia, myalgia.

Overdose and treatment
Although data specific to torsemide overdosage are lacking, signs and symptoms would probably reflect excessive pharmacologic effect: dehydration, hypovolemia, hypotension, hyponatremia, hypokalemia, hypochloremic alkalosis, and hemoconcentration. Treatment should consist of fluid and electrolyte replacement.

☑ Special considerations
- Tinnitus and hearing loss (usually reversible) have been observed after rapid I.V. injection of other loop diuretics and also have been noted after oral torsemide administration. Inject drug slowly over 2 minutes; single doses should not exceed 200 mg.
- In patients with CV disease, especially those receiving cardiac glycosides, diuretic-induced hypokalemia may be a risk factor for the development of arrhythmias. The risk of hypokalemia is greatest in patients with hepatic cirrhosis, brisk diuresis, inadequate oral intake of electrolytes, or concomitant therapy with corticosteroids or corticotropin. Perform periodic monitoring of serum potassium and other electrolytes.
- Excessive diuresis may cause dehydration, blood-volume reduction, and possibly thrombosis and embolism, especially in elderly patients. Monitor fluid intake and output, serum electrolyte levels, blood pressure, weight, and pulse rate during rapid diuresis and routinely with chronic use.

Patient education
- Encourage patient to follow a high-potassium diet, including citrus fruits, tomatoes, bananas, dates, and apricots.
- Instruct patient to take torsemide in the morning to prevent nocturia.
- Advise patient to change positions slowly to prevent dizziness.
- Inform patient to report ringing in ears immediately because this may indicate toxicity.
- Tell patient to call before taking OTC medications.
- Advise patient to take protective measures against exposure to sunlight or ultraviolet light.

Geriatric use
- Special dosage adjustment usually is not necessary. However, elderly patients are at greater risk for dehydration, blood-volume reduction, and possibly thrombosis and embolism with excessive diuresis.

Pediatric use
- Safety and effectiveness in children under age 18 have not been established.

Breast-feeding
- It is not known if torsemide is excreted in breast milk. Use caution when administering drug to breast-feeding women.

tramadol hydrochloride
Ultram

Pharmacologic classification: synthetic derivative
Therapeutic classification: analgesic
Pregnancy risk category C

How supplied
Available by prescription only
Tablets: 50 mg

Indications, route, and dosage
Moderate to moderately severe pain
Adults: 50 to 100 mg P.O. q 4 to 6 hours, p.r.n. Maximum dosage, 400 mg/day.
✦ ***Dosage adjustment.*** In patients with creatinine clearance below 30 ml/minute, increase dosing interval to q 12 hours; maximum daily dosage, 200 mg.

In patients with cirrhosis, recommended dose is 50 mg q 12 hours.

Pharmacodynamics
Analgesic action: Mechanism of action is unknown. It is a centrally acting synthetic analgesic compound that is not chemically related to opiates but is thought to bind to opioid receptors and inhibit reuptake of norepinephrine and serotonin.

Pharmacokinetics
- *Absorption:* Tramadol is almost completely absorbed. Mean absolute bioavailability of a 100-mg dose is about 75%.
- *Distribution:* Tramadol is about 20% bound to plasma protein; may cross the blood-brain barrier.
- *Metabolism:* Tramadol is extensively metabolized.
- *Excretion:* About 30% of a dose of tramadol is excreted unchanged in urine and 60% as metabolites. Half-life of drug is about 6 to 7 hours.

Contraindications and precautions
Contraindicated in patients with hypersensitivity to drug or acute intoxication with alcohol, hypnotics, centrally acting analgesics, opioids, or psychotropic drugs. Use cautiously in patients at risk for seizures or respiratory depression; in those with increased intracranial pressure or head injury, acute abdominal conditions, impaired renal or hepatic function; and in patients physically dependent on opioids.

Interactions
Carbamazepine increases tramadol metabolism. Patients receiving chronic carbamazepine therapy at dosages up to 800 mg daily may require up to twice the recommended dose of tramadol. *CNS de-*

pressants produce additive effects. Use together with caution. Dosage of tramadol may need to be reduced. *MAO inhibitors* and *neuroleptic drugs* increase the risk of seizures. Monitor patient closely.

Effects on diagnostic tests
Tramadol may increase creatinine clearance and liver enzyme levels, decrease hemoglobin levels, and cause proteinuria.

Adverse reactions
CNS: *dizziness, vertigo, headache, somnolence, CNS stimulation, asthenia,* anxiety, confusion, coordination disturbance, euphoria, nervousness, sleep disorder, ***seizures.***
CV: vasodilation.
EENT: visual disturbances.
GI: *nausea, constipation, vomiting,* dyspepsia, dry mouth, diarrhea, abdominal pain, anorexia, flatulence.
GU: urine retention, urinary frequency, menopausal symptoms.
Respiratory: ***respiratory depression.***
Skin: *pruritus,* diaphoresis, rash.
Other: malaise, hypertonia.

Overdose and treatment
Serious potential consequences are respiratory depression and seizures. Because naloxone will reverse some, but not all, of the symptoms caused by tramalol overdosage, supportive therapy is recommended. Hemodialysis removes only a small percentage of drug.

☑ Special considerations
- Monitor patient's CV and respiratory status and stop dose if respirations decrease or rate is below 12 breaths/minute or if patient exhibits signs of respiratory depression.
- Constipation is a common adverse effect and may require laxative therapy.
- For better analgesic effect, give drug before patient has intense pain.
- Monitor patient at risk for seizures closely; drug has been reported to reduce seizure threshold.
- Monitor patient for drug dependence. Because drug dependence similar to codeine or dextropropoxyphene can occur, the potential for abuse exists.

Patient education
- Instruct patient to take drug only as prescribed and not to alter dosage or dosage interval without medical approval.
- Caution ambulatory patient about getting out of bed or walking. Warn outpatient to avoid driving and other potentially hazardous activities that require mental alertness until adverse CNS effects of drug are known.
- Advise patient not to take OTC medications unless instructed because drug interactions can occur.

Geriatric use
- Use cautiously in elderly patients because serum concentrations are slightly elevated and the elimination half-life of drug is prolonged. Do not exceed daily dose of 300 mg in patients over age 75.

Pediatric use
- Safety and effectiveness in children under age 16 have not been established.

Breast-feeding
- Use of drug in breast-feeding women is not recommended because its safety has not been established.

trandolapril
Mavik

Pharmacologic classification: ACE inhibitor
Therapeutic classification: antihypertensive
Pregnancy risk category C (D second and third trimesters)

How supplied
Available by prescription only
Tablets: 1 mg, 2 mg, 4 mg

Indications, route, and dosage
Hypertension
Adults: In patient not taking a diuretic, initially 1 mg for the nonblack patient and 2 mg for the black patient P.O. once daily. If control is not adequate, dosage can be increased at intervals of at least 1 week. Maintenance dosage ranges from 2 to 4 mg daily for most patients; there is little experience with doses of more than 8 mg. Patients receiving once-daily dosing at 4 mg may use b.i.d. dosing.

For patient receiving a diuretic, initially 0.5 mg P.O. once daily. Subsequent dosage adjustment made based on blood pressure response.

Pharmacodynamics
Antihypertensive action: Unknown. Drug action is thought to result primarily from inhibition of circulating and tissue ACE activity, thereby reducing angiotensin II formation, decreasing vasoconstriction, decreasing aldosterone secretion, and increasing plasma renin. Decreased aldosterone secretion leads to diuresis, natriuresis, and a small increase in serum potassium.

Pharmacokinetics
- *Absorption:* Absolute bioavailability after oral administration of trandolapril is about 10% for trandolapril and 70% for its metabolite, trandolaprilat.
- *Distribution:* Drug is about 80% protein-bound.
- *Metabolism:* Drug is metabolized by the liver to the active metabolite, trandolaprilat, and at least seven other metabolites.
- *Excretion:* Trandolapril is about 66% excreted in feces; 33% in urine. Elimination half-lives of trandolapril and trandolaprilat are about 6 and 10 hours, respectively, but like all ACE inhibitors, trandolaprilat also has a prolonged terminal elimination phase.

Contraindications and precautions
Contraindicated in patients with hypersensitivity to drug and history of angioedema related to previous treatment with an ACE inhibitor. Drug is not recommended for use in pregnant women. Use cautiously in patients with impaired renal function, heart failure, or renal artery stenosis.

Interactions
Diuretics increase risk of excessive hypotension. Stop diuretic or lower dose of trandolapril. Trandolapril increases serum *lithium* levels and lithium toxicity. Avoid concomitant use. *Potassium-sparing diuretics, potassium supplements,* and *sodium substitutes containing potassium* increase the risk of hyperkalemia. Monitor serum potassium closely.

Effects on diagnostic tests
Trandolapril may cause minor elevations in creatinine clearance and BUN. Elevations of liver enzymes and uric acid may also occur.

Adverse reactions
CNS: dizziness, headache, fatigue, drowsiness, insomnia, paresthesia, vertigo, anxiety.
CV: chest pain, ***AV first-degree block,*** bradycardia, edema, flushing, hypotension, palpitations.
EENT: epistaxis, throat inflammation, upper respiratory tract infection.
GI: diarrhea, dyspepsia, abdominal distention, abdominal pain or cramps, constipation, vomiting, pancreatitis.
GU: urinary frequency, impotence, decreased libido.
Hematologic: ***neutropenia,*** leukopenia.
Respiratory: dry, persistent, tickling, nonproductive cough; dyspnea.
Skin: rash, pruritus, pemphigus.
Other: ***anaphylactoid reactions, angioedema,*** hyperkalemia, hyponatremia.

Overdose and treatment
Although no information is available, it is thought that the effects of overdosage are similar to other ACE inhibitor overdosage, with hypotension being the main adverse reaction. Because the hypotensive effect of trandolapril is achieved through vasodilation and effective hypovolemia, it is reasonable to treat trandolapril overdose by infusion of 0.9% NaCl solution. In addition, renal function and serum potassium should be monitored. Trandolaprilat is removed by hemodialysis.

☑ Special considerations
- Monitor for hypotension. Excessive hypotension can occur when drug is given with diuretics. If possible, diuretic therapy should be discontinued 2 to 3 days before starting trandolapril to decrease potential for excessive hypotensive response. If trandolapril does not adequately control blood pressure, diuretic therapy may be reinstituted with care.
- Assess patient's renal function before and periodically throughout therapy. Monitor serum potassium levels.
- Other ACE inhibitors have been associated with agranulocytosis and neutropenia. Monitor CBC with differential counts before therapy, especially in patients who have collagen vascular disease with impaired renal function.
- Angioedema associated with involvement of the tongue, glottis, or larynx may be fatal because of airway obstruction. Appropriate therapy, such as S.C. epinephrine 1:1,000 (0.3 to 0.5 ml) and equipment to ensure a patent airway, should be readily available.
- If jaundice develops, discontinue drug because, although rare, ACE inhibitors have been associated with a syndrome of cholestatic jaundice, fulminant hepatic necrosis, and death.

Patient education
- Advise patient to report signs of infection (such as fever and sore throat) and the following signs or symptoms: easy bruising or bleeding; swelling of tongue, lips, face, eyes, mucous membranes, or extremities; difficulty swallowing or breathing; and hoarseness.
- Tell patient to avoid sodium substitutes; these products may contain potassium, which can cause hyperkalemia.
- Light-headedness can occur, especially during the first few days of therapy. Tell patient to rise slowly to minimize this effect and to report symptoms. If syncope occurs, tell patient to stop taking drug and notify the health care provider immediately.
- Instruct patient to use caution in hot weather and during exercise. Inadequate fluid intake, vomiting, diarrhea, and excessive perspiration can lead to light-headedness and syncope.
- Tell female patient to report suspected pregnancy immediately. Drug will need to be discontinued.

Pediatric use
- Safety and effectiveness in children have not been established.

Breast-feeding
- It is not known if drug is excreted in breast milk; it should not be given to breast-feeding women.

tranylcypromine sulfate
Parnate

Pharmacologic classification: MAO inhibitor
Therapeutic classification: antidepressant
Pregnancy risk category C

How supplied
Available by prescription only
Tablets: 10 mg

Indications, route, and dosage
Severe depression, ◊ panic disorder
Adults: 30 mg P.O. daily in divided doses. Increase in 10-mg increments daily q 1 to 3 weeks; maximum daily dosage, 60 mg.

Pharmacodynamics

Antidepressant action: Endogenous depression is thought to result from low CNS concentrations of neurotransmitters, including norepinephrine and serotonin. Tranylcypromine acts by inhibiting effects of MAO, an enzyme that normally inactivates amine-containing substances, thus increasing concentration and activity of these agents.

Pharmacokinetics

- *Absorption:* Rapidly and completely absorbed from the GI tract. Peak serum levels occur at 1 to 3 hours; onset of therapeutic activity may not occur for 3 to 4 weeks.
- *Distribution:* Not fully understood. Dosage adjustments are determined by therapeutic response and adverse reaction profile.
- *Metabolism:* Drug is metabolized in the liver.
- *Excretion:* Excreted primarily in urine within 24 hours; some drug is excreted in feces via the biliary tract. Half-life, 2½ hours (relatively short); enzyme inhibition is prolonged and unrelated to half-life.

Contraindications and precautions

Contraindicated in patients receiving MAO inhibitors or dibenzazepine derivatives; sympathomimetics (including amphetamines); some CNS depressants (including narcotics and alcohol); selective serotonin reuptake inhibitors; antihypertensive, diuretic, antihistaminic, sedative or anesthetic drugs; bupropion hydrochloride, buspirone hydrochloride, dextromethorphan, meperidine; cheese or other foods with a high tyramine or tryptophan content; or excessive quantities of caffeine.

Also contraindicated in patients with a confirmed or suspected cerebrovascular defect, CV disease, hypertension, or history of headache and in those undergoing elective surgery.

Use cautiously in patients with renal disease, diabetes, seizure disorders, Parkinson's disease, or hyperthyroidism; in those at risk for suicide; and in patients receiving antiparkinsonian drugs or spinal anesthetics.

Interactions

Concomitant use of tranylcypromine with *amphetamines, ephedrine, phenylephrine, phenylpropanolamine,* or *related drugs* may result in serious CV toxicity; most *OTC cold, hay fever,* and *weight-reduction products* contain these drugs. Circulatory collapse and death have occurred after administration of *meperidine.* Concomitant use with *disulfiram* may cause tachycardia, flushing, or palpitations.

Concomitant use with *general or spinal anesthetics,* which are normally metabolized by MAO inhibitors, may cause severe hypotension and excessive CNS depression. Tranylcypromine should be discontinued for at least 1 week before using these agents.

Tranylcypromine decreases effectiveness of *local anesthetics* (such as *lidocaine, procaine*), resulting in poor nerve block. *Cocaine* or *local anesthetics containing vasoconstrictors* should be avoided. Use cautiously and in reduced dosage with *alcohol, barbiturates* and *other sedatives, narcotics,* and *dextromethorphan.* Wait at least 2 weeks before switching to *tricyclic antidepressants.*

Effects on diagnostic tests

Drug therapy elevates liver function tests and urinary catecholamine levels.

Adverse reactions

CNS: *dizziness,* headache, anxiety, agitation, paresthesia, drowsiness, weakness, numbness, tremor, jitters, confusion.
CV: *orthostatic hypotension, tachycardia,* paradoxical hypertension, palpitations.
EENT: blurred vision, tinnitus.
GI: dry mouth, *anorexia,* nausea, diarrhea, constipation, abdominal pain.
GU: impotence, SIADH, urine retention, impaired ejaculation.
Hematologic: anemia, leukopenia, ***agranulocytosis, thrombocytopenia.***
Skin: rash.
Other: edema, hepatitis, muscle spasm, myoclonic jerks, chills.

Overdose and treatment

Signs and symptoms of tranylcypromine overdose include exacerbations of adverse reactions or an exaggerated response to normal pharmacologic activity; such signs and symptoms become apparent slowly (24 to 48 hours) and may persist for up to 2 weeks. Agitation, flushing, tachycardia, hypotension, hypertension, palpitations, increased motor activity, twitching, increased deep tendon reflexes, seizures, hyperpyrexia, cardiorespiratory arrest, or coma may occur. Death has occurred with doses of 350 mg.

Treat symptomatically and supportively: give 5 to 10 mg of phentolamine I.V. push for hypertensive crisis; treat seizures, agitation, or tremors with I.V. diazepam, tachycardia with beta blockers, and fever with cooling blankets. Monitor vital signs and fluid and electrolyte balance. Sympathomimetics (such as norepinephrine and phenylephrine) are contraindicated in hypotension because of MAO inhibitors.

☑ Special considerations

Besides those relevant to all *MAO inhibitors,* consider the following recommendations.

- Consider the inherent risk of suicide until significant improvement of depressive state occurs. Closely supervise high-risk patients during initial drug therapy. To reduce risk of suicidal overdose, prescribe the smallest quantity of tablets consistent with good management.
- Tranylcypromine may have a more rapid onset of antidepressant effect compared with other MAO inhibitors (7 to 10 days versus 21 to 30 days). MAO activity also returns rapidly to pretreatment values.

Patient education

- Warn patient to avoid taking alcohol and other CNS depressants or self-prescribed medications, such as cold, hay fever, or diet preparations without medical approval.

- To minimize daytime sedation, tell patient to take drug at bedtime.
- Explain that many foods and beverages containing tyramine or tryptophan (such as wines, beer, cheeses, preserved fruits, meats, and vegetables) may interact with drug. A list of foods to avoid can be obtained from the hospital dietary department or pharmacy.
- Tell patient to avoid hazardous activities that require alertness until full effect of drug on the CNS is known.
- Inform patient to lie down after taking drug and avoid abrupt postural changes, especially when arising to prevent dizziness induced by orthostatic blood pressure changes.
- Tell patient to take drug exactly as prescribed, not to double dose if a dose is missed, and not to stop taking drug abruptly. Patient should promptly report any adverse reactions. Dosage reduction can relieve most adverse reactions.
- Advise patient to store drug safely away from children.

Geriatric use
- Drug is not recommended for patients over age 60.

Pediatric use
- Drug is not recommended for patients under age 16.

Breast-feeding
- Safety has not been established. Use drug with caution.

trazodone hydrochloride
Desyrel

Pharmacologic classification: triazolopyridine derivative
Therapeutic classification: antidepressant
Pregnancy risk category C

How supplied
Available by prescription only
Tablets: 50 mg, 100 mg
Tablets (film-coated): 50 mg, 100 mg
Dividose tablets: 150 mg, 300 mg

Indications, route, and dosage
Depression
Adults: Initial dosage is 150 mg daily in divided doses, which can be increased by 50 mg/day q 3 to 4 days. Average dosage ranges from 150 mg to 400 mg/day. Maximum dosage, 400 mg/day in outpatients; 600 mg/day in hospitalized patients.
◊ ***Aggressive behavior***
Adults: 50 mg P.O. b.i.d.
◊ ***Panic disorder***
Adults: 300 mg P.O. daily.

Pharmacodynamics
Antidepressant action: Trazodone is thought to exert its antidepressant effects by inhibiting reuptake of norepinephrine and serotonin in CNS nerve terminals (presynaptic neurons), which results in increased concentration and enhanced activity of these neurotransmitters in the synaptic cleft. Trazodone shares some properties with tricyclic antidepressants: It has antihistaminic, alpha-blocking, analgesic, and sedative effects as well as relaxant effects on skeletal muscle. Unlike tricyclic antidepressants, however, trazodone counteracts the pressor effects of norepinephrine, has limited effects on the CV system and, in particular, has no direct quinidine-like effects on cardiac tissue; it also causes relatively fewer anticholinergic effects. Trazodone has been used in patients with alcohol dependence to decrease tremors and to alleviate anxiety and depression. Adverse reactions are somewhat dose-related; incidence increases with higher dosage levels.

Pharmacokinetics
- *Absorption:* Drug is well absorbed from the GI tract after oral administration. Peak effect occurs in 1 hour. Concomitant ingestion of food delays absorption, extends peak effect of drug to 2 hours, and increases amount of drug absorbed by 20%.
- *Distribution:* Widely distributed in the body; drug does not concentrate in any particular tissue, but small amounts may appear in breast milk. About 90% is protein-bound. Proposed therapeutic drug levels have not been established. Steady state plasma levels are reached in 3 to 7 days, and onset of therapeutic activity occurs in 7 days.
- *Metabolism:* Trazodone is metabolized by the liver; more than 75% of metabolites are excreted within 3 days.
- *Excretion:* Mostly excreted in urine; rest is excreted in feces via the biliary tract.

Contraindications and precautions
Contraindicated during initial recovery phase of MI or in patients with hypersensitivity to drug. Use cautiously in patients with cardiac disease and in those at risk for suicide.

Interactions
Additive effects are likely after concomitant use of trazodone with *antihypertensive drugs*, such as *clonidine, guanabenz, guanadrel, guanethidine, methyldopa,* and *reserpine* (hypotension); and with *CNS depressants,* such as *alcohol, analgesics, barbiturates, narcotics, tranquilizers,* and *anesthetics* (oversedation).

Trazodone may increase serum levels of *digoxin* and *phenytoin.*

Effects on diagnostic tests
Trazodone may prolong conduction time (elongation of QT and PR intervals, flattened T waves on ECG); it also may elevate liver function tests, decrease WBC counts, and alter serum glucose levels.

Adverse reactions
CNS: *drowsiness, dizziness,* nervousness, fatigue, confusion, tremor, weakness, hostility, anger, night-

mares, vivid dreams, headache, insomnia, ***generalized tonic-clonic seizures.***
CV: orthostatic hypotension, tachycardia, hypertension, syncope, shortness of breath.
EENT: blurred vision, tinnitus, nasal congestion.
GI: dry mouth, dysgeusia, constipation, nausea, vomiting, anorexia.
GU: urine retention; priapism, possibly leading to impotence; decreased libido; hematuria.
Hematologic: anemia.
Skin: rash, urticaria.
Other: diaphoresis.

Overdose and treatment

The most common signs and symptoms of drug overdose are drowsiness and vomiting; other signs and symptoms include orthostatic hypotension, tachycardia, headache, shortness of breath, dry mouth, and incontinence. Coma may occur.

Treatment is symptomatic and supportive and includes maintaining airway, and stabilizing vital signs and fluid and electrolyte balance. Induce emesis if gag reflex is intact; follow with gastric lavage (begin with lavage if emesis is unfeasible) and activated charcoal to prevent further absorption. Forced diuresis may aid elimination. Dialysis is usually ineffective.

☑ Special considerations

- Consider the inherent risk of suicide until significant improvement of depressive state occurs. Closely monitor high-risk patients during initial drug therapy. To reduce risk of suicidal overdose, prescribe the smallest quantity of tablets consistent with good management.
- Administering trazodone with food helps to prevent GI upset and increases absorption.
- Adverse effects are more common when dosages exceed 300 mg/day.
- 150-mg tablet may be broken on the scoring to obtain doses of 50 mg, 75 mg, or 100 mg.
- Tolerance to adverse effects (especially sedative effects) usually develops after 1 to 2 weeks of treatment.
- Trazodone has been used in alcohol dependence to decrease tremors and relieve anxiety and depression. Dosages range from 50 to 75 mg daily.
- Drug has fewer adverse cardiac and anticholinergic effects than tricyclic antidepressants.
- Drug may cause prolonged painful erections that may require surgical correction. Consider carefully before prescribing for male patients, especially those who are sexually active.
- Do not withdraw drug abruptly. However, discontinued drug at least 48 hours before surgical procedures.
- Sugarless chewing gum or hard candy or ice may relieve dry mouth.
- Monitor blood pressure because hypotension may occur.

Patient education

- Tell patient that full effects of drug may not become apparent for up to 2 weeks after therapy begins.
- Tell patient to take drug exactly as prescribed and not to double dose for missed ones, not to share drug with others, and not to discontinue drug abruptly.
- Inform patient that drug may cause drowsiness or dizziness; instruct patient not to participate in activities that require mental alertness until full effects of drug are known.
- Tell patient to avoid alcoholic beverages or medicinal elixirs while taking drug.
- Warn patient to store drug safely away from children.
- Suggest taking drug with food or milk if it causes stomach upset.
- To prevent dizziness, tell patient to lie down for about 30 minutes after taking the medication and avoid sudden postural changes, especially rising to upright position.
- Tell patient that sugarless chewing gum or sugarless hard candy may relieve dry mouth.
- Advise patient to report unusual effects immediately and to report prolonged, painful erections, sexual dysfunction, dizziness, fainting, or rapid heartbeat. He should regard an involuntary erection lasting more than 1 hour as a medical emergency.

Geriatric use

- Elderly patients usually require lower initial dosages; they are more likely to develop adverse reactions. However, it may be preferred in elderly patients because it has fewer adverse cardiac effects.

Pediatric use

- Drug is not recommended for children under age 18.

tretinoin (systemic)

Vesanoid

Pharmacologic classification: retinoid
Therapeutic classification: antineoplastic
Pregnancy risk category D

How supplied

Available by prescription only
Capsules: 10 mg

Indications, route, and dosage

Induction of remission in patients with acute promyelocytic leukemia (APL), French-American-British classification M3 (including the M3 variant), characterized by the presence of the t(15,17) translocation or the presence of PML/RAR alpha gene who are refractory to, or who have relapsed from, anthracycline chemotherapy or for whom anthracycline-based chemotherapy is contraindicated
Adults and children age 1 and older: 45 mg/m^2/day P.O. administered as two evenly divided doses until complete remission is documented. Discontinue therapy 30 days after achievement of complete remission or after 90 days of treatment, whichever occurs first.

Pharmacodynamics

Antineoplastic action: Exact mechanism of action of tretinoin is unknown. Tretinoin produces an initial maturation of primitive promyelocytes derived from the leukemic clone, followed by a repopulation of bone marrow and peripheral blood by normal, polyclonal hematopoietic cells.

Pharmacokinetics

- *Absorption:* Well absorbed from the GI tract.
- *Distribution:* About 95% is bound to plasma protein.
- *Metabolism:* Drug may induce its own metabolism.
- *Excretion:* Excreted in urine and feces.

Contraindications and precautions

Contraindicated in patients with known hypersensitivity to retinoids or parabens, which are used as preservatives in the gelatin capsule. Do not use in pregnant or breast-feeding women.

Interactions

Potential for alteration in pharmacokinetics exists when given concomitantly with *drugs that induce or inhibit hepatic cytochrome P-450 3A*. When administered within 1 hour of *ketoconazole*, increased tretinoin mean plasma area under the curve has been reported.

Effects on diagnostic tests

None reported.

Adverse reactions

CNS: cerebral hemorrhage, dizziness, *paresthesia, headache, anxiety, insomnia, depression, confusion,* ***cerebral hemorrhage***, intracranial hypertension, agitation, hallucination, abnormal gait, agnosia, aphasia, asterixis, cerebellar edema, cerebellar disorders, ***seizures, coma,*** CNS depression, dysarthria, encephalopathy, facial paralysis, hemiplegia, hyporeflexia, hypotaxia, no light reflex neurologic reaction, spinal cord disorder, tremor, leg weakness, unconsciousness, dementia, forgetfulness, somnolence, slow speech.
CV: *chest discomfort,* ***arrhythmias,*** *hypotension, hypertension, phlebitis, edema,* ***cardiac failure, cardiac arrest, MI,*** enlarged heart, heart murmur, ischemia, ***stroke,*** myocarditis, pericarditis, secondary cardiomyopathy.
EENT: *ear fullness, visual disturbances, ocular disorders,* hearing loss.
GI: *GI hemorrhage, nausea, vomiting, anorexia, abdominal pain, GI disorders, diarrhea, constipation, dyspepsia, abdominal distention,* hepatosplenomegaly, hepatitis, ulcer, unspecified liver disorder.
GU: *renal insufficiency,* ***acute renal failure,*** micturition frequency, dysuria, renal tubular necrosis, enlarged prostate.
Hematologic: leukocytosis, *hemorrhage, DIC.*
Respiratory: *pneumonia, upper respiratory tract disorders, dyspnea, respiratory insufficiency, pleural effusion, crackles, expiratory wheezing,* lower respiratory tract disorders, pulmonary infiltrate, bronchial asthma, pulmonary or larynx edema, unspecified pulmonary disease, pulmonary hypertension.
Skin: *flushing, skin mucous membrane dryness, pruritus, decreased sweating, alopecia, skin changes.*
Other: *fever, infections, malaise, shivering, peripheral edema, pain, weight increase, injection site reactions, weight decrease, myalgia, bone pain, mucositis,* flank pain, cellulitis, facial edema, fluid imbalance, pallor, lymph disorder, acidosis, hypothermia, ascites, bone inflammation, hypercholesterolemia, hypertriglyceridemia, elevated liver function study results.

Overdose and treatment

No information available. Overdosage with other retinoids has been associated with transient headache, facial flushing, cheilosis, abdominal pain, dizziness, and ataxia. These signs and symptoms have quickly resolved without apparent residual effects.

☑ Special considerations

- Because patients with APL are generally at high risk and can have severe adverse reactions to tretinoin, administer drug in a facility with laboratory and supportive services sufficient to monitor drug tolerance and protect and maintain patients compromised by drug toxicity.
- About 25% of patients given drug during clinical studies have experienced retinoic acid–APL syndrome, which is characterized by fever, dyspnea, weight gain, radiographic pulmonary infiltrates, and pleural or pericardial effusions. This syndrome has occasionally been accompanied by impaired myocardial contractility and episodic hypotension with or without concomitant leukocytosis. Some patients have died because of progressive hypoxemia and multiorgan failure. The syndrome generally occurs during the first month of therapy. Treatment with high-dose steroids at the first signs of the syndrome appear to reduce morbidity and mortality.
- Monitor CBC and platelet counts regularly. Patients with high WBC counts at diagnosis are at greater risk for having further rapid increases in WBC counts. Rapidly evolving leukocytosis is associated with a higher risk of life-threatening complications.
- Monitor patient, especially children, for signs and symptoms of pseudotumor cerebri. Early signs and symptoms of pseudotumor cerebri include papilledema, headache, nausea, vomiting, and visual disturbances.
- Monitor cholesterol and triglyceride levels and liver function studies.
- Maintain supportive care, such as infection control and bleeding precautions, and provide prompt treatment.
- Ensure that pregnancy testing and contraception counseling are repeated monthly throughout tretinoin therapy.

Patient education

- Inform female patient that a pregnancy test is required within 1 week before tretinoin therapy. When possible, therapy will be delayed until a negative

result is obtained. Also tell female patient that effective contraception must be used during therapy and for 1 month following discontinuation of drug. Contraception must be used even when there is history of infertility or menopause unless a hysterectomy has been performed. Tell patient that two forms of contraception should be used simultaneously unless abstinence is the chosen method. If pregnancy is suspected, tell patient to report this immediately.
- Instruct patient on infection control and bleeding precautions. Tell patient to report signs or symptoms of infection (fever, sore throat, fatigue) or bleeding (easy bruising, nosebleeds, bleeding gums, melena) occur. Also tell patient to record temperature daily.

Pediatric use
- Safety and effectiveness in children under age 1 have not been established.

Breast-feeding
- It is not known if drug is excreted in breast milk. Because of the potential for serious adverse reactions in breast-fed infants, drug should not be given to breast-feeding women.

tretinoin (topical)
Renova, Retin-A, Retin-A Micro

Pharmacologic classification: vitamin A derivative
Therapeutic classification: antiacne
Pregnancy risk category C

How supplied
Available by prescription only
Cream: 0.025%, 0.05%, 0.1%
Gel: 0.025%, 0.01%
Solution: 0.05%
Microsphere gel: 0.1%

Indications, route, and dosage
Acne vulgaris (especially grades I, II, and III)
Adults and children: Clean affected area and lightly apply solution once daily h.s. or as directed.
◊ ***Treatment of photodamaged skin (wrinkles)***
Adults: 0.05% solution or 0.025% to 0.1% cream applied daily for at least 4 months.

Pharmacodynamics
Antiacne action: Mechanism of action of tretinoin has not been determined; however, it appears that tretinoin acts as a follicular epithelium irritant, preventing horny cells from sticking together and therefore inhibiting the formation of additional comedones.

Pharmacokinetics
- *Absorption:* Limited with topical use.
- *Distribution:* None.
- *Metabolism:* None.
- *Excretion:* Minimal amount is excreted in the urine.

Contraindications and precautions
Contraindicated in patients with known hypersensitivity to vitamin A or retinoic acid. Use cautiously in patients with eczema. Avoid contact of drug with eyes, mouth, angles of the nose, mucous membranes, or open wounds. Avoid use of topical preparations containing high concentrations of alcohol, menthol, spices, or lime because they may cause skin irritation. Avoid use of medicated cosmetics on treated skin.

Interactions
Concomitant use with the following *topical agents* should be undertaken with caution because of the possibility of interactions: *benzoyl peroxide, resorcinol, salicylic acid,* or *sulfur.*

Effects on diagnostic tests
None reported.

Adverse reactions
Skin: peeling, erythema, blisters, crusting, hyperpigmentation and hypopigmentation, contact dermatitis.

Note: Discontinue drug if sensitization or extreme redness and blistering of skin occur.

Overdose and treatment
No information available. Stop use and rinse area thoroughly. Oral ingestion of drug may lead to the same adverse effects as those associated with excessive oral intake of vitamin A.

☑ Special considerations
- Make sure that patient knows how to use medication and is aware of time required for clinical effect; therapeutic effect normally occurs in 2 to 3 weeks but may take 6 weeks or more. Relapses generally occur within 3 to 6 weeks of stopping medication.
- Do not use drug in patients who cannot or will not minimize sun exposure.
- Although tretinoin microsphere gel was developed to minimize dermal irritation, the skin of some individuals may become excessively dry, red, swollen, blistered, or crusted.

Patient education
- Advise patient to apply sparingly to thoroughly clean, dry skin to minimize irritation, and to wash face with mild soap no more than once or twice daily. Stress importance of thorough removal of dirt and makeup before application and of hand washing after each use, but warn against use of strong, medicated, or perfumed cosmetics, soaps, or skin cleansers.
- Explain that application of medication may cause a temporary feeling of warmth. If discomfort occurs, tell patient to decrease amount, but not to discontinue medication.
- Stress that initial exacerbation of inflammatory lesions is common and that redness and scaling (usually occurring in 7 to 10 days) are normal skin responses; these disappear when medication is decreased or discontinued.

• If severe local irritation develops, advise patient to stop drug temporarily and readjust dosage when irritation or inflammation subsides.
• Caution patient to keep exposure to sunlight or ultraviolet rays to a minimum and, if sunburned, to delay therapy until sunburn fades. If patient cannot avoid exposure to sunlight, recommend using a sunscreen with a sun protection factor of 15 or higher and wearing protective clothing.

triamcinolone (systemic)
Aristocort, Kenacort

triamcinolone acetonide
Kenalog, Triam-A

triamcinolone diacetate
Amcort, Aristocort, Aristocort Forte, Aristocort Intralesional, Articulose-L.A., Cenocort Forte, Kenacort, Triam-Forte, Triamolone 40, Tristoject

triamcinolone hexacetonide
Aristospan Intra-articular, Aristospan Intralesional

Pharmacologic classification: glucocorticoid
Therapeutic classification: anti-inflammatory, immunosuppressant
Pregnancy risk category C

How supplied
Available by prescription only
triamcinolone
Tablets: 1 mg, 2 mg, 4 mg, 8 mg
Syrup: 2 mg/ml, 4 mg/ml
triamcinolone acetonide
Injection: 10 mg/ml, 40 mg/ml suspension
triamcinolone diacetate
Injection: 25 mg/ml, 40 mg/ml suspension
triamcinolone hexacetonide
Injection: 5 mg/ml, 20 mg/ml suspension

Indications, route, and dosage
Adrenal insufficiency
triamcinolone
Adults: 4 to 12 mg P.O. daily, in single or divided doses.
Children: 117 mcg/kg or 3.3 mg/m² P.O. daily, in single or divided doses.
Severe inflammation or immunosuppression
triamcinolone
Adults: 8 to 16 mg P.O. daily, in single or divided doses.
Children: 416 mcg to 1.7 mg/kg or 12.5 to 50 mg/m² P.O. daily, in single or divided doses.
triamcinolone acetonide
Adults: Initially, 60 mg I.M. Additional doses of 20 to 100 mg may be given p.r.n. at 6-week intervals. Alternatively, administer 2.5 to 15 mg intra-articularly, or up to 1 mg intralesionally p.r.n.
Children age 6 to 12: 0.03 to 0.2 mg/kg I.M. at 1- to 7-day intervals.
triamcinolone diacetate
Adults: 40 mg I.M. once weekly; or 2 to 40 mg intra-articularly, intrasynovially, or intralesionally q 1 to 8 weeks; or 4 to 48 mg P.O. divided q.i.d.
Children: 0.117 to 1.66 mg/kg/day P.O. divided q.i.d.
triamcinolone hexacetonide
Adults: 2 to 20 mg intra-articularly q 3 to 4 weeks p.r.n.; or up to 0.5 mg intralesionally per square inch of skin.
Tuberculosis meningitis
triamcinolone
Adults: 32 to 48 mg P.O. daily.
Edematous states
triamcinolone
Adults: 16 to 48 mg P.O. daily.
Collagen diseases
triamcinolone
Adults: 30 to 48 mg P.O. daily.
Dermatologic disorders
triamcinolone
Adults: 8 to 16 mg P.O. daily.
Allergic states
triamcinolone
Adults: 8 to 12 mg P.O. daily.
Ophthalmic diseases
triamcinolone
Adults: 12 to 40 mg P.O. daily.
Respiratory diseases
triamcinolone
Adults: 16 to 48 mg P.O. daily.
Hematologic diseases
triamcinolone
Adults: 16 to 60 mg P.O. daily.
Neoplastic diseases
triamcinolone
Adults: 16 to 100 mg P.O. daily.

Pharmacodynamics
Anti-inflammatory action: Triamcinolone stimulates the synthesis of enzymes needed to decrease the inflammatory response. It suppresses the immune system by reducing activity and volume of the lymphatic system, thus producing lymphocytopenia (primarily of T lymphocytes), decreases immunoglobulin and complement concentrations, decreases passage of immune complexes through basement membranes, and possibly depresses reactivity of tissue to antigen-antibody interactions.

Triamcinolone is an intermediate-acting glucocorticoid. The addition of a fluorine group in the molecule increases the anti-inflammatory activity, which is five times more potent than an equal weight of hydrocortisone. It has essentially no mineralocorticoid activity.

Triamcinolone may be administered orally. The diacetate and acetonide salts may be administered by I.M., intra-articular, intrasynovial, intralesional or sublesional, and soft-tissue injection. The diacetate suspension is slightly soluble, providing a prompt onset of action and a longer duration of effect (1 to 2 weeks). Triamcinolone acetonide is relatively insoluble and slowly absorbed. Its extended duration of action lasts for several weeks. Triamcinolone hexacetonide is relatively insoluble, is absorbed slowly, and has a prolonged action of 3 to 4 weeks. Do not administer any of the parenteral suspensions I.V.

Pharmacokinetics

• *Absorption:* Absorbed readily after oral administration. After oral and I.V. administration, peak effects occur in about 1 to 2 hours. The suspensions for injection have variable onset and duration of action, depending on whether they are injected into an intra-articular space or a muscle, and on the blood supply to that muscle.
• *Distribution:* Drug is removed rapidly from the blood and distributed to muscle, liver, skin, intestines, and kidneys. It is extensively bound to plasma proteins (transcortin and albumin). Only the unbound portion is active. Adrenocorticoids are distributed into breast milk and through the placenta.
• *Metabolism:* Drug is metabolized in the liver to inactive glucuronide and sulfate metabolites.
• *Excretion:* The inactive metabolites and small amounts of unmetabolized drug are excreted by the kidneys. Insignificant quantities of drug are also excreted in feces. Biologic half-life of triamcinolone is 18 to 36 hours.

Contraindications and precautions

Contraindicated in patients with hypersensitivity to any component of the formulation or systemic fungal infections.

Use cautiously in patients with GI ulcer, renal disease, hypertension, osteoporosis, diabetes mellitus, hypothyroidism, cirrhosis, diverticulitis, nonspecific ulcerative colitis, recent intestinal anastomosis, thromboembolic disorders, seizures, myasthenia gravis, heart failure, tuberculosis, ocular herpes simplex, emotional instability, or psychotic tendencies.

Interactions

When used concomitantly, triamcinolone rarely may decrease the effects of *oral anticoagulants.*

Glucocorticoids increase the metabolism of *isoniazid* and *salicylates*; cause hyperglycemia, requiring dosage adjustment of *insulin* or *oral antidiabetic agents* in diabetic patients; and may enhance hypokalemia associated with *diuretic* or *amphotericin B* therapy. The hypokalemia may increase the risk of toxicity in patients concurrently receiving *cardiac glycosides.*

Barbiturates, phenytoin, and *rifampin* may cause decreased corticosteroid effects because of increased hepatic metabolism. *Antacids, cholestyramine,* and *colestipol* decrease the effect of triamcinolone by absorbing the corticosteroid, decreasing the amount absorbed.

Concomitant use with *estrogens* may reduce the metabolism of triamcinolone by increasing the concentration of transcortin. The half-life of the corticosteroid is then prolonged because of increased protein-binding. Concomitant administration of *ulcerogenic drugs* such as *NSAIDs* may increase the risk of GI ulceration.

Effects on diagnostic tests

Triamcinolone suppresses reactions to skin tests; causes false-negative results in the nitroblue tetrazolium test for systemic bacterial infections; decreases ^{131}I uptake and protein-bound iodine concentrations in thyroid function tests; may increase glucose and cholesterol levels; may decrease serum potassium, calcium, T_3, and T_4 levels; and may increase urine glucose and calcium levels.

Adverse reactions

Most adverse reactions to corticosteroids are dose- or duration-dependent.

CNS: *euphoria, insomnia,* psychotic behavior, pseudotumor cerebri, vertigo, headache, paresthesia, ***seizures.***
CV: ***heart failure, thromboembolism,*** hypertension, edema, ***arrhythmias,*** thrombophlebitis.
EENT: cataracts, glaucoma.
Endocrine: menstrual irregularities, cushingoid state (moonface, buffalo hump, central obesity).
GI: *peptic ulceration,* GI irritation, increased appetite, pancreatitis, nausea, vomiting.
Skin: delayed wound healing, acne, various skin eruptions.
Other: muscle weakness, osteoporosis, hirsutism, susceptibility to infections; hypokalemia, hyperglycemia, and carbohydrate intolerance; growth suppression in children; ***acute adrenal insufficiency with increased stress (infection, surgery, or trauma) or abrupt withdrawal after long-term therapy.***

After abrupt withdrawal, rebound inflammation, fatigue, weakness, arthralgia, fever, dizziness, lethargy, depression, fainting, orthostatic hypotension, dyspnea, anorexia, hypoglycemia. ***After prolonged use, sudden withdrawal may be fatal.***

Overdose and treatment

Acute ingestion, even in massive doses, is rarely a clinical problem. Toxic signs and symptoms rarely occur if drug is used for less than 3 weeks, even at large doses. However, chronic use causes adverse physiologic effects, including suppression of the hypothalamic-pituitary-adrenal axis, cushingoid appearance, muscle weakness, and osteoporosis.

☑ Special considerations

Recommendations for use of triamcinolone and for care and teaching of patients during therapy are the same as those for all *systemic adrenocorticoids.*

Pediatric use

• Chronic use of adrenocorticoids or corticotropin in children and adolescents may delay growth and maturation.

triamcinolone acetonide (oral and nasal inhalant)

Azmacort, Nasacort

Pharmacologic classification: glucocorticoid
Therapeutic classification: anti-inflammatory, antiasthmatic
Pregnancy risk category C

How supplied

Available by prescription only
Oral inhalation aerosol: 100 mcg/metered spray, 240 doses/inhaler
Nasal aerosol: 55 mcg/metered spray

Indications, route, and dosage

Steroid-dependent asthma

Adults: 2 inhalations t.i.d. or q.i.d. Maximum dosage, maximum of 16 inhalations daily.

Children age 6 to 12: 1 or 2 inhalations t.i.d. or q.i.d. Maximum dosage, 12 inhalations daily.

Rhinitis, allergic disorders, inflammatory conditions, nasal polyps

Adults: 2 sprays in each nostril daily; may increase dosage to maximum of 4 sprays per nostril daily, if needed.

Pharmacodynamics

Anti-inflammatory action: Glucocorticoids stimulate the synthesis of enzymes needed to decrease the inflammatory response. Triamcinolone acetonide is used as an oral inhalant to treat bronchial asthma in patients who require corticosteroids to control symptoms.

Pharmacokinetics

- *Absorption:* Systemic absorption from the lungs is similar to oral administration. Peak levels are attained in 1 to 2 hours.
- *Distribution:* After oral inhalation, 10% to 25% of drug is distributed to the lungs; rest is swallowed or deposited within the mouth. After nasal use, only a small amount reaches systemic circulation.
- *Metabolism:* Drug is metabolized mainly by the liver. Some that reaches the lungs may be metabolized locally.
- *Excretion:* The major portion of a dose is eliminated in feces. Biologic half-life of triamcinolone is 18 to 36 hours.

Contraindications and precautions

Oral form is contraindicated in patients hypersensitive to any component of the formulation and in those with status asthmaticus. Nasal form is contraindicated in patients with hypersensitivity or untreated localized infections.

Use oral form cautiously in patients with tuberculosis of the respiratory tract; untreated fungal, bacterial, or systemic viral infections; or ocular herpes simplex and in those receiving corticosteriods. Use both forms with caution in breast-feeding women.

Interactions

None reported.

Effects on diagnostic tests

None reported.

Adverse reactions

Most adverse reactions to corticosteroids are dose- or duration-dependent.

EENT: dry or irritated nose or throat, hoarseness.
Respiratory: cough, wheezing (with oral form).
Other: *oral candidiasis,* dry or irritated tongue or mouth, facial edema (with oral form).

Overdose and treatment

No information available.

☑ Special considerations

Recommendations for use of triamcinolone and for care and teaching of patients during therapy are the same as those for all *inhalant adrenocorticoids.*

Patient education

- Instruct patient to rinse mouth or gargle after inhaler use.

Pediatric use

- Safety and effectiveness have not been established for children under age 12 for nasal aerosol and under age 6 for oral aerosol.

Breast-feeding

- Use drug with caution in breast-feeding women.

triamcinolone acetonide (topical)

Aristocort, Flutex, Kenalog, Kenalog in Orabase, Triacet, Triaderm*

Pharmacologic classification: topical adrenocorticoid
Therapeutic classification: anti-inflammatory
Pregnancy risk category C

How supplied

Available by prescription only
Cream, ointment: 0.025%, 0.1%, 0.5%
Lotion: 0.025%, 0.1%
Paste: 0.1%

Indications, route, and dosage

Inflammation of corticosteroid-responsive dermatoses

Adults and children: Apply cream, ointment, or lotion sparingly once to four times daily. Apply paste to oral lesions by pressing a small amount into lesion without rubbing until thin film develops. Apply b.i.d. or t.i.d. after meals and h.s.

Pharmacodynamics

Anti-inflammatory action: Glucocorticoids stimulate the synthesis of enzymes needed to decrease the inflammatory response. Triamcinolone acetonide is a synthetic fluorinated corticosteroid. The 0.5% cream and ointment are recommended only for dermatoses refractory to treatment with lower concentrations.

Pharmacokinetics

- *Absorption:* Drug absorption depends on potency of preparation, amount applied, and nature of skin at application site. It ranges from about 1% in areas with a thick stratum corneum (such as the palms, soles, elbows, and knees) to as high as 36% in areas of the thinnest stratum corneum (face, eyelids, and genitals). Absorption increases in areas of skin damage, inflammation, or occlusion. Some systemic absorption of steroids occurs, especially through the oral mucosa.
- *Distribution:* After topical application, drug is distributed throughout the local skin layer. Drug ab-

sorbed into circulation is rapidly distributed into muscle, liver, skin, intestines, and kidneys.
- *Metabolism:* After topical administration, drug is metabolized primarily in the skin. The small amount that is absorbed into systemic circulation is metabolized primarily in the liver to inactive compounds.
- *Excretion:* Inactive metabolites are excreted by the kidneys, primarily as glucuronides and sulfates, but also as unconjugated products. Small amounts of the metabolites are also excreted in feces.

Contraindications and precautions
Contraindicated in patients hypersensitive to drug.

Interactions
None reported.

Effects on diagnostic tests
None reported.

Adverse reactions
Skin: burning, pruritus, irritation, dryness, erythema, folliculitis, hypertrichosis, hypopigmentation, acneiform eruptions, perioral dermatitis, allergic contact dermatitis, *maceration, secondary infection, atrophy, striae, miliaria* (with occlusive dressings).
Other: ***hypothalamic-pituitary-adrenal axis suppression***, Cushing's syndrome, hyperglycemia, glycosuria.

Overdose and treatment
No information available.

☑ Special considerations
Recommendations for use of triamcinolone, for care and teaching of patients during therapy, and for use in elderly patients, children, and breast-feeding women are the same as those for all *topical adrenocorticoids.*

triamterene
Dyrenium

Pharmacologic classification: potassium-sparing diuretic
Therapeutic classification: diuretic
Pregnancy risk category B

How supplied
Available by prescription only
Capsules: 50 mg, 100 mg

Indications, route, and dosage
Diuresis
Adults: Initially, 100 mg P.O. b.i.d. after meals. Total daily dosage should not exceed 300 mg.

Pharmacodynamics
Diuretic action: Triamterene acts directly on the distal renal tubules to inhibit sodium reabsorption and potassium excretion, reducing the potassium loss associated with other diuretic therapy.

Triamterene is commonly used with other more effective diuretics to treat edema associated with excessive aldosterone secretion, hepatic cirrhosis, nephrotic syndrome, and heart failure.

Pharmacokinetics
- *Absorption:* Drug is absorbed rapidly after oral administration, but the extent varies. Diuresis usually begins in 2 to 4 hours. Diuretic effect may be delayed 2 to 3 days if used alone; maximum antihypertensive effect may be delayed 2 to 3 weeks.
- *Distribution:* Drug is about 67% protein-bound.
- *Metabolism:* Metabolized by hydroxylation and sulfation.
- *Excretion:* Drug and its metabolites are excreted in urine; half-life of triamterene is 100 to 150 minutes.

Contraindications and precautions
Contraindicated in patients receiving other potassium-sparing agents, such as spirolactone or amiloride hydrochloride, and in those with hypersensitivity to drug, anuria, severe or progressive renal disease or dysfunction, severe hepatic disease, or hyperkalemia. Use cautiously in patients with impaired hepatic function or diabetes mellitus and in elderly or debilitated patients.

Interactions
Triamterene may potentiate the hypotensive effects of other *antihypertensive agents;* this may be used to therapeutic advantage.

Triamterene increases the hazard of hyperkalemia when administered with *other potassium-sparing diuretics, ACE inhibitors (captopril, enalapril), potassium supplements, potassium-containing medications (parenteral penicillin G),* or *salt substitutes.*

NSAIDs, such as *ibuprofen* or *indomethacin,* may alter renal function and thus affect potassium excretion. Diuretics may decrease *lithium* clearance.

Cimetidine may increase the bioavailability of triameterene and decrease its renal clearance and hydroxylation.

Effects on diagnostic tests
Drug therapy may interfere with enzyme assays that use fluorometry such as serum quinidine determinations.

Adverse reactions
CNS: dizziness, weakness, fatigue, headache.
CV: hypotension.
GI: dry mouth, nausea, vomiting, diarrhea.
Hematologic: megaloblastic anemia related to low folic acid levels, ***thrombocytopenia.***
Skin: photosensitivity, rash.
Other: ***anaphylaxis, hyperkalemia,*** muscle cramps, transient elevation in BUN or creatinine levels, acidosis, interstitial nephritis, hypokalemia, azotemia, jaundice, increased liver enzyme abnormalities.

Overdose and treatment
Clinical signs include those indicative of dehydration and electrolyte disturbance.

Treatment is supportive and symptomatic. For recent ingestion (less than 4 hours), empty stomach by induced emesis or gastric lavage. In severe hyperkalemia (more than 6.5 mEq/L), reduce serum potassium levels with I.V. sodium bicarbonate or glucose with insulin. A cation exchange resin, sodium polystyrene sulfonate (Kayexalate), given orally or as a retention enema, may also reduce serum potassium levels.

☑ Special considerations

Recommendations for the use of triamterene and for care and teaching of the patient during therapy are the same as those for all *potassium-sparing diuretics.*

Geriatric use

- Elderly and debilitated patients require close observation because they are more susceptible to drug-induced diuresis and hyperkalemia. Reduced dosages may be indicated.

Pediatric use

- Use with caution; children are more susceptible to hyperkalemia.

Breast-feeding

- Drug may be excreted in breast milk; safety during breast-feeding has not been established.

triazolam

Halcion

Pharmacologic classification: benzodiazepine
Therapeutic classification: sedative-hypnotic
Controlled substance schedule IV
Pregnancy risk category X

How supplied

Available by prescription only
Tablets: 0.125 mg, 0.25 mg

Indications, route, and dosage

Insomnia

Adults under age 65: 0.125 to 0.25 mg P.O. h.s. (0.5 mg P.O. h.s. only in exceptional patients; maximum dose, 0.5 mg).
Adults over age 65: 0.125 mg P.O. h.s. May give up to 0.25 mg.

Pharmacodynamics

Sedative-hypnotic action: Triazolam depresses the CNS at the limbic and subcortical levels of the brain. It produces a sedative-hypnotic effect by potentiating the effect of the neurotransmitter gamma-aminobutyric acid on its receptor in the ascending reticular activating system, which increases inhibition and blocks both cortical and limbic arousal.

Pharmacokinetics

- *Absorption:* Drug is well absorbed through the GI tract after oral administration. Peak levels occur in 1 to 2 hours. Onset of action occurs at 15 to 30 minutes.
- *Distribution:* Distributed widely throughout the body. Drug is 90% protein-bound.
- *Metabolism:* Metabolized in the liver primarily to inactive metabolites.
- *Excretion:* Metabolites of triazolam are excreted in urine. Half-life of triazolam ranges from approximately 1½ to 5½ hours.

Contraindications and precautions

Contraindicated in patients with hypersensitivity to benzodiazepines and during pregnancy. Use cautiously in patients with impaired renal or hepatic function, chronic pulmonary insufficiency, sleep apnea, mental depression, suicidal tendencies, or history of drug abuse.

Interactions

Triazolam potentiates the CNS depressant effects of *alcohol, antidepressants, antihistamines, barbiturates, general anesthetics, MAO inhibitors, narcotics,* and *phenothiazines.* Enhanced amnestic effects have been reported when combined with *alcohol* (even in small amounts).

Concomitant use with *cimetidine* and possibly *disulfiram* causes diminished hepatic metabolism of triazolam, which increases its plasma concentration.

Heavy smoking accelerates triazolam metabolism, thus lowering clinical effectiveness.

Benzodiazepines may decrease the therapeutic effects of *levodopa.*

Triazolam may decrease serum levels of *haloperidol.*

Erythromycin decreases clearance of triazolam.

Effects on diagnostic tests

Drug therapy may elevate liver function test results. Minor changes in EEG patterns, usually low-voltage, fast activity, may occur during and after triazolam therapy.

Adverse reactions

CNS: *drowsiness, dizziness, headache,* rebound insomnia, amnesia, light-headedness, lack of coordination, mental confusion, depression, nervousness, ataxia.
GI: nausea, vomiting.
Other: physical or psychological dependence.

Overdose and treatment

Clinical manifestations of overdose include somnolence, confusion, hypoactive reflexes, dyspnea, labored breathing, hypotension, bradycardia, slurred speech, unsteady gait or impaired coordination and, ultimately, coma.

Support blood pressure and respiration until drug effects subside; monitor vital signs. Flumazenil, a specific benzodiazepine antagonist, may be useful. Mechanical ventilatory assistance via endotracheal tube may be required to maintain a patent airway and support adequate oxygenation. Use I.V. fluids and vasopressors, such as dopamine and phenylephrine, to treat hypotension as needec. If patient is conscious, induce emesis. Use gastric lavage if ingestion was recent, but only if an endotracheal tube is present to prevent aspiration. After emesis or lavage, administer activated charcoal with a cathartic as a single dose. Do not use barbiturates if excitation occurs. Dialysis is of limited value.

☑ Special considerations

Besides those relevant to all *benzodiazepines,* consider the following recommendations.
- Monitor hepatic function studies to prevent toxicity
- Onset of sedation or hypnosis is rapid; patient should be in bed when taking triazolam.
- Store in a cool, dry place away from light.

Patient education
- Instruct patient not to take OTC drugs or to change medication regimen without medical approval.
- As necessary, teach safety measures to prevent injury such as gradual position changes.
- Suggest other measures to promote sleep, such as drinking warm fluids, listening to quiet music, not drinking alcohol near bedtime, exercising regularly, and maintaining a regular sleep pattern.
- Advise patient that rebound insomnia may occur after stopping drug.
- To prevent falls, encourage safety precautions at start of therapy.
- Advise patient of the potential for physical and psychological dependence.
- Advise female patient to report suspected pregnancy immediately.

Geriatric use
- Elderly patients are more susceptible to CNS depressant effects of triazolam. Use with caution.
- Lower doses are usually effective in elderly patients because of decreased elimination.
- Elderly patients who receive triazolam require supervision with ambulation and activities of daily living during initiation of therapy or after an increase in dose.

Pediatric use
- Safe use in patients under age 18 has not been established.

Breast-feeding
- Triazolam is excreted in breast milk. A breast-fed infant may become sedated, have feeding difficulties, or lose weight. Avoid use in breast-feeding women.

trientine hydrochloride
Syprine

Pharmacologic classification: chelating agent
Therapeutic classification: heavy metal antagonist
Pregnancy risk category C

How supplied
Available by prescription only
Capsules: 250 mg

Indications, route, and dosage
Wilson's disease in patients who are intolerant of penicillamine
Adults: 750 to 1,250 mg in doses divided b.i.d. to q.i.d. Maximum dosage, 2 g/day.
Children under age 12: 500 to 750 mg in doses divided b.i.d. to q.i.d. Maximum dosage, 1,500 mg/day.

Pharmacodynamics
Chelating action: Trientine forms a soluble complex with free serum copper that is renally excreted, removing excess copper.

Pharmacokinetics
- *Absorption:* Well absorbed after oral administration.
- *Distribution:* Unknown.
- *Metabolism:* None.
- *Excretion:* Excreted in urine as unchanged drug or a trientine-copper complex.

Contraindications and precautions
Contraindicated in patients with hypersensitivity to drug, rheumatoid arthritis, biliary cirrhosis, and cystinuria.

Interactions
Concomitant ingestion of trientine with *mineral supplements,* especially *iron,* reduces absorption of drug.

Effects on diagnostic tests
None reported.

Adverse reactions
Hematologic: iron-deficiency anemia.
Other: hypersensitivity reactions (rash), systemic lupus erythematosus.

Overdose and treatment
Data on effects of overdose are unavailable. Treat symptomatically.

☑ Special considerations
- Drug is designed for use only in patients unable to tolerate penicillamine, which remains the standard therapy for Wilson's disease.
- Daily dosage may be increased if clinical response is inadequate or free serum copper level remains above 20 mcg/dl.
- Observe patient for signs or symptoms of hypersensitivity, such as asthma, fever, or skin eruptions; monitor all patients for iron-deficiency anemia.
- For optimal therapeutic effect, give drug 1 hour before or 2 hours after meals and at least 1 hour apart from other drugs, food, or milk.

Patient education
- Explain disease process and rationale for therapy, stress importance of compliance with low-copper diet and follow-up visits.

- Tell patient how and when to take drug; especially advise patient to swallow capsule whole (not to open or chew), and to drink 8 oz (240 ml) of water with each dose.
- Advise patient to take temperature nightly for the first month of treatment and to report fever or skin eruptions.
- Explain that drug causes contact dermatitis; if accidental contact occurs, tell patient to wash area with water promptly.
- Advise patient to take drug on empty stomach, at least 1 hour before meals or 2 hours after meals and at least 1 hour apart from other drugs, food, or milk.

Pediatric use

- Safety and efficacy in children have not been established; use drug with caution.

Breast-feeding

- It is unknown whether drug crosses into breast milk. Use with caution in breast-feeding women.

triethanolamine polypeptide oleate-condensate

Cerumenex

Pharmacologic classification: oleic acid derivative
Therapeutic classification: ceruminolytic
Pregnancy risk category C

How supplied

Available by prescription only
Otic solution: 10% in 6-ml and 12-ml bottle with dropper

Indications, route, and dosage

Impacted cerumen
Adults and children: Fill ear canal with solution, and insert cotton plug. After 15 to 30 minutes, flush ear with warm water using a soft rubber bulb ear syringe. Do not expose ear canal to solution for more than 30 minutes.

Pharmacodynamics

Ceruminolytic action: Emulsifies and disperses accumulated cerumen.

Pharmacokinetics

- *Absorption:* No information available.
- *Distribution:* No information available.
- *Metabolism:* No information available.
- *Excretion:* No information available.

Contraindications and precautions

Contraindicated in perforated eardrum, otitis media, and otitis externa.

Interactions

None reported.

Effects on diagnostic tests

None reported.

Adverse reactions

EENT: ear erythema or itching.
Skin: severe eczema.

Overdose and treatment

Clinical manifestations of overdose include vomiting and diarrhea, which, if protracted, may lead to fluid and electrolyte abnormalities. Evaluate patient for oral burns. Spontaneous emesis often occurs; if not, significant ingestion may not have occurred. Activated charcoal or a cathartic are unnecessary.

Ocular exposure may result in transient eye irritation but usually no permanent damage. Treat eye exposure by irrigation with large amounts of tepid water for at least 15 minutes. Treat dermal exposure by washing the exposed area.

☑ Special considerations

- To determine allergic potential, do patch test: Place 1 drop of drug on inner forearm, then cover with small bandage; read in 24 hours. If reaction (redness, swelling) occurs, do not use drug.
- Moisten cotton plug with drug before insertion.
- Keep container closed and away from moisture.
- Avoid touching ear with dropper.

Patient education

- Advise patient not to exceed prescribed dosage and to avoid touching the ear with the dropper.
- Teach patient correct application and storage.

trifluoperazine hydrochloride

Apo-Trifluoperazine*, Novo-Flurazine*, Solazine*, Stelazine, Terfluzine*

Pharmacologic classification: phenothiazine (piperazine derivative)
Therapeutic classification: antipsychotic, antiemetic
Pregnancy risk category C

How supplied

Available by prescription only
Tablets (regular and film-coated): 1 mg, 2 mg, 5 mg, 10 mg
Oral concentrate: 10 mg/ml
Injection: 2 mg/ml

Indications, route, and dosage

Anxiety states
Adults: 1 to 2 mg P.O. b.i.d. Increase dosage p.r.n., but do not exceed 6 mg/day.
Schizophrenia and other psychotic disorders
Adults: For outpatients, 1 to 2 mg P.O. b.i.d., increased p.r.n. For hospitalized patients, 2 to 5 mg P.O. b.i.d.; may increase gradually to 40 mg daily. For I.M. injection, 1 to 2 mg q 4 to 6 hours, p.r.n.
Children age 6 to 12 (hospitalized or under close supervision): 1 mg P.O. daily or b.i.d.; may increase dosage gradually to 15 mg daily. Alternatively, administer 1 mg I.M. once or twice daily.

Pharmacodynamics

Antipsychotic action: Trifluoperazine is thought to exert its antipsychotic effects by postsynaptic blockade of CNS dopamine receptors, thereby inhibiting dopamine-mediated effects; antiemetic effects are attributed to dopamine receptor blockade in the medullary chemoreceptor trigger zone. Trifluoperazine has many other central and peripheral effects; it produces alpha and ganglionic blockade and counteracts histamine- and serotonin-mediated activity. Its most prevalent adverse reactions are extrapyramidal; it has less sedative and autonomic activity than aliphatic and piperidine phenothiazines.

Pharmacokinetics

- *Absorption:* Rate and extent of absorption vary with route of administration: Oral tablet absorption is erratic and variable, with onset of action ranging from ½ to 1 hour; oral concentrate absorption is much more predictable. I.M. drug is absorbed rapidly.
- *Distribution:* Distributed widely in the body, including breast milk. Drug is 91% to 99% protein-bound. Peak effect occurs in 2 to 4 hours; steady state serum levels are achieved within 4 to 7 days.
- *Metabolism:* Metabolized extensively by the liver, but no active metabolites are formed; duration of action is about 4 to 6 hours.
- *Excretion:* Mostly excreted in urine via the kidneys; some is excreted in feces via the biliary tract.

Contraindications and precautions

Contraindicated in patients with hypersensitivity to phenothiazines or in patients experiencing coma, CNS depression, bone marrow suppression, or liver damage. Use cautiously in elderly or debilitated patients; in those exposed to extreme heat; and in patients with CV disease, seizure disorders, glaucoma, or prostatic hyperplasia.

Interactions

Concomitant use of trifluoperazine with *sympathomimetics,* including *epinephrine, phenylephrine, phenylpropanolamine,* and *ephedrine* (commonly found in nasal sprays), and *appetite suppressants* may decrease their stimulatory and pressor effects. Using *epinephrine* as a pressor agent in patients taking trifluoperazine may result in epinephrine reversal or further lowering of blood pressure.

Trifluoperazine may inhibit blood pressure response to *centrally acting antihypertensive drugs,* such as *clonidine, guanabenz, guanadrel, guanethidine, methyldopa,* and *reserpine.* Additive effects are likely after concomitant use of trifluoperazine with *CNS depressants,* including *alcohol, analgesics, barbiturates, narcotics, tranquilizers, anesthetics (general, spinal, epidural),* and *parenteral magnesium sulfate* (oversedation, respiratory depression, and hypotension); *antiarrhythmic agents, disopyramide, procainamide,* and *quinidine* (increased incidence of arrhythmias and conduction defects); *atropine* and *other anticholinergic drugs,* including *antidepressants, antihistamines, MAO inhibitors, meperidine, phenothiazines,* and *antiparkinsonian agents* (oversedation, paralytic ileus, visual changes, and severe constipation); *nitrates* (hypotension); and *metrizamide* (increased risk of seizures).

Beta-blocking agents may inhibit trifluoperazine metabolism, increasing plasma levels and toxicity.

Concomitant use of trifluoperazine with *propylthiouracil* increases risk of agranulocytosis; concomitant use with *lithium* may result in severe neurologic toxicity with an encephalitis-like syndrome and in decreased therapeutic response to trifluoperazine.

Pharmacokinetic alterations and subsequent decreased therapeutic response to trifluoperazine may follow concomitant use with *phenobarbital* (enhanced renal excretion), *aluminum-* and *magnesium-containing antacids* and *antidiarrheals* (decreased absorption), *caffeine,* and *heavy smoking* (increased metabolism).

Trifluoperazine may antagonize therapeutic effect of *bromocriptine* on prolactin secretion; it also may decrease the vasoconstricting effects of *high-dose dopamine* and may decrease effectiveness and increase toxicity of *levodopa* (by dopamine blockade). Trifluoperazine may inhibit metabolism and increase toxicity of *phenytoin.*

Effects on diagnostic tests

Drug causes false-positive test results for urine porphyrins, urobilinogen, amylase, and 5-hydroxyindoleacetic acid levels from darkening of urine by metabolites; it also causes false-positive urine pregnancy results in tests using human chorionic gonadotropin as the indicator.

Trifluoperazine elevates tests for liver function and protein-bound iodine and causes quinidine-like effects on ECG.

Adverse reactions

CNS: *extrapyramidal reactions, tardive dyskinesia,* pseudoparkinsonism, dizziness, drowsiness, insomnia, fatigue, headache.
CV: *orthostatic hypotension,* tachycardia, ECG changes.
EENT: ocular changes, *blurred vision.*
GI: *dry mouth, constipation,* nausea.
GU: *urine retention.*
Hematologic: transient leukopenia, ***agranulocytosis.***
Hepatic: cholestatic jaundice.
Skin: *photosensitivity,* allergic reactions, pain at I.M. injection site, sterile abscess, rash.
Other: weight gain; rarely, ***neuroleptic malignant syndrome*** (fever, tachycardia, tachypnea, profuse diaphoresis), menstrual irregularities, gynecomastia, inhibited lactation.

After abrupt withdrawal of long-term therapy: gastritis, nausea, vomiting, dizziness, tremor, feeling of warmth or cold, diaphoresis, tachycardia, headache, insomnia, anorexia, muscle rigidity, altered mental status, and evidence of autonomic instability.

Overdose and treatment

CNS depression is characterized by deep, unarousable sleep and possible coma, hypotension or hypertension, extrapyramidal symptoms, dystonia, abnormal involuntary muscle movements, agitation, seizures, arrhythmias, ECG changes, hypothermia or hyperthermia, and autonomic nervous system dysfunction.

Treatment is symptomatic and supportive and includes maintaining vital signs, airway, stable body temperature, and fluid and electrolyte balance.

Do not induce vomiting: Drug inhibits cough reflex, and aspiration may occur. Use gastric lavage, then activated charcoal and sodium chloride cathartics; dialysis is usually ineffective. Regulate body temperature as needed. Treat hypotension with I.V. fluids: *Do not give epinephrine.* Treat seizures with parenteral diazepam or barbiturates; arrhythmias with parenteral phenytoin (1 mg/kg with rate titrated to blood pressure); extrapyramidal reactions with benztropine at 1 to 2 mg or parenteral diphenhydramine at 10 to 50 mg.

☑ Special considerations

Besides those relevant to all *phenothiazines,* consider the following recommendations.

- Other agents such as benzodiazepines are preferred for the treatment of anxiety. When drug is given for anxiety, do not exceed 6 mg daily for longer than 12 weeks. Some clinicians recommend using drug only for psychosis.
- Administer I.M. injection deep in the upper outer quadrant of the buttock. Massaging the area after administration may prevent formation of abscesses. I.M. injection may cause skin necrosis; do not extravasate.
- Solution for injection may be slightly discolored. Do not use if excessively discolored or a precipitate is evident. Contact pharmacist.
- Monitor blood pressure before and after parenteral administration.
- Shake concentrate before administration.
- Chewing sugarless gum or hard candy or ice may help relieve dry mouth.
- Worsening anginal pain has been reported in patients receiving trifluoperazine; however, ECG reactions are less common with drug than with other phenothiazines.
- Liquid and injectable formulations may cause a rash after contact with skin.
- Drug may cause pink to brown discoloration of urine or blue-grey skin.
- Drug is associated with a high incidence of extrapyramidal symptoms and photosensitivity reactions. Patient should avoid exposure to sunlight or heat lamps.
- Monitor regularly for abnormal body movements (at least once every 6 months).
- Oral formulations may cause stomach upset. Administer with food or fluid.
- Concentrate must be diluted in 2 to 4 oz (60 to 120 ml) of liquid, preferably water, carbonated drinks, fruit juice, tomato juice, milk, or pudding.
- Protect liquid formulation from light.

Patient education

- Explain risks of dystonic reactions, akathisia, and tardive dyskinesia, and tell patient to report abnormal body movements.
- Explain that many drug interactions are possible. Tell patient to seek medical approval before taking *any* self-prescribed medication.
- Tell patient that adverse reactions may be alleviated by a dosage reduction. Instruct him to report difficulty urinating, sore throat, dizziness, or fainting; male patients should be warned about inhibited ejaculation.
- Warn patient against hazardous activities that require alertness until the effect of drug is established. Reassure patient that sedative effects usually subside in several weeks.
- Tell patient to avoid sun exposure and wear sunscreen when going outdoors to prevent photosensitivity reactions. (Explain that heat lamps and tanning beds also may cause burning of the skin or skin discoloration.)
- Warn patient to avoid extremely hot or cold baths and exposure to temperature extremes, sunlamps, and tanning beds; drug may cause thermoregulatory changes.
- Tell patient to take drug exactly as prescribed and not to double dose for missed doses, stop taking drug abruptly, or share drug with others.
- Advise patient to store medication in a safe place, away from children.
- Tell patient to avoid alcohol and other medications that may cause excessive sedation.
- Inform patient that sugarless candy or gum, ice chips, or artificial saliva may relieve dry mouth.

Geriatric use

- Elderly patients tend to require lower doses, titrated to effect. Adverse effects, especially tardive dyskinesia and other extrapyramidal effects and hypotension, are more likely to develop in such patients.

Pediatric use

- Not recommended for children under age 6.

Breast-feeding

- Drug may enter breast milk. Potential benefits to the mother should outweigh the potential harm to the infant.

trifluridine

Viroptic

Pharmacologic classification: fluorinated pyrimidine nucleoside
Therapeutic classification: antiviral
Pregnancy risk category C

How supplied

Available by prescription only
Ophthalmic solution: 1%

Indications, route, and dosage

Primary keratoconjunctivitis and recurrent epithelial keratitis caused by herpes simplex virus types I and II

Adults: 1 drop instilled into the affected eye q 2 hours while patient is awake, to maximum of 9 drops daily until reepithelialization of the corneal ulcer occurs; then, 1 drop q 4 hours (minimum, 5 drops daily) for an additional 7 days.

Pharmacodynamics

Antiviral action: Exact mechanism of action is unknown, but drug appears to interfere with DNA synthesis, preventing viral cell replication; it is active against herpes simplex virus types I and II and vaccinia virus.

Pharmacokinetics

- *Absorption:* Intraocular penetration occurs after topical administration; however, appreciable systemic absorption does not occur. Inflammation may enhance penetration.
- *Distribution:* Unknown.
- *Metabolism:* Unknown.
- *Excretion:* Half-life of trifluridine is approximately 12 to 18 minutes.

Contraindications and precautions

Contraindicated in patients hypersensitive to drug.

Interactions

None reported.

Effects on diagnostic tests

None reported.

Adverse reactions

EENT: *stinging on instillation,* edema of eyelids, increased intraocular pressure, epithelial keratopathy, superficial punctate keratopathy, stromal edema, irritation, keratitis sicca.
Other: hypersensitivity reactions.

Overdose and treatment

The toxicity of ingested trifluridine is unknown; if large quantities are ingested, use general measures, such as emesis, lavage, or a cathartic, to remove drug from the GI tract. Treat dermal exposure by washing the area with soap and water. Observe patient closely for possible signs and symptoms.

☑ Special considerations

- Consider another form of therapy if improvement does not occur after 7 days or if complete reepithelialization does not occur after 14 days of treatment.
- Drug should not be used for more than 21 consecutive days because of potential for ocular toxicity.
- Keep drug refrigerated; gradually bring to room temperature before use.

Patient education

- Reassure patient that mild local irritation of the conjunctiva and cornea that occurs when solution is instilled is usually temporary.
- Warn patient not to exceed recommended dosage and frequency of administration.
- Caution patient to report if improvement is not seen in 7 days or if condition worsens or irritation occurs.
- Tell patient the correct way to instill eyedrops and not to touch eye or surrounding area with dropper.
- Instruct patient not to share washcloths and towels with family members during treatment period.

trihexyphenidyl hydrochloride

Apo-Trihex*, Artane, Artane Sequels, Trihexane, Trihexy-2, Trihexy-5

Pharmacologic classification: anticholinergic
Therapeutic classification: antiparkinsonian
Pregnancy risk category C

How supplied

Available by prescription only
Tablets: 2 mg, 5 mg
Capsules (sustained-release): 5 mg
Elixir: 2 mg/5 ml

Indications, route, and dosage

Idiopathic parkinsonism

Adults: 1 mg P.O. on first day, 2 mg on second day, then increase 2 mg q 3 to 5 days until total of 6 to 10 mg is given daily. Usually given t.i.d. with meals and, if needed, q.i.d. (last dose should be before bedtime). Postencephalitic parkinsonism may require 12 to 15 mg total daily dosage. Patients receiving levodopa may need 3 to 6 mg daily.

Drug-induced parkinsonism

Adults: 5 to 15 mg daily.

Pharmacodynamics

Antiparkinsonian action: Trihexyphenidyl blocks central cholinergic receptors, helping to balance cholinergic activity in the basal ganglia. It may also prolong the effects of dopamine by blocking dopamine reuptake and storage at central receptor sites.

Pharmacokinetics

- *Absorption:* Rapidly absorbed after oral administration. Onset of action occurs within 1 hour.
- *Distribution:* Drug crosses the blood-brain barrier; little else is known about its distribution.
- *Metabolism:* Exact metabolic fate is unknown. Duration of effect is 6 to 12 hours.
- *Excretion:* Excreted in the urine as unchanged drug and metabolites.

Contraindications and precautions

Contraindicated in patients hypersensitive to drug. Use cautiously in patients with impaired renal, cardiac, or hepatic function, glaucoma, obstructive disease of the GI or GU tract, or prostatic hyperplasia.

Interactions

Concomitant use with *amantadine* may amplify anticholinergic adverse effects of trihexyphenidyl, causing confusion and hallucinations. Concomitant use with *haloperidol* or *phenothiazines* may decrease the antipsychotic effectiveness of these drugs, possibly from direct CNS antagonism; concomitant *phenothiazine* use also increases the risk of anticholinergic adverse effects.

Concomitant use with *CNS depressants,* such as *tranquilizers, sedative-hypnotics,* and *alcohol,* increases sedative effects of trihexyphenidyl. When used with *levodopa,* dosage of both drugs may need adjustment because of synergistic anticholinergic effects and possible enhanced GI metabolism of *levodopa* from reduced gastric motility and delayed gastric emptying. *Antacids* and *antidiarrheals* may decrease absorption of trihexyphenidyl.

Effects on diagnostic tests
None reported.

Adverse reactions
CNS: nervousness, dizziness, headache, hallucinations, drowsiness, weakness.
CV: tachycardia.
EENT: blurred vision, mydriasis, increased intraocular pressure.
GI: *dry mouth, nausea,* constipation, vomiting.
GU: urinary hesitancy, urine retention.

Overdose and treatment
Clinical effects of overdose include central stimulation followed by depression, with such psychotic symptoms as disorientation, confusion, hallucinations, delusions, anxiety, agitation, and restlessness. Peripheral effects may include dilated, nonreactive pupils; blurred vision; flushed, dry, hot skin; dry mucous membranes; dysphagia; decreased or absent bowel sounds; urine retention; hyperthermia; headache; tachycardia; hypertension; and increased respiration.

Treatment is primarily symptomatic and supportive, as needed. Maintain patent airway. If the patient is alert, induce emesis (or use gastric lavage) and follow with sodium chloride cathartic and activated charcoal to prevent further drug absorption. In severe cases, physostigmine may be administered to block antimuscarinic effects of trihexyphenidyl. Give fluids, as needed, to treat shock; diazepam to control psychotic symptoms; and pilocarpine (instilled into the eyes) to relieve mydriasis. If urine retention occurs, catheterization may be necessary.

☑ Special considerations
Besides those relevant to all *anticholinergics,* consider the following recommendations.
- Store drug in tight containers.
- Monitor patient for urinary hesitancy.
- Arrange for gonioscopic evaluation and close intraocular pressure monitoring, especially in patients over age 40.
- Tolerance may develop to drug, necessitating higher doses.

Patient education
- Tell patient to avoid activities that require alertness until CNS effects of drug are known.
- Advise patient to report signs of urinary hesitation or urine retention.
- Tell patient to relieve dry mouth with cool drinks, ice chips, sugarless gum, or hard candy.

Geriatric use
- Use caution when administering drug to elderly patients. Lower doses are indicated.

Breast-feeding
- Drug may be excreted in breast milk, possibly resulting in infant toxicity. Breast-feeding women should avoid drug. Drug may also decrease milk production.

trimeprazine tartrate
Panectyl*, Temaril

Pharmacologic classification: phenothiazine-derivative antihistamine
Therapeutic classification: antipruritic
Pregnancy risk category NR

How supplied
Available by prescription only
Tablets: 2.5 mg
Spansule capsules (sustained-release): 5 mg
Syrup: 2.5 mg/5 ml (5.7% alcohol)

Indications, route, and dosage
Pruritus
Adults and children age 12 and older: 2.5 mg P.O. q.i.d.; or (timed-release) 5 mg P.O. q 12 hours.
Children age 6 to 11: One spansule capsule (5 mg) daily. Spansule capsules are not recommended for children under age 6.
Children age 3 to 5: 2.5 mg P.O. h.s. or t.i.d., p.r.n.
Infants age 6 months to 2 years: 1.25 mg P.O. h.s. or t.i.d., p.r.n.

Pharmacodynamics
Antipruritic action: Antihistamines compete for H_1-receptor sites by binding to cellular receptors; they prevent access of histamine and suppress histamine-induced allergic symptoms, even though they do not prevent its release.

Pharmacokinetics
- *Absorption:* Well absorbed. After oral administration, onset of action in 15 to 60 minutes, with peak effect in 1 to 2 hours and duration of 3 to 6 hours.
- *Metabolism:* Hepatic biotransformation.
- *Distribution:* Unknown.
- *Excretion:* Renal.

Contraindications and precautions
Contraindicated in patients with hypersensitivity to drug or other phenothiazines, acute asthma, coma, CNS depression, or bone marrow depression; in neonates or premature infants; in acutely ill or dehydrated children; and in breast-feeding patients.

Use cautiously in children under age 12; in patients with angle-closure glaucoma, prostatic hyperplasia, stenosing peptic ulcer, or pyloroduodenal or bladder neck obstruction; and in those receiving MAO inhibitors.

Interactions
MAO inhibitors interfere with the detoxification of antihistamines and phenothiazines and thus prolong and intensify their central depressant and anticholinergic effects; added sedation and CNS depression may occur when trimeprazine is used con-

comitantly with other *CNS depressants,* including *alcohol, barbiturates, sleeping aids, tranquilizers,* and *antianxiety agents.* Concomitant use with *beta blockers* and *antihypertensives* produces additive effects of both drugs.

Phenothiazines potentiate the CNS depressant and analgesic effect of *narcotics;* the phenothiazine activity of trimeprazine is potentiated by *nylidrin hydrochloride, oral contraceptives, progesterone,* and *reserpine.*

Do not give *epinephrine* to reverse trimeprazine-induced hypotension; partial *adrenergic blockade* may cause further hypotension. Trimeprazine blocks dopamine receptors and inhibits the antiparkinsonian effect of *levodopa.*

Effects on diagnostic tests

Discontinue drug 4 days before diagnostic skin tests to avoid preventing, reducing, or masking positive test response. Drug may cause false-positive or false-negative urine pregnancy test results.

Adverse reactions

CNS: drowsiness, dizziness, confusion, headache, restlessness, tremor, irritability, insomnia, paradoxical excitation.
CV: hypotension, palpitations, tachycardia.
GI: anorexia, nausea, vomiting, *dry mouth and throat.*
GU: urinary frequency, urine retention.
Hematologic: ***agranulocytosis,*** leukopenia.
Skin: urticaria, rash, *photosensitivity.*

Overdose and treatment

Clinical manifestations of overdose may include either CNS depression (sedation, reduced mental alertness, apnea, and CV collapse) or CNS stimulation (insomnia, hallucinations, tremors, or seizures). Anticholinergic symptoms, such as dry mouth, flushed skin, fixed and dilated pupils, and GI symptoms, are common, especially in children. The manufacturer warns against inducing emesis because dystonic reaction of head and neck may result in aspiration of vomitus. Use gastric lavage followed by activated charcoal. Treat hypotension with vasopressors, and control seizures with diazepam or phenytoin I.V. *Do not give stimulants.*

☑ Special considerations

Besides those relevant to all *antihistamines,* consider the following recommendations.

- Increased requirements for riboflavin may occur.
- Monitor patients on prolonged therapy for CV, hematologic, and hepatic function and for neurologic or ophthalmologic effects.

Patient education

- Warn patient about risk of photosensitivity; recommend sunscreen, and advise patient to report skin reactions immediately.
- Instruct patient to store drug in a tightly closed container away from direct sunlight and heat.

Geriatric use

- Elderly patients may experience more frequent and severe adverse effects with drug than with other antihistamines because of its phenothiazine structure. Elderly patients are usually more sensitive to adverse effects of antihistamines and are especially likely to experience a greater degree of dizziness, sedation, hyperexcitability, dry mouth, and urine retention than younger patients. Symptoms usually respond to a decrease in dosage.

Pediatric use

- Contraindicated for use in neonates; infants and children under age 6 may experience paradoxical hyperexcitability.

Breast-feeding

- Antihistamines such as trimeprazine should not be used during breast-feeding. Many of these drugs are secreted in breast milk, exposing the infant to risks of unusual excitability; premature infants are at particular risk for seizures.

trimethobenzamide hydrochloride

Arrestin, Stemetic, Tebamide, T-Gen, Ticon, Tigan, Tiject-20, Trimazide

Pharmacologic classification: ethanolamine-related antihistamine
Therapeutic classification: antiemetic
Pregnancy risk category C

How supplied

Available by prescription only
Capsules: 100 mg, 250 mg
Suppositories: 100 mg, 200 mg
Injection: 100 mg/ml

Indications, route, and dosage

Nausea and vomiting (treatment)
Adults: 250 mg P.O. t.i.d. or q.i.d.; or 200 mg I.M. or P.R. t.i.d. or q.i.d.
Children weighing 30 to 90 lb (14 to 41 kg): 100 to 200 mg P.O. or P.R. t.i.d. or q.i.d.
Children weighing under 30 lb: 100 mg P.R. t.i.d. or q.i.d.

Pharmacodynamics

Antiemetic action: Trimethobenzamide is a weak antihistamine with limited antiemetic properties. Its exact mechanism of action is unknown. Drug effects may occur in the chemoreceptor trigger zone of the brain; however, drug apparently does not inhibit direct impulses to the vomiting center.

Pharmacokinetics

- *Absorption:* Approximately 60% of an oral dose is absorbed. After oral administration, action begins in 10 to 40 minutes; after I.M. administration, in 15 to 35 minutes.
- *Distribution:* Unknown.
- *Metabolism:* Approximately 50% to 70% of dose is metabolized, probably in the liver.
- *Excretion:* Drug is excreted in urine and feces. After oral administration, duration of effect is 3 to 4 hours; after I.M. administration, 2 to 3 hours.

Contraindications and precautions
Contraindicated in patients with hypersensitivity to drug. Suppositories are contraindicated in patients hypersensitive to benzocaine hydrochloride or similar local anesthetic. Use cautiously in children.

Interactions
Alcohol and other *CNS depressants,* including *tricyclic antidepressants, antihypertensives, phenothiazines,* and *belladonna alkaloids,* may increase trimethobenzamide toxicity.

Effects on diagnostic tests
None reported.

Adverse reactions
CNS: *drowsiness,* dizziness (in large doses), headache, disorientation, depression, parkinsonian-like symptoms, ***coma, seizures.***
CV: hypotension.
GI: diarrhea.
Hepatic: jaundice.
Other: hypersensitivity reactions (pain, stinging, burning, redness, swelling at I.M. injection site); blurred vision; muscle cramps.

Overdose and treatment
Signs and symptoms of overdose may include severe neurologic reactions, such as opisthotonos, seizures, coma, and extrapyramidal reactions. Discontinue drug and provide supportive care.

☑ Special considerations
- Give I.M. dose by deep injection into upper outer gluteal quadrant to minimize pain and local irritation.
- Record frequency and volume of vomiting; observe patient for signs and symptoms of dehydration.
- Drug may be less effective against severe vomiting than other agents.
- Drug has little or no value in treating motion sickness.

Patient education
- Warn patient to avoid hazardous activities that require alertness because drug may cause drowsiness, and to avoid consuming alcohol to prevent additive sedation.
- Instruct patient to report persistent vomiting.
- Instruct patient using suppositories to remove foil and, if necessary, to moisten suppository with water for 10 to 30 seconds before inserting; tell patient to store suppositories in refrigerator.

Geriatric use
- Use drug with caution in elderly patients because they may be more susceptible to adverse CNS effects.

Pediatric use
- Use drug with caution in children. Do not administer to children with viral illness because drug may contribute to development of Reye's syndrome.

trimethoprim
Proloprim, Trimpex

Pharmacologic classification: synthetic folate antagonist
Therapeutic classification: antibiotic
Pregnancy risk category C

How supplied
Available by prescription only
Tablets: 100 mg, 200 mg

Indications, route, and dosage
Treatment of uncomplicated urinary tract infections
Adults: 100 mg P.O. q 12 hours or 200 mg q 24 hours for 10 days. Drug is not recommended for children under age 12.
◇ ***Prophylaxis of chronic and recurrent urinary tract infections***
Adults: 100 mg P.O. h.s. for 6 weeks to 6 months.
◇ ***Traveler's diarrhea***
Adults: 200 mg P.O. b.i.d. for 3 to 5 days.
◇ **Pneumocystis carinii**
Adults: 20 mg/kg P.O. in four divided doses in conjunction with dapsone 100 mg daily for 21 days.
✦ ***Dosage adjustment.*** In patients with renal failure and creatinine clearance of 10 to 50 ml/minute, increase dosage interval to q 18 hours. If creatinine clearance is below 10 ml/minute, give q 24 hours.

Pharmacodynamics
Antibacterial action: By interfering with action of dihydrofolate reductase, drug inhibits bacterial synthesis of folic acid. Drug is effective against many gram-positive and gram-negative organisms, including most Enterobacteriaceae organisms (except *Pseudomonas*), *Proteus mirabilis, Klebsiella,* and *Escherichia coli.*

Trimethoprim is usually bactericidal.

Pharmacokinetics
- *Absorption:* Drug is absorbed quickly and completely, reaching peak serum levels in 1 to 4 hours.
- *Distribution:* Widely distributed. Approximately 42% to 46% of dose is plasma protein-bound.
- *Metabolism:* Less than 20% of dose is metabolized in the liver.
- *Excretion:* Most of dose is excreted in the urine via filtration and secretion. In patients with normal renal function, elimination half-life is 8 to 11 hours; in patients with impaired renal function, half-life is prolonged.

Contraindications and precautions
Contraindicated in patients with hypersensitivity to drug and in those with documented megaloblastic anemia caused by folate deficiency. Use cautiously in patients with folate deficiency and impaired hepatic or renal function (especially those with creatinine clearance of 15 ml/minute or less).

Interactions
When used concomitantly, trimethoprim may inhibit *phenytoin* metabolism, causing increased serum phenytoin levels.

Effects on diagnostic tests
Liver enzyme levels and renal function indices (BUN and serum creatinine levels) may increase during trimethoprim therapy.

Adverse reactions
GI: *epigastric distress, nausea, vomiting,* glossitis.
Hematologic: ***thrombocytopenia,*** leukopenia, megaloblastic anemia, methemoglobinemia.
Skin: *rash, pruritus,* exfoliative dermatitis.
Other: fever.

Overdose and treatment
Clinical effects of acute overdose include nausea, vomiting, dizziness, headache, confusion, and bone marrow depression. Treatment includes gastric lavage and supportive measures. Urine may be acidified to enhance drug elimination.

Clinical effects of chronic toxicity caused by prolonged high-dose therapy include bone marrow depression, leukopenia, thrombocytopenia, and megaloblastic anemia. Treatment includes drug discontinuation and administration of leucovorin—3 to 6 mg I.M. daily for 3 days or 5 to 15 mg P.O. daily until normal hematopoiesis returns.

☑ Special considerations
- Obtain specimen for culture and sensitivity tests before starting therapy.
- Drug is usually used with other antibiotics (especially sulfamethoxazole) because resistance develops rapidly when used alone.
- If patient is receiving drug concomitantly with phenytoin, monitor serum phenytoin levels.
- Advanced age, malnourishment, pregnancy, debilitation, renal impairment, and prolonged high-dose therapy increase risk of hematologic toxicity, as does concomitant therapy with folate antagonistic drugs (such as phenytoin).
- Sore throat, fever, pallor, and purpura may be early signs and symptoms of serious blood disorders. Monitor blood counts regularly.

Patient education
- Instruct patient to continue taking drug as directed, until it is completed, even if feeling better.
- Advise patient to report signs or symptoms of blood disorders (sore throat, fever, pallor, and purpura) immediately.

Geriatric use
- Elderly patients may be more susceptible to hematologic toxicity.

Pediatric use
- Safety in children under age 2 months has not been established; effectiveness in children under age 12 has not been established.

Breast-feeding
- Drug is excreted in breast milk; alternative feeding method is recommended during therapy with trimethoprim.

trimetrexate glucuronate
Neutrexin

Pharmacologic classification: dihydrofolate reductase inhibitor
Therapeutic classification: antimicrobial/antineoplastic
Pregnancy risk category D

How supplied
Injection: 25-mg vials

Indications, route, and dosage
Treatment of patients with **Pneumocystis carinii** ***pneumonia who have exhibited serious (severe or life-threatening) intolerance to both co-trimoxazole and pentamidine (hospital use only)***
Adults: Dosage and indication vary with protocol. Administer 45 mg/m² I.V. bolus daily for 21 days, with leucovorin (20 mg/m² I.V. or P.O. daily).

Dose modification or discontinuation is needed for patients with hematologic toxicity.

Pharmacodynamics
Dihydrofolate reductase inhibiting action: In vitro, the affinity of trimetrexate for pneumocystis dihydrofolate reductase is about 1,500 times that of trimethoprim. Unlike methotrexate, trimetrexate is highly lipophilic and is passively taken up by and concentrated in protozoan cells.

Pharmacokinetics
- *Absorption:* No data are available regarding oral bioavailability.
- *Distribution:* Drug distributes rapidly after I.V. administration.
- *Metabolism:* Probably metabolized by the liver; at least two metabolites (one active) have been identified.
- *Excretion:* Excreted in bile and urine.

Contraindications and precautions
Contraindicated during pregnancy and in patients with hypersensitivity to trimetrexate, methotrexate, or leucovorin. Use cautiously in patients with impaired hematologic, renal, or hepatic function and in women of childbearing age.

Interactions
Trimetrexate plasma concentrations may be altered with coadministration of *erythromycin, fluconazole, ketoconazole, rifabutin,* and *rifampin. Drugs that inhibit the P450 enzyme system* may elicit important drug interactions that may alter plasma concentrations of trimetrexate.

Effects on diagnostic tests
None reported.

Adverse reactions
CNS: peripheral neuropathy.
GI: nausea, vomiting, stomatitis.
Hematologic: ***neutropenia, thrombocytopenia, anemia.***
Hepatic: hepatotoxicity.
Skin: rash.

Overdose and treatment
Although no information is available, clinical effects are expected to be similar to those of methotrexate.

Methotrexate overdose produces myelosuppression, anemia, nausea, vomiting, dermatitis, alopecia, and melena.

Specific treatment information is unavailable, but calcium levocovorin would probably serve as an appropriate treatment. Contact the manufacturer (Warner-Lambert) for further information.

☑ Special considerations
- Avoid I.M. injections in patients with thrombocytopenia.
- Store intact vials in refrigerator.
- Reconstitute with 5% dextrose injection or sterile water for injection to yield concentration of 12.5 mg/ml; solution should appear pale greenish yellow. Observe for particulate matter. Do not use if cloudiness or precipitate appears in the solution.
- Dilute further with 5% dextrose injection to yield concentration of 0.25 to 2 mg/ml. Administer over 60 minutes.
- I.V. line should be flushed with 10 ml 5% dextrose injection before and after administration.
- Incompatible with chloride-containing solutions (including 0.9% NaCl). Only D_5W is recommended for infusions.
- After reconstitution, solution is stable under refrigeration or at room temperature for up to 24 hours.
- Dosage adjustments may be necessary in patients with altered hepatic or renal function.
- Continue leucovorin for 72 hours after last dose of trimetrexate.

trimipramine maleate
Surmontil

Pharmacologic classification: tricyclic antidepressant
Therapeutic classification: antidepressant, antianxiety
Pregnancy risk category C

How supplied
Available by prescription only
Capsules: 25 mg, 50 mg, 100 mg

Indications, route, and dosage
Depression
Adults: For outpatients, give 75 mg/day in divided doses and increase to 200 mg/day; maintenance dose, 50 to 150 mg/day. Dosage for inpatients is 100 mg/day in divided doses and increased p.r.n. Maximum daily dosage, 300 mg.
Adolescents and elderly patients: 50 to 100 mg/day.

Pharmacodynamics
Antidepressant action: Trimipramine is thought to exert its antidepressant effects by equally inhibiting reuptake of norepinephrine and serotonin in CNS nerve terminals (presynaptic neurons), which results in increased concentration and enhanced activity of these neurotransmitters in the synaptic cleft. Trimipramine also has anxiolytic effects and inhibits gastric acid secretion.

Pharmacokinetics
- *Absorption:* Absorbed rapidly from the GI tract after oral administration.
- *Distribution:* Distributed widely in the body. Drug is 90% protein-bound. Peak effect occurs in 2 hours; steady state within 7 days.
- *Metabolism:* Metabolized by the liver; a significant first-pass effect may explain variability of serum levels in different patients taking the same dosage.
- *Excretion:* Mostly excreted in urine; some excreted in feces via the biliary tract.

Contraindications and precautions
Contraindicated during acute recovery phase of MI, in patients with hypersensitivity to drug, or in those receiving MAO inhibitor therapy within 14 days.

Use cautiously in adolescents; in elderly or debilitated patients; in those receiving thyroid medications; and in those with CV disease, increased intraocular pressure, hyperthyroidism, impaired hepatic function, or history of seizures, urine retention, or angle-closure glaucoma.

Interactions
Concomitant use of trimipramine with *sympathomimetics,* including *epinephrine, phenylephrine, phenylpropanolamine,* and *ephedrine* (commonly found in nasal sprays) may increase blood pressure; use with *warfarin* may increase PT and cause bleeding.

Concomitant use with *thyroid medication, pimozide,* and *antiarrhythmic agents (disopyramide, procainamide, quinidine)* may increase incidence of arrhythmias and conduction defects.

Trimipramine may decrease hypotensive effects of centrally acting antihypertensive drugs, such as *clonidine, guanabenz, guanadrel, guanethidine, methyldopa,* and *reserpine.*

Concomitant use with *disulfiram* or *ethchlorvynol* may cause delirium and tachycardia.

Additive effects are likely after concomitant use of trimipramine with *CNS depressants,* including *alcohol, analgesics, barbiturates, narcotics, tranquilizers,* and *anesthetics* (oversedation); *atropine* and *other anticholinergic drugs,* including *antihistamines, meperidine, phenothiazines,* and *antiparkinsonian agents* (oversedation, paralytic ileus, visual changes, and severe constipation); and *metrizamide* (increased risk of seizures).

Barbiturates and *heavy smoking* induce trimipramine metabolism and decrease therapeutic efficacy; *haloperidol* and *phenothiazines* decrease its metabolism, decreasing therapeutic efficacy; *beta blockers, cimetidine, methylphenidate, oral contraceptives,* and *propoxyphene* may inhibit trimipramine metabolism, increasing plasma levels and toxicity.

Effects on diagnostic tests
Drug may prolong conduction time (elongation of QT and PR intervals, flattened T waves on ECG); it also may elevate liver function test levels, decrease WBC counts, and alter serum glucose levels. Trimipramine may alter PT.

Adverse reactions
CNS: *drowsiness, dizziness,* paresthesia, ataxia, hallucinations, delusions, anxiety, agitation, insomnia, tremor, weakness, confusion, headache, EEG changes, ***seizures,*** extrapyramidal reactions.
CV: *orthostatic hypotension,* tachycardia, hypertension, ***arrhythmias, heart block, MI, stroke.***
EENT: *blurred vision,* tinnitus, mydriasis.
GI: *dry mouth, constipation,* nausea, vomiting, anorexia, paralytic ileus.
GU: *urine retention.*
Skin: rash, urticaria, photosensitivity.
Other: *diaphoresis,* hypersensitivity reaction.

After abrupt withdrawal of long-term therapy: nausea, headache, malaise (does not indicate addiction).

Overdose and treatment
The first 12 hours after acute ingestion are a stimulatory phase characterized by excessive anticholinergic activity (agitation, irritation, confusion, hallucinations, parkinsonian symptoms, seizure, urine retention, dry mucous membranes, pupillary dilation, constipation, and ileus). This is followed by CNS depressant effects, including hypothermia, decreased or absent reflexes, sedation, hypotension, cyanosis, and cardiac irregularities (including tachycardia, conduction disturbances, and quinidine-like effects on the ECG).

Severity of overdose is best indicated by prolongation of QRS interval beyond 100 mseconds, which usually represents a serum level in excess of 1,000 ng/ml; serum levels are generally not helpful. Metabolic acidosis may follow hypotension, hypoventilation, and seizures.

Treatment is symptomatic and supportive and includes maintaining airway, stable body temperature, and fluid and electrolyte balance. Induce emesis with ipecac if patient is conscious; follow with gastric lavage and activated charcoal to prevent further absorption. Dialysis is of little use. Physostigmine given I.V. slowly has been used to reverse most of the CV and CNS effects of overdosage. Treat seizures with parenteral diazepam or phenytoin; arrhythmias with parenteral phenytoin or lidocaine; and acidosis with sodium bicarbonate. *Do not give barbiturates*—these may enhance CNS and respiratory depressant effects.

☑ Special considerations
Besides those relevant to all *tricyclic antidepressants,* consider the following recommendations.
- Consider the inherent risk of suicide until significant improvement of depressive state occurs. Closely monitor high-risk patients during initial drug therapy. To reduce risk of suicidal overdose, prescribe the smallest quantity of capsules consistent with good management.
- May give the full dosage at bedtime to offset daytime sedation.
- Drug also has been used to decrease gastric acid secretion in peptic ulcer disease. The safety and efficacy of trimipramine maleate in peptic ulcer disease has not been established.
- Watch for bleeding because drug may cause alterations in PT.
- Do not withdraw drug abruptly. However, it should be discontinued at least 48 hours before surgical procedures.
- Tolerance generally develops to the sedative effects of drug.
- Manic or hypomanic episodes may occur in some patients, especially those with cyclic-type disorders, when taking trimipramine.

Patient education
- Advise patient to take full dosage at bedtime to minimize daytime sedation.
- Explain that full effects of drug may not become apparent for up to 4 to 6 weeks after therapy begins.
- Tell patient to take drug exactly as prescribed; not to take double doses for missed ones; not to discontinue drug suddenly; and not to share drug with others.
- Warn patient that drug may cause drowsiness or dizziness. Tell him to avoid activities that require mental alertness until the full effects of drug are known.
- Warn patient not to drink alcoholic beverages or medicinal elixirs while taking drug.
- Tell patient to store drug safely away from children.
- Suggest taking drug with food or milk if it causes stomach upset and to ease dry mouth with sugarless chewing gum, hard candy, or ice.
- To prevent dizziness, advise patient to lie down for about 30 minutes after each dose and to avoid abrupt postural changes, especially when rising to an upright position.
- Tell patient to report adverse reactions promptly, especially confusion, movement disorders, rapid heartbeat, dizziness, fainting, or difficulty urinating.

Geriatric use
- Recommended starting dose for elderly patients is 25 mg. Such patients may be more vulnerable to adverse cardiac effects.

triprolidine hydrochloride
Myidyl

Pharmacologic classification: alkylamine antihistamine derivative
Therapeutic classification: antihistamine (H_1-receptor antagonist)
Pregnancy risk category C

How supplied
Available with or without a prescription
Tablets: 2.5 mg
Syrup: 1.25 mg/5 ml

Indications, route, and dosage

Colds and allergy symptoms

Adults and children age 12 and older: 2.5 mg P.O. q 4 to 6 hours; maximum daily dosage, 10 mg.
Children age 6 to 11: 1.25 mg q 4 to 6 hours; maximum daily dosage, 5 mg.
Children age 4 to 5: 0.9 mg q 6 to 8 hours; maximum daily dosage, 3.75 mg.
Children age 2 to 3: 0.6 mg q 6 to 8 hours; maximum daily dosage, 2.5 mg.
Infants age 4 months to 2 years: 0.3 mg q 4 to 6 hours; maximum daily dosage, 1.25 mg.

Pharmacodynamics

Antihistamine action: Antihistamines compete with histamine for H_1-receptor sites on the smooth muscle of the bronchi, GI tract, uterus, and large blood vessels; by binding to cellular receptors, they prevent access of histamine and suppress histamine-induced allergic symptoms, even though they do not prevent its release.

Pharmacokinetics

- *Absorption:* Well absorbed from the GI tract; it has a rapid onset of action, with peak effects occurring in about 3½ hours and a duration of about 12 hours.
- *Distribution:* Not fully known; drug is distributed to the lungs, spleen, and kidneys.
- *Metabolism:* Metabolized by the liver.
- *Excretion:* Half-life is about 2 to 6 hours.

Contraindications and precautions

Contraindicated in patients with hypersensitivity to drug or acute asthma and in neonates, premature infants, and breast-feeding patients.

Use with caution in patients with increased intraocular pressure, angle-closure glaucoma, hyperthyroidism, CV disease, hypertension, bronchial asthma, prostatic hyperplasia, bladder neck obstruction, or stenosing peptic ulcer and in children under age 12.

Interactions

MAO inhibitors interfere with the detoxification of antihistamines and thus prolong and intensify their central depressant and anticholinergic effects; added CNS depression may occur when triprolidine is given concomitantly with other *CNS depressants,* such as *alcohol, barbiturates, sleeping aids, tranquilizers,* and *antianxiety agents.*

Triprolidine may diminish the effects of *sulfonylureas* and may partially counteract the anticoagulant effects of *heparin.*

Effects on diagnostic tests

Discontinue drug 4 days before diagnostic skin tests; antihistamines can prevent, reduce, or mask positive skin response to the test.

Adverse reactions

CNS: *drowsiness, dizziness,* confusion, restlessness, insomnia, headache, *sedation, sleepiness, incoordination,* fatigue, anxiety, nervousness, tremor, ***seizures,*** *stimulation.*
CV: hypotension, palpitations, tachycardia.
EENT: *dry nose and throat.*
GI: anorexia, diarrhea or constipation, nausea, vomiting, *dry mouth,* epigastric distress.
GU: urinary frequency, urine retention.
Hematologic: hemolytic anemia, ***thrombocytopenia, agranulocytosis.***
Skin: urticaria, rash, photosensitivity, diaphoresis.
Other: ***anaphylactic shock,*** chills, thickening of bronchial secretions.

Overdose and treatment

Clinical manifestations of overdose may include either CNS depression (sedation, reduced mental alertness, apnea, and CV collapse) or CNS stimulation (insomnia, hallucinations, tremors, or seizures). Anticholinergic signs and symptoms, such as dry mouth, flushed skin, fixed and dilated pupils, and GI symptoms, are common, especially in children.

Treat overdose by inducing emesis with ipecac syrup (in conscious patient), followed by activated charcoal to reduce further drug absorption. Use gastric lavage if patient is unconscious or ipecac fails. Treat hypotension with vasopressors, and control seizures with diazepam or phenytoin. *Do not give stimulants.*

☑ Special considerations

Besides those relevant to all *antihistamines,* consider the following recommendation.

- Triprolidine has a low incidence of drowsiness.

Patient education

- Recommendations for teaching of patients are the same as those for all *antihistamines.*

Geriatric use

- Elderly patients are usually more sensitive to adverse effects of antihistamines and are especially likely to experience a greater degree of dizziness, sedation, hyperexcitability, dry mouth, and urine retention than younger patients. Signs and symptoms usually respond to a decrease in medication dosage.

Pediatric use

- Drug is not indicated for use in premature or newborn infants; infants and children under age 6 may experience paradoxical hyperexcitability.

Breast-feeding

- Antihistamines such as triprolidine should not be used during breast-feeding. Many of these drugs are secreted in breast milk, exposing the infant to risks of unusual excitability; premature infants are at particular risk for seizures.

troglitazone

Rezulin

Pharmacologic classification: thiazolidinedione
Therapeutic classification: antidiabetic
Pregnancy risk category B

How supplied
Available by prescription only
Tablets: 200 mg, 400 mg

Indications, route, and dosage
As monotherapy for patients with type 2 diabetes mellitus not controlled with diet alone
Adults: Initially, 400 mg P.O. once daily; may increase to 600 mg after 1 month if needed. For patients not responding to 600 mg after 1 month, drug should be discontinued and alternative therapeutic options taken.
In combination with sulfonylureas in patients with type 2 diabetes mellitus
Adults: Initially, 200 mg P.O. once daily; continue current sulfonylurea dose. Increase dosage after 2 to 4 weeks p.r.n. to maximum dose of 600 mg/day. Sulfonylurea dose may have to be lowered.
Adjunct to diet and insulin therapy in patients with type 2 diabetes mellitus whose hyperglycemia is inadequately controlled
Adults: Initially, for patients on insulin therapy, continue with current insulin dose and begin concomitant therapy with 200 mg P.O. once daily, taken with a meal. Dosage may be increased after 2 to 4 weeks p.r.n. Usual daily dose, 400 mg; maximum recommended daily dose, 600 mg. Insulin dose may be decreased by 10% to 25% when fasting glucose levels are below 120 mg/dl in patients receiving both troglitazone and insulin.

Pharmacodynamics
Antidiabetic action: Troglitazone lowers blood glucose by improving target cell response to insulin. Action is dependent on presence of insulin for activity. It also decreases hepatic glucose output and increases insulin-dependent glucose disposal in skeletal muscle. Its mechanism of action is thought to involve binding to nuclear receptors that regulate the transcription of a number of insulin responsive genes critical for the control of glucose and lipid metabolism.

Pharmacokinetics
- *Absorption:* Rapidly absorbed after oral administration, with peak plasma concentrations occurring within 2 to 3 hours. Food increases absorption from 30% to 85%. Steady-state plasma levels are reached in 3 to 5 days.
- *Distribution:* Extensively bound (over 99%) to serum albumin. Volume of distribution after multiple doses is 10.5 to 26.5 L/kg of body weight.
- *Metabolism:* Metabolized to three major metabolites.
- *Excretion:* Excreted as metabolites in the feces (85%) and the urine (3%). Plasma elimination half-life is 16 to 34 hours.

Contraindications and precautions
Contraindicated in patients with known hypersensitivity to drug and in patients with type 1 diabetes or diabetic ketoacidosis. Use cautiously in patients with hepatic disease and class III or IV cardiac status. Troglitazone should not be initiated in patients with ALT levels over 1.5 times the upper limit of normal.

Interactions
Cholestyramine reduces absorption of troglitazone by 70%; avoid concomitant administration. Coadministration with *oral contraceptives* may cause reduced plasma concentrations of hormones, resulting in loss of contraceptive properties. Additional form of contraception is recommended.

Effects on diagnostic tests
Drug may cause transient elevations in AST and ALT levels, small changes in serum lipid levels, and small decreases in hemoglobin levels, hematocrit, and neutrophil counts.

Adverse reactions
CNS: asthenia, dizziness, *headache.*
CV: peripheral edema.
EENT: pharyngitis, rhinitis.
GI: diarrhea, ***hepatitis, jaundice,*** nausea.
GU: urinary tract infection.
Musculoskeletal: back pain.
Other: accidental injury, ***death,*** *infection, pain.*

Overdose and treatment
No information available.

☑ Special considerations
- Drug does not stimulate insulin secretion; do not use to treat patients with type 1 diabetes or ketoacidosis.
- When used concomitantly with insulin, monitor patient for hypoglycemia. Insulin dose may need to be reduced.
- Before starting therapy, investigate and address secondary causes of poor glycemic control (including infection and poor injection technique).
- Monitor glucose levels, especially during increased stress, such as infection, fever, surgery, and trauma because insulin requirements may change.
- Monitor serum transaminase levels at baseline and every month for the first 8 months, then every 2 months for the remainder of the first year of troglitazone therapy. Continue checking serum transaminase levels periodically thereafter.
- If patient has jaundice or ALT rises above 3 times the upper limit of normal, then discontinue troglitazone.
- In premenopausal anovulatory women, drug treatment may result in resumption of ovulation increasing risk of pregnancy.
- Rare cases of severe idiosyncratic hepatocellular injury have been reported. The injury is usually reversible, but very rare cases of hepatic failure, including death, have been reported. Injury has occurred after both short- and long-term troglitazone treatment.

Patient education
- Advise patient to report signs or symptoms, such as nausea, vomiting, abdominal pain, fatigue, anorexia or dark urine, which may indicate hepatitis or hepatic failure and require immediate attention.
- Instruct patient about nature of diabetes, importance of following treatment, avoiding infection, and adhering to specific diet, weight reduction, exer-

cise, and personal hygiene programs. Explain how and when to perform self-monitoring of blood glucose level, teach signs of hypoglycemia and hyperglycemia, and explain what to do if those conditions occur. Include responsible family members in teaching.
- Tell patient that drug should be taken with a meal. If a dose is missed, take it with the next meal. If a dose is missed on one day, he should not double the dose on the following day.
- Tell patient that drug may cause resumption of ovulation in premenopausal anovulatory women, causing an increased risk for pregnancy.
- Instruct patient to carry medical identification at all times.
- Advise patient to use additional methods of contraception if taking oral contraceptives.

Geriatric use
- No differences in safety and efficacy were observed in patients over age 65 and younger patients.

Pediatric use
- Safety and effectiveness in pediatric patients have not been established.

Breast-feeding
- In animal studies, troglitazone was excreted in breast milk. Avoid use of drug in breast-feeding women.

troleandomycin
Tao

Pharmacologic classification: macrolide antibiotic
Therapeutic classification: antibiotic
Pregnancy risk category C

How supplied
Available by prescription only
Capsules: 250 mg
Suspension: 125 mg/ml

Indications, route, and dosage
Pneumonia or respiratory tract infection caused by sensitive pneumococci or group A beta-hemolytic streptococci
Adults: 250 to 500 mg P.O. q 6 hours.
Children: 125 to 250 mg P.O. q 6 hours.

Pharmacodynamics
Antibacterial action: Drug inhibits bacterial protein synthesis by binding to 50S ribosomal subunit. It produces bacteriostatic effects on susceptible bacteria, including gram-positive cocci and bacilli and a few gram-negative organisms *(Haemophilus influenzae, Neisseria gonorrhoeae,* and *N. meningitidis*).

Pharmacokinetics
- *Absorption:* Absorbed rapidly but incompletely. Peak serum levels occur in approximately 2 hours.
- *Distribution:* Drug is distributed widely to body fluids, except to CSF.
- *Metabolism:* Metabolized in the liver.
- *Excretion:* Drug is excreted in the bile, feces, and urine (10% to 25%).

Contraindications and precautions
Contraindicated in patients with known hypersensitivity to drug. Use cautiously to patients with hepatic dysfunction.

Interactions
When used concomitantly, troleandomycin may decrease clearance of *carbamazepine, methylprednisolone,* and *theophylline* possibly causing toxicity. (Clinical significance of decreased clearance of methylprednisolone is questionable; however, some clinicians recommend lower doses of the steroid.) Concomitant use with *ergotamine* may precipitate severe ischemic reactions and peripheral vasospasms. Concomitant use with *oral contraceptives* may cause marked cholestatic jaundice.

Effects on diagnostic tests
Liver function test results may show increased enzyme levels, and eosinophilia and leukocytosis may occur during troleandomycin therapy.

Adverse reactions
GI: *abdominal cramps, discomfort,* vomiting, diarrhea.
Hepatic: cholestatic jaundice.
Skin: urticaria, rash.
Other: ***anaphylaxis.***

Note: Discontinue drug if liver function test values increase or if signs or symptoms of cholestatic hepatitis occur.

Overdose and treatment
No information available.

☑ Special considerations
- Obtain culture and sensitivity tests before starting therapy.
- If patient is receiving drug concomitantly with theophylline or carbamazepine, closely monitor serum theophylline or carbamazepine levels and assess patient frequently for signs and symptoms of theophylline or carbamazepine toxicity.
- Know that patient receiving drug concomitantly with methylprednisolone may require reduced doses.
- Monitor total serum bilirubin and AST, ALT, and serum alkaline phosphatase levels.
- Repeated courses of therapy or therapy exceeding 2 weeks may lead to allergic cholestatic hepatitis, as indicated by jaundice, right upper abdominal quadrant pain, fever, nausea, vomiting, eosinophilia, and leukocytosis.

Patient education
- Instruct patient to continue taking drug as directed, even if feeling better.
- For best absorption, advise patient to take drug on an empty stomach 1 hour before or 2 hours after meals, with full glass of water.

• Instruct patient to report abdominal pain or nausea immediately.

tromethamine

Tham

Pharmacologic classification: sodium-free organic amine
Therapeutic classification: systemic alkalinizer
Pregnancy risk category C

How supplied

Available by prescription only
Injection: 18 g/500 ml

Indications, route, and dosage

Correction of metabolic acidosis (associated with cardiac bypass surgery or with cardiac arrest)

Adults: Dosage depends on base deficit. Calculate as follows: ml of 0.3 molar tromethamine solution required = body weight in kilograms X base deficit in mEq/L. Total dosage should be administered over at least 1 hour and should not exceed 500 mg/kg for an adult.

Usual dose of a 0.3 M solution (3.6 to 10.8 g tromethamine) may be administered into a large peripheral vein. If the chest is open, 55 to 165 ml of a 0.3 M solution (2 to 6 g tromethamine) has also been injected into the ventricular cavity (*not into the cardiac muscle*).

For systemic acidosis during cardiac bypass surgery, usual single dose of a 0.3 M solution is 9 ml/kg (324 mg/kg tromethamine) or about 500 ml (18 g tromethamine) for most adults.

To titrate the excess acidity of stored blood used to prime the pump-oxygenator during cardiac bypass surgery

Adults: Add 14 to 70 ml of 0.3 M solution to each 500 ml of blood, depending on pH of blood.

Pharmacodynamics

Systemic alkalinizing action: Tromethamine, as a weak base, acts as a proton acceptor to prevent or correct acidosis; drug reduces hydrogen ion concentration. It also acts as a weak osmotic diuretic, increasing the flow of alkaline urine.

Pharmacokinetics

• *Absorption:* Absorption is immediate because drug is available for I.V. use only.
• *Distribution:* At pH of 7.4, about 25% of drug is un-ionized; this portion may enter cells to neutralize acidic ions of intracellular fluid.
• *Metabolism:* None.
• *Excretion:* Drug is rapidly excreted renally as the bicarbonate salt.

Contraindications and precautions

Contraindicated in patients with anuria, uremia, or chronic respiratory acidosis or during pregnancy (except in acute, life-threatening situations). Use cautiously in patients with renal disease and poor urine output.

Interactions

Concomitant use with other *respiratory* or *CNS depressants* may cause cumulative respiratory depression.

Effects on diagnostic tests

Tromethamine alters serum electrolyte levels. Transient decreases in blood glucose concentrations may occur.

Adverse reactions

Respiratory: *respiratory depression.*
Other: hypoglycemia, ***hyperkalemia*** (with decreased urine output), venospasm; I.V. thrombosis; inflammation, necrosis, and sloughing (if extravasation occurs); hemorrhagic hepatic necrosis.

Overdose and treatment

Clinical signs of overdose include respiratory or systemic alkalosis, arrhythmias secondary to hypokalemia, respiratory depression, and hypoglycemia. Stop drug and correct pH; use decreased ventilation and systemic acidifiers if necessary. Treat hypokalemia cautiously with potassium (serum potassium levels increase with correction of alkalosis), and hypoglycemia with I.V. glucose as needed.

☑ Special considerations

• Monitor vital signs, blood pH levels, carbon dioxide tension, and bicarbonate, glucose, and electrolyte levels before, during, and after infusion.
• Administer drug by slow I.V. into the largest antecubital vein or via a large needle, indwelling catheter, or pump-oxygenator. Check infusion site frequently to avoid extravasation of solution and prevent tissue damage. If extravasation occurs, aspirate as much fluid as possible. Infiltrating area with 1% procaine hydrochloride to which hyaluronidase has been added to help with extravasation and venospasm. Local injection of phentolamine can be used to reverse venospasm.

Geriatric use

• Patients with severe renal dysfunction or chronic respiratory acidosis are at increased risk with tromethamine; use drug with caution.

Pediatric use

• Use drug cautiously; severe hepatic necrosis has occurred in infants and neonates after administration of a 1.2 M solution through the umbilical vein.

tropicamide

I-Picamide, Mydriacyl, Ocu-Tropic, Tropicacyl

Pharmacologic classification: anticholinergic
Therapeutic classification: cycloplegic, mydriatic
Pregnancy risk category C

How supplied

Available by prescription only
Ophthalmic solution: 0.5%, 1%

Indications, route, and dosage

Cycloplegic refractions

Adults and children: Instill 1 or 2 drops of 0.5% or 1% solution in each eye; repeat in 5 minutes.

Fundus examinations

Adults and children: Instill 1 or 2 drops of 0.5% or 1% solution in each eye 15 to 20 minutes before examination. May repeat q 30 minutes if necessary.

Apply light finger pressure on lacrimal sac for 1 minute after instillation to minimize systemic absorption. Care should be taken to avoid contamination of the dropper tip.

Pharmacodynamics

Mydriatic action: Anticholinergic action prevents the sphincter muscle of the iris and the muscle of the ciliary body from responding to cholinergic stimulation, producing pupillary dilation (mydriasis) and paralysis of accommodation (cycloplegia).

Pharmacokinetics

- *Absorption:* Peak effect usually occurs in 20 to 40 minutes.
- *Distribution:* Unknown.
- *Metabolism:* Unknown.
- *Excretion:* Recovery from cycloplegic and mydriatic effects usually occurs in about 6 hours.

Contraindications and precautions

Contraindicated in patients with shallow anterior chamber and angle-closure glaucoma or hypersensitivity to drug. Use cautiously in elderly patients.

Interactions

None significant.

Effects on diagnostic tests

None reported.

Adverse reactions

CNS: confusion, somnolence, hallucinations, behavioral disturbances in children.

EENT: *transient eye stinging on instillation,* increased intraocular pressure, hyperemia, irritation, conjunctivitis, edema, *blurred vision, photophobia, dry throat.*

GI: dry mouth.

Skin: dryness.

Overdose and treatment

Clinical manifestations of overdose include dry, flushed skin; dry mouth; dilated pupils; delirium; hallucination; tachycardia; and decreased bowel sounds. Treat accidental ingestion with emesis or activated charcoal. Use physostigmine to antagonize anticholinergic activity of tropicamide in severe toxicity and propranolol to treat symptomatic tachyarrhythmias unresponsive to physostigmine.

☑ Special considerations

- Tropicamide is the shortest-acting cycloplegic, but its mydriatic effect is greater than its cycloplegic effect.

Patient education

- Advise patient to protect eyes from bright illumination for comfort.
- Instruct patient not to touch the dropper tip to any surface and to replace cap after use to avoid contamination.

Geriatric use

- Use with caution in elderly patients to avoid triggering undiagnosed narrow-angle glaucoma.

Pediatric use

- Infants and small children may be especially susceptible to CNS disturbances from systemic absorption. Psychotic reactions, behavioral disturbances, and cardiopulmonary collapse have been reported in children.

Breast-feeding

- No data available; however, tropicamide should be used with extreme caution during breast-feeding because of the potential for CNS and cardiopulmonary effects in infants.

trovafloxacin mesylate

Trovan Tablets

alatrofloxacin mesylate

Trovan I.V.

Pharmacologic classification: fluoroquinolone derivative
Therapeutic classification: antibiotic
Pregnancy risk category C

How supplied

Available by prescription only
Tablets: 100 mg, 200 mg
Injection: 5 mg/ml, in 40 ml (200 mg) and 60 ml (300 mg) vials

Indications, route, and dosage

For the treatment of infections caused by susceptible microorganisms, the following dosages are administered once every 24 hours:

Gynecologic and pelvic infections, complicated intra-abdominal and postsurgical infections

Adults: 300 mg I.V. daily followed by 200 mg P.O. daily for 7 to 14 days.

Nosocomial pneumonia

Adults: 300 mg I.V. daily followed by 200 mg P.O. daily for 10 to 14 days.

Community-acquired pneumonia

Adults: 200 mg P.O. or I.V. daily followed by 200 mg P.O. daily for 7 to 14 days.

Complicated skin and diabetic foot infections

Adults: 200 mg P.O. or I.V. daily followed by 200 mg P.O. daily for 10 to 14 days.

Surgical prophylaxis (colorectal, abdominal and vaginal hysterectomy)

Adults: 200 mg P.O. or I.V as a single dose 30 minutes to 4 hours before surgery.

Acute sinusitis, chronic prostatitis, cervicitis, and pelvic inflammatory disease (mild to moderate)

Adults: 200 mg P.O. daily for 5 days (cervicitis), 10 days (acute sinusitis), 14 days (pelvic inflammatory disease), or 28 days (chronic prostatitis).

Uncomplicated urinary tract infections, uncomplicated skin and skin structure infections, bacterial bronchitis, uncomplicated gonorrhea

Adults: 100 mg P.O. daily for 7 to 10 days (3 days for urinary tract infection, single dose for gonorrhea).

✦ ***Dosage adjustment.*** Dosage adjustments are unnecessary when switching from I.V. to oral forms. An adjustment in dosage is not needed in patients with renal impairment; however, in patients with mild to moderate hepatic disease (cirrhosis), the following dosage reductions are recommended: reduce 300 mg I.V. to 200 mg I.V., reduce 200 mg I.V. or P.O. to 100 mg I.V. or P.O.; no reduction needed for 100 mg P.O.

Pharmacodynamics

Antibiotic action: Trovafloxacin is related to the fluoroquinolones with in vitro activity against a wide range of gram-positive and gram-negative aerobic and anaerobic microorganisms. The bactericidal action of trovafloxacin results from inhibition of DNA gyrase and topoisomerase IV, two enzymes involved in bacterial replication.

Pharmacokinetics

- *Absorption:* Drug is well absorbed after oral administration with an absolute bioavailability of approximately 88%. Peak serum concentrations occur about 1 hour after oral administration, and steady state levels are obtained by the third day of oral or I.V. administration.
- *Distribution:* Widely and rapidly distributed throughout the body, resulting in significantly higher tissue concentrations than in plasma or serum. Mean plasma protein bound fraction is approximately 76%. Trovafloxacin is found in measurable concentrations in breast milk.
- *Metabolism:* Primarily metabolized by conjugation although there is minimal oxidative metabolism by cytochrome P-450. Approximately 13% of a dose appears in the urine as the glucuronide ester and 9% as the N-acetyl metabolite.
- *Excretion:* Primary route of elimination is fecal. Approximately 50% of an oral dose (43% in feces and 6% in urine) is excreted as unchanged drug.

Contraindications and precautions

Contraindicated in patients with hypersensitivity to trovafloxacin, alatrovafloxacin, or other quinolone antimicrobials. Use cautiously in patients with history of seizures, psychosis, or increased intracranial pressure.

Interactions

The bioavailability of trovafloxacin is significantly reduced following concomitant administration of *aluminum-, magnesium-,* and *iron-containing preparations* such as *antacids* and *vitamin-minerals.* Concomitant administration of *sucralfate* and *I.V. morphine* also produce significant reductions in trovafloxacin plasma levels. Minor interactions that are probably not clinically significant include plasma level reductions by *calcium carbonate, omeprazole,* and *caffeine.*

Effects on diagnostic tests

None reported.

Adverse reactions

CNS: *dizziness,* light-headedness, headache, ***seizures.***
GI: diarrhea, nausea, vomiting, abdominal pain, pseudomembranous colitis.
GU: vaginitis.
Hematologic: ***bone marrow aplasia (anemia, thrombocytopenia, leukopenia).***
Hepatic: elevated hepatic transaminases.
Musculoskeletal: arthralgia, arthropathy, myalgia.
Skin: pruritis, rash, injection site reaction (I.V), photosensitivity.

Overdose and treatment

Trovafloxacin has a low order of acute toxicity. Clinical signs include decreased activity and respiration, ataxia, ptosis, tremors, and seizures. Treat by emptying the stomach and providing symptomatic and supportive treatment. Drug is not efficiently removed by hemodialysis.

☑ Special considerations

- Changes in laboratory values during trovafloxacin therapy did not produce clinical abnormalities, and levels generally returned to normal 1 to 2 months after discontinuation of therapy.
- Perform periodic assessment of liver function because drug increases ALT, AST, and alkaline phosphatase levels.
- Oral form is less cost-effective and carries less risk; both forms have similar clinical efficacy and pharmacokinetics. Patients started with I.V. therapy may be switched to oral therapy when clinically indicated and at the discretion of the health care provider.
- Drug can be given as a single daily dose without regard for food.
- As with other quinolones, neurologic complications such as seizures, psychosis, or increased intracranial pressure may occur. Monitor patients with these preexisting conditions closely.
- Safety and efficacy of prolonged treatment (over 4 weeks) have not been studied.
- After dilution, I.V. drug should be administered as a 60-minute infusion. Compatible I.V. solutions are D_5W, 0.45% NaCl, 5% dextrose and 0.45% NaCl, 5% dextrose and 0.2% NaCl, and 5% dextrose and lactated Ringer's.

Patient education

- Inform patient that drug may be taken without regard to meals; however, tell him to take sucralfate, antacids containing citric acid buffered with sodium citrate, or products containing iron, aluminum, or magnesium (vitamin-minerals, antacids) at least 2 hours before or after a trovafloxacin dose.
- Advise patient who experiences lightheadedness or dizziness to take drug with meals or at bedtime.
- Warn patient to avoid excessive sunlight or artificial ultraviolet light.

- Instruct patient to discontinue treatment, refrain from exercise, and seek medical advice if pain, inflammation, or rupture of a tendon occurs.
- Advise patient to discontinue treatment at first sign of rash, hives, difficulty swallowing or breathing, or other symptoms suggesting an allergic reaction and to seek medical help immediately.
- Instruct patient to report severe diarrhea because this could indicate pseudomembraneous colitis.

Geriatric use
- At recommended doses, drug is as well tolerated and efficacious in patients age 65 and over as in younger patients.

Pediatric use
- Safety and effectiveness in children under age 18 have not been established.

Breast-feeding
- Drug is excreted in breast milk in measurable concentrations. Because of unknown effects in infants, the risks of therapy and breast-feeding should be evaluated.

tuberculosis skin test antigens

tuberculin purified protein derivative (PPD)
Aplisol, Tubersol

tuberculin cutaneous multiple-puncture device
Aplitest (PPD), Mono-Vacc Test (Old Tuberculin), Sclavo-Test PPD, Tine Test (Old Tuberculin), Tine Test PPD

Pharmacologic classification: Mycobacterium tuberculosis and *Mycobacterium bovis* antigen
Therapeutic classification: diagnostic skin test antigen
Pregnancy risk category C

How supplied
Available by prescription only
tuberculin PPD
Injection (intradermal): 1 tuberculin unit/0.1 ml, 5 tuberculin units/0.1 ml, 250 tuberculin units/0.1 ml
tuberculin cutaneous multiple-puncture device
Test: 25 devices/pack

Indications, route, and dosage
Diagnosis of tuberculosis; evaluation of immunocompetence in patients with cancer or malnutrition
Adults and children: Intradermal injection of 5 tuberculin units/0.1 ml.

A single-use, multiple-puncture device is used for determining tuberculin sensitivity. All multiple-puncture tests are equivalent to or more potent than 5 tuberculin units of PPD.

Adults and children: Apply the unit firmly and without any twisting to the upper one third of the forearm for approximately 3 seconds; this ensures stabilizing the dried tuberculin B in the tissue lymph. Exert enough pressure to ensure that all four tines have entered the skin of the test area and a circular depression is visible.

Pharmacodynamics
Diagnosis of tuberculosis: Administration to a patient with a natural infection with *M. tuberculosis* usually results in sensitivity to tuberculin and a delayed hypersensitivity reaction (after administration of old tuberculin or PPD). The cell-mediated immune reaction to tuberculin in tuberculin-sensitive individuals, which results mainly from cellular infiltrates of the dermis of the skin, usually causes local edema.

Evaluation of immunocompetence in patients with cancer or malnutrition: PPD is given intradermally with three or more antigens to detect anergy, the absence of an immune response to the test. The reaction may not be evident. Injection into a site subject to excessive exposure to sunlight may cause a false-negative reaction.

Pharmacokinetics
- *Absorption:* When PPD is injected intradermally or when a multiple-puncture device is used, a delayed hypersensitivity reaction is evident in 5 to 6 hours and peaks in 48 to 72 hours.
- *Distribution:* Injection must be given intradermally or by skin puncture; an S.C. injection invalidates the test.
- *Metabolism:* Not applicable.
- *Excretion:* Not applicable.

Contraindications and precautions
Severe reactions to tuberculin PPD are rare and usually result from extreme sensitivity to the tuberculin. Inadvertent S.C. administration of PPD may result in a febrile reaction in highly sensitized patients. Old tubercular lesions are not activated by administration of PPD.

Interactions
When PPD antigen is used 4 to 6 weeks after immunization with *live* or *inactivated viral vaccines,* the reaction to tuberculin may be suppressed. False-negative reactions may also occur if test is used in patients receiving *systemic corticosteroids* or *aminocaproic acid.*

Topical alcohol theoretically may inactivate the PPD antigen and invalidate the test.

Effects on diagnostic tests
None reported.

Adverse reactions
Other: Local pain, pruritus, vesiculation, ulceration, or necrosis in some tuberculin-sensitive patients; hypersensitivity (immediate reaction may occur at the test site in the form of a wheal or flare that lasts less than a day, which should not interfere with the PPD test reading at 48 to 72 hours); ***anaphylaxis;*** Arthus reaction.

Overdose and treatment
No information available.

☑ Special considerations
tuberculin PPD
- Obtain a history of allergies and previous skin test reactions before administration of the test.
- Epinephrine 1:1,000 should be available to treat rare anaphylactic reaction.
- Intradermal injection should produce a bleb 6 to 10 mm in diameter on skin. If bleb does not appear, retest at a site at least 5 cm from the initial site.
- Read test in 48 to 72 hours. An induration of 10 mm or greater is a significant reaction in patients who are not suspected to have tuberculosis and who have not been exposed to active tuberculosis, indicating present or past infection. An induration of 5 mm or more is significant in patients with AIDS or in those suspected to have tuberculosis or who have recently been exposed to active tuberculosis. An induration of 5 to 9 mm is inconclusive in patients not suspected of having been exposed or having tuberculosis infection; therefore, test should be repeated if there is more than 10 mm of erythema without induration. The amount of induration at the site, not the erythema, determines the significance of the reaction.

For either test, keep a record of the administration technique, manufacturer and tuberculin lot number, date and location of administration, date test is read, and the size of the induration in millimeters.

Multiple-puncture device
- Obtain history of allergies, especially to acacia (contained in the Tine Test as stabilizer), and reactions to skin tests.
- Report all known cases of tuberculosis to appropriate public health agency.
- Reaction may be depressed in patients with malnutrition, immunosuppression, or miliary tuberculosis.
- Read test at 48 to 72 hours. Measure the size of the largest induration in millimeters. A large reaction may cause the area around the puncture site to be indistinguishable.

Positive reaction: If vesiculation is present, the test may be interpreted as positive if induration is greater than 2 mm, but consider further diagnostic procedures.

Negative reaction: Induration is less than 2 mm. There is no reason to retest the patient unless the person is a contact of a patient with tuberculosis or there is clinical evidence of the disease.

Diagnosis of tuberculosis: PPD administration to a patient with a natural infection with *M. tuberculosis* usually results in sensitivity to tuberculin and a delayed hypersensitivity reaction after administration of old tuberculin or PPD. The cell-mediated immune reaction to tuberculin in tuberculin-sensitive individuals is seen as erythema and induration, which mainly results from cellular infiltrates of the dermis of the skin, usually causing local edema.

Diagnosis of immunocompetence in patients with such conditions as cancer or malnutrition: PPD is given intradermally with three or more antigens (such as Multitest CMI) to detect anergy.

- No evidence to date of adverse effects to fetus has been seen. The benefits of the test are thought to outweigh the potential risks to the fetus.

Patient education
- Advise patient to report unusual adverse effects. Explain that induration will disappear in a few days.
- Reinforce the benefits of treatment if test is positive for tuberculosis.

Geriatric use
- Elderly patients not having a cell-mediated immune reaction to the test may be anergic or they may test negative.

Breast-feeding
- There appears to be no risk to breast-feeding infants.

tubocurarine chloride
Tubarine*

Pharmacologic classification: nondepolarizing neuromuscular blocker
Therapeutic classification: skeletal muscle relaxant
Pregnancy risk category C

How supplied
Available by prescription only
Injection: 3 mg/ml parenteral

Indications, route, and dosage
Adjunct to general anesthesia to induce skeletal muscle relaxation, facilitate intubation, and reduce fractures and dislocations
Dose depends on anesthetic used, individual needs, and response. Doses listed are representative and must be adjusted. Dosage may be calculated on the basis of 0.165 mg/kg.
Adults: Initially, 6 to 9 mg I.V. or I.M., followed by 3 to 4.5 mg in 3 to 5 minutes if needed. Additional doses of 3 mg may be given if needed during prolonged anesthesia.
To assist with mechanical ventilation
Adults: Initially, 0.0165 mg/kg I.V. or I.M. (average 1 mg), then adjust subsequent doses to patient's response.
To weaken muscle contractions in pharmacologically or electrically induced seizures
Adults: Initially, 0.165 mg/kg I.V. or I.M. slowly. As a precaution, 3 mg less than the calculated dose should be administered initially.
Diagnosis of myasthenia gravis
Adults: Single I.V. or I.M. dose of 0.004 to 0.033 mg/kg.

Pharmacodynamics
Skeletal muscle relaxant action: Tubocurarine prevents acetylcholine from binding to receptors on motor end-plate, thus blocking depolarization. Tubocurarine has histamine-releasing and ganglionic-blocking properties and is usually antagonized by anticholinesterase agents.

Pharmacokinetics

• *Absorption:* After I.V. injection, onset of muscle relaxation is rapid and peaks within 2 to 5 minutes. Duration is dose-related; effects usually begin to subside in 20 to 30 minutes. Paralysis may persist for 25 to 90 minutes. Subsequent doses have longer durations. After I.M. injection, onset of paralysis is unpredictable (10 to 25 minutes); duration is dose related.
• *Distribution:* After I.V. injection, drug is distributed in extracellular fluid and rapidly reaches its site of action. After tissue compartment is saturated, drug may persist in tissues for up to 24 hours; 40% to 45% is bound to plasma proteins, mainly globulins.
• *Metabolism:* Tubocurarine undergoes N-demethylation in the liver.
• *Excretion:* Approximately 33% to 75% of a dose is excreted unchanged in urine in 24 hours; up to 11% is excreted in bile.

Contraindications and precautions

Contraindicated in patients with hypersensitivity to drug and in those for whom histamine release is a hazard (asthmatic patients).

Use cautiously in elderly or debilitated patients; in those with impaired hepatic or pulmonary function, hypothermia, respiratory depression, myasthenia gravis, myasthenic syndrome of lung cancer or bronchiogenic carcinoma, dehydration, thyroid disorders, collagen diseases, porphyria, electrolyte disturbances, fractures, or muscle spasms; and in patients undergoing cesarean section.

Interactions

Concomitant use with *aminoglycoside antibiotics, clindamycin, lincomycin, polymyxin antibiotics, general anesthetics, local anesthetics, beta-adrenergic blockers, calcium salts, furosemide, parenteral magnesium salts, depolarizing neuromuscular blocking agents, other nondepolarizing neuromuscular blocking agents, quinidine* or *quinine, thiazide diuretics*, or *other potassium-depleting drugs* may enhance or prolong tubocurarine-induced neuromuscular blockade.

Respiratory depressant effects may be increased by *opioid analgesics, quinidine,* and *quinine.*

Effects on diagnostic tests

None reported.

Adverse reactions

CV: hypotension, ***arrhythmias, cardiac arrest,*** bradycardia.
Respiratory: ***respiratory depression or apnea, bronchospasm.***
Other: profound and prolonged muscle relaxation, hypersensitivity reactions, idiosyncrasy, residual muscle weakness, increased salivation.

Overdose and treatment

Clinical manifestations of overdose include apnea or prolonged muscle paralysis, which can be treated with controlled ventilation. Use a peripheral nerve stimulator to monitor effects and to determine nature and degree of blockade. Anticholinesterase agents may antagonize tubocurarine. Atropine given before or concurrently with the antagonist counteracts its muscarinic effects.

☑ Special considerations

• The margin of safety between therapeutic dose and dose causing respiratory paralysis is small.
• Monitor respirations closely for early symptoms of paralysis.
• Allow effects of succinylcholine to subside before giving tubocurarine.
• Measure and record intake and output.
• Decrease dose if inhalation anesthetics are used.
• Use only fresh solution. Discard if discolored.
• Do not mix with barbiturates or other alkaline solutions in same syringe.
• I.V. administration requires direct medical supervision. Drug should be given I.V. slowly over 60 to 90 seconds or I.M. by deep injection in deltoid muscle. Tubocurarine is usually administered by I.V. injection, but if patient's veins are inaccessible, drug may be given I.M. in same dosage as given I.V.
• Assess baseline tests of renal function and serum electrolyte levels before drug administration. Electrolyte imbalance (particularly potassium and magnesium) can potentiate effects of drug.
• Keep airway clear. Have emergency respiratory support equipment readily available.
• Be prepared for endotracheal intubation, suction, or assisted or controlled respiration with oxygen administration. Have available atropine and the antagonists neostigmine or edrophonium (cholinesterase inhibitors). A nerve stimulator may be used to evaluate recovery from neuromuscular blockade.
• Muscle paralysis follows drug administration in sequence: jaw muscles, levator eyelid muscles and other muscles of head and neck, limbs, intercostals and diaphragm, abdomen, trunk. Facial and diaphragm muscles recover first, then legs, arms, shoulder girdle, trunk, larynx, hands, feet, pharynx. Muscle function is usually restored within 90 minutes. Patient may find speech difficult until muscles of head and neck recover.
• Monitor blood pressure, vital signs, and airway until patient recovers from drug effects. Ganglionic blockade (hypotension), histamine liberation (increased salivation, bronchospasm), and neuromuscular blockade (respiratory depression) are known effects of tubocurarine.
• After neuromuscular blockade dissipates, watch for residual muscle weakness.
• Renal dysfunction prolongs drug action. Peristaltic action may be suppressed. Check for bowel sounds.
• Test of myasthenia gravis is considered positive if drug exaggerates muscle weakness.
• Drug does not affect consciousness or relieve pain; assess patient's need for analgesic or sedative.

Geriatric use

• Administer cautiously to elderly patients.

Pediatric use

• Administer cautiously to children.

Breast-feeding
- It is unknown whether drug is excreted in breast milk. Use with caution in breast-feeding women.

typhoid vaccine

Pharmacologic classification: vaccine
Therapeutic classification: bacterial vaccine
Pregnancy risk category C

How supplied
Available by prescription only
Oral vaccine: enteric-coated capsules of 2 to 6 X 10^9 colony-forming units of viable *Salmonella typhi* Ty-21a and 5 to 10 X 10^9 bacterial cells of nonviable *S. typhi* Ty-21a
Injection: suspension of killed Ty-2 strain of *S. typhi;* provides 8 units/ml in 5-ml, 10-ml, and 20-ml vials
Powder for suspension: killed Ty-2 strain of *S. typhi;* provides 8 units/ml in 50-dose vial with 20 ml diluent/dose

Indications, route, and dosage
Primary immunization (exposure to typhoid carrier or foreign travel planned to area endemic for typhoid fever)
Parenteral
Adults and children over age 9: 0.5 ml S.C.; repeat in 4 or more weeks.
Infants and children age 6 months to 9 years: 0.25 ml S.C.; repeat in 4 or more weeks.
Booster
Adults and children over age 10: 0.5 ml S.C. or 0.1 ml intradermally q 3 years.
Infants and children age 6 months to 10 years: 0.25 ml S.C. or 0.1 ml intradermally q 3 years.
Oral
Adults and children over age 6: Primary immunization—1 capsule on alternate days (for example, days 1, 3, 5, 7) for four doses. Booster—repeat primary immunization regimen q 5 years.

Pharmacodynamics
Typhoid fever prophylaxis action: Vaccine promotes active immunity to typhoid fever in 70% to 90% of patients vaccinated.

Pharmacokinetics
- *Absorption:* Duration of vaccine-induced immunity is at least 2 years.
- *Distribution:* No information available.
- *Metabolism:* No information available.
- *Excretion:* No information available.

Contraindications and precautions
Contraindicated in immunosuppressed patients and in those with hypersensitivity to vaccine. Vaccination should be deferred in patients with acute illness. Also, oral vaccine should not be given to patients with acute GI distress (diarrhea or vomiting).

Interactions
Concomitant use of typhoid vaccine with *corticosteroids* or *immunosuppressants* may impair the immune response to this vaccine. *Sulfonamides* and *other anti-infectives active against S. typhi* may inhibit multiplication of the bacterial strain from the live attenuated oral vaccine, which may prevent the development of a protective immune response. Concomitant use of *phenytoin* may decrease antibody response to S.C. typhoid vaccine.

Effects on diagnostic tests
None reported.

Adverse reactions
CNS: headache.
GI: nausea, abdominal cramps, vomiting.
Skin: rash, urticaria, swelling, pain, inflammation (at injection site).
Other: *fever,* malaise, ***anaphylaxis,*** myalgia.

Overdose and treatment
No information available.

☑ Special considerations
- Obtain a thorough history of allergies and reactions to immunizations.
- Have epinephrine solution 1:1,000 available to treat allergic reactions.
- Shake vial thoroughly before withdrawing dose.
- Store injection at 36° to 50° F (2° to 10° C). Do not freeze.
- Store oral capsules at 36° to 46° F (2° to 8° C).

Patient education
- Tell patient what to expect after vaccination: pain and inflammation at the injection site, fever, malaise, headache, nausea, or difficulty breathing. These reactions occur in most patients within 24 hours and may persist for 1 to 2 days. Recommend acetaminophen for fever.
- Encourage patient to report adverse reactions.
- Tell patient traveling to an area where typhoid fever is endemic to select food and water carefully. Vaccination is not a substitute for careful selection of food.
- Inform patient that not all recipients of typhoid vaccine are fully protected. Travelers should take all necessary precautions to avoid infection.
- Advise patient that it is essential that all four doses of oral vaccine be taken at the prescribed alternate-day interval to obtain a maximal protective immune response.
- Tell patient to take oral vaccine capsule about 1 hour before a meal with a cold or lukewarm (not exceeding body temperature) drink and to swallow the capsule as soon as possible after placement in the mouth. Remind patient not to chew the capsule.

Pediatric use
- Parenteral typhoid vaccine is not indicated for those under age 6 months. Oral typhoid vaccine is not indicated for children under age 6.

Breast-feeding
• It is unknown whether typhoid vaccine is distributed into breast milk. Use with caution in breast-feeding women.

typhoid Vi polysaccharide vaccine
Typhim Vi

Pharmacologic classification: vaccine
Therapeutic classification: bacterial vaccine
Pregnancy risk category C

How supplied
Available by prescription only
Injection: 0.5-ml syringe, 20-dose vial, 50-dose vial

Indications, route, and dosage
Active immunization against typhoid fever
Adults and children age 2 and older: 0.5 ml I.M. as a single dose. Reimmunization is recommended q 2 years with 0.5 ml I.M. as a single dose, if needed.

Pharmacodynamics
Antibacterial vaccine action: Typhoid Vi polysaccharide vaccine promotes active immunity to typhoid fever.

Pharmacokinetics
Because of the low incidence of typhoid fever in the United States, efficacy studies have not been feasible.
• *Absorption:* Antibody levels usually remain elevated for 12 months after vaccination.
• *Distribution:* No information available.
• *Metabolism:* No information available.
• *Excretion:* No information available.

Contraindications and precautions
Contraindicated in patients with hypersensitivity to any component of vaccine. Do not use to treat typhoid fever or give to those who are chronic typhoid carriers. Use cautiously in patients with thrombocytopenia or bleeding disorders and in those taking an anticoagulant because bleeding may occur following an I.M. injection in these individuals.

Interactions
None significant.

Effects on diagnostic tests
None reported.

Adverse reactions
CNS: *headache.*
GI: nausea, diarrhea, vomiting.
Other: *local injection site pain or tenderness, induration, erythema* at injection site; *malaise,* myalgia, fever.

Overdose and treatment
No information available.

☑ Special considerations
• Delay administration of vaccine, if possible, in patients with febrile illnesses.
• Although anaphylaxis is rare, keep epinephrine readily available to treat anaphylactoid reactions.
• If vaccine is administered to immunosuppressed persons or persons receiving immunosuppressive therapy, the expected immune response may not be obtained.
• Persons who should receive the vaccine include persons traveling to or living in areas of higher endemicity for typhoid fever.
• Administer as an I.M. injection into the deltoid region in adults and in the deltoid or the vastus lateralis in children. It should not be administered in the gluteal region or areas where there may be a nerve trunk. Never inject I.V.

Patient education
• Advise patient to take all necessary precautions to avoid contact with or ingestion of contaminated food and water.
• Inform patient that immunization should be given at least 2 weeks before expected exposure. Although an optimal reimmunization schedule has not been established, reimmunization with a single dose for U.S. travelers every 2 years, if exposure to typhoid fever is possible, is recommended at this time.

Pediatric use
• Safety and effectiveness in patients under age 2 have not been established.

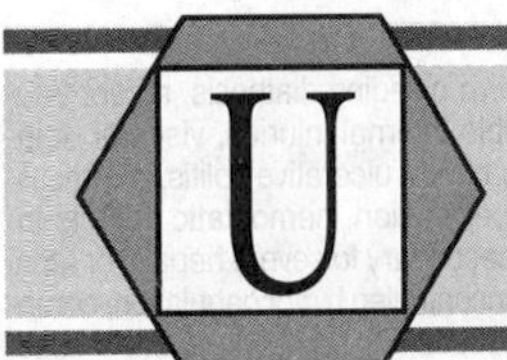

urea (carbamide)
Ureaphil

Pharmacologic classification: carbonic acid salt
Therapeutic classification: osmotic diuretic
Pregnancy risk category C

How supplied
Available by prescription only
Injectable: 40-g vial

Indications, route, and dosage
Reduction of intracranial or intraocular pressure
Adults: 1 to 1.5 g/kg as a 30% solution given by slow I.V. infusion over 1 to 2½ hours.
Children over age 2: 0.5 to 1.5 g/kg by slow I.V. infusion.
Children under age 2: As little as 0.1 g/kg by slow I.V. infusion may be given. Maximum dosage, 4 ml/minute.

Maximum daily adult dosage, 120 g. To prepare 135 ml of 30% solution, mix contents of a 40-g vial of urea with 105 ml of D_5W or $D_{10}W$ with 10% invert sugar in water. Each milliliter of 30% solution provides 300 mg of urea.

◊ SIADH
Adults: 80 g as a 30% solution I.V. over 6 hours.

◊ Diuresis
Adults and children over age 2: 500 mg to 1.5 g/kg as a 30% solution given by slow I.V. infusion over 30 minutes to 2 hours.
Children under age 2: 100 mg to 1.5 g/kg as a 30% solution given by slow I.V. infusion over 30 minutes to 2 hours.

Pharmacodynamics
Diuretic action: Urea elevates plasma osmolality, enhancing the flow of water into extracellular fluid such as blood, and reducing intracranial and intraocular pressure.

Pharmacokinetics
- *Absorption:* I.V. urea produces diuresis and maximal reduction of intraocular and intracranial pressure within 1 to 2 hours; even though drug is administered I.V., it is hydrolyzed and absorbed from the GI tract.
- *Distribution:* Urea distributes into intracellular and extracellular fluid, including lymph, bile, and CSF.
- *Metabolism:* Hydrolyzed in the GI tract by bacterial urease.
- *Excretion:* Excreted by the kidneys.

Contraindications and precautions
Contraindicated in patients with severely impaired renal function, marked dehydration, frank hepatic failure, active intracranial bleeding, and sickle-cell disease with CNS involvement. Use cautiously in patients with cardiac disease or impaired renal or hepatic function and in pregnant or breast-feeding women.

Interactions
Urea may enhance renal excretion of *lithium* and lower serum lithium levels.

Effects on diagnostic tests
Urea therapy alters electrolyte balance.

Adverse reactions
CNS: *headache,* syncope, disorientation.
GI: *nausea, vomiting.*
Other: irritation or necrotic sloughing with extravasation.

Overdose and treatment
Clinical signs of overdose include unusually elevated BUN levels, polyuria, cellular dehydration, hypotension, and CV collapse. Discontinue infusion and institute supportive measures.

☑ Special considerations
Besides those relevant to all *osmotic diuretics,* consider the following recommendations.
- Avoid rapid I.V. infusion, which may cause hemolysis or increased capillary bleeding. Also avoid extravasation, which may cause reactions ranging from mild irritation to necrosis.
- Do not administer through the same infusion line as blood.
- Do not infuse into leg veins; this may cause phlebitis or thrombosis, especially in elderly patients.
- Watch for hyponatremia or hypokalemia (muscle weakness, lethargy); such signs may indicate electrolyte depletion before serum levels are reduced.
- Maintain adequate hydration; monitor fluid and electrolyte balance.
- Monitor BUN levels frequently in patients with renal disease.
- Indwelling urinary catheter should be used in comatose patients to ensure bladder emptying. Use of an hourly urometer collection bag facilitates accurate measurement of urine output.
- If satisfactory diuresis does not occur in 6 to 12 hours, urea should be discontinued and renal function reevaluated.
- Use only freshly reconstituted urea for I.V. infusion; solution turns to ammonia when left standing. Use within minutes of reconstitution.

• Urea has been used orally on an investigational basis for migraine prophylaxis, acute sickle-cell crisis prevention, and the correction of SIADH.
• Mix with carbonated beverages, jelly, or jam to disguise unpleasant flavor.

Geriatric use
• Elderly or debilitated patients will require close observation and may require lower dosages. Excessive diuresis promotes rapid dehydration and hypovolemia, hypokalemia, and hyponatremia.

Breast-feeding
• Safety has not been established.

urokinase
Abbokinase, Abbokinase Open-Cath

Pharmacologic classification: thrombolytic enzyme
Therapeutic classification: thrombolytic enzyme
Pregnancy risk category B

How supplied
Injection: 5,000 IU/ml unit-dose vial; 250,000-IU/vial

Indications, route, and dosage
Lysis of acute massive pulmonary emboli and of pulmonary emboli accompanied by unstable hemodynamics
Adults: For I.V. infusion only by constant infusion pump; priming dose: 4,400 IU/kg over 10 minutes, followed with 4,400 IU/kg hourly for 12 hours.
Coronary artery thrombosis
Adults: 6,000 IU/minute of urokinase intra-arterial via a coronary artery catheter until artery is maximally opened, usually within 15 to 30 minutes; however, drug has been administered for up to 2 hours. Average total dose, 500,000 IU.
Venous catheter occlusion
Adults: Instill 5,000 IU into occluded line.

Pharmacodynamics
Thrombolytic action: Urokinase promotes thrombolysis by directly activating conversion of plasminogen to plasmin.

Pharmacokinetics
• *Absorption:* Urokinase is not absorbed from GI tract; plasminogen activation begins promptly after infusion or instillation; adequate activation of fibrinolytic system occurs in 3 to 4 hours.
• *Distribution:* Rapidly cleared from circulation; most drug accumulates in kidney and liver.
• *Metabolism:* Rapidly metabolized by the liver.
• *Excretion:* Small amount is eliminated in urine and bile. Half-life is 10 to 20 minutes; longer in patients with hepatic dysfunction. Anticoagulant effect may persist for 12 to 24 hours after the infusion is discontinued.

Contraindications and precautions
Contraindicated in patients with active internal bleeding, history of CVA, aneurysm, arteriovenous malformation, known bleeding diathesis, recent trauma with possible internal injuries, visceral or intracranial malignancy, ulcerative colitis, diverticulitis, severe hypertension, hemostatic defects including those secondary to severe hepatic or renal insufficiency, uncontrolled hypocoagulation, chronic pulmonary disease with cavitation, subacute bacterial endocarditis or rheumatic valvular disease, and recent cerebral embolism, thrombosis, or hemorrhage.

Also contraindicated during pregnancy and first 10 days postpartum; within 10 days after intra-arterial diagnostic procedure or any surgery (liver or kidney biopsy, lumbar puncture, thoracentesis, paracentesis, or extensive or multiple cutdowns); or within 2 months after intracranial or intraspinal surgery.

I.M. injections and other invasive procedures are contraindicated during urokinase therapy.

Interactions
Concomitant use with *anticoagulants* may cause hemorrhage; *heparin* must be stopped and its effects allowed to diminish. It may also be necessary to reverse effects of *oral anticoagulants* before beginning therapy.

Concomitant use with *aspirin, indomethacin, phenylbutazone,* or *other drugs affecting platelet activity* increases risk of bleeding; do not use together.

Aminocaproic acid inhibits urokinase-induced activation of plasminogen.

Effects on diagnostic tests
Drug increases thrombin time, activated partial thromboplastin time, and PT; drug sometimes moderately decreases hematocrit.

Adverse reactions
CV: ***reperfusion arrhythmias.***
Hematologic: ***bleeding.***
Respiratory: ***bronchospasm,*** minor breathing difficulties.
Other: phlebitis at injection site, fever, rash, ***anaphylaxis.***

Overdose and treatment
Clinical manifestations of overdose include signs of potentially serious bleeding: bleeding gums, epistaxis, hematoma, spontaneous ecchymoses, oozing at catheter site, increased pulse, and pain from internal bleeding. Discontinue drug and restart when bleeding stops.

☑ Special considerations
Besides those relevant to all *thrombolytic enzymes,* consider the following recommendation.
• To reconstitute I.V. solution, add 5.2 ml sterile water for injection; dilute further with 0.9% NaCl injection or 5% dextrose injection before infusion. Don't use bacteriostatic water, which contains preservatives. A catheter-clearing product is available in a Univial, containing 5,000 IU urokinase with the proper diluent. Discard unused portion; product contains no preservatives.
• Although not approved by the FDA, urokinase is commonly used in peripheral arterial occlusions.

Geriatric use

• Patients age 75 or older have a greater risk of cerebral hemorrhage because they are more apt to have preexisting cerebrovascular disease.

ursodiol (ursodeoxycholic acid)

Actigall

Pharmacologic classification: bile acid
Therapeutic classification: gallstone solubilizing agent
Pregnancy risk category B

How supplied

Available by prescription only
Capsules: 300 mg

Indications, route, and dosage

Dissolution of radiolucent gallbladder stones; to increase the flow of bile in patients with bile duct prosthesis or stents

Adults: 8 to 10 mg/kg/day given in two or three divided doses.

Ursodiol is indicated for patients with radiolucent, noncalcified, gallbladder stones smaller than 20 mm in greatest diameter in whom elective cholecystectomy is not feasible because of increased surgical risk related to systemic disease, advanced age, or idiosyncratic reaction to anesthesia; or because the patient has refused surgery.

Pharmacodynamics

Gallstone dissolving action: Ursodiol, an agent intended for dissolution of radiolucent gallstones, is a naturally occurring bile acid found in small quantities in normal human bile and in larger quantities in the biles of certain species of bears. Ursodiol suppresses hepatic synthesis and secretion of cholesterol and also inhibits intestinal absorption of cholesterol. It has little inhibitory effect on synthesis and secretion into bile of endogenous bile acids and does not appear to affect phospholipid secretion into bile.

Ursodiol also appears to solubilize cholesterol.

Pharmacokinetics

• *Absorption:* About 90% of a therapeutic dose is absorbed in the small bowel after oral administration.

• *Distribution:* After absorption, ursodiol enters the portal vein and is extracted from portal blood by the liver ("first pass" effect) where it is conjugated with either glycine or taurine and is then secreted into the hepatic bile ducts. Ursodiol in bile is concentrated in the gallbladder and expelled into the duodenum in gallbladder bile via the cystic and common ducts by gallbladder contractions provoked by physiologic responses to eating. Small quantities of ursodiol appear in the systemic circulation.

• *Metabolism:* Metabolized by the liver. A small portion of orally administered drug undergoes bacterial degradation with each cycle of enterohepatic circulation. Ursodiol can be both oxidized and reduced, yielding either 7-keto-lithocholic acid or lithocholic acid, respectively.

• *Excretion:* Very small amounts are excreted in the urine. Free ursodiol, 7-keto-lithocholic acid, and lithocholic acid are relatively insoluble in aqueous media, and larger proportions of these compounds are excreted via the feces. Eighty percent of lithocholic acid formed in the small bowel is excreted in the feces; the 20% that is absorbed is sulfated in the liver to relatively insoluble lithocholyl conjugates that are excreted into bile and lost in feces. Absorbed 7-keto-lithocholic acid is stereospecifically reduced in the liver to chenodiol. Reabsorbed free ursodiol is reconjugated by the liver.

Contraindications and precautions

Contraindicated in patients hypersensitive to ursodiol or other bile acids and in those with chronic hepatic disease, unremitting acute cholecystitis, cholangitis, biliary obstruction, gallstone-induced pancreatitis, or biliary fistula.

Interactions

Concurrent use of *estrogens, oral contraceptives,* and *clofibrate* (and perhaps other *lipid-lowering drugs*) that increase hepatic cholesterol secretion and encourage cholesterol gallstone formation may counteract the effectiveness of ursodiol. *Aluminum-based antacids* adsorb bile acids in vitro and interfere with the action of ursodiol by reducing its absorption. *Cholestyramine* and *colestipol* may interfere with the action of ursodiol by reducing its absorption.

Effects on diagnostic tests

None reported.

Adverse reactions

CNS: headache, fatigue, anxiety, depression, sleep disorders.
EENT: rhinitis.
GI: nausea, vomiting, dyspepsia, metallic taste, abdominal pain, biliary pain, cholecystitis, diarrhea, constipation, stomatitis, flatulence.
Respiratory: cough.
Skin: pruritus, rash, dry skin, urticaria, hair thinning, diaphoresis.
Other: arthralgia, myalgia, back pain.

Overdose and treatment

The most likely manifestation of severe overdose with ursodiol would probably be diarrhea. Treatment includes symptomatic and supportive measures.

☑ Special considerations

• Gallbladder stone dissolution with ursodiol treatment requires months of therapy. Complete dissolution may not occur, and recurrence of stones is possible within 5 years in up to 50% of patients. Carefully select patients for therapy, and consider alternative therapies. Safety of use of ursodiol beyond 24 months is not established.

• Monitor gallstone response. Obtain ultrasound images of the gallbladder at 6-month intervals for first year of ursodiol therapy. If gallstones appear to have dissolved, continue therapy and confirm dissolution on a repeat ultrasound within 1 to 3 months. Most patients who achieve complete stone dissolution show partial or complete dissolution at first on-treatment reevaluation. If partial stone dissolution does not occur by 12 months, eventual dissolution is unlikely.

- Partial stone dissolution occurring within 6 months of therapy appears to be associated with a greater than 70% chance of eventual complete stone dissolution with further treatment; partial dissolution within 1 year of therapy indicates a 40% probability of complete dissolution.
- Consider that some patients may never require therapy. Patients with silent or minimally symptomatic stones develop moderate to severe symptoms or gallstone complications at a rate between 2% and 6% per year; 7% to 27% in 5 years. The rate is higher for patients already having symptoms.
- Cholecystectomy offers immediate and permanent stone removal but carries a high risk in some patients.
- Surgical risk varies as a function of age and the presence of other disease. About 5% of cholecystectomized patients have residual symptoms of retained common duct stones.

Geriatric use

- Age, sex, weight, degree of obesity, and serum cholesterol level are not related to the chance of stone dissolution with ursodiol.

Pediatric use

- Safety and efficacy have not been established.

Breast-feeding

- It is not known if ursodiol is excreted in breast milk. Use with caution in breast-feeding women.

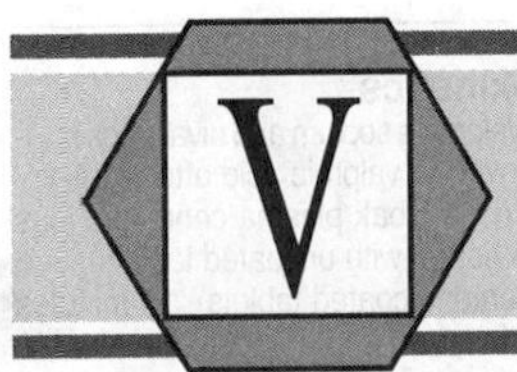

valacyclovir hydrochloride

Valtrex

Pharmacologic classification: synthetic purine nucleoside
Therapeutic classification: antiviral
Pregnancy risk category B

How supplied

Available by prescription only
Caplets: 500 mg

Indications, route, and dosage

Treatment of herpes zoster in immunocompetent patients
Adults: 1 g P.O. t.i.d. daily for 7 days.
Treatment of initial episode of genital herpes
Adults: 1 g P.O. b.i.d. for 10 days.
Treatment of recurrent genital herpes in immunocompetent patients
Adults: 500 mg P.O. b.i.d. for 5 days.
✦ ***Dosage adjustment.*** Base dosage adjustments in renally impaired patients on creatinine clearance levels.

Pharmacodynamics

Antiviral action: Valacyclovir rapidly becomes converted to acyclovir. Acyclovir becomes incorporated into viral DNA and inhibits viral DNA polymerase, thus inhibiting viral multiplication.

Pharmacokinetics

- *Absorption:* Rapidly absorbed from the GI tract. Absolute bioavailability of drug is about 54.5%.
- *Distribution:* Valacyclovir's protein binding ranges from 13.5% to 17.9%.
- *Metabolism:* Drug is rapidly and nearly completely converted to acyclovir and L-valine by first-pass intestinal or hepatic metabolism.
- *Excretion:* Excreted in urine and feces. Half-life of drug is about 2.5 to 3.3 hours.

Contraindications and precautions

Contraindicated in patients with hypersensitivity or intolerance to valacyclovir, acyclovir, or any component of the formulation and in immunocompromised patients. Use cautiously in patients with impaired renal function and in those receiving other nephrotoxic drugs.

Interactions

Cimetidine and *probenecid* reduce the rate, but not the extent, of valacyclovir to acyclovir and reduce the renal clearance of acyclovir, thus increasing acyclovir blood levels. Monitor patient for possible toxicity.

Effects on diagnostic tests

None reported.

Adverse reactions

CNS: *headache,* dizziness.
GI: *nausea,* vomiting, diarrhea, constipation, abdominal pain, anorexia.
Other: asthenia.

Overdose and treatment

There is no report of overdosage. However, precipitation of acyclovir in renal tubules may occur when the solubility (2.5 mg/ml) is exceeded in the intratubular fluid. If acute renal failure and anuria occur, hemodialysis may be helpful until renal function is restored.

☑ Special considerations

- Glaxo-Wellcome, the manufacturer, maintains an ongoing registry of women exposed to drug during pregnancy. Follow-up studies to date have not shown an increased risk for birth defects in infants born to patients exposed to drug during pregnancy. Health care providers are encouraged to report such exposures to the registrar at (800) 722-9292, extension 58465.
- Initiate therapy at first signs or symptoms of an episode, preferably within 24 hours after their onset.
- Thrombotic thrombocytopenic purpura and hemolytic uremic syndrome have occurred resulting in death in some patients with advanced infection with HIV, and also in bone marrow transplant and renal transplant recipients participating in clinical trials of valacyclovir.

Patient education

- Inform patient that valacyclovir may be taken without regard to meals.
- Advise patient about signs and symptoms of herpes infection (such as rash, tingling, itching, and pain), and advise him to call immediately if they occur. Treatment should be initiated as soon as possible after symptoms appear and is most effective when initiated within 48 hours of the onset of zoster rash.

Geriatric use

- Dosage adjustment may be necessary in elderly patients based on underlying renal status.

Pediatric use

- Safety and effectiveness in children have not been established.

Breast-feeding
• It is unknown if drug is excreted in breast milk. Therefore, its use in breast-feeding women is not recommended.

valproic acid
Depakene, Epival*

divalproex sodium
Depakote, Depakote Sprinkle

valproate sodium
Depacon

Pharmacologic classification: carboxylic acid derivative
Therapeutic classification: anticonvulsant
Pregnancy risk category D

How supplied
Available by prescription only
valproic acid
Capsules: 250 mg
Syrup: 250 mg/5 ml
divalproex sodium
Tablets (enteric-coated): 125 mg, 250 mg, 500 mg
Capsules (sprinkle): 125 mg
valproate sodium
Injection: 5 ml single-dose vials

Indications, route, and dosage
Simple and complex absence seizures and mixed seizure types, ◊ tonic-clonic seizures
Adults and children: P.O.—Initially, 15 mg/kg P.O. daily, divided b.i.d. or t.i.d.; may increase by 5 to 10 mg/kg daily at weekly intervals up to a maximum of 60 mg/kg daily, divided b.i.d. or t.i.d. The b.i.d. dosage is recommended for the enteric-coated tablets.

Note: Dosages of divalproex sodium (Depakote) are expressed as valproic acid.

Adults and children: I.V.—Initially 10 to 15 mg/kg/day as a 60-minute I.V. infusion (rate 20 mg/minute or less). The dosage may increase by 5 to 10 mg/kg daily at weekly intervals up to a maximum of 60 mg/kg daily. Drug should be diluted in at least 50 ml of compatible diluent. Use of valproate sodium injection for periods of more than 14 days has not been studied. Patients should be switched to oral products as soon as it is clinically feasible.

Mania
Adults: 750 mg P.O. in divided doses (divalproex sodium).

◊ Status epilepticus refractory to I.V. diazepam
Adults: 400 to 600 mg P.O. in divided doses.

Pharmacodynamics
Anticonvulsant action: Valproic acid's mechanism of action is unknown; effects may be from increased brain levels of gamma-aminobutyric acid (GABA), an inhibitory transmitter. Valproic acid also may decrease GABA's enzymatic catabolism. Onset of therapeutic effects may require a week or more. Valproic acid may be used with other anticonvulsants.

Pharmacokinetics
• *Absorption:* Valproate sodium and divalproex sodium quickly convert to valproic acid after administration of oral dose; peak plasma concentrations occur in 1 to 4 hours (with uncoated tablets), 3 to 5 hours (with enteric-coated tablets), 15 minutes to 2 hours (with syrup) and immediately with I.V. administration; bioavailability of drug is same for all dosage forms.
• *Distribution:* Valproic acid is distributed rapidly throughout the body; drug is 80% to 95% protein-bound.
• *Metabolism:* Valproic acid is metabolized by the liver.
• *Excretion:* Valproic acid is excreted in urine; some drug is excreted in feces and exhaled air. Breast milk levels are 1% to 10% of serum levels.

Contraindications and precautions
Contraindicated in patients with hypersensitivity to drug. Use cautiously in patients with history of hepatic dysfunction.

Do not administer valproate sodium injection to patients with hepatic disease or significant hepatic dysfunction.

Interactions
Valproic acid may potentiate effects of *MAO inhibitors* and *other CNS antidepressants* and of *oral anticoagulants.* Besides additive sedative effects, valproic acid increases serum levels of *phenobarbital, phenytoin,* and *primidone;* such combinations may cause excessive somnolence and require careful monitoring.

Concomitant use with *clonazepam* may cause absence seizures and should be avoided.

Effects on diagnostic tests
Valproic acid may cause false-positive test results for urinary ketones; it also may cause abnormalities in liver function test results. Valproic acid reportedly alters thyroid function tests but clinical importance of this is not known.

Adverse reactions
Because drug usually is used in combination with other anticonvulsants, adverse reactions reported may not be caused by valproic acid alone.
CNS: *sedation,* emotional upset, depression, psychosis, aggressiveness, hyperactivity, behavioral deterioration, muscle weakness, tremor, ataxia, headache, dizziness, incoordination.
EENT: nystagmus, diplopia.
GI: *nausea, vomiting, indigestion,* diarrhea, abdominal cramps, constipation, increased appetite and weight gain, anorexia, ***pancreatitis.*** (*Note:* lower incidence of GI effects occur with divalproex sodium.)
Hematologic: ***thrombocytopenia,*** increased bleeding time, petechiae, bruising, eosinophilia, ***hemorrhage, leukopenia,*** bone marrow suppression.
Hepatic: *elevated liver enzymes,* ***toxic hepatitis.***
Skin: rash, alopecia, pruritus, photosensitivity, erythema multiforme.

Overdose and treatment

Symptoms of overdose include somnolence and coma.

Treat overdose supportively: maintain adequate urinary output, and monitor vital signs and fluid and electrolyte balance carefully. Naloxone reverses CNS and respiratory depression but also may reverse anticonvulsant effects of valproic acid. Hemodialysis and hemoperfusion have been used.

☑ Special considerations

- Evaluate liver function, platelet count, and PT at baseline and monthly intervals—especially during first 6 months.
- Therapeutic range of drug is 50 to 100 mcg/ml.
- Do not withdraw drug abruptly.
- Tremors may indicate need for dosage reduction.
- Administer drug with food to minimize GI irritation. Enteric-coated formulation may be better tolerated.
- When switching from oral to I.V. route, total daily dose I.V. should be equivalent to the oral daily dose with the same frequency of dose. Monitor plasma concentration and make dosage adjustments as needed.
- Administer I.V. as 60-minute infusion with rate not exceeding 20 mg/minute.

Patient education

- Advise patient not to discontinue drug suddenly, not to alter dosage without medical approval, and to call before changing brand or using generic drug as therapeutic effect may change.
- Tell patient to swallow tablets or capsules whole to avoid local mucosal irritation and, if necessary, to take with food but not carbonated beverages because tablet may dissolve before swallowing, causing irritation and unpleasant taste.
- Warn patient to avoid alcohol while taking drug because it may decrease drug's effectiveness and increase CNS adverse effects.
- Advise patient to avoid tasks that require mental alertness until CNS sedative effects are determined. Drowsiness and dizziness may occur. Bedtime administration of drug may minimize CNS depression.
- Teach patient signs and symptoms of hypersensitivity and adverse effects and need to report them.
- Encourage patient to wear a Medic Alert bracelet or necklace, listing drug and seizure disorders, while taking anticonvulsants.

Geriatric use

- Elderly patients eliminate drug more slowly; lower dosages are recommended.

Pediatric use

- Valproic acid is not recommended for use in children under age 2; this age-group is at highest risk of adverse effects. Reportedly, hyperexcitability and aggressiveness have occurred in a few children.

Breast-feeding

- Valproic acid appears in breast milk in concentration levels from 1% to 10% of serum concentrations. Alternate feeding method is recommended during therapy.

valsartan

Diovan

Pharmacologic classification: angiotensin II antagonist
Therapeutic classification: antihypertensive
Pregnancy risk category X

How supplied

Available by prescription only
Capsules: 80 mg, 160 mg

Indications, route, and dosage

Hypertension, used alone or in combination with other antihypertensives

Adults: Initially, 80 mg P.O. once daily as monotherapy in patients who are not volume depleted. Blood pressure reduction should occur in 2 to 4 weeks. If additional antihypertensive effect is needed, may increase dosage to 160 or 320 mg daily or add diuretic. (Addition of diuretic has greater effect than dosage increases beyond 80 mg.) Usual dosage range, 80 to 320 mg daily.

Pharmacodynamics

Antihypertensive action: Blocks the binding of angiotensin II to receptor sites in vascular smooth muscle and the adrenal gland, which inhibits the pressor effects of the renin-angiotensin system.

Pharmacokinetics

- *Absorption:* Absolute bioavailability is approximately 25%. Peak plasma concentration is reached 2 to 4 hours after dosing.
- *Distribution:* Drug does not distribute extensively into tissues; it is highly bound to serum proteins (95%)—mainly to serum albumin.
- *Metabolism:* Only about 20% is metabolized. The enzyme(s) responsible for valsartan metabolism have not been identified, but do not appear to be cytochrome P-450 enzymes.
- *Excretion:* Excreted primarily through the feces (83% of dose) and about 13% in the urine. Average elimination half-life is about 6 hours.

Contraindications and precautions

Contraindicated in patients with known hypersensitivity to drug. Use cautiously in patients with renal or hepatic disease.

Interactions

Diuretics may increase risk of excessive hypotension. Assess fluid status before starting concomitant therapy.

Effects on diagnostic tests

Neutropenia was observed in 1.9% of patients and 4.4% of patients experienced greater than 20% increases in serum potassium.

...erse reactions

...: dizziness, headache.
... abdominal pain, diarrhea, nausea.
...matologic: ***neutropenia.***
Musculoskeletal: arthralgia.
Respiratory: cough, pharyngitis, rhinitis, sinusitis, upper respiratory infection.
Other: edema, fatigue, hyperkalemia, viral infection.

Overdose and treatment

Limited data are available. The most likely symptoms would be hypotension and tachycardia; bradycardia could occur from parasympathetic (vagal) stimulation. If symptomatic hypotension should occur, supportive treatment should be instituted.

☑ Special considerations

- Excessive hypotension can occur when drug is given with high doses of diuretics. Correct volume and salt depletions before initiating therapy.
- Do not use in pregnant patients because fetal and neonatal morbidity and death may occur.

Patient education

- Advise patient on birth control methods.
- Tell female patient to call if pregnancy occurs; drug will need to be discontinued.
- Tell patient drug may be taken without regard for food.

Geriatric use

- Although no overall difference in efficacy or safety was observed, greater sensitivity of some older individuals cannot be ruled out.

Pediatric use

- Safety and effectiveness have not been established.

Breast-feeding

- It is not known if drug is excreted in breast milk; use with caution.

vancomycin hydrochloride

Lyphocin, Vancocin, Vancoled

Pharmacologic classification: glycopeptide
Therapeutic classification: antibiotic
Pregnancy risk category C

How supplied

Available by prescription only
Pulvules: 125 mg, 250 mg
Powder for oral solution: 1-g, 10-g bottles
Powder for injection: 500-mg, 1-g, 5-g vials; 10-g pharmacy bulk package

Indications, route, and dosage

Severe staphylococcal infections when other antibiotics are ineffective or contraindicated
Adults: 500 mg I.V. q 6 hours, or 1 g q 12 hours.
Children: 40 mg/kg I.V. daily, divided q 6 hours.
Neonates: Initially, 15 mg/kg; then, 10 mg/kg I.V. daily, divided q 12 hours for first week of life; then q 8 hours up to age 1 month.
Antibiotic-associated pseudomembranous and staphylococcal enterocolitis
Adults: 125 to 500 mg P.O. q 6 hours for 7 to 10 days.
Children: 40 mg/kg P.O. daily, divided q 6 to 8 hours for 7 to 10 days. Do not exceed 2 g/day in children.
Endocarditis prophylaxis for dental, GI, biliary, and GU instrumentation procedures; surgical prophylaxis in patients allergic to penicillin
Adults: 1 g I.V., given slowly over 1 hour, starting 1 hour before procedure. In high-risk patients, dose may be repeated in 8 to 12 hours.
Children: 20 mg/kg, if child weighs less than 60 lb (27 kg); adult dose, if child weighs more than 60 lb. In high-risk patients, dose may be repeated in 8 to 12 hours.
✦ ***Dosage adjustment.*** In patients with renal failure, adjust dosage or frequency of administration based on degree of renal impairment, severity of infection, and susceptibility of causative organism. Base dosage on serum concentrations of drug.

Recommended initial dose is 15 mg/kg. Subsequent doses should be adjusted p.r.n. Some clinicians use the following schedule.

Serum creatinine level (mg/dl)	Dosage in adults
< 1.5	1 g q 12 hr
1.5 to 5	1 g q 3 to 6 days
> 5	1 g q 10 to 14 days

Pharmacodynamics

Antibacterial action: Vancomycin is bactericidal by hindering cell-wall synthesis and blocking glycopeptide polymerization. Its spectrum of activity includes many gram-positive organisms, including those resistant to other antibiotics. It is useful for *Staphylococcus epidermidis* and methicillin-resistant *S. aureus.* It is also useful for penicillin-resistant *S. pneumococcus.*

Pharmacokinetics

- *Absorption:* Minimal systemic absorption occurs with oral administration. (However, drug may accumulate in patients with colitis or renal failure.)
- *Distribution:* Distributed widely in body fluids, including pericardial, pleural, ascitic, synovial, and placental fluid. It will achieve therapeutic levels in CSF in patients with inflamed meninges. Therapeutic drug levels are 18 to 26 mcg/ml for 2-hour, postinfusion peaks; 5 to 10 mcg/ml for preinfusion troughs (however, these values may vary, depending on laboratory and sampling time).
- *Metabolism:* Unknown.
- *Excretion:* When administered parenterally, drug is excreted renally, mainly by filtration. When administered orally, drug is excreted in feces. In patients with normal renal function, plasma half-life is 6 hours; in those with creatinine clearance of 10 to 30 ml/minute, plasma half-life is about 32 hours; if

creatinine clearance is below 10 ml/minute, plasma half-life is 146 hours.

Contraindications and precautions
Contraindicated in patients with hypersensitivity to drug. Use cautiously in patients with impaired renal or hepatic function, preexisting hearing loss, or allergies to other antibiotics; in those receiving other neurotoxic, nephrotoxic, or ototoxic drugs; and in patients over age 60.

Interactions
When used concomitantly, vancomycin may have additive nephrotoxic effects with *other nephrotoxic drugs* such as *aminoglycosides, amphotericin B, capreomycin, cisplatin, colistin, methoxyflurane,* and *polymyxin B.*

Effects on diagnostic tests
BUN and serum creatinine levels may increase, and neutropenia and eosinophilia may occur during vancomycin therapy.

Adverse reactions
EENT: tinnitus, ototoxicity.
GI: nausea.
GU: nephrotoxicity.
Hematologic: ***neutropenia.***
Skin: "red-neck" syndrome with rapid I.V. infusion (maculopapular rash on face, neck, trunk, and extremities).
Other: chills, fever, ***anaphylaxis,*** superinfection, pain or thrombophlebitis at injection site, hypotension, wheezing, dyspnea.

Overdose and treatment
There is limited information available on the acute toxicity of vancomycin. Treatment includes providing supportive care and maintaining glomerular filtration rate. Hemodialysis and hemoperfusion have been used.

☑ Special considerations
- Obtain culture and sensitivity tests before starting therapy (unless drug is being used for prophylaxis).
- To prepare drug for oral administration, reconstitute as directed in manufacturer's instructions. Reconstituted solution remains stable for 2 weeks when refrigerated.
- To prepare drug for I.V. injection, reconstitute 500 mg with 10 ml or 1 g with 20 ml of sterile water for injection, to yield 50 mg/ml. Withdraw desired dose and further dilute to 100 to 250 ml with 0.9% NaCl solution or D_5W; 1 g should be diluted with at least 200 ml of diluent. Infuse over at least 60 minutes to avoid adverse effects related to rapid infusion rate. Initial reconstituted solution remains stable for 14 days when refrigerated.
- Do not give I.M. because drug is highly irritating.
- Monitor blood counts and BUN, serum creatinine, and drug levels.
- If patient develops maculopapular rash on face, neck, trunk, and upper extremities, slow infusion rate.
- If patient has preexisting auditory dysfunction or requires prolonged therapy, auditory function tests may be indicated before and during therapy.
- Hemodialysis and peritoneal dialysis remove only minimal drug amounts. Patients receiving these treatments need usual dose once every 5 to 7 days.

Patient education
- If patient is taking drug orally, remind him to continue taking it as directed, even if he feels better.
- Advise patient not to take antidiarrheal agents concomitantly with drug except as prescribed.
- Instruct patient to call promptly if he develops ringing in the ears.

Geriatric use
- Elderly patients may be more susceptible to drug's ototoxic effects. Monitor serum levels closely and adjust dosage as needed.

Breast-feeding
- Drug is excreted in breast milk. Use with caution in breast-feeding women.

varicella virus vaccine, live
Varivax

Pharmacologic classification: vaccine
Therapeutic classification: viral vaccine
Pregnancy risk category C

How supplied
Available by prescription only
Injection: Single-dose vial containing 1,350 plaque-forming units of Oka/Merck varicella virus

Indications, route, and dosage
Prevention of varicella-zoster (chickenpox) infections
Adults and children age 13 and older: Administer 0.5 ml S.C. followed by a second dose of 0.5 ml 4 to 8 weeks later.
Children age 1 to 12: 0.5 ml S.C. as a single dose.

Pharmacodynamics
Antiviral vaccine action: Varicella virus vaccine prevents chickenpox by inducing the production of antibodies to varicella-zoster virus.

Pharmacokinetics
- *Absorption:* Antibodies are usually detectable 4 to 6 weeks after S.C. injection. Varicella antibodies have been detected 99.5% of the time 4 years postvaccination.
- *Distribution:* No information available.
- *Metabolism:* No information available.
- *Excretion:* No information available.

Contraindications and precautions
Contraindicated in patients hypersensitive to drug; in those with history of anaphylactoid reaction to neomycin, blood dyscrasia, leukemia, lymphomas, neoplasms affecting bone marrow or lymphatic system, primary and acquired immunosuppressive states, active untreated tuberculosis, or any febrile

respiratory illness or other active febrile infection; and in pregnant patients.

Interactions

Blood products and *immune globulin* may inactivate vaccine. Defer vaccination for at least 5 months following blood or plasma transfusions or administration of immune globulin or *varicella-zoster immune globulin. Immunosuppressants* increase risk of severe reactions to live-virus vaccines. Postpone routine vaccination. Reye's syndrome has been reported with use of *salicylates.* Avoid use of salicylates for 6 weeks after varicella infections.

Effects on diagnostic tests

None reported.

Adverse reactions

Other: *fever, injection site reactions (swelling, redness, pain, rash),* varicella-like rash.

Overdose and treatment

No information available.

☑ Special considerations

- To reconstitute vaccine, withdraw 0.7 ml of diluent into the syringe. Inject the contents of the syringe into the vial of lyophilized vaccine and gently agitate to mix thoroughly. Administer immediately after reconstitution. Discard if not used within 30 minutes.
- Have epinephrine available for potential anaphylactoid reaction.
- Vaccine has been safely and effectively used in combination with measles, mumps, and rubella vaccine.
- Vaccine appears to be less effective in adults compared with children.
- Studies are underway to determine the incidence of herpes zoster, which may occur following a latent period.
- Vaccine contains a live attenuated virus. Children who develop a rash may be capable of transmitting the virus.

Patient education

- Inform patient or parents of adverse reactions associated with vaccine.
- Caution women of childbearing age to call if pregnancy is suspected before receiving vaccine. Pregnancy should be avoided for 3 months after receiving vaccine.

Pediatric use

- A safety study protocol program is available for children and adolescents (age 12 to 17) with acute lymphocytic leukemia. Clinicians can enroll patients in this program by contacting Bio-Pharm Clinical Services at (215) 283-0897.
- Safety and efficacy have not been established for children under age 1.

Breast-feeding

- It is not known if varicella vaccine virus is excreted in breast milk; use cautiously in breast-feeding women.

varicella-zoster immune globulin (VZIG)

Pharmacologic classification: immune serum
Therapeutic classification: varicella-zoster prophylaxis
Pregnancy risk category C

How supplied

Available by prescription only
Injection: 10% to 18% solution of the globulin fraction of human plasma containing 125 units of varicella-zoster virus antibody in 2.5 ml or less

Indications, route, and dosage

Passive immunization of susceptible patients, primarily immunocompromised patients after exposure to varicella (chickenpox or herpes zoster)
Adults and children: 125 units per 10 kg of body weight I.M., to a maximum of 625 units. Higher doses may be needed in immunocompromised adults.

Pharmacodynamics

Postexposure prophylaxis: This agent provides passive immunity to varicella-zoster virus.

Pharmacokinetics

- *Absorption:* After I.M. absorption, the persistence of antibodies is unknown, but protection should last at least 3 weeks. Protection is sufficient to prevent or lessen the severity of varicella infections.
- *Distribution:* No information available.
- *Metabolism:* No information available.
- *Excretion:* No information available.

Contraindications and precautions

Contraindicated in patients with thrombocytopenia, coagulation disorders, or history of severe reaction to human immune serum globulin or thimerosal.

Interactions

Concomitant use of VZIG with *corticosteroids* or *immunosuppressants* may interfere with the immune response to this immune globulin. Whenever possible, avoid using these agents during the postexposure immunization period.

Also, VZIG may interfere with the immune response to *live virus vaccines* (for example, those for *measles, mumps,* and *rubella*). Do not administer live virus vaccines within 3 months after or 2 weeks before administering VZIG. If it becomes necessary to administer VZIG and a live virus vaccine concomitantly, confirm seroconversion with follow-up serologic testing.

Effects on diagnostic tests

None reported.

Adverse reactions

GI: GI distress.
Respiratory: respiratory distress.
Other: ***anaphylaxis***, discomfort at injection site, malaise, headache, rash, ***angioedema, angioneu-***

rotic edema, nephrotic syndrome, fever, myalgia, chest tightness.

Overdose and treatment
No information available.

☑ Special considerations
• Obtain a thorough history of allergies and reactions to immunizations.
• Epinephrine solution 1:1,000 should be available to treat allergic reactions.
• VZIG is recommended primarily for immunodeficient patients under age 15 and certain infants exposed in utero, although use in other patients (especially immunocompromised patients of any age, normal adults, pregnant women, and premature and full-term infants) should be considered on a case-by-case basis. It is not routinely recommended for use in immunocompetent pregnant women because chickenpox is much less severe than in immunosuppressed patients. Moreover, it will not protect the fetus.
• Although usually used only in children under age 15, VZIG may be administered to adults if necessary.
• Administer only by deep I.M. injection. Never administer I.V. Use the gluteal muscle in infants and small children and the deltoid or anterolateral thigh in adults and larger children.
• For maximum benefit, administer VZIG within 96 hours of presumed exposure.
• Store unopened vials between 36° and 46° F (2° and 8° C). Do not freeze.

Patient education
• Explain that patient's chances of AIDS or hepatitis from VZIG are very small.
• Tell patient that he may experience some local pain, swelling, and tenderness at the injection site. Recommend acetaminophen to alleviate these minor effects.
• Encourage patient to report severe reactions.

Breast-feeding
• It is unknown whether VZIG is distributed into breast milk. Use cautiously in breast-feeding women.

vasopressin (antidiuretic hormone [ADH])
Pitressin Synthetic

Pharmacologic classification: posterior pituitary hormone
Therapeutic classification: antidiuretic hormone, peristaltic stimulant, hemostatic
Pregnancy risk category B

How supplied
Available by prescription only
Injection: 0.5-ml and 1-ml ampules and vials, 20 units/ml

Indications, route, and dosage
Nonnephrogenic, nonpsychogenic diabetes insipidus
Adults: 5 to 10 units I.M. or S.C. b.i.d. to q.i.d., p.r.n.
Children: 2.5 to 10 units I.M. or S.C. b.i.d. to q.i.d., p.r.n.
Postoperative abdominal distention
Adults: 5 units I.M. initially, then q 3 to 4 hours, increasing dosage to 10 units, if needed. Reduce dosage for children proportionately.
To expel gas before abdominal X-ray
Adults: Inject 5 to 15 units S.C. at 2 hours, then again at 30 minutes before X-ray. Enema before first dose may also help to eliminate gas.
Upper GI tract hemorrhage
Adults: 0.2 to 0.4 units/minute I.V. or 0.1 to 0.5 units/minute intra-arterially.

Pharmacodynamics
Antidiuretic action: Vasopressin is used as an antidiuretic to control or prevent signs and complications of neurogenic diabetes insipidus. Acting primarily at the renal tubular level, vasopressin increases cAMP, which increases water permeability at the renal tubule and collecting duct, resulting in increased urine osmolality and decreased urinary flow rate.

Peristaltic stimulant action: Used to treat postoperative abdominal distention and to facilitate abdominal radiographic procedures, vasopressin induces peristalsis by directly stimulating contraction of smooth muscle in the GI tract.

Hemostatic action: In patients with GI hemorrhage, vasopressin, administered I.V. or intra-arterially into the superior mesenteric artery, controls bleeding of esophageal varices by directly stimulating vasoconstriction of capillaries and small arterioles.

Pharmacokinetics
• *Absorption:* Vasopressin is destroyed by trypsin in the GI tract and must be administered intranasally or parenterally.
• *Distribution:* Drug is distributed throughout the extracellular fluid, with no evidence of protein-binding.
• *Metabolism:* Most of dose is destroyed rapidly in the liver and kidneys.
• *Excretion:* Approximately 5% of an S.C. dose is excreted unchanged in urine after 4 hours. Duration of action after I.M. or S.C. administration is 2 to 8 hours. Half-life, 10 to 20 minutes.

Contraindications and precautions
Contraindicated in patients with chronic nephritis accompanied by nitrogen retention. Use cautiously in patients with seizure disorders, migraine headache, asthma, CV or renal disease, heart failure, goiter with cardiac complications, arteriosclerosis, or fluid overload; in children and elderly or pregnant patients; or in preoperative or postoperative patients who are polyuric.

Interactions
Concomitant use of vasopressin with *carbamazepine, chlorpropamide,* or *clofibrate* may po-

tentiate vasopressin's antidiuretic effect; use with *alcohol, demeclocycline, epinephrine, heparin, lithium,* or *norepinephrine* may decrease antidiuretic effect.

Effects on diagnostic tests
None reported.

Adverse reactions
CNS: tremor, headache, vertigo.
CV: angina in patients with vascular disease; vasoconstriction, ***arrhythmias, cardiac arrest,*** myocardial ischemia, circumoral pallor, decreased cardiac output.
GI: abdominal cramps, nausea, vomiting, flatulence.
Other: ***water intoxication*** (drowsiness, listlessness, headache, confusion, weight gain, ***seizures, coma***), hypersensitivity reactions (urticaria, angioedema, ***bronchoconstriction, anaphylaxis***), diaphoresis, cutaneous gangrene.

Overdose and treatment
Clinical manifestations of overdose include drowsiness, listlessness, headache, confusion, anuria, and weight gain (water intoxication). Treatment requires water restriction and temporary withdrawal of vasopressin until polyuria occurs. Severe water intoxication may require osmotic diuresis with mannitol, hypertonic dextrose, or urea, either alone or with furosemide.

☑ Special considerations
Besides those relevant to all *posterior pituitary hormones,* consider the following recommendations.
- Establish baseline vital signs and intake and output ratio at the initiation of therapy.
- Monitor patient's blood pressure twice daily. Watch for excessively elevated blood pressure or lack of response to drug, which may be indicated by hypotension. Also monitor fluid intake and output and daily weight.
- Question patient with abdominal distention about passage of flatus and stool.
- A rectal tube will facilitate gas expulsion after vasopressin injection.
- Observe for signs of early water intoxication—drowsiness, listlessness, headache, confusion, and weight gain—to prevent seizures, coma, and death.
- Never inject during first stage of labor; this may cause ruptured uterus.
- Use extreme caution to avoid extravasation because of risk of necrosis and gangrene.

Patient education
- Tell patient to drink one or two glasses of water with each dose of vasopressin. This reduces the adverse reactions of unusual paleness, nausea, abdominal cramps, and vomiting.
- Teach patient how to maintain a fluid intake and output record.
- Show patient how to check the expiration date.
- Tell patient to call immediately if the following symptoms occur: chest pain, confusion, fever, hives, rash, headache, problems with urination, seizures, weight gain, unusual drowsiness, wheezing, trouble with breathing, or swelling of face, hands, feet, or mouth.
- Encourage patient to rotate injection sites.

Geriatric use
- Elderly patients show increased sensitivity to the effects of vasopressin. Use with caution.

Pediatric use
- Children show increased sensitivity to the effects of vasopressin. Use with caution.

Breast-feeding
- Use caution when administering to breast-feeding women.

vecuronium bromide
Norcuron

Pharmacologic classification: nondepolarizing neuromuscular blocker
Therapeutic classification: skeletal muscle relaxant
Pregnancy risk category C

How supplied
Available by prescription only
Injection: 10 mg (with or without diluent), 20 mg (without diluent)

Indications, route, and dosage
Adjunct to anesthesia, to facilitate intubation, and to provide skeletal muscle relaxation during surgery or mechanical ventilation
Dose depends on anesthetic used, individual needs, and response. Doses are representative and must be adjusted.
Adults and children age 10 and over: Initially, 0.08 to 0.10 mg/kg I.V. bolus. Higher initial doses (up to 0.3 mg/kg) may be used for rapid onset. Maintenance doses of 0.010 to 0.015 mg/kg within 25 to 40 minutes of initial dose should be administered during prolonged surgical procedures. Maintenance doses may be given q 12 to 15 minutes in patients receiving balanced anesthetic.

Pharmacodynamics
Skeletal muscle relaxant action: Vecuronium prevents acetylcholine from binding to receptors on motor end-plate, thus blocking depolarization. Vecuronium exhibits minimal CV effects and does not appear to alter heart rate or rhythm, systolic or diastolic blood pressure, cardiac output, systemic vascular resistance, or mean arterial pressure. It has little or no histamine-releasing properties.

Pharmacokinetics
- *Absorption:* After I.V. administration of 0.08 to 0.1 mg/kg, onset of action occurs within 1 minute; action peaks at 3 to 5 minutes. The duration is about 25 to 40 minutes depending on anesthetic used, dose, and number of doses given.
- *Distribution:* After I.V. administration, drug is distributed in extracellular fluid and rapidly reaches its site of action. It is 60% to 90% plasma protein-

bound. Volume of distribution is decreased in children under age 1 and may be decreased in elderly patients.
- *Metabolism:* Drug undergoes rapid and extensive hepatic metabolism.
- *Excretion:* Drug and its metabolites appear to be primarily excreted in feces by biliary elimination; also excreted in urine.

Contraindications and precautions
Contraindicated in patients with hypersensitivity to bromides. Use cautiously in patients with altered circulation caused by CV disease and edematous states, hepatic disease, severe obesity, bronchogenic carcinoma, electrolyte disturbances, or neuromuscular diseases and in the elderly.

Interactions
Concomitant use with *aminoglycosides, clindamycin, lincomycin, polymyxin antibiotics, furosemide, parenteral magnesium salts, depolarizing neuromuscular blocking agents, other nondepolarizing neuromuscular blocking agents, quinidine or quinine, thiazide diuretics, other potassium-depleting drugs,* and *general anesthetics* (decrease dose by 15%, especially with *enflurane* and *isoflurane*) may increase vecuronium-induced neuromuscular blockade. Concomitant use with *anticholinesterase agents* may also antagonize effects of vecuronium. Concomitant use with *narcotic (opioid) analgesics* may increase central respiratory depression.

Effects on diagnostic tests
None reported.

Adverse reactions
Respiratory: ***prolonged, dose-related respiratory insufficiency or apnea.***
Other: skeletal muscle weakness.

Overdose and treatment
Clinical manifestations of overdose include prolonged duration of neuromuscular blockade, skeletal muscle weakness, decreased respiratory reserve, low tidal volume, and apnea. Treatment is supportive and symptomatic. Keep airway clear and maintain adequate ventilation.

Use peripheral nerve stimulator to determine and monitor the degree of blockade. Give anticholinesterase agent (edrophonium, neostigmine, or pyridostigmine) to reverse neuromuscular blockade and atropine or glycopyrrolate to overcome muscarinic effects.

☑ Special considerations
- Administer by rapid I.V. injection or I.V. infusion. Do not give I.M.
- Reconstitute using diluent supplied by manufacturer (bacteriostatic water for injection) or a compatible solution (such as 0.9% NaCl, D_5W, sterile water for injection, 5% dextrose in 0.9% NaCl, or lactated Ringer's) to produce a solution containing 1 mg/ml or 2 mg/ml.
- Diluent supplied by manufacturer contains benzyl alcohol, which is not intended for use in newborns.
- Do not mix in same syringe or give through same needle as barbiturates or other alkaline solutions.
- Protect solution from light.
- After reconstitution, solution should be stored in refrigerator or at room temperature not exceeding 86° F (30° C). Do not use if discolored. Discard unused portion after 24 hours. When reconstituted with supplied bacteriostatic water, solution can be stored for 5 days.
- Have emergency respiratory support equipment immediately available.
- Assess baseline serum electrolyte levels, acid-base balance, and renal and hepatic function before administration.
- Peripheral nerve stimulator may be used to identify residual paralysis during recovery and is especially useful during administration to high-risk patients.
- After procedure, monitor vital signs at least every 15 minutes until patient is stable, then every 30 minutes for next 2 hours. Monitor airway and pattern of respirations until patient has recovered from drug effects. Anticipate problems with ventilation in obese patients and those with myasthenia gravis or other neuromuscular disease.
- Evaluate recovery from neuromuscular blockade by checking strength of hard grip, ability to breathe naturally, to take deep breaths and cough, to keep eyes open, and to lift head keeping mouth closed.
- Drug does not relieve pain or affect consciousness; if indicated, assess need for analgesic or sedative.

Geriatric use
- Administer cautiously to elderly patients.

Pediatric use
- Safety and efficacy have not been established in infants under age 7 weeks. Infants age 7 weeks to 1 year are more sensitive to neuromuscular blocking effects; less frequent administration may be necessary. Higher doses may be needed in children age 1 to 9.

Breast-feeding
- It is unknown if drug is excreted in breast milk. Use with caution in breast-feeding women.

venlafaxine hydrochloride
Effexor, Effexor XR

Pharmacologic classification: neuronal serotonin, norepinephrine, and dopamine reuptake inhibitor
Therapeutic classification: antidepressant
Pregnancy risk category C

How supplied
Available by prescription only
Capsules (extended-release): 37.5 mg, 75 mg, 150 mg
Tablets: 25 mg, 37.5 mg, 50 mg, 75 mg, 100 mg

Indications, route, and dosage

Depression

Adults: Initially, 75 mg P.O. daily, in two or three divided doses with food. Increase dosage as tolerated and needed in increments of 75 mg/day at intervals of no less than 4 days. For moderately depressed outpatients, usual maximum dosage is 225 mg/day; in certain severely depressed patients, dosage may be as high as 350 mg/day. For extended-release capsules, 75 mg P.O. daily, in a single dose. For some patients, it may be desirable to start at 37.5 mg P.O. daily for 4 to 7 days before increasing to 75 mg daily. Dosage may be increased at increments of 75 mg/day q 4 days to a maximum of 225 mg/day.

✦ ***Dosage adjustment.*** Reduce dosage by 50% in patients with impaired hepatic function. In patients with moderate renal impairment (glomerular filtration rate of 10 to 70 ml/minute), total daily dosage should be reduced by 25%. In hemodialysis patients, reduce dose by 50% and withhold drug until after dialysis treatment.

Note: Discontinue drug in patient who develops seizures

Pharmacodynamics

Antidepressant action: Venlafaxine is thought to potentiate neurotransmitter activity in the CNS. Preclinical studies have shown that venlafaxine and its active metabolite, O-desmethylvenlafaxine (ODV), are potent inhibitors of neuronal serotonin and norepinephrine reuptake and weak inhibitors of dopamine reuptake.

Pharmacokinetics

- *Absorption:* Approximately 92% is absorbed after oral administration.
- *Distribution:* Drug is approximately 25% to 29% protein-bound in plasma.
- *Metabolism:* Drug is extensively metabolized in the liver, with ODV being the only major active metabolite.
- *Excretion:* Approximately 87% of dose is recovered in urine within 48 hours (5% as unchanged venlafaxine, 29% as unconjugated ODV, 26% as conjugated ODV, and 27% as minor inactive metabolites).

Contraindications and precautions

Contraindicated in patients hypersensitive to drug and within 14 days of MAO inhibitor therapy. Use cautiously in patients with impaired renal or hepatic function, diseases or conditions that could affect hemodynamic responses or metabolism, or history of seizures or mania.

Interactions

MAO inhibitors may precipitate a syndrome similar to neuroleptic malignant syndrome when used with venlafaxine. Do not start venlafaxine within 14 days of discontinuing therapy with an MAO inhibitor, and do not start MAO inhibitor therapy within 7 days of stopping venlafaxine.

Concurrent administration of *cimetidine* and venlafaxine should be done with caution in elderly patients and in patients with hepatic dysfunction or preexisting hypertension; use of these agents together could cause a more pronounced increase in venlafaxine concentration. For the same reason, caution is advised when administering venlafaxine concomitantly with *CNS-active drugs.*

Effects on diagnostic tests

None reported.

Adverse reactions

CNS: *headache, somnolence, dizziness, nervousness, insomnia,* anxiety, tremor, abnormal dreams, paresthesia, agitation.
CV: hypertension, vasodilation.
EENT: blurred vision.
GI: *nausea, constipation,* vomiting, *dry mouth, anorexia,* diarrhea, dyspepsia, flatulence.
GU: *abnormal ejaculation,* impotence, urinary frequency, impaired urination.
Other: *diaphoresis, asthenia,* weight loss, rash, yawning, chills, infection.

Overdose and treatment

Symptoms may range from none (most commonly) to somnolence, generalized seizures, and prolongation of the QT interval.

Treatment should consist of general measures used in managing any antidepressant overdose (ensuring an adequate airway, providing oxygenation and ventilation, monitoring cardiac rhythm and vital signs). General supportive and symptomatic measures also are recommended. Use of activated charcoal, induction of emesis, or gastric lavage should be considered. No specific antidotes are known for venlafaxine overdose.

☑ Special considerations

- Because drug is associated with sustained increases in blood pressure, regular monitoring of blood pressure is recommended. For patients who experience a sustained increase in blood pressure while receiving venlafaxine, either dose reduction or discontinuation should be considered.
- Monitor patients with major affective disorders because drug may activate mania or hypomania.
- When discontinuing drug therapy after more than 1 week, taper dose. If patient has received drug for at least 6 weeks gradually taper dosage over 2 weeks.

Patient education

- Caution patient not to operate hazardous machinery until drug's effects are known.
- Advise female patient to call if pregnancy is planned or suspected during therapy.
- Instruct patient to call before taking other medications, including OTC preparations, because of potential interactions.
- Tell patient to avoid alcohol while taking venlafaxine.
- Instruct patient to report rash, hives, or a related allergic reaction.

Pediatric use

- Safety and effectiveness in children under age 18 have not been established.

Breast-feeding
- Use cautiously in breast-feeding patients.

verapamil hydrochloride
Calan, Calan SR, Isoptin, Isoptin SR, Verelan

Pharmacologic classification: calcium channel blocker
Therapeutic classification: antianginal, antihypertensive, antiarrhythmic
Pregnancy risk category C

How supplied
Available by prescription only
Tablets: 40 mg, 80 mg, 120 mg
Tablets (sustained-release): 120 mg, 180 mg, 240 mg
Capsules (sustained-release): 120 mg, 180 mg, 240 mg
Injection: 2.5 mg/ml

Indications, route, and dosage
Management of Prinzmetal's or variant angina or unstable or chronic, stable angina pectoris
Adults: Initial dose of 80 to 120 mg P.O. t.i.d. Dosage may be increased at weekly intervals. Some patients may require up to 480 mg daily.
Supraventricular tachyarrhythmias
Adults: 0.075 to 0.15 mg/kg (5 to 10 mg) I.V. push over 2 minutes. If no response occurs, give a second dose of 10 mg (0.15 mg/kg) 15 to 30 minutes after the initial dose.
Children age 1 to 15: 0.1 to 0.3 mg/kg (2 to 5 mg) as I.V. bolus over 2 minutes. Dose should not exceed 5 mg. Dose may be repeated in 30 minutes if no response occurs (should not exceed 10 mg).
Children under age 1: 0.1 to 0.2 mg/kg (0.75 to 2 mg) as I.V. bolus over 2 minutes. Dose may be repeated in 30 minutes if no response occurs.
Control of ventricular rate in digitalized patients with chronic atrial flutter or fibrillation
Adults: 240 to 320 mg P.O. daily in three to four divided doses.
Hypertension
Adults: Usual starting dose is 80 mg P.O. t.i.d. Daily dose may be increased to 360 to 480 mg.

Initiate therapy with sustained-release capsules at 180 mg (240 mg for Verelan) daily in the morning. A starting dose of 120 mg may be indicated in people who may have an increased response to verapamil. Adjust dosage based on clinical effectiveness 24 hours after dosing. Increase by 120 mg daily until a maximum dose of 480 mg daily is given. Sustained-release capsules should be given only once daily. Antihypertensive effects are usually seen within the first week of therapy. Most patients respond to 240 mg daily.

Pharmacodynamics
Antianginal action: Verapamil manages unstable and chronic stable angina by reducing afterload, both at rest and with exercise, thereby decreasing oxygen consumption. It also decreases myocardial oxygen demand and cardiac work by exerting a negative inotropic effect, reducing heart rate, relieving coronary artery spasm (via coronary artery vasodilation), and dilating peripheral vessels. The net result of these effects is relief of angina-related ischemia and pain. In patients with Prinzmetal's variant angina, verapamil inhibits coronary artery spasm, resulting in increased myocardial oxygen delivery.

Antihypertensive action: Verapamil reduces blood pressure mainly by dilating peripheral vessels. Its negative inotropic effect blocks reflex mechanisms that lead to increased blood pressure.

Antiarrhythmic action: Verapamil's combined effects on the SA and AV nodes help manage arrhythmias. Drug's primary effect is on the AV node; slowed conduction reduces the ventricular rate in atrial tachyarrhythmias and blocks reentry paths in paroxysmal supraventricular arrhythmias.

Pharmacokinetics
- *Absorption:* Absorbed rapidly and completely from the GI tract after oral administration; however, only about 20% to 35% of drug reaches systemic circulation because of first-pass effect. When administered orally, peak effects occur within 1 to 2 hours with conventional tablets and within 4 to 8 hours with sustained-release preparations. When administered I.V., effects occur within minutes after injection and usually persist about 30 to 60 minutes (although they may last up to 6 hours). Therapeutic serum levels are 80 to 300 ng/ml.
- *Distribution:* Steady-state distribution volume in healthy adults ranges from about 4.5 to 7 L/kg but may increase to 12 L/kg in patients with hepatic cirrhosis. Approximately 90% of circulating drug is bound to plasma proteins.
- *Metabolism:* Drug is metabolized in the liver.
- *Excretion:* Excreted in the urine as unchanged drug and active metabolites. Elimination half-life is normally 6 to 12 hours and increases to as much as 16 hours in patients with hepatic cirrhosis. In infants, elimination half-life may be 5 to 7 hours.

Contraindications and precautions
Contraindicated in patients with hypersensitivity to drug; severe left ventricular dysfunction; cardiogenic shock; second- or third-degree AV block or sick sinus syndrome except in presence of functioning pacemaker; atrial flutter or fibrillation and accessory bypass tract syndrome; severe heart failure (unless secondary to verapamil therapy); and severe hypotension. In addition, I.V. verapamil is contraindicated in patients receiving I.V. beta-adrenergic blocking agents and in those with ventricular tachycardia.

Use cautiously in the elderly and in patients with impaired renal or hepatic function or increased intracranial pressure.

Interactions
Concomitant use of verapamil with *beta blockers* may cause additive effects leading to heart failure, conduction disturbances, arrhythmias, and hypotension, especially if high beta-blocker doses are used, if drugs are administered I.V., or if the patient has moderately severe to severe heart failure, severe cardiomyopathy, or recent MI.

Concomitant use of oral verapamil with *digoxin* may increase serum digoxin concentration by 50% to 75% during the first week of therapy. Concomitant use with *antihypertensives* may lead to combined antihypertensive effects, resulting in clinically significant hypotension. Concomitant use with *drugs that attenuate alpha-adrenergic response* (such as *prazosin and methyldopa*) may cause excessive blood pressure reduction. Concomitant use with *disopyramide* may cause combined negative inotropic effects; with *quinidine* to treat hypertrophic cardiomyopathy, may cause excessive hypotension; with *carbamazepine,* may cause increased serum carbamazepine levels and subsequent toxicity; with *flecainide,* may add to negative inotropic effect and prolong AV conduction; with *neuromuscular blocking agents,* may potentiate their action; with *rifampin,* may substantially reduce verapamil's oral bioavailability. Verapamil therapy may inhibit the clearance and increase the plasma levels of *theophylline.*

Verapamil may increase serum levels of *cyclosporine. Phenobarbital* may increase verapamil clearance. Verapamil may increase sensitivity of *lithium* effects. Use cautiously with *inhalation anesthetics* to avoid excessive CV depression; verapamil may prolong intoxicating effects of *alcohol.*

Effects on diagnostic tests
None reported.

Adverse reactions
CNS: dizziness, headache, asthenia.
CV: *transient hypotension,* ***heart failure,*** pulmonary edema, bradycardia, AV block, ***ventricular asystole, ventricular fibrillation,*** peripheral edema.
GI: *constipation,* nausea.
Hepatic: elevated liver enzymes.
Skin: rash.

Overdose and treatment
Clinical effects of overdose are primarily extensions of adverse reactions. Heart block, asystole, and hypotension are the most serious reactions and require immediate attention.

Treatment may include administering I.V. isoproterenol, norepinephrine, epinephrine, atropine, or calcium gluconate in usual doses. Adequate hydration should be ensured.

In patients with hypertrophic cardiomyopathy, alpha-adrenergic agents, including methoxamine, phenylephrine, and metaraminol, should be used to maintain blood pressure. (Isoproterenol and norepinephrine should be avoided.) Inotropic agents, including dobutamine and dopamine, may be used if necessary.

If severe conduction disturbances, such as heart block and asystole, occur with hypotension that does not respond to drug therapy, cardiac pacing should be initiated immediately, with CPR measures as indicated.

In patients with Wolff-Parkinson-White or Lown-Ganong-Levine syndrome and a rapid ventricular rate caused by hemodynamically significant antegrade conduction, synchronized cardioversion may be used. Lidocaine and procainamide may be used as adjuncts.

☑ Special considerations
- If verapamil is initiated in patient receiving carbamazepine, a 40% to 50% reduction in carbamazepine dosage may be necessary. Monitor patient closely for signs of toxicity.
- Reduce dosage in patients with renal or hepatic impairment.
- If patient is receiving I.V. verapamil, monitor ECG and blood pressure continuously.
- If verapamil is added to therapy of patient receiving digoxin, reduce digoxin dose by half and monitor subsequent serum drug levels.
- During long-term combination therapy with verapamil and digoxin, monitor ECG periodically to observe for AV block and bradycardia.
- Obtain periodic liver function tests.
- Use reduced dosage in patients with severely compromised cardiac function and those receiving beta blockers. Monitor closely.
- Discontinue disopyramide 48 hours before starting verapamil therapy and do not reinstitute until 24 hours after verapamil has been discontinued.
- Generic sustained-release verapamil tablets may be substituted only for Isoptin SR and Calan SR, not Verelan capsules. The capsule formulation should be given only once daily. When using sustained-release tablets, doses over 240 mg should be given b.i.d.

Patient education
- Instruct patient to report signs of heart failure, such as swelling of hands and feet or shortness of breath.
- Urge patient who is receiving nitrate therapy while verapamil dose is being titrated to comply with prescribed therapy.

Geriatric use
- Elderly patients may require lower doses. In elderly patients, administer I.V. doses over at least 3 minutes to minimize risk of adverse effects.

Pediatric use
- Currently, only the I.V. form is indicated for use in pediatric patients to treat supraventricular tachyarrhythmias.

Breast-feeding
- Drug is excreted in breast milk. To avoid possible adverse effects in infants, discontinue breast-feeding during therapy.

vidarabine (adenine arabinoside)
Vira-A

Pharmacologic classification: purine nucleoside
Therapeutic classification: antiviral
Pregnancy risk category C

How supplied
Available by prescription only
Ophthalmic ointment: 3% in 3.5-g tube (equivalent to 2.8% vidarabine)

Indications, route, and dosage
Acute keratoconjunctivitis and recurrent epithelial keratitis caused by herpes simplex virus types 1 and 2
Adults and children: Administer ½" (1.3 cm) ointment into lower conjunctival sac five times daily at 3-hour intervals.

Pharmacodynamics
Antiviral action: Vidarabine is an adenine analogue. Its exact mechanism of action is unknown; presumably it involves inhibition of DNA polymerase and viral replication by incorporation into viral DNA.

Pharmacokinetics
- *Absorption:* No systemic absorption occurs with ophthalmic use.
- *Distribution:* Only trace amounts of drug are detected in the aqueous humor if the cornea is intact.
- *Metabolism:* Metabolized into the active metabolite arabinosyl-hypoxanthine.
- *Excretion:* Unknown.

Contraindications and precautions
Contraindicated in patients with hypersensitivity to drug or with sterile trophic ulcers. Use cautiously in patients receiving corticosteroids.

Interactions
None reported.

Effects on diagnostic tests
None reported.

Adverse reactions
EENT: temporary burning, itching, mild irritation, pain, lacrimation, foreign body sensation, conjunctival injection, punctal occlusion, sensitivity, superficial punctate keratitis, photophobia.
Other: hypersensitivity reactions.

Overdose and treatment
No information available.

☑ Special considerations
- Drug proves effective only if patient has at least minimal immunocompetence.
- Definitive diagnosis of herpes simplex conjunctivitis should be made before administration of ophthalmic form.

Patient education
- Warn patient who is receiving ophthalmic ointment not to exceed recommended frequency or duration of therapy. Instruct him to wash hands before and after applying ointment, and warn him against allowing tip of tube to touch eye or surrounding area.
- Advise patient to wear sunglasses if photosensitivity occurs.
- Instruct patient to store ophthalmic ointment in tightly sealed, light-resistant container.

vinblastine sulfate (VLB)
Velban, Velbe*, Velsar

Pharmacologic classification: vinca alkaloid (cell cycle–phase specific, M phase)
Therapeutic classification: antineoplastic
Pregnancy risk category D

How supplied
Available by prescription only
Injection: 10-mg vials (lyophilized powder), 10 mg/10 ml vials

Indications, route, and dosage
Dosage and indications may vary. Check current literature for recommended protocol.
Breast or testicular cancer, Hodgkin's and malignant lymphomas, choriocarcinoma, lymphosarcoma, neuroblastoma, lung cancer, mycosis fungoides, histiocytosis, Kaposi's sarcoma
Adults: 0.1 mg/kg or 3.7 mg/m² I.V. weekly or q 2 weeks. May be increased in weekly increments of 50 mcg/kg or 1.8 to 1.9 mg/m² to maximum dose of 0.5 mg/kg or 18.5 mg/m² I.V. weekly, based on response. Dose should not be repeated if WBC count falls below 4,000/mm³.
Children: 2.5 mg/m² I.V. as a single dose every week, increased weekly in increments of 1.25 mg/m² to maximum of 7.5 mg/m².

Pharmacodynamics
Antineoplastic action: Vinblastine exerts its cytotoxic activity by arresting the cell cycle in the metaphase portion of cell division, resulting in a blockade of mitosis. Drug also inhibits DNA-dependent RNA synthesis and interferes with amino acid metabolism, inhibiting purine synthesis.

Pharmacokinetics
- *Absorption:* Absorbed unpredictably across the GI tract after oral administration and therefore must be given I.V.
- *Distribution:* Distributed widely into body tissues. Drug crosses the blood-brain barrier but does not achieve therapeutic concentrations in the CSF.
- *Metabolism:* Metabolized partially in the liver to an active metabolite.
- *Excretion:* Excreted primarily in bile as unchanged drug. A smaller portion is excreted in urine. Plasma elimination of vinblastine is described as triphasic, with half-lives of 3.7 minutes, 1.6 hours, and 24.8 hours for the alpha, beta, and terminal phases, respectively.

Contraindications and precautions
Contraindicated in patients with severe leukopenia, granulocytopenia (unless result of disease being treated), or bacterial infection. Use cautiously in patients with hepatic dysfunction.

Interactions

Concomitant use with *phenytoin* may result in lower plasma phenytoin levels requiring increased dosage of phenytoin. Concomitant use of *mitomycin* has produced acute shortness of breath and severe bronchospasm. Concomitant use with *erythromycin* may cause toxicity of vinblastine.

Effects on diagnostic tests

Drug therapy may increase blood and urine concentrations of uric acid.

Adverse reactions

CNS: depression, *paresthesia, peripheral neuropathy and neuritis, numbness, loss of deep tendon reflexes, muscle pain and weakness,* ***seizures, CVA,*** headache.
CV: hypertension, ***MI.***
EENT: pharyngitis.
GI: *nausea, vomiting,* ulcer, bleeding, *constipation, ileus, anorexia,* diarrhea, *weight loss,* abdominal pain, *stomatitis.*
Hematologic: *anemia,* ***leukopenia*** (nadir occurs days 4 to 10 and lasts another 7 to 14 days), ***thrombocytopenia.***
Respiratory: ***acute bronchospasm,*** shortness of breath.
Skin: vesiculation.
Other: reversible alopecia, *irritation, phlebitis,* cellulitis, necrosis with extravasation.

Overdose and treatment

Clinical manifestations of overdose include stomatitis, ileus, mental depression, paresthesia, loss of deep reflexes, permanent CNS damage, and myelosuppression.

Treatment is usually supportive and includes transfusion of blood components and appropriate symptomatic therapy.

☑ Special considerations

- To reconstitute drug, use 10 ml of preserved 0.9% NaCl injection to yield a concentration of 1 mg/ml.
- Drug may be administered by I.V. push injection over 1 minute into the tubing of a freely flowing I.V. infusion.
- Dilution into larger volume is not recommended for infusion into peripheral veins. This method increases risk of extravasation. Drug may be administered as an I.V. infusion through a central venous catheter.
- Give an antiemetic before administering drug to reduce nausea.
- Do not administer more frequently than every 7 days to allow review of effect on leukocytes before administration of next dose. Leukopenia may develop.
- Reduced dosage may be required in patients with liver disease.
- After administering drug, monitor for life-threatening acute bronchospasm reaction. This reaction is most likely to occur in patient also receiving mitomycin.
- Prevent uric acid nephropathy with generous oral fluid intake and administration of allopurinol.
- Treat extravasation with liberal injection of hyaluronidase into the site, followed by warm compresses to minimize the spread of the reaction. (Some clinicians treat extravasation with cold compresses.) Prepare hyaluronidase by adding 3 ml of 0.9% NaCl solution to the 150-unit vial.
- Give laxatives as needed. Stool softeners may be used prophylactically.
- Do not confuse vinblastine with vincristine or the investigational agent vindesine.
- Drug is less neurotoxic than vincristine.

Patient education

- Encourage adequate fluid intake to increase urine output and facilitate excretion of uric acid.
- Reassure patient that therapeutic response is not immediate. Adequate trial is 12 weeks.
- Advise patient to avoid exposure to people with infections and to report signs of infection or unusual bleeding immediately.
- Reassure patient that hair should grow back after treatment has ended.

Geriatric use

- Patients with cachexia or ulceration of the skin (which is more common in elderly patients) may be more susceptible to leukopenic effect of drug.

Breast-feeding

- It is not known if drug distributes into breast milk. However, because of risk of serious adverse reactions, mutagenicity, and carcinogenicity in infants, breast-feeding is not recommended.

vincristine sulfate

Oncovin, Vincasar PFS, Vincrex

Pharmacologic classification: vinca alkaloid (cell cycle–phase specific, M phase)
Therapeutic classification: antineoplastic
Pregnancy risk category D

How supplied

Available by prescription only
Injection: 1 mg/1 ml, 2 mg/2 ml, 5 mg/5 ml multiple-dose vials; 1 mg/1 ml, 2 mg/2 ml preservative-free vials

Indications, route, and dosage

Dosage and indications may vary. Check current literature for recommended protocol.

Acute lymphoblastic and other leukemias; Hodgkin's disease; lymphosarcoma; reticulum cell, osteogenic, and other sarcomas; neuroblastoma; rhabdomyosarcoma; Wilms' tumor; lung and ◊ breast cancer

Adults: 10 to 30 mcg/kg I.V. or 0.4 to 1.4 mg/m² I.V. weekly.

Children: 2 mg/m² I.V. weekly. Maximum single dose (adults and children), is 2 mg.

Children weighing under 22 lb (10 kg) or body surface area below 1 m²: 0.05 mg/kg once weekly.

✦ ***Dosage adjustment.*** Reduce dose by 50% in patients with direct serum bilirubin concentration exceeding 3 ml/dl or other evidence of significant hepatic impairment.

Pharmacodynamics

Antineoplastic action: Vincristine exerts its cytotoxic activity by arresting the cell cycle in the metaphase portion of cell division, resulting in a blockade of mitosis. Drug also inhibits DNA-dependent RNA synthesis and interferes with amino acid metabolites, inhibiting purine synthesis.

Pharmacokinetics

- *Absorption:* Drug is absorbed unpredictably across the GI tract after oral administration and therefore must be given I.V.
- *Distribution:* Rapidly and widely distributed into body tissues and is bound to erythrocytes and platelets. Drug crosses the blood-brain barrier but does not achieve therapeutic concentrations in the CSF.
- *Metabolism:* Drug is extensively metabolized in the liver.
- *Excretion:* Drug and its metabolites are primarily excreted into bile. A smaller portion is eliminated through the kidneys. The plasma elimination of vincristine is described as triphasic, with half-lives of about 4 minutes, 2¼ hours, and 85 hours for the distribution, second, and terminal phases, respectively.

Contraindications and precautions

Contraindicated in patients hypersensitive to drug or who have the demyelinating form of Charcot-Marie-Tooth syndrome. Do not give to patients who are concurrently receiving radiation therapy through ports that include the liver. Use cautiously in patients with hepatic dysfunction, neuromuscular disease, or infection.

Interactions

Concomitant use of vincristine increases the therapeutic effect of *methotrexate.* This interaction may be used to therapeutic advantage; it allows a lower dose of methotrexate, reducing the potential for methotrexate toxicity. Concomitant use with other *neurotoxic drugs* increases neurotoxicity through an additive effect.

Asparaginase decreases the hepatic clearance of vincristine. *Calcium channel blockers* enhance vincristine accumulation in cells. Concomitant use with *digoxin* decreases digoxin levels; monitor serum digoxin levels. Use with *mitomycin* may possibly increase the frequency of bronchospasm and acute pulmonary reactions.

Concurrent use with *phenytoin* may decrease plasma phenytoin levels; therefore, dosage adjustments may be needed.

Effects on diagnostic tests

Drug therapy may increase blood and urine concentrations of uric acid. Because WBC and platelet counts may decrease, frequently monitor blood counts.

Adverse reactions

CNS: *peripheral neuropathy,* sensory loss, *loss of deep tendon reflexes, paresthesia, wristdrop and footdrop,* ***seizures, coma,*** headache, ataxia, cranial nerve palsies, *jaw pain,* hoarseness, vocal cord paralysis, *muscle weakness and cramps*—some neurotoxicities may be permanent.
CV: hypotension, hypertension.
EENT: diplopia, optic and extraocular neuropathy, ptosis, photophobia, transient cortical blindness, optical atrophy.
GI: diarrhea, *constipation, cramps,* ileus that mimics surgical abdomen, paralytic ileus, *nausea, vomiting,* anorexia, weight loss, dysphagia, ***intestinal necrosis,*** *stomatitis.*
GU: urine retention, syndrome of inappropriate antidiuretic hormone, dysuria, acute uric acid neuropathy, polyuria.
Hematologic: anemia, ***leukopenia, thrombocytopenia.***
Respiratory: ***acute bronchospasm,*** dyspnea.
Other: *reversible alopecia,* fever, severe local reaction with extravasation, *phlebitis,* cellulitis at injection site, hyponatremia.

Overdose and treatment

Clinical manifestations of overdose include alopecia, myelosuppression, paresthesias, neuritic pain, motor difficulties, loss of deep tendon reflexes, nausea, vomiting, and ileus.

Treatment is usually supportive and includes transfusion of blood components, antiemetics, enemas for ileus, phenobarbital for seizures, and other appropriate symptomatic therapy. Administration of calcium leucovorin at a dosage of 15 mg I.V. every 3 hours for 24 hours, then every 6 hours for 48 hours may help protect cells from the toxic effects of vincristine.

☑ Special considerations

- Drug may be administered by I.V. push injection over 1 minute into the tubing of a freely flowing I.V. infusion.
- Dilution into larger volumes is not recommended for infusion into peripheral veins; this method increases risk of extravasation. Drug may be administered as an I.V. infusion through a central venous catheter.
- Necrosis may result from extravasation. Manufacturer recommends treatment with cold compresses and prompt administration of 150 units of intradermal hyaluronidase, sodium bicarbonate, and local injection of hydrocortisone, or a combination of these treatments. However, some clinicians prefer to treat extravasation only with warm compresses.
- After administering, monitor for life-threatening bronchospasm reaction. It is most likely to occur in patients also receiving mitomycin.
- Because of potential for neurotoxicity, do not give drug more than once weekly. Children are more resistant to neurotoxicity than adults. Neurotoxicity is dose-related and usually reversible; reduce dose if symptoms of neurotoxicity develop.
- Monitor for neurotoxicity by checking for depression of Achilles tendon reflex, numbness, tingling,

footdrop or wristdrop, difficulty in walking, ataxia, and slapping gait. Also check ability to walk on heels. Patient should have support during walking.
- Prevent uric acid nephropathy with generous oral fluid intake and administration of allopurinol. Alkalinization of urine may be required if serum uric acid concentration is increased.
- Monitor patient's bowel function. Give patient stool softener, laxative, or water before dosing. Constipation may be an early sign of neurotoxicity.
- Reduced dosage may be required in patients with obstructive jaundice or liver disease.
- Do not confuse vincristine with vinblastine or the investigational agent vindesine.
- Vials of 5 mg are for multiple-dose use only. Do not administer entire vial to patient as single dose.
- Drug may cause SIADH secretion. Treatment requires fluid restriction and a loop diuretic.
- Management of patients mistakenly receiving intrathecal vincristine is a medical emergency. Prognosis is generally poor.

Patient education
- Encourage adequate fluid intake to increase urine output and facilitate excretion of uric acid.
- Tell patient to call regarding use of laxatives if constipation or stomach pain occurs.
- Assure patient that hair growth should resume after treatment is discontinued.

Geriatric use
- Elderly patients who are weak or bedridden may be more susceptible to neurotoxic effects.

Breast-feeding
- It is not known if drug distributes into breast milk. However, because of risk of serious adverse reactions, mutagenicity, and carcinogenicity in the infant, breast-feeding is not recommended.

vinorelbine tartrate
Navelbine

Pharmacologic classification: semisynthetic vinca alkaloid
Therapeutic classification: antineoplastic
Pregnancy risk category D

How supplied
Available by prescription only
Injection: 10 mg/ml in 1-ml and 5-ml single-use vials

Indications, route, and dosage
Alone or as adjunct therapy with cisplatin for first-line treatment of ambulatory patients with nonresectable advanced non-small cell lung cancer (NSCLC); alone or with cisplatin in stage IV of NSCLC; with cisplatin in stage III of NSCLC
Adults: 30 mg/m² I.V. weekly. In combination treatment, same dosage used along with 120 mg/m² of cisplatin, given on days 1 and 29, then q 6 weeks.
✦ ***Dosage adjustment.*** Adjust dose based on hematologic toxicity or hepatic insufficiency.

Pharmacodynamics
Antineoplastic action: Vinorelbine exerts its antineoplastic effect by disrupting microtubule assembly, which disrupts spindle formation and prevents mitosis.

Pharmacokinetics
- *Absorption:* Vinorelbine is only given I.V.
- *Distribution:* Vinorelbine binding to plasma constituents ranges from 79.6% to 91.2%. It demonstrates high binding to human platelets and lymphocytes.
- *Metabolism:* Drug undergoes substantial hepatic metabolism.
- *Excretion:* About 18% is excreted in urine and 46% is excreted in feces. Terminal phase half-life averages 27.7 to 43.6 hours.

Contraindications and precautions
Contraindicated in patients with pretreatment granulocyte counts below 1,000 cells/m³. Use with extreme caution in patients whose bone marrow may have been compromised by previous exposure to radiation or chemotherapy or whose bone marrow is still recovering from previous chemotherapy. Also use cautiously in patients with impaired hepatic function.

Interactions
Vinorelbine tartrate increases risk of bone marrow suppression when used concomitantly with *cisplatin.* Monitor patient's hematologic status closely. *Mitomycin* may cause pulmonary reactions. Monitor patient's respiratory status closely.

Effects on diagnostic tests
None reported.

Adverse reactions
GI: *nausea, vomiting, anorexia, diarrhea, constipation, stomatitis.*
Hematologic: ***bone marrow suppression (agranulocytosis,*** LEUKOPENIA, ***thrombocytopenia,*** anemia).
Hepatic: *abnormal liver function tests, bilirubinemia.*
Respiratory: dyspnea.
Skin: *alopecia,* rash, *injection pain or reaction.*
Other: *peripheral neuropathy, asthenia,* jaw pain, *fatigue,* myalgia, SIADH, chest pain, arthralgia.

Overdose and treatment
The primary anticipated complications of overdosage are bone marrow suppression and peripheral neurotoxicity. Treatment includes general supportive measures and appropriate blood transfusions and antibiotics as needed. There is no known antidote.

☑ Special considerations
- Check patient's granulocyte count before initiating therapy (should be 1,000 cells/mm³ or more for drug to be administered).
- Dilute drug before administration. Administer I.V. over 6 to 10 minutes into the side port of a free-flowing I.V. closest to the I.V. bag, followed by flush-

ing with at least 75 to 125 ml of D_5W or 0.9% NaCl solution.

- Avoid extravasation when administering vinorelbine because drug can cause considerable irritation, localized tissue necrosis, and thrombophlebitis. If extravasation occurs, stop immediately and inject remaining dosage portion into a new vein.
- Adjust dosage based on hematologic toxicity or hepatic insufficiency, whichever results in a lower dose. Reduce dosage by 50% if patient's granulocyte count falls below 1,500 cells/mm^3 but exceeds 1,000 cells/mm^3. If three consecutive doses are skipped because of granulocytopenia, stop further drug therapy.
- Drug may be a contact irritant and the solution must be handled and administered with care. Use gloves. Avoid inhalation of vapors and contact with skin or mucous membranes, especially the eyes. If contact occurs, wash with copious amounts of water for at least 15 minutes.
- Monitor patient closely for hypersensitivity reactions.
- Monitor patient's peripheral blood count and bone marrow to guide effects of therapy.

Patient education

- Instruct patient not to take other drugs, including OTC preparations, unless instructed.
- Instruct patient to report signs and symptoms of infection (fever, chills, malaise) because drug has immunosuppressive activity.
- Tell patient to avoid becoming pregnant during therapy.

Pediatric use

- Safety and effectiveness in children have not been established.

Breast-feeding

- It is not known if drug is excreted in breast milk. Because of risk of adverse effects in the breast-fed infant, do not use drug in breast-feeding women.

vitamin A (retinol)

Aquasol A, Del-Vi-A, Palmitate-A 5000

Pharmacologic classification: fat-soluble vitamin
Therapeutic classification: vitamin
Pregnancy risk category A (X if dose exceeds RDA)

How supplied

Available by prescription only
Tablets: 10,000 IU
Capsules: 25,000 IU, 50,000 IU
Injection: 2-ml vials (50,000 IU/ml with 0.5% chlorobutanol, polysorbate 80, butylated hydroxyanisole, and butylated hydroxytoluene)

Available without a prescription, as appropriate
Drops: 30 ml with dropper (5,000 IU/0.1 ml)
Capsules: 10,000 IU
Tablets: 5,000 IU

Indications, route, and dosage

Severe vitamin A deficiency with xerophthalmia

Adults and children over age 8: 500,000 IU P.O. daily for 3 days, then 50,000 IU P.O. daily for 14 days, then maintenance dosage of 10,000 to 20,000 IU P.O. daily for 2 months, followed by adequate dietary nutrition and RDA vitamin A supplements.

Severe vitamin A deficiency

Adults and children over age 8: 100,000 IU P.O. or I.M. daily for 3 days, then 50,000 IU P.O. or I.M. daily for 14 days, then maintenance dosage of 10,000 to 20,000 IU P.O. daily for 2 months, followed by adequate dietary nutrition and RDA vitamin A supplements.

Children age 1 to 8: 17,500 to 35,000 IU I.M. daily for 10 days.

Infants under age 1: 7,500 to 15,000 IU I.M. daily for 10 days.

Note: The RDA for vitamin A is as follows:

Infants		
age 6 to 12 months	375 RE	1,875 IU
birth to 6 months	375 RE	1,875 IU
Children		
age 7 to 10	700 RE	3,500 IU
age 4 to 6	500 RE	2,500 IU
age 1 to 3	400 RE	2,000 IU
Males		
age 11 and over	1,000 RE	5,000 IU
Females		
age 11 and over	800 RE	4,000 IU
Pregnant	800 RE	4,000 IU
Breast-feeding	1,300 RE (1st 6 months)	6,500 IU
	1,200 RE (2nd 6 months)	6,000 IU

RE = retinol equivalents; IU = combination of retinol and beta-carotene.

Pharmacodynamics

Metabolic action: One IU of vitamin A is equivalent to 0.3 mcg of retinol or 0.6 mcg of beta-carotene. Beta-carotene, or provitamin A yields retinol after absorption from the intestinal tract.

Retinol's combination with opsin, the red pigment in the retina, helps form rhodopsin, which is necessary for visual adaptation to darkness. Vitamin A prevents growth retardation and preserves the integrity of the epithelial cells. Vitamin A deficiency is characterized by nyctalopia (night blindness), keratomalacia (necrosis of the cornea), keratinization and drying of the skin, low resistance to infection, growth retardation, bone thickening, diminished cortical steroid production, and fetal malformations.

Pharmacokinetics

• *Absorption:* In normal doses, vitamin A is absorbed readily and completely if fat absorption is normal. Larger doses, or regular doses in patients with fat malabsorption, low protein intake, or hepatic or pancreatic disease, may be absorbed incompletely. Because vitamin A is fat-soluble, absorption requires bile salts, pancreatic lipase, and dietary fat.
• *Distribution:* Vitamin A is stored (primarily as palmitate) in Kupffer's cells of the liver. Normal adult liver stores are sufficient to provide vitamin A requirements for 2 years. Lesser amounts of retinyl palmitate are stored in the kidneys, lungs, adrenal glands, retinas, and intraperitoneal fat. Vitamin A circulates bound to a specific alpha$_1$ protein, retinol-binding protein (RBP). Blood level assays may not reflect liver storage of vitamin A because serum levels depend partly on circulating RBP. Liver storage should be adequate before discontinuing therapy. Vitamin A is distributed into breast milk. It does not readily cross the placenta.
• *Metabolism:* Metabolized in the liver.
• *Excretion:* Retinol (fat-soluble) is conjugated with glucuronic acid and then further metabolized to retinal and retinoic acid. Retinoic acid is excreted in feces via biliary elimination. Retinal, retinoic acid, and other water-soluble metabolites are excreted in urine and feces. Normally, no unchanged retinol is excreted in urine, except in patients with pneumonia or chronic nephritis.

Contraindications and precautions

Oral form contraindicated in patients with malabsorption syndrome; if malabsorption is from inadequate bile secretion, oral route may be used with concurrent administration of bile salts (dehydrocholic acid).

Also contraindicated in those with hypervitaminosis A and hypersensitivity to any ingredient in product. I.V. route contraindicated except for special water-miscible forms intended for infusion with large parenteral volumes. I.V. push of vitamin A of any type also contraindicated (anaphylaxis or anaphylactoid reactions and death have resulted).

Use cautiously in pregnant patients.

Interactions

Concomitant use of vitamin A with *oral contraceptives* significantly increases the vitamin's plasma levels.

Prolonged use of *mineral oil* may interfere with the intestinal absorption of vitamin A. Concomitant use with *cholestyramine* may decrease the absorption of vitamin A by decreasing bile acids and preventing the micellar phase in the GI lumen. Daily vitamin A supplements have been recommended during long-term cholestyramine therapy.

Use with *neomycin* may decrease vitamin A absorption. Large doses of vitamin A may interfere with the hypoprothrombinemic effect of *warfarin.*

Because of potential for additive adverse effects, patients receiving *retinoids* (such as *etretinate* or *isotretinoin*) should avoid concomitant use of vitamin A.

Effects on diagnostic tests

Vitamin A therapy may falsely increase serum cholesterol level readings by interfering with the Zlatkis-Zak reaction. Vitamin A has also been reported to falsely elevate bilirubin determinations.

Adverse reactions

Adverse reactions usually occur only with toxicity.
CNS: irritability, headache, ***increased intracranial pressure,*** fatigue, lethargy, malaise.
EENT: papilledema, exophthalmos.
GI: anorexia, epigastric pain, vomiting, polydipsia.
GU: hypomenorrhea, polyuria.
Hepatic: jaundice, hepatomegaly, ***cirrhosis,*** elevated liver enzymes.
Musculoskeletal: slow growth, decalcification, hypercalcemia, periostitis, premature closure of epiphyses, migratory arthralgia, cortical thickening over the radius and tibia.
Skin: alopecia; dry, cracked, scaly skin; pruritus; lip fissures; erythema; inflamed tongue, lips, and gums; massive desquamation; increased pigmentation; night sweats.
Other: splenomegaly, ***anaphylactic shock.***

Overdose and treatment

In cases of acute toxicity, increased intracranial pressure develops within 8 to 12 hours; cutaneous desquamation follows in a few days. Toxicity can follow a single dose of 25,000 IU/kg, which in infants would represent about 75,000 IU and in adults over 2 million IU.

Chronic toxicity results from administration of 4,000 IU/kg for 6 to 15 months. In infants (age 3 to 6 months) this would represent about 18,500 IU/day for 1 to 3 months; in adults, 1 million IU/day for 3 days, 50,000 IU/day for more than 18 months, or 500,000 IU/day for 2 months.

To treat toxicity, discontinue vitamin A administration if hypercalcemia persists; administer I.V. NaCl solution, prednisone, and calcitonin, if indicated. Perform liver function tests to detect possible liver damage.

☑ Special considerations

• Safety of amounts exceeding 5,000 IU/day (oral) or 6,000 IU/day (parenteral) during pregnancy is not known.
• In any dietary deficiency, multiple vitamin deficiency should be suspected.
• Give vitamin A concurrently with bile salts to patients with malabsorption caused by inadequate bile secretion.
• Vitamin A given by I.V. push is contraindicated because it can cause anaphylaxis and death.
• Use special water-miscible form of vitamin A when adding to large parenteral volumes.

Patient education

• Explain that patient must avoid prolonged use of mineral oil while taking drug because mineral oil

reduces vitamin A absorption in the intestine.
- Tell patient not to exceed recommended dosage.
- Instruct patient to report promptly symptoms of overdose (nausea, vomiting, anorexia, malaise, drying or cracking of skin or lips, irritability, headache, or loss of hair) and to discontinue drug immediately if they occur.
- Teach patient to consume adequate protein, vitamin E, and zinc, which, along with bile, are necessary for vitamin A absorption.
- Tell patient to store vitamin A in a tight, light-resistant container.

Geriatric use
- Liquid preparations are available to adminster by nasogastric tube.

Pediatric use
- Liquid preparations may be mixed with fruit juice or cereal.

Breast-feeding
- Vitamin A is distributed into breast milk. The RDA of vitamin A for breast-feeding women in the United States is 1,300 and 1,200 RE for the first 6 months and second 6 months, respectively. Unless the maternal diet is grossly inadequate, infants can usually obtain sufficient vitamin A from breast-feeding. The effect of large maternal dosages of vitamin A on breast-fed infants is unknown.

vitamin E (alpha tocopherol)
Amino-Opti-E, Aquasol E, E-200 IU Softgels, E-400 IU in a water-soluble base, E-1000 IU Softgels, E-Complex-600, E-Vitamin Succinate, Vita-Plus E

Pharmacologic classification: fat-soluble vitamin
Therapeutic classification: vitamin
Pregnancy risk category A (C if greater than RDA)

How supplied
Available without prescription, as appropriate
Capsules: 50 IU, 100 IU, 200 IU, 400 IU, 500 IU, 600 IU, 1,000 IU
Tablets: 100 IU, 200 IU, 400 IU, 500 IU, 600 IU, 1,000 IU
Tablets (chewable): 100 IU, 200 IU, 400 IU
Oral solution: 50 IU/ml

Indications, route, and dosage
Vitamin E deficiency in premature infants and in patients with impaired fat absorption (including patients with cystic fibrosis); biliary atresia
Adults: 60 to 75 IU P.O. daily, depending on severity. Maximum dosage, 300 IU/day.
Children: 1 unit/kg P.O. daily.
Premature neonates: 5 units P.O. daily.
Full-term neonates: 5 units P.O. per liter of formula.

Note: The RDA for vitamin E is as follows:
Infants up to age 6 months: 4 TE.
Children age 6 months to 1 year: 6 TE.
Children age 1 to 3: 9 TE.
Children age 4 to 10: 10 TE.
Males over age 11: 15 TE.
Females over age 11: 12 TE.
Pregnant women: 15 TE.
Breast-feeding women: First 6 months, 18 TE; over 6 months, 16 TE.

TE is alpha tocopherol equivalent (equal to 1 mg d-alpha-tocopherol or 1.49 IU).

Pharmacodynamics
Nutritional action: As a dietary supplement, the exact biochemical mechanism is unclear, although it is believed to act as an antioxidant. Vitamin E protects cell membranes, vitamin A, vitamin C (ascorbic acid), and polyunsaturated fatty acids from oxidation. It also may act as a cofactor in enzyme systems, and some evidence exists that it decreases platelet aggregation.

Pharmacokinetics
- *Absorption:* GI absorption depends on the presence of bile. Only 20% to 60% of the vitamin obtained from dietary sources is absorbed. As dosage increases, the fraction of vitamin E absorbed decreases.
- *Distribution:* Distributed to all tissues and is stored in adipose tissue.
- *Metabolism:* Vitamin E is metabolized in the liver by glucuronidation.
- *Excretion:* Excreted primarily in bile. Some enterohepatic circulation may occur. Small amounts of the metabolites are excreted in urine.

Contraindications and precautions
No known contraindications. Use cautiously in patients with liver or gallbladder disease.

Interactions
Concomitant use of vitamin E with *cholestyramine, colestipol, mineral oil,* or *sucralfate* may increase vitamin E requirements.

Vitamin E may have *anti-vitamin K effects;* patients receiving *oral anticoagulants* may be at risk for hemorrhage after large doses of vitamin E.

Effects on diagnostic tests
None reported.

Adverse reactions
None reported with recommended dosages. Hypervitaminosis E symptoms include fatigue, weakness, nausea, headache, blurred vision, flatulence, diarrhea.

Overdose and treatment
Clinical manifestations of overdose include a possible increase in blood pressure. Treatment is generally supportive.

☑ Special considerations
- Give concurrently with bile salts if patient has malabsorption caused by lack of bile.
- Vitamin E has been used investigationally to prevent retrolental fibroplasia and bronchopulmonary

dysplasia in neonates, to prevent periventricular hemorrhage in premature infants, and to decrease the severity of hemolytic anemia in infants.

Patient education

- Inform patient about dietary sources of vitamin E.
- Tell patient to store vitamin E in a tight, light-resistant container.
- Instruct patient to swallow capsules whole and not to crush or chew them.

vitamin K derivatives

phytonadione

AquaMEPHYTON, Konakion, Mephyton

Pharmacologic classification: vitamin K
Therapeutic classification: blood coagulation modifier
Pregnancy risk category C (X if used in third trimester or near term)

How supplied

Available by prescription only
Tablets: 5 mg
Injection (aqueous colloidal solution): 2 mg/ml, 10 mg/ml
Injection (aqueous dispersion): 2 mg/ml, 10 mg/ml

Indications, route, and dosage

Hypoprothrombinemia secondary to vitamin K malabsorption or drug therapy, or when oral administration is desired and bile secretion is inadequate
Adults: 5 to 10 mg P.O. daily, or titrated to patient's requirements.
Hypoprothrombinemia secondary to vitamin K malabsorption, drug therapy, or excess vitamin A
Adults: 2 to 25 mg P.O. or parenterally, repeated and increased up to 50 mg, if necessary.
Children: 5 to 10 mg P.O. or parenterally.
Infants: 2 mg P.O. or parenterally.

Note: When I.V. administration is considered unavoidable, the drug should be injected very slowly, not exceeding 1 mg/minute.

Hypoprothrombinemia secondary to effect of oral anticoagulants
Adults: 2.5 to 10 mg P.O., S.C., or I.M., based on PT, repeated, if necessary, 12 to 48 hours after oral dose or 6 to 8 hours after parenteral dose. In emergency, give 10 to 50 mg slow I.V., rate not to exceed 1 mg/minute, repeated q 6 to 8 hours, p.r.n.
Prevention of hemorrhagic disease in neonates
Neonates: 0.5 to 1 mg S.C. or I.M. immediately after birth, repeated in 2 to 3 weeks, if needed, especially if mother received oral anticoagulants or long-term anticonvulsant therapy during pregnancy.
Prevention of hypoprothrombinemia related to vitamin K deficiency in long-term parenteral nutrition
Adults: 5 to 10 mg I.M. weekly.
Children: 2 to 5 mg I.M. weekly.

Note: The RDA for vitamin K is as follows:
Infants up to age 6 months: 5 mcg.
Children age 6 months to 1 year: 10 mcg.
Children age 1 to 3: 15 mcg.
Children age 4 to 6: 20 mcg.
Children age 7 to 10: 30 mcg.
Males age 11 to 14: 45 mcg.
Males age 15 to 18: 65 mcg.
Males age 19 to 24: 70 mcg.
Males over age 24: 80 mcg.
Females age 11 to 14: 45 mcg.
Females age 15 to 18: 55 mcg.
Females age 19 to 24: 60 mcg.
Females over age 24: 65 mcg.
Pregnant or breast-feeding women: 65 mcg.

Pharmacodynamics

Coagulation modifying action: Vitamin K is a lipid-soluble vitamin that promotes hepatic formation of active prothrombin and several other coagulation factors (specifically factors II, VII, IX, and X).

Phytonadione (vitamin K_1) is a synthetic form of vitamin K and is also lipid-soluble. Vitamin K does not counteract the action of heparin.

Pharmacokinetics

- *Absorption:* Phytonadione requires the presence of bile salts for GI tract absorption. Once absorbed, vitamin K enters the blood directly. Onset of action after I.V. injection is more rapid, but of shorter duration, than that occurring after S.C. or I.M. injection.
- *Distribution:* Vitamin K concentrates in the liver for a short time. Action of parenteral phytonadione begins in 1 to 2 hours; hemorrhage is usually controlled within 3 to 6 hours, and normal prothrombin levels are achieved in 12 to 14 hours. Oral phytonadione begins to act within 6 to 10 hours.
- *Metabolism:* Metabolized rapidly by the liver; little tissue accumulation occurs.
- *Excretion:* Data are limited. High concentrations occur in feces; however, intestinal bacteria can synthesize vitamin K.

Contraindications and precautions

Contraindicated in patients with hypersensitivity to drug.

Interactions

Broad-spectrum antibiotics (especially *cefamandole, cefoperazone,* and *cefotetan*) may interfere with the actions of vitamin K, producing hypoprothrombinemia.

Mineral oil inhibits absorption of oral vitamin K; give drugs at well-spaced intervals, and monitor result. Vitamin K antagonizes the effects of *oral anticoagulants*; patients receiving these agents should take vitamin K only for severe hypoprothrombinemia.

Effects on diagnostic tests

Phytonadione can falsely elevate urine steroid levels.

Adverse reactions

CNS: headache, dizziness, convulsive movements.
CV: transient hypotension after I.V. administration, rapid and weak pulse, ***arrhythmias.***
GI: nausea, vomiting.
Skin: diaphoresis, flushing, erythema, urticaria, pruritus, allergic rash.
Other: ***bronchospasm,*** dyspnea, cramplike pain, ***anaphylaxis and anaphylactoid reactions*** (usually after too-rapid I.V. administration), pain, swelling, hematoma at injection site.
Neonates: hyperbilirubinemia, ***fatal kernicterus, severe hemolytic anemia.***

Note: Discontinue drug if allergic or severe CNS reactions appear.

Overdose and treatment

Excessive doses of vitamin K may cause hepatic dysfunction in adults; in neonates and premature infants, large doses may cause hemolytic anemia, kernicterus, and death. Treatment is supportive.

☑ Special considerations

- Check particular product for approved routes of administration.
- If severity of condition warrants I.V. infusion, mix with preservative-free 0.9% NaCl, D_5W, or dextrose 5% in 0.9% NaCl solution. Monitor for flushing, weakness, tachycardia, and hypotension; shock may follow. Deaths have occurred.
- Monitor PT to determine effectiveness.
- Monitor patient response, and watch for adverse effects; failure to respond to vitamin K may indicate coagulation defects or irreversible hepatic damage.
- Excessive use of vitamin K may temporarily defeat oral anticoagulant therapy; higher doses of oral anticoagulant or interim use of heparin may be required.
- Phytonadione for hemorrhagic disease in infants causes fewer adverse reactions than do other vitamin K analogues; phytonadione is the vitamin K analogue of choice to treat an oral anticoagulant overdose.
- Patients receiving phytonadione who have bile deficiency require concomitant use of bile salts to ensure adequate absorption.

Patient education

- For patients receiving oral form, explain rationale for drug therapy; stress importance of complying with medical regimen and keeping follow-up appointments. Tell patient to take a missed dose as soon as possible, but not if it is almost time for next dose, and to report missed doses.

Pediatric use

- Do not exceed recommended dose. Hemolysis, jaundice, and hyperbilirubinemia in newborns, particularly premature infants, may be related to vitamin K administration.

Breast-feeding

- Vitamin K is not excreted in breast milk. However, use with caution.

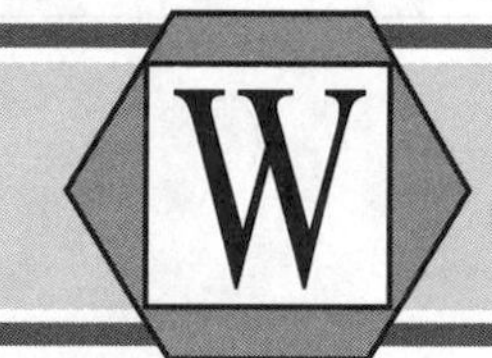

warfarin sodium

Coumadin, Panwarfin

Pharmacologic classification: coumarin derivative
Therapeutic classification: anticoagulant
Pregnancy risk category X

How supplied

Available by prescription only
Tablets: 1 mg, 2 mg, 2.5 mg, 4 mg, 5 mg, 7.5 mg, 10 mg
Injection: 5 mg/vial

Indications, route, and dosage

Pulmonary emboli, deep vein thrombosis, MI, rheumatic heart disease with heart valve damage, atrial arrhythmias
Adults: Initially, 2 to 5 mg P.O.; then daily PT and INR are used to establish optimal dose. Usual maintenance dosage, 2 to 10 mg P.O. daily.

Pharmacodynamics

Anticoagulant action: Warfarin inhibits vitamin K-dependent activation of clotting factors II, VII, IX, and X, which are formed in the liver; it has no direct effect on established thrombi and cannot reverse ischemic tissue damage. However, warfarin may prevent additional clot formation, extension of formed clots, and secondary complications of thrombosis.

Pharmacokinetics

- *Absorption:* Rapidly and completely absorbed from the GI tract.
- *Distribution:* Drug is highly bound to plasma protein, especially albumin; it crosses placenta but does not appear to accumulate in breast milk.
- *Metabolism:* Warfarin is hydroxylated by liver into inactive metabolites.
- *Excretion:* Metabolites are reabsorbed from bile and excreted in urine. Half-life of parent drug is 1 to 3 days, but highly variable. Because therapeutic effect is relatively more dependent on clotting factor depletion (factor X has half-life of 40 hours), PT will not peak for 1½ to 3 days despite use of a loading dose. Duration of action is 2 to 5 days—more closely reflecting drug's half-life.

Contraindications and precautions

Contraindicated in pregnant patients; in patients with bleeding or hemorrhagic tendencies, GI ulcerations, severe hepatic or renal disease, severe uncontrolled hypertension, subacute bacterial endocarditis, threatened abortion, eclampsia, preeclampsia, regional or lumbar block anesthesia, polycythemia vera, and vitamin K deficiency; in those in whom diagnostic tests or therapeutic procedures have potential for uncontrolled bleeding; in unsupervised patients with senility, alcoholism, psychosis, or lack of cooperation; and after recent eye, brain, or spinal cord surgery.

Use cautiously in patients with diverticulitis, colitis, hypertension, hepatic or renal disease, drainage tubes in any orifice, infectious disease or disturbance of intestinal flora, trauma, surgery resulting in large exposed surface, indwelling catheters, known or suspected deficiency in protein C or S, heart failure, severe diabetes, vasculitis, polycythemia vera, concurrent use of NSAIDs, or risk of hemorrhage and during lactation.

Interactions

Oral anticoagulants interact with many drugs; thus, changes in drug regimen, including use of *OTC compounds,* require careful monitoring. The most significant interactions follow.

Concomitant use with *amiodarone, anabolic steroids, chloramphenicol, cimetidine, clofibrate, dextrothyroxine, metronidazole,* and *other thyroid preparations, salicylates, streptokinase, urokinase, disulfiram,* or *sulfonamides* markedly increases warfarin's anticoagulant effect; avoid concomitant use.

Concomitant use with *ethacrynic acid, indomethacin, mefenamic acid, phenylbutazone,* or *sulfinpyrazone* increases warfarin's anticoagulant effect and causes severe GI irritation (may be ulcerogenic); avoid concomitant use when possible.

Concomitant use with *allopurinol, cefamandole, cefoperazone, cefotetan, danazol, diflunisal, erythromycin, glucagon, heparin, miconazole, quinidine, sulindac,* or *vitamin E* increases warfarin's anticoagulant effects. Monitor carefully.

Concomitant use with *glutethimide* or *rifampin* causes decreased anticoagulant effect of major significance and should be avoided. *Barbiturates* may inhibit anticoagulant effect for several weeks after barbiturate withdrawal, and fatal hemorrhage can occur after cessation of barbiturate effect; if barbiturates are withdrawn, reduce anticoagulant dose.

Concomitant use with *carbamazepine, corticosteroids, ethchlorvynol, griseofulvin, oral contraceptives,* and *vitamin K* may cause decreased anticoagulant effect; monitor carefully. *Cholestyramine* decreases warfarin's anticoagulant effect when used close together; administer 6 hours after warfarin.

Concomitant use with *chloral hydrate* may increase or decrease warfarin's anticoagulant effect; monitor therapy carefully and avoid when possible. Acute *alcohol intoxication* increases warfarin's anticoagulant effect, and *chronic alcohol abuse* decreases anticoagulant effect but may predispose patient to bleeding problems.

Effects on diagnostic tests
Warfarin prolongs both PT and partial thromboplastin time; it may enhance uric acid excretion, elevate serum transaminase levels, increase LD activity, and cause false-negative serum theophylline levels.

Adverse reactions
GI: anorexia, nausea, vomiting, cramps, *diarrhea*, mouth ulcerations, sore mouth.
GU: hematuria.
Hematologic: ***hemorrhage*** (with excessive dosage).
Hepatic: hepatitis, elevated liver function tests, jaundice.
Skin: dermatitis, urticaria, necrosis, gangrene, alopecia, *rash.*
Other: *fever.*

Overdose and treatment
Clinical manifestations of overdose vary with severity and may include internal or external bleeding or skin necrosis of fat-rich areas, but most common sign is hematuria. Excessive prolongation of PT or minor bleeding mandates withdrawal of therapy; withholding one or two doses may be adequate in some cases. Treatment to control bleeding may include oral or I.V. phytonadione (vitamin K_1) and, in severe hemorrhage, fresh frozen plasma or whole blood. Use of phytonadione may interfere with subsequent oral anticoagulant therapy.

☑ Special considerations
- Store drug in light-resistant containers at controlled room temperature (59° to 86° F [15° to 30° C]). After reconstitution, warfarin injection is stable for 4 hours at controlled room temperature.
- Discard solution that contains a precipitate.

Patient education
- Warn patient to avoid taking OTC products containing aspirin, other salicylates, or drugs that may interact with the anticoagulant, causing an increase or decrease in action of drug, and to seek medical approval before stopping or starting medication.
- Advise patient not to substantially alter daily intake of leafy green vegetables (asparagus, broccoli, cabbage, lettuce, turnip greens, spinach, or watercress) or of fish, pork or beef liver, green tea, or tomatoes. These foods contain vitamin K and widely varying daily intake may alter anticoagulant effect of warfarin.
- Instruct patient to inform all his health care providers (including dentists) about use of warfarin.

Geriatric use
- Elderly patients are more susceptible to effects of anticoagulants and are at increased risk of hemorrhage; this may be caused by altered hemostatic mechanisms or age-related deterioration of hepatic and renal functions.

Pediatric use
- Infants, especially neonates, may be more susceptible to anticoagulants because of vitamin K deficiency.

Breast-feeding
- Although drug does not appear to accumulate in breast milk, it should be used with caution in breast-feeding women.

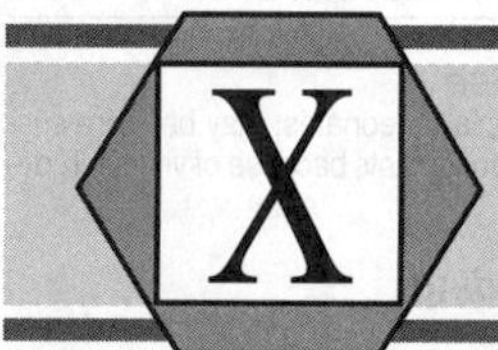

xylometazoline hydrochloride
Chlorohist-LA, Otrivin

Pharmacologic classification: sympathomimetic
Therapeutic classifications: decongestant, vasoconstrictor
Pregnancy risk category C

How supplied
Available without a prescription
Nasal drops: 0.05%, 0.1% (pediatric use)
Nasal spray: 0.1%

Indications, route, and dosage
Nasal congestion
Adults and children over age 12: Apply 2 or 3 drops or sprays of 0.1% solution to nasal mucosa q 8 to 10 hours, not to exceed three times in 24 hours.
Infants and children age 6 months to 12 years: Apply 2 or 3 drops or 1 spray of 0.05% solution to nasal mucosa q 8 to 10 hours, not to exceed three times in 24 hours.
Infants under age 6 months: 1 drop of 0.05% solution in each nostril q 6 hours p.r.n. under medical direction.

Pharmacodynamics
Decongestant action: Acts on alpha-adrenergic receptors in nasal mucosa to produce constriction, thereby decreasing blood flow and nasal congestion.

Pharmacokinetics
- *Absorption:* No information available.
- *Distribution:* No information available.
- *Metabolism:* No information available.
- *Excretion:* No information available.

Contraindications and precautions
Contraindicated in patients with hypersensitivity to drug or acute-closure glaucoma. Use cautiously in patients with hyperthyroidism, cardiac disease, hypertension, diabetes mellitus, and advanced arteriosclerosis.

Interactions
When used concomitantly with *tricyclic antidepressants*, xylometazoline may potentiate the pressor effects of tricyclic antidepressants if significant systemic absorption occurs.

Effects on diagnostic tests
None reported.

Adverse reactions
EENT: transient burning, stinging; dryness or ulceration of nasal mucosa; sneezing; rebound nasal congestion, irritation (with excessive or long-term use).

Overdose and treatment
Clinical manifestations of overdose include somnolence, sedation, sweating, CNS depression with hypertension, bradycardia, decreased cardiac output, rebound hypotension, CV collapse, depressed respirations, coma.

Because of rapid onset of sedation, emesis is not recommended in therapy unless given early. Activated charcoal or gastric lavage may be used initially. Monitor vital signs and ECG. Treat seizures with I.V. diazepam.

☑ Special considerations
- Monitor carefully for adverse effects in patients with CV disease, diabetes mellitus, or hyperthyroidism.
- Nasal spray is less likely to cause systemic absorption and is more effective if 3 to 5 minutes elapse between sprays and nose is cleared before next spray.

Patient education
- Tell patient that drug should only be used for short-term relief of symptoms, no longer than 3 to 5 days.
- Teach patient how to use correctly. Have patient hold head upright and sniff spray briskly. Only one person should use dropper bottle or nasal spray.
- Caution patient not to exceed recommended dosage to avoid rebound congestion.
- Tell patient to report insomnia, dizziness, weakness, tremor, or irregular heartbeat.

Geriatric use
- Use with caution in elderly patients with cardiac disease, diabetes mellitus, or poorly controlled hypertension.

Pediatric use
- Children may be prone to greater systemic absorption, with resultant increase in adverse effects.

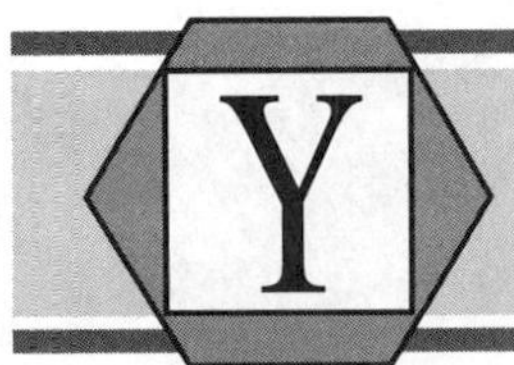

yellow fever vaccine

YF-Vax

Pharmacologic classification: vaccine
Therapeutic classification: viral vaccine
Pregnancy risk category C

How supplied

Available by prescription only
Injection: live, attenuated 17D yellow fever virus in 1-dose, 5-dose, 20-dose, and 100-dose vials, with diluent; supplied only to designated yellow fever vaccination centers authorized to issue yellow fever vaccination certificates

Indications, route, and dosage

Primary vaccination
Adults and children over age 6 months: 0.5 ml deep S.C. Booster dosage, 0.5 ml S.C. q 10 years.

Pharmacodynamics

Yellow fever prophylaxis: Vaccine promotes active immunity to yellow fever.

Pharmacokinetics

- *Absorption:* Immunity usually develops within 7 to 10 days and lasts for 10 years or longer.
- *Distribution:* No information available.
- *Metabolism:* No information available.
- *Excretion:* No information available.

Contraindications and precautions

Contraindicated in immunosuppressed patients; in those with cancer, gamma globulin deficiency, or hypersensitivity to chickens or eggs; and in those receiving corticosteroid or radiation therapy. Also contraindicated during pregnancy and in infants under age 9 months, except in high-risk areas. Information regarding these areas can be obtained from the Centers for Disease Control and Prevention, Division of Vector-Borne Infectious Diseases, at (970) 221-6400.

Interactions

Concomitant use of yellow fever vaccine with *corticosteroids* or other *immunosuppressants* may impair the immune response to the vaccine. Vaccination should be deferred for 2 months after a *blood or plasma transfusion.*

Administration of yellow fever and *cholera vaccines* simultaneously or 1 to 3 weeks apart may result in lower than normal antibody responses to both vaccines.

Effects on diagnostic tests

None reported.

Adverse reactions

Other: ***anaphylaxis,*** *fever, malaise,* myalgia, headache, mild swelling, pain (at injection site).

Overdose and treatment

No information available.

☑ Special considerations

- Obtain a thorough history of allergies, especially to eggs, and of reactions to immunizations.
- Epinephrine solution 1:1,000 should be available to treat allergic reactions.
- Do not administer yellow fever vaccine less than 1 month before or after immunization with other live virus vaccines except for live, attenuated measles virus vaccine; BCG vaccine and hepatitis B vaccine may also be given concurrently.
- Whenever possible, administer cholera and yellow fever vaccines at least 3 weeks apart; however, if time constraints require it, they may be given simultaneously.
- Because of theoretical risk of maternal-fetal transmission of infection through vaccination, do not give yellow fever vaccine to pregnant women unless they are at high risk of exposure in an epidemic focus. There are no data that exhibit teratogenicity, or ill effects in the fetus following maternal immunization.
- Reconstitute vaccine only with diluent provided. Follow package insert for reconstitution directions. Swirl and agitate reconstituted vial; do not shake vigorously to avoid foaming of the suspension. Use vaccine within 60 minutes of preparation.
- Unreconstituted vials must be stored between −22° and 41° F (−30° and 5° C). Do not use unless shipping case contains some dry ice upon arrival.
- Discard unused reconstituted vaccine.

Patient education

- Tell patient that pain or swelling at the injection site and fever or general malaise may occur. Recommend acetaminophen to alleviate fever.
- Encourage patient to report adverse reactions.
- Inform patient about need for revaccination in 10 years to maintain his traveler's vaccination certificate.

Pediatric use

- Never give vaccine to children under age 4 months. Vaccination of children age 4 to 9 months may be needed in high-risk areas or when travel to high-risk areas cannot be postponed and a high level of protection against mosquito exposure is not feasible.

Breast-feeding

- It is unknown if vaccine occurs in breast milk. Use with caution in breast-feeding women.

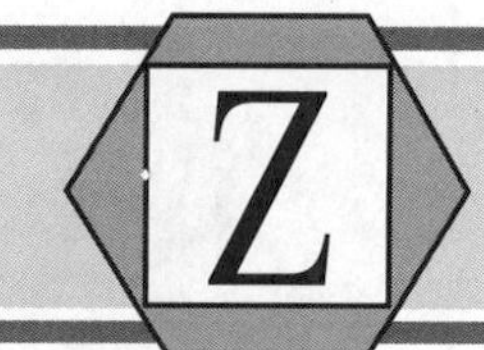

zafirlukast

Accolate

Pharmacologic classification: leukotriene receptor antagonist
Therapeutic classification: antiasthmatic
Pregnancy risk category B

How supplied

Available by prescription only
Tablets: 20 mg

Indications, route, and dosage

Prophylaxis and chronic treatment of asthma
Adults and children age 12 and older: 20 mg P.O. b.i.d. taken 1 hour before or 2 hours after meals.

Pharmacodynamics

Antiasthma action: Selectively competes for leukotriene receptor (LTD_4 and LTE_4) sites, blocking inflammatory action.

Pharmacokinetics

- *Absorption:* Rapidly absorbed following oral administration. Peak plasma concentrations are achieved 3 hours after dosing.
- *Distribution:* Over 99% is protein bound to plasma proteins, predominantly albumin.
- *Metabolism:* Extensively metabolized through the cytochrome P-450 2C9 (CYP 2C9) system. Drug also inhibits the CYP 3A4 and CYP 2C9 isoenzymes.
- *Excretion:* Primarily excreted in feces. Mean terminal half-life, approximately 10 hours.

Contraindications and precautions

Contraindicated in patients with known hypersensitivity to drug or its components. Use cautiously in patients with hepatic impairment and in the elderly.

Interactions

Aspirin causes increased plasma levels of zafirlukast. Concurrent use with *erythromycin* and *theophylline* causes decreased plasma levels of zafirlukast. Concomitant use with *warfarin* causes increased PT; monitor PT and INR levels, and adjust dosage of anticoagulant.

Although no formal drug interactions have been found, administer *astemizole, carbamazepine, cisapride, cyclosporine, dihydropyridine calcium channel blockers, phenytoin,* and *tolbutamide,* and with caution because these drugs are metabolized by CYP 2C9 and CYP 3A4 isoenzymes respectively.

Effects on diagnostic tests

Drug may elevate liver enzymes.

Adverse reactions

CNS: asthenia, dizziness, *headache.*
GI: abdominal pain, diarrhea, dyspepsia, nausea, vomiting.
Musculoskeletal: back pain, myalgia.
Other: accidental injury, fever, increased ALT, infection, pain.

Overdose and treatment

There is no experience with zafirlukast overdose in humans. Should an overdose occur, treat patient symptomatically and provide supportive measures as required. If indicated, remove unabsorbed drug from the GI tract.

☑ Special considerations

- Drug is not indicated for the reversal of bronchospasm in acute asthma attacks.
- Drug is known to be an inhibitor of CYP 3A4 and CYP 2C9 in vitro; it is reasonable to use appropriate clinical monitoring when drugs metabolized by this isoenzyme system are administered together.

Patient education

- Tell patient that drug is used for chronic treatment of asthma and to keep taking drug even if his symptoms disappear.
- Advise patient to continue taking other antiasthma drugs as prescribed.
- Instruct patient not to take drug with food. Drug should be taken 1 hour before or 2 hours after meals.

Geriatric use

- Drug clearance is reduced in the elderly; use with caution.

Pediatric use

- Safety and effectiveness in children under age 12 have not been established.

Breast-feeding

- Do not administer drug in breast-feeding women because it occurs in breast milk.

zalcitabine (dideoxycytidine, ddC)

Hivid

Pharmacologic classification: nucleoside analogue
Therapeutic classification: antiviral
Pregnancy risk category C

How supplied

Available by prescription only
Tablets (film-coated): 0.375 mg, 0.75 mg

Indications, route, and dosage

Patients with advanced HIV infection (CD4 count below 300 cells/mm³) who have demonstrated significant clinical or immunologic deterioration

Adults weighing 66 lb (30 kg) or more: 0.75 mg P.O. q 8 hours. Can be taken with zidovudine (200 mg P.O. q 8 hours).

✦ ***Dosage adjustment.*** May be necessary in patients with impaired renal function (creatinine clearance below 55 ml/minute). In adults with renal failure, refer to following dosing chart.

Creatinine clearance (ml/min)	Dose
> 40	0.75 mg P.O. q 8 hr
10 to 40	0.75 mg P.O. q 12 hr
< 10	0.75 mg P.O. q 24 hr

Pharmacodynamics

Antiviral action: Zalcitabine is active against HIV. Within cells, it is converted by cellular enzymes into its active metabolite, dideoxycytidine 5′-triphosphate. It inhibits the replication of HIV by blocking viral DNA synthesis. The drug inhibits reverse transcriptase by acting as an alternative for the enzyme's substrate, deoxycytidine triphosphate.

Pharmacokinetics

- *Absorption:* Mean absolute bioavailability is above 80%; administering drug with food decreases the rate and extent of absorption.
- *Distribution:* Steady-state volume of distribution is 0.534 ± 0.127 L/kg. Drug enters the CNS.
- *Metabolism:* Drug does not appear to undergo significant hepatic metabolism; phosphorylation to the active form occurs within cells.
- *Excretion:* Excretion is primarily by the kidneys; about 70% of a dose appears in urine within 24 hours. Mean elimination half-life, 2 hours.

Contraindications and precautions

Contraindicated in patients with hypersensitivity to drug or any component of the formulation. Use cautiously in patients with preexisting peripheral neuropathy, impaired renal function, hepatic failure, and history of pancreatitis, heart failure, or cardiomyopathy.

Interactions

Concomitant use with *drugs that cause peripheral neuropathy* (such as *chloramphenicol, cisplatin, dapsone, disulfiram, ethionamide, glutethimide, gold salts, hydralazine, iodoquinol, isoniazid, metronidazole, nitrofurantoin, phenytoin, ribavirin, vincristine*) may increase risk of peripheral neuropathy.

Drugs that may impair renal function may also increase risk of zalcitabine-induced adverse effects; these drugs include *aminoglycosides, amphotericin,* and *foscarnet.* Concomitant use with pentamidine is not recommended because of the risk of pancreatitis. Cimetidine and probenecid decrease elimination of zalcitabine.

Effects on diagnostic tests

Toxic effects of drug may cause abnormalities in several laboratory tests, including CBC, leukocyte count, reticulocyte count, granulocyte count, hemoglobin, platelet count, AST, ALT, and alkaline phosphatase.

Adverse reactions

CNS: *peripheral neuropathy, headache, fatigue,* dizziness, confusion, ***seizures,*** impaired concentration, amnesia, insomnia, mental depression, tremor, hypertonia, anxiety.
EENT: pharyngitis, cough, ocular pain, abnormal vision, ototoxicity, nasal discharge.
GI: nausea, vomiting, diarrhea, abdominal pain, anorexia, constipation, stomatitis, esophageal ulcer, glossitis.

Overdose and treatment

There is little experience with acute overdosage. It is unknown if drug is dialyzable. Treat symptomatically.

During early clinical trials, patients exposed chronically to doses about six times higher than the current recommended dosage experienced peripheral neuropathy within 10 weeks; patients exposed to twice the recommended dosage experienced peripheral neuropathy within 12 weeks.

☑ Special considerations

- If drug is discontinued because of toxicity, resume recommended dosage for zidovudine alone, which is 100 mg every 4 hours.
- If symptoms indicating peripheral neuropathy occur, discontinue drug if symptoms are bilateral and persist beyond 72 hours. If these symptoms persist or worsen beyond 1 week, permanently withdraw drug. However, if all findings relevant to peripheral neuropathy have resolved to minor symptoms, drug may be reintroduced at 0.375 mg P.O. every 8 hours.
- In clinical trials in which drug was the only treatment, peripheral neuropathy occurred in 17% to 31% of patients. The peripheral neuropathy seen with zalcitabine therapy is a sensorimotor neuropathy, initially characterized by numbness and burning in the extremities. If drug is not withdrawn, symptoms can progress to sharp, shooting pain or severe, continuous burning pain requiring narcotic analgesics and may or may not be reversible.
- Women of childbearing age should use an effective contraceptive while taking drug.

Patient education

- Make sure patient understands that drug doesn't cure HIV infection and that he can still transmit HIV. Opportunistic infections may continue to occur despite use of drug. Review safe sex practices with the patient.
- Tell patient that drug may cause peripheral neuropathy and life-threatening pancreatitis. Review

signs and symptoms of these reactions, and instruct patient to report them immediately.

Pediatric use

- Safety and efficacy in children under age 13 have not been established.

Breast-feeding

- It is unknown if drug is excreted in breast milk. Because of risk of transmitting the virus, HIV-positive women should not breast-feed.

zidovudine (AZT)

Retrovir

Pharmacologic classification: thymidine analogue
Therapeutic classification: antiviral
Pregnancy risk category C

How supplied

Capsules: 100 mg
Syrup: 50 mg/5 ml
Injection: 10 mg/ml

Indications, route, and dosage

Symptomatic HIV, AIDS, or advanced AIDS-related complex

Adults and children over age 12: 100 mg P.O. q 4 hours (600 mg daily dose). Or administer by I.V. infusion 1 mg/kg (at a constant rate over 1 hour) q 4 hours for total of 6 mg/kg/day.
Children age 3 months to 12 years: 180 mg/m^2 q 6 hours (720 mg/m^2/day). Do not exceed 200 mg q 6 hours.

Asymptomatic HIV infection (CD4 count below 500/mm^3)

Adults and children over age 12: 100 mg P.O. q 4 hours while awake (for total of five doses or 500 mg daily). Alternatively, administer 1 mg/kg I.V. over 1 hour q 4 hours while awake (5 mg/kg daily).
Children age 3 months to 12 years: 180 mg/m^2 q 6 hours (720 mg/m^2 P.O. daily) in divided doses q 6 hours. Do not exceed 200 mg q 6 hours.

Maternal-fetal transmission of HIV

Adults: Maternal dosing: Give 100 mg P.O. q 4 hours while awake (for total of five doses daily) until onset of labor. During labor and delivery, administer 2 mg/kg I.V. over 1 hour followed by a continuous infusion of 1 mg/kg/hour until clamping of the umbilical cord. Infant dosing: 2 mg/kg P.O. q 6 hours starting 12 hours after birth and continuing until 6 weeks of age.

✦ ***Dosage adjustment.*** Because drug is partially removed by dialysis, dosage adjustment may be required in affected patients. Dosage adjustment may also be warranted in patients with decreased liver function.

Pharmacodynamics

Antiviral action: Zidovudine is converted intracellularly to an active triphosphate compound that inhibits reverse transcriptase (an enzyme essential for retroviral DNA synthesis), thereby inhibiting viral replication. When used in vitro, drug inhibits certain other viruses and bacteria; however, this has undetermined clinical significance.

Pharmacokinetics

- *Absorption:* Absorbed rapidly from the GI tract. Average systemic bioavailability is 65% of dose (drug undergoes first-pass metabolism).
- *Distribution:* Preliminary data reveal good CSF penetration. Approximately 36% of dose is plasma protein-bound.
- *Metabolism:* Metabolized rapidly to an inactive compound.
- *Excretion:* Parent drug and metabolite are excreted by glomerular filtration and tubular secretion in the kidneys. Urine recovery of parent drug and metabolite is 14% and 74%, respectively. Elimination half-lives of these compounds is 1 hour.

Contraindications and precautions

Contraindicated in patients with hypersensitivity to drug. Use cautiously in patients in advanced stages of HIV and in those with severe bone marrow suppression, renal insufficiency, or hepatomegaly, hepatitis, or other risk factors for hepatic disease.

Interactions

When used concomitantly with *drugs that are nephrotoxic or that affect bone marrow function or formation of bone marrow elements* (such as *amphotericin B, dapsone, doxorubicin, flucytosine, ganciclovir, interferon, pentamidine, vinblastine, vincristine*), zidovudine may increase the risk of drug toxicity. Concomitant use with *probenecid* may impair elimination of zidovudine.

Effects on diagnostic tests

Drug may cause depression of formed elements (erythrocytes, leukocytes, and platelets) in peripheral blood.

Adverse reactions

CNS: *headache,* ***seizures,*** paresthesia, *malaise,* insomnia, *dizziness,* somnolence.
GI: *nausea, anorexia, abdominal pain, vomiting,* constipation, *diarrhea,* dyspepsia.
Hematologic: ***severe bone marrow suppression (resulting in anemia), agranulocytosis, thrombocytopenia.***
Skin: *rash.*
Other: myalgia, diaphoresis, *fever, asthenia,* taste perversion.

Overdose and treatment

No information available.

☑ Special considerations

- Optimum duration of treatment, as well as dosage for optimum effectiveness and minimum toxicity, is not yet known.
- Monitor CBC and platelet count at least every 2 weeks. Significant anemia (hemoglobin less than 7.5 g/dl or reduction of over 25% of baseline) or significant neutropenia (granulocyte count below 750 cells/mm^3 or reduction of more than 50% from baseline) may require interruption of zidovudine therapy until evidence of bone marrow recovery oc-

curs. In patients with less severe anemia or neutropenia, a reduction in zidovudine dosage may be adequate.
- I.V. dosage equivalent to 100 mg P.O. every 4 hours is approximately 1 mg/kg I.V. every 4 hours.
- Observe patient for signs and symptoms of opportunistic infection (including pneumonia, meningitis, and sepsis).
- Store undiluted injection, capsules, and syrup at room temperature (77° F [25° C]); protect from light. Dilute I.V. form to less than 4 mg/ml with D_5W before administering. Do not mix with protein-containing solutions. To minimize potential for microbial contamination, administer within 8 hours of mixing if left at room temperature or within 24 hours if refrigerated (36° to 46° F [2° to 8° C]).
- Drug does not cure HIV infection or AIDS but may reduce morbidity resulting from opportunistic infections and thus prolong the patient's life.

Patient education
- Because drug frequently causes a low RBC count, advise patient that they may need blood transfusions or epoetin alfa therapy during treatment.
- Teach patient about the disease, ways to prevent disease transmission, rationale for drug therapy, and drug's limitations.
- Teach patient about proper drug administration. When drug must be taken every 4 hours around-the-clock, explain the importance of maintaining an adequate blood level and suggest ways to avoid missing doses, such as using an alarm clock.
- Inform patient about importance of follow-up medical visits to evaluate for adverse effects and to monitor clinical status.
- Instruct patient how to recognize adverse drug effects and to report them immediately.
- Warn patient not to take other drugs for AIDS (especially from the "street") without medical approval.
- Make sure patient understands that drug therapy does not reduce his ability to transmit HIV infection.

Breast-feeding
- To avoid transmitting HIV to the infant, HIV-positive women should not breast-feed.

zileuton
Zyflo Filmtab

Pharmacologic classification: 5-lipoxygenase inhibitor
Therapeutic classification: antiasthmatic
Pregnancy risk category C

How supplied
Available by prescription only
Tablets: 600 mg

Indications, route, and dosage
Prophylaxis and chronic treatment of asthma
Adults and children age 12 and older: 600 mg P.O. q.i.d.

Pharmacodynamics
Antiasthmatic action: Inhibits enzyme responsible for the formation of leukotrienes, thus reducing inflammatory response.

Pharmacokinetics
- *Absorption:* Rapidly absorbed with oral administration (mean time to peak concentrations is 1.7 hours).
- *Distribution:* Apparent volume of distribution is 1.2 L/kg. Drug is 93% bound to plasma proteins, primarily albumin.
- *Metabolism:* Zileuton is oxidatively metabolized by the cytochrome P-450 system. Several active and inactive metabolites of zileuton have been identified.
- *Excretion:* Elimination of drug is predominantly via metabolism with a mean terminal half-life of 2½ hours.

Contraindications and precautions
Contraindicated in patients with known hypersensitivity to drug or its components and in those with active hepatic disease or transaminase elevations at least three times the normal upper limit. Use with caution in patients with hepatic impairment or history of heavy alcohol use.

Interactions
Coadministration with *propranolol* and *other beta blockers* may increase beta-blocker effect. Monitor patient and reduce dosage of beta blocker.

Coadministration with *theophylline* decreases theophylline clearance (on average, serum theophylline concentrations double); reduce theophylline dose and monitor serum levels. Coadministration with *warfarin* increases PT. Monitor PT and INR and adjust dosage of anticoagulant.

Use cautiouly when administered concurrently with *drugs that are metabolized by the CYP 3A4 isoenzyme (astemizole, dihydropyridine calcium channel blockers, cisapride, cyclosporine, estradiol, ethinyl, prednisone).*

Effects on diagnostic tests
Drug may elevate liver enzymes and temporarily lower WBC count.

Adverse reactions
CNS: asthenia, dizziness, *headache*, insomnia, nervousness, somnolence.
CV: chest pain.
EENT: conjunctivitis.
GI: abdominal pain, constipation, dyspepsia, flatulence, nausea.
GU: urinary tract infection, vaginitis.
Hematologic: leukopenia.
Musculoskeletal: arthralgia, hypertonia, myalgia, neck pain and rigidity.
Skin: pruritus.
Other: accidental injury, fever, lymphadenopathy, malaise, pain.

Overdose and treatment
Acute overdosage with zileuton is limited. Drug is not removed by dialysis. If overdose occurs, treat

patient symptomatically and provide supportive measures. If indicated, eliminate unabsorbed drug by emesis or gastric lavage.

☑ Special considerations

- Drug is not indicated for use in the reversal of bronchospasm in acute asthma attacks.
- Obtain baseline liver enzyme levels and monitor periodically.

Patient education

- Tell patient that drug is used for chronic treatment of asthma and to continue taking drug even if his symptoms disappear.
- Caution patient that drug is not a bronchodilator and should not be used to treat an acute asthma attack.
- Advise patient to continue taking other antiasthmatic drugs.
- Instruct patient to call if the short-acting bronchodilator is effective in relieving symptoms.
- Tell patient to call immediately if signs and symptoms of hepatic dysfunction develop (right upper quadrant pain, nausea, fatigue, pruritus, jaundice, malaise).
- Advise patient to avoid alcohol and to seek approval before taking OTC or new prescription drugs.

Pediatric use

- Safety and effectiveness in children under age 12 have not been studied.

Breast-feeding

- It is not known if drug is excreted in breast milk. Use with caution.

zinc

Orazinc, Verazinc, Zinc 15, Zinc-220, Zincate

zinc sulfate (ophthalmic)

Eye-Sed

Pharmacologic classification: trace element; miscellaneous anti-infective
Therapeutic classification: nutritional supplement; topical anti-infective
Pregnancy risk category C

How supplied

Available by prescription only
Injection: 10 ml (1 mg/ml), 30 ml (1 mg/ml with 0.9% benzyl alcohol), 5 ml (5 mg/ml); 10 ml (5 mg/ml), 50 ml (1 mg/ml)
Tablets: 220 mg (50 mg zinc)
Capsules: 220 mg (50 mg zinc)

Available without a prescription, as appropriate
Tablets: 110 mg (25 mg zinc), 200 mg (47 mg zinc)
Capsules: 110 mg (25 mg zinc), 220 mg (50 mg zinc)
Solution: 15 ml (0.217%)

Indications, route, and dosage

RDA of zinc is 15 mg/day P.O. for adults and 0.3 mg/kg/day P.O. for children.

Metabolically stable zinc deficiency
Adults: 2.5 to 4 mg/day I.V.; add 2 mg/day for acute catabolic states.

Stable zinc deficiency with fluid loss from the small bowel
Adults: Add 12.2 mg/L of total parenteral nutrition solution or 17.1 mg/kg of stool output.

Zinc deficiency
Children under age 5: 100 mcg/kg/day I.V.
Premature infants: 300 mcg/kg/day I.V.

For relief of minor eye irritation
Adults: 1 to 2 drops ophthalmic solution into the eye b.i.d. to q.i.d. Patients are advised to report irritation that persists for more than 3 days.

Pharmacodynamics

Metabolic action: Zinc serves as a cofactor for more than 70 different enzymes. It facilitates wound healing, normal growth rates, and normal skin hydration and helps maintain the senses of taste and smell.

Adequate zinc provides normal growth and tissue repair. In patients receiving total parenteral nutrition with low plasma levels of zinc, dermatitis has been followed by alopecia. Zinc is an integral part of many enzymes important to carbohydrate and protein mobilization of retinal-binding protein.

Zinc sulfate ophthalmic solution exhibits astringent and weak antiseptic activity, which may result from precipitation of protein by the zinc ion and by clearing mucus from the outer surface of the eye. Drug has no decongestant action and produces mild vasodilation.

Pharmacokinetics

- *Absorption:* Zinc sulfate is absorbed poorly from the GI tract; only 20% to 30% of dietary zinc is absorbed. After administration, zinc resides in muscle, bone, skin, kidney, liver, pancreas, retina, prostate, and, particularly, RBCs and WBCs. Zinc binds to plasma albumin, alpha-2 macroglobulin, and some plasma amino acids including histidine, cysteine, threonine, glycine, and asparagine.
- *Distribution:* Major zinc stores are in the skeletal muscle, skin, bone, and pancreas.
- *Metabolism:* Zinc is a cofactor in many enzymatic reactions. It is required for the synthesis and mobilization of retinal binding protein.
- *Excretion:* After parenteral administration, 90% of zinc is excreted in the stool, urine, and sweat. After oral use, the major route of excretion is secretion into the duodenum and jejunum. Small amounts are also excreted in the urine (0.3 to 0.5 mg/day) and in sweat (1.5 mg/day).

Contraindications and precautions

Parenteral use of zinc sulfate is contraindicated in patients with renal failure or biliary obstruction (and requires caution in all patients); monitor zinc plasma levels frequently. Do not exceed prescribed doses. In patients with renal dysfunction or GI malfunction, trace metal supplements may need to be reduced, adjusted, or omitted. Hypersensitivity may result. Routine use of zinc supplementation during pregnancy is not recommended.

Administering *copper* in the absence of zinc or administering zinc in the absence of copper may result in decreased serum levels of either element. When only one trace element is needed, it should be added separately and serum levels monitored closely. To avoid overdosage, administer multiple trace elements only when clearly needed. In patients with extreme vomiting or diarrhea, extreme amounts of trace element replacement may be needed. Excessive intake in healthy persons may be deleterious.

Interactions

Concomitant use of oral zinc sulfate with *fluoroquinolones* and *tetracycline* will impair antibiotic absorption. When zinc sulfate ophthalmic solution is used with *sodium borate*, precipitation of zinc borate may occur; *glycerin* may prevent this interaction. Zinc sulfate ophthalmic solution has a dehydrating effect on *methylcellulose suspensions*, causing precipitation of *methylcellulose*. Zinc sulfate ophthalmic solution may also precipitate acacia and certain proteins.

Effects on diagnostic tests

None reported.

Adverse reactions

CNS: restlessness.
GI: distress and irritation, nausea, vomiting with high doses, gastric ulceration, diarrhea.
Skin: rash.
Other: dehydration.

Overdose and treatment

Clinical manifestations of severe toxicity include hypotension, pulmonary edema, diarrhea, vomiting, jaundice, and oliguria. Dosage must be discontinued and support measures begun.

☑ Special considerations

- Results may not appear for 6 to 8 weeks in zinc-depleted patients.
- Zinc decreases the absorption of tetracyclines.
- Monitor for severe vomiting and dehydration, which may indicate overdose.
- Calcium supplements may confer a protective effect against zinc toxicity.
- Because of potential for infusion phlebitis and tissue irritation, an undiluted direct injection must not be administered into a peripheral vein.
- Do not exceed prescribed dosage of oral zinc; if oral zinc is administered in single 2-g doses, emesis will occur.
- If ophthalmic use causes increasing irritation, discontinue use.

Patient education

- Tell patient not to take zinc with dairy products, which can reduce zinc absorption.
- Teach patient how to instill ophthalmic solution and to prevent contamination. Tell him to avoid contacting the lip of the container with other surface and to tightly close the container after use.
- Warn patient about self-medication with zinc sulfate ophthalmic solution, which should not continue longer than 3 days. Patient should report increased irritation or redness.
- Warn patient that GI upset may occur after oral administration but may be diminished if zinc is taken with food. Patients must avoid foods high in calcium, phosphorus, or phytate during zinc therapy.

---

zolmitriptan

Zomig

Pharmacologic classification: selective 5-hydroxytryptamine receptor agonist
Therapeutic classification: antimigraine
Pregnancy risk category C

How supplied

Available by prescription only
Tablets: 2.5 mg, 5 mg

Indications, route, and dosage

Treatment of acute migraine headaches with or without aura

Adults: Initially, 2.5 mg P.O. or lower. A dose lower than 2.5 mg can be achieved by manually breaking a 2.5 mg tablet in half. If headache returns after initial dose, a second dose may be given after 2 hours. Maximum dose is 10 mg in 24-hour period.

✦ ***Dosage adjustment.*** In patients with liver disease, use doses under 2.5 mg.

Pharmacodynamics

Antimigraine action: Zolmitriptan binds with high affinity to human recombinant 5-HT_{1D} and 5-HT_{1B} receptors aborting migraine headaches by causing constriction of cranial blood vessels and inhibition of pro-inflammatory neuropeptide release.

Pharmacokinetics

- *Absorption:* Well-absorbed after oral administration with peak plasma concentration occurring in 2 hours. Mean absolute bioavailability is approximately 40%.
- *Distribution:* Apparent volume of distribution is 7 L/kg. Plasma protein binding is 25%.
- *Metabolism:* Drug is converted to an active N-desmthyl metabolite. Time to maximum concentration for the metabolite is 2 to 3 hours. Mean elimination half-life of zolmitriptan and the active N-desmethyl metabolite is 3 hours.
- *Excretion:* Mean total clearance is 31.5 ml/minute/kg of which one-sixth is renal clearance. The renal clearance is greater than the glomerular filtration rate, suggesting renal tubular secretion. Approximately 65% of the dose is excreted in the urine and 30% in the feces.

Contraindications and precautions

Contraindicated in patients with hypersensitivity to drug or its components; in those with uncontrolled hypertension, ischemic heart disease (angina pectoris, history of MI or documented silent ischemia), or other significant heart disease (including Wolff-Parkinson-White syndrome).

Avoid use within 24 hours of other 5-HT_1 agonists, ergot-containing medications, or within 2 weeks of discontinuing MAO inhibitor therapy. Also avoid use in patients with hemiplegic or basilar migraine.

Use cautiously in patients with liver disease and in pregnant or breast-feeding women.

Interactions
Cimetidine doubles the half-life of zolmitriptan. *Ergot-containing drugs* may cause additive vasospastic reactions. *Fluoxetine, fluvoxamine, paroxetine,* and *sertraline* may cause weakness, hyperreflexia, and incoordination. *MAO inhibitors* increase plasma concentrations of zolmitriptan.

Effects on diagnostic tests
None reported.

Adverse reactions
CNS: somnolence, vertigo, *dizziness,* hyperesthesias, paresthesias, asthenia.
CV: palpitations, pain or heaviness in chest, *pain, tightness, or pressure in the neck, throat, or jaw.*
GI: dry mouth, dyspepsia, dysphagia, nausea.
Musculoskeletal: myalgia.
Skin: sweating.
Other: warm or cold sensations.

Overdose and treatment
No specific antidote exists. If severe intoxication occurs, intensive care procedures are recommended including establishing and maintaining a patent airway ensuring adequate oxygenation and ventilation, and monitoring and support of the CV system. The effect of hemodialysis or peritoneal dialysis on the plasma levels of zolmitriptan is unknown.

☑ Special considerations
- Monitor blood pressure in patients with liver disease.
- Drug is not intended for prophylactic therapy of migraine headaches or for use in hemiplegic or basilar migraines.
- Safety has not been established for cluster headaches.
- Know that although not reported in clinical trials, serious cardiac events, including some that have been fatal, have occurred rarely following use of 5-HT_1 agonists. Events reported have included coronary artery vasospasm, transient myocardial ischemia, MI, ventricular tachycardia, and ventricular fibrillation.

Patient education
- Tell patient that drug is intended to relieve the symptoms of migraines, not to prevent them.
- Advise patient to take drug only as prescribed and not to take a second dose unless instructed. If a second dose is indicated and approved by the health care provider, take it 2 hours after initial dose.
- Advise patient to report pain or tightness in the chest or throat, heart throbbing, rash, skin lumps, or swelling of the face, lips, or eyelids at once.
- Caution patient to avoid drug if pregnancy is being planned or suspected.
- Remind patient that drug should not be taken with other migraine agents.

Geriatric use
- Although the pharmacokinetic disposition is similar to that seen in younger adults, there is no information in this population because patients over 65 were excluded from clinical trials.

Pediatric use
- Safety and effectiveness have not been established

Breast-feeding
- It is not known if drug occurs in breast milk. Use with caution when administering to breast-feeding women.

zolpidem tartrate
Ambien

Pharmacologic classification: imidazopyridine
Therapeutic classification: hypnotic
Controlled substance schedule IV
Pregnancy risk category B

How supplied
Available by prescription only
Tablets: 5 mg, 10 mg

Indications, route, and dosage
Short-term management of insomnia
Adults: 10 mg P.O. immediately before bedtime.
✦ ***Dosage adjustment.*** In elderly or debilitated patients or patients with hepatic insufficiency, 5 mg P.O. immediately before bedtime.

Maximum daily dosage, 10 mg.

Pharmacodynamics
Hypnotic action: While zolpidem is a hypnotic agent with a chemical structure unrelated to benzodiazepines, barbiturates, or other drugs with known hypnotic properties, it interacts with a gamma-aminobutyric acid (GABA)-benzodiazepine or omega-receptor complex and shares some of the pharmacologic properties of the benzodiazepines. It exhibits no muscle relaxant or anticonvulsant properties.

Pharmacokinetics
- *Absorption:* Absorbed rapidly from the GI tract with a mean peak concentration time of 1.6 hours. Food delays drug absorption.
- *Distribution:* Protein-binding of zolpidem is about 92.5%.
- *Metabolism:* Zolpidem is converted to inactive metabolites in the liver.
- *Excretion:* Primarily eliminated in the urine; elimination half-life is about 2.6 hours.

Contraindications and precautions

No known contraindications. Use cautiously in patients with conditions that could affect metabolism or hemodynamic response and in those with decreased respiratory drive, depression, or history of alcohol or drug abuse.

Interactions

Other *CNS depressants* and *ethanol* enhance the CNS depression of zolpidem. Concomitant use should be avoided.

Effects on diagnostic tests

None reported.

Adverse reactions

CNS: daytime drowsiness, light-headedness, abnormal dreams, amnesia, dizziness, *headache*, hangover, sleep disorder, lethargy, depression.
CV: palpitations.
EENT: sinusitis, pharyngitis, dry mouth.
GI: nausea, vomiting, diarrhea, dyspepsia, constipation, abdominal pain.
Skin: rash.
Other: back or chest pain, flulike symptoms, hypersensitivity reactions, myalgia, arthralgia.

Overdose and treatment

Symptoms may range from somnolence to light coma. CV and respiratory compromise also may occur. General symptomatic and supportive measures should be used, along with immediate gastric lavage when appropriate. I.V. fluids should be administered as needed. Flumazenil may be useful. Hypotension and CNS depression should be monitored and treated. Sedatives should be withheld after zolpidem overdosage even if excitation occurs.

☑ Special considerations

- Observe patients with history of addiction to or abuse of drugs or alcohol because they are at risk of habituation and dependence.
- Limit drug therapy to 7 to 10 days; reevaluate patient if drug is to be taken for over 2 weeks.
- Because sleep disturbance may be the presenting manifestation of a physical or psychiatric disorder, initiate symptomatic treatment of insomnia only after careful evaluation of patient.
- Zolpidem has CNS-depressant effects similar to other sedative-hypnotic drugs. Because of its rapid onset of action, drug should be given immediately before going to bed.
- Dosage adjustments may be necessary when drug is given with other CNS-depressant agents because of the potentially additive effects.
- Prevent hoarding or self-overdosing by hospitalized patients who are depressed, suicidal, or known to abuse drug.

Patient education

- Tell patient not to take drug with or immediately after a meal.
- Stress importance of taking drug only as prescribed; inform patient of potential drug dependency associated with hypnotics taken for long periods.
- Inform patient that tolerance may occur if drug is taken for more than a few weeks.
- Warn patient against use of alcohol or other sleep medications during therapy to avoid serious adverse effects.
- Caution patient to avoid activities that require alertness, such as driving a car, until adverse CNS effects of drug are known.
- Tell patient not to increase dosage and to call if he feels drug is no longer effective.

Geriatric use

- Impaired motor or cognitive performance after repeated exposure or unusual sensitivity to sedative-hypnotics may occur in elderly patients. Recommended dosage is 5 mg rather than 10 mg.

Pediatric use

- Safety and effectiveness in children under age 18 have not been established.

Breast-feeding

- Use of drug in breast-feeding women is not recommended.

Pharmacologic classes

adrenergics, direct and indirect acting

albuterol sulfate, arbutamine hydrochloride, bitolterol mesylate, brimonidine tartrate, dobutamine hydrochloride, dopamine hydrochloride, ephedrine, ephedrine hydrochloride, ephedrine sulfate, epinephrine, epinephrine bitartrate, epinephrine hydrochloride, epinephryl borate, isoetharine hydrochloride, isoetharine mesylate, isoproterenol, isoproterenol hydrochloride, isoproterenol sulfate, metaproterenol sulfate, metaraminol bitartrate, naphazoline hydrochloride, norepinephrine bitartrate, phenylephrine hydrochloride, pirbuterol acetate, pseudoephedrine hydrochloride, pseudoephedrine sulfate, ritodrine hydrochloride, salmeterol xinafoate, terbutaline sulfate, tetrahydrozoline hydrochloride, xylometazoline hydrochloride

Beta-receptor activation is associated with the activation of adenylate cyclase and the accumulation of cAMP; the cellular consequences of alpha-receptor activation are less well understood.

Alpha$_1$ receptors are located on smooth muscle and glands and are excitatory; alpha$_2$ receptors are prejunctional regulatory receptors in the CNS and postjunctional receptors in many peripheral tissues. Beta$_1$ receptors are located in cardiac tissues and are excitatory; beta$_2$ receptors are located primarily on smooth muscle and glands and are inhibitory.

Adrenergic drugs may mimic the naturally occurring catecholamines norepinephrine, epinephrine, and dopamine or may function by stimulating the release of norepinephrine.

Pharmacology

Most actions of clinically useful adrenergic agents involve peripheral excitatory actions on glands and vascular smooth muscle; cardiac and CNS excitatory actions; peripheral inhibitory actions on smooth muscle of the bronchial tree and blood vessels supplying skeletal muscles and gut; and metabolic and endocrine effects. Because different tissues respond in varying degrees to adrenergic agonists, differences in the actions of catecholamines are attributed to the presence of different receptor types within the tissues (alpha and beta).

Clinical indications and actions

Most agents act on two or more receptor sites; the net effect is the sum of alpha and beta activity. Dopaminergic and serotonergic activity may occur, possibly stimulating receptors in the CNS to release histamine.

Temporary appetite suppression is another effect, often resulting in a reboundlike weight gain after patient develops tolerance to the anorexic effect, or after withdrawal of the drug. Other uses include support of blood pressure, suppression of urinary incontinence and enuresis, and relief from pain of dysmenorrhea.

Hypotension

Alpha agonists (norepinephrine, metaraminol, phenylephrine, and pseudoephedrine) cause arteriolar and venous constriction, resulting in increased blood pressure. This action helps support blood pressure in hypotension and in management of serious allergic conditions. Topical formulations are used to induce local vasoconstriction (decongestion), arrest superficial hemorrhage (styptic), stimulate radial smooth muscle of the iris (mydriasis), and (with local anesthetics) localize anesthesia and prolong duration of action. Ophthalmic preparations reduce aqueous humor production and increase uveoscleral outflow.

Cardiac stimulation

Beta$_1$ agonists (dobutamine) act primarily in the heart, producing a positive inotropic effect. Because they increase heart rate, enhance AV conduction, and increase the strength of the heartbeat, beta$_1$ agonists may be used to restore heartbeat in cardiac arrest and for heart block in syncopal seizures (not treatment of choice), or to treat acute heart failure and cardiogenic or other types of shock. Their use in shock is somewhat controversial, because beta$_1$ agonists induce lipolysis (increase of free fatty acids in plasma), which promotes a metabolic acidosis, and because they favor arrhythmias, which pose a special threat in cardiogenic shock.

Bronchodilation

Beta$_2$ agonists (albuterol, bitolterol, isoetharine, metaproterenol, and terbutaline) act primarily on smooth muscle of the bronchial tree, vasculature, intestines, and uterus. They also induce hepatic and muscle glycogenolysis, which results in hyperglycemia (sometimes useful in insulin overdose) and hyperlactic acidemia.

Some are used as bronchodilators, some as vasodilators. They are also used to relax the uterus, to delay delivery in premature labor, and for dysmenorrhea. Some degree of cardiostimulation may occur, because all beta$_2$ agonists have some degree of beta$_1$ activity.

Shock

Dopamine is currently the only commercially available sympathomimetic with significant dopaminergic activity, although some other sympathomimetics appear to act on dopamine receptors in the CNS. Dopamine receptors are prominent in the periphery (splanchnic and renal vasculature), where they mediate vasodilation, which is useful in treating shock and acute heart failure. Renal vasodilation may induce diuresis.

Overview of adverse reactions

Patients known to be more sensitive to the effects of these drugs include elderly persons, infants, and patients with thyrotoxicosis or CV disease.

The alpha agonists commonly produce CV reactions. An excessive increase in blood pressure is a major adverse reaction of systemically administered alpha agonists. Exaggerated pressor response may occur in hypertensive or elderly patients, which may evoke vagal reflex responses resulting in bradycardia and AV block. Alpha agonists also interfere with lactation and may cause nausea, vomiting, sweating, piloerection, rebound congestion or miosis, difficult urination, and headache. Ophthalmic use may cause mydriasis, photophobia, burning, stinging, and blurring.

The beta agonists most frequently cause tachycardia, palpitations, and other arrhythmias. Their other effects include premature atrial and ventricular contractions; tachyarrhythmias, and myocardial necrosis. Reflex tachycardia and palpitations occur with $beta_2$ agonists because of decreased blood pressure.

Metabolic reactions to beta agonists include hyperglycemia, increased metabolic rate, hyperlactic acidosis, and local and systemic acidosis (decreased bronchodilator response).

Respiratory reactions include increased perfusion of nonfunctioning portions of lungs (COPD); mucus plugs may develop due to increased mucus secretion. Other reactions include tremors, vertigo, insomnia, sweating, headache, nausea, vomiting, and anxiety.

The centrally acting adrenergics have similar effects, which may also be associated with dry mouth, flushing, diarrhea, impotence, hyperthermia (excessive doses), agitation, anorexia, dizziness, dyskinesia, and changes in libido. Chronic use of adrenergics in children may cause endocrine disturbances that arrest growth; however, growth usually rebounds after withdrawal of drug.

☑ Special considerations

Parenteral preparations

- If used as a pressor agent, correct fluid volume depletion before administration. Adrenergics are not a substitute for blood, plasma, fluid, or electrolytes.
- Monitor blood pressure, pulse, and respiratory and urinary output carefully during therapy.
- Tachyphylaxis or tolerance may develop after prolonged or excessive use.

For inhalation therapy

- The preservative sodium bisulfite is present in many adrenergic formulations. Patients with a history of allergy to sulfites should avoid preparations that contain this preservative.
- Administer when patient arises in morning and before meals to reduce fatigue by improving ventilation.
- For unknown reasons, paradoxical airway resistance (manifested by sudden increase in dyspnea) may result from repeated excessive use of isoetharine. If this occurs, patient should discontinue drug and use alternative therapy (such as epinephrine).
- Adrenergic inhalation may be alternated with other drug administration (steroids, other adrenergics) if necessary, but should not be administered simultaneously because of danger of excessive tachycardia.
- Do not use discolored or precipitated solutions.
- Protect solutions from light, freezing, and heat. Store at controlled room temperature.
- Systemic absorption, though infrequent, can follow applications to nasal and conjunctival membranes. If symptoms of systemic absorption occur, patient should stop the drug.
- Prolonged or too-frequent use may cause tolerance to bronchodilating and cardiac stimulant effect. Rebound bronchospasm may follow end of drug effect.

Patient education

Inhalation

- Instruct patient in correct use of nebulizer and warn to use lowest effective dose.
- Explain that overuse of adrenergic bronchodilators may cause tachycardia, headache, nausea and dizziness, loss of effectiveness, possible paradoxical reaction, and cardiac arrest.
- Tell patient to call if bronchodilator causes dizziness, chest pain, or lack of therapeutic response to usual dose.
- Tell patient to avoid other adrenergic medications unless they are prescribed.
- Inform patient that saliva and sputum may appear pink after inhalation treatment.
- Instruct patient to begin treatment with first symptoms of bronchospasm.
- Caution patient to keep spray away from eyes.
- Tell patient not to discard drug applicator. Refill units are available.

Nasal

- Instruct patient to blow nose gently (with both nostrils open) to clear nasal passages well, before administration of medication.
- Instruct patient on proper method of instillation.

– Drops: Tell patient to tilt head back while sitting or standing up, or to lie on bed with head over side. Stay in position a few minutes to permit medication to spread through nose.

– Spray: With head upright, squeeze bottle quickly and firmly to produce 1 or 2 sprays into each nostril; wait 3 to 5 minutes, blow nose, and repeat dose.

– Jelly: Place in each nostril and sniff it well back into nose.

Ophthalmic

- To avoid excessive systemic absorption, tell patient to apply pressure to lacrimal sac during and for 1 to 2 minutes after instillation of drops.
- Inform patient that after instillation of ophthalmic preparation, pupils of eyes will be very large and eyes may be more sensitive to light than usual. Advise patient to use dark glasses until pupils return to normal.
- Warn patient to use drug only as directed.
- Instruct to call if no relief or condition worsens.
- Tell patient to store drug away from heat and light and out of reach of children.

Geriatric use

- Elderly patients may be more sensitive to therapeutic and adverse effects of some adrenergics and may require lower doses.

Pediatric use

- Lower doses of adrenergics are recommended for use in children.

Breast-feeding

- The use of adrenergics during breast-feeding usually is not recommended.

Representative combinations

Ephedrine sulfate with guaifenesin and theophylline: Bronkolixir; with guaifenesin, theophylline, and phenobarbital: Bronkotabs; with belladonna extract, boric acid, zinc oxide, beeswax, and cocoa butter: Wyanoids Relief Factor.

Epinephrine with benzalkonium chloride: Glaucon; with pilocarpine: E-Pilo.

Isoproterenol hydrochloride with phenylephrine bitartrate: Duo-Medihaler.

Naphazoline with antazoline phosphate, boric acid, phenylmercuric acetate, and carbonate anhydrous: Vasocon-A Solution; with pheniramine maleate: Naphcon-A; with phenylephrine hydrochloride, pyrilamine maleate, and phenylpropanolamine hydrochloride: 4-Way Long Lasting Spray; with polyvinyl alcohol: Albalon.

Pseudoephedrine with chlorpheniramine maleate: Chlor-Trimeton; with codeine phosphate and guaifenesin: Alamine Expectorant, Deproist Expectorant with Codeine, Guiatussin DAC, Isoclor Expectorant, Novahistine Expectorant, Robitussin-DAC; with dextromethorphan and acetaminophen: Contac Severe Cold and Flu Nighttime; with dextromethorphan, acetaminophen, and guaifenesin: Vicks 44M Cough, Cold, and Flu Relief; with dextrompheniramine: Disophrol, Drixoral; with dexchlorpheniramine: Polaramine; with guaifenesin: Robitussin-PE, Zephrex; with hydrocordone bitartrate: De-Tuss, Detussin Liquid, Entuss-D, Tussend; with triprolidine: Actagen, Actamin, Actifed, Allerfrim Tablets, Aprodine, Cenafed Plus, Triposed. See also *antihistamines, barbiturates,* and *xanthine derivatives.*

adrenocorticoids (systemic)

Glucocorticoids: **betamethasone, betamethasone sodium phosphate, betamethasone sodium phosphate and betamethasone acetate, cortisone acetate, dexamethasone, dexamethasone acetate, dexamethasone sodium phosphate, hydrocortisone, hydrocortisone acetate, hydrocortisone cypionate, hydrocortisone sodium phosphate, hydrocortisone sodium succinate, methylprednisolone, methylprednisolone acetate, methylprednisolone sodium succinate, prednisolone, prednisolone acetate, prednisolone sodium phosphate, prednisolone tebutate, prednisone, triamcinolone, triamcinolone acetonide, triamcinolone diacetate, triamcinolone hexacetonide**

Mineralocorticoid: **fludrocortisone acetate**

Active adrenocortical extracts were first prepared in 1930; by 1942, chemists had isolated 28 steroids from the adrenal cortex.

The adrenocortical hormones are classified according to their activity into two groups: the mineralocorticoids and the glucocorticoids. The mineralocorticoids regulate electrolyte homeostasis. The glucocorticoids regulate carbohydrate, lipid, and protein metabolism; inflammation; and the body's immune responses to diverse stimuli. Many corticosteroids exert both kinds of activity.

Pharmacology

The corticosteroids dramatically affect almost all body systems. They are thought to act by controlling the rate of protein synthesis; they react with receptor proteins in the cytoplasm of sensitive cells to form a steroid-receptor complex. Steroid receptors have been identified in many tissues. The steroid-receptor complex migrates into the nucleus of the cell, where it binds to chromatin. Information carried by the steroid of the receptor protein directs the genetic apparatus to transcribe RNA, resulting in the synthesis of specific proteins that serve as enzymes in various biochemical pathways. Because the maximum pharmacologic activity lags behind peak blood concentrations, corticosteroids' effects may result from modification of enzyme activity rather than from direct action by the drugs.

Mineralocorticoids act renally at the distal tubules to enhance the reabsorption of sodium ions (and thus water) from the tubular fluid into the plasma, and the urinary excretion of both potassium and hydrogen ions. The primary features of excess mineralocorticoid activity are positive sodium balance and expansion of the extracellular fluid volume; normal or slight increase in the concentration of sodium in the plasma; hypokalemia; and alkalosis. In contrast, deficiency of mineralocorticoids produces sodium loss, hyponatremia, hyperkalemia, contraction of the extracellular fluid volume, and cellular dehydration.

Clinical indications and actions

Inflammation

A major pharmacologic use of the glucocorticoids is treatment of inflammation. The anti-inflammatory effects depend on the direct local action of the steroids. Glucocorticoids decrease the inflammatory response by stabilizing leukocyte lysosomal membranes, which prevent the release of destructive acid hydrolases from leukocytes; inhibiting macrophage accumulation in inflamed areas; reducing leukocyte adhesion to the capillary endothelium; reducing capillary wall permeability and edema formation; decreasing complement components; antagonizing histamine activity and release of kinin from substrates; reducing fibroblast proliferation, collagen deposition, and subsequent scar tissue formation; and by other unknown mechanisms.

Immunosuppression

The full mechanisms of immunosuppressive actions are unknown. Glucocorticoids reduce activity and volume of lymphatic system, producing lymphocytopenia, decreasing immunoglobulin and complement concentrations, decreasing passage of immune complexes through basement membranes, and possibly depressing reactivity of tissue to antigen-antibody interaction.

Adrenal insufficiency

Combined mineralocorticoid and glucocorticoid therapy is used in treating adrenal insufficiency and in salt-losing forms of congenital adrenogenital syndrome.

Rheumatic and collagen diseases; other severe diseases

Glucocorticoids are used to treat rheumatic and collagen diseases (arthritis, polyarteritis nodosa, systemic lupus erythematosus); thyroiditis; severe dermatologic diseases, such as pemphigus, exfoliative dermatitis, lichen planus, and psoriasis; allergic reactions; ocular disorders (such as inflammations); respiratory diseases (asthma, sarcoidosis, lipid pneumonitis); hematologic diseases (autoimmune hemolytic anemia, idiopathic thrombocytopenia); neoplastic diseases (leukemias, lymphomas); and GI diseases (ulcerative colitis, regional enteritis, celiac disease). Other indications include myasthenia gravis, organ transplants, nephrotic syndrome, and septic shock.

◊ ***Acute spinal cord injury***

Large I.V. doses of glucocorticoids, when given shortly after injury, may improve motor and sensory function in patients with acute spinal cord injury.

Overview of adverse reactions

Suppression of the hypothalamic-pituitary-adrenal (HPA) axis is the major effect of systemic therapy with corticosteroids. When administered in high doses or for prolonged therapy, the glucocorticoids suppress release of corticotropin from the pituitary gland; subsequently, the adrenal cortex stops secreting endogenous corticosteroids. The degree and duration of HPA axis suppression produced by the drugs is highly variable among patients and depends on the dose, frequency and time of administration, and duration of therapy.

Patients with a suppressed HPA axis resulting from exogenous glucocorticoid administration who abruptly discontinue therapy may experience severe withdrawal symptoms such as fever, myalgia, arthralgia, malaise, anorexia, nausea, desquamation of skin, orthostatic hypotension, dizziness, fainting, dyspnea, and hypoglycemia. Therefore, corticosteroid therapy should always be withdrawn gradually.

Adrenal suppression may persist for as long as 12 months in patients who have received large doses for prolonged periods. Until complete recovery occurs, patients subjected to stress may show signs and symptoms of adrenal insufficiency and may need glucocorticoid and mineralocorticoid replacement therapy.

Cushingoid symptoms, the effects of excessive glucocorticoid therapy, may develop in patients receiving large doses of glucocorticoids over several weeks or longer. These include moon face, central obesity, striae, hirsutism, acne, ecchymoses, hypertension, osteoporosis, muscle atrophy, sexual dysfunction, diabetes, cataracts, hyperlipidemia, peptic ulcer, increased susceptibility to infection, and fluid and electrolyte imbalances.

Other adverse reactions to normal or high dosages of corticosteroids may include CNS effects (euphoria, insomnia, psychotic behavior, pseudotumor cerebri, mental changes, nervousness, restlessness); CV effects (heart failure, hypertension, edema); GI effects (peptic ulcer, irritation, increased appetite); metabolic effects (hypokalemia, sodium retention, fluid retention, weight gain, hyperglycemia, osteoporosis); dermatologic effects (delayed wound healing, acne, skin eruptions, muscle atrophy, striae); and immunosuppression (increased susceptibility to infection).

☑ Special considerations

- Watch for sudden patient weight gain, edema, change in blood pressure, or change in electrolyte status.
- During times of physiologic stress (trauma, surgery, infection), patient may require additional steroids and may experience signs of steroid withdrawal; patients who were previously steroid-dependent may need systemic corticosteroids to prevent adrenal insufficiency.
- Reduce drug gradually in long-term therapy. Rapid reduction may cause withdrawal symptoms.
- Be aware of patient's psychological history and watch for behavioral changes.
- Observe for infection or delayed wound healing.

Patient education

- Be sure that patient understands need to take the adrenocorticoid as prescribed. Give him instructions on what to do if a dose is inadvertently missed.
- Warn patient not to stop drug abruptly.
- Inform patient of therapeutic and adverse effects of drug and tell to report complications right away.
- Tell patient to carry medical identification card noting need for more adrenocorticoids during stress.

Geriatric use

- Many elderly patients have conditions that could easily be aggravated by corticosteroid therapy. Elderly patients have a reduced ability to metabolize and eliminate drugs; monitor closely.

Pediatric use

- Long-term administration of pharmacologic dosages of glucocorticoids in children may retard bone growth. Manifestations of adrenal suppression in children include retardation of linear growth, delayed weight gain, low plasma cortisol concentrations, and lack of response to corticotropin stimulation. Alternate-day therapy is recommended to minimize growth suppression.

Breast-feeding

- Women who are taking pharmacologic dosages of corticosteroids should not breast-feed.

Representative combinations

Betamethasone sodium phosphate with betamethasone acetate: Celestone Soluspan.

Dexamethasone sodium phosphate with lidocaine hydrochloride: Decadron with Xylocaine.

adrenocorticoids (nasal and oral inhalation)

Nasal: beclomethasone dipropionate, budesonide, dexamethasone sodium phosphate, flunisolide, fluticasone propionate, triamcinolone acetonide

Oral: beclomethasone dipropionate, budesonide, dexamethasone sodium phosphate, flunisolide, triamcinolone acetonide

Topical administration through oral aerosol and nasal spray delivers adrenocorticoids to sites of inflammation in the nasal passages or the tracheobronchial tree. Because smaller doses are administered, less drug is absorbed systemically, with fewer systemic adverse effects.

Pharmacology

Inhaled glucocorticoid is absorbed through the nasal mucosa or through the trachea, bronchi, and alveoli. The anti-inflammatory effects of the glucocorticoids depend on the direct local action of the steroid. Glucocorticoids stimulate transcription of messenger RNA in individual cell nuclei to synthesize enzymes that decrease inflammation. These enzymes stimulate biochemical pathways that decrease the inflammatory response by stabilizing leukocyte lysosomal membranes, which prevent the release of destructive acid hydrolases from leukocytes; inhibiting macrophage accumulation in inflamed areas; reducing leukocyte adhesion to the capillary endothelium; reducing capillary wall permeability and edema formation; decreasing complement components; antagonizing histamine activity and release of kinin from substrates; reducing fibroblast proliferation, collagen deposition, and scar tissue formation; and by other unknown mechanisms.

Clinical indications and actions

Nasal inflammation

Nasal solutions are used to relieve symptoms of seasonal or perennial rhinitis when antihistamines and decongestants are ineffective; to treat inflammatory conditions of the nasal passages; and to prevent recurrence after surgical removal of nasal polyps.

Chronic bronchial asthma

Aerosols treat chronic bronchial asthma not controlled by bronchodilators and other nonsteroidal drugs.

Overview of adverse reactions

Nasal: Local sensations of nasal burning and irritation occur in about 10% of patients; sneezing attacks immediately after the nasal application in about 10% of patients; and transient mild nosebleeds in 10% to 15% of patients, but it is unknown whether this is an effect

of the nasal solution or of the dryness it induces in the nasal passages. Localized candidal infections of the nose or pharynx have occurred rarely.
Oral: Localized infections with *Candida albicans* or *Aspergillus niger* have occurred commonly in the mouth and pharynx and occasionally in the larynx.
Systemic: Systemic absorption may occur, potentially leading to hypothalamic-pituitary-adrenal (HPA) axis suppression. This is more likely with large doses or with combined nasal and oral corticosteroid therapy.
Other: Hypersensitivity reactions are possible. Also, some patients may be intolerant of the fluorocarbon propellants in the preparations.

☑ Special considerations

- Full therapeutic benefit requires regular use and is usually evident within a few days, although a few patients may require up to 3 weeks of therapy for maximum benefit. Therapy should be discontinued in the absence of significant symptomatic improvement within recommended time frame (varies per drug used).
- Use of nasal or oral inhalation therapy may allow a patient to discontinue systemic corticosteroid therapy.
- After the desired clinical effect is obtained, maintenance dose should be reduced to the smallest amount necessary to control symptoms.
- Drug should be discontinued if the patient develops signs of systemic absorption (including Cushing's syndrome, hyperglycemia, or glucosuria), mucosal irritation or ulceration, hypersensitivity, or infection. (If antifungals or antibiotics are being used with corticosteroids and the infection does not respond immediately, discontinue corticosteroids until the infection is controlled.)

Patient education

For patients using a *nasal* inhaler

- Instruct patient to use only as directed. Inform him that full therapeutic effect is not immediate but requires regular use of inhaler.
- Encourage patient with blocked nasal passsages to use an oral decongestant 30 minutes before intranasal corticosteroid administration to ensure adequate penetration. Advise patient to clear nasal passages of secretions before using the inhaler.
- Instruct patient to clean inhaler according to manufacturer's instructions.

For patients using an *oral* inhaler

- Instruct patient to use only as directed.
- Advise patient receiving bronchodilators by inhalation to use the bronchodilator before the corticosteroid to enhance penetration of the corticosteroid into the bronchial tree. He should wait several minutes to allow time for the bronchodilator to relax the smooth muscle.
- Instruct patient to hold breath for a few seconds to enhance placement and action of the drug and to wait 1 minute before taking subsequent puffs of medication.
- Tell patient to rinse mouth with water after using the inhaler to decrease the chance of oral fungal infections. Tell him to check nasal and oral mucous membranes frequently for signs of fungal infection.
- Instruct patient to clean inhaler properly.
- Warn asthmatic patient not to increase use of corticosteroid inhaler during a severe asthma attack, but to call for adjustment of therapy, possibly by adding a systemic steroid.

For patients using *either* type of inhaler

- Tell patient to report decreased response; dosage adjustment or discontinuation of drug may be needed.
- Instruct patient to observe for adverse effects, and if fever or local irritation develops, to discontinue use and report the effect promptly.

Geriatric use

- Many elderly patients have conditions that could be aggravated by the excessive use of corticosteroid inhalant therapy. Elderly patients have a reduced ability to metabolize and eliminate drugs; monitor closely for adverse effects.

Pediatric use

- In children, nasal or oral inhalant corticosteroid therapy may be successfully substituted for systemic corticosteroid therapy. However, the risk of HPA axis suppression and Cushing's syndrome still exists.

Breast-feeding

- Use with caution in breast-feeding women.

Representative combinations

None.

adrenocorticoids (topical)

alclometasone dipropionate, amcinonide, betamethasone benzoate, betamethasone dipropionate, betamethasone valerate, clobetasol propionate, clocortolone pivalate, desonide, desoximetasone, dexamethasone, dexamethasone sodium phosphate, diflorasone diacetate, fluocinolone acetonide, fluocinonide, flurandrenolide, fluticasone propionate, halcinonide, halobetasol propionate, hydrocortisone, hydrocortisone acetate, hydrocortisone butyrate, hydrocortisone valerate, methylprednisolone acetate, triamcinolone acetonide

Since topical hydrocortisone was introduced in the 1950s, numerous analogues have been developed to provide a wide range of potencies in creams, ointments, lotions, and gels.

Pharmacology

The anti-inflammatory effects of topical glucocorticoids depend on the direct local action of the steroid. Although the exact mechanism of action is unclear, many researchers believe that glucocorticoids stimulate transcription of messenger RNA in individual cell nuclei to synthesize enzymes that decrease inflammation. These enzymes stimulate biochemical pathways that decrease the inflammatory response by stabilizing leukocyte lysosomal membranes, which prevents the release of destructive acid hydrolases from leukocytes; inhibiting macrophage accumulation in inflamed areas; reducing leukocyte adhesion to the capillary endothelium; reducing capillary wall permeability and edema formation; decreasing complement components; antagonizing histamine activity and release of kinin from substrates; reducing fibroblast proliferation, collagen deposition, and subsequent scar tissue formation; and by other unknown mechanisms.

Topical corticosteroids are minimally absorbed systemically and cause fewer adverse effects than systemically administered corticosteroids. Fluorinated derivatives are absorbed to a greater extent than other topical steroids. The degree of absorption depends on the site of application, the amount applied, the relative potency, the presence of an occlusive dressing (may increase penetration by 10%), the condition of the skin, and the vehicle carrying the drug. Topical corticosteroids

COMPARATIVE POTENCY OF TOPICAL CORTICOSTEROIDS

Topical corticosteroid preparations can be grouped according to relative anti-inflammatory activity. The following list arranges groups of topical corticosteroids in decreasing order of potency (based mainly on vasoconstrictor assay or clinical effectiveness in psoriasis). Preparations within each group are approximately equivalent.

GROUP	DRUG	CONCENTRATION (%)
I	betamethasone dipropionate (Diprolene)	0.05
	betamethasone dipropionate (Diprolene AF)	0.05
	clobetasol propionate (Temovate)	0.05
	diflorasone diacetate (Psorcon)	0.05
II	amcinonide (Cyclocort)	0.1
	betamethasone dipropionate ointment (Diprosone)	0.05
	desoximetasone (Topicort)	0.05, 0.25
	diflorasone diacetate (Florone, Maxiflor)	0.05
	fluocinonide (Lidex)	0.05
	fluocinonide gel	0.05
	halcinonide (Halog)	0.1
III	betamethasone benzoate gel	0.025
	betamethasone dipropionate cream (Diprosone)	0.05
	betamethasone valerate ointment (Valisone)	0.1
	diflorasone diacetate cream (Florone, Maxiflor)	0.05
	triamcinolone acetonide cream (Aristocort)	0.5
IV	desoximetasone (Topicort LP)	0.05
	fluocinolone acetonide (Synalar-HP)	0.2
	fluocinolone acetonide ointment (Synalar)	0.025
	flurandrenolide (Cordran)	0.05
	fluticasone propionate (Cutivate)	0.005, 0.05
	triamcinolone acetonide ointment (Aristocort, Kenalog)	0.1
V	betamethasone benzoate cream	0.025
	betamethasone dipropionate lotion (Diprosone)	0.05
	betamethasone valerate cream or lotion (Valisone)	0.1
	fluocinolone acetonide cream (Synalar)	0.025
	flurandrenolide (Cordran)	0.05
	thydrocortisone butyrate (Locoid)	0.1
	thydrocortisone valerate (Westcort)	0.2
	triamcinolone acetonide cream or lotion (Kenalog)	0.1
VI	alclometasone dipropionate (Aclovate)	0.05
	desonide (Tridesilon)	0.05
	fluocinolone acetonide solution (Synalar)	0.01

are used to relieve pruritus, inflammation, and other signs of corticosteroid-responsive dermatoses.

Ointments are preferred for dry, scaly areas; solutions, gels, aerosols, and lotions for hairy areas. Creams can be used for most areas except those in which dampness may cause maceration. Gels and lotions can be used for moist lesions; however, gels may contain alcohol, which can dry and irritate the skin. The topical preparations are classified by potency into six groups: group I is the most potent, group VI the least potent. (See *Comparative potency of topical corticosteroids.*)

Clinical indications and actions

Inflammatory disorders of skin and mucous membranes

The topical adrenocorticoids relieve inflammatory and pruritic skin disorders, including localized neurodermatitis, psoriasis, atopic or seborrheic dermatitis, the inflammatory phase of xerosis, anogenital pruritus, discoid lupus erythematosus, lichen planus, granuloma annulare, and lupus erythematosus.

These drugs may also relieve irritant or allergic contact dermatitis; however, relief of acute dermatosis may require systemic adrenocorticoids.

Rectal disorders responsive to this class of drugs include ulcerative colitis, cryptitis, inflamed hemorrhoids, post-irradiation or factitial proctitis, and pruritus ani.

Oral lesions, such as nonherpetic oral inflammatory and ulcerative lesions and routine gingivitis, may respond to treatment with topical adrenocorticoids.

OTC formulations of the topical corticosteroids are indicated for minor skin irritation such as itching; rash due to eczema, dermatitis, insect bites, poison ivy, poison oak, or poison sumac; or dermatitis due to exposure to soaps, detergents, cosmetics, and jewelry.

Overview of adverse reactions

Local effects include burning, itching, irritation, dryness, folliculitis, striae, miliaria, acne, perioral dermatitis, hypopigmentation, hypertrichosis, allergic contact dermatitis, secondary infection, and atrophy.

Systemic absorption may occur leading to hypothalamic-pituitary-adrenal (HPA) axis suppression.

The risk of adverse reactions increases with the use of occlusive dressings or more potent steroids, in patients with liver disease, and in children (because of their greater ratio of skin surface to body weight).

Prolonged application around the eyes may lead to cataracts or glaucoma.

☑ Special considerations

Method for applying topical preparations

- Wash hands before and after applying the drug.
- Gently clean the area of application. Washing or soaking the area before application may increase drug penetration.
- Apply sparingly in a light film; rub in lightly. Avoid contact with eyes, unless using an ophthalmic product.
- Avoid prolonged application in areas near the eyes, genitals, rectum, on the face, and in skin folds. High-potency topical corticosteroids are more likely to cause striae and atrophy in these areas because of their higher rates of absorption.
- Monitor response. Observe area of inflammation.
- Do not apply occlusive dressings over topical steroids. However, if unavailable, minimize adverse reactions by using occlusive dressing intermittently. Do not leave it in place longer than 16 hours each day.
- Stop drug if patient develops signs of systemic absorption.

Patient education

- Instruct patient on use of drug.
- Instruct patient to discontinue drug and report local or systemic adverse reactions, worsening condition, or persistent symptoms.
- Warn patient not to use OTC topical products other than those specifically recommended.
- Tell patient to apply a missed dose as soon as it is remembered, and continue on with his regular schedule of application. However, if it is almost time for the next application, tell him to wait and continue with regular schedule. He should not apply a double dose.

Geriatric use

- In elderly patients, loss of collagen may lead to friable and transparent skin with increased epidermal permeability to water and certain chemicals. In these patients, topically applied drugs such as steroid creams may have a greater effect locally. Elderly patients also have a reduced ability to metabolize and eliminate drugs and may have higher plasma drug levels and more adverse reactions. Monitor these patients closely.

Pediatric use

- To minimize the risk, limit topical corticosteroid therapy in children to the minimum amount necessary for therapeutic efficacy. Advise parents not to use tight-fitting diapers or plastic pants on a child being treated in the diaper area, because such garments may serve as occlusive dressings.

Breast-feeding

- Topical corticosteroids should be used with caution in breast-feeding women.

Representative combinations

Betamethasone with clotrimazole: Lotrisone.

Betamethasone dipropionate with clotrimazole: Lotrisone.

Dexamethasone with neomycin sulfate: Neo-Decadron Cream; with neomycin sulfate and polymyxin B sulfate: Dexacidin Ointment.

Fluocinolone acetonide with neomycin: Neo-Synalar.

Flurandrenolide with neomycin: Cordran.

Hydrocortisone with iodoquinol: Vytone Cream; with iodochlorhydroxyquin: Vioform-Hydrocortisone Cream, AP, Corque Cream, Hysone; with neomycin: Hydrocortisone-Neomycin, Neo-Cortef; with pramoxine: Pramosone, Zone-A Forte; with neomycin and polymyxin B: Cortisporin Cream; with neomycin, bacitracin, and polymyxin B sulfate: Cortisporin Ointment; with neomycin sulfate and polymyxin B sulfate: Cortisporin; with dibucaine: Corticaine; with pyrilamine maleate, pheniramine maleate, and chlorpheniramine maleate: HC Derma-Pax; with benzoyl peroxide and mineral oil: Vanoxide-HC; with lidocaine and glycerin: Lida-Mantle-HC; with sulfur and salicylic acid: Therac Lotion.

Methylprednisolone with neomycin: Neo-Medrol Acetate.

Triamcinolone acetonide with nystatin: Mykacet, Myco II, Myco-Biotic II, Mycogen II, Mycolog-II, Myco-Triacet II, Mytrex, Nystatin-Triamcinolone Acetonide, N.G.T.; with neomycin, gramicidin, and nystatin: Myco-Triacet II, Tri-Statin II.

alpha-adrenergic blockers

carvedilol, dihydroergotamine mesylate, doxazosin mesylate, ergotamine tartrate, phentolamine mesylate, prazosin hydrochloride, tamsulosin hydrochloride, terazosin hydrochloride, tolazoline hydrochloride

Drugs that block the effects of peripheral neurohormonal transmitters (norepinephrine, epinephrine, and related sympathomimetic amines) on adrenergic receptors in various effector systems are designated as adrenergic blocking agents. As adrenoreceptors are classified into two subtypes—alpha and beta—so too are the blocking agents. Essentially, those agents that antagonize mydriasis, vasoconstriction, nonvascular smooth muscle excitation, and other adrenergic responses caused by alpha receptor stimulation are termed alpha-adrenergic blockers.

Pharmacology

Nonselective alpha antagonists

Ergotamine, phentolamine, and tolazoline antagonize both $alpha_1$ and $alpha_2$ receptors. Generally, alpha blockade results in tachycardia, palpitations, and increased secretion of renin due to the abnormally large amounts of norepinephrine (transmitter "overflow") released from adrenergic nerve endings as a result of the concurrent blockade of $alpha_1$ and $alpha_2$ receptors. The effects of norepinephrine are clinically counterproductive to the major uses of nonselective alpha blockers, which include treating peripheral vascular disorders such as Raynaud's disease, acrocyanosis, frostbite, acute arterial occlusion, phlebitis, phlebothrombosis, diabetic gangrene, shock, and pheochromocytoma.

Selective alpha antagonists

$Alpha_1$ blockers have readily observable effects and are currently the only alpha-adrenergic agents with known clinical uses. They decrease vascular resistance and increase venous capacitance, thereby lowering blood pressure and causing pink warm skin, nasal and scleroconjunctival congestion, ptosis, postural and exercise hypotension, mild to moderate miosis, and interference with ejaculation. They also relax nonvascular smooth muscle, notably in the prostate capsule, thereby reducing urinary symptoms in men with benign prostatic hyperplasia (BPH). Because $alpha_1$ blockers do not block $alpha_2$ receptors, they do not cause transmitter overflow. In theory, $alpha_1$ blockers should be useful in the same conditions as nonselective alpha blockers; however, doxazosin, prazosin, and terazosin are approved only for treating hypertension. Terazosin also is approved in treatment of prostatic outflow obstruction secondary to BPH.

$Alpha_2$ blockers produce more subtle physiologic effects and currently have no therapeutic applications. Yohimbine is one such agent.

Clinical indications and actions

Peripheral vascular disorders

Alpha-adrenergic blocking agents are indicated for treating peripheral vascular disorders, including Raynaud's disease, acrocyanosis, frostbite, acute atrial occlusion, phlebitis, and diabetic gangrene. Dihydroergotamine and ergotamine have been used to treat vascular headaches. Prazosin has been used to treat Raynaud's disease. Phentolamine is indicated to treat dermal necrosis caused by extravasation of norepinephrine, dopamine, or phenylephrine (alpha agonists).

Hypertension

Tolazoline is indicated to treat persistent pulmonary hypertension in neonates. Prazosin, carvedilol, doxazosin, and terazosin are used in managing essential hypertension. Phentolamine is used to control hypertension and is a useful adjunct in surgical treatment of pheochromocytoma.

BPH

Terazosin, tamsulosin, and doxazosin are used to control mild to moderate urinary obstructive symptoms in men with BPH.

Overview of adverse reactions

Nonselective alpha antagonists typically cause orthostatic hypotension, tachycardia, palpitations, fluid retention (from excess renin secretion), nasal and ocular congestion, and aggravation of the signs and symptoms of respiratory infection. Use of these agents is contraindicated in patients with severe cerebral and coronary atherosclerosis and in those with renal insufficiency.

Selective alpha antagonists may cause severe orthostatic hypotension and syncope, especially with the first dose; most common adverse effects of $alpha_1$ blockade are dizziness, headache, and malaise.

☑ Special considerations

- Monitor vital signs, especially blood pressure.
- Administer dose at bedtime to reduce potential of dizziness or light-headedness.
- To avoid first-dose syncope, begin with small dose.

Patient education

- Warn patient about postural hypotension. Tell him to avoid sudden changes to upright position.
- Tell patient to promptly report dizziness or irregular heartbeat.
- Advise patient to take dose at bedtime to reduce potential for dizziness or light-headedness.
- Warn patient to avoid driving and other hazardous tasks that require mental alertness until effects of medication are established.
- Reassure patient that adverse effects, including dizziness, should lessen after several doses.
- Tell patient that the alcohol use, excessive exercise, prolonged standing, and exposure to heat will intensify adverse effects.
- Advise patient of the reason for taking the medication (hypertension versus BPH).

Geriatric use

- Hypotensive effects may be more pronounced in the elderly.

Representative combinations

None.

aminoglycosides

amikacin sulfate, gentamicin sulfate, kanamycin sulfate, neomycin sulfate, netilmicin sulfate, streptomycin sulfate, tobramycin sulfate

Aminoglycoside antibiotics were discovered during the search for drugs to treat serious penicillin-resistant, gram-negative infections. Streptomycin, derived from soil actinomycetes, was the first therapeutically useful aminoglycoside. Bacterial resistance to this prototype and adverse reactions soon led to the development of kanamycin, gentamicin, neomycin, netilmicin, tobramycin, and amikacin.

The basic structure of aminoglycosides is a hexose nucleus joined to at least two amino sugars by glycosidic linkage, hence the name aminoglycosides.

Aminoglycosides share certain pharmacokinetic properties, such as poor oral absorption, poor CNS penetration, and renal excretion, as well as serious adverse reactions and toxicity; their clinical use may require close monitoring of serum levels.

Pharmacology

Aminoglycosides are bactericidal. They bind directly and irreversibly to 30S ribosomal subunits, inhibiting bacterial protein synthesis. Bacterial resistance to aminoglycosides may be from decreased bacterial cell wall permeability, low affinity of the drug for ribosomal binding sites, or enzymatic degradation by microbial enzymes.

Aminoglycosides are active against many aerobic gram-negative organisms and some aerobic gram-positive organisms; they do not kill fungi, viruses, or anaerobic bacteria.

Gram-negative organisms susceptible to aminoglycosides include *Acinetobacter, Citrobacter, Enterobacter, Escherichia coli, Klebsiella,* indole-positive and indole-negative *Proteus, Providencia, Pseudomonas aeruginosa, Salmonella, Serratia,* and *Shigella.* Streptomycin is active against *Brucella, Calymmatobacterium granulomatis, Pasteurella multocida,* and *Yersinia pestis.*

Susceptible aerobic gram-positive organisms include *Staphylococcus aureus* and *S. epidermidis.* Streptomycin is active against *Nocardia, Erysipelothrix,* and some mycobacteria, including *Mycobacterium tuberculosis, M. marinum,* and certain strains of *M. kansasii* and *M. leprae.*

Aminoglycosides are not systemically absorbed after oral administration to patients with intact GI mucosa and, with few exceptions, are used parenterally for systemic infections; intraventricular or intrathecal administration is necessary for CNS infections. Kanamycin and neomycin are given orally for bowel sterilization.

Aminoglycosides are distributed widely throughout the body after parenteral administration; CSF concentrations are minimal even in patients with inflamed meninges. Over time, aminoglycosides accumulate in body tissue, especially the kidney and inner ear, causing drug saturation. The drug is released slowly from these tissues. Most aminoglycosides are minimally pro-

AMINOGLYCOSIDES: RENAL FUNCTION AND HALF-LIFE

As the chart shows, the aminoglycosides, which are excreted by the kidneys, have significantly prolonged half-lives in patients with end-stage renal disease. Knowing this can help you assess the patient's potential for drug accumulation and toxicity. Nephrotoxicity, a major hazard of therapy with aminoglycosides, is clearly linked to serum concentrations that exceed the therapeutic concentrations listed in the chart below. Therefore, monitoring peak and trough levels is essential for safe use of these drugs.

	HALF-LIFE		THERAPEUTIC CONCENTRATIONS (mcg/ml)	
DRUG AND ADMINISTRATION	NORMAL RENAL FUNCTION	END-STAGE RENAL DISEASE	PEAK	TROUGH
amikacin I.M., I.V.	2 to 3 hr	24 to 60 hr	16 to 32	< 10
gentamicin I.M., I.V., topical	2 hr	24 to 60 hr	4 to 8	< 2
kanamycin I.M., I.V., topical	2 to 3 hr	24 to 60 hr	15 to 40	< 10
neomycin P.O., topical	2 to 3 hr	12 to 24 hr	Not applicable	Not applicable
netilmicin I.M., I.V.	2 to 2.7 hr	< 10 hr	6 to 10	< 4
streptomycin I.M., I.V.	2.5 hr	100 hr	20 to 30	Not applicable
tobramycin I.M., I.V., topical	2 to 2.5 hr	24 to 60 hr	4 to 8	< 2

tein-bound, and are not metabolized. They do not penetrate abscesses well.

Aminoglycosides are excreted primarily in urine, chiefly by glomerular filtration; neomycin is chiefly excreted unchanged in feces when taken orally. Elimination half-life ranges between 2 and 4 hours and is prolonged in patients with decreased renal function. (See *Aminoglycosides: Renal function and half-life.*)

Clinical indications and actions

Infection caused by susceptible organisms

Aminoglycosides are used as sole therapy for:

- infections caused by susceptible aerobic gram-negative bacilli, including septicemia; postoperative, pulmonary, intra-abdominal, and urinary tract infections; and infections of skin, soft tissue, bones, and joints
- infections from aerobic gram-negative bacillary meningitis (not susceptible to other antibiotics); because of poor CNS penetration, drugs are given intrathecally or intraventricularly (in ventriculitis).

Aminoglycosides are combined with other antibacterials in many other types of infection, including:

- serious staphylococcal infections (with an antistaphylococcal penicillin)
- serious *P. aeruginosa* infections (with such drugs as an antipseudomonal penicillin or cephalosporin)
- enterococcal infections, including endocarditis (with such drugs as penicillin G, ampicillin, or vancomycin)
- as initial empiric therapy in febrile, leukopenic compromised host (with an antipseudomonal penicillin and/or cephalosporin)
- serious *Klebsiella* infections (with a cephalosporin)
- nosocomial pneumonia (with a cephalosporin)
- anaerobic infections involving *Bacteroides fragilis* (with such drugs as clindamycin, metronidazole, cefoxitin, doxycycline, chloramphenicol, or ticarcillin)
- tuberculosis (concomitant use of parenteral kanamycin or streptomycin with other antitubercular agents).

Overview of adverse reactions

Systemic reactions: Ototoxicity and nephrotoxicity are the most serious complications of aminoglycoside therapy. Ototoxicity involves both vestibular and auditory functions and usually is related to persistently high serum drug levels. Damage is reversible only if detected early and if drug is discontinued promptly.

Any aminoglycoside may cause usually reversible nephrotoxicity. The damage results in tubular necrosis. Mild proteinuria and casts are early signs of declining renal function; elevated serum creatinine levels follow several days after the decline has begun. Nephrotoxicity usually begins on day 4 to 7 of therapy and appears to be dose-related.

Neuromuscular blockade results in skeletal weakness and respiratory distress similar to that seen with the use of neuromuscular blocking agents like tubocurarine and succinylcholine.

Oral aminoglycoside therapy most often causes nausea, vomiting, and diarrhea. Less common adverse reactions include hypersensitivity reactions (ranging from mild rashes, fever, and eosinophilia to fatal anaphylaxis); hematologic reactions include hemolytic anemia, transient neutropenia, leukopenia, and thrombocytopenia. Transient elevations of liver function values also occur.

Local reactions: Parenterally administered forms of aminoglycosides may cause vein irritation, phlebitis, and sterile abscess.

☑ Special considerations

- Do not give an aminoglycoside to patient with history of hypersensitivity reactions to any aminoglycoside.
- Obtain results of culture and sensitivity tests before giving first dose.
- Monitor vital signs, electrolyte levels, and renal function studies before and during therapy; be sure patient is well hydrated to minimize chemical irritation of renal tubules; watch for signs of declining renal function.
- Keep peak serum levels and trough serum levels at recommended concentrations, especially in patients with decreased renal function. Draw blood for peak level 1 hour after I.M. injection (30 minutes to 1 hour after I.V. infusion); for trough level, draw sample just before the next dose. Time and date all blood samples. Do not use heparinized tube to collect blood samples; it interferes with results.
- Evaluate patient's hearing before and during therapy; monitor for complaints of tinnitus, vertigo, or hearing loss.
- Avoid concomitant use of aminoglycosides with other ototoxic or nephrotoxic drugs.
- Usual duration of therapy is 7 to 10 days; if no response occurs in 3 to 5 days, drug should be discontinued and cultures repeated for reevaluation of therapy.
- Closely monitor patients on long-term therapy—especially elderly and debilitated patients and others receiving immunosuppressant or radiation therapy—for possible bacterial or fungal superinfection; monitor especially for fever.
- Do not add or mix other drugs with I.V. infusions—particularly penicillins, which will inactivate aminoglycosides; the two groups are chemically and physically incompatible. If other drugs must be given I.V., temporarily stop infusion of primary drug.
- Oral aminoglycoside may be absorbed systemically in patients with ulcerative GI lesions; significant absorption may endanger patients with decreased renal function.

Oral and parenteral administration

- Too-rapid I.V. administration may cause neuromuscular blockade. Infuse I.V. drug continuously or intermittently over 30 to 60 minutes for adults, 1 to 2 hours for infants; dilution volume for children is determined individually.
- Solutions should always be clear, colorless to pale yellow (in most cases, darkening indicates deterioration), and free of particles; do not give solutions containing precipitates or other foreign matter.
- Amikacin, gentamicin (without preservatives), kanamycin, and tobramycin have been administered intrathecally or intraventricularly. Some clinicians prefer intraventricular administration to ensure adequate CSF levels in the treatment of ventriculitis.

Patient education

- Tell patient signs and symptoms of hypersensitivity and other adverse reactions to aminoglycosides.
- Teach signs and symptoms of bacterial or fungal superinfection to elderly and debilitated patients and others with low resistance from immunosuppressants or irradiation; emphasize need to report them promptly.

Geriatric use

- Elderly patients often have decreased renal function and, thus, are at greater risk for nephrotoxicity; they often require lower drug dosage and longer dosing intervals. They are also susceptible to ototoxicity and superinfection.

Pediatric use

- Half-life of aminoglycosides is prolonged in neonates and premature infants because of immaturity of their renal systems; dosage alterations may be necessary in infants and children.

Breast-feeding

- Recommend an alternative feeding method during therapy.

Representative combinations

Neomycin with polymyxin B sulfates and bacitracin: Neosporin, Mycitracin, Foille Plus; with polymyxin B sulfates and gramicidin: Neosporin; with polymyxin B sulfates and hydrocortisone: Cortisporin, Drotic, Octicair, Otocort; with dexamethasone sodium phosphate: Neo-Decadron; with flurandrenolide: Cordran SP.

See also *topical adrenocorticoids.*

androgens

danazol, fluoxymesterone, methyltestosterone, testosterone, testosterone cypionate, testosterone enanthate, testosterone propionate, testosterone transdermal system

Testosterone is the endogenous androgen (male sex hormone). The testosterone esters (cypionate, enanthate, propionate), methyltestosterone, and fluoxymesterone are synthetic derivatives with greater potency or longer duration of action than testosterone.

Pharmacology

Testosterone promotes maturation of the male sexual organs and the development of secondary sexual characteristics (facial and body hair, vocal cord thickening). Testosterone also causes the growth spurt of adolescence and terminates growth of the long bones by closing the epiphyses (growth plates at the ends of bones). Testosterone promotes retention of calcium, nitrogen, phosphorus, sodium, and potassium and enhances anabolism (tissue building). Through negative feedback on the pituitary, exogenously administered testosterone (and other androgenic drugs) decreases endogenous testosterone production and to some degree inhibits spermatogenesis in males. Androgens repeatedly stimulate production of erythrocytes, apparently by enhancing the production of erythropoietic stimulating factor.

Clinical indications and actions

Androgen deficiency

Androgens (testosterone, all testosterone esters, methyltestosterone, fluoxymesterone) are indicated to treat androgen deficiency resulting from testicular failure or castration, or gonadotropin or luteinizing hormone releasing hormone deficiency of pituitary origin. Methyltestosterone and testosterone cypionate are also indicated to treat male climacteric symptoms and impotence when these are caused by androgen deficiency.

Delayed male puberty

All androgens may be used to stimulate the onset of puberty when it is significantly delayed and psychological support proves insufficient.

Breast cancer

Testosterone, all testosterone esters, and fluoxymesterone are indicated for palliative treatment of metastatic breast cancer in women during the first 5 postmenopausal years. Androgens also may be used in premenopausal women with metastatic disease if the tumor is hormone-responsive.

Postpartum breast engorgement

Fluoxymesterone, testosterone, methyltestosterone, and testosterone propionate are indicated to treat painful postpartum breast engorgement in non-breast-feeding women.

Hereditary angioedema

Danazol is indicated in the prophylaxis of angioedema attacks.

Endometriosis

Danazol is indicated for palliative treatment of endometriosis. Danazol relieves pain and helps resolve endometrial lesions in 30% to 80% of patients who receive it. Endometriosis usually recurs 8 to 12 months after danazol is discontinued.

Fibrocystic breast disease

Danazol is indicated for palliative treatment of fibrocystic breast disease unresponsive to simple therapy. It usually relieves pain before it reduces nodularity. Fibrocystic breast disease recurs in about half of patients treated successfully with danazol, usually 1 year after discontinuing the drug.

Overview of adverse reactions

The most common adverse effects associated with androgen therapy are extensions of the hormonal action. In males, frequent and prolonged erections, bladder irritability (causing frequent urination), and gynecomastia (swelling or tenderness of breast tissue) may occur. In females, clitoral enlargement, deepening of the voice, growth of facial or body hair, unusual hair loss, and irregular or absent menses may occur. Note that virilization, including hirsutism, deepening of voice, or clitoral enlargement may be irreversible even with prompt discontinuation of the drug. Oily skin or acne occurs commonly in both sexes.

Metabolic adverse effects include retention of fluid and electrolytes (occasionally resulting in edema), increased serum calcium levels (hypercalcemia may occur, especially in women receiving the drug for breast cancer metastatic to bone), decreased blood glucose levels, and increased serum cholesterol levels.

Long-term administration of androgens may cause loss of libido and suppression of spermatogenesis in males. Serious, although rare, hepatic dysfunction, including hepatic necrosis and hepatocellular carcinoma, has been reported in prolonged androgen administration.

☑ Special considerations

- Do not administer androgens to males with breast or prostatic cancer, or symptomatic prostatic hypertrophy; to patients with severe cardiac, renal, or hepatic disease; or to patients with undiagnosed abnormal genital bleeding.
- Do not administer androgens during pregnancy because they may cause masculinization of female fetus.
- Hypercalcemia symptoms may be difficult to distinguish from symptoms of the condition being treated unless anticipated and thought of as a cluster. Hypercalcemia is most likely to occur in women with breast cancer, particularly when metastatic to bone.
- Priapism in males indicates that dosage is excessive.
- Yellowing of the sclera of the eyes or of skin may indicate hepatic dysfunction resulting from administration of androgens.

Patient education

- Warn patient against using androgens to improve athletic performance. Androgens are now classified as Schedule III controlled substances and their distribution is regulated by the Drug Enforcement Agency.
- Tell patient to report GI upset.
- Tell patient that virilization, including hirsutism, deepening of voice, or clitoral enlargement, may not be reversible.
- Explain to female patients that medication may cause menstrual cycle irregularities in premenopausal women and withdrawal bleeding in postmenopausal women.

Geriatric use

- Elderly male patients receiving androgens may be at increased risk for prostatic hypertrophy and prostatic carcinoma. Androgens are contraindicated in the presence of prostatic hypertrophy with obstruction because they can aggravate this condition.

Pediatric use

- Observe children receiving androgens carefully for excessive virilization and precocious puberty. Androgen therapy may cause premature epiphyseal closure and short stature. Regular X-ray examinations of hand bones may be used to monitor skeletal maturation during therapy.

Breast-feeding

- The degree of androgen excretion in breast milk is unknown. Because androgens may induce premature sexual development (in males) or virilization (in females), women who are receiving androgens should not breast-feed their infants.

Representative combinations

Fluoxymesterone with ethinyl estradiol: Halodrin.

Testosterone cypionate with estradiol cypionate: De-Comberol, depAndrogyn, Depo-Testadiol, Depotestogen, Duo-Cyp, Duratestin, Menoject-L.A., Test-Estro Cypionate.

Testosterone enanthate with estradiol valerate: Andrest 90-4, Andro-Estro 90-4, Androgyn L.A., Duo-Gen L.A., Duogex L.A.*, Neo-Pause*, Teev, Valertest No. 1.

angiotensin-converting enzyme (ACE) inhibitors

benazepril hydrochloride, captopril, enalapril maleate, fosinopril sodium, lisinopril, moexipril hydrochloride, quinapril hydrochloride, ramipril, trandolapril

ACE inhibitors are used to manage hypertension, and most are used to treat heart failure. Captopril is indicated for the prevention of diabetic nephropathy, and captopril and lisinopril are useful in improving survival in patients after an MI.

Pharmacology

ACE inhibitors prevent the conversion of angiotensin I to angiotensin II, a potent vasoconstrictor. Besides decreasing vasoconstriction, and thus reducing peripheral arterial resistance, inhibition of angiotensin II decreases adrenocortical secretion of aldosterone. This results in decreased sodium and water retention and extracellular fluid volume.

Clinical indications and actions

Hypertension, heart failure

ACE inhibitors are used to treat hypertension; their antihypertensive effects are secondary to decreased peripheral resistance and decreased sodium and water retention.

ACE inhibitors are used to manage heart failure; they decrease systemic vascular resistance (afterload) and pulmonary capillary wedge pressure (preload). They are also used post-MI to decrease mortality.

Overview of adverse reactions

The most common adverse effects of therapeutic doses of ACE inhibitors are headache, fatigue, hypotension, tachycardia, dysgeusia, proteinuria, hyperkalemia, rash, cough, and angioedema of the face and extremities. Severe hypotension may occur at toxic drug levels. ACE inhibitors should be used cautiously in patients with impaired renal function or serious autoimmune disease, and in patients taking other drugs known to depress WBC count or immune response.

☑ Special considerations

- Discontinue diuretic therapy 2 to 3 days before beginning ACE inhibitor therapy to reduce risk of hypotension; if drug does not adequately control blood pressure, reinstate diuretics.
- Periodically monitor WBC counts.
- Lower dosage is necessary in patients with impaired renal function.
- Use potassium supplements with caution because ACE inhibitors may cause potassium retention.
- Discontinue ACE inhibitors if pregnancy is detected. Drug may harm or cause fetal death during the second or third trimesters.

Patient education

- Tell patient that the agents may cause a dry, persistent, tickling cough; it is reversible when therapy is discontinued.
- Tell patient to report feelings of light-headedness, especially in first few days, so dose can be adjusted; signs of infection such as sore throat and fever because drugs may decrease WBC count; facial swelling or difficulty breathing because drugs may cause angioedema; and loss of taste, which may necessitate discontinuation of drug.
- Advise patient to avoid sudden position changes to minimize orthostatic hypotension.
- Warn patient to seek medical approval before taking OTC cold preparations.
- Tell patient to call if troublesome cough develops.
- Instruct patient to promptly report pregnancy.
- Tell patient not to take potassium-containing salt substitutes without medical approval.

Geriatric use

- Elderly patients may need lower doses because of impaired drug clearance.

Pediatric use

- Safety and efficacy of ACE inhibitors in children have not been established; use only if potential benefit outweighs risk.

Breast-feeding

- Captopril and enalapril are distributed into breast milk. An alternative feeding method is recommended during therapy.

Representative combinations

Captopril with hydrochlorothiazide: Capozide.

Benazepril hydrochloride with amlodipine: Lotrel; with hydrochlorothiazide: Lotensin HCT.

Enalapril with hydrochlorothiazide: Vaseretic.

Lisinopril with hydrochlorothiazide: Prinzide, Zestoretic.

anticholinergics

***Belladonna alkaloids:* atropine sulfate, hyoscyamine sulfate, scopolamine hydrobromide**

***Synthetic quaternary anticholinergics:* glycopyrrolate, ipratropium bromide, mepenzolate bromide, propantheline bromide**

***Tertiary synthetic (antispasmodic) derivative:* dicyclomine hydrochloride, tolterodine tartrate**

***Antiparkinsonian agents:* benztropine mesylate, biperiden hydrochloride, biperiden lactate, trihexyphenidyl hydrochloride**

Anticholinergics are used to treat various spastic conditions, including acute dystonic reactions, muscle rigidity, parkinsonism, and extrapyramidal disorders. They also are used to reverse neuromuscular blockade, to prevent nausea and vomiting resulting from motion sickness, as adjunctive treatment for peptic ulcer disease and other GI disorders, and preoperatively to decrease secretions and block cardiac reflexes. Belladonna alkaloids are naturally occurring anticholinergics that have been used for centuries. Many semisynthetic alkaloids and synthetic anticholinergic compounds are available; however, most offer few advantages over naturally occurring alkaloids.

Pharmacology

Anticholinergics competitively antagonize the actions of acetylcholine and other cholinergic agonists within the parasympathetic nervous system. Lack of specificity for site of action increases the hazard of adverse effects in association with therapeutic effects.

Antispasmodics are structurally similar to anticholinergics; however, their anticholinergic activity usually occurs only at high doses. They are believed to directly relax smooth muscle.

Clinical indications and actions

Hypersecretory conditions

Many anticholinergics (atropine, belladonna leaf, glycopyrrolate, hyoscyamine, levorotatory alkaloids of belladonna, and mepenzolate) are used therapeutically for their antisecretory properties; these properties derive from competitive blockade of cholinergic receptor sites, causing decreased gastric acid secretion, salivation, bronchial secretions, and sweating.

GI tract disorders

Some anticholinergics (atropine, belladonna leaf, glycopyrrolate, hyoscyamine, levorotatory alkaloids of belladonna, mepenzolate, and propantheline), as well as the antispasmodics dicyclomine and oxyphencyclimine, treat spasms and other GI tract disorders. These drugs competitively block acetylcholine's actions at cholinergic receptor sites. Antispasmodics presumably act by a nonspecific, direct spasmolytic action on smooth muscle. These agents are useful in treating pylorospasm, ileitis, and irritable bowel syndrome.

Sinus bradycardia

Atropine is used to treat sinus bradycardia caused by drugs, poisons, or sinus node dysfunction. It blocks normal vagal inhibition of the SA node and causes an increase in heart rate.

Dystonia and parkinsonism

Biperiden, benzotropine, and trihexyphenidyl hydrochloride are used to treat acute dystonic reactions and drug-induced extrapyramidal adverse effects. They act centrally by blocking cholinergic receptor sites, balancing cholinergic activity with dopamine.

Perioperative use

Atropine, glycopyrrolate, and hyoscyamine are used postoperatively with anticholinesterase agents to reverse nondepolarizing neuromuscular blockade. These agents block muscarinic effects of anticholinesterase agents by competitively blocking muscarinic receptor sites.

Atropine, glycopyrrolate, and scopolamine are used preoperatively to decrease secretions and block cardiac vagal reflexes. They diminish secretions by competitively inhibiting muscarinic receptor sites; they block cardiac vagal reflexes by preventing normal vagal inhibition of the SA node.

Motion sickness

Scopolamine is effective in preventing nausea and vomiting associated with motion sickness. Its exact mechanism of action is unknown, but it is thought to affect neural pathways originating in the labyrinth of the ear.

Overview of adverse reactions

Dry mouth, decreased sweating or anhidrosis, headache, mydriasis, blurred vision, cycloplegia, urinary hesitancy and retention, constipation, palpitations, and tachycardia most commonly occur with therapeutic doses and usually disappear once the drug is discontinued. Signs of drug toxicity include CNS signs resembling psychosis (disorientation, confusion, hallucinations, delusions, anxiety, agitation, and restlessness) and such peripheral effects as dilated, nonreactive pupils; blurred vision; hot, dry, flushed skin; dry mucous membranes; dysphagia; decreased or absent bowel sounds; urine retention; hyperthermia; tachycardia; hypertension; and increased respiration.

☑ Special considerations

- Monitor patient's vital signs, urine output, visual changes, and for signs of impending toxicity.
- Constipation may be relieved by stool softeners or bulk laxatives.
- The safety of anticholinergic therapy during pregnancy has not been determined. Use by pregnant women is indicated only when drug's benefits outweigh potential risks to the fetus.

Patient education

- Teach patient how and when to take drug.
- Warn patient to avoid driving and other hazardous tasks if he experiences dizziness, drowsiness, or blurred vision.
- Advise patient to avoid alcoholic beverages, because they may cause additive CNS effects.
- Advise patient to consume plenty of fluids and dietary fiber to help avoid constipation.
- Tell patient to promptly report dry mouth, blurred vision, rash, eye pain, or significant changes in urine volume, or pain or difficulty on urination.
- Warn patient that drug may cause increased sensitivity or intolerance to high temperatures, resulting in dizziness.
- Instruct patient to report confusion and rapid or pounding heartbeat.
- Advise female patient to report pregnancy or intent to conceive.
- Warn patient to avoid OTC agents such as Benadryl or Nytol (also have anticholinergic activity).

Geriatric use

- Administer cautiously to elderly patients. Lower doses are usually indicated. Patients over age 40 may be more sensitive to the effects of these drugs.

Pediatric use

- Safety and effectiveness have not been established.

Breast-feeding

- Some anticholinergics may be excreted in breast milk, possibly resulting in infant toxicity. Breast-feeding women should avoid these drugs. Anticholinergics may decrease milk production.

Representative combinations

Atropine with meperidine: Atropine/Demerol injection; with scopolamine hydrobromide (hyoscine hydrobromide), hyoscyamine sulfate, and phenobarbital: Antispasmodic Elixir, Donnatal No. 2, Phenobarbital with Belladonna Alkaloids Elixir, Bellalphen, Donnatal, Haponal, Kinesed, Spasmolin; with scopolamine hydrobromide (hyoscine hydrobromide), hyoscyamine sulfate, kaolin, pectin, sodium benzoate, alcohol, and powdered opium: Donnagel-PG; with phenazopyridine, hyoscyamine, and scopolamine: Urogesic; with hyoscyamine, methenamine, phenyl salicylate, methylene blue, and benzoic acid: Urised; with scopalamine hydrobromide, hyoscyamine hydrobromide, and phenobarbital: Barbidonna No. 2 Tablets, Barbidonna Tablets, Belladonna Alkaloids with Phenobarbital Tablets, Barophen, Donnamor, Donnapine, Donnatal Extentabs, Hyosophen Tablets, Malatal Tablets, Spasmophen, Spasquid, Susano.

Belladonna alkaloids with ergotamine tartrate, caffeine, and phenacetin: Wigraine; with phenobarbital: Chardonna-2, Butibel Elixir; with powdered opium: B&O Supprettes No. 15A, B&O Supprettes No. 16A.

Belladonna extract with butabarbital: Butibel.

Hyoscyamine sulfate with phenobarbital: Levsin with Phenobarbital Tablets, Levsin-PB, Bellacane Tablets.

antihistamines

astemizole, azelastine hydrochloride, brompheniramine maleate, cetirizine hydrochloride, chlorpheniramine maleate, clemastine fumarate, cyclizine hydrochloride, cyclizine lactate, cyproheptadine hydrochloride, dimenhydrinate, diphenhydramine hydrochloride, loratadine, meclizine hydrochloride, promethazine hydrochloride, trimeprazine tartrate, triprolidine hydrochloride

Antihistamines, synthetically produced H_1-receptor antagonists, were discovered in the late 1930s and proliferated rapidly during the next decade. They have many applications related specifically to chemical structure, their widespread use testifying to their versatility and relative safety. Some antihistamines are used primarily to treat rhinitis or pruritus, whereas others are used more often for their antiemetic and antivertigo effects; still others are used as sedative-hypnotics, local anesthetics, and antitussives.

Pharmacology

Antihistamines are structurally related chemicals that compete with histamine for H_1-receptor sites on the smooth muscle of the bronchi, GI tract, uterus, and large blood vessels, binding to the cellular receptors and preventing access and subsequent activity of histamine. They do not directly alter histamine or prevent its release.

Clinical indications and actions

Allergy

Most antihistamines (azelastine, brompheniramine, chlorpheniramine, clemastine, cyproheptadine, diphenhydramine, promethazine, and triprolidine) are used to treat allergic symptoms, such as rhinitis and urticaria. By preventing access of histamine to H_1-receptor sites, they suppress histamine-induced allergic symptoms.

Pruritus

Cyproheptadine, hydroxyzine, methdilazine, and trimeprazine are used systemically. It is believed that these drugs counteract histamine-induced pruritus by a combination of peripheral effects on nerve endings and local anesthetic and sedative activity.

Diphenhydramine is used topically to relieve itching associated with minor skin irritation. Structurally related to local anesthetics, this compound prevents initiation and transmission of nerve impulses.

Vertigo, nausea, and vomiting

Cyclizine, dimenhydrinate, and meclizine are used only as antiemetic and antivertigo agents; their antihistaminic activity has not been evaluated. Diphenhydramine and promethazine are used as antiallergic and antivertigo agents and as antiemetics and antinauseants. Although the mechanisms are not fully understood, antiemetic and antivertigo effects probably result from central antimuscarinic activity.

Sedation

Diphenhydramine and promethazine are used for their sedative action; the mechanism of antihistamine-induced CNS depression is unknown.

Suppression of cough

Diphenhydramine syrup is used as an antitussive. The cough reflex is suppressed by a direct effect on the medullary cough center.

Dyskinesia

The central antimuscarinic action of diphenhydramine reduces drug-induced dyskinesias and parkinsonism through inhibition of acetylcholine (anticholinergic effect).

Overview of adverse reactions

At therapeutic dosage levels, all antihistamines except astemizole and loratadine are likely to cause drowsiness and impaired motor function during initial therapy. Also, their anticholinergic action usually causes dry mouth and throat, blurred vision, and constipation. Antihistamines that are also phenothiazines such as promethazine may cause other adverse effects, including cholestatic jaundice (thought to be a hypersensitivity reaction) and may predispose patients to photosensitivity; patients taking such drugs should avoid prolonged exposure to sunlight.

Toxic doses elicit a combination of CNS depression and excitation as well as atropine-like symptoms, including sedation, reduced mental alertness, apnea, CV collapse, hallucinations, tremors, seizures, dry mouth, flushed skin, and fixed, dilated pupils. Toxic effects reverse when medication is discontinued. Used appropriately, in correct dosages, antihistamines are safe for prolonged use.

☑ Special considerations

- Do not use antihistamines during an acute asthma attack because they may not alleviate the symptoms, and antimuscarinic effects can cause thickening of secretions.
- Use antihistamines with caution in elderly patients and in those with increased intraocular pressure, hyperthyroidism, CV or renal disease, diabetes, hypertension, bronchial asthma, urine retention, prostatic hypertrophy, bladder neck obstruction, or stenosing peptic ulcers.
- Monitor blood counts during long-term therapy; watch for signs of blood dyscrasias.
- Reduce GI distress by giving antihistamines with food; give sugarless gum, sour hard candy, or ice chips to relieve dry mouth; increase fluid intake (if allowed) or humidify air to decrease adverse effect of thickened secretions.
- If tolerance develops to one antihistamine, another may be substituted.
- Know that some antihistamines may mask ototoxicity from high doses of aspirin and other salicylates.
- Astemizole may cause QT interval prolongation and ventricular arrhythmias in patients receiving concomitant therapy with ketoconazole, itraconazole, or erythromycin.

Patient education

- Advise patient to take drug with meals or snack to prevent gastric upset and to use any of the following measures to relieve dry mouth: warm water rinses, artificial saliva, ice chips, or sugarless gum or candy. He should avoid overusing mouthwash, which may add to dryness (alcohol content) and destroy normal flora.
- Warn patient to avoid hazardous activities, such as driving a car or operating machinery, until extent of CNS effects are known and to seek medical approval before using alcoholic beverages, tranquilizers, sedatives, pain relievers, or sleeping medications.
- Warn patient to stop taking antihistamines 4 days before diagnostic skin tests, to preserve accuracy of tests.

Geriatric use

- Elderly patients are usually more sensitive to adverse effects of antihistamines and are especially likely to experience a greater degree of dizziness, sedation, hypotension, and urine retention.

Pediatric use

- Children, especially those under age 6, may experience paradoxical hyperexcitability with restlessness, insomnia, nervousness, euphoria, tremors, and seizures.

Breast-feeding

- Antihistamines should not be used during breast-feeding.

Representative combinations

Carbinoxamine maleate with pseudoephedrine and dextromethorphan: Carbodec DM, Pseudo-Car DM, Rondec-DM, Tussafed; with pseudoephedrine hydrochloride: Rondec, Rondec-TR; with pseudoephedrine and guaifenesin: Brexin L.A.

Chlorpheniramine with phenylephrine and phenylpropanolamine: Naldecon; with dextromethorphan: Vicks Formula 44 Cough Mixture; with codeine and guaifenesin: Tussar SF; with acetaminophen: Coricidin Tablets; with pseudoephedrine and dextromethorphan: Rhinosyn-DM; with pseudoephedrine, dextromethorphan, and acetaminophen: Co-Apap; with phenylpropanolamine: Contac 12-hour, Ornade, Resaid S.R., Triaminic-12, Dura-Vent; with pseudoephedrine hydrochloride: Cophene No. 2, Rescon Capsules, Chlordrine S.R., Chlorphendrine SR, Colfed-A, Duralex, Klerist-D, Kronofed-A, N-D Clear, Pseudo-Clor, Rescon-ED, Time-Hist, Chlorpheniramine Maleate/Pseudoephedrine HCl.

Diphenhydramine with pseudoephedrine: Benadryl Decongestant, Benylin DM; with acetaminophen: Tylenol Severe Allergy.

Promethazine with codeine: Phenergan with codeine; with dextromethorphan: Phenergan with Dextromethorphan; with phenylephrine: Phenergan VC; with phenylephrine and codeine: Phenergan VC with codeine.

Pyrilamine maleate with codeine: Tricodene Cough and Cold; with phenylephrine and codeine; Codimal; with phenylephrine and dextromethorphan: Codimal DM; with phenylephrine, dextromethorphan, and acetaminophen: Robitussin Night Relief; with phenylephrine and hydrocodone: Codimal; with phenylpropanolamine, chlorpheniramine maleate, and dextromethorphan: Tricodene Forte, Tricodene NN, Triminol Cough.

Triprolidine with pseudoephedrine and codeine: Actifed with Codeine, CoActifed*, Pseudodine C Cough; with pseudoephedrine: Actagen, Actifed, Allerfrin, Novafed, Triacin-C, Triafed with Codeine, Trifed-C, Trifed-C Cough, Triofed, Triposed.

barbiturates

amobarbital, amobarbital sodium, butabarbital sodium, mephobarbital, phenobarbital, pentobarbital sodium, phenobarbital sodium, primidone, secobarbital sodium

Barbituric acid was compounded more than 100 years ago in 1864. The first hypnotic barbiturate, barbital, was introduced into medicine in 1903. Although barbiturates have been used extensively as sedative-hypnotics and antianxiety agents, benzodiazepines are the current drugs of choice for sedative-hypnotic effects. Phenobarbital remains an effective anticonvulsant therapy. A few short-acting barbiturates are used as general anesthetics.

Pharmacology

Barbiturates are structurally related compounds that act throughout the CNS, particularly in the mesencephalic reticular activating system, which controls the CNS arousal mechanism. Barbiturates decrease both presynaptic and postsynaptic membrane excitability.

The exact mechanism(s) of action of barbiturates at these sites is not known, nor is it clear which cellular and synaptic actions result in sedative-hypnotic effects. Barbiturates can produce all levels of CNS depression, from mild sedation to coma to death. Barbiturates exert their effects by facilitating the actions of gamma-aminobutyric acid (GABA). Barbiturates also exert a central effect, which depresses respiration and GI motility. The principal anticonvulsant mechanism of action is reduction of nerve transmission and decreased excitability of the nerve cell. Barbiturates also raise the seizure threshold.

Clinical indications and actions

Seizure disorders

Phenobarbital is used in the prophylactic treatment and acute management of seizure disorders. It is used mainly in tonic-clonic (grand mal) and partial seizures. At anesthetic doses, all barbiturates have anticonvulsant activity. Phenobarbital is an effective parenteral agent for status epilepticus (with airway support).

Barbiturates suppress the spread of seizure activity produced by epileptogenic foci in the cortex, thalamus, and limbic systems by enhancing the effects of GABA.

Sedation, hypnosis

Most currently available barbiturates are used as sedative-hypnotics for short-term (up to 2 weeks) treatment of insomnia because of their nonspecific CNS effects.

Barbiturates are not used routinely as sedatives. Barbiturate-induced sleep differs from physiologic sleep by decreasing the rapid-eye-movement sleep cycles.

Preanesthesia sedation

Barbiturates are also used as preanesthetic sedatives.

Overview of adverse reactions

Drowsiness, lethargy, vertigo, headache, and CNS depression are common with barbiturates. After hypnotic doses, a hangover effect, subtle distortion of mood, and impairment of judgment or motor skills may continue for many hours. After a decrease in dosage or discontinuation of barbiturates used for hypnosis, rebound insomnia or increased dreaming or nightmares may occur. Barbiturates cause hyperalgesia in subhypnotic doses. Hypersensitivity reactions (rash, fever, serum sickness) are not common, and are more likely to occur in patients with a history of asthma or allergies to other drugs; reactions include urticaria, rash, angioedema, and Stevens-Johnson syndrome. Barbiturates can cause paradoxical excitement at low doses, confusion in elderly patients, and hyperactivity in children. High fever, severe headache, stomatitis, conjunctivitis, or rhinitis may precede skin eruptions. Because of the potential for fatal consequences, discontinue barbiturates if dermatologic reactions occur.

Withdrawal symptoms may occur after as little as 2 weeks of uninterrupted therapy. Symptoms of abstinence usually occur within 8 to 12 hours after the last dose, but may be delayed up to 5 days. They include weakness, anxiety, nausea, vomiting, insomnia, hallucinations, and possibly seizures.

☑ Special considerations

- Dosage of barbiturates must be individualized.
- Parenteral solutions are highly alkaline and contain organic solvents (propylene glycol); infuse at 100 mg/minute or less; avoid extravasation, which may cause local tissue damage and tissue necrosis; inject I.V. or deep I.M. only. Do not exceed 5 ml per I.M. injection site to avoid tissue damage.
- Too-rapid I.V. administration of barbiturates may cause respiratory depression, apnea, laryngospasm, or hypotension. Have resuscitative measures available. Assess I.V. site for signs of infiltration or phlebitis.
- Drug may be given P.R. if oral or parenteral route is inappropriate.
- Assess level of consciousness before and frequently during therapy to evaluate effectiveness of drug. Monitor neurologic status for possible alterations or deteriorations. Monitor seizure character, frequency, and du-

ration for changes. Institute seizure precautions, as necessary.
- Check vital signs frequently, especially during I.V. administration.
- Assess patient's sleeping patterns before and during therapy to ensure effectiveness of drug.
- Institute safety measures—side rails, assistance when out of bed, call light within reach—to prevent falls and injury.
- Consider airway support during I.V. administration.
- Anticipate possible rebound confusion and excitatory reactions in patient.
- Assess bowel elimination patterns; monitor for complaints of constipation. Advise diet high in fiber, if indicated.
- Monitor PT carefully in patients taking anticoagulants; dosage of anticoagulant may require adjustment to counteract possible interaction.
- Abrupt discontinuation may cause withdrawal symptoms; discontinue slowly.
- Death is common with an overdose of 2 to 10 g; it may occur at much smaller doses if alcohol is also ingested.
- Avoid administering barbiturates to patients with status asthmaticus.
- Barbiturates should be used cautiously, if at all, in patients who are mentally depressed or have suicidal tendencies or history of drug abuse.

Patient education
- Warn patient to avoid concurrent use of other drugs with CNS depressant effects, such as antihistamines, analgesics, and alcohol, because they will have additive effects and result in increased drowsiness. Instruct patient to seek medical approval before taking OTC cold or allergy preparations.
- Caution patient not to change dose or frequency without medical approval; abrupt discontinuation of medication may trigger rebound insomnia, with increased dreaming, nightmares, or seizures.
- Warn patient against driving and other hazardous tasks that require alertness while taking barbiturates. Instruct him in safety measures to prevent injury.
- Be sure patient understands that barbiturates are capable of causing physical or psychological dependence (addiction), and that these effects may be transmitted to the fetus; withdrawal symptoms can occur in neonates whose mothers took barbiturates in the third trimester.
- Instruct patient to report skin eruption or other marked adverse effect.
- Explain that a morning hangover is common after therapeutic use of barbiturates.

Geriatric use
- Elderly patients and patients receiving subhypnotic doses may experience hyperactivity, excitement, or hyperalgesia. Use with caution.

Pediatric use
- Premature infants are more susceptible to the depressant effects of barbiturates because of immature hepatic metabolism. Children receiving barbiturates may experience hyperactivity, excitement, or hyperalgia.

Breast-feeding
- Barbiturates are excreted in breast milk and may result in infant CNS depression. Use with caution.

Representative combinations
Amobarbital with secobarbital: Tuinal 100 mg Pulvules, Tuinal 200 mg Pulvules.

Butabarbital with acetaminophen: Sedapap; with belladonna: Butibel.

Phenobarbital with CNS stimulants: Bronkolixir, Bronkotabs, Quadrinal; with ergotamine tartrate: Bellergal-S; with phenytoin: Dilantin Kapseals; with aminophylline and ephedrine hydrochloride: Mudrane; with belladonna: Chardonna-2, Butibel, Butibel Elixir; with atropine: Antrocol; with hyoscyamine: Levsin-PB, Levsin and Phenobarbital, Bellacane; with ASA and codeine phosphate: Phenaphen with Codeine No. 3, Phenaphen with Codeine No. 4; with atropine, hyoscyamine, and scopolamine hydrobromide: Donnatal, Donnatol No. 2, Donnamor, Donnapine, Donnatal Extentabs, Barbidonna, Barophen, Hyosophen, Kinesed, Spasmophen, Spasquid, Susano, Barbidonna No. 2, Belladonna Alkoids with Phenobarbital Tablets, Malatal, Antispasmodic Elixir, Hyoscyamine Compound, Phenobarbital with Belladonna Alkaloids Elixir.

Pentobarbital sodium with ephedrine: Ephedrine and Nembutal Sodium; with ergotamine tartrate and caffeine: Cafergot-PB.

See also *anticholinergics (belladonna alkaloids)*.

benzodiazepines

alprazolam, chlordiazepoxide hydrochloride, clonazepam, clorazepate dipotassium, diazepam, estazolam, flurazepam hydrochloride, lorazepam, midazolam hydrochloride, oxazepam, quazepam, temazepam, triazolam

Benzodiazepines, synthetically produced sedative-hypnotics, gained popularity in the early 1960s, replacing barbiturates as the treatment of choice for anxiety, convulsive disorders, and sedation. These drugs are preferred over barbiturates because therapeutic doses produce less drowsiness, respiratory depression, and impairment of motor function and toxic doses are less likely to be fatal.

Pharmacology
Benzodiazepines are a group of structurally related chemicals that selectively act on polysynaptic neuronal pathways throughout the CNS. Their precise sites and mechanisms of action are not completely known. However, the benzodiazepines enhance or facilitate the action of gamma-aminobutyric acid (GABA), an inhibitory neurotransmitter in the CNS. All of the benzodiazepines have CNS-depressant activities; however, individual derivatives act more selectively at specific sites, allowing them to be subclassified into five categories based on their predominant clinical use.

Clinical indications and actions
Seizure disorders
Four of the benzodiazepines (diazepam, clonazepam, clorazepate, and parenteral lorazepam) are used as anticonvulsants. Their anticonvulsant properties are derived from an ability to suppress the spread of seizure activity produced by epileptogenic foci in the cortex, thalamus, and limbic systems by enhancing presynaptic inhibition. Clonazepam is useful in the adjunctive treatment of petit mal variant (Lennox-Gastaut syndrome), myoclonic, or akinetic seizures. Parenteral diazepam is indicated to treat status epilepticus.

Anxiety, tension, and insomnia
Most benzodiazepines (alprazolam, chlordiazepoxide, clorazepate, diazepam, estazolam, flurazepam, lorazepam, oxazepam, quazepam, temazepam, and tri-

azolam) are useful as antianxiety agents or sedative-hypnotic agents. They have a similar mechanism of action: they are believed to facilitate the effects of GABA in the ascending reticular activating system, increasing inhibition and blocking both cortical and limbic arousal.

They are used to treat anxiety and tension that occur alone or as an adverse effect of a primary disorder. They are not recommended for tension associated with everyday stress. The choice of a specific benzodiazepine depends on individual metabolic characteristics of the drug. For instance, in patients with depressed renal or hepatic function, alprazolam, lorazepam, or oxazepam may be selected because they have a relatively short duration of action and have no active metabolites.

The sedative-hypnotic properties of chlordiazepoxide, clorazepate, diazepam, lorazepam, and oxazepam make these the drugs of choice as preoperative medication and as an adjunct in the rehabilitation of alcoholics.

Surgical adjuncts for conscious sedation or amnesia

Diazepam, midazolam, and lorazepam have amnesic effects. The mechanism of such action is not known. Parenteral administration before such procedures as endoscopy or elective cardioversion causes impairment of recent memory and interferes with the establishment of memory trace, producing anterograde amnesia.

Skeletal muscle spasm, tremor

Because oral forms of diazepam and chlordiazepoxide have skeletal muscle relaxant properties, they are often used to treat neurologic conditions involving muscle spasms and tetanus. The mechanism of such action is unknown, but they are believed to inhibit spinal polysynaptic and monosynaptic afferent pathways.

Overview of adverse reactions

Therapeutic dosage of the benzodiazepines usually causes drowsiness and impaired motor function, which should be monitored early in treatment. It may or may not be persistent. GI discomfort, such as constipation, diarrhea, vomiting, and changes in appetite, with urinary alterations also have been reported. Visual disturbances and CV irregularities also are common. Continuing problems with short-term memory, confusion, severe depression, shakiness, vertigo, slurred speech, staggering, bradycardia, shortness of breath or difficulty breathing, and severe weakness usually indicate a toxic dose level. Prolonged or frequent use of benzodiazepines can cause physical dependency and withdrawal syndrome when use is discontinued.

☑ Special considerations

- Assess level of consciousness and neurologic status before and frequently during therapy for changes. Monitor for paradoxical reactions, especially early in therapy.
- Assess sleep patterns and quality. Institute seizure precautions. Assess for changes in seizure character, frequency, or duration.
- Assess vital signs frequently during therapy. Significant changes in blood pressure and heart rate may indicate impending toxicity.
- Administer with milk or immediately after meals to prevent GI upset. Give antacid, if needed, at least 1 hour before or after dose to prevent interaction and ensure maximum drug absorption and effectiveness.
- Monitor renal and hepatic function periodically to ensure adequate drug removal and prevent cumulative effects.
- As needed, institute safety measures—raised side rails and ambulatory assistance—to prevent injury. Anticipate possible rebound excitement reactions.
- After prolonged use, abrupt discontinuation may cause withdrawal symptoms; discontinue gradually.

Patient education

- Warn to avoid use of alcohol or other CNS depressants, such as antihistamines, analgesics, MAO inhibitors, antidepressants, and barbiturates, to prevent additive depressant effects.
- Caution patient to take drug as prescribed and not to give medication to others. Tell him not to change the dose or frequency and to call before taking OTC cold or allergy preparations that may potentiate CNS depressant effects.
- Warn patient to avoid activities requiring alertness and good psychomotor coordination until the CNS response to the drug is determined. Instruct him in safety measures to prevent injury.
- Tell patient to avoid using antacids, which may delay drug absorption, unless prescribed.
- Be sure patient understands that benzodiazepines are capable of causing physical and psychological dependence with prolonged use.
- Warn patient not to stop taking the drug abruptly to prevent withdrawal symptoms after prolonged therapy.
- Tell patient that smoking decreases drug's effectiveness. Encourage him to stop smoking during therapy.
- Tell patient to report adverse effects. These are often dose-related and can be relieved by dosage adjustments.
- Inform female patient of childbearing age who is taking drug to report if she suspects pregnancy or intends to become pregnant during therapy.

Geriatric use

- Because they are sensitive to their CNS effects, elderly patients receiving benzodiazepines require lower doses. Use with caution.
- Parenteral administration of these drugs is more likely to cause apnea, hypotension, bradycardia, and cardiac arrest in elderly patients.
- Geriatric patients may show prolonged elimination of benzodiazepines, except possibly of oxazepam, lorazepam, temazepam, and triazolam.

Pediatric use

- Because children, particularly very young ones, are sensitive to the CNS depressant effects of benzodiazepines, caution must be exercised. A neonate whose mother took a benzodiazepine during pregnancy may exhibit withdrawal symptoms.
- Use of benzodiazepines during labor may cause neonatal flaccidity.

Breast-feeding

- The breast-fed infant of a mother who uses a benzodiazepine drug may show sedation, feeding difficulties, and weight loss. Safe use has not been established.

Representative combinations

Chlordiazepoxide with amitriptyline hydrochloride: Limbitrol DS; with clidinium bromide: Librax; with esterified estrogens: Menrium.

beta-adrenergic blockers

$beta_1$ blockers: acebutolol, atenolol, betaxolol hydrochloride, bisoprolol, esmolol, metoprolol tartrate

$beta_1$ and $beta_2$ blockers: carteolol hydrochloride, carvedilol, labetalol, levobunolol hydrochloride, metipranolol hydrochloride, nadolol, penbutolol sulfate, pindolol, propranolol, sotalol, timolol maleate

Beta-adrenergic blocking agents were first used in the early 1960s; they are now widely used to treat hypertension, angina pectoris, and arrhythmias. These agents are well tolerated by most patients.

Pharmacology

Beta blockers are chemicals that compete with beta agonists for available beta-receptor sites; individual agents differ in their ability to affect beta receptors. Some available agents are considered nonselective; that is, they block both $beta_1$ receptors in cardiac muscle and $beta_2$ receptors in bronchial and vascular smooth muscle. Several agents are cardioselective and in lower doses primarily inhibit $beta_1$ receptors. Some beta blockers have intrinsic sympathomimetic activity and simultaneously stimulate and block beta receptors, decreasing cardiac output; still others also have membrane-stabilizing activity, which affects cardiac action potential. (See *Comparing beta-adrenergic blockers.*)

Clinical indications and actions

Hypertension

Most beta blockers are used to treat hypertension. Although the exact mechanism of their antihypertensive effect is unknown, the action is thought to result from decreased cardiac output, decreased sympathetic outflow from the CNS, and suppression of renin release.

Angina

Propranolol, atenolol, nadolol, and metoprolol are used to treat angina pectoris; they decrease myocardial oxygen requirements through the blockade of catecholamine-induced increases in heart rate, blood pressure, and the extent of myocardial contraction.

Arrhythmias

Propranolol, acebutolol, sotalol, and esmolol are used to treat arrhythmias; they prolong the refractory period of the AV node and slow AV conduction.

Glaucoma

The mechanism by which betaxolol, levobunolol, metipranolol, and timolol reduce intraocular pressure is unknown, but the drug effect is at least partially caused by decreased production of aqueous humor.

MI

Timolol, propranolol, atenolol, and metoprolol are used to prevent MI in susceptible patients.

Migraine prophylaxis

Propranolol and timolol are used to prevent recurrent attacks of migraine and other vascular headaches. The exact mechanism by which propranolol and timolol decrease the incidence of migraine headache attacks is unknown, but it is thought to result from inhibition of vasodilation of cerebral vessels.

Other uses

Some beta blockers have been used as antianxiety agents, as adjunctive therapy of bleeding esophageal varices or pheochromocytomas, and to treat portal hypertension or essential tremors. Carvedilol is used to treat heart failure with cardiac glycosides, diuretics, or ACE inhibitors.

Overview of adverse reactions

Therapeutic doses may cause bradycardia, fatigue, and dizziness; some cause other CNS disturbances, such as nightmares, depression, memory loss, or hallucinations. Impotence, cold extremities, and elevated cholesterol levels may also occur. Severe hypotension, bradycardia, heart failure, or bronchospasm usually indicates toxic dosage levels.

COMPARING BETA-ADRENERGIC BLOCKERS

DRUG	HALF-LIFE (hr)	LIPID SOLUBILITY	MEMBRANE-STABILIZING ACTIVITY	INTRINSIC SYMPATHOMIMETIC ACTIVITY
Nonselective				
carteolol	6	Low	0	++
carvedilol	7 to 10	High	Not known	0
labetalol	6 to 8	Moderate	0	0
metipranolol	4	Low to moderate	0	0
nadolol	20	Low	0	0
penbutolol	5	High	0	+
pindolol	3 to 4	Moderate	+	+++
propranolol	4	High	++	0
timolol	4	Low to moderate	0	0
$Beta_1$-selective				
acebutolol	3 to 4	Low	+	+
atenolol	6 to 7	Low	0	0
betaxolol	14 to 22	Low	+	0
esmolol	0.15	Low	0	0
metoprolol	3 to 7	Moderate	*	0

* Only in higher-than-usual doses.

☑ Special considerations

- Check apical pulse rate daily. Monitor BP, ECG, and heart rate and rhythm frequently; be alert for progression of AV block or severe bradycardia.
- Weigh patients with heart failure regularly; watch for gains of more than 5 lb (2.27 kg) per week.
- Signs of hypoglycemic shock are masked; watch diabetic patients for sweating, fatigue, and hunger.
- Do not discontinue these drugs before surgery for pheochromocytoma; before any surgical procedure, notify anesthesiologist that patient is taking a beta-adrenergic blocking agent.
- Glucagon may be prescribed to reverse signs and symptoms of beta blocker overdose.
- Do not prescribe for patients with asthma.

Patient education

- Explain rationale for therapy, and emphasize importance of taking as prescribed, even when feeling well.
- Warn patient that abrupt discontinuation can exacerbate angina or precipitate MI.
- Teach patient to minimize dizziness from orthostatic hypotension by taking dose at bedtime, and by rising slowly and avoiding sudden position changes.
- Advise patient to seek medical approval before taking OTC cold preparations.

Geriatric use

- Elderly patients may require lower maintenance doses of beta-adrenergic blocking agents; they also may experience enhanced adverse effects.

Pediatric use

- Safety and efficacy of beta-adrenergic blocking agents in children have not been established; they should be used only if potential benefit outweighs risk.

Breast-feeding

- Beta-adrenergic blocking agents are distributed into breast milk. Recommendations for breast-feeding vary with individual drugs.

Representative combinations

Atenolol with chlorthalidone: Tenoretic.

Bisoprolol with hydrochlorothiazide: Ziac Tablets.

Metoprolol with hydrochlorothiazide: Lopressor HCT.

Pindolol with hydrochlorothiazide: Viskazide.

Propranolol hydrochloride with hydrochlorothiazide: Inderide, Inderide LA.

Timolol with hydrochlorothiazide: Timolide.

calcium channel blockers

amlodipine besylate, bepridil hydrochloride, diltiazem hydrochloride, felodipine, isradipine, nicardipine hydrochloride, nifedipine, nimodipine, nisoldipine, verapamil hydrochloride

Calcium channel blockers (also called slow channel calcium antagonists or slow channel blockers) were introduced in the United States in the early 1980s. They have become increasingly popular as a treatment for classic and variant angina and are now the preferred drugs for Prinzmetal's variant angina (vasospastic angina). They have been used as antihypertensives. Verapamil has proved effective in the acute treatment of supraventricular tachycardias (SVTs). (See *Comparing oral calcium channel blockers.*)

Pharmacology

The main physiologic action of calcium channel blockers is to inhibit calcium influx across the slow channels of myocardial and vascular smooth muscle cells. By inhibiting calcium influx into these cells, calcium channel blockers reduce intracellular calcium concentrations. This, in turn, dilates coronary arteries, peripheral arteries, and arterioles, and slows cardiac conduction.

When used to treat Prinzmetal's variant angina, calcium channel blockers inhibit coronary spasm, increasing oxygen delivery to the heart. Peripheral artery dilation leads to a decrease in total peripheral resistance; this reduces afterload, which, in turn, decreases myocardial oxygen consumption. Inhibition of calcium influx into the specialized cardiac conduction cells (specifically, those in the SA and AV nodes) slows conduction through the heart. This effect is most pronounced with verapamil and diltiazem.

Clinical indications and actions

Angina

Calcium channel blockers are useful in managing Prinzmetal's variant angina, chronic stable angina, and unstable angina. In Prinzmetal's variant angina, they inhibit spontaneous and ergonovine-induced coronary spasm, thereby increasing coronary blood flow and maintaining myocardial oxygen delivery. In unstable and chronic stable angina, their effectiveness presumably stems from their ability to reduce afterload.

Arrhythmias

Of the calcium channel blockers, verapamil and diltiazem have the greatest effect on the AV node, slowing the ventricular rate in atrial fibrillation or flutter and converting SVT to normal sinus rhythm.

Hypertension

Because they dilate systemic arteries, most of these agents are useful in mild to moderate hypertension.

Other uses

Calcium channel blockers (especially verapamil) may also prove to be effective as a hypertrophic cardiomyopathy therapy adjunct by improving left ventricular outflow as a result of negative inotropic effects and possibly improved diastolic function. They have been used to treat migraine headaches, peripheral vascular disorders, and as adjunctive therapy in the treatment of esophageal spasm.

Overview of adverse reactions

Verapamil may cause adverse effects on the conduction system, including bradycardia and various degrees of heart block, exacerbate heart failure and hypotension after rapid I.V. administration. Prolonged oral verapamil therapy may cause constipation.

Adverse effects of nifedipine include hypotension, reflex tachycardia, peripheral edema, flushing, lightheadedness, and headache.

Diltiazem most commonly causes anorexia, nausea, various degrees of heart block, bradycardia, heart failure, and peripheral edema.

☑ Special considerations

- Monitor cardiac rate and rhythm and blood pressure carefully when initiating therapy or increasing dose.
- Concomitant use of calcium supplements may decrease the effectiveness of calcium channel blockers.
- Use cautiously in patients with impaired left ventricular function.

Patient education

- Tell patient not to abruptly discontinue drug; gradual dosage reduction may be necessary.

COMPARING ORAL CALCIUM CHANNEL BLOCKERS

DRUG	ONSET OF ACTION	PEAK SERUM LEVEL	HALF-LIFE	THERAPEUTIC SERUM LEVEL
bepridil	1 hr	2 to 3 hr	24 hr	1 to 2 ng/ml
diltiazem	15 min	30 min	3 to 4 hr	50 to 200 ng/ml
felodipine	2 to 5 hr	2.5 to 5 hr	11 to 16 hr	Unknown
nicardipine	20 min	1 hr	8.6 hr	28 to 50 ng/ml
nifedipine	5 to 30 min	30 min to 2 hr	2 to 5 hr	25 to 100 ng/ml
nimodipine	Unknown	< 1 hr	1 to 2 hr	Unknown
verapamil	30 min	1 to 2.2 hr	6 to 12 hr	80 to 300 ng/ml

- Instruct patient to report irregular heartbeat, shortness of breath, swelling of hands and feet, pronounced dizziness, constipation, nausea, or hypotension.
- Warn patient not to double dose.

Geriatric use

- Use with caution because the half-life of calcium channel blockers may be increased as a result of decreased clearance.

Pediatric use

- Adverse hemodynamic effects of parenteral verapamil have been observed in neonates and infants. Safety and effectiveness of diltiazem and nifedipine have not been established.

Breast-feeding

- Calcium channel blocking agents (verapamil and diltiazem) may be excreted in breast milk. To avoid possible adverse effects in infants, breast-feeding should be discontinued during therapy with these drugs.

Representative combinations

Amlodipine and benazepril hydrochloride: Lotrel.

cephalosporins

First-generation cephalosporins: **cefadroxil, cefazolin sodium, cephalexin monohydrate, cephalothin sodium, cephradine**

Second-generation cephalosporins: **cefaclor, cefamandole nafate, cefmetazole sodium, cefonicid sodium, cefotetan disodium, cefoxitin sodium, cefprozil, ceftibuten, cefuroxime axetil, cefuroxime sodium**

Third-generation cephalosporins: **cefdinir, cefixime, cefoperazone sodium, cefotaxime sodium, cefpodoxime proxetil, ceftazidime, ceftizoxime sodium, ceftriaxone sodium**

Fourth-generation cephalosporin: **cefepime hydrochloride**

Cephalosporins are beta-lactam antibiotics first isolated in 1948 from the fungus *Cephalosporium acremonium.* Their mechanism of action is similar to that of penicillins, but their antibacterial spectra differ.

Pharmacology

Cephalosporins are chemically and pharmacologically similar to penicillin; their structure contains a beta-lactam ring, a dihydrothiazine ring, and side chains, and they act by inhibiting bacterial cell wall synthesis, causing rapid cell lysis. (See *Comparing cephalosporins,* page 1122.)

The sites of action for cephalosporins are enzymes known as penicillin-binding proteins (PBP). The affinity of certain cephalosporins for PBP in various microorganisms helps explain the differing spectra of activity in this class of antibiotics.

Bacterial resistance to beta-lactam antibiotics is conferred most significantly by production of beta-lactamase enzymes (by both gram-negative and gram-positive bacteria) that destroy the beta-lactam ring and thus inactivate cephalosporins; decreased cell wall permeability and alteration in binding affinity to PBP also contribute to bacterial resistance.

Cephalosporins are bactericidal; they act against many gram-positive and gram-negative bacteria, and some anaerobic bacteria; they do not kill fungi or viruses.

First-generation cephalosporins act against many gram-positive cocci, including penicillinase-*producing Staphylococcus aureus* and *S. epidermidis; Streptococcus pneumoniae,* group B streptococci, and group A beta-hemolytic streptococci; susceptible gram-negative organisms include *Klebsiella pneumoniae, Escherichia coli, Proteus mirabilis,* and *Shigella.*

Second-generation cephalosporins are effective against all organisms attacked by first-generation drugs and have additional activity against *Branhamella catarrhalis, Haemophilus influenzae, Enterobacter, Citrobacter, Providencia, Acinetobacter, Serratia,* and *Neisseria; Bacteroides fragilis* is susceptible to cefotetan and cefoxitin.

Third-generation cephalosporins are less active than first- and second-generation drugs against gram-positive bacteria, but more active against gram-negative organisms, including those resistant to first- and second-generation drugs; they have the greatest stability against beta-lactamases produced by gram-negative bacteria. Susceptible gram-negative organisms *include E. coli, Klebsiella, Enterobacter, Providencia, Acinetobacter, Serratia, Proteus, Morganella,* and *Neisseria;* some third-generation drugs are active against *B. fragilis* and *Pseudomonas.*

COMPARING CEPHALOSPORINS

DRUG AND ROUTE	ELIMINATION HALF-LIFE (hr)		SODIUM (mEq/g)	CSF PENETRATION
	NORMAL RENAL FUNCTION	END-STAGE RENAL DISEASE		
cefaclor P.O.	**0.5 to 1**	3 to 5.5	No data available	No
cefadroxil P.O.	1 to 2	20 to 25	No data available	No
cefamandole I.M., I.V.	0.5 to 2	12 to 18	3.3	No
cefazolin I.M., I.V.	1.2 to 2.2	12 to 50	2.0 to 2.1	No
cefepime I.M., I.V.	2	Unknown	No data available	Yes
cefixime P.O.	3 to 4	11.5	No data available	Unknown
cefmetazole I.V.	1.2	Unknown	2	Unknown
cefonicid I.M., I.V.	3.5 to 5.8	100	3.7	No
cefoperazone I.M., I.V.	1.5 to 2.5	3.4 to 7	1.5	Sometimes
cefotaxime I.M., I.V.	1 to 1.5	11.5 to 56	2.2	Yes
cefotetan I.M., I.V.	2.8 to 4.6	13 to 35	3.5	No
cefoxitin I.M., I.V.	0.5 to 1	6.5 to 21.5	2.3	No
cefpodoxime P.O.	2 to 3	9.8	No data available	Unknown
cefprozil P.O.	1 to 1.5	5.2 to 5.9	No data available	Unknown
ceftazidime I.M., I.V.	1.5 to 2	35	2.3	Yes
ceftibuten P.O.	2.4	Unknown	No data available	Unknown
ceftizoxime I.M., I.V.	1.5 to 2	30	2.6	Yes
ceftriaxone I.M., I.V.	5.5 to 11	15.7	3.6	Yes
cefuroxime I.M., I.V.	1 to 2	15 to 22	2.4	Yes
cephalexin P.O.	0.5 to 1	7.5 to 14	No data available	No
cephalothin I.M., I.V.	0.5 to 1	19	2.8	No
cephapirin I.M., I.V.	0.5 to 1	1.0 to 1.5	2.4	No
cephradine P.O., I.M., I.V.	0.5 to 2	8 to 15	6	No

The fourth-generation cephalosporin, cefepime, is active against a wide range of gram-positive and gram-negative bacteria. Susceptible gram-negative organisms include *Enterobacter spp., E. coli, K. pneumoniae, P. mirabilis,* and *Pseudomonas aeruginosa;* susceptible gram-positive organisms include *S. aureus* (methicillin-susceptible strains only), *S. pneumoniae,* and *Streptococcus pyogenes* (Lancefield's Group A streptococci).

Oral absorption of cephalosporins varies widely; many must be given parenterally. Most are distributed widely into the body, the actual amount varying with individual drugs. CSF penetration by first- and second-generation drugs is minimal; third-generation drugs achieve much greater penetration; and although the fourth-generation drug, cefepime, is known to cross the blood-brain barrier, it is not known to what degree. Cephalosporins cross the placenta. Degree of metabolism varies with individual drugs; some are not metabolized at all, and others are extensively metabolized.

Cephalosporins are excreted primarily in urine, chiefly by renal tubular effects; elimination half-life ranges from ½ to 10 hours in patients with normal renal function. Some drug is excreted in breast milk. Most cephalosporins can be removed by hemodialysis or peritoneal dialysis. Patients on dialysis may require dosage adjustment.

Clinical indications and actions

Infection caused by susceptible organisms

Parenteral cephalosporins: Cephalosporins are used to treat serious infections of the lungs, skin, soft tissue, bones, joints, urinary tract, blood (septicemia), abdomen, and heart (endocarditis).

Third-generation cephalosporins (except moxalactam and cefoperazone) and the second-generation drug cefuroxime are used to treat CNS infections caused by susceptible strains of *N. meningitidis, H. influenzae,* and *S. pneumoniae;* meningitis caused by *E. coli* or *Klebsiella* can be treated by ceftriaxone, cefotaxime, or ceftizoxime.

First-generation, and some second-generation, cephalosporins also can be given prophylactically to reduce postoperative infection after surgical procedures classified as contaminated or potentially contaminated; third-generation drugs are not usually indicated.

Penicillinase-producing *N. gonorrhoeae* can be treated with cefoxitin, cefotaxime, ceftriaxone, ceftizoxime, or cefuroxime.

Oral cephalosporins: Cephalosporins can be used to treat otitis media and infections of the respiratory tract, urinary tract, and skin and soft tissue.

Overview of adverse reactions

Hypersensitivity reactions range from mild rash, fever, and eosinophilia to fatal anaphylaxis, and are more common in patients with penicillin allergy. Hematologic reactions include positive direct and indirect antiglobulin (Coombs' test), thrombocytopenia or thrombocythemia, transient neutropenia, reversible leukopenia, adverse renal effects, nausea, vomiting, diarrhea, abdominal pain, glossitis, dyspepsia, tenesmus, and minimal elevation of liver function test results.

Local venous pain and irritation are common after I.M. injection; such reactions occur more often with higher doses and long-term therapy.

Disulfiram-type reactions occur when cefamandole, cefoperazone, moxalactam, cefonicid, or cefotetan are administered within 48 to 72 hours of alcohol ingestion.

Bacterial and fungal superinfection results from suppression of normal flora.

☑ Special considerations

- Review patient's history of allergies.
- Monitor continuously for possible hypersensitivity reactions or other untoward effects.
- Monitor renal function studies; dosages of certain cephalosporins must be lowered in patients with severe renal impairment. In decreased renal function, monitor BUN levels, serum creatinine levels, and urine output for significant changes.
- Monitor PT and platelet counts and assess patient for signs of hypoprothrombinemia, which may occur, with or without bleeding, during therapy with cefamandole, cefepime, cefoperazone, cefonicid, or cefotetan, usually in elderly, debilitated, or malnourished patients.
- Monitor patients on long-term therapy for possible bacterial and fungal superinfection, especially elderly, and debilitated patients, and others receiving immunosuppressants or radiation therapy.
- Monitor susceptible patients receiving sodium salts of cephalosporins for possible fluid retention; consult individual drug entry for sodium content.
- Cephalosporins cause false-positive results in urine glucose tests using cupric sulfate solutions (Benedict's reagent or Clinitest); glucose oxidase tests are not affected. Consult individual drug entries for other possible test interactions.

Administration

- Give cephalosporins at least 1 hour before giving bacteriostatic antibiotics (tetracyclines, erythromycins, and chloramphenicol); these drugs inhibit bacterial cell growth, decreasing cephalosporin uptake by bacterial cell walls.
- Give oral cephalosporin at least 1 hour before or 2 hours after meals for maximum absorption.
- Refrigerate oral suspensions; shake well before administering to assure correct dosage.
- Administer I.M. dose deep into large muscle mass (gluteal or midlateral thigh); rotate injection sites.
- Do not add or mix other drugs with I.V. infusions—particularly aminoglycosides, which will be inactivated if mixed with cephalosporins; if other drugs must be given I.V., temporarily stop infusion of primary drug.
- Adequate dilution of I.V. infusion and rotation of the site every 48 hours help minimize local vein irritation; use of small-gauge needle in larger available vein may be helpful.

Patient education

- Explain disease process and rationale for therapy.
- Teach signs and symptoms of hypersensitivity and other adverse reactions, and emphasize need to report any unusual effects.
- Teach signs and symptoms of bacterial and fungal superinfection to elderly and debilitated patients and others with low resistance from immunosuppressants or irradiation; emphasize need to report them promptly.
- Warn patient not to ingest alcohol in any form within 72 hours of treatment with cefamandole, cefoperazone, moxalactam, cefonicid, or cefotetan.
- Advise patient to add yogurt or buttermilk to diet to prevent intestinal superinfection resulting from suppression of normal intestinal flora.
- Advise diabetic patients to monitor urine glucose level with Diastix, Chemstrip uG, or glucose enzymatic test strip and not to use Clinitest.
- Tell to take oral drug with food if GI irritation occurs.
- Be sure patient understands how and when to take drug; urge patient to complete entire prescribed regimen, to comply with instructions for around-the-clock dosage, and to keep follow-up appointments.

• Counsel patient to check expiration date of drug, how to store drug, and to discard unused drug.

Geriatric use

• Use with caution; elderly patients are susceptible to superinfection and to coagulopathies. Elderly patients commonly have renal impairment and may require lower dosage of cephalosporins.

Pediatric use

• Serum half-life is prolonged in neonates and in infants up to age 1.

Breast-feeding

• Cephalosporins are excreted in breast milk; use with caution in breast-feeding women.

Representative combinations

None.

diuretics, loop

bumetanide, ethacrynate sodium, ethacrynic acid, furosemide, torsemide

Loop diuretics are sometimes referred to as high-ceiling diuretics because they produce a peak diuresis greater than that produced by other agents. Loop diuretics are particularly useful in edema associated with heart failure, hepatic cirrhosis, and renal disease. Ethacrynic acid was synthesized during the search for compounds that might interact with renal sulfhydryl groups like mercurial diuretics. Unfortunately, ethacrynic acid is associated with ototoxicity and a higher incidence of GI reactions and is therefore used less frequently. Structurally similar to furosemide, bumetanide is approximately 40 times more potent. Torsemide is the newest loop diuretic. (See *Comparing loop diuretics.*)

Pharmacology

Loop diuretics inhibit sodium and chloride reabsorption in the ascending loop of Henle, thus increasing renal excretion of sodium, chloride, and water; like thiazide diuretics, loop diuretics increase excretion of potassium. Loop diuretics produce greater maximum diuresis and electrolyte loss than thiazide diuretics.

Clinical indications and actions

Edema

Loop diuretics effectively relieve edema associated with heart failure. They may be useful in patients refractory to other diuretics; because furosemide and bumetanide may increase glomerular filtration rate, they are useful in patients with renal impairment. I.V. loop diuretics are used adjunctively in acute pulmonary edema to decrease peripheral vascular resistance. Loop diuretics also are used to treat edema associated with hepatic cirrhosis and nephrotic syndrome.

Hypertension

Loop diuretics are used in patients with mild to moderate hypertension, although thiazides are the initial diuretics of choice in most patients. Loop diuretics are preferred in patients with heart failure or renal impairment; used I.V., they are a helpful adjunct in managing hypertensive crises.

Overview of adverse reactions

The most common adverse effects associated with therapeutic doses of loop diuretics are metabolic and electrolyte disturbances (particularly potassium depletion), hypochloremic alkalosis, hyperglycemia, hyperuricemia, and hypomagnesemia. Rapid parenteral administration of loop diuretics may cause hearing loss (including deafness) and tinnitus. High doses may produce profound diuresis, leading to hypovolemia and CV collapse.

☑ Special considerations

• Monitor blood pressure and pulse rate (especially during rapid diuresis), establish baseline values before therapy, and watch for significant changes.
• Advise safety measures for all ambulatory patients until response to the diuretic is known.
• Establish baseline and periodically review CBC, including WBC count; serum electrolytes; carbon dioxide; magnesium; BUN and creatinine levels; and results of liver function tests.
• Administer diuretics in the morning so major diuresis occurs before bedtime. To prevent nocturia, do not prescribe diuretics for use after 6 p.m.
• Consider possible dosage adjustment in the following circumstances: reduced dosage for patients with hepatic dysfunction; increased dosage in patients with renal impairment, oliguria, or decreased diuresis (inadequate urine output may result in circulatory overload, causing water intoxication, pulmonary edema, and heart failure); increased doses of insulin or oral hypoglycemics in diabetic patients; and reduced dosages of other antihypertensive agents.
• Monitor for signs of excessive diuresis: hypotension, tachycardia, poor skin turgor, and excessive thirst.
• Monitor patient for edema and ascites.
• Patients taking digitalis glycosides are at increased risk of digitalis toxicity from potassium depletion.
• Patients with hepatic disease are especially susceptible to diuretic-induced electrolyte imbalance; in extreme cases, stupor, coma, and death can result.

Patient education

• Explain the rationale for therapy and diuretic effect of these drugs (increased volume and frequency of urination).
• Teach patient signs of adverse effects, especially hypokalemia (weakness, fatigue, muscle cramps, paresthesias, confusion, nausea, vomiting, diarrhea, headache, dizziness, or palpitations), and importance of reporting such symptoms promptly.
• Advise patient to eat potassium-rich foods.
• Tell patient to report increased edema or weight or excess diuresis (more than 2-lb [0.9-kg] weight loss per day).
• With initial doses, caution patient to change position slowly, especially when rising to upright position, to prevent dizziness from orthostatic hypotension.
• Instruct patient to call at once if chest, back, or leg pain; shortness of breath; or dyspnea occurs.
• Inform patient that photosensitivity may occur in some patients. Caution patient to take protective measures, such as sunscreens and protective clothing, against exposure to ultraviolet light or sunlight.

Geriatric use

• Elderly and debilitated patients require close observation, because they are more susceptible to drug-induced diuresis. In elderly patients, excessive diuresis can quickly lead to dehydration, hypovolemia, hy-

COMPARING LOOP DIURETICS

DRUG AND ROUTE	ONSET	PEAK	DURATION	USUAL DOSAGE
bumetanide				
I.V.	≤ 5 min	15 to 45 min	4 to 6 hr	0.5 to 1 mg ≤ t.i.d
P.O.	30 to 60 min	1 to 2 hr	4 to 6 hr	0.5 to 2 mg/day
ethacrynic acid				
I.V.	≤ 5 min	¼ to ½ hr	2 hr	50 mg/day
P.O.	≤ 30 min	2 hr	6 to 8 hr	50 to 100 mg/day
furosemide				
I.V.	≤ 5 min	⅓ to 1 hr	2 hr	20 to 40 mg q 2 hr, p.r.n.
P.O.	30 to 60 min	1 to 2 hr	6 to 8 hr	20 to 80 mg ≤ b.i.d.
torsemide				
I.V.	≤ 10 min	≤ 60 min	6 to 8 hr	5 to 20 mg/day
P.O.	≤ 60 min	60 to 120 min	6 to 8 hr	5 to 20 mg/day

pokalemia, and hyponatremia and may cause circulatory collapse. Reduced dosages may be indicated.

Pediatric use

- Use loop diuretics with caution in neonates. The usual pediatric dose can be used, but dosage intervals should be extended.

Breast-feeding

- Do not use loop diuretics in breast-feeding women.

Representative combinations

None.

diuretics, osmotic

glycerin, isosorbide, mannitol, urea

Osmotic diuretics are used to reduce intraocular and intracranial pressure. Most clinicians prefer mannitol because it is relatively less toxic and more stable in solution. Mannitol is approved for prevention and, adjunctively, for treatment of acute renal failure or oliguria.

Pharmacology

Osmotic diuretics elevate osmotic pressure of the glomerular filtrate, thereby hindering tubular reabsorption of solutes and water and promoting renal excretion of water, sodium, potassium, chloride, calcium, phosphorus, magnesium, and uric acid. Osmotic diuretics also elevate osmotic pressure in blood and promote the shift of intracellular water into the blood.

Clinical indications and actions

Acute renal failure or oliguria

Mannitol is used to prevent and treat the oliguric phase of acute renal failure. It enhances renal blood flow by its osmotic diuretic effect and by vasodilating effects.

Reduction of intracranial pressure

Mannitol and urea reduce intracranial pressure and control cerebral edema caused by trauma or disease and during surgery by drawing water from cells (including those in the brain and CSF) into the blood. A rebound effect may occur 12 hours after the administration of urea.

Reduction of intraocular pressure

Osmotic diuretics are used to reduce intraocular pressure when it cannot be reduced by other means; these drugs are especially useful in acute angle-closure glaucoma, in absolute or secondary glaucoma, and before surgery. Their osmotic effect draws fluid from the anterior chamber of the eye, reducing intraocular pressure. Urea, unlike mannitol, penetrates the eye and may cause a rebound increase in intraocular pressure if plasma urea levels fall below that in the vitreous humor. Because urea penetrates the eye, it should not be used when irritation is present.

Drug intoxication

Mannitol is used alone or with other diuretics to enhance urinary excretion of toxins, including aspirin, some barbiturates, bromides, imipramine, and lithium. Besides promoting diuresis, mannitol maintains renal blood flow.

Overview of adverse reactions

The most severe adverse effects associated with mannitol are fluid and electrolyte imbalance. Circulatory overload may follow administration of mannitol to patients with inadequate urine output. The most common adverse reactions associated with other osmotic diuretics are headache, nausea, and vomiting; a rebound increase in intraocular pressure also may occur.

☑ Special considerations

- Maintain adequate hydration. Monitor fluid and electrolyte balance.
- Monitor I.V. infusion site for inflammation.
- Patient should have frequent mouth care or fluids as appropriate to relieve thirst.
- In patients with urethral catheter, an hourly urometer collection bag should be used to facilitate accurate measurement of urine output.

Patient education
- Tell patient he may feel thirsty or experience mouth dryness, and emphasize importance of drinking only the amount of fluids provided.
- With initial doses, warn patient to change position slowly, especially when rising to an upright position, to prevent dizziness from orthostatic hypotension.
- Instruct patient to call immediately if he experiences chest, back, or leg pain; shortness of breath; or apnea.

Geriatric use
- Elderly or debilitated patients will require close observation and may require lower dosages. In elderly patients, excessive diuresis can quickly lead to dehydration, hypovolemia, hypokalemia, and hyponatremia.

Breast-feeding
- Safety has not been established.

Representative combinations
None.

diuretics, potassium-sparing

amiloride hydrochloride, spironolactone, triamterene

Potassium-sparing diuretics are less potent than many others; in particular, amiloride and triamterene have little clinical effect when used alone. However, they protect against potassium loss and are used with more potent diuretics. Spironolactone, an aldosterone antagonist, is particularly useful in patients with edema and hypertension associated with hyperaldosteronism.

Pharmacology
Amiloride and triamterene act directly on the distal renal tubules, inhibiting sodium reabsorption and potassium excretion, thereby reducing potassium loss. Spironolactone competitively inhibits aldosterone at the distal renal tubules, also promoting sodium excretion and potassium retention.

Clinical indications and actions
Edema

All potassium-sparing diuretics are used to manage edema associated with hepatic cirrhosis, nephrotic syndrome, and heart failure.

Hypertension

Amiloride and spironolactone are used to treat mild and moderate hypertension; the exact mechanism is unknown. Spironolactone may block the effect of aldosterone on arteriolar smooth muscle.

Diagnosis of primary hyperaldosteronism

Because spironolactone inhibits aldosterone, correction of hypokalemia and hypertension is presumptive evidence of primary hyperaldosteronism.

Overview of adverse reactions
Hyperkalemia is the most important adverse reaction; it may occur with all drugs in this class and could lead to arrhythmias. Other adverse reactions include nausea, vomiting, headache, weakness, fatigue, bowel disturbances, cough, and dyspnea.

Potassium-sparing diuretics are contraindicated in patients with serum potassium levels above 5.5 mEq/L, in those receiving other potassium-sparing diuretics or potassium supplements, and in patients with anuria, acute or chronic renal insufficiency, diabetic nephropathy, or known hypersensitivity to the drug. They should be used cautiously in patients with severe hepatic insufficiency because electrolyte imbalance may precipitate hepatic encephalopathy, and in patients with diabetes, who are at increased risk of hyperkalemia.

☑ Special considerations
- Monitor for hyperkalemia and arrhythmias; measure serum potassium and other electrolyte levels frequently, and check for significant changes. Monitor the following at baseline and periodic intervals: CBC including WBC count, carbon dioxide, BUN, and creatinine levels and, especially, liver function studies.
- Monitor vital signs, intake and output, weight, and blood pressure daily; check patient for edema, oliguria, or lack of diuresis, which may indicate drug tolerance.
- Monitor patient with hepatic disease in whom mild drug-induced acidosis may be hazardous; watch for mental confusion, lethargy, or stupor. Patients with hepatic disease are especially susceptible to diuretic-induced electrolyte imbalance; in extreme cases, coma and death can result.
- Administer diuretics in morning to ensure that major diuresis occurs before bedtime. To prevent nocturia, do not prescribe diuretics for use after 6 p.m.
- Establish safety measures for ambulatory patients until response is known; diuretics may cause orthostatic hypotension, weakness, ataxia, and confusion.
- Consider possible dosage adjustments in the following circumstances: reduced dosage for patients with hepatic dysfunction and for those taking other antihypertensive agents; increased dosage in patients with renal impairment; and changes in insulin requirements in diabetic patients.
- Monitor for other signs of toxicity.

Patient education
- Explain signs and symptoms of possible adverse effects and importance of reporting unusual effect.
- Tell to report increased edema or weight or excess diuresis (more than 2-lb [0.9-kg] weight loss per day) and to record weight each morning after voiding and before dressing and breakfast, using same scale.
- Teach how to minimize dizziness from orthostatic hypotension by avoiding sudden postural changes.
- Advise patient to avoid potassium-rich food and potassium-containing salt substitutes or supplements, which increase the hazard of hyperkalemia.
- Advise patient to take drug at same time each morning to avoid interrupted sleep from nighttime diuresis.
- Advise patient to take drug with or after meals to minimize GI distress.
- Caution patient to avoid hazardous activities, such as driving or operating machinery, until response to drug is known.
- Tell patient to seek medical approval before taking OTC drugs; many contain sodium and potassium and can cause electrolyte imbalance.

Geriatric use
- Elderly and debilitated patients require close observation because they are more susceptible to drug-induced diuresis and hyperkalemia. Reduced dosages may be indicated.

Pediatric use
- Use drugs with caution; children are more susceptible to hyperkalemia.

Breast-feeding
- Safety has not been established; drug may be excreted in breast milk.

Representative combinations

Amiloride with hydrochlorothiazide: Moduretic.

Spironolactone with hydrochlorothiazide: Aldactazide.

Triamterene with hydrochlorothiazide: Dyazide, Maxzide.

diuretics, thiazide

bendroflumethiazide, chlorothiazide, hydrochlorothiazide, methyclothiazide

diuretics, thiazide-like

chlorthalidone, indapamide, metolazone

Thiazide diuretics were discovered and synthesized as an outgrowth of studies on carbonic anhydrase inhibitors. Until the 1950s, organic mercurials were the only effective diuretics available; though potent, they were also toxic. Introduction of the thiazides in 1957 proved a major advance because these were the first potent, and safe, diuretics.

Pharmacology

Thiazide diuretics interfere with sodium transport across tubules of the cortical diluting segment of the nephron, thereby increasing renal excretion of sodium, chloride, water, potassium, and calcium.

The exact mechanism of thiazides' antihypertensive effect is unknown; however, it is thought to be partially caused by direct arteriolar dilatation. Thiazides initially decrease extracellular fluid volume, plasma volume, and cardiac output; extracellular fluid volume and plasma volume revert to near baseline levels in several weeks but remain slightly below normal. Cardiac output returns to normal or slightly above. Total body sodium remains slightly below pretreatment levels. Peripheral vascular resistance is initially elevated but falls below pretreatment levels with chronic diuretic therapy. (See *Comparing thiazides*.)

In patients with diabetes insipidus, thiazides cause a paradoxical decrease in urine volume and increase in renal concentration of urine, possibly because of sodium depletion and decreased plasma volume, which leads to an increase in renal water and sodium reabsorption.

Clinical indications and actions

Edema

Thiazide diuretics are used to treat edema associated with right-sided heart failure, mild to moderate left-sided heart failure, and nephrotic syndrome and, with spironolactone, to treat edema and ascites secondary to hepatic cirrhosis.

Efficacy and toxicity profiles of thiazide and thiazide-like diuretics are equivalent at comparable dosages; the single exception is metolazone, which may be more effective in patients with impaired renal function. Usually, thiazide diuretics are less effective than loop diuretics in patients with renal insufficiency.

Hypertension

Thiazide diuretics are commonly used for initial management of all degrees of hypertension. Used alone, they reduce mean blood pressure by only 10 to 15 mm Hg; in mild hypertension, thiazide diuresis alone will usually reduce blood pressure to desired levels. However, in moderate to severe hypertension that does not respond to thiazides alone, combination therapy with another antihypertensive agent is necessary.

Diabetes insipidus

In diabetes insipidus, thiazides cause a paradoxical decrease in urine volume; urine becomes more concentrated, possibly because of sodium depletion and decreased plasma volume. Thiazides are particularly effective in nephrogenic diabetes insipidus.

Overview of adverse reactions

Therapeutic doses of thiazide diuretics cause electrolyte and metabolic disturbances, the most common being potassium depletion; patients may require dietary supplementation.

Other abnormalities include hypochloremic alkalosis, hypomagnesemia, hyponatremia, hypercalcemia, hyperuricemia, elevated cholesterol levels, and hyperglycemia. Overdose of thiazides may produce lethargy that can progress to coma within a few hours.

☑ Special considerations

- Thiazides and thiazide-like diuretics (except metolazone) are ineffective in patients with a glomerular filtration rate below 25 ml per minute.
- Because thiazides may cause adverse lipid effects, consider an alternative agent in patients with significant hyperlipidemia.
- Monitor intake and output, weight, and serum electrolyte levels regularly.
- Monitor serum potassium levels; consult dietitian to provide high-potassium diet. Foods rich in potassium include citrus fruits, tomatoes, bananas, dates, and apricots. Watch for signs of hypokalemia (for example, muscle weakness or cramps). Patients also taking a cardiac glycoside have an increased risk of digitalis toxicity from the potassium-depleting effect of these diuretics.
- Thiazides may be used with potassium-sparing diuretics or potassium supplements to prevent potassium loss.

COMPARING THIAZIDES

Under most conditions, thiazide diuretics differ mainly in duration of action.

DRUG	EQUIVALENT DOSE	ONSET	PEAK	DURATION
bendroflumethiazide	5 mg	Within 2 hr	4 hr	6 to 12 hr
chlorothiazide	500 mg	Within 2 hr	4 hr	6 to 12 hr
hydrochlorothiazide	50 mg	Within 2 hr	4 to 6 hr	6 to 12 hr
methyclothiazide	5 mg	Within 2 hr	4 to 6 hr	24 hr

- Monitor blood glucose values in diabetic patients. Thiazides may cause hyperglycemia and a need to adjust insulin or oral hypoglycemic doses.
- Monitor serum creatinine and BUN levels regularly. Drug is not as effective if these levels are more than twice normal.
- Monitor blood uric acid levels, especially in patients with history of gout; these agents may cause an increase in uric acid levels.
- Prescribe for use in morning to prevent nocturia.
- Antihypertensive effects persist for approximately 1 week after discontinuation of drug.

Patient education

- Explain rationale of therapy and diuretic effects of these drugs (increased volume and frequency of urination).
- Instruct patient to report joint swelling, pain, or redness; these signs may indicate hyperuricemia.
- Warn patient to call immediately if signs of electrolyte imbalance occur; these include weakness, fatigue, muscle cramps, paresthesias, confusion, nausea, vomiting, diarrhea, headache, dizziness, and palpitations.
- Tell patient to report increased edema, excess diuresis, or weight loss (more than a 2-lb [0.9-kg] weight loss per day); advise him to record weight each morning after voiding and before dressing and breakfast, using the same scale.
- Advise patient to take drug with food to minimize gastric irritation; to eat potassium-rich foods; and not to add salt to other foods. Recommend use of salt substitutes.
- Counsel patient to avoid smoking because nicotine increases blood pressure.
- Tell patient to seek medical approval before taking OTC drugs.
- Warn patient about photosensitivity reactions.

With initial doses

- Caution patient to change position slowly, especially when rising to upright position, to prevent dizziness from orthostatic hypotension.
- Instruct patient to call immediately if chest, back, or leg pain; shortness of breath; or dyspnea occurs.
- Tell patient to take drug only as prescribed and at the same time each day, to prevent nighttime diuresis and interrupted sleep.

Geriatric use

- Elderly and debilitated patients require close observation and may require reduced dosages. They are more sensitive to excess diuresis because of age-related changes in CV and renal function. In elderly patients, excess diuresis can quickly lead to dehydration, hypovolemia, hyponatremia, hypomagnesemia, and hypokalemia.

Pediatric use

- Safety and effectiveness have not been established for all thiazide diuretics.

Breast-feeding

- Thiazides are distributed in breast milk; safety and effectiveness in breast-feeding women have not been established.

Representative combinations

Chlorthalidone with atenolol: Tenoretic, Atenolol/Chlorthalidone Tablets; with reserpine: Regroton.

Hydrochlorothiazide with bisoprolol: Ziac Tablets; with deserpidine: Oreticyl; with guanethidine monosulfate: Esimil; with hydralazine: Apresazide, Hydrochlorothiazide/Hydralazine Caps; with hydralazine hydrochloride and reserpine: Hydrap-ES Tablets, Marpres Tablets, Tri-Hydroserpine Tablets with methyldopa: Aldoril, Methyldopa and Hydrochlorothiazide Tablets; with propranolol: Inderide, Propranolol/Hydrochlorothiazide Tablets; with reserpine: Hydrochlorothiazide/Reserpine Tablets, Hydropine, Hydropres, Hydro-Serp, Hydroserpine, Hydrotensin, Mallopres; with hydralazine and reserpine: Ser-Ap-Es, Unipres; with spironolactone: Aldactazide; with timolol maleate: Timolide; with triamterene: Dyazide, Maxzide; with amiloride hydrochloride: Moduretic.

Hydroflumethiazide with reserpine: Salutensin Tablets.

estrogens

chlorotrianisene, dienestrol, diethylstilbestrol, diethylstilbestrol diphosphate, esterified estrogens, estradiol, estradiol cypionate, estradiol valerate, estrogen and progestin, estrogenic substances (conjugated), estropipate, ethinyl estradiol

Estrogens were first discovered in the urine of humans and animals in 1930. Since that time, numerous synthetic modifications of the naturally occurring estrogen molecules and completely synthetic estrogenic compounds have been developed.

Estrogens have several uses: in treating the symptoms of menopause, atrophic vaginitis, breast cancer, and other diseases; in the prophylaxis of osteoporosis; and as contraceptives when used in combination with progestins.

Pharmacology

Conjugated estrogens and estrogenic substances are normally obtained from the urine of pregnant mares. Other estrogens are manufactured synthetically. Of the six naturally occurring estrogens in humans, three (estradiol, estrone, and estriol) are present in significant quantities.

The estrogens promote the development and maintenance of the female reproductive system and secondary sexual characteristics. Estrogens inhibit the release of pituitary gonadotropins and also have various metabolic effects, including retention of fluid and electrolytes, retention and deposition in bone of calcium and phosphorus, and mild anabolic activity.

Estrogens and estrogenic substances administered as drugs have effects related to endogenous estrogen's mechanism of action. They can mimic the action of endogenous estrogen when used as replacement therapy or produce such useful effects as inhibiting ovulation or inhibiting growth of certain hormone-sensitive cancers.

Use of estrogens is not without risk. Long-term use is associated with an increased incidence of endometrial cancer, gallbladder disease, and thromboembolic disease. Elevations in blood pressure often occur as well.

Clinical indications and actions

Moderate to severe vasomotor symptoms of menopause

Endogenous estrogens are markedly reduced in concentration after menopause. This commonly results in vasomotor symptoms, such as hot flashes and dizziness. Chlorotrianisene, diethylstilbestrol, estradiol cypionate, and ethinyl estradiol serve to mimic the action of endogenous estrogens in preventing these symptoms.

Atrophic vaginitis; kraurosis vulvae
Chlorotrianisene and diethylstilbestrol stimulate development, cornification, and secretory activity in vaginal tissues.

Carcinoma of the breast
Conjugated estrogens, diethylstilbestrol, esterified estrogens, estradiol, and ethinyl estradiol inhibit the growth of hormone-sensitive cancers in certain carefully selected male and postmenopausal female patients.

Carcinoma of the prostate
Chlorotrianisene, conjugated estrogens, diethylstilbestrol, esterified estrogens, estradiol, estradiol valerate, and ethinyl estradiol inhibit growth of hormone-sensitive cancer tissue in males with advanced disease.

Prophylaxis of postmenopausal osteoporosis
Conjugated estrogens replace or augment activity of endogenous estrogen in causing calcium and phosphate retention and preventing bone decalcification.

Contraception
Estrogens are also used in combination with progestins for ovulation control to prevent conception.

Overview of adverse reactions

Acute reactions: changes in menstrual bleeding patterns (spotting, prolongation or absence of bleeding), abdominal cramps, swollen feet or ankles, bloated sensation (fluid and electrolyte retention), breast swelling and tenderness, weight gain, nausea, loss of appetite, headache, photosensitivity, loss of libido.

With chronic administration: increased blood pressure (sometimes into the hypertensive range), thromboembolic disease, cholestatic jaundice, benign hepatomas, endometrial carcinoma (rare). Risk of thromboembolic disease increases markedly with cigarette smoking, especially in women over age 35.

☑ Special considerations

- Do not use estrogens in patients with thrombophlebitis or thromboembolic disorders; cancer of the breast, reproductive organs, or genitals; or undiagnosed abnormal genital bleeding.
- Use with caution in hypertension, asthma, mental depression, bone disease, blood dyscrasias, gallbladder disease, migraine, seizures, diabetes mellitus, amenorrhea, heart failure, hepatic or renal dysfunction, or a family history of breast or genital tract cancer. Development or worsening of these conditions may require discontinuation of the drug.
- Give patient package insert describing estrogen adverse reactions, and also provide verbal explanation.
- Advise the pathologist if patient is receiving estrogen therapy when specimen is sent.
- Closely monitor patients with diabetes mellitus for loss of diabetes control.
- If patient is receiving a warfarin-type anticoagulant, monitor PT for anticoagulant dosage adjustment.
- Stop drug immediately if pregnancy occurs during therapy because it may adversely affect the fetus.
- Estrogen therapy is usually administered cyclically. The drugs are usually given once daily for 3 weeks, followed by 1 week without the drugs, and then this regimen is repeated as necessary.

Patient education

- Warn to report adverse reactions immediately.
- Tell male patient on long-term therapy about possible gynecomastia and impotence.
- Explain to patients on cyclic therapy for postmenopausal symptoms that, although withdrawal bleeding may occur in week off drug, fertility has not been restored; ovulation does not occur.
- Diabetic patients should report symptoms of hyperglycemia or glycosuria.
- Tell women who are planning to breast-feed not to take estrogens.

Geriatric use

- Postmenopausal women with long-term estrogen use have an increased risk of endometrial cancer if they have a uterus. This risk can be reduced by adding a progestin to the regimen.

Pediatric use

- Because of the effects of estrogen on epiphyseal closure, estrogens should be used with caution in adolescents whose bone growth is not complete.

Breast-feeding

- Estrogens are contraindicated in breast-feeding women.

Representative combinations

Estradiol cypionate with testosterone cypionate and chlorobutanol: Depo-testadiol, Duo-cyp, Menoject, testosterone cypionate and estradiol cypionate, depAndrogyn, Depotestogen, Duratestrin, T-E Cypionates, Test-Estro Cypionate.

Estradiol valerate with testosterone enanthate: Deladumone, Delatestadiol, Teev, Testosterone Enanthate and Estradiol Valerate Injection, Valertest.

Estrogen with methyltestosterone: Estratest, Estratest H.S.

Estrogenic substances (conjugated) with meprobamate: Milprem, PMB; with methyltestosterone: Premarin with methyltestosterone; with medroxyprogesterone: Premphase, Prempro.

Esterified estrogens with chlordiazepoxide: Menrium.

Ethinyl estradiol with norethindrone: Brevicon, Genora 1/35, Jenest, Loestrin Fe 1.5/30, ModiCon, Nelova1/35E, Ortho-Novum 1/35, Ortho-Novum 7/7/7, Ortho-Novum 10/11; with norgestimate: Cyclen; with ethynodiol diacetate: Demulen 1/35, Demulen 1/50; with desogestrel: Desogen, Marvelon; with norgestrel: Lo/Ovral, Ovral; with levonorgestrel: Levlen, Min-Ovral, Nordette, Tri-Levlen, Triphasil, Triquilar.

Ethynodiol diacetate with ethinyl estradiol: Demulen 1/35, Demulen 1/50.

histamine (H)$_2$-receptor antagonists

cimetidine, famotidine, nizatidine, ranitidine, rantidine bismuth citrate

The introduction of H_2-receptor antagonists has revolutionized the treatment of peptic ulcer disease. These drugs structurally resemble histamine and competitively inhibit histamine's action on gastric H_2 receptors. Cimetidine, approved for clinical use in 1977, is the prototype of this class.

Pharmacology

All H_2-receptor antagonists inhibit histamine's action at H_2 receptors in gastric parietal cells, reducing gastric acid output and concentration regardless of the stimulatory agent (histamine, food, insulin, caffeine) or basal conditions.

Clinical indications and actions

Duodenal ulcer

Cimetidine, famotidine, nizatidine, and ranitidine, are used to treat acute duodenal ulcer and to prevent ulcer recurrence. Ranitidine bismuth citrate is used in combination with clarithromycin to treat active duodenal ulcer associated with *Helicobacter pylori* infection.

Gastric ulcer

Cimetidine famotidine, nizatidine, and ranitidine are indicated for acute gastric ulcer. However, the benefits of long-term therapy (over 8 weeks) with these drugs remain unproven.

Hypersecretory states

Cimetidine, famotidine, nizatidine, and ranitidine are used to treat hypersecretory states such as Zollinger-Ellison syndrome. Because patients with these conditions require much higher doses than patients with peptic ulcer disease, they may experience more pronounced adverse effects.

Reflux esophagitis

Cimetidine, famotidine, nizatidine, and ranitidine are used to provide short-term relief from gastroesophageal reflux in patients who don't respond to conventional therapy (lifestyle changes, antacids, diet modification). They act by raising the stomach pH. Some clinicians prefer to combine the H_2-receptor antagonist with metoclopramide, but further study is necessary to confirm effectiveness of the combination.

◇ ***Stress ulcer prophylaxis***

Cimetidine, famotidine, nizatidine, and ranitidine are used to prevent stress ulcers in critically ill patients, particularly those in intensive care units. However, this remains an unlabeled (FDA unapproved) indication; some health care providers prefer intensive antacid therapy for such patients.

◇ ***Other uses***

H_2-receptor antagonists have been used for a number of other unlabeled indications, including short-bowel syndrome, prophylaxis for allergic reactions to I.V. contrast medium, and to eradicate *H. pylori* in treatment of peptic ulcers. Ranitidine bismuth citrate in combination with clarithromycin is used to treat *H. pylori.*

Overview of adverse reactions

H_2-receptor antagonists rarely cause adverse reactions. However, mild transient diarrhea, neutropenia, dizziness, fatigue, arrhythmias, and gynecomastia have been reported.

Cimetidine may inhibit hepatic enzymes, thereby impairing the metabolism of certain drugs. Ranitidine may also produce this effect, but to a lesser extent. Famotidine and nizatidine have not been shown to inhibit hepatic enzymes or drug clearance.

☑ Special considerations

- Give single daily dose at bedtime, twice-daily doses morning and evening, and multiple doses with meals and at bedtime. Most clinicians prefer the once-daily dosage at bedtime regimen for improved compliance.
- When administering drugs I.V., do not exceed recommended infusion rates because this may increase the risk of adverse CV effects. Continuous I.V. infusion may yield better suppression of acid secretion.
- Because antacids may decrease drug absorption, give them at least 1 hour apart from H_2-receptor antagonists.
- Know that patients with renal disease may require a modified schedule.
- Avoid discontinuing these drugs abruptly.
- Many investigational uses for these drugs (particularly cimetidine) are being evaluated. Ranitidine bismuth citrate should not be prescribed alone for the treatment of active duodenal ulcers.
- Symptomatic response to therapy does not rule out gastric malignancy.

Patient education

- Instruct patient to avoid smoking during drug therapy because smoking stimulates gastric acid secretion and worsens the disease.

Geriatric use

- Use caution when administering these drugs to elderly patients because of the increased risk of adverse reactions, particularly those affecting the CNS. Dosage adjustment is required in patients with impaired renal function.

Pediatric use

- Safety and efficacy have not been established.

Breast-feeding

- H_2-receptor antagonists may be secreted in breast milk. Ratio of risk to benefit must be considered.

Representative combinations

None.

hydantoin derivatives

fosphenytoin sodium, mephenytoin, phenytoin, phenytoin sodium

Hydantoins, of which phenytoin is the prototype, are used primarily to control tonic-clonic and partial seizures. Parenteral phenytoin and fosphenytoin are used for treatment of status epilepticus, prevention and treatment of seizures during neurosurgery, and as a short-term substitute for oral phenytoin therapy. Fosphenytoin, unlike phenytoin, may be administered I.M. when I.V. access is either not feasible or unavailable. Mephenytoin is used to treat partial seizures refractory to less toxic agents. Mephenytoin is more likely to produce fatal blood dyscrasias than either ethotoin or phenytoin but is less likely to cause ataxia, gingival hyperplasia, hypertrichosis, or GI distress.

Pharmacology

The hydantoins exert their anticonvulsant effects by inhibiting the spread of seizure activity in the motor cortex; they stabilize seizure threshold against hyperexcitability produced by excessive stimulation and decrease post-tetanic potentiation that accompanies abnormal focal discharge.

Phenytoin's antiarrhythmic effects are similar to those produced by quinidine or procainamide; it improves AV conduction, especially that depressed by digitalis glycosides, and prolongs the effective refractory period. (See *Comparing selected anticonvulsants.*)

Clinical indications and actions

Seizure disorders

Hydantoins are used to control grand mal (tonic-clonic) and psychomotor seizures; parenteral phenytoin and fosphenytoin are used to control status epilepticus and seizures occurring during neurosurgery and in patients who cannot receive oral therapy. Mephenytoin is used

COMPARING SELECTED ANTICONVULSANTS

The chart below lists some common anticonvulsant drugs and their various indications.

DRUGS	INDICATIONS	THERAPEUTIC SERUM LEVELS	TIME TO REACH STEADY STATE
carbamazepine	• tonic-clonic seizures • partial seizures • mixed seizures	6 to 14 mcg/ml	2 to 4 days
clonazepam	• absence seizures • myoclonic seizures • akinetic seizures	20 to 80 ng/ml	5 to 10 days
clorazepate	• partial seizures	Not established	5 to 10 days
diazepam	• status epilepticus	Not established	Not applicable
ethosuximide	• absence seizures	40 to 100 mcg/ml	4 to 7 days
gabapentin	• partial seizures	Not established	2 to 4 days
lamotrigine	• partial seizures	Not established	2 to 3 days
mephenytoin	• tonic-clonic seizures • complex partial seizures • simple partial seizures	25 to 40 mcg/ml	Not established
methsuximide	• absence seizures	10 to 40 mcg/ml	8 to 16 hours
phenobarbital	• status epilepticus • tonic-clonic seizures	10 to 40 mcg/ml	14 to 21 days
phenytoin	• status epilepticus • tonic-clonic seizures • complex partial seizures	10 to 20 mcg/ml	5 to 10 days
primidone	• tonic-clonic seizures • partial seizures	5 to 12 mcg/ml (primidone) 10 to 40 mcg/ml (phenobarbital)	4 to 7 days
trimethadione	• absence seizures	700 to 800 mcg/ml	2 to 5 days
valproic acid	• absence seizures • simple and complex partial seizures	50 to 100 mcg/ml	5 to 7 days

only for focal, jacksonian, and psychomotor seizures and in patients with refractory seizures.

◊ ***Arrhythmias***

Phenytoin is also used to counteract arrhythmias, especially those produced by digitalis glycosides. However, this is an unlabeled (Food and Drug Administration unapproved) use.

Overview of adverse reactions

The most common adverse reactions to hydantoins involve the CNS and are dose-related, especially drowsiness, headache, ataxia, and dizziness. Other reactions include GI irritation, itching, numbness, tingling, severe dermatologic and hematopoietic reactions, lymphadenopathy, gingival hyperplasia, and hepatotoxicity.

☑ Special considerations

- Monitor liver function and hematologic studies.
- Observe patient closely during therapy for possible adverse effects. Hydantoins may cause gingival hyperplasia; good oral hygiene and gum care are essential to minimize effects.
- Hemodynamic monitoring is required with I.V. administration. Elevated serum concentration may promote seizure activity.
- Discontinue hydantoins slowly over 6 weeks; abrupt discontinuation may cause status epilepticus.
- Drug interactions are frequently a problem, primarily with hepatically cleared drugs, such as chloramphenicol, digitoxin, isoniazid, and griseofulvin; be especially alert for toxic symptoms or breakthrough seizures in patients taking these drugs.

Patient education

- Tell patient not to use alcohol while taking drug because it may decrease drug's effectiveness and may increase CNS adverse reactions.

• Advise patient to avoid hazardous tasks that require mental alertness until degree of CNS sedative effect is determined.
• Tell patient to take oral drug with food if GI distress occurs.
• Teach patient signs and symptoms of hypersensitivity, hepatic dysfunction, and blood dyscrasia and to call immediately if the following occur: sore throat, fever, bleeding, easy bruising, lymphadenopathy, or rash.
• Tell to call immediately if pregnancy is suspected.
• Warn patient never to discontinue drug suddenly or without medical supervision.
• Encourage patient to wear a medical identification bracelet or necklace, listing drug and seizure disorders, while taking anticonvulsants.
• Caution patient to consult pharmacist before changing brand or using generic drug; effect may change.
• Explain that drug may increase gum growth and sensitivity (gingival hyperplasia); teach proper oral hygiene and urge patient or parent to establish good mouth care.
• Assure patient that pink or reddish brown discoloration of urine is normal and harmless.

Geriatric use
• Use anticonvulsant drugs with caution. Elderly patients metabolize and excrete all drugs more slowly and may obtain therapeutic effect from lower dosages.

Pediatric use
• Be sure to administer only dosage forms prepared for pediatric use.

Breast-feeding
• Hydantoin anticonvulsants are excreted in breast milk; women should discontinue breast-feeding while taking these drugs.

Representative combinations
Phenytoin with phenobarbital: Dilantin sodium with phenobarbital.

nitrates

amyl nitrite, isosorbide dinitrate, isosorbide mononitrate, nitroglycerin

Nitrates have been recognized as effective vasodilators for more than 100 years. The best known drug of this group, nitroglycerin, remains the therapeutic mainstay for classic and variant angina. With the availability of a commercial I.V. nitroglycerin form, the drug's use in reducing afterload and preload in various cardiac disorders has generated renewed enthusiasm. Various other dosage forms of nitroglycerin and of the other nitrates also are available, thereby improving and extending their clinical usefulness.

Pharmacology
Nitrates' major pharmacologic property is vascular smooth muscle relaxation, resulting in generalized vasodilation. Venous effects predominate; however, nitroglycerin produces dose-dependent dilatation of both arterial and venous beds. Decreased peripheral venous resistance results in venous pooling of blood and decreased venous return to the heart (preload); decreased arteriolar resistance reduces systemic vascular resistance and arterial pressure (afterload). These vascular effects lead to reduction of myocardial oxygen consumption, promoting a more favorable oxygen supply:demand ratio. (Although nitrates reflexively increase heart rate and myocardial contractility, reduced ventricular wall tension results in a net decrease in myocardial oxygen consumption.) In the coronary circulation, nitrates redistribute circulating blood flow along collateral channels and preferentially increase subendocardial blood flow, improving perfusion to the ischemic myocardium.

Nitrates relax all smooth muscle—not just vascular smooth muscle—regardless of autonomic innervation, including bronchial, biliary, GI, ureteral, and uterine smooth muscle.

Clinical indications and actions
Angina pectoris
By relaxing vascular smooth muscle in both the venous and arterial beds, nitrates cause a net decrease in myocardial oxygen consumption; by dilating coronary vessels, they lead to redistribution of blood flow to ischemic tissue. Although systemic and coronary vascular effects may vary slightly, depending on which nitrate is used, both smooth muscle relaxation and vasodilation probably account for nitrates' value in treating angina. Because individual nitrates have similar pharmacologic and therapeutic properties, the best nitrate to use in a specific situation depends mainly on the onset of action and duration of effect required.

Sublingual nitroglycerin is considered the drug of choice to treat acute angina pectoris because of its rapid onset of action, relatively low cost, and well-established effectiveness. Lingual or buccal nitroglycerin and other rapidly acting nitrates (amyl nitrite and sublingual or chewable isosorbide dinitrate) also may prove useful for this indication. Amyl nitrite is rarely used because it is expensive, inconvenient, and carries a high risk of adverse effects. Sublingual, lingual, or buccal nitroglycerin or sublingual or chewable isosorbide dinitrate typically prove effective in circumstances likely to provoke an angina attack.

Long-acting nitrates and beta-adrenergic blockers usually are considered the drugs of choice in the prophylactic management of angina pectoris. Nitrates with a relatively long duration of effect include oral preparations of isosorbide mononitrate, pentaerythritol tetranitrate, and oral or topical nitroglycerin.

The effectiveness of oral nitrates is debatable, although isosorbide dinitrate and nitroglycerin generally are now considered effective. However, the effectiveness of pentaerythritol tetranitrate and of topical nitroglycerin preparations have not been fully determined. Some experts believe oral nitrates are ineffective or less effective than rapidly acting I.V. nitrates in reducing frequency of angina and increasing exercise tolerance. Also, prolonged use of oral nitrates may cause cross-tolerance to sublingual nitrates.

I.V. nitroglycerin may be used to treat unstable angina pectoris, Prinzmetal's angina, and angina pectoris in patients who have not responded to recommended doses of nitrates or a beta-adrenergic blocker.

Sedatives may be useful in the adjunctive management of angina pectoris associated with psychogenic factors. However, if combination therapy is required, each drug should be adjusted individually; fixed combinations of oral nitrates and sedatives should be avoided.

Acute MI
The hemodynamic effects of I.V., sublingual, or topical nitroglycerin may prove beneficial in treating left ventricular failure and pulmonary congestion associated with acute MI. However, the drugs' effects on morbidi-

ty and mortality in patients with these conditions is controversial.

I.V., sublingual, and topical nitroglycerin and isosorbide dinitrate are effective adjunctive agents in managing acute and chronic heart failure. Sublingual administration can quickly reverse the signs and symptoms of pulmonary congestion in acute pulmonary edema; however, the I.V. form may control hemodynamic status more accurately.

Overview of adverse reactions

Headache is most common early in therapy; it may be severe, but usually diminishes rapidly. Postural hypotension, dizziness, weakness, transient flushing may occur. In patients sensitive to hypotensive effects, nausea, vomiting, weakness, restlessness, pallor, cold sweats, tachycardia, syncope, or CV collapse may occur. Dosage reduction may control GI upset; therapy should be discontinued if blurred vision, dry mouth, or rash develops. Tolerance and dependence can occur with repeated, prolonged use.

Tolerance to both the vascular and antianginal effects of the drugs can develop, and cross-tolerance between the nitrates and nitrites has been demonstrated. Tolerance is associated with a high or sustained plasma drug concentration and occurs with oral, I.V., and topical therapy. It rarely occurs with intermittent sublingual use. However, patients taking oral isosorbide dinitrate or topical nitroglycerin have not exhibited cross-tolerance to sublingual nitroglycerin.

To prevent tolerance, the lowest effective dose and an intermittent dosing schedule should be used. A nitrate-free interval of 10 to 12 hours daily may also be helpful.

☑ Special considerations

Oral dosage form

- Provide a dosage regimen that incorporates a 10- to 12-hour nitrate-free interval.
- Best absorption will occur if taken on an empty stomach (1 hour before or 2 hours after meals) and with a full glass of water.
- Dosage should be titrated to patient response. Patients should avoid switching brands after they are stabilized on a particular formulation.

Buccal dosage form

- The tablet should be placed between the upper lip or cheek and gum.
- Dissolution rate varies, but will usually range from 3 to 5 hours. Hot liquids will increase dissolution rate and should be avoided.
- Patient should not use buccal form at bedtime because of risk of aspiration.

Sublingual dosage form

- Only the sublingual and translingual forms should be used to relieve acute angina attack. Although a burning sensation was formerly an indication of drug's potency, many current preparations do not produce this sensation.

Translingual spray

- Only the sublingual and translingual forms should be used to relieve acute angina attack. The translingual form should be sprayed onto or under the tongue. Patient should not inhale the spray.

Topical dosage form

- To apply ointment, spread in uniform thin layer to any hairless part of the skin except distal parts of arms and legs, because absorption will not be maximal at these sites. Do not rub in. Cover with plastic film to aid absorption and to protect clothing. If using Tape-Surrounded Appli-Ruler (TSAR) system, keep TSAR on skin to protect patient's clothing and ensure that ointment remains in place. If serious adverse reactions develop in patients using ointment or transdermal system, remove product at once or wipe ointment from skin. Be sure to avoid contact with ointment.
- Be sure to remove transdermal patch before defibrillation. Because of the patch's aluminum backing, electric current may cause patch to explode.
- Do not coadminister with sildenafil (Viagra).

Patient education

- Instruct patient to avoid alcohol while taking nitrates, because severe hypotension and CV collapse may occur.
- Instruct patient to sit when taking nitrates, to prevent injury from transient episodes of dizziness, syncope, or other signs of cerebral ischemia that the drug may cause.
- Advise patient to treat headache with aspirin or acetaminophen.
- Tell patient to report blurred vision, dry mouth, or persistent headache.
- Warn patient not to stop taking drug abruptly, because this may cause withdrawal symptoms.

Pediatric use

- Safety and effectiveness of nitrates in children have not been established.

Breast-feeding

- Excretion into breast milk is unknown. Use with caution.

Representative combinations

None.

nonsteroidal anti-inflammatory drugs (NSAIDs)

diclofenac sodium, diflunisal, etodolac, fenoprofen calcium, flurbiprofen sodium, ibuprofen, indomethacin, indomethacin sodium trihydrate, ketoprofen, ketorolac tromethamine, nabumetone, naproxen, naproxen sodium, oxaprozin, piroxicam, sulindac

NSAIDs are a growing class of drugs that are prescribed widely for their analgesic and anti-inflammatory effects; some members of this class have an antipyretic effect.

Pharmacology

The analgesic effect of NSAIDs may result from interference with the prostaglandins involved in pain. Prostaglandins appear to sensitize pain receptors to mechanical stimulation or to other chemical mediators. NSAIDs inhibit synthesis of prostaglandins peripherally and possibly centrally. Their anti-inflammatory action may also contribute indirectly to their analgesic effect.

Like the salicylates, the anti-inflammatory effects of NSAIDs may result in part from inhibition of prostaglandin synthesis and release during inflammation. The exact mechanism has not been established, but the anti-inflammatory effect of NSAIDs correlates with their ability to inhibit prostaglandin synthesis.

Clinical indications and actions

Pain, inflammation, and fever

NSAIDs are used principally for symptomatic relief of mild to moderate pain and inflammation. These agents usually provide temporary relief of mild to moderate pain, especially that associated with inflammation. NSAIDs are used to treat low-intensity pain of headache, arthralgia, myalgia, neuralgia, and mild to moderate pain from dental or surgical procedures or dysmenorrhea.

Oral NSAIDs are also used for long-term treatment of rheumatoid arthritis, juvenile arthritis, and osteoarthritis. In osteoarthritis, NSAIDs are used primarily for analgesia. NSAIDs offer only symptomatic treatment for rheumatoid conditions, and do not reverse or arrest the disease process. NSAIDs reduce pain, stiffness, swelling, and tenderness.

Overview of adverse reactions

Adverse reactions to oral NSAIDs chiefly involve the GI tract, particularly erosion of the gastric mucosa. Most common symptoms are dyspepsia, heartburn, epigastric distress, nausea, and abdominal pain. GI symptoms usually occur in the first few days of therapy, and often subside with continuous treatment. They can be minimized by administering NSAIDs with meals or food, antacids, or large quantities of water or milk.

CNS adverse effects (headache, dizziness, drowsiness) may also occur. Flank pain with other signs and symptoms of nephrotoxicity has occasionally been reported. Fluid retention may aggravate preexisting hypertension or heart failure. NSAIDs should not be used in patients with renal insufficiency.

☑ Special considerations

- Use NSAIDs cautiously in patients with history of GI disease, increased risk of GI bleeding, or decreased renal function.
- Patients with known "triad" symptoms (aspirin hypersensitivity, rhinitis or nasal polyps, and asthma) are at high risk of bronchospasm.
- NSAIDs may mask the signs and symptoms of acute infection.
- Administer oral NSAIDs with a full 8-oz (240-ml) glass of water to assure adequate passage into stomach.
- Tablets may be crushed and mixed with food or fluids to aid swallowing, and with antacids to minimize gastric upset.
- Monitor for signs and symptoms of bleeding. Assess bleeding time if surgery is required.
- Monitor ophthalmic and auditory function before and periodically during therapy to prevent toxicity.
- Monitor CBC, platelets, PT, and hepatic and renal function studies periodically to detect abnormalities.
- Use of an NSAID with an opioid analgesic has an additive effect. Use of lower doses of the opioid analgesic may be possible.

Patient education

- Tell patient to take medication with 8 oz (240 ml) of water 30 minutes before or 2 hours after meals, or with food or milk if gastric irritation occurs.
- Explain that taking drug as directed is necessary to achieve the desired effect; 2 to 4 weeks of treatment may be needed before benefit is seen.
- Advise patients on chronic NSAID therapy to arrange for monitoring of laboratory parameters, especially BUN, serum creatinine, liver function tests, and CBC.
- Warn patients with current rectal bleeding or history of rectal bleeding to avoid using rectal NSAID suppositories. Because they must be retained in the rectum for at least 1 hour, they may cause irritation and bleeding.
- Warn pregnant patient to avoid the use of all NSAIDs, especially during the third trimester, when prostaglandin inhibition may cause prolonged gestation, dystocia, and delayed parturition.
- Warn patient that use of alcoholic beverages while on NSAID therapy may cause increased GI irritation and, possibly, GI bleeding.

Geriatric use

- Patients over age 60 may be more susceptible to the toxic effects of NSAIDs because of decreased renal function, resulting in NSAID accumulation.
- The effects of NSAIDs on renal prostaglandins may cause fluid retention and edema, a significant drawback for elderly patients, especially those with heart failure.

Pediatric use

- Do not use long-term NSAID therapy in children under age 14; safety has not been established.

Breast-feeding

- Most NSAIDs are distributed into breast milk; NSAID therapy is not recommended during breast-feeding.

Representative combinations

None.

opioids

alfentanil hydrochloride, codeine phosphate, codeine sulfate, difenoxin hydrochloride, diphenoxylate hydrochloride, fentanyl citrate, hydromorphone hydrochloride, levomethadyl acetate hydrochloride, meperidine hydrochloride, methadone hydrochloride, morphine sulfate, oxycodone hydrochloride, oxymorphone hydrochloride, propoxyphene hydrochloride, propoxyphene napsylate, remifentanil hydrochloride, sufentanil citrate

Opioids, previously called narcotic agonists, are usually understood to include natural and semisynthetic alkaloid derivatives from opium and their synthetic surrogates, whose actions mimic those of morphine. Most of these drugs are classified as Schedule II by the Federal Drug Enforcement Agency, because they have a high potential for addiction and abuse. Until relatively recently, opioids were used indiscriminately for analgesia and sedation and to control diarrhea and cough. (See *Comparing opioids.*)

Pharmacology

Opioids act as agonists at specific opiate receptor binding sites in the CNS and other tissues; these are the same receptors occupied by endogenous opioid peptides (enkephalins and endorphins) to alter CNS response to painful stimuli. Opiate agonists do not alter the cause of pain, but only the patient's perception of the pain; they relieve pain without affecting other sensory functions. Opiate receptors are present in highest concentrations in the limbic system, thalamus, striatum, hypothalamus, midbrain, and spinal cord.

Opioids produce respiratory depression by a direct effect on the respiratory centers in the brain stem, re-

COMPARING OPIOIDS

DRUG	ROUTE	ONSET	PEAK	DURATION
alfentanil	I.V.	Immediate	Not available	Not available
codeine	I.M., P.O., S.C.	15 to 30 min	30 to 60 min	4 to 6 hr
fentanyl	I.M., I.V.	7 to 8 min	Not available	1 to 2 hr
hydrocodone	P.O.	30 min	60 min	4 to 6 hr
hydromorphone	I.M., I.V., S.C. P.O., P.R.	15 min 30 min	30 min 60 min	4 to 5 hr 4 to 5 hr
meperidine	I.M. P.O. S.C.	10 to 15 min 15 to 30 min 10 to 15 min	30 to 50 min 60 min 40 to 60 min	2 to 4 hr 2 to 4 hr 2 to 4 hr
methadone	I.M., P.O., S.C.	30 to 60 min	30 to 60 min	4 to 6 hr*
morphine	I.M. P.O., P.R. S.C.	≤ 20 min ≤ 20 min ≤ 20 min	30 to 60 min ≤ 60 min 50 to 90 min	3 to 7 hr 3 to 7 hr 3 to 7 hr
oxycodone	P.O.	15 to 30 min	30 to 60 min	4 to 6 hr
oxymorphone	I.M., S.C. I.V. P.R.	10 to 15 min 5 to 10 min 15 to 30 min	30 to 60 min 30 to 60 min 30 to 60 min	3 to 6 hr 3 to 6 hr 3 to 6 hr
propoxyphene	P.O.	20 to 60 min	2 to 2½ hr	4 to 6 hr
remifentanil	I.V.	Immediate	Not available	Not available
sufentanil	I.V.	1.3 to 3 min	Not available	Not available

*Due to cumulative effects, duration of action increases with repeated doses.

sulting in decreased sensitivity and responsiveness to increases in carbon dioxide tension. These drugs' antitussive effects are mediated by a direct suppression of the cough reflex center. They cause nausea, probably by stimulation of the chemoreceptor trigger zone in the medulla oblongata; through orthostatic hypotension, which causes dizziness; and possibly by increasing vestibular sensitivity.

Opioids also cause drowsiness, sedation, euphoria, dysphoria, mental clouding, and EEG changes; higher than usual analgesic doses cause anesthesia. Most opioids cause miosis, although meperidine and its derivatives may also cause mydriasis or no pupillary change.

Because opioids decrease gastric, biliary, and pancreatic secretions and delay digestion, constipation is a common adverse reaction. At the same time, these drugs increase tone in the biliary tract and may cause biliary spasms. Some patients may have no biliary effects, whereas others may have biliary spasms that increase plasma amylase and lipase levels up to 15 times the normal values.

Opioids increase smooth muscle tone in the urinary tract and induce spasms, causing urinary urgency. These drugs have little CV effect in a supine patient, but may cause orthostatic hypotension when the patient assumes upright posture. These drugs are also associated with manifestations of histamine release or peripheral vasodilation, including pruritus, flushing, red eyes, and sweating. These effects are often mistakenly attributed to allergy and should be evaluated carefully.

The opiates can be divided chemically into three groups: phenanthrenes (codeine, hydrocodone, hydromorphone, morphine, oxycodone, and oxymorphone); phenylheptylamines (levomethadyl, methadone, and propoxyphene); and phenylpiperidines (alfentanil, diphenoxylate, fentanyl, meperidine, and remifentanil, sufentanil). If a patient is hypersensitive to an opioid, agonist-antagonist, or antagonist of a given chemical group, use extreme caution in considering the use of another agent from the same chemical group; however, a drug from the other groups might be well tolerated.

Some of the opioids are well absorbed after oral or rectal administration; others must be administered parenterally. I.V. dosing is the most rapidly effective and reliable; absorption after I.M. or S.C. dosing may be erratic. Opioids vary in onset and duration of action; they are removed rapidly from the bloodstream and distributed, in decreasing order of concentration, into skeletal muscle, kidneys, liver, intestinal tract, lungs, spleen, and brain; they readily cross the placenta.

Opioids are metabolized mainly in the microsomes in the endoplasmic reticulum of the liver (first-pass effect) and also in the CNS, kidneys, lungs, and placenta. They undergo conjugation with glucuronic acid, hydrolysis, oxidation, or N-dealkylation. They are excreted primarily in the urine; small amounts are excreted in the feces.

Clinical indications and actions

The opioids produce varying degrees of analgesia and have antitussive, antidiarrheal, and sedative effects. Clinical response is dose-related and varies with each patient.

Analgesia

Opioids may be used in the symptomatic management of moderate to severe pain associated with acute and some chronic disorders, including renal or biliary colic, MI, acute trauma, postoperative pain, or terminal cancer. They also may be used to provide analgesia during diagnostic and orthopedic procedures and during labor. Drug selection, route of administration, and dosage depend on a variety of factors. For example, in mild pain, oral therapy with codeine or oxycodone usually suffices. In acute pain of known short duration, such as that associated with diagnostic procedures or orthopedic manipulation, a short-acting drug such as meperidine or fentanyl is effective. These drugs are often given to alleviate postoperative pain, but because they influence CNS function, take special care to monitor the course of recovery and to detect early signs of complications. Opioids are commonly used to manage severe, chronic pain associated with terminal cancer; this requires careful evaluation and titration of drug used and dosage and route of administration.

Pulmonary edema

Morphine, meperidine, oxymorphone, hydromorphone, and other similar drugs have been used to relieve anxiety in patients with dyspnea associated with acute pulmonary edema and acute left ventricular failure. These drugs should not be used to treat pulmonary edema resulting from a chemical respiratory stimulant. Opioids decrease peripheral resistance, causing pooling of blood in the extremities and decreased venous return, cardiac workload, and pulmonary venous pressure; blood is thus shifted from the central to the peripheral circulation.

Preoperative sedation

Routine use of opioids for preoperative sedation in patients without pain is not recommended because it may cause complications during and after surgery. To allay preoperative anxiety, a barbiturate or benzodiazepine is equally effective, with a lower incidence of postoperative vomiting.

Anesthesia

Certain opioids, including alfentanil, fentanyl, remifentanil, and sufentanil, may be used for induction of anesthesia, as an adjunct in the maintenance of general and regional anesthesia, or as a primary anesthetic agent in surgery.

Cough suppression

Some opioids, most commonly codeine and its derivative, hydrocodone, are used as antitussives to relieve dry, nonproductive cough.

Diarrhea

Diphenoxylate and other opioids are used as antidiarrheal agents. All opioids cause constipation to some degree; however, only a few are indicated for this use. Usually, opiate antidiarrheals are empirically combined with antacids, absorbing agents, and belladonna alkaloids in commercial preparations.

Overview of adverse reactions

Respiratory depression and, to a lesser extent, circulatory depression (including orthostatic hypotension) are the major hazards of treatment with opioids. Rapid I.V. administration increases the incidence and severity of these serious adverse effects. Respiratory arrest, shock, and cardiac arrest have occurred. It is likely that equianalgesic doses of individual opiates produce a comparable degree of respiratory depression, but its duration may vary. Other adverse CNS effects include dizziness, visual disturbances, mental clouding or depression, sedation, coma, euphoria, dysphoria, weakness, faintness, agitation, restlessness, nervousness, seizures, and, rarely, delirium and insomnia. Adverse effects seem to be more prevalent in ambulatory patients and those not experiencing severe pain. Adverse GI effects include nausea, vomiting, and constipation, as well as increased biliary tract pressure that may result in biliary spasm or colic. Tolerance, psychological dependence, and physical dependence (addiction) may follow prolonged, high-dose therapy (more than 100 mg of morphine daily for more than 1 month).

Use opiate agonists with extreme caution during pregnancy and labor, because they readily cross the placenta. Premature infants appear especially sensitive to their respiratory and CNS depressant effects when used during delivery.

Opiate agonists have a high potential for addiction and should always be administered with caution in patients prone to physical or psychic dependence. The agonist-antagonists have a lower potential for addiction and abuse, but the liability still exists.

☑ Special considerations

- Administer with extreme caution to patients with head injury, increased intracranial pressure, seizures, asthma, COPD, alcoholism, prostatic hypertrophy, severe hepatic or renal disease, acute abdominal conditions, arrhythmias, hypovolemia, or psychiatric disorders, and to elderly or debilitated patients. Reduced doses may be necessary.
- Keep resuscitative equipment and a narcotic antagonist (naloxone) available. Be prepared to provide support of ventilation and gastric lavage.
- Parenteral administration of opiates provides better analgesia than oral administration. I.V. administration should be given by slow injection, preferably in diluted solution. Rapid I.V. injection increases the incidence of adverse effects.
- Parenteral injections by I.M. or S.C. route should be given cautiously to patients who are chilled, hypovolemic, or in shock, because decreased perfusion may lead to accumulation of the drug and toxic effects. Rotate I.M. or S.C. injection sites to avoid induration.
- A regular dosage schedule (rather than "as needed for pain") is preferred to alleviate the symptoms and anxiety that accompany pain.
- Duration of respiratory depression may be longer than the analgesic effect. Monitor patient closely with repeated dosing.
- With chronic administration, evaluate patient's respiratory status before each dose. Because severe respiratory depression may occur (especially with accumulation from chronic dosing), watch for respiratory rate below the patient's baseline level. Evaluate patient for restlessness, which may be a sign of compensatory response for hypoxia.
- Opiates or agonist-antagonists may cause orthostatic hypotension in ambulatory patients. Have the patient sit or lie down to relieve dizziness or fainting.
- Because opiates depress respiration when they are used postoperatively, encourage patient turning, coughing, and deep breathing to avoid atelectases.
- If gastric irritation occurs, give oral products with food; food delays absorption and onset of analgesia.
- Opiates may obscure the signs and symptoms of an acute abdominal condition or worsen gallbladder pain.

- The antitussive activity of opiates is used to control persistent, exhausting cough or dry, nonproductive cough.
- The first sign of tolerance to the therapeutic effect of opioid agonists or agonist-antagonists is usually a shortened duration of effect.
- Administration of an opiate to a woman shortly before delivery may cause respiratory depression in the neonate. Monitor closely and be prepared to resuscitate.
- Preservative-free morphine (Astramorph, Duramorph) is available for epidural or intrathecal use.

Patient education

- Instruct patient to use drug with caution and to avoid hazardous activities that require full alertness and coordination.
- Tell patient to avoid ingestion of alcohol when taking opioid agonists, because it will cause additive CNS depression.
- Explain that constipation may result from taking an opiate. Suggest measures to increase dietary fiber content, or recommend a stool softener.
- If patient's condition allows, instruct patient to breathe deeply, cough, and change position every 2 hours to avoid respiratory complications.
- Encourage patient to void at least every 4 hours to avoid urine retention.
- Tell the patient to take drug as prescribed and to call if significant adverse effects occur.
- Tell patient not to increase dosage if he is not experiencing the desired effect, but to call for prescribed dosage adjustment.
- Instruct the patient not to double dose. Tell him to take a missed dose as soon as he remembers unless it is almost time for the next dose. If this is the case, he should skip the missed dose and go back to the regular dosage schedule.
- Tell patient to call immediately for emergency help if he thinks he or someone else has taken an overdose.
- Explain signs of overdose to patient and his family.

Geriatric use

- Lower doses are usually indicated for elderly patients, who may be more sensitive to the therapeutic and adverse effects of drug.

Pediatric use

- Safety and effectiveness in children have not been established.

Breast-feeding

- Codeine, meperidine, methadone, morphine, and propoxyphene are excreted in breast milk and should be used with caution in breast-feeding women. Methadone has been shown to cause physical dependence in breast-feeding infants of women maintained on methadone.

Representative combinations

Codeine with acetaminophen: Phenaphen with codeine, Tylenol with codeine, Capital with codeine, Aceta with codeine, Acetaminophen with Codeine Oral Solution, Acetaminophen with Codeine Tablets, Margesic No. 3, Tylenol with Codeine No. 4, Phenaphen with Codeine No. 4; with caffeine: Fioricet with codeine; with calcium iodide and alcohol: Calcidrine.

Codeine phosphate with guaifenesin: Cheracol, Guiatuss AC, Guiatussin with Codeine Liquid, Mytussin AC, Robitussin A-C, Tolu-Sed Cough; with iodinated glycerol: Tussi-Organidin NR; with triprolidine hydrochloride and pseudoephedrine hydrochloride: Actifed with Codeine.

Codeine with aspirin: Empirin with codeine, Aspirin with Codeine No. 3, Aspirin with Codeine No. 4.

Codeine and aspirin with caffeine and butalbital: Fiorinal with Codeine; with carisoprodol: Soma Compound with Codeine.

Dihydrocodeine with acetaminophen and caffeine: Synalgos-DC.

Fentanyl with droperidol: Innovar, Fentanyl Citrate and Droperidol.

Hydrocodone bitartrate with acetaminophen: Anexsia 5/500 Tablets, Anexsia 7.5/650 Tablets, Anexsia 10/660 Tablets, Bancap HC, Dolacet, Duocet, Hydrocet, Lorcet-HD, Lorcet Plus, Zydone, Lortab, Lortab Elixir, Co-Gesic, Damason-P, Hydrogesic, Hy-Phen, Vicodin, Vicodin ES, Hydrocodone Bitartrate and Acetaminophen Tablets; with aspirin: Lortab ASA, Panasal 5/500; with aspirin and caffeine: Damason-P; with aspirin, acetaminophen, and caffeine: Hyco-Pap; with guaifenesin: Hycotuss Expectorant Syrup (with alcohol); with guaifenesin and pseudoephedrine hydrochloride: Detussin Expectorant, Entuss-D; with guaifenesin and phenindamine tartrate: P-V-Tussin tablets; with guaifenesin and phenylephrine: Donatussin DC; with potassium guaiacosulfonate: Codiclear DH, Entuss-D Liquid; with pseudoephedrine hydrochloride: Detussin Liquid; with homatropine methylbromide: Hycodan; with phenylephrine hydrochloride and pyrilamine maleate: Codimal DH; with phenylpropanolamine hydrochloride: Hycomine; with phenylephrine hydrochloride, pyrilamine maleate, chlorpheniramine maleate salicylamide, citric acid, and caffeine: Citra Forte; with pheniramine maleate, pyrilamine maleate, potassium citrate, and ascorbic acid: Citra forte; with phenylephrine hydrochloride, phenylpropanolamine hydrochloride, pheniramine maleate, pyrilamine maleate, and alcohol: Ru-Tuss with hydrocodone; with guaifenesin and alcohol: S-T forte; with phenyltoloxamine: Tussionex.

Hydromorphone with guaifenesin: Dilaudid Cough.

Meperidine with promethazine: Mepergan, Mepergan Fortis; with atropine sulfate: Atropine and Demerol Injection.

Oxycodone hydrochloride with acetaminophen: Tylox, Roxicet, Roxicet 5/500 Caplets, Roxicet Oral Solution, Oxycodone with Acetaminophen Capsules, Roxilox Capsules, Oxycocet*, Percocet, Percocet-Demi; with aspirin: Oxycodone with Aspirin Tablets, Roxiprin Tablets; with oxycodone terephthalate and aspirin: Percodan, Percodan-Demi.

Propoxyphene with acetaminophen: Lorcet, Wygesic, Darvocet-N, Propacet 100, Propoxyphene Napsylate and Acetaminophen, E-Lor Tablets, Genagesic.

Propoxyphene napsylate with acetaminophen: Darvocet-N 50, Darvocet-N 100, Propocet 100; with aspirin: Propoxyphene HCl Compound Capsules; with aspirin and caffeine: Darvon Compound, Propoxyphene Compound, PC-CAP.

opioid (narcotic) agonist-antagonists

buprenorphine hydrochloride, butorphanol tartate, nalbuphine hydrochloride, pentazocine hydrochloride

The term "narcotic (or opiate) agonist-antagonist" is somewhat imprecise. This class of drugs has varying degrees of agonist and antagonist activity. These drugs

* Canada only

◇ Unlabeled clinical use

are potent analgesics, with somewhat less addiction potential than the pure narcotic agonists.

Pharmacology

The detailed pharmacology of these drugs is poorly understood. Each agent is believed to act on different opiate receptors in the CNS to a greater or lesser degree, thus yielding slightly different effects. Like the opioid agonists, these drugs can be divided into related chemical groups. Buprenorphine, butorphanol, and nalbuphine are phenanthrenes, like morphine, whereas pentazocine falls into a unique class, the benzmorphans.

Clinical indications and actions

Pain

Opioid agonist-antagonists are primarily used as analgesics, particularly in patients at high risk for drug dependence or abuse. Some are used as preoperative or preanesthetic medication, to supplement balanced anesthesia or to relieve prepartum pain.

Overview of adverse reactions

Major hazards of agonist-antagonists are respiratory depression, apnea, shock, and cardiopulmonary arrest, possibly causing death. All opioid agonist-antagonists can cause respiratory depression, but the severity of such depression each drug can cause has a "ceiling"; for example, each drug depresses respiration to a certain point, but increased doses do not depress it further. All of the opioid agonist-antagonists have been reported to cause withdrawal symptoms after abrupt discontinuation of long-term use; they appear to have some addiction potential, but less than that of the pure opioid agonists.

CNS effects are the most common adverse reactions and may include drowsiness, sedation, light-headedness, dizziness, hallucinations, disorientation, agitation, euphoria, dysphoria, insomnia, confusion, headache, tremor, miosis, seizures, and psychic dependence. CV reactions may include tachycardia, bradycardia, palpitations, chest wall rigidity, hypertension, hypotension, syncope, and edema. GI reactions may include nausea, vomiting, and constipation (most common), dry mouth, anorexia, and biliary spasms (colic). Other effects include urine retention or hesitancy, decreased libido, flushing, rash, pruritus, and pain at the injection site.

Opioid agonist-antagonists can produce morphine-like dependence and thus have abuse potential. Psychic and physiologic dependence with drug tolerance can develop upon chronic repeated administration. Patients with dependence or tolerance to narcotic agonist-antagonists usually present with an acute abstinence syndrome or withdrawal signs and symptoms, of which the severity is related to the degree of dependence, abruptness of withdrawal, and the drug used.

Commonly, signs and symptoms of withdrawal are yawning, lacrimation, and sweating (early); mydriasis, piloerection, flushing of face, tachycardia, tremor, irritability, and anorexia (intermediate); and muscle spasms, fever, nausea, vomiting, and diarrhea (late).

☑ Special considerations

- Opioid agonist-antagonists are contraindicated in patients with known hypersensitivity to any drug of the same chemical group. Use these drugs with extreme caution in patients with supraventricular arrhythmias; avoid or administer drug with extreme caution in patients with head injury or increased intracranial pressure, because neurologic parameters are obscured; during pregnancy and labor, because drug crosses placenta readily (premature infants are especially sensitive to respiratory and CNS depressant effects of opioid agonist-antagonists).
- Use opioid agonist-antagonists cautiously in patients with renal or hepatic dysfunction, because drug accumulation or prolonged duration of action may occur; in patients with pulmonary disease (asthma, COPD) because drug depresses respiration and suppresses cough reflex; in patients undergoing biliary tract surgery because drug may cause biliary spasm; in patients with convulsive disorders because drug may precipitate seizures; in elderly and debilitated patients, who are more sensitive to both therapeutic and adverse drug effects; and in patients prone to physical or psychic addiction because of the high risk of addiction to this drug.
- Opioid agonist-antagonists have a lower potential for abuse than do opioid agonists, but the risk still exists.
- The opioid agonist-antagonists, as well as the opioids, antagonists, can reverse the desired effects of opioids; thus, members of different pharmacologic groups (for example, meperidine and buprenorphine) should not be prescribed at the same time.
- Always keep resuscitative equipment and an opioid antagonist (naloxone) available. Be prepared to provide ventilation and gastric lavage.
- Parenteral administration of opioid agonist-antagonists provides better analgesia than does oral dosing. I.V. dosing should be given by very slow injections, preferably in diluted solution. Rapid I.V. injection increases the incidence of adverse effects.
- Give I.M. or S.C. injections cautiously to patients who are chilled, hypovolemic, or in shock, because decreased perfusion may lead to accumulation.
- Before administration, visually inspect all parenteral products for particles and discoloration and note the strength of the solution.
- Patient tolerance may develop to the opiate agonist activity but does not develop to opiate antagonist activity.
- A regular dosing schedule (rather than "as needed for pain") is preferable to alleviate the symptoms and anxiety that accompany pain.
- The duration of respiratory depression may be longer than the analgesic effect. Monitor patient closely with repeated dosing.
- During chronic administration, regularly evaluate the patient's respiratory status. Because severe respiratory depression may occur (especially with accumulation on chronic dosing), watch for respiratory rate that is less than the patient's baseline respiratory rate. Also evaluate patient for restlessness, which may be a compensatory response to hypoxia.
- Opioid agonist-antagonists may cause orthostatic hypotension in ambulatory patients. Have patient sit or lie down to relieve dizziness or fainting.
- Because opioid agonist-antagonists can depress respiration when used postoperatively, strongly encourage patient turning, coughing, and deep breathing to avoid atelectases. Monitor respiratory status.
- Oral opioid agonist-antagonists may be taken with food to prevent gastric irritation. Food will delay absorption and the onset of analgesia.
- Opioid agonist-antagonists may obscure the signs and symptoms of an acute abdominal condition or worsen gallbladder pain.

- The first sign of tolerance to the therapeutic effect of opioid agonist-antagonists is usually a reduced duration of effect.
- Administering an opiate agonist-antagonist to the mother shortly before delivery may cause respiratory depression in the neonate. Monitor infant closely and be prepared to resuscitate.

Patient education
- Warn ambulatory patient to be cautious when performing tasks that require alertness, such as driving, if they are taking an opioid agonist-antagonist.
- Warn patient not to stop taking an opioid agonist-antagonist abruptly if he has been taking it for a prolonged period or at a high dose.
- Tell patient not to increase dosage if it is not producing the desired effect, but to call for prescribed dosage adjustment.
- Tell patient to avoid ingesting alcohol when taking opioid agonist-antagonists, because additive CNS depression will occur.
- Tell patient that constipation may result. Suggest measures to increase dietary fiber content or recommend a stool softener.
- Instruct patient not to double dose. Tell him to take a missed dose as soon as he remembers unless it is almost time for next dose. If this is the case, tell him to skip the missed dose and go back to regular dosage schedule.
- Tell patient to call for emergency help if he thinks he or someone else has taken an overdose.
- Explain signs of overdose to patient and to his family.
- Instruct patient to breathe deeply, cough, and change position every 2 hours to avoid respiratory complications.
- Encourage patient to void at least every 4 hours to avoid urine retention.
- Tell patient to take drug as prescribed and to promptly report significant adverse effects.
- Inform the female patient taking an opioid agonist-antagonist to call promptly if she is planning or suspects pregnancy; warn her that her fetus may become addicted to the drug.

Geriatric use
- Lower doses are usually indicated for elderly patients, who may be more sensitive to the therapeutic and adverse effects of these drugs.

Pediatric use
- Neonates may be more susceptible to the respiratory depressant effects of opiate agonist-antagonists.

Breast-feeding
- These drugs are usually not recommended for use in breast-feeding women.

Representative combinations
Pentazocine with acetaminophen: Talacen; with aspirin: Talwin Compound; with naloxone: Talwin Nx.

penicillins

***Natural penicillins:* penicillin G benzathine, penicillin G potassium, penicillin G procaine, penicillin G sodium, penicillin V potassium**

***Aminopenicillins:* amoxicillin trihydrate with clavulanate potassium, ampicillin, ampicillin sodium with sulbactam sodium, ampicillin trihydrate**

***Penicillinase-resistant penicillins:* cloxacillin sodium, dicloxacillin sodium, methicillin sodium, nafcillin sodium, oxacillin sodium**

***Extended spectrum penicillins:* carbenicillin indanyl sodium, mezlocillin sodium, piperacillin sodium, piperacillin sodium with tazobactam sodium, ticarcillin disodium, ticarcillin with clavulanate potassium**

Penicillins are very effective antibiotics with low toxicity. Their activity was first discovered by Sir Alexander Fleming in 1928, but they were not developed for use against systemic infections until 1940. Penicillin is naturally derived *from Penicillium chrysogenum.* New synthetic derivatives are created by chemical reactions that modify their structure, resulting in increased GI absorption, resistance to destruction by beta-lactamase (penicillinase), and a broader spectrum of susceptible organisms.

Pharmacology
The basic structure of penicillin is a thiazolidine ring connected to a beta-lactam ring that contains a side chain. This nucleus is the main structural requirement for antibacterial activity; modifications of the side chain alter penicillin's antibacterial and pharmacologic effects.

Penicillins are generally bactericidal. They inhibit synthesis of the bacterial cell wall, causing rapid cell lysis, and are most effective against fast-growing susceptible bacteria.

The sites of action for penicillins are enzymes known as penicillin-binding proteins (PBP). The affinity of certain penicillins for PBP in various microorganisms helps explain differing spectra of activity in this class of antibiotics.

Bacterial resistance to beta-lactam antibiotics is conferred most significantly by bacterial production of beta-lactamase enzymes, which destroy the beta-lactam ring and thus inactivate penicillin; decreased cell wall permeability and alteration in binding affinity to PBP also contribute to such resistance.

Oral absorption of penicillin varies widely; the most acid labile is penicillin G. Side-chain modifications in penicillin V, ampicillin, amoxicillin, and other orally administered penicillins are more stable in gastric acid and permit better absorption from the GI tract. (See *Comparing penicillins,* pages 1140 and 1141.)

Penicillins are distributed widely throughout the body; CSF penetration is minimal but is enhanced in patients with inflamed meninges. Most penicillins are only partially metabolized. With the exception of nafcillin, penicillins are excreted primarily in urine, chiefly through renal tubular effects; nafcillin undergoes en-

COMPARING PENICILLINS

DRUG	ROUTE	ADULT DOSAGE	FREQUENCY	PENICILLINASE-RESISTANT
amoxicillin	P.O.	250 to 500 mg 3 g with 1 g probenecid for gonorrhea	q 8 hr Single dose	No
amoxicillin/ clavulanate potassium	P.O.	250 mg 500 mg	q 8 hr q 12 hr	Yes
ampicillin	I.M., I.V. P.O.	2 to 14 g daily 250 to 500 mg 2.5 g with 1 g probenecid (for gonorrhea)	Divided doses given q 4 to 6 hr q 6 hr Single dose	No
ampicillin sodium/ sulbactam sodium	I.M., I.V.	1.5 to 3 g	q 6 to 8 hr	Yes
carbenicillin	P.O.	382 to 764 mg	q 6 hr	No
cloxacillin	P.O.	250 mg to 1 g	q 6 hr	Yes
dicloxacillin	P.O.	125 to 500 mg	q 6 hr	Yes
methicillin	I.M., I.V.	1 to 2 g	q 4 to 6 hr	Yes
mezlocillin	I.M., I.V.	3 to 4 g	q 4 to 6 hr	No
nafcillin	I.M., I.V. P.O.	250 mg to 2 g 500 mg to 1 g	q 4 to 6 hr q 6 hr	Yes
oxacillin	I.M., I.V. P.O.	250 mg to 2 g 500 mg to 1 g	q 4 to 6 hr q 6 hr	Yes
penicillin G benzathine	I.M.	1.2 to 2.4 million units	Single dose	Yes
penicillin G potassium	I.M., I.V.	200,000 to 4 million units	q 4 hr	No
penicillin G procaine	I.M.	600,000 to 1.2 million units 4.8 million units with 1 g probenecid (for syphilis)	q 1 to 3 days Single dose for primary, secondary, and early latent syphilis; weekly for 3 weeks for late latent syphilis	No
penicillin G sodium	I.M., I.V.	200,000 to 4 million units	q 4 hr	No
penicillin V potassium	P.O.	250 to 500 mg	q 6 to 8 hr	No
piperacillin	I.M., I.V.	100 to 300 mg/kg daily	Divided dose given q 4 to 6 hr	No
piperacillin sodium/ tazobactam sodium	I.V.	3.375 g	q 6 hr	Yes

COMPARING PENICILLINS *(continued)*

DRUG	ROUTE	ADULT DOSAGE	FREQUENCY	PENICILLINASE-RESISTANT
ticarcillin	I.M., I.V.	150 to 300 mg/kg daily	Divided doses given q 3 to 6 hr	No
ticarcillin/clavulanate potassium	I.V.	3.1 g	q 4 to 6 hr	Yes

terohepatic circulation and is excreted chiefly through the biliary tract.

Clinical indications and actions

Infection caused by susceptible organisms

• Natural penicillins. Penicillin G is the prototype of this group; derivatives such as penicillin V are more acid stable and thus better absorbed by the oral route. All natural penicillins are vulnerable to inactivation by beta-lactamase–producing bacteria. Natural penicillins act primarily against gram-positive organisms.

Clinical indications for natural penicillins include streptococcal pneumonia, enterococcal and nonenterococcal Group D endocarditis, diphtheria, anthrax, meningitis, tetanus, botulism, actinomycosis, syphilis, relapsing fever, Lyme disease, and others. Natural penicillins are used prophylactically against pneumococcal infections, rheumatic fever, bacterial endocarditis, and neonatal Group B streptococcal disease.

Susceptible aerobic gram-positive cocci include *Staphylococcus aureus;* nonenterococcal Group D streptococci, Groups A, B, D, G, H, K, L, and M streptococci, Streptococcus viridans; and enterococcus (usually in combination with an aminoglycoside). Susceptible aerobic gram-negative cocci include *Neisseria meningitidis* and non-penicillinase–producing *N. gonorrhoeae.*

Susceptible aerobic gram-positive bacilli include *Corynebacterium* (both diphtheria and opportunistic species), *Listeria,* and *Bacillus anthracis.* Susceptible anaerobes include *Peptococcus, Peptostreptococcus, Actinomyces, Clostridium, Fusobacterium, Veillonella,* and non-beta-lactamase–producing strains of *S. pneumoniae.*

Susceptible spirochetes include *Treponema pallidum, T. pertenue, Leptospira,* and *Borrelia recurrentis* and possibly *Borrelia burgdorferi.*

• Aminopenicillins (amoxicillin and ampicillin) offer a broader spectrum of activity including many gram-negative organisms. Like natural penicillins, aminopenicillins are vulnerable to inactivation by penicillinase. They are primarily used to treat septicemia, gynecologic infections, and infections of the urinary, respiratory, and GI tracts, and skin, soft tissue, bones, and joints. Their activity spectrum includes *Escherichia coli, Proteus mirabilis, Shigella, Salmonella, S. pneumoniae, N. gonorrhoeae, Haemophilus influenzae, Staphylococcus aureus, S. epidermidis* (non-penicillinase–producing *Staphylococcus*), and *Listeria monocytogenes.*

• Penicillinase-resistant penicillins (cloxacillin, dicloxacillin, oxacillin, and nafcillin) are semisynthetic penicillins designed to remain stable against hydrolysis by most staphylococcal penicillinases and thus are the drugs of choice against susceptible penicillinase-producing staphylococci. They also retain activity against most organisms susceptible to natural penicillins. Clinical indications are much the same as for aminopenicillins.

• Extended-spectrum penicillins (carbenicillin, mezlocillin, piperacillin, and ticarcillin), as their name implies, offer a wider range of bactericidal action than the other three classes, are used in hard-to-treat gram-negative infections, and are usually given in combination with aminoglycosides. They are used most often against susceptible strains of *Enterobacter, Klebsiella, Citrobacter, Serratia, Bacteroides fragilis, and Pseudomonas aeruginosa:* their gram-negative spectrum also includes *Proteus vulgaris, Providencia rettgeri,* and *Morganella morganii.* These penicillins are also vulnerable to destruction by beta-lactamase or penicillinases.

Overview of adverse reactions

Systemic reactions: Hypersensitivity reactions range from mild rash, fever, and eosinophilia to fatal anaphylaxis. Hematologic reactions include hemolytic anemia, transient neutropenia, leukopenia, and thrombocytopenia.

Certain adverse reactions are more common with specific classes of penicillin: bleeding episodes are usually seen at high-dose levels of extended-spectrum penicillins; acute interstitial nephritis is reported most often with methicillin; GI adverse effects are most common with but not limited to ampicillin. High doses, especially of penicillin G, irritate the CNS in patients with renal disease, causing confusion, twitching, lethargy, dysphagia, seizures, and coma. Hepatotoxicity is most common with penicillinase-resistant penicillins; hyperkalemia and hypernatremia with extended-spectrum penicillins.

Jarisch-Herxheimer reaction can occur when penicillin G is used in secondary syphilis; it presents as chills, fever, headache, myalgia, tachycardia, malaise, sweating, hypotension, and sore throat and is attributed to release of endotoxin following spirochete death.

Local reactions: Local irritation from parenteral therapy may be severe enough to require discontinuation of the drug or administration by subclavian catheter if drug therapy is to continue.

☑ Special considerations

• Assess patient's history of allergies.

• Keep in mind that a negative history for penicillin hypersensitivity does not preclude future allergic reactions; monitor patient continuously for possible allergic reactions or other untoward effects.

• Reduce dosage in patients with renal impairment based on creatinine clearance and manufacturer's guidelines.

• Assess level of consciousness, neurologic status, and renal function when high doses are used, because excessive blood levels can cause CNS toxicity.

- Monitor vital signs, electrolytes, and renal function studies; monitor body weight for fluid retention with extended-spectrum penicillins for possible hypokalemia or hypernatremia.
- Coagulation abnormalities, even frank bleeding, can follow high doses, especially of extended-spectrum penicillins; monitor PT and platelet counts, and assess patient for signs of occult or frank bleeding.
- Monitor patients on long-term therapy for possible superinfection, especially elderly and debilitated patients and others receiving immunosuppressants or radiation therapy; monitor closely, especially for fever.

Oral and parenteral administration

- Give penicillins at least 1 hour before giving bacteriostatic antibiotics (tetracyclines, erythromycins, and chloramphenicol); these drugs inhibit bacterial cell growth, decreasing rate of penicillin uptake by bacterial cell walls.
- Give oral penicillin at least 1 hour before or 2 hours after meals to enhance gastric absorption; food may or may not decrease absorption.
- Refrigerate oral suspensions; shake well before administering, to assure correct dosage.
- Administer I.M. dose deep into large muscle mass (gluteal or midlateral thigh); rotate injection sites to minimize tissue injury; do not inject more than 2 g of drug per injection site. Apply ice to injection site for pain.
- Do not add or mix other drugs with I.V. infusions—particularly aminoglycosides, which will be inactivated if mixed with penicillins; they are chemically and physically incompatible. If other drugs must be given I.V., temporarily stop infusion of primary drug.
- Infuse I.V. drug continuously or intermittently (over 30 minutes) and assess I.V. site frequently to prevent infiltration or phlebitis; rotate infusion site q 48 hours; intermittent I.V. infusion may be diluted in 50 to 100 ml sterile water, 0.9% NaCl solution, D_5W, D_5W and 0.45% NaCl, or lactated Ringer's solution.

Patient education

- Explain disease process and rationale for therapy.
- Teach signs and symptoms of hypersensitivity and other adverse reactions, and emphasize need to report unusual reactions.
- Teach signs and symptoms of bacterial and fungal superinfection to patients, especially elderly and debilitated patients and others with low resistance from immunosuppressants or irradiation; emphasize need to report signs of infection.
- Be sure patient understands how and when to take drugs; urge him to complete entire prescribed regimen, to comply with instructions for around-the-clock dosage, and to keep follow-up appointments.
- Counsel patient to check expiration date of drug and to discard unused drug and not give it to family members or friends.

Geriatric use

- Use with caution; elderly patients are susceptible to superinfection.
- Many elderly patients have renal impairment, which decreases excretion of penicillins; lower the dosage in elderly patients who have diminished creatinine clearance.

Pediatric use

- Specific dosage recommendations have been established for most penicillins.

Breast-feeding

- Consult individual drug recommendations.

Representative combinations

Amoxicillin with clavulanate potassium: Augmentin.

Ampicillin with probenecid: Polycillin-PRB, Probampacin.

Ampicillin sodium with sulbactam sodium: Unasyn.

Ampicillin trihydrate with probenecid: Polycillin-PRB, Principen with Probenecid, Probampacin.

Penicillin G benzathine with penicillin G procaine: Bicillin C-R, Bicillin C-R 900/300.

Piperacillin sodium with tazobactam sodium: Zosyn.

Ticarcillin disodium with clavulanate potassium: Timentin.

phenothiazines

Aliphatic derivatives: chlorpromazine hydrochloride, promethazine hydrochloride, trimeprazine tartrate

Piperazine derivatives: fluphenazine hydrochloride, perphenazine, prochlorperazine, trifluoperazine hydrochloride

Piperidine derivatives: mesoridazine besylate, thioridazine

Thioxanthene: thiothixene

The phenothiazines were originally synthesized by European scientists seeking aniline-like dyes in the late 1800s. Several decades later, in the 1930s, promethazine was identified and found to have sedative, antihistaminic, and narcotic-potentiating effects. Chlorpromazine was synthesized in the 1950s; this drug proved to have many effects, among them strong antipsychotic activity.

Pharmacology

Phenothiazines are classified in terms of chemical structure: the aliphatic agent (chlorpromazine) has a greater sedative, hypotensive, allergic, and convulsant activity; the piperazines (perphenazine, prochlorperazine, fluphenazine, and trifluoperazine) are more likely to produce extrapyramidal symptoms; the piperidines (thioridazine and mesoridazine) have intermediate effects. Thioxanthenes are chemically similar to phenothiazines, and pharmacologically similar to piperazine phenothiazines. Promethazine is a derivative that has antihistamine qualities.

All antipsychotics have fundamentally similar mechanisms of action; they are believed to function as dopamine antagonists, blocking postsynaptic dopamine receptors in various parts of the CNS; their antiemetic effects result from blockage of the chemoreceptor trigger zone. They also produce varying degrees of anticholinergic and alpha-adrenergic receptor blocking actions. The drugs are structurally similar to tricyclic antidepressants (TCAs) and share many adverse reactions.

All antipsychotics have equal clinical efficacy when given in equivalent doses; choice of specific therapy is determined primarily by the individual patient's response and adverse reaction profile. A patient who does not respond to one drug may respond to another.

Onset of full therapeutic effects requires 6 weeks to 6 months of therapy; therefore, dosage adjustment is recommended at not less than weekly intervals.

Clinical indications and actions

Psychoses

The phenothiazines (except promethazine and trimeprazine) and thiothixene are indicated to treat agitated psychotic states. They are especially effective in controlling hallucinations in schizophrenic patients, the manic phase of manic-depressive illness, and excessive motor and autonomic activity.

Nausea and vomiting

Chlorpromazine, perphenazine, and prochlorperazine are effective in controlling severe nausea and vomiting induced by CNS disturbances. They do not prevent motion sickness or vertigo.

◊ ***Anxiety***

Chlorpromazine, mesoridazine, promethazine, prochlorperazine, and trifluoperazine also may be used for short-term treatment of moderate anxiety in selected nonpsychotic patients, for example, to control anxiety before surgery.

Severe behavior problems

Chlorpromazine and thioridazine are indicated to control combativeness and hyperexcitability in children with severe behavior problems. They also are used in hyperactive children for short-term treatment of excessive motor activity with labile moods, impulsive behavior, aggressiveness, attention deficit, and poor tolerance of frustration. Mesoridazine is used to manage hypersensitivity and to promote cooperative behavior in patients with mental deficiency and chronic brain syndrome.

Tetanus

Chlorpromazine is an effective adjunct in treating tetanus.

Porphyria

Because of its effects on the autonomic nervous system, chlorpromazine is effective in controlling abdominal pain in patients with acute intermittent porphyria.

Intractable hiccups

Chlorpromazine has been used to treat patients with intractable hiccups. The mechanism is unknown.

Neurogenic pain

Fluphenazine is a useful adjunct, managing selected chronic pain states.

Allergies and pruritus

Because of their potent antihistaminic effects, many of these drugs (including promethazine and trimeprazine) are used to relieve itching or symptomatic rhinitis.

Overview of adverse reactions

Phenothiazines may produce extrapyramidal symptoms (dystonic movements, torticollis, oculogyric crises, parkinsonian symptoms) from akathisia during early treatment, to tardive dyskinesia after long-term use.

In rare cases, a neuroleptic malignant syndrome resembling severe parkinsonism may occur; it consists of rapid onset of hyperthermia, muscular hyperreflexia, marked extrapyramidal and autonomic dysfunction, arrhythmias, and sweating.

Other adverse reactions are similar to those seen with TCAs, including sedative and anticholinergic effects, orthostatic hypotension, reflex tachycardia, fainting, dizziness, arrhythmias, anorexia, nausea, vomiting, abdominal pain, local gastric irritation, seizures, endocrine effects, hematologic disorders, ocular changes, skin eruptions, and photosensitivity. Allergic manifestations are usually marked by elevation of liver enzymes progressing to obstructive jaundice.

The piperidine derivatives have the most pronounced CV effects; the piperazine derivatives have the least. Parenteral administration is often associated with CV effects because of more rapid absorption. Seizures are common with aliphatic derivatives.

☑ Special considerations

- Phenothiazines are contraindicated in patients with known hypersensitivity to phenothiazines and related compounds.
- Use with caution in patients with cardiac disease (arrhythmias, heart failure, angina pectoris, valvular disease, or heart block).
- Also use cautiously in patients with encephalitis, Reye's syndrome, head injury, epilepsy, or other seizure disorders.
- Use phenothiazines cautiously in patients with glaucoma, prostatic hypertrophy, paralytic ileus, urine retention, hepatic or renal dysfunction, Parkinson's disease, pheochromocytoma, and hypocalcemia.
- Check vital signs regularly for decreased blood pressure (especially before and after parenteral therapy) or tachycardia; observe patient carefully for other adverse reactions.
- Check intake and output for urine retention or constipation, which may require dosage reduction.
- Monitor bilirubin levels weekly for first 4 weeks; monitor CBC, ECG (for quinidine-like effects), liver and renal function studies, electrolyte levels (especially potassium), and eye examinations at baseline and periodically thereafter, especially in patients on long-term therapy.
- Observe patient for mood changes to monitor progress; benefits may not be apparent for several weeks.
- Monitor for involuntary movements. Check patient receiving prolonged treatment at least once every 6 months.
- Do not withdraw drug abruptly; although physical dependence does not occur with antipsychotic drugs, rebound exacerbation of psychotic symptoms may occur, and many drug effects persist.
- Carefully follow manufacturer's instructions for reconstitution, dilution, administration, and storage of drugs; slightly discolored liquids may or may not be all right to use. Check with pharmacist.

Patient education

- Explain rationale and anticipated risks and benefits of therapy, and that full therapeutic effect may not occur for several weeks.
- Teach signs and symptoms of adverse reactions and importance of reporting unusual effects, especially involuntary movements.
- Tell patient to avoid beverages and drugs containing alcohol, and not to take other drugs (especially CNS depressants) including OTC products without medical approval.
- Instruct diabetic patients to monitor blood glucose because drug may alter insulin needs.
- Teach patient how and when to take drug, not to increase dose without medical approval, and never to discontinue drug abruptly; suggest taking full dose at bedtime if daytime sedation is troublesome.
- Advise patient to lie down for 30 minutes after first dose (1 hour if I.M.) and to rise slowly from sitting or supine position to prevent orthostatic hypotension.
- Warn patient to avoid tasks requiring mental alertness and psychomotor coordination such as driving until full effects of drug are established; emphasize that sedative effects will lessen after several weeks.
- Drugs are locally irritating; advise patient to take drug with milk or food to minimize GI distress. Warn that oral concentrates and solutions will irritate skin, and tell pa-

tient not to crush or open sustained-release products, but to swallow them whole.

- Warn patient that photosensitivity reactions (burns and abnormal hyperpigmentation) may occur.
- Tell patient to avoid exposure to extremes of heat or cold, because of risk of hypothermia or hyperthermia induced by alteration in thermoregulatory function.
- Explain that phenothiazines may cause pink to brown discoloration of urine.

Geriatric use

- Lower doses are indicated in geriatric patients, who are more sensitive to therapeutic and adverse effects, especially cardiac toxicity, tardive dyskinesia, and other extrapyramidal effects. Titrate dosage to patient response.

Pediatric use

- Unless otherwise specified, antipsychotics are not recommended for children under age 12; be careful when using phenothiazines for nausea and vomiting because acutely ill children (suffering from chickenpox, measles, CNS infections, dehydration) are at greatly increased risk of dystonic reactions.

Breast-feeding

- If possible, patient should not breast-feed while taking antipsychotics; most phenothiazines are excreted in breast milk and have a direct effect on prolactin levels. Benefit to mother must outweigh hazard to infant.

Representative combinations

None.

pituitary hormones, posterior

desmopressin acetate, oxytocin, vasopressin (antidiuretic hormone)

In 1954, the structure of antidiuretic hormone was determined and its synthesis achieved. The following year, duVigneaud was awarded the Nobel prize for his work. The drugs in this class are used to treat postoperative ileus, diabetes insipidus, and upper GI hemorrhage and to stimulate expulsion of gas before pyelography. Oxytocin is used in labor and delivery.

Pharmacology

Endogenous vasopressin and oxytocin are secreted by the hypothalamus and stored in the posterior pituitary. Vasopressin is found in all mammals except swine. Desmopressin, an analogue of vasopressin, was synthesized in 1967.

Posterior pituitary preparations have oxytocic and vasopressor activity. Posterior pituitary powder is obtained from the dried posterior lobe of the pituitary of domesticated animals used by humans for food. These drugs increase cAMP, thereby increasing water reabsorption in the kidneys, causing increased urine osmolality and decreased urinary flow rate. Desmopressin also increases factor VIII activity by causing the release of endogenous factor VIII from plasma stores. Oxytocin causes contraction of uterine smooth muscle (increasing amplitude and frequency of contractions) and myoepithelial cells surrounding breast alveoli (causing milk ejection).

Clinical indications and actions

Diabetes insipidus

Vasopressin, desmopressin, and posterior pituitary hormone are used to control or prevent signs and complications of neurogenic diabetes insipidus. Acting primarily at the renal tubular level, they increase cAMP, which increases water permeability at the renal tubule and collecting duct, causing increased urine osmolality and decreased urinary flow rate.

Postoperative abdominal distention and abdominal radiographic procedures

Vasopressin and posterior pituitary hormone induce peristalsis by directly stimulating smooth muscle contraction in the GI tract.

GI hemorrhage

Vasopressin has been used I.V. or intra-arterially into the superior mesenteric artery to temporarily control bleeding of esophageal varices by directly stimulating capillaries and small arterioles, causing vasoconstriction. Posterior pituitary hormone, I.M. or S.C., also is used as an aid to achieve hemostasis in surgery and in the presence of esophageal varices.

Hemophilia A and von Willebrand's disease

Desmopressin increases Factor VIII activity by releasing endogenous Factor VIII from plasma storage sites.

Induction and augmentation of labor

Oxytocin is used to induce labor in prolonged pregnancies (greater than 42 weeks' gestation) and in complicated term or near-term pregnancies (hypertension, antepartum bleeding, preeclampsia, eclampsia, or premature rupture of membranes in which spontaneous labor does not ensue).

Overview of adverse reactions

Adverse effects of posterior pituitary hormones commonly reflect excessive oxytoxic or vasopressor activity and may include abdominal and uterine smooth muscle cramping, chest pain, and hypertension. Anaphylaxis and other hypersensitivity reactions may occur.

☑ Special considerations

- Use with caution in patients with coronary artery insufficiency or hypertensive CV disease.
- Adjust fluid intake to reduce risk of water intoxication and sodium depletion, especially in young or old patients.
- Overdose may cause oxytocic or vasopressor activity. If patient develops uterine cramps, increased GI activity, fluid retention, or hypertension, withhold drug until effects subside. Furosemide may be used if fluid retention is excessive.
- Some patients may have difficulty measuring and inhaling drug into nostrils. Teach patient correct method of administration.

Representative combinations

None.

progestins

hydroxyprogesterone caproate, medroxyprogesterone acetate, megestrol acetate, norethindrone, norethindrone acetate, norgestrel, progesterone

Progesterone is the endogenous progestin, secreted by the corpus luteum within the female ovary. Several synthetic progesterone derivatives with greater potency or duration of action have been synthesized. Some of these derivatives also possess weak androgenic or estrogenic activity. The progestins are used to treat dysfunctional uterine bleeding and certain cancers. They also are used as contraceptives, either alone or in combination with estrogens.

Pharmacology

Progesterone causes secretory changes in the endometrium, changes in the vaginal epithelium, increases in body temperature, relaxation of uterine smooth muscle, stimulation of growth of breast alveolar tissue, inhibition of gonadotropin release from the pituitary, and withdrawal bleeding (in the presence of estrogens). The synthetic progesterone derivatives have these properties as well.

Clinical indications and actions

Hormonal imbalance, female

Hydroxyprogesterone, medroxyprogesterone, norethindrone, and progesterone are indicated to treat amenorrhea and dysfunctional uterine bleeding resulting from hormonal imbalance. Hydroxyprogesterone also is indicated to produce desquamation and a secretory endometrium.

Endometriosis

Norethindrone and norethindrone acetate are indicated to treat endometriosis.

Carcinoma

Hydroxyprogesterone, medroxyprogesterone, and megestrol are indicated in the adjunctive and palliative treatment of certain types of metastatic tumors. They are not considered primary therapy. See individual agents for specific indications.

Contraception

Norethindrone and norgestrel are approved for use with estrogens or alone as oral contraceptives.

Progestins are no longer indicated to detect pregnancy (because of teratogenicity) or to treat threatened or habitual abortion, for which they are not effective.

Overview of adverse reactions

The most common adverse effect is a change in menstrual bleeding pattern, ranging from spotting or breakthrough bleeding to complete amenorrhea. Other reactions include breast tenderness and secretion, weight changes, increases in body temperature, edema, nausea, acne, somnolence, insomnia, hirsutism, hair loss, depression, cholestatic jaundice, and allergic reactions (rare). Some patients taking parenteral progestins have also suffered localized reactions at the injection site.

☑ Special considerations

- Progestins are contraindicated during pregnancy and in patients with thromboembolic disorders, breast cancer, undiagnosed abnormal vaginal bleeding, or severe hepatic disease.
- Use cautiously in patients with diabetes mellitus, cardiac or renal disease, seizure disorder, migraine, or mental depression.
- Give oil injections deep I.M. in gluteal muscles. I.M. injections may be painful; observe injection site for sterile abscess formation.
- Do not use progestins in breast-feeding patients, except for Depo-Provera which is indicated for breast-feeding women after 6 weeks.
- Glucose tolerance may be altered in diabetic patients. Monitor patient closely because antidiabetic medication may need to be adjusted.
- When used as an oral contraceptive, progestins are administered daily without interruption, regardless of menstrual cycle.
- Use of progestins may lead to gingival bleeding and hyperplasia.
- A patient who is exposed to progestins during the first 4 months of pregnancy or who becomes pregnant while receiving the drug should be informed of the potential risks to the fetus.
- Because oral contraceptive combinations contain progestins, the precautions associated with oral contraceptives should be considered in patients receiving progestins.

Patient education

- Tell patient that GI distress may subside with use (after a few cycles).
- Instruct patient receiving progestins to have a full physical examination, including a gynecologic examination and a Papanicolaou test, every 6 to 12 months.
- Advise patient to discontinue therapy and call immediately if migraine or visual disturbances occur, or if sudden severe headache or vomiting develops.
- Teach patient how to perform breast self-examination.
- Tell patient to call promptly if period is missed or unusual bleeding occurs; and to call and discontinue drug immediately if pregnancy is suspected.
- Advise patient who misses a dose to take the missed dose as soon as possible or omit it; and not to double dose.
- Advise patient who misses a dose when used as a contraceptive to discontinue the drug and use an alternative contraception method until period begins or pregnancy is ruled out.
- Inform patient that drug may cause possible dental problems (tenderness, swelling, or bleeding of gums). Advise patient to brush and floss teeth, massage gums, and have dentist clean teeth regularly. She should check with dentist if there are questions about care of teeth or gums or if tenderness, swelling, or bleeding of gums is noticed.
- Advise patient to use extra care to avoid pregnancy when starting use of drug as an oral contraceptive and for at least 3 months after discontinuing it.
- Advise patient to keep an extra 1-month supply available.
- Tell patient to keep tablets in original container.
- Emphasize importance of not giving medication to anyone else.

Representative combinations

Hydroxyprogesterone caproate with estradiol valerate: Hylutin.

Norethindrone acetate with ethinyl estradiol: Brevicon, Loestrin 1.5/30, Loestrin Fe 1.5/30, Loestrin 21 1/20, Loestrin Fe 1/20, Modicon, Norinyl 1 + 35, Ortho 1/35*, Ortho 7/7/7*, Ortho 10/11*, Ortho-Novum 7/7/7, Ovcon-35, Ovcon-50, Tri-Norinyl; with mestranol: Norinyl 1/50, Ortho-Novum 0.5/35*, Ortho-Novum 1/50, Ortho-Novum 1/35.

Norgestrel with ethinyl estradiol: Lo/Ovral, Ovral.

salicylates

aspirin, choline magnesium trisalicylate, choline salicylate, magnesium salicylate, salsalate

Salicylates provide temporary relief of mild to moderate pain, especially pain associated with inflammation, and as prophylaxis for MI. Widely prescribed, these drugs are the standard of comparison and evaluation for other nonnarcotic analgesics, NSAIDs, and antipyretic drugs.

Pharmacology

Salicylates produce analgesic, anti-inflammatory, and antipyretic effects through action of the salicylate moiety; dissociation or hydrolysis to salicylic acid is not required for pharmacologic effects.

Salicylates may act peripherally by inhibiting the enzyme cyclooxygenase, thus decreasing formation of the prostaglandins involved in pain and inflammation. These prostaglandins appear to sensitize pain receptors to mechanical stimulation or to other chemical mediators. These drugs may also act centrally, possibly in the hypothalamus. The anti-inflammatory action of the salicylates, also related to prostaglandin inhibition, may contribute to their analgesic effect. The exact mechanism of the latter effect is unknown.

Salicylates lower body temperature principally by inhibiting synthesis and release of the prostaglandins that mediate the effect of endogenous pyrogens on the hypothalamus. Also, salicylates produce a centrally mediated dilation of peripheral blood vessels, enhancing heat dissipation and sweating. Salicylates rarely decrease body temperature in afebrile patients.

Clinical indications and actions

Salicylates are used principally for the symptomatic relief of mild to moderate pain, inflammation, and fever.

Pain

Salicylates are most effective in treating low-intensity pain of headache, arthralgia, myalgia, and neuralgia. They may also relieve mild to moderate pain from dental and surgical procedures, dysmenorrhea, and rheumatic fever.

Inflammation

Salicylates are commonly used for initial long-term treatment of rheumatoid arthritis, juvenile arthritis, and osteoarthritis. It is important to note that in rheumatoid conditions, these agents offer only symptomatic relief, reducing pain, stiffness, swelling, and tenderness. They do not reverse or arrest the disease process.

Fever

Use of salicylates in fever is nonspecific and does not influence the course of the underlying disease.

Overview of adverse reactions

Most common symptoms are dyspepsia, heartburn, epigastric distress, nausea, and abdominal pain. The incidence and severity of GI bleeding are exposure related. Nephrotoxicity may occur, especially in the elderly.

Chronic salicylate intoxication (salicylism) may occur with prolonged therapy, at high doses. Signs and symptoms include tinnitus, hearing loss, hepatotoxicity, moderate to severe noncardiogenic edema, and adverse renal effects.

Salicylate-induced bronchospasm, with or without urticaria and angioedema, may occur in patients with hypersensitivity to these drugs, particularly those with the "triad" of aspirin sensitivity, rhinitis or nasal polyps, and asthma. A significant incidence of cross-reactivity has been observed with tartrazine; 5% of allergic patients also exhibit cross-sensitivity with acetaminophen.

☑ Special considerations

- Use salicylates with caution in patients with history of GI disease (especially peptic ulcer disease), increased risk of GI bleeding, or decreased renal function.
- Tablets may be chewed, broken, or crumbled and administered with food or fluids to aid swallowing. Uncoated plain aspirin tablets allowed to remain in contact with mucous membranes of the mouth and aspirin chewing gum have produced mucosal erosions and mouth ulcerations.
- Patient should take 8 oz (240 ml) of water or milk with salicylates to ensure passage into stomach. Patient should sit up for 15 to 30 minutes after taking salicylates to prevent lodging of salicylate in esophagus.
- Administer antacids, if prescribed, with salicylates except enteric-coated forms. Separate doses of antacids and enteric-coated salicylates by 1 to 2 hours to ensure adequate absorption.
- Monitor vital signs frequently, especially temperature.
- Salicylates may mask the signs and symptoms of acute infection (fever, myalgia, erythema); carefully evaluate patients at risk for infections, such as those with diabetes.
- Monitor CBC, platelets, PT, BUN, serum creatinine, and liver function studies periodically during salicylate therapy to detect abnormalities.
- Avoid use for 1 week prior to surgery.
- Assess for signs and symptoms of potential hemorrhage, such as petechiae, bruising, coffee ground vomitus, and black tarry stools.
- Reduce dosage if fever or illness causes fluid depletion.

Patient education

- Tell patient to take tablet or capsule forms of medication with 8 oz (240 ml) of water and not to lie down for 15 to 30 minutes after swallowing drug.
- Tell patient to take drug 30 minutes before or 2 hours after meals, or with food or milk if gastric irritation occurs.
- Explain that taking drug as directed is necessary to achieve the desired effect; 2 to 4 weeks of treatment may be needed before benefit is seen.
- Advise patients on chronic salicylate therapy to arrange for monitoring of laboratory parameters, especially BUN, serum creatinine, liver function tests, CBC, and PT.
- Warn patients with current case or history of rectal bleeding to avoid using salicylate suppositories. The latter must be retained in the rectum for at least 1 hour and could cause irritation and bleeding.
- Warn patient of childbearing age to avoid use of all salicylates. Pregnant patients should avoid all salicylates, especially during the third trimester, when prostaglandin inhibition can adversely affect fetal CV development.
- Advise patient to avoid taking aspirin-containing medications or NSAIDs such as ibuprofen without medical approval.
- Warn patient that use of alcoholic beverages with salicylates may cause increased GI irritation and possibly GI bleeding.
- Tell patient to take a missed dose as soon as he remembers, unless it is almost time for next dose; then skip the missed dose and return to regular schedule.
- Tell patient not to take these medications for more than 10 consecutive days unless otherwise directed.

Geriatric use

- Patients over age 60 may be more susceptible to the toxic effects of salicylates because of possible impaired renal function.
- Effects of salicylates on renal prostaglandins may cause fluid retention and edema, a significant disadvantage in elderly patients, especially those with heart failure.

Pediatric use

- Use with caution because children may be more susceptible to toxic effects of salicylates.

• Because of epidemiologic association with Reye's syndrome, the Centers for Disease Control and Prevention recommend that children with chickenpox or flulike symptoms not be given salicylates.
• Do not use long-term salicylate therapy in children under age 14; safety has not been established.
• Generally, children should not take salicylates more than five times or for more than 5 days.

Breast-feeding

• Salicylates are distributed into breast milk and should be avoided during breast-feeding.

Representative combinations

Aspirin with magnesium hydroxide and aluminum hydroxide: Arthritis Pain Formula; with magnesium oxide and aluminum hydroxide: Cama Arthritis Pain Reliever; with magnesium hydroxide, aluminum hydroxide, and calcium carbonate: Magnaprin, Ascriptin, Ascriptin A/D, Magnaprin Arthritis Strength; with magnesium oxide, magnesium carbonate, and calcium carbonate: Bufferin; with magnesium carbonate and aluminum glycinate: Bufferin Extra-Strength, Arthritis Strength Bufferin; with magnesium oxide, magnesium carbonate, and calcium carbonate: Tri-Buffered Bufferin; with magnesium carbonate and aluminum glycinate: Buffex; with magnesium salicylate and choline salicylate: Trilisate Tablets, Trilisate Liquid; with caffeine: Anacin, Anacin Maximum Strength, Cope, Gensan, C2, Instantine; with acetaminophen and caffeine: Gelpirin, Supac, Buffets II, Vanquish Caplets, Pain Reliever, Extra Strength Excedrin, Goody's Extra-Strength Tablets; with salicylamide and caffeine: BC Powder; with butabarbital: Axotal; with caffeine and butabarbital: Fiorinal; with acetaminophen, salicylamide, and caffeine: S-A-C, Saleto; with meprobamate: Equagesic, Meprogesic Q, Micrainin Tablets.

Salicylic acid with sulfur: Sebulex, Fostex Medicated Cleansing, Meted.

See also *opioids.*

sulfonamides

co-trimoxazole (trimethoprim-sulfamethoxazole), sulfadiazine, sulfamethoxazole, sulfasalazine, sulfisoxazole

Sulfonamides were the first effective drugs used to treat systemic bacterial infections. The prototype, sulfanilamide, was discovered in 1908 and first used clinically in 1933. Since then, many derivatives have been synthesized, and many therapeutic milestones have been reached, including improved solubility of sulfonamides in urine (which reduces renal toxicity) and discovery of the advantages of combinations such as triple sulfa and, especially, of combined trimethoprim and sulfamethoxazole (co-trimoxazole). Development of other major antibiotics has reduced the clinical impact of sulfonamides; however, introduction of the combination agent co-trimoxazole has increased their usefulness in certain infections.

Pharmacology

Sulfonamides are bacteriostatic. Their mechanism of action correlates directly with the structural similarities they share with para-aminobenzoic acid. They inhibit biosynthesis of folic acid, which is needed for cell growth; susceptible bacteria are those that synthesize folic acid.

Sulfonamides are well absorbed from the GI tract after oral administration, except for sulfasalazine, which is absorbed minimally by the oral route. Sulfonamides are distributed widely into tissues and fluids, including pleural, peritoneal, synovial, and ocular fluids; some, including sulfisoxazole, penetrate CSF. Sulfonamides readily cross the placenta and are found in low concentrations in breast milk. Sulfonamides are metabolized by the liver and the parent drug and metabolites are excreted in urine by glomerular filtration. Hemodialysis removes both sulfamethoxazole and sulfisoxazole, but peritoneal dialysis removes only sulfisoxazole.

Clinical indications and actions

Bacterial infections

When first introduced, sulfonamides were active against many gram-positive and gram-negative organisms; over time, many bacteria have become resistant. Currently, sulfonamides are active against some strains of staphylococci, streptococci, *Nocardia asteroides* and *brasiliensis, Clostridium tetani* and *perfringens, Bacillus anthracis, Escherichia coli,* and *Neisseria gonorrhoeae* and *meningitidis.* Resistance to sulfonamides is common if therapy continues beyond 2 weeks; resistance to one sulfonamide usually means cross-resistance to others.

Sulfonamides are used to treat urinary tract infections caused by *E. coli, Proteus mirabilis* and *vulgaris, Klebsiella, Enterobacter,* and *Staphylococcus aureus,* and genital lesions caused by *Haemophilus ducreyi* (chancroid). They are the drugs of choice in nocardiosis, usually with surgical drainage or combined with other antibiotics, including ampicillin, erythromycin, cycloserine, or minocycline. Sulfonamides also are used to treat otitis media and may be used as alternative therapy to tetracyclines against *Chlamydia trachomatis* (lymphogranuloma venereum). Sulfadiazine is used to eradicate meningococci from the nasopharynx of asymptomatic carriers of *N. meningitidis.*

◇ Co-trimoxazole is used to treat infections of the urinary tract, respiratory tract, and ear; to treat chronic bacterial prostatitis; and to prevent recurrent urinary tract infection in women and "traveler's diarrhea."

Parasitic infections

Sulfonamides combined with pyrimethamine are used to treat toxoplasmosis; certain sulfonamides are combined with quinine and pyrimethamine to treat chloroquine-*resistant Plasmodium falciparum* malaria.

Co-trimoxazole is also used to treat *Pneumocystis carinii* pneumonia.

Inflammations

Sulfasalazine, used to treat inflammatory bowel disease, is cleaved in the intestine to sulfapyridine and 5-aminosalicylic acid.

Overview of adverse reactions

Sulfonamides cause adverse reactions affecting many organs and systems. Many are considered to be caused by hypersensitivity, including the following: rash, fever, pruritus, erythema multiforme, erythema nodosum, Stevens-Johnson syndrome, Lyell's syndrome, exfoliative dermatitis, photosensitivity, joint pain, conjunctivitis, leukopenia, and bronchospasm. Hematologic reactions include granulocytopenia, thrombocytopenia, agranulocytosis, hypoprothrombinemia, and, in G6PD deficiency, hemolytic anemia. Renal effects usually result from crystalluria (precipitation of the sulfonamide in the renal system). GI reactions include anorexia, stomatitis, pancreatitis, diarrhea, and folic acid malabsorption. Oral therapy commonly causes nausea and vomiting. Hepatotoxicity and CNS reactions (dizziness, confusion, headache, ataxia, drowsiness, and insomnia) are rare.

☑ Special considerations

• Assess patient's history of allergies; do not give a sulfonamide to patient with history of hypersensitivity reactions to sulfonamides or to other drugs containing sulfur.
• Sulfonamides are also contraindicated in patients with severe renal or hepatic dysfunction, or porphyria; during pregnancy at term and during breast-feeding. Sulfonamides may cause kernicterus in infants, because they displace bilirubin at the binding site, cross the placenta, and are excreted in breast milk. Do not use in infants under age 2 months (except in the treatment of congenital toxoplasmosis as adjunctive therapy with pyrimethamine).
• Administer sulfonamides with caution to patients with the following conditions: mild to moderate renal or hepatic impairment; urinary obstruction, because of the risk of drug accumulation; severe allergies; asthma; blood dyscrasia; or G6PD deficiency.
• Monitor continuously for possible hypersensitivity reactions or other untoward effects; patients with AIDS have a much higher incidence of adverse reactions.
• Obtain results of cultures and sensitivity tests before giving first dose, but therapy may begin before laboratory tests are complete; check test results periodically to assess drug efficacy. Monitor urine cultures, CBCs, and urinalysis before and during therapy.
• Monitor patients on prolonged for superinfection, especially elderly and debilitated patients and others receiving immunosuppressants or radiation therapy.
• Sulfonamides may interact with other drugs (oral anticoagulants, cyclosporine, digoxin, folic acid, hydantoins, methotrexate, and sulfonylureas) and may alter test results; consult individual drug entries for possible test interactions.

Administration

• Give oral dosage with full glass (8 oz [240 ml]) of water, and force fluids to 12 to 16 glasses/day depending on the agent; patient's urine output should be at least 1,500 ml/day.
• Follow manufacturer's directions for reconstitution, dilution, and storage of drugs; check expiration dates.
• Give oral sulfonamide at least 1 hour before or 2 hours after meals for maximum absorption.
• Shake oral suspensions well before administering to ensure correct dosage.

Patient education

• Teach signs and symptoms of hypersensitivity and other adverse reactions, and emphasize need to report these; specifically urge patient to report bloody urine, difficulty breathing, rash, fever, chills, or severe fatigue.
• Teach signs and symptoms of bacterial and fungal superinfection to elderly and debilitated patients and others with low resistance from immunosuppressants or irradiation; emphasize need to report them.
• Advise diabetic patient that sulfonamides may increase effects of oral hypoglycemic and not to monitor urine glucose levels with Clinitest; sulfonamides alter results of tests using cupric sulfate.
• Advise patient to avoid exposure to direct sunlight because of risk of photosensitivity reaction.
• Tell patient to take oral drug with a full glass of water and to drink at least 12 to 16 8-oz (240-ml) glasses of water daily depending on the agent; explain that tablet may be crushed and swallowed with water to ensure maximal absorption.
• Be sure patient understands how and when to take drugs; urge him to complete entire prescribed regimen, to comply with instructions for around-the-clock dosage, and to keep follow-up appointments.
• Teach patient to check expiration date of drug and how to store drug, and to discard unused drug.
• For sulfasalazine, inform patient to take with food if GI irritation occurs and tell him that it may cause an orange-yellow discoloration of the urine or skin and may permanently stain soft contact lenses yellow.
• Photosensitization may occur; therefore, caution patient to take protective measures (for example, sunscreen, protective clothing) against exposure to ultraviolet light or sunlight until tolerance is determined.

Geriatric use

• Use with caution; elderly patients are susceptible to bacterial and fungal superinfection, are at greater risk of folate deficiency anemia after sulfonamide therapy, and commonly are at greater risk of renal and hematologic effects because of diminished renal function.

Pediatric use

• Sulfonamides are contraindicated in infants under age 2 months, unless there is no therapeutic alternative.
• Give sulfonamides with caution to children with fragile X chromosome associated with mental retardation because they are vulnerable to psychomotor depression from folate depletion.

Breast-feeding

• Because sulfonamides are excreted into breast milk, a decision should be made whether to discontinue breast-feeding or to discontinue the drug, taking into account the importance of the drug to the mother. Premature infants, infants with hyperbilirubinemia, and those with G6PD deficiency are at risk for kernicterus.

Representative combinations

Sulfadiazine with sulfamerazine and sulfamethazine: Triple Sulfa.

Sulfamethizole with oxytetracycline hydrochloride and phenazopyridine: Urobiotic-250; with sulfathiazole, sulfacetamide, sulfabenzamide, and urea: Triple Sulfa, V.V.S., Trysul, Gyne-Sulf, Sultrin, Triple Sulfa.

Sulfamethoxazole with phenazopyridine hydrochloride: Azo Gantanol, Azo-Sulfamethoxazole; with trimethoprim: Bactrim, Cotrim, Co-Trimoxazole, Septra, SMZ-TMP.

Sulfisoxazole with erythromycin ethylsuccinate: Pediazole; with phenazopyridine hydrochloride: Azo Gantrisin.

Sulfadoxine with pyrimethamine: Fansidar.

sulfonylureas

acetohexamide, chlorpropamide, glimepiride, glipizide, glyburide, tolazamide, tolbutamide

In 1942, a sulfonamide, an antibacterial agent, was discovered to have hypoglycemic effects. Subsequent experiments showed that this drug did not exert similar effects in pancreatectomized animals. Later, tolbutamide was introduced and soon became popular for managing certain diabetic patients. Sulfonylureas are useful only in patients with mild to moderately severe type 2, or non-insulin-dependent diabetes mellitus (NIDDM). These drugs can be used only in patients with functioning beta cells of the pancreas.

COMPARING ORAL ANTIDIABETIC AGENTS

Typically, sulfonylureas have similar actions and produce similar effects. They differ mainly in duration of action and dosage.

SULFONYLUREAS	USUAL DAILY DOSAGE	ONSET	ACTION PEAK	DURATION
First generation				
acetohexamide (Dymelor)	500 mg once daily or b.i.d.	1 hr	2 hr	12 to 24 hr
chlorpropamide (Diabenese)	250 mg once daily	1 hr	3 to 6 hr	60 hr
tolazamide (Tolinase)	250 mg once daily or b.i.d.	4 to 6 hr	6 to 10 hr	12 to 24 hr
tolbutamide (Orinase)	1,000 mg b.i.d. or t.i.d.	½ to 1 hr	4 to 8 hr	6 to 12 hr
Second generation				
glimepiride (Amaryl)	1 to 4 mg once daily	1 hr	2 to 3 hr	24 hr
glipizide (Glucotrol)	5 mg once daily	1 to 1½ hr	2 to 3 hr	10 to 24 hr
glyburide (DiaBeta, Micronase)	5 mg once daily	2 hr	3 to 4 hr	24 hr

Pharmacology

The sulfonylurea antidiabetic agents are sulfonamide derivatives that exert no antibacterial activity.

Sulfonylureas lower blood glucose levels by stimulating insulin release from the pancreas. These agents work only in the presence of functioning beta cells in the islet tissue of the pancreas. After prolonged administration, they produce hypoglycemia through significant extrapancreatic effects, including reduction of hepatic glucose production and enhanced peripheral sensitivity to insulin. The latter may result from an increase in the number of insulin receptors or from changes in events after insulin binding. (See *Comparing oral antidiabetic agents.*)

The sulfonylureas are divided into first-generation agents (chlorpropamide) and second-generation agents (glyburide, glipizide, and glimepiride). Although their mechanisms of action are similar, the second-generation agents carry a more lipophilic side chain, are more potent, and cause fewer adverse reactions. Their most important differences are their durations of action.

Clinical indications and actions

Diabetes mellitus, non-insulin-dependent

Sulfonylureas are used to manage mild to moderately severe, stable, nonketotic NIDDM that cannot be controlled by diet alone. Sulfonylureas stimulate insulin release from the pancreas. After long-term therapy, extrapancreatic hypoglycemic effects include reduced hepatic glucose production, an increased number of insulin receptors, and changes in insulin binding.

◇ ***Neurogenic diabetes insipidus***

Although an unlabeled indication, chlorpropamide has been used in selected patients to treat neurogenic diabetes insipidus. The drug appears to potentiate the effect of minimal levels of antidiuretic hormone.

Overview of adverse reactions

Dose-related adverse effects, which are usually not serious and respond to decreased dosage, include headache, nausea, vomiting, anorexia, heartburn, weakness, and paresthesia. Hypoglycemia may follow excessive dosage, increased exercise, decreased food intake, or consumption of alcohol. Signs and symptoms of overdose include anxiety, chills, cold sweats, confusion, cool pale skin, difficulty concentrating, drowsiness, excessive hunger, headache, nausea, nervousness, rapid heartbeat, shakiness, unsteady gait, weakness, and unusual fatigue.

☑ Special considerations

- Administer sulfonylureas 30 minutes before the morning meal for once-daily dosing, or 30 minutes before the morning and evening meals for twice-daily dosing.
- Contraindicated in patients with juvenile-onset, brittle, or severe diabetes; diabetes mellitus adequately controlled by diet; and maturity-onset diabetes complicated by ketosis, acidosis, diabetic coma, Raynaud's gangrene, renal or hepatic impairment, or thyroid or other endocrine dysfunction.
- Use cautiously in patients with sulfonamide hypersensitivity.
- Do not use sulfonylurea antidiabetic agents in pregnant patients because of prolonged, severe hypoglycemia lasting from 4 to 10 days in neonates born to mothers taking these drugs. Also, use of insulin permits more rigid control of blood glucose levels, which should reduce the incidence of congenital abnormalities, mortality, and morbidity caused by abnormal glucose levels.
- Monitor patients transferring from insulin therapy to a sulfonylurea agent for urine glucose and ketones at least three times daily, before meals; emphasize the need for

testing a double-voided specimen. Patients may require hospitalization during such changes in therapy.
- Know that patients transferring from another sulfonylurea (except chlorpropamide) usually need no transition period.
- NIDDM patients may require insulin therapy during periods of increased stress, such as infection, fever, surgery, or trauma. Monitor patients closely for hyperglycemia in these situations.

Patient education
- Teach patient about the nature of his disease.
- Emphasize importance of following therapeutic regimen and adhering to specific diet, weight reduction, exercise, and personal hygiene recommendations. He also should know how to avoid infections, test for glycosuria and ketonuria, and know signs and symptoms of hypoglycemia (fatigue, excessive hunger, profuse sweating, and numbness of extremities) and hyperglycemia (excessive thirst or urination and excessive urine glucose or ketones).
- Be sure patient knows that therapy relieves symptoms but does not cure the disease.
- Discourage patient from consuming moderate to large amounts of alcohol while taking sulfonylureas; disulfiram-type reactions are possible.

Geriatric use
- Elderly patients and those with renal insufficiency may be more sensitive to these agents because of decreased metabolism and excretion. They usually require lower dosages and should be closely monitored.
- Hypoglycemia may be more difficult to recognize in elderly patients, although it usually causes neurologic symptoms in such patients. Agents with prolonged duration of action should be avoided in elderly patients.

Pediatric use
- Oral antidiabetic agents are not effective in insulin-dependent (type 1, juvenile-onset) diabetes mellitus.

Breast-feeding
- Oral antidiabetic agents are excreted in breast milk in minimal amounts and may cause hypoglycemia in the breast-feeding infant.

Representative combinations
None.

tetracyclines

demeclocycline hydrochloride, doxycycline hyclate, minocycline hydrochloride, oxytetracycline hydrochloride, tetracycline hydrochloride

Tetracycline antibiotics were discovered during the random screening of soil samples for antibiotic-producing microorganisms. The prototype, chlortetracycline, was discovered in 1948; tetracycline was developed in 1952. Structural modifications that enhanced both antibacterial activity and pharmacokinetic parameters led to development of doxycycline in 1966 and minocycline in 1972.

Usually well-tolerated with few serious adverse effects, tetracyclines have an unusually broad spectrum of antibacterial activity, including gram-negative and gram-positive anaerobic and aerobic bacteria, *Chlamydia,* and protozoa; longer-acting tetracyclines have enhanced activity against *Chlamydia* and *Legionella.*

Demeclocycline has a higher incidence of severe photosensitivity reactions; also, because of its renal effects, it is rarely prescribed for clinical use, although it is used investigationally to treat SIADH secretion.

Pharmacology
Tetracyclines are bacteriostatic but may be bactericidal against certain organisms. They bind reversibly to 30S and 50S ribosomal subunits, inhibiting bacterial protein synthesis. Bacterial resistance to tetracyclines is usually mediated by plasmids (R-factor resistance), which decrease bacterial cell wall permeability; this is the most important cause of resistance by staphylococci, streptococci, most aerobic gram-negative organisms, and *Pseudomonas aeruginosa.* With two exceptions, cross-resistance occurs with all tetracyclines; doxycycline is active against *Bacteroides fragilis,* and minocycline is active against *Staphylococcus aureus.*

Tetracyclines attack many pathogens; they are not antifungal or antiviral.

Susceptible gram-positive organisms *include Bacillus anthracis, Actinomyces israelii, Clostridium perfringens, C. tetani, Listeria monocytogenes,* and *Nocardia.* Initial but transient activity exists against staphylococci and streptococci; infections caused by these organisms are usually treated with other drugs.

Susceptible gram-negative organisms *include Neisseria meningitidis, Pasteurella multocida, Legionella pneumophila, Brucella, Vibrio cholerae, Yersinia enterocolitica, Y. pestis, Bordetella pertussis, Haemophilus influenzae, H. ducreyi, Campylobacter fetus, Shigella,* and many other common pathogens.

Other susceptible organisms include *Rickettsia akari, R. typhi, R. prowazekii, R. tsutsugamushi, Coxiella burnetii, Chlamydia trachomatis, C. psittaci, Mycoplasma pneumoniae, M. hominis, Leptospira, Treponema pallidum, T. pertenue,* and *Borrelia recurrentis.*

Tetracyclines are absorbed systemically after oral administration, chiefly from the duodenum; with the exception of doxycycline and minocycline, absorption is decreased by food, milk, and divalent and trivalent cations. Oral absorption of tetracyclines is affected by chelation with certain minerals such as calcium (doxycycline is least involved); chelation causes tetracyclines to localize in bones and teeth. Because of hepatotoxicity and thrombophlebitis, only doxycycline and, to a lesser extent, minocycline, are used I.V.

Tetracyclines occur widely into body tissues and fluid, but CSF penetration is minimal; lipid-soluble minocycline and doxycycline penetrate fluids and tissues better; all tetracyclines cross the placenta.

Tetracyclines are excreted primarily in urine, chiefly by glomerular filtration; some drug is excreted in breast milk, and some inactivated drug is excreted in feces. Unlike other tetracyclines, minocycline undergoes enterohepatic circulation and is excreted in feces.

Oxytetracycline is moderately hemodialyzable; other tetracyclines are removed only minimally by hemodialysis or peritoneal dialysis.

Clinical indications and actions
Bacterial, antiprotozoal, rickettsial, and fungal infections
Tetracyclines are used as first-line therapy for chlamydial infections and are the drugs of choice for lymphogranuloma venereum, nonlymphogranuloma venereum strains *of C. trachomatis* in sexually transmitted diseases, psittacosis, and nongonococcal urethritis if the primary pathogen is *probably M. hominis* or *C. trachomatis.* They are also the drugs of choice for rickettsial infections (Rocky Mountain spotted fever,

scrub and endemic typhus, rickettsial pox, and Q fever) and brucellosis. Tetracyclines also are used to treat infections caused by *Campylobacter*, mycoplasma pneumonia (after Legionnaire's disease is ruled out), pertussis, and cholera (in United States only).

Tetracyclines are second-line drugs in therapy of syphilis, actinomycosis, listeriosis, chancroid, and infections caused by *Pasteurella multocida* and *Yersinia pestis*. They also provide economical prophylaxis in chronic pulmonary disease.

Tetracyclines are used orally to treat inflammatory acne vulgaris, topically for mild to moderate inflammatory acne, and as eyedrops for superficial eye infections, inclusion conjunctivitis, and prophylaxis of ophthalmia neonatorum.

Individual tetracyclines are more effective against certain species or strains of a particular organism.

◊ ***Diuretic agent in SIADH***

Demeclocycline causes diuresis by blocking antidiuretic hormone-induced reabsorption of water in the distal convoluted tubules and collecting ducts of the kidney.

Sclerosing agent

Parenteral tetracycline hydrochloride has been administered by intracavitary injection as a sclerosing agent in pleural or pericardial effusion. Parenteral doxycycline hyclate has been used as a sclerosing agent to control pleural effusions associated with metastatic tumors.

Overview of adverse reactions

The most common adverse effects of tetracyclines involve the GI tract and are dose related. Among them are anorexia; flatulence; nausea; vomiting; bulky, loose stools; epigastric burning; and abdominal discomfort.

Hypersensitivity reactions are infrequent; they manifest as urticaria, rash, pruritus, eosinophilia, and exfoliative dermatitis.

Photosensitivity reactions may be severe; they commonly occur with demeclocycline, rarely with minocycline.

Renal effects are minor and include occasional elevations in BUN levels (without rise in serum creatinine level) and a reversible diabetes insipidus syndrome (reported only with demeclocycline); renal failure has been attributed to Fanconi's syndrome after use of outdated tetracycline.

Rare adverse effects include hepatotoxicity (often in pregnant women receiving more than 2 g/day I.V.), leukocytosis, thrombocytopenia, hemolytic anemia, leukopenia, neutropenia, and atypical lymphocytes. There have also been reports of vaginal candidiasis, microscopic thyroid discoloration (after chronic use), light-headedness, dizziness, drowsiness, vein irritation (after I.V. use), and permanent discoloration of teeth, in children under age 8.

Drug use with oral contraceptives can decrease contraceptive's effectiveness and increase the risk of pregnancy.

☑ Special considerations

- Assess patient's allergic history; do not give tetracycline antibiotics to patient with history of hypersensitivity reactions to other tetracyclines; monitor patient continuously for this and other adverse reactions.
- Obtain results of cultures and sensitivity tests before giving first dose, but do not delay therapy; check cultures periodically to assess drug efficacy.
- Monitor vital signs, electrolytes, and renal function studies before and during therapy.
- Check expiration dates. Outdated tetracyclines may cause nephrotoxicity.
- Monitor for bacterial and fungal superinfection, especially in elderly, debilitated, and other patients who are receiving immunosuppressants or radiation therapy; watch especially for oral candidiasis. If symptoms occur, discontinue drug.
- Tetracyclines may interfere with certain laboratory tests; consult individual drug entry.

Administration

- Give oral drugs 1 hour before or 2 hours after meals for maximum absorption; do not give with food, milk or other dairy products, sodium bicarbonate, iron compounds, or antacids, which may impair absorption.
- Give water with and after oral drug to facilitate passage to stomach because incomplete swallowing can cause severe esophageal irritation; do not administer within 1 hour of bedtime, to prevent esophageal reflux.
- Follow manufacturer's directions for reconstitution and storage; keep product refrigerated and out of light.
- Avoid I.V. use of drug in patients with decreased renal function.
- I.V. use of tetracyclines in pregnancy or in patients with renal impairment, especially when dosage exceeds 2 g/day, can cause hepatic failure.
- Monitor I.V. injection sites and rotate routinely to reduce local irritation. I.V. use may cause severe phlebitis.

Patient education

- Explain disease process and rationale for therapy.
- Teach signs and symptoms of adverse reactions, and emphasize need to report these promptly; urge patient to report unusual effects.
- Teach signs and symptoms of bacterial and fungal superinfection to elderly and debilitated patients and others with low resistance from immunosuppressants or irradiation.
- Advise patients using oral contraceptives to use a back-up method of contraception during drug therapy.
- Advise patient to avoid direct sunlight and to use a sunscreen to prevent photosensitivity reactions.
- Tell patient to take oral tetracyclines with a full glass (8 oz [240 ml]) of water (to facilitate passage to the stomach) 1 hour before or 2 hours after meals for maximum absorption, and not less than 1 hour before bedtime (to prevent irritation from esophageal reflux).
- Emphasize that taking drug with food, milk or other dairy products, sodium bicarbonate, or iron compounds may interfere with absorption. Tell him to take antacids 3 hours after tetracycline.
- Stress importance of completing prescribed regimen exactly as ordered and keeping follow-up appointments.
- Tell patient that doxycycline and monocycline may be taken with food.
- Instruct patient to check expiration date before use.

Geriatric use

- Some elderly patients have decreased esophageal motility; use tetracyclines cautiously and monitor for local irritation from slowly passing oral dosage forms. Elderly patients are more susceptible to superinfection.

Pediatric use

- Do not use in children under age 8 unless there is no alternative. Tetracyclines can cause permanent discoloration of teeth, enamel hypoplasia, and a reversible decrease in bone calcification.
- Reversible decreases in bone calcification have been reported in infants.

Breast-feeding

- Avoid use of tetracyclines by breast-feeding women.

Representative combinations

Oxytetracycline with polymyxin B sulfate: Terramycin with polymyxin B, Terramycin topical ointment.

Oxytetracycline hydrochloride with phenazopyridine hydrochloride and sulfamethizole: Urobiotic-250.

Tetracycline hydrochloride with citric acid: Achromycin V.

thrombolytic enzymes

alteplase, anistreplase, reteplase (recombinant), streptokinase, urokinase

When a thrombus obstructs a blood vessel, permanent damage to the ischemic area may occur before the body can dissolve the clot. Thrombolytic agents were developed in the hope that speeding lysis of the clot would prevent permanent ischemic damage. Thrombolytic activity attributable to streptokinase was described in 1933; this compound's effects have since been studied on various kinds of clots. It is not clear whether such agents significantly reduce thrombosis-induced ischemic damage in all situations for which the drugs are currently used. (See *Comparing thrombolytic enzymes.*)

Pharmacology

Streptokinase is a proteinlike substance produced by group C beta-hemolytic streptococci; urokinase is an enzyme isolated from human kidney tissue cultures. Alteplase is a tissue-type plasminogen activator synthesized by recombinant DNA technology. Anistreplase is anisoylated streptokinase-plasminogen activated complex; it is a fibrinolytic enzyme (plasminogen) plus activator complex (streptokinase) with the activator temporarily blocked by an anisoyl group. Reteplase is a recombinant-plasminogen activator. Thrombolytic enzymes act to lyse clots chiefly by converting plasminogen to plasmin; in contrast, anticoagulants act by preventing thrombi from developing. Thrombolytics are more likely to produce clinical bleeding than are oral anticoagulants.

Clinical indications and actions

Thrombosis, thromboembolism

Alteplase, streptokinase, and urokinase are used to treat acute pulmonary thromboembolism; streptokinase and urokinase are used to treat deep vein thrombosis, acute arterial thromboembolism, or acute coronary arterial thrombosis and to clear arteriovenous cannula occlusion and venous catheter obstruction. Anistreplase, alteplase, reteplase, streptokinase, and urokinase are indicated in acute MI. These agents are administered in an attempt to lyse coronary artery thrombi, which may result in improved ventricular function and decreased risk of heart failure. Alteplase is used in the management of acute ischemic stroke.

Overview of adverse reactions

Adverse reactions to these agents are essentially an extension of their actions; hemorrhage is the most common adverse effect. These agents cause bleeding twice as often as does heparin. Streptokinase is more likely

COMPARING THROMBOLYTIC ENZYMES

Thrombolytic enzymes dissolve clots by accelerating the formation of plasmin by activated plasminogen. Plasminogen activators, found in most tissues and body fluids, help plasminogen (an inactive enzyme) convert to plasmin (an active enzyme), which dissolves the clot.

Two thrombolytic enzymes — streptokinase and urokinase — have been widely used; two enzymes — tissue plasminogen activator (TPA or alteplase) and anistreplase — have recently been added to current use. The newest addition is reteplase. Doses of these enzymes may vary according to the patient's condition.

DRUG	ACTION	INITIAL DOSE	MAINTENANCE THERAPY
alteplase	Directly converts plasminogen to plasmin	I.V. bolus: 6 to 10 mg over 1 to 2 min	I.V. infusion: 50 to 54 mg/hr over 1st hr; 20 mg (20 ml/hr over next 2 hr, then discontinue
anistreplase	Directly converts plasminogen to plasmin	I.V. push: 30 units over 2 to 3 min	Not necessary
reteplase	Enhances the cleavage of plasminogen to generate plasmin	Double I.V. bolus injection of 10 + 10 units	Not necessary
streptokinase	Indirectly activates plasminogen, which converts to plasmin	Intracoronary bolus: 15,000 to 20,000 IU I.V. bolus: none needed	Intracoronary infusion: 2,000 to 4,000 IU/min over 60 min; I.V. infusion: 1,500,000 units over 60 min
urokinase	Directly converts plasminogen to plasmin	Intracoronary bolus: none needed	Intracoronary infusion: 2,000 units/lb/hr (4,400 units/kg/hr); rate of 15 ml of solution/hr for total of 12 hr (total volume shouldn't exceed 200 ml)

to cause an allergic reaction than urokinase. Information regarding hypersensitivity to alteplase is limited.

☑ Special considerations

- Thrombolytic therapy requires medical supervision with continuous clinical and laboratory monitoring.
- Thrombolytics act only on fibrin clots, not those formed by a precipitated drug.
- Follow instructions for reconstitution precisely and pass solution through a filter 0.45 microns or smaller to remove filaments in the solution; do not use dextran concomitantly because it can interfere with coagulation as well as blood typing and crossmatching.
- Obtain pretherapy baseline determinations of thrombin time, activated partial thromboplastin time, PT, INR, hematocrit, and platelet count for subsequent blood monitoring. Monitor laboratory studies on a flowsheet in patient's chart. During systemic thrombolytic therapy, as in pulmonary embolism or venous thrombosis, PT, INR, or thrombin time after 4 hours of therapy should be approximately twice the pretreatment value.
- Keep venipuncture sites to a minimum; apply pressure dressings for at least 15 minutes to prevent bleeding and hematoma. For arterial puncture (except intracoronary), use upper extremities, which are more accessible for pressure dressings; apply pressure for at least 30 minutes after arterial puncture.
- Administer drugs by infusion pump to ensure accuracy; I.M. injections are contraindicated during therapy because of increased risk of bleeding at the injection site.
- Check vital signs frequently. Monitor for blood pressure alterations in excess of 25 mm Hg and any change in cardiac rhythm; check pulses, color, and sensitivity of extremities every hour; monitor for excessive bleeding every 15 minutes for first hour, every 30 minutes for second through eighth hours; then at least once every 8 hours. Stop therapy if bleeding is evident; pretreatment with heparin or drugs affecting platelets increases risk.
- Monitor for hypersensitivity as well as hemorrhage: keep available typed and crossmatched packed RBCs and whole blood, aminocaproic acid to treat bleeding, and corticosteroids to treat allergic reactions.
- Keep involved extremity in straight alignment to prevent bleeding from infusion site. Establish precautions to prevent injury and avoid unnecessary handling of patient because bruising is likely.
- At end of infusion, flush remaining dose from pump tubing with I.V. 5% dextrose or normal saline solution.
- Continuous heparin infusion usually is started with the prescribed thrombolytic.
- Before using thrombolytic to clear an occluded catheter, try to gently aspirate or flush with heparinized saline solution. Avoid forcible flushing or vigorous suction, which could rupture the catheter or expel the clot into the circulation.
- When treating MI or CVA, the sooner treatment is administered, the greater the benefit.

Patient education

- Explain rationale for treatment and procedure, and necessity for bed rest.
- Ask patient to be alert for signs of bleeding.
- When using these drugs to clear catheter, tell patient to exhale and hold breath at any time catheter is not connected, to prevent air entering the open catheter.

Geriatric use

- Patients age 75 or older are at greater risk of cerebral hemorrhage, because they are more apt to have preexisting cerebrovascular disease.

Pediatric use

- Safe use in children has not been established.

Breast-feeding

- Safe use has not been established.

Representative combinations

None.

thyroid hormones

levothyroxine sodium, liothyronine sodium, liotrix, thyroid USP (desiccated), thyrotropin (TSH)

The thyroid gland was first described by Wharton in 1656. In 1891, Murray was the first to treat hypothyroidism by injecting an extract of the thyroid gland. The next year, the extract was found to be effective orally. Thyroid hormones are used for treating hypothyroidism (myxedema, cretinism), nontoxic goiter, and (with antithyroid drugs) thyrotoxicosis and as a diagnostic aid.

Thyroid hormone synthesis is regulated by thyroid-stimulating hormone (TSH) secreted by the anterior pituitary. TSH secretion is controlled by a feedback mechanism and by thyrotropin-releasing hormone from the hypothalamus. Thyroid hormone, which contains T_3 and T_4, is stored in the thyroid as thyroglobulin. The amounts of T_3 and T_4 released into circulation are regulated by TSH. T_4 is the major component of normal secretions of the thyroid gland and is the major determinant of normal thyroid function. Most of T_3 (about 80%) is derived from T_4 by deiodination in peripheral tissues. About 35% of secreted T_4 is monodeiodinated peripherally to T_3. In normal human thyroid tissue, the T_4:T_3 ratio is 10:1 to 15:1; in a hyperthyroid patient, the ratio is about 5:1.

Pharmacology

Thyroid hormones include natural (thyroid USP and thyroglobulin) and synthetic T_4, liothyronine, and liotrix) derivatives. The thyroid hormones have catabolic and anabolic effects and influence normal metabolism, growth, and development. Thyroid hormones affect all organ systems and are vital to normal CNS function.

TSH increases iodine uptake by the thyroid and increases formation and release of thyroid hormone. TSH is isolated from bovine anterior pituitary glands.

Clinical indications and actions

Hypothyroidism (myxedema, cretinism, or replacement therapy)

All drugs in this class (except TSH) are used to treat hypothyroidism; drug of choice is T_4. Dessicated thyroid is rarely used. These hormones affect protein and carbohydrate metabolism, promote gluconeogenesis, increase use and mobilization of glycogen stores, stimulate protein synthesis, and regulate cell growth and differentiation. The major effect of exogenous thyroid hormones is to increase the metabolic rate of tissue.

Nontoxic goiter

T_4, liotrix, liothyronine, and thyroid USP are used to suppress TSH secretion in treating simple goiter.

Diagnostic uses

T_4 is used in the T_3 suppression test to differentiate suspected hyperthyroidism from euthyroidism in patients with borderline or high ^{131}I uptake values. TSH increases iodine uptake by the thyroid and increases formation and release of thyroid hormone.

Thyrotoxicosis

T_4, liotrix, and thyroid USP are used with antithyroid agents to prevent goitrogenesis and hypothyroidism.

Because thyroid hormones have wide-ranging metabolic effects and are possibly dangerous, they are not indicated for relief of mental and physical sluggishness, irritability, depression, nervousness, and ill-defined pains; to treat obesity in patients with normal thyroid function; to treat metabolic insufficiency not associated with thyroid insufficiency; or to treat menstrual disorders or male infertility not associated with hypothyroidism.

Overview of adverse reactions

Adverse reactions to thyroid hormones are extensions of their pharmacologic properties. Signs of overdose include nervousness, insomnia, tremor, tachycardia, palpitations, nausea, headache, fever, and sweating.

☑ Special considerations

- Thyroid hormone dosage varies widely among patients. Treatment should start at the lowest level, titrating to higher doses according to patient's symptoms and laboratory data, until euthyroid state is reached.
- Administer thyroid hormones at the same time each day. Morning dosage is preferred to prevent insomnia.
- Monitor pulse rate and blood pressure.
- Monitor PT; patients taking anticoagulants usually require lower doses.
- Signs of thyrotoxicosis or inadequate dosage therapy include diarrhea, fever, irritability, listlessness, rapid heartbeat, vomiting, or weakness.
- Do not use thyroid medication for weight reduction.

Patient education

- Advise patient to call at once if signs or symptoms of overdose or of aggravated CV disease occur.

Geriatric use

- In patients over age 60, initial hormone replacement dosage should be 25% less than the usual recommended starting dosage.

Pediatric use

- During first few months of therapy, children may suffer partial, but temporary, hair loss.

Breast-feeding

- Minimal levels occur in breast milk. No problems have been noted in infants.

Representative combinations

None.

tricyclic antidepressants (TCAs)

amitriptyline hydrochloride, amoxapine, clomipramine hydrochloride, desipramine hydrochloride, doxepin hydrochloride, imipramine hydrochloride, imipramine pamoate, nortriptyline hydrochloride, trimipramine maleate

The inherent mood-elevating activity of tricyclic antidepressants (TCAs) was discovered during research with iminodibenzyl, a compound originally investigated for sedative, analgesic, antihistaminic, and antiparkinsonian effects. Clinical trials in 1958 with the class prototype, imipramine, found no antipsychotic activity, but showed marked mood-elevating effects.

Pharmacology

Although the precise mechanism of their CNS effects is not established, TCAs may exert their effects by inhibiting reuptake of the neurotransmitters norepinephrine and serotonin in CNS nerve terminals (presynaptic neurons), resulting in increased concentration and enhanced activity of neurotransmitters in the synaptic cleft. TCAs also have antihistaminic, sedative, anticholinergic, vasodilatory, and quinidine-like effects; the drugs are structurally similar to phenothiazines and share similar adverse reactions.

Individual TCAs differ somewhat in their degree of CNS inhibitory effect. The tertiary amines (amitriptyline, doxepin, imipramine, and trimipramine) exert greater sedative effects; tertiary amines and protriptyline have more profound effects on cardiac conduction, whereas desipramine has the least anticholinergic activity. All of the currently available TCAs have equal clinical efficacy when given in equivalent therapeutic doses; choice of specific therapy is determined primarily by pharmacokinetic properties and the patient's adverse reaction profile. Patients may respond to some TCAs and not others; if a patient does not respond to one drug, another should be tried.

Clinical indications and actions

Depression

TCAs are used to treat major depression and dysthymic disorder. Depressed patients who are also anxious are helped most by the more sedating agents: doxepin, imipramine, and trimipramine. Protriptyline has a stimulant effect that evokes a favorable response in withdrawn depressed patients; only maprotiline has Food and Drug Administration approval for use in depression mixed with anxiety.

Obsessive-compulsive disorder (OCD)

Clomipramine is used in the treatment of OCD.

Enuresis

Imipramine is used for enuresis in children over age 6.

Severe, chronic pain

TCAs, especially amitriptyline, desipramine, doxepin, imipramine, and nortriptyline, are useful in the management of severe chronic pain.

Overview of adverse reactions

Adverse reactions to TCAs are similar to those seen with phenothiazine antipsychotic agents, including varying degrees of sedation, anticholinergic effects, and orthostatic hypotension. The tertiary amines have the strongest sedative effects; tolerance to these effects usually develops in a few weeks. Protriptyline has the least sedative effect (and may be stimulatory), but shares with the tertiary amines the most pronounced effects on blood pressure and cardiac tissue. Maprotiline and amoxapine are most likely to cause seizures, especially in overdose situations. Desipramine has a greater margin of safety in patients with prostatic hypertrophy, paralytic ileus, glaucoma, and urine retention because of its relatively low level of anticholinergic activity.

☑ Special considerations

- TCAs impair ability to perform tasks requiring mental alertness such as driving a car.
- Check vital signs regularly for decreased blood pressure or tachycardia; observe patient carefully for adverse reactions and report changes. Check ECG in patients over age 40 before initiating therapy. Consider

having patient take the first dose in the office to allow close observation for adverse reactions.
- Check for anticholinergic adverse reactions, which may require dosage reduction.
- Caregiver should be sure patient swallows each dose of drug when given; as depressed patients begin to improve, they may hoard pills for suicide attempt.
- Observe patients for mood changes to monitor progress; benefits may not occur for several (3 to 6) weeks.
- Do not withdraw full dose of drug abruptly; gradually reduce dosage over a period of weeks to avoid rebound effect or other adverse reactions.
- Carefully follow manufacturer's instructions for reconstitution, dilution, and storage of drugs.
- Investigational uses include treating peptic ulcer, migraine prophylaxis, and allergy. Potential toxicity has, to date, outweighed most advantages.
- Because suicidal overdosage with TCAs is commonly fatal, prescribe only small amounts. If possible, entrust a reliable family member with the medication and warn him to store drug safely away from children.

Patient education
- Explain rationale for therapy and anticipated risks and benefits; also explain that full therapeutic effect may not occur for several weeks.
- Teach signs and symptoms of adverse reactions and the importance of reporting them.
- Tell patient to avoid beverages and drugs containing alcohol and not to take other drugs (including OTC products) without medical approval.
- Teach patient how and when to take drug, not to increase dosage without medical approval, and never to discontinue drug abruptly.
- Tell patient to lie down for 30 minutes after first dose and to rise slowly to avoid orthostatic hypotension.
- Advise taking drug with milk or food to minimize GI distress; suggest taking full dose at bedtime if daytime sedation is troublesome.
- Urge diabetic patients to monitor blood glucose, as drug may alter insulin needs.
- Advise patient to avoid tasks that require mental alertness until full effect of drug is determined.
- Warn patient that excessive exposure to sunlight, heat lamps, or tanning beds may cause burn and abnormal hyperpigmentation.
- Recommend sugarless gum or hard candy, artificial saliva, or ice chips to relieve dry mouth.
- Advise patient that unpleasant adverse effects (except dry mouth) generally diminish over time.

Geriatric use
- Use lower doses because these patients are more sensitive to both therapeutic and adverse effects of TCAs.

Pediatric use
- TCAs are not advised for children under age 12.

Breast-feeding
- Safety in breast-feeding has not been established.

Representative combinations
Amitriptyline hydrochloride with perphenazine: Etrafon, Triavil; with chlordiazepoxide: Limbitrol.

vitamins

***Fat-soluble:* vitamin A (retinol), vitamin A acid (retinoic acid), vitamin D, vitamin D_2 (ergocalciferol), vitamin D_3 (calcipotriene), vitamin E, vitamin K (phytonadione)**

***Water-soluble:* vitamin B_1 (thiamine), vitamin B_2 (riboflavin), vitamin B_3 (niacin), vitamin B_6 (pyridoxine), vitamin B_9 (folic acid, folacin), vitamin B_{12} (cyanocobalamin), vitamin C (ascorbic acid)**

Vitamins are chemically unrelated organic compounds that are required for normal growth and maintenance of metabolic functions. Because the body is unable to synthesize many vitamins, it must obtain them from exogenous sources. Vitamins do not furnish energy and are not essential building blocks for the body; however, they are essential for the transformation of energy and for the regulation of metabolic processes.

Vitamins are classified as fat-soluble or water-soluble, and the Food and Nutrition Board of the National Research Council determines the RDAs for each. These allowances represent amounts that will provide adequate nutrition in most healthy persons; they are not minimum requirements. Note that a diet that includes ample intake of the four basic food groups will provide sufficient quantities of vitamins. If needed, vitamins should be used as an adjunct to a regular diet and not as a food substitute.

Controversy has existed for years over the vitamin issue. Some argue that vitamin supplementation is unnecessary; some advise moderate supplementation; still others advocate the use of megavitamins. The public should be warned against self-medication with vitamins because the safety and efficacy of their chronic use have not been established.

Pharmacology
Vitamins are available as single drugs or in combination with several other vitamins with or without minerals, trace elements, iron, fluoride, or other nutritional supplements. Often, diets deficient in one vitamin are also deficient in other vitamins of similar dietary source. Malabsorption syndromes also affect the usage of several vitamins as do certain disease states that increase metabolic rates. Therefore, multiple vitamin therapy may prove rational and useful in these situations.

Fat-soluble vitamins are absorbed with dietary fats and stored in the body in moderate amounts; they are not normally excreted in urine. Chronic ingestion leads to excessive build-up of these agents and toxicity.

Water-soluble vitamins are not stored in the body in any appreciable amounts and are excreted in urine. These agents seldom cause toxicity in patients with normal renal function.

Both types of vitamins are needed for the maintenance of normal structure and metabolic functions of the body. (See *Recommended daily allowances for adults age 23 to 50*, page 1156.)

Clinical indications and actions
Vitamin deficiency or malabsorption; conditions of metabolic stress

Vitamin supplementation is required when deficiencies exist, in malabsorption syndrome, in hypermetabolic disease states, during pregnancy and lactation, and in the elderly, alcoholics, or dieters. Multiple vitamins may

RECOMMENDED DAILY ALLOWANCES FOR ADULTS AGE 23 TO 50

VITAMIN	MALES	FEMALES	PREGNANT FEMALES	LACTATING FEMALES*
A	1,000 mcg	800 mcg	800 mcg	1,300 mcg
B_1	1.5 mg	1.1 mg	1.5 mg	1.6 mg
B_2	1.7 mg	1.3 mg	1.6 mg	1.8 mg
B_6	2 mg	1.6 mg	2.2 mg	2.1 mg
B_{12}	2 mcg	2 mcg	2.2 mcg	2.6 mcg
C	60 mg	60 mg	70 mg	95 mg
D	200 IU	200 IU	400 IU	400 IU
E	10 IU	8 IU	10 IU	12 IU
K	80 mcg	65 mcg	65 mcg	65 mcg
folic acid	200 mcg	180 mcg	400 mcg	280 mcg
niacin	19 mg	15 mg	17 mg	20 mg

*First 6 months.

be indicated for patients taking oral contraceptives, estrogens, prolonged antibiotic therapy, isoniazid, or for patients receiving prolonged total parenteral nutrition.

Persons with increased metabolic requirements such as infants and those suffering severe injury, trauma, major surgery, or severe infection also require supplementation. Prolonged diarrhea, severe GI disorders, malignancy, surgical removal of sections of GI tract, obstructive jaundice, cystic fibrosis, and other conditions leading to reduced or poor absorption are indications for multiple vitamin therapy. Refer to individual agents for specific indications.

Overview of adverse reactions

Common adverse reactions seen with both vitamins include nausea, vomiting, diarrhea, tiredness, weakness, headache, loss of appetite, rash, and itching.

☑ Special considerations

- Monitoring may be required. See specific vitamin entries for details.
- Vitamins containing iron may cause constipation and black, tarry stools.
- Excessive fluoride supplements can result in hypocalcemia and tetany.
- Give with food or after meals to reduce GI distress associated with vitamin therapy.
- Vitamins are not food substitutes. Stress importance of adequate dietary intake of four basic food groups.

Patient education

- Stress importance of adequate dietary intake of food pyramid. Vitamins are not food substitutes.
- Tell patient to take vitamins only as directed, not to exceed RDA, and to take with food, milk, or after meals to reduce chance of stomach upset.
- Store vitamins away from heat and light, and out of small children's reach.
- Warn patient that vitamins with iron may cause constipation and black, tarry stools.
- Tell patient to read all label directions. Warn him not to take large doses unless prescribed.
- Inform patient that liquid vitamins may be mixed with food or juice.
- Advise patient not to refer to vitamins or other drugs as candy and to avoid taking them indiscriminately.

Pediatric use

- RDAs vary with age. Excessive amounts of vitamins, particularly in neonates, may be toxic.

Breast-feeding

- RDAs may be increased in breast-feeding women.

Representative combinations

The following list includes selected combinations that are available only by prescription.

B vitamins (oral) niacin (B_3), pantothenic acid (B_5), pyridoxine (B_6), and cyanocobalamin (B_{12}), with folic acid (B_9), iron, manganese, zinc, and 13% alcohol: Megaton Elixir; with thiamine (B_1), riboflavin (B_2), ferric pyrophosphate, and 15% alcohol: Senilezol Liquid; with thiamine (B_1), riboflavin (B_2), ascorbic acid, and folic acid: Berocca, B-Plex, Strovite, B-C with folic acid; with thiamine (B_1), riboflavin (B_2), ascorbic acid, folic acid, and biotin: Nephrocaps.

B vitamins (parenteral) with riboflavin (B_2), niacin (B_3), pantothenic acid (B_5), pyridoxine (B_6), and ascorbic acid: Becomject-100.

Multivitamins (oral) vitamins E, thiamine (B_1), riboflavin (B_2), niacin (B_3), pantothenic acid (B_5), pyridoxine (B_6), cyanocobalamin (B_{12}), ascorbic acid, and folic acid: Cefol Filmtabs; with vitamins A, D, E, thiamine (B_1), riboflavin (B_2), niacin (B_3), pantothenic acid (B_5), pyridoxine (B_6), cyanocobalamin (B_{12}), ascorbic acid, iron, and folic acid: Unicomplex-T&M Tablets, Cerovite Jr., Quintabs-M, Centrum Jr. with Iron, Monocaps, Unicap Sr., Hi-Po-Vites.

Multivitamins (parenteral) vitamins A, D, E, thiamine (B_1), riboflavin (B_2), niacin (B_3), pantothenic acid (B_5), pyridoxine (B_6), cyanocobalamin (B_{12}), ascorbic acid, biotin, and folic acid: Berocca Parenteral Nutrition, M.V.I.-12.

Multivitamins with fluoride (oral) vitamins A, D, thiamine (B_1), riboflavin (B_2), niacin (B_3), pantothenic acid (B_5), pyridoxine (B_6), cyanocobalamin (B_{12}), ascorbic acid, folic acid, and fluoride: Polyvitamin Fluoride, Mulvidren-F Softab Tablets, Polytabs-F; vitamins A, D, E, thiamine (B_1), riboflavin (B_2), niacin (B_3), pyridoxine (B_6), cyanocobalamin (B_{12}), ascorbic acid, folic acid, and fluoride: Poly-Vi-Flor, Florvite, Vi-Daylin/F.

Physician assistants' prescribing authority by state

The prescribing authority of physician assistants (PAs) is constantly changing as regulations are either continually implemented or in the process of being passed. Consult the respective state board for the most current laws and regulations on the prescribing authority for PAs. As of August 1998, PAs held the prescribing authorities indicated by the map below.

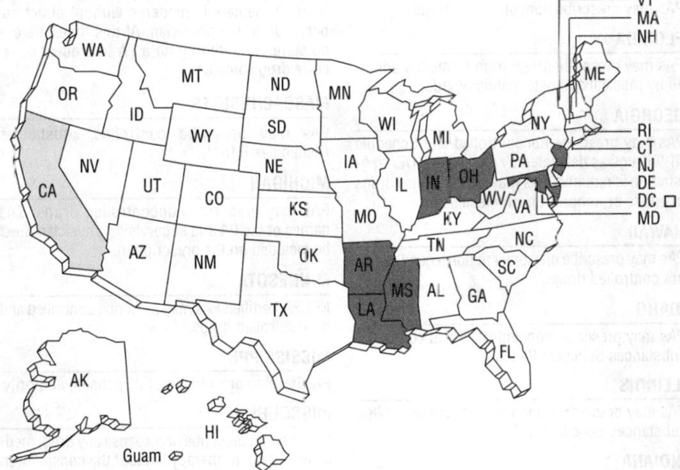

KEY:

- No physician signature required.
- Written prescription transmittal orders.
- Physician signature required.

ALABAMA

PAs may prescribe noncontrolled drugs from board-approved formulary.

ALASKA

PAs may prescribe Schedule III to V controlled substances. The prescription must be written and signed by PA and include the collaborating physician's name and Drug Enforcement Administration (DEA) number.

ARIZONA

PAs may prescribe noncontrolled and controlled drugs. However, Schedule II and III drugs are limited to a 72-hour supply and Schedule IV and V drugs to a 34-day supply. Refills cannot be prescribed and DEA registration is required. Except for samples, dispensed drugs must be prepackaged by physician or pharmacist.

ARKANSAS

PAs do not have prescribing or dispensing authority.

CALIFORNIA

PAs may administer or provide medications to a patient, or transmit orally or in writing on a patient's record or in a transmittal order, a prescription from a supervising physician based on protocol or on patient-specific order. Prescriptions for controlled substances may not be transmitted without a patient-specific order from the physician. PAs may hand the patient a properly labeled drug prepackaged by pharmacist, physician, or manufacturer. Medical records containing a prescription must be countersigned by supervising physician within 7 days.

COLORADO

PAs may prescribe controlled and noncontrolled substances using the supervising physician's forms. All drugs dispensed by PAs must be unit doses prepackaged by pharmacist or physician.

CONNECTICUT

PAs may prescribe noncontrolled and controlled (Schedule IV-V) drugs and dispense drugs in outpatient or nonprofit clinics. They may also order Schedule II and III drugs for inpatients.

(continued)

Physician assistants' prescribing authority by state *(continued)*

DELAWARE

PAs may prescribe therapeutic drugs (Schedule II-V and legend drugs) as delegated by the physician, consistent with board rules.

DISTRICT OF COLUMBIA

PAs may prescribe noncontrolled drugs.

FLORIDA

PAs may prescribe drugs from formulary adopted by medical and osteopathic boards.

GEORGIA

PAs may prescribe noncontrolled and Schedule III-V drugs as delegated by physicians. DEA registration is required. PAs may also dispense drugs in public or nonprofit health facilities.

HAWAII

PAs may prescribe only prescription legend drugs, not controlled drugs.

IDAHO

PAs may prescribe noncontrolled and controlled substances Schedule III-V.

ILLINOIS

PAs may prescribe noncontrolled and controlled substances Schedule III-V.

INDIANA

PAs have no prescribing authority. PAs may only use or dispense drugs prescribed or approved by the supervising physician. They may not dispense controlled substances.

IOWA

PAs may prescribe controlled substances (except Schedule II stimulants and depressants) and dispense drugs under certain conditions.

KANSAS

PAs may verbally (by telephone) transmit a prescription for Schedule III to V controlled substance (Schedule II drug only in emergency). Prescription for noncontrolled substances may be transmitted verbally (by phone) or in writing. Prescription-only drugs may be supplied to patients if directly ordered by the physician, authorized in written protocol, or in an emergency.

KENTUCKY

PAs can prescribe for legend drugs.

LOUISIANA

PAs have no prescribing or dispensing authority.

MAINE

PAs may prescribe and dispense drugs and medical devices, including Schedules III-V controlled substances. DEA registration is required.

MARYLAND

PAs may write medication orders in either a hospital, correctional facility, or a public health clinic and only pursuant to that institution's policy. All medication orders are reviewed and countersigned by the supervising physician within 48 hours if the care is rendered without direct supervision of the physician. At this time, there is no statutory authority for a PA to request or receive drug samples.

MASSACHUSETTS

PAs may prescribe controlled substances (Schedules II to V).

MICHIGAN

PAs may prescribe noncontrolled drugs. The names of the PA and supervising physician must be included on the prescription.

MINNESOTA

NCCPA-certified PAs may prescribe controlled and noncontrolled drugs.

MISSISSIPPI

PAs have no prescribing or dispensing authority.

MISSOURI

PAs may not prescribe or dispense any drug, medicine, device, or therapy without the consultation of the supervising physician. Regulations to clarify prescriptive authority are pending.

MONTANA

PAs may prescribe and dispense drugs, including Schedule II-V controlled substances, as delegated by a physician. Schedule II controlled substances are limited to a 34-day supply.

NEBRASKA

PAs prescribe medications under the supervision of a physician. PAs may prescribe medications, including 72-hour supply of Schedule II controlled substances, in the supervising physician's name if authority is assigned by that physician.

NEVADA

With board approval, PAs may prescribe and dispense noncontrolled and controlled (Schedule II-V) drugs and devices as required by the supervising physician. Registration with pharmacy board required.

NEW HAMPSHIRE

PAs may prescribe noncontrolled and controlled (Schedule II-V) drugs. They must pass pharmacy law examination.

NEW JERSEY

PAs may prescribe medications, other than controlled substances, only in an inpatient setting and must provide specific information on the prescription blanks with required physician signature.

NEW MEXICO

PAs may prescribe, administer, and distribute Schedules II-V under direction of the supervising physician and within parameters of board-approved formulary and guidelines.

NEW YORK

PAs may write and sign prescriptions for non-controlled and controlled substances Schedule III-V on the prescription blanks of the supervising physician.

NORTH CAROLINA

PAs may prescribe controlled drugs in Schedules I-V (Schedule II and III limited to 7-day supply). Pharmacy Board approval required for compounding and dispensing drugs.

NORTH DAKOTA

PAs may prescribe Schedule III to V controlled substances. They may also dispense prepackaged medications (Schedules IV and V and noncontrolled substances) prepared by pharmacist acting on the physician's written order and labeled to show names of PA and physician. Dispensing must be authorized by and within preestablished guidelines of the supervising physician.

OHIO

PAs do not have prescribing or dispensing authority.

OKLAHOMA

PAs may transmit oral or written prescriptions for noncontrolled drugs on board-approved formulary.

OREGON

PAs may prescribe drugs, including Schedule III to V controlled substances, as determined by the physician and approved by board. DEA registration is required. PAs may apply for emergency dispensing authority for medications prepackaged by pharmacist.

PENNSYLVANIA

PAs may prescribe and dispense drugs from a formulary which excludes parenterals except insulin and allergy kits. PAs may prescribe Schedule III-V drugs, which are limited to a 30-day supply unless they are for chronic conditions.

RHODE ISLAND

PAs may prescribe drugs, including Schedule V. They must register with the state drug control office and DEA.

SOUTH CAROLINA

PAs may prescribe drugs, including Schedule V controlled substances.

SOUTH DAKOTA

PAs may prescribe drugs, including Schedules II-V substances. Schedule II drugs are limited to a 48-hour supply.

TENNESSEE

PAs may prescribe noncontrolled drugs.

TEXAS

PAs may sign or complete presigned prescription blanks if delegated this task under standing orders. Limited to medically underserved areas, practices with preponderance of medically indigent patients, a physician's primary practice site, hospital, or other location or when physician is present.

UTAH

PAs may prescribe noncontrolled and controlled Schedule II-V drugs. Any limitations on prescribing may be made in the delegation agreement. Prescriptions for Schedule II and III medications require chart cosignature.

VERMONT

PAs may prescribe drugs, including Schedule II-V, authorized by physician in job description and the formulary.

VIRGINIA

PAs may prescribe noncontrolled drugs and devices on board-approved formulary.

WASHINGTON

Certified PAs may write and sign prescriptions, including controlled substances in Schedules II to V; using the supervisor's DEA number with suffix or own number. PAs may dispense medications from office supplies (for osteopathic PAs), limited to 48-hour supply.

WEST VIRGINIA

PAs with 2 years of experience who have completed board-approved pharmacology course and maintain NCCPA certification may prescribe controlled (Schedule III to V) and noncontrolled drugs from formulary. Schedule III drugs are limited to 72-hour supply. DEA registration is required. PAs may dispense samples and, under certain conditions, legend drugs.

WISCONSIN

PAs may prepare prescription order for controlled substances Schedule II-V in situations specified in written protocols and, when practical, after consultation with the physician. The physician must review and sign records within certain time limits.

WYOMING

Physicians may delegate prescribing (including Schedules III-V) to PAs; dispensing of prepackaged drugs in rural areas is allowed when pharmacy services are unavailable. The supervising physician's DEA number must be used when prescribing controlled substances.

Selected analgesic combination products

Many common analgesics are combinations of two or more generic drugs. The following chart details these drugs and their components in two categories: nonnarcotic analgesics and narcotic and opioid analgesics.

TRADE NAME	GENERIC DRUG COMBINATION
Nonnarcotic analgesics	
Allerest No-Drowsiness Tablets, Coldrine, Ornex No Drowsiness Caplets, Sinus-Relief Tablets, Sinutab Without Drowsiness	• acetaminophen 325 mg • pseudoephedrine hydrochloride 30 mg
Amaphen, Anoquan, Butace, Endolor, Esgic, Femcet, Fioricet, Medigesic, Repan, Tencet, Two-Dyne	• acetaminophen 325 mg • caffeine 40 mg • butalbital 50 mg
Anacin, Gensan, PAC analgesic	• aspirin 400 mg • caffeine 32 mg
Arthritis Foundation Nighttime, Midol PM	• acetaminophen 500 mg • diphenhydramine 25 mg
Ascriptin	• aspirin 325 mg • magnesium hydroxide 50 mg • aluminum hydroxide 50 mg • calcium carbonate 50 mg
Ascriptin A/D	• aspirin 325 mg • magnesium hydroxide 75 mg • aluminum hydroxide 75 mg • calcium carbonate 75 mg
Cama Arthritis Pain Reliever	• aspirin 500 mg • magnesium oxide 150 mg • aluminum hydroxide 125 mg
COPE	• aspirin 421 mg • caffeine 32 mg • magnesium hydroxide 50 mg • aluminum hydroxide 25 mg
Doan's P.M. Extra Strength	• magnesium salicylate 500 mg • diphenhydramine 25 mg
Excedrin Extra Strength	• aspirin 250 mg • acetaminophen 250 mg • caffeine 65 mg
Excedrin P.M. Caplets	• acetaminophen 500 mg • diphenhydramine citrate 38 mg
Fiorinal, Isollyl Improved, Lanorinal	• aspirin 325 mg • caffeine 40 mg • butalbital 50 mg
Midrin	• isometheptene mucate 65 mg • dichloralphenazone 100 mg • acetaminophen 325 mg
Phrenilin	• acetaminophen 325 mg • butalbital 50 mg
Phrenilin Forte	• acetaminophen 650 mg • butalbital 50 mg

*Available in Canada only.

TRADE NAME	GENERIC DRUG COMBINATION
Nonnarcotic analgesics *(continued)*	
Sinus Excedrin Extra Strength	• acetaminophen 500 mg • pseudoephedrine hydrochloride 30 mg
Sinutab Regular*	• acetaminophen 325 mg • chlorpheniramine 2 mg • pseudoephedrine hydrochloride 30 mg
Sinutab Maximum Strength	• acetaminophen 500 mg • pseudoephedrine hydrochloride 30 mg • chlorpheniramine maleate 2 mg
Tecnal*	• aspirin 330 mg • caffeine 40 mg • butalbital 50 mg
Tencon	• acetaminophen 650 mg • butalbital 50 mg
Vanquish	• aspirin 227 mg • acetaminophen 194 mg • caffeine 33 mg • aluminum hydroxide 25 mg • magnesium hydroxide 50 mg
Narcotic and opioid analgesics	
222*	• aspirin 375 mg • codeine phosphate 8 mg • caffeine citrate 30 mg
282*	• aspirin 375 mg • codeine phosphate 15 mg • caffeine citrate 30 mg
292*	• aspirin 375 mg • codeine phosphate 30 mg • caffeine citrate 30 mg
692*	• aspirin 375 mg • propoxyphene hydrochloride 65 mg • caffeine 30 mg
A.C. & C.*	• aspirin 325 mg • codeine phosphate 8 mg • caffeine 15 mg
Aceta with Codeine, Empracet-30*, Emtec-30*	• acetaminophen 300 mg • codeine phosphate 30 mg
Anacin With Codeine*	• aspirin 325 mg • codeine phosphate 8 mg • caffeine 32 mg
Capital with Codeine, Tylenol with Codeine Elixir	• acetaminophen 120 mg • codeine phosphate 12 mg/5 ml
Darvocet-N 50	• acetaminophen 325 mg • propoxyphene napsylate 50 mg
Darvocet-N 100, Propacet 100	• acetaminophen 650 mg • propoxyphene napsylate 100 mg

(continued)

* Available in Canada only.

Selected analgesic combination products *(continued)*

TRADE NAME	GENERIC DRUG COMBINATION
Narcotic and opioid analgesics *(continued)*	
Darvon-N Compound*	• aspirin 375 mg • propoxyphene napsylate 100 mg • caffeine 30 mg
Darvon-N With A.S.A.*	• aspirin 325 mg • propoxyphene napsylate 100 mg
E-Lor, Wygesic	• acetaminophen 650 mg • propoxyphene hydrochloride 65 mg
Empirin With Codeine No. 3	• aspirin 325 mg • codeine phosphate 30 mg
Empirin With Codeine No. 4	• aspirin 325 mg • codeine phosphate 60 mg
Empracet-30*	• acetaminophen 300 mg • codeine phosphate 30 mg
Empracet-60*	• acetaminophen 300 mg • codeine phosphate 60 mg
Endodan*, Oxycodan*, Percodan*	• aspirin 325 mg • oxycodone hydrochloride 5 mg
Endocet*, Oxycocet*	• acetaminophen 325 mg • oxycodone hydrochloride 5 mg
Fioricet/Codeine	• acetaminophen 325 mg • butalbital 50 mg • caffeine 40 mg • codeine phosphate 30 mg
Fiorinal With Codeine	• aspirin 325 mg • butalbital 50 mg • caffeine 40 mg • codeine phosphate 30 mg
Innovar Injection	• droperidol 2.5 mg • fentanyl citrate 0.05 mg/ml
Lenoltec With Codeine No. 1*, Novogesic C8*	• acetaminophen 300 mg • codeine phosphate 8 mg • caffeine 15 mg
Lorcet 10/650	• acetaminophen 650 mg • hydrocodone bitartrate 10 mg
Lortab 2.5/500	• acetaminophen 500 mg • hydrocodone bitartrate 2.5 mg
Lortab 5/500	• acetaminophen 500 mg • hydrocodone bitartrate 5 mg
Lortab 7.5/500	• acetaminophen 500 mg • hydrocodone bitartrate 7.5 mg
Percocet	• acetaminophen 325 mg • oxycodone hydrochloride 5 mg
Percodan-Demi	• aspirin 325 mg • oxycodone hydrochloride 2.25 mg • oxycodone terephthalate 0.19 mg

*Available in Canada only.

TRADE NAME	GENERIC DRUG COMBINATION
Narcotic and opioid analgesics *(continued)*	
Percodan-Demi*	• aspirin 325 mg • oxycodone hydrochloride 2.5 mg
Percodan, Roxiprin	• aspirin 325 mg • oxycodone hydrochloride 4.5 mg • oxycodone terephthalate 0.38 mg
Phenaphen/Codeine No. 3	• acetaminophen 325 mg • codeine phosphate 30 mg
Phenaphen/Codeine No. 4	• acetaminophen 325 mg • codeine phosphate 60 mg
Propoxyphene Napsylate/Acetaminophen	• propoxyphene napsylate 100 mg • acetaminophen 650 mg
Roxicet	• acetaminophen 325 mg • oxycodone hydrochloride 5 mg
Roxicet 5/500	• acetaminophen 500 mg • oxycodone hydrochloride 5 mg
Roxicet Oral Solution	• acetaminophen 325 mg • oxycodone hydrochloride 5 mg/5 ml
Talacen	• acetaminophen 650 mg • pentazocine hydrochloride 25 mg
Talwin Compound	• aspirin 325 mg • pentazocine hydrochloride 12.5 mg
Tylenol With Codeine No. 2	• acetaminophen 300 mg • codeine phosphate 15 mg
Tylenol With Codeine No. 3	• acetaminophen 300 mg • codeine phosphate 30 mg
Tylenol With Codeine No. 4	• acetaminophen 300 mg • codeine phosphate 60 mg
Tylox	• acetaminophen 500 mg • oxycodone hydrochloride 5 mg
Vicodin	• acetaminophen 500 mg • hydrocodone bitartrate 5 mg
Vicodin ES	• acetaminophen 750 mg • hydrocodone bitartrate 7.5 mg

* Available in Canada only.

Topical drugs

Numerous drugs are used to treat topical conditions. This chart shows commonly used topical drugs and their indications, dosages, and actions. It also outlines key considerations related to topical administration of the drugs.

	DRUG	INDICATIONS AND DOSAGE
Antibacterials and antifungals	**alcohol, ethyl and isopropyl**	*To disinfect skin, instruments, and ampules:* disinfect, p.r.n. Isopropyl alcohol is superior to ethyl alcohol as an anti-infective (70%). *Antipyresis:* apply 25% solution. *Anhidrosis:* apply 50% solution p.r.n.
	hydrogen peroxide (PerOxyl)	*Cleaning wounds:* use 1.5% to 3% solution, p.r.n. *Mouthwash for necrotizing ulcerative gingivitis:* gargle with 3% solution, p.r.n. *Cleaning minor wounds or irritations of the mouth or gums:* use 1.5% gel, p.r.n. *Cleaning douche:* use 2% solution q.i.d., p.r.n.
Antiseptics and germicidals	**benzalkonium chloride** (Benza, Zephiran Chloride)	*Preoperative disinfection of unbroken skin:* apply 1:750 tincture or spray. *Disinfection of mucous membranes and denuded skin:* apply 1:10,000 to 1:5,000 aqueous solution. *Irrigation of vagina:* instill 1:5,000 to 1:2,000 aqueous solution. *Irrigation of deep infected wounds:* instill 1:20,000 to 1:3,000 aqueous solution. *Irrigation of urinary bladder and urethra:* 1:5,000 to 1:20,000 aqueous solution.
	chlorhexidine gluconate (Hibiclens, Hibistat, Peridex)	*Surgical hand scrub, hand wash, hand rinse, skin wound cleanser:* use 0.5% to 4% strength, p.r.n. *Gingivitis:* use 0.12% strength (Peridex oral rinse), p.r.n.
	hexachlorophene (pHisoHex, Septisol)	*Surgical scrub, bacteriostatic skin cleanser:* use 0.23% to 3% concentrations, p.r.n.
	iodine	*Preoperative disinfection of skin (small wounds and abraded areas):* apply p.r.n.
	povidone-iodine (ACU-dyne, Aerodine, Betadine, Betagen, Biodine, Efodine, Iodex, Operand, Polydine)	*Preoperative skin preparation and scrub; germicide for surface wounds; postoperative application to incisions; prophylactic application to urinary meatus of catheterized patients; miscellaneous disinfection:* apply p.r.n., or use as scrub p.r.n.
Keratolytics	**podophyllum resin** (Pod-Ben 25, Podocon)	*Venereal warts:* apply podophyllum resin preparation to the lesion, cover with waxed paper, and bandage. The first application should remain on skin for 30 to 40 minutes; subsequent applications may last 1 to 4 hours, depending on lesion and patient's condition. Wash lesion to remove medication. Repeat at weekly intervals, if indicated. *Multiple superficial epitheliomatosis and keratosis:* apply daily with applicator and allow to dry. Remove necrotic tissue before each application.
	salicylic acid (Calicylic, Compound W, DuoFilm, Freezone, Gordofilm, Hydrisalic, Keralyt, Occlusal, Off-Ezy, Sal-Acid, Wart-Off)	*Scaling dermatoses, hyperkeratosis, calluses, warts:* apply to affected area and cover with occlusive dressing at night.
Protectants	**benzoin tincture compound**	*Demulcent and protectant (cutaneous ulcers, bedsores, cracked nipples, fissures of lips and anus):* apply locally once daily or b.i.d.
	zinc oxide with calamine and gelatin (Dome-Paste)	*Protectant (lesions or injuries of lower legs or arms):* wrap the wet bandage in place and retain for about 1 week. Dome-Paste, in 3" to 4" bandages, can be applied directly to arm or leg.
Wet dressings, soaks	**aluminum acetate, aluminum sulfate** (Boropak Powder, Burow's Solution, Domeboro Powder)	*Mild skin irritation from exposure to soaps, chemicals, diaper rash, acne, eczema:* apply p.r.n. *Skin inflammation, contact dermatoses:* mix powder or tablet with 1 pint of lukewarm water. Apply to loose dressing q 15 to 30 minutes for 4 to 8 hours.

ACTION	SPECIAL CONSIDERATIONS
Antibacterial effect through reduction of surface tension of bacterial cell walls, inhibiting bacterial growth. Also antipyretic and astringent effects.	• Avoid contact with eyes and mucous membranes. • Contraindicated in patients taking disulfiram if used over large surface area. • Do not apply to open wounds.
Antibacterial effect through oxidation.	• Do not instill into closed body cavities or abscesses because released gas cannot escape. • Store in tightly capped, dark container in cool, dry place. • Do not confuse with peroxide (6% to 20%) used for bleaching hair.
Cationic surface action producing bacteriostatic or bactericidal effect, depending on the concentration used.	• Do not use with occlusive dressings or packs. • Inactivated by anionic compounds such as soap. • Rinse area thoroughly after each application. • Skin inflammation and irritation may require lower concentration or discontinuation.
Persistent antimicrobial effect against gram-negative and gram-positive bacteria.	• Avoid contact with eyes, ears, and mucous membranes. Rinse well if drug enters eyes or ears. • May cause deafness if drug enters middle ear.
Bacteriostatic effect against staphylococci and other gram-positive bacteria, probably due to inhibition of bacterial membrane-bound enzymes.	• Do not use on broken skin, skin lesions, burns, wounds, or under occlusive dressings. Do not use around eyes or mucous membranes. • Discontinue promptly if CNS irritability occurs. • Rinse thoroughly after use. • Do not use in infants; use cautiously in children.
Germicidal effect against bacteria, fungi, and viruses, probably due to disruption of microorganism proteins.	• Do not cover after application to avoid irritation. • Iodine stains skin and clothing. • Toxic if ingested; sodium thiosulfate is antidote.
Germicidal effect against bacteria, fungi, and viruses; has same action as iodine without its irritating effects.	• Contraindicated in patients with known sensitivity to iodine. • Do not use around eyes; do not use full-strength solution on mucous membranes. May stain skin and mucous membranes. • Avoid using solution that contains a detergent when treating open wounds.
Caustic and erosive action from disruption of epithelial cell division.	• Should not be used in pregnant patients. • May be toxic if applied to large surface area or applied too frequently. • Wash hands thoroughly after applying. • Protect surrounding area with petrolatum. • Wash off thoroughly with soap and water after prescribed time. • May cause abnormal pigmentation. • To be applied by a health care provider only.
Causes desquamation of cornified epithelium by increasing hydration.	• Do not use on birthmarks, moles, or areas with hair follicle involvement. • Do not use in aspirin-sensitive patients. • Hydrate skin for at least 5 minutes before application. • Apply emollient to surrounding skin for protection. • Wash off thoroughly after overnight use.
Protects skin from external environment by coating action.	• Clean and dry area before applying. • Useful in protection of skin from adhesive.
Protects skin by forming occlusive barrier.	• Watch for signs of infection. • Warn patient not to shower or bathe with gel on. • Remove by soaking in warm water. Remove all of previous application before reapplying. • Apply with nap of hair to avoid folliculitis. • Do not use with constrictive bandage.
Reduces friction and provides soothing relief through astringent action.	• Avoid use around eyes and mucous membranes. • Do not use with occlusive dressings. • Discontinue if irritation occurs.

Immunization schedule

The current childhood immunization schedule as approved by the American Academy of Family Physicians, the American Academy of Pediatrics, and the Advisory Committee on Immunization Practices encompasses recent changes in recommendations. The schedule may be appropriately altered with the use of currently licensed combination vaccines.

The following chart includes important information to consider when immunizing children.

<table>
<tr><th rowspan="2">Vaccine</th><th colspan="11">Age</th></tr>
<tr><th>Birth</th><th>1 mo.</th><th>2 mos.</th><th>4 mos.</th><th>6 mos.</th><th>12 mos.</th><th>15 mos.</th><th>18 mos.</th><th>4-6 yrs.</th><th>11-12 yrs.</th><th>14-16 yrs.</th></tr>
<tr><td rowspan="2">Hepatitis B[1]</td><td colspan="3">Hep B-1</td><td></td><td></td><td></td><td></td><td></td><td></td><td></td><td></td></tr>
<tr><td></td><td colspan="3">Hep B-2</td><td colspan="4">Hep B-3</td><td></td><td>Hep B</td><td></td></tr>
<tr><td>Diphtheria and tetanus toxoids and acellular pertussis[2] (DTaP, DTP)</td><td></td><td></td><td>DTaP or DTP</td><td>DTaP or DTP</td><td>DTaP or DTP</td><td></td><td colspan="2">DTaP or DTP</td><td>DTaP or DTP</td><td colspan="2">Td</td></tr>
<tr><td>Haemophilus influenzae type b[3]</td><td></td><td></td><td>Hib</td><td>Hib</td><td>Hib</td><td colspan="2">Hib</td><td></td><td></td><td></td><td></td></tr>
<tr><td>Poliovirus[4]</td><td></td><td></td><td>Polio</td><td>Polio</td><td></td><td colspan="3">Polio</td><td>Polio</td><td></td><td></td></tr>
<tr><td>Measles, mumps, rubella[5]</td><td></td><td></td><td></td><td></td><td></td><td colspan="2">MMR</td><td></td><td>MMR</td><td>or MMR</td><td></td></tr>
<tr><td>Varicella virus[6]</td><td></td><td></td><td></td><td></td><td></td><td colspan="3">Var</td><td></td><td>Var</td><td></td></tr>
</table>

Range of acceptable ages for vaccination.

"Catch-up" vaccination.

[1]Hepatitis B: Children and adolescents who were not immunized against hepatits B in infancy may begin the series at any time. The series should be initiated or completed at age 11 or 12 in any child who has not previously received three doses of hepatitis B. The 2nd dose should be administered at least 1 month after the 1st dose, and the 3rd dose should be given at least 4 months after the 1st dose and at least 2 months after the 2nd dose.

Infants born to hepatitis B surface antigen (HBsAG)-negative mothers should receive 2.5 mcg of Recombivax HB (Merck) or 10 mcg of Engerix-B (SmithKline Beecham) at birth. The 2nd dose is given at least 1 month after the 1st.

Infants born to HBsAg-positive mothers should receive 0.5 ml of hepatitis B immune globulin (HBIG) within 12 hours of birth, and either 5 mcg of Recombivax HB (Merck) or 10 mcg of Engerix-B (SmithKline Beecham) at a separate site. The 2nd dose is given at age 1 to 2 months and the 3rd dose at age 6 months.

Infants born to mothers with unknown HBsAG status should receive 5 mcg of Recombivax HB (Merck) or 10 mcg of Engerix-B (SmithKline Beecham) within 12 hours of birth. Blood should be drawn at the time of delivery to determine the mother's HBsAg status. If positive, the baby should receive 0.5 ml of HBIG as soon as possible and no later than age 1 week. The dosage and timing of subsequent vaccine doses should be based upon the mother's HBsAg status.

[2]DTP: DTaP is the recommended vaccine for all doses in the series. Children who have received one or more doses of the whole-cell DTP may complete the series with DTaP. To combat compliance issues in patients who are unlikely to return at age 15 to 18 months, the 4th dose of the vaccine may be given as early as age 12 months, as long as 6 months have elapsed since the 3rd dose. Td is recommended at age 11 to 12, provided that at least 5 years have elapsed since the last dose of DTP, DTaP, or DT. Routine Td boosters are recommended every 10 years for adults.

[3]*H. influenzae* type b: Three H. influenzae type b (Hib) vaccines are licensed for use in infants. They are given at age 2, 4, 6, and 12 to 15 months unless the PRP-OMP (PedvaxHIB [Merck]) is used, in which case a dose at age 6 months is not necessary. Any Hib conjugate vaccine may be used as a booster dose at age 12 to 15 months.

[4]Poliovirus: Two poliovirus vaccines are currently licensed for use. The inactivated poliovirus vaccine (IPV), and the oral poliovirus vaccine (OPV), may be given according to the following schedules:

IPV at age 2 and 4 months; OPV at age 12 to 18 months and age 4 to 6.
IPV at age 2, 4, 12 to 18 months, and 4 to 6.
OPV at age 2, 4, 6 to 18 months, and 4 to 6.

OPV should not be used in immunocompromised children or those in close contact with immunocompromised persons.

[5]Measles, mumps, rubella: The 2nd dose is recommended at age 4 to 6 before school entry, or age 11 or 12. The 2nd dose may be administered at any visit, as long as both doses are given at or after age 12 months, and at least 1 month has elapsed between the 1st and 2nd doses.

[6]Varicella virus: Varicella vaccine may be administered on or after age 12 months to any child who lacks a reliable history of varicella. Any child who has not been previously vaccinated and does not have a reliable history of chickenpox should receive the vaccine at age 11 or 12. Children age 13 or older must be given two doses of the vaccine at least 1 month apart.

Creatinine clearance calculations

In adults with stable renal function, the following formulas will provide a reliable estimate of creatinine clearance (Cl_{cr}) except:

Patients with falsely low serum creatinine (such as paraplegic patients with muscle wasting) will give an artificially high predicted Cl_{cr}.

Patients with rapidly increasing serum creatinine (over 0.5 to 0.7 mg/dl/day) will give an unreliable estimate of Cl_{cr}.

Adults (age 18 and older)

Method 1*:

Estimated creatinine clearance, Cl_{cr} (ml/minute):

$$\text{Male } Cl_{cr} = \frac{(140 - \text{age})\ (\text{IBW})}{(72)\ (\text{Scr})}$$

Female Cl_{cr} = (Estimated male Cl_{cr}) (0.85)

where age = in years

IBW = ideal body weight in kilograms:

IBW (Male) = 50 + [(2.3) (height in inches over 5 feet)]

IBW (Female) = 45.5 + [(2.3) (height in inches over 5 feet)]

Note: The use of the patient's IBW is recommended except when the patient's actual body weight is less than IBW.

S_{cr} = Serum creatinine in mg/dl

Method 2†:

Estimated creatinine clearance, Cl_{cr} (ml/minute/1.73 m^2):

$$\text{Male } Cl_{cr} = \frac{98 - [(0.8)\ (\text{age} - 20)]}{S_{cr}}$$

Female Cl_{cr} = (Estimated male Cl_{cr}) (0.90)

where age is in years, S_{cr} is serum creatinine in mg/dl.

*Cockroft, D.W., and Gault, M.H. "Prediction of Creatinine Clearance From Serum Creatinine," *Nephron* 16:31, 1976.

†Jelliffe, R.W. "Creatinine Clearance: Bedside Estimate," *Ann Intern Med* 79:604, 1973.

Therapeutic drug monitoring guidelines

Many drugs require certain laboratory tests to be monitored. This chart lists which tests should be followed for selected drugs.

DRUG	LABORATORY TEST MONITORED	THERAPEUTIC RANGES OF TEST
aminoglycoside antibiotics (amikacin, gentamicin, tobramycin)	Serum amikacin peak trough Serum gentamicin/tobramycin peak trough Serum creatinine	20 to 25 mcg/ml 5 to 10 mcg/ml 4 to 8 mcg/ml 1 to 2 mcg/ml 0.6 to 1.3 mg/dl
amphotericin B	Serum creatinine BUN Serum electrolytes (especially potassium and magnesium) Liver function tests CBC with differential and platelets	0.6 to 1.3 mg/dl 7 to 18 mg/dl Potassium: 3.5 to 5 mEq/L Magnesium: 1.7 to 2.1 mEq/L Sodium: 135 to 145 mEq/L Chloride: 98 to 106 mEq/L † *
antibiotics	WBC with differential Cultures and sensitivities	*
biguanides (Metformin)	Serum creatinine Fasting serum glucose Glycosolated hemoglobin CBC	0.6 to 1.3 mg/dl 65 to 110 mg/dl 5.5 to 8.5% of total hemoglobin *
clozapine	WBC with differential	*
digoxin	Serum digoxin Serum electrolytes (especially potassium, magnesium, and calcium) Serum creatinine	0.5 to 2 ng/ml Potassium: 3.5 to 5 mEq/L Magnesium: 1.7 to 2.1 mEq/L Sodium: 135 to 145 mEq/L Chloride: 98 to 106 mEq/L Calcium: 8.6 to 10 mg/dl 0.6 to 1.3 mg/dl
diuretics	Serum electrolytes Serum creatinine BUN Uric acid Fasting serum glucose	Potassium: 3.5 to 5 mEq/L Magnesium: 1.7 to 2.1 mEq/L Sodium: 135 to 145 mEq/L Chloride: 98 to 106 mEq/L Calcium: 8.6 to 10 mg/dl 0.6 to 1.3 mg/dl 7 to 18 mg/dl 2 to 7 mg/dl 65 to 110 mg/dl
erythropoietin	Hematocrit	Female: 36% to 48% Male: 42% to 52%
gemfibrozil	Serum lipids	Total cholesterol: < 200 mg/dl LDL: < 130 mg/dl HDL: female: 40 to 85 mg/dl male: 37 to 70 mg/dl Triglycerides: 40 to 160 mg/dl
heparin	Activated partial thromboplastin time (APTT)	1.5 to 2 times control

* For areas marked with an asterisk, the following values can be used:

Hemoglobin: Female: 12 to 16 g/dl
Male: 14 to 18 g/dl
Hematocrit: Female: 37% to 48%
Male: 42% to 52%
RBCs: 4 to 5.5 x 10^6/mm^3
WBCs: 5 to 10 x 10^3/mm^3

Differential: Neutrophils: 45% to 74%
Bands: 0% to 4%
Lymphocytes: 16% to 45%
Monocytes: 4% to 10%
Eosinophils: 0% to 7%
Basophils: 0% to 2%

MONITORING GUIDELINES

Wait until the administration of the third dose to check drug levels. Check peak level 30 minutes after the end of I.V. infusion or 60 minutes after I.M. administration. Check trough level just before administration of next dose. Adjust dose if necessary and re-check after three doses. Serum creatinine can be used to determine renal function, which is useful in calculating individualized dosing.

Monitor serum creatinine, BUN, and serum electrolytes at least weekly during therapy. Blood counts and liver function tests should also be monitored regularly during therapy.

Obtain a follow-up on specimen cultures and sensitivities to determine the causative agent of the infection and the best treatment. Monitor WBC with differential weekly during therapy.

Check renal function and hematologic parameters before initiation of therapy and at least annually thereafter. In the presence of impaired renal function, metformin may cause lactic acidosis and should not be used. Monitor response to therapy with periodic evaluations of fasting glucose and glycosolated hemoglobin. Home glucose monitoring by the patient can also be very useful.

Obtain WBC with differential before initiating therapy, weekly during therapy, and 4 weeks after discontinuation.

Serum digoxin levels should be checked at least 12 hours after the administration of the last dose, preferably 24 hours after the last dose. For monitoring maintenance therapy, levels should be checked at least 1 to 2 weeks after the initiation or a change of therapy. Adjustments in therapy should be made based on entire clinical picture, not solely on drug levels. Electrolytes and renal function should also be checked periodically during therapy.

Baseline and periodic determinations of serum electrolytes, serum calcium, BUN, uric acid, and serum glucose should be performed to monitor fluid and electrolyte balance.

With the initiation of therapy and after any dosage change, monitor the hematocrit twice weekly for 2 to 6 weeks until stabilized in the target range and a maintenance dose determined. The hematocrit should be monitored at regular intervals thereafter.

If response is not adequate after 3 months, withdraw therapy. Patient must be fasting to measure triglycerides.

When given by continuous I.V. infusion, check APTT every 4 hours in the early stages of therapy. When given by deep S.C. injection, check APTT 4 to 6 hours after injection.

(continued)

† For areas marked with a dagger, the following values can be used:

ALT: 7 to 56 U/L
AST: 5 to 40 U/L
Alkaline phosphotase: 17 to 142 U/L
LD: 60 to 220 U/L
GGTP: < 40 U/L
Total bilirubin: 0.2 to 1 mg/dl

Therapeutic drug monitoring guidelines *(continued)*

DRUG	LABORATORY TEST MONITORED	THERAPEUTIC RANGES OF TEST
HMG-CoA reductase inhibitors (fluvastatin, lovastatin, pravastatin, simvastatin)	Serum lipids Liver function tests	Total cholesterol: < 200 mg/dl LDL: < 130 mg/dl HDL: female: 40 to 85 mg/dl male: 37 to 70 mg/dl Triglycerides: 40 to 160 mg/dl †
insulin	Fasting serum glucose Glycosylated hemoglobin	65 to 110 mg/dl 5.5% to 8.5% of total hemoglobin
lithium	Serum lithium Serum creatinine CBC Serum electrolytes (especially potassium and sodium) Fasting serum glucose Thyroid function tests	0.8 to 1.2 mEq/L 0.6 to 1.3 mg/dl * Potassium: 3.5 to 5 mEq/L Magnesium: 1.7 to 2.1 mEq/L Sodium: 135 to 145 mEq/L Chloride: 98 to 106 mEq/L 65 to 110 mg/dl TSH: 0.2 to 5.4 microU/mL T_3: 80 to 200 ng/dl T_4: 5.4 to 11.5 mcg/dl
phenytoin	Serum phenytoin CBC	10 to 20 mcg/ml *
potassium chloride	Serum potassium	3.5 to 5 mEq/L
procainamide	Serum procainamide Serum N-acetylprocainamide CBC	4 to 8 mcg/ml (procainamide) 5 to 30 mcg/ml (combined procainamide and NAPA) *
quinidine	Serum quinidine CBC Liver function tests Serum creatinine Serum electrolytes (especially potassium)	2 to 6 mcg/ml * † 0.6 to 1.3 mg/dl Potassium: 3.5 to 5 mEq/L Magnesium: 1.7 to 2.1 mEq/L Sodium: 135 to 145 mEq/L Chloride: 98 to 106 mEq/L
sulfonylureas	Fasting serum glucose Glycosylated hemoglobin	65 to 110 mg/dl 5.8% to 8.5% of total hemoglobin
theophylline	Serum theophylline	10 to 20 mcg/ml
thyroid hormone	Thyroid function tests	TSH: 0.2 to 5.4 microU/ml T_3: 80 to 200 ng/dl T_4: 5.4 to 11.5 mcg/dl
vancomycin	Serum vancomycin Serum creatinine	20 to 40 mcg/ml (peak) 5 to 10 mcg/ml (trough) 0.6 to 1.3 mg/dl
warfarin	International Normalized Ratio (INR)	For acute MI, atrial fibrillation, treatment of pulmonary embolism, prevention of systemic embolism, tissue heart valves, valvular heart disease, or prophylaxis or treatment of venous thrombosis: 2 to 3 For mechanical prosthetic valves or recurrent systemic embolism: 3 to 4.5

* For areas marked with an asterisk, the following values can be used:

Hemoglobin: Female: 12 to 16 g/dl
Male: 14 to 18 g/dl
Hematocrit: Female: 37% to 48%
Male: 42% to 52%
RBCs: 4 to 5.5 x 10^6/mm³
WBCs: 5 to 10 x 10^3/mm³

Differential: Neutrophils: 45% to 74%
Bands: 0% to 4%
Lymphocytes: 16% to 45%
Monocytes: 4% to 10%
Eosinophils: 0% to 7%
Basophils: 0% to 2%

MONITORING GUIDELINES

If adequate response is not achieved within 6 weeks, consider change in therapy. Liver function tests should be determined at baseline, 6 to 12 weeks after the initiation of therapy or any increase in dose, and periodically thereafter.

Monitor response to therapy with evaluations of serum glucose and glycosolated hemoglobin. Glycosolated hemoglobin is a good measure of long-term control. Home glucose monitoring by the patient is also useful for measuring compliance and response.

Obtain serum lithium levels immediately before next dose. Levels should be checked twice weekly until stable. Once at steady state, levels may be obtained weekly and, when the patient is on the appropriate maintenance dose, levels may be monitored every 2 to 3 months. Serum creatinine, CBC, serum electrolytes, fasting serum glucose, and thyroid function tests should be performed before initiating therapy and periodically during therapy.

Check serum phenytoin levels immediately before next dose, 2 to 4 weeks after initiation of therapy or dose adjustment. Obtain a CBC at baseline and monthly early in therapy. If toxic effects appear at therapeutic levels, the measured level should be adjusted for hypoalbuminemia or renal impairment — both increase free drug levels.

Check level weekly after initiation of oral replacement therapy until stable, and every 3 to 6 months thereafter.

Measure procainamide levels 6 to 12 hours after the start of a continuous infusion, or immediately prior to the next oral dose. Combined (procainamide and NAPA) levels can be used as an index of toxicity when renal impairment exists. CBC should be obtained periodically during longer-term therapy.

Obtain levels immediately before next oral dose, 30 to 35 hours after initiation of therapy or dosage change. Obtain periodic blood counts, liver and kidney function tests, and serum electrolytes.

Monitor response to therapy with periodic evaluations of fasting glucose and glycosolated hemoglobin. Home glucose monitoring by the patient is a good measure of compliance and response.

Obtain serum quinidine levels immediately before next dose of sustained-release oral product, at least 2 days after initiation or change of therapy.

Monitor thyroid function tests every 2 to 3 weeks until appropriate maintenance dose is determined.

Serum vancomycin levels may be checked with the third dose administered (at the earliest). Peak levels should be drawn ½ hour after the completion of an I.V. infusion. Trough levels should be drawn immediately before the administration of the next dose. Renal function can be used to adjust dosing and intervals.

Obtain daily INR beginning 3 days after initiation of therapy, continue until therapeutic goal is achieved, monitor periodically thereafter. Also check levels 7 days after any change in warfarin dose or concomitant, potentially interacting therapy.

† For areas marked with a dagger, the following values can be used:

ALT: 7 to 56 U/L
AST: 5 to 40 U/L
Alkaline phosphotase: 17 to 142 U/L
LD: 60 to 220 U/L
GGTP: < 40 U/L
Total bilirubin: 0.2 to 1 mg/dl

Therapeutic management guidelines: Cancer pain

Managing a patient with cancer-related pain involves regular assessment, a step-up approach to analgesic use, and the empowerment of patients or their caregivers to control pain therapy. Pain control options should be individualized according to the specific needs of each patient, family, and setting. Analgesics should be administered on time using a logical, coordinated effort on the part of the entire health care team.

Schedule administration of analgesics at regular intervals. Add "break-through" doses (⅓ of the scheduled dose) as needed. Use oral route for analgesics whenever possible. Rectal or transdermal routes may be used during periods of nausea or vomiting.

The patient should be assessed for pain at regular intervals, after each new report of pain, and after each administration of an analgesic or adjuvant drug, such as hydroxyzine, dexamethasone, or trazodone. Adjuvant drugs enhance the analgesic effects of opioids, treat conditions that may exacerbate pain, or provide independent analgesia for specific types of pain. These agents may be used at any point in pain therapy.

This diagram illustrates the steps in the management of an adult patient with cancer-related pain.

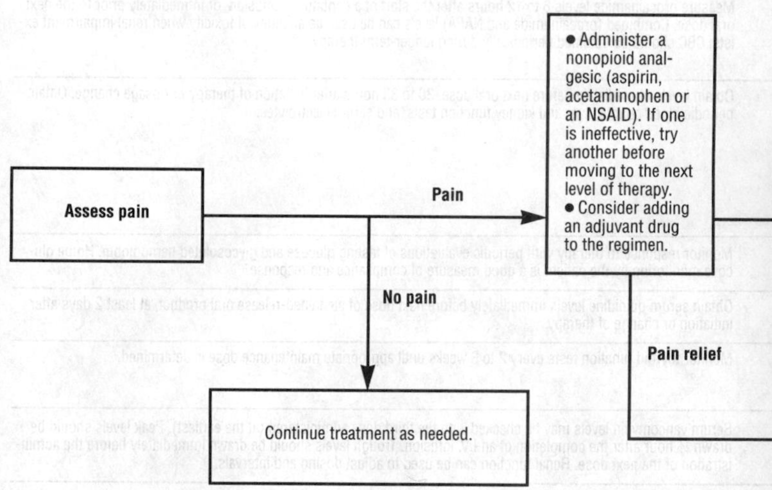

Based on guidelines from the Agency for Health Care Policy and Research (AHCPR). (AHCPR. *Management of Cancer Pain: Adults*. No. 94-0593. Rockville, MD: U.S. Department of Health and Human Services Public Health Service Agency for Health Care Policy and Research, 1994.)

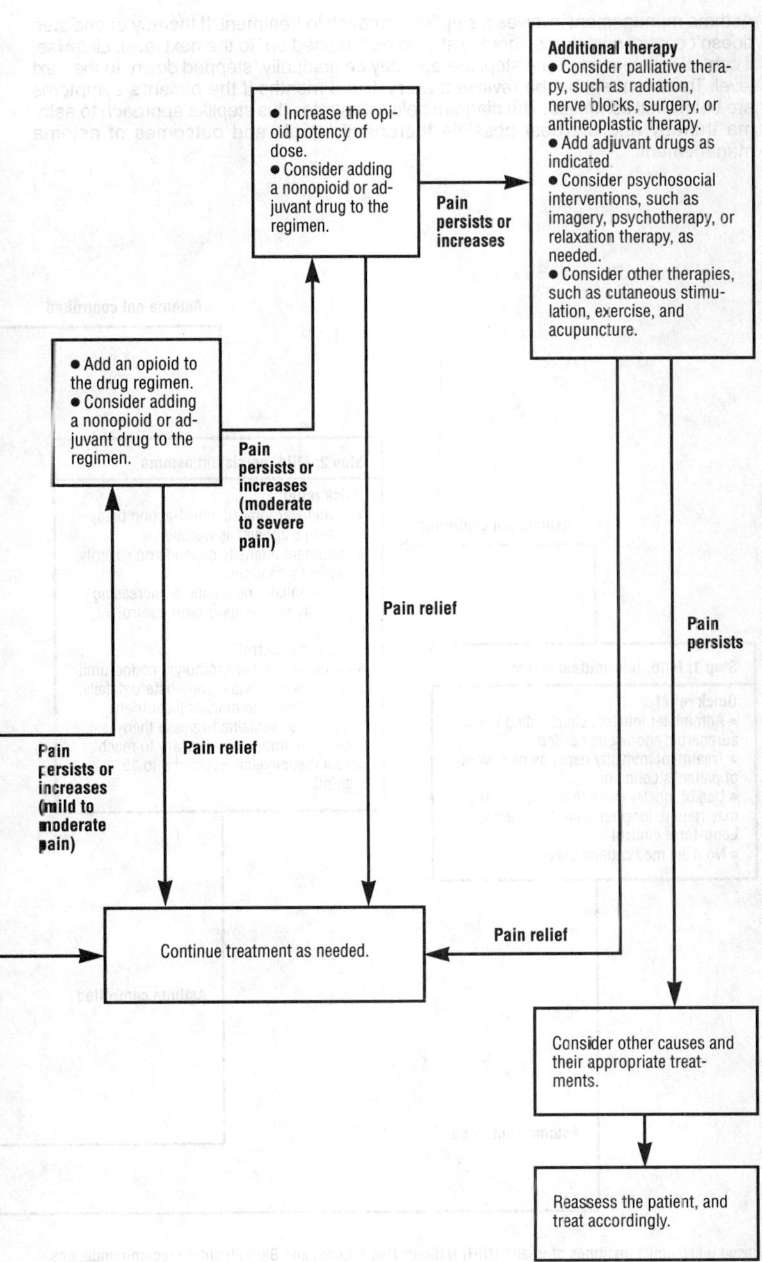
• Add an opioid to the drug regimen.
• Consider adding a nonopioid or adjuvant drug to the regimen.
Pain persists or increases (moderate to severe pain)
• Increase the opioid potency of dose.
• Consider adding a nonopioid or adjuvant drug to the regimen.
Pain persists or increases
Additional therapy
• Consider palliative therapy, such as radiation, nerve blocks, surgery, or antineoplastic therapy.
• Add adjuvant drugs as indicated.
• Consider psychosocial interventions, such as imagery, psychotherapy, or relaxation therapy, as needed.
• Consider other therapies, such as cutaneous stimulation, exercise, and acupuncture.
Pain relief
Pain persists
Pain persists or increases (mild to moderate pain)
Pain relief
Continue treatment as needed.
Pain relief
Consider other causes and their appropriate treatments.
Reassess the patient, and treat accordingly.

Therapeutic management guidelines: Asthma

Asthma management involves a steplike approach to treatment. If therapy at one step doesn't control symptoms, therapy should be "stepped up" to the next level. Likewise, if control is achieved at one step, therapy may be gradually "stepped down" to the next level. Treatment should be reviewed every 1 to 6 months if the patient's symptoms are being well controlled. The diagram below illustrates this steplike approach to asthma therapy and the best possible therapeutic goals and outcomes of asthma management.

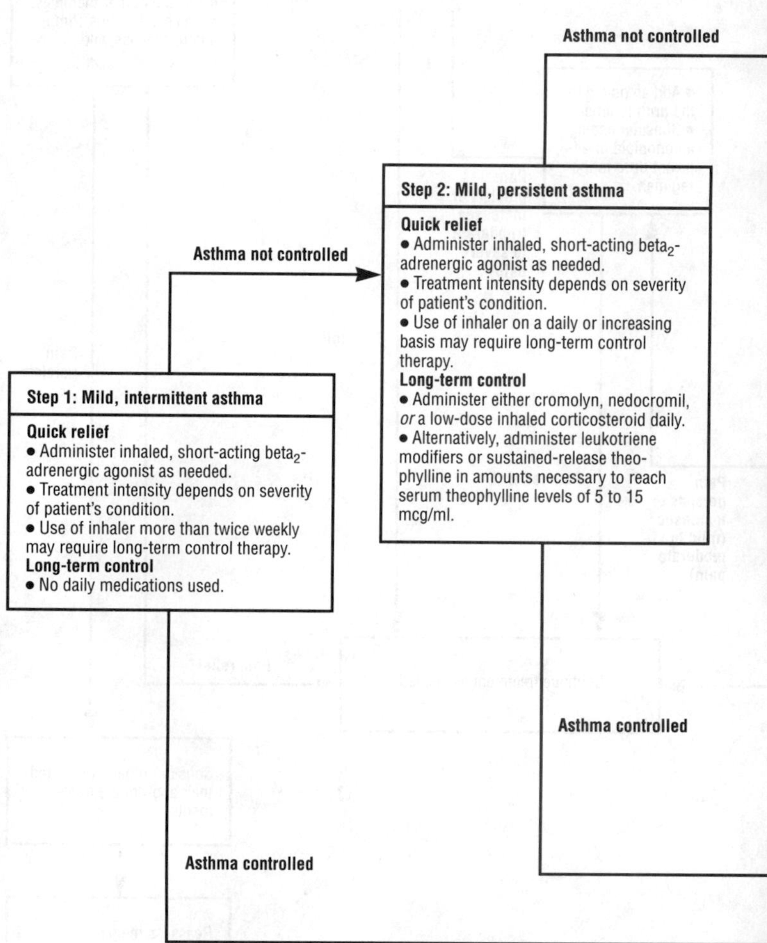

Based on National Institutes of Health (NIH) National Heart, Lung, and Blood Institute recommendations for asthma management. (*Guidelines for the Diagnosis and Management of Asthma.* NIH pub. 97-4051. Washington, D.C.: U.S. Government Printing Office, April, 1997.)

Step 4: Severe, persistent asthma

Quick relief
- Administer inhaled, short-acting beta$_2$-adrenergic agonist as needed.
- Treatment intensity depends on severity of patient's condition.
- Use of inhaler on a daily or increasing basis may require long-term control therapy.

Long-term control
- Administer daily doses of a high-dose inhaled corticosteroid *and* a long-acting beta$_2$-adrenergic agonist (or sustained-release theophylline or a long-acting beta$_2$-adrenergic agonist in tablet form) *and* 2 mg/kg/day of long-term oral corticosteroids (maximum daily dose, 60 mg).

Asthma not controlled

Step 3: Moderate, persistent asthma

Quick relief
- Administer inhaled, short-acting beta$_2$-adrenergic agonist as needed.
- Treatment intensity depends on severity of patient's condition.
- Use of inhaler on a daily or increasing basis may require long-term control therapy.

Long-term control
- Administer daily doses of either a medium-dose inhaled corticosteroid alone *or* a low-to-medium–dose inhaled corticosteroid and a long-acting inhaled beta$_2$-adrenergic agonist (or sustained-release theophylline or a long-acting beta$_2$-adrenergic agonist in tablet form). (Combination therapy is preferred for managing nighttime symptoms.)
- If needed, administer medium-to-high–dose inhaled corticosteroid and either a long-acting, inhaled beta$_2$-adrenergic agonist, sustained-release theophylline, or a long-acting beta$_2$-adrenergic agonist in tablet form.

Asthma controlled

Asthma controlled

Therapeutic goals
- Prevention of chronic and bothersome symptoms, such as coughing or shortness of breath in the early morning, at night, or following exertion.
- Maintenance of normal or nearly normal pulmonary function.
- Maintenance of normal activity, including exercise and other physical activity.
- Prevention of recurrent episodes of asthma and minimal need for treatment in an emergency department or hospital.
- Fulfillment of the patient's and family's expectations of care.

Therapeutic management guidelines: Status epilepticus

Status epilepticus is defined as a period of continuous seizure activity lasting longer than 30 minutes or as the occurrence of two or more successive seizures without return of consciousness between them. The diagram on these pages illustrates recommended treatment options for status epilepticus in adults.

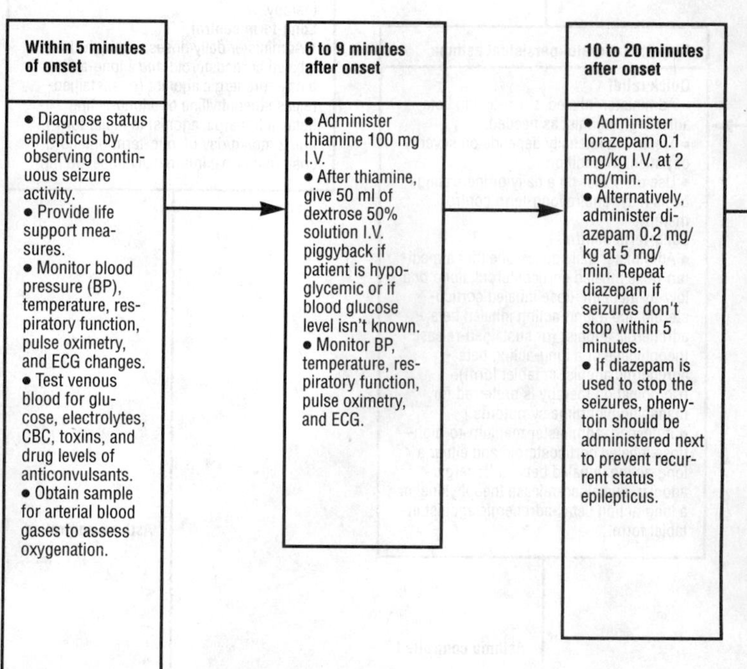

Based on recommendations of the Epilepsy Foundation of America's Working Group on Status Epilepticus. ("Treatment of Convulsive Status Epilepticus," *JAMA* 270(7): 854-59, 1993.)

21 to 60 minutes after onset

- Administer phenytoin 15 to 20 mg/kg I.V. at a rate not to exceed 50 mg/min by I.V. bolus or I.V. piggyback in normal saline solution. Final concentration should not exceed 5 mg/ml. Flush catheter with saline before and after administration.
- Or, administer fosphenytoin 15 to 20 mg PE (phenytoin sodium equivalent)/kg I.V. at a rate not to exceed 150 mg PE/min by I.V. bolus or I.V. piggyback in normal saline solution or dextrose 5% in water.
- Monitor for changes in ECG, BP, and respiratory function. If changes occur, decrease infusion rate.

→

More than 60 minutes after onset

- If status epilepticus doesn't stop with phenytoin 20 mg/kg, administer additional doses of phenytoin 5 mg/kg I.V. to maximum cumulative dose of 30 mg/kg.
- If status epilepticus persists, administer phenobarbital 20 mg/kg I.V. at 60 mg/min. Monitor BP and respiratory function.

→ **Status epilepticus persists** →

- Obtain neurologic consultation.
- Consider initiating barbiturate-induced coma using phenobarbital or pentobarbital I.V.
- Monitor vital signs continuously.
- Provide ventilatory assistance and vasopressors as needed.

Therapeutic management guidelines: Hypertension

Hypertension in adults is generally categorized according to a person's risk of developing hypertension-related diseases. Optimal blood pressure (below 120 mm Hg systolic and 80 mm Hg diastolic) is associated with the lowest cardiovascular risk. Other categories include normal (below 130 mm Hg systolic and 85 mm Hg diastolic), high-normal (130 to 139 mm Hg systolic or 85 to 89 mm Hg diastolic), or hypertension.

Hypertension is further classified as stage 1 (140 to 159 mm Hg systolic or 90 to 99 mm Hg diastolic), stage 2 (160 to 179 mm Hg systolic or 100 to 109 mm Hg diastolic), or stage 3 (180 mm Hg or above systolic or 110 mm Hg or above diastolic). The diagram below illustrates recommended treatment options for hypertension.

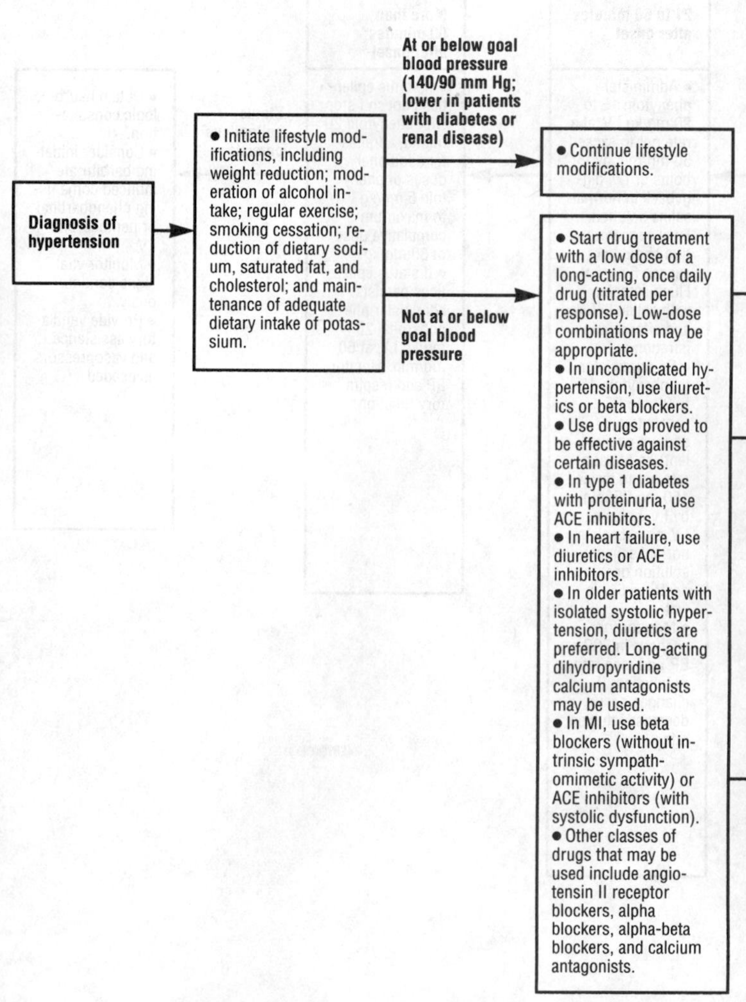

Based on recommendations of the Sixth Report of the Joint National Committee on Prevention, Detection, Evaluation, and Treatment of High Blood Pressure. (*Arch Intern Med* 157(21):2413-46, 1997.)

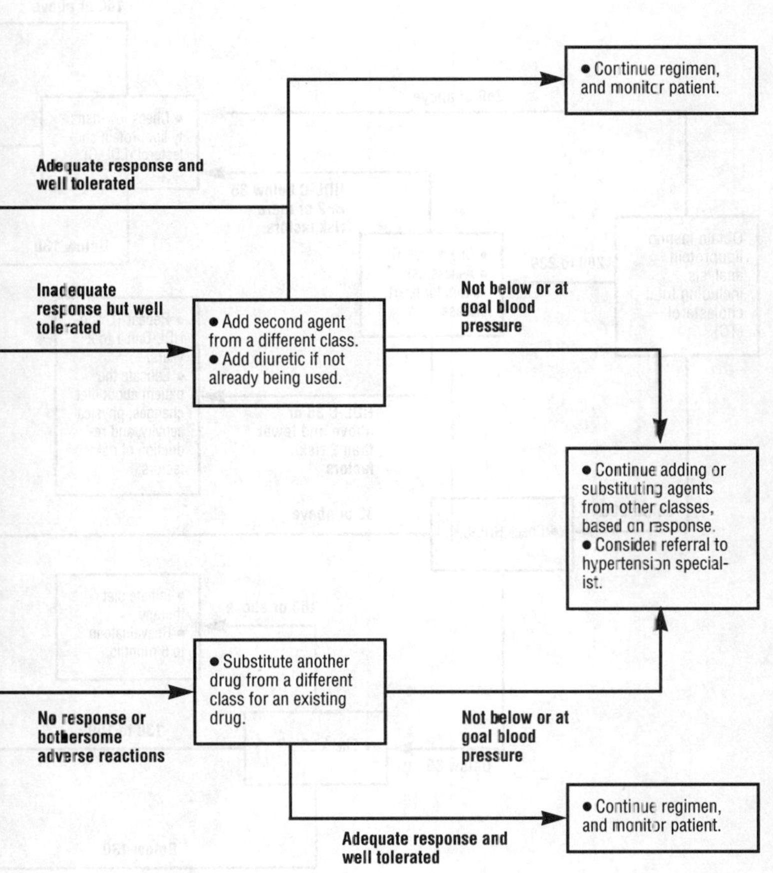
Adequate response and well tolerated
• Continue regimen, and monitor patient.
Inadequate response but well tolerated
• Add second agent from a different class.
• Add diuretic if not already being used.
Not below or at goal blood pressure
• Continue adding or substituting agents from other classes, based on response.
• Consider referral to hypertension specialist.
No response or bothersome adverse reactions
• Substitute another drug from a different class for an existing drug.
Not below or at goal blood pressure
• Continue regimen, and monitor patient.
Adequate response and well tolerated

Therapeutic management guidelines: Dyslipidemia without evidence of heart disease

Heart disease in adults can be prevented by primary measures, used for adults without current evidence of heart disease. All adults 20 years and older should be tested for serum cholesterol levels at least every 5 years. Results of lipoprotein levels and the number of patient risk factors involved help to determine treatment options.

Risk factors include being a male age 45 or older; being a female age 55 or older; having premature menopause without estrogen replacement therapy; a history of MI or sudden death before age 55 in father or other immediate male relative; a history of MI before age 65 in mother or other immediate female relative; current cigarette smoking; the presence of hypertension or diabetes mellitus; or having a low high-density lipoprotein cholesterol (HDL-C) level (below 35 mg/dl).

The diagram here illustrates the steps in primary prevention in adults without evidence of heart disease. All cholesterol levels are measured in mg/dl.

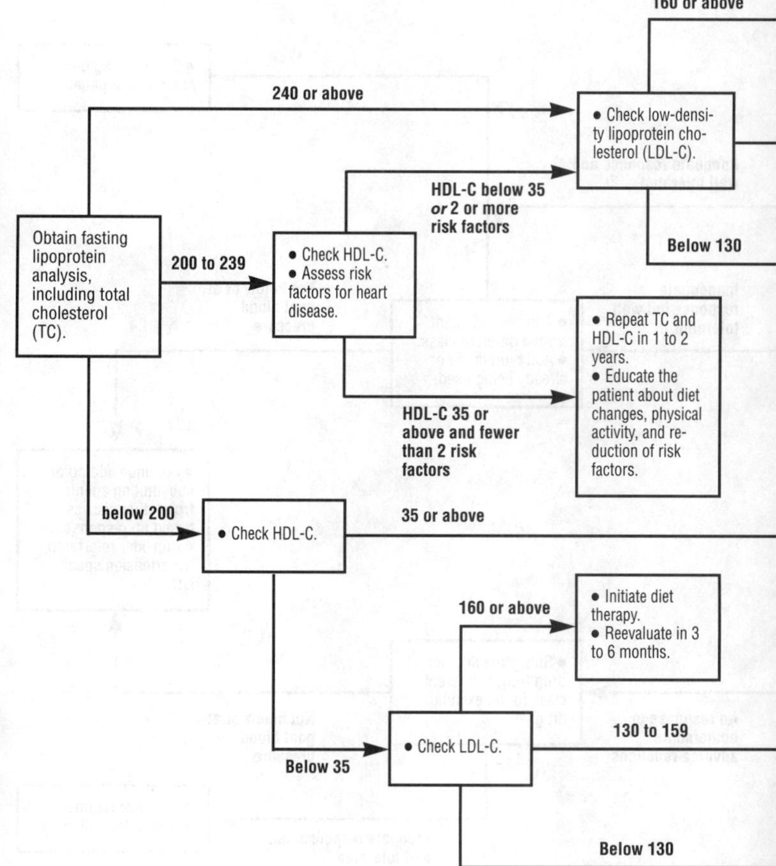

Based on recommendations of the Second Report of the National Cholesterol Education Program Expert Panel on Detection, Evaluation, and Treatment of High Blood Cholesterol in Adults. (*JAMA* 269(23): 3015-23, 1993.)

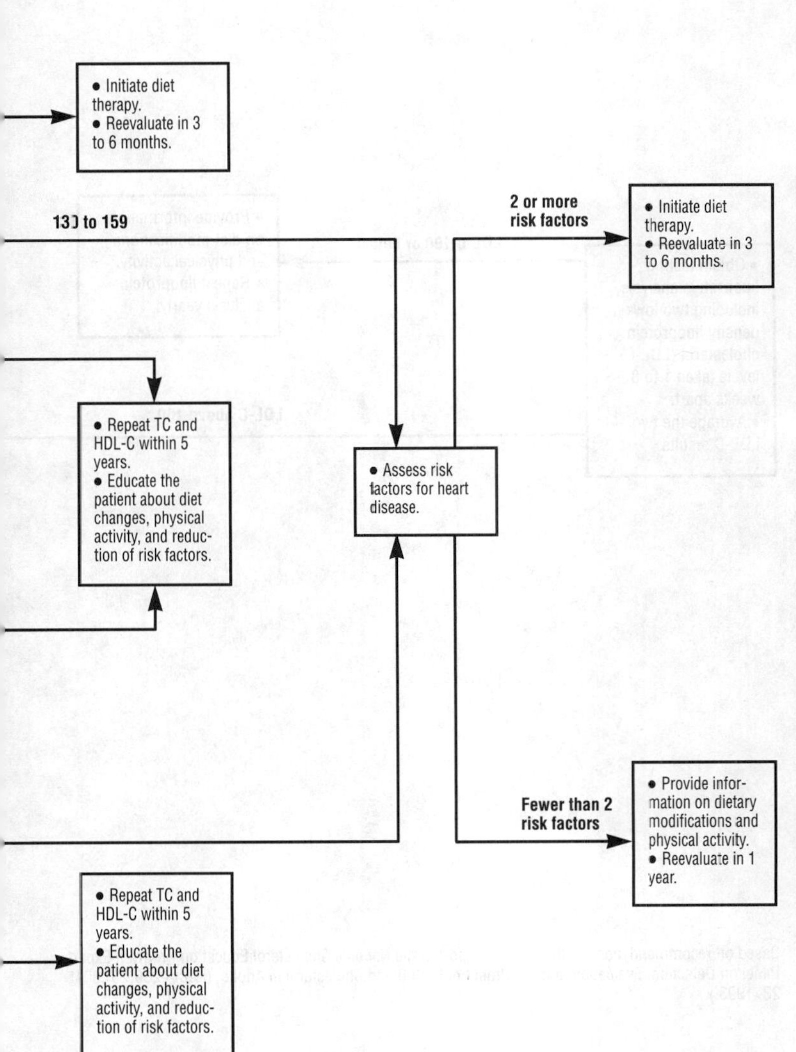
• Initiate diet therapy.
• Reevaluate in 3 to 6 months.
130 to 159
2 or more risk factors
• Initiate diet therapy.
• Reevaluate in 3 to 6 months.
• Repeat TC and HDL-C within 5 years.
• Educate the patient about diet changes, physical activity, and reduction of risk factors.
• Assess risk factors for heart disease.
Fewer than 2 risk factors
• Provide information on dietary modifications and physical activity.
• Reevaluate in 1 year.
• Repeat TC and HDL-C within 5 years.
• Educate the patient about diet changes, physical activity, and reduction of risk factors.

Therapeutic management guidelines: Dyslipidemia with evidence of heart disease

Secondary prevention of heart disease in adults—used for those with current evidence of heart disease—involves on-going assessment of the patient's lipoprotein levels ; instruction in diet, activity, and risk factors; and appropriate diet and pharmacologic treatment. A lowering of cholesterol levels through diet and drug therapies is associated with a reduction not only in recurrent heart disease but also in total mortality rates.

The diagram here illustrates the steps in secondary prevention in adults with evidence of heart disease. All cholesterol levels are measured in mg/dl.

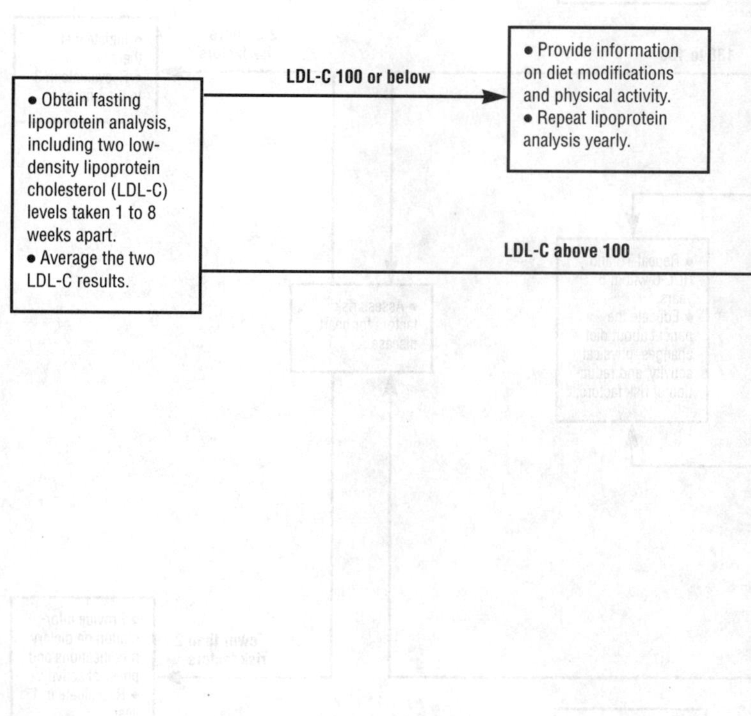

Based on recommendations of the Second Report of the National Cholesterol Education Program Expert Panel on Detection, Evaluation, and Treatment of High Blood Cholesterol in Adults. (*JAMA* 269(23):3015-23, 1993.)

- Conduct complete health assessment.
- Evaluate patient for secondary causes of high LDL-C.
- Check for presence of familial disorders.
- Consider influence of risk factors for heart disease.
- Determine necessary treatment, if any.

→

Initiate diet therapy if:

- LDL-C is 160 or above and patient has fewer than 2 risk factors without evidence of heart disease.
- LDL-C is 130 or above and patient has 2 or more risk factors without evidence of heart disease.
- LDL-C is above 100 and patient has evidence of heart disease.

Initiate drug therapy if:

- LDL-C is 190 or above and patient has fewer than 2 risk factors without evidence of heart disease.
- LDL-C is 160 or above and patient has 2 or more risk factors without evidence of heart disease.
- LDL-C is 130 or above and patient has evidence of heart disease.

Pharmaceutical companies and their drug information contact numbers

Company	Main number	Medical product information number	Web site address
Abbott Laboratories	(847) 937-6100	(800) 633-9110	www.abbott.com
Alcon Laboratories, Inc.	(817) 293-0450	(800) 757-9195	www.alconlabs.com
Allergan, Inc.	(714) 246-4500		www.allergan.com
ALRA Laboratories, Inc.	(800) 248-ALRA		
ALZA Pharmaceuticals	(800) 634-8977		www.alza.com
Amgen, Inc.	(800) 447-1000	(800) 772-6436	www.amgen.com
Astra Merck, Inc.	(800) 942-0424	(800) 236-9933	www.astramerck.com
Baker Norton	(800) 347-4774		
Baxter Heathcare Co.	(818) 956-3200	(818) 507-5496	www.baxter.com
Bayer Co. Pharmaceutical	(800) 468-0894		www.bayerus.com
Allergy	(509) 489-5656		www.bayer-ag.de
Biological	(510) 705-5000		
Beach Pharmaceuticals	(813) 839-6565		
Bedford Laboratories	(800) 521-5169		
Beiersdorf, Inc.	(203) 563-5800	(800) 537-1063	www.beiersdorf.com
Berlex Laboratories	(973) 694-4100		www.berlex.com
Beutlich LP Pharmaceuticals	(800) 238-8542		www.beutlich.com
Blansett Pharmacal	(501) 758-8635		
Boehringer Ingelheim	(203) 798-9988	(800) 243-0127	www.boehringer-ingelheim.com
Braintree Laboratories	(800) 874-6756		www.braintreelabs.com
Bristol-Myers Squibb Co.	(609) 897-2000	(800) 321-1335	www.bms.com
Westwood-Squibb	(800) 333-0950		
Carnrick Laboratories	(973) 267-2670		www.carnick.com
Carter Wallace	(609) 655-6000		www.astelin.com
Cetylite Industries, Inc.	(800) 257-7740		www.cetylite.com
Chiron Therapeutics	(510) 655-8730	(800) 244-7668	www.chiron.com
Dupont Pharmaceuticals	(302) 922-5000		www.dupontmerck.com
Dura Pharmaceuticals, Inc.	(619) 457-2553		www.durapharm.com
Duramed Pharmaceuticals, Inc.	(513) 731-9900		duramed@duramed.com
Eli Lilly & Co.	(800) 545-5979		www.lilly.com
Ferring Pharmaceuticals	(888) 793-6367		www.ferringusa.com
The Feilding Pharmaceutical Co., Inc.	(314) 567-5462		www.feildingcompany.com
Flemming and Co.	(314) 343-8200		ao.@flemingandcompany.com
Forest Pharmaceuticals, Inc.	(314) 344-8870		
Fujisawa Healthcare, Inc.	(847) 317-8800	(800) 727-7003	www.fujisawausa.com
Galderma Laboratories, Inc.	(817) 263-2600		www.galderma.com
Gate Pharmaceuticals	(215) 256-8400		www.tuzapharmusa.com
Glaxo Wellcome, Inc.	(800) 5-GLAXO-5	(800) 334-0089	www.glaxowellcome.com
Glenwood Palisades	(800) 237-9083		www.glenwood-llc.com
Heel/BHI, Inc.	(800) 621-7644	(800) 621-7644	www.heelbhi.com
Hoechst Marion Roussel USA	(800) 362-7466	(800) 633-1610	www.hmri.com
ICN Pharmaceuticals, Inc.	(800) 556-1937		www.icnpharm.com
Immunex Corp.	(800) 466-8639		www.immunex.com
Ion Laboratories, Inc.	(817) 589-7257		
Janssen Pharmaceutica, Inc.	(800) JANSSEN		
Key Pharmaceuticals	(908) 298-4000	(800) 526-4099	www.schering-plough.com
Knoll Pharmaceutical Co.	(800) 526-1072	(800) 526-0221	www.basf.com
3M Pharmaceuticals	(800) 328-0255	(612) 733-8045	www.mmm.com
Marlyn Neutraceuticals	(800) 4-MARLYN		www.naturallyvitamins.com
McNeil Consumer Products Co.	(215) 233-7000		www.tylenol.com
Medeva Pharmaceuticals	(716) 274-5300		www.medeva.com
Merck & Co., Inc.	(800) 672-6372	(800) 672-6372	www.merck.com
Merz Pharmaceuticals	(336) 856-2003		
Mission Pharmaceutical Co.	(210) 533-7118		
Monarch Pharmaceuticals	(800) 546-4906		www.monarchpharm.com
Monsanto	(847) 982-7000	(800) 323-4204	www.monsanto.com
Muro Pharmaceutical, Inc.	(800) 225-0974		

Company	Main number	Medical product information number	Web site address
Mylan Pharmaceuticals	(800) 82-Mylan		www.mylan.com
Neutrogena	(310) 642-1150	(800) 217-1136	www.neutrogena.com
Novartis	(973) 503-7500		www.novartis.com
Novartis Pharmaceuticals	(888) 669-6682		www.novartis.com
Novartis Professional Services	(800) 452-0051		www.novartis.com
Novo Nordisk Pharmaceuticals	(609) 987-5800		www.novo.dk
Novopharm USA, Inc.	(847) 882-4200		www.novopharmusa.com
Ohemeda Pharmaceutical	(800) 262-3784 (voice box tech. support)		www.baxter.com
Organon, Inc.	(800) 631-1253		
Ortho Biotech, Inc.	(800) 325-7504		www.j&j.com
Ortho-McNeil Pharmaceutical Co.	(800) 682-6532	(800) 682-6532	www.j&j.com
Ortho Dermatological Division	(800) 426-7762	(800) 426-7762	www.j&j.com
Paddock Laboratories	(800) 328-5113		www.paddocklabs.com
Par Pharmaceutical, Inc.	(800) 828-9393		www.parpharm.com
Parke-Davis	(800) 223-0432	(800) 223-0432	
Pasteur Meriuex Connaught Rhone Poulenc Group	(800) 822-2463	(800) VACCINE	www.us.pmc-vacc.com
Pedinol Pharmacal, Inc.	(516) 293-9500		
Person & Covey, Inc.	(800) 423-2341		
Pfizer Consumer Health Care	(973) 887-2100	(800) 438-1985	www.pfizer.com
Pfizer, Inc./Labs Division	(800) 438-1985	(800) 438-1985	www.pfizer.com
Pharmaceutical Associates, 2055, Inc.	(800) 845-8210		
Pharmacia & Upjohn Co.	(616) 833-8244	(800) 253-8600	www.pnu.com\pres.-info.htm
Procter & Gamble Pharmaceutical, Inc.	(800) 836-0658	(800) 836-0658	www.pg.com
The Purdue Fredrick Co.	(203) 853-0123		www.pharma.com
Respa Pharmaceuticals	(630) 462-9986		
Rhone-Poulenc Rorer	(610) 454-8000	(800) 727-6737	www.rp-rorer.com
Rhône-Poulenc Rorer Pharmaceuticals, Inc.	(610) 454-8110	(800) 340-7502	www.rp-rorer.com
Richwood Shirer Co., Inc.	(606) 282-2100		www.shiregroup.com
Roche Pharmaceuticals	(973) 235-5000	(800) 526-6367	www.roche.com
Ross Products Division	(800) 624-7677	(800) 227-5767	www.healthanswers.com www.abbott.com
Roxane Laboratories, Inc.	(800) 848-0120		www.roxane.com
Rystan Co., Inc.	(973) 256-3737		
Sanofi Winthrop Pharmaceuticals, Inc.	(212) 551-4000	(800) 446-6267	
Savage Laboratories	(516) 454-7677		
Scandipharm, Inc.	(205) 991-8085		www.scandipharm.com
Schering-Plough	(908) 298-4000	(800) 526-4099	www.allergy-relief.com
Schwarz Pharma, Inc.	(800) 558-5114		www.schwarzpharma.com
G.D. Searle & Co.	(800) 323-4204		www.searlehealthnet.com
Serono Laboratories	(800) 283-8088		www.seronousa.com
Smith Kline Beecham Consumer Health Care	(800) Beecham		www.sb.com
Smith Kline Beecham Pharmaceuticals	(800) 366-8900		www.sb.com
Solvay Pharmaceuticals, Inc.	(770) 578-9000		www.solvay.com
Star Pharmaceuticals, Inc.	(954) 971-9704		www.starpharm.com
Stiefel Laboratories, Inc.	(305) 443-3800	(800) 327-3858	www.stiefel-labs.com
Syntex Puerto Rico, Inc.	(800) 526-6367	(800) 526-6367	www.roche.com
TAP Pharmaceuticals, Inc.	(800) 622-2011	(800) 622-2011	www.abbott.com
Teva Pharmaceuticals USA	(888) TEVA-USA		www.tevapharmusa.com
Tyson and Associates, Inc.	(800) 318-9766		
US Bioscience, Inc.	(800) 872-4672	(800) 872-4672	www.usbio.com
Upsher-Smith Laboratories, Inc.	(800) 654-2299		www.upsher-smith.com
Warner Chilcott, Inc.	(800) 521-8813	(800) 521-8813	www.wclabs.com
Warner Wellcome	(800) 524-2624		www.warner-lambert.com
WE Pharmaceuticals, Inc.	(760) 788-9155		www.weez.com
Wyeth-Ayerst Laboratories	(800) 934-5556	(800) 934-5556	www.ahp.com

Acknowledgments

We would like to thank the following companies for granting us permission to include their drugs in the full-color photoguide.

Abbott Laboratories
Biaxin®
Depakote®
Depakote® Sprinkle
E.E.S.®
Ery-Tab®
Erythrocin Stearate Filmtab®
Erythromycin Base Filmtab®
Hytrin®
Ogen®
PCE®

American Home Products Corporation
Micro-K Extencaps®

Astra Pharmaceuticals
Prilosec®
Toprol XL®

Bayer Corporation
Adalat®
Cipro®

Bristol-Myers Squibb Company
BuSpar®
Capoten®
Cefzil®
cephalexin
Duricef®
Estrace®
Pravachol®
Sumycin®
Trimox®

DuPont Pharmaceuticals Company
Coumadin®
Sinemet®
Sinemet® CR

Eli Lilly and Company
Axid®
Ceclor®
Darvocet-N® 100
Lorabid®
Prozac®

Endo Pharmaceuticals, Inc.
Percocet®

ESI Lederle Inc.
atenolol

Ethex Corporation
potassium chloride

Forest Pharmaceutical, Inc.
Lorcet® 10/650

Glaxo Wellcome, Inc.
Ceftin®
Lanoxin®
Zantac®
Zantac® EFFERdose®
Zovirax®

Hoechst Marion Roussel
Allegra®
Altace®
Carafate®
Cardizem®
Cardizem® CD
DiaBeta®
Lasix®
Trental®

Janssen Pharmaceutica, Inc.
Hismanal®
Propulsid®

Jones Pharma
Levoxyl®

Knoll Pharmaceutical Company
E-Mycin®
ibuprofen
Synthroid®
Vicodin®
Vicodin ES®

Lederle Pharmaceutical Division of American Cyanamid Co.
Suprax®

McNeil PPC, Inc.
Motrin®

Medeva Pharmaceuticals
methylphenidate hydrochloride

Merck & Co., Inc.
Cozaar®
Fosamax®
Mevacor®
Pepcid®
Prinivil®
Vasotec®
Zocor®

Mylan Pharmaceuticals, Inc.
amitriptyline hydrochloride
cimetidine
cyclobenzaprine hydrochloride
doxepin hydrochloride
furosemide
glipizide
naproxen

Mylan Pharmaceuticals, Inc. *(continued)*
propoxyphene napsylate with acetaminophen

Novartis Pharmaceuticals Corporation
DynaCirc®
Fiorinal® with Codeine
Pamelor®

Novopharm USA, Inc., Division of Novopharm Limited
amoxicillin trihydrate

Ortho-McNeil Pharmaceutical
Floxin®
Tylenol® with Codeine No. 3
Ultram®

Pfizer, Inc.
Cardura®
Diflucan®
Glucotrol®
Glucotrol XL®
Norvasc®
Procardia XL®
Zithromax®
Zoloft®
Zyrtec®

Pharmacia & Upjohn
Deltasone®
Glynase®
Halcion®
Micronase®
Provera®
Xanax®

Proctor and Gamble Pharmaceuticals, Inc.
Macrobid®

Rhône-Poulenc Rorer Pharmaceuticals, Inc.
Dilacor XR®
Lozol®
Slo-bid™Gyrocaps®

Roche Laboratories, Inc.
Bumex®
Klonopin®
Naprosyn®
Ticlid®
Toradol®
Valium®

Roxane Laboratories, Inc.
Roxicet™

Schein Pharmaceutical, Inc.
nortriptyline hydrochloride

Schering-Plough Corporation
Claritin®
K-Dur®
Theo-Dur®

Schwarz Pharma, Inc.
Verelan

G.D. Searle & Company
Ambien®
Calan®
Daypro®

SmithKline Beecham Pharmaceuticals
Amoxil®
Augmentin®
Compazine®
Compazine® Spansule®
Dyazide®
Paxil®
Relafen®
Tagamet®

Warner-Lambert Company
Accupril®
Dilantin®
Dilantin® Kapseals®
Lopid®
Nitrostat®

Watson Laboratories, Inc.
hydrocodone bitartrate and acetaminophen

Wyeth-Ayerst Laboratories
Ativan®
Cordarone®
Effexor®
Inderal®
Lodine®
Oruvail®
Premarin®

Zeneca Pharmaceuticals
Nolvadex®
Tenormin®
Zestril®

Zenith Goldline Pharmaceuticals
verapamil hydrochloride

Index

t refers to a table; **boldface** refers to full-color photographs.

t refers to a table; **boldface** refers to full-color photographs.

B

t refers to a table; **boldface** refers to full-color photographs.

C

t refers to a table; **boldface** refers to full-color photographs.

t refers to a table; **boldface** refers to full-color photographs.

t refers to a table; **boldface** refers to full-color photographs.

E

H

t refers to a table; **boldface** refers to full-color photographs.

t refers to a table; **boldface** refers to full-color photographs.

t refers to a table; **boldface** refers to full-color photographs.

t refers to a table; **boldface** refers to full-color photographs.

N

t refers to a table; **boldface** refers to full-color photographs.

t refers to a table; **boldface** refers to full-color photographs.

t refers to a table; **boldface** refers to full-color photographs.

t refers to a table; **boldface** refers to full-color photographs.

X

Y

Z